Volume 1

Jubb, Kennedy, and Palmer's

Pathology of Domestic Animals

FIFTH EDITION

For Elsevier:

Commissioning Editor: Joyce Rodenhuis
Development Editor: Rita Demetriou-Swanwick
Editorial Assistant: Louisa Welch
Project Manager: Anne Dickie
Designer: Andy Chapman
Illustrations: Merlyn Harvey

Volume 1

Jubb, Kennedy, and Palmer's

Pathology of Domestic Animals

FIFTH EDITION

Edited by

M. Grant Maxie

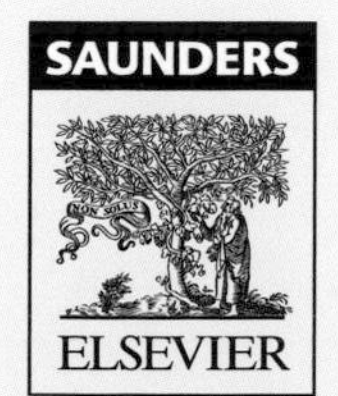

Edinburgh London New York Oxford Philadelphia St Louis Sydney Toronto 2007

ELSEVIER
SAUNDERS

An imprint of Elsevier Limited

First published 1963
Second edition 1970
Third edition 1985
Fourth edition 1993
Fifth edition 2007

Volume 1
ISBN 13 – 978 0 7020 2784 0
ISBN 10 – 0 7020 2784 7

3 volume set
ISBN 13 – 978 0 7020 2823 6
ISBN 10 – 0 7020 2823 1

British Library Cataloguing in Publication Data
A catalogue record for this book is available from the British Library

Library of Congress Cataloging in Publication Data
A catalog record for this book is available from the Library of Congress

Notice

Knowledge and best practice in this field are constantly changing. As new research and experience broaden our knowledge, changes in practice, treatment and drug therapy may become necessary or appropriate. Readers are advised to check the most current information provided (i) on procedures featured or (ii) by the manufacturer of each product to be administered, to verify the recommended dose or formula, the method and duration of administration, and contraindications. It is the responsibility of the practitioner, relying on their own experience and knowledge of the patient, to make diagnoses, to determine dosages and the best treatment for each individual patient, and to take all appropriate safety precautions. To the fullest extent of the law, neither the publisher nor the author assumes any liability for any injury and/or damage.

The Publisher

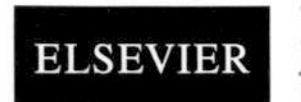

Printed in China

Contents of Volumes 1–3

VOLUME 1

CHAPTER

VOLUME 2

VOLUME 3

Contributors

VOLUME 1

Pamela E. Ginn *BS, DVM, Diplomate ACVP*
Department of Infectious Diseases and Pathobiology
College of Veterinary Medicine
University of Florida
Gainesville, Florida
USA

Joanne E. K. L. Mansell *DVM, MS, Diplomate ACVP*
Department of Veterinary Pathobiology
College of Veterinary Medicine
Texas A&M University
College Station, Texas
USA

M. Grant Maxie *DVM, PhD, Diplomate ACVP*
Animal Health Laboratory
Laboratory Services Division
University of Guelph
Guelph, Ontario
Canada

Pauline M. Rakich *DVM, PhD, Diplomate ACVP*
Athens Veterinary Diagnostic Laboratory
College of Veterinary Medicine
University of Georgia
Athens, Georgia
USA

Keith Thompson *BVSc, PhD, Diplomate ACVP*
Pathobiology Section
Institute of Veterinary, Animal and Biomedical Sciences
Massey University
Palmerston North
New Zealand

Beth A. Valentine *DVM, PhD, Diplomate ACVP*
Oregon State University
College of Veterinary Medicine
Corvallis, Orlando
USA

John F. Van Vleet *DVM, PhD, Diplomate ACVP*
School of Veterinary Medicine
Purdue University
West Lafayette, Indiana
USA

Brian P. Wilcock *DVM, PhD*
Histovet Surgical Pathology
Guelph, Ontario
Canada
(Formerly: Department of Pathobiology, Ontario Veterinary College, University of Guelph, Canada)

Sameh Youssef *BVSc, MVSc, PhD, DVSc, Diplomate ACVP*
Animal Health Laboratory
Laboratory Services Division
University of Guelph
Guelph, Ontario
Canada

VOLUME 2

Dale C. Baker *DVM, PhD, Diplomate ACVP, Diplomate ABT*
Department of Toxicology and Pathology
Portola Pharmaceuticals, Inc.
South San Francisco, California
USA
(Formerly: Department of Pathology, Colorado State University, USA)

Ian K. Barker *DVM, PhD*
Department of Pathobiology
Ontario Veterinary College
University of Guelph
Guelph, Ontario
Canada

Corrie C. Brown *DVM, PhD, Diplomate ACVP*
Department of Pathology
College of Veterinary Medicine
University of Georgia
Athens, Georgia
USA

Jeff L. Caswell *DVM, DVSc, PhD, Diplomate ACVP*
Department of Pathobiology
Ontario Veterinary College
University of Guelph
Guelph, Ontario
Canada

Jennifer A. Charles *BVSc, MVS, Diplomate ACVP*
Department of Veterinary Science
Faculty of Veterinary Science
University of Melbourne
Werribee, Victoria
Australia

M. A. (Tony) Hayes *BVSc, PhD, Diplomate ACVP*
Department of Pathobiology
Ontario Veterinary College
University of Guelph
Guelph, Ontario
Canada

M. Grant Maxie *DVM, PhD, Diplomate ACVP*
Animal Health Laboratory
Laboratory Services Division
University of Guelph
Guelph, Ontario
Canada

Shelley J. Newman *DVM, DVSc, Diplomate ACVP*
Department of Pathology
College of Veterinary Medicine
University of Tennessee
Knoxville, Tennessee
USA

Margaret J. Stalker *DVM, PhD, Diplomate ACVP*
Department of Pathobiology
Ontario Veterinary College
University of Guelph
Guelph, Ontario
Canada

Kurt J. Williams *DVM, PhD, Diplomate ACVP*
Department of Pathobiology and Diagnostic Investigation
College of Veterinary Medicine
Michigan State University
East Lansing, Michigan
USA

VOLUME 3

Charles C. Capen *DVM, PhD, Diplomate ACVP*
Department of Veterinary Biosciences
Ohio State University
Columbus, Ohio
USA

Robert A. Foster *BVSc, PhD, MACVSc, Diplomate ACVP*
Department of Pathobiology
Ontario Veterinary College
University of Guelph
Guelph, Ontario
Canada

Patricia A. Gentry *PhD*
Department of Biomedical Sciences
Ontario Veterinary College
University of Guelph
Guelph, Ontario
Canada

Philip W. Ladds *BVSc, MVSc, PhD, FACVSc, FRCPath, Diplomate ACVP*
Goonellabah, New South Wales
Australia

M. Grant Maxie *DVM, PhD, Diplomate ACVP*
Animal Health Laboratory
Laboratory Services Division
University of Guelph
Guelph, Ontario
Canada

Richard B. Miller *DVM, PhD, Diplomate ACVP*
School of Veterinary Medicine
Ross University
St. Kitts, West Indies

Wayne F. Robinson *BVSc, MVSc, PhD, Diplomate ACVP, MACVSc*
Vice Chancellor's Office
University of Ballarat
Ballarat, Victoria
Australia

Donald H. Schlafer *DVM, PhD, Diplomate ACVP, Diplomate ACVM, Diplomate ACT*
Department of Biomedical Sciences
College of Veterinary Medicine
Cornell University
Ithaca, New York
USA

V. E. O. (Ted) Valli *DVM, PhD, Diplomate ACVP*
Department of Pathobiology
College of Veterinary Medicine
University of Illinois at Urbana-Champaign
Urbana, Illinois
USA

Preface

It was an honor to be asked by Drs. Jubb, Kennedy, and Palmer to assume the editorship of *Pathology of Domestic Animals*. I studied from the first edition in Saskatoon as a DVM student, used the second edition as a working pathologist, and encouraged production of, and contributed to, the third and fourth editions. I'm delighted to have been able to be part of this continuum. In this age of instantaneous global communication and virtually universal access to databases through powerful search engines, does the need continue for such print versions of textbooks? I firmly believe that printed books continue to serve a useful function, partly through their portability and ease of use, but primarily through provision of a measured overview of important topics, with the relevance of competing topics put into perspective by authorities in the field. In particular, this latest edition of these volumes is offered as a comprehensive, and we hope beneficial, overview of the diseases of the major domestic mammals.

The literature and knowledge of veterinary pathology have grown tremendously since publication of the fourth edition in 1993. However, the foundations of these volumes remain sound, and are firmly rooted in the detailed descriptions of gross and histologic pathology recorded by Jubb and Kennedy in the first edition. Etiologies and pathogeneses have been clarified over time, with the major revisions of the fifth edition involving the addition of knowledge gained from molecular biology. Diseases dating from antiquity, such as tuberculosis, are still with us, diseases thought to be under control, such as leptospirosis, have re-emerged as significant concerns, and new diseases and agents have evolved, such as porcine circovirus-associated disease caused by *Porcine circovirus 2*. I hope that we have captured significant changes, and have synthesized this new knowledge to provide a balanced overview of all topics covered. Keeping pace with changing agents and their changing impacts is of course a never-ending challenge. We have used current anatomical and microbial terminology, based on internationally accepted reference sources, such as the Universal Virus Database of the International Committee on Taxonomy of Viruses http://www.ncbi.nlm.nih.gov/ICTVdb/index.htm. Microbial taxonomy is, of course, continually evolving, and classifications and names of organisms can be expected to be updated as newer phylogenetic analyses are reported.

My thanks to the primary contributors to the 5th edition for their rigorous perusal of the literature in their areas of interest, for their addition of insightful information to their chapters, and for their inclusion of many new figures. Additional contributors are acknowledged in individual chapters, but I also offer my thanks to others who have labored in the background and provided helpful suggestions and advice, including Dr. Ron Slocombe (University of Melbourne) and Dr. Murray Hazlett (University of Guelph). The chapter format of the 5th edition is similar to previous editions, with the exception of including Peritoneum within the Alimentary system chapter. We have attempted to improve readability and usability by increased use of highlighting of text (boldfacing, italicization), use of bullet points, and updating of the graphic design, including reorganization of tables of contents. The complete index to all 3 volumes is printed in each volume, again as an aid to readers. Of necessity, bibliographies have been pruned to save space, with references being presented as entry points to the literature through computerized search and retrieval systems embodied in major databases, such as PubMed.

My thanks to Elsevier, and formerly Academic Press, for their help and support throughout this project, with particular thanks to Rita Demetriou-Swanwick (Associate Editor, Health Professions) and Joyce Rodenhuis (Commissioning Editor, Veterinary Medicine). Louisa Welch (Editorial Assistant, Health Sciences) has done a fine job of assembling permissions for use of previously published material. We have attempted to contact all contributors of figures from previous editions, and apologize to any that we were unable to contact or overlooked. My sincere thanks to Sue Nicholls, Senior Production Editor, Keyword Group Ltd, for her diligent checking and cross-checking of text and figures, and for her coordination of copyeditors, typesetters, and proofreaders.

Grant Maxie,
Guelph, Ontario, 2006

Dedication

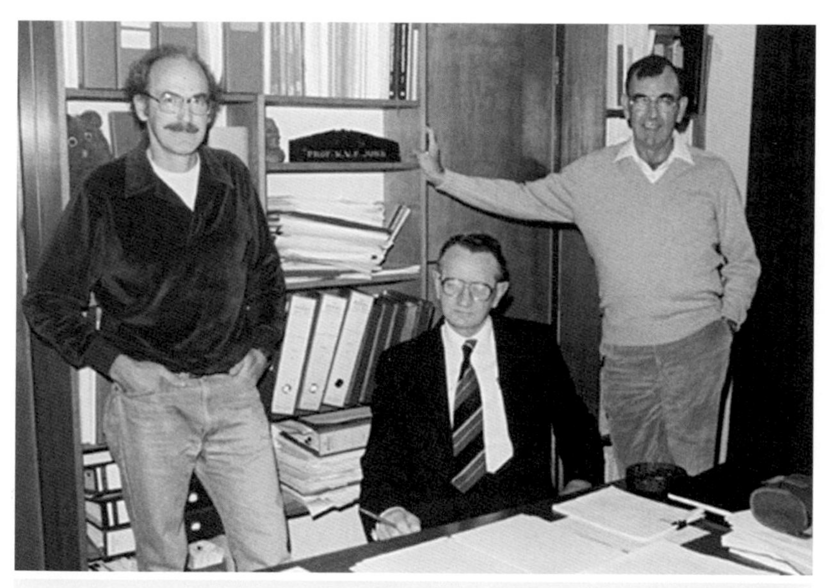

Drs. Palmer, Jubb, and Kennedy, while working on the 3rd edition, Melbourne, 1983. (Courtesy of University of Melbourne.)

These volumes are dedicated to
Drs. Kenneth V. F. Jubb, Peter C. Kennedy,
and Nigel C. Palmer, and to my family –
Laura, Kevin, and Andrea.

1 Bones and joints

Keith Thompson

Diseases of bones

ACKNOWLEDGMENTS

This update of Chapter 1 is based on the foundation developed in previous editions by Dr Ken Jubb and, more recently, Dr Nigel Palmer. It is an honor to follow in their footsteps. I am grateful to the many pathologists who have contributed illustrations to this chapter, in particular Dr Rob Fairley. Significant contributions have also come from the transparency collections of pathology departments at Ontario Veterinary College, Texas A&M University, Massey University, North Carolina State University, Ohio State University, University of California-Davis, and Western College of Veterinary Medicine.

Diseases of bones

GENERAL CONSIDERATIONS

Bone is a highly specialized connective tissue, its properties depending largely on the unique nature of its extracellular matrix. In addition to providing mechanical support and protecting key organ systems from traumatic injury, bone is intimately involved in the homeostasis of calcium, an essential cation in a wide range of bodily functions. In spite of their apparent inertia, *bones are dynamic organs, undergoing constant remodeling throughout life*. Even in mature individuals, bone tissue is continually undergoing localized resorption and replacement in response to the demands of mineral homeostasis and alterations in mechanical forces. The dynamic nature of bones is well illustrated by their impressive powers of repair following injury.

Because of the difficulties associated with processing mineralized tissue, the study of bones, both by researchers and diagnosticians, has lagged behind that of most other organ systems. The skeleton is seldom examined in detail during routine necropsy and it is highly likely that many disorders go undiagnosed. Even in cases where a bone disease is suspected, many veterinary pathologists do not feel confident in their approach to making a diagnosis. *Familiarity with the gross and microscopic anatomy of bones, factors regulating bone formation and resorption, and an understanding of the responses of bone to injury are key to an appreciation of the pathogenesis and pathology of bone diseases*. The initial sections of this chapter will therefore focus on these aspects and outline an approach to examining the skeleton at necropsy.

STRUCTURE AND FUNCTION OF BONE TISSUE

Cellular elements

Bone tissue consists of four cell types: *osteoblasts, osteocytes, lining cells, and osteoclasts*. The first three are derived from primitive

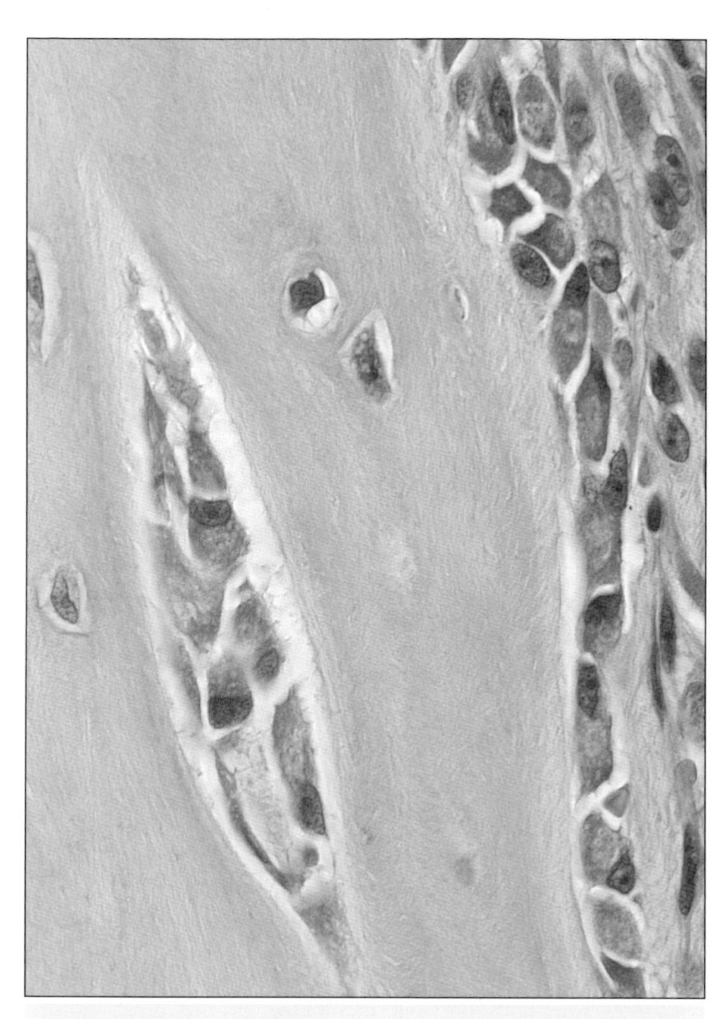

Figure 1.1 Active osteoblasts at a site of rapid bone formation in a newborn kitten. Note the eccentric nuclei, basophilic cytoplasm and prominent Golgi zone in many of the cells. Some osteoblasts have surrounded themselves with osteoid to become osteocytes.

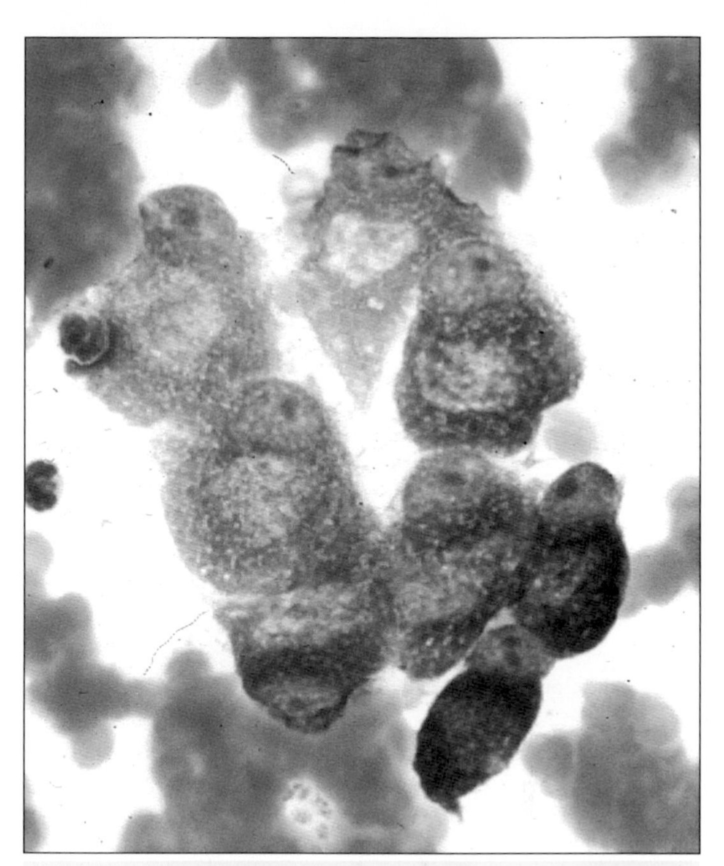

Figure 1.2 Active osteoblasts in a cytological preparation showing the characteristic eccentric nucleus, basophilic cytoplasm and prominent Golgi zone.

osteoprogenitor cells of mesenchymal origin, which are present in bone as well as other tissues, and which can be induced to differentiate into osteoblasts under the influence of appropriate paracrine and autocrine stimuli. Osteoclasts are derived from hematopoietic stem cells, probably of the monocyte series.

Osteoblasts *are responsible for manufacturing osteoid*, the organic component of bone matrix. Active osteoblasts, which line surfaces where bone formation is occurring, have abundant rough endoplasmic reticulum and a prominent Golgi apparatus, reflecting their role in protein synthesis. Histologically they appear as plump, cuboidal cells with basophilic cytoplasm, their nuclei sometimes being polarized away from the adjacent bone surface (Fig. 1.1). The typical morphologic features of osteoblasts are often more easily appreciated in cytologic preparations (Fig. 1.2). Not only do osteoblasts produce the osteoid, *they play a role in initiating its mineralization*, although the mechanism is not fully understood. The membranes of osteoblasts are rich in alkaline phosphatase, which appears to be involved in mineralization of both osteoid and cartilage. The high level of alkaline phosphatase activity measured normally in the serum of rapidly growing young animals presumably reflects the intense osteoblastic activity that is occurring in the developing skeleton. There is mounting evidence that the osteoblast is the central cell through which bone resorption and formation are mediated. In addition to osteoid, they produce an array of *regulatory factors* that are deposited in bone matrix and which play a critical role in bone remodeling.

Inactive osteoblasts, or **bone-lining cells**, are flattened cells with few organelles that cover endosteal bone surfaces that are undergoing neither formation nor resorption. Although barely visible in histological sections, these are the most abundant cells on the endosteal surface of the adult skeleton and link with each other to *form a functional barrier* between the extracellular fluid compartment of bone tissue and that of surrounding tissues. Bone-lining cells are believed to be involved in calcium homeostasis by regulating the exchange of calcium and other ions, such as sodium and magnesium, between bone fluid and extracellular fluid, under the influence of parathyroid hormone. It is likely that bone-lining cells can produce osteoid and contribute to bone deposition should the demand arise at a site of previous inactivity. Endosteal osteoprogenitor cells may be residents of this population of bone-lining cells.

During active bone formation, about 10–20% of osteoblasts at regular intervals along a bone-forming surface surround themselves with osteoid and become **osteocytes** (see Fig. 1.1). *These are the most abundant cells of bone tissue, residing in small spaces (lacunae) within the mineralized matrix.* Newly formed osteocytes retain some morphological and functional characteristics of osteoblasts, but as they mature and become embedded deeper in the mineralized matrix, the amount of rough endoplasmic reticulum in their cytoplasm is reduced considerably and they develop features more typical of phagocytic cells. Osteocytes maintain contact with adjacent osteocytes, and with bone-lining cells or osteoblasts on the surface, by a network of branching cytoplasmic processes extending through *canaliculi*. In routinely stained histological sections, the canaliculi are not visible and only the nuclei of osteocytes are usually apparent.

Osteocytes are thought to be capable of producing and resorbing bone in their immediate vicinity, thereby decreasing or increasing the size of their lacunae. This process is known as *osteocytic osteolysis*. The perilacunar bone matrix is less heavily mineralized and more labile than that in other areas. The action of osteocytes on this perilacunar bone is believed to be important in regulating the concentration of calcium and other minerals in the bone fluid compartment. Because of the large surface area of mineralized bone exposed to either osteocytes or their canaliculi, significant quantities of calcium can be mobilized from this source very rapidly in response to the demands of calcium homeostasis. Although osteocytes can enlarge their lacunae by resorbing perilacunar bone matrix, this process of osteocytic osteolysis does not play a significant role in structural modifications of bones, or in the development of bone lesions associated with disease processes.

Osteocytes probably survive for several years in the mature skeleton but eventually die, leaving empty lacunae. The gradual loss of osteocytes is presumably a normal phenomenon, compensated by the construction of new bone as part of the remodeling process that occurs throughout life. In disease states in which bone necrosis is a feature, there is no immediate loss in structural integrity of the dead bone tissue, but efforts to remove the remaining mineralized matrix and replace it with new bone suggest that its function is impaired.

Osteoclasts *are primarily responsible for resorption of bone tissue*. They are probably related to monocytes and macrophages, which are capable of resorbing bone in vitro, but are sufficiently different histochemically to suggest that they may possess a distinct stem cell. Osteoclasts are rich in acid phosphatase and a range of other acid hydrolases, packaged in primary lysosomes. The acid phosphatase isoenzyme present in osteoclasts is tartrate-resistant, unlike the tartrate-sensitive acid phosphatase found in monocytes and macrophages. Osteoclasts are easily recognizable histologically as large, multinucleated cells with eosinophilic cytoplasm, typically situated on bone surfaces and often within shallow pits called **Howship's lacunae**. The presence of Howship's lacunae on a bone surface is convincing evidence of previous resorption at that site, even if no osteoclasts are present at the time of observation. Although not always apparent histologically, osteoclasts involved in active bone resorption have a highly specialized "ruffled" or brush border contiguous with the bone surface (Fig. 1.3). A clear zone adjacent to the brush border is free of organelles but contains actin-like filaments, which may assist in anchoring the cell to the bone matrix. This attachment of active osteoclasts to the bone surface is an essential requirement for resorption to occur, as is the activity of a specific intracellular, membrane-bound tyrosine kinase. Deletion of the gene coding for this enzyme in mice has been shown to induce osteopetrosis, a disease characterized by defective osteoclastic activity.

During **osteoclastic bone resorption**, an acid environment is created in the narrow space between the cell and the bone surface. Hydrogen and bicarbonate ions are generated from carbon dioxide and water by the action of carbonic anhydrase II on the brush border membrane of osteoclasts. An ATP-mediated proton pump, also located on the brush border membrane, actively transfers hydrogen ions into the extracellular space. The acidity of the local environment not only induces demineralization of the bone, it enhances the activity of the acid hydrolases released from osteoclasts when primary lysosomes fuse with the cell membrane of the brush border. Fragments of degraded matrix are endocytosed by osteoclasts and further digested within secondary lysosomes.

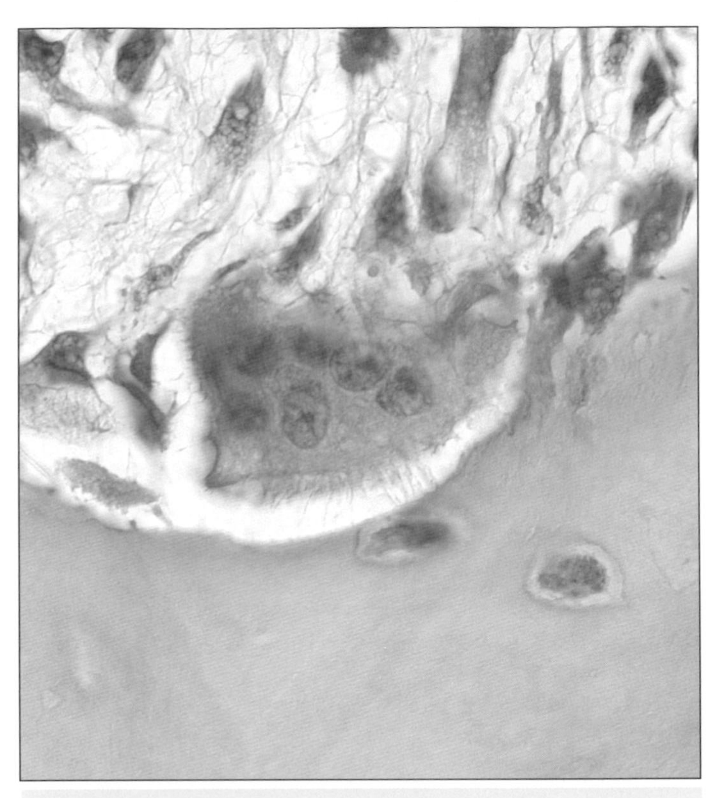

Figure 1.3 Multinucleated osteoclast in a shallow pit (Howship's lacuna) on a bone surface undergoing resorption. Note the ruffled border of the osteoclast adjacent to the bone.

The potential rate of removal of bone by osteoclasts is much greater than the rate of formation by osteoblasts. An individual osteoclast can erode approximately 400 μm^3 of bone, and travel 100 μm across a bone surface, per hour. As a result, localized or generalized removal of bone during the normal physiological processes of modeling and remodeling, or in disease states, can occur very rapidly.

Once osteoclasts have completed their required phase of resorption, they most likely undergo apoptosis and disappear from resorption sites. This is characterized by condensation of nuclear chromatin, loss of the ruffled border and detachment from the bone surface. Drugs that inhibit bone resorption have been shown to induce osteoclast apoptosis both in vitro and in vivo. Importantly, parathyroid hormone promotes the survival of osteoclasts and in cases of either nutritional or renal hyperparathyroidism, surviving osteoclasts are found in medullary spaces mixed with fibroblastic elements. The abnormal persistence of osteoclasts in these sites is an important aid to the diagnosis of these conditions.

Bone matrix

Bone matrix consists of an *organic component, called* **osteoid**, *and an inorganic component comprised predominantly of hydroxyapatite crystals*. The main constituent of osteoid (approximately 90%) is **type I collagen**, which is also the predominant form of collagen in tendons, ligaments, dentine, and the ocular sclera. Each collagen molecule consists of three polypeptide chains assembled into a triple helix, which is a highly stable configuration, resistant to proteolytic degradation, and which forms the basic unit of all collagenous structures. The strength of bone and other collagenous structures is due in part to the manner in which individual collagen molecules are aggregated into fibrils, with each fibril overlapping its neighbor by about one quarter of its length. This creates a characteristic banding pattern, clearly evident on transmission electron microscopy. The tensile strength of collagenous structures is further enhanced by intermolecular cross-links, which form by the oxidative deamination of either lysyl or hydroxylysyl residues under the influence of the copper-dependent enzyme lysyl oxidase. The number of these cross-links in bone collagen is greater than that of the collagen types found in soft tissues. Interference with the formation of cross-links, as occurs in copper deficiency or certain toxicity diseases (see below), may significantly alter the mechanical properties of bone and other connective tissues.

Several *noncollagenous proteins* are also produced by osteoblasts and form part of the organic matrix of bone. The most abundant of these is **osteonectin**, a phosphoprotein that interacts with both type I collagen and hydroxyapatite, and has been shown to facilitate the mineralization of type I collagen in vitro. Osteonectin concentration is highest in mature bone, especially in areas with the highest degree of mineralization. **Osteocalcin**, also referred to as *bone Gla protein* because of its γ-carboxyglutamic acid (Gla) residues, is also abundant in bone, accounting for up to 10% of total noncollagenous proteins. Its synthesis by osteoblasts is vitamin K-dependent and is stimulated by 1,25 dihydroxyvitamin D. Osteocalcin is deposited in osteoid shortly before mineralization and binds strongly to calcium ions and to hydroxyapatite, suggesting that it is important in the mineralization process. There is also evidence to suggest that it may be involved in the recruitment of osteoclasts to sites of bone resorption or remodeling. Interestingly, depletion of osteocalcin concentration to less than 1% of normal in rats fed warfarin is not accompanied by a reduction in the mechanical strength of bone. Osteocalcin is also found in plasma, where it serves as a marker for osteoblastic activity. A second Gla-containing protein, *matrix Gla protein*, occurs in bone as well as several other tissues. Its function is not known but it appears early in skeletal development when osteocalcin levels are still low, suggesting a possible role in bone development.

The **proteoglycans** of bone matrix are considerably smaller and less abundant than those found in cartilage matrix, possessing a relatively small protein core and only one or two glycosaminoglycan (chondroitin sulfate) side-chains. The bone proteoglycans are concentrated near the mineralization front where they are believed to play a *key role in the organization and mineralization of the matrix*. During this process, the protein core is degraded, leaving the chondroitin sulfate side-chains, which persist in the mineralized matrix of bone.

Several other noncollagenous proteins have been detected in bone matrix, including *osteopontin*, a sialoprotein that binds strongly to hydroxyapatite, and many other glycoproteins and phosphoproteins whose functions are unknown.

Bone matrix also contains a *variety of growth factors* that are capable of inducing mitogenic responses in a range of cell types, including bone cells. These factors, which probably play an important role in bone development, modeling and remodeling, especially at the local level, include: bone morphogenetic proteins, fibroblast growth factors, platelet-derived growth factors, insulin-like growth factors, and transforming growth factors β.

The **inorganic (mineral) component** of bone matrix is known to consist largely of **hydroxyapatite** $[Ca_{10}(PO_4)_6(OH)_2]$, but its structure and properties are poorly understood. In addition to calcium and phosphate, bone mineral contains considerable quantities of *carbonate, magnesium, sodium and zinc*, not all of which are available for exchange. *Fluoride* is also present in small amounts in bone matrix. Ultrastructurally, hydroxyapatite is present in bone matrix either as thin, needle-like crystals oriented in the same direction as collagen fibrils, or as an amorphous, granular phase, depending on the type of bone.

Matrix mineralization

The mineralization of skeletal tissues is a highly complex process, and is only partly understood. In organ systems throughout the body, extracellular tissue fluids in equilibrium with plasma are supersaturated with respect to hydroxyapatite. Many also contain type I collagen similar to that in bone, but mineralization does not normally occur. This is most likely due to the presence of potent inhibitors, which must be enzymatically degraded before mineralization can be initiated. In bone, the selective and localized degradation of such inhibitors, and the synthesis by osteoblasts of unique molecules that promote mineralization, could account for the orderly manner in which mineral deposition occurs in this tissue. However, the presence of substrates that promote nucleation at humoral solute concentrations is also required.

There is no doubt that **matrix vesicles**, *tiny extracellular organelles originating as cytoplasmic blebs from osteoblasts, chondrocytes and odontoblasts*, play an important role in initiating the mineralization process, particularly in cartilage undergoing endochondral ossification. These vesicles are rich in calcium-binding phospholipids and proteins, alkaline phosphatase, pyrophosphatases, phospholipase A_2 and in metalloproteinases that degrade proteoglycans, potential inhibitors of mineralization. Although the mechanism is still uncertain, the initial nucleation of hydroxyapatite crystals occurs on the inner surface of matrix vesicle membranes, at least in mineralizing cartilage matrix. Phospholipids in vesicles are believed to sequester calcium, while pyrophosphatases and metalloproteinases inactivate local inhibitors and alkaline phosphatase generates phosphates, allowing mineralization to proceed.

Although mineral deposition in some tissues such as growth plate cartilage appears to be mediated almost exclusively by matrix vesicles, this is not the case for bone matrix. Unlike cartilage, where mineralization of collagen fibrils does not occur, hydroxyapatite crystals are deposited in the type I collagen fibrils of bone. Evidence suggests however that collagen fibrils alone are not capable of initiating primary nucleation. The adsorption to collagen of bone-specific noncollagenous proteins such as osteonectin and osteocalcin, both of which are strong binders of Ca^{2+} ions, may create appropriate sites for nucleation. Once initiated, the mineral spreads in an orderly manner throughout collagen fibers until the entire aqueous space of the fiber is filled with hydroxyapatite crystals. The mineralization of individual fibers occurs rapidly, as evidenced by the sharp division between highly and sparsely mineralized matrix at the junction between mineralized bone and osteoid seams.

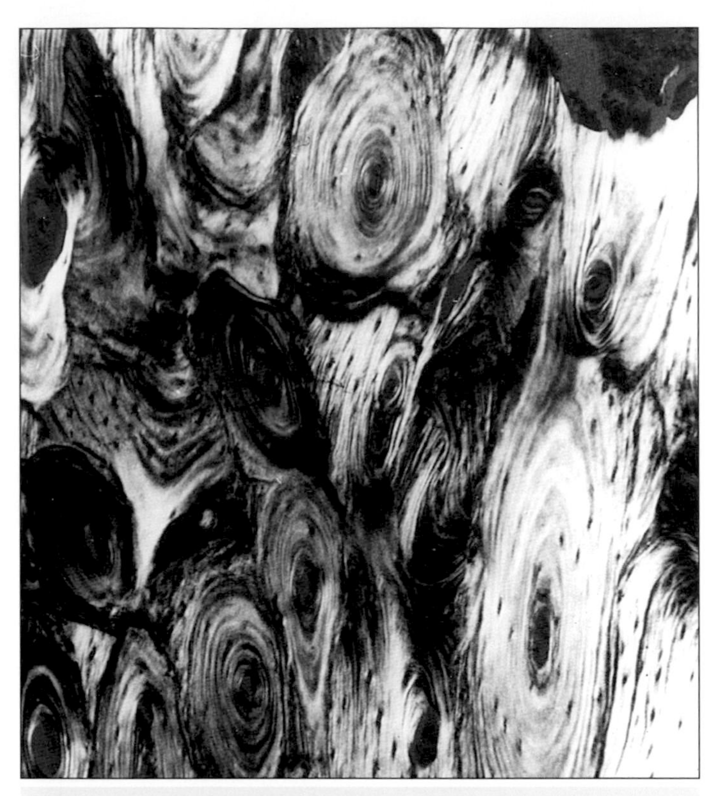

Figure 1.4 Transverse (slightly oblique) section of cortical bone viewed under polarized light to show the **osteons or Haversian systems**, which consist of concentric lamellae of bone surrounding a central vascular canal.

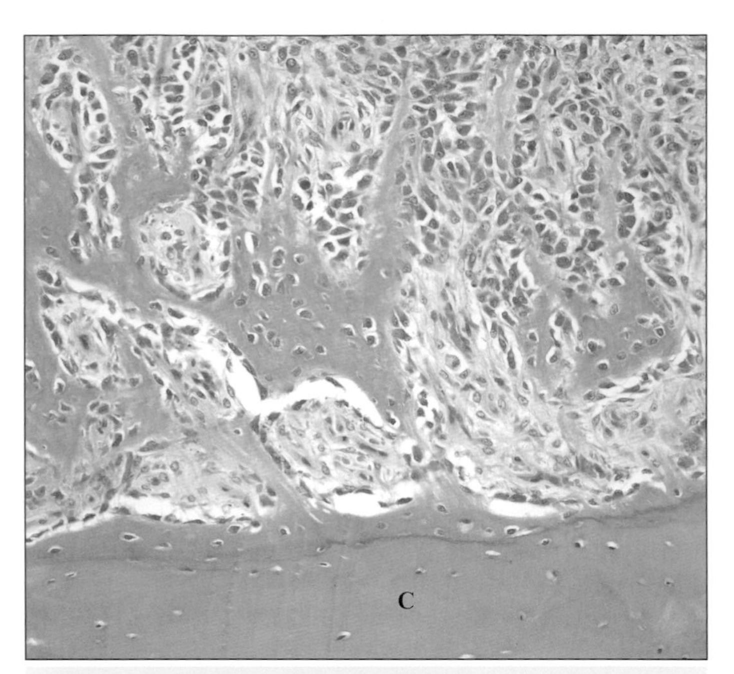

Figure 1.5 Trabeculae of **woven bone** emerging from the cortex (C) beneath an elevated periosteum. The osteocytes in the woven bone are more numerous than in the mature lamellar bone of the cortex and are irregularly distributed. The matrix of the woven bone is slightly more basophilic than that of the mature bone.

Osteoid does not become mineralized for 5–10 days after deposition. As a result, *a thin layer of unmineralized osteoid*, the **osteoid seam**, covers the surfaces where bone is being formed. Although not always apparent histologically in decalcified tissue sections, the osteoid seam is usually more eosinophilic than previously mineralized bone tissue and, in lamellar bone, separated from it by *a basophilic line*, the **mineralization front**. The osteoid seam may be 5–15 μm in depth, depending on its rate of formation. Once mineralization of osteoid begins, it occurs very rapidly, with over 60% of the matrix becoming mineralized almost immediately. However, the remaining deposition of mineral is a slow cumulative process that can take weeks to complete.

Structural organization of bone tissue

Although the cellular elements of bone tissue, and the basic composition of the matrix, are relatively constant, there is variation in the organization of these components both at the macroscopic and microscopic level. The adult skeleton consists predominantly of mature **lamellar bone**, where the collagen fibers of the bone matrix are oriented in parallel layers. This pattern is clearly apparent in histological sections viewed under polarized light (Fig. 1.4). Osteocytes are present in small slit-like lacunae between layers in a regular pattern, their distribution reflecting the orderly manner in which osteoblasts manufacture lamellar bone. In dense cortical bone, the lamellae are organized into **osteons** or **Haversian systems**, consisting of concentric lamellae surrounding a central vascular canal (Fig. 1.4). *Osteons run longitudinally through the cortex and are cemented together by interstitial lamellae.* The trabecular or spongy bone of medullary cavities consists of variable numbers of lamellae arranged parallel to the surface rather than organized into osteons.

The alternating pattern of birefringent and nonbirefringent layers in lamellar bone has traditionally been interpreted as reflecting a 90° switch in orientation of collagen fibers between successive layers, creating a structure with physical strength similar to plywood. This model has remained unquestioned since the early 20th century, but has been challenged by recent studies using scanning electron microscopy. An alternative model proposes that lamellar bone consists of alternating layers of collagen-rich (dense) and collagen-poor (loose) lamellae, only the former showing birefringence.

A variant of lamellar bone is often seen on the weight-bearing aspects of long bones of rapidly growing animals, especially young ruminants. In these areas, the outer cortex is often arranged in laminar arrays rather than conventional Haversian systems, and is known as **laminar bone**.

In the developing fetus, and at sites of rapid bone formation during postnatal life, the *collagen fibers in bone matrix are arranged in a haphazard, interwoven fashion*. This immature form of bone tissue is referred to as **woven bone**, or coarse-bundle bone. Its matrix is more basophilic than that of lamellar bone and the osteocytes are larger, more numerous, and are irregularly arranged (Fig. 1.5). During skeletal maturation and remodeling, woven bone is resorbed and replaced with lamellar bone, which has greater strength, but it is seen in adults at sites where bone is produced rapidly in response to injury, inflammation or neoplasia. Fracture calluses invariably contain this form of bone tissue, as do bone-forming tumors.

A third type of bone, **chondroid bone**, arises directly from fibrocartilaginous origins and is found in ossifying tendon sheaths, of bone derived from neural crest origins and probably from some mixed tumors.

Formation of cranial bones

The pathology of the cranial bones often differs from bones elsewhere in the body, and some of the cranial bones may be spared in disorders that affect other bones. This is probably due to the complex origins of the cranial bones. The base of the cranium develops from a hyaline cartilage model that mineralizes and subsequently undergoes endochondral ossification. The remainder of the cranial bones and also the facial bones arise from mesenchyme directly by the process of intramembranous bone formation. Experimental studies using chimeric chick embryos and transgenic mice indicate that neural crest cells populate the sutures of membranous cranial bones, contribute to tooth morphogenesis and the formation of odontoblasts, dentine and cementum of teeth, and in the formation of the mandible and its cartilaginous articulation with the temporal bones. Chondroid bone that develops from neural crest cells populates the cranial bone sutures, and also forms as an intermediate step in the formation of intramembranous skull bones. Sutures remain as active sites of intramembranous bone production, and are probably the site of origin for the distinctive tumor that arises in the skull, the multilobular tumor of bone.

The embryology and development of the vertebral column is also complex, and in most vertebrae there are eight separate ossification centers. However, the atlas and axis differ in their structure and development.

Bibliography

Chai Y. et al. Fate of the mammalian cranial neural crest during tooth and mandibular morphogenesis. Development 2000;127:1671–1694.

Lengele B. et al. Embryonic origin and fate of chondroid tissue and secondary cartilages in the avian skull. Anat Rec 1996;246:377–393.

Morriss-Kay GM. Derivation of the mammalian skull vault. J Anat 2001;199:143–151.

Regulation of bone formation and resorption

The regulation of bone cell function is accomplished by the action of a variety of systemic hormones and the local action of cytokines, which not only influence the recruitment and action of differentiated osteoblasts and osteoclasts, but also may stimulate the proliferation of their precursors. A list of systemic and local factors involved in bone remodeling is presented in Table 1.1.

Systemic hormones known to have either direct or indirect effects on the skeleton include: parathyroid hormone, 1,25-dihydroxyvitamin D_3, calcitonin, glucocorticoids, growth hormone, insulin, sex steroids, and thyroid hormones. **Parathyroid hormone** (PTH) is a potent activator of osteoclastic bone resorption, but its action appears to be mediated through osteoblasts or bone-lining cells as PTH receptors have been identified on osteoblasts but not osteoclasts. Furthermore, in vitro studies have demonstrated that the activation of osteoclasts by PTH depends on the presence of osteoblasts. The TNF-family molecule RANK-L (receptor activator of NF-kappaB ligand) has recently been identified as an essential signal in osteoclast development, activation, and survival. RANK-L is highly expressed in areas of bone remodeling and at sites of pathological bone loss in a variety of disease states in man and animals.

Osteoclasts are poorly able to resorb unmineralized bone matrix and since a thin layer of osteoid covers all bone surfaces, except those undergoing resorption, this layer must be removed before resorption can be initiated. Osteoblasts also may be involved in this process through activation of a latent form of collagenase, the synthesis and secretion of which are enhanced by PTH. In addition to its effect on bone resorption, PTH has been shown experimentally both to inhibit and stimulate bone formation, depending on the duration of administration and the dose rate. High doses cause increased bone resorption leading to fibrous osteodystrophy. In contrast, low and intermittent doses of PTH that are too small to affect serum calcium concentration have been shown to promote bone formation and increase bone mineral density. This anabolic effect of PTH is mediated through inhibition of apoptosis of osteoblasts and osteocytes, thereby increasing their lifespan.

Table 1.1 Factors controlling bone remodeling

Systemic factors	Local factors
Polypeptide hormones • Parathyroid hormone • Calcitonin • Insulin • Growth hormone **Steroid hormones** • Vitamin D (1,25-dihydroxyvitamin D_3 • Sex hormones • Corticosteroids **Thyroid hormones**	**Cytokines** • Interleukins (IL-1, IL-6, IL-11) • Insulin-like growth factors (IGF-I, IGF-II) • Transforming growth factors (TGF-β) • Bone morphogenetic proteins • Fibroblast growth factors • Platelet-derived growth factor • Tumor necrosis factors • Interferons • Colony stimulating factors (M-CSF, GM-CSF) **Prostaglandins** • Prostaglandin E2 **Nitric oxide**

Like PTH, **1,25-dihydroxyvitamin D_3** ($1,25(OH)_2D_3$), *the active form of vitamin D_3, is a potent stimulator of osteoclastic bone resorption*. It promotes the differentiation and fusion of osteoclast progenitors and activates mature osteoclasts, probably by a mechanism similar to, but independent of, PTH. Receptors for $1,25(OH)_2D_3$ do not occur on osteoclasts but are present on osteoblasts, supporting the involvement of osteoblasts in mediating osteoclastic resorption triggered by $1,25(OH)_2D_3$. The effect of $1,25(OH)_2D_3$ on bone formation is complex, but it appears to be required for normal bone growth and mineralization. This effect on mineralization is partly related to maintaining adequate serum concentrations of calcium and phosphorus, but evidence for a direct effect of $1,25(OH)_2D_3$ on mineralization has been provided by experiments in mice and rats. The synthesis of osteocalcin by osteoblasts is stimulated by $1,25(OH)_2D_3$, but there is confusion over the exact role of this peptide hormone and other metabolites of vitamin D_3 on bone formation.

Calcitonin *has a direct, but transient, inhibitory effect on osteoclastic bone resorption* but does not appear to influence bone formation. Following exposure to calcitonin, active osteoclasts rapidly lose their ruffled border and become physically separated from the underlying bone surface. There is also an inhibitory effect on osteoclast formation through reduced proliferation of progenitor cells and reduced differentiation of committed precursors. Calcitonin is capable of inhibiting PTH-induced bone resorption in vitro, but the mechanism and significance of this action is unclear.

Insulin does not regulate bone resorption but *plays an important role in the synthesis of bone matrix, and in cartilage formation*. As such, it has a major influence on normal skeletal growth. Rather than influence bone cell replication, insulin stimulates bone matrix synthesis by differentiated osteoblasts. **Growth hormone** promotes longitudinal growth of bones in immature individuals and appositional bone growth in adults, but its action is indirect, being mediated through insulin-like growth factors produced by the liver.

Glucocorticoids *have a significant catabolic effect on the skeleton* through actions on both osteoblasts and osteoclasts. There is direct inhibition of osteoblastic activity, thereby reducing bone formation, and an indirect enhancement of osteoclastic resorption. The latter is probably due to inhibition of enteric calcium absorption and impaired renal tubular calcium reabsorption, leading to reduced serum ionized calcium concentration and secondary hyperparathyroidism. Reduction in bone mass is a recognized sequel to long-term corticosteroid therapy both in human and animal patients.

Estrogens and **androgens** appear to be *important regulators of skeletal growth and maturation*. Androgen receptors are present on osteoblasts, but at low densities. During puberty, androgens stimulate bone growth, while in male adults they are involved in the maintenance of the skeleton. Androgens do not affect osteoclasts directly, but may inhibit bone resorption indirectly by inhibiting the recruitment of osteoclast precursors from bone marrow. A significant effect of estrogens appears to be to inhibit bone resorption. Immediately after menopause, a decline in circulating estrogen levels in some women is accompanied by a rapid acceleration in bone loss, leading to osteoporosis. Treatment of postmenopausal women with estrogen has been shown to significantly reduce the risk of osteoporosis-related fractures. Estrogen may inhibit bone resorption by reducing the synthesis of cytokines such as interleukin-6, although the exact mechanism is unknown.

Thyroid hormones are important for normal skeletal development, primarily through *stimulation of cartilage growth*, but they also stimulate bone resorption. In human patients, accelerated bone resorption in hyperthyroidism may result in hypercalcemia and increased risk of osteoporosis. Hypothyroidism during fetal development has been linked to congenital abnormalities of the skeleton in animals. Reduced longitudinal bone growth, delayed ossification and impaired bone resorption were reported in lambs following fetal thyroidectomy, while delayed ossification of carpal bones in newborn foals has been described in association with hyperplastic goiter.

In addition to the range of systemic hormones capable of influencing bone formation and resorption, several locally produced **growth regulatory factors** or **cytokines** with paracrine, autocrine, or juxtacrine functions have been identified. In fact, these factors are likely to be more important than the systemic hormones in initiating physiologic bone resorption and remodeling, which occurs in discrete localities throughout the skeleton. Many of these growth factors become stored in the matrix and their release in active form during future episodes of bone resorption may stimulate the differentiation and proliferation of osteoblast precursors. They can be grouped into distinct families based on their action and target cell, but there is considerable overlap and redundancy in their activities.

The **insulin-like growth factors** (IGF-I and IGF-II) are growth hormone-dependent polypeptides produced by several tissues, including bone. *They are known to have powerful systemic and local effects on bone formation and maintenance of bone mass.* IGF-I, which is more potent than IGF-II, stimulates the proliferation of osteoblast precursors and enhances matrix synthesis by differentiated osteoblasts. It also inhibits the degradation of bone collagen, most likely by inhibiting the expression of interstitial collagenase by osteoblasts. The synthesis of IGF-I is stimulated by PTH and other agents that stimulate cAMP in bone cells, but is inhibited by glucocorticoids. The reduced bone mass that occurs in association with glucocorticoid excess may be due in part to this inhibition of IGF-I.

Transforming growth factor-β (TGF-β), another family of polypeptide hormones produced both in bone and other tissues, *has powerful effects on both osteoclasts and osteoblasts, and probably plays a key role in bone remodeling*. During bone resorption, TGF-βs are released from the bone matrix in active form. They inhibit the proliferation and differentiation of osteoclast precursors, as well as the activity of mature osteoclasts. TGF-βs also stimulate the replication of osteoblast progenitors, increase collagen synthesis by differentiated osteoblasts and induce osteoblast chemotaxis in vitro.

Bone morphogenetic proteins (BMPs) are a *large subgroup of signaling molecules* within the TGF-β superfamily and have been the subject of intense research in recent years. Approximately 30 different BMPs with overlapping expression patterns have been identified. BMP-specific antagonists, such as noggin and chordin, have also been identified. BMPs appear early in embryogenesis and are involved in the induction of bone and cartilage development during organogenesis. They stimulate osteoblast differentiation and have a unique property of inducing heterotopic bone formation in vivo. This has led to considerable interest in the possible therapeutic use of BMPs in disease conditions where enhanced bone formation is desirable.

Acidic and basic **fibroblast growth factors** (FGFs) also have been shown to *stimulate bone formation* but, unlike TGF-βs, they do not influence bone resorption. FGFs probably generate additional osteoblast precursors, leading to increased numbers of differentiated osteoblasts, and are effective in stimulating new bone formation to restore bone mass. Abnormalities in FGF receptors have been identified in human patients with certain inherited skeletal disorders, including achondroplasia. **Platelet-derived growth factor** (PDGF) is a *potent stimulator of new bone formation, but also promotes bone resorption*.

Estrogen depletion induced by ovariectomy in a rat model markedly increases the synthesis of **interleukin-6** (IL-6) and **interleukin-11** (IL-11) by osteoblasts or their precursors in the bone marrow stroma. *These cytokines appear to play a crucial role in the recruitment, proliferation, and differentiation of osteoclast progenitors that eventually lead to reduced bone mass in estrogen deficiency*. Further support is derived from studies in mice following deletion of the IL-6 gene. Unlike normal controls, mice lacking the IL-6 gene do not show any reduction in bone mass after ovariectomy. **Interleukin-1** (IL-1) and **tumor necrosis factor-α** (TNF-α) are related cytokines that act synergistically on bone and also have been implicated in the pathogenesis of postmenopausal osteoporosis. Both are potent stimulators of osteoclastic activity in vitro and in vivo and may be involved in mediating focal bone resorption in certain inflammatory disorders. Unlike other cytokines, **γ-interferon** does not stimulate bone resorption. In fact, it selectively inhibits the resorption stimulated by IL-1 and TNF, probably through inhibition of prostaglandin synthesis. **Osteoprotegerin** (OPG), a newly described receptor-like protein, is a member of the TNF receptor family, and acts as a decoy receptor for RANK-L. Its major role appears to be in regulating bone remodeling through a negative effect on the maturation and activation of osteoclasts.

Several **colony-stimulating factors** (CSFs) influence bone resorption by regulating the proliferation and differentiation of osteoclast precursors. Their importance is highlighted by studies in mice with the *op/op* variant of osteopetrosis, where there is impaired production of macrophage colony-stimulating factor (M-CSF or CSF-1). A decrease in osteoclast formation, leading to reduced bone resorption and osteopetrosis, can be reversed transiently by the administration of M-CSF. Granulocyte macrophage colony-stimulating factor (GM-CSF) can also increase osteoclast differentiation from their precursors, thereby promoting bone resorption. Osteoblasts are capable of secreting GM-CSF following exposure to bacterial endotoxin or PTH.

Prostaglandins (PGs), in particular those of the E series, are another group of *important mediators of local bone resorption*. They are characterized by restricted, local activity before being rapidly degraded, making studies of their in vivo action extremely difficult. Consequently, their precise role has not been determined. PGE_2 appears to directly stimulate osteoclastic activity and may be a mediator of bone resorption regulated by osteoblasts. Local production of PGE_2 in response to inflammation, mechanical trauma, or neoplasia is likely to contribute to the bone resorption that is often associated with such conditions. PGE_2 has also been linked to the bone resorption and hypercalcemia associated with certain malignancies.

Nitric oxide, generated by the nitric oxide synthase group of enzymes, may be an important mediator of bone cell function. In vitro studies have revealed a biphasic effect on bone resorption. At low concentrations, nitric oxide potentiates IL-1-induced osteoclastic bone resorption, suggesting that small amounts of nitric oxide may be required for normal osteoclast activity. In contrast, high concentrations of nitric oxide strongly inhibit bone resorption both in organ cultures and in cultures of isolated osteoclasts. This inhibitory effect appears to be due to apoptosis of osteoclast progenitors, induced by the action of nitric oxide derived from osteoblasts. The effect of nitric oxide on osteoblast function is less clear, although estrogen has been shown to stimulate nitric oxide synthase activity in both endothelial cells and osteoblasts, suggesting a possible role of nitric oxide in mediating the protective effects of estrogen on bone. At high concentrations, nitric oxide inhibits osteoblast growth and differentiation. This provides a possible explanation for the reduced bone formation and osteoporosis that occurs in association with certain inflammatory conditions. The role of nitric oxide in vivo has yet to be established, but there is increasing evidence to support its role as an important regulator of bone turnover.

Remodeling of bone tissue

Throughout postnatal life, old or defective bone is constantly being replaced with new bone tissue by a process of **remodeling**. This occurs at a local level and involves the coordinated activities of osteoclasts and osteoblasts in so-called **bone remodeling units**, presumably mediated by a complex interaction between systemic hormones and locally acting cytokines. The remodeling sequence starts with activation of osteoblasts (probably bone-lining cells) by external signals such as hormones, cytokines, or growth factors to induce accelerated formation of osteoclasts from their precursors. The osteoclasts attach to the bone surface, seal it off from the extracellular space, and resorb bone matrix and mineral. Then follows a reversal phase during which resorption ceases, the osteoclasts detach from the bone and disappear, probably by apoptosis. Osteoblasts are attracted by an unknown mechanism to the resorption site where they deposit new bone.

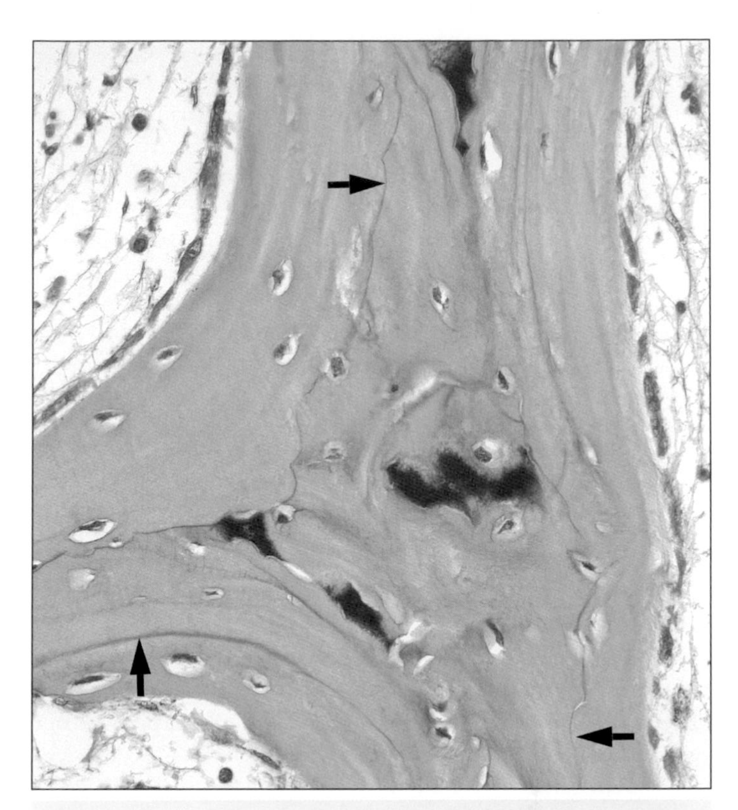

Figure 1.6 Cementing lines in a segment of trabecular bone. The smoothly contoured lines (vertical arrow) are referred to as **resting lines** and indicate sites at which bone formation had ceased for a period then recommenced. The scalloped lines (horizontal arrows) are **reversal lines** and reflect previous resorption, followed by deposition of new bone.

In the cortex, activated osteoclasts form a "cutting cone" which bores longitudinally through the dense, primary bone, creating a *resorption canal*. As the canal advances, it becomes lined by osteoblasts, which fill the space with concentric layers of new lamellar bone, creating a *secondary osteon or Haversian system*. This process provides a mechanism for on-going internal replacement of cortical bone without altering its gross form or function. Remodeling of trabecular bone follows a similar sequence, but from the trabecular surface, without the formation of resorption canals.

In histological sections, the separate units of secondary bone that form during remodeling can be distinguished from each other, and from adjacent primary bone, by the presence of deeply basophilic **cementing lines** (Fig. 1.6). These lines are created by the deposition of a thin layer of highly mineralized, collagen-free matrix at sites where bone resorption or formation ceases. Two types of cementing lines are recognized. Those with a scalloped appearance are termed **reversal lines**, and indicate a site where previous bone resorption had occurred, then new bone deposited in its place. Smoothly contoured cementing lines, or **resting lines**, mark sites where bone formation ceased for a period, then re-commenced. The number and pattern of cementing lines may provide useful information on the recent history of an area of bone, in particular regarding the rate of turnover.

Markers of bone remodeling

Although not used routinely in veterinary medicine, various **markers of bone remodeling** or turnover can be measured in serum or urine and may add support to a clinical diagnosis, or be of value in research. *Serum alkaline phosphatase activity is a well-recognized indicator of osteoblastic activity*, increased levels occurring in diseases characterized by increased bone formation such as hyperparathyroidism. Its diagnostic value is limited however by the fact that high levels are also detected normally in rapidly growing young animals. Furthermore, other isoforms of alkaline phosphatase are commonly used as indicators of cholestatic liver disease in several species and hyperadrenocorticism in dogs. Another potentially useful indicator of osteoblastic activity is *serum osteocalcin*. Approximately 10–25% of the osteocalcin synthesized by osteoblasts escapes into the circulation and serum concentrations are proportional to the rate of osteoid synthesis.

Bone resorption, associated with increased osteoclastic activity, is reflected by increased serum activity of *tartrate-resistant acid phosphatase*, an enzyme released by osteoclasts during the degradation of bone matrix. Increased urinary concentration of *hydroxyproline* has long been considered a marker of bone resorption, but this amino acid is present in all types of collagen, not just the type I collagen of bone, and cannot therefore be considered specific. Recent interest has focused on measurement of urinary concentrations of the *pyridinium cross-links* that bind the nontriple helical portions of one collagen molecule to another. Of these molecules, hydroxylysyl pyridinoline is the most abundant, but is less specific for type I collagen than deoxypyridinoline. Both can be detected in urine as either free or peptide-bound forms using commercially available kits.

In dogs, horses, rats and humans, considerable diurnal variations in the serum and urinary concentrations of bone markers have been demonstrated. This may reflect circadian rhythms in the rates of bone formation and resorption. There has been increasing interest in such markers of bone resorption in human medicine as indicators of post-menopausal bone loss or monitoring the effectiveness of antiresorptive therapy, but their application in animals is still largely confined to research.

Bibliography

Allen MJ, et al. Serum markers of bone metabolism in dogs. Am J Vet Res 1998;59:250–254.

Anderson HC. Molecular biology of matrix vesicles. Clin Orthop 1995;314:266–288.

Athanasou NA. Current concepts review: Cellular biology of bone-resorbing cells. J Bone Joint Surg 1996;78A:1096–1107.

Boyce BF, et al. Recent advances in bone biology provide insight into the pathogenesis of bone diseases. Lab Invest 1999;79:83–94.

Boyle WJ, Lacey DL. Osteoprotegerin. In: Canalis E ed. Skeletal Growth Factors. Philadelphia, PA: Lippincott Williams & Wilkins, 2000:365–374.

De Ricqles A, et al. Comparative microstructure of bone. In: Hall BK, ed. Bone: Bone Matrix and Bone Specific Products. Boca Raton, FL: CRC Press, 1991;3:1–78.

Goldring SR, Goldring MB. Cytokines and skeletal physiology. Clin Orthop 1996:324:13–23.

Hodgkinson A, Thompson T. Measurement of the fasting urinary hydroxyproline: creatinine ratio in normal adults and its variation with age and sex. J Clin Pathol 1984;35:807–811.

Horowitz MC. The role of cytokines in bone remodeling. J Clin Densitometry 1998;1:187–198.

Kawabata M, Miyazono K. Bone morphogenetic proteins. In: Canalis E, ed. Skeletal Growth Factors. Philadelphia, PA: Lippincott Williams & Wilkins, 2000:269–290.

Kleerekoper M. Biochemical markers of bone remodeling. Am J Med Sci 1996;312:270–277.

Lian JB, et al. Bone formation: osteoblast lineage cells, growth factors, matrix proteins and the mineralization process. In: Favus MJ, ed. Primer on the Metabolic Bone Diseases and Disorders of Mineral Metabolism. 4th ed. Philadelphia, PA: Lippincott Williams & Wilkins, 1999:14–29.

Liesegang A, et al. Diurnal variation in concentrations of various markers of bone metabolism in dogs. Am J Vet Res 1999;60:949–953.

Marks SC, Popoff SN. Bone cell biology: The regulation of development, structure and function in the skeleton. Am J Anat 1988;183:1–44.

Marotti G. Morphological and quantitative aspects of bone formation and mineralization. In: Pecile A, de Bernard B, eds. Bone Regulatory Factors. Morphology, Biochemistry, Physiology and Pharmacology. New York, London: Plenum Press, 1990:39–53.

Mohan S, Baylink DJ. Bone growth factors. Clin Orthop 1991;263:30–48.

Mundy GR. Regulation of bone formation by bone morphogenetic proteins and other growth factors. Clin Orthop 1996;323:24–28.

Mundy GR. Bone remodeling. In: Favus MJ, ed. Primer on the Metabolic Bone Diseases and Disorders of Mineral Metabolism. 4th ed. Philadelphia, PA: Lippincott Williams & Wilkins, 1999:30–38.

Parfitt AM. Cellular basis of bone remodeling. Calcif Tiss Int 1984;36:S37–45.

Raisz LG, Kream BE. Regulation of bone formation. New Engl J Med 1983;309:29–89.

Schenk RK, Hofstetter W, Felix R. Morphology and chemical composition of connective tissue: bone. In: Royce PM, Steinmann B, eds. Connective Tissue and its Heritable Disorders. Molecular, Genetic and Medical Aspects. 2nd ed. New York: Wiley-Liss, 2002:67–120.

Suda T, et al. Regulation of osteoclast function. J Bone Min Res 1997;12:869–879.

Theill LE, et al. RANK-L and RANK: T cells, bone loss and mammalian evolution. Ann Rev Immunol 2002;20:795–823.

Vaes G. Cellular biology and biochemical mechanism of bone resorption. Clin Orthop 1988;231: 239–271.

Vanderschueren D, Bouillon R. Androgens and bone. Calcif Tissue Int 1995;56:341–346.

van't Hof RJ, Ralston SH. Nitric oxide's function in bone cells. Curr Opin Orthop 1997;8:19–24.

Ectopic mineralization and ossification

Extraskeletal deposition of either amorphous calcium phosphate or hydroxyapatite crystals, referred to as **ectopic** or **heterotopic mineralization** (calcification), occurs in a range of disease conditions, and must be differentiated from **ectopic ossification**, where the mineral is deposited in the form of bone tissue.

Three main forms of ectopic mineralization are recognized in animals: metastatic, dystrophic, and idiopathic. **Metastatic mineralization** is a frequent complication of disease conditions associated with hypercalcemia and/or hyperphosphatemia, such as vitamin D toxicity, hypercalcemia of malignancy, primary hyperparathyroidism and uremia. In dogs, direct precipitation of mineral occurs when the *calcium-phosphate solubility product*, expressed in mg/dL, persistently exceeds 60. The mineral deposited in metastatic mineralization typically occurs in the outer medullary region of the kidney, the fundus of the stomach, and the lungs, all of which are involved in acid secretion and possess a local alkaline environment favoring mineral precipitation. Other favored sites include the media of large arteries and the elastic tissue of the endocardium, but the reason for such predilection is not clear.

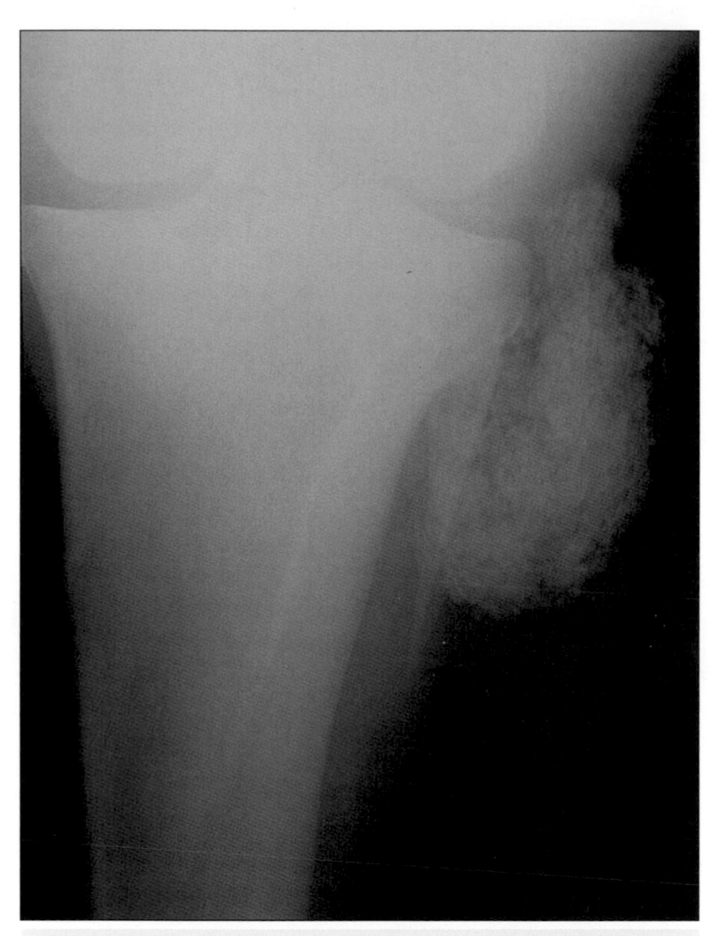

Figure 1.7 Tumoral calcinosis in a horse. A large, discrete mass lateral to the femoro-tibial joint contains multiple radiodense deposits.

Dystrophic mineralization occurs in association with *damaged tissue* rather than an elevated calcium-phosphate solubility product, probably due to the release or establishment of cellular components with nucleation properties following injury. Examples include mineral deposition in the caseous lesions of bovine tuberculosis and caprine paratuberculosis, and the mineralization of muscle fibers in animals with nutritional myodegeneration.

Idiopathic forms of ectopic mineralization occur in a variety of unrelated disease syndromes, including **calcinosis cutis**, which is characterized by widespread mineralization of dermal elastic fibers in association with hyperadrenocorticism, and **tumoral calcinosis** (*calcinosis circumscripta*), where tumor-like nodules of ectopic mineralization develop in soft tissues, often close to joints. Tumoral calcinosis in horses usually occurs in animals about 2–4 years of age, and 90% of lesions develop on the lateral aspect of the stifle (Fig. 1.7). The lesions may be single or multiple and are sometimes attached to the joint capsule, but not to the overlying skin. They usually appear as hard, well-circumscribed, nonpainful, subcutaneous swellings ranging in size from about 3–12 cm in diameter. Individual lesions consist of a tough, outer, fibrous capsule with collagenous trabeculae dividing the interior into numerous variable-sized locules consisting of finely granular, chalky white accumulations of calcium salts, surrounded by a rim of granulomatous inflammation cells. The lesions usually do not cause lameness and do not recur after surgical removal. Tumoral calcinosis in humans is also characterized by deposition of mineral in locular masses adjacent to major joints, particularly the shoulder and hip. Autosomal recessive inheritance is suggested to account for approximately one third of human cases, and hyperphosphatemia is often present, but the pathogenesis is unknown.

In dogs, the manifestations of calcinosis circumscripta are variable, and show breed preferences. In German Shepherds, the lesions are generally solitary, occurring most often in the skin near pressure points, but multiple lesions occur in some dogs, often attached to tendons, joint capsules, or the periosteum. Involvement of the vertebral processes of C-4 and C-5 was reported in three 5–6-month-old Great Dane puppies from the same litter, suggesting the possibility of a familial etiology. The lesions are usually nonpainful and nonprogressive, but may cause clinical signs if they interfere with the function of adjacent structures. For example, spinal cord compression caused by paravertebral calcinosis circumscripta occurred in two young dogs of different breeds. Although the pathogenesis is not known, repetitive trauma has been suggested as a predisposing factor, at least in some cases with skin involvement. Trauma is less likely to be responsible for lesions associated with vertebrae or involving the tongue, as has been reported.

A syndrome characterized by calcium hydroxyapatite deposition in the spinal canal of young Great Dane puppies has been reported to cause paraplegia and incoordination. Mineral deposition may also be present in joints and soft tissues of affected pups. In one report, the condition occurred in two litters of related Great Danes and was considered familial.

Ectopic ossification refers to the *formation of nonneoplastic trabecular bone in extraosseous sites*, presumably following the induction of pluripotential stem cells by appropriate growth factors. In most cases, ectopic bone is detected as an incidental finding at necropsy without an obvious predisposing cause. Typical sites include the pulmonary connective tissue of dogs and cattle, and the cervical and lumbosacral dura mater of aged dogs (ossifying pachymeningitis). Ectopic ossification also occurs in the supporting connective tissue of certain tumors in dogs, particularly mammary carcinomas, where it is very common, and to a lesser extent in thyroid and salivary carcinomas.

Specific disease entities associated with widespread ossification of soft tissues have been described both in human patients and animals and may involve overexpression or dysregulation of bone morphogenetic proteins. The temptation with such diseases in animals is to classify them according to the human syndrome that they most closely resemble. Such comparisons are usually subjective and may not be appropriate in all cases. A syndrome resembling human **fibrodysplasia ossificans progressiva** has been described in several cats and occasionally in the dog, although some of these cases more closely resemble myositis ossificans. In cats, the disease is characterized by *progressive, symmetrical, hyperplasia and ossification of connective tissue in the subcutis and epimysium of the neck, dorsum and limbs.* Affected cats have ranged in age from 5 months to 6 years. A feature of the disease in humans, and in some reported cases in animals, is the formation of bone in soft tissue sites by the process of endochondral ossification. In the 5-month-old cat referred to above, there was massive thickening of joint capsules and synovial membranes of several limb joints with disorganized hyaline cartilage (Fig. 1.8A, B). There was bilateral involvement of carpal and stifle joints in addition to several metatarsophalangeal and interphalangeal joints. Many foci of endochondral ossification were scattered throughout the hyperplastic

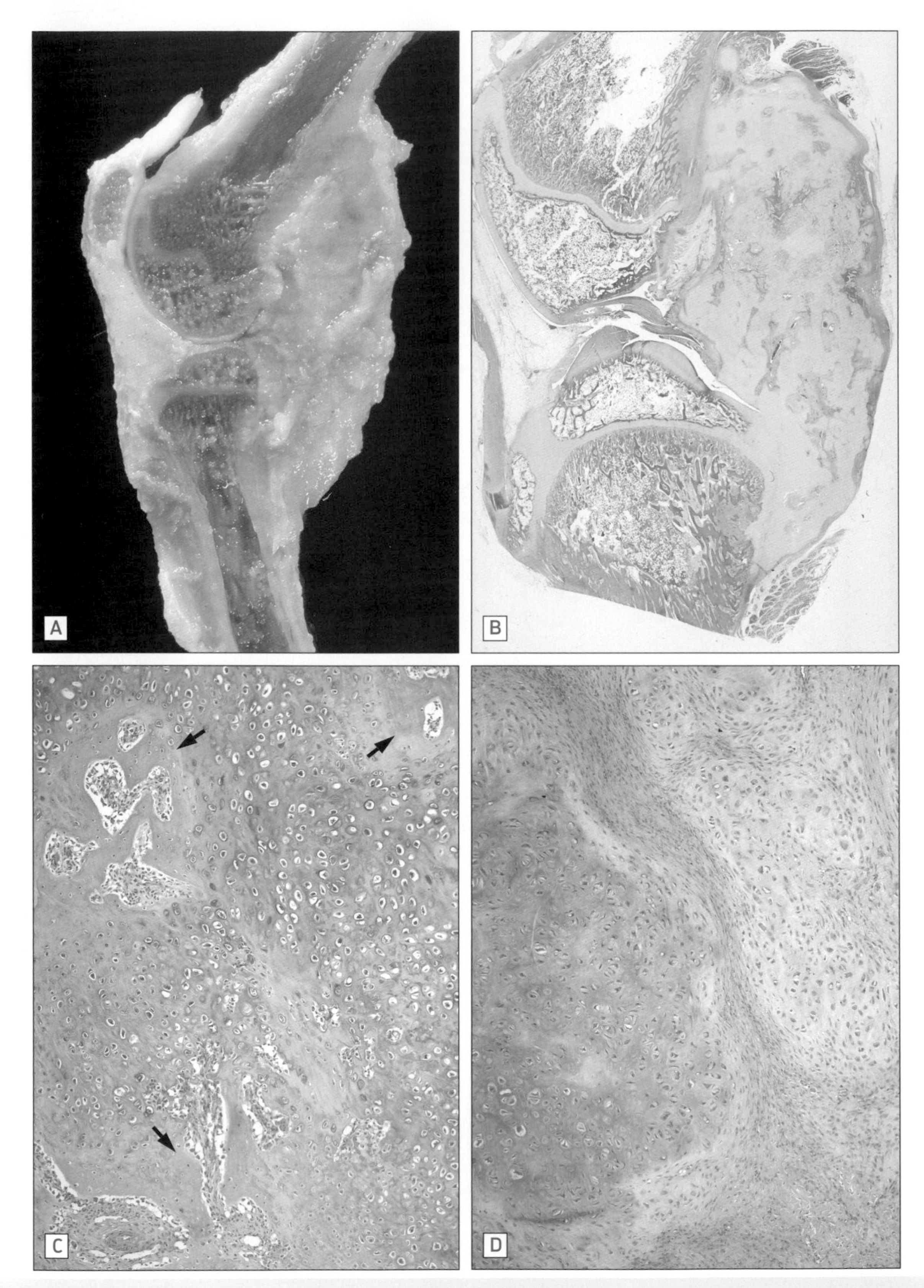

Figure 1.8 Fibrodysplasia ossificans progressiva in a 5-month-old kitten. **A.** Left stifle joint showing massive thickening of the joint capsule on the caudal aspect of the joint with tissue resembling cartilage. Similar lesions involved the right stifle, and several other limb joints. **B.** Subgross preparation of the same lesion, showing a cartilaginous mass bridging the stifle joint and attaching to the cortex of the adjacent femur and tibia in the region of the capsular insertions. **C.** Microscopically, the lesion consists of disorganized hyaline cartilage containing many plump chondrocytes and undergoing multifocal endochondral ossification (arrows). **D.** Biopsy of an early lesion from the same kitten, showing proliferating nodules of disorganized hyaline cartilage with features suggestive of chondrosarcoma.

cartilage, which, in some areas, had microscopic features suggestive of chondrosarcoma (Fig. 1.8C, D). The disease in man is associated with overexpression of at least one of the BMPs and is inherited as an autosomal dominant trait. Although there is no evidence of a genetic etiology in cats, there have been too few reported cases for this to be established.

Myositis ossificans has also been reported in cats and in a dog, but differs from fibrodysplasia ossificans in being *localized and asymmetric.* The lesions characteristically possess a peripheral zone of orderly maturation from fibrous tissue to mineralized osteoid, which is gradually replaced by lamellar bone. The prognosis following surgical removal is very good. Trauma is considered the initiating factor in most human cases of myositis ossificans, and the same probably applies to animals. Ossification of a hematoma may be the mechanism in some cases.

Generalized forms of myositis ossificans have been reported in cats and pigs but may have been more appropriately classified as fibrodysplasia ossificans. The disease in pigs was familial, occurring at 2–6 months of age in 34 of 115 offspring of an affected boar, and was characterized by widespread ossification of soft tissues, especially around vertebrae. The boar had developed similar lesions at 9 months of age.

Ectopic bone may form in lesions that have been mineralized for an extended period, possibly due to metaplasia of cells involved in the initial process of mineralization. This may account for the disseminated foci of metaplastic bone that form occasionally in the skin of dogs with hyperadrenocorticism and calcinosis cutis. Alternatively, the cutaneous osseous metaplasia in such cases may be due to local production of specific growth factors, including TGF-β, FGFs, and BMPs, by inflammatory cells in the dermis. TGF-β has been found in large quantities in inflammatory disorders of the skin of human patients with osteoma cutis, a condition similar to that described in dogs, and has been associated with the differentiation of fibroblastic cells into osteoblasts.

Where ectopic bone forms in close association with or becomes attached to a bone, differentiation of the lesion from a fracture callus or a parosteal osteosarcoma may prove difficult. Depending on its stage of maturation, a fracture callus is likely to contain remnants of cartilage or chondro-osseous bone, while *ectopic bone is composed exclusively of trabecular bone.* In parosteal osteosarcoma, the spaces between trabeculae will be populated with mesenchymal cells showing features of malignancy, rather than a single layer of osteoblasts lined up along the surface of bone trabeculae.

Bibliography

Aaron DN, et al. Report of an unusual case of ectopic ossification and review of the literature. J Am Anim Hosp Assoc 1985;21:819–829.

Bone DL, McGavin MD. Myositis ossificans in the dog: A case report and review. J Am Anim Hosp Assoc 1985;21:135–138.

Ellison GW, Norrdin RW. Multicentric periarticular calcinosis in a pup. J Am Vet Med Assoc 1980;177:542–546.

Frazier KS, et al. Multiple cutaneous metaplastic ossification associated with iatrogenic hyperglucocorticoidism. J Vet Diagn Invest 1998;10:303–307.

Goulden BE, O'Callaghan MW. Tumoral calcinosis in the horse. N Z Vet J 1980;28:217–219.

Lewis DG, Kelly DF. Calcinosis circumscripta in dogs as a cause of spinal ataxia. J Small Anim Pract 1990;31:35–37.

Seibold HR, Davis CL. Generalized myositis ossificans (familial) in pigs. Pathol Vet 1967;4:79–88.

Shore EM, et al. Osteogenic induction in hereditary disorders of heterotopic ossification. Clin Orthop Rel Res 1999;374:303–316.

Waldron D, et al. Progressive ossifying myositis in a cat. J Am Vet Med Assoc 1985;187:64–65.

Warren HB, Carpenter JL. Fibrodysplasia ossificans in three cats. Vet Pathol 1984;21:495–499.

Wünchmann A, et al. Calcium hydroxylapatite deposition disease in a Great Dane puppy. Vet Pathol 2000;37:346–349.

BONES AS ORGANS

Development and anatomy

There are two distinct processes by which bone formation occurs in the developing fetus. *Flat bones of the skull develop by* **intramembranous ossification**. Mesenchymal progenitor cells migrate from the neural crest to form condensations at specific, highly vascular, sites in the head region and some other flat bones, where they differentiate directly into osteoblasts and produce anastomosing trabeculae of woven bone. These centers of ossification expand by on-going osteoblastic differentiation of mesenchymal cells at the periphery and apposition of new bone on the surface of trabeculae, to form a plate. A fibrous layer, *the periosteum*, separates the developing membrane bone from adjacent tissues and controls its shape. Individual bones of the developing skull are separated by connective tissue **sutures** until growth ceases, at which time a bony union forms. With maturity, the woven bone is remodeled and replaced by lamellar bone. Intramembranous bone formation also occurs at the periosteal surfaces of all bones during growth.

Most bones of the skeleton, including those of the limbs, vertebral column, pelvis, and base of the skull, develop by **endochondral ossification**. In this process, condensations of primitive mesenchymal cells differentiate into chondrocytes and produce crude cartilage models of the adult bone destined to form at that site. An avascular fibrous layer, the perichondrium, surrounds each cartilage model. As expansion of the model continues by interstitial growth, chondrocytes near the center become hypertrophic, and the matrix undergoes mineralization. Meanwhile, the perichondrium becomes invaded with capillaries, converting it into a periosteum, and a narrow cuff of bone forms by intramembranous ossification around the mid-shaft region of the developing bone. Capillaries and osteoclasts then invade the hypertrophic cartilage from the periosteum and establish a vascular network. Preosteoblasts also enter with the invading capillaries and differentiate into osteoblasts, which deposit osteoid on remnants of the mineralized cartilage, creating a **primary ossification center**. This process of endochondral ossification continues as the chondrocytes at either end of the developing bone continue to proliferate and the model expands in length and width. Once the bone reaches a certain stage of development, **secondary ossification centers** appear at one or both ends (depending on the bone), and expand by endochondral ossification to form the **epiphyses** of long bones. As the epiphyses expand, they remain separated from the primary ossification center, now occupying the **diaphysis** and **metaphysis** of the developing bone, by the **physis** or **growth plate**. Limited growth in size of the epiphysis continues by endochondral ossification beneath

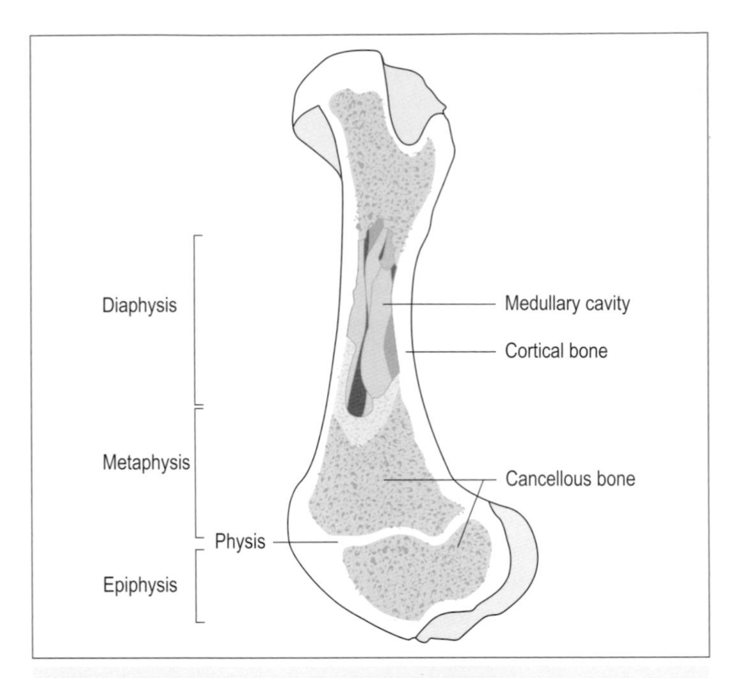

Figure 1.9 Drawing of the femur from a newborn calf, illustrating the **gross anatomy and terminology** of the different regions.

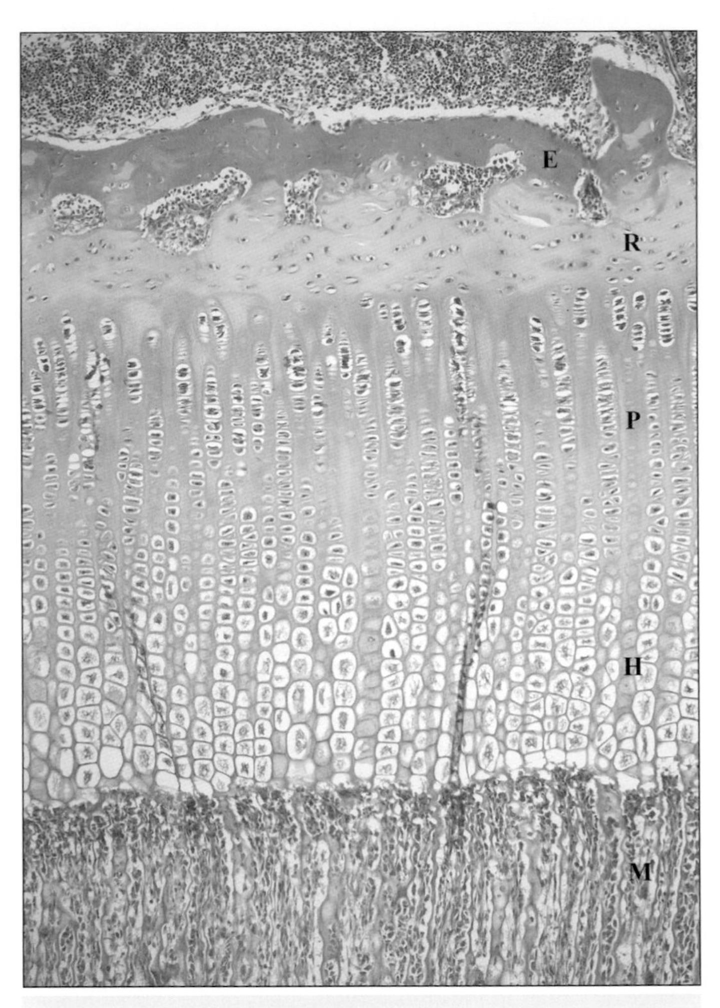

Figure 1.10 Physis or growth plate of a young animal showing the reserve (R), proliferative (P), and hypertrophic (H) zones. The reserve zone is anchored to trabecular bone of the epiphysis (E). Also note the abrupt transition from the hypertrophic zone of the physis to the metaphysis (M).

the articular cartilage at the articular–epiphyseal cartilage complex. The epiphyseal side of the growth plate soon becomes capped by a layer of trabecular bone, preventing further growth from that side, but proliferation of chondrocytes in the growth plate and endochondral ossification on the metaphyseal side continues until maturity. The gross anatomy and terminology of a developing long bone, in this case the femur of a newborn calf, is illustrated in Figure 1.9.

During active bone growth, *the hyaline cartilage of the growth plate is organized into three easily recognizable zones* (Fig. 1.10). A **reserve**, or **resting zone**, with irregularly dispersed chondrocytes and pale-staining matrix, is anchored to the trabecular bone of the epiphysis. The chondrocytes in this zone have the lowest concentration of intracellular ionized calcium, but the matrix has the highest concentration of type-II collagen. In the **proliferative zone**, the chondrocytes are tightly packed into longitudinal columns, the cell at the top being the progenitor cell for longitudinal growth of each column. The chondrocytes in this zone are actively dividing, accumulating glycogen, and synthesizing matrix proteoglycans. The columns of chondrocytes are separated by deeply basophilic cartilage matrix rich in aggregated proteoglycans, which inhibit mineralization in spite of the presence of matrix vesicles. Within columns, only thin matrix septa separate individual chondrocytes. The chondrocytes of the **hypertrophic zone** become enlarged, but remain metabolically active and are responsible for preparing the matrix for mineralization. They rely on anaerobic glycolysis for energy production because of the distance from epiphyseal blood vessels, which terminate at the top of the proliferative zone, and the inability of oxygen to diffuse from the metaphysis through the mineralized matrix of the lower hypertrophic zone. The energy is used primarily in the accumulation, storage, then release of calcium as part of the mineralization process. The lower region of the hypertrophic zone is commonly referred to as the *zone of degeneration*, as the chondrocytes appear to have separated from the pericellular matrix and become degenerate in sections prepared for histology and electron microscopy by routine methods. Following the development of more sophisticated techniques for preparing sections of cartilage for transmission electron microscopy, this concept has been challenged. Rather than being degenerate, these chondrocytes appear to be highly differentiated cells capable of synthesizing type-X collagen, chondrocalcin and other macromolecules that, together with matrix vesicles, are likely to be involved in initiating matrix mineralization. Mineralization of the cartilage matrix occurs in the deepest layer of the hypertrophic zone and is an essential event in the process of endochondral ossification. This mineralized layer is not evident in histological sections prepared after demineralization. The transition from growth plate to metaphysis is abrupt, and is designated by the last intact layer of chondrocytes.

Around the perimeter of the growth plate there is a wedge-shaped groove of cells, termed the **ossification groove of Ranvier**. The cells in this groove proliferate and are responsible for increasing the diameter of the physis during growth. A dense layer of fibrous tissue, the **perichondrial ring of LaCroix**, surrounds the groove of Ranvier and is continuous with the fibrous layer of the periosteum. As such, it provides strong mechanical support at the bone–cartilage junction of the growth plate, an area that is prone to injury in fast-growing young animals.

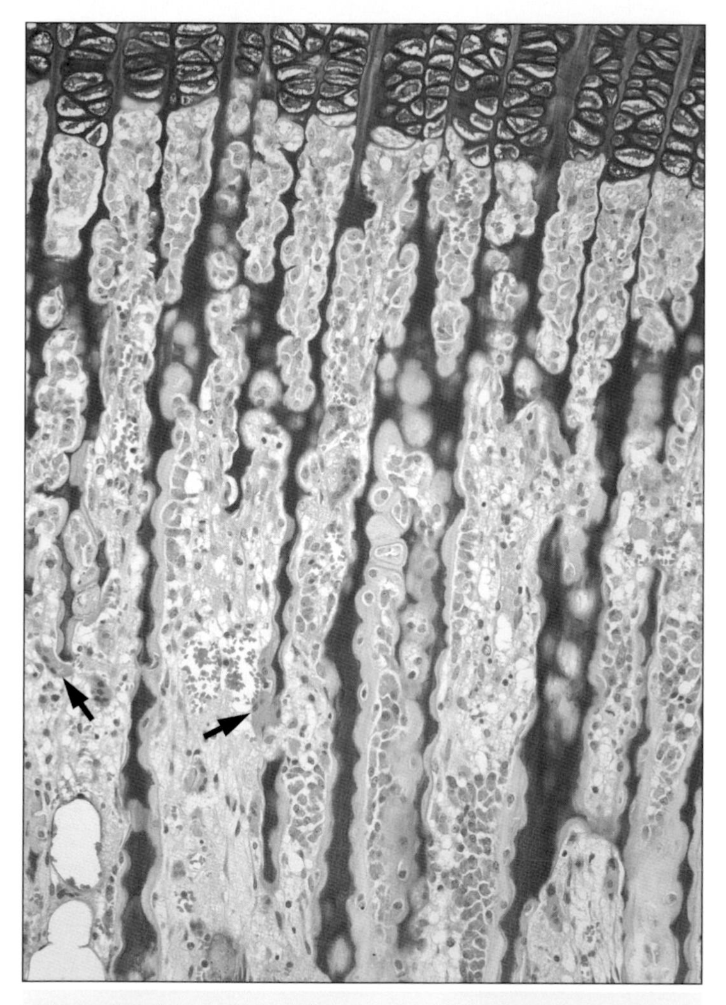

Figure 1.11 Primary spongiosa in a rapidly growing young animal. Basophilic spicules of calcified cartilage matrix extending into the metaphysis at right angles to the growth plate, form a lattice on which osteoblasts are lining up and depositing osteoid. Osteoclasts (arrows) are resorbing some trabeculae from the medullary end.

From the metaphyseal side of the growth plate, osteoclasts attack the mineralized cartilage matrix and rapidly remove the delicate transverse septa between individual chondrocytes within columns, allowing vascular invasion. The thicker longitudinal septa of mineralized cartilage matrix between columns of chondrocytes are not resorbed at this stage. Instead, they provide a framework on which newly differentiated osteoblasts line up and deposit a layer of woven bone (Fig. 1.11). *This lattice of trabeculae, with a basophilic core of mineralized cartilage covered by a thin, eosinophilic layer of bone is termed the* **primary spongiosa**. Trabeculae of the primary spongiosa extend at right angles to the direction of the growth plate, but deeper in the metaphysis, the trabeculae are remodeled by the coordinated action of osteoclasts and osteoblasts and are realigned in directions most suited to withstanding the mechanical forces acting on the bone. During this process, the cartilage cores and woven bone of the primary spongiosa are largely removed and replaced by thicker trabeculae of lamellar bone, which form the **secondary spongiosa**. While growth in length of a bone is continuing from the growth plate, osteoclastic resorption of trabeculae occurs at the metaphyseal–diaphyseal junction in order to *create the medullary cavity*.

The thickness of a growth plate is relatively constant across the width of the bone and is proportional to its rate of growth. So too is the distance to which trabeculae of the primary spongiosa extend into the metaphysis before they are remodeled. As growth slows, the different layers within the growth plate become narrow, and a transverse layer of trabecular bone forms on the metaphyseal side. The cartilage of the growth plate is then replaced with a bony scar, which is gradually remodeled into trabecular bone, blurring the margin between the epiphysis and metaphysis. The timing of growth plate closure varies both between and within bones and is controlled to a large degree by androgens and estrogens, but it is likely that nutritional factors can also play a role. In the radius, the distal growth plate remains open longer, and contributes significantly more to the length of the bone, than the proximal growth plate. In the humerus, femur, and tibia, the opposite is true. *The fastest-growing growth plates are the ones that are most likely to suffer damage due to trauma or nutritional imbalances*, and are therefore worthwhile sites to examine at necropsy, and to sample for histopathology.

The growth in width of the diaphysis in young animals occurs by intramembranous ossification beneath the **periosteum**, *which covers the surface of bones except at their articular ends and at insertion points of muscles and tendons*. The periosteum has a tough outer fibrous layer and a more cellular inner layer, *the cambium*, which contributes preosteoblasts for new bone formation (Fig. 1.12). Where muscle fibers and tendons insert onto bones, dense collagen fibers termed **Sharpey's fibers** become embedded in the bone matrix. The periosteum has a rich supply of nerve endings and blood vessels. *The inner bone surface is lined by a thin layer of osteogenic cells called the* **endosteum**.

Regulation of physeal growth

Many of the systemic hormones and local growth factors that regulate the formation and resorption of bone tissue also influence growth plate function. Their effect may be on a particular zone of the growth plate, and may vary with the age of the animal. **Growth hormone** and its mediators, the **insulin-like growth factors** (IGF-I and IGF-II), act throughout all zones of the growth plate, but **IGF** receptors are most abundant in the proliferative zone, implying a strong influence on cellular proliferation and hence longitudinal growth. **Thyroid hormones** are essential for cartilage growth and the maturation of chondrocytes, and appear to act synergistically with IGF-I. Deficiency of thyroid hormones leads to growth retardation and cretinism. **PTH** acts primarily on the proliferative and upper hypertrophic zones of the growth plate, and has a direct mitogenic effect on chondrocytes, as well as stimulating proteoglycan synthesis. It enhances the mitogenic effect of local growth factors. **Calcitonin** has been shown to accelerate chondrocyte maturation and matrix mineralization. The primary influence of **glucocorticoids** on the growth plate is to inhibit chondrocyte differentiation and proliferation. In young animals, excessive glucocorticoids from either endogenous or exogenous sources result in growth retardation. At physiological concentrations, **androgens** are anabolic factors, stimulating proteoglycan synthesis by chondrocytes in young animals, but they also stimulate mineralization in the growth plate. High doses of androgens actually depress growth and accelerate growth plate closure. **Estrogens**, in general, exhibit an inhibitory effect on longitudinal bone growth, excessive levels leading to premature closure of growth plates.

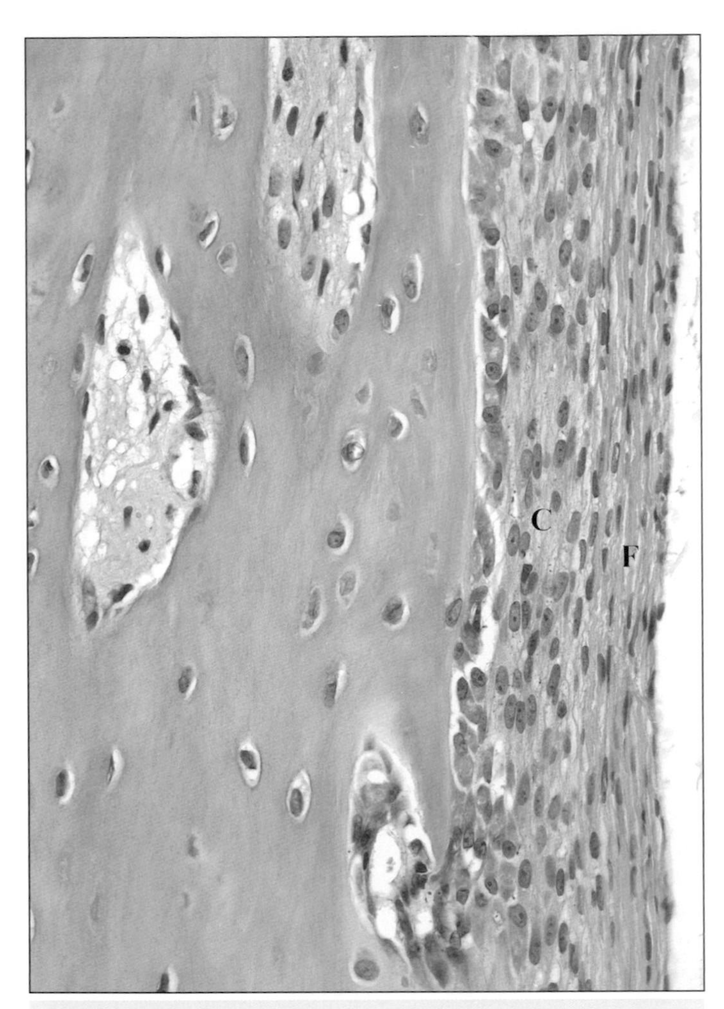

Figure 1.12 Periosteum in an actively growing young animal. Note the outer fibrous layer (F) and the cambium layer (C) containing primitive mesenchymal cells. A single layer of active osteoblasts lines the bone surface.

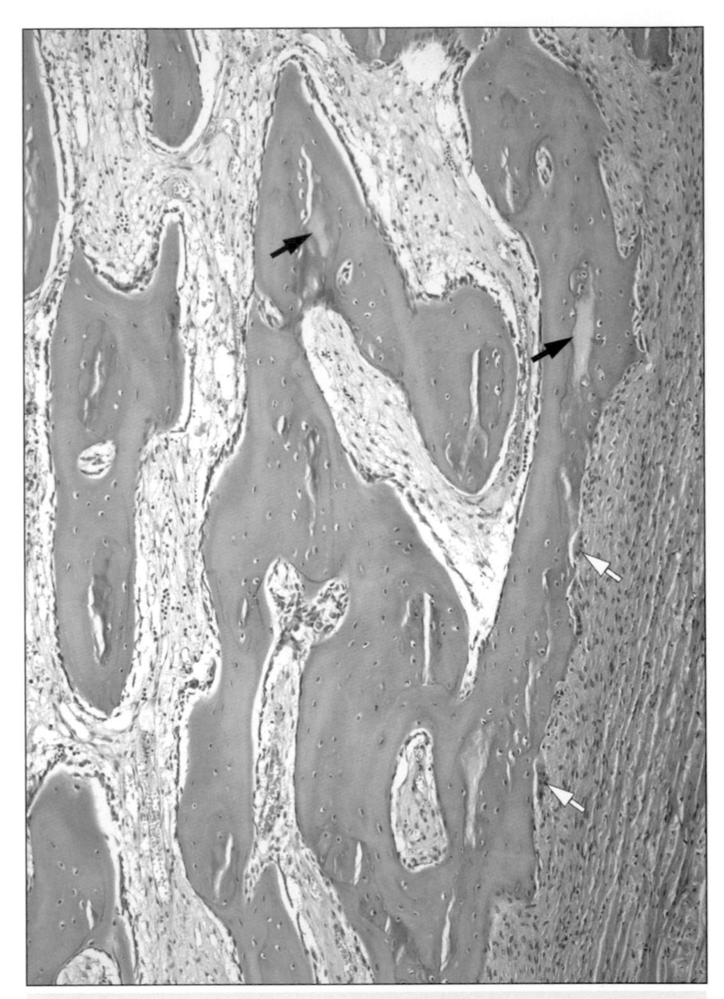

Figure 1.13 Architectural modeling in the metaphysis of a long bone during growth in length. In order to maintain the flare in the metaphyseal region, osteoclasts (white arrows) resorb bone at the periosteal surface, while osteoblasts actively deposit bone along trabeculae of the primary and secondary spongiosa. Trabecular bone of endochondral origin is thus converted into dense cortical bone. The spicules of mineralized cartilage (black arrows) derived from the growth plate persist until the cortex is remodeled.

Replication of chondrocytes is stimulated by several local growth factors, including **TGF-β**, **FGF**, and **epidermal growth factor** (EGF). TGF-β, in addition to its role as a regulator of bone formation, is also involved in the formation of cartilage, and has been shown to be a potent inhibitor of interleukin-1, which induces degradation of growth plate chondrocytes. **Prostaglandins** are present at low levels in the growth plate and although they have been shown to inhibit alkaline phosphatase activity and collagen synthesis while stimulating proteoglycan synthesis, their overall effect on growth plate function in unclear.

Modeling

In order to establish the unique shape of a long bone, extensive architectural **modeling** *occurs throughout the growth phase.* As the bone increases in size, the diameter of the diaphysis increases by deposition of new bone beneath the periosteum and resorption from the endosteal surface. However, growth in length is more complex and involves the coordinated actions of osteoclasts and osteoblasts operating on different bone surfaces. The diameter of most long bones is greatest at the level of the growth plate, then tapers through the metaphyseal region to its narrowest region in the diaphysis. This basic funnel shape is maintained during growth in length by continual osteoclastic resorption beneath the periosteum around the circumference of the metaphysis, thereby reducing its diameter. Meanwhile, osteoblasts rapidly deposit new bone within tunnels between the peripheral trabeculae of the primary and secondary spongiosa, converting it into dense cortical bone (Fig. 1.13). During this process, spicules of mineralized cartilage originating from the growth plate become incorporated into the cortex and will remain there until they are removed by remodeling.

The peripheral metaphysis of a growing long bone is therefore an area of intense osteoclastic and osteoblastic activity. The cortex is relatively porous, consisting of trabecular bone undergoing compaction, and there is extensive peritrabecular fibrosis. This must be borne in mind when examining histological sections from such areas in young animals with suspected metabolic bone diseases, particularly fibrous osteodystrophy.

The normal curvature present in some bones is produced during growth by a modeling process referred to as **osseous drift**, whereby the shaft of a bone moves on its long axis. This is accomplished by successive waves of osteoblastic and osteoclastic activity beneath appropriate periosteal and endosteal surfaces of the diaphyseal cortex,

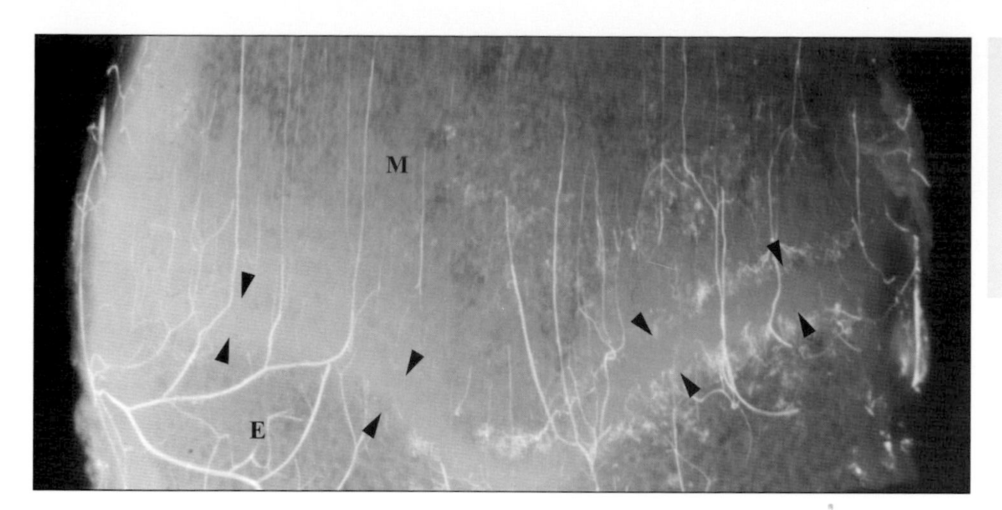

Figure 1.14 Transphyseal blood vessels. Cabinet radioangiogram of a 2 mm thick slice of decalcified distal 3rd metacarpal bone from a 13-day-old foal. The physis is between the arrowheads. The arterial blood supply to this area had been injected with radio-opaque dye immediately after death. Numerous transphyseal arteries can be seen crossing from the epiphysis (E) to the metaphysis (M). (Courtesy of EC Firth.)

presumably under the influence of both genetic and mechanical forces, leading to the formation of laminar bone deposits. The same process is involved in efforts to correct shape abnormalities in long bones resulting from malunited fractures, or other acquired defects altering the mechanical forces acting on a bone.

Bones respond to increased usage during the growth phase by an increase in bone mass, particularly in the density and thickness of the cortex. In adults, increased mechanical usage does not increase bone mass, but can decrease remodeling and conserve the amount of bone already present.

Blood supply

The blood supply to bones is derived from arteries entering the medullary cavity through foramina in the cortices of the diaphysis, metaphysis, and epiphysis, as well as periosteal arteries. In young growing animals, **nutrient arteries** supply the diaphyseal marrow and most of the central area of the metaphysis, while **metaphyseal arteries** supply the peripheral regions. Terminal branches from these vessels pass vertically towards the metaphyseal surface of the growth plate, where they end in fenestrated capillary loops immediately below the last intact transverse septum of the mineralized cartilage matrix. At this point they turn back sharply into wide-bore venules characterized by low flow rate. Some terminal branches of the nutrient and metaphyseal arterial systems anastomose with each other but they do not penetrate the growth plate.

Epiphyseal arteries supply the epiphyses or secondary centers of ossification and small branches pass through narrow cartilage canals in the reserve zone of the growth plate to terminate at the start of the proliferative zone. This is the only source of oxygen and nutrients to the growth plate as no blood vessels terminate in the hypertrophic zone. Further branches of the epiphyseal artery pass to the undersurface of the overlying articular cartilage, where they form vascular loops similar to those on the metaphyseal side of growth plates, and participate in endochondral ossification.

Transphyseal blood vessels have been identified in newborn animals of several species (Fig. 1.14), but their function remains obscure. Most evidence suggests that the direction of arterial flow in these vessels is from the epiphysis to the metaphysis, but that venous flow occurs in the opposite direction. Transphyseal blood vessels do not provide nutrients to the growth plate but may enhance the blood supply to the metaphysis during the rapid growth phase in very young animals. At sites where transphyseal vessels enter the metaphysis, they are surrounded by cartilage projections, which might be expected to strengthen the union between the epiphysis and metaphysis at a time when the growth plate is highly susceptible to shear forces. These vessels may also be involved in certain diseases of bones, such as osteomyelitis, where they provide a possible route for spread of infection across the growth plate. The periphery of the growth plate is supplied by perichondrial arteries to the perichondrial ring of LaCroix, and by metaphyseal arteries.

The blood supply to the bone cortex in young animals is predominantly derived from the endosteal surface by way of nutrient arteries, and the flow of blood within the cortex is centrifugal. Arterial blood enters Haversian systems of the cortex through capillaries communicating with medullary sinusoids, but venous drainage occurs through the periosteal surface. With age, the cortex becomes increasingly dependent on **periosteal arteries** for its blood supply.

Bibliography

Baron R. Anatomy and ultrastructure of bone. In: Favus MJ, ed. Primer on Metabolic Bone Disease. 3rd ed. Philadelphia, New York: Lippincott-Raven, 1996:3–10.

Brookes M. Morphology and distribution of blood vessels and blood flow in bone. In: Schoutens A, et al, eds. Bone Circulation and Vascularization in Normal and Abnormal Conditions. NATO ASI Series, New York, London: Plenum Press, 1993:19–28.

Firth EC, Hodge H. Physeal form of the long bones of the foal. Res Vet Sci 1997;62:217–221.

Firth EC, Poulos PW. Blood vessels in the developing growth plate of the equine distal radius and metacarpus. Res Vet Sci 1982;33:159–166.

Goyal HO, et al. Growth rates at the extremities of limb bones in young horses. Can Vet J 1981;22:31–33.

Hunziker EB, et al. Cartilage ultrastructure after high pressure freezing, freeze substitution, and low temperature embedding. I. Chondrocyte ultrastructure. Implications for the theories of mineralization and vascular invasion. J Cell Biol 1984;227:267–276.

Ianotti JP. Growth plate physiology and pathology. Orthop Clin North Am 1990;21:1–17.

Frost HM. Review article. Mechanical determinants of bone modeling. Metab Bone Dis Rel Res 1982;4:217–229.

POSTMORTEM EXAMINATION OF THE SKELETON

Of all organ systems, the skeleton is perhaps the most neglected during postmortem examination, even by experienced pathologists. Most organs are examined as part of the routine necropsy technique, but examination of the skeleton is more often confined to those occasions where the clinical history clearly indicates a skeletal problem. As a result, many skeletal disorders are likely to be missed. Furthermore, lack of familiarity with the normal appearance of skeletal structures commonly leads to misinterpretation in cases where a skeletal disease is suspected and a detailed examination of the skeleton is performed.

Gross examination

Complete examination of the skeleton is both impractical and unnecessary. A standard procedure for examining the skeleton should include an assessment of the shape, flexibility and breaking strength of readily accessible bones, such as ribs, cranium and key limb bones during routine necropsy. *No skeletal examination is complete without sectioning one or two representative long bones longitudinally* to reveal the growth plates, the thickness of the cortex, and the amount and density of trabecular bone in metaphyseal and epiphyseal regions. When the clinical history suggests the possibility of a skeletal disorder, a more detailed assessment is required. Antemortem radiographs are a valuable component of the gross examination in such cases and may highlight areas requiring special attention. The pathologist should insist on viewing them before commencing the necropsy. Radiographs of lesions identified during necropsy, either in the form of whole bones or sawn slabs, can also provide valuable information on the extent and severity of bone lysis or demineralization, but is an insensitive indicator of diffuse bone loss, as occurs in osteoporosis.

The manifestations of generalized skeletal diseases are likely to be most severe in certain bones. Even within bones, some regions may be affected more severely than others. For example, lesions associated with metabolic bone diseases, such as rickets and fibrous osteodystrophy, will be most marked at sites of rapid bone formation. The growth plates of the distal radius, proximal humerus, distal femur, and proximal tibia should therefore be targeted for gross and histological examination. Costochondral junctions of the largest ribs are also useful sites to examine in such cases. In osteoporosis, the depletion of trabecular bone is more rapid than that of cortical bone, presumably due to the greater surface area available for resorption in trabecular bone tissue.

Histological techniques and stains

Bone specimens for histological processing should be sawn at approximately 5 mm thickness and immersed in neutral buffered formalin. Other than in a few specialist laboratories equipped to prepare undemineralized bone sections, the specimens must then be demineralized prior to sectioning. In most laboratories, this involves the use of *commercial decalcifying agents*, usually consisting of strong acid solutions, which induce decalcification within 24–48 h. In the interests of section quality, the specimen should not be left in the decalcifying fluid any longer than necessary. It is important that bone slabs are no thicker than 5 mm, in order to minimize the time they spend in the fluid. The endpoint for decalcification can be judged by probing the tissue with a needle or by radiography. The decalcified tissue should be immersed in flowing tap water for 2–4 h to remove the acid, which would otherwise interfere with staining procedures. Although strong decalcifying solutions will allow the rapid preparation of sections for diagnostic purposes, they will also cause more tissue damage and may therefore impair interpretation. *Slower decalcification* in a chelating solution such as ethylene-diamine tetra-acetic acid (EDTA), will take approximately 7 days, but enables the preparation of higher-quality histological sections.

The *preparation of undecalcified sections* requires the use of plastic embedding media, such as methyl methacrylate, and a heavy-duty sledge microtome. Several useful staining methods for undemineralized bone sections are available, including hematoxylin and eosin, Von Kossa, and Villanueva's bone stain.

Hematoxylin and eosin is also a good general-purpose stain for routine histological examination of demineralized bone sections, allowing clear differentiation of bone and cartilage matrices, and providing adequate cellular detail. However, it does not reliably allow assessment of the thickness of osteoid seams, which is of diagnostic significance in diseases such as rickets or osteomalacia. These seams generally appear pale orange/pink, in contrast to the slightly more basophilic bone that was previously mineralized, but the distinction is often too subtle or variable to allow confident interpretation. The Masson's trichrome method is another useful general-purpose stain for bone sections, but has similar limitations with regard to identifying osteoid seams. Staining methods that allow identification of unmineralized osteoid in demineralized sections have been published (see Ralis and Ralis, 1975 and Tripp and MacKay, 1972 in bibliography) and, although not used routinely, can be easily performed in laboratories that are unable to cut undemineralized sections.

Preparation artifacts in histological sections

Because of the difficulty in preparing histological sections from bones, artifactual changes are often present and could be misinterpreted as lesions. During the process of sawing bones prior to demineralization, multiple small, irregular-sized fragments of *bone "sawdust"* and soft-tissue debris often become embedded in spaces between bone trabeculae (Fig. 1.15). Such fragments are commonly misinterpreted as necrotic bone. Rinsing the cut surface of the bone under running water, and gently brushing it before fixation, can minimize this artifact. Since the fragments will be most abundant near sawn surfaces, further trimming of the face to be sectioned, after demineralization, will further reduce them. In a section where "sawdust" is a problem, slicing deeper into the paraffin block is likely to yield cleaner sections for examination.

The heat generated by a band saw, or power drill in the case of bone biopsies, may create coagulative changes, resembling early ischemic necrosis, along the edges of the specimen. Overexposure to strong acid solutions during decalcification inhibits the staining of nucleic acids by hematoxylin, and of collagen by eosin, resulting in poor cellular detail and difficulties in interpretation.

Another common histological artifact is the presence of empty clefts between bone surfaces and the soft tissues of the marrow cavity. This reflects the much greater shrinkage of the soft tissues, when compared to bone, during

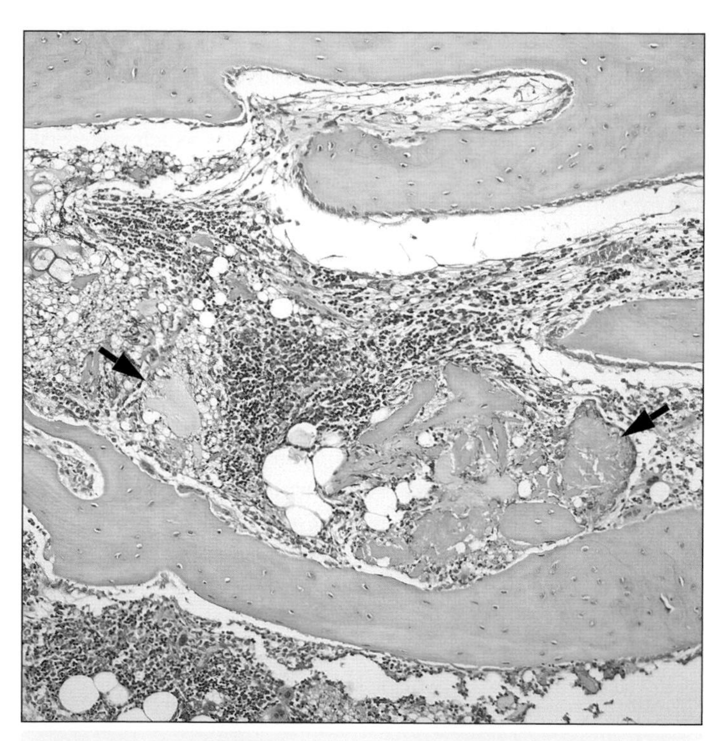

Figure 1.15 The multiple small fragments of bone and cartilage (arrows) embedded in the marrow spaces between trabeculae are **artifacts of sawing** ("sawdust") and should not be misinterpreted as lesions. Such artifacts are commonly present if sections are prepared too close to a sawn surface.

fixation in formalin. Consequently, osteoblasts or osteoclasts lining the bone surface may become separated from their site of activity. However, where bone resorption has been occurring, the surface of the bone will have a characteristic scalloped appearance. Also, bone does not adhere to microscope slides as well as soft tissues of the marrow spaces and may become dislodged, leaving large spaces lined by osteoblasts. These could be misinterpreted as vascular spaces.

Other laboratory techniques

The use of technetium labeling to identify areas of metabolically active bone, detected by scintigraphy, has dramatically improved the ability to detect bone abnormalities in the live animal. This technique greatly assists in locating multifocal lesions, such as the spread of metastatic disease within the skeleton, and although widely used in human medicine, has a relatively limited use for this purpose in animals.

A variety of other techniques may be used in the study of bones, but most are confined to the research laboratory. **Bone ash** measurements have historically been performed in animals with suspected metabolic bone diseases, but are of limited value for routine diagnosis because of the variability between individual bones and the lack of reliable reference ranges for animals of different age groups. More sophisticated and accurate methods for determining **bone density**, such as dual energy X-ray absorptiometry (DEXA scanning), have been developed for assessing bone mineral density in human patients, but are not readily available to most veterinary pathologists.

Microradiography of thick sections provides an indication of the pattern and degree of mineralization within the bone. Sections of bone, 60–100 μm thick, are placed in close contact with X-ray film and exposed. This creates an image of the bone section, which can be examined microscopically in association with histological sections prepared from the same slab.

The periodic administration to growing animals of **fluorescent markers**, which are deposited at sites of active mineralization, allows objective measurement of the rate of bone formation in physiological and disease states. The most commonly used marker is the antibiotic **tetracycline**, which fluoresces bright yellow when examined in undemineralized sections under UV light. Since the marker is only deposited at sites of active mineralization, a thin fluorescent line results from each dose. The distance is measured between lines representing sequential periods of exposure to the marker, and the rate of bone formation estimated.

Bibliography

Anderson C. Manual for the Examination of Bone. Boca Raton, Florida: CRC Press, 1982.

Bauer TW, Stulberg BN. The histology of osteonecrosis and its distinction from histologic artifacts. In: Schoutens A, et al, eds. Bone Circulation and Vascularization in Normal and Pathological Conditions. New York, London: Plenum Press, 1993:283–292.

Boivin G, et al. Transmission electron microscopy of bone tissue. Acta Orthop Scand 1990;61:170–180.

Hahn M, et al. Undecalcified preparation of bone tissue: Report of technical experience and new methods. Virchows Arch (A) Pathol Anat 1991;418:1–7.

Hassager C, Christiansen C. Measurement of bone mineral density. Calcif Tissue Int 1995;57:1–5.

Parfitt AM, et al. Bone histomorphometry: Standardization of nomenclature, symbols and units. Report of the ASBMR histomorphometry nomenclature committee. J Bone Min Res 1987;2:595–610.

Ralis, ZA, Ralis HM. A simple method for demonstration of osteoid in paraffin sections. Med Lab Tech 1975;32:203–213.

Tothill P. Methods of bone mineral measurement. Phys Med Biol 1989;34:543–572.

Tripp EJ, MacKay EH. Silver staining of bone prior to decalcification of osteoid in sections. Stain Tech 1972;47:129–136.

Villaneuva AR, Lundin KD. A versatile new mineralized bone stain for simultaneous identification of tetracycline and osteoid seams. Stain Technol 1989;64:129–137.

RESPONSE TO MECHANICAL FORCES AND INJURY

The cells of bone tissue are capable of the same basic cellular responses as most other tissues, including *atrophy, hypertrophy, hyperplasia, metaplasia, neoplasia, degeneration, and necrosis*. Bones have an excellent capacity for repair or modification in response to a wide range of injurious stimuli or changes in mechanical demand. Depending on the stimulus, the response may be localized or generalized but, in general, the magnitude of skeletal response is greater in young growing animals than in adults. If the response is generalized, it is likely to be most prominent at sites of rapid bone growth or modeling.

Mechanical forces

Bone adapts or remodels in response to the mechanical demands placed upon it. According to **Wolff's law**, *it is deposited at sites where it is required and resorbed where it is not*. For example, trabeculae in the epiphyseal and metaphyseal regions of long bones are aligned in directions which best reflect the compressive forces associated with weight bearing, and the tension associated with muscle insertions. In young individuals, increased mechanical stress on the skeleton increases the density of metaphyseal trabecular bone and the thickness of cortices. Increased mechanical usage in adults does not lead to an increase in bone mass, but reduces remodeling activity and conserves the amount of bone already present. Decreased activity accelerates bone loss by removing the inhibition of remodeling, and reduces formation, leading to a net reduction in bone mass.

Reduced mechanical stress on bones due to partial or complete immobilization, as occurs during fracture repair, leads to increased resorption, resulting in decreased bone strength and stiffness. If an implant, such as a metal plate, remains attached to a bone after a fracture has repaired, it will share the mechanical load with the bone. The bone will then atrophy in proportion to the decreased load and its strength will be greatly reduced. For this reason, *rigid implants should be removed soon after a fracture has healed*. Such implants may also trigger the development of an osteosarcoma at the site (see below), providing further reason for their removal.

Prolonged weightlessness associated with space travel has also been shown to result in decreased bone mass in weight-bearing bones. In contrast, increased mechanical stress associated with strenuous exercise has been associated with increased bone density.

Growth plate damage

In young growing animals, the growth plate is the weakest structure in the ends of long bones and is prone to traumatic injury resulting from shearing forces, compressive forces, or, in the case of traction epiphyses (e.g., lesser trochanter of the femur), excessive tension. In general, *the fastest growing growth plates are the most susceptible to injury*, the distal radial physis being the most commonly affected. Undulations in the growth plates of some bones increase their resistance to separation in response to shearing forces.

The consequences of growth plate injury depend on several factors, including the nature of the lesion, its location, the age of the animal and the status of the blood supply. Growth plates subjected primarily to traction consist at least partly of fibrocartilage, which imparts increased resistance to tensile forces. Such growth plates are sometimes referred to as **apophyses**.

Complete separation through the growth plate, referred to as **epiphyseolysis** (or "slipped epiphysis"), is a relatively common sequel to severe trauma or horizontal shear forces acting in the region of the bone–growth plate interface. The separation almost invariably occurs through the hypertrophic zone, where the cell volume is greatest and the matrix, which provides strength to the physis, is relatively sparse. Providing the epiphyseal vasculature has not been disrupted, the prognosis for this type of fracture is very good as the proliferative zone of the growth plate, and its blood supply, are likely to remain intact. However, epiphyseolysis of the capital femoral epiphysis, which may be associated with birth trauma in calves and occurs with some frequency in growing foals and puppies, may result in avascular necrosis of the femoral head. This reflects the greater risk of vascular damage as the nutrient vessels to the proximal femoral epiphysis travel along the neck of the femur and traverse the rim of the growth plate. The vessels supplying most other long bone epiphyses enter the bone at some distance from the growth plate and are protected by the periosteum or the fibrous layer of the joint capsule. A syndrome characterized by physeal dysplasia and slipped capital femoral epiphysis has been described recently in cats (4.5–24 months of age), most of which were male and obese. The Siamese breed was over-represented. In affected cats, the physeal cartilage was abnormally thick and chondrocytes were in disorganized clusters surrounded by abundant matrix. A similar syndrome is recognized in adolescent, overweight boys. Epiphyseolysis of the femoral head also occurs in pigs and deer as a manifestation of osteochondrosis, where there is likely to be an underlying weakness in the growth plate. Slipped capital femoral epiphysis must be distinguished from Legg–Calvé–Perthes disease and fractures through the femoral neck.

The *most common type of physeal fracture* reported in dogs, cats, horses, and humans, is characterized by extension of the fracture along the growth plate for a variable distance, then out through the metaphysis, leaving a triangular fragment of metaphyseal bone still attached to the growth plate. As with complete epiphyseolysis, the prognosis for further growth is very good. In contrast, fractures that cross the growth plate, with displacement of the fragments, will lead to the formation of a bony bridge between the metaphysis and epiphysis, precluding further growth in length at that site.

It is relatively common for epiphyseal separations, similar to those described above, to be induced during postmortem examination of young animals when limb joints are disarticulated forcefully. Such "fractures" are not accompanied by hemorrhage and are therefore easily distinguished from antemortem epiphyseolysis.

Growth plates of major limb bones, particularly the distal radius and ulna, are also susceptible to crushing injuries caused by compressive forces transmitted through the epiphysis. Such injuries, if severe enough, damage the epiphyseal blood supply as well as chondrocytes in the proliferating zone, leading to cessation of growth. *When the lesion is confined to one side of the growth plate, as it often is, continued growth on the other side leads to* **angular limb deformity**.

In dogs, *premature closure of the distal ulnar growth plate* is a common cause of limb deformity. Shearing forces acting on this growth plate result in crushing injury rather than epiphyseolysis, because of its conical shape, and are therefore more likely to result in retarded growth. If the growth plate of the adjacent radius escapes injury, the required synchrony between the two bones during development will be disturbed. Shortening of the limb will be accompanied by cranial bowing of the radius, valgus deformity, and outward rotation of the carpal and metacarpal bones.

Angular limb deformities ("bent leg") have been associated with a range of disease syndromes in several species, and are not always due to growth plate lesions. These will be discussed separately in a later section of this chapter.

Detachment of the ischial tuberosity from the pelvis is a well-recognized entity in young breeding sows, resulting in acute lameness. The separation, which may be bilateral, usually occurs between 8 and 14 months of age, prior to the closure of the apophyseal growth plate between the tuber ischiadicum and the rest of the ischium. The tuber ischiadicum serves as the origin for the semitendinosus and semimembranosus muscles, and as an attachment for the sacrotuberous ligament. As such, it is subject to considerable traction force and any weakness in the growth plate, as may occur in osteochondrosis, predisposes it to fracture.

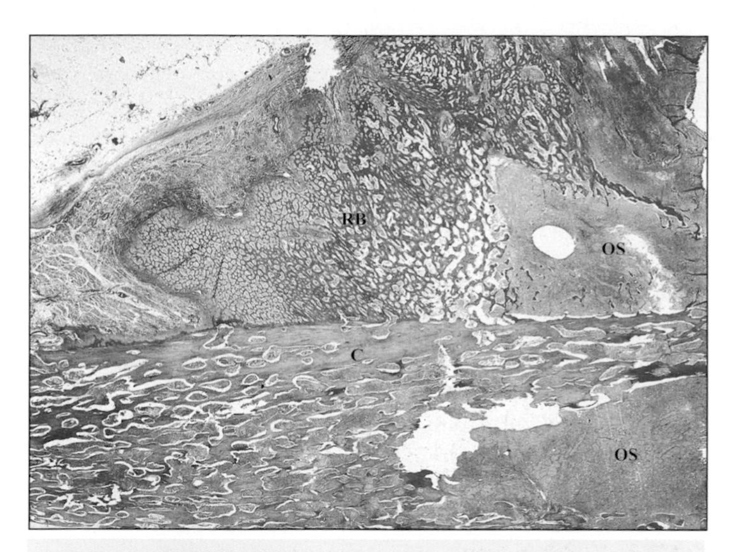

Figure 1.16 Reactive bone (RB) forming a so-called **"Codman's triangle"** beneath an elevated periosteum in a dog with osteosarcoma. The cortex (C) is porous due to tumor invasion. Sheets of tumor cells (OS) fill the medullary cavity and are replacing the sub-periosteal new bone in some areas.

Periosteal damage

Periosteal damage due to trauma stimulates rapid formation of new or **reactive bone** following activation and proliferation of osteoblast progenitors in the cambium layer. Trabeculae of woven bone extend from the underlying bone surface at acute angles, and can be readily distinguished histologically from the mature lamellar bone of the cortex (see Fig. 1.5). Separation of the periosteum from the bone surface by hemorrhage, inflammatory exudate, or neoplasia, or following surgical intervention, is also followed by *sub-periosteal new bone formation.* A pyramid-shaped region of new bone, referred to as **Codman's triangle**, may form beneath the periosteum in association with osteosarcoma (Fig. 1.16), but can also occur in association with other bone lesions, such as osteomyelitis. The mechanism of periosteal new bone formation is not clear, but it often precedes actual involvement of the periosteum by an underlying osteosarcoma or inflammatory process, suggesting that it may involve either local circulatory disturbances or the release of growth factors in response to bone resorption.

Localized outgrowths of new bone beneath the periosteum are referred to as **exostoses**. Depending on their size, and the inciting cause, they may either persist or gradually be removed by remodeling.

Fracture repair

Bone fractures are very common in animals and occur either when a bone is subjected to a mechanical force beyond that to which it is designed to withstand, or when there is an *underlying disease process that has reduced its normal breaking strength.* The latter is referred to as a **pathological fracture** and unless the predisposing disorder is corrected then the repair process is unlikely to be successful. The possibility of a localized bone disease (e.g., neoplasia or osteomyelitis) or a generalized disorder (e.g., fibrous osteodystrophy or osteoporosis) should always be considered if bone fracture has occurred without evidence of trauma.

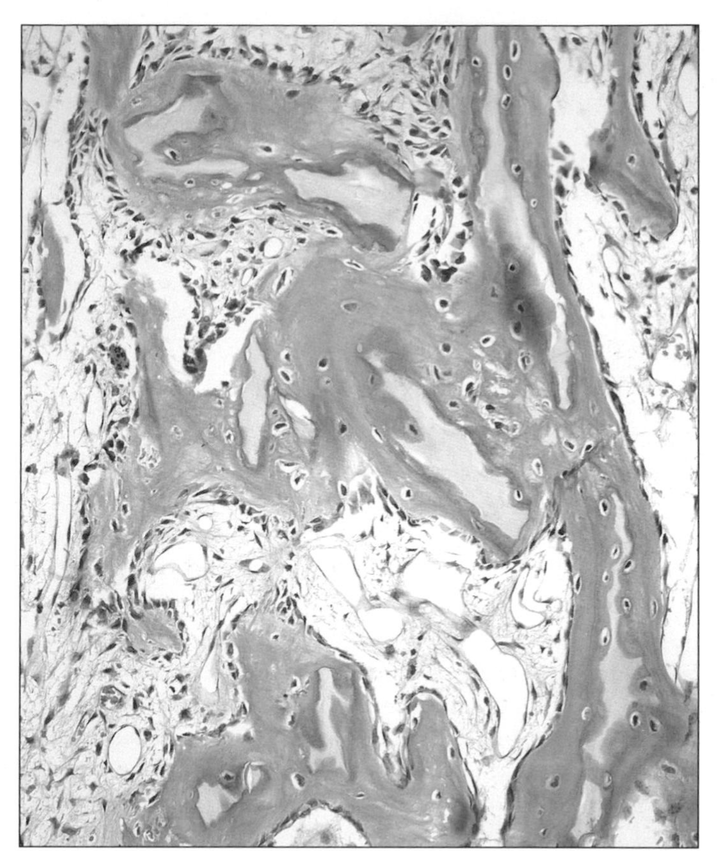

Figure 1.17 Trabecular microfractures in a calf with **osteogenesis imperfecta**. Note the abnormal alignment of cartilage cores in adjacent trabeculae that have been incorporated in a microcallus.

Types of fractures

Fractures are classified as **simple,** if there is a clean break separating the bone into two parts, or **comminuted**, if several fragments of bone exist at the fracture site. When one segment of bone is driven into another the fracture is referred to as an **impacted** fracture, and when there is a break in the overlying skin, usually due to penetration by a sharp fragment of bone, the fracture is referred to as **compound**. If there has been minimal separation between the fractured bone ends, and the periosteum remains intact, the lesion is classified as a **greenstick** fracture. An **avulsion** fracture occurs when there is excessive trauma at sites of ligamentous or tendinous insertions and a fragment of bone is torn away.

Microscopic fractures of individual trabeculae, or localized segments of cortical bone, also occur and are referred to as **microfractures**. Trabecular microfractures can sometimes be detected in histological sections by the abnormal alignment of their cartilage cores, which are normally situated at right angles to the growth plate, and parallel to the cartilage cores of adjacent trabeculae (Fig. 1.17). Such microfractures must however be differentiated from artifactual alterations in trabecular alignment that may occur when a bone is being sawn during processing. Once trabeculae have lost their cartilage core through remodeling this does not apply, and since the direction of remodeled trabeculae is less predictable, detection of microfractures is more difficult. *Multiple microfractures involving several adjacent trabeculae without gross displacement of the bone ends are referred to as* **infractions**. These are sometimes seen

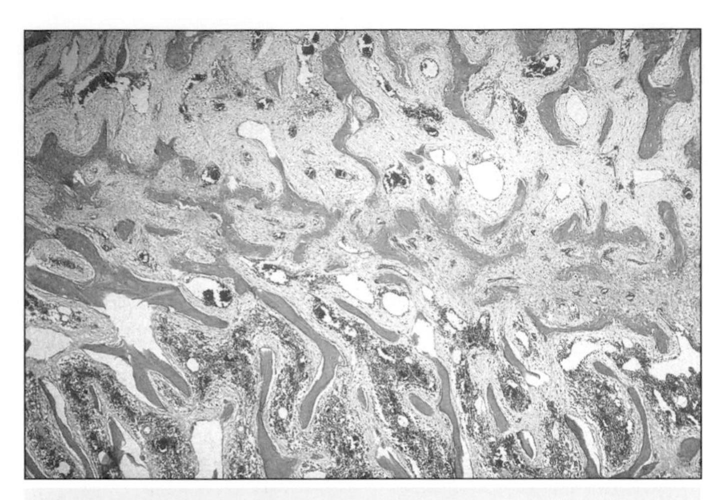

Figure 1.18 Infraction line in the metaphysis of a young pig with fibrous osteodystrophy. The abnormal alignment of trabeculae across the center of the field represents a band of healed trabecular microfractures.

in association with weight bearing on bones weakened by an underlying disease process, such as fibrous osteodystrophy (Fig. 1.18). Repeated bone trauma associated with strenuous exercise may lead to a **stress** fracture in the cortex of a limb bone. This represents the accumulation of several cortical microfractures, rather than a single traumatic event, and is typically seen in the dorsal or dorsomedial cortex of metacarpal III in young racehorses when they first enter training (see below).

Process of fracture repair

Unlike most other tissues, bone is capable of repair by regeneration rather than scar formation and successful repair of a fracture can return the bone both to its original shape and strength. The process of fracture repair follows a consistent pattern, but can be modified by methods of stabilization and by interfering factors, such as infection or the presence of an underlying bone disease.

The initial event in uncomplicated fracture repair is the *formation of a hematoma* between the bone ends. With disruption of the blood supply, *ischemic necrosis of bone* and other tissues in the vicinity of the fracture is inevitable. An *acute inflammatory response* is triggered by mediators released from the hematoma and from necrotic tissues. Inhibition of this inflammatory phase by anti-inflammatory drugs has been shown to interfere with the natural process of fracture repair. Although neutrophils and macrophages are the first cells to arrive at the fracture site, mesenchymal cells from the medullary cavity, endosteum, and cambium layer of the periosteum rapidly proliferate in and around the hematoma, forming a **callus** consisting initially of loose connective tissue. Subperiosteal new bone formation commences on the bone surface adjacent to the bone ends while primitive mesenchymal cells in the fracture gap differentiate into chondroblasts and replace the loose connective tissue with chondroid matrix. Meanwhile, osteoclasts appear and start to remove the dead bone. Osteoblasts producing new bone have been identified ultrastructurally in the medullary callus as early as 24 hours after fracture. Evidence suggests that at least some of these osteoblasts may be derived from transformed endothelial cells from capillaries and small venules in the vicinity of the fracture.

The early callus, consisting predominantly of hyaline cartilage, forms very rapidly and serves to anchor the fractured bone ends, allowing limited function while the repair process continues. As revascularization of the fracture site occurs, endochondral ossification within the callus leads to progressive replacement of the cartilage by trabeculae of woven bone. The *development of a bony callus* further stabilizes the fracture and allows a return to normal function, although the repair process continues. The *final phase* may take several months, or even years, and *involves the replacement of woven bone in the callus with mature lamellar bone*, and modeling of the callus to eventually restore the bone to its original shape. Once this process is completed, the strength of the bone will also be returned to its previous state. Modeling of the callus is more rapid in young animals than in adults and is more likely to result in complete resolution. In adults, residual changes such as persistence of medullary trabeculae and thickening of the periosteal bone surface are likely to persist at the fracture site.

The size of a fracture callus is proportional to the amount of movement between the fractured bone ends. Where there is considerable movement, callus formation will be exuberant, and may create diagnostic problems for the pathologist, especially in cases where the clinical history is incomplete and radiographs of the lesion are not available. In the early stages of callus formation the abundance of pleomorphic spindle cells, sometimes exhibiting primitive osteoid formation, can easily be misinterpreted as an osteosarcoma in biopsy specimens (Fig. 1.19). As the callus matures, a more organized pattern develops, with osteoblasts lining up along trabeculae of woven bone and the cells between trabeculae appearing less primitive. It must be remembered that an underlying osteosarcoma could have predisposed the bone to fracture and the two processes may in fact be present.

In fractures in which the separated ends have been perfectly aligned, and rigidly immobilized by metal plates or other methods of fixation, callus formation is minimal, or even nonexistent. The repair process in this situation is more protracted as it relies on the process of internal remodeling, whereby resorption canals form across the fracture line in the apposed cortices and new osteons are created. This is referred to as **primary cortical healing**.

There seems little doubt that local and systemic regulators of bone growth influence fracture repair, but their precise role has yet to be determined. Platelet-derived growth factor, transforming growth factor-β, fibroblast growth factor and bone morphogenetic proteins are released from the hematoma and necrotic bone soon after a bone fractures. These factors are important in regulating normal bone formation and resorption (see above) and are believed to play an important role in the modulation and coordination of callus formation during fracture repair. The possible therapeutic use of such growth factors in enhancing fracture repair is an exciting area of current research.

Complications of fracture repair

The repair process does not always proceed smoothly. In comminuted fractures, *fragments of necrotic bone that are too large for removal by osteoclastic resorption may persist at the site and interfere with the healing process*. Such bone fragments are referred to as **sequestrae**. The repair of compound fractures may be delayed by the development of bacterial osteomyelitis following contamination of the fracture site through the open skin wound. Failure to control the

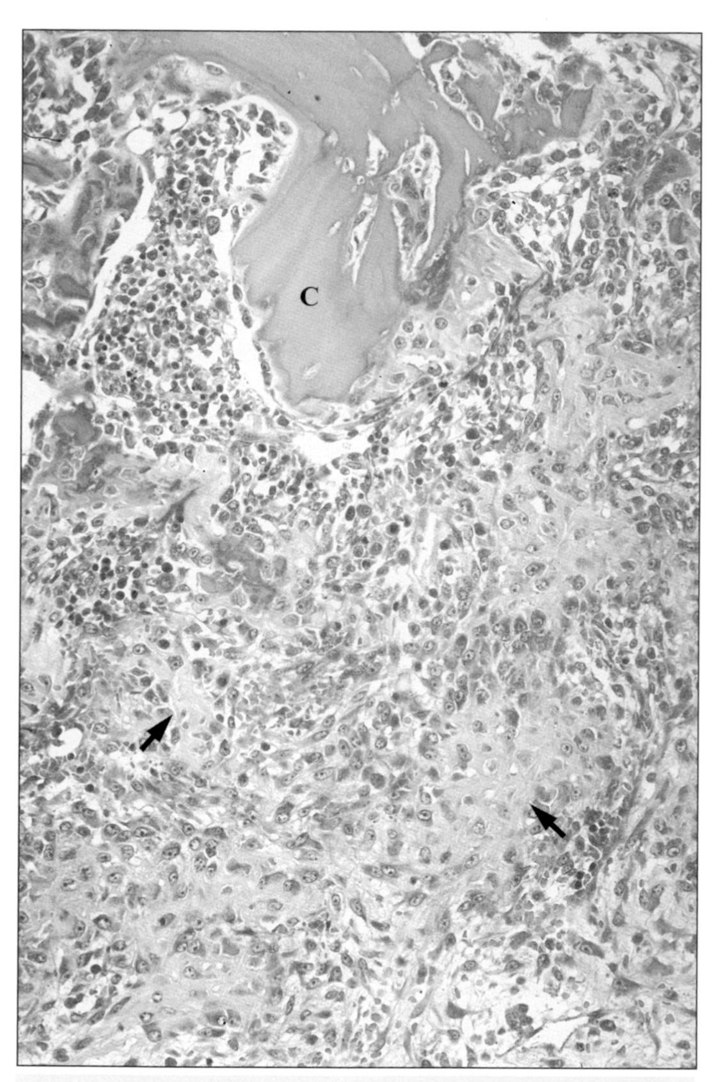

Figure 1.19 Repairing fracture at 1 week. Disorganized condensations of plump mesenchymal cells are producing osteoid (arrows) in a manner similar to that which occurs in some osteosarcomas. A fragment of preexisting cortical bone (C) is still present and serves as an attachment site for some of the newly formed bone spicules.

infection in the early stages will interfere with new bone formation and the resorption of dead bone. If the infection becomes chronic, new bone may form at the margin of healthy and diseased tissue in an attempt to wall off the infected area. The result may be the development of a large callus containing pockets of infection or fistulae surrounded by granulation tissue and trabecular bone. Any large fragments of bone engulfed by the inflammatory process are likely to persist as sequestrae, causing irritation, delayed healing, or nonhealing.

Excessive movement between bone ends during the repair process may inhibit the formation of a bony callus by continually disrupting attempts at revascularization. This favors the formation of cartilage and fibrous tissue and may lead to the development of a false joint or **pseudoarthrosis** at the fracture site. A pseudoarthrosis may also develop if soft tissues separate the fractured bone ends or if persistent infection inhibits callus formation.

Generalized skeletal disorders or deficiencies of nutrients crucial to bone formation will inevitably delay or prevent fracture repair, and must be corrected if normal healing is to proceed. Certain drugs, for example corticosteroids, can also interfere with bone healing.

Stress-related lesions in horses

A spectrum of stress-related lesions, including **bucked shins** and **incomplete cortical fractures**, *commonly affect the dorsal cortex of the third metacarpal bone in young sport horses*, particularly Thoroughbreds or Quarter Horses, undergoing intensive training for their first season of racing. Estimations of prevalence for bucked shins vary from 30–90% of all young horses in training. *Incomplete cortical fractures (so-called saucer fractures)* usually occur several months after the initial signs of bucked shins. Both lesions affect the left third metacarpal bone more often than the right, but they may be bilateral.

Bucked shins is characterized by the formation of smoothly contoured foci of periosteal new bone on the dorsal aspect of the metacarpal bone, accompanied by pain and swelling. For many years, bucked shins was considered to be the result of fatigue injuries leading to microfractures in the dorsal cortex of the metacarpal bone, with subsequent callus formation. This seems unlikely, as the extent of new bone formation is in excess of what would be expected as a response to such microfractures with negligible bone displacement and instability. Recent studies have suggested an alternative hypothesis. According to this hypothesis, repeated high-strain fatigue during training or racing decreases bone stiffness. This *then induces the formation of reactive bone on the periosteal surface in an effort to increase the inertial properties of the bone and increase its resistance to bending*, as would be predicted by Wolff's law.

Incomplete cortical fractures (stress or saucer fractures) seldom occur in horses that have not previously had bucked shins, suggesting that the conditions are related, but only about 12% of horses with bucked shins eventually develop such fractures. They usually occur 6–12 months after the onset of bucked shins and involve the periosteal new bone that forms on the dorsal or dorsolateral aspect of the third metacarpal. Until this bone is remodeled and strengthened, it is susceptible to fatigue injury during the high-strain cyclic loading associated with training or racing. Failure of the bone may be in the form of many small saucer-shaped stress fractures, extending part way into the cortex before returning to the surface.

Stress-related lesions are often found incidentally in the **distal condyles** of the third **metacarpal** and **metatarsal** bones of Thoroughbred racehorses. Linear defects in the articular cartilage adjacent to the sagittal ridge are closely related to increased density of the subchondral bone and to intense focal remodeling of the bone immediately adjacent to the articular defects. These changes are presumably a response to increased strain associated with training and may predispose to condylar fractures.

Bibliography

Brighton CT, Hunt RM. Early histological and ultrastructural changes in medullary fracture callus. J Bone Joint Surg Am 1991;73-A:832–846.

Cornell CN, Lane JM. Newest factors in fracture healing. Clin Orthop 1992;277:297–311.

Craig LE. Physeal dysplasia with slipped capital femoral epiphysis in 13 cats. Vet Pathol 2001;38:92–97.

Done SH, et al. Detachment of the ischial tuberosity in sows. Vet Rec 1979;105:520–523.

Einhorn TA. The cell and molecular biology of fracture healing. Clin Orthop 1998;355S:S7–S21.

Fretz PB. Angular limb deformities in foals. Vet Clin North Am 1980;2:125–150.

Hamilton GF, et al. Slipped capital femoral epiphysis in calves. J Am Vet Med Assoc 1978;172: 1318–1322.

Ianotti JP. Growth plate physiology and pathology. Orthop Clin North Am 1990;21:1–17.

Joyce ME, et al. Transforming growth factor-β in the regulation of fracture repair. Orthop Clin North Am 1990;21:199–209.

Marretta SM, Schrader SC. Physeal injuries in the dog: a review of 135 cases. J Am Vet Med Assoc 1983;182:708–710.

Nordin M, Frankel VH. Biomechanics of bone. In: Nordin M, Frankel VH, eds. Basic Biomechanics of the Musculoskeletal System. 2nd ed., Philadelphia, London: Lea and Febiger, 1989, 3–29.

Nunamaker DM. Metacarpal stress fractures. In: Nixon AJ, ed. Equine Fracture Repair. 1996: 195–199.

Riggs CM, et al. Pathology of the distal condyles of the third metacarpal and third metatarsal bones of the horse. Equine Vet J 1999;31:140–148.

SKELETAL DYSPLASIAS

A variety of genetic abnormalities primarily affecting bone formation or remodeling have been reported in humans and domestic animals. These are collectively known as skeletal dysplasias and are *usually associated with short stature, abnormally shaped bones, and/or increased bone fragility*. Not surprisingly, human skeletal dysplasias have been subjected to much greater scientific scrutiny than those in animals, leading to the development of detailed and sometimes confusing systems of classification, based on their radiographic appearance, the bones involved, age of onset, or pathogenesis. A comprehensive international classification system for skeletal dysplasias, proposed in 1991, includes well over 100 entities. Advances in molecular biology will inevitably lead to the development of a more precise classification system based on the actual genetic defect. Already, the mutations underlying several human skeletal dysplasias have been identified and it is now apparent that some disorders previously thought to be separate entities, are merely examples of variable expression of the same genetic defect. Skeletal dysplasias of animals are seldom investigated in as much detail as their human counterparts and classification is often imprecise, but it is clear that a similar range of conditions exist, creating opportunities for the development of potentially useful animal models. Studies in animals, particularly laboratory mice, are already proving valuable in helping to identify the molecular basis of inherited disorders of the skeleton and other body systems. Such studies may also generate new information on the role of specific proteins in bone function and physiology.

The diversity of skeletal dysplasias reflects the complexity of the processes involved in bone formation and remodeling, and the large number of genes required for normal development. In some dysplasias the entire skeleton is involved, while in others the defect is confined to individual bones or regions within bones. The terminology generally reflects either the distribution of lesions or the nature of the defect. Some examples of commonly used terms are listed in Table 1.2.

Most skeletal dysplasias in animals are usually either lethal or semi-lethal, but the gene frequency of some disorders in some breeds, has reached surprisingly high levels. This most likely reflects either inbreeding, or excessive use of a sire carrying a defective gene. The latter has clearly been responsible for the very high prevalence reached by certain genetic diseases in cattle, where artificial breeding is widely practiced.

Table 1.2 Terminology of some congenital abnormalities in skeletal development

Term	Nature of the defect
Generalized	
• Achondroplasia	— absence of cartilage development
• Chondrodysplasia	— Disordered cartilage development
• Osteogenesis imperfecta	— Genetic defect in type-I collagen formation characterized by osteopenia and excessive bone fragility
• Osteopetrosis	— Persistence of primary and/or secondary spongiosa due to defect in osteoclastic bone resorption.
• Skeletal dysplasia	— Disordered skeletal development
Head	
• Brachycephalic	— Shortening of the head
• Brachygnathia	— Abnormally short jaw (inferior or superior)
• Campylognathia	— Harelip
• Palatoschisis	— Cleft palate
• Prognathia	— Abnormal projection of the jaw
Spine	
• Kyphosis	— Abnormal dorsal curvature of the spinal column
• Lordosis	— Abnormal ventral curvature of the spinal column
• Scoliosis	— Lateral deviation in the spinal column
Limbs	
• Amelia	— Absence of one or more limbs
• Hemimelia	— Absence of the distal part of a limb
• Micromelia	— Presence of abnormally small limbs
• Notomelia	— Accessory limb attached to the back
• Peromelia	— Congenital deformity of the limbs
• Phocomelia	— Absence of the proximal portion of one or more limbs
Digits	
• Adactyly	— Absence of a digit
• Dactylomegaly	— Abnormally large digits
• Ectrodactyly	— Partial or complete absence of a digit
• Polydactyly	— Presence of supernumerary digits
• Polypodia	— Presence of supernumerary feet
• Syndactyly	— Fusion of digits

Not all skeletal abnormalities are caused by genetic defects. Exposure of developing fetuses to certain toxic principles, mineral deficiencies, or infectious agents at appropriate stages of gestation can create skeletal lesions virtually indistinguishable from those with a genetic etiology. For the veterinary pathologist, it is as important to accurately determine the cause of the problem as it is to characterize the lesions. Otherwise valuable stud animals may be slaughtered unnecessarily or teratogenic agents may go undetected. In this section, discussion will focus on those skeletal dysplasias of domestic animals that are known, or strongly believed, to be genetic in origin. Acquired skeletal abnormalities will be discussed in a later section.

Bibliography

Beighton P, et al. International classification of osteochondrodysplasias. Am J Med Genet 1992;44:223–229.

Greene HJ, et al. Congenital defects in cattle. Irish Vet J 1973;27:37–45.

Sillence DO, et al. Morphologic studies in the skeletal dysplasias. A review. Am J Pathol 1979;96:811–870.

Generalized skeletal dysplasias

Several important generalized disorders of bones are recognized in animals, all of them having analogous human counterparts. The underlying defect may lie in the formation of cartilage, thus affecting all bones that form by endochondral ossification. Such disorders are referred to as **chondrodysplasias** and affected individuals, no matter what the species, usually *show various degrees of dwarfism*. The term **achondroplasia** is often used in place of chondrodysplasia to describe diseases characterized by *disproportionate dwarfism*, especially in human medicine, and although it is less accurate, the term is entrenched in the literature. Alternatively, the defect may involve the synthesis of a specific component of bone matrix, e.g., type I collagen, as occurs in **osteogenesis imperfecta**. A defect in bone remodeling is the mechanism involved in another group of skeletal dysplasias, the **osteopetroses**. Only those disorders reported in domestic animals are included in this section but from time to time, the veterinary pathologist will be confronted with bone deformities that do not resemble any of the syndromes currently recognized in animals. In such cases, reference to the substantial human literature on skeletal dysplasias may be useful.

Chondrodysplasias

The *dwarfism of the chondrodysplasias is disproportionate*, in contrast to the proportionate or primordial dwarfism associated with somatotropin deficiency. Primordial dwarfism is usually inherited as a recessive trait and is well recognized in horses and dogs, where it forms the basis of several distinct breeds, e.g., Miniature Poodle. The chondrodystrophic dog breeds, e.g., Dachshund, Pekingese, and Basset Hound, are actually variant forms of disproportionate dwarfs. These forms of chondrodysplasia are inherited as polygenic traits associated with defects in hormone receptors, matrix components, or chondrocyte regulatory factors, and differ from the less "desirable" chondrodysplasias discussed below, which are believed to be caused by single gene defects.

Cartilage grows by both interstitial proliferation and surface apposition. Longitudinal growth of the cartilage model in the fetus, and at growth plates in young animals, relies primarily on interstitial proliferation of chondrocytes, while transverse growth occurs by interstitial growth and apposition. In some chondrodysplasias, appositional growth is normal but interstitial growth of cartilage is defective, resulting in premature closure of growth plates and reduced length of long bones. The intersphenoid, spheno-occipital, and interoccipital synchondroses at the base of the skull also develop by interstitial proliferation of chondrocytes and close prematurely in such disorders. In some chondrodysplastic calves, bony ridges project into the cranial cavity, possibly due to early fusion of the spheno-occipital synchondrosis and altered growth in this region of the skull. Although there is hypoplasia of basocranial bones and impaired development of the ethmoids and turbinates, the mandible, which enlarges by appositional growth, develops normally, leading to prognathia inferior. As the brain continues to grow, the cranium becomes domed and hydrocephalus may develop. The spinal column is shorter than normal due to reduced length of individual vertebrae, as are the ribs, but costochondral junctions may be enlarged since the cartilage expands by appositional growth.

The underlying molecular defects in most chondrodysplasias of animals have yet to be determined but their identification will eventually provide a more precise system of classification than is currently possible. In human achondroplasia, the most common form of heritable disproportionate dwarfism in people, the cartilage lacks a receptor for a growth factor as a result of a mutation in the gene encoding fibroblast growth factor receptor 3 (FGFR3). Such discoveries provide clues for investigating the mechanisms of chondrodysplasias in animals and may lead to the development of valuable animal models for assessing treatment options in human patients.

Chondrodysplasias of cattle

Several phenotypic forms of inherited chondrodysplasia occur in different breeds of cattle, and are broadly classified on the basis of their morphological characteristics into *"bulldog," Telemark, "snorter" (brachycephalic), and long-headed (dolichocephalic) types.* Because of the range of syndromes, it is likely that more than one gene locus is involved, or at least that there are different modifying alleles influencing the expression of a major gene.

The most severe form of bovine chondrodysplasia is the lethal **bulldog type**, which occurs in the Dexter and Holstein breeds, and possibly in Charolais and Jersey. Dexter cattle are considered short-legged derivatives of the Kerry breed, originating from Ireland, and are gaining in popularity in many countries because of the desirability of small, easily managed cattle for "lifestyle" farms. Some short-legged Dexters are heterozygous for an *incompletely dominant gene* which, when homozygous, gives rise to a bulldog calf. Bulldog calves may be carried to full term but are usually aborted before the seventh month of gestation and may not be detected by the owner. In all cases, they possess severe, relatively consistent, skeletal abnormalities. As well as being *much smaller than normal for the stage of pregnancy, they have extremely short limbs, which are usually rotated, a domed head with retruded muzzle and protruding mandible, and a large ventral abdominal hernia* (Fig. 1.20A). The tongue is of normal size so protrudes markedly, and the hard palate is absent. The shortened limb bones consist of mushroom-shaped, cartilaginous epiphyses separated by a short, central segment of diaphyseal bone. Histologically, the long bones lack distinct growth plates. Instead, the physeal cartilage consists of densely packed chondrocytes showing no orderly arrangement into columns (Fig. 1.20B), and a fibrillar intercellular matrix surrounding large, vascular, cartilage canals. Due to defective endochondral ossification at growth plates there is little growth in the length of long bones and no distinct primary or secondary spongiosa (Fig. 1.20B). In contrast, intramembranous ossification beneath the periosteum appears to proceed normally and contributes disproportionately to the bone volume (Fig. 1.20C). Holstein bulldog calves are similar to those of the Dexter breed, *but in Holsteins, the defect is characterized by autosomal recessive inheritance* rather than as an incomplete dominant. The defective gene coding for chondrodysplasia in Dexter cattle has recently been identified, and a test for carriers is now commercially available.

The **Telemark lethal** form of bovine chondrodysplasia is inherited as an *autosomal recessive trait* and, as such, the heterozygous parents are phenotypically normal. Affected calves are born alive but cannot stand, and die of suffocation shortly after birth. The head and facial abnormalities are similar to those of bulldog calves, and the limbs, although not quite as short as in bulldog calves, are much shorter than normal and rotated to varying degrees. A similar

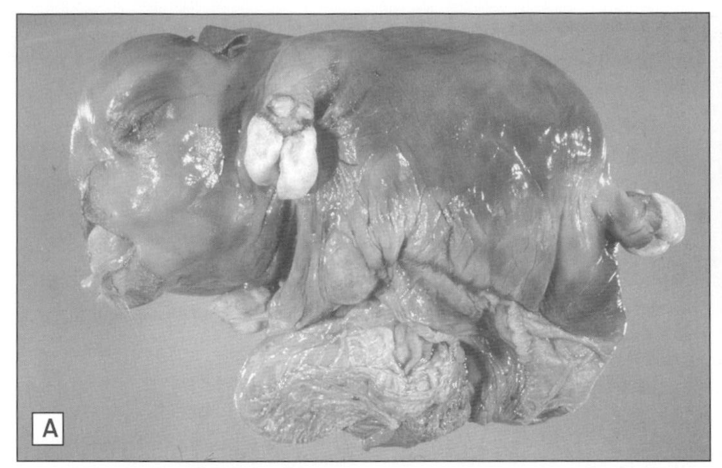

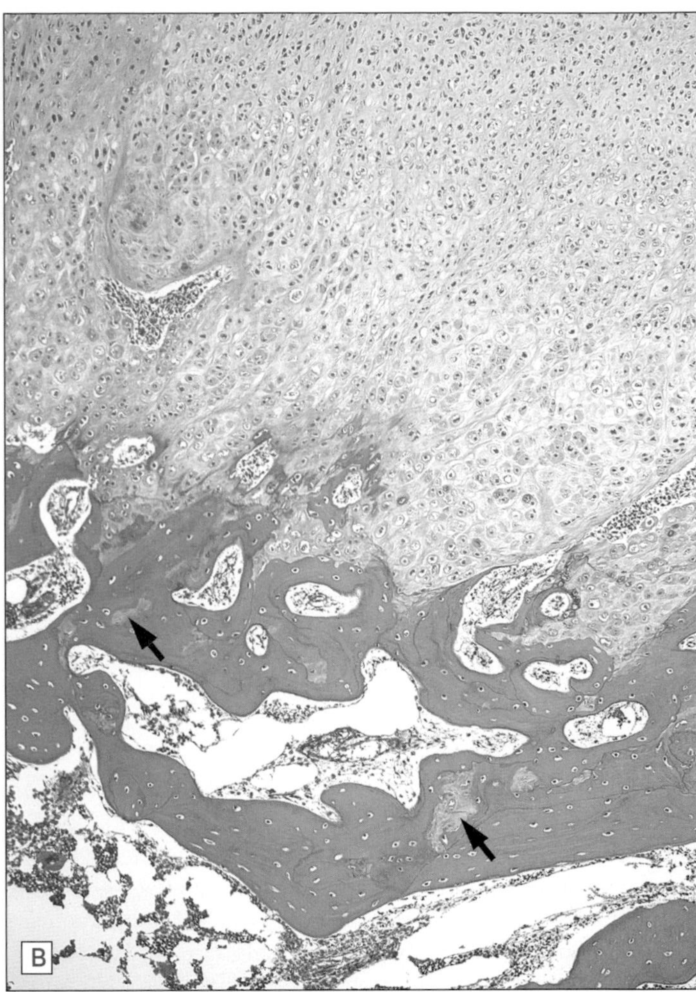

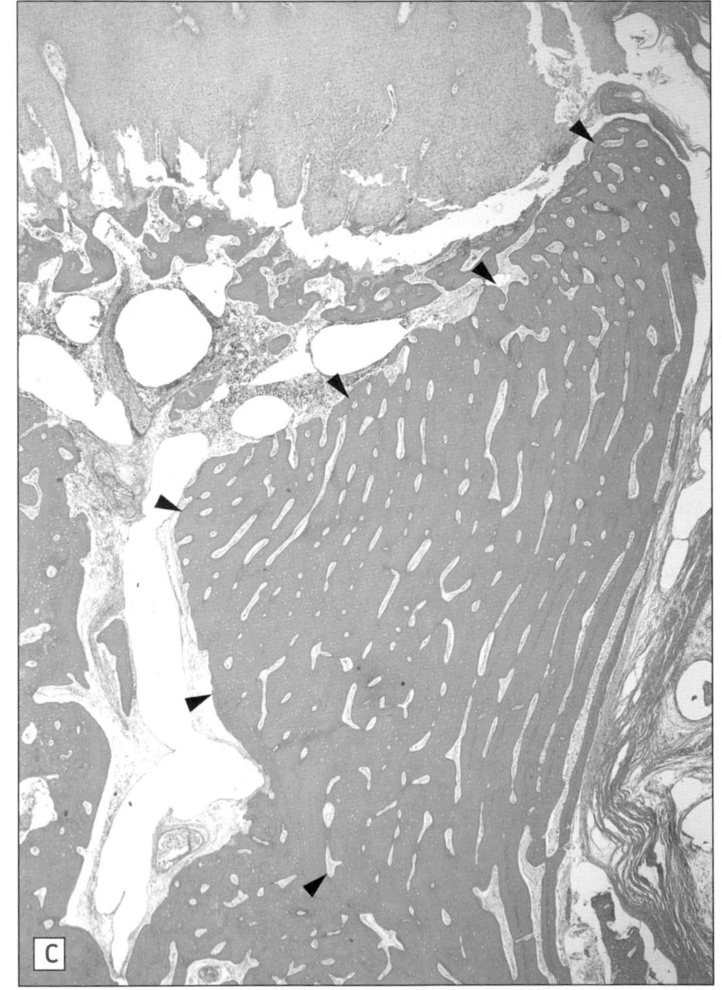

Figure 1.20 Bovine chondrodysplasia. **A.** Aborted Dexter bulldog calf with extremely short, rotated limbs, retruded muzzle, protruding mandible and tongue and umbilical hernia. (Courtesy of RW Cook and PA Windsor.) **B.** Physeal and metaphyseal regions of a long bone from a Dexter bulldog calf. There is no arrangement of chondrocytes into a recognizable growth plate. The metaphysis is markedly abbreviated and consists of thick bony trabeculae incorporating only occasional cartilage spicules (arrows). **C.** Longitudinal low-power view of part of a major long bone from the same calf. The arrowheads delineate the intramembranous bone of periosteal origin, which greatly exceeds the volume of bone derived from endochondral ossification at the growth plates. (Microscope slides courtesy of RW Cook.)

disorder, characterized by autosomal recessive inheritance, occurs in Jersey cattle, but shows much greater phenotypic variability. The lesions in Jerseys may include a short, broad head, deformed mandible, cleft palate, and short, spiraled limbs, but many calves have mild lesions and are viable.

Brachycephalic ("snorter") type dwarfism was common in the Hereford breed in North America and New Zealand during the late 1940s and early 1950s, but also occurred in other beef breeds, especially the Angus. Although inherited as an *autosomal recessive trait*, the defect appears to be partially expressed in heterozygotes, which are slightly smaller and more compact than normal. Selection for this phenotype most likely facilitated the spread of the chondrodysplasia gene in these traditional beef breeds and accounted for the high gene frequency. With a change in emphasis towards a larger frame score in beef cattle, and the introduction of programs to eliminate the defective gene, *snorter dwarfism is now rare.*

Snorter dwarfism is a much milder form of chondrodysplasia than the bulldog and Telemark types, but *affected calves have a short, broad head with bulging forehead, retruded upper jaw and a slightly protruding mandible* (Fig. 1.21). The eyes are prominent and laterally displaced. The vertebral column is shortened and the ventral borders of individual vertebrae are flattened, a useful diagnostic feature

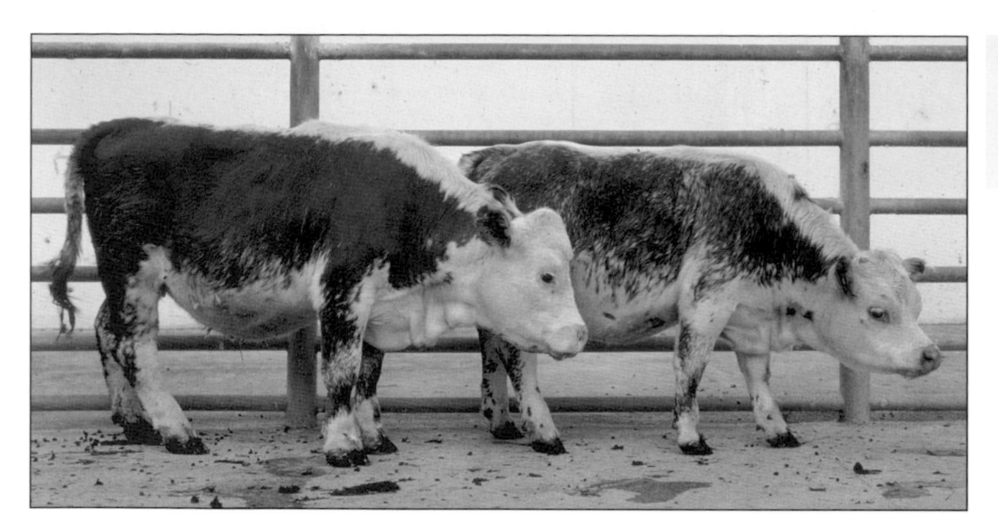

Figure 1.21 Bovine chondrodysplasia. Two brachycephalic ("snorter") dwarf Hereford calves with characteristic short stature, domed forehead, retruded upper jaw and distended abdomen. (Courtesy of RD Jolly.)

visible radiographically in young calves. Chronic ruminal tympany is a feature of snorter dwarfs, possibly as a result of reduced intra-abdominal space and impaired eructation. There is premature closure of basocranial synchondroses leading to compression of the cerebellum and shortening of the brain stem. The distal limb bones are proportionately shorter than proximal bones, the metacarpi showing the greatest degree of shortening. Interestingly, the width of long bones from brachycephalic dwarfs is comparable to, or greater than, that of normal calves. *The ratio of total metacarpal length to diaphyseal diameter is therefore a useful diagnostic indicator of this form of dwarfism.* In snorter dwarfs the ratio is usually 4.0 or less, but in normal animals it is greater than 4.5. Histological changes in the growth plates of snorter dwarfs are relatively mild and are not of diagnostic value. The microscopic organization of growth plates into their different zones is normal, but the columns of palisading chondrocytes are shorter, less hypertrophied and more irregular.

Long-headed or **dolichocephalic** dwarfs are slightly larger than snorter dwarfs, but the main difference is that *the head is proportionately much longer and tapers to a narrow muzzle.* Affected animals may have crooked limbs, slow growth rate and are unthrifty. Another form of chondrodysplasia, considered to be *rhizomelic* in type, occurs in Japanese Brown cattle. Lesions are confined to the long bones of the limbs and are associated with degenerative changes in growth plates and disordered endochondral ossification.

Proportionate dwarfism has been reported in an estimated 21 of 63 (33%) progeny from a clinically normal purebred Charolais bull. The miniature calves were derived both from Charolais cows and crossbred cows of diverse breeding, over several years. Affected calves weighed from 5–16 kg at birth and were born 2 weeks or more premature, with a high proportion dead at birth. Other than their small size, there were no anatomical differences between the miniature and normal calves sired by the bull. The condition was considered to be inherited as an *autosomal dominant trait*, probably resulting from a new mutation in the bull's primordial germ cells. This would explain the fact that the bull was clinically normal, and that less than 50% of its progeny were affected.

Bibliography

Agerholm JS, Arnbjerg J, Andersen O. Familial chondrodysplasia in Holstein calves. J Vet Diagn Invest 2004;16:293–298.

Harper PAW, et al. Chondrodysplasia in Australian Dexter cattle. Aust Vet J 1998;76:199–202.

Jayo MJ. Bovine dwarfism: clinical, biochemical, radiological and pathological aspects. J Vet Med A 1987;34:161–177.

Jones JM, Jolly RD. Dwarfism in Hereford cattle: a genetic, morphological and biochemical study. N Z Vet J 1982;30:185–189.

Moritomo Y, et al. Morphological changes of epiphyseal plate in the long bone of chondrodysplastic dwarfism in Japanese Brown cattle. J Vet Med Sci 1992;54:453–459.

Shiang R, et al. Mutations in the transmembrane domain of FGFR3 cause the most common genetic form of dwarfism, achondroplasia. Cell 1994;78:335–337.

Chondrodysplasias of sheep

The most common, and potentially important, form of hereditary chondrodysplasia in sheep is **spider lamb syndrome**, *a semi-lethal condition of Suffolk and Hampshire sheep.* Spider lambs were first recognized in North America in the late 1970s and the defect has since been introduced to Australia and New Zealand with imported Suffolk genetic material. The trait is characterized by *autosomal recessive inheritance with complete penetrance*, but with variation in expressivity between individuals. The prevalence of spider lamb syndrome in North America has reached a much higher level than would normally be expected for a semi-lethal genetic disorder, possibly due to selection for long-legged animals heterozygous for the "spider" gene.

Lambs with spider syndrome may be aborted or stillborn, but most are born alive showing skeletal deformities of variable severity. Some appear clinically normal at birth but develop typical signs of the disease within their first month of life, including *disproportionately long limbs and neck, shallow body, scoliosis and/or kyphosis* (Fig. 1.22A), *sternal deformity, and valgus deformity of the forelimbs below the carpus, creating a "knock-kneed" appearance.* Hindlimb deformities may also be present, but are less severe than those involving the forelimbs. Facial deformities, including Roman nose (Fig. 1.22A), deviated nasal septum and shortening of the maxilla are common, but not consistent. The deformities of the limbs and spinal column become progressively more severe with age. *Diagnosis is best confirmed by demonstrating characteristic radiographic changes in the elbow, sternum, and shoulder.* Multiple, irregular islands of ossification are present consistently at these sites and there is malalignment and displacement of sternebrae.

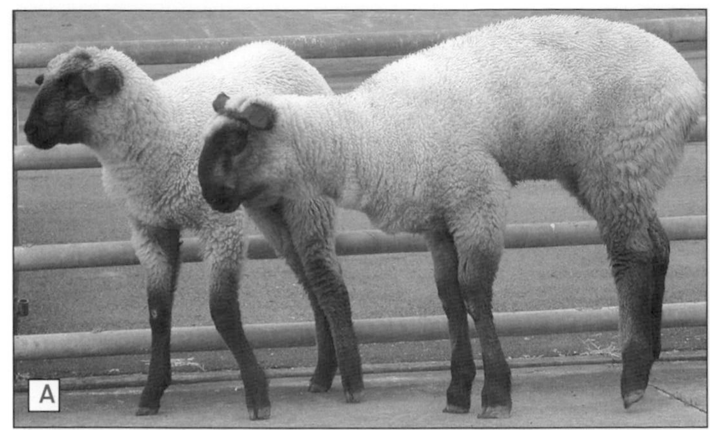

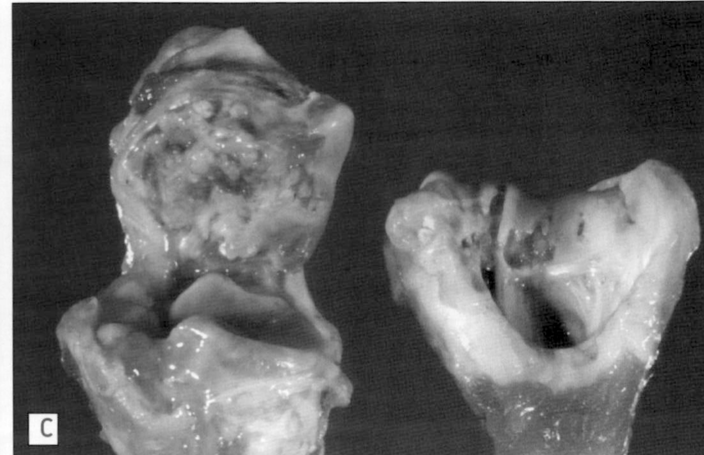

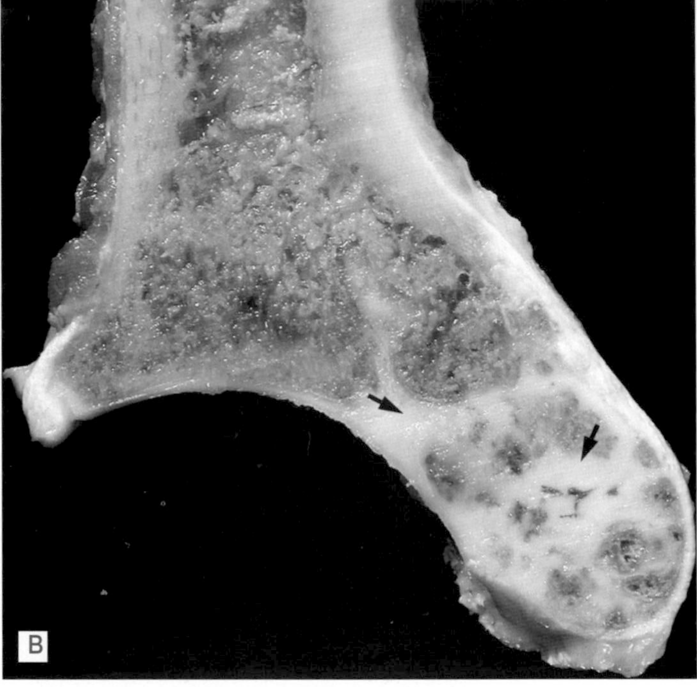

Figure 1.22 Spider lamb syndrome. **A.** Affected lambs with long legs, straight hocks and lumbar kyphosis. One has a pronounced Roman nose. Both lambs had severe valgus deformity of the hind limbs giving a "cow-hocked" appearance but this is not evident in this image. **B.** Distal scapula showing persistent islands and bands of cartilage (arrows) surrounding multiple small ossification centers in the supraglenoid tubercle. **C.** Severe degeneration of the elbow joint in an affected lamb. The olecranon is thickened and there is loss of articular cartilage with irregular pitting of the subchondral bone in the trochlear notch. The humeral condyle is devoid of articular cartilage and the subchondral bone is pitted.

In addition to the changes described above, other gross lesions may be detected at necropsy. In particular, there is *elongation of occipital condyles in a craniocaudal direction*, sometimes with erosion of the articular cartilage and dorsal deviation of the sternum between the second and sixth sternebrae. The caudal sternebrae often fail to fuse across the midline. Cervical and thoracic vertebral bodies contain excessive quantities of cartilage with disorganized arrangement, often accompanied by abnormalities in shape and symmetry. The olecranon and distal scapula also contain an excess of cartilage surrounding the multiple, irregular-shaped islands of ossification (Fig. 1.22B). Severe degenerative arthropathy, particularly involving the atlanto-occipital, elbow (Fig. 1.22C), and carpal joints, is present in lambs older than 3 months.

Histologically, the changes reflect abnormal development of ossification centers in bones developing by endochondral ossification. Multiple small ossification centers develop in nodules of hypertrophic cartilage but they fail to coalesce and expand in normal fashion towards articular surfaces (Fig. 1.23). The lack of subchondral bone predisposes to degenerative arthropathy. The proliferative and hypertrophic zones of growth plates in vertebrae and long bones are irregularly thickened and tongues of cartilage extend into the metaphysis or epiphysis. Chondrocyte columns in growth plates are often irregular. An interesting feature of the disease is that the ossification centers most severely affected are those that develop around the time of birth. Those that complete their development in utero, where they are not subjected to the mechanical forces of weight bearing and locomotion, appear normal. The lesions associated with spider lamb syndrome therefore may reflect the influence of mechanical stress on a defective cartilage model. This could help to explain the variable expressivity that is such a feature of the disease.

A *point mutation in ovine FGFR3* has been identified as the underlying defect in spider lamb syndrome. The gene encoding this receptor has largely been cloned and sequenced, and an accurate test for detecting heterozygous individuals is now available.

Chondrodysplastic syndromes characterized by **disproportionate dwarfism** do occur in sheep, but are rare. The best known of these is the *Ancon mutant*, which at one time gained popularity as a breed for its inability to jump walls. Although the breed is now extinct, the defect has reappeared on odd occasions, presumably due to new mutations. The Ancon abnormality is a *mesomelic, short-limbed dwarfism* caused by premature closure of certain growth plates.

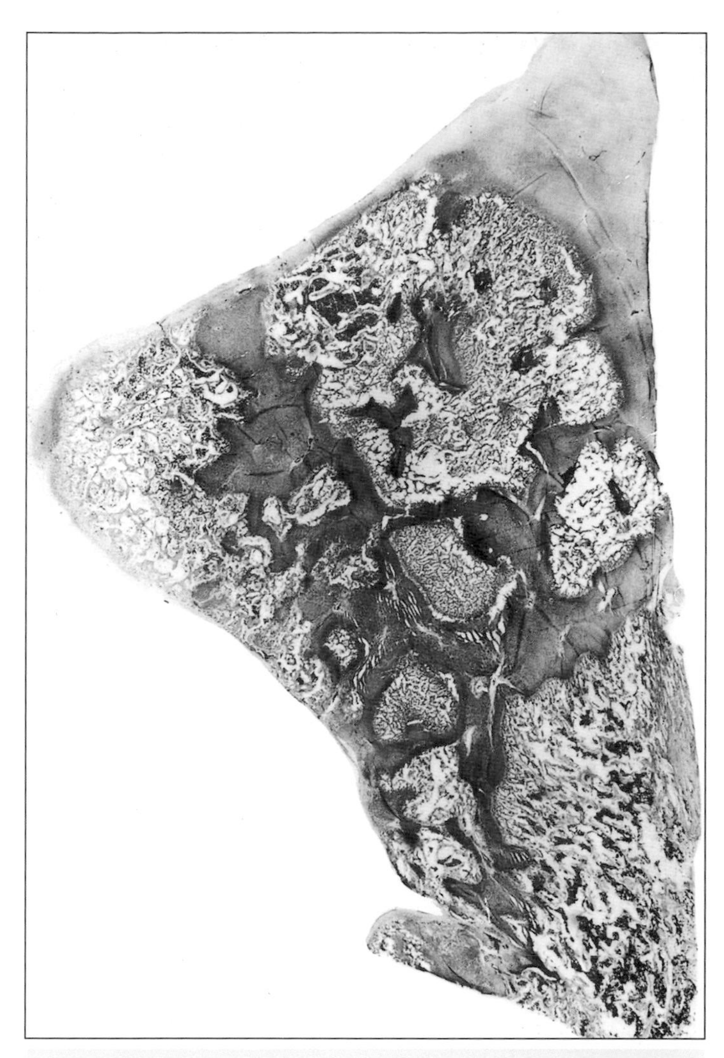

Figure 1.23 Subgross preparation of the olecranon from a **spider lamb** showing multiple ossification centers separated by irregular bands of cartilage.

Another form of chondrodysplasia reported in South Country Cheviot sheep in Scotland, was characterized by ectrodactyly, domed forehead and protruding eyes, together with shortened ears and tail. The syndrome was believed to be of genetic origin with recessive inheritance, but this was not proven.

A severe form of dwarfism affecting 27 of 110 lambs born to 70 mixed-breed ewes occurred in the United Kingdom. Most affected lambs were alive at birth but died within a few minutes. The abnormalities included a domed head, shortened nose, short, paddle-like limbs, narrow thorax, and swollen abdomen, and were said to resemble bulldog calves. Recessive inheritance could be eliminated due to the high incidence of affected lambs and the genetic diversity of the ewe flock. It is possible that a new, dominant mutation occurred in primordial germ cells of a ram in the flock.

A chondrodysplasia characterized by *dwarfism and varus deformity of the forelimbs* has recently been recognized in **Texel sheep** in New Zealand. The syndrome is inherited as an *autosomal recessive trait, but with variable expression*. Affected lambs appear normal at birth, but by 2–4 weeks of age show evidence of reduced growth rate, shortened neck and legs, varus forelimb deformities and a wide-based stance. Severely affected lambs show progressive reluctance to walk and often die within the first 4 months of life. In such cases, the articular cartilage on major weight-bearing surfaces of the hip and shoulder joints may be completely eroded, exposing the subchondral bone. The trachea is flaccid, sometimes kinked, and tracheal rings are partially flattened. *Histologically, there is disorganization of chondrocytes in articular and physeal cartilage and multiple foci of chondrolysis*, which sometimes coalesce to form large clefts. The matrix surrounding chondrocytes has an abnormal fibrillar and granular appearance. Similar microscopic changes are present in tracheal cartilage, confirming the generalized nature of the chondrodysplasia.

Chondrodysplasias of pigs

Disproportionate dwarfism was reported in three litters of Danish Landrace pigs sired by the same boar. The abnormalities were confined to the long bones of the limbs, and were most severe in the forelimbs. The bones of the skull and axial skeleton were unaffected. Signs of the disease were first apparent at 1–2 weeks of age and became more apparent with time. By weaning, affected pigs had an abnormal gait due to loose attachment of the limbs to the body and excessive mobility of joints. Few of them reached breeding age. Histologically, the growth plates had reduced thickness of the proliferative zone and irregularity of the hypertrophic zone, but the chondrocytes within each zone appeared normal. The disorder was inherited as an autosomal recessive trait.

In another report of dwarfism in pigs, almost 100 of 800 juvenile pigs developed gait abnormalities and marked shortening of limb bones, especially those of the hindlimb. The reduced length of limbs was due to premature closure of growth plates. The skull and axial skeleton were unaffected. In spite of the very high incidence, autosomal recessive inheritance was suspected.

Dwarfism also occurs in pig with vitamin A toxicosis (see later) but the lesions are more widespread than in this heritable form of chondrodysplasia, affecting vertebral bodies as well as limb bones.

Bibliography

Beever JE, et al. Spider lamb syndrome is caused by a point mutation in ovine fibroblast growth factor receptor 3. Proc XXVI Int Conf Anim Gen: International Society for Animal Genetics, 1998:81.

Duffell SJ, et al. Skeletal abnormality of sheep: clinical, radiological and pathological account of occurrence of dwarf lambs. Vet Rec 1985;117:571–576.

Jensen PT, et al. Hereditary dwarfism in pigs. Nord Vet Med 1984;36:32–37.

Kaman J, et al. Congenital disproportional chondrodysplasia in pigs. Acta Vet Brno 1991;60:237–251.

Oberbauer AM, et al. Developmental progression of the spider lamb syndrome. Small Rum Res 1995;18:179–184.

Rook JS, et al. Diagnosis of hereditary chondrodysplasia (spider lamb syndrome) in sheep. J Am Vet Med Assoc 1988;193:713–718.

Shelton M. A recurrence of the Ancon dwarf in merino sheep. J Hered 1968;59:267–268.

Thompson KG, et al. Chondrodysplasia of Texel sheep – a new disease of suspected genetic aetiology. NZ Vet J 2003;51:45–46.

Vanek JA, et al. Radiographic diagnosis of hereditary chondrodysplasia in newborn lambs. J Am Vet Med Assoc 1989;194:244–248.

Chondrodysplasias of dogs

A variety of different forms of inherited chondrodysplasia are recognized in dogs of different breeds. Some are clinically apparent at birth

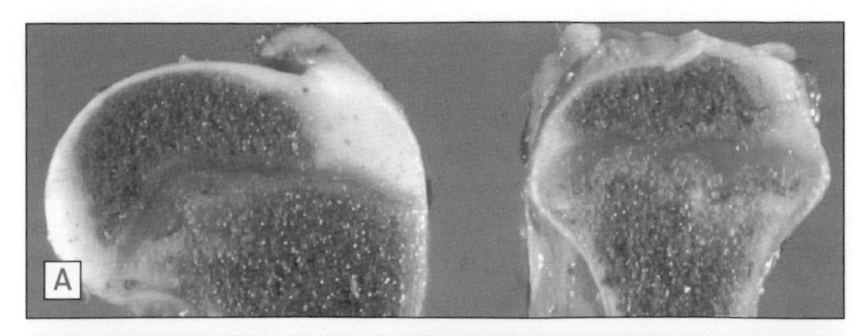

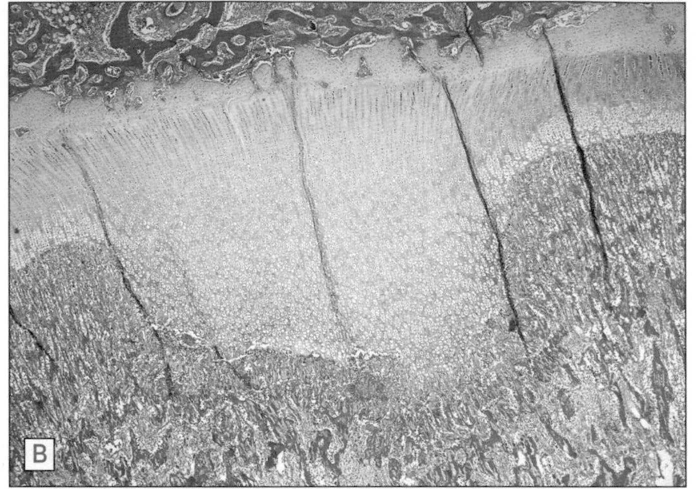

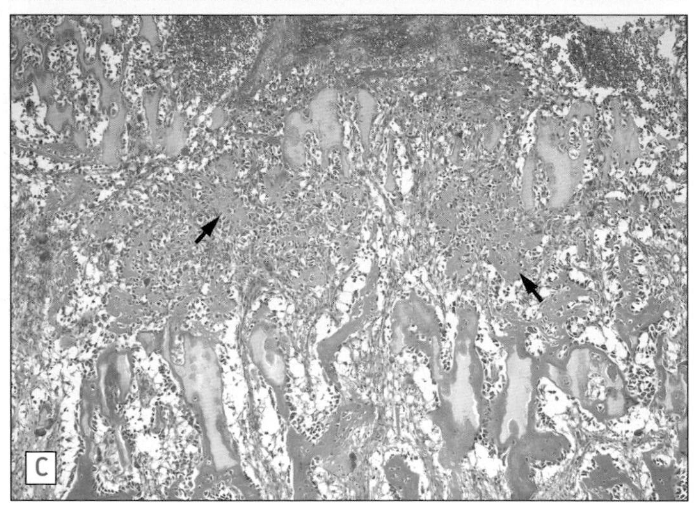

Figure 1.24 Alaskan Malamute chondrodysplasia. **A.** Proximal humerus (left) and distal radius of an affected pup showing irregular thickening of the physes. **B.** Marked, segmental thickening of the hypertrophic zone in the physis of an Alaskan Malamute pup with chondrodysplasia. **C.** Primary spongiosa immediately beneath a thickened segment of physis in the same Malamute pup. Note the disruption of the normal trabecular architecture and replacement by proliferating osteoblasts producing disorganized spicules of osteoid (arrows). An area of hemorrhage is present closer to the physis.

but others are not manifest for several weeks. **Chondrodysplasia in the Alaskan Malamute** is characterized by *disproportionate, short-legged dwarfism*, and *autosomal recessive inheritance* with complete penetrance and variable expression. At birth, the growth plates of affected puppies appear normal radiographically. Radiographic changes are apparent as early as 7–10 days of age but are more pronounced after 3 weeks. Similarly, there is little difference in growth plate and metaphyseal histology between dwarf and normal Malamutes at birth. During growth, the changes become marked, suggesting that mechanical force is required in order to create the clinical and pathological changes. Irregular thickening of growth plates in the limb bones is a feature of the disease (Fig. 1.24A). Broad tongues of hypertrophic cartilage extend into the metaphysis in close proximity to healing trabecular microfractures (Fig. 1.24B, C). Disruption of the metaphyseal blood supply, leading to impaired vascular invasion of the developing growth plate, is considered responsible for the physeal thickenings. *The lesions bear a remarkable resemblance to rickets*, both grossly and in demineralized bone sections, but the mineralization of cartilage is normal. Abnormal endochondral ossification occurs throughout the body, but *the most striking lesions occur in the distal ulna and radius*, resulting in enlarged carpal regions and valgus deformity of the forelimbs. This most likely reflects the proportionately greater weight-bearing responsibility of the forelimbs compared to the hindlimbs, and the greater susceptibility to injury. A reduction in the hydroxyproline content of cartilage, and in the stability of type II collagen cross-links, has been demonstrated in dwarf Alaskan Malamutes, the collagen defect possibly increasing the susceptibility of trabeculae in the primary spongiosa to fractures. Hemolytic anemia characterized by stomatocytosis, macrocytosis, and increased concentration of sodium within erythrocytes, accompanies the chondrodysplasia in this breed. Heterozygotes have intermediate hemoglobin concentrations, suggesting that this manifestation of the syndrome is inherited as an incompletely dominant trait.

Chondrodysplasia in the Norwegian Elkhound is a *disproportionate, short-legged dwarfism* similar to the disease in Malamutes but with significant morphologic differences. In Elkhounds, the vertebral bodies are also shortened and there is a marked reduction in the width of the proliferative zone in growth plates. *A highly distinctive feature is the presence of one or more large, intracytoplasmic inclusions in the chondrocytes of all zones* (Fig. 1.25). The inclusions stain deep blue by the Alcian Blue-periodic acid-Schiff method at pH 1.0 and 2.6. Inclusions that escape from degenerate chondrocytes persist and lie free in lacunae. The cell columns in the zone of hypertrophy and degeneration are generally disorganized and separated by wide matrix bars. Trabeculae in the primary spongiosa are coarse and shortened, with many horizontal bridges and thick osteoid seams. No inclusions are present in osteoblasts or osteocytes.

Chondrodysplasia in the English Pointer has been reported in the United Kingdom and Australia in related dogs. Inheritance appears to be *autosomal recessive*. Affected puppies are smaller than their normal littermates and develop locomotory abnormalities, including a bunny-hopping gait. Some also have inferior prognathism. Growth plates are irregularly thickened due to increased width of the hypertrophic zone, but the lesion varies in severity between different bones. Increased mineralization of laryngeal and tracheal cartilage occurs in some affected animals. At around 10 weeks of age, articular cartilages appear normal but by 16–18 weeks, there are abnormalities in the cartilage of all major limb joint, including wrinkles, projections and sometimes fibrillation. In the epiphyseal cartilage beneath these lesions there are irregular cavities containing degenerate chondrocytes and strands of collagen. Severe degenerative arthropathy develops in some joints.

Chondrodysplasia in the Great Pyrenees also appears to be inherited as *an autosomal recessive trait*. Affected pups are normal at birth but by 2 weeks they are shorter and lighter than their littermates. Mature dwarfs are less than half of normal size. Radiographic abnormalities are restricted to the metaphyses of long bones and vertebrae and are characterized by *delayed ossification*. Histologically, chondrocyte columns in growth plates are disorganized and many chondrocytes contain cytoplasmic vacuoles that consist of dilated cisternae of rough endoplasmic reticulum. Metaphyseal trabeculae are thicker than normal and are often joined by lateral bridges.

Pseudoachondroplastic dysplasia, a disease of **Miniature Poodles**, was originally named epiphyseal dysplasia. Inheritance of the trait is *probably autosomal recessive*. The disease is not apparent at birth but by 2–3 weeks of age affected pups are noticeably smaller than their normal littermates and have difficulty standing and walking. The skull is usually normal but mild inferior prognathism may be present. Vertebral bodies are short and show delayed ossification, costal cartilages are longer than normal and costochondral junctions are enlarged (Fig. 1.26). Severely affected pups have dorsoventral flattening of the rib cage, presumably due to persistent recumbency. The limb bones are also short, particularly those of the forelimbs, and possess enlarged epiphyses which are sometimes flared over the metaphyses (Fig. 1.27). Histologically, the cartilage matrix is sparse and lacks basophilia. Chondrocytes vary in size and are sometimes clumped together in enlarged lacunae. Chondrocyte

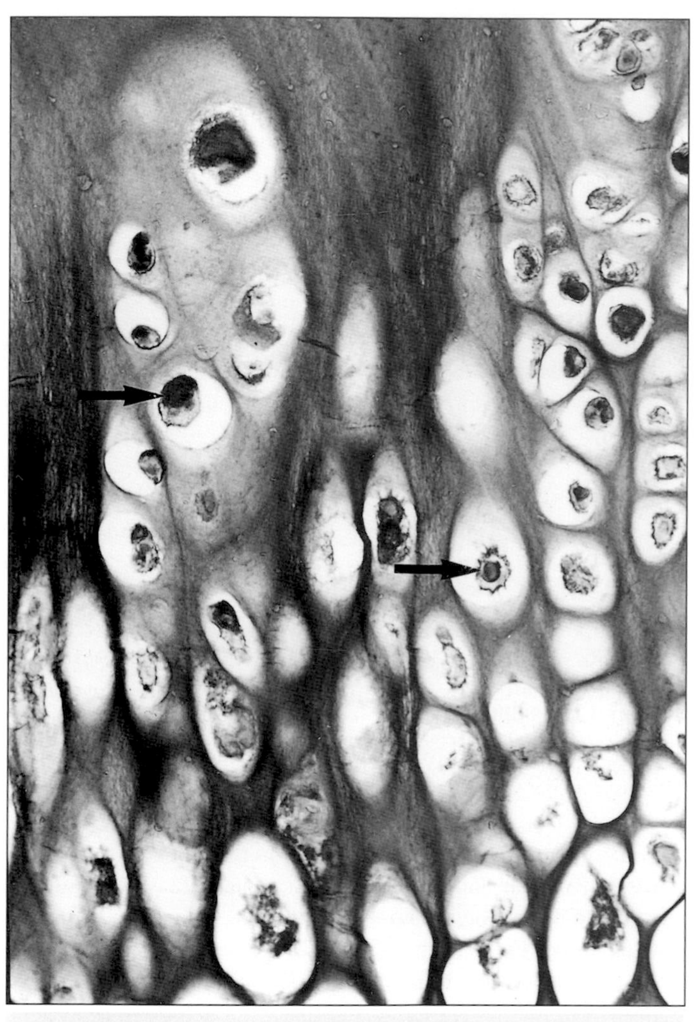

Figure 1.25 Norwegian Elkhound chondrodysplasia. Inclusion bodies in chondrocytes (arrows). (Courtesy of SA Bingel.)

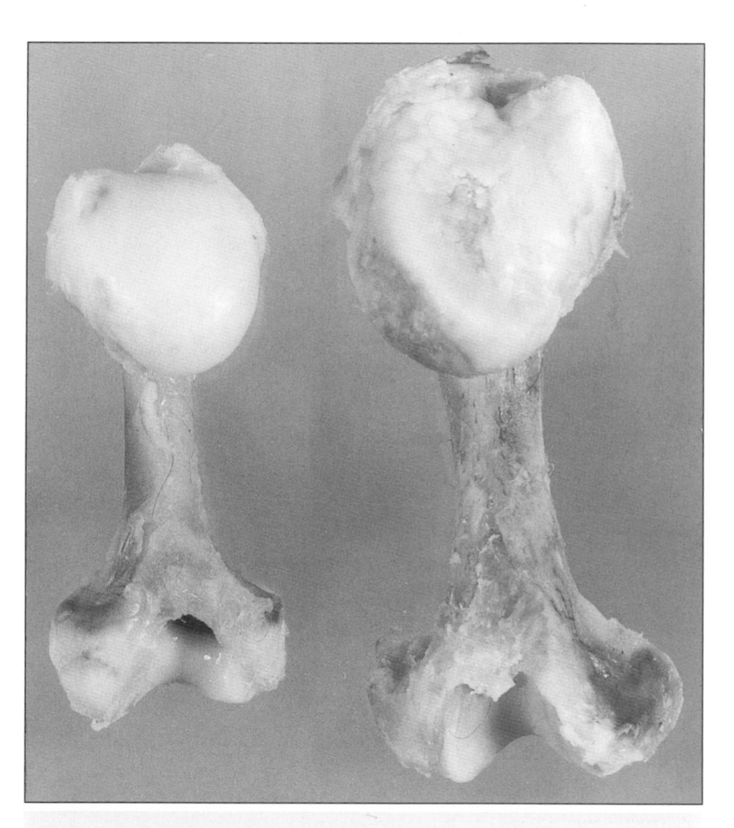

Figure 1.27 Pseudoachondroplastic dysplasia in Miniature Poodle. Humerus of immature and mature dogs. The articular cartilage of the humeral head in the adult dog is degenerate.

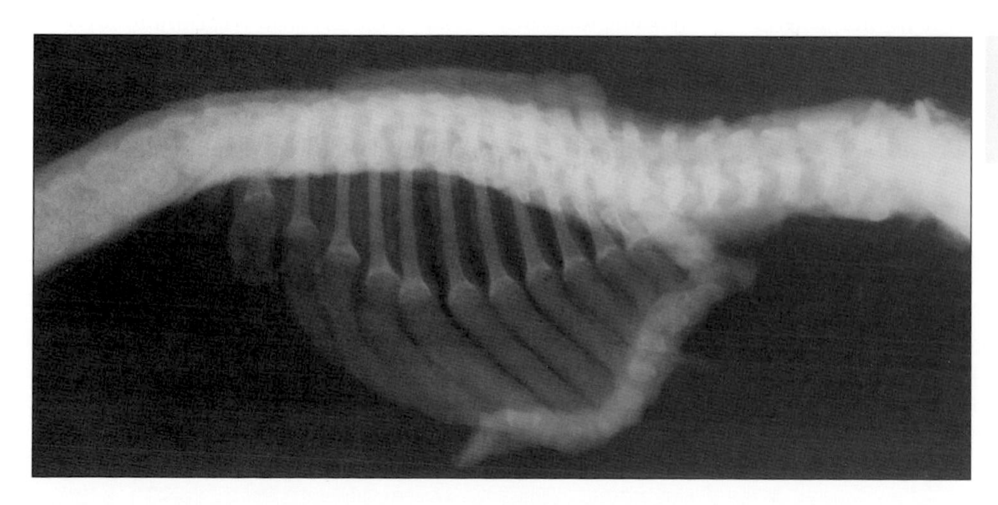

Figure 1.26 Pseudoachondroplastic dysplasia in Miniature Poodle. Thoracic radiograph showing enlarged costochondral junctions, long costal cartilages, and shortened vertebrae.

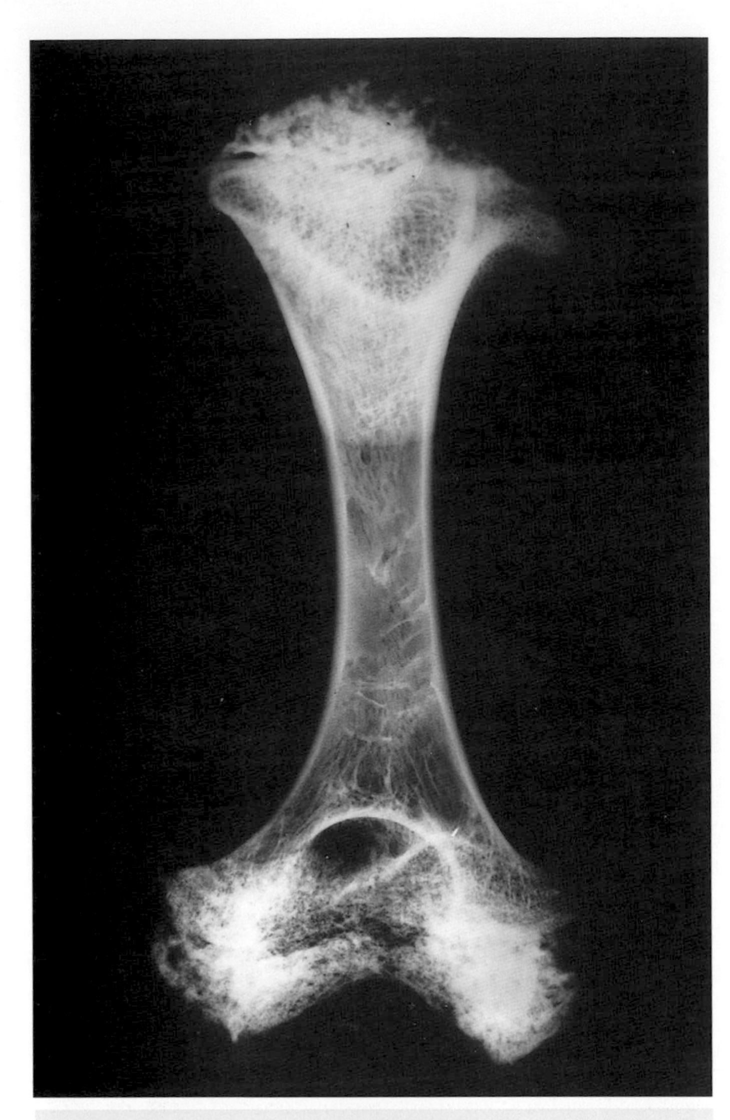

Figure 1.28 Pseudoachondroplastic dysplasia in Miniature Poodle. Radiograph of humerus showing irregular, multifocal development of ossification centers, creating a stippled appearance.

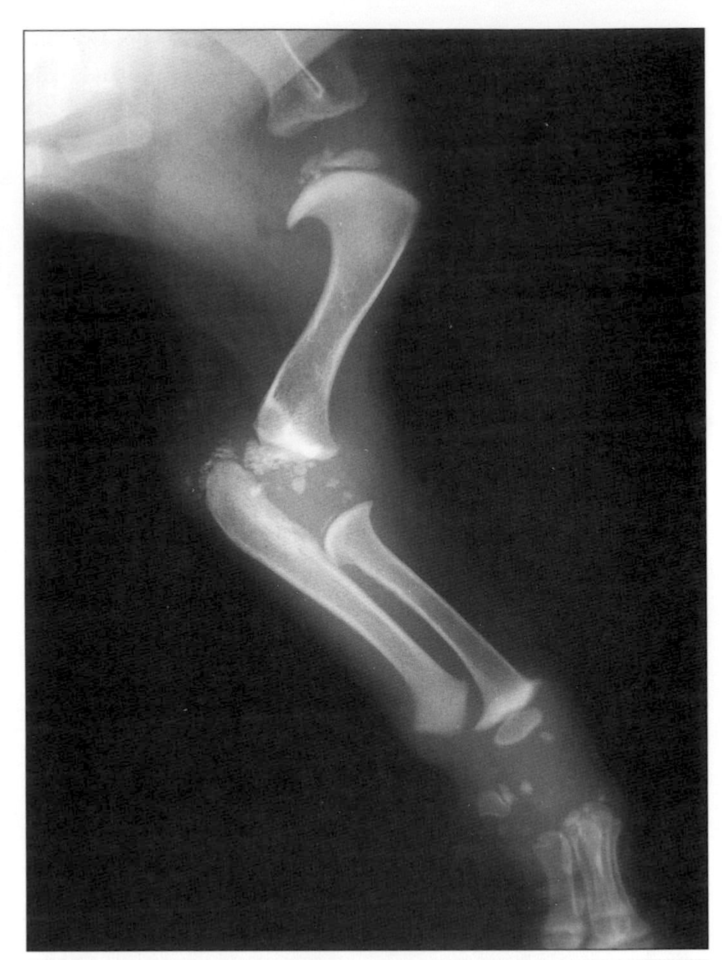

Figure 1.29 Multiple epiphyseal dysplasia in a Beagle dog. Forelimb radiograph showing stippled epiphyses in shoulder, elbow and carpal regions. (Courtesy of GP Rasmussen.)

columns in growth plates are irregular and the proliferative zone is abnormal. Ossification centers develop later than normal and are multifocal, creating a stippled appearance radiographically in affected pups (Fig. 1.28). By 2 years of age, ossification is complete and the long bones are only half to two-thirds normal length. Interestingly, the lumbar vertebrae are longer than in normal dogs of the same age. Degenerative arthropathy and spondylosis may develop in pups less than a year of age. *The underlying defect in cartilage matrix formation not only causes defective endochondral ossification, but also results in abnormal formation of the trachea and nasal septum.* Collagen synthesis is normal but the defect appears to involve decreased sulfation of glycosaminoglycans.

Multiple epiphyseal dysplasia is a rare condition of **Beagle dogs**, probably inherited as an *autosomal recessive trait.* Affected puppies walk with a swaying gait but, in adults, lameness is only apparent after exercise. The earliest radiographic signs are not visible until 3 weeks of age and consist of *stippled epiphyseal mineralization* (Fig. 1.29), especially in the tarsal and carpal bones, the femoral, humeral, metacarpal and metatarsal epiphyses, and in the bodies of the sixth and seventh lumbar vertebrae. By 5 months the stippling is no longer apparent, having been incorporated into the normal ossification centers. The abnormal foci of epiphyseal mineralization develop in a specific subarticular zone of the epiphyses. The initial lesion is a floccular accumulation of chondroitin sulfate and glycoprotein in chondrocyte lacunae. As adjacent lacunae coalesce and liquefy to form cysts, their contents mineralize. The stippled radiographic appearance of epiphyses resembles that of pseudoachondroplastic dysplasia of Miniature Poodles but the histologic changes are distinct.

Osteochondrodysplasia in the Scottish Deerhound becomes apparent at around 4–5 weeks of age, with affected puppies showing exercise intolerance and retarded growth. These pups go on to develop a bunny-hopping gait, kyphosis, marked bowing of the limbs, and joint laxity. Mature dogs have shortened, porotic long bones, shortened vertebrae, distorted carpal and tarsal bones, incongruencies of hip and elbow joints, and enlargement of muscle attachment sites. Growth plates are irregular in width and physeal–metaphyseal junctions are uneven. Histologically, there are islands of basophilic, vacuolated chondrocytes in epiphyses, but physeal and metaphyseal lesions are intermittent. Physes contain some areas that are virtually normal, in addition to areas that are narrow and hypocellular, or lack proliferative or hypertrophic zones. A characteristic feature is the *presence of periodic acid-Schiff-positive, diastase-resistant cytoplasmic inclusions in proliferative and hypertrophic chondrocytes.* The metaphyses may consist of normal primary and secondary spongiosa in some areas, while elsewhere the trabeculae are thin, sparse and largely replaced by fibrovascular connective tissue. The irregularity of the physeal and metaphyseal lesions may reflect localized trauma. The condition is probably inherited as an *autosomal recessive trait.*

A syndrome with combined **ocular and skeletal dysplasia** occurs in the **Labrador Retriever** and **Samoyed** breeds. The bone lesions are confined to the appendicular skeleton and include *shortening of the limb bones, valgus deformity of the carpi, and abnormally shaped radii and ulnas.* Affected dogs have a *characteristic "downhill" conformation* due to more severe involvement of the forelimbs. In some dogs, the coronoid processes are ununited and there is hypoplasia of both the coronoid and anconeal processes, but these changes may be incidental as they also occur as separate defects in these breeds. Retained cartilage cores may be present in the distal ulna. Although clinical evidence of dwarfism may not be evident until about 8 weeks of age, *a radiographic image-classification system allows identification of affected puppies at birth.* The ocular lesions in both breeds consist of *cataracts and retinal detachment.* In Retrievers, there is also retinal dysplasia. The ocular and skeletal lesions appear to be inherited together, but the defective gene has recessive effects on the skeleton and incomplete dominance on the eye. Heterozygotes therefore possess mild eye lesions but a clinically normal skeleton.

Chondrodysplasias of cats

There are *few reports* of chondrodysplasias in cats. One report describes a severe form in a stillborn kitten *in association with homozygous Pelger–Huët anomaly.* The kitten was small and had a dome-shaped skull, flattened face, and protruding tongue. Vertebrae were shortened, as were ribs and long bones of the limbs. The limbs were thickened and had broad, mushroom-shaped epiphyses. Growth plates were incompletely formed with partial or irregular ossification at the center of the physis, and more normal peripheral regions. A live littermate, which was heterozygous for the Pelger–Huët anomaly, also had skeletal abnormalities, including pectus excavatum, lordosis, shortened vertebral bodies, and flared distal radial metaphyses. The skeletal lesions in the stillborn kitten were very similar to those seen in rabbits with homozygous Pelger–Huët anomaly.

A *possible metaphyseal chondrodysplasia* was also diagnosed in two unrelated kittens with shortened limbs, bowed forelimbs, marked widening of the growth plates and flaring of the metaphyses. The most severe growth plate lesions were present in the distal radius and proximal humerus. The radiographic changes in growth plates initially led to a diagnosis of rickets, but neither kitten responded to treatment and there was no evidence of defective mineralization. One kitten had two siblings with similar limb deformities and its probable sire was also known to have short, deformed forelimbs, suggesting a genetic etiology.

An osteochondrodysplasia characterized by a short, thick, inflexible tail and misshapen distal limbs with extensive new bone formation on the plantar aspect of the tarsi and metatarsi, is reported in **Scottish Fold** cats. Other abnormalities in affected cats include irregularity in the size and shape of tarsal, carpal, metatarsal, and metacarpal bones, phalanges, and caudal vertebrae, narrowing of joint spaces, progressive new bone formation around distal limb joints and diffuse osteopenia of adjacent bones. Histologically, there is evidence of defective endochondral ossification in physes and beneath articular cartilages. Cartilage columns in physes are disorganized and there is irregular thickening of physeal cartilage. Islands of cartilage may also extend from articular cartilage into epiphyses. Lesions can be detected in kittens as young as 7 weeks of age, but the bony changes are slowly progressive and may not be detected for several years. Originally, it was thought that affected cats were homozygous for the Fd (fold-eared) gene and resulted only from matings between fold-eared cats. Recent evidence suggests that the disease can also develop in heterozygous Scottish Folds and that significant lesions may be present in such animals as early as 6 months of age.

Bibliography

Bingel SA, Sande RD. Chondrodysplasia in five Great Pyrenees. J Am Vet Med Assoc 1994;205:845–848.

Bingel SA, et al. Chondrodysplasia in the Alaskan Malamute. Characterization of proteoglycans dissociatively extracted from dwarf growth plates. Lab Invest 1985;53:479–485.

Breur GJ, et al. Clinical, radiographic, pathologic and genetic features of osteochondrodysplasia in Scottish deerhounds. J Am Vet Med Assoc 1989;195:606–612.

Carrig CB, et al. Growth of the radius and ulna in Labrador Retriever dogs with ocular and skeletal dysplasia. Vet Radiol 1990;31:165–168.

Gunn-Moore DA, et al. Unusual metaphyseal disturbance in two kittens. J Small Anim Pract 1996;37:583–590.

Latimer KS, et al. Homozygous Pelger-Huët anomaly and chondrodysplasia in a stillborn kitten. Vet Pathol 1988;25:325–328.

Malik R, et al. Osteochondrodysplasia in Scottish Fold cats. Aust Vet J 1999;77:85–92.

Meyers VN, et al. Short-limbed dwarfism and ocular defects in the Samoyed dog. J Am Vet Med Assoc 1983;183:975–979.

Rasmussen PG. Multiple epiphyseal dysplasia in a litter of Beagle puppies. J Small Anim Pract 1971;12:91–96.

Sande RD, Bingel SA. Animal models of dwarfism. Vet Clin North Am: Small Anim Pract 1982;13:71–89.

Whitbread TJ, et al. An inherited enchondrodystrophy in the English Pointer dog. A new disease. J Small Anim Pract 1983;24:399–411.

Zhu D, et al. Canine bone shape analysis by use of a radiographic image-classification system. Am J Vet Res 1992;53:1090–1095.

Osteogenesis imperfecta

Osteogenesis imperfecta is one of the most frequently observed inherited connective tissue disorders of humans, but *occurs rarely in domestic animals.* The disease is characterized by *excessive bone fragility*, which in severe cases may result in multiple intrauterine fractures, marked skeletal deformity, and either stillbirth or perinatal death. Milder forms may be inapparent at birth but lead to an increased incidence of postnatal fractures and bowing of the limbs. Other abnormalities may include fragile, opalescent teeth (dentinogenesis imperfecta), joint laxity, and blue sclerae. Based on clinical features and mode of inheritance, *at least four distinct forms of osteogenesis imperfecta are recognized in human patients.* Most human cases of osteogenesis imperfecta are inherited as autosomal dominant traits and represent new mutations, although rare recessive forms also exist. A quantitative or qualitative defect in type I collagen is the molecular basis of the disease and may be due to one of many mutations in either of the two genes, *COL1A1* or *COL1A2*, that code for the $\alpha 1$ and $\alpha 2$ chains, respectively. Type I collagen is the

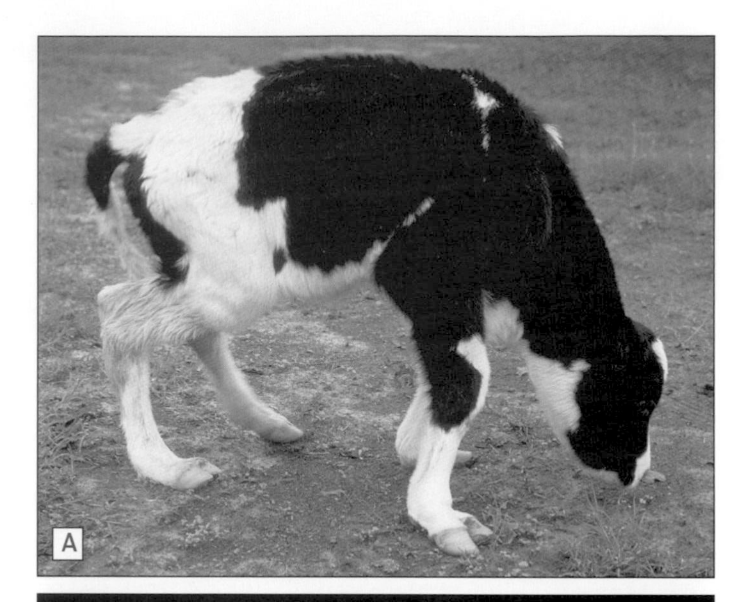

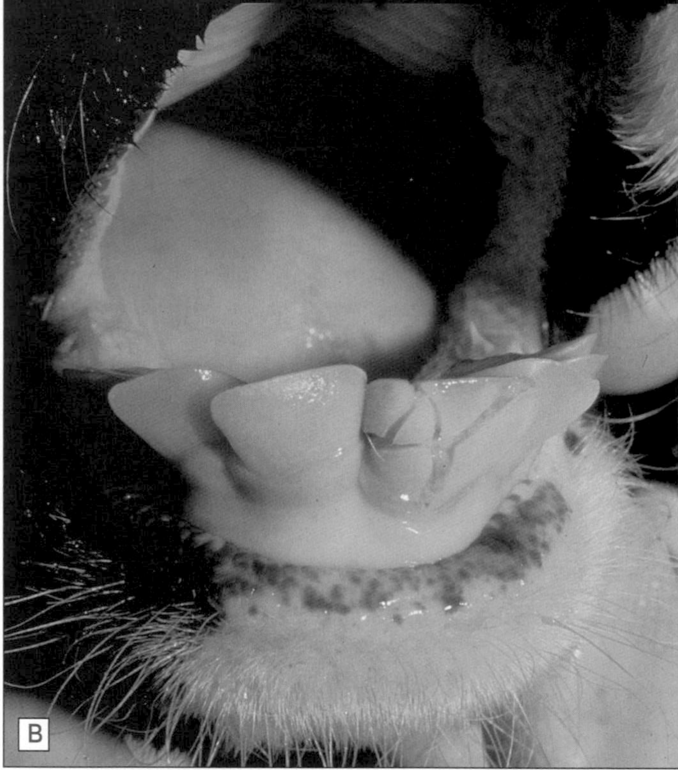

Figure 1.30 Bovine osteogenesis imperfecta. A. Affected Holstein calf, 2 weeks old. Because of excessive joint laxity, the calf has a crouched stance and its pasterns almost touch the ground. **B.** Fractured incisor tooth due to dentinal dysplasia in the same calf.

predominant collagen type in bone, dentin, ligaments, tendons, and in the ocular sclera, thus accounting for the characteristic distribution of lesions.

Most reports of osteogenesis imperfecta in animals are in calves and lambs and appear analogous to the most severe form of the disease in humans. In **cattle**, the disease has occurred in Australia, the US, and Denmark in the offspring of three clinically normal, unrelated **Holstein-Friesian** bulls, and in **Charolais** calves in Denmark. A single crossbred **Hereford** calf with osteogenesis imperfecta has been identified in New Zealand. There is convincing evidence to support an *autosomal dominant* mode of inheritance, at least in Holstein-Friesian cattle, although the percentage of calves affected from the three Holstein-Friesian bulls varied from approximately 9% to 44%. This presumably reflects different degrees of gonadal mosaicism following mutations in the germ cell lines of each bull. The manifestations of the disease in each report in calves have been similar, but minor variations exist, suggesting that different mutations may be involved. Affected calves are usually born alive and are of normal size, but most are unable to stand due to marked hypermobility of the joints and, in some cases, the presence of limb fractures. Some affected Holstein-Friesian calves are able to stand and can walk with difficulty, but have a characteristic crouched stance with pasterns almost touching the ground (Fig. 1.30A). As in some forms of the human disease, calves with osteogenesis imperfecta have dentinal dysplasia characterized by small, translucent pink-gray teeth, which are barely erupted at birth and may fracture in calves that survive for a few weeks (Fig. 1.30B). In some calves the sclerae are distinctly blue, but this is more evident during postmortem examination following enucleation of the eye. Skin fragility is not a feature of the disease in calves.

The main findings during *postmortem examination* relate to the skeleton. *Although the bones are essentially normal in shape, they are extremely brittle* and can usually be broken with little effort. Acute fractures are common in the mandibles and major limb bones; the latter probably occurring during attempts to stand. Severely affected calves may have multiple, well-developed calluses on their ribs (Fig. 1.31A), indicating intrauterine fractures. In spite of their fragility, the cortices of long bones are similar in thickness to those of normal calves but the volume of trabecular bone in metaphyses and epiphyses is reduced and shows a finer, denser pattern. In calves that have stood and walked, infraction lines may be present in the epiphysis and metaphysis of major limb bones (Fig. 1.31B). These represent bands of healing trabecular microfractures presumably resulting from trauma during weight bearing. Tendons are thinner than normal and discolored pink.

Histologically, osteoblastic activity appears normal but calcified cartilage spicules in the primary spongiosa are lined by only a thin layer of basophilic bone matrix and there is little osteoclastic resorption or realignment of trabeculae. Infractions and trabecular microfractures are common (see Fig. 1.17). Bone cortices are porous due to incomplete compaction of primary osteons and consist predominantly of deeply basophilic woven bone with few lamellae (Fig. 1.32A, B). The dentin in affected calves is basophilic, coarsely laminated and approximately one fifth as thick as in control calves. Dentinal tubules are irregularly oriented and reduced in number, and there is an undulating margin with the pulp cavity. The sclera is approximately one half of normal thickness. Ultrastructurally, collagen fibrils in the tendons, dentin, sclera, and skin of affected calves are significantly narrower than normal.

Chemical analysis of bone from Holstein-Friesian calves with osteogenesis imperfecta has provided evidence that *different mutations are involved*. In bone tissue from both American and Australian calves there is reduced size of apatite crystals and a decrease in the amount of type I collagen and proteoglycans. The *main difference is in the concentration of osteonectin*, which is normal in the Australian calves with osteogenesis imperfecta, but only 10% of normal in the affected American calves. Phosphophoryn, a dentin-specific protein, and an osteonectin-like protein of dentin are also markedly deficient in these calves.

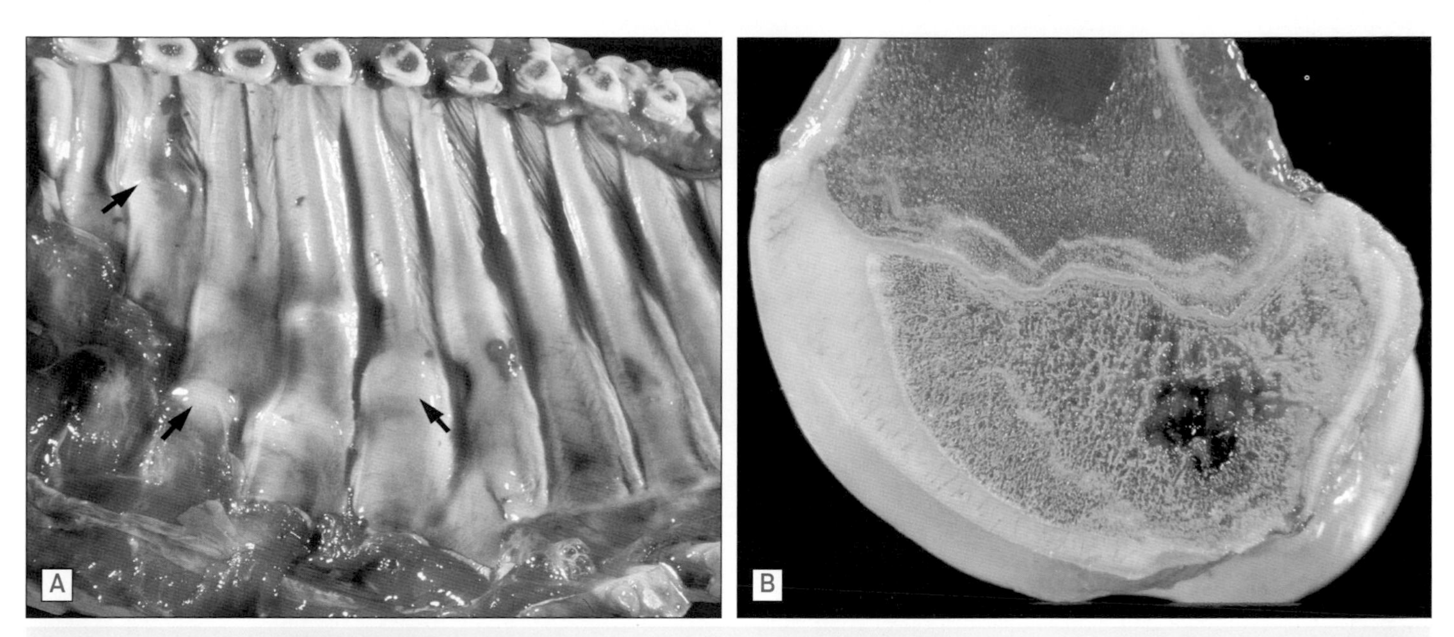

Figure 1.31 Bovine osteogenesis imperfecta. **A.** Several mature calluses (arrows) on the ribs of a newborn calf, indicating intrauterine fractures due to extreme bone fragility. **B.** Distal femur from a calf that had survived for a couple of weeks and had walked. Multiple infraction lines are present in the epiphysis and metaphysis. The cancellous bone is more porous than normal.

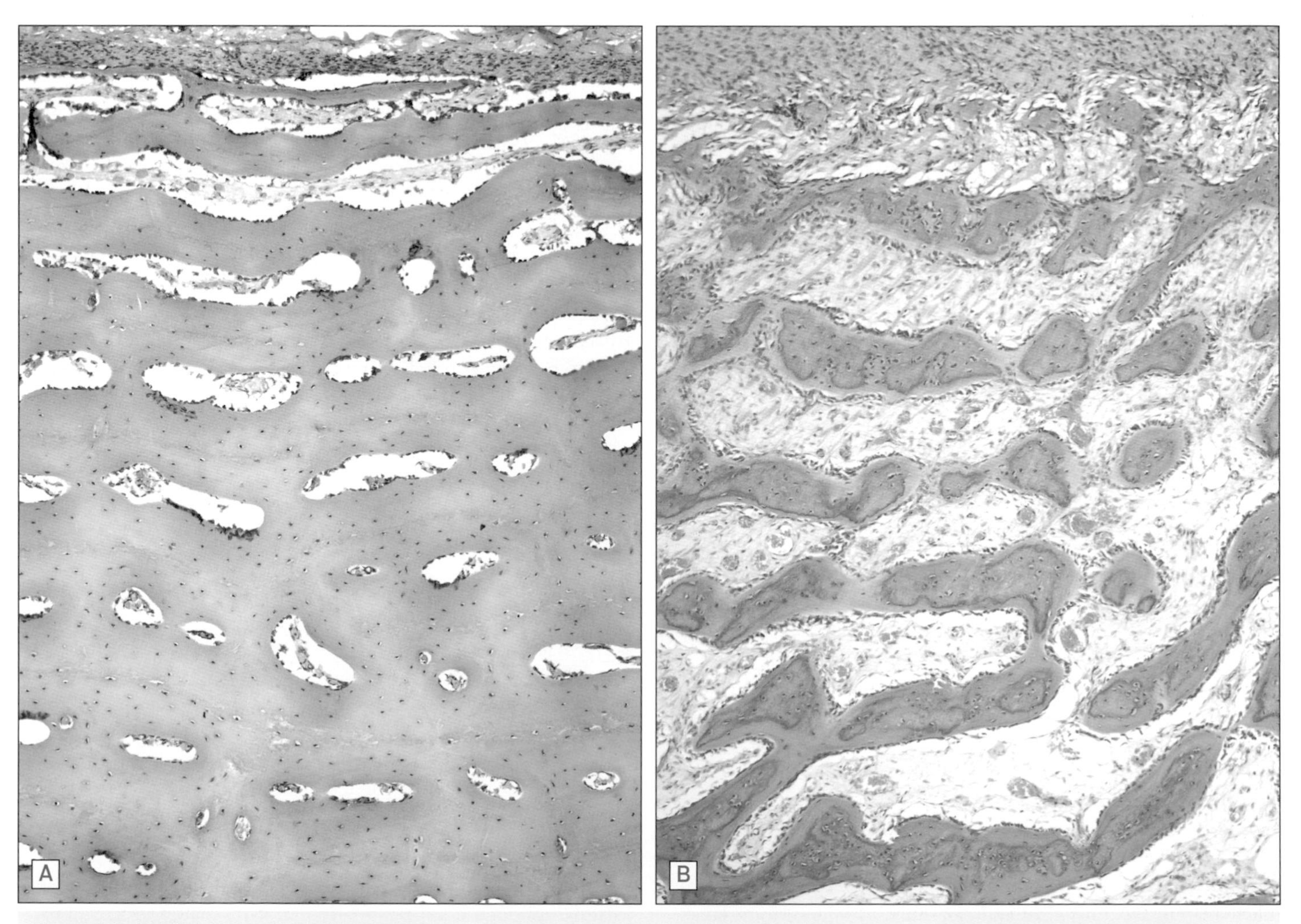

Figure 1.32 Bovine osteogenesis imperfecta. **A.** Microscopic view of periosteum and developing cortical bone in a **normal newborn calf**. **B.** Similar view of the developing cortex in an **affected calf** showing basophilic spicules of woven bone and minimal compaction by the addition of lamellar bone.

Skin fragility is not reported in calves with osteogenesis imperfecta, but Belgian calves with dermatosparaxis do have skeletal lesions. These calves are deficient in the activity of procollagen *N*-peptidase, an enzyme involved in the conversion of procollagen to collagen. Although the bones are grossly normal and not prone to spontaneous fractures, they are abnormally brittle when processed. Histologically, the cortical bone of periosteal origin is disorganized and hypermineralized, while that derived from compaction of the chondro–osseous complex is normal. **Arachnomelia**, a lethal defect in German Simmental and Brown Swiss-Braunvieh cattle, is also accompanied by increased bone fragility but affected calves also have arthrogryposis, distortion of the vertebral column and brachygnathia inferior, in addition to cardiovascular anomalies. The limbs are long and distorted, and the bones have very narrow diaphyses.

In **sheep**, severe forms of osteogenesis imperfecta have occurred in two flocks in New Zealand and one in the United Kingdom. In both New Zealand reports, one of which involved the **Romney** breed, affected lambs died either during parturition or soon after. The Romney lambs had a domed head (Fig. 1.33A) with brachygnathia inferior, dark blue sclerae, fragile, pink teeth, and marked joint laxity. A feature of the disease in Romneys, which involved about 50 lambs, was the presence of marked skin fragility. This has not been described in any of the other reports of osteogenesis imperfecta in humans or animals. Using DNA fingerprinting, the defect was traced to one of five clinically normal Romney rams being used in the flock and a suspicion of *dominant inheritance* was confirmed by test-matings with unrelated ewes of a different breed. In affected lambs, the bones could be easily bent or cut with a knife and were often abnormally shaped with thickened diaphyseal regions (Fig. 1.33B). Most lambs had recent fractures surrounded by hemorrhage and older (in utero) fractures with poorly formed calluses, especially involving the ribs. Microscopic changes are similar to those described in calves with osteogenesis imperfecta, but more severe. Persistent trabeculae of calcified cartilage, lined by a thin layer of basophilic bone, extend from growth plates deep into the diaphyses of long bones, filling the marrow cavities (Fig. 1.34A, B). Osteoclastic resorption of the primary spongiosa is impaired, and there is no formation of a recognizable secondary spongiosa. The cortices are extremely porous, but thicker than normal, and consist of narrow, basophilic trabeculae separated by loose connective tissue. There is no evidence of compaction into normal cortical bone.

Similar gross and microscopic bone lesions occurred in lambs from the other New Zealand flock, together with tooth abnormalities and skin fragility. The breed of these sheep was not disclosed and the mode of inheritance not determined, but circumstantial evidence favors a dominant trait. The United Kingdom outbreak occurred in lambs of the **Clun Forest** breed. These lambs often survived parturition and were bright and alert, but usually could not stand. Blue sclerae were reported but there was no mention of tooth abnormalities. Multiple recent and intrauterine bone fractures were present in most lambs, and the histological lesions in bone closely resembled those seen in the New Zealand lambs.

A milder form of osteogenesis imperfecta is described in **Barbados Blackbelly** sheep. Although fractures occur in utero, affected lambs are born alive and can stand, in spite of joint laxity. The teeth of these lambs are normal. Autosomal recessive inheritance is suspected in this breed.

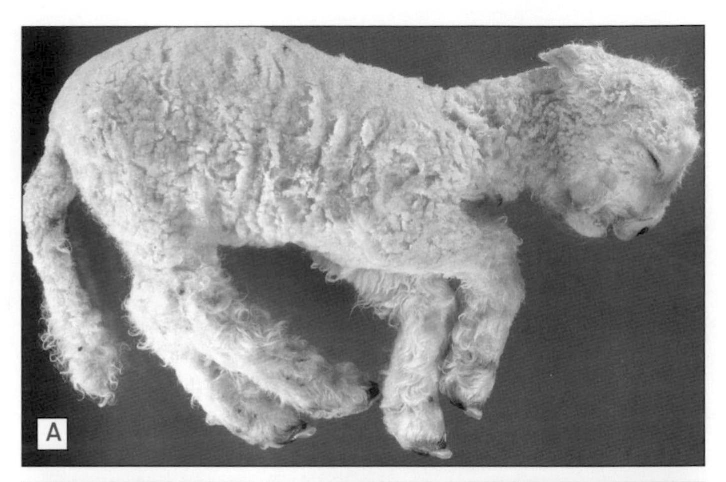

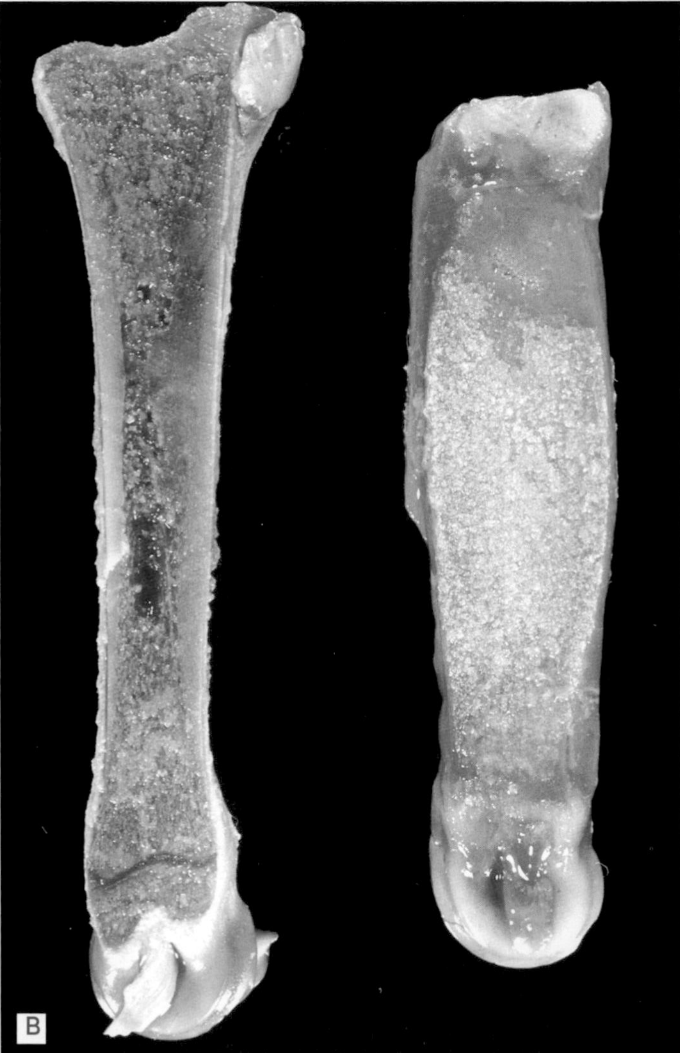

Figure 1.33 Ovine osteogenesis imperfecta in Romney lamb. **A.** Note the domed forehead and brachygnathia inferior. **B.** Sagittal sections of metatarsal bones from a **normal newborn lamb** (left) and a **lamb with osteogenesis imperfecta**. The bone from the affected lamb is shorter, has a thickened diaphysis and no medullary cavity.

Osteogenesis imperfecta has been described in **puppies** and **kittens**, although it appears likely that early reports of the disease in these species were misdiagnoses of fibrous osteodystrophy caused by nutritional secondary hyperparathyroidism. More recently,

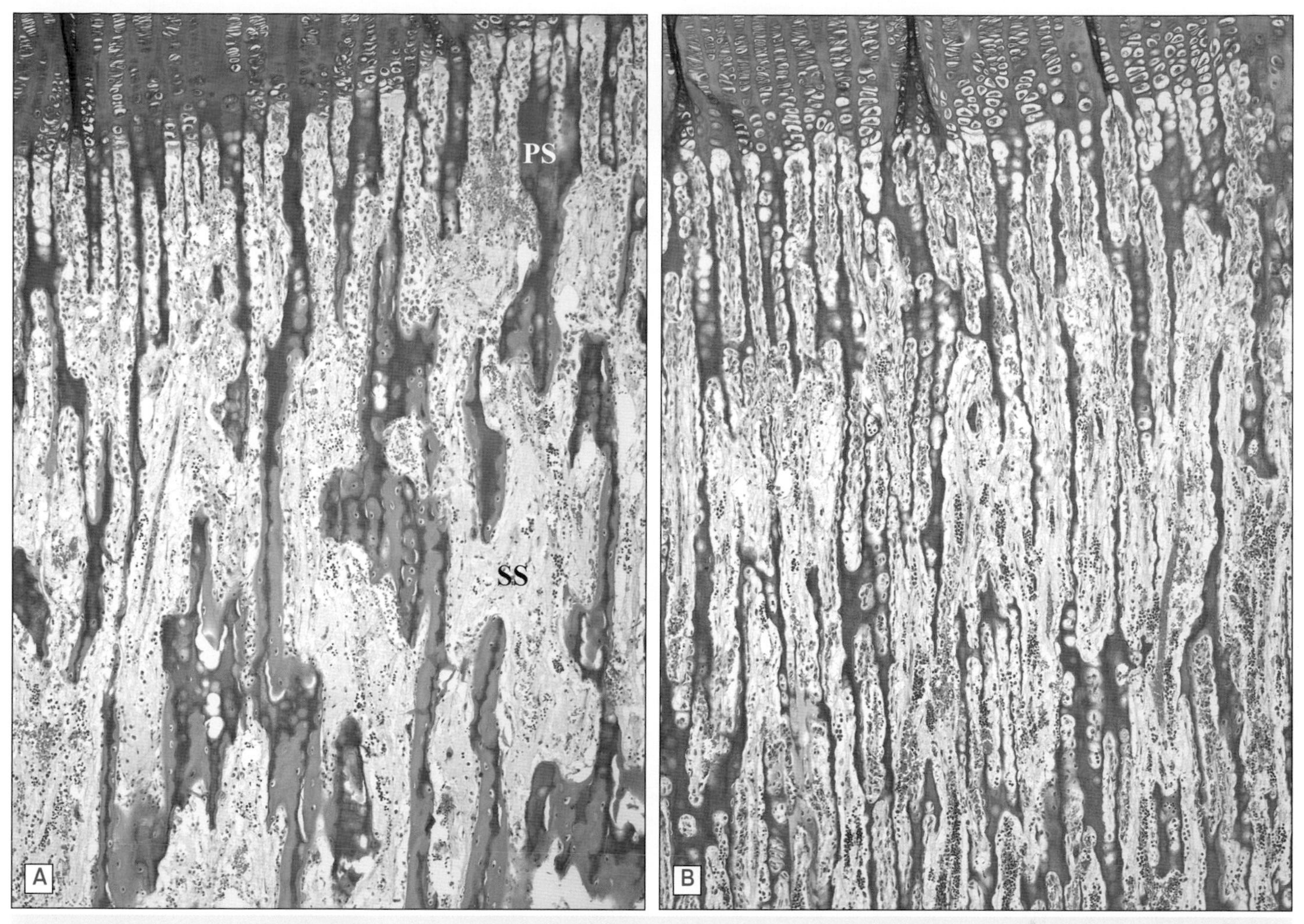

Figure 1.34 Ovine osteogenesis imperfecta. **A.** Metaphysis from a long bone of a **normal newborn lamb** showing primary spongiosa (PS) and secondary spongiosa (SS). **B.** Similar microscopic field from a **newborn lamb with osteogenesis imperfecta**. The primary spongiosa persists deep into the metaphysis and consists of delicate trabeculae lined by a thin layer of basophilic bone.

convincing cases have been recognized in both species. Multiple bone and tooth fractures, together with joint laxity, were reported in 2/4 and 3/6 pups from two litters of **Dachshunds** sired by the same dog. The disease was apparent from 3–4 weeks of age and histologic lesions in bone and dentine resembled those described in calves and lambs with osteogenesis imperfecta. Isolated cases of osteogenesis imperfecta have also occurred in **Golden Retriever, Beagle**, and **Standard Poodle** pups. Defective type I collagen formation was demonstrated in these three breeds using cultured skin fibroblasts. The disease was also diagnosed in a 12-week-old **domestic longhair** kitten that developed multiple spontaneous fractures of long bones. The kitten also had fractured teeth. Histologic examination of bones revealed a marked reduction in the quantity of cortical bone, most of which was woven bone, and an absence of well-developed osteons. These cases of osteogenesis imperfecta in the puppies and kitten appear analogous to the milder forms of the disease in humans.

Bibliography

Angerholm JS, et al. Osteogenesis imperfecta in Holstein-Friesian calves. J Med Vet 1994;A41: 128–138.

Arthur DG, et al. Lethal osteogenesis imperfecta and skin fragility in newborn New Zealand Romney lambs. NZ Vet J 1992;40:112–116.

Brem G, et al. Zum Auftreten des Arachnomelie-Syndroms in der Brown-Swiss Braunvieh Population Bayerns. Berl Munch Tierarztl Wschr 1984;97:393–397.

Byres PH. Disorders of collagen biosynthesis and structure. In: Scriver CR, et al, eds. The Metabolic and Molecular Bases of Inherited Disease. 8th ed. New York: McGraw-Hill, 2001:5241–5285.

Campbell BG, et al. Clinical signs and diagnosis of osteogenesis imperfecta in three dogs. J Am Vet Med Assoc 1997;211:183–187.

Cassella JP, et al. A morphological and ultrastructural study of bone in osteogenesis imperfecta. Calcif Tiss Int 1996;58:155–165.

Cohn LA, Meuten DJ. Bone fragility in a kitten: An osteogenesis imperfecta-like syndrome. J Am Vet Med Assoc 1990;197:98–100.

Denholm LJ, Cole WG. Heritable bone fragility, joint laxity and dysplastic dentin in Friesian calves: a bovine syndrome of osteogenesis imperfecta. Aust Vet J 1983;60:9–17.

Dhem A, et al. Bone in dermatosparaxis. I. Morphologic analysis. Calcif Tissue Res 1976;21: 29–36.

Fisher LW, et al. Two bovine models of osteogenesis imperfecta exhibit decreased apatite crystal size. Calcif Tissue Int 1987;40:282–285.

Gertner JM, Root L. Osteogenesis imperfecta. Orthop Clin North Am 1990;21:151–162.

Jensen PT, et al. Congenital osteogenesis imperfecta in Charolais cattle. Nord Vet Med 1976;28:304–308.

Seeliger F, et al. Osteogenesis imperfecta in two litters of Dachshunds. Vet Pathol 2003;40:530–539.

Osteopetrosis

Osteopetrosis, or "*marble bone disease*," is a group of rare disorders occurring in humans, as well as in laboratory and domestic animals, characterized by *defective osteoclastic bone resorption and the accumulation of primary spongiosa in marrow cavities*. Two main forms of the disease are recognized in humans – a severe, recessively inherited, *lethal (malignant) form* with lesions present at birth, and a *dominant (benign) form* which becomes manifest later in life. Intermediate forms also exist. *In animals, most descriptions of osteopetrosis appear analogous to the malignant form and autosomal recessive inheritance is suspected in most cases.* Because of the complexity of osteoclast differentiation and function there are many points at which bone resorption can be interrupted, thus accounting for the clinical and morphologic variability associated with the osteopetroses. In some forms, osteoclasts are present in abundance but are incapable of resorbing bone, while in others osteoclasts are either absent or markedly reduced in number. For example, in the *op/op* osteopetrotic mouse, a deficiency in macrophage specific growth factor (M-CSF or CSF-1) results in an absence of osteoclasts. The disorder in these mice can be successfully treated with M-CSF. Deficiency of carbonic anhydrase II causes osteopetrosis in humans by interfering with the intracellular generation of protons by osteoclasts. Affected individuals have abundant osteoclasts, but acidification of the microenvironment at the cell–bone interface is not possible and resorption cannot occur. Patients with this form of osteopetrosis also have renal tubular acidosis and cerebral mineralization, reflecting a systemic deficiency of the enzyme.

In **cattle**, osteopetrosis is best studied in the **Angus** breed, where it is inherited as an *autosomal recessive trait*. Affected calves are small, premature (250–275 days of gestation) and usually stillborn. Clinically, they show brachygnathia inferior, impacted molar teeth and protruding tongue (Fig. 1.35A, B). The long bones are shorter than normal and easily fractured. Radiographically, the medullary cavities are dense, without clear differentiation between the cortex and medulla. Vertebrae are shortened, frontal and parietal bones are thick, and the bones of the cranial base are thick and dense. On cut surface, *the metaphyses and diaphyses of long bones, are filled with dense, unresorbed cones of primary spongiosa extending from the metaphysis to the center of the diaphysis* (Fig. 1.36A). In spite of their increased density, the bones are more fragile than normal and fractures are sometimes detected at necropsy. The fragility is much less marked than in osteogenesis imperfecta. Although the skeletal lesions of osteopetrosis are generalized, they vary in expression throughout the body. Nutrient foramina are either absent or hypoplastic. As a result of the abnormalities of the skull, the cerebral hemispheres are rectangular with flattened dorsal surfaces, the cerebellum is partially herniated through the foramen magnum, and optic nerves are hypoplastic.

Histologically, growth plates are essentially normal but metaphyses are relatively avascular. Dense chondro-osseous tissue, consisting of cartilage matrix lined by a thin layer of woven bone, occupies the medulla (Fig. 1.36B). Osteoclasts are rare and when present, appear to be inactive. *Failure to replace the primary spongiosa and its associated woven bone with thicker trabeculae of mature lamellar bone, presumably accounts for the increased fragility of osteopetrotic bones.* Cortical bone is apparently normal. In the brain, mineralized vessel walls and/or neurons may be found in the thalamus, cerebellum, meninges, choroid plexus, and around the aqueduct of Sylvius.

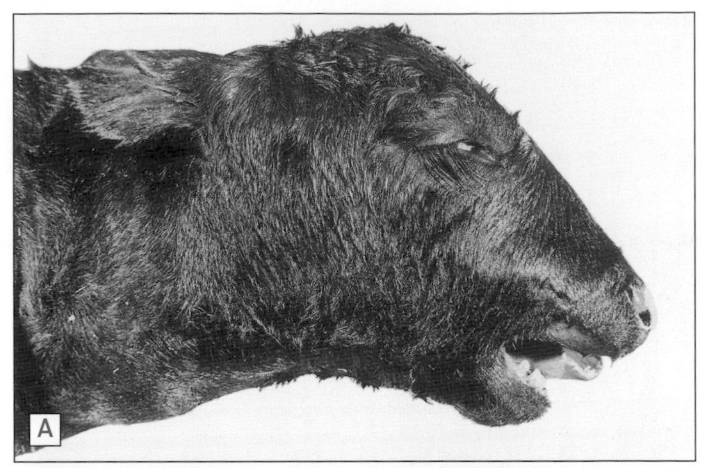

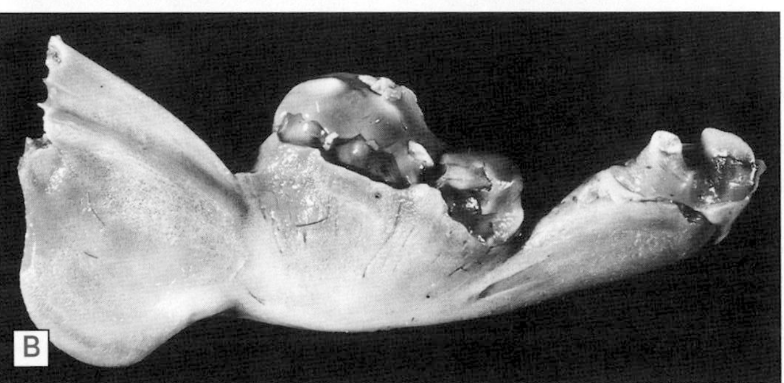

Figure 1.35 Bovine osteopetrosis. A. Stillborn Angus calf with inferior brachygnathia. **B.** Impacted molars in deformed, fragile mandible from the same calf.

Osteopetrosis of **Hereford** and **Simmental** breeds resembles that of Angus calves in most respects, including mode of inheritance, but in affected Herefords the frontal bones are markedly thickened and filled with cystic spaces. The domed forehead of these calves could be misinterpreted as hydrocephalus unless the skull is sectioned. An outbreak of an osteopetrosis-like disorder involving five of 16 Angus and Angus-Charolais cross fetuses has been reported but was associated with multiple skeletal deformities, including arthrogryposis and kyphoscoliosis in addition to frontal bone lesions similar to those of osteopetrosis in Hereford calves. Although a genetic etiology was suspected, the more likely possibility of a teratogenic agent was not excluded. In particular, infection of fetuses or young calves with ***Bovine viral diarrhea virus*** is capable of causing zonal osteopetrosis-like lesions, most likely secondary to transitory virus-induced osteoclast depletion. Acquired osteopetrosis-like lesions with varying degrees of metaphyseal sclerosis may also occur in association with ***Canine distemper virus*** infection in pups and in **lead poisoning** (see below).

A syndrome characterized by *persistence of the secondary spongiosa, perhaps analogous to metaphyseal dysplasia*, a rare human osteosclerotic disorder, was reported in three aborted or neonatal Hereford, Holstein, and Japanese Black calves. The macroscopic and histologic changes in these calves differed from those of osteopetrosis and

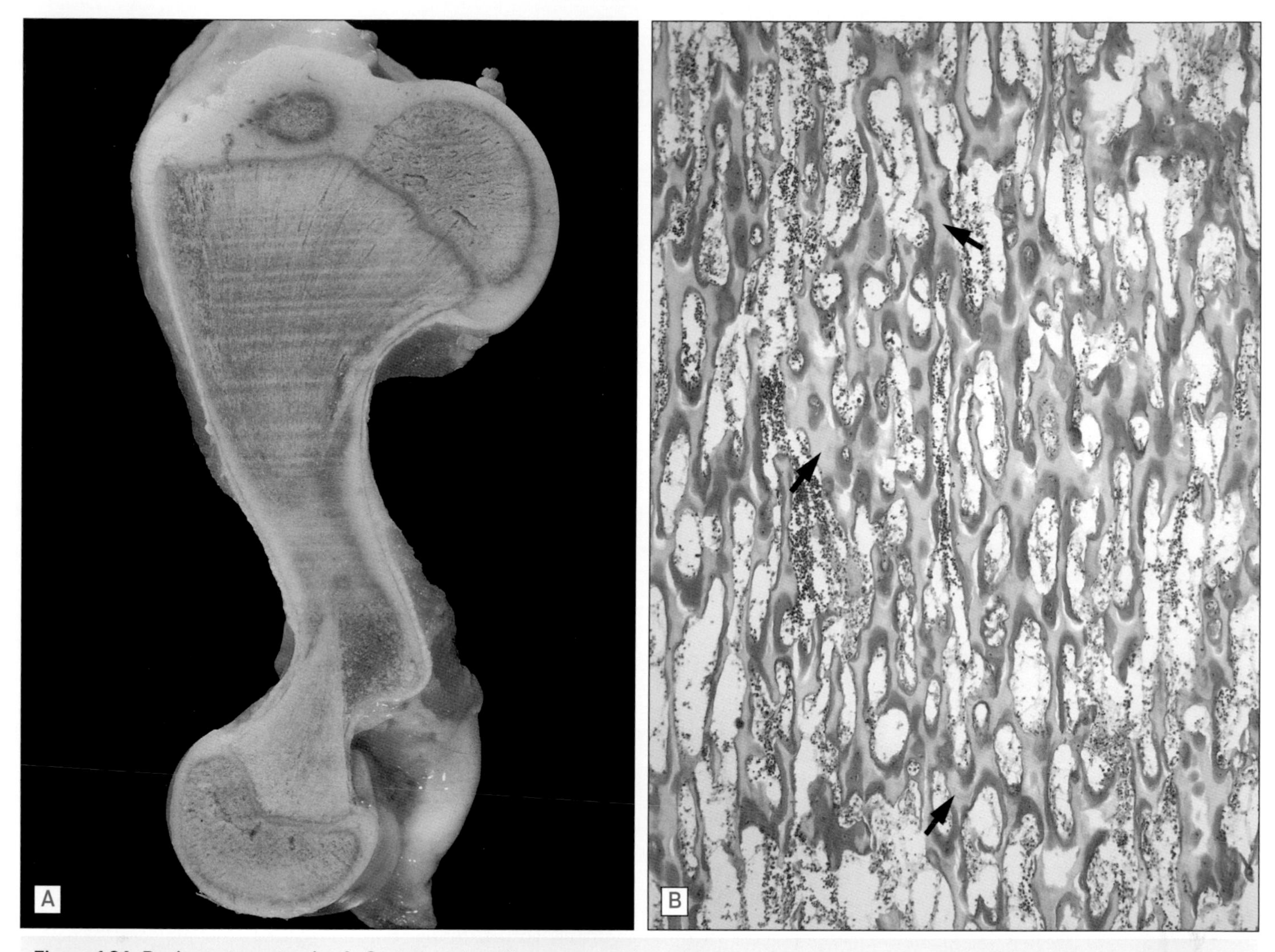

Figure 1.36 Bovine osteopetrosis. **A.** Sagittal section of humerus showing unresorbed cones of primary spongiosa extending from the proximal and distal growth plates into the diaphysis. No medullary cavity is evident. (Courtesy of RA Fairley.) **B.** Section of metaphysis showing a dense lattice of delicate interconnected trabeculae consisting of cartilage matrix (arrows) covered by a thin layer of bone.

their significance is questionable. In two of the calves, the shape of the bones was essentially normal and there was no mention of fragility. Osteoclast numbers were not reduced but those present were thin and inactive. Such subtle skeletal abnormalities could be much more common than is currently recognized, as without radiography or longitudinal sectioning of long bones they would remain undetected.

Osteopetrosis in **horses** with clinical, radiographic and pathologic features similar to the severe lethal form in Angus calves has been reported in four **Peruvian Paso foals** and one **Appaloosa**. Affected foals are of normal size at birth and are born alive but unable to stand. Brachygnathia inferior is a consistent finding and there is malpositioning and impaction of the teeth, reflecting the requirement of osteoclastic activity for normal tooth eruption. Long bones and vertebrae contain medullary cones of primary spongiosa extending from the physis to the center of the diaphysis, filling the medullary cavity (Fig. 1.37). The fragility of the bones is illustrated by the presence of multiple rib fractures, some of which probably occur in utero. Histologic changes are similar to those described for Angus calves except for the presence of normal to increased numbers of osteoclasts in affected foals. The osteoclasts appear larger than normal but no ruffled border is evident ultrastructurally, *suggesting a functional defect in osteoclasts as the basis of the disease in foals.* Although the total number of cases is small, it is likely that the disease in Peruvian Paso horses is inherited as an autosomal recessive trait.

Osteopetrosis has also been reported in an inbred captive herd of **white-tailed deer**. In addition to marked brachygnathia inferior, impacted teeth and protruding tongue, affected fawns had characteristic radiodense bones and calluses on several ribs, indicating in utero fractures.

In **dogs**, osteopetrosis is reported in three neonatal **Dachshund** puppies from the same litter. Their bones were of normal size and shape but had increased fragility. Isolated cases in an **Australian Shepherd** and a **Pekingese** were diagnosed at 12 months and 30 months of age respectively. Both dogs developed severe myelophthisic anemia.

In **cats**, osteopetrosis has been associated with chronic vitamin D toxicosis and subsequent to infection with *Feline leukemia virus*. Increased density of vertebrae and thickening of the cortices of long bones characterized an osteopetrosis-like disorder in two adult

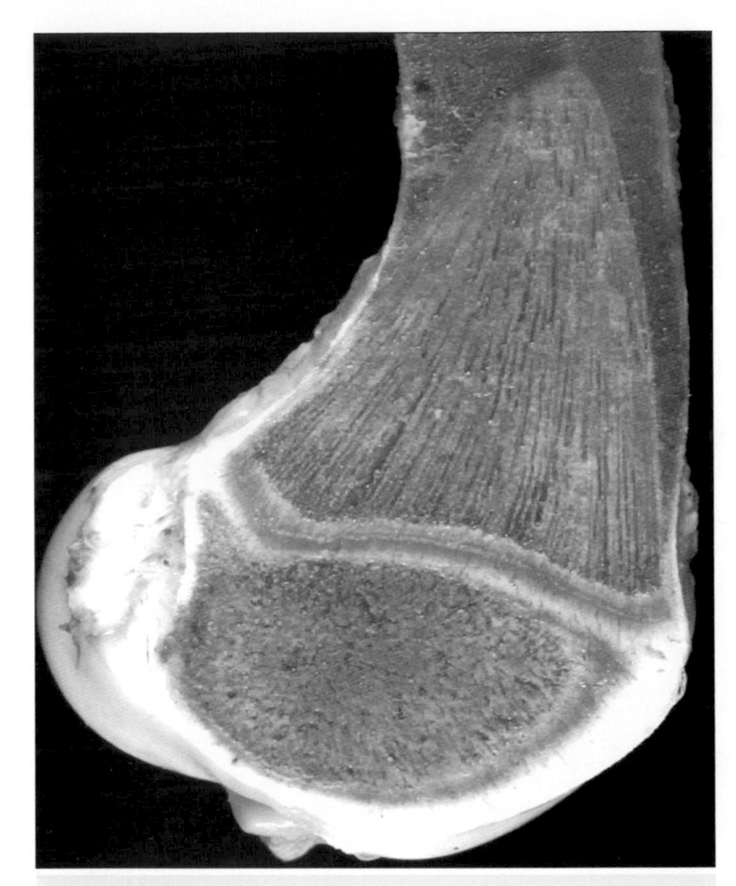

Figure 1.37 Equine osteopetrosis. Distal femur of an affected foal. Note the cone of unresorbed primary spongiosa extending into the metaphysis from the physis. (Courtesy of MW Leach.)

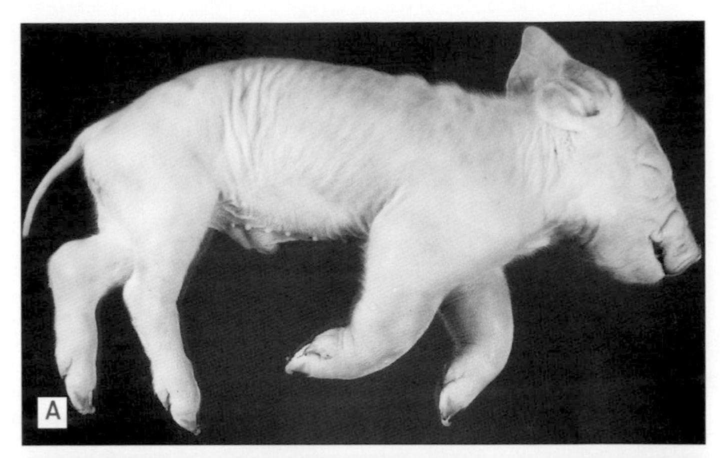

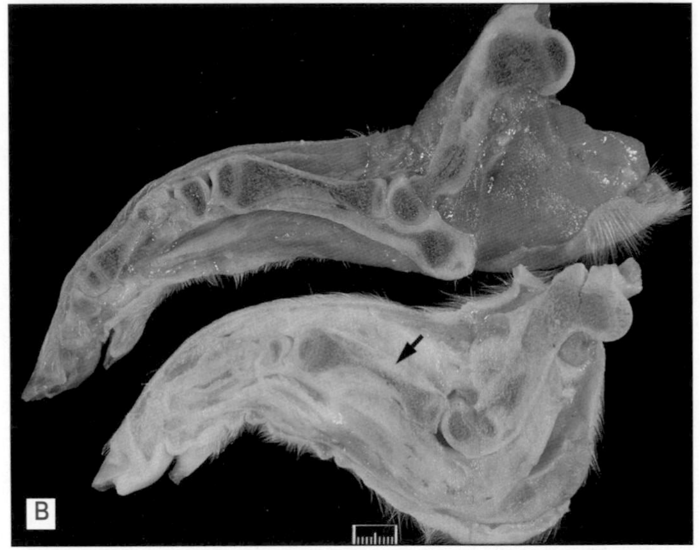

Figure 1.38 Porcine congenital hyperostosis. A. Marked swelling of both forelegs and less severe involvement of the left hindleg. **B.** Comparison of forelegs from a normal (above) and affected piglet. The radius of the affected limb is thickened due to increased periosteal bone (arrow). There is extensive edema and swelling of soft tissues throughout the entire limb. (Courtesy of RA Fairley.)

cats. The shape and size of the bones were normal. This syndrome, and that in the Australian Shepherd and Pekingese dogs, may be analogous to one of the benign forms of human osteopetrosis, or could be acquired lesions of undetermined pathogenesis.

Bibliography

Berry CR, et al. Radiographic and pathologic features of osteopetrosis in two Peruvian Paso foals. Vet Radiol Ultrasound 1994;35:355–361.

Kramers P, et al. Osteopetrosis in cats. J Small Anim Pract 1988;29:153–164.

O'Brien SE, et al. Osteopetrosis in an adult dog. J Am Vet Med Assoc 1987;23:213–216.

Ojo SA, et al. Osteopetrosis in two Hereford calves. J Am Vet Med Assoc 1975;166:781–783.

Scruggs DW, et al. Osteopetrosis, anaemia, thrombocytopenia, and marrow necrosis in beef calves naturally infected with bovine virus diarrhea virus. J Vet Diagn Invest 1995;7:555–559.

Smits BS, Bubenik GA. Congenital osteopetrosis in white-tailed deer. J Wildlife Dis 1990;26:567–571.

Umemura T, et al. Persistence of secondary spongiosa in three calves. Vet Pathol 1988;25:312–314.

Whyte MP. Sclerosing bone dysplasias. In: Favus MJ, ed. Primer on the Metabolic Bone Disease and Disorders of Mineral Metabolism. 4th ed. Philadelphia, PA: Lippincott Williams & Wilkins, 1999:367–383.

Wolf DC, Van Alstine WG. Osteopetrosis in five fetuses from a single herd of 16 cows. J Vet Diagn Invest 1989;1:262–264.

Congenital hyperostosis

Congenital hyperostosis (*cortical hyperostosis, diaphyseal dysplasia*) is a rare disease of newborn **pigs**. Affected piglets are either stillborn or die within the first few days of life, and show various degrees of thickening of one or more forelimbs (Fig. 1.38A), and sometimes the hindlimbs as well. The thickened limbs are hard and may be up to twice their normal size. The radius and ulna are the most severely affected and in some cases are the only bones involved. Grossly, *a thick layer of extracortical bone extends along the diaphyses* (Fig. 1.38B). Marked edema of the surrounding soft tissues contributes to the thickness of the limb. Histologically, radiating trabeculae of woven bone extend from the surface of apparently normal cortical bone beneath a thickened periosteum (Fig. 1.39A) containing multiple layers of active osteoblasts. The periosteum merges with edematous, poorly vascular connective tissue containing scattered, stellate fibroblasts, which infiltrate adjacent muscle bundles and the overlying dermis (Fig. 1.39B). No lesions are found in bones of the axial skeleton.

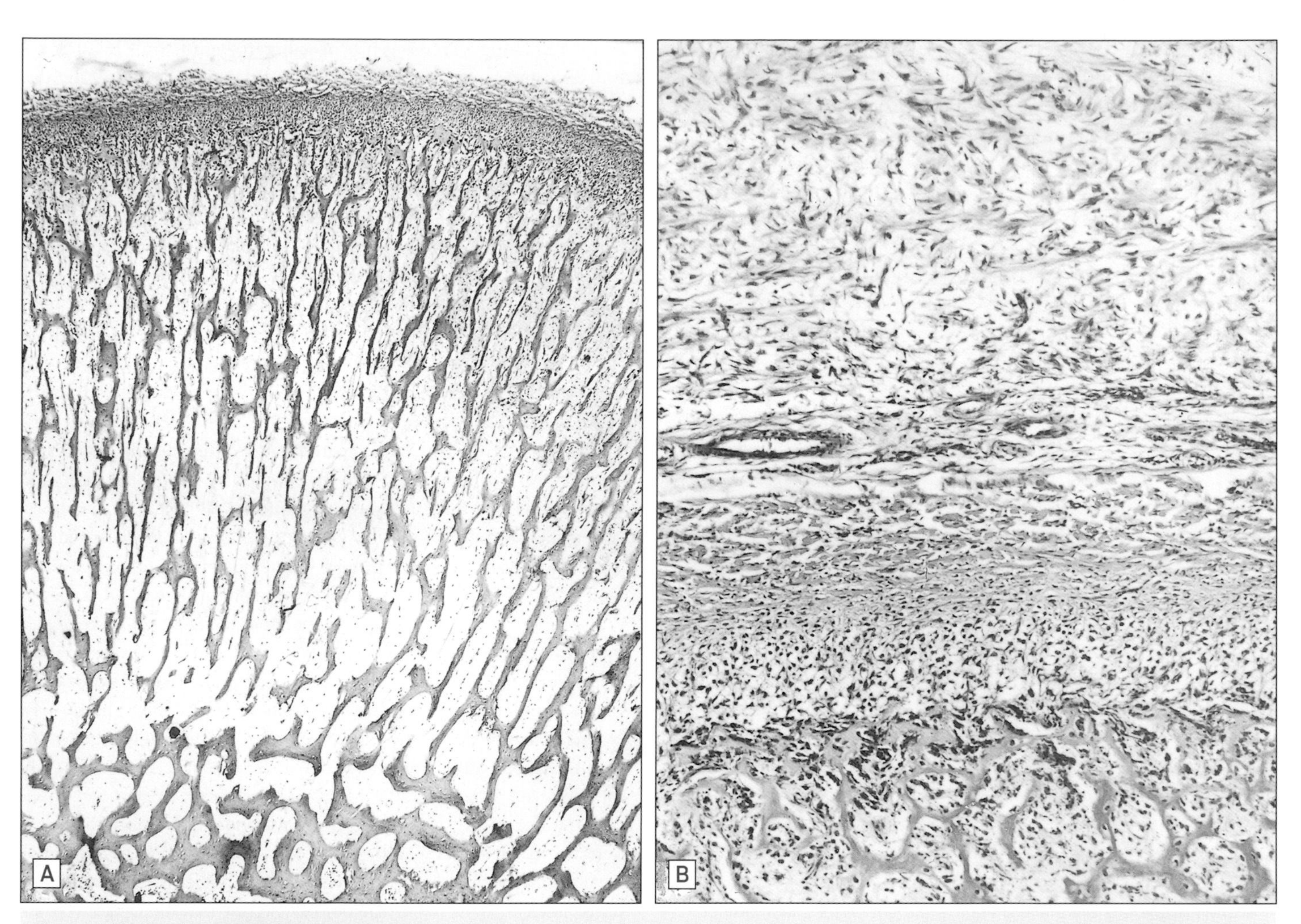

Figure 1.39 Porcine congenital hyperostosis. A. Transverse section of bone showing radiating trabeculae of woven bone extending out from the cortex beneath a thickened periosteum. **B.** Closer view of reactive bone forming at the periosteal surface. The surrounding muscle is edematous, myofibers are atrophic and there are many stellate fibroblasts throughout.

Congenital hyperostosis of pigs is believed to be inherited as an autosomal recessive trait, but this has not been proven. In fact, the disease may not be inherited at all. The pathogenesis is not known, but the periosteal reaction is consistent with prolonged edema caused by a local circulatory disturbance. Arteriosclerotic lesions in small arteries and arterioles have been identified in vessels supplying the radioulnar region in affected piglets, supporting the possibility that the mechanism may involve localized hypertensive changes, perhaps due to abnormal intrauterine positioning of the fetus.

Infantile cortical hyperostosis, or Caffey's disease, is a disease of children, which resembles congenital hyperostosis of pigs. The disease may be congenital but more often develops in infancy and is characterized by extensive periosteal new bone formation at multiple sites, most commonly the mandible, clavicle, and long bones, including those of the forearm. However, the human syndrome is self-limiting and regresses over several years. A hyperostotic disease similar to infantile cortical hyperostosis was reported in a **West Highland White Terrier** dog that had periosteal new bone formation involving the pelvis, scapulae, humeri, ulnae, femora, radii, and tibiae when it was destroyed at 22 months of age.

Osteochondromatosis

Osteochondromatosis, also known as *multiple cartilaginous exostosis*, is a skeletal dysplasia characterized by the formation of single or multiple tumor-like exostoses. In humans, dogs, and horses, the disease is inherited as an *autosomal dominant trait*. In dogs, the lesions usually are not present at birth but arise in young animals on the surface of endochondral bones adjacent to physes or subarticular growth cartilages, and continue to enlarge until the skeleton matures. In affected horses, the lesions are often present at birth and tend to be bilaterally symmetrical. Because of their tumor-like appearance, these lesions are discussed in more detail in the section on cartilage-forming tumors (Tumors and tumor-like lesions of bones, p. 119).

Idiopathic multifocal osteopathy

This syndrome, characterized by *multifocal absence of bone in the skull, cervical vertebrae, and proximal regions of the radius, ulna and femur*, has recently been reported in four **Scottish Terriers**. Three of the four dogs were related, suggesting a genetic etiology. It was not clear whether the disorder was acquired or congenital as the abnormalities were not detected until the dogs were young adults, by which time the lesions were well developed. The localized areas of absent bone were replaced with fibrous tissue but whether this reflects abnormal development of the bone, or lysis of bone and replacement fibrosis, is not clear. Histological evidence of osteolysis was present in one case, supporting the latter option. A similar condition characterized by multicentric bone lysis and replacement fibrosis occurs in humans where it is referred to as *Winchester syndrome or "vanishing bone disease."*

Bibliography

Baker JR. Bone disease in a dog similar to infantile cortical hyperostosis. Vet Rec 1975;97:74–75.

Dickson GR, et al. An investigation of vanishing bone disease. Bone 1990;11:205–210.

Hay CW. Idiopathic multifocal osteopathy in four Scottish Terriers (1991–1996). J Am Animal Hosp Assoc 1999;35:62–67.

Roels S, et al. Localised arteriosclerotic changes in congenital hyperostosis in pigs. Vet Rec 1996;139:446–447.

Snook SS, King NW. Familial infantile cortical hyperostosis (Caffey's disease) in Rhesus monkeys. Vet Pathol 1989;26:274–277.

Localized skeletal dysplasias

Skeletal dysplasias characterized by localized anomalies of the appendicular or axial skeleton are included in this section, together with discussion of the vertebral abnormalities associated with wobbler syndrome in dogs and horses.

Limb dysplasias

The most frequent malformations of the limbs are the localized chondrodysplasias seen in chondrodystrophoid breeds of dog. These are inherited as polygenic traits and are mediated by variations in receptor activities for hormones and other factors that regulate the proliferation of physeal chondrocytes. The defect is usually confined to the distal bones, producing the sort of dwarfism seen in such breeds as the Basset Hound and Dachshund. In some breeds, such as the Pekingese, chondrocytes of neural crest origin are also involved and there are basocranial abnormalities. In other breeds, such as the Boston Terrier and Boxer, only the basocranium is affected, the limbs being of normal length. The cartilage abnormality may also involve the intervertebral disks, the central or perinuclear portions of which develop as immature hyaline cartilage with only a gradual transition at the periphery towards the normal laminated fibrocartilage of the annulus fibrosus. Such disks are predisposed to degeneration of the hyaline cartilage followed by herniation of the disks (see disk degeneration and spondylosis, p. 154).

A wide range of defects of the limbs and/or digits has been reported in domestic animals, often as isolated cases of unknown etiology. Rather than attempt to present a comprehensive list, discussion in this section will focus on those conditions known or suspected to be genetic in origin.

Syndactyly, a defect characterized by *partial or complete fusion of functional digits*, occurs in several breeds of cattle, including Holstein-Friesian, Angus, Chianina, Hereford, Simmental, German Red Pied, Indian Hariana, and Japanese native cattle. Inheritance in cattle is *autosomal recessive with incomplete penetrance and variable expression.* The disorder became very common in the Holstein-Friesian breed following extensive use of a heterozygous bull by artificial breeding, but is rare in other breeds. In Holstein-Friesians, the disorder seldom affects all four digits. The right forelimb is most frequently affected, followed by the left forelimb then the right hindlimb. In contrast, the defect in Angus cattle usually affects all four digits. *The lesions of syndactyly may vary from complete horizontal fusion of paired phalanges to fusion of only one or none of the phalanges, but fusion of interdigital soft tissues.* Vertical fusion of phalanges is reported in some affected Angus cattle. The production of affected calves from Angus-Holstein matings suggests that the same gene locus is involved, at least in these breeds, but differences in the manifestations of syndactyly between affected Angus and Holstein-Friesian calves suggests the existence of two recessive alleles. In the Holstein-Friesian breed, syndactyly is linked to increased susceptibility to hyperthermia and affected cattle often die of heat stress. Syndactyly has been reported in Shorthorn cattle in association with **dactylomegaly**, a form of club foot (talipes). The condition was characterized by various degrees of dew claw enlargement. Syndactyly is also reported in pigs, where it is presumed to be caused by a simple dominant gene, and occasionally in sheep and dogs.

Incomplete fusion of the paw is reported in dogs and cats and referred to as **ectrodactyly**. In cats, a *dominant gene* with variable expressivity is responsible and the defect is bilateral. In dogs, dominant inheritance is likely and the defect is usually unilateral. The cleft in the paw extends to the level of the metacarpals, and occasionally reaches the carpus. Various other limb defects may accompany the ectrodactyly, including aplasia or hypoplasia of carpal and metacarpal bones, duplication of digits, fusion of metacarpals, and elbow joint luxation. Syndromes characterized by total or partial absence of phalanges have been reported as ectrodactyly in calves and lambs. These defects differ from the disease in cats and dogs and may be better termed **adactyly**, a condition characterized by the *absence of phalanges* and reported as a possible inherited defect in Southdown lambs.

Polydactyly *is an increase in the number of digits.* The anomaly is observed in all species but is perhaps best known in *cats, dogs, horses, and cattle.* Polydactyly is an inherited trait in various bovine breeds but the inheritance pattern is poorly understood. In most cases, it is the medial digit (digit 2) that is duplicated and although all four feet may be affected, the anomaly is more frequently confined to the forelimbs. A polygenic mode of inheritance requiring a dominant gene at one locus and two recessive genes at another is postulated in Simmental cattle. In horses, two forms of polydactyly occur. The *common, atavistic type* features an extra medial digit, usually involving a forelimb, which articulates with a second metacarpal. *The rare, teratogenic form* is characterized by duplication of bones distal to the fetlock joint, producing a cloven hoof. In goats, a Shami buck with two extra digits on both hindlegs sired a doe kid with a similar defect, suggesting a genetic etiology. An inherited syndrome of multiple skeletal defects including polydactyly and syndactyly together with cleft palate, shortened tibia, brachygnathism, and scoliosis occurred in a family of Australian Shepherd Dogs. An X-linked lethal gene was suspected. Polydactyly is also reported in pigs where it is usually associated with cleft palate and is believed, but not proven, to be inherited.

Hemimelia *refers to the partial absence of one or more limbs* and occurs as a recessively inherited lethal defect in Galloway calves. Affected calves have bilateral agenesis of the tibial bones and patellae. Other bones of the hindlimbs are apparently normal, highlighting the localized nature of the defect. A similar syndrome characterized by tibial hemimelia, meningocele, retained testicles and abdominal hernia is reported in Shorthorn calves and is also believed to be transmitted as an autosomal recessive trait. Bilateral tibial hypoplasia has been reported in a Simmental calf. A recessively inherited form of hemimelia involving distal forelimbs is reported in Chihuahua dogs. The abnormality may be either transverse, in which case the entire forearm is absent, or paraxial, where there is aplasia of only some metacarpals and digits. Paraxial hemimelia with bilateral agenesis of radial bones is reported in goat kids. In lambs, hemimelia characterized by incomplete development of distal limbs has been reported but in one "outbreak" was most likely due to ingestion of lupin alkaloids by pregnant ewes, rather than a genetic defect.

Peromelia, a term sometimes used synonymously with hemimelia, has been used to describe a syndrome characterized by *agenesis of distal parts of the limbs in Angora goats*. Affected kids lack the phalanges and parts of the metacarpus or metatarsus on one or more limbs. Autosomal recessive inheritance is suspected. In isolated cases where the distal limb is absent, it is important to exclude the possibility that the missing component was accidentally ingested by the dam when she was eating the placenta. This is most likely to occur in goats. *Congenital absence of one or more limbs*, **amelia**, has been reported in a foal and a calf.

Skull

Brachygnathia inferior, *shortening of the mandibles*, and **brachygnathia superior**, *shortening of the maxillae*, may occur alone or in combination with other skeletal defects. Brachygnathia inferior is commonly encountered in otherwise normal domestic animals and, while not life-threatening, is considered an undesirable characteristic. Genetic and teratogenic etiologies have been suggested and both are likely to occur. Brachygnathia superior occurs in association with degenerative joint disease as a lethal genetic defect in Angus calves. In addition to brachygnathia superior, affected calves have other skull changes similar to those of brachycephalic dogs and degenerative changes are present in articular cartilage throughout the body. The nature of the underlying defect is not known, but histologically there is degeneration of cartilage matrix and necrosis of chondrocytes in articular cartilage.

Sternum

Lateral curvature of the sternum occurs in association with vertebral scoliosis, especially when the latter shows simultaneous torsion. *Retraction of the caudal sternebrae and xiphoid* is seen in lambs and calves, and is apparently due to shortness of the tendinous portions of the diaphragm. *Clefts of the sternum* may occur as isolated defects, but are usually accompanied by ectopia cordis or form part of the defect known as *schistosomus reflexus*. In this syndrome, there is lordosis, dorsal reflection of the ribs with more-or-less total eventration, nonunion of the pelvic symphysis and dorsal reflection of the pelvic bones. *Sternal deformity* also occurs in "spider lamb" chondrodysplasia.

Ribs

Costal abnormalities are usually secondary to malformation of the vertebral column or sternum. Absent or fused ribs correspond to absent or fused vertebrae and may accompany severe scoliosis.

Pelvis

Lesions of the lumbosacral region, arising from abnormalities of the notochord failing to give rise to appropriate dermatomes, occur in humans and lead to various abnormalities often collectively termed the **caudal regression syndrome**. Abnormalities of this derivation result in lumbosacral agenesis, as seen in English bulldogs, but often are accompanied by anorectal abnormalities, urogenital anomalies, various anomalies of the spinal cord, and in humans the development of a variety of tumors and cysts. These include yolk sac cysts, cysts of urogenital origin, lipomas, teratomas, and nephroblastomas. The sacrum may be absent, or it may be hypoplastic or deviated in association with absence of the coccygeal vertebrae. Hypoplastic chondrodysplasia of the coccygeal vertebrae is a characteristic of French bulldogs and occurs occasionally, with kinking of the remnants, in cattle and cats. Malformations of the sacrum accompany other severe spinal defects. The pubic bones are separated and may be absent, in association with ectropion of the bladder.

Bibliography

Al-Ani FK, et al. Polydactyly in Shami breed goats in Jordan. Small Rum Res 1997;26:177–179.

Alonso RA, et al. An autosomal recessive form of hemimelia in dogs. Vet Rec 1982;110: 128–129.

Baum KH, et al. Radial agenesis and ulnar hypoplasia in two caprine kids. J Am Vet Med Assoc 1985;186:170–171.

Braund KG, et al. Morphological studies of the canine intervertebral disk. The assignment of the Beagle to the chondroplastic classification. Res Vet Sci 1975;19:167–172.

Chapman VA, Zeiner FN. The anatomy of polydactylism in cats with observations on genetic control. Anat Rec 1961;141:205–217.

DeBowes RM, Leipold HW. Anterior amelia. J Equine Vet Sci 1984;4:133–135.

Doige CE, et al. Tibial hypoplasia in a calf. Can Vet J 1978;19:230–233.

Dore MAP. Teratogenic polydactyly in a halfbred foal. Vet Rec 1989;125:375–376.

Feuston MH, Scott WJ. Cadmium-induced forelimb ectrodactyly: A proposed mechanism of teratogenesis. Teratology 1985;32:407–419.

Gruneberg H, Huston K. The development of bovine syndactylism. J Embryol Exp Morph 1965;19:251–259.

Hawkins CD, et al. Hemimelia and low marking percentage in a flock of Merino ewes and lambs. Aust Vet J 1983;60:22–24.

Hawkins CD, Grandage J. Dactylomegaly, a type of club foot (talipes) in a herd of Shorthorn cattle. Aust Vet J 1983;60:55–56.

Hiraga T, et al. Anatomical findings of apodia in a calf. J Vet Med Sci 1991;53:1125–1127.

Hughes EH. Polydactyly in swine. J Hered 1935;26:415–418.

Huston K, Wearden S. Congenital taillessness in cattle. J Dairy Sci 1958;41:1359–1370.

Jayo M, et al. Brachygnathia superior and degenerative joint disease: a new lethal syndrome in Angus calves. Vet Pathol 1987;24:148–155.

Johnson JL, et al. Characterization of bovine polydactyly. Bovine Pract 1982;3:7–14.

Lapointe J-M, et al. Tibial hemimelia, meningocele and abdominal hernia in Shorthorn cattle. Vet Pathol 2000;37:508–511.

Leipold HW, et al. Ectrodactyly in two beef calves. Am J Vet Res 1969;30:1689–1692.

Leipold HW, et al. Adactylia in Southdown lambs. J Am Vet Med Assoc 1972;160: 1002–1003.

Leipold HW, et al. Hereditary syndactyly in Angus cattle. J Vet Diagn Invest 1998;10:247–254.

Lewis RE, Van Sickle DC. Congenital hemimelia (agenesis) of the radius in a dog and a cat. J Am Vet Med Assoc 1970;156:1892–1897.

Martig J, et al. Deforming ankylosis of the coffin joint in calves. Vet Rec 1972;91:307–310.
Modransky P, et al. Unilateral phalangeal dysgenesis and navicular bone agenesis in a foal. Equine Vet J 1987;19:347–349.
Montgomery M, Tomlinson J. Two cases of ectrodactyly and congenital elbow luxation in the dog. J Am Anim Hosp Assoc 1985;21:781–785.
Nordby JE, et al. The etiology and inheritance of inequalities in the jaws of sheep. Anat Rec 1945;92:235–254.
Ojo SA, et al. Tibial hemimelia in Galloway calves. J Am Vet Med Assoc 1974;165:548–550.
Ojo SA, et al. Syndactyly in Holstein-Friesian, Hereford, and crossbred Chianina cattle. J Am Vet Med Assoc 1975;166:607–609.
Stanek C, Hantak E. Bilateral atavistic polydactyly in a colt and its dam. Equine Vet J 1986;18: 76–79.
Vaughan LC, France C. Abnormalities of the volar and plantar sesamoid bones in Rottweilers. J Small Anim Pract 1986;27:551–558.

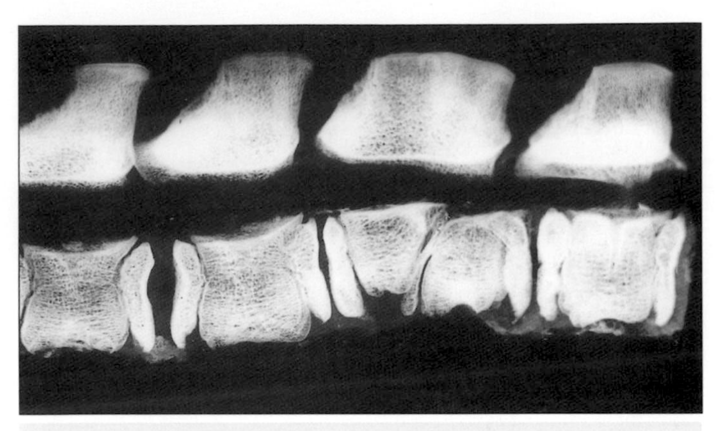

Figure 1.40 Block vertebra. Two vertebral bodies are incompletely separated and their dorsal processes are fused.

Vertebrae

The development of the vertebrae and intervertebral disks is a complex process involving interactions between ectodermal and mesodermal elements. Defects can arise from errors at many stages of development and, because of the proximity of the spinal cord, the consequences are often serious. **Spina bifida** *results from defective closure of dorsal vertebral laminae in a segment of the vertebral column*. It has been reported in several different breeds of cattle and there is some evidence to support autosomal recessive inheritance. Teratogenic agents acting early in pregnancy can no doubt produce similar lesions. The lesions vary markedly in severity and are often accompanied by defects in the overlying skin, meningocele, and sometimes myelodysplasia. The defect may occur at virtually any level of the vertebral column but appears to favor the lumbar and sacral regions. Various nonskeletal defects have been described in association with spina bifida, including arthrogryposis, due to spinal damage and defective innervation of some muscle groups, fusion of the kidneys, unilateral aplasia of one uterine horn, atresia ani, and kyphoscoliosis.

Perosomus elumbus, a rare congenital defect characterized by *agenesis of the lumbosacral spinal cord and vertebrae*, is reported in cattle, sheep, and pigs. In two affected Hereford calves, the spinal column terminated at the last thoracic vertebra. Both calves had arthrogryposis of the hindlimbs and one also had other skeletal defects, including absence of some ribs, unilateral agenesis of the scapula and humerus, and polydactyly involving one leg. The absence of the lumbar spinal cord in affected cattle is associated with extreme muscle atrophy and replacement with adipose tissue. In an affected stillborn Holstein heifer calf, the skeletal abnormalities were accompanied by anomalies in the urogenital system and distal colon/rectum. It has been suggested, but not proven, that perosomus elumbus in Holstein cattle is inherited.

Block vertebra *results from improper segmentation of the somites in the embryo, resulting in complete or partial fusion of adjacent vertebrae* (Fig. 1.40). The fused structure may be equal to or shorter than the pair of vertebrae it replaces. There are usually no clinical signs. **Butterfly vertebrae** are so called because of the *appearance of the indented vertebral end plates on ventrodorsal radiographs*. The cause is *persistence of notochord*, or a sagittal cleft of notochord, that leads to a dorsoventral, sagittal cleft in the vertebral body. The halves may spread laterally but the condition is usually an incidental radiographic finding in screw-tailed dogs such as Bulldogs, Pugs, and Boston Terriers. **Hemivertebrae** may arise as a result of displacement and inappropriate fusion of somites. In this case, *one member of a pair of somites fuses diagonally with a somite cranial or caudal to it*, forming a vertebra but leaving the other members of the pairs to persist as hemivertebrae.

Complex vertebral malformation is a lethal congenital defect of Holstein calves characterized by shortening of the cervical and thoracic vertebral column due to multiple hemivertebrae, fused and misshapen vertebrae, and scoliosis. Affected calves are smaller than normal, sometimes born premature, and consistently show symmetrical arthrogryposis of the forelimbs. The hindlimbs may also show mild arthrogryposis. Approximately 50% have heart malformations, including ventricular septal defects and dextraposition of the aorta. A genetic etiology is suspected. Two common ancestral sires were identified in the pedigrees of 18 affected calves in Denmark and it is suggested that one is a carrier. Both are former elite sires of US origin and it is possible therefore that the defect is present in several countries. There is one recent report of the syndrome in the USA.

Subluxations, fusions, and other anomalies of cervical vertebrae are described with developmental disturbances of joints.

Cervical vertebral stenotic myelopathy (wobbler syndrome)

Cervical vertebral stenotic myelopathy (cervical vertebral malformation, cervicospinal arthropathy, wobbler syndrome) is a neurological disease characterized by slow, progressive, ataxia of the hindlimbs, and occasionally the forelimbs, due to compression or stretching of the spinal cord as a result of a primary abnormality in the vertebral column. The syndrome occurs most commonly in horses and large breeds of dog, particularly Great Danes and Doberman Pinschers. In both species, male animals are affected much more often than females, and rapid growth is an apparent predisposing factor. The vertebral lesions reported in horses and dogs with the disease are similar, suggesting a common pathogenesis. In both species there are two pathologic syndromes, *cervical vertebral instability* and *cervical static stenosis*, the former damaging the cord only when the neck is extended or flexed, the latter resulting in cord compression no matter what position the neck is in. Usually the onset is insidious, but vague signs are often exacerbated following trauma or strenuous activity. The disease in

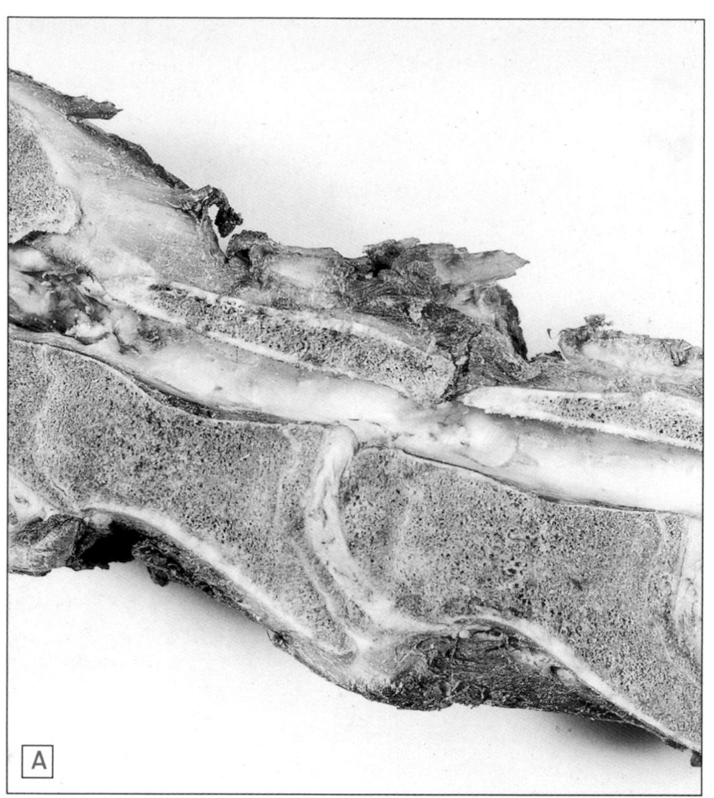

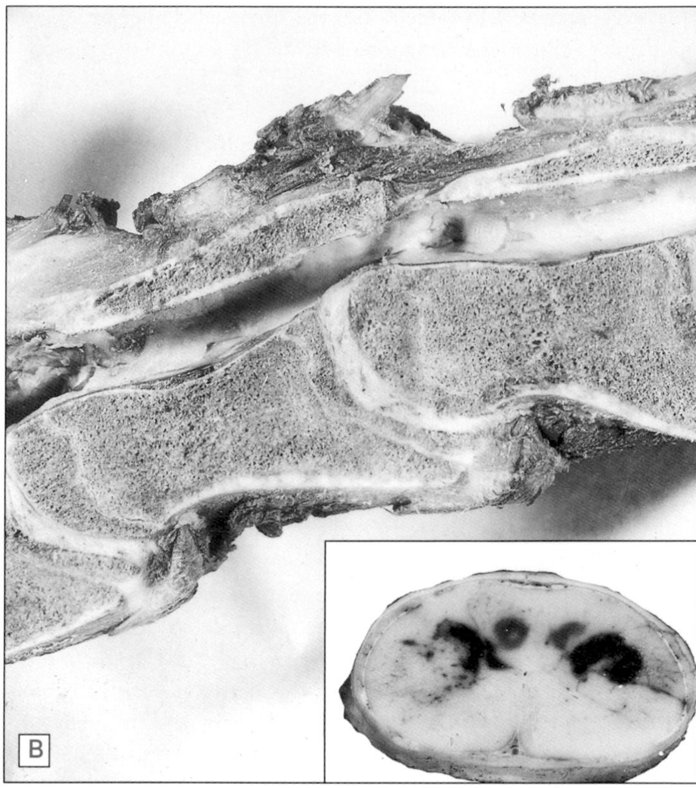

Figure 1.41 Cervical vertebral stenotic myelopathy. C-3 and C-4 from a "wobbler" horse. **A.** Neck extended. **B.** Neck ventroflexed to show stenosis of the spinal canal. Malacia of cervical cord is illustrated in the inset.

horses is not progressive, but if the signs are severe, recovery does not occur.

In **horses**, cervical vertebral stenotic myelopathy occurs most often in *Thoroughbreds* and *Quarter Horses*. **Cervical vertebral instability** usually affects fast growing young horses 8–18 months of age and is associated with lesions in the region of C-3 to C-5. The lesions vary and are not always easy to detect at necropsy, especially since the problem may only be apparent when the neck is ventroflexed (Fig. 1.41A, B). In a few cases, a lip may be palpated on the dorsal border of the vertebral body, apparently due to expansion of the cranial epiphysis. More often, a distinct lip is not palpable, but a mid-sagittal section of affected vertebrae shows that the floor of the spinal canal angles upwards and the roof angles downwards to produce a funnel-shaped canal with cranial stenosis. Occasionally, the cranial articular processes of the vertebral bodies project in a ventro-medial direction and impinge upon the spinal canal, compressing the dorsolateral parts of the cord. In a small proportion of cases, increased mobility of adjacent cervical vertebrae, which allows subluxation is apparently responsible for the cord compression. Although the lesions in cervical vertebral instability occur most often at C-3 to C-5, other vertebrae may also be affected, and more than one lesion may be present in a single animal.

Articular facets of vertebrae in horses with cervical vertebral instability often contain lesions typical of the degenerative arthropathy that follows osteochondrosis (see below). These lesions may be accompanied by osteophytic outgrowths at the articular margin, altering the size and shape of the facet and occasionally encroaching on the spinal canal. Similar changes can however be found in many clinically normal horses and their presence in a wobbler must be interpreted with caution. Asymmetry of articular facets is also present in many affected horses (Fig. 1.42), but this too is of questionable significance, since many clinically normal horses have similar changes. In some affected horses, there is also evidence for osteochondrosis affecting vertebral growth plates in the cervical

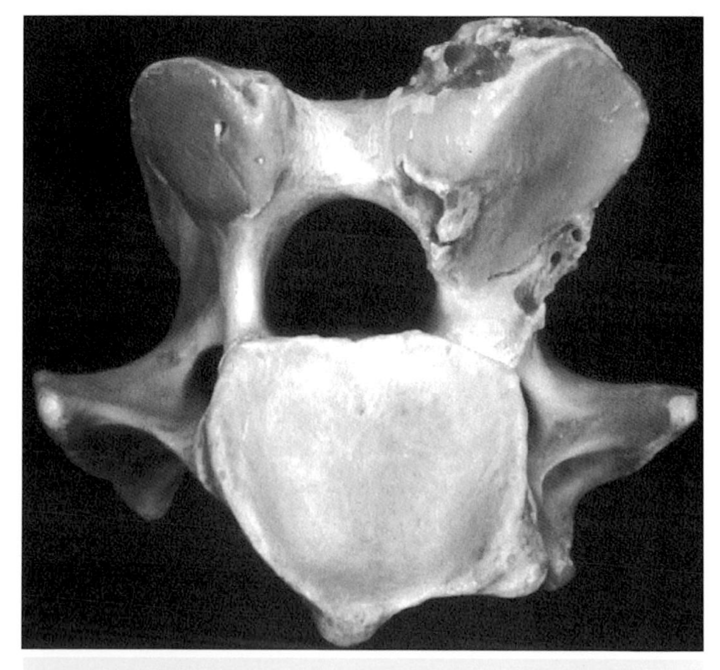

Figure 1.42 Asymmetry of articular facets in a "wobbler" horse. (Courtesy of JD Baird.)

region. Nonetheless, in some horses the spinal cord injury is likely to be due to vertebral malalignment created by asymmetry of articular facets.

The fundamental cause of cervical vertebral instability in horses is not clear. There is growing evidence that the multiple genetic factors that permit rapid growth, and the dietary excesses that encourage it, are responsible. In particular, the *ad libitum feeding of high-protein, high-energy rations to weanlings to produce maximum-sized yearlings seems to be the major influence.* Such feeding practices are commonly associated with osteochondrosis and many affected horses have lesions of this disease, but the significance of this to the overall incidence of cervical vertebral instability is presently undetermined.

Cervical static stenosis, the second, less common form of cervical vertebral stenotic myelopathy, usually occurs in large male horses between 1 and 4 years of age and is caused primarily by *thickening of the ligamentum flavum and the dorsal lamina of the vertebral arches.* The spinal cord is compressed by the encroachment of these structures on the spinal canal. Histologically, there is increased fibrocartilage at the attachment of the ligamentum flavum to the dorsal lamina, and deposition of fibrovascular tissue both in the ligamentum and the contiguous joint capsule. The thickening of the dorsal lamina is due to osteosclerosis, with the dense trabeculae being formed by compaction of the fibrocartilage of the ligamentum flavum. Degenerative arthropathy of articular facets is usually present and, although its severity is not correlated with the severity of signs, it may be the result of a primary vertebral instability that also subjects the ligaments and laminae to abnormal mechanical forces. The osteosclerosis and development of fibrocartilage are consistent with increased forces and joint movement. Compression of the spinal cord by synovial cysts has also been reported.

In the final analysis, *interpretation of osseous lesions depends on their linkage with spinal cord degeneration.* There is variation in the suddenness and the severity of cord injury, and in the immediate pathogenesis of injury, which may occur directly by pressure on the nervous tissues, or indirectly if local blood vessels are compromised. Thus, there may be one or more primary foci of softening in the cervical cord with Wallerian degeneration of the ascending and descending tracts. Careful examination of the cord, with the dura mater reflected, sometimes reveals a slight depression in the contour of the nervous tissue at the affected site. Sometimes, the primary foci of malacia are visible after fixation as brown areas in the gray matter, usually adjacent to an articulation (Fig. 1.41B). The fixed cord should be sliced at intervals of no more than 2 mm, otherwise a lesion may be missed. Histologic examination is necessary to confirm and demonstrate lesions.

Microscopically, there is more-or-less extensive demyelination in the cord. In severe cases with gross lesions, hemorrhagic and necrotic foci can be found in the gray matter in either the ventral or lateral horns, and may be either unilateral or bilateral. Even when lesions are absent from the gray matter, the primary focus or foci are visible in short segments of the white matter, which shows the moth-eaten appearance typical of demyelination. In the primary foci there are ragged microcavitations, which represent areas of liquefactive necrosis. Many adjacent degenerate fibers are swollen and basophilic. About the primary focus, demyelination may be present in all tracts while *cranial to the focus, the lesions can be seen in ascending fibers, most of which are in the dorsolateral funiculi. Caudal to the focus the demyelination is primarily in the ventral and ventrolateral funiculi*, symmetrical on either side of the ventromedian fissure, and extending as far as the lumbar region in some animals. As a consequence of localized edema, often there is striking astrocytosis in chronic lesions and cells are increased both in number and size, becoming gemistocytic in type.

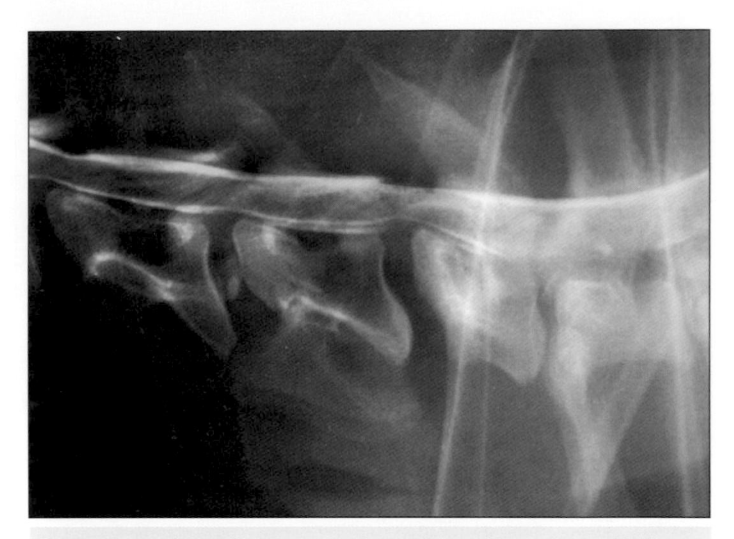

Figure 1.43 Caudal cervical spondylomyelopathy in a Doberman Pinscher. Myelogram showing compression of the spinal cord at the cranial opening of C-7. The body of this vertebra is malformed. (Courtesy of HM Burbidge.)

There are many similarities between cervical vertebral stenotic myelopathy in **dogs** and the disease in horses. The *age of onset varies from a few weeks to several years* although, in general, Great Danes develop signs at an earlier age than Dobermans. There is mounting evidence for an *inherited predisposition*, although overnutrition and abnormal biomechanical forces involving cervical vertebrae have also been suggested as contributing factors. *A variety of anatomical or functional abnormalities have been described in affected dogs, usually in the region of C-6 to C-7.* Malformation of vertebrae, including stenosis of the cranial opening (Fig. 1.43), degeneration and asymmetry of articular facets, and misshapen vertebral bodies caused by early closure of the dorsal part of the caudal physis with elongation of the ventral part of the body, are detected in some affected dogs. Instability of cervical vertebrae, particularly of those that are misshapen, is also reported but is difficult to assess objectively. There is no doubt that some cases of wobbler syndrome in dogs are caused by alterations in the supporting ligaments rather than the vertebrae. In one study, the most common cause of spinal cord compression in dogs was considered to be hyperplasia of the ligamentum flavum with protrusion into the spinal canal. Compression of the cord by the bulging ligament is greatest when the neck is extended and is relieved when the neck undergoes traction or full flexion.

Stenosis of the cervical vertebral canal also occurs in **sheep** and although little is known about the syndrome in this species, it is probably linked to heavy feeding and perhaps the trauma associated with fighting.

Bibliography

Agerholm JS, et al. Complex vertebral malformation in Holstein calves. J Vet Diagn Invest 2001;13:283–289.

Agerhom JS, et al. Morphological variation of "complex vertebral malformation" in Holstein calves. J Vet Diagn Invest 2004;16:548–553.

Bailey CS. An embryological approach to the clinical significance of congenital vertebral and spinal cord abnormalities. J Am Anim Hosp Assoc 1975;11:426–434.
Burbidge HM. A review of wobbler syndrome in the Doberman Pinscher. Aust Vet Pract 1995;25:147–156.
Dennis SM. Perosomus elumbis in sheep. Aust Vet J 1975;51:135–136.
Doige CE. Spina bifida in a calf. Can Vet J 1975;16:22–25.
Fisher LF, et al. Spinal ataxia in a horse caused by a synovial cyst. Vet Pathol 1981;18:407–410.
Jones CJ. Perosomus elumbis (vertebral agenesis and arthrogryposis) in a stillborn Holstein calf. Vet Pathol 1999;36:64–70.
Lewis DG. Cervical spondylomyelopathy ("wobbler" syndrome) in the dog: A study based on 224 cases. J Small Anim Pract 1989;30:657–665.
McFarland LZ. Spina bifida with myelomeningocele in a calf. J Am Vet Med Assoc 1959;134: 32–34.
Olsson S-E, et al. Dynamic compression of the cervical spinal cord. A myelographic and pathologic investigation in Great Dane dogs. Acta Vet Scand 1982;23: 65–78.
Palmer AC, et al. Stenosis of the cervical vertebral canal in a yearling ram. Vet Rec 1981;109:53–55.
Powers BE, et al. Pathology of the vertebral column of horses with cervical static stenosis. Vet Pathol 1986;23:392–399.
Stewart RH, et al. Frequency and severity of osteochondrosis in horses with cervical stenotic myelopathy. Am J Vet Res 1991;52:873–879.
Tarvin G, Prata RG. Lumbosacral stenosis in dogs. J Am Vet Med Assoc 1977;177:154–159.

GENETIC DISEASES INDIRECTLY AFFECTING THE SKELETON

Lysosomal storage diseases

The lysosomal storage diseases are a large group of inherited or acquired deficiencies in the activity of specific lysosomal enzymes, culminating in the accumulation of otherwise digestible substrates in the lysosomal system of various cell types. Although many such diseases have been reported in domestic animals, only the mucopolysaccharidoses and the gangliosidoses affect the skeleton. In both groups of diseases there are lesions of greater significance in other organ systems, particularly the central nervous system (see Vol. 1, Nervous system).

The **mucopolysaccharidoses** (MPS) are characterized by the *accumulation of partially catabolized glycosaminoglycans in lysosomes* and, in human medicine, are classified on the basis of the specific enzyme defect and clinical phenotype as MPS I through MPS VII (with several subgroups):

- **MPS I** (Hurler's syndrome), caused by a deficiency of α-L-iduronidase,
- **MPS VI** (Maroteaux-Lamy syndrome), caused by arylsulfatase-B deficiency, and
- **MPS VII**, caused by β-glucuronidase deficiency.

All three have all been associated with skeletal deformities in **cats**.

MPS VI occurs in Siamese cats where it is inherited as an autosomal recessive trait. By 2 months of age the typical features of the syndrome, including broad flattened face, small ears, diffuse corneal clouding, large forepaws, and pectus excavatum are evident. Radiographic lesions are present in the axial and distal skeleton by 6 months of age and are progressive. Most affected cats have symmetrical epiphyseal dysplasia, short stature, and develop degenerative joint disease. Thoracic vertebral bodies are short and there are fusions of cervical and lumbar vertebrae, absence or dysplasia of cervical and thoracic vertebral spinous processes, and increased width of intervertebral spaces. The ribs broaden at the costochondral junctions. In older animals, the epiphyses and metaphyses of long bones are distorted by bony proliferation, and articular surfaces are irregular. Some animals develop posterior ataxia and paresis at less than a year of age due to compression of the spinal cord by osteophytes, which project into the vertebral canal between T-12 and L-2. Affected kittens can be recognized at 1 week of age by their excessive concentrations of urinary dermatan sulfate. Metachromatic granules are present in the cytoplasm of circulating neutrophils. *Microscopic abnormalities in the skeleton are centered on articular and physeal cartilage.* Growth plates have poorly organized proliferative zones, lack of column formation in hypertrophic zones, disorganized zones of mineralization, and uneven chondro–osseous junctions. Chondrocytes are swollen with abundant, finely vacuolated cytoplasm. Osteoclast numbers in the primary spongiosa are reduced. Membrane-bound cytoplasmic inclusions are present in hepatocytes, bone marrow granulocytes, vascular smooth muscle cells and fibroblasts of the skin, heart valves, and cornea. This disease of cats closely resembles MPS VI of human patients.

Feline MPS I is reported in domestic shorthaired cats and most likely has an autosomal recessive mode of inheritance. The bony lesions in this disease are milder than those of MPS VI and are not accompanied by epiphyseal dysplasia of long bones. Nor are there metachromatic granules in circulating neutrophils. Although the number of cases is small, cats with MPS I appear to have a high incidence of meningiomas. Only *isolated cases of MPS VII* are reported in domestic shorthaired cats but the skeletal lesions are severe and resemble those of MPS VI.

MPS I also occurs in **Plott Hounds**, probably as an autosomal recessive trait. Affected dogs are stunted and develop progressive lameness in addition to diffuse, bilateral corneal opacity. A feature of the canine disease is the development of *severe degenerative joint disease* with extensive periarticular bone proliferation. Cytologic evaluation of synovial fluid may reveal mononuclear and multinucleated cells containing abundant basophilic granules (on Wright-Giemsa stain). Allogeneic bone marrow transplantation of irradiated dogs reduces the neurovisceral lesions of MPS I but the effect is minimal in chondrocytes, except those near the articular surface.

GM_1 gangliosidosis *occurs in cats, calves, sheep, and dogs, and is due to a deficiency of beta-galactosidase.* In sheep, there is a concomitant deficiency of α-neuraminidase. In dogs, skeletal lesions are present in **English Springer Spaniels** but in the Beagle, only the neurovisceral changes are present. Also, the stored undegraded oligosaccharides differ between the two breeds. In both breeds, the trait is autosomal recessive. Affected Springers develop neurologic signs at 4–6 months. Skeletal lesions may include proportional dwarfism with frontal bossing and hypertelorism, irregular intervertebral spaces, and degenerative changes in the femoral and tibial articular cartilages.

A storage-like disease with visceral and skeletal (but not neural) involvement occurred in a **Rhodesian Ridgeback dog**. The dog was lame from an early age and showed multiple osteolytic lesions in radiographs of long bones and vertebrae. Osteoarthritic changes, especially in the elbow, hip, and stifle, were accompanied by marked enlargement of acetabular and olecranon fossae. The liver, lymph nodes, and synovial villi were enlarged due to accumulation of cells with abundant vacuolated cytoplasm. Similar cells were seen in endocrine glands and vertebrae. The stored material, which appeared to be confined to the monocyte–macrophage system and synovial lining cells, was not identified but was variably oil red O-positive.

Congenital erythropoietic porphyria

Red-brown discoloration of the teeth and bones, caused by a recessively inherited defect in porphyrin metabolism, is reported in several breeds of cattle, including Hereford, Holstein, Ayrshire, Shorthorn, and Jamaica Red and Black. A deficiency of uroporphyrin III cosynthetase leads to the accumulation of uroporphyrin I and coproporphyrin I in blood, bone, and a variety of other tissues. The urine may also be red-brown or turn red on exposure to sunlight. The action of sunlight on porphyrins accumulated in the skin results in photodynamic dermatitis. The teeth, bones, and urine of affected animals show bright cherry-red fluorescence on exposure to ultraviolet light in a darkened room. Congenital erythropoietic protoporphyria in Limousin cattle, caused by a deficiency of the mitochondrial enzyme ferrochelatase, is associated with photosensitivity but no discoloration of the bones or teeth.

Inherited forms of porphyria associated with discoloration of the bones and teeth have been reported in cats and Duroc pigs, but the enzyme defect is unknown.

Acquired porphyria with pink discoloration of bones was recognized at slaughter in approximately 300 of 390 *crossbred lambs in Australia*. Similar "outbreaks" have also occurred in lambs and young deer in New Zealand. The discoloration was most prominent in the cortex of long bones and fluoresced on exposure to ultraviolet light, but teeth were not affected. On cut surfaces of long bones in a sample of affected lambs and deer, the pink discoloration was confined to areas of bone that had formed in the weeks prior to death, in particular the outer cortex. This reflects the fact that *porphyrins are only deposited at sites of active mineralization.* In congenital porphyria, the constant availability of porphyrins during dental and skeletal mineralization results in diffuse discoloration of all mineralized tissues. The extraction of coproporphyrin and protoporphyrin from the bones of lambs in the Australian outbreak suggested an enzyme block towards the end of the heme synthetic pathway, most likely induced by a toxin. Although lead toxicity can induce porphyrin accumulation, no lead was detected in affected lambs. Toxicity caused by some chlorinated hydrocarbons can also result in impaired heme synthesis and the detection of 1,2,4-trichlorobenzene in fat samples supported this possibility in the lambs. This compound is a *major metabolite of lindane*, an organochlorine insecticide that was widely used in parts of Australia and New Zealand before being banned. The occurrence of acquired porphyria in grazing animals may therefore reflect environmental contamination due to leakage from chemical dumpsites.

Bibliography

Abreu S, et al. Growth plate pathology in feline mucopolysaccharidosis VI. Calcif Tiss Int 1995;57:185–190.

Alroy J, et al. Neurovisceral and skeletal GM_1-gangliosidosis in dogs with β-galactosidase deficiency. Science 1985;229:470–472.

Breider MA, et al. Long-term effects of bone marrow transplantation in dogs with mucopolysaccharidosis I. Am J Pathol 1989;134:677–692.

Haskins ME, McGrath JT. Meningiomas in young cats with mucopolysaccharidosis I. J Neuropath Exp Neurol 1983;42:664–670.

Nichol AW, et al. Porphyrin accumulation in sheep bones associated with 1,2,4-trichlorobenzene. Bull Environm Contam 1981;27:72–78.

Schultheiss PC, et al. Mucoploysaccharidosis VII in a cat. Vet Pathol 2000;37:502–505.

Scott DW, et al. Dermatohistopathologic changes in bovine congenital porphyria. Cornell Vet 1979;69:145–158.

Shull RM, et al. Canine α-L-iduronidase deficiency. A model of mucopolysaccharidosis I. Am J Pathol 1982;109:244–248.

Yamashita C, et al. Congenital porphyria in swine. Jap J Vet Sci 1980;42:353–360.

ACQUIRED ABNORMALITIES IN SKELETAL GROWTH, DEVELOPMENT, AND REMODELING

Bone growth and maturation is a complex process, requiring an interaction between genetic factors, local and systemic hormones, dietary nutrients, and mechanical forces. Anything that interferes with the synthesis of proteoglycans or collagen by chondroblasts or osteoblasts, the differentiation of precursor cells, or the resorption of bone by osteoclasts can result in a skeletal abnormality. The expression of an abnormality depends on many factors, including the phase of skeletal development that is altered, the severity of the defect, the age of the animal at the time of the insult, and how long it persists. As a result, the range of possible skeletal defects is huge, and a single etiology may vary considerably in its manifestations.

An accurate etiological diagnosis is not always possible in an animal with a skeletal defect, particularly since the inciting cause is often no longer present at the time of examination. In many cases the pathologist is presented with lesions reflecting an insult that occurred several weeks or months earlier and can only speculate as to its cause. It may not even be possible to determine with confidence whether a defect is genetic or acquired. Such decisions should not be taken lightly as they can greatly influence the actions of the owner, sometimes leading to unnecessary culling of related animals, resulting in considerable wastage of valuable breeding stock. *Many teratogenic agents have been shown to mimic genetic diseases of the skeleton and other organ systems*, and unless there is clear evidence that the problem is inherited, or it resembles an established genetic disorder, any temptation to attribute a genetic etiology should be resisted.

The term "*developmental orthopedic disease*" has been used to encompass a complex and important group of skeletal problems in horses, including osteochondrosis, subchondral cystic lesions, physeal dysplasia, wobbler syndrome, acquired angular limb deformities, flexural deformities, and cuboidal bone deformities. These disorders are associated with abnormalities in endochondral ossification at either the articular/epiphyseal cartilage complex or the growth plate of developing bones, but their etiology and pathogenesis are obscure. Although a genetic component is suspected, at least in some of these conditions, most appear to have a multifactorial etiology that includes nutritional and biomechanical factors. Rather than discuss the developmental orthopedic diseases as a group they will be included as separate entities in this chapter, reflecting the fact that although some of them may be different manifestations of the same underlying problem, their clinical and pathological presentation varies. Although osteochondrosis is a disorder of endochondral ossification, its clinical and pathological

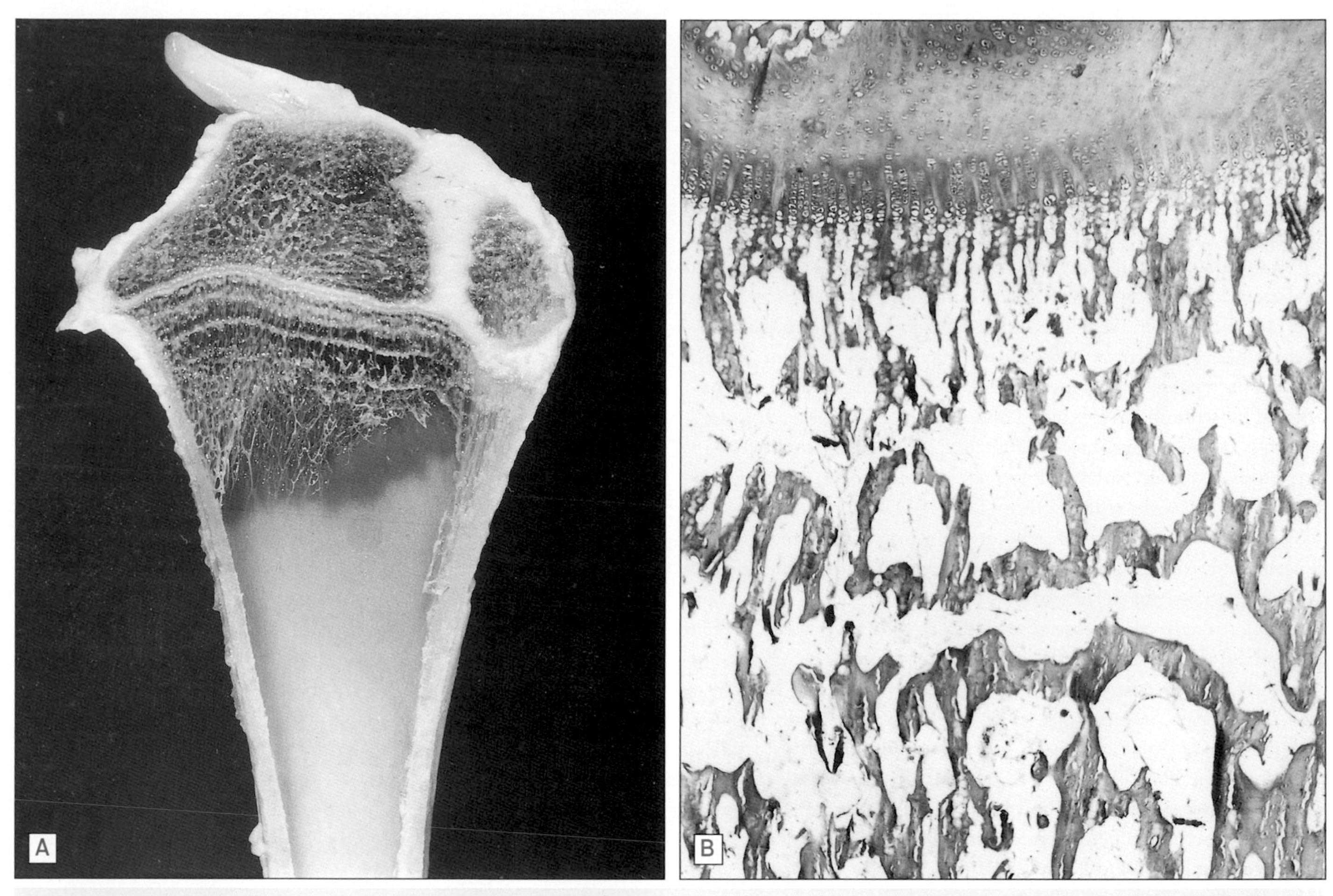

Figure 1.44 Growth arrest lines A. Proximal tibia from a lamb with osteoporosis. Several growth arrest lines are parallel to the physis. **B.** Microscopic section showing the **transverse trabeculae** that form during periods of growth arrest. These are left behind in the metaphysis once growth at the physis

manifestations in most species relate principally to its effect on joints, and is therefore included in a later section (Developmental diseases of joints).

Nutritional imbalances and toxins affecting skeletal growth

Bone development by endochondral ossification is sensitive to quantitative and qualitative alterations in nutrition, both in fetal and postnatal life. *Malnutrition or starvation*, if severe enough, will retard longitudinal bone growth, resulting in narrow growth plates that may become sealed by a horizontal plate of bone on the metaphyseal side. If the nutritional abnormality is corrected, physeal growth will resume and the plate of bone will be displaced into the metaphysis, persisting for some time as a radiographically and grossly visible **growth arrest line**, parallel to the growth plate. The presence of several parallel lines of transverse trabeculae (Fig. 1.44A, B) indicates recurrent episodes of retarded growth. Growth arrest lines are often accompanied by osteoporosis due to reduced bone formation and increased resorption in response to starvation, and the contents of the marrow cavity may be gelatinous due to serous atrophy of medullary adipose tissue. *Growth arrest lines may be detected in fetuses*, in which case they imply either defective maternal nutrition or retarded fetal development due to some other cause, such as intrauterine infection. Similar, but less well-defined lines in the metaphysis also occur in fetuses and in postnatal animals in association with certain infectious or toxic agents that interfere with osteoclastic resorption of the primary or secondary spongiosa and must be differentiated from growth arrest lines. These bands of metaphyseal sclerosis are discussed later in this section.

Overnutrition, in particular chronic excess of dietary calcium, in rapidly growing young dogs of large breeds, has been linked to a range of skeletal disorders, including osteochondrosis, metaphyseal osteopathy, and hip dysplasia. It is proposed that hypercalcitoninism, secondary to persistent stimulation by gastrointestinal hormones and post-prandial elevations in plasma calcium concentration, causes impaired osteoclastic activity and defective bone remodeling. The possibility that this may impair the development of bony foramina and predispose to conditions such as wobbler syndrome and eosinophilic panosteitis has been suggested, but remains to be proven.

Deficiencies or excesses of specific nutrients, including minerals and vitamins, can have a major impact on the developing skeleton. So too can a variety of toxic principles, primarily of plant origin, that an animal is exposed to during skeletal development. These will be discussed in some detail in this section, drawing comparisons between different animal species where appropriate. The so-called metabolic bone diseases, rickets, osteomalacia, fibrous osteodystrophy, and osteoporosis, caused by deficiencies or imbalances of vitamin D, calcium, or phosphorus, are discussed in detail in a later section of this chapter.

Mineral imbalances

Manganese is an essential trace element in animals, being required for the activation of xylosyltransferase, the first enzyme in the biosynthetic pathway of sulfated glycosaminoglycans. *A deficiency of manganese causes decreased production and increased degradation of cartilage glycosaminoglycans* and therefore potentially affects all bones that develop by endochondral ossification.

Manganese deficiency has been incriminated as the cause of skeletal deformities in newborn calves and other farmed livestock in several countries. The deficiency does not appear to affect adult animals but calves born to cows fed on manganese-deficient rations during pregnancy may show various degrees of **skeletal deformity**. The syndrome resembles that described as "*crooked calf disease*," which is discussed in more detail below under "Plant toxicities." In one study, pregnant cows fed 183 mg of manganese per day produced normal calves whereas those fed 115–123 mg manganese per day produced calves with deformities of the limbs, including reduced length and breaking strength of humeri, enlarged joints, and twisted legs. Similar skeletal defects occur in lambs and kids. The reduced breaking strength of bones in this syndrome may reflect the fact that manganese is necessary for the glycosylation of collagen as well as in the synthesis of cartilage glycosaminoglycans.

In New Zealand, manganese deficiency was incriminated in a naturally occurring "outbreak" of **chondrodystrophy** involving 32 purebred Charolais calves to various degrees. Because of severe drought, the pregnant cows had been fed a diet of apple pulp and corn silage, both of which are low in manganese. The calves had short limbs with enlarged joints, and collapsed tracheas with thick cartilage rings. The limb bones were short and had large mushroom-shaped epiphyses (Fig. 1.45). Microscopic lesions included irregular alignment and degeneration of physeal chondrocytes, absence of hypertrophic cells, and degeneration of matrix with unmasking of collagen fibers. Calves with mild lesions that were able to walk gradually recovered, but their legs remained bent and shortened for several months.

Manganese deficiency is also suggested as a possible cause of unusual skeletal deformities in calves from several properties in western Canada. **Congenital spinal stenosis** and myelomalacia, together with focal premature closure of growth plates, malformations of the cranial base and shortening of long bones characterize the syndrome. The spinal stenosis appears to be the result of flaring of the ends of vertebral bodies and protrusion of vertebral articular processes. Focal closure of growth plates is found in the offspring of manganese-deficient rats.

Congenital skeletal malformations in 47 Holstein calves on a property in South Africa were also suggested as being due to manganese deficiency, but the evidence was not convincing. Affected calves were small and showed variable joint laxity, doming of the forehead, brachygnathia superior, and shortening of their long bones. These outbreaks of skeletal deformities highlight the difficulty in establishing a definitive etiologic diagnosis in a disease that is not discovered until several months after the initial damage has occurred.

There is no doubt that **copper deficiency** influences skeletal development, but full appreciation of the range of manifestations and the mechanisms involved is lacking. The role of copper deficiency in **osteoporosis** and its association with **osteochondrosis** in some species are discussed further elsewhere in this chapter. *As a component of the enzyme lysyl oxidase, copper is required for cross-linkage of collagen molecules.* This is an important step in strengthening the matrix elements of bone tissue, cartilage, and other connective tissues that rely on collagen for support. It is not surprising therefore that increased fragility of bone, and possibly cartilage, is a feature of copper deficiency. Studies in dogs and swine have demonstrated reduced osteoblastic activity in animals with copper deficiency, leading to narrow cortices of long bones and reduced deposition of bone on persistent spicules of mineralized cartilage in the primary spongiosa. These metaphyseal changes resemble those of vitamin C deficiency, which is not surprising since both deficiencies interfere with collagen synthesis and cross-linkage.

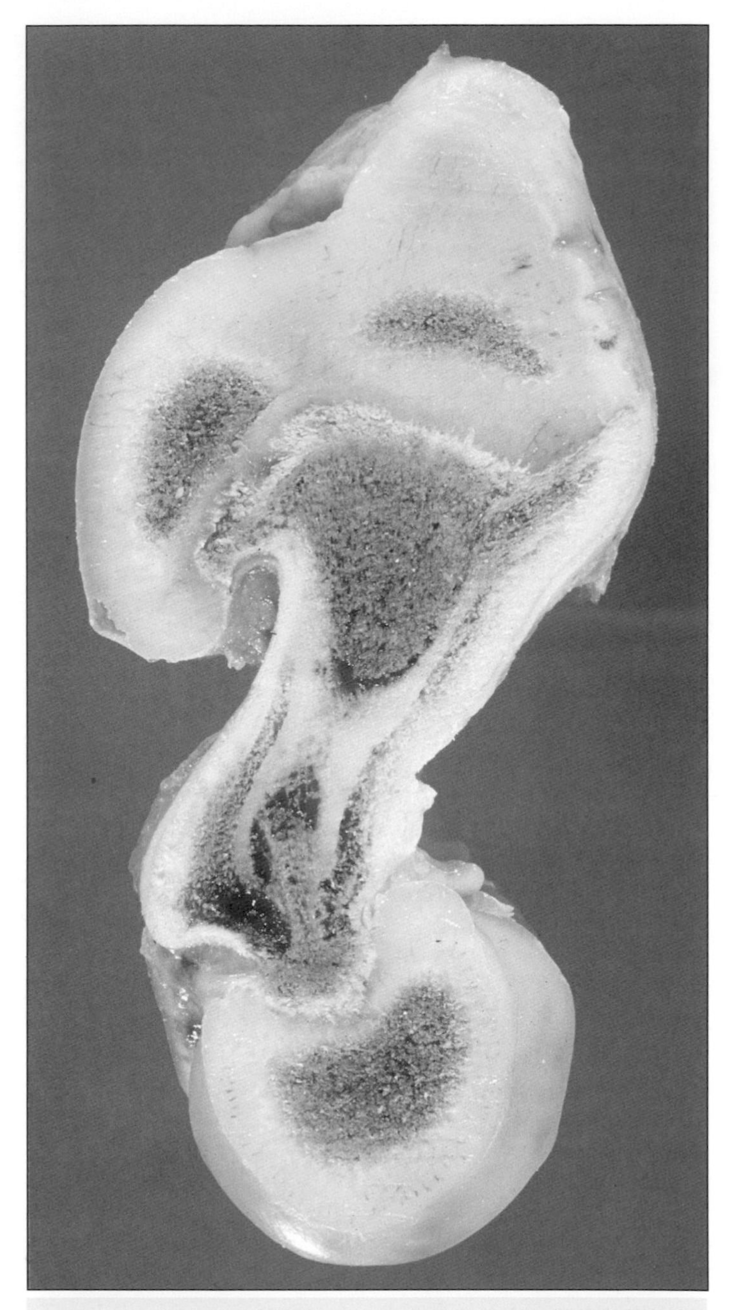

Figure 1.45 Chondrodystrophy in a newborn calf caused by intrauterine **manganese deficiency**. The humerus is considerably shorter than normal and the epiphyses are excessively large in comparison.

In calves, foals, pigs, and dogs, copper deficiency has been associated with grossly visible focal thickenings in rapidly growing growth plates. These foci consist of *retention of hypertrophic zone chondrocytes*, which protrude into the metaphysis, but the mechanism for this lesion in copper deficiency is not clear. It is possible that the stress of weight bearing causes microfractures of fragile trabeculae in the primary spongiosa with local disruption of the metaphyseal blood supply and impaired invasion of the mineralized cartilage. A similar mechanism has been proposed for the focal thickening of growth plates observed in chondrodystrophic Alaskan Malamutes and for the physeal thickening seen in some cases of osteochondrosis. In support of this hypothesis, trabecular microfractures, adjacent to foci of physeal thickening, are described in copper-deficient swine, calves, and foals, but it is seldom possible to accurately assign cause and effect in natural cases as the lesions are frequently too advanced to provide clues as to their origin. Whatever the mechanism, *these growth plate lesions bear a strong resemblance, grossly and histologically, to those of rickets and osteochondrosis*. Differentiation from rickets may be further complicated by the possibility of spontaneous long-bone fractures in copper-deficient animals due to osteoporosis and increased bone fragility.

Physeal changes are not a feature of copper deficiency in lambs. In one report, lambs with experimentally induced copper deficiency developed osteoporosis, but no lesions were detected in growth plates. Nor are there any descriptions of growth plate thickening in sheep with natural copper deficiency, suggesting either a species difference, or the fact that lambs, because of their lower bodyweight, are less likely to develop trabecular microfractures than foals, calves, or pigs.

Copper deficiency may be either *primary*, due to inadequate dietary copper, or *secondary* to increased dietary levels of copper antagonists, but the mechanisms vary between species. Absorption of copper is reduced by the presence of divalent cations such as zinc, iron, and cadmium that compete with copper for a common transport mechanism. Zinc may also induce the formation of metallothionine, a protein that binds copper in the intestine, liver, and kidney and reduces its availability. Phytates in the carbohydrate diets may form insoluble ligands with copper and prevent its absorption. Skeletal lesions consistent with osteochondrosis are described in pigs and foals fed experimental diets high in zinc, and in foals grazing pastures contaminated with zinc close to industrial plants. The possibility of a direct toxic effect of zinc on developing bone or cartilage must be considered, but a secondary effect through induction of copper deficiency is favored.

Calves and lambs grazing pastures containing high levels of *molybdenum* have developed skeletal lesions consistent with copper deficiency. This is believed to be due to the formation of thiomolybdates in the sulfide-rich environment of the rumen and *induction of secondary copper deficiency*. Thiomolybdates do not form in the digestive tract of nonruminants, providing a possible explanation for the higher tolerance of monogastric species to dietary molybdenum. However, although dietary molybdenum has little effect on copper uptake in horses, skeletal lesions resembling those of copper deficiency have been reproduced in rats and rabbits fed on rations with high levels of molybdenum.

Molybdenosis in sheep is associated with *epiphysiolysis of the greater trochanter and sub-periosteal hemorrhages of long bones*, leading to formation of bony excrescences. Sub-periosteal new bone formation at sites of muscle and tendon insertion has also been described in rats fed a low-copper diet supplemented with tetrathiomolybdate. In feedlot cattle, molybdenum poisoning caused weight loss and animals died over many months despite a short exposure to toxic levels, with both severe nephrosis and hepatotoxicity found in fatal cases. Although it has been suggested that bone lesions, at least in lambs, may be due to molybdenum toxicity rather than copper deficiency, the latter seems to be a better option. In ruminants, molybdenum may also interfere with the metabolism of sulfur, and affect ruminal microflora. Weakening of connective tissues with tearing of insertion sites due to reduced strength of tendons and ligaments would not be surprising in copper-deficient animals with reduced cross-linkage of collagen. The formation of reactive bone would be an expected response to periosteal elevation induced by hemorrhage at such sites. In affected animals, the other commonly associated lesions of copper deficiency are absent, so the exact pathogenesis of bone lesions in molybdenosis remains uncertain.

Fluorine is an essential trace element but, when present in chronic excess, is capable of inducing *characteristic dental and/or bony changes*. **Fluorosis** *is the term used to denote chronic fluoride toxicity*. All species are susceptible but because of the manner in which chronic poisoning occurs, *fluorosis is most common in herbivorous animals*. Discussion here is based on fluorosis in cattle, which are more susceptible than sheep and horses and for which the abnormalities are better described.

Toxic levels may be obtained from subsurface waters, especially where *rock phosphate* is plentiful. Rock phosphates vary considerably in their fluoride content, and chronic poisoning has been observed in cattle and sheep given rock phosphates as "licks." Contamination of pastures adjacent to *mineral ore refineries* may also cause toxicity, either directly or by uptake of fluorine by plants, since fluorine is volatile at high temperatures and is part of the gaseous and particulate effluent of many industrial processes. *Dust from volcanic eruptions* also contains abundant fluorides. Because of the widespread distribution of fluorine in nature, many animals obtain small non-toxic doses, partly from drinking water and partly from wind-blown dust, which settles on pasture.

Fluoride is removed rapidly from the blood, by renal excretion and deposition in bones and teeth. A small amount is deposited in soft tissues. Some fluorine crosses the placental barrier and although plasma levels are lower in fetal than maternal circulation, under certain circumstances fetal fluorosis may develop. Evidence regarding fluorine levels in milk is conflicting. The deposition of fluoride in bone may be functionally comparable to that of other elements, such as lead and strontium, and *may represent a detoxification mechanism*. Unless the intake of fluoride is very low, there is a steady accumulation of the element since it is deposited as calcium fluoride or fluorapatite, which are of low solubility. Many normal cattle have 600–900 μg/g in their bones but fetal lesions apparently occur at concentrations as low as 100–200 μg/g. Evidence of fluorosis does not develop in older cattle until the concentration reaches 2500–3000 μg/g. A level of 40–60 mg/kg (dry matter) in feed will produce such concentrations in the bone of cattle after 2–3 years. In general, the toxicity of fluorine depends on the aqueous solubility of the compound fed; sodium compounds are more soluble and more toxic than calcium compounds.

Fluoride toxicity is enhanced by poor nutrition, and alleviated somewhat by high dietary intakes of calcium and aluminum. While ingesting toxic levels of fluorine, urine of cattle usually contains

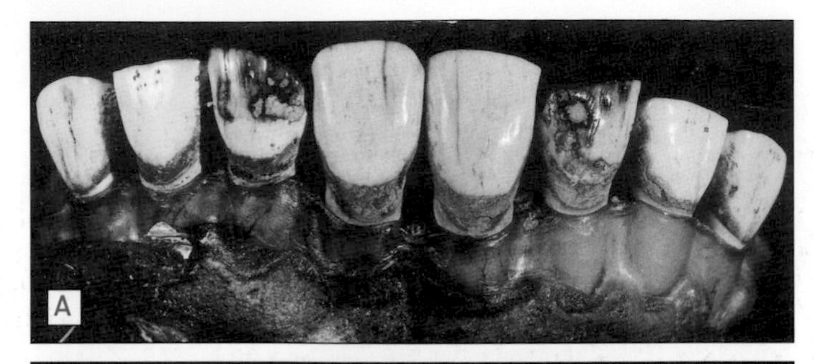

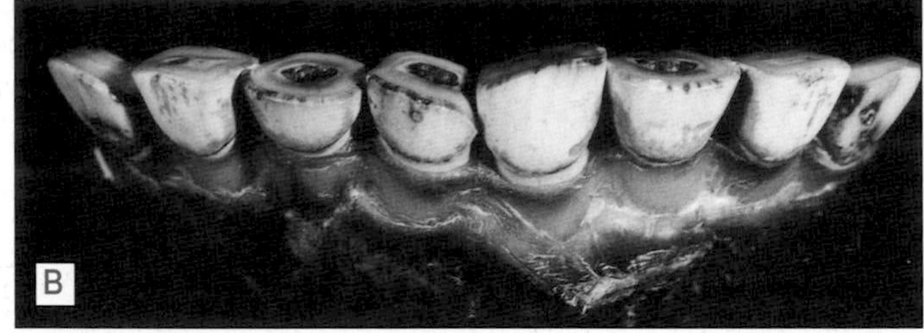

Figure 1.46 Fluorosis. (Courtesy of JL Shupe.) **A.** Dark brown discoloration and hypoplasia of enamel in the incisors of a cow. The variable involvement of the teeth reflects variation in levels of the toxin during enamel formation. **B.** Accelerated wear of incisor teeth in a cow with fluorosis.

10 μg/g or more although high urinary concentrations may persist for some time after excess fluorine is removed from the diet. Plasma fluorine is also elevated during periods of exposure but declines a few days after fluorine is removed from the diet.

The characteristic changes of severe fluorosis occur in teeth and bones and are accompanied by shifting lameness, loss of production, and a variety of nonspecific signs of debility. **Dental lesions** develop only if intoxication occurs while teeth are in the developmental stages and enamel is forming. Ameloblasts and odontoblasts are extremely sensitive to fluorine, which causes them to produce a matrix that mineralizes abnormally and is reduced in quality and quantity. In particular, *the outer layer of enamel is hypomineralized*. The incremental lines in the enamel are disrupted and the normal subsurface pigment band of bovine incisors is distorted.

The mildest macroscopic evidence of dental fluorosis is the *presence of small foci with a dry, chalky appearance compared to the normal glistening surface of enamel*. These mottled areas are readily visible as opacities when the tooth is transilluminated. In more severe cases, *all the enamel in affected teeth may be chalky, opaque and show various degrees of yellow, dark brown, or black discoloration* (Fig. 1.46A), *which is virtually pathognomonic for fluorosis*. Affected teeth show accelerated wear (Fig. 1.46B) and may develop chip fractures. In chronic cases, they may be worn to the gum line. The pigment is present in the enamel layer and possibly in the dentin, and may reflect oxidation of the organic matrices of the teeth. Unlike the pigment of food stains and tartar, it is not limited to the surface and cannot be removed by scraping. Hypoplasia of enamel may occur in severe fluorosis and is evident as punctate pits or as horizontal grooves, usually most prominent on the lateral aspect of the tooth. The horizontal disposition of the grooves and pits is attributable to periodic interference with mineralization of enamel during odontogenesis.

Although the fetus does not accumulate high levels of fluorine, under some circumstances lesions may develop in the deciduous teeth of calves exposed during gestation. Microscopically the odontoblasts are disorganized and have vacuolated cytoplasm. There is excessive predentin and formation of globular dentin. Fibrosis of the pulp cavity with ectopic bone formation is also seen. Lesions in permanent teeth, especially those that are last to erupt, are much more common, those that erupt first showing little or no damage. In cattle, the permanent teeth are sensitive to fluorosis from about 6–36 months of age. The most severe effects occur when exposure coincides with initiation of crown formation. In areas of endemic fluorosis, where ingestion of the element is more-or-less continuous, the lateral incisors of cattle show the most obvious lesions and, together with the second premolars and second and third molars, the most severe lesions. Lesions of similar severity should be present in teeth that develop simultaneously. These associations include the first incisor with the second molar, second incisor with the third molar, and the third incisor with the second premolar. Lesions in the second incisor must be severe before lesions are prominent in the third molar, and in general, incisor abrasion develops prior to molar abrasion. Lesions may develop in the fourth incisor in the absence of changes in other teeth.

The bone lesions of fluorine toxicity, **osteofluorosis**, are generalized but not uniform and, in severe cases, are characterized grossly by the formation of *periosteal hyperostoses*, which give the macerated bones a chalky roughened appearance (Fig. 1.47A, B, C). Lesions occur first on the medial surface of the proximal third of the metatarsal and later on the mandible, metacarpals, and ribs. The pelvis, vertebrae, and other bones of the distal limbs are also affected. In chronically affected cattle, fracture of the digital bones in the medial claw is common, leading to lameness and a preference for affected animals to stand cross-legged. A similar pattern of development occurs in horses. Although exostoses often develop at sites of tendinous or fascial insertions, this is not the rule and the reasons for their occurrence and distribution are unknown. Endostoses seldom occur in farm animals. Articular surfaces are normal, and lameness is due to involvement of the periosteum, encroachment of osteophytes on tendons and ligaments and, in some cases, to mineralization and even ossification of the latter structures. Fluorine is incorporated into bone matrix during mineralization and will therefore be most abundant in young animals at sites of active formation but is also deposited in older animals during remodeling. Exposure of cattle after 3 years of age may therefore produce osteofluorosis but not dental fluorosis.

Depending on the level of exposure to fluoride, and its concentration in bone, the bones may appear grossly and radiographically normal. A characteristic microscopic feature that may be detected in ground bone sections in such cases is the presence of brown discoloration of osteons, similar to that in enamel. The discoloration is apparently due to the effect of fluoride on osteoblasts, and its extent depends on the rates of bone growth or remodeling. Both endosteal and periosteal osteoblasts are affected and produce an abnormal matrix, which mineralizes abnormally. Sections of cortex may have a mottled appearance with some lamellae in some osteons showing discoloration and others appearing normal, depending on whether they were exposed to toxic levels of fluorine during formation. In fetuses, brown mottling of lamellar bone occurs at much lower concentrations of fluorine than in older cattle.

At *highly toxic levels*, the gross lesions of osteofluorosis occur rapidly. Not only is any new bone abnormal, preformed bone is apparently

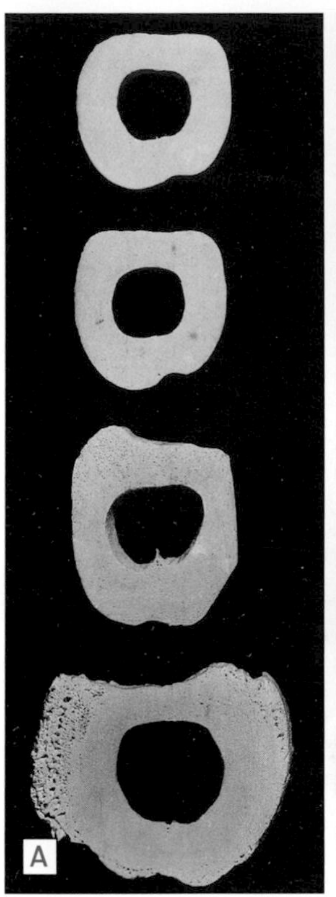

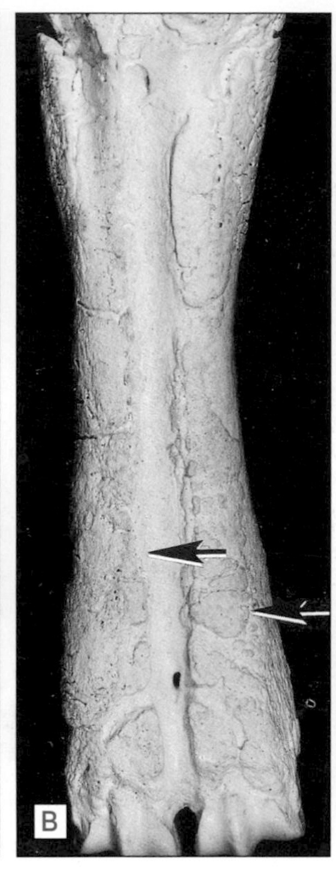

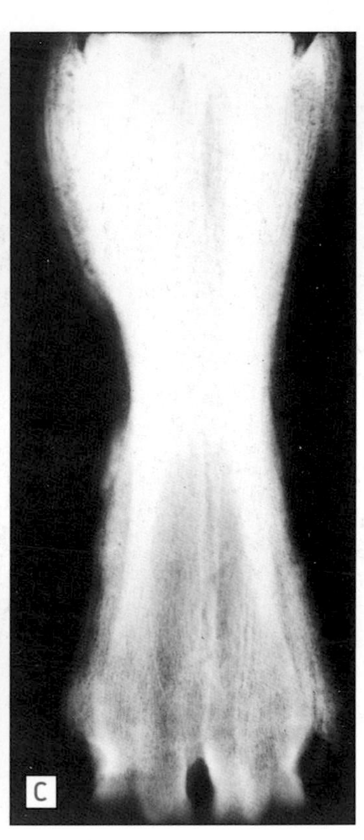

Figure 1.47 Chronic osteofluorosis in a cow. (Courtesy of JL Shupe.) **A.** Transverse sections of the diaphysis of metatarsals from cattle with increasing severity of osteofluorosis (top to bottom). Note the increased thickness of the cortex due to periosteal new bone formation. **B. Extensive periosteal new bone formation** (arrows) on the metatarsal bone. **C.** Radiograph of a metatarsal from an affected animal illustrating the extent of the periosteal hyperostosis.

altered in its mechanical properties and has a reduced life span. The rate of remodeling is correspondingly increased both for fluoridated normal bone and for bone formed under the influence of fluoride. The medullary cavity is enlarged and resorption spreads progressively outward through the cortex, and may involve the laminar periosteal bone. Resorption cavities may be excavated much more rapidly than they can be refilled, and the cortex becomes porotic. The impaired mechanical properties induce periosteal reinforcement with laminar bone or, if the need is greater and the deposition of new bone more rapid, by coarse woven cancellous bone. When fluoride levels are very high, the new matrices produced are abnormal and remain unmineralized, as in osteomalacia.

In young, growing dogs and pigs, and presumably in other species, fluorine intoxication produces lesions, which, in many respects, resemble rickets. This is presumably due to inhibition of mineralization when fluorine is present in high doses. The ends of long bones and the costochondral junctions are enlarged while physes are usually increased in depth, softer than normal, and yield to the pressure of weight bearing. The change at osteochondral junctions appears to be due to continued proliferation of chondrocytes, which fail to mature and align themselves. Associated with immaturity, there is a reduced amount of cartilaginous matrix and, although this appears to mineralize normally, albeit intermittently, the mineralized spicules are thin and fragile. The wide seams of osteoid that are deposited are poorly and irregularly mineralized.

Lead toxicity is better recognized for its effects on the nervous system, but also causes bone lesions. *The characteristic lesion is a band of sclerosis, referred to as a* **"lead line,"** visible radiographically and grossly in the metaphysis of developing bones. This is a relatively early morphological lesion in children with lead poisoning, and also occurs in animals (Fig. 1.48A). The sclerosis is due to persistence of mineralized cartilage trabeculae in the metaphysis (Fig. 1.48B) because of impaired osteoclastic resorption. Microscopically, many osteoclasts are present but they may be separated from the surface of bone trabeculae (Fig. 1.48C) and appear poorly able to degrade mineralized matrix. Some osteoclasts may contain *acid-fast intranuclear inclusions*. Ultrastructurally, a large amount of mineralized cartilage matrix is present in the cytoplasm of osteoclasts suggesting a defect in intracellular processing of the matrix. The metaphyseal sclerosis associated with lead toxicity radiographically and grossly resembles that seen in association with some cases of canine distemper viral infection and intrauterine *Bovine viral diarrhea virus* infection, both of which may interfere with osteoclast function or number.

Bibliography

Bridges CH, Moffitt PG. Influence of variable content of dietary zinc on copper metabolism of weanling foals. Am J Vet Res 1990;51:275–280.

Doige CE, et al. Congenital spinal stenosis in beef calves in western Canada. Vet Pathol 1990;27:16–25.

Eamans GJ, et al. Skeletal abnormalities in young horses associated with zinc toxicity and hypocuprosis. Aust Vet J 1984;61:205–207.

Editorial. Continuing controversy over dietary fluoride tolerance for dairy cattle. Fluoride 1987;20:101–103.

Eisenstein R, Kawanoue S. The lead line in bone-a lesion apparently due to chondroclastic indigestion. Am J Pathol 1975;80:309–316.

Follis RH, et al. Studies on copper metabolism XVIII. Skeletal changes associated with copper deficiency in swine. Bull Johns Hopkins Hosp 1955;97:405–409.

Gunson DE, et al. Environmental zinc and cadmium pollution associated with generalized osteochondrosis, osteoporosis and nephrocalcinosis in horses. J Am Vet Med Assoc 1982;180:295–299.

Hedhammer A, et al. Overnutrition and skeletal disease: an experimental study in growing Great Dane dogs. Cornell Vet Suppl 1974;5:11–160.

Hurtig M, et al. Correlative study of defective cartilage and bone growth in foals fed a low-copper diet. Equine Vet J 1993;Suppl 16:66–73.

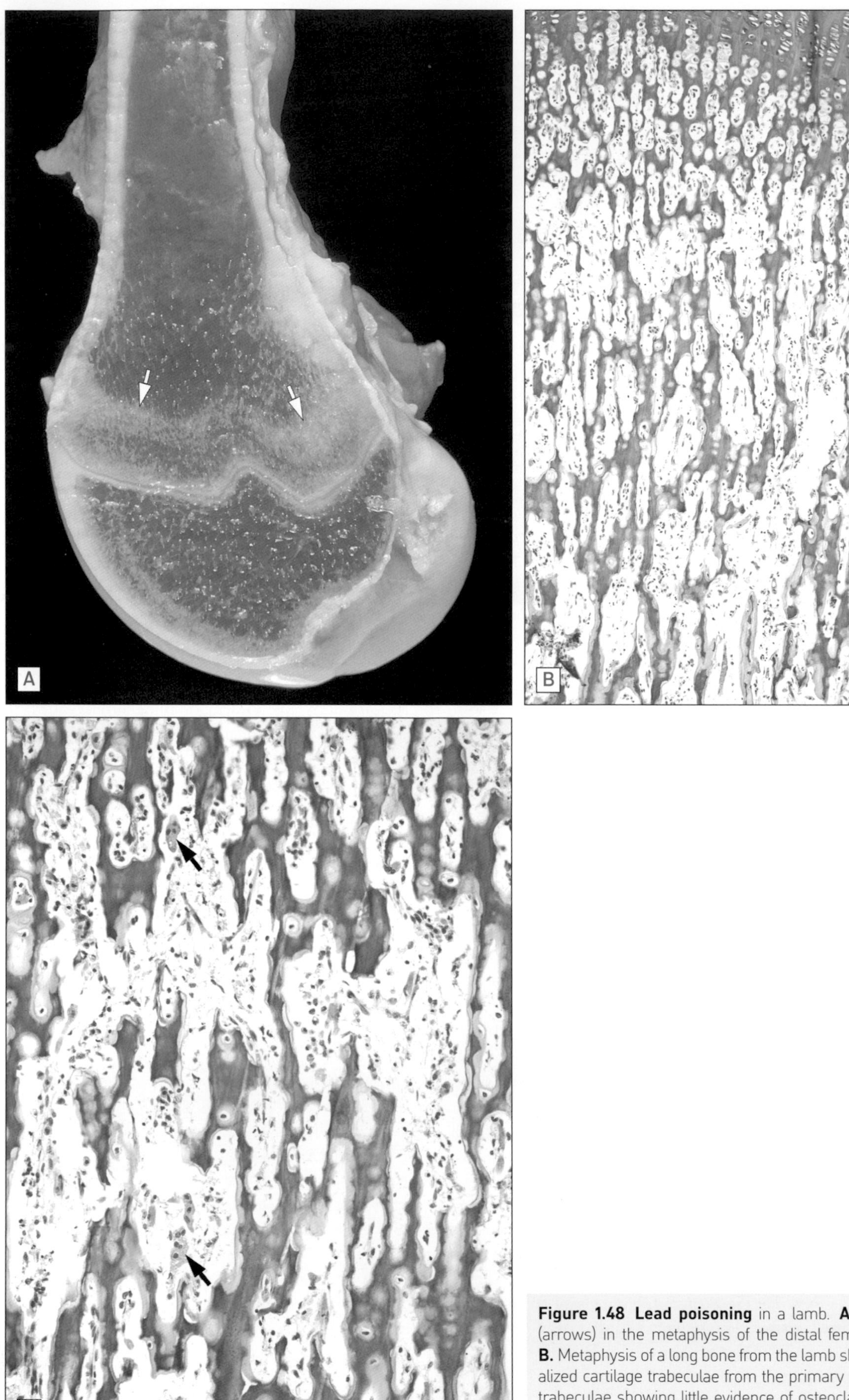

Figure 1.48 Lead poisoning in a lamb. **A.** Note the band of sclerosis (arrows) in the metaphysis of the distal femur. (Courtesy of RA Fairley.) **B.** Metaphysis of a long bone from the lamb showing persistence of mineralized cartilage trabeculae from the primary spongiosa. **C.** Closer view of trabeculae showing little evidence of osteoclastic resorption, even though several osteoclasts are present (arrows).

Kragstrup J, et al. Experimental osteo-fluorosis in the domestic pig: A histomorphometric study of vertebral trabecular bone. J Dental Res 1984;63: 885–889.
Lucas PA, et al. The effect of vitamin A deficiency and fluoride on glycosaminoglycan metabolism in bone. Conn Tiss Res 1984;13:17–26.
Maylin GA, et al. Fluoride intoxication in dairy calves. Cornell Vet 1987;77: 84–98.
Orr JP, McKenzie GC. Unusual skeletal deformities in calves in a Saskatchewan beef herd. Can Vet J 1981;22:121–125.
Pitt M, et al. Molybdenum toxicity in sheep: epiphysiolysis, exostoses and biochemical changes. J Comp Pathol 1980;90:567–576.
Platt BS, Stewart, RJC. Transverse trabeculae and osteoporosis in bones in experimental protein-calorie deficiency. Br J Nutr 1962;16:483–495.
Pond WG, et al. Bone pathology without cardiovascular lesions in pigs fed high zinc and low copper diet. Nutr Res 1990;10:871–885.
Shearer TR, et al. Bovine dental fluorosis: histologic and physical characteristics. Am J Vet Res 1978;39:597–602.
Shupe JL, et al. Relationship of cheek tooth abrasion to fluoride-induced permanent incisor lesions in livestock. Am J Vet Res 1987;48:1498–1503.
Smart ME, et al. Copper deficiency in calves in northcentral Manitoba. Can Vet J 1980;21:349–352.
Spence JA, et al. A sequential study of the skeletal abnormalities which develop in rats given a small dietary supplement of ammonium tetrathiomolybdate. J Comp Pathol 1980;90:139–153.
Spence JA, et al. Morphology and radio-opaque lines in bones of foetal lambs: the effects of maternal nutrition. J Comp Path 1982;92:317–329.
Staley GP, et al. Congenital skeletal malformations in Holstein calves associated with putative manganese deficiency. J South Afr Vet Assoc 1994;65:73–78.
Suttle NF, et al. Osteoporosis in copper-depleted lambs. J Comp Pathol 1972;82:93–97.

Vitamin imbalances

Deficiencies and excesses of vitamins A and D can significantly influence skeletal development and remodeling, as can deficiency of vitamin C. The skeletal manifestations of imbalances in these vitamins will be discussed here, except for vitamin D deficiency, which will be included with the metabolic bone diseases because of its role in the etiology of rickets and osteomalacia.

Vitamin A in the diet originates from both plant and animal sources. Retinyl esters of animal origin are hydrolyzed in the gut to retinol, which is bound to lipid and absorbed, then re-esterified and transported to the liver. Retinol is transported from the liver to target tissues bound to a specific transport protein, retinol-binding protein, an α1-globulin. Provitamins such as carotenes and carotenoids of plant origin are absorbed in the small intestine, where a molecule of β-carotene, for example, can be converted enzymatically in epithelial cells to two molecules of retinaldehyde (retinal). Most of this is reduced to the alcohol form, retinol. A small proportion of retinaldehyde is oxidized to retinoic acid, which is not converted to retinol in the body and is not stored in the liver. Instead, it is excreted in bile and urine after being transported in plasma bound to albumin. Retinol is essentially synonymous with vitamin A since it, or its derivatives, can supply all the requirements for reproduction, vision, and growth supplied by the vitamin. Retinoic acid, and its natural and synthetic derivatives, are classified as retinoids. These compounds do not support the visual functions of vitamin A and only some of its reproductive functions.

The functions of vitamin A, other than that of retinal in relation to vision (see Vol. 1, Eye and ear), are incompletely understood. *Retinol and retinoic acid stimulate the activity of osteoclasts*, causing them to increase their acid phosphatase content and resorb bone. *Development and differentiation of epithelial structures and bone are sustained by retinol, retinyl esters, retinal, and retinoic acid*, but the mechanisms are unclear. It is postulated that retinol and retinoids may either act as carriers of sugar for glycoprotein biosynthesis or function through a specific receptor protein. The metabolically active form is also unknown – the model of 11-*cis*-retinal in the rhodopsin cycle does not apply to other functions. Retinyl phosphate, retinoic acid, or some other metabolite, may be the active compound.

Vitamin A deficiency *occurs in cattle and pigs fed unsupplemented rations of grain and/or old hay*. Yellow corn, new hay, and fresh silage are adequate sources of carotene but potency decreases with storage. Animals grazing green pasture or crops are unlikely to suffer from vitamin A deficiency, but dry summer pastures may be deficient. Although deficiency of vitamin A affects many tissues, the emphasis here is on the skeletal manifestations and their sequelae. *The underlying skeletal abnormality in vitamin A deficiency involves defective remodeling of membranous bone, presumably due to the stimulatory effect of vitamin A on osteoclastic activity*. Consequently, there is asynchrony between the developing central nervous system and the bones of the skull and spinal column. Failure of the cranial cavity and spinal canal to enlarge sufficiently to accommodate the brain, cranial nerves, and spinal cord results in secondary changes in the central nervous system and a variety of nervous signs. Membrane bones in other locations, including the periosteal surface of long bones, are also affected and may develop a coarse profile, but these changes are not significant clinically.

In the cranium, the defect is particularly severe in the bones of the caudal fossa, and *the cerebellum may herniate into the foramen magnum*. In puppies with vitamin A deficiency, deafness is a prominent sign because of changes in the internal auditory meatus, while affected *calves and pigs develop blindness due to narrowing of the optic foramina and compression of optic nerves*. The basis for these variations between species is not clear but lesions are modified according to the severity of the deficiency and the stage of skeletal growth. Spinal nerve roots, especially those in the cervical cord, may herniate into the intervertebral foramina, although the lesions are not always bilaterally symmetrical.

The pathogenesis of the asynchrony in development between the nervous system and skeleton is complex and is related to altered patterns of drift in bones that are growing during the period of deficiency. Normally osteoclasts are responsive to vitamin A, and in the cranium of deficient animals, there is inadequate resorption of endosteal bone. Often, bone is produced at sites where resorption should be occurring thus exacerbating the retarded expansion of the cranial cavity and the various foramina. Endochondral bone does not appear to be directly influenced by vitamin A deficiency.

The nervous signs in growing animals with vitamin A deficiency may be related to cranial and spinal nerve degeneration and to hydrocephalus. The hydrocephalus probably is due mainly to decreased absorption of cerebrospinal fluid into the blood, a process that occurs in the arachnoid granulations and villi. The granulations are located in the tentorium cerebelli, which is severely affected by the thickening that occurs in the dura mater in vitamin A deficiency. Hypersecretion of cerebrospinal fluid with vitamin A deficiency also contributes to the development of hydrocephalus.

Clinical signs of deficiency in growing cattle may include edema of the brisket and limbs, irreversible blindness, night blindness, and the neurologic effects of increased intracranial pressure. Growing pigs may show incoordination and posterior paresis. Pigs less than a week old may be affected if maternal supplies are low but signs usually are seen in older animals. Gross neurologic lesions include osseous thickening of the tentorium cerebelli, cerebral edema and coning of the cerebellum. Microscopically, there is Wallerian degeneration in the spinal cord and brain (see Vol. 1, Nervous system).

The most characteristic extraskeletal lesion of vitamin A deficiency is squamous metaplasia of various glandular or ductular epithelia. *In cattle, squamous metaplasia of the parotid salivary duct is virtually pathognomonic for vitamin A deficiency*, but this resolves within a few weeks following correction of the deficiency. In vitamin A-deficient pigs, focal squamous metaplasia in the urinary bladder may be grossly visible as 1–2 mm light-yellow nodules on the mucosa.

The effect of vitamin A deficiency on dental development is well studied in the continuously growing incisors of rats and guinea pigs, but not in teeth of other species. Inadequate differentiation and spatial organization of odontoblasts lead to irregular formation of poor-quality dentin. Ameloblastic differentiation is also suboptimal and results in enamel hypoplasia. In addition, undifferentiated ameloblasts invade the dental pulp where they induce the odontoblasts to form concretions.

Vitamin A deficiency, like excess, is **teratogenic**, and swine and large Felidae appear to be very susceptible. Abortions, stillbirths, and a variety of lesions, including subcutaneous edema, microphthalmia, retinal dysplasia, hypotrichosis, supernumerary ears, polydactyly, arthrogryposis, cleft palate, pulmonary hypoplasia, diaphragmatic hernia, hepatic cysts, and cardiac, renal, and gonadal malformations may occur in the offspring of vitamin A-deficient swine. Hydrocephalus, and protrusions of spinal cord through intervertebral foramina, may also occur. The frontal and parietal bones may be thin and the basioccipital bone thicker than normal. The latter bone is also thickened in neonatal calves from vitamin A-deficient dams, as are the squamous occipital, basisphenoid and presphenoid bones. Stillbirths, and congenital blindness, incoordination and thickened carpal joints are also seen in calves as well as hydrocephalus, with herniation of cerebellar vermis through the foramen magnum, constriction and degeneration of optic nerves, and retinal dysplasia.

Vitamin A toxicity is well recognized as a cause of skeletal disease in man and animals. Natural cases of toxicity usually follow an accidental overdose with vitamin A concentrate or excessive feeding of diets containing high concentrations of the vitamin, such as liver. Depending on the age and species of animal, and the duration and level of exposure to excess vitamin A, *the manifestations of toxicity may include physeal damage, osteoporosis, or the development of exostoses (osteophytes)*. High concentrations of carotenes in green feed oats may predispose to rickets in lambs through inhibition of vitamin D activity.

The **physeal lesions** of vitamin A toxicity are characterized by reduced chondrocyte proliferation and reduced size of hypertrophic chondrocytes, resulting in narrowing of growth plates. Loss of proteoglycans and unmasking of collagen fibers occur, and sometimes with high doses there is complete destruction of segments of growth plates. Rapidly growing physes, especially those subjected to the greatest compressive forces are most likely to show changes, resulting in reduced length of certain long bones. In organ culture, vitamin A inhibits chondrocyte proliferation and reduces RNA and protein synthesis. Lysis of matrix may be the result of destabilization of lysosomal membranes with the release of acid proteases that attack matrix proteins.

The **osteoporosis** of vitamin A toxicity is associated with decreased numbers of osteoblasts and fewer, thinner osteoid seams than normal, and is most severe in cortical bone and some of the membranous bones of the skull. Periosteal bone formation is more severely affected than endosteal and intracortical formation. In long bones, this results in thin cortices, reduced diaphyseal diameter and an exaggerated metaphyseal flare. Metaphyseal trabeculae tend to be reduced in number but thicker than normal. Hypervitaminosis A interferes with cell differentiation in the embryonic skeleton and may have similar effects on osteoblasts in postnatal bone. The decrease in osteoid production also suggests a direct toxic effect on osteoblasts. The osteoporosis may be exacerbated by continued bone resorption, osteoclasts apparently being less sensitive than osteoblasts to the effects of increased vitamin A. Fractures are not a feature of vitamin A toxicity in farm animals and pets as they are in some laboratory species. Osteoporosis is reversible in animals removed from diets high in vitamin A but the physeal damage is permanent and the consequences emphasized with time.

The *formation of exostoses* in association with vitamin A toxicity is often extensive. The pathogenesis of this lesion is not clear but may be associated with fragility of periosteal attachments, and provoked by tensions and minor trauma.

Toxicity associated with *single, large doses of vitamin A* has been recognized in pigs and calves. In baby **pigs** given excess vitamin A orally as part of disease prevention programs, a characteristic syndrome develops. Grossly there is shortening of long bones and prolongation of the traction epiphyses of the tibial tuberosity, the greater trochanter of the femur, and the humeral tuberosity. Rotation of epiphyses, particularly those of the distal femur and proximal and distal humerus, is also described, and tarsal and carpal bones may be distorted. The medial and lateral metatarsal bones, and to a lesser extent the metacarpal bones, may be of different lengths. Pigs treated shortly after birth show an abnormal gait and possess noticeably short legs by 6–8 weeks of age. The condition occurs with as little as twice the recommended dose of vitamin A. *The basis for the gross lesions is destruction and focal closure of growth plates.* Continued growth of the intact parts of the physis, and superimposed adaptational deformities, account for the characteristic appearance of the bones.

Similar lesions occur in **kittens** given daily oral doses of 40–100 μg/g body weight of vitamin A for 4 to 5 weeks, followed by a 6–15 week recovery period. The metacarpal lesions tend to be more severe than in piglets, the tibial lesions are similar, while those in the distal femur and other sites are less severe.

In 7-week-old **pigs** given about 20 μg/g body weight for 5 weeks then killed, osteoporosis is prominent. Lesions are especially severe in the squamous occipital bone, which may be so thin that the cerebellum can be crushed by manual pressure to the overlying skin. The long bones are short and fragile with thin cortices, flared metaphyses, and typical physeal lesions, but the latter are less severe than at higher dose rates and gross deformities do not occur. Exostoses may be present, especially near the insertion of the brachialis muscle on the proximal radius.

Vitamin A toxicity has been incriminated as the cause of **"hyena disease"** in **calves**. This unusual form of dwarfism is characterized

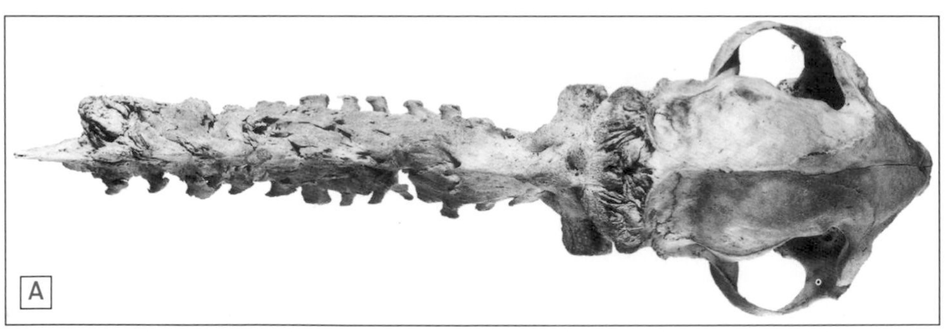

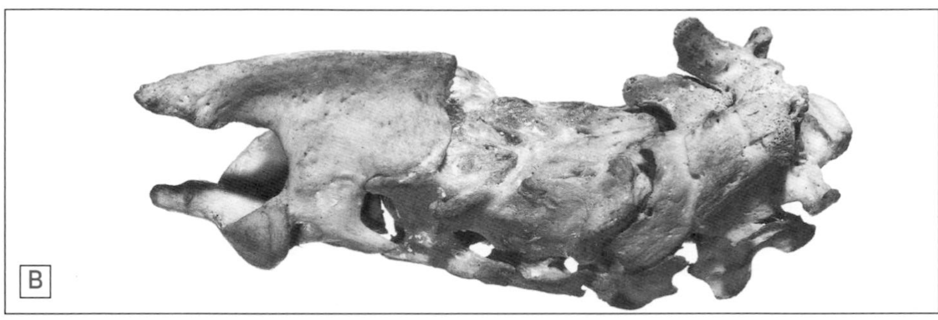

Figure 1.49 Vitamin A toxicity in a cat. **A, B.** Dorsal and lateral views of cervical vertebrae showing extensive exostoses leading to ankylosis. (Courtesy of AA Seawright.)

by *relative underdevelopment of the caudal body structures* due to premature closure of growth plates, particularly in the pelvic limbs, and has been associated with the injection of newborn calves with vitamins A and D. Affected calves have a characteristic "bunny-hopping" gait and a sloped back with small hindquarters, resembling a hyena. Although the lesions are most severe in the bones of the pelvic limbs and lumbosacral vertebrae, the pectoral limbs are also affected. Physes are narrow, but many focal triangular projections of physeal cartilage may protrude into the metaphysis. Administration of excess vitamin A to calves has been shown to induce premature mineralization of physeal cartilage leading to early closure of growth plates and impaired longitudinal bone growth, supporting vitamin A toxicity as the cause of hyena disease. An autoimmune mechanism associated with *Bovine viral diarrhea virus* has also been suggested but is not supported by convincing evidence.

Osteophyte formation is the hallmark of prolonged exposure to excess vitamin A in many species and is the outstanding feature of *chronic vitamin A poisoning in* **cats**, producing the syndrome referred to as **deforming cervical spondylosis**. The syndrome results from prolonged feeding of bovine livers to adult cats, which ordinarily contain large amounts of vitamin A when derived from grazing animals. The disease was common in Australia and Uruguay where beef livers are plentiful and relatively cheap, but also occurs sporadically in other countries when domestic cats are given unconventional diets. In young growing cats, this same diet would be expected to result in fibrous osteodystrophy because of the imbalance in calcium and phosphorus.

Deforming cervical spondylosis is typically *seen in cats after 2 years of age* and is characterized by postural changes, cervical ankylosis and forelimb lameness, sometimes accompanied by cutaneous hyperesthesia or anesthesia. The vertebral lesions are similar to those of mucopolysaccharidosis VI but the age of the cat should prevent confusion. *Extensive confluent exostoses develop, especially on the dorsal and lateral aspects of the cervical vertebrae and sometimes on the occipital bone.* In general, the exostoses do not encroach on the neural canal and only occasionally involve ventral aspects of the vertebrae (Fig. 1.49A, B). The intervertebral foramina are considerably altered in shape and reduced in size, causing compression and degeneration of nerves leading to denervation atrophy of muscles. Exostoses occasionally occur on the cranial thoracic vertebrae and may be accompanied by similar outgrowths on the sternum and fixation of the ribs. Periarticular osteophytes also occur about the proximal joints of one or both forelimbs and, if extensive, may cause fixation of the shoulder and elbow joints, usually in the flexed position. Lumbar vertebrae and pelvic limbs are seldom affected. The osteophytes consist initially of either osteocartilaginous tissue that overgrows joints and causes ankylosis, or of woven bone that develops at the site of muscle insertions and extends into the perimysium. Later, the woven bone and cartilage are replaced by lamellar bone. The stress on cervical intervertebral joints associated with regular grooming probably accounts for the concentration of exostoses in the cervical region of cats. In animals with chronic lesions, patches of ungroomed fur may develop in inaccessible sites. Interestingly, cats fed bovine liver tend to have higher and more persistently elevated plasma vitamin A concentration than cats supplemented with the vitamin, even at a higher equivalent dosage.

Oral and dental lesions, including hypermobility and loss of incisor teeth, may also occur in older cats in association with vitamin A toxicity and cervical spondylosis, but it is difficult to determine whether the changes are primary or secondary. Liver has a low calcium content, which could lead to resorption of alveolar bone, but excess vitamin A causes dental lesions even when dietary calcium is normal.

Several *other lesions* are associated with vitamin A toxicity. In some species, including humans, rats, rabbits, and dogs, it causes *ectopic mineralization* in internal organs. In cattle, pigs, and dogs there is decreased cerebrospinal fluid pressure and, in calves at least, this is associated with *thinning of the fibrous cap of arachnoid granulations*. Vitamin A is stored in the liver in *Ito cells*, which increase in size with dietary excess. Peliosis-like changes in the liver, in addition to hemorrhages around joints and hair loss, are reported in people with hypervitaminosis A. *Alopecia and dermatitis* are features of toxicity in horses.

Like vitamin A deficiency, *excess vitamin A is* **teratogenic**, the effects depending to some extent on dose, stage of gestation, and the compound administered. Teratogenicity is increased by protein or protein-energy malnutrition. Vitamin A is used extensively to treat skin disease in people and to a lesser extent in dogs. The half-life of some retinoids is many months, and anomalies in children exposed in utero are well recognized, but are not reported in puppies. *Experimental hypervitaminosis A during pregnancy produces defects in many systems in a variety of animals.* Vitamin A toxicity was incriminated as the cause of continued high prevalence of cleft palate and lip, pulmonary hypoplasia, and abortions near term in a swine herd. The problem in this herd ceased following reduction of vitamin A supplementation to normal levels. The mechanism of teratogenesis is unknown, but excess vitamin A in the embryo inhibits chondrogenesis and osteogenesis, possibly by modifying the differentiation of mesenchyme.

Vitamin D is essential for normal bone development, in particular mineralization of cartilage during endochondral ossification and of newly formed osteoid, but in excess, it is highly toxic. **Vitamin D toxicity** may result from accidental over-supplementation of young animals, ingestion of plants that contain the active form of the vitamin, or accidental ingestion of rodenticide containing cholecalciferol (vitamin D_3). The potency of the latter toxin is illustrated by the fact that cats and dogs may be poisoned by ingesting the carcasses of poisoned rats. Cats appear to be more sensitive to vitamin D toxicity than dogs. When administered as one or two massive doses shortly before parturition, vitamin D appears to prevent postparturient hypocalcemia ("milk fever") in cows but mineralization of soft tissues may result, particularly in pregnant Jersey cows, and in this breed its use is contraindicated. Vitamin D is stored in muscle and fat, and meat from vitamin D-treated "downer cows" is a potential hazard to dogs and cats. Significant amounts of vitamin D may be secreted in milk, and soft tissue mineralization in suckling puppies has been attributed to high dietary levels in the bitch.

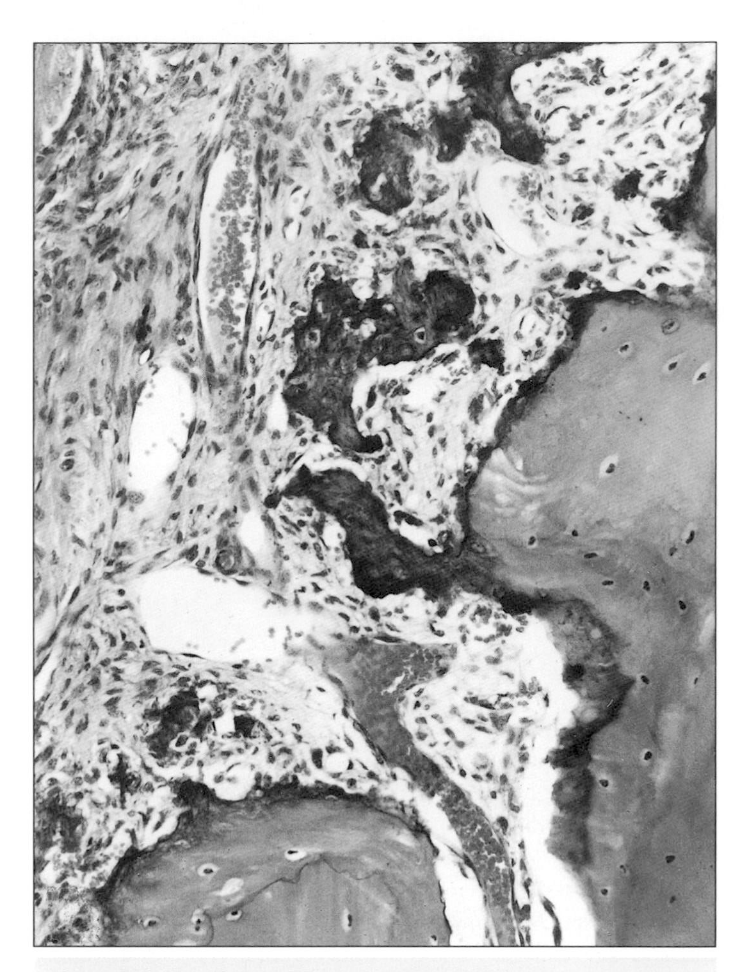

Figure 1.50 Vitamin D toxicity. Intensely basophilic bone matrix deposited on surface of trabeculae and in marrow spaces.

Several plants, including *Solanum malacoxylon* (syn. *glaucum*, *glaucophyllum*), *Cestrum diurnum* and *Trisetum flavescens* cause diseases similar to hypervitaminosis D in grazing animals in various parts of the world (see Enteque seco and Manchester wasting disease, in Vol. 3, Endocrine glands). Traditionally, vitamin D_2 (ergocalciferol) is regarded as the plant form of vitamin D, but *the toxic principle in these plants is 1,25-dihydroxycholecalciferol-glycoside*. Lesions in poisoned animals are indistinguishable from those produced by excess vitamin D. Other calcinogenic plants in which the active principle is less well defined include *Solanum torvum*, *S. verbascifolium*, possibly *S. esuriale*, and *Dactylis glomerata*. Alfalfa (*Medicago sativa*) contains vitamin D_3 in addition to vitamin D_2.

The *mechanism of vitamin D toxicity* is related primarily to its effect on increasing calcium absorption from the intestine, mobilizing it from bone and reducing its excretion by the kidney. The end result is *hypercalcemia* together with *hyperphosphatemia*, which, if persistent, will lead to widespread mineralization of soft tissues, in particular the kidneys, gastric mucosa, lungs, endocardium, and arterial walls. Death from renal failure is likely to occur before noticeable changes develop in the skeleton. In fact, there are few reports of the skeletal lesions of vitamin D toxicity in animals.

The skeletal changes in hypervitaminosis D may be characterized by either sclerosis or rarefaction, depending on the level of dietary calcium and the pattern of exposure. An early response in bone is widespread, intense osteoclastic activity, which may remove most of the primary spongiosa and cause active resorption in other sites. With continued administration, the matrix produced by osteoblasts accumulates, sometimes in large amounts and in a distinctive pattern. It often has a tangled fibrillary arrangement and appears somewhat mucoid, floccular, and intensely basophilic (Fig. 1.50). Osteoblasts are abundant. Mineralization of this basophilic matrix is delayed but it is gradually converted to a relatively homogeneous eosinophilic substance resembling osteoid. Initially, the maturation of the matrix is local and irregular in distribution, and is unrelated to normal patterns of osteogenesis. If toxicity is prolonged, the abnormal matrices continue to accumulate and virtually obliterate the marrow spaces. This produces a mosaic of basophilic and acidophilic matrix, and newly formed woven bone. *The presence of abundant basophilic matrix is virtually pathognomonic for vitamin D toxicity* and is valuable diagnostically when plasma levels of the vitamin are not known.

Vitamin D poisoning is usually associated with intermittent toxic doses of the vitamin. This results in surges of osteoblastic activity during periods of withdrawal with rapid production of large amounts of abnormal matrix. This matrix may slowly mature and mineralize, but the process is hastened by further administration of the vitamin. With continued intermittent administration of vitamin D, there are further cycles of matrix deposition, maturation, and mineralization. *Broad, basophilic, resting lines separate the layers of bone produced in each cycle.* Necrosis of osteocytes occurs with high doses of vitamin D and groups of empty lacunae are often present in cortical bone and in the center of trabeculae.

Virtually all bones are affected to some extent in vitamin D toxicity, but *the outstanding changes occur in long bones, especially in the ends where growth is most rapid.* The epiphyses are usually normal and appear to escape even the resorptive changes. The growth plates are also normal. The lesions involve the metaphyseal spongiosa and extend well into the diaphysis to fill the medullary cavity. Little active bone marrow remains and is gradually replaced by dilated veins and loose fibrous tissue, which is sparsely populated with hematopoietic cells. Areas of sclerosis may alternate with transverse bands of resorption, indicating intermittent toxicity. Active resorption of primary spongiosa may be accompanied by an intense neutrophilic reaction. Both the periosteum and endosteum are involved, and new periosteal bone contributes to the thickness of the metaphysis. Usually, the perichondrium is not affected, but sometimes it produces new cartilage and bone. In addition, there is rapid metaplastic bone formation in the thickened fibrous layer of the periosteum, producing a collar of new bone around the metaphysis.

Vitamin D deficiency is discussed in the section Metabolic bone diseases (Rickets and osteomalacia).

Vitamin C (ascorbic acid) is a co-factor for the enzymes prolyl and lysyl hydroxylase, which are required for the hydroxylation of proline and lysine during collagen synthesis, and is also an important antioxidant. In **vitamin C deficiency**, *there is reduction or failure in the secretion and deposition of collagen.* Furthermore, the deficiency of hydroxylysine results in impaired formation of intermolecular cross-links and any collagen that is produced is of reduced strength. Vitamin C also promotes the differentiation of osteoblasts from their progenitors and the hypertrophy of chondrocytes, both of which are critical to the process of endochondral ossification. Most mammals synthesize ascorbic acid from glucose via glucuronic acid and gulonic acid. Some species, including humans, certain nonhuman primates, and guinea pigs, lack the hepatic microsomal enzyme L-gulonolactone oxidase and, in the absence of a dietary source of ascorbic acid, develop **scurvy**. The disease normally does not occur in other species except as a result of genetic defects in vitamin C synthesis. *A spontaneous mutation involving L-gulonolactone oxidase is recorded in pigs.* The defect in pigs is inherited as an autosomal recessive trait and homozygous recessive piglets develop classic scorbutic lesions shortly after weaning. Maternal milk is a rich source of vitamin C and prevents signs of deficiency prior to weaning. A similar defect is also recognized in ODS rats.

The lesions of scurvy in guinea pigs with dietary vitamin C deficiency and in pigs with an inherited deficiency of L-gulonolactone oxidase are similar, although the lesions described in pigs are more severe. This probably reflects the complete absence of vitamin C in affected pigs, and the effect of greater body mass on weakened connective tissues. In guinea pigs, a dietary deficiency of vitamin C may be partial rather than absolute, or may be sporadic, and the bone lesions therefore vary in severity. Pigs with inherited L-gulonolactone oxidase deficiency are normal at birth but lose condition, become reluctant to stand or move, and develop swellings around their joints. Gross lesions are dominated by *sub-periosteal accumulations of clotted blood* around the shafts of the long bones, the scapulas, the bones of the head, especially the mandible, and on the ribs. The metaphyses are fragile, discolored by hemorrhage and separate easily from the adjacent physes. Similar hemorrhages occur around major joints, along costochondral junctions and on mandibles of affected guinea pigs. The bones are osteopenic and fragile. Subclinical scurvy in guinea pigs is accompanied by such nonspecific signs as diarrhea, weight loss, and dehydration, and may be more common than is generally appreciated as the early bone lesions may not be detected clinically or on gross postmortem examination.

The most characteristic microscopic lesion of scurvy is in the metaphysis. *Naked spicules of calcified cartilage, derived from the zone of provisional calcification in the growth plate, persist as a "scorbutic lattice"* (Fig. 1.51A, B). The layer of bone that is normally deposited on this cartilage framework by active osteoblasts is absent or deficient. Osteoblasts are sparse and appear to have lost their polarity. The marrow cavity may be filled with a population of poorly differentiated mesenchymal cells showing little if any collagen formation (Fig. 1.51B). In some cases, apparently normal bone trabeculae are present in the secondary spongiosa, representing bone formed during a period when dietary vitamin C was adequate. The cartilage spicules of the scorbutic lattice do not have the strength of normal trabeculae. Microfractures or infractions associated with hemorrhage and fibrin, but with little evidence of normal repair (Fig. 1.51A, B), are often present. Mechanical forces no doubt influence the development of such lesions.

Physes are generally thin and contain a reduced number of chondrocytes, poorly organized into columns. Cortices of long bones are thin and the periosteum may be elevated with hemorrhage or thin, irregular spicules of basophilic, woven bone separated by loose connective tissue.

The cartilage spicules of the scorbutic lattice have a high mineral content and may be visible radiographically as a radiodense band in the metaphysis.

Early suggestions that vitamin C deficiency may be a cause of metaphyseal osteopathy (hypertrophic osteodystrophy) in young dogs have been refuted. Dogs are capable of manufacturing their own vitamin C and although there are radiographic similarities between scurvy and metaphyseal osteopathy, the histologic lesions are quite different.

Bibliography

Biesalski HK. Comparative assessment of the toxicology of vitamin A and retinoids in man. Toxicology 1989;57:117–161.

Boland RL. Plants as a source of vitamin D_3 metabolites. Nutr Rev 1986;44:1–8.

Carrigan MJ, et al. Hypovitaminosis A in pigs. Aust Vet J 1988;65:159–160.

Clarke GL, et al. Subclinical scurvy in the guinea pig. Vet Pathol 1980;17:40–44.

Clark L. Growth rates of epiphyseal plates in normal kittens and kittens fed excess vitamin A. J Comp Pathol 1973;83:447–460.

Doige CE, Schoonderwoerd M. Dwarfism in a swine herd: Suspected vitamin A toxicosis. J Am Vet Med Assoc 1988;193:691–693.

Fooshee SK, Forrester SD. Hypercalcemia secondary to cholecalciferol rodenticide toxicosis in two dogs. J Am Vet Med Assoc 1990;8:1265–1268.

Geelen JAG. Hypervitaminosis A induced teratogenesis. CRC Crit Rev Toxicol 1979;351–375.

Grey RM, et al. Pathology of skull, radius and rib in hypervitaminosis A. Pathol Vet 1965;2:446–467.

Harrington DD, Page EH. Acute vitamin D_3 toxicosis in horses: Case reports and experimental studies of the comparative toxicity of vitamins D_2 and D_3. J Am Vet Med Assoc 1983;182:1358–1369.

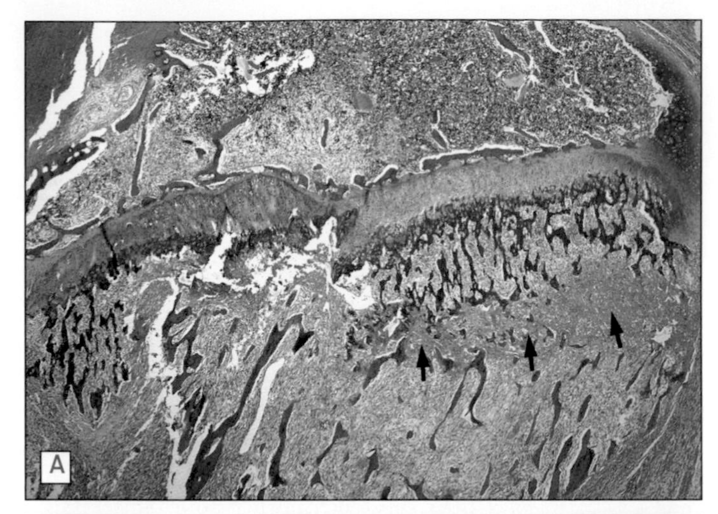

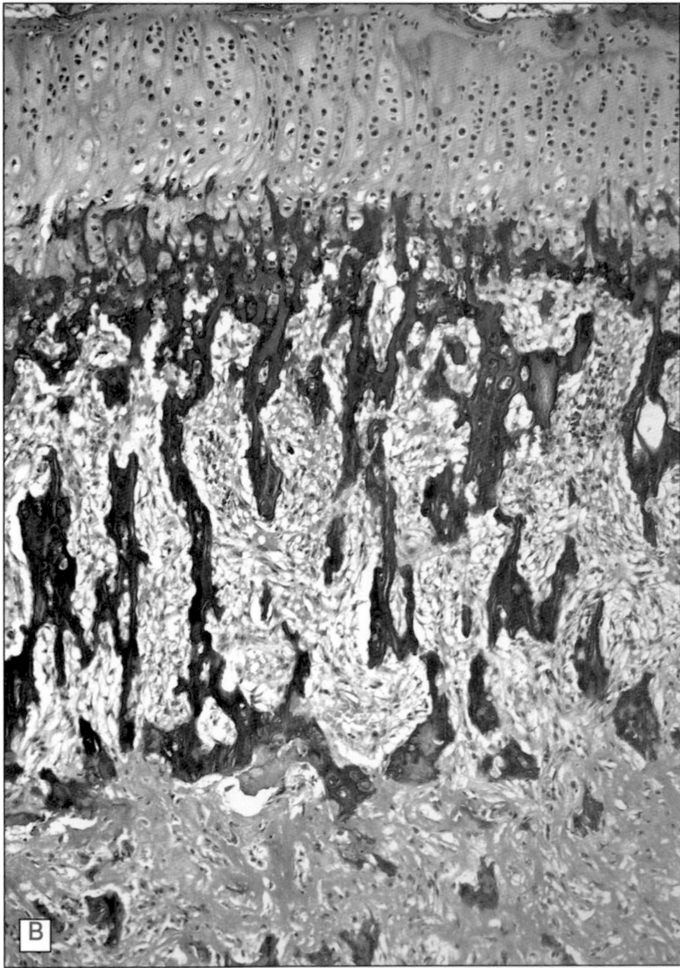

Figure 1.51 Scurvy. **A.** Physis and metaphysis from an affected guinea pig. Note the basophilic spicules of cartilage matrix without osteoid deposition in the area of the primary spongiosa. This is referred to as a "scorbutic lattice." Trabeculae in the secondary spongiosa do possess an osteoid layer, indicating that the deficiency of vitamin C is relatively recent. An infraction line (arrows) between the primary and secondary spongiosa reflects the fragility of bone trabeculae. **B.** Closer view of physis and **"scorbutic lattice"** in the same guinea pig. The calcified cartilage spicules are devoid of an osteoid layer and no osteoblasts are apparent. The spaces between trabeculae are filled with poorly differentiated mesenchymal cells. Trabecular fragments surrounded by fibrin at the bottom of the illustration form part of the infraction shown in (**A**). There is no evidence of repair.

Hayes KC, Cousins RJ. Vitamin A deficiency and bone growth I. Altered drift patterns. Calc Tiss Res 1970;6:120–132.

Hayes KC, et al. The fine structure of vitamin A deficiency II. Arachnoid granulations and CSF pressure. Brain 1971;94:213–224.

Howerth EW. Fatal soft tissue calcification in suckling puppies. J South Afr Vet Assoc 1983;54:21–24.

Jensen PT, et al. Congenital ascorbic acid deficiency in pigs. Acta Vet Scand 1983;24:392–402.

Littledike ET, Horst RL. Vitamin D_3 toxicity in dairy cows. J Dairy Sci 1982;65:749–759.

MacKay RJ, et al. Focal premature physeal closure (hyena disease) in calves. J Am Vet Med Assoc 1992;201:902–905.

Paulsen ME, et al. Blindness and sexual dimorphism associated with vitamin A deficiency in feedlot cattle. J Am Vet Med Assoc 1989;194:933–937.

Rosa FW, et al. Teratogen update: Vitamin A congeners. Teratology 1986;33:355–364.

Seawright AA, Hrdlicka J. Pathogenetic factors in tooth loss in young cats on a high daily oral intake of vitamin A. Aust Vet J 1974;50:133–141.

Simesen MG, et al. Hypervitaminosis D in sheep. An experimental study. Acta Vet Scand 1978;19:588–600.

Van der Lugt JJ, Prozesky L. The pathology of blindness in newborn calves caused by hypovitaminosis A. Onderstepoort J Vet Res 1989;56:99–109.

Vieth R. The mechanisms of vitamin D toxicity. Bone Mineral 1990;11:267–272.

Woodard JC, et al. Pathogenesis of vitamin (A and D)-induced premature growth-plate closure in calves. Bone 1997;21:171–182.

Plant toxicities

Many plant species are known, or suspected, to cause skeletal abnormalities, either by inducing a teratogenic effect on the developing fetus, or influencing skeletal remodeling in young growing animals. Those with a teratogenic action typically exert their influence early in pregnancy and require ingestion by the dam during a specific stage of fetal development. The classic example is ***Veratrum californicum*** (false hellebore, wild corn, or skunk cabbage), which causes **cyclopia** (Fig. 1.52) in the progeny of ewes that consume the plant on day 14 of gestation. Similar anomalies also occur in calves and kids whose dams are fed the plant at this stage of gestation, when the neural groove has formed and the first cranial somites are developing. Ingestion of *V. californicum* by pregnant ewes near day 29 produces marked shortening of the metacarpals, metatarsals, and tibiae, and sometimes the radii, while tracheal and laryngeal stenosis occurs in the offspring of ewes ingesting the plant on or about day 31 of gestation. There is variation in the degree of susceptibility, but lesions are usually bilaterally symmetrical and twins tend to be affected equally. Fusion of metacarpals may result in postnatal bowing of the legs and fusion or deformities of joints may cause **arthrogryposis**. Obviously not all ewes will graze the plant at precisely the same time of gestation and in a natural outbreak the changes detected in affected lambs would be expected to include a range of abnormalities. Prolonged gestation is also a feature of malformed fetal lambs and embryonic losses may be substantial. Death of about 17% of embryos occurs with maternal ingestion of *V. californicum* on days 19–21 of gestation, and up to 75% of embryos when the plant is ingested on day 14.

Ingestion of *V. californicum* by *pregnant cows* between days 12 and 30 of gestation may induce a range of anomalies, including cleft palate, harelip, brachygnathia, hypermobility of hock joints, and

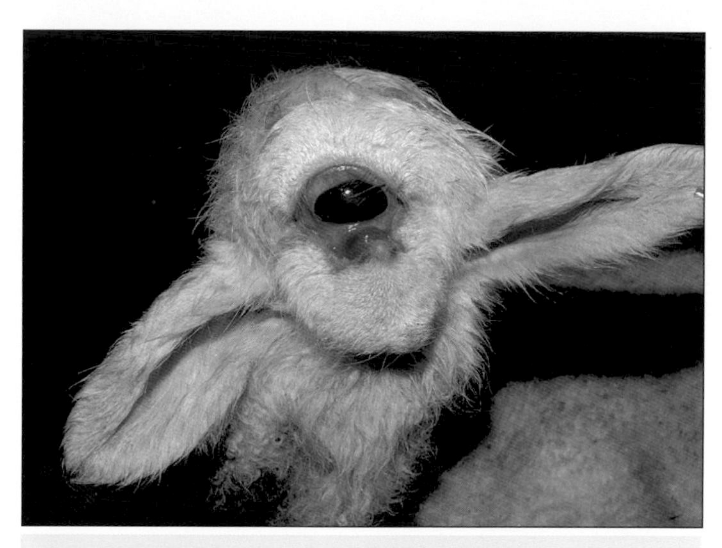

Figure 1.52 Cyclopia in a lamb. This deformity has been associated with ingestion of *Veratrum californicum* by pregnant ewes at around day 14 of gestation.

syndactyly and reduced number of coccygeal vertebrae. The length and diameter of all limb bones may be reduced, or the changes may be restricted to the metacarpals and metatarsals. Between days 30–36 of gestation, the teratogens selectively inhibit growth in length of the metacarpal and metatarsal bones.

V. californicum contains several steroidal alkaloids, the most active being cyclopamine, cycloposine, and jervine. *Cyclopamine is most abundant in the plant and is responsible for the craniofacial defects*, but the cause of the other anomalies is unknown.

A syndrome referred to as **crooked-calf disease** occurs when pregnant cows ingest certain **wild lupins**, including *Lupinus caudatus, L. sericeus,* and *L. formosus*, especially between days 40 and 80 of gestation. Malformation of the limbs, notably the forelimbs, is the most common alteration, but the axial skeleton may also be involved. *The limb abnormalities consist of flexion contracture and arthrogryposis associated with disordered growth of joints*, in addition to shortening and variable rotation of the bones. *Torticollis, and either scoliosis or kyphosis are common*, involvement of the thoracic spine being associated with costal deformities. There are various subtle and often asymmetric changes in the skull, where *the most definable malformations are cleft palate, or brachygnathia superior*. Affected calves are usually born alive and may survive, depending on the nature and severity of their malformations, but growth is retarded and the malformations persist, often becoming more severe with age. Neuromuscular structure and function are regarded as normal, or at least not primarily responsible for the skeletal deformity. No remarkable or consistent histological changes are reported in crooked calves.

Lupins contain several alkaloids, some of which are teratogenic. The quinolizidine alkaloid *anagyrine* is present in *L. caudatus* and *L. sericeus* and is almost certainly a teratogen. In *L. formosus* the piperidine alkaloid *ammodendrine* may be responsible. Inhibition of fetal movement caused by a sedative or anesthetic effect of the alkaloids may be the basis for the skeletal deformities. Alternatively, secondary effects of direct toxicity to the dam may be involved; sustained uterine contractions producing deformities in the fetus have been suggested. *Lupinus caudatus* (tailcup lupine) does not produce lesions in fetal lambs or kids, suggesting differences between cattle and other species in the metabolism of anagyrine.

Lupins cause two other distinct diseases in animals; a nervous disorder associated with the alkaloids in bitter lupins (see Vol. 1, Nervous system) and a mycotoxicosis caused by *Phomopsis leptostromiformis* (see Vol. 2, Liver and biliary system).

Conium maculatum (poison hemlock, European hemlock, spotted hemlock) is toxic to various species and causes a syndrome characterized by excitation and subsequent depression. There are five piperidine alkaloids in *C. maculatum*, the major ones being *coniine and γ-coniceine*. Both are thought to be toxic, and the latter teratogenic. Cattle are most susceptible, and there is decreasing susceptibility through sheep, horses, and pigs. *Conium maculatum* is also teratogenic, especially for cattle, with pigs being less susceptible and sheep relatively resistant. The plant causes *arthrogryposis and spinal deformities in the offspring of sows and cows* when fed between days 43–53 and 55–75 of gestation, respectively. *Cleft palate* occurs in the offspring of pigs exposed to the plant between days 30–45 and goats exposed between days 30 and 60 of gestation. *Carpal flexure* occurred in lambs and kids when *Conium* was fed to pregnant ewes and goats from days 30–60 of gestation, but resolved spontaneously as they grew.

Nicotiana tabacum (burley tobacco) causes arthrogryposis and sometimes brachygnathia and kyphosis in piglets exposed to the plant in utero. ***Nicotiana glauca*** (wild tree tobacco) causes similar lesions and also produces arthrogryposis and spinal deformities in calves exposed between days 45–75 of gestation. The teratogen is an α-substituted piperidine alkaloid, anabasine, which is present also in *N. tabacum*. It produces the lesions when given between days 43 and 53 of gestation and causes cleft palate when administered between days 30 and 37.

Jimsonweed (*Datura stramonium*) and **wild black cherry** (*Prunus serotina*) are suspected teratogens in sows, both being linked to *arthrogryposis*.

Various etiologies, including plant toxicities, have been incriminated in a limb deformity syndrome of lambs referred to as **"bent leg."** In Australia, the syndrome has been associated with ingestion of *Trachymene ochracea* (white parsnip), *T. cyanantha* and *T. glaucifolia* (wild parsnip) by ewes, which preferentially graze the inflorescence of *Trachymene* sp. The toxic principle is unknown, but the deformity may either be congenital, due to exposure of lambs in utero, or may develop during postnatal growth, probably following exposure of lambs through the milk. Gross deformities are usually most prominent in the forelimbs, and include outward bowing, flexion, and lateral rotation of the carpal joints and medial or lateral rotation of the fetlocks. Similar syndromes are described in New Zealand (where it is called **"bowie"**) and South Africa, but plant toxicities are not suspected. In both of these conditions, calcium deficiency and osteoporotic bone disease play a major role in the weakening and deformity that develop. Further discussion of these syndromes is included later in this chapter under the heading "Angular limb deformity."

Outbreaks of congenital limb deformity and abortion have been reported in cattle, sheep, and horses in association with ingestion of **locoweed** (species of *Astragalus* and *Oxytropis*) by pregnant animals. The abnormalities include *brachygnathia, contracture or over-extension of joints, limb rotations, osteoporosis, and bone fragility*. The toxic agent responsible for the skeletal defects is not known but is most likely unrelated to that responsible for the neurological manifestations of locoweed toxicity (see Vol. 1, Nervous system), which inhibits the lysosomal enzyme α-mannosidase, inducing a lysosomal storage disease.

The leguminous plant ***Lathyrus odoratus*** (sweet pea) contains the amino acid β-aminopropionitrile, which inhibits lysyl oxidase and interferes with the formation of intermolecular cross-links in collagen and elastin. Skeletal deformities have been produced experimentally when the plant was fed to young rats, but natural disease associated with ingestion by grazing animals is unlikely.

Fetal ankylosis and abortion are recorded in foals whose dams graze **hybrid sorghum and Sudan grass** (*Sorghum sudanense*) during days 20–50 of gestation, and a similar association has been made in cattle. The lesions in foals involve many joints but are not well described. It is not clear whether the foals have ankylosis or arthrogryposis.

Other toxicities

Overdosing of ewes with the anthelmintic **parbendazole** between days 12–24 of gestation may produce skeletal abnormalities in a high proportion of lambs. Neurologic lesions may also be present (see Vol. 1, Nervous system). The skeletal malformations include compression and/or fusion of vertebral bodies, fusion of proximal ribs, curvature of long bones, hypoplasia of articular surfaces and absence of various bones such as ulna, humerus, and metacarpals. Lesions are reliably reproduced by a double dose of the drug and may even occur with less than twice the recommended dose.

A range of fetal abnormalities, including twisted limbs, brachygnathia inferior, and arthrogryposis is reported in several sheep flocks in New Zealand where ewes had been affected by **nitrate toxicity** during early pregnancy. The ewes had been fed during the winter on crops containing high levels of nitrate and although the evidence to incriminate nitrate toxicity as the cause of fetal abnormalities was circumstantial, the possible involvement of agents such as pestivirus and *Akabane virus* was excluded. The problem occurred on seven properties and the incidence of abnormal lambs varied from 1 to 11%.

Bibliography

Abbot LC, et al. Crooked calf disease: A histological and histochemical examination of eight affected calves. Vet Pathol 1986;23:734–740.

Clark L, et al. Observations on the pathology of bent leg of lambs in south-western Queensland. Aust Vet J 1975;51:4–10.

Crowe MW, Swerczek TW. Congenital arthrogryposis in offspring of sows fed tobacco (*Nicotiana tabacum*). Am J Vet Res 1974;35:1071–1073.

Dyson DA, Wrathall AE. Congenital deformities in pigs possibly associated with exposure to hemlock (*Conium maculatum*). Vet Rec 1977;100:241–242.

Gumbrell RC. Nitrate poisoning and foetal abnormalities in sheep. Surveillance 1990;17:10–11.

James LF. Syndromes of locoweed poisoning in livestock. Clin Toxicol 1972;5:567–573.

Keeler RF. Alkaloid teratogens from *Lupinus, Conium, Veratrum* and related genera. In: Keeler RF, et al. eds. Effects of Poisonous Plants on Livestock. New York: Academic Press, 1978:397–408.

Keeler RF. Early embryonic death in lambs induced by *Veratrum californicum*. Cornell Vet 1990;80:203–207.

Leipold HW, et al. Congenital arthrogryposis associated with ingestion of jimsonweed by pregnant sows. J Am Vet Med Assoc 1973;162:1059–1060.

McIlwraith CW, James LF. Limb deformities in foals associated with ingestion of locoweed by mares. J Am Vet Med Assoc 1982;181:255–258.

Morgan SE, et al. Sorghum cystitis ataxia syndrome in horses. Vet Human Toxicol 1990;32:582. (References to teratogenicity)

Panter KE, Keeler RF. Quinolizidine and piperidine alkaloid teratogens from poisonous plants and their mechanism of action in animals. Vet Clinics North Am 1993;9:33–40.

Panter KE, et al. Congenital skeletal malformations and cleft palate induced in goats by ingestion of *Lupinus, Conium* and *Nicotiana* species. Toxicon 1990;12:1377–1385. (Review with references to other species)

Philbey AW. *Trachymene glaucifolia* associated with bentleg in lambs. Aust Vet J 1990;67:468.

Prozesky L, et al. Paralysis in lambs caused by overdosing with parbendazole. Onderstepoort J Vet Res 1981;48:159–167.

Selby LA, et al. Outbreak of swine malformations associated with the wild black cherry, *Prunus serotina*. Arch Environ Health 1971;22:496–501.

Skeletal anomalies of unknown etiology

A syndrome of neonatal foals, characterized by **thyroid hyperplasia** *accompanied by* **musculoskeletal deformities,** has been recognized in western Canada for several years. The skeletal abnormalities include mandibular prognathia, flexural deformities of the forelimbs, ruptured common and deep digital extensor tendons, and delayed ossification of carpal and tarsal bones. In some affected foals, abnormal development of carpal bones, especially the third carpal, is considered to cause angular limb deformity. Lesions typical of osteochondrosis are sometimes present on articular surfaces of carpal bones, perhaps secondary to delayed ossification and increased susceptibility to injury during weight bearing. Hyperplasia of the thyroid gland is a consistent finding in affected foals, and similar abnormalities have been reproduced in partially thyroidectomized foals, but the etiology is not known. Unlike iodine deficiency goiter, the thyroid glands in foals with this syndrome usually are only slightly enlarged, if at all, and could easily be overlooked if not examined microscopically. The syndrome is not genetic and it is considered that *some factor in the feed, perhaps a mycotoxin or plant toxin,* is responsible for interfering with thyroid function, leading to skeletal and other changes normally associated with hypothyroidism. Exposure to cruciferous plants may be responsible.

A syndrome characterized by the birth of deformed calves with a range of abnormalities including joint laxity, disproportionate dwarfism, and sometimes varus or valgus forelimb deformities is well recognized in the western United States, Canada, and Australia. Severely affected calves walk on the palmar and plantar surfaces of their phalanges and some have brachygnathia superior. Originally called **"acorn calves"** because the defect was attributed to ingestion of acorns by pregnant cows, this etiology has now been dispelled, but the name persists in the literature. In Canada, the disease has been referred to as **congenital joint laxity and dwarfism.** Although the actual cause is not known, nutritional deficiency or possibly ingestion of a toxin by the dam, probably between 3 and 6 months of gestation, is suspected. Up to 10% of calves may be affected in herds grazing native pastures of foothills in the western United States. Similar environmental conditions occur in Australia, but the disease incidence tends to be lower, and in Canada where 2–40% of calves in a herd may be affected. The calves usually survive but do not prosper.

In Canada the disease is produced by feeding grass/legume silage during gestation and prevented by adding hay and grain to the silage ration. Timothy grass, fed as silage, produces the disease while timothy from the same fields fed as hay does not. It is suspected that fermentation of silage leading to production of mycotoxins, in particular those from *Fusarium*, is responsible.

Other, isolated examples of generalized abnormalities do occur sporadically. For example, forelimb abnormalities, resembling human "thalidomide babies," affected up to 29% of beef calves in two herds in Australia. There was an axial malformation in one calf and congenital blindness in another, but otherwise the lesions were restricted to the forelimbs. The scapulae were present and usually completely cartilaginous, but distal portions of the limbs were either vestigial or absent. A teratogen was suspected but health and management records provided no clues.

A disproportionate dwarfism in two dairy Shorthorn siblings also occurred in Australia, and was characterized by marked shortening of the pelvic limbs, mild shortening of pectoral limbs, and a normal axial skeleton. Retardation of growth in the femurs, tibias, and metatarsals was prominent, and there was deformity of the femorotibial joints. The calves were affected at birth, suggesting that this syndrome may be *different from hyena disease* (see above), which may be a manifestation of vitamin A toxicity. In hyena disease, the abnormality is usually not apparent until 3–4 months of age.

Bibliography

Allen AL, et al. The effects of partial thyroidectomy on the development of the equine fetus. Equine Vet J 1998;30:53–59.

Barry MR, Murphy WJB. Acorn calves in the Albury district of New South Wales. Aust Vet J 1964;40:195–201.

Carrig CB, et al. Disproportionate dwarfism in two bovine siblings. Vet Radiol 1981;22:78–82.

Harbutt PR, et al. Congenital forelimb abnormalities in calves. Aust Vet J 1965;41:173–177.

McLaughlan BG, Doige CE. A study of ossification of the carpal and tarsal bones in normal and hypothyroid foals. Can Vet J 1982;23:164–168.

Angular limb deformity

Angular limb deformities are relatively common in young animals of several domestic species, particularly in fast-growing breeds. In many cases, the deformity can be traced to an asymmetric lesion involving an active growth plate, such as the distal radius, but growth plate damage is not always the underlying cause, and even when it is, the etiology is often not apparent. Abnormal development of carpal or tarsal bones is also reported as causing limb deformities, especially in horses, as has joint instability due to laxity of supporting structures. *Lateral deviation* of the limb distal to the affected growth plate or joint is referred to as a **valgus deformity** and *medial deviation* as a **varus deformity**.

In **horses**, angular limb deformities occur primarily in young foals and are included with a group of disorders referred to as *developmental orthopedic diseases*. A variety of congenital and acquired lesions have been identified in foals with limb deformities and in many cases it is not possible to determine which changes are primary and which are secondary. The abnormality is often centered on the carpal, tarsal, or fetlock joints. Many foals are born with weakness of the supporting periarticular tissues of these joints and have minor structural abnormalities in the osteochondral junctions of developing joint surfaces or the physes of adjacent bones. These minor defects are often clinically manifest as angular limb deformities at birth but most resolve spontaneously within the first week or two of life. During this period, the periarticular attachments strengthen and any regions of physis or developing joint surface that are subjected to extra strain or compressive force during locomotion or weight bearing compensate by an increase in the rate of endochondral ossification. This allows correction of most minor structural abnormalities. If the deformity is more severe, the compensatory mechanisms are exceeded and the deformity will persist without intervention.

Congenital **defects in carpal and tarsal bones** are reported as a *cause of angular limb deformity in newborn foals*. The bones may be abnormal in size or contour, or may possess osteochondrosis-like lesions, both of which can alter the alignment of bones within the joint and therefore the angle of the lower limb. As described above, these lesions may occur in association with other musculoskeletal abnormalities and thyroid hyperplasia. Delayed ossification of affected bones due to hypothyroidism is suggested as a possible mechanism. Even in foals with no evidence of hypothyroidism, the bones of the carpus and tarsus vary considerably in their degree of ossification at birth. In premature foals, or foals with inadequate mineralization of these bones, any minor conformational defects associated with joint laxity may become permanent due to abnormal compression and plastic deformation of the thick cartilaginous layer.

Physeal lesions are occasionally present at birth but are more often the cause of acquired angular limb deformities during the first 6 months of life. *Physes are the weakest structure in the developing ends of long bones and are very susceptible to injury.* In rapidly growing young foals, physeal lesions may also occur as a manifestation of osteochondrosis. The physes most at risk of both trauma and osteochondrosis are those that grow most rapidly, such as the distal radius. Other common sites are the distal physes of the metacarpals and metatarsals, the distal physis of the tibia and the proximal physis of the first phalanx. Such lesions, if detected radiographically as thickened foci in the growth plate, are *often termed "physitis" or "epiphysitis,"* both of which create the misleading impression that they are primarily inflammatory. *These are essentially clinical terms and should not be used by pathologists.* Although many lesions of this type resolve spontaneously without causing clinical disease, some will predispose to angular limb deformity. Microscopically, the lesions of "physitis" reflect focal disruption of endochondral ossification and resemble those associated with osteochondrosis. Septic infection of bone in young foals may also involve physes, causing destruction of the growth cartilage (Fig. 1.53) (see osteomyelitis, in Inflammatory diseases of bones). Foals that survive such infections may develop angular limb deformity.

In **dogs**, angular limb deformity is most commonly associated with *premature closure of the distal ulnar physis*, which is particularly susceptible to trauma, presumably because of its conical shape. If the physis of the adjacent radius continues to grow, the resultant asynchrony will induce valgus deformity. The syndrome occurs most often in large breeds but is described as an autosomal recessive trait in the Skye Terrier. Less frequently, angular limb deformity in young pups results from a lesion in either the proximal or distal physis of the radius, the latter being the most common. Such lesions may be due to a fracture through the hypertrophic zone of the

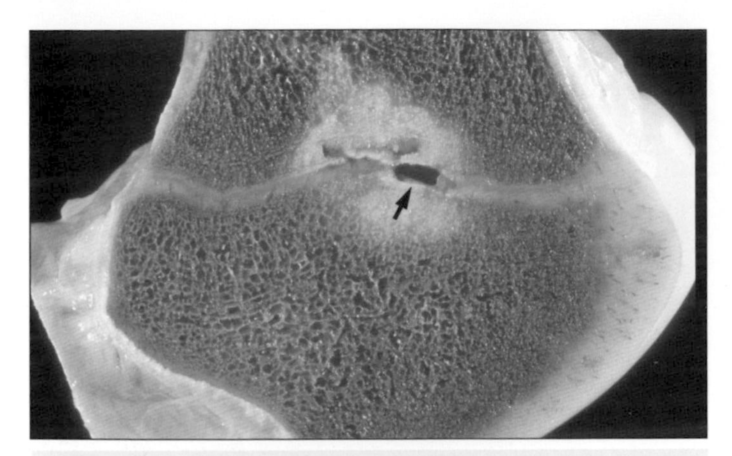

Figure 1.53 Septic physitis and osteomyelitis causing disruption of the distal femoral growth plate in a young foal. Had the foal survived, there would have been fusion between the epiphysis and metaphysis in the area of physeal disruption (arrow) possibly leading to angular limb deformity.

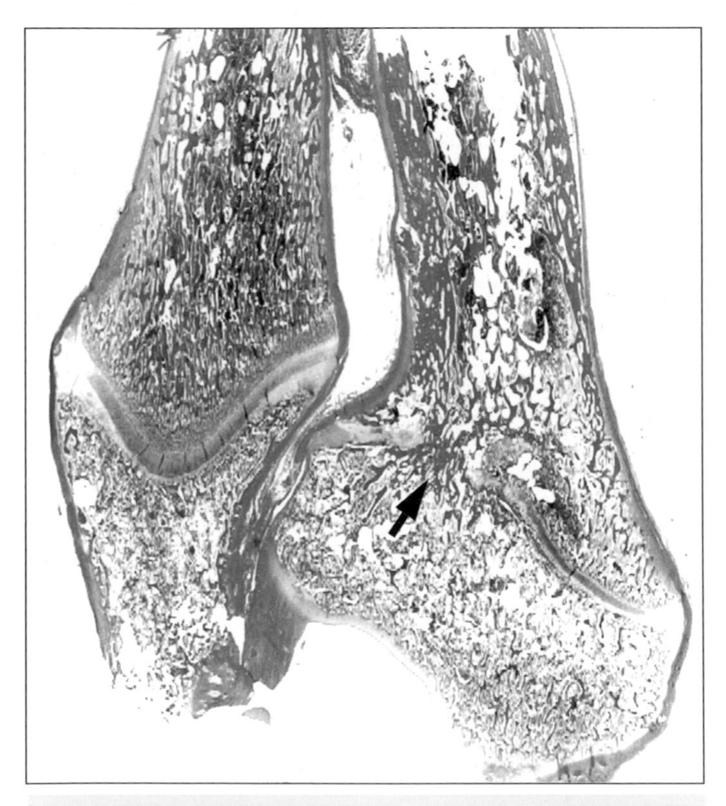

Figure 1.54 Distal radius and ulna from a pup with **angular limb deformity** secondary to traumatic damage to the radial physis. One side of the physis has been destroyed and is penetrated by thick bony trabeculae (arrow). Fusion of the epiphysis and metaphysis on this side has prevented further growth, while growth has continued from the undamaged segment of physis, resulting in angular deformity. (Courtesy of DH Read.)

growth plate, or to a crushing force transmitted through the epiphyseal bone. If the injury affects just one side of the growth plate, and growth continues on the other side, angular deformity will result (Fig. 1.54). Premature closure of the distal tibial physis, resulting in curvature of the tibia/fibula, also occurs occasionally in pups.

In large dogs, especially Great Danes, *closure of the distal ulnar growth plate can be confused with retarded endochondral ossification* (retained endochondral cartilage core). Although the clinical manifestations are often similar, the underlying lesion and its pathogenesis are different. The lesion is bilateral, often clinically silent, and may heal uneventfully. Large retained cores are more likely to interfere with longitudinal growth of the ulna and cause angular deformity. The lesion consists of a cone-shaped mass of unmineralized hypertrophic cartilage with its base at the center of the ulnar growth plate and its apex projecting into the metaphysis (Fig. 1.55A, B). The periphery of the plate is normal. The cause of the abnormality is not known but it could be a manifestation of osteochondrosis, or perhaps due to a temporary interruption or insufficiency in the metaphyseal blood supply. Retained cartilage in the distal ulna occurred in nine of nine pups in two successive litters of captive Mackenzie Valley timber wolves and was associated with limb deformities in all animals.

Angular limb deformity is also described in young, rapidly growing **sheep**, in different parts of the world and is often referred to as **"bent leg"** or **"bowie."** It is relatively common in ram lambs in feedlots, but also occurs in pasture-fed lambs. The forelimbs are affected more frequently than the hindlimbs and the deformity be either unilateral or bilateral, and either valgus or varus (Fig. 1.56A). The etiology is not known, but there is a *strong association with high-energy rations and rapid growth*, suggesting a nutritional component. Dietary imbalances of calcium and phosphorus have been implicated but not proven. One outbreak involved approximately 100 of 160 lambs, 6–9 weeks of age, some of which had been implanted with an anabolic hormone to increase growth rate. Bowie was common in sheep grazing unimproved hill country in New Zealand during the 1950s, involving up to 40% of lambs on some properties, but is now rare. The etiology was never identified but superphosphate topdressing was partially effective in controlling the disease.

Most reports of angular limb deformity in sheep describe gross and microscopic lesions in the *fast-growing physis of the distal radius*, and to a lesser extent in the *distal metacarpals or metatarsals*. The lesions typically consist of *focal or segmental thickening of the physis* (Fig. 1.56B) due to expansion of the hypertrophic zone with extension into the proximal metaphysis. These lesions closely resemble the physeal manifestations of osteochondrosis in foals and pigs, a syndrome that also occurs in rapidly growing young animals, predominantly males (see later in this chapter), and it is likely that the etiology and pathogenesis are similar. Although rickets may also produce similar lesions, there is no evidence of impaired provisional mineralization of cartilage in animals with bent leg, or of reduced bone strength, as would be expected in rickets.

Angular limb deformity is also described in young **goats**, especially those of *fast-growing dairy breeds*, when fed concentrate rations. Males are affected more often than females. The signs of deformity usually are first noticed around the time of weaning at 2–3 months of age, but occasionally in kids only a few days old. Many affected kids recover spontaneously by the time they are 5 months old. *Focal thickening of the physes of the distal radius or distal metacarpal is the characteristic gross lesion* and microscopically these consist of persistent hypertrophic chondrocytes. The syndrome is probably analogous to that in lambs and may be a manifestation of osteochondrosis.

In contrast, limb deformities reported in **llamas** and **fallow deer** have been in animals that are in poor condition and small for their age, suggesting a different mechanism. In llamas, the deformity is almost invariably valgus and centered on the distal radial physis. Radiographic evidence suggests that the deformities in this species

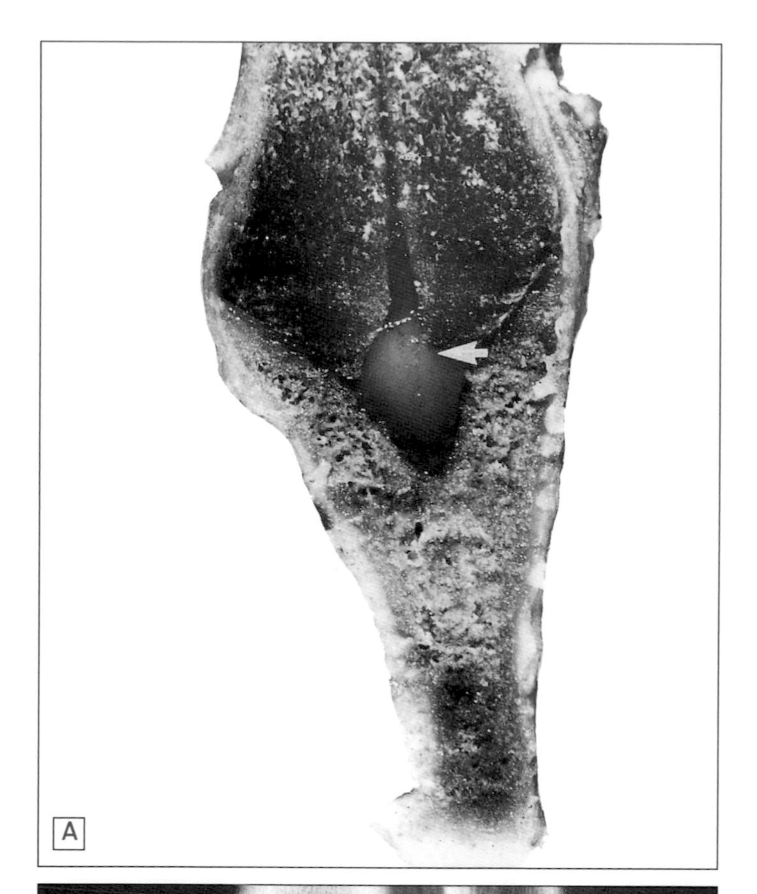

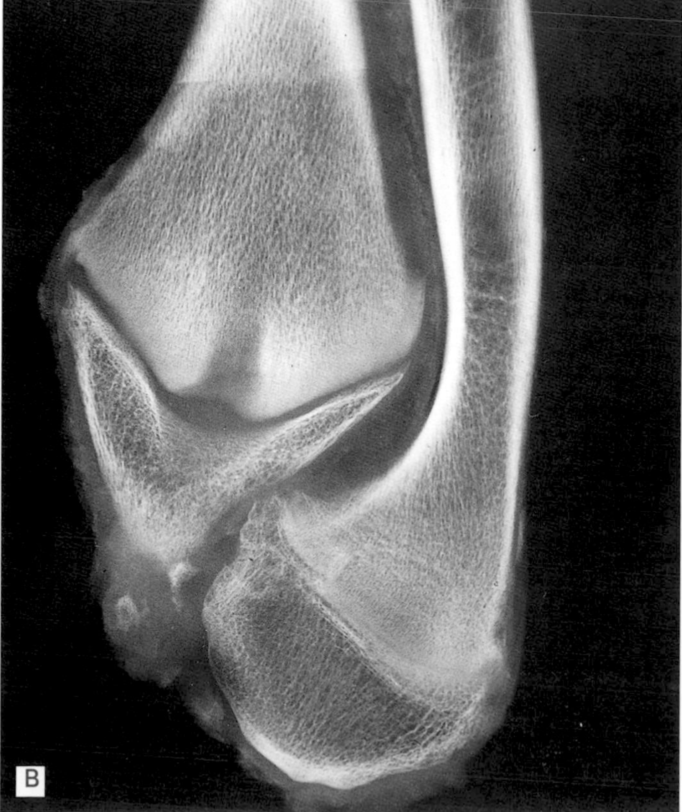

Figure 1.55 Retained cartilage core in the distal ulna of a dog. **A.** A mass of unresorbed physeal cartilage (arrow) projects into the metaphysis. **B.** Slab radiograph showing retained cartilage core in distal ulna of a dog with angular limb deformity secondary to reduced growth from the ulna physis.

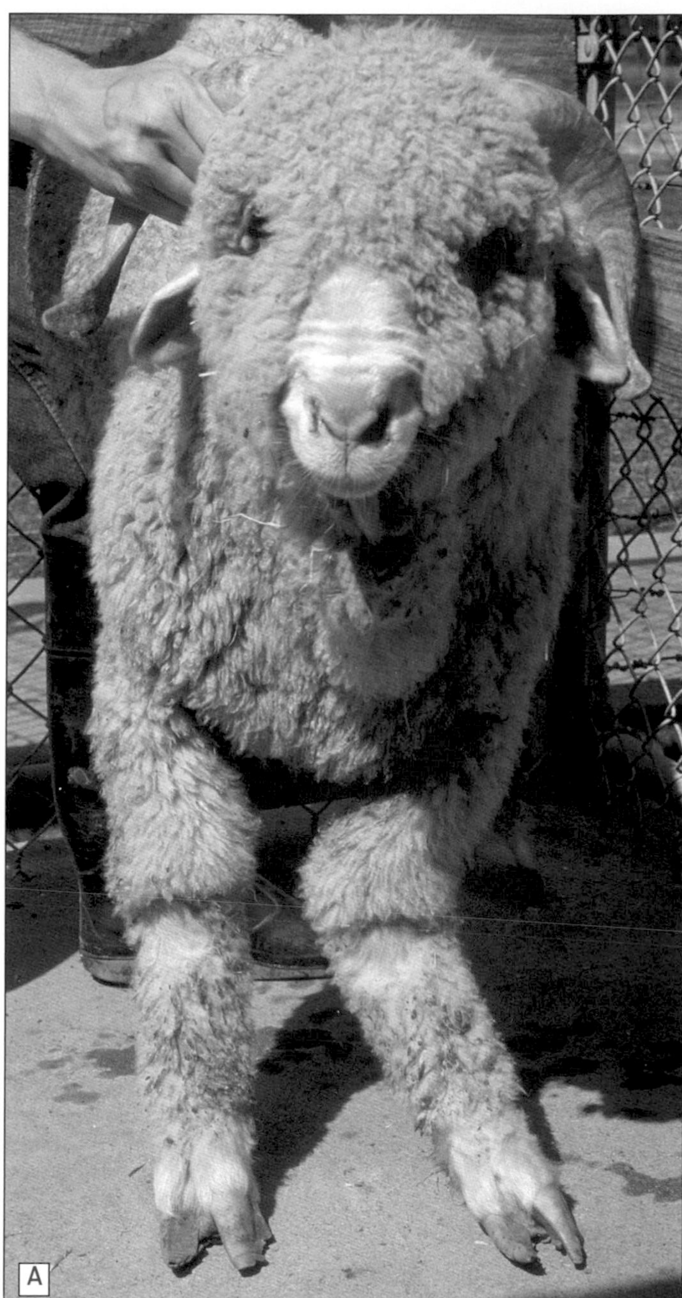

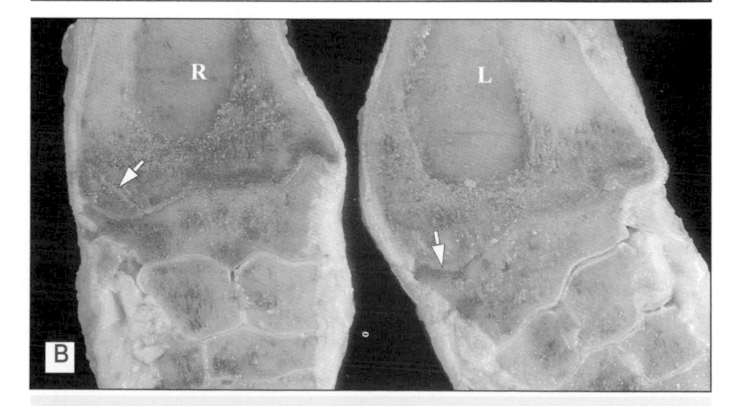

Figure 1.56 Angular limb deformity in a sheep. **A.** Varus deformity of the right foreleg and valgus deformity of the left in a young Rambouillet ram. **B.** Distal radial physes from the same ram. Note the focal duplication of the physeal cartilage (arrow) in the right leg (R) and focal thickening of the physis (arrow) in the left leg (L). In both legs, the physeal abnormalities are on the side that has grown more.

are due to premature closure of the distal ulnar physis, as occurs in dogs. In one report describing several cases of limb deformity in an inbred group of llamas, a genetic etiology was suggested, but not proven. A high incidence of limb deformity was recorded in fallow deer from a large deer park in the United Kingdom. In these animals, the lesion was usually centered on the distal metacarpal or metatarsal physes. Thickening of the physes was seen radiographically and grossly only in deer less than 1 year of age, while deformities were detected only in older deer whose growth plates had fused. In addition to the physeal lesions, some affected deer had widened metaphyses. Also, young deer in the park had previously been found with spontaneous fractures, suggesting the possibility of a metabolic bone disease, such as rickets. *The physeal lesions of rickets could predispose to angular limb deformity* and may have been involved on this property. Such physeal lesions could also be involved in angular limb deformities in llamas as camelids appear to be more susceptible to rickets than other grazing ruminants, especially when farmed at low altitudes (see p. 76).

Bibliography

Auer JA, et al. Angular limb deformity in foals part II. Developmental factors. Compend Contin Educ Pract Vet 1983;5:S27–S35.

Carrig CB. Growth abnormalities of the canine radius and ulna. Vet Clin North Am: Small Anim Pract 1983;13:91–115.

Chapman DI, et al. Deformities of the metacarpus and metatarsus in fallow deer (*Dama dama* L.) J Comp Path 1984;94:77–91.

Fitch LWN. Osteodystrophic diseases of sheep in New Zealand II-"bowie" or "bent-leg". NZ Vet J 1954;2:118–122.

Henney LHS, Gambardella PC. Premature closure of the ulnar physis in the dog: A retrospective clinical study. J Am An Hosp Ass 1989;25:573–581.

McErlean BA, McAllister H. Osteodystrophy in unweaned lambs. Irish Vet J 1982;36:39–41.

Ossent P, et al. Retained cartilage in the ulnar metaphysis with deformation of the forelegs in two litters of captive wolves. Zbl Veterinaermed A 1984;30: 241–250.

Paul-Murphy JR, et al. Radiographic findings in young llamas with forelimb valgus deformities: 28 cases (1980–1988). J Am Vet Med Assoc 1991;198:2107–2111.

Ramadan RO, Vaughan LC. Disturbance in the growth of the tibia and femur in dogs. Vet Rec 1979;104:433–435.

Vandewater A, Olmstead ML. Premature closure of the distal radial physis in the dog. A review of eleven cases. Vet Surg 1983;12:7–12.

Effect of infectious agents on skeletal development and remodeling

Various infectious agents, in particular viruses, have been shown to infect bone cells and induce abnormalities in the developing skeleton. Infectious agents causing inflammatory changes in bones are discussed in a later section (see Inflammatory diseases of bones). Discussion here is confined to those infectious agents that influence skeletal development *by directly influencing the activity of bone cells*.

The ***Bovine viral diarrhea virus*** (BVDV) has been associated with the formation of zones of metaphyseal sclerosis parallel to the growth plate, referred to as **growth retardation lattices**, in aborted calves following maternal infection (Fig. 1.57A, B). These lattices consist of zones of persistent primary spongiosa with increased cross-connections between cartilage spicules (Fig. 1.57C), presumably reflecting transient periods of impaired osteoclastic activity. Similar zonal **osteopetrosis-like lesions** have also been linked to type 2 BVDV infection in older calves, up to 4 months of age. In these calves, a dense lattice of persistent primary spongiosa adjacent to growth plates contrasted sharply with the apparently normal trabecular arrangement deeper in the metaphysis. The paucity of osteoclasts detected histologically in affected calves, and reduced cellularity of marrow spaces, suggests that *viral destruction of osteoclasts*, or osteoclast precursors, is a likely mechanism for the lesion. It is possible that some cases of osteopetrosis in calves where there is widespread persistence of the secondary spongiosa might be caused by intrauterine viral infection but no specific agent has been incriminated.

Classical swine fever virus, which is closely related to BVDV, causes similar lesions in pigs that survive the acute phase of the disease.

Growth retardation lattices similar to those described in calves have been observed in association with natural and experimental infection by ***Canine distemper virus*** (Fig. 1.58), and in cats infected with ***Feline herpesvirus***. In experimental infections in weanling dogs, viral antigen was demonstrated by immunocytochemistry in osteoclasts, osteoblasts, and less often in osteocytes, from about day 5 to day 41 after infection. Viral antigen was most abundant in bone cells of the primary spongiosa and was strongly correlated with osseous changes, which were most prominent between days 26 and 32 post-infection. Impaired osteoclastic resorption of the primary spongiosa was considered the likely pathogenesis and was supported by the detection of necrotic osteoclasts. The lesions were transitory and resolved once viral antigen disappeared.

The term "growth retardation lattice" has become widely used for lesions of the type described here and in association with lead poisoning, but it creates a misleading impression of the nature of the lesion and *could easily be confused with "growth arrest lines."* The lattice of persistent primary or secondary spongiosa that comprises the former lesion is the result of reduced osteoclastic activity, not reduced growth of the bone. Physeal cartilage is not necessarily affected and growth in length of the bones may be continuing normally. In contrast, growth arrest lines, as discussed earlier in this section, occur when physeal growth ceases then commences again later. *The two lesions differ both in pathogenesis and in microscopic appearance, and should not be confused.*

Toxigenic strains of ***Pasteurella multocida*** cause osteoblast necrosis and are associated with the development of atrophic rhinitis in pigs.

Bibliography

Baumgärtner W, et al. Histologic and immunocytochemical characterization of canine distemper-associated metaphyseal bone lesions in young dogs following experimental infection. Vet Pathol 1995;32:702–709.

Done JT, et al. Bovine virus diarrhea-mucosal disease virus: pathogenicity for the fetal calf following maternal infection. Vet Rec 1980;106:473–479.

Scruggs DW, et al. Osteopetrosis, anemia, thrombocytopenia, and marrow necrosis in beef calves naturally infected with bovine virus diarrhea virus. J Vet Diagn Invest 1995;7:555–559.

Wolf DC, Van Alstine WG. Osteopetrosis in five fetuses from a single herd of 16 cows. J Vet Diagn Invest 1989;1:262–264.

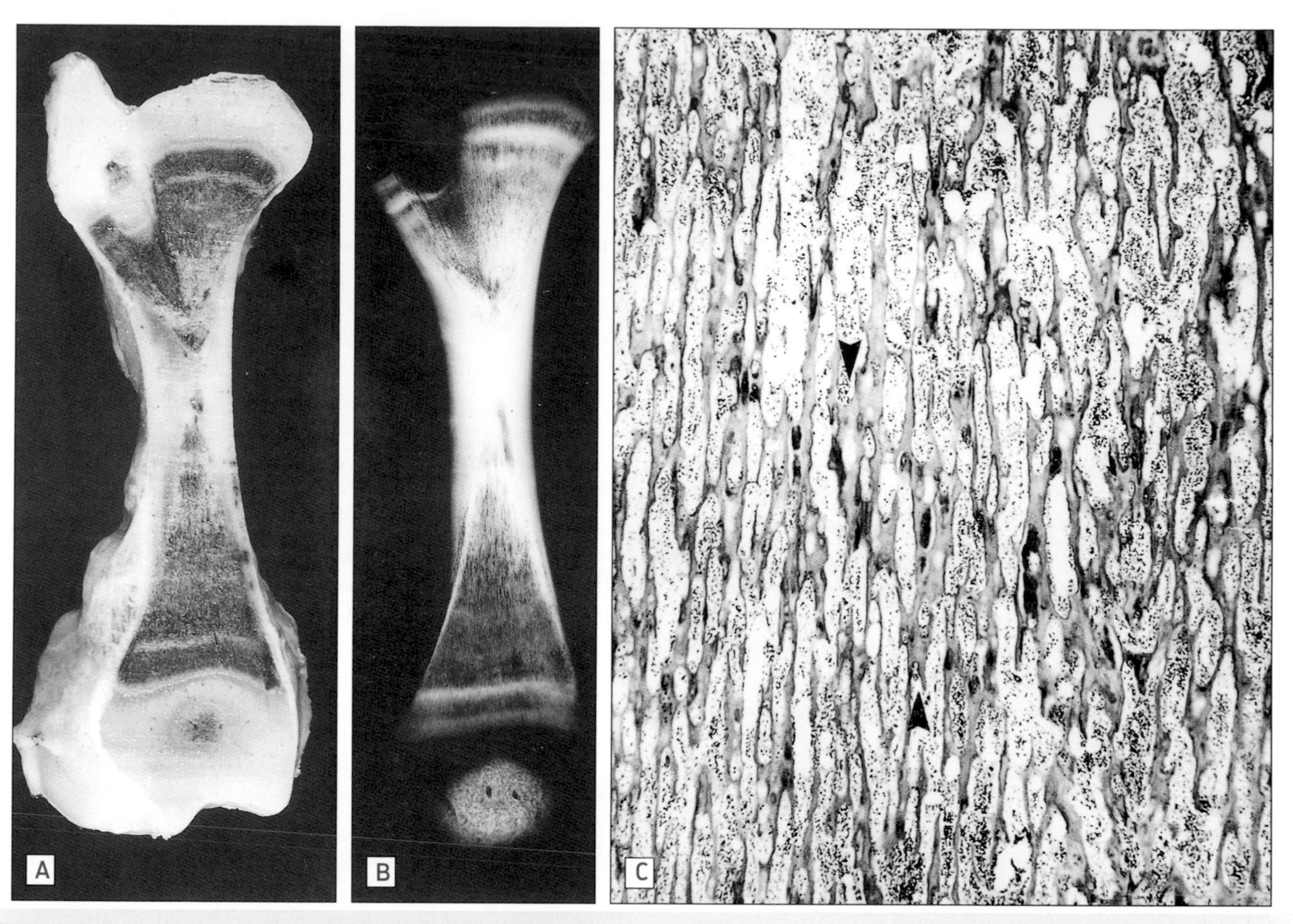

Figure 1.57 Bovine fetus. Intrauterine ***Bovine viral diarrhea virus* infection**. **A.** Narrow sclerotic bands in the metaphyses and relative persistence of medullary bone. **B.** Radiograph of (**A**) showing increased radiographic density of the metaphyseal bands and diaphysis. **C.** Histological preparation of the metaphysis, showing persistence of the primary spongiosa and a poorly defined zone (between arrowheads) where there are increased numbers of cross-connections between cartilage spicules. This corresponds to the sclerotic band seen grossly and radiographically.

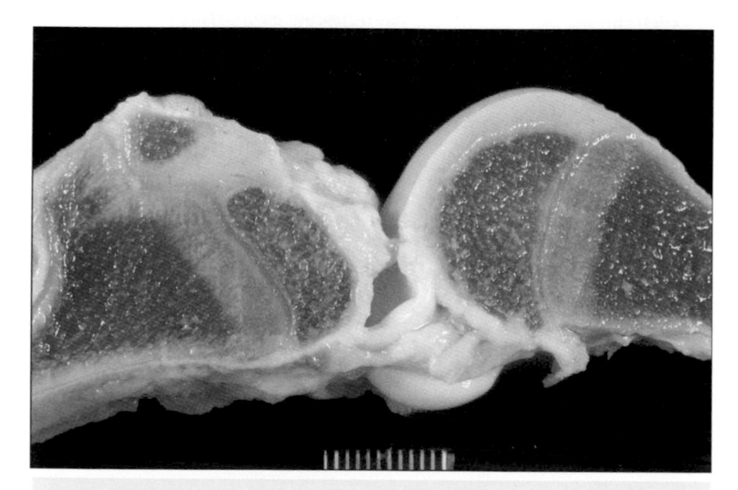

Figure 1.58 ***Canine distemper virus* infection** in a pup. Note the thick bands of metaphyseal sclerosis adjacent to the physes in the distal femur and proximal tibia. (Courtesy of TM Monticello.)

METABOLIC BONE DISEASES

Metabolic bone diseases, also referred to as **osteodystrophies**, *are the result of disturbed bone growth, modeling, or remodeling due to either nutritional or hormonal imbalances.* Because of the complexity of the processes involved in bone development, errors may occur at many stages, the consequences varying with the nature and severity of the imbalance. Genetic defects involving specific enzymes or receptors critical to the activity of hormones or cells participating in bone formation are also reported as causing metabolic bone disease in man and animals, but these are rare. The manifestations of metabolic bone diseases are generally most severe in young animals where the skeleton is undergoing rapid turnover, but lesions also occur in adults due to an effect on the quality or quantity of bone formed during remodeling. In addition to variations with age, there are variations between species in the manifestations of dietary mineral imbalances.

Metabolic bone diseases are traditionally classified as **rickets, osteomalacia, fibrous osteodystrophy**, or **osteoporosis**. Although these are distinct morphological entities with characteristic pathogenesis and lesions, *they can occur in combination in the same individual*. This may create confusion diagnostically. Furthermore, *their etiology can vary between species*. For example, calcium deficiency in sheep is likely to result in osteoporosis, but in a rapidly growing pig, fibrous osteodystrophy is a more likely result. Also, each of these disorders can be caused by more than one dietary or endocrine imbalance. The distinguishing features of each entity, together with their etiology, pathogenesis, and occurrence in different species are discussed in detail below. The term **osteopenia** is often used to describe syndromes associated with increased radiolucency of bone, but makes no inference as to its quality. As such, it includes osteoporosis, where only the quantity of bone is abnormal, as well as osteomalacia, fibrous osteodystrophy, and osteogenesis imperfecta, where the bone is not only reduced, it is abnormal in quality.

Since bone matrix is composed largely of calcium and phosphate ions in the form of hydroxyapatite crystals, any dietary or physiological factors affecting the metabolism of calcium and/or phosphorus can interfere with the formation of bone tissue and cause an osteodystrophy. Because of the importance of these two elements in bone formation, and hence in the etiology of metabolic bone diseases, a brief review of their homeostasis is presented below. Vitamin D and parathyroid hormone are integral components of homeostatic control mechanisms for calcium and phosphorus and their role also is discussed.

Metabolic bone diseases can usually be treated successfully, providing the problem is recognized early enough and there are no lasting effects caused by pathologic fractures or disruption of growth plates in young, growing animals. However, in cases where severe generalized osteoporosis has developed, insufficient bone surfaces may remain to allow appositional bone deposition to proceed and affected animals remain susceptible to hypocalcemic crises and the deleterious effects of chronically weakened bones. In production animals, an early and accurate diagnosis is important if significant economic loss is to be avoided. This requires a good history, recognition of species differences and an ability to accurately interpret radiographic and/or pathologic alterations. Whenever possible, more than one affected animal should be examined as the lesions may vary in severity between animals even if they are being fed the same ration. *It is important to examine and sample bones from several sites, particularly those that are showing obvious abnormalities and those from sites of rapid growth or movement. This includes the physes of the distal radius, proximal humerus, proximal tibia, distal femur, and costochondral junctions of the largest ribs.*

In reality, metabolic bone diseases seldom result from a deficiency of a single dietary nutrient. *More often, there is either a deficiency of several nutrients or a dietary imbalance in the ratio of calcium and phosphorus.* Diseases of other organ systems, especially gastrointestinal disorders that cause malabsorption, can affect the skeleton by reducing the absorption of essential minerals or vitamins. Metabolic bone disease also occurs in humans and animals in association with renal failure, due to interference with mineral metabolism and reduced synthesis of 1,25-dihydroxyvitamin D. This will be discussed in more detail below. Hepatobiliary and pancreatic disorders can, at least potentially, predispose to osteodystrophy through impaired absorption of vitamin D and other nutrients, but this is seldom recognized in domestic animals.

Calcium and phosphorus homeostasis

Calcium and phosphorus are required for a variety of essential bodily functions in addition to those involving skeletal development. *Approximately 99% of the calcium in the body is present in the skeleton as hydroxyapatite, the remaining 1% being contained in extracellular fluids and soft tissues.* The concentration of calcium in extracellular fluids and in the cytosol must be kept within narrow limits in order to maintain critical functions such as muscle contraction, neuromuscular irritability, blood coagulation, and mineralization of bone matrix. A small fraction of the calcium in bone (about 1%) is freely exchangeable with the extracellular fluid compartment. The skeleton is therefore an important storage site for calcium, providing a readily available source should dietary levels become temporarily deficient. Phosphorus is also a component of hydroxyapatite in bone matrix but, like calcium, has other essential functions; in particular the generation and transfer of cellular energy. *Approximately 85% of the phosphorus in the body is included in the skeleton.*

There are *three distinct fractions of calcium* in extracellular fluids (including plasma); an ionized fraction (about 50%), a protein-bound fraction (about 40%), and calcium complexed to other ions such as citrate and phosphate (about 10%). The *ionized fraction of calcium (Ca^{2+}) is the physiologically active form* and is tightly controlled by the actions of parathyroid hormone, 1,25-dihydroxyvitamin D and calcitonin on the intestinal tract, skeleton and, to a lesser extent, the kidney. Most of the protein-bound calcium is bound to albumin and plasma concentrations vary with the concentrations of plasma albumin. The binding of calcium to albumin is highly pH-dependent. Acute acidosis decreases binding and increases ionized calcium concentrations, while acute alkalosis increases binding and reduces the concentration of ionized calcium in plasma and extracellular fluids. Such alterations in ionized calcium are seldom reflected in the total serum calcium concentrations routinely measured by diagnostic laboratories.

Inorganic phosphate also exists in ionized, protein-bound, and complexed forms in plasma. The protein-bound fraction is relatively small (about 10%), but 35% of plasma phosphate is complexed to sodium, calcium, and magnesium, the remaining 55% being ionized. The predominant form of ionized phosphate in plasma is the divalent anion HPO_4^{2+}. Plasma phosphorus concentration is controlled by the action of parathyroid hormone and 1,25-dihydroxyvitamin D on the kidney and intestinal tract, but the control mechanisms are not as precise as for calcium. Consequently, plasma phosphorus concentration varies more widely than calcium, and is more easily influenced by diet, age, sex, pH, and various hormones. An inverse relationship exists between plasma ionized phosphate and plasma ionized calcium concentrations, *an increase in phosphate resulting in a reduction in ionized calcium.*

Parathyroid hormone (PTH) is intimately involved in the regulation of ionized calcium and phosphate concentrations in plasma through its action on specific cells in bone and kidneys, and indirectly on the intestine:

- stimulates the release of calcium and phosphate from bone by osteoclastic resorption,
- stimulates reabsorption of calcium and inhibits reabsorption of phosphate from renal glomerular filtrate,
- stimulates renal synthesis of 1,25-dihydroxyvitamin D from 25-dihydroxyvitamin D, thereby increasing intestinal absorption of calcium and phosphate.

The parathyroid gland responds to any decrease in the concentration of plasma-ionized calcium by releasing PTH. *The net effect of PTH is to increase plasma-ionized calcium and reduce plasma phosphate concentrations.* Once the ionized calcium has been restored to an acceptable level, PTH secretion is halted. Although PTH releases phosphate from bone, together with calcium, the increased loss of phosphate in the urine under the influence of PTH results in a net decrease in plasma phosphate. Osteoclasts do not possess receptors for PTH but are stimulated indirectly through increased expression of RANK-L by osteoblasts under the influence of PTH. This functional linkage between osteoblasts and osteoclasts may account for the concurrent increase in osteoblastic and osteoclastic activity in the bones of animals with hyperparathyroidism. PTH also reduces expression of osteoprotegerin, an inhibitor of osteoclast maturation and activation, and is closely involved in regulating the formation of the active form of vitamin D through its action on renal 1α-hydroxylase. Interestingly, intermittent, low doses of PTH have been shown to have a powerful anabolic effect on bone, creating new opportunities for treating osteoporosis in human patients.

Vitamin D is biologically inert, but undergoes two successive hydroxylations, in the liver and kidney, to form the *active hormone 1,25-dihydroxyvitamin D*, which acts in concert with PTH in maintaining plasma ionized calcium concentrations. 1,25-dihydroxyvitamin D has various actions on target organs:

- enhances absorption of calcium and phosphate from the small intestine,
- stimulates release of calcium and phosphate from bone by osteoclastic resorption,
- enhances phosphate reabsorption from glomerular filtrate.

In the intestine, 1,25-dihydroxyvitamin D increases the efficiency of calcium absorption from about 10% to 70%, probably by stimulating the local production of calcium-binding protein, although several mechanisms may be involved. Phosphorus absorption in the intestine is also increased by 1,25-dihydroxyvitamin D. *The principal action of 1,25-dihydroxyvitamin D on bone is to enhance calcium mobilization when the dietary levels are inadequate to maintain normal plasma-ionized calcium concentrations.* This requires the presence of both 1,25-dihydroxyvitamin D and PTH and is achieved by inducing the differentiation of osteoclasts from monocytic stem cells in the bone marrow as well as stimulating osteocytic osteolysis. In the absence of vitamin D metabolites, osteoid is poorly mineralized and calcium cannot be efficiently mobilized by osteoclasts. Although vitamin D is considered essential for normal mineralization of bone matrix, there is uncertainty whether this is a direct effect or mediated through maintenance of adequate extracellular concentrations of calcium and phosphorus. In addition to its effects on bone, 1,25-dihydroxyvitamin D has other biological effects, including inhibiting the synthesis of PTH and interleukin 2, and enhancing the secretion of insulin and thyroid-stimulating hormone. In vitro, 1,25-dihydroxyvitamin D has been shown to induce monocytes to differentiate into osteoclast-like multinucleated giant cells.

Vitamin D exists in two forms, *vitamin D_2 and vitamin D_3*, both of which have similar potency in humans and domestic animals. Some species however, such as New World primates (Cebus monkeys, tamarins (*Saguinus* spp.)), can utilize only vitamin D_3, while in chickens vitamin D_3 has about ten times greater potency than vitamin D_2. *Vitamin D_2 (ergocalciferol)* is of dietary origin, being present predominantly in yeasts and plants. *Vitamin D_3 (cholecalciferol)* may also be derived from dietary sources, especially fatty fish and cod liver oil, but most is formed in the skin following photochemical conversion of 7-dehydrocholesterol by energy derived from solar ultraviolet light with wavelengths from 290–315 nm (ultraviolet B). The previtamin D_3 formed by this process is then transformed into vitamin D_3 over a period of a few hours by heat-induced isomerization. Latitude, time of day, and season can all have a dramatic effect on vitamin D_3 production in the skin due to lessening of the intensity of ultraviolet light when the sun is at lower angles. At higher latitudes, sunlight is incapable of stimulating vitamin D_3 synthesis in the skin during the winter months. Furthermore, dark-skinned people require longer exposure to sunlight than people with light skin to manufacture the same amount of vitamin D_3. The same most likely applies to animals, and a dense hair coat is likely to reduce cutaneous vitamin D_3 synthesis even further. In fact, there is doubt that vitamin D is synthesized at all in the skin of dogs and cats. The need for carnivores to manufacture their own vitamin D is perhaps obviated by the ample supply of this fat-soluble vitamin in their usual diet.

Once formed in the skin, vitamin D_3 is transported to the circulation where it is bound to an α-1-globulin. Vitamin D_2 or D_3 absorbed from the intestine is transported in chylomicrons, reflecting its lipid solubility. Vitamin D from either source is transported to the liver where it is converted to 25-hydroxyvitamin D by the addition of a hydroxyl group. This is the major form of vitamin D in circulation. Since the reaction of the hepatic enzyme vitamin D-25-hydroxylase is not closely regulated, the concentration of 25-hydroxyvitamin D in circulation reflects the level of cutaneous vitamin D_3 formation and/or dietary levels of vitamin D. Measurements of 25-hydroxyvitamin D in plasma are therefore used to determine whether an individual has adequate or deficient vitamin D status.

The most active form of vitamin D is 1,25-dihydroxyvitamin D, which is formed by the addition of a second hydroxyl group to 25-hydroxyvitamin D under the direction of 25-hydroxyvitamin D-1α-hydroxylase. This reaction occurs predominantly in mitochondria of renal proximal tubular epithelial cells and is closely regulated by circulating concentrations of PTH and inorganic phosphorus. In pregnant animals, 1,25-dihydroxyvitamin D is also formed in the placenta, from where it may become involved in fetal bone and mineral metabolism. Synthesis of 1,25-dihydroxyvitamin D is stimulated directly by high PTH and low phosphorus, and indirectly by low ionized calcium, which acts through PTH. Once formed, 1,25-dihydroxyvitamin D also induces negative feedback on its own synthesis. When plasma phosphorus and ionized calcium concentrations are adequate, and PTH levels are low, 25-hydroxyvitamin D is converted to either 24,25-dihydroxyvitamin D or 1,24,25-trihydroxyvitamin D. These biologically inert metabolites are considered to represent the initial steps in biodegradation pathways.

Calcitonin also plays an important role in calcium and phosphorus homeostasis, and in bone metabolism. Produced by thyroidal C-cells, and secreted in response to increased concentrations of plasma-ionized calcium, *the main biological function of calcitonin is to inhibit osteoclastic bone resorption.* Within minutes of calcitonin administration, osteoclasts shrink and reduce their bone-resorbing activity. As a result, the release of calcium from bone is inhibited and plasma calcium returns to normal.

Osteoporosis

Osteoporosis is easily the most common of the metabolic bone diseases, both in man and animals. Rather than being a specific disease, *osteoporosis is a lesion characterized by a reduction in the quantity of bone, the quality of which is normal.* In effect, osteoporosis represents an imbalance between bone formation and resorption in favor of the latter, resulting in bone that is structurally normal but with reduced breaking strength. Strictly speaking, all osteoporoses should be

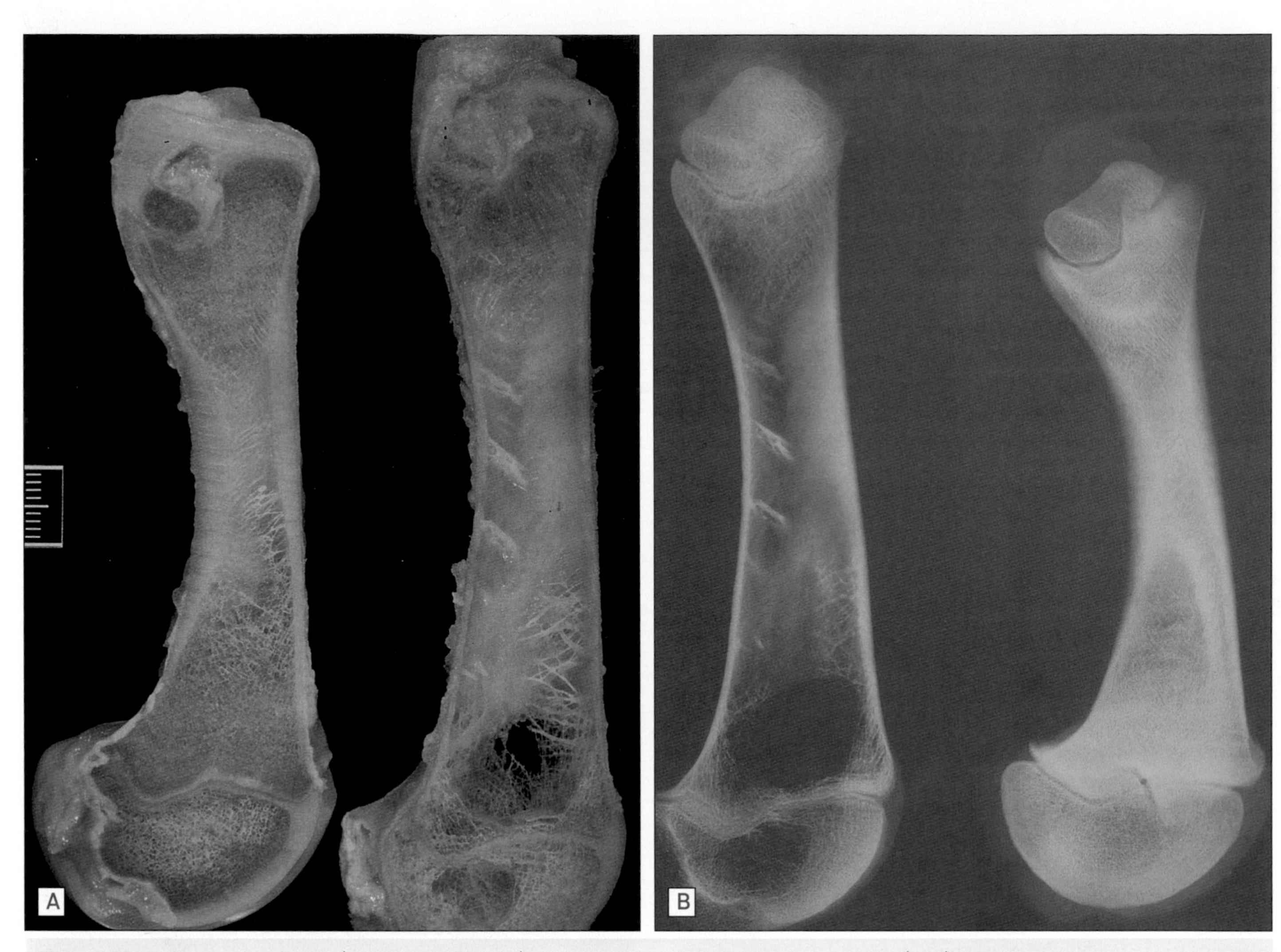

Figure 1.59 Osteoporosis in a pig. (Courtesy of RA Fairley.) **A.** Femur from a pig with severe osteoporosis (right) compared to that of a normal pig. Note the marked depletion of cancellous bone in the metaphyses and epiphyses and the very thin cortices in the affected pig. **B.** Radiograph of the same two bones (positions reversed) showing marked differences in the quantity of cancellous and cortical bone.

called osteopenias pending qualitative assessment of the bone tissue but, for practical purposes, this seldom occurs. Some diseases, for example osteogenesis imperfecta, are characterized by a reduction in bone quality as well as an alteration in bone mass and should not therefore be referred to as osteoporosis, even though the skeleton may appear porotic radiographically and show marked fragility.

The development of a negative balance between bone formation and resorption is recognized as a *normal part of the aging process* in man and animals. Osteoporosis could therefore be considered a natural phenomenon, but there are several physiological situations and disease states that either accelerate bone loss or increase bone resorption, leading to premature depletion of the skeleton. Those of most importance in animals are discussed in detail below.

Many mild cases of osteoporosis in animals remain undetected, even at postmortem examination, as the shape of individual bones is not altered and unless there have been pathological fractures, lameness is not likely to have been observed clinically. The *occurrence of a bone fracture without evidence of excessive trauma may be the first indication that an animal, or human, is suffering from osteoporosis.* In farmed livestock, there may be an unusually high incidence of fractures in the herd or flock, suggesting increased bone fragility.

Confirmation of osteoporosis can be difficult, especially when the degree of bone depletion is relatively mild. Routine radiographic procedures are insensitive in the early stages of osteoporosis as approximately 30–50% of skeletal calcium must be lost before the change can be reliably detected by this method. For this reason, and because of the importance of osteoporosis in human patients, *new diagnostic techniques* have been developed for its early recognition and quantitation. These techniques, which include photon absorptiometry, dual-energy X-ray absorptiometry, ultrasonography, magnetic resonance imaging, and computed tomography, are not widely used for the diagnosis of osteoporosis in animals. *Subjective assessment of the cut surface of bones at necropsy will allow diagnosis of advanced cases of osteoporosis*, but knowledge of what is normal for an animal of the age and species in question is essential, especially when the changes are equivocal. Radiography of isolated bones can detect much smaller alterations in bone density than whole-body radiographs, but comparison with an age-matched control may still be necessary before osteoporosis can be diagnosed with confidence. When it is important to be sure of the diagnosis, objective measurement of radiographs, or use of one of the more precise imaging techniques mentioned above, is recommended. Objective measurement of histological parameters such as bone volume, trabecular thickness, osteoid volume, osteoblastic and osteoclastic activity and bone mineral apposition rate is commonly used by medical pathologists (see review by Bullough et al.), but *histomorphometry* remains largely a research tool in veterinary pathology. *Bone ash measurements* have been traditionally used for the diagnosis of osteoporosis in animals and although they may provide information on the matrix–mineral relationship, reliable reference ranges are seldom available and interpretation of results is difficult. Because the ratio of calcium to phosphorus is fixed in deposits of hydroxyapatite within bone, bone ash samples do not identify low calcium or low phosphorus as causes for osteopenic bone disease, merely that the matrix to mineral ratio is abnormal.

Osteoporosis in human subjects is defined as bone mass 2.5 standard deviations below the young adult mean. In animals, such precise data are not available and the cut-off point between a normal and osteoporotic skeleton is somewhat arbitrary. For this reason, the diagnosis tends to be restricted to cases where there is an obvious reduction in bone mass.

Gross lesions of osteoporosis are generally most marked in bones, or areas of bones, which consist predominantly of *cancellous bone*, presumably because trabecular bone has a greater surface area to volume ratio than cortical bone and is resorbed more rapidly. Vertebral bodies in particular are affected early in the disease in human patients and animals with osteoporosis and may contain pathological fractures. Flat bones of the skull, scapula, ilium, and the ribs may also be severely affected and the breaking strength of the ribs, as assessed during necropsy, may be noticeably reduced. Cancellous bone in the metaphyses and epiphyses of long bones may be reduced in amount and more porous than normal (Fig. 1.59A, B). Trabeculae that are most concerned with transmission of weight-bearing stress are relatively spared and may become more prominent. Thickened trabeculae extending partially or completely across the medullary cavity may be present in the metaphysis or diaphysis of human patients and animals with chronic osteoporosis (Fig. 1.60). The pathogenesis of these *so-called reinforcement lines or bone bars* is uncertain but they may represent an attempt to reinforce weakened bones at locations of particular biomechanical stress. In most forms of osteoporosis, an exception being disuse osteoporosis (see below), cortical bone is resorbed most rapidly from the endosteal surface and along vascular channels. In advanced stages, the medullary cavities of affected long bones are enlarged and the cortices thin (Fig. 1.59A, B). Osteoporotic bones are usually light and fragile, but an accompanying reduction in soft tissue mass and muscular power in many cases tends to preserve the skeleton against stress fractures.

Histological examination of severely osteoporotic bones will not necessarily yield information of diagnostic value, as the depletion of bone tissue is likely to have been clearly established on the basis of either radiography or gross examination. However, it may allow assessment of bone quality, thus allowing differentiation from other metabolic bone diseases and certain other forms of osteopenia. Furthermore, *although it is not likely to allow an etiologic diagnosis, histology may provide an indication of the pathogenesis of bone loss.* For example, there is evidence that osteoporosis evolving from increased resorption is characterized by a decline in trabecular numbers, while in osteoporosis caused by decreased formation there are normal numbers of thin trabeculae. Quantitative histomorphometry may be of value in the diagnosis of osteoporosis in equivocal cases, but this is essentially a research tool rather than one to be used in routine diagnosis.

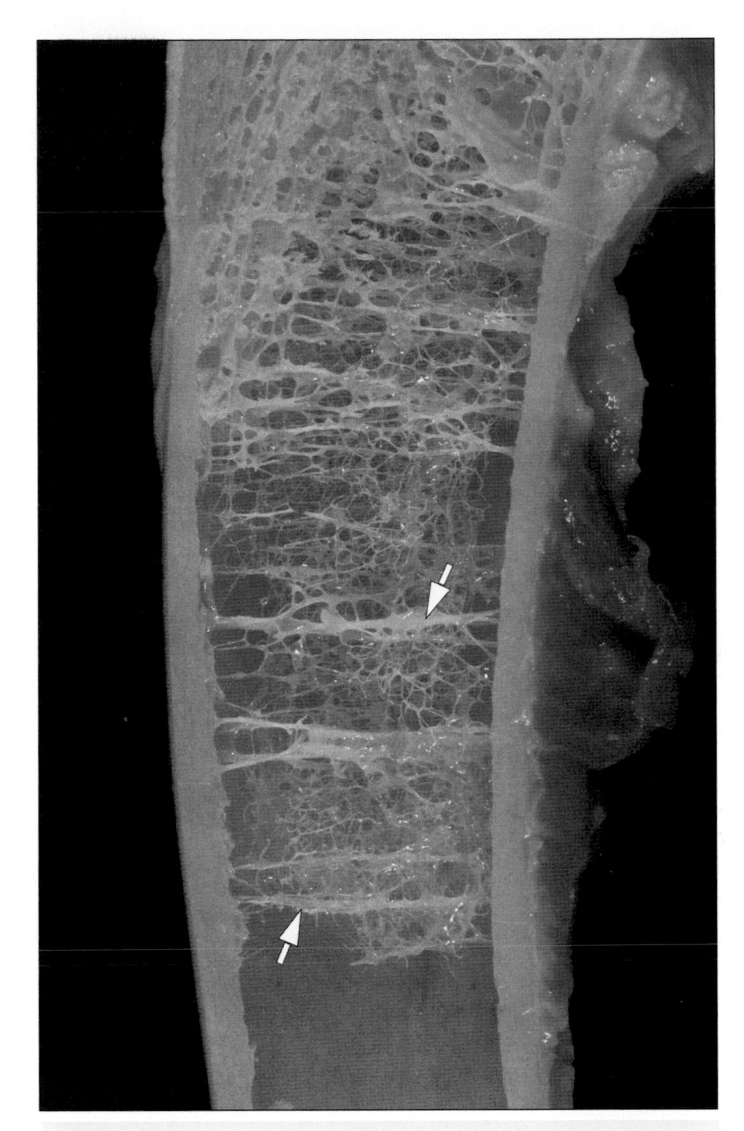

Figure 1.60 Osteoporosis in a dog. Narrow cortices, depletion of cancellous bone and formation of transverse reinforcement trabeculae (arrows), in a dog with chronic osteoporosis. (Courtesy of RA Fairley.)

In severely osteoporotic young animals, the hypertrophic zone of the growth cartilages may be narrowed or absent and when growth ceases, the physis is sealed by a plate of bone (Fig. 1.61A, B). Microscopically, trabeculae are reduced in number and/or size and often are fractured. Depending on the cause of the osteoporosis, evidence of abnormal activity of osteoblasts and/or osteoclasts is present. Intracortical resorption in long bones occurs along vascular channels and is produced by teams of osteoclasts working parallel to the long axes of the bones, the so-called *cutting cones*. Intracortical resorption is functionally important because a small loss of compact bone has a greater effect on bone stiffness than a comparable loss of cancellous bone.

Postmenopausal osteoporosis is the most important form of osteoporosis in human patients and, although the etiology is multifactorial, estrogen deficiency around the time of menopause is believed to play a significant role. Estrogen indirectly inhibits osteoclastic bone resorption through inhibition of interleukin-1 synthesis by peripheral blood monocytes. After estrogen withdrawal, interleukin-1 enhances the production of interleukin-6, a potent stimulator of

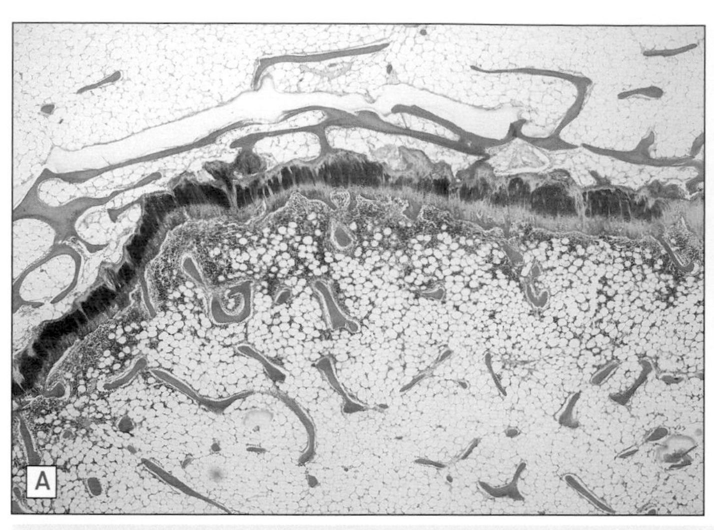

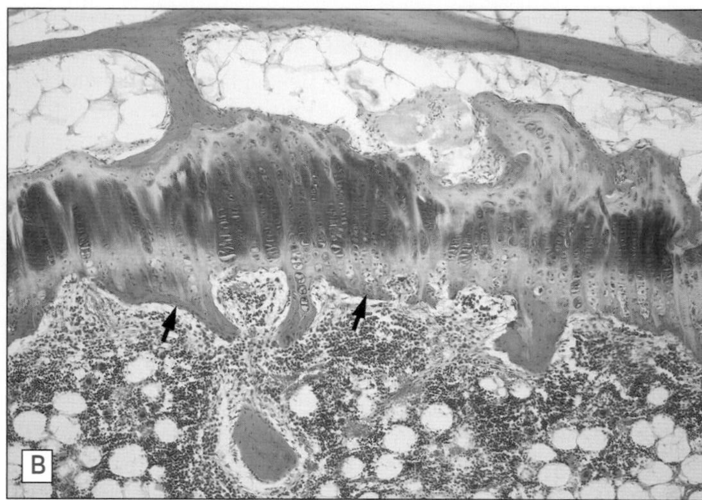

Figure 1.61 Osteoporosis: physeal closure. **A.** Narrowing of the physis and marked deficiency of trabecular bone in the epiphysis and metaphysis of a young pig with severe osteoporosis. **B.** Closer view of the physis in the same animal, showing almost complete absence of hypertrophic chondrocytes and sealing of the metaphyseal side of the physis with narrow plates of bone (arrows). Occasional plump trabeculae extend for a sort distance into the metaphysis.

osteoclastic activity. The inhibitory effect of estrogen on bone resorption may also involve promotion of osteoclast apoptosis by this hormone. This has been demonstrated both in vitro and in vivo and appears to be mediated by TGF-β. An equivalent form of osteoporosis is not currently recognized in animals but there are several other possible causes, many of which are discussed below.

Senile osteoporosis is common in humans and occurs in other animals, but *seldom appears as a clinical problem in veterinary medicine*. This may reflect the considerably shorter lifespan of most domestic animals when compared with humans, although in reality, it is often difficult for the veterinary pathologist to distinguish between the effects of age and other factors that might contribute to reduced skeletal mass in old animals. Beagle dogs aged 7–8 years have approximately 8% less bone tissue in their forelimbs than do young adults, but this reduction is not clinically significant.

Most cases of osteoporosis in animals, especially farm animals, are **nutritional** in origin and may be due to deficiency of a specific nutrient, such as calcium, phosphorus, or copper, or to **starvation**, where there is restricted intake of an otherwise balanced ration. Starvation is relatively common in grazing animals in areas prone to drought or due to overstocking in seasons when pasture growth is below expectations. Poor-quality milk replacers fed to young calves or other young animals may also result in starvation due to inadequate digestibility and absorption of nutrients. In starved animals, the mechanism of osteoporosis is complex, but the lack of dietary protein and energy most likely contribute, either directly or indirectly.

The *effects of starvation* on the skeleton are greater in young growing animals than in adults. Growth of the skeleton is retarded and may cease during periods of starvation due to reduced production of bone matrix. The physes are narrower than normal and the chondrocytes are small, with a relative increase in the amount of cartilage matrix. Thin, widely spaced bone trabeculae are present on the epiphyseal side of the physis, and the metaphyseal side may be sealed by a narrow, horizontal plate of bone (Fig. 1.61B), indicating cessation of growth. As a result, the epiphyseal and metaphyseal sides of the growth plate may appear similar. The cortical and trabecular bone of the diaphyses is reduced in amount. In some cases, characteristic transverse trabeculae may be evident grossly and microscopically in the metaphysis (see Fig. 1.44A, B). These **growth arrest lines**, which differ from the reinforcement lines referred to above, result from intermittent cessation and reactivation of physeal growth and represent a succession of sealing layers from the physis. Transverse radiodense striations also develop in limb bones of fetuses from ewes on a low plane of nutrition. In these lambs, there may be considerable variation in the number of arrest lines between littermates, the number of lines being correlated positively with retardation of fetal size and skeletal maturity. Serous atrophy of medullary adipose tissue is a common feature of starvation-induced osteoporosis in animals (Fig. 1.62).

The *pathogenesis of starvation osteoporosis* in terms of remodeling imbalance is not completely defined. The histologic appearance of inactive osteoblasts, and *a priori* reasoning, both *suggest that deficient bone formation is responsible*. Support for this hypothesis is derived from findings in dogs with malabsorption syndrome, in which tetracycline-labeled sites of bone formation are sparse or absent. The level of bone resorption during starvation is not known.

Severe undernutrition also has a profound effect on tooth development. Delayed formation and eruption of the whole dentition, with a relatively greater delay in the growth of the jaws, leads to overcrowding of the teeth, especially the permanent molars. This causes malocclusion and malalignment of teeth, and there is partial or complete elimination of the diastemata between incisors and canines, and between canines and deciduous molars. Nutritional rehabilitation allows rapid growth of jaws and teeth but malocclusion of permanent dentition persists and often there is abnormal development of parts of some teeth.

Uncomplicated **calcium deficiency**, in the presence of optimum dietary levels of phosphorus and vitamin D, causes osteoporosis experimentally in mature and immature animals, but rarely if ever occurs as a natural disease. In gilts, **lactational osteoporosis** occurs when rations marginally deficient in calcium, and with normal or excess phosphorus, are fed over extended periods during gestation and/or lactation. Generalized osteoporosis, and a tendency to fracture vertebrae, femurs, and phalanges, characterizes the condition.

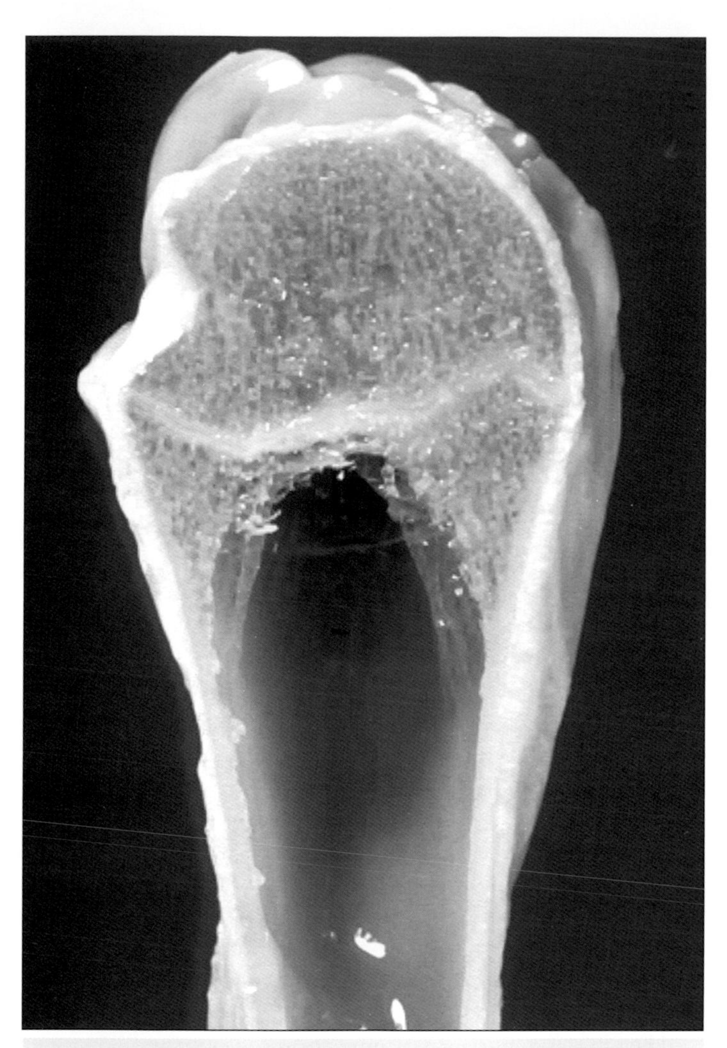

Figure 1.62 Starvation-induced osteoporosis in a lamb. Marked depletion of metaphyseal cancellous bone, thin cortices, and serous atrophy of medullary adipose tissue.

Significant losses associated with lactational osteoporosis occur in some swine herds. The condition may be complicated by disuse osteoporosis caused by confinement in farrowing crates, or by other dietary deficiencies and affected animals may have microscopic evidence of concurrent fibrous osteodystrophy.

The *osteoporosis induced by calcium deficiency is due to excess bone resorption* as a result of increased activity of parathyroid hormone following a reduction in plasma-ionized calcium concentration. In adult animals, the bone loss probably results from an increase in the activation of new remodeling sites. Cortical bone is lost through increased endosteal resorption and, in severe calcium deficiency, intracortical resorption as well. In both adult and growing animals, there is severe loss of cancellous bone, especially in bones with a high trabecular component such as vertebrae. In immature metaphyses, the primary spongiosa may be removed completely, so that there is no framework remaining for the production of secondary spongiosa.

Unless the deficiency is extremely severe, physeal growth and mineralization of cartilage are normal. Osteoid seams are of normal width and frequency, and mineralization occurs normally. *Rickets is not a feature of uncomplicated calcium deficiency* because calcium resorption from bone ensures that this mineral is not a limiting factor at sites of mineralization. In mature animals, calcium deficiency is usually asymptomatic, but in the young, trabecular microfractures, infractions, and complete fractures of bones may occur in both the axial and appendicular skeleton, and animals may die suddenly from hypocalcemic crises when stressed. Parathyroid glands are slightly enlarged due to hyperplasia, and fibrous osteodystrophy sometimes develops, but is less florid than in the osteodystrophy of calcium deficiency induced by phosphorus excess or vitamin D deficiency.

Prolonged calcium deficiency causes dental abnormalities in sheep, including delayed eruption, and increased susceptibility to wear due to mild enamel hypoplasia. When adequate calcium becomes available, superior brachygnathia develops because of inadequate repair of the upper skull compared to the mandible.

Classically, **phosphorus deficiency** *produces osteomalacia in adults and rickets in growing animals, both under natural and experimental conditions. However, under some circumstances it causes osteoporosis.* The reasons for this are not clear, but it may be related to the anorexia that often accompanies phosphorus deficiency, the age and growth rate of the animals, and the severity and duration of phosphorus deficiency. It is not clear whether osteoporosis and osteomalacia are interconvertible or whether osteoporosis is a stage in the development of osteomalacia.

Osteoporosis is recognized as a feature of naturally occurring and experimental **copper deficiency** in lambs, calves, foals, pigs, and dogs. As a component of the enzyme lysyl oxidase, *copper is required for the cross-linkage of collagen and elastin.* Deficiency of this enzyme is probably responsible for the reduced osteoblastic activity observed in swine and dogs with copper deficiency, while the impaired cross linkage of collagen in bone matrix most likely accounts for the increased bone fragility in copper-deficient animals when compared to animals with osteoporosis of other causes.

The bone lesions associated with primary and secondary copper deficiency are discussed earlier in this chapter in the section Mineral imbalances and will not be repeated here. It should be mentioned however that *the gross and microscopic bone lesions of copper deficiency may resemble the lesions of rickets and osteochondrosis.* In fact, there is increasing evidence, at least in some species, that copper deficiency is a cause of, or predisposing factor in, osteochondrosis.

Osteoporosis is often present in animals with severe **gastrointestinal parasitism**, most likely *secondary to malabsorption.* However, there is convincing evidence that subclinical parasitism may also cause osteoporosis, probably by a different mechanism. In one study, continuous dosing of lambs with *Trichostrongylus colubriformis* between 4 and 7 months of age produced a mineral osteoporosis characterized by a reduction in cortical and trabecular bone. This was accompanied by a reduction in the length and volume of bones, and in their degree of mineralization. Some animals showed widened osteoid seams on trabeculae and physeal changes suggestive of concurrent rickets. The lambs had low plasma phosphorus concentrations and normal plasma calcium, suggesting that the bone lesions were due to an induced phosphorus deficiency, although the possible effect of increased corticosteroid production on bone formation was also considered. In goats infused with a subclinical dose of *Trichostrongylus colubriformis* in another study, concurrent subclinical coccidial infection was shown to have an additive effect. Recently, trichostrongyle infections have been shown to lower the concentration of phosphorus carrier proteins in the intestinal mucosa, leading to phosphorus malabsorption in parasitized animals.

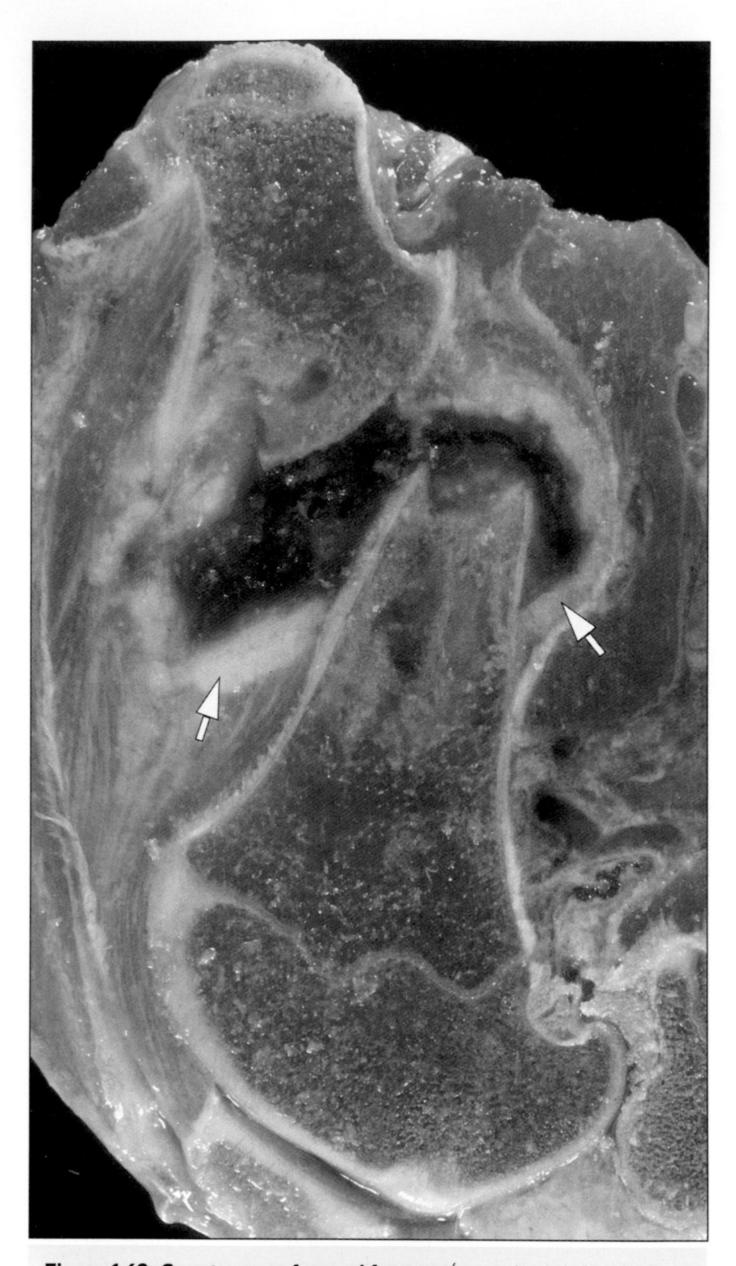

Figure 1.63 Spontaneous femoral fracture (approximately 1 week duration) in a heavily parasitized young sheep with **severe osteoporosis**. Note the thin cortices and porous cancellous bone. There is hemorrhage and early callus formation (arrows) between the malaligned bone ends.

Subclinical infection of lambs with *Ostertagia circumcincta* has also been shown to produce osteoporosis. This was a *matrix osteoporosis*, mediated apparently through restrictions in the availability of protein and energy for matrix deposition. Reduced bone volume was a consistent finding, but there was no effect on growth plates and the length of bones was normal. In calves infected experimentally with *Ostertagia* spp., the utilization of phosphorus is adversely affected.

The *importance of parasite-induced osteoporosis in grazing animals is unknown* but it is undoubtedly much more common than is recognized and may be responsible for some of the unexplained cases of spontaneous bone fractures encountered in cattle and sheep (Fig. 1.63).

Osteoporosis is a complication of **inflammatory bowel disease** in humans and has been described in dogs with **malabsorption syndrome**, but the mechanism is unknown. Reduced intake and/or absorption of vitamin D and calcium have been suggested as a possible mechanism for the osteoporosis in human patients with ulcerative colitis or Crohn's disease. So too has corticosteroid therapy, which is often used in such patients and is well known as a cause of osteoporosis, but recent human studies have failed to demonstrate a link between corticosteroid therapy and inflammatory bowel disease. The generation of proinflammatory cytokines such as interleukin-1 and interleukin-6, both of which induce bone resorption and inhibit its formation, may play an important role in the osteoporosis associated with inflammatory bowel diseases of humans, and may also be important in various parasitic and other enteric diseases of animals. Recent evidence that activated T lymphocytes may play a role in local or systemic bone loss through the production of RANK-L has provided an alternative hypothesis for the osteoporosis of inflammatory bowel disease.

Corticosteroid-induced osteoporosis is common in humans and its occurrence in animals may be underestimated. Moderate doses of corticosteroids inhibit both the synthesis of collagen by pre-existing osteoblasts and the differentiation of osteoblasts from their precursor cells, resulting in *decreased apposition rate*. In addition to their effect on bone formation, corticosteroids have been shown to *stimulate osteoclastic bone resorption*, resulting in a generalized loss of skeletal mass. Indirect effects of corticosteroids on the skeleton are mediated through reduced calcium absorption in the intestine and reduced calcium reabsorption in renal tubules, both of which would be expected to enhance bone resorption through secondary hyperparathyroidism. Interference with vitamin D metabolism has also been implicated in the development of corticosteroid-induced osteoporosis but the evidence from various studies is conflicting.

The clinical importance of osteoporosis in dogs and other animal species with *spontaneous and iatrogenic hyperadrenocorticism* is not clear as few studies have been reported, but hyperadrenocorticism is considered one of the most common causes of generalized osteopenia observed radiographically in dogs. In one study, a 25% reduction in mean trabecular bone volume was detected in Beagle dogs with clinical hyperadrenocorticism. In addition, a significant reduction in osteoblast number and the amount of osteoid lining trabecular surfaces was also demonstrated in Beagles with subclinical hyperadrenocorticism. Reduced bone formation in these dogs did not appear to be accompanied by increased osteoclastic activity.

Other causes of *generalized osteoporosis* in humans and domestic animals include **vitamin A toxicity**, **hyperthyroidism,** and chronic **metabolic acidosis**. The immunosuppressive agent **cyclosporin** and certain **anticonvulsant drugs** (e.g., phenobarbital, diphenylhydantoin, and carbamazepine) have also been associated with osteoporosis in human patients.

Disuse osteoporosis is a loss of bone mass due to muscular inactivity and reduced weight bearing. It may be localized, following paralysis or fracture of a limb, or more generalized in association with prolonged recumbency or inactivity. *Bones that normally carry the greatest loads suffer the greatest proportional loss in mass from disuse.* Measurable loss of mineral occurs in horses that have a limb cast for prolonged periods. The mechanism of disuse osteoporosis is not clear but it does occur in immobilized parathyroidectomized animals, indicating that it is *not PTH-dependent*, and is seen in human fetuses with neuromuscular disease.

In experimental long-term disuse osteoporosis of the forelimb in young adult Beagle dogs, the lesion develops in several stages. The first is marked by rapid loss of tissue, which reduces the bone mass by about 16% in 6 weeks. This results from imbalanced resorption on endosteal, periosteal, and intracortical surfaces, and may be due to nonspecific activation of numerous remodeling sites. This is followed by an increase in bone mass from 8–12 weeks after immobilization, presumably as a result of net bone formation at activated remodeling sites, and the bone mass approaches normal. In the period between 8–12 and 24–32 weeks following immobilization, there is slower bone loss, 80–90% of which is subperiosteal bone. The reduction in bone mass may reach 30–50% of normal and be maintained at this level. The distal bones of the limb lose more bone than the proximal, but in all cases the subperiosteal bone is diminished.

The effects of remobilization on disuse osteoporosis are not clearly defined. Recovery from relatively short periods of immobilization does occur but the age of the patient influences the response. The effect of weightlessness associated with prolonged space travel is well documented and the loss of bone strength remains for a prolonged period after returning to normal gravity.

Bibliography

Adachi JD. Corticosteroid-induced osteoporosis. Am J Med Sci 1997;313:41–49.
Andreassen H, et al. Inflammatory bowel disease and osteoporosis. Scand J Gastroenterol 1997;32:1247–1255.
Audran M, Kumar R. The physiology and pathophysiology of vitamin D. Mayo Clin Proc 1985;60:851–866.
Bjarnason I, et al. Reduced bone density in patients with inflammatory bowel disease. Gut 1997;40:228–233.
Breslau NA. Calcium, magnesium, and phosphorus: intestinal absorption. In: Favus MJ, ed. Primer on Metabolic Bone Diseases and Disorders of Mineral Metabolism. 3rd ed. Philadelphia, New York: Lippincott-Raven, 1996:41–49.
Buckingham SHW, Jeffcott LB. Osteopenic effects of forelimb immobilization in horses. Vet Rec 1991;128:370–373.
Bullough PG, et al. The tissue diagnosis of metabolic bone disease. Role of histomorphometry. Orthop Clinics North Am 1990;21:65–79.
Coop RL, et al. *Ostertagia circumcincta* infection of lambs, the effect of different intakes of larvae on skeletal development. J Comp Pathol 1981;91:521–530.
Doige CE. Pathological findings associated with locomotory disturbances in lactating and recently weaned sows. Can J Comp Med 1982;46:1–6.
High WB, et al. Effects of thyroxine on cortical bone remodeling in adult dogs. Amer J Pathol 1981;102:438–446.
Holick MF. Vitamin D: photobiology, metabolism, mechanism of action, and clinical applications. In: Favus MJ, ed. Primer on Metabolic Bone Diseases and Disorders of Mineral Metabolism. 3rd ed. Philadelphia, New York: Lippincott-Raven, 1996:74–81.
Jaworski ZFG, et al. Effect of long-term immobilisation on the pattern of bone loss in older dogs. J Bone Joint Surg [Br] 1980;62:104–110.
Kronenberg HM. Parathyroid hormone: mechanism of action. In: Favus MJ, ed. Primer on Metabolic Bone Diseases and Disorders of Mineral Metabolism. 3rd ed. Philadelphia, New York: Lippincott-Raven, 1996:68–70.
Kunkle BN, et al. Osteopenia with decreased bone formation in Beagles with malabsorption syndrome. Calcif Tissue Int 1982;34:396–402.
Mazess RB. On aging and bone loss. Clin Orthop 1982;165:239–252.
Norrdin RW, et al. Trabecular bone morphometry in Beagles with hyperadrenocorticism and adrenal adenomas. Vet Pathol 1988;25:256–264.
Platt BS, Stewart RJC. Transverse trabeculae and osteoporosis in bones in experimental protein-calorie deficiency. Br J Nutr 1962;16:483–495.
Poppi DP, et al. Calcium and phosphorus absorption in lambs exposed to *Trichostrongylus colubriformis*. J Comp Pathol 1985;95:458–462.
Theill LE, et al. RANK-L and RANK: T cells, bone loss and mammalian evolution. Ann Rev Immunol 2002;20:795–823.
Wenham G. A radiographic study of the changes in skeletal growth and development of the foetus caused by poor nutrition in the pregnant ewe. Br Vet J 1981;137:176–187.

Rickets and osteomalacia

It is convenient to consider these two diseases together as they have *a similar etiology and pathogenesis, differing only in the age at which they occur.* **Rickets** is a disease of the developing skeleton in young animals and is accompanied *by abnormal endochondral ossification at growth plates, in addition to defective bone formation.* Its expression is greatly influenced by the level of physical activity undertaken; sedentary animals are less likely to suffer from fractures, infractions, and joint collapse. **Osteomalacia** occurs only in adults and although there are no lesions associated with growth cartilages, *the bone changes are the same as those that occur in rickets.* Both diseases occur in all domestic animal species and wildlife, but there are differences between species in the circumstances under which they occur, and in the most likely cause.

The pathogenesis of both rickets and osteomalacia involves **defective mineralization**. In young animals with rickets, this includes cartilage matrix at sites of endochondral ossification, as well as newly formed osteoid. In adults, where skeletal growth by endochondral ossification is no longer occurring, the defective mineralization affects only the osteoid formed during skeletal remodeling. The nature of the lesions varies, depending on the etiology, the age and growth rate of the animal, and the duration of the disease process. Furthermore, the dietary abnormality may involve a deficiency of more than one nutrient. As a result, the macroscopic and microscopic changes are not always classical, and the lesions may overlap with those of the other metabolic bone diseases. Accurate diagnosis on the basis of morphology alone may therefore be difficult.

Anything that interferes with the mineralization of cartilage or bone matrix may cause rickets or osteomalacia, but *most cases in animals result from dietary deficiencies of either vitamin D or phosphorus.* It is still uncertain whether the protective effect of 1,25-dihydroxyvitamin D against rickets is mediated by a direct effect on matrix mineralization or whether it is based on maintenance of adequate extracellular ionized calcium concentrations. The role of 1,25-dihydroxyvitamin D in matrix mineralization may involve its action in stimulating the synthesis of noncollagenous proteins such as osteocalcin, which is thought to be required for normal mineralization.

Vitamin D deficiency may occur in grazing animals where the combination of relatively high latitudes and temperate climates allows them to be pastured for much of the year. Such conditions occur in parts of the United Kingdom, South America, New Zealand, and southern Australia. Photobiosynthesis is a more important source of vitamin D than diet in grazing animals, but may be inadequate during the winter months in some regions. When the winter sun is at an angle of less than 30 degrees to the horizontal, the short-wavelength ultraviolet rays required for the activation of 7-dehydrocholesterol in the skin are reflected by the atmosphere and dermal synthesis of previtamin D_3 is impaired. Mature grass and sun-cured hay are relatively good alternative sources of vitamin

D_2, but the levels present in immature pasture are likely to be inadequate. This may be further compounded by the anti-vitamin D activity of carotenes present in lush pasture and green cereal crops. The extra demands of pregnancy and lactation during winter and early spring may also contribute significantly to the development of clinical osteomalacia. *It is likely that many grazing animals are vitamin D deficient for a period during the winter*, but clinical rickets or osteomalacia are only likely to develop if the deficiency is marked or persists for longer than usual. Problems may also occur if vitamin D deficiency is combined with deficiencies of other essential nutrients, such as phosphorus or copper.

Sheep appear to be more susceptible to vitamin D deficiency than **cattle**, possibly because a dense fleece covers much of their skin. Not surprisingly, the concentration of vitamin D in blood increases following shearing. **Alpacas** and **llamas** *may be even more susceptible to vitamin D deficiency than sheep*. Rickets has been diagnosed in young camelids in New Zealand, South Australia, and northern regions of the USA. The disease occurs during winter months and is accompanied by low blood concentrations of both 25-hydroxyvitamin D and phosphorus. In the New Zealand report, lambs grazing the same pasture had normal serum phosphorus concentrations and the phosphorus content of the pasture was normal. Vitamin D deficiency was considered the most likely etiology, the low serum phosphorus concentrations being secondary to reduced absorption of phosphorus from the intestine. The natural environment for alpacas and llamas is at high altitude near the equator, where solar irradiation is intense. Their dense fiber and pigmented skin may have evolved as a protective mechanism to prevent excessive solar irradiation reaching the skin. This could prove to be a disadvantage in animals moved to lower altitudes, especially at latitudes with limited solar irradiation during the winter.

Dietary deficiency of vitamin D also occurs in housed animals, particularly **piglets** and **calves** (at higher latitudes), due to lack of sunlight and errors in the formulation of rations. Piglets grow rapidly and are weaned early. If exposed to rachitogenic diets while the cartilages are still growing rapidly, the lesions tend to be florid. Vitamin D deficiency rickets occurs only rarely in **pups** and **kittens**, even though neither species seems capable of manufacturing vitamin D in their skin. The widespread availability of balanced commercial diets has reduced the likelihood of deficient rations being fed to dogs and cats, although inadequate rations are occasionally incriminated in the etiology of osteodystrophies in pups, as indicated in a report of rickets in a litter of Greyhounds. In the presence of adequate dietary levels of calcium and phosphorus, the vitamin D requirements of dogs appear to be very low. The vitamin D concentration of canine milk is very low, but deficiency in neonatal pups is unlikely, providing sufficient vitamin D has been stored in the liver of the pups during pregnancy.

Phosphorus deficiency *is well established as a cause of rickets and osteomalacia*, although the exact mechanism is uncertain. Presumably, the delayed mineralization in phosphorus-deficient animals reflects inadequate extracellular concentrations of the phosphate ions essential for the formation of hydroxyapatite. *Rickets and osteomalacia due to phosphorus deficiency are uncommon, but do occur in animals grazing pastures low in phosphorus*. There are many areas of the world, including South America, South Africa, northern Australia, and New Zealand, where soil phosphorus levels are very low and successful livestock production requires application of phosphorus either to the soil or the animals. Supplementation of individual animals is often not practical, but the problem can be prevented by regular applications of phosphorus-containing fertilizers. Reduced fertilizer use in an effort to cut production costs has led to an increased incidence of rickets, osteomalacia, and other diseases associated with phosphorus deficiency in some countries. **Cattle** appear to be more susceptible than **sheep** to phosphorus deficiency, while **horses** seem to be remarkably resistant. Rickets has also been diagnosed in farmed red **deer** grazing phosphorus deficient pastures in New Zealand. Phosphorus-deficiency rickets is not recognized in piglets but hypophosphatemia may be a complication of vitamin D deficiency.

Signs of phosphorus deficiency develop slowly, especially in the mature skeleton, and many animals with subclinical osteomalacia no doubt remain undiagnosed. Clinical disease is most likely to occur in cows where the deficiency is exacerbated by the extra demands of pregnancy or lactation. Such animals lose condition, develop transient, shifting lameness, and show an increased susceptibility to fractures. They may crave phosphorus-rich materials, and *osteophagia and pica are characteristic signs of the deficiency*. Fertility can be severely reduced and estrum may be irregular, inapparent, or absent. Newborn calves are of normal size and development (at the expense of their dams) but while suckling, their growth is subnormal, and this is accentuated after weaning. Growth is also aberrant in that maturity is delayed and deficient animals appear long and lean, and have a rough hair coat. Hypophosphatemia develops early but also returns to normal rapidly if the animals are supplemented. Serum calcium concentrations are usually normal or increased. The presence of normal serum phosphorus concentration in an animal with osteodystrophy does not therefore exclude phosphorus deficiency as the cause. The poorly mineralized bone is removed only slowly and will persist until well after the underlying dietary deficiency has been corrected.

Dietary phosphorus deficiency is virtually impossible in carnivores because of the high levels of phosphorus normally present in their rations. In fact, excess dietary phosphorus resulting in nutritional secondary hyperparathyroidism and fibrous osteodystrophy is relatively common in pups and kittens.

Calcium is also required for mineralization but there is doubt that uncomplicated calcium deficiency is capable of inducing rickets. Since any decrease in extracellular concentrations of ionized calcium is rapidly corrected by the actions of PTH and 1,25-dihydroxyvitamin D on bone and small intestine, *calcium is unlikely to be a limiting factor at sites of mineralization. Persistent dietary deficiency or unavailability of calcium is more likely to lead to fibrous osteodystrophy or osteoporosis* (depending on age and species) due to hyperparathyroidism and excessive bone resorption. Hypocalcemia does not occur until the advanced stages of calcium deficiency, by which time skeletal growth will be retarded and any effect on growth plates reduced. It is important to recognize however, that vitamin D deficiency will be accompanied by hypocalcemia due to impaired resorption of calcium from bone and absorption from the small intestine. The skeletal lesions of vitamin D deficiency in young animals would therefore be expected to include changes characteristic of both rickets and fibrous osteodystrophy. In contrast, lesions attributable to hyperparathyroidism should not complicate phosphorus-deficiency rickets or osteomalacia. More likely, chronic phosphorus deficiency will be accompanied by anorexia, and the skeletal changes may therefore reflect a combination of osteomalacia and osteoporosis.

Interestingly, calcium deficiency has been shown to induce a deficiency of vitamin D in rats. The mechanism is not certain, but evidence suggests that increased secretion of PTH in calcium deficiency stimulates increased production of 1,25-dihydroxyvitamin D, which acts directly or indirectly to enhance inactivation of 25-hydroxyvitamin D in the liver. This may explain the concurrent development of vitamin D deficiency in certain human disorders characterized by hyperparathyroidism, including gastrointestinal disease, chronic liver disease, and anticonvulsant therapy.

Several other, less common, causes of rickets and osteomalacia are recognized in man and animals. These include two types of **vitamin D-dependent rickets** (types I and II) caused by inborn errors in vitamin D metabolism. **Type I** is caused by a defect in the renal enzyme 1α-hydroxylase, which converts 25-hydroxyvitamin D to 1,25-dihydroxyvitamin D in proximal tubules. The disease is inherited as an *autosomal recessive trait* in people and pigs, and sporadic cases have been suspected in dogs and cats. The disease is characterized by high levels of serum parathyroid hormone and 25-hydroxyvitamin D but low or undetectable levels of 1,25-dihydroxyvitamin D. Affected pigs are clinically normal until 4–6 weeks of age, but then plasma calcium and phosphate levels fall and alkaline phosphatase activity rises. Florid rickets develops over the next 3–4 weeks and the pigs die unless treated. **Type II** vitamin D-dependent rickets, which is also more appropriately called **hereditary vitamin D-resistant rickets**, is due to a defect in 1,25-dihydroxyvitamin D receptor-effector systems in the cells of target organs. The disease occurs in people, and possibly in the common marmoset, *Callithrix jacchus*. These animals, like other New World monkeys, cannot utilize vitamin D_2 but, in addition, require unusually large amounts of vitamin D_3 and have very high levels of plasma 1,25-dihydroxyvitamin D without hypercalcemia. Despite the elevated 1,25-dihydroxyvitamin D, some marmosets develop a bone disease with features of rickets.

Hypophosphatemic vitamin D-resistant rickets (renal hypophosphatemic rickets) is characterized by hypophosphatemia, normocalcemia, decreased renal tubular reabsorption of phosphate, and skeletal deformities. Plasma 1,25-dihydroxyvitamin D levels are inappropriately low. Hypophosphatemia results from impaired renal reabsorption and intestinal absorption of phosphorus. Combined treatment with 1,25-dihydroxyvitamin D to depress parathyroid hormone and thus phosphaturia, and phosphate has beneficial effects on bone lesions. The disease is inherited as an X-linked dominant trait in children and in mice. Hypophosphatemic vitamin D-resistant rickets and osteomalacia have also been associated with various neoplasms in human patients. The mechanism is unknown but is thought to involve production by the tumor of a humoral substance that interferes with phosphate absorption in renal proximal tubules. This syndrome has yet to be reported in animals but could easily be missed both clinically and at necropsy.

Rickets and osteomalacia are recognized in human patients with **gastrointestinal malabsorption** resulting from chronic disorders of the small bowel, hepatobiliary system, or pancreas. Since vitamin D is fat soluble, any interference with the digestion or absorption of fat would be expected to reduce dietary vitamin D absorption and predispose to deficiency. Reduced absorption of calcium in malabsorption syndromes may enhance the efficiency of vitamin D, as outlined above. Although the same would be expected to occur in animals, there are no reports. This may reflect less complete radiographic and pathologic evaluation of the skeleton in animals with such diseases or the fact that affected animals do not live long enough for the skeletal lesions to become manifest clinically.

Rickets has been reproduced experimentally in rats by the addition of **iron** to a normal, nonrachitogenic diet. *Iron interferes with the absorption of phosphorus* and high dietary levels may induce phosphorus deficiency. High dietary levels of other phosphorus antagonists, such as **calcium** and **aluminum**, might also be expected to induce phosphorus-deficiency rickets. Lesions resembling osteomalacia have been observed in cattle ingesting high concentrations of **fluoride**, which *interferes with mineralization* when incorporated into bone matrix.

Animals with *rickets* are generally stiff or lame, and in severe cases are reluctant to stand. The limbs, especially the forelimbs, may be bowed. Swelling of the carpals and other joints, due to enlarged ends of long bones, may lead to an initial suspicion of arthritis. Varus or valgus deformity may be present, reflecting asymmetric involvement of growth plates. Affected pigs may stand with a hunched back, walk on the tips of their toes, or adopt a dog-sitting position. Knuckling of the carpus is also described in pigs with rickets. In many animals however, the clinical signs are mild and nonspecific.

Macroscopic lesions of rickets are most prominent at sites of rapid growth, including metaphyseal and epiphyseal regions of long bones and costochondral junctions of the large middle ribs. Enlargement of costochondral junctions is a classic feature of the human disease and is referred to as the "*rachitic rosary*." Costochondral junctions are normally prominent in fast-growing young animals and any enlargement must be interpreted with caution. In rickets, the metaphysis of the rib is often wider than the cartilaginous portion and on sagittal section, the chondro–osseous junction is irregular, with tongues of unresorbed cartilage extending into the metaphysis (Fig. 1.64A). The normal architecture of the metaphysis is replaced by a mixture of disorganized trabeculae, irregular tongues and islands of cartilage, fibrous tissue, and sometimes hemorrhage (Fig. 1.64B). Loss of the normal trabecular arrangement in the metaphysis is best appreciated radiographically, at least in severe cases (Fig. 1.65). Similar changes may be evident in sagittal sections of long bones (Figs 1.66A, B; 1.67A, B), especially at sites of most rapid growth, such as distal radius, proximal humerus, distal femur, and both ends of the tibia. Metacarpal and metatarsal physes are also likely to show gross changes (Fig. 1.68). The severity of lesions between different physes may vary considerably, even within the same animal, and although the disease is systemic, the physeal lesions are often multifocal rather than diffuse. This emphasizes the importance of examining sagittal sections of several bones during postmortem examination. The enlargement of the ends of long bones is due partly to flaring of the metaphysis and partly to compression caused by weight bearing on metaphyseal bone of reduced strength. Also, there is accumulation of poorly mineralized osteoid, which is not removed efficiently by osteoclasts.

Focal thickening of physeal cartilage, similar to that observed in rickets is also described in osteochondrosis in various species, and in the inherited dwarfism of Alaskan Malamute dogs. In rickets however, the physeal lesions are generally accompanied by evidence of bone fragility, including trabecular disruption, hemorrhage, and infractions. Pathological fractures may be present in the limbs, ribs, or vertebrae in severe cases. When the deficiency is relatively recent but severe, a distinct zone where abnormal bone formation commenced may be present in the metaphysis (Fig. 1.64A). This reflects a change from adequate to inadequate dietary phosphorus or vitamin D and

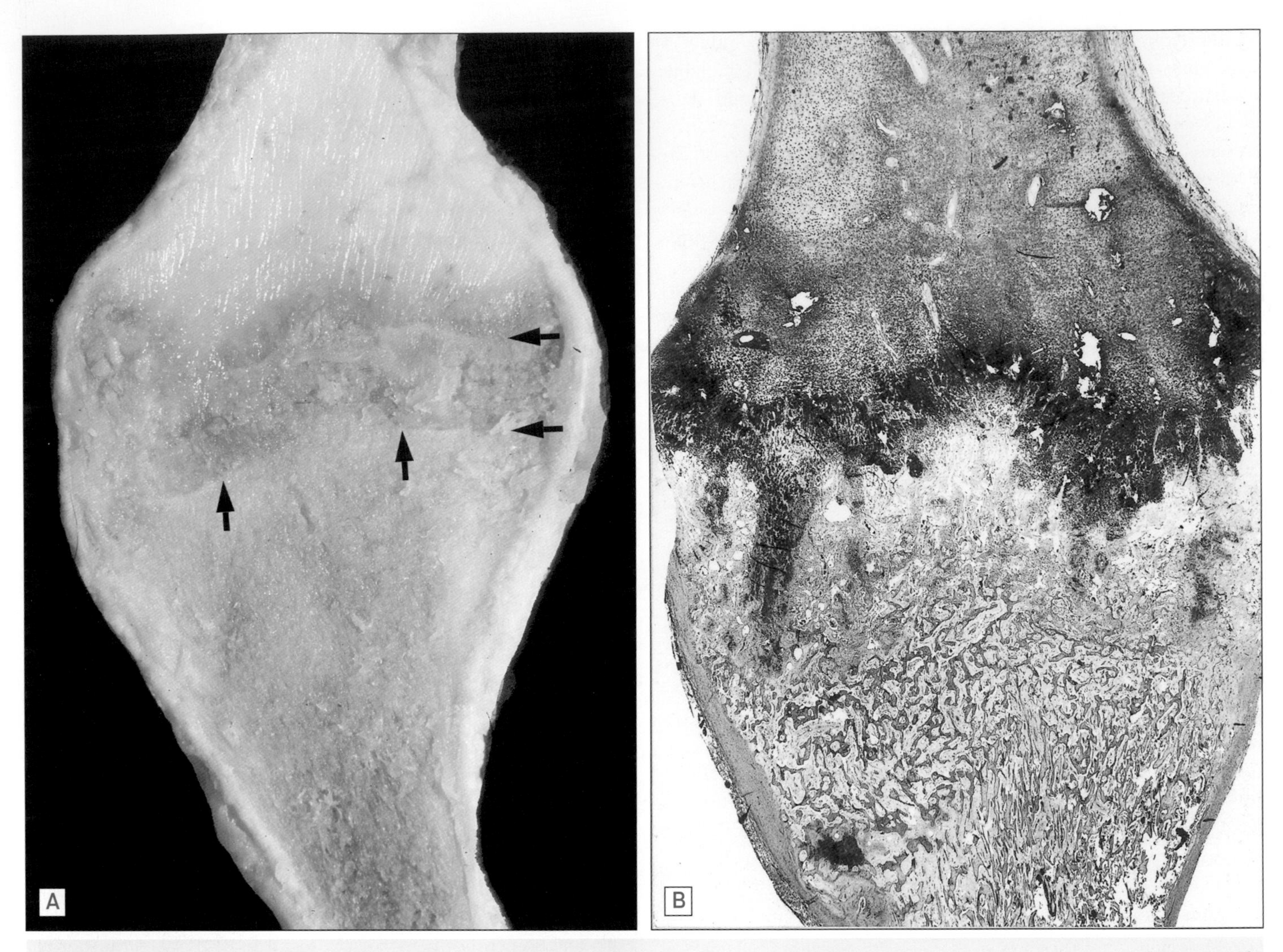

Figure 1.64 Rickets, bovine. **A.** Phosphorus deficiency rickets in a 1-year-old steer. Swelling of metaphysis at the costochondral junction and disruption of normal architecture in the zone between the horizontal arrows. Broad tongues of cartilage extend into the metaphysis from the physeal cartilage. The stage at which defective bone formation commenced is indicated by the vertical arrows. **B.** Subgross preparation of costochondral junction from a calf with rickets showing irregular tongues of cartilage remaining in the metaphysis and disorganization of metaphyseal bone.

may be of value in relating the disease to a particular change in diet or environment.

Endochondral ossification occurring beneath articular cartilage is also abnormal in animals with rickets, but since the rate of epiphyseal bone formation is slower than that of the metaphysis, the lesions are milder. The articular cartilage may be irregularly thickened and in severe cases, there may be infolding and irregularity of the articular surface due to collapse of weakened subchondral bone. These articular lesions of rickets occur most often in pigs, but also occur in association with fibrous osteodystrophy, and tend to involve large, weight-bearing joints such as the shoulder and hip. Similar macroscopic lesions occur in the articular cartilage of pigs with osteochondrosis, but since this disease is not associated with defective bone formation, the subchondral bone does not collapse.

In mild rickets, the lesions may not be apparent grossly or radiographically. Furthermore, reduced growth rate in animals with phosphorus-deficiency rickets may reduce the severity of lesions. In such cases, histology is essential for confirmation.

The microscopic lesions of rickets reflect the failure of mineralization of cartilage at sites of endochondral ossification, and of osteoid deposited during bone growth and remodeling. Mineralization of cartilage matrix is a critical event in the process of endochondral ossification at physes and appears to be functionally coupled with vascular invasion from the metaphyseal side. As the physeal cartilage becomes mineralized, the hypertrophic chondrocytes degenerate, the narrow septa between adjacent cells are broken down and capillary sprouts derived from metaphyseal vessels invade their vacant lacunar spaces. These invading capillaries are accompanied by osteoprogenitor cells, which differentiate into osteoblasts and deposit osteoid on the spicules of mineralized cartilage, which previously separated the columns of chondrocytes. Experiments in vitamin D-deficient rachitic rats demonstrated that metaphyseal angiogenesis and invasion of physeal cartilage is halted or impaired. Within 96 hours of vitamin D repletion, the metaphyseal vasculature returns to normal and capillary sprouts recommence invasion of the physeal cartilage.

Persistence of hypertrophic chondrocytes at sites of endochondral ossification, both at physes and beneath articular cartilage, is the hallmark of rickets in histological preparations. The lesions are often irregular and are usually accompanied by disruption of the underlying trabecular bone. As the cartilage continues to accumulate, its growth rate slows, possibly

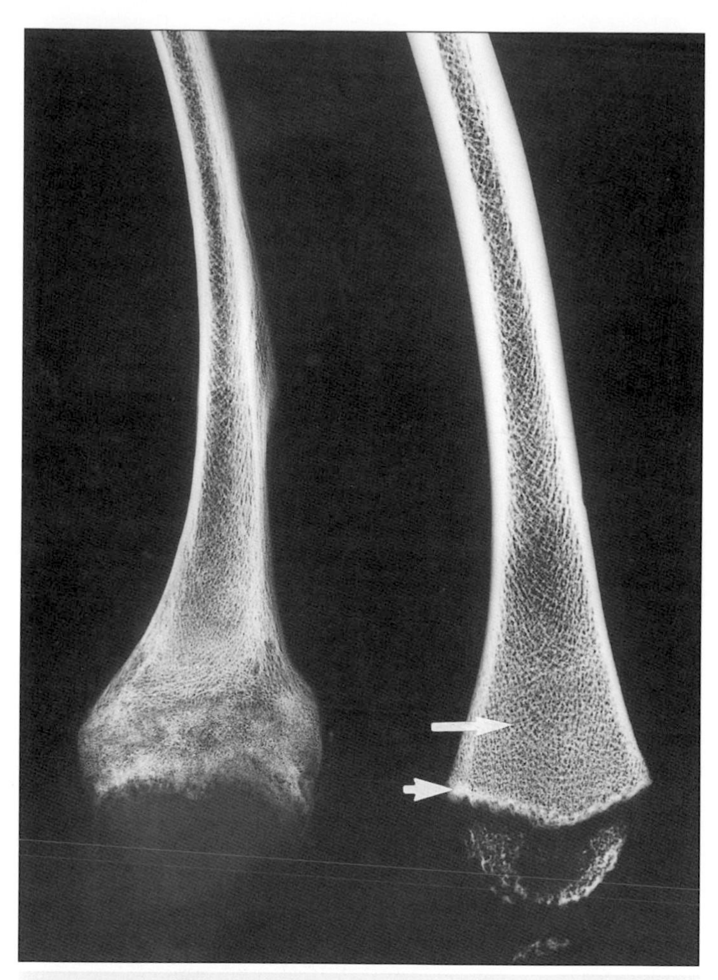

Figure 1.65 Rickets, calf. Normal rib on right. There is metaphyseal swelling and disorganization of trabecular bone in the rachitic bone. Note the regular trabecular pattern in the primary (short arrow) and secondary spongiosa (long arrow) in the normal rib.

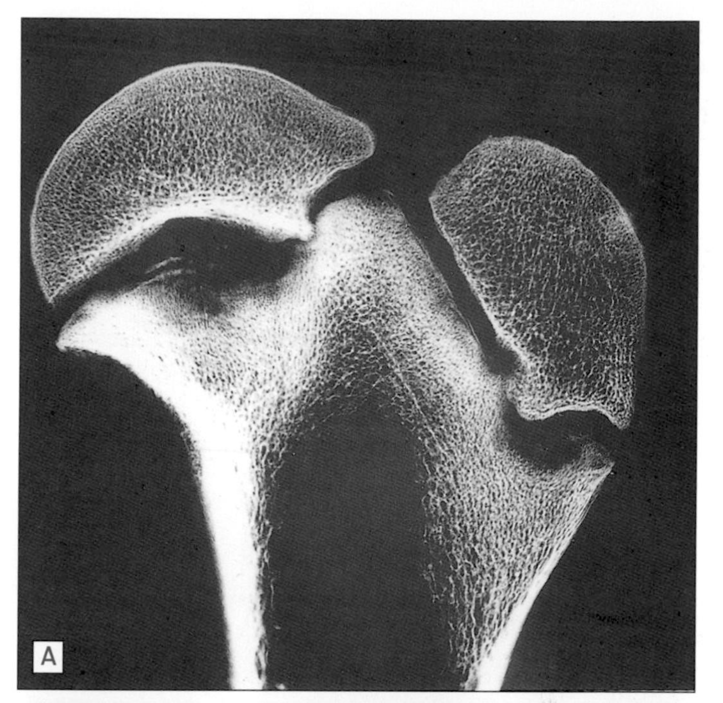

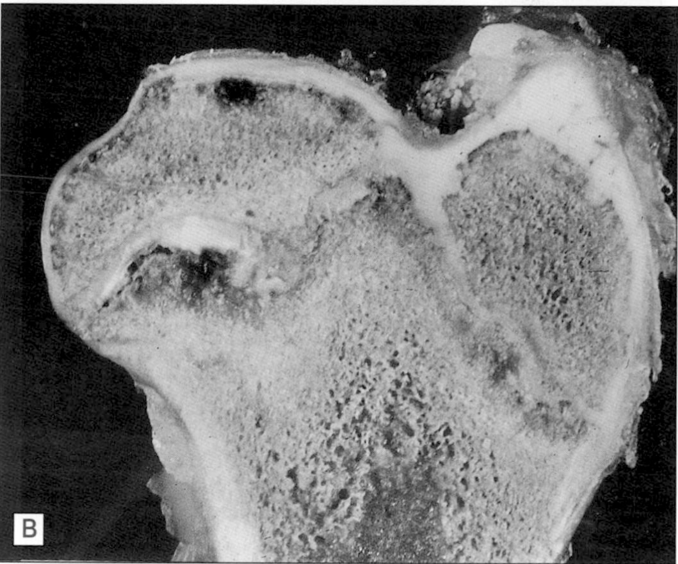

Figure 1.66 Rickets, pig. **A.** Slab radiograph of proximal femur showing increased depth of physeal cartilage. **B.** Proximal femur showing irregular thickening of the physes in addition to hemorrhage and disruption of trabeculae in metaphyses. Also note the collapse of the articular cartilage of the femoral head and abnormalities in the subchondral bone. (Courtesy of PA Taylor.)

because of inadequate diffusible nutrient, and the hypertrophic cells form irregular clumps instead of the characteristic columns. Some of these clumps are bypassed by the irregular ingrowth of vascular and osteogenic tissue and ultimately come to lie in the metaphysis as unmineralized clusters of hypertrophic chondrocytes surrounded by osteoid (Fig. 1.69A, B). Occasionally, the persistent tongues of cartilage degenerate and are replaced by connective tissue, in which metaplastic osteoid forms. Degenerate cartilage, which loses its basophilia and stains like osteoid, is sometimes referred to as pseudo- or cartilaginous osteoid. If the dietary deficiency is corrected, plates of rachitic cartilage may become undermined by invading vessels and stranded in the metaphysis, forming a grossly visible, translucent band parallel to the growth plate.

Metaphyseal trabeculae are thicker than normal, irregular in shape and may be partly covered by seams of unmineralized osteoid (Fig. 1.70A). Trabecular microfractures are common. Infractions (incomplete fractures) in various stages of repair are also relatively common and reflect the fragility of the trabeculae (Fig. 1.70B). *In vitamin D deficiency, the histologic lesions may have features of fibrous osteodystrophy in addition to rickets*, because of the hypocalcemia and secondary hyperparathyroidism. In such cases, osteoblastic and osteoclastic activity are prominent and trabeculae are separated by loose fibrous connective tissue, even in areas distant from repairing infractions. A combination of rickets and fibrous osteodystrophy can, at least in theory, also occur in association with chronic renal disease (see Fibrous osteodystrophy section below) due to renal secondary hyperparathyroidism and impaired renal synthesis of 1,25-dihydroxyvitamin D. However, in animals with renal disease the lesions of fibrous osteodystrophy generally predominate.

Cortical bone is also affected in rickets, but the lesions are generally overshadowed by those involving growth plates. Grossly, the diaphyses of long bones may appear shorter and thicker than normal with a narrow medullary cavity. In spite of their increased thickness, the cortices are more susceptible to weight-bearing trauma and, in severe cases may be soft, bent, or contain pathological fractures.

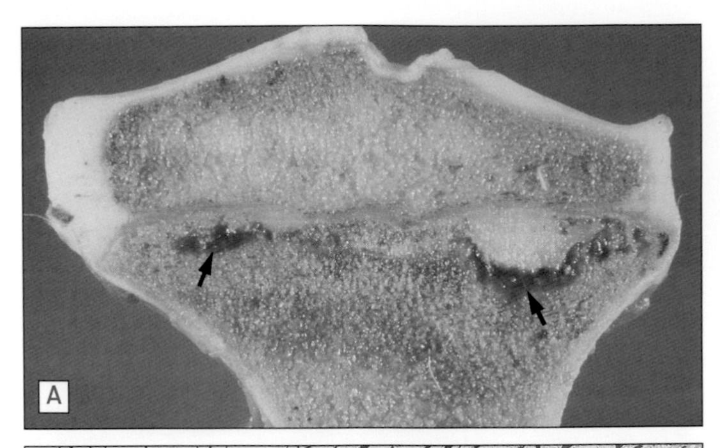

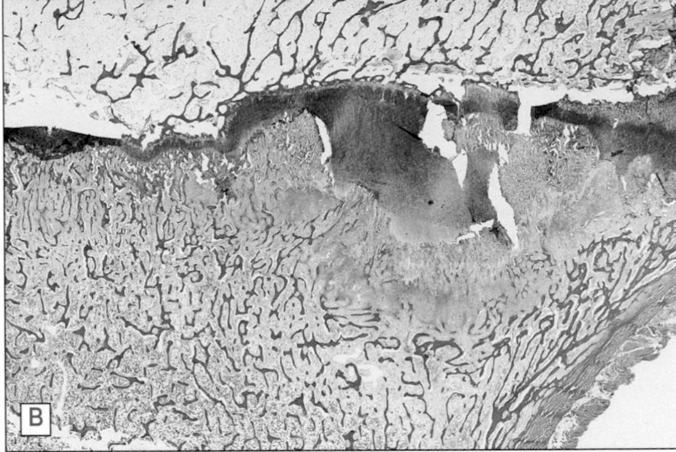

Figure 1.67 Rickets, pig. **A.** Massive, focal thickening of the physis in the proximal tibia. The dark areas, which appear gelatinous grossly (arrows), indicate trabecular disruption and replacement with highly vascular fibrous connective tissue. **B.** Subgross photograph of the same specimen showing the thickened physeal cartilage and replacement of trabecular bone in the underlying metaphysis with repair tissue.

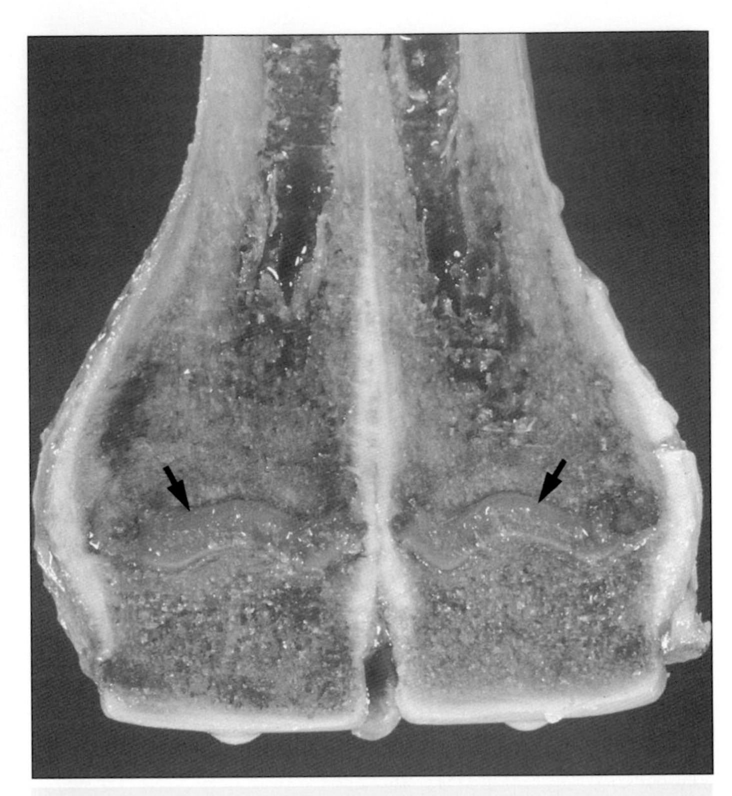

Figure 1.68 Rickets, alpaca. The physes of the distal metacarpal bone (arrows) are diffusely thickened and bulging from the cut surface.

Histologically, a layer of poorly mineralized osteoid may accumulate within partly filled Haversian systems and on the periosteal surface.

Osteoid seams are best illustrated in undemineralized sections, but can be appreciated in demineralized sections stained with hematoxylin and eosin as pale, eosinophilic matrix against the darker staining bone tissue that was previously mineralized (Fig. 1.70A). Special stains for demonstrating unmineralized osteoid in demineralized sections (see page 18) can be of value but are not used routinely and sections may be difficult to interpret in the absence of controls. *It is important to recognize that osteoid seams are not pathognomonic for rickets and osteomalacia.* Nor are they invariably present. They also may occur in other syndromes at sites of rapid bone formation rather than due to delayed mineralization.

The **lesions of osteomalacia** *are similar to those of rickets but since they occur in adult animals, growth plates are not involved.* Osteomalacic bones have reduced resistance to pressure and tension, and increased susceptibility to the stress and strain of ordinary activity. As a result, there is *excessive deposition of matrix where mechanical stimuli are strongest*, such as at insertions of tendons and fascia, places of angulation and curvature, and on stress-oriented epiphyseal trabeculae. When the disease is advanced, the *bones fracture readily*, the marrow cavity is expanded and may extend into the epiphysis, and the cortex is thin, spongy and soft. In affected cattle, fractures are most common in the ribs, pelvis, and long bones, while in pigs they occur most often in the vertebral column. *Deformities* are often present, including kyphosis or lordosis, medial displacement of the acetabula with compression of pubic bones, twisting of the ilia, and narrowing of the pelvis. The ribs and transverse processes of the lumbar vertebrae droop so that the thorax is narrowed and flattened and the sternum prominent. Collapse of articular surfaces and degeneration of cartilages is sometimes observed and tendons may separate from their attachments. In long-standing cases of osteomalacia, cachexia and anemia are often present.

The *histological changes of osteomalacia reflect the inadequate mineralization of osteoid formed during remodeling*, the lesions resembling those in the cortex of animals with rickets. In many cases, particularly those caused by phosphorus deficiency, osteoporosis associated with concurrent deficiency of protein and other nutrients is superimposed. The lesions develop slowly but in advanced cases, trabeculae are reduced in size and number, and the cortices are thin and porous. Osteoid covers the trabeculae and lines the expanded Haversian canals. Localized accumulations of osteoid occur at sites of mechanical stress.

Bibliography

Barnes JE, Jephcott BR. Phosphorus deficiency in cattle in the Northern Territory and its control. Aust Vet J 1955;31:302–311.

Bonniwell MA, et al. Rickets associated with vitamin D deficiency in young sheep. Vet Rec 1988;122:386–388.

Brock JF, Diamond LK. Rickets in rats by iron feeding. J Pediat 1934;4:442–453.

Christakos S, et al. Vitamin D-dependent calcium binding proteins: Chemistry, distribution, functional considerations, and molecular biology. Endocrine Rev 1989;10:3–26.

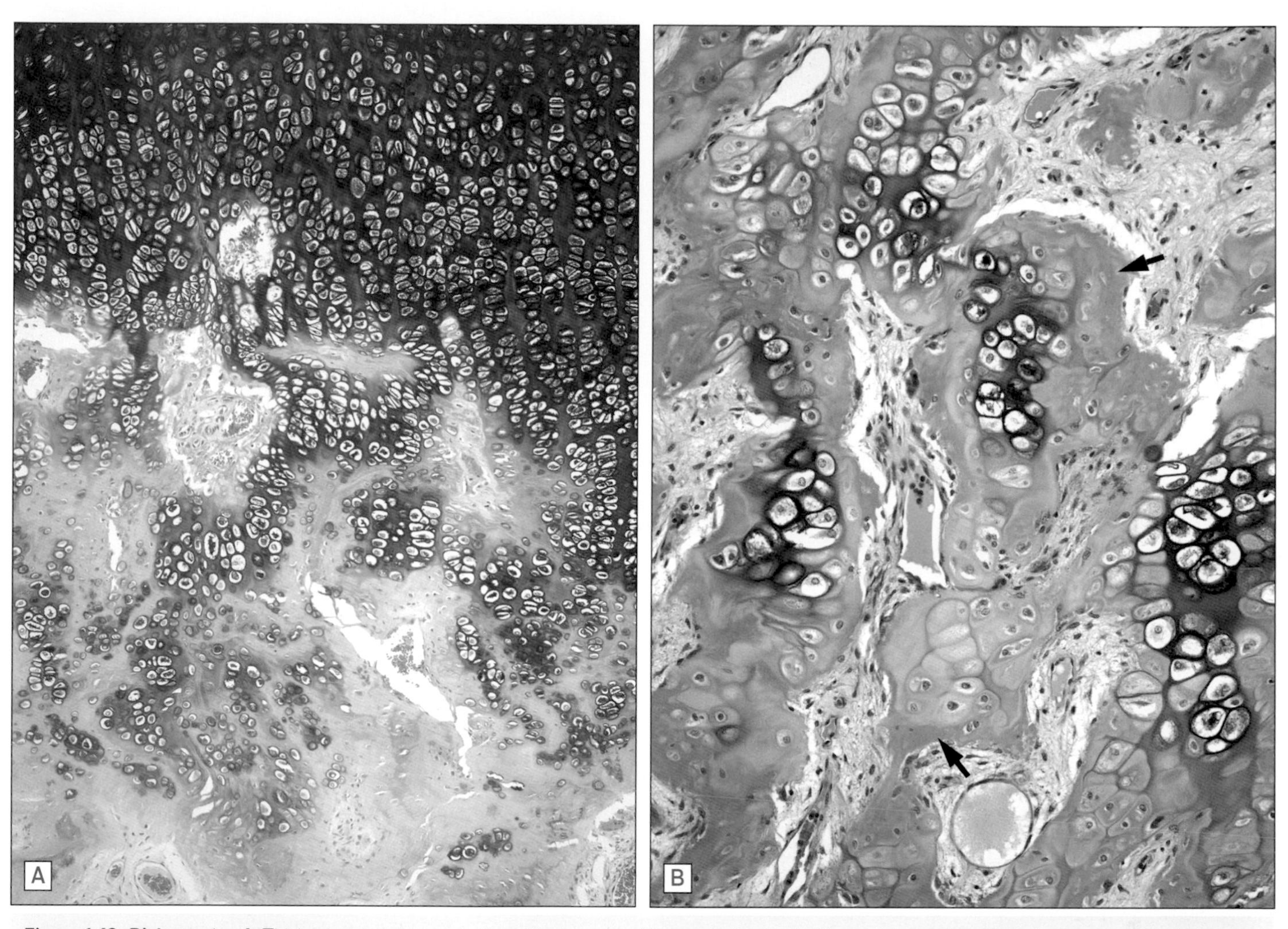

Figure 1.69 Rickets, pig. **A.** Thickening and disorganization of the hypertrophic zone in the physis. Metaphysis consists of persistent tongues and islands of hypertrophic chondrocytes surrounded by a thick layer of osteoid. **B.** High-power view of metaphysis showing clusters of hypertrophic chondrocytes, some of which are degenerate, surrounded in some areas by seams of unmineralized osteoid (arrows).

Clements MR, et al. A new mechanism for indexed vitamin D deficiency in calcium deprivation. Nature 1987;325:62–65.

Freeman S, McLean FC. Experimental rickets. Blood and tissue changes in puppies receiving diets very low in phosphorus with and without vitamin D. Arch Pathol 1941;32:387–408.

Gershoff SN, et al. The effect of vitamin D-deficient diets containing various Ca:P ratios on cats. J Nutr 1957;63:79–92.

Grant AB. Carotene: a rachitogenic factor in green-feeds. Nature Lond 1953;172:627.

Hill FI, et al. Rickets in alpacas (*Lama pacos*) in New Zealand. N Z Vet J 1994;42:229–232.

How KL, et al. Dietary vitamin D dependence of dog and cat due to inadequate cutaneous synthesis of vitamin D. General Comp Endocrinol 1994; 96:12–18.

Hunter WL, et al. Rearrangement of the metaphyseal vasculature of the rat growth plate in rickets and rachitic reversal: A model of vascular arrest and angiogenesis renewed. Anat Rec 1991;229:453–461.

Johnson KA, et al. Vitamin D-dependent rickets in a Saint Bernard dog. J Small Anim Pract 1988;29:657–666.

Judson GJ, Feakes A. Vitamin D doses for alpacas (*Lama pacos*). Aust Vet J 1999;77:310–315.

Kealy RD, et al. Some observations on the dietary vitamin D requirements of weanling pups. J Nutr 1991;121:S66–S69.

Malik R, et al. Rickets in a litter of racing Greyhounds. J Small Anim Pract 1997;38:109–114.

Mankin HJ. Rickets, osteomalacia and renal osteodystrophy. An update. Orthop Clinics North Am 1990;21:81–96.

Nisbet DI, et al. Osteodystrophic diseases of sheep. II. Rickets in young sheep. J Comp Pathol 1966;76:159–169.

Pepper TA, et al. Rickets in growing pigs and response to treatment. Vet Rec 1978;103:4–8.

Pitt MJ. Rickets and osteomalacia. In: Resnick D, ed. Diagnosis of Bone and Joint Diseases. 3rd ed. vol 4. Philadelphia: W. B. Saunders, 1994:1885–1922.

Pointillart A, et al. Effects of vitamin D on calcium regulation in vitamin-D-deficient pigs given a phytate-phosphorus diet. Br J Nutrition 1986;56: 661–669.

Shupe JL, et al. Clinical signs and bone changes associated with phosphorus deficiency in beef cattle. Am J Vet Res 1988;49:1629–1636.

Smith BSW, Wright H. Relative contributions of diet and sunshine to the overall vitamin D status of the grazing ewe. Vet Rec 1984;115:537–538.

Van Saun RJ, et al. Evaluation of vitamin D status of llamas and alpacas with hypophosphatemic rickets. J Am Vet Med Assoc 1996;209:1128–1133.

Winkler I, et al. Absence of renal 25-hydroxy-cholecalciferol-1-hydroxylase activity in a pig strain with vitamin D-dependent rickets. Calcif Tiss Int 1986;38:87–94.

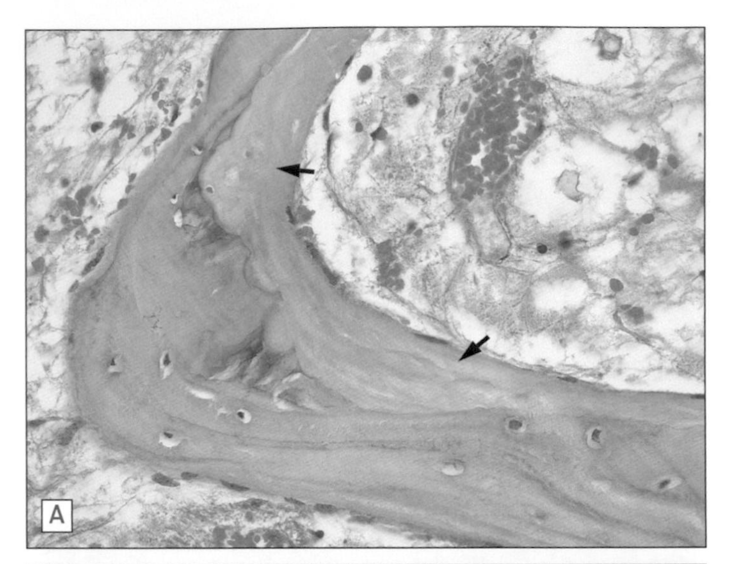

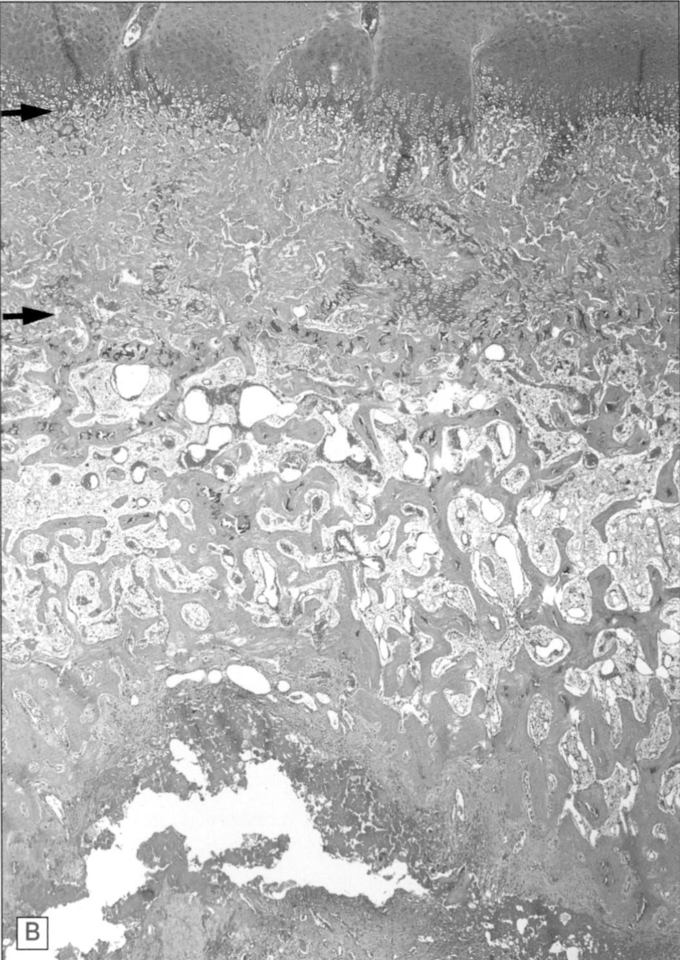

Figure 1.70 Rickets, due to phosphorus deficiency, in a farmed red deer. **A.** Pale-staining osteoid seam (arrows) on the surface of a metaphyseal trabecula. Note the scalloped reversal line separating the osteoid seam from the underlying mineralized bone, indicating previous osteoclastic resorption at the site. **B.** Low-power view of costochondral junction from the same deer showing an irregular line of recent trabecular fractures deep in the metaphysis. Note the disruption of trabecular architecture and persistent islands of cartilage in the primary and secondary spongiosa (between arrows).

Yamaguchi A, et al. Bone in the marmoset: A resemblance to vitamin D-dependent rickets, Type II. Calcif Tiss Int 1986;39:22–27.

Fibrous osteodystrophy

Fibrous osteodystrophy (osteodystrophia fibrosa, osteitis fibrosa cystica) is a relatively common metabolic bone disease characterized by extensive bone resorption accompanied by proliferation of fibrous tissue and poorly mineralized, immature bone. The pathogenesis involves persistent elevation of plasma PTH and the lesion can be considered to represent the skeletal manifestation of primary or secondary hyperparathyroidism. Different animal species vary in their susceptibility to fibrous osteodystrophy and, to some degree, in the distribution of lesions. Horses, pigs, dogs, cats, ferrets, and goats are often affected, as are reptiles and New World nonhuman primates, but the disease is rare in sheep and cattle.

Primary hyperparathyroidism *is usually the result of a functional parathyroid gland adenoma* (see Vol. 3, Endocrine glands). This occurs rarely in adult dogs and there are isolated reports in horses and cattle. Hereditary primary hyperparathyroidism associated with diffuse parathyroid hyperplasia was also reported in a litter of German Shepherd puppies with fibrous osteodystrophy. *In primary hyperparathyroidism, autonomous secretion of PTH results in persistent hypercalcemia and hypophosphatemia*, the latter reflecting increased urinary clearance of phosphate. This differs from secondary hyperparathyroidism where plasma total calcium concentrations are usually either normal or slightly decreased and, depending on the cause, plasma phosphorus concentrations are either normal or increased. The persistent hypercalcemia in primary hyperparathyroidism is generally accompanied by *polydipsia/polyuria, muscular weakness, and widespread mineralization of soft tissues*. Affected animals may succumb to the effects of *nephrocalcinosis* before the skeletal changes are severe enough to become clinically apparent. The skeletal changes in the German Shepherd pups with primary hyperparathyroidism (discussed below) were more severe than those described in adult dogs with functional parathyroid adenomas. This probably reflects the more rapid turnover of bone in young animals. Generalized bone resorption also occurs in **pseudohyperparathyroidism** or **hypercalcemia of malignancy** caused by the production of parathyroid-related hormone by tumors such as malignant lymphoma and apocrine gland adenocarcinoma of the anal sac. However, although increased osteoclastic activity and reduced trabecular bone volume have been demonstrated by histomorphometric techniques, the bone lesions are usually mild and are not apparent clinically or even radiographically.

Secondary hyperparathyroidism is a much more common cause of fibrous osteodystrophy in animals than primary hyperparathyroidism and *may be due to either chronic renal disease or a dietary imbalance of calcium and phosphorus*. PTH secretion is stimulated by a reduction in plasma-ionized calcium, whatever the cause, and if the stimulus persists then generalized bone resorption results. **Renal secondary hyperparathyroidism** occurs most often in dogs, and occasionally in cats, as a complication of chronic renal failure. Impaired glomerular filtration in animals with renal failure leads to progressive hyperphosphatemia due to reduced renal clearance of phosphate. Hypocalcemia develops as a result of the inverse relationship between plasma-ionized phosphate and calcium concentrations, and stimulates the release of PTH. In addition, chronic renal disease may result in impaired formation of 1,25-dihydroxyvitamin D, thereby reducing calcium absorption from the intestine and contributing further to the hypocalcemia. This combination of secondary hyperparathyroidism and deficient synthesis of 1,25-dihydroxyvitamin D in animals and humans with renal failure may give rise to a bone disease with features of both fibrous osteodystrophy and osteomalacia. For this reason, the disorder is often referred to by the more general term, **renal osteodystrophy**.

Nutritional secondary hyperparathyroidism *may be due to a simple dietary deficiency of calcium, excess dietary phosphorus, or to a deficiency of vitamin D.* As discussed previously in this chapter, vitamin D deficiency alone is also a cause of rickets or osteomalacia, but reduced calcium absorption from the intestine in animals with vitamin D deficiency often results in concurrent fibrous osteodystrophy. Excess dietary phosphorus may cause fibrous osteodystrophy even in animals receiving adequate dietary calcium. Increased plasma phosphate concentration, resulting from increased intestinal absorption of phosphorus, depresses plasma-ionized calcium and indirectly stimulates the release of PTH.

In practice, *nutritional secondary hyperparathyroidism is most often caused by diets containing low calcium and a relatively high concentration of phosphorus* and, with the exception of horses, affects young, rapidly growing animals. Horses seem to be remarkably sensitive to the effects of high-phosphorus diets and relatively resistant to the effects of rations low in phosphorus. In all species, there are several factors that influence the development and the severity of lesions in secondary hyperparathyroidism. These include the degree to which dietary calcium is deficient and, perhaps more importantly, the degree to which dietary phosphorus is in excess. Although the efficiency of calcium absorption decreases markedly at high intakes, that of phosphorus seems to be unchanged. Furthermore, over a wide range of intakes, plasma calcium concentration is more sensitive to dietary phosphorus than to dietary calcium.

Differences between species in the susceptibility, likely etiology, and distribution of lesions in fibrous osteodystrophy are discussed below in some detail.

In the **horse**, the disease occurs at any time after weaning but the prevalence, and possibly the susceptibility, declines after about the seventh year. Horses require a calcium:phosphorus ratio of approximately 1:1. Diets in which the calcium:phosphorus ratio is 1:3 or wider, can result in osteodystrophia fibrosa depending to some extent on individual and familial susceptibility, and on alternative sources of calcium, such as drinking water. The condition usually occurs after maintenance for some months on diets consisting largely of grain, corn, and grain by-products such as bran, hence the term "bran-disease." Fibrous osteodystrophy also occurs in horses grazing tropical grasses high in oxalate, even though dietary calcium and phosphorus are normal. Prevalences of 10–15% occur in Sri Lanka and the Philippines. The problem is also reported in northern Australia and southern states of the USA. Lush pastures are most hazardous, some containing as much as 7.8% oxalate on a dry weight basis. Those with total oxalate over 0.5% and calcium:oxalate ratios below 0.5 are potentially dangerous because oxalate binds the calcium and makes it unavailable for absorption. Several grasses, including *Setaria sphacelata*, *Cenchrus ciliaris* (buffel grass), *Brachiaria mutica* (para grass), *Digitaria decumbens* (pangola grass), and *Panicum* spp., contain sufficient oxalate to produce clinical disease. Renal secondary hyperparathyroidism is not reported in horses as renal failure in this species typically results in hypercalcemia rather than hypocalcemia.

The *clinical signs and gross lesions* of fibrous osteodystrophy generally develop more rapidly in young, growing horses due to their increased rate of bone formation and remodeling. Early signs consist of minor changes in gait, stiffness, transient and shifting lameness, and lassitude. Loss of appetite with progressive cachexia and anemia develop later. The anemia may be due to depression of erythropoiesis by parathyroid hormone or its metabolites. *The most characteristic feature is bilateral swelling of the bones of the skull* (Fig. 1.71A), including both the maxillae and mandibles, hence the term "*big-head*." The bony swelling begins along the alveolar margins of the mandibles, producing cylindrical thickenings and reducing the intermandibular space. The molar margins of the maxillae then begin to swell and the enlargement spreads to involve the palate, the remainder of the maxillae, and the lacrimal and zygomatic bones. In severe cases (Fig. 1.71B), the nasal and frontal bones are also swollen. Initially, the swellings are soft but later they harden. Involvement of the palate reduces the nasal passages and may cause dyspnea. Palatine and mandibular thickening causes reduction of the buccal cavity and mastication is impaired. The teeth loosen and are partially buried or may exfoliate, and the softened bone yields to pressure, further impairing prehension and mastication. The food may be swallowed unchewed or allowed to drop out of the mouth. The face may be continually wet from occlusion of the lacrimal canals. In advanced cases, the enlargement of the head may be extreme and although the swelling is invariably bilateral, it is not always symmetrical.

Gross lesions in the remainder of the skeleton indicate advanced disease. In such cases, the scapulae may be thickened and curved so that the shoulder joint is displaced forward and the trunk droops in the pectoral girdle, giving undue prominence to the sternum. The vertebral column curves downwards, sometimes upwards, and the arch of the ribs is reduced. There is an increased susceptibility to *fractures* and to avulsion of ligaments. *Detachment of ligaments and tendons* occurs chiefly in the lower limbs. Some animals escape the fractures and ligamentous detachments and pass into *cachectic recumbency* but multiple fractures may occur if such animals are forced to rise. Radiography of affected bones may show generalized osteopenia, but not until the relatively advanced stages of the disease. Macerated bones from severely affected animals are finely cancellous or pumice-like and may be brittle and crumbly. The weight of the macerated bones may be less than 50% of normal.

Severe cases of fibrous osteodystrophy in horses are now rare and animals with facial swelling due to nutritional secondary hyperparathyroidism are seldom seen. Milder forms of the disease, however, may still be a cause of poorly defined lameness and could perhaps predispose to spontaneous fractures of sesamoid bones or phalanges in racehorses in training, which are fed rations high in grain.

Serum concentrations of calcium and phosphate are of limited value in the diagnosis of nutritional secondary hyperparathyroidism in horses, although a slight increase in serum phosphate is reported as a common finding in affected horses. Serum concentrations of PTH are likely to be of more diagnostic value and the test has been validated for use in horses. Increased urinary fractional clearance of phosphorus is also considered a sensitive indicator of secondary hyperparathyroidism. In one survey, abnormally high phosphorus clearance ratios were detected in 87.5% of racehorses in Hong Kong, suggesting that subclinical hyperparathyroidism is relatively common.

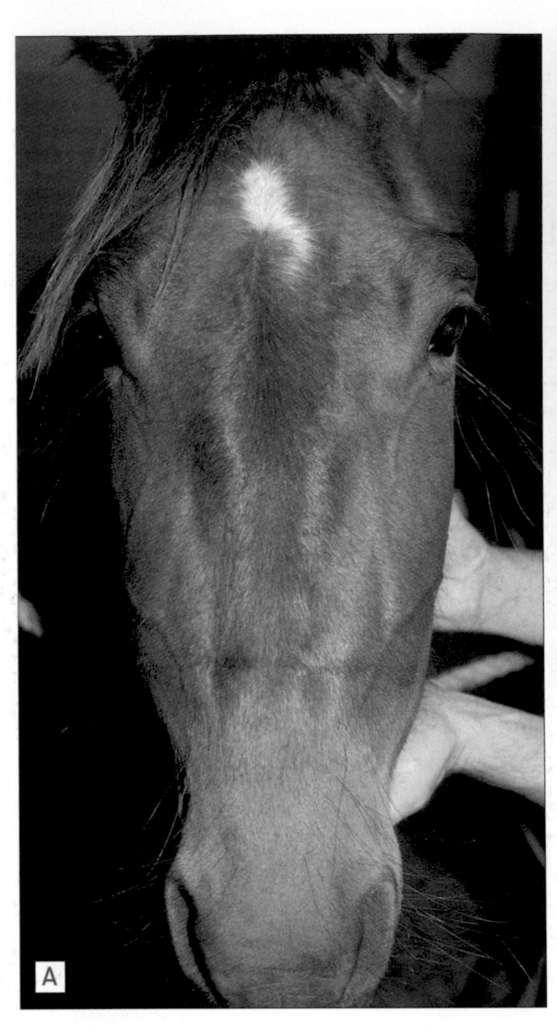

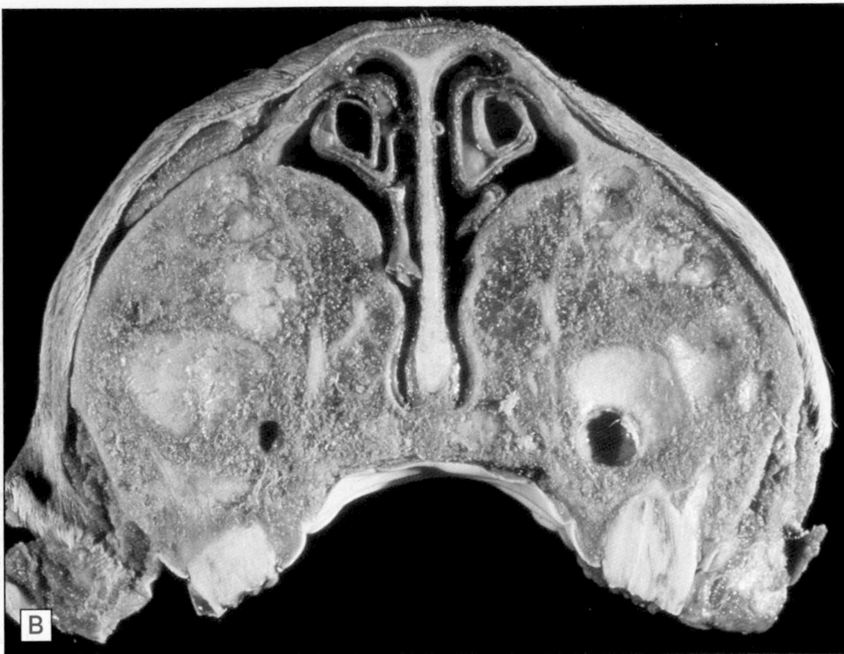

Figure 1.71 Fibrous osteodystrophy, horse. **A.** Bilateral swelling of maxillary bones. **B.** Marked, bilateral swelling of maxillary bones with obliteration of maxillary sinuses and attenuation of nasal passages. (Courtesy of PC Stromberg.)

In **swine**, *fibrous osteodystrophy usually occurs in young growing animals fed unsupplemented grain rations*. The disease also accompanies rickets in association with vitamin D deficiency. Clinical signs include stiffness, reluctance to rise and, in severe cases, lameness. Some affected animals may develop enlargement of the skull similar to that seen in horses. The mandibles may be affected first, and sometimes are the only site of gross lesions, but in other cases, the basocranium is also enlarged. Sometimes, the mouth cannot be closed and the tongue protrudes because of the swelling of the jaws and the shortness of the mandibular rami. The teeth are mobile and often deeply and obliquely embedded in the fibro-osseous connective tissue. Radiographically, there is a generalized reduction in bone density.

At necropsy, the ribs may bend or snap with little effort. Recent or healing pathological fractures are often present. Articular surfaces of major joints may be irregular and focally depressed due to collapse of subchondral bone (Fig. 1.72). Growth plates are of normal thickness, except in cases caused by vitamin D deficiency where rickets and fibrous osteodystrophy occur concurrently.

Severe fibrous osteodystrophy is relatively common in **goats** fed rations high in concentrates, but there are no convincing reports of the disease in either **sheep** or **cattle**, suggesting species variation in susceptibility. In goats, fibro-osseous enlargement of the mandibles and maxillae is a characteristic clinical feature (Fig. 1.73). Respiratory distress may be present due to encroachment by swollen maxillary bones on the nasal cavity. The relative severity of lesions in bones of the skull in goats and certain other species may be related to the mechanical stimulus associated with chewing. The bones of the limbs are also affected in goats with fibrous osteodystrophy and may be markedly bowed.

In **dogs** and **cats**, nutritional secondary hyperparathyroidism is usually caused by *diets consisting largely or entirely of meat or offal*. The calcium content of such diets is low and the calcium:phosphorus ratio very wide. For example, the calcium content of cardiac and skeletal muscle is approximately 10 mg/100 g and the ratio of calcium to phosphorus approximately 1:20. The calcium:phosphorus ratio of liver is approximately 1:50. The ideal ratio is about 1:1, and skeletal abnormalities develop when ratios are 1:2 or greater. Supplementation of all-meat diets with appropriate levels of calcium corrects the imbalance and prevents fibrous osteodystrophy.

Clinical signs of nutritional secondary hyperparathyroidism usually begin a few weeks after weaning. Kittens fed exclusively on beef heart develop signs of fibrous osteodystrophy within 4 weeks. In both kittens and puppies, signs of the disease are progressive and include reluctance to move, hindlimb lameness and incoordination. Enlargement of facial bones is uncommon. Affected animals become depressed and may develop sudden lameness due to infractions of long bones or vertebrae, the latter resulting in paralysis. Callus formation at fracture sites does occur but consists primarily of fibrous tissue with little evidence of mineralization. Radiographically there is generalized, often marked, osteopenia (Fig. 1.74). Fibrous osteodystrophy in cats has been inappropriately referred to as osteogenesis imperfecta in the early veterinary literature because of the osteopenia and

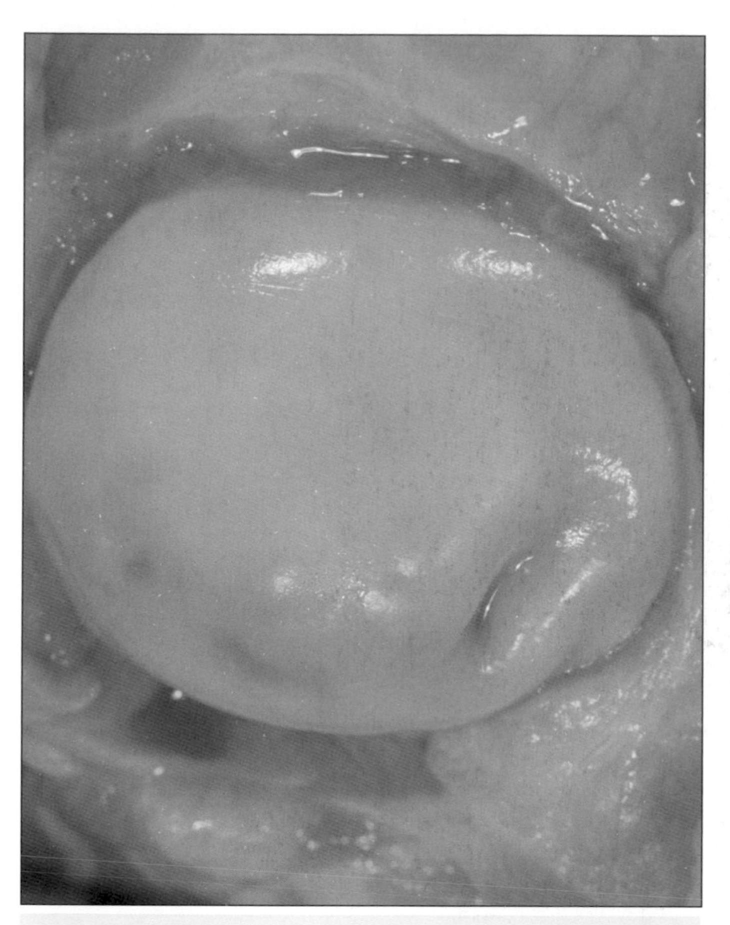

Figure 1.72 Fibrous osteodystrophy, pig. Irregular articular surface of humeral head due to collapse of subchondral bone. (Courtesy of RA Fairley.)

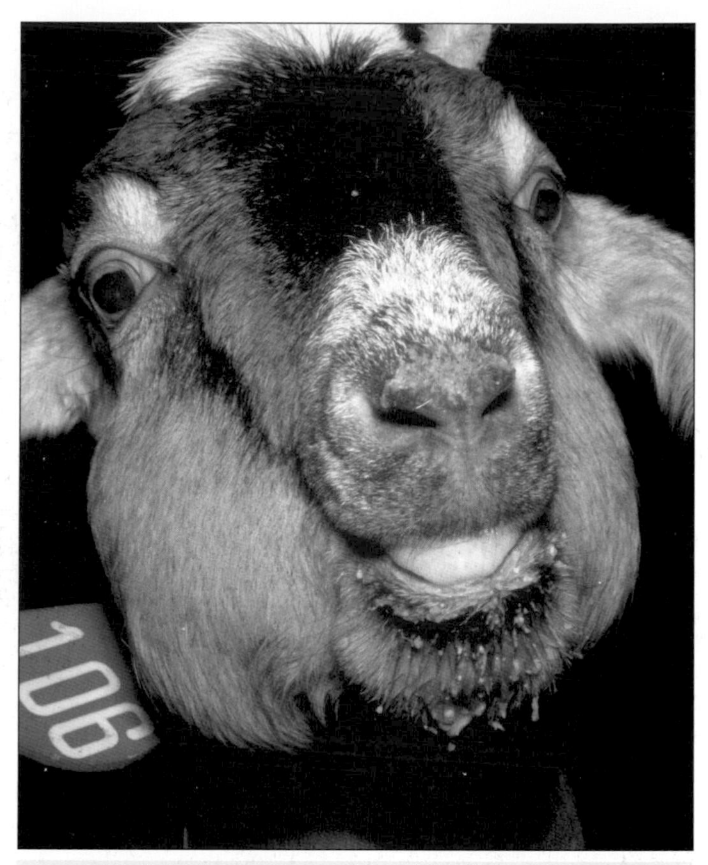

Figure 1.73 Fibrous osteodystrophy, goat. Bilateral swelling of maxillary bones and mandibles.

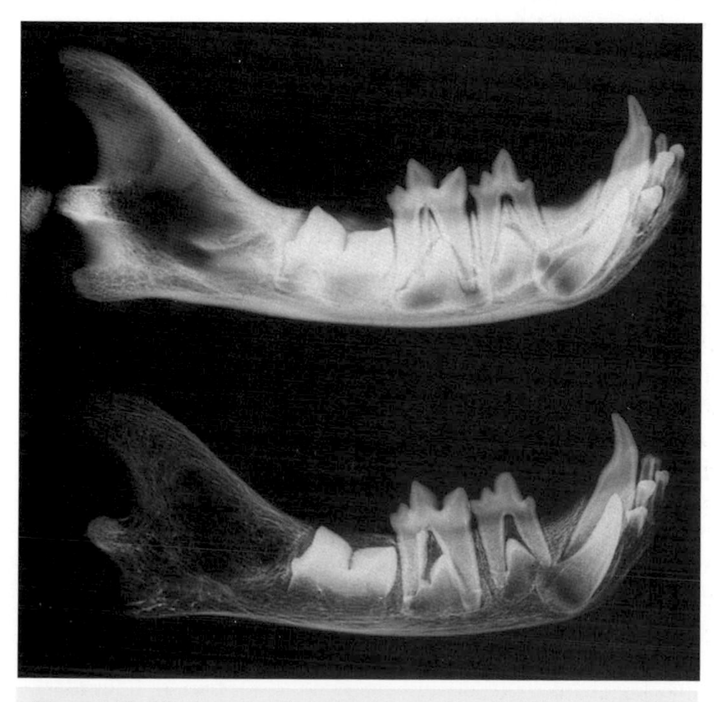

Figure 1.74 Fibrous osteodystrophy, kitten. Mandible from a normal kitten (top) and a kitten with fibrous osteodystrophy. Note the marked, diffuse rarefaction in the affected kitten and the loss of alveolar bone.

bone fragility. Osteogenesis imperfecta has however been diagnosed in the cat and remains a differential for fibrous osteodystrophy.

Renal secondary hyperparathyroidism may occur in adult dogs with renal failure, but the skeletal lesions are usually of secondary importance to the manifestations of uremia. Resorption of alveolar socket bone and loss of lamina dura dentes occurs early in the disease and may be evident radiographically. As the disease progresses, there is accelerated resorption of cancellous bones of the maxilla and mandibles, occasionally resulting in soft, pliable mandibles (so-called "*rubber jaw*"). Skull bones may have a moth-eaten appearance due to localized areas of accentuated resorption. Facial hyperostosis is a feature of some dogs with renal secondary hyperparathyroidism, but usually occurs in dogs with familial renal disease that develop slowly progressive renal failure from a young age. In such dogs, there is symmetrical enlargement of the head due to marked swelling of the maxillae and mandibles. The bones are firm rather than hard and can usually be cut with a knife. Focal red-brown areas of recent or old hemorrhage may be evident on cut surface. Young dogs with renal osteodystrophy may also have enlarged costochondral junctions and irregularly thickened physes, reflecting concurrent rickets due to impaired formation of 1,25-dihydroxyvitamin D.

In the German Shepherd pups with *hereditary primary hyperparathyroidism*, clinical signs were apparent by 2 weeks of age and included stunted growth, muscular weakness, and polydipsia/polyuria. Diffuse reduction in bone density was detected radiographically. At necropsy, the long bones were fragile and had narrow cortices. Facial bones were not enlarged but firm, pale yellow, swollen regions in the

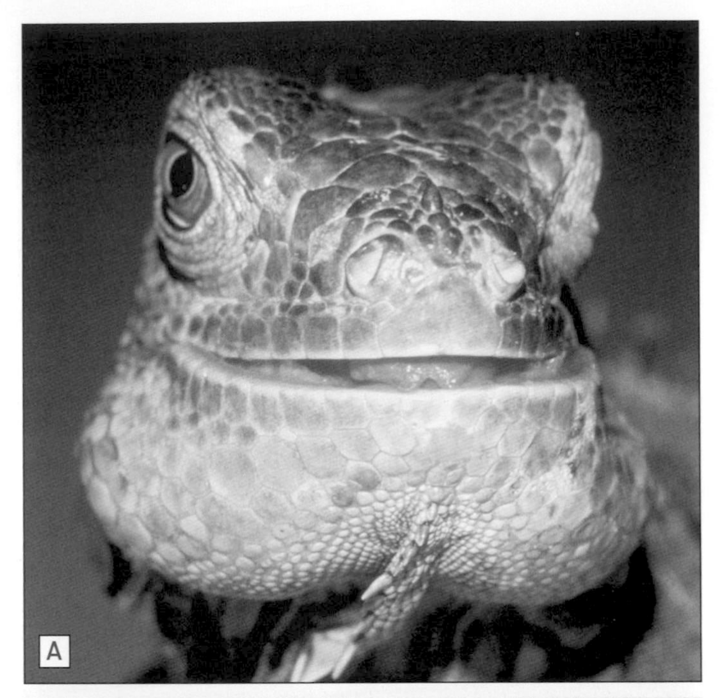

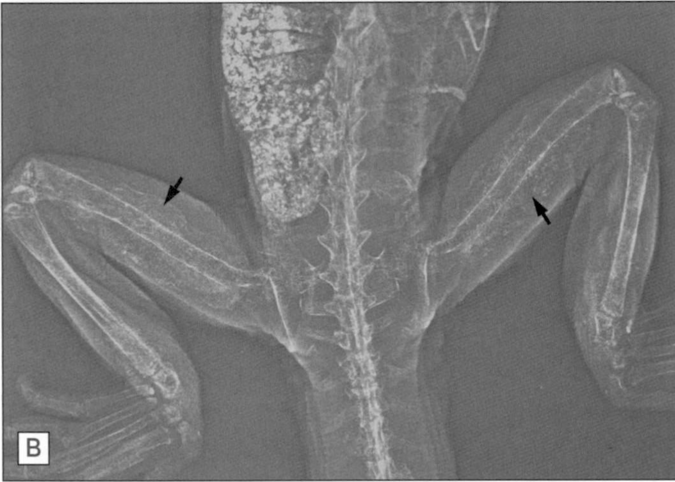

Figure 1.75 Fibrous osteodystrophy, iguana. **A.** Bilateral mandibular swelling. **B.** Xeroradiograph of the hindlegs and spine of the same iguana. The cortices of long bones are very thin and there is extensive periosteal new bone formation, particularly along the femurs (arrows).

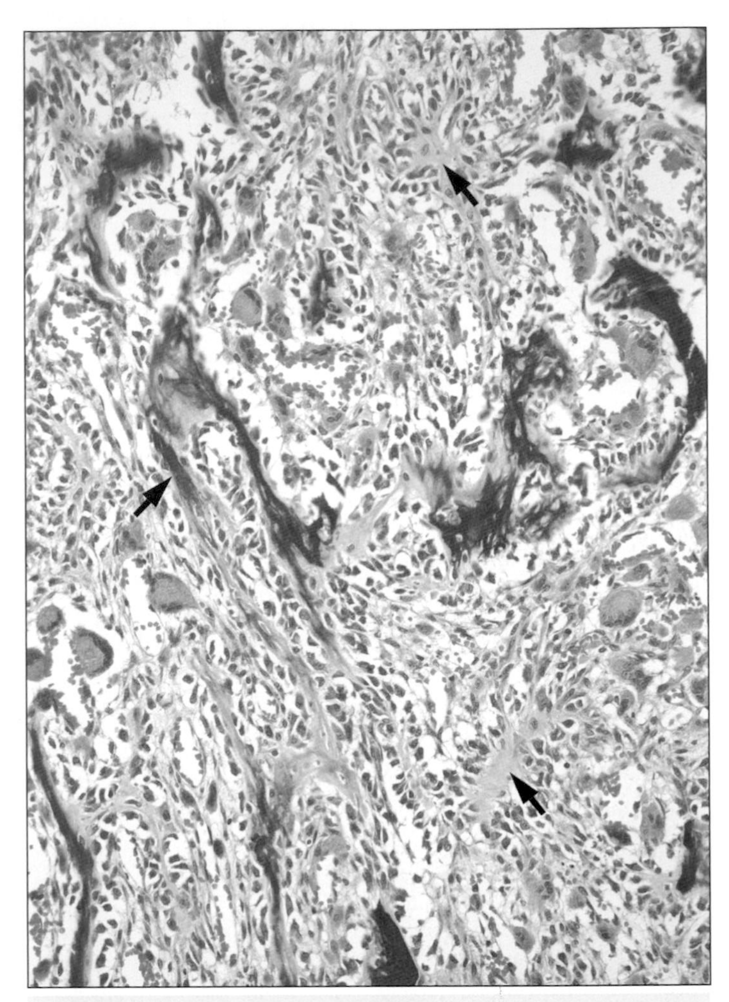

Figure 1.76 Fibrous osteodystrophy, ferret. Undemineralized section stained by the Von Kossa method and counterstained with hematoxylin and eosin. Highly reactive osteoblasts are forming delicate spicules of poorly mineralized or unmineralized bone (arrows). Many large osteoclasts are also present.

metaphyses of the ribs extended 2–3 cm along the shaft from close to costochondral junctions. Similar swollen segments were also present in the diaphyses of some ribs.

Fibrous osteodystrophy was reported in a strain of German Shepherd pups in Japan and although the possibility of a familial increase in susceptibility was suggested, the syndrome was apparently due to nutritional secondary hyperparathyroidism and was not analogous to the hereditary primary hyperparathyroidism referred to above.

Nutritional secondary hyperparathyroidism is relatively common in **reptiles** fed on diets that are either high in phosphorus (e.g., meat) or low in calcium (e.g., fruits, vegetables). Typically, there is thickening and softening of the bones of the skull and limbs, and a reduction in radiographic bone density (Fig. 1.75A, B).

The **microscopic features** *of fibrous osteodystrophy are similar in all domestic animal species and are characterized by increased osteoclastic bone resorption, marked fibroplasia, and increased osteoblastic activity with formation of immature woven bone.* These are also features of normal bone during development, and can be found in other disease processes. For example, longitudinal growth of long bones in rapidly growing young animals is accompanied by prominent osteoclastic and osteoblastic activity and intertrabecular fibrosis in the peripheral metaphyses as part of the normal modeling process. Such areas must be avoided when examining bone for histological evidence of fibrous osteodystrophy. Repairing fractures at certain stages of maturity, and diseases associated with hyperostosis (discussed elsewhere in this chapter), may also be confused with fibrous osteodystrophy if histological sections are examined without an awareness of their exact location and an adequate clinical and/or radiographic knowledge of the case.

The lesions of fibrous osteodystrophy vary between different bones, depending on their rate of turnover, and with the stage of the disease process. It is important therefore to examine several sections from different parts of the skeleton, particularly those areas that are growing most rapidly. In early lesions, the increase in bone resorption is reflected by increased numbers of plump, active osteoclasts, often within Howship's lacunae along the surface of bone trabeculae. Osteoblastic activity is also prominent (Fig. 1.76) and it is not unusual to find

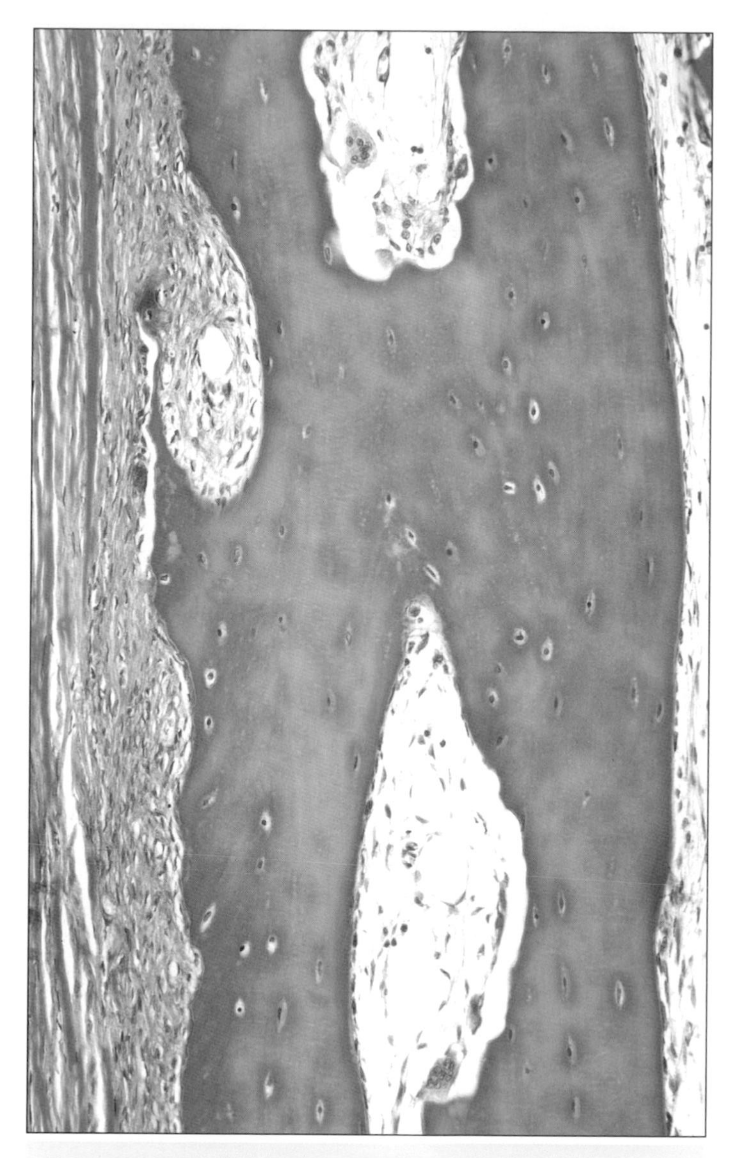

Figure 1.77 Fibrous osteodystrophy, kitten. Large resorption cavities in the cortex. Osteoclasts and Howship's lacunae indicate active resorption.

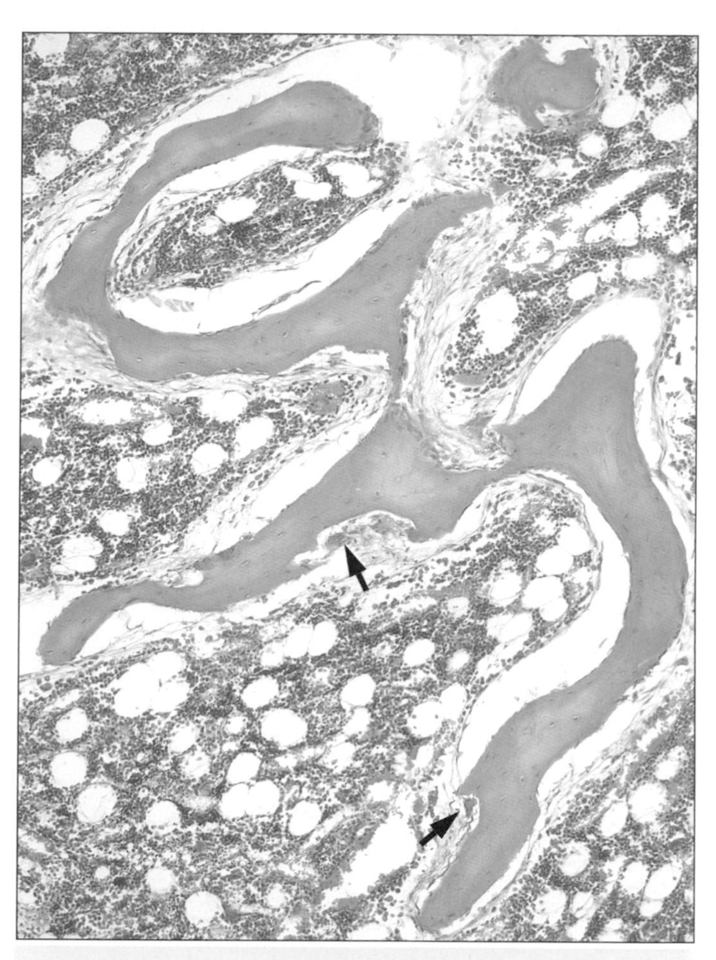

Figure 1.78 Fibrous osteodystrophy, pig. Early lesion with peritrabecular fibrosis and osteoclastic resorption (arrows).

bone trabeculae being resorbed on one side while new bone is being added to the other. Wide osteoid seams may be present at sites of rapid bone formation, especially in renal osteodystrophy where there may be concurrent rickets or osteomalacia due to deficient renal synthesis of 1,25-dihydroxyvitamin D. Resorption cavities lined by osteoclasts may be present in cortical bone (Fig. 1.77), and even within trabeculae, providing convincing evidence for exaggerated bone resorption. Lightly fibrillar connective tissue initially surrounds trabeculae undergoing resorption (Fig. 1.78), but later progresses to fill the intertrabecular spaces. As the disease progresses, *mature trabecular and cortical bone are extensively replaced by a combination of loose fibrous connective tissue and irregular trabeculae of poorly mineralized or unmineralized woven bone*, which may encroach on the medullary cavity and expand peripherally to elevate the periosteum (Fig. 1.79). The compact bone of the cortex is resorbed from endosteal and periosteal surfaces, and from within. In advanced lesions, only porous remnants of the original cortex may remain (Fig. 1.79). The soft, swollen mandibles and maxillae in animals with facial hyperostosis consist of highly cellular fibrous connective tissue surrounding delicate trabeculae of poorly mineralized woven bone (Fig. 1.80A, B). Osteoclastic activity may be largely absent in such advanced lesions, or remain in isolated pockets where remnants of the original bone are still being resorbed. In the absence of an adequate history or gross description, such lesions could be confused with benign or malignant bone tumors, or perhaps a fracture callus. Cyst-like cavities are sometimes present, possibly secondary to localized hemorrhage, and there may be sufficient hemosiderin in some areas to cause brown discoloration grossly.

Growth plates are histologically normal in fibrous osteodystrophy unless there is concurrent rickets or interference with vascular invasion due to trabecular fractures in the adjacent metaphysis. Premature resorption of the primary spongiosa is a feature of fibrous osteodystrophy in young, growing animals. The primary spongiosa normally consists of delicate trabeculae extending into the metaphysis at right angles to the growth plate and containing a central core of mineralized cartilage. In fibrous osteodystrophy, the newly formed trabeculae are resorbed almost as rapidly as they form and are replaced by disorganized spicules of woven bone lacking the cartilage core (Fig. 1.81). The spicules are often lined by osteoclasts and/or active osteoblasts, two to three cells deep, and are separated by a moderate amount of fibrous connective tissue.

In severe cases, articular cartilage of weight-bearing joints is often herniated into the epiphysis, causing an irregular articular surface. This is the result of osteoclastic resorption of the calcified zone of

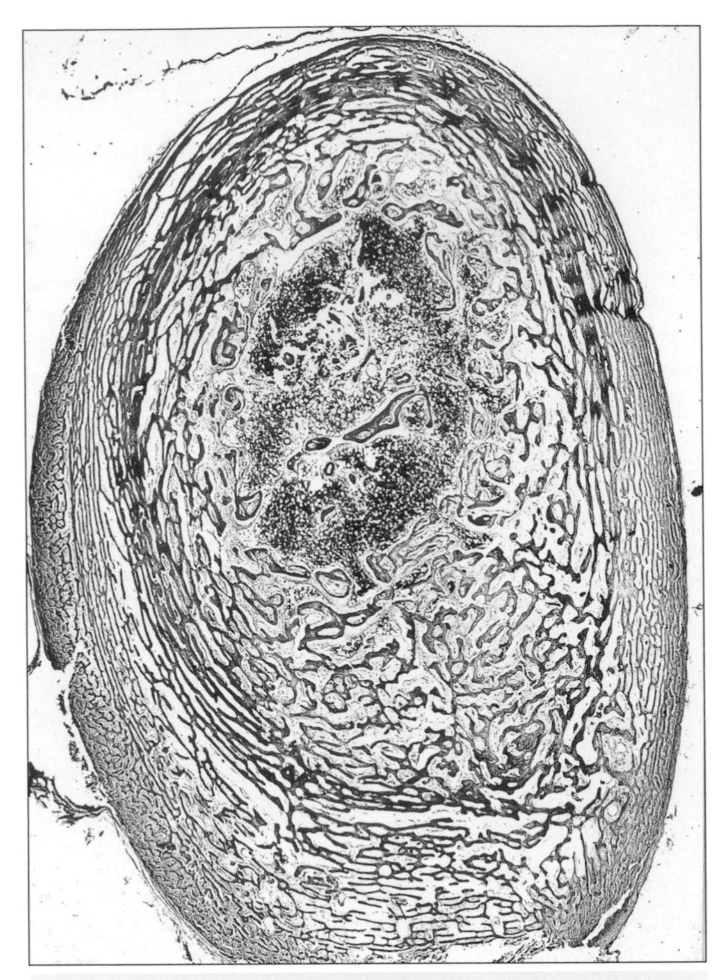

Figure 1.79 Fibrous osteodystrophy, pig. Transverse, subgross section of humeral diaphysis in an advanced lesion. Rarefaction of original and proliferation of new bone on medullary and periosteal surfaces.

articular cartilage, as well as resorption and collapse of subchondral epiphyseal bone.

In humans with renal failure, histologic lesions of osteomalacia are a prominent feature, but in dogs with renal secondary hyperparathyroidism, fibrous osteodystrophy predominates. An inherited disease known as Albright's syndrome appears as fibrous osteodystrophy in children, and in some children a phosphorus-losing nephropathy has been identified. Even in relatively young pups, histologic evidence of rickets is unlikely because the characteristic physeal lesions of rickets require relatively rapid growth and pups with renal failure generally grow poorly. *The lesions of renal osteodystrophy in dogs are usually most severe in the bones of the skull.* Histologic evidence of bone resorption by numerous large osteoclasts is prominent, particularly around teeth where the alveolar bone may be removed completely (Fig. 1.80A). Although facial hyperostosis occurs in some cases, osteopenia is more common in dogs with renal failure. Increased bone resorption on endosteal and periosteal surfaces is not balanced by formation, resulting in reduced cortical thickness.

Bibliography

Andrews AH, et al. Osteodystrophia fibrosa in young goats. Vet Rec 1983;112:404–406.

Colussi G, et al. Bone and joints alterations in uremic patients. Role of parathyroid hormone. Contributions Nephrology 1990;77:157–167.

Cushner HM, Adams ND. Review: Renal osteodystrophy – pathogenesis and treatment. Am J Med Sci 1986;29:264–275.

David JB, et al. Equine nutritional secondary hyperparathyroidism. Compend Contin Educ Pract Vet 1997;19:1380–1386.

Doige CE, et al. Influence of calcium and phosphorus on growth and skeletal development of growing swine. Can J Anim Sc 1975;55:147–164.

Feinfeld DA, Sherwood LM. Parathyroid hormone and 1,25(OH)$_2$D$_3$ in chronic renal failure. Kid Int 1988;33:1049–1058.

Goodman WG, et al. Renal osteodystrophy in adults and children. In: Favus MJ, ed. Primer on the Metabolic Bone Diseases and Disorders of Mineral Metabolism. 4th ed. Philadelphia, Lippincott Williams & Wilkins, 1999:347–363.

Kawaguchi K, et al. Nutritional secondary hyperparathyroidism occurring in a strain of German Shepherd puppies. Jpn J Vet Res 1993;41:89–96.

Mason DK, et al. Diagnosis, treatment and prevention of nutritional secondary hyperparathyroidism in Thoroughbred racehorses in Hong Kong. Equine Pract 1988;10:10–17.

Norrdin RW, Shih MS. Profiles of cortical remodeling sites in longitudinal rib sections of Beagles with renal failure and parathyroid hyperplasia. Metab Bone Dis Rel Res 1983;5:353–359.

Ronen N, et al. Clinical and biochemical findings and parathyroid hormone concentrations in three horses with secondary hyperparathyroidism. J South Afr Vet Assoc 1992;63:134–136.

Roussel AJ, et al. Radioimmunoassay for parathyroid hormone in equids. Am J Vet Res 1987;48:586–588.

Spencer GR. Porcine lactational osteoporosis. Am J Pathol 1975;95:270–280.

Storts RW, Koestner A. Skeletal lesions associated with a dietary calcium and phosphorus imbalance in the pig. Am J Vet Res 1965;26:280–294.

Thompson KG, et al. Primary hyperparathyroidism in German Shepherd dogs: a disorder of probable genetic origin. Vet Pathol 1984;21:370–376.

Villafane F, et al. Bone remodeling in chronic renal failure in perinatally irradiated Beagles. Calcif Tiss Res 1977;23:171–178.

OSTEONECROSIS

Like any living tissue, *bone will die when deprived of its blood supply.* This is referred to as **osteonecrosis**, or the synonymous term **osteosis**. In animals, bone ischemia is most often associated with trauma, particularly fractures, where vascular disruption to part of the fractured bone is inevitable. Osteonecrosis also occurs in many acute inflammatory diseases of bones, where the periosteal or myeloid vascular supplies may be disrupted by exudate accumulating either beneath the periosteum or between trabecular bone in marrow spaces. In such cases, the presence of a *large fragment of necrotic bone,* or **sequestrum**, often proves to be a major hindrance to successful repair. This is discussed in more detail in the following section Inflammatory diseases of bones. Other causes of ischemic necrosis of bone, or **bone infarction**, include infiltrating neoplasms, thromboembolism and peripheral vasoconstriction in association with ergotism, fescue foot, or chronic anemia. Severely dehydrated animals in cold climates may also develop peripheral vasoconstriction and necrosis of bone, together with ischemic necrosis of other tissues in peripheral regions. As a rule, regions of bone that are served by end-arteries and have poor collateral circulation, such as the femoral head, are most prone to nonseptic osteonecrosis.

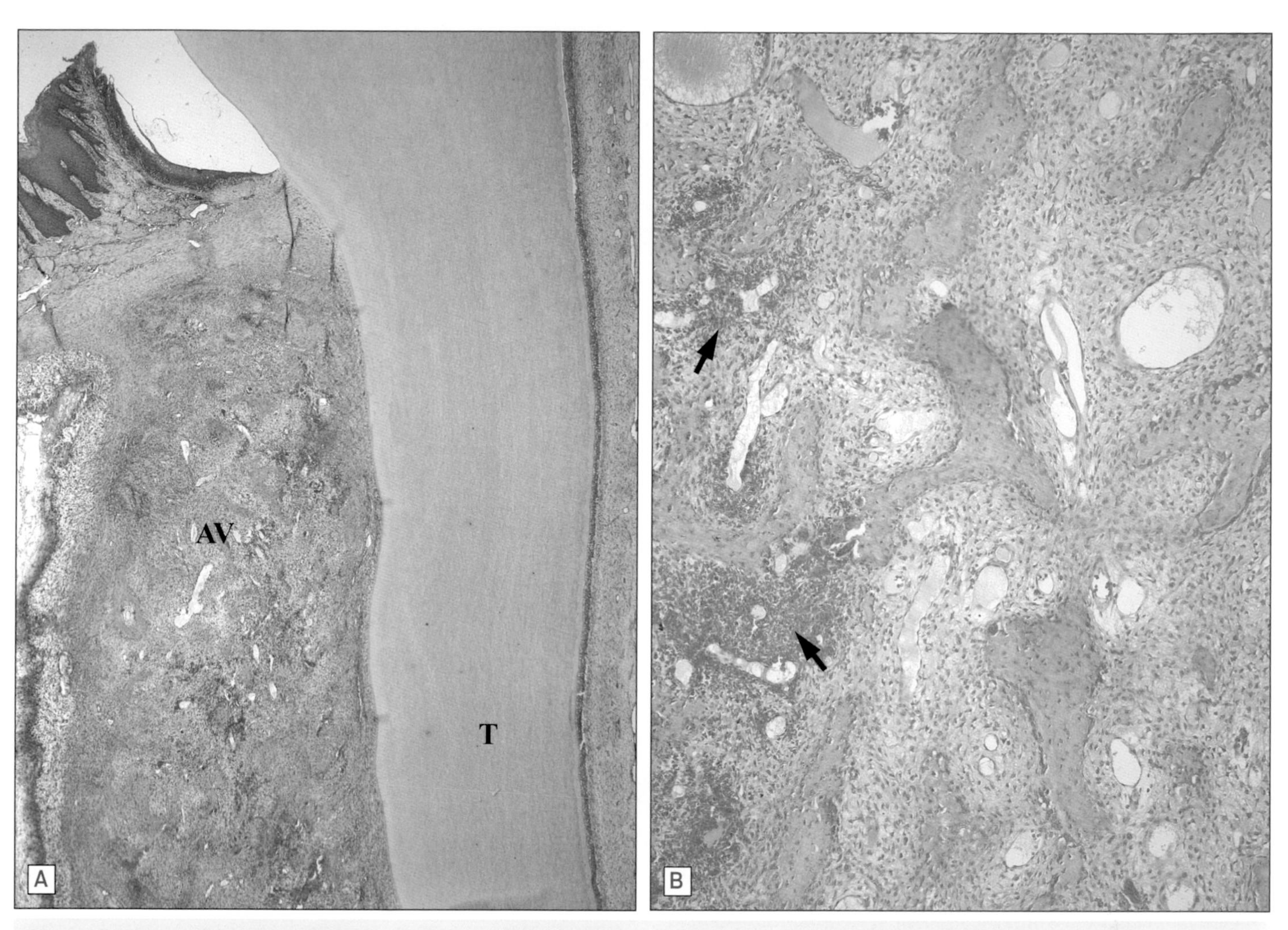

Figure 1.80 Fibrous osteodystrophy, dog. **A.** Section of tooth (T) and alveolar bone (AV) from a young dog with renal secondary hyperparathyroidism. The normally dense alveolar bone has been completely replaced by disorganized trabecular bone and fibrous connective tissue. **B.** Higher-power view showing the irregular trabeculae of woven bone surrounded by highly cellular fibrous connective tissue. The trabeculae are surrounded by active osteoblasts and occasional osteoclasts. Foci of hemorrhage (arrows) are also present.

In humans, bone infarction occurs in association with steroid therapy, alcoholism, hyperviscosity, hemoglobinopathies, and in divers or tunnel workers who work in dysbaric conditions. **Steroid-induced bone necrosis** is believed to be secondary to fat embolism of small blood vessels and although it can occur in many locations, lesions are found most often in the femoral head, distal femur, and proximal humerus. In animals, bone necrosis has been induced experimentally in rabbits and horses, but its prevalence in association with routine steroid therapy is unknown. The availability of sensitive imaging tools such as MRI now provides an opportunity to investigate the occurrence of bone infarcts in animals on long-term steroid therapy. Fat embolism is also believed to be involved in the pathogenesis of alcohol-induced osteonecrosis in humans. Although alcoholism is not a problem in animals, other causes of impaired lipid metabolism that do occur in animals might be expected to predispose to bone infarction. Dysbaric osteonecrosis is caused by the lodgment of nitrogen gas emboli in subarticular bone and medullary cavities following rapid decompression.

Necrosis of bone and bone marrow is described in calves with the juvenile form of sporadic lymphosarcoma. Infarcts of various sizes are found both in vertebral bodies and long bones (see Fig. 1.124A). The pathogenesis of the lesion is not known but may involve vascular obstruction due to increased intra-osseous pressure associated with neoplastic infiltration of the bone marrow.

A possible sequel to bone infarction is the *development of osteosarcoma.* Multiple bone infarcts have been associated with the formation of osteosarcoma in breeds of dog not usually susceptible to this tumor (e.g., Miniature Schnauzer). The reparative process triggered by the infarcts may be responsible for initiating the malignancy, similar to the proposed mechanism of tumor induction at sites of fracture repair and osteomyelitis in dogs and cats (see below).

Morphology and fate of necrotic bone

In the early stages, necrotic bone is often impossible to recognize on gross examination. Furthermore, its mineral composition will be unaltered and its radiographic appearance will therefore resemble that of normal healthy bone. *The earliest recognizable alteration is usually a change in the periosteum to a dull, dry, parchment-like sheath, which can be detached easily.* This contrasts with the normal periosteum and cortical surface, which is smooth, white, glistening, and firmly adherent, except where muscles and fascia are inserted. The sharp contrast in

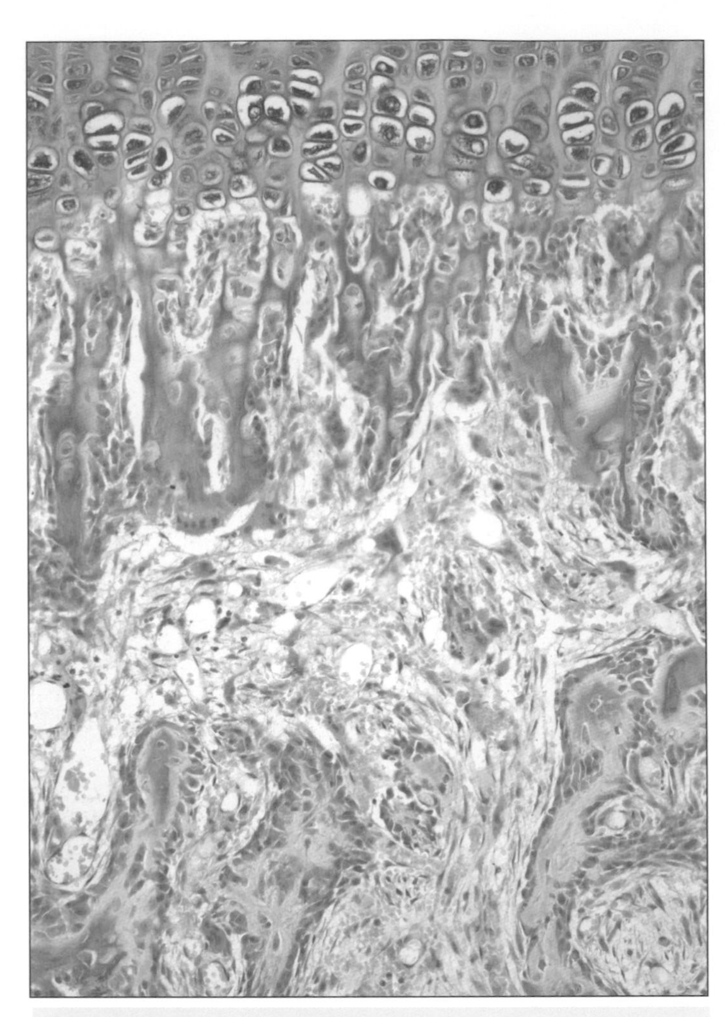

Figure 1.81 Fibrous osteodystrophy, kitten. Physis is normal, but there is premature osteoclastic resorption of trabeculae in the primary spongiosa and replacement with disorganized spicules of woven bone.

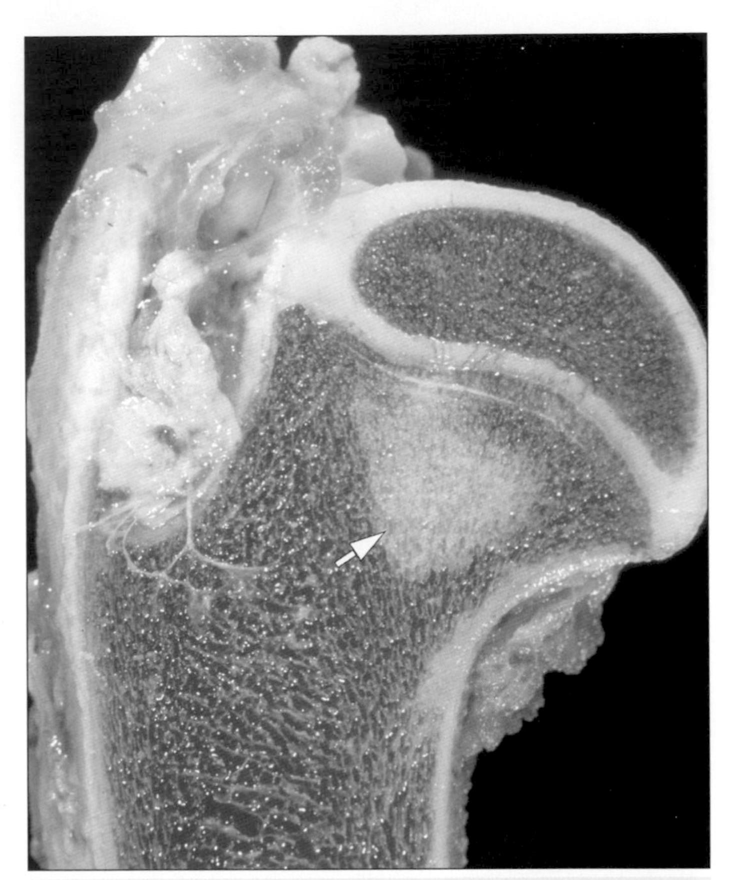

Figure 1.82 Necrosis of bone in the metaphysis of a young foal with **acute osteomyelitis**. The necrotic bone (arrow) is much paler than the surrounding hematopoietic bone marrow.

color between a pale tan area of ischemia and the adjacent areas of normal marrow is an early indication of necrosis during gross examination, especially in young animals where the marrow is red due to active hematopoiesis (Fig. 1.82). Necrotic bone is slowly but progressively resorbed by osteoclasts, but these cells can only gain access to areas where the blood supply is intact and oxygen tension is maintained. Within a few weeks, evidence of the resorptive process will be apparent grossly as a margin of fibrous connective tissue separates the necrotic bone from adjacent viable bone. The necrotic bone may remain chalky white or become light brown.

Microscopically, zones of empty lacunae due to loss of osteocytes characterize necrotic bone (Fig. 1.83), but pyknotic nuclei from dead osteocytes may take anywhere from 2 days to 4 weeks to disappear. Hematopoietic tissue in the marrow cavity will show evidence of necrosis within 2 to 3 days after ischemia and can therefore provide an early indication, but adipose tissue is more resistant to ischemia and will not show evidence of necrosis for about 5 days. If an ischemic event is only transient, then there may be death of hematopoietic cells and perhaps osteocytes, but not adipocytes. Gas gangrene occasionally develops in the necrotic bones of livestock, but is rare in companion animals. The discovery of scattered empty lacunae in a section of bone does not justify a diagnosis of osteonecrosis as this may reflect normal turnover or even be an artifact of preparation. Prolonged immersion in acidic demineralizing solutions can also mimic osteocyte death. In osteonecrosis, all the lacunae in an area of bone should be empty, and the contents of the marrow cavity should be necrotic. Sometimes, focal dystrophic calcification occurs in the necrotic medullary fat.

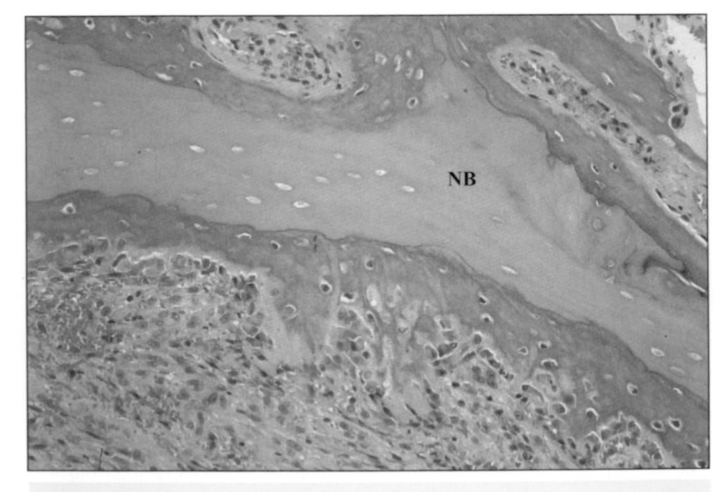

Figure 1.83 Necrotic bone surrounded by new, woven bone at a **fracture site** in a cat. Note the empty lacunae in the necrotic bone (NB) and the more basophilic matrix of the new bone. The necrotic bone has a scalloped margin, reflecting a period of osteoclastic resorption before the new bone was deposited on its surface.

The fate of necrotic bone depends on several factors, the most important being its volume, whether it is accompanied by sepsis, and whether it is in contact with viable tissue. In pyogenic infections of bone, sequestration is a common problem and usually has serious implications. The prognosis is more favorable if the necrotic bone is at a site that is both sterile and has good collateral circulation, and the volume of necrotic bone is small. In such cases, a zone of granulation tissue develops at the interface between the necrotic and viable tissue. This encroaches on the dead tissue and over a period of several weeks, the necrotic fat is replaced with collagenous connective tissue. *Osteoblasts derived from local progenitor cells begin to deposit seams of new woven bone on the remnants of necrotic bone* (Fig. 1.83). This new bone is sharply demarcated from the necrotic bone, which will usually be lamellar, and can be easily distinguished by its increased basophilia and the presence of viable osteocytes. Meanwhile, osteoclasts are recruited to the site and commence removal of the necrotic bone that is being used as a framework for deposition of new bone. This repair process, sometimes referred to as "*creeping substitution*," therefore involves the gradual resorption of dead bone at the same time that it is being replaced by new bone. Eventually, the new woven bone will be replaced with lamellar bone, but until such remodeling is complete, the combination of woven bone and partly resorbed dead bone may not be strong enough to withstand the forces of weight bearing, and the fragile, repairing trabeculae may collapse.

When the volume of necrotic bone is small, and is not in an area predisposed to further damage during the repair process, resolution is likely to be uncomplicated and complete. In fact, many such events probably occur throughout life but do not become clinically apparent. Repetitive injury at the same site may lead to an exaggerated response with formation of local exostoses.

The healing process is more complex when the necrotic bone is separated from viable connective tissue, as occurs frequently with necrosis or detachment of the periosteum. In such lesions, resorption of necrotic bone may still be complete if its volume is small, but if a relatively large volume of cortical bone is involved, sequestration may occur. Even when infection is not present, the sequestrum may interfere with the healing process by acting as a foreign body. *Attempts to wall off the sequestrum will lead to the formation of a layer of granulation tissue and reactive bone, the latter being referred to as an* **involucrum** (Fig. 1.84).

The efficacy of the collateral circulation is another important factor in the likely outcome of osteonecrosis. When the nutrient artery is occluded, large areas of the bone marrow become necrotic, along with the adjacent cancellous and compact bone. If the damage is restricted to the diaphyseal extremities, the prognosis is more favorable as this region has a dual blood supply of osseous origin – from the nutrient vessels on the diaphyseal side, and from the vessels of the joint capsule and ligaments on the epiphyseal side – as well as that from adjacent soft tissues.

As a rule, *the collateral circulation in cortical bone is inefficient* because, in spite of abundant anastomoses, the vessels are small and because they are confined within narrow canals, they are incapable of effective compensatory dilation. The resting and proliferative cartilage of the major growth plates depends on the epiphyseal circulation, while the sinusoidal circulation of the primary spongiosa is derived from metaphyseal vessels and is vulnerable to trauma. In contrast, the articular cartilages are relatively insensitive to regional ischemia since their nutrient supply is obtained by diffusion from the synovial fluid.

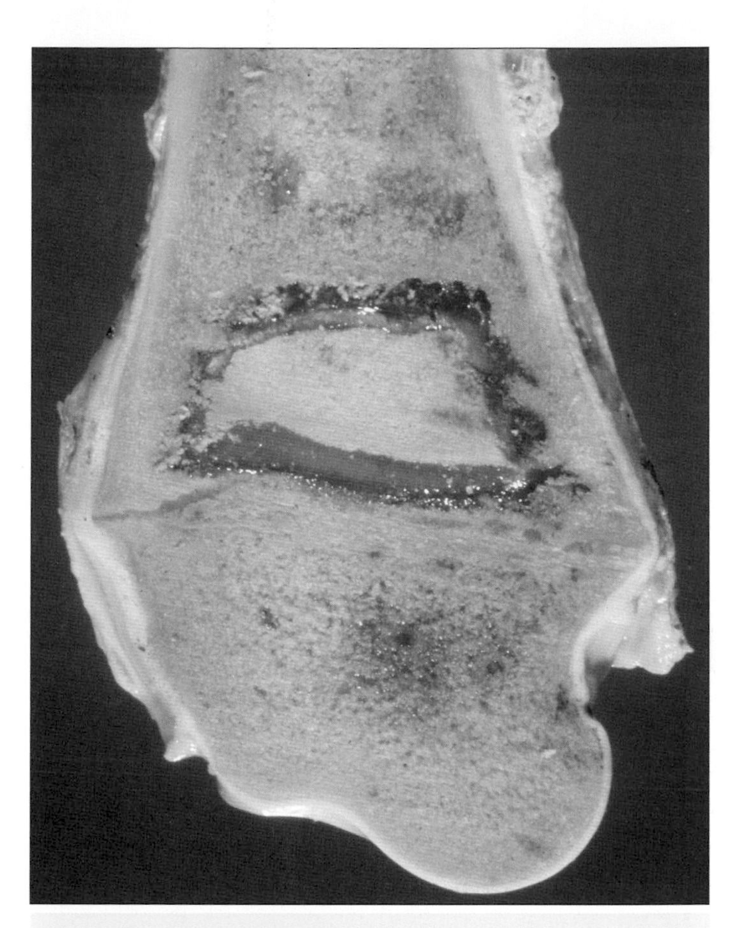

Figure 1.84 Large sequestrum surrounded by an involucrum of granulation tissue in the distal radius of a foal with salmonellosis.

Osseous sequestration is a relatively common sequel to distal limb wounds in horses, the most common sites being the proximal half of the third metatarsal bone and the third metacarpal bone. Although the initial event may be traumatic, it is likely that the introduction of infection to the site predisposes to sequestration, rather than reduced peripheral cortical circulation alone. Sequestra may be detected at about 14 days after injury, when there is some separation from adjacent viable bone and early formation of an involucrum.

Legg–Calvé–Perthes disease

This disease, characterized by *avascular necrosis of the femoral head*, is a well-recognized entity in children but also occurs with some frequency in dogs, especially smaller breeds. Miniature Poodles are particularly susceptible, as are West Highland white and Yorkshire Terriers, and there is evidence to suggest that the disease is inherited as an *autosomal recessive trait*. Avascular necrosis of the femoral head may also occur in other breeds of dog, and in other species, as a result of fractures of the femoral head, but such cases should not be confused with Legg–Calvé–Perthes disease which has a different pathogenesis. Clinically, the disease has an insidious onset, usually between 4 and 8 months of age, and is bilateral in approximately 15% of cases. There is no obvious sex or leg preference in dogs, unlike children where boys are affected five times more frequently than girls.

Anatomical and experimental evidence supports the theory that *the osteonecrosis in Legg–Calvé–Perthes disease is initiated by one or more episodes of ischemia*. As maturation takes place, the developing blood

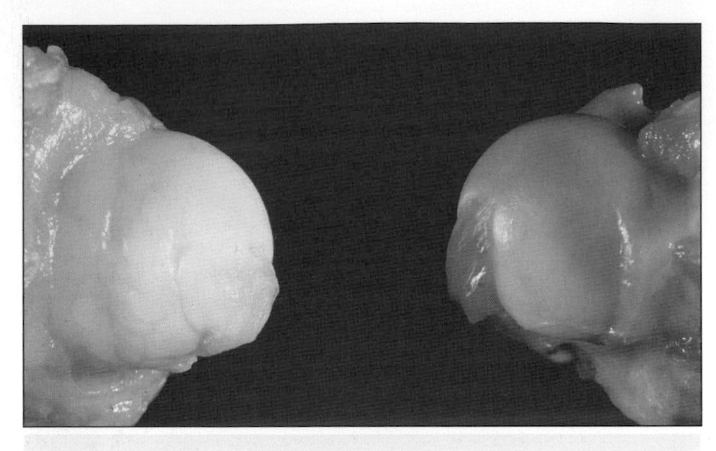

Figure 1.85 Legg–Calvé–Perthes disease in a dog. The articular surface of the femoral head on the left is irregular due to collapse of necrotic subchondral bone. The unaffected femoral head from the same dog is included for comparison. (Courtesy of MW Leach.)

vessels supplying the femoral head are progressively incorporated into fibro-osseous canals, which offer protection as they travel along the femoral neck. In highly susceptible Miniature Poodles, the incorporation of vessels into these canals is delayed, or is incomplete, in contrast to mongrels, where the vessels run mainly intra-osseously. In experimental studies, even a relatively slight degree of intracapsular tamponade produces lesions similar to those in the naturally occurring disease, probably by occluding the veins that drain the femoral head. A transient increase in intra-articular pressure caused by an effusion associated with synovitis or trauma would therefore be expected to interfere with venous drainage from the femoral head and produce the natural disease.

In the early stages of the disease, the shape of the femoral head, and the outlines of the articular cartilage and physis appear grossly and radiographically normal, even though the subchondral bone may be necrotic. If the area of necrosis is small, and the vascular supply is quickly re-established, healing may occur uneventfully. When the subchondral infarct is more extensive, *continued weight-bearing leads to fracture and collapse of the necrotic trabecular bone and flattening of the femoral head* (Fig. 1.85), predisposing to degenerative arthropathy. The physis of the femoral head is also disrupted in some cases, presumably due to interruption of its epiphyseal blood supply at the time of the initial insult.

The repair process involves initial revascularization and proliferation of mesenchymal cells from the margin of the necrotic area, followed by deposition of woven bone on the remnants of necrotic trabeculae. Gradually, the dead bone is removed by osteoclasts and eventually the woven bone is replaced by lamellar bone.

Bibliography

Doige CE. Bone and bone marrow necrosis associated with the calf form of sporadic bovine leukosis. Vet Pathol 1987;24:186–188.

Dubielzig RR, et al. Bone sarcomas associated with multifocal medullary bone infarction in dogs. J Am Vet Med Assoc 1981;179:64–68.

Firth EC. Bone sequestration in horses and cattle. Aust Vet J 1987;64:65–69.

Glade MJ, Krook L. Glucocorticoid-induced inhibition of osteolysis and the development osteopetrosis, osteonecrosis and osteoporosis. Cornell Vet 1982;72:76–91.

Gold EW, et al. Corticosteroid-induced avascular necrosis: an experimental study in rabbits. Clin Orthop 1978;135:272–280.

Kawai K, et al. Fat necrosis of osteocytes as a causative factor in idiopathic osteonecrosis in heritable hyperlipemic rabbits. Clin Orthop 1980;153:273–282.

Kemp HBS. Perthes' disease in rabbits and puppies. Clin Orthop 1986;209:139–159.

Mickelson MR, et al. Legg-Calvé-Perthes disease in dogs: a comparison to human Legg-Calvé-Perthes disease. Clin Orthop 1981;157:287–300.

Moens Y, et al. Bone sequestration as a consequence of limb wounds in the horse. Vet Radiol 1980;21:40–44.

Olsson S-E, et al. Coxa plana-vara and femoral capital fractures in the dog. J Am An Hosp Assoc 1985;21:563–571.

Robinson R. Legg-Calvé-Perthes disease in dogs: genetic aetiology. J Small Anim Pract 1992;33:275–276.

Slichter SJ, et al. Dysbaric osteonecrosis: A consequence of intravascular bubble formation, endothelial damage, and platelet thrombosis. J Lab Clin Med 1981;98:568–590.

INFLAMMATORY DISEASES OF BONES

Inflammation of bones inevitably originates in vascular areas of either the medullary cavity or the periosteum and is referred to as either **osteomyelitis** or **periostitis** respectively. **Osteitis** is a more general term for inflammation of bones, but is used less frequently. Most inflammatory diseases of bones are caused by bacterial infections, although mycotic and viral agents can also infect bones. *Bacterial osteomyelitis is particularly common and important in domestic animals* and will be discussed in some detail below, as will other forms of infectious osteitis.

Noninfectious osteitis also occurs, usually in response to local periosteal injury, and typically results in the formation of **exostoses**. This may be due to a single insult if there is damage to the periosteum or to repeated minor trauma. Tearing of ligamentous insertions will often induce local periostitis and the development of exostoses or osteophytes. Small exostoses may be completely resorbed if the stimulus is removed, but larger ones may be converted from woven to lamellar bone and persist indefinitely. These often remain clinically inapparent but may interfere with the function of adjacent structures, such as tendons or ligaments, as occurs in some cases of "splints" on the second and fourth metacarpal bones of horses. There is evidence to suggest that traumatic injury to the periosteum may predispose to bacterial osteitis at the site, even if the overlying skin is intact. The mechanism is uncertain but damage to adjacent tissues may increase their susceptibility to infection. More extensive periostitis, particularly involving vertebrae, is reported in dogs in association with parasitic myositis caused by *Hepatozoon americanum* infection. Presumably, the periosteum is reacting to the release of inflammatory mediators or other factors in response to the presence of parasitic stages in muscle fibers.

Bacterial infections of bones

Bacterial infections of bones are very common in animals, especially young horses and ruminants. Since the route of infection is *usually hematogenous*, most are centered on the medullary cavity and are referred to as osteomyelitis. There is little doubt that bacterial osteomyelitis is far more common than is diagnosed, as affected animals often die of septicemia before the bone lesions become evident and the skeleton is generally not closely examined at necropsy unless clinical signs have suggested a skeletal disorder.

During bacteremia or septicemia, bacteria can become localized in many organs and at many sites. In bones, there is a strong predilection for sites of active endochondral ossification within the metaphyses and epiphyses of long bones and vertebral bodies. This reflects the unique nature of the vascular architecture at the physis, and at the equivalent site in expanding epiphyses. Capillaries invading the mineralized cartilage make sharp loops before opening into wider sinusoidal vessels that communicate with the medullary veins. The capillaries are fenestrated, thus permitting ready escape of bacteria into the bone marrow. Furthermore, sluggish circulation in the sinusoidal system, and the relative inefficiency of the phagocytic cells lining it, also tend to favor the development and persistence of infection. Experiments in rabbits have suggested that trauma, or some other factor that alters the metaphyseal environment, enhances the establishment of bone infection in animals with bacteremia. Thus, *a combination of physeal, metaphyseal, or epiphyseal injury and concurrent bacteremia or septicemia may be involved in the pathogenesis of hematogenous osteomyelitis.* Localization of bacteria in the vessels of cartilage canals is also common in hematogenous infections of young animals. As the skeleton matures, the vascular morphology at chondro–osseous junctions alters to make it less suitable for bacterial localization. In fact, there is probably only a narrow window during which bacteria, be they derived from umbilical infections in colostrum-deprived animals, or from infections in the respiratory or alimentary tracts, are able to establish in bones. The clinical manifestations of osteomyelitis may not develop until several months later when the bone lesion becomes extensive enough to cause pain, disfigurement of the bone, or perhaps result in a pathological fracture.

Some bacteria appear to have a predilection for localization within bone. This probably reflects the fact that *certain bacteria* (e.g., *Staphylococcus aureus*) *possess receptors to bone surface proteins,* such as sialoproteins and collagen. It is possible that trauma makes binding sites on these proteins more accessible to bacterial receptors. This might account for the frequent establishment of bone infection at sites of blunt trauma, even when the skin surface has remained intact. Once bound to bone proteins, *S. aureus* bacteria surround themselves with a thick mucopolysaccharide glycocalyx, which allows tighter adhesion to the bone surface and favors persistence of the infection by protecting the organisms from host defense mechanisms and inhibiting the penetration of antibiotics. Other bacteria that commonly establish in bones (e.g., *Salmonella* spp.) may possess similar mechanisms of survival.

At sites of bacterial infection, cytokines such as tumor necrosis factor, interleukin-1, and prostaglandin E_2 released from inflammatory cells activate *bone resorption by osteoclasts*. There is also evidence that inflammatory cells themselves may be able to resorb bone.

There are several possible sequelae to hematogenous bacterial infection of bone. The initial response is characterized by *edema and acute purulent inflammation*. Many infections are probably eliminated spontaneously by host defenses at this early stage, perhaps assisted by prompt and vigorous treatment with specific antibacterial agents. If the infection is not eliminated it may become segregated by fibrous inflammatory tissue and woven bone, with development of a *metaphyseal or epiphyseal abscess* (*Brodie's abscess*). Alternatively, the exudate may percolate through the adjacent marrow cavity causing necrosis of soft tissues and trabecular bone. These early lesions appear grossly as discrete areas of pallor, sharply demarcated from the normal red bone marrow (Fig. 1.82). *Resorption of necrotic trabecular bone* from the edge of the lesion, and *proliferation of granulation tissue*, results in separation of the necrotic, infected bone from adjacent viable tissues (Fig. 1.84). It is not unusual to find several foci of osteomyelitis in different bones within the same animal (Fig. 1.86A), or even within the same bone. Osteoclasts or inflammatory cells

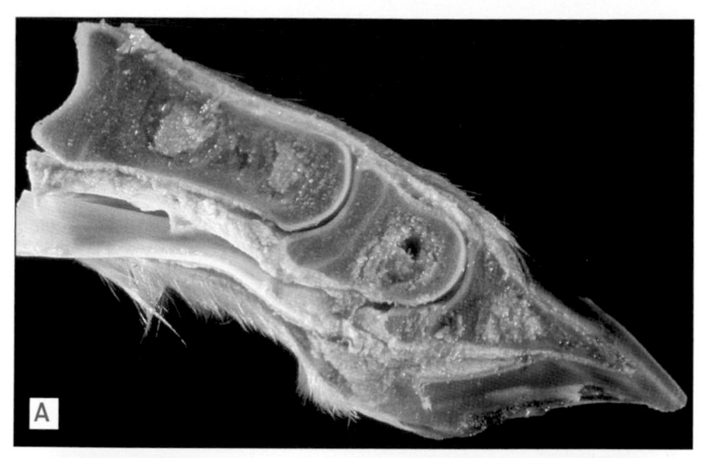

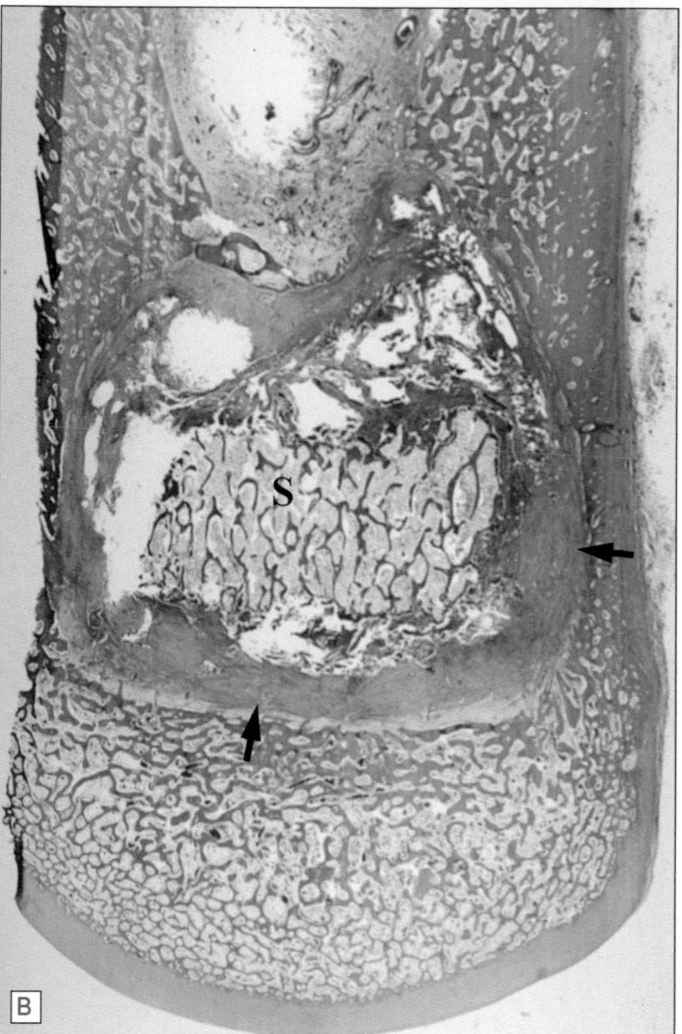

Figure 1.86 Osteomyelitis in a foal with salmonellosis. **A.** All three digits contain large sequestra. **B.** Sequestrum in the distal metaphysis of P-1 from the same foal. Note the thick involucrum of granulation tissue (arrows) surrounding the sequestrum of necrotic cancellous bone (S).

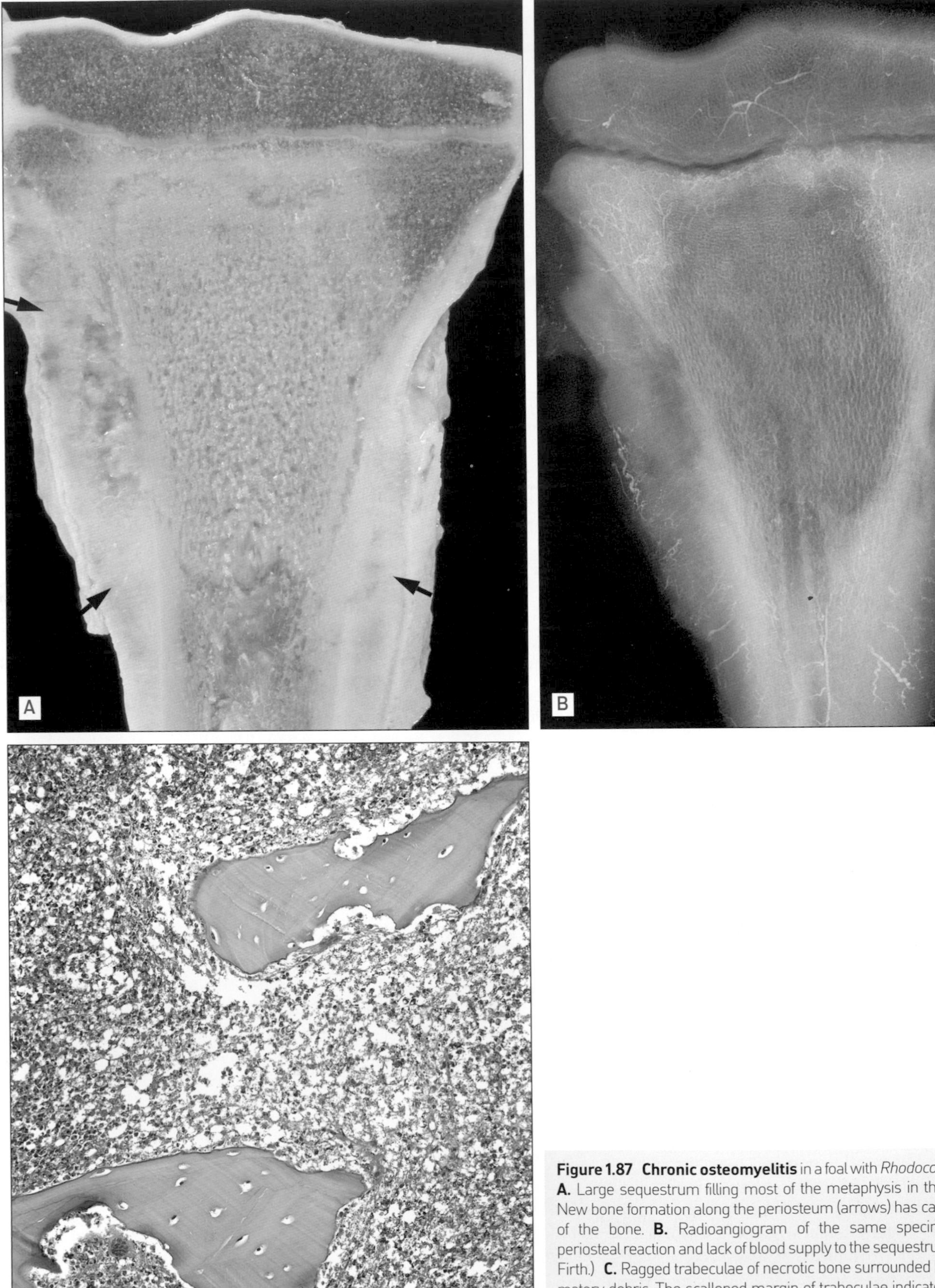

Figure 1.87 Chronic osteomyelitis in a foal with *Rhodococcus equi* infection. **A.** Large sequestrum filling most of the metaphysis in the proximal radius. New bone formation along the periosteum (arrows) has caused enlargement of the bone. **B.** Radioangiogram of the same specimen showing the periosteal reaction and lack of blood supply to the sequestrum. (Courtesy of EC Firth.) **C.** Ragged trabeculae of necrotic bone surrounded by necrotic inflammatory debris. The scalloped margin of trabeculae indicates previous osteoclastic resorption.

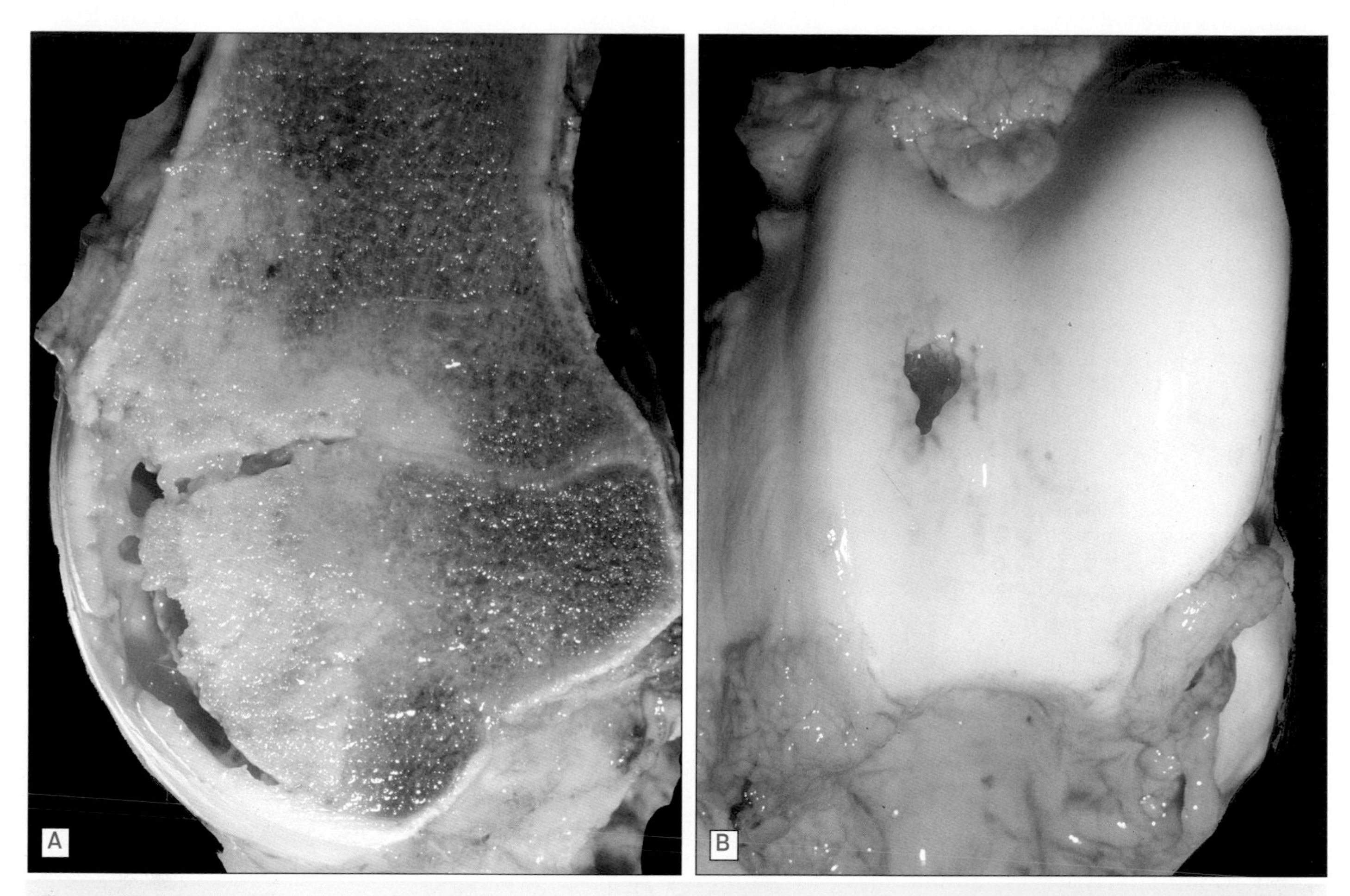

Figure 1.88 Osteomyelitis, foal. *Salmonella typhimurium* infection. **A.** Extensive destruction of subchondral bone in the distal femur. The infection has spread to involve much of the epiphysis, as well as the physis and part of the metaphysis. **B.** Same lesion prior to sectioning, showing communication with the stifle joint through a focal defect in the trochlear groove.

may resorb small foci of necrotic bone, but larger foci, which become separated from a viable vascular supply, persist as **sequestra**, harboring bacteria and interfering with the repair process. *Granulation tissue or reactive bone, which often forms a layer around sequestra* (Figs 1.84; 1.86A, B) is referred to as an **involucrum**.

The physis usually prevents the spread of infection from the metaphysis to the epiphysis, but transphyseal blood vessels in very young animals may transmit infection from one side to the other. In such cases, the physis is usually involved in the septic inflammatory process and is destroyed locally (see Fig. 1.53). The cortex is relatively porous in young animals and offers little resistance to the spread of infection, which penetrates through vascular canals to the periosteum. If cortical penetration occurs within the attachment of a joint capsule, then *septic arthritis* may result but, more commonly, a *subperiosteal abscess* develops. Disruption or thrombosis of the blood supply from the metaphysis to the inner portion of the cortex, together with periosteal elevation and interference with periosteal blood vessels, causes *segmental cortical necrosis and formation of sequestra*. In severe cases of bacterial osteomyelitis, there may be locally extensive necrosis and sequestration of metaphyseal and cortical bone, with an exuberant involucrum formed beneath an elevated periosteum, resulting in swelling and disfigurement of the bone (Fig. 1.87A, B).

The *predilection sites* for long bone lesions of osteomyelitis vary in distribution between species. There is also some variation in the bacteria involved and in the age distribution of affected animals. In **foals**, osteomyelitis seldom occurs after 4 months of age and the lesions occur more often in the secondary ossification centers of the epiphyses than the metaphysis. *Most infections establish immediately beneath the thickest part of the articular cartilage*, particularly in the caudal aspect of the lateral and medial femoral condyles, dorsal to the weight-bearing articular surface. Other common sites for epiphyseal localization of infection in foals include the distal intermediate ridge of the tibia, medial styloid process of the radius, and the proximal humerus, but many other sites also may be involved. The vascular arrangement at sites of thickened cartilage is characterized by an increased arterial supply and greater sinusoidal filling than in areas where the articular cartilage is thinner. If the infection becomes established, there may be extensive destruction of subchondral bone with underrunning of the articular cartilage (Fig. 1.88A, B). The inflammation may progress to involve much of the epiphysis and may communicate with the joint space through defects in the overlying cartilage.

Metaphyseal lesions in foals are most common at sites where the physis deviates greatest from a horizontal plane. Approximately 70% of foals with bacterial osteomyelitis, including virtually all of those with epiphyseal lesions, also have septic arthritis. This may reflect either concurrent establishment of infection in the synovium during bacteremia, or direct spread from bone. The bacteria most commonly involved in foals with osteomyelitis are *Escherichia coli*,

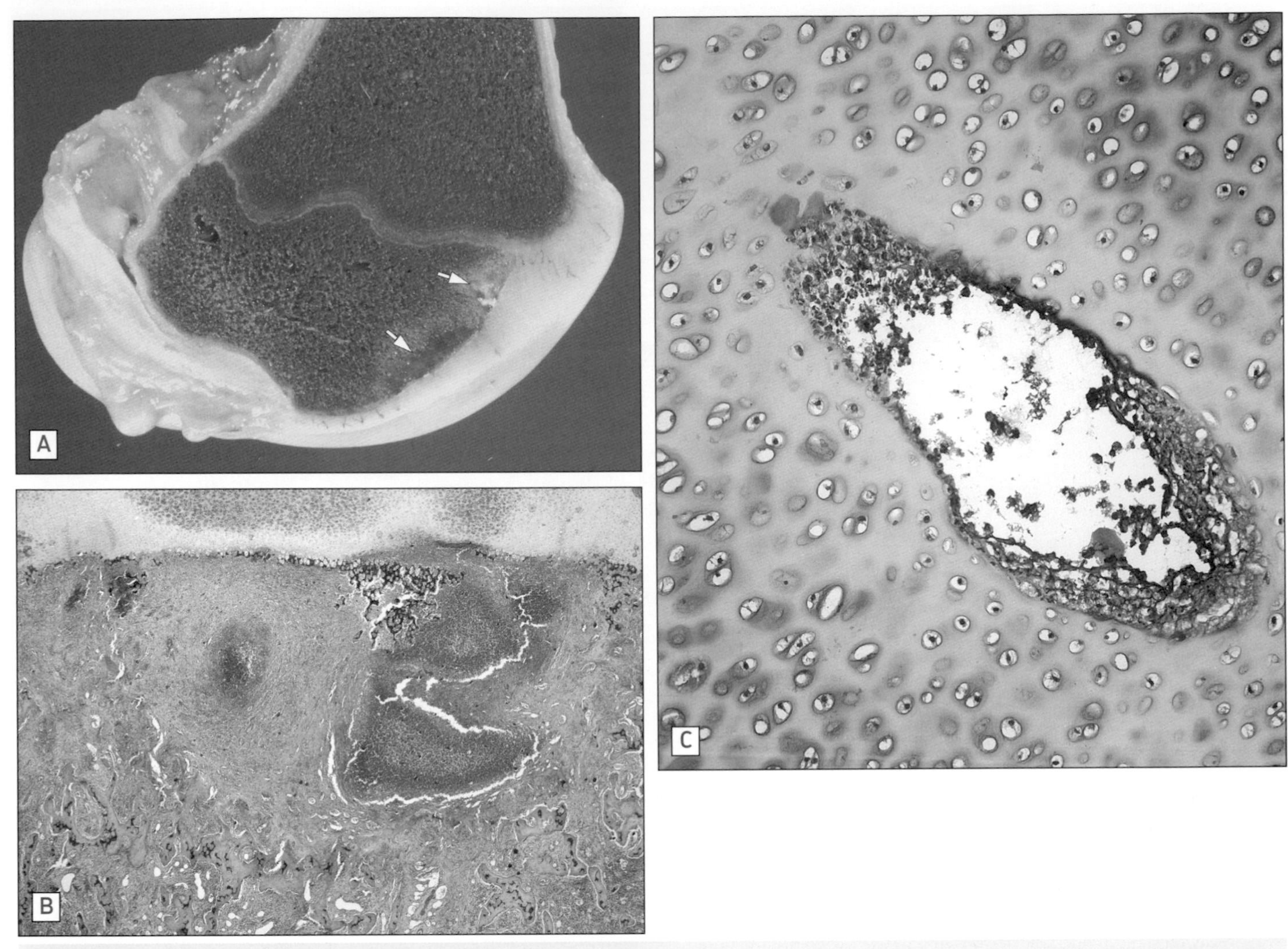

Figure 1.89 Subacute, suppurative osteomyelitis in the epiphysis of the distal femur in a calf. **A.** Foci of suppuration and trabecular destruction (arrows) immediately beneath the articular surface of the trochlear groove. The calf also had polyarthritis (see Fig. 1.154A, B) **B.** Low-power microscopic view showing foci of intense, suppurative inflammation and effacement of epiphyseal trabecular bone immediately beneath the articular cartilage. The pale areas of cartilage are degenerate. **C.** Cartilage canal in the same calf, showing destruction of vascular structures and replacement with necrotic debris.

Streptococcus spp., *Salmonella* spp., *Klebsiella* spp., and *Rhodococcus equi*. Hematogenous osteomyelitis of the tarsal bones, usually in association with infectious arthritis, is reported as an entity in young foals less than a month of age.

In **cattle**, hematogenous osteomyelitis is not confined to young animals, as it is in foals. In one study, the age range in cattle was 2 weeks to 5 years. *Metaphyseal osteomyelitis* in this study occurred at many sites in long bones, but particularly the distal metacarpus, metatarsus, radius, and tibia. *Epiphyseal osteomyelitis* occurred most often in the distal femoral condyle, distal radius and in the patella, and was usually associated with infection by *Salmonella* spp. In contrast, metaphyseal infections were most often caused by *Arcanobacterium pyogenes*. The *Salmonella* spp. infections were almost invariably in calves less than 3 months of age, while *Arcanobacterium pyogenes* usually affected cattle older than 6 months. As in foals, septic osteomyelitis generally accompanies bacterial arthritis in calves (Fig. 1.89A). Hematogenous osteomyelitis and arthritis also frequently occur together in young **lambs**, **goats**, and **deer**, and are associated with a range of organisms.

Histological changes in bacterial osteomyelitis are predictable, but depend on the causative agent and the stage of infection. *Acute osteomyelitis* in young animals may be distinguished from active myelopoiesis by the presence of fibrin, and a dense population of neutrophils and necrotic cells in the primary spongiosa, where hematopoietic tissue is usually absent. Inappropriate or excessive osteoclastic resorption of bone trabeculae is another characteristic microscopic feature and there may be necrosis of physeal or articular cartilage. In the epiphysis, inflammatory foci typically start immediately beneath the articular cartilage resulting in local destruction of subchondral trabecular bone (Fig. 1.89B). Degeneration or necrosis of the overlying articular cartilage is common in young animals with hematogenous bacterial osteomyelitis due to septic embolism or thrombosis of blood vessels in cartilage canals (Fig. 1.89C). In *chronic osteomyelitis*, marrow spaces between necrotic, partly resorbed bone trabeculae may be filled with necrotic debris (Fig. 1.87C), fibrous connective tissue, or a mixed population of inflammatory cells. A thick layer of granulation tissue infiltrated with neutrophils may surround larger areas of necrotic bone, with prominent osteoclastic activity at the margins. Proliferation of connective tissue and woven bone in chronic lesions may create difficulty in distinguishing the reaction from neoplasia, especially in biopsy specimens where the sample is small and perhaps not representative. The presence of neutrophils and plasma cells amongst the reactive bone and connective tissue supports a diagnosis of chronic osteomyelitis. Osteomyelitis secondary to a compound fracture may present a considerable diagnostic challenge, as the inflammatory changes will be superimposed on the proliferative components of fracture repair. In such cases, the history and radiographic changes are indispensable.

Hematogenous bacterial osteomyelitis is rare in **dogs** but may occur in pups that survive canine parvovirus infection, or other diseases associated with short-term or persistent neutropenia. A myelokathexis-like syndrome in Border Collie pups, characterized by persistent neutropenia, is typically accompanied by hematogenous osteomyelitis involving the metaphyses of several long bones. More often, bacterial osteomyelitis in dogs and **cats** is a *complication of compound fractures, wound contamination during open fracture repair, bite wounds, or gunshot injury*. Staphylococci, especially *Staphylococcus intermedius*, and streptococci are the most common organisms involved, although mixed infections including gram-negative bacteria, such as *Escherichia coli* and *Proteus* spp., also occur. Because of the association with fractures, osteomyelitis in dogs is most common in long bones of the appendicular skeleton, particularly the femur. Foreign material implanted traumatically beneath the skin, or surgical implants, may act as a nidus for infection. The surfaces of such implants are soon coated with matrix and serum proteins, fibronectin, and carbohydrates. Cell membrane receptors on staphylococci and some other gram-positive bacteria bind with fibronectin, while anaerobes and gram-negative bacteria attach less firmly via pili and fimbriae. In addition, the mucopolysaccharide glycocalyx produced by staphylococci and other gram-positive aerobes protects them from phagocytosis, antibodies, and may even alter the action of some antibiotics. Even after apparent resolution, bacterial infections of bone may recur as a result of proliferation of bacteria that have survived within the glycocalyx or in fragments of necrotic bone.

Vertebral osteomyelitis is a relatively common manifestation of bacterial osteomyelitis in horses and farmed livestock. Most cases probably result from hematogenous spread of infection to the bones during the neonatal period in animals with inadequate passive immunity. Bacteria may enter via the umbilicus, respiratory tract, digestive tract, or perhaps via the placenta immediately before parturition. In piglets and lambs, tail biting and tail docking respectively are believed to provide a portal of entry for bacteria in at least some cases of vertebral osteomyelitis. Following localization in the epiphysis or metaphysis of a vertebral body, or adjacent to a growth plate in a developing vertebral arch, the infection causes progressive destruction and weakening of the affected vertebral bone. As in long bones, sequestration and abscessation may occur. The *most common sequela is pathological fracture and collapse of affected vertebrae* with dorsal displacement of pus and necrotic bone fragments into the spinal canal (Fig. 1.90). Such an event is accompanied by the sudden onset of neurological signs caused by compression of the spinal cord. The severity and nature of the clinical signs will depend on the segment of cord involved and the degree of damage. In cases where vertebral fracture does not occur, the suppurative process may permeate the cortex in any direction, spreading to involve the pleura or peritoneum, the spinal muscles, or protrude as an encapsulated abscess into the spinal canal and cause partial compression of the cord. If the infection is contained or does not result in cord compression it may go undetected, or be found incidentally at slaughter.

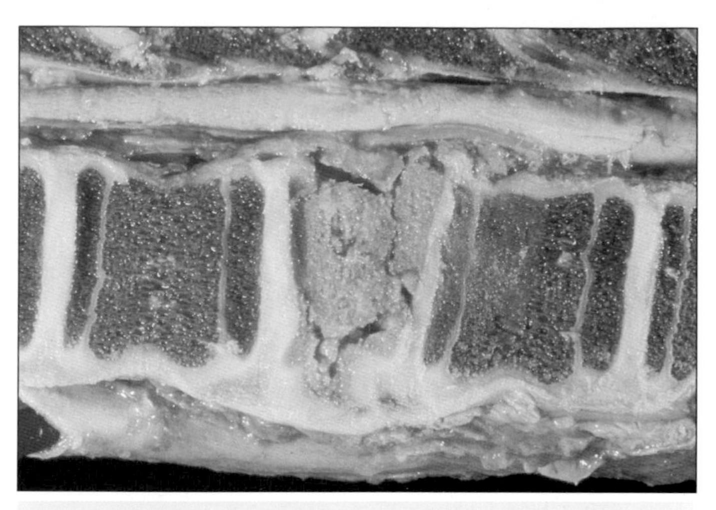

Figure 1.90 Vertebral osteomyelitis, calf. *Escherichia coli* infection. The vertebral body is completely necrotic and has collapsed. Several fragments have been forced into the spinal canal, compressing the cord. (Courtesy of PC Stromberg.)

Arcanobacterium pyogenes is the most common causative organism in vertebral osteomyelitis in most species, but a range of other bacteria may be involved. These include: *Escherichia coli, Salmonella typhimurium,* staphylococci, streptococci, and *R. equi* in foals; tuberculosis in older horses; *Fusobacterium necrophorum* in calves; *Mannheimia (Pasteurella) haemolytica, F. necrophorum,* and staphylococci in sheep; and *Erysipelothrix rhusiopathiae*, staphylococci, and streptococci in pigs. In one survey of cervico-thoracic vertebral osteomyelitis in calves, *Salmonella dublin* was isolated from eight of ten cases at postmortem. The lesions in this study all involved one or more of the vertebrae between C5 and T1. In regions where brucellosis is endemic in swine, *Brucella suis* may produce vertebral lesions as a sequel to diskospondylitis.

In dogs, bacterial osteomyelitis has been linked to penetration of grass seeds. Since the lesions are confined to the lumbar region, it is suggested that the grass seeds have most likely been ingested and penetrate the intestinal wall, perhaps at the caudal duodenal flexure, and ascend in the mesoduodenum to the lumbar vertebrae. Possible sequelae include sublumbar abscessation, osteomyelitis, and fistulation to the skin of the flank.

Localized bacterial periostitis is often associated with primary inflammatory conditions in adjacent tissues. Examples include infections of the feet of cattle with *F. necrophorum* ("footrot"), necrotic stomatitis of cattle caused by the same organism, infections of the paranasal sinuses as an extension from perforating injuries, bite wounds that produce cellulitis or abscesses, chronic paronychia and pressure sores over bony prominences. Penetrating wounds of the hoof in cattle or horses may also spread to involve the adjacent third phalanx.

Atrophic rhinitis of pigs, induced by exposure to toxins from certain strains of *Pasteurella multocida,* is associated with mixed bacterial infections and rhinitis. Absorption of the toxins leads to localized osteonecrosis of turbinate bones, and affected bones may lyse completely, leaving no substrate for repair (see Vol. 2, Respiratory system). A similar lytic condition may affect the turbinates of dogs.

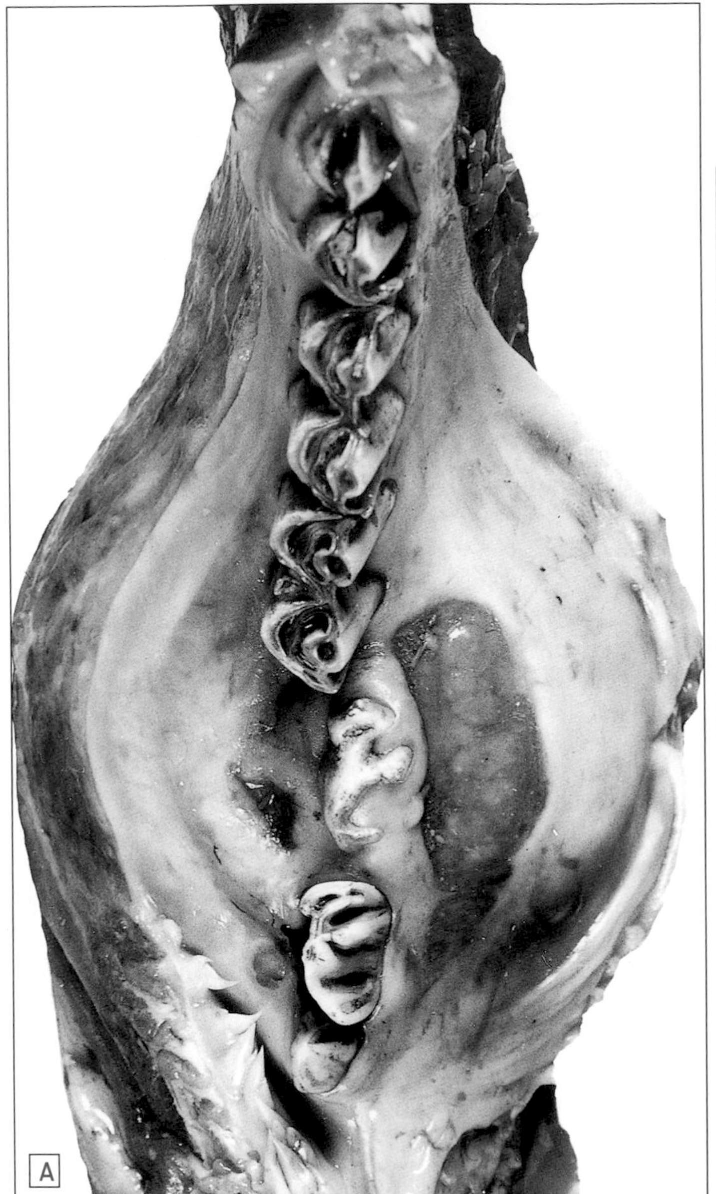

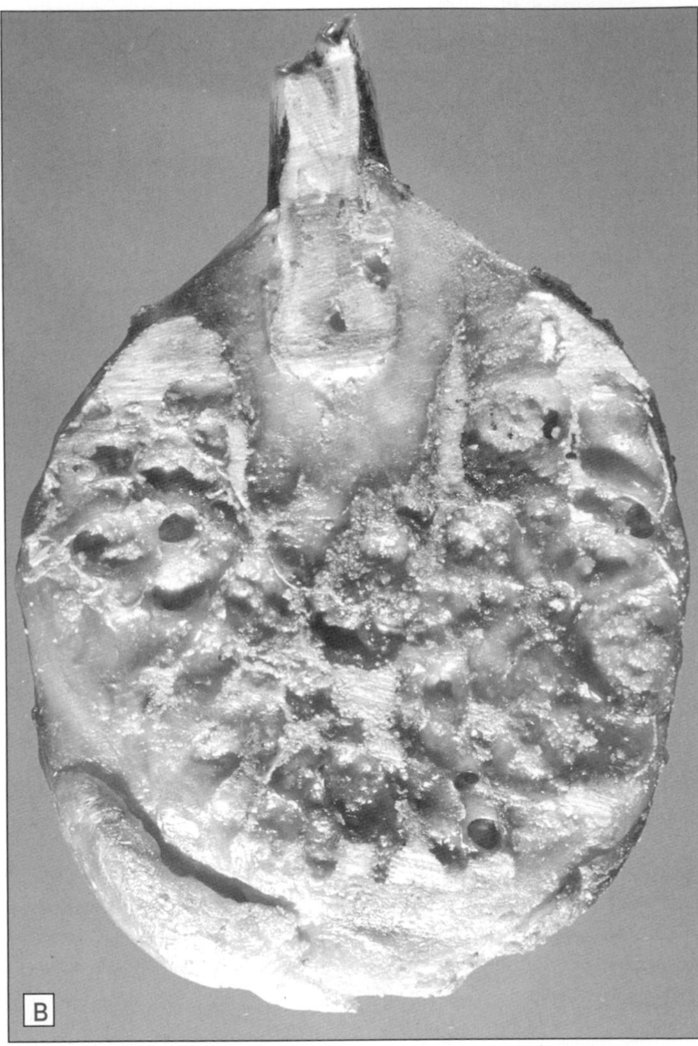

Figure 1.91 Mandibular osteomyelitis, cow. *Actinomyces bovis* infection. **A.** The mandible is markedly swollen. There is gingival ulceration and displacement of a tooth. **B.** Section through mandible showing "honeycomb" appearance caused by pockets of inflammatory tissue surrounded by reactive bone.

Mandibular osteomyelitis is primarily a disease of cattle caused by *Actinomyces bovis*, but occasionally occurs in horses, pigs, deer, sheep, and dogs. In cattle, the disease is known as **actinomycosis** or **"lumpy jaw**," and *the classic lesion is confined to the mandible.* The maxilla is rarely involved and the organism rarely spreads even to regional lymph nodes, which, although large and indurated, are not infected. *A. bovis* is probably an obligate parasite of the oropharyngeal mucosa in a number of animal species, and most infections involve the buccal tissues. The organism is not particularly virulent, and in most, perhaps all cases, the surface tissues must be injured by some other agent or by a foreign body for invasion to occur. The osteomyelitis follows direct extension of the infection from the gums and periodontium. Extension to the periosteum causes actinomycotic periostitis, and the infection may not progress any further. Similar lesions may be produced by *A. pyogenes*. *Actinomyces bovis* may invade bone directly though the periosteum, but *osteomyelitis usually develops from periodontitis*, presumably via lymphatics, which drain into the mandibular bone. Once in the bone, *A. bovis* causes a chronic, pyogranulomatous inflammatory reaction. Suppurative tracts permeate the medullary spaces leading to multiple foci of bone resorption and proliferation. Large sequestra do not develop, even when the cortex is invaded, probably because of the slow, progressive nature of the disease. Fistulae often extend into the overlying soft tissue and may discharge through the skin or mucous membranes. Periosteal proliferation is excessive and the bone may become enormously enlarged (Fig. 1.91A), the normal architecture of the mandible being destroyed. The teeth in the affected portion of the jaw become loosened, lost, or buried in granulation tissue. On cut surface, the affected mandible has a "honeycomb" appearance with reactive bone surrounding pockets of inflammatory tissue (Fig. 1.91B). Fragments of necrotic trabecular bone accumulate in purulent exudate as "bone sand." The pus is also likely to contain many 1–2-mm diameter, soft,

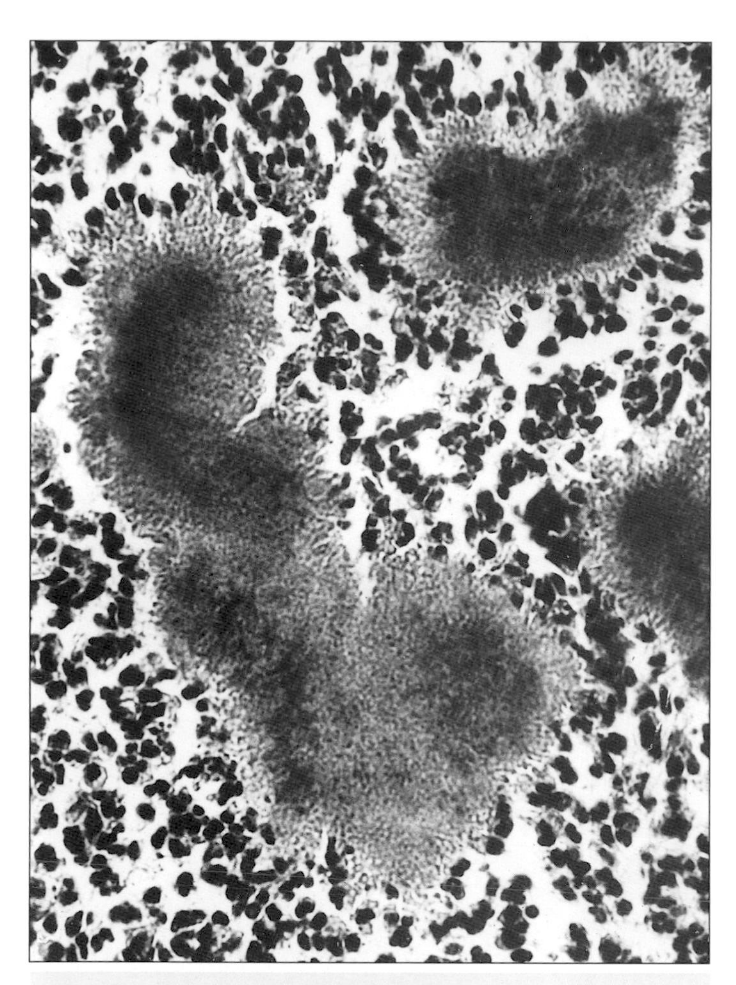

Figure 1.92 Colonies of *Actinomyces bovis* with characteristic club formation. The colonies are surrounded by neutrophils.

light yellow granules referred to as "sulfur granules." These consist of an internal mass of tangled, gram-positive filaments mixed with some bacillary and coccoid forms, and a periphery consisting of closely packed, club-shaped, gram-negative bodies (Fig. 1.92).

A similar tissue reaction, accompanied by club-colonies, occurs in association with some other bacteria, in particular *Actinobacillus lignieresi*, but the colonies in actinomycosis are much larger and the clubs are smaller and less discrete than in actinobacillosis. Furthermore, actinobacillosis is a disease of soft tissues rather than bone. *Fusobacterium necrophorum* and a variety of nonspecific bacteria may cause osteomyelitis by direct spread from periodontitis, but the lesions are usually more destructive and less proliferative than with *Actinomyces bovis*.

Mandibular osteomyelitis associated with loosening or loss of molar teeth (Fig. 1.93A) is sometimes detected in ill-thrifty **sheep** in the absence of other likely causes of weight loss, and may be a more important problem than is currently recognized in commercial sheep flocks. Grass awns or other plant matter may be wedged into pockets between teeth and the alveolar bone (Fig. 1.93B), providing a route of entry for opportunistic bacteria into the mandible.

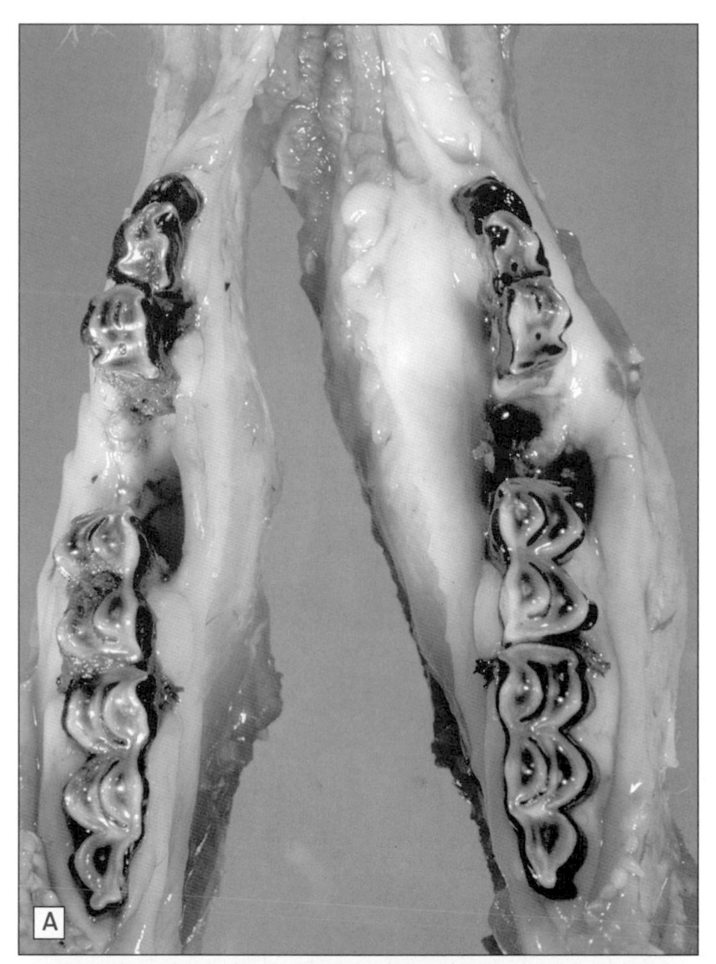

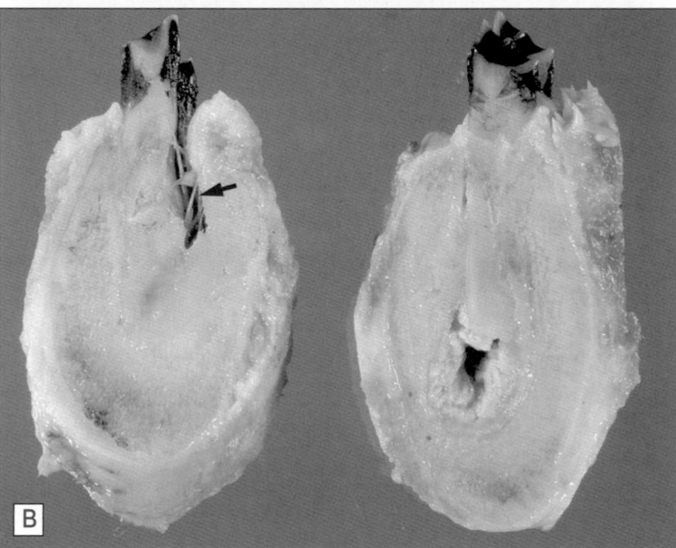

Figure 1.93 Mandibular osteomyelitis, sheep. **A.** Bilateral loss of individual molar teeth and swelling of the mandible on the right. **B.** Sections through swollen mandible shown in (**A**). Note the plant material (arrow) wedged between the tooth and adjacent bone in one section and the lytic focus filled with necrotic debris near the base of the tooth in the other.

Mycotic infections of bones

Mycotic infections of bone are less common than those caused by bacteria but certain pathogenic fungi, in particular the yeasts *Coccidioides immitis, Blastomyces dermatitidis, Cryptococcus neoformans*, and *Histoplasma capsulatum* may cause osteomyelitis following inhalation of spores and hematogenous dissemination. Multiple bones may be involved and the lesions may vary from lytic to highly proliferative, depending on the stage of the disease and the immune status of the host. Histologically, *the inflammatory response is pyogranulomatous*

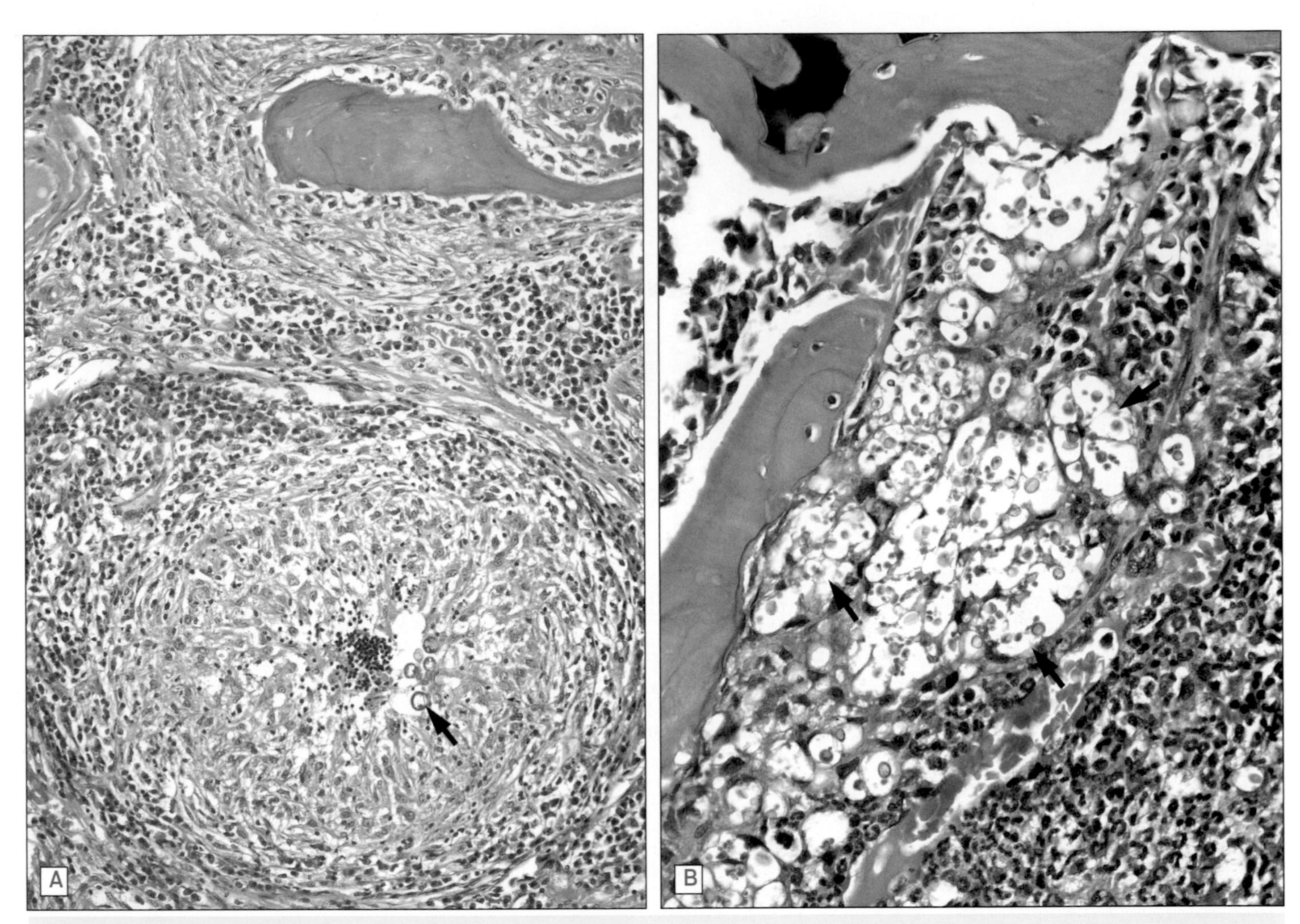

Figure 1.94 Mycotic osteomyelitis, dog. **A.** *Coccidioides immitis* infection. Focus of pyogranulomatous inflammation containing occasional organisms (arrow) and surrounded by a mantle of plasma cells. **B.** *Cryptococcus neoformans* infection. Numerous clusters of organisms with characteristic thick capsule (arrows) in marrow spaces of the rib.

(Fig. 1.94A) and is generally confined to the medullary cavity, at least in the early stages. The organisms can usually be detected readily, especially in cryptococcosis, where the host response may be minimal, perhaps reflecting impaired immunity (Fig. 1.94B). Lesions may also be present in a range of other tissues in animals with systemic mycoses and the presence of bone involvement may be overlooked.

Paecilomyces sp., a saprophyte in soil and decaying organic material, is generally considered nonpathogenic but is occasionally reported to cause osteomyelitis in dogs in association with systemic infection. The bone lesions may be multifocal and lytic, resembling plasma cell myeloma radiographically and grossly, especially when vertebral bodies are involved. Alternatively, they may be associated with extensive periosteal new bone formation leading to marked thickening of long bones (Fig. 1.95A, B). *Aspergillus* infections occasionally cause osteomyelitis in dogs, less so in other species. Other fungi, such as *Pithium insidiosum,* localize sporadically in bone and cause osteomyelitis.

Viral infections of bones

Several viruses are known to cause distinctive lesions in bones. Zones of metaphyseal sclerosis may be associated with ***Canine distemper virus*** infection and the **pestiviruses** of **bovine viral diarrhea** and ***Classical swine fever***, presumably due to destruction of osteoclasts or their precursors. This has been discussed in more detail earlier in this chapter.

***Canine adenovirus* type I** infection in pups may be accompanied by grossly visible metaphyseal hemorrhages at costochondral junctions due to virus-induced injury to endothelial cells, some of which contain characteristic intranuclear inclusion bodies. Necrosis of all cellular elements in the metaphysis also occurs, possibly due to ischemia, but there are no reports of residual lesions.

Feline herpesvirus causes necrosis in the turbinate bones of germ-free cats following intranasal inoculation, and produces necrosis in the metaphyses and periosteum of growing bones when administered intravenously. Sites of active osteogenesis are most susceptible. The virus infects osteoprogenitor cells, osteoblasts, osteoclasts, and endothelial cells, all of which may contain intranuclear inclusions.

Medullary sclerosis may occur in cats infected with ***Feline leukemia virus***, and is associated with nonregenerative anemia (see Vol. 3, Hematopoietic system). It is not clear whether the osteosclerosis is a direct result of the viral infection or is secondary to chronic anemia or hypoxia. Myelofibrosis may also be a feature of this infection.

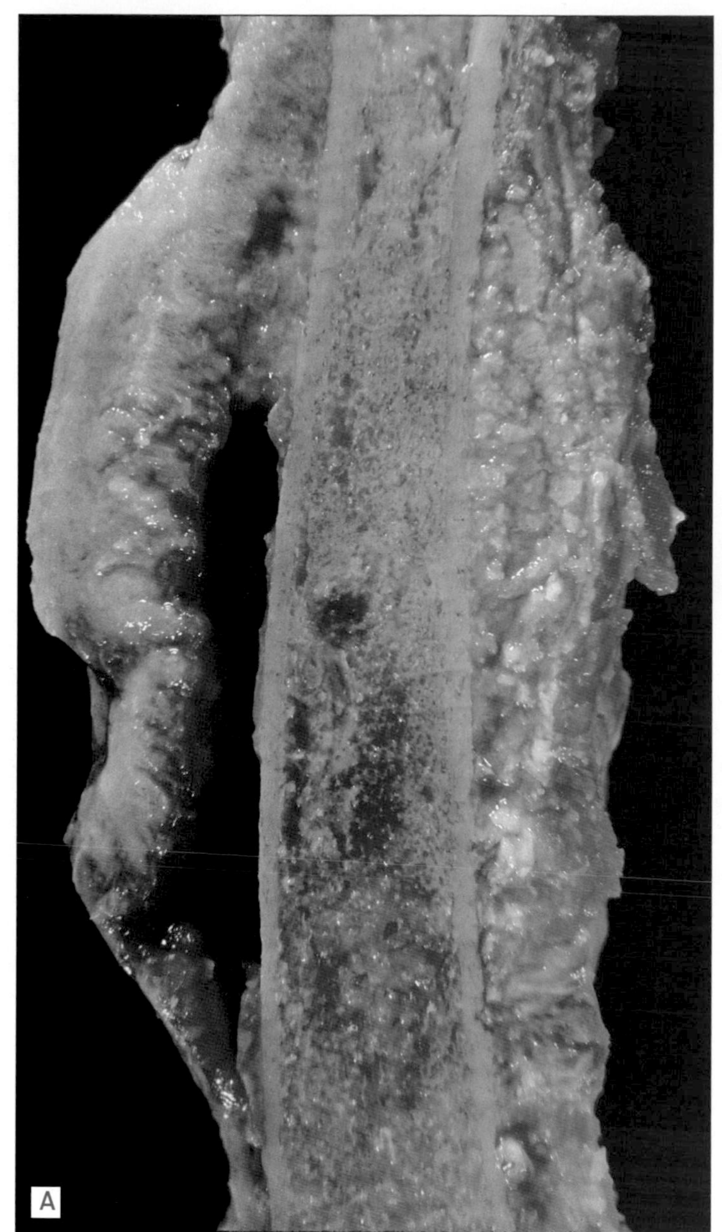

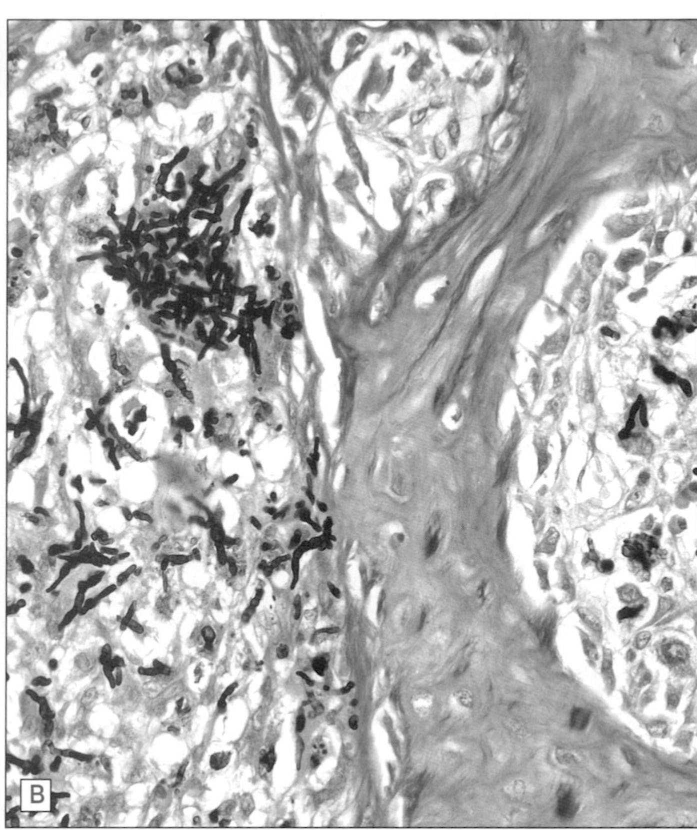

Figure 1.95 Mycotic osteomyelitis, dog. *Paecilomyces* sp. **A.** Extensive periosteal new bone formation along the femoral diaphysis. A cavity has formed between the new bone and the cortex on one side. **B.** Clusters of fine, silver-positive, fungal hyphae adjacent to woven bone trabecula.

Bibliography

Alfaro AA, Mendoza L. Four cases of equine bone lesions caused by *Pithium insidiosum*. Equine Vet J 1990;22:295–297.

Allan FJ, et al. Neutropenia with a probable hereditary basis in Border Collies. N Z Vet J 1996;44:62–72.

Finley GG. A survey of vertebral abscesses in domestic animals in Ontario. Can Vet J 1975;16:114–117.

Firth EC. Bone sequestration in horses and cattle. Aust Vet J 1987;64:65–69.

Firth EC, Goedegebuure SA. The site of focal osteomyelitis lesions in foals. Vet Quart 1988;10:99–108.

Firth EC, Poulos PW. Vascular characteristics of the cartilage and subchondral bone of the distal radial epiphysis of the young foal. N Z Vet J 1993;41:73–77.

Healey AM, et al. Cervico-thoracic vertebral osteomyelitis in 14 calves. Vet J 1997;154:227–232.

Hoover EA, Kociba GJ. Bone lesions in cats with anemia induced by feline leukemia virus. J Natl Cancer Inst 1974;53:1277–1284.

Jang SS, et al. Paecilomycosis in a dog. J Am Vet Med Assoc 1971;159:1775–1779.

Johnson KA. Osteomyelitis in dogs and cats. J Am Vet Med Assoc 1994;205: 1882–1887.

Johnston DE, Summers BA. Osteomyelitis of the lumbar vertebrae in dogs caused by grass-seed foreign bodies. Aust Vet J 1971;47:289–294.

Markel MD, et al. Vertebral body osteomyelitis in the horse. J Am Vet Med Assoc 1986;188:632–634.

Mee AP, et al. Canine distemper virus transcripts detected in the bone cells of dogs with metaphyseal osteopathy. Bone 1993;14:59–67.

Norden CW. Lessons learned from animal models of osteomyelitis. Rev Infect Dis 1988;10:103–110.

Whalen JL, et al. A histological study of acute hematogenous osteomyelitis following physeal injuries in rabbits. J Bone Joint Surg 1988;70A:1383–1392.

Metaphyseal osteopathy

Although *the cause of canine metaphyseal osteopathy is unknown*, and a variety of noninfectious etiologies have been proposed, the disease

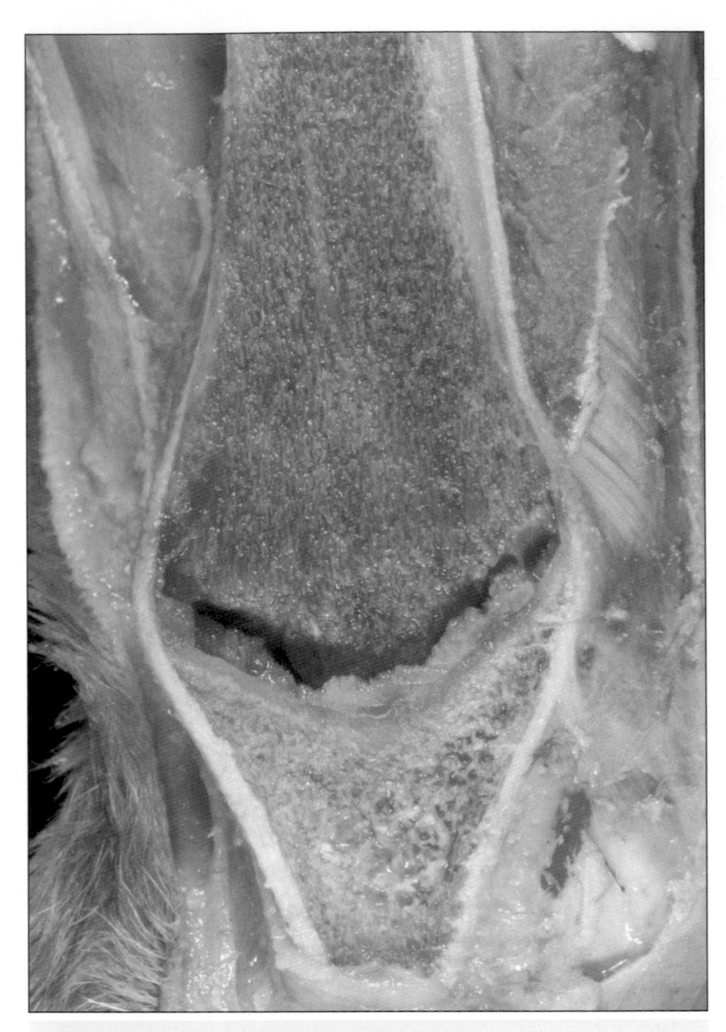

Figure 1.96 Metaphyseal osteopathy, dog. Acute lesion showing an infraction line through weakened trabeculae in the primary spongiosa of the distal ulna. (Courtesy of DJ Meuten.)

is included here amongst inflammatory diseases of bones because of the nature of the early lesions and increasing evidence that it is a manifestation of infectious osteomyelitis and periostitis. The disease is commonly referred to as "*hypertrophic osteodystrophy*" but *this term implies a metabolic rather than an inflammatory origin and should be discontinued*. Similarly, the term "skeletal scurvy" is purely historic and is inappropriate.

Metaphyseal osteopathy is a *disease of young growing dogs*, mainly those of large and giant breeds, although Weimaraners are over-represented in published reports. Affected dogs are usually 3–6 months of age at the time of initial presentation and typically show signs of fever, anorexia and severe lameness associated with swelling and pain of the metaphyseal regions of long bones. Some animals are reported to show diarrhea, or some other clinical abnormality, 7–10 days prior to the onset of fever. The *distal radius and ulna* are usually most severely affected but all fast-growing bones including ribs may be involved. Bones distal to the tarsus and carpus are usually spared. Radiographs taken early in the disease show alternating radiodense and radiolucent zones in the metaphysis parallel to the physis, and there is often lipping of the metaphyseal margins. Acute lesions are characterized grossly by a narrow band of pallor in the primary spongiosa adjacent to rapidly growing physes. Infractions

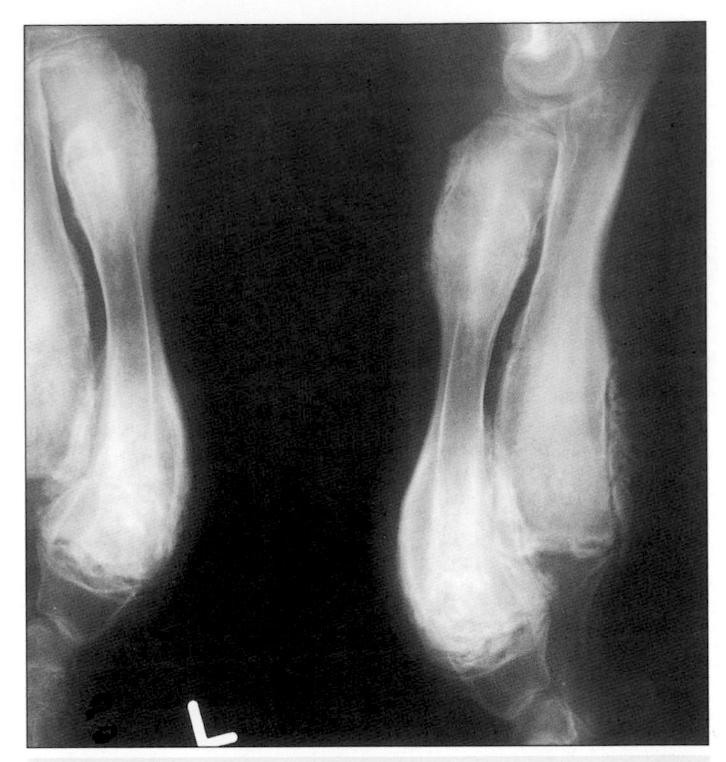

Figure 1.97 Metaphyseal osteopathy, dog. Radiograph of chronic lesion with extensive periosteal reaction involving the radius and ulna.

(antemortem or postmortem) may be present through the primary spongiosa of some bones (Fig. 1.96) reflecting the fragility of the trabeculae in these areas of acute inflammation.

In most cases, the lesion does not progress but in others, periosteal and extraperiosteal ossification develops and the ends of the long bones become swollen and hard. Occasionally these swellings are extensive and involve almost two-thirds of the length of the bone, excluding only the mid-diaphysis and epiphyses (Fig. 1.97). The lesions are *usually bilaterally symmetrical*. Remissions and exacerbations may occur over a period of weeks to months and, rarely, a chronically affected dog dies or, more commonly, is killed for humane reasons. Most animals recover completely without, or in spite of, treatment and the excess metaphyseal bone is gradually removed.

The *histologic lesions* in acute cases are characteristic. The growth plates and primary spongiosa are structurally normal but there is *persistence of the calcified cartilage lattice of the primary spongiosa and intense intertrabecular, suppurative inflammation with necrosis and disappearance of osteoblasts* (Fig. 1.98A, B). Deposition of osteoid on the calcified cartilage spicules of the primary spongiosa is absent and the delicate trabeculae frequently fracture. Osteoclastic activity is prominent in some areas. The suppurative inflammation and necrosis of marrow contents may extend throughout much of the metaphysis and fibrin thrombi may be present in small blood vessels. Aggregates of segmented neutrophils are often present in the periosteum, associated with hemorrhages, as well as in cartilage canals of the epiphyses, and in bones such as vertebrae, mandibles, and turbinates. Enamel hypoplasia associated with inflammation of the dental crypt may also occur.

If the disease progresses, periosteal and extraperiosteal woven bone may develop in areas of previous hemorrhage and inflammation, eventually forming a collar of bone around metaphyses. At the same

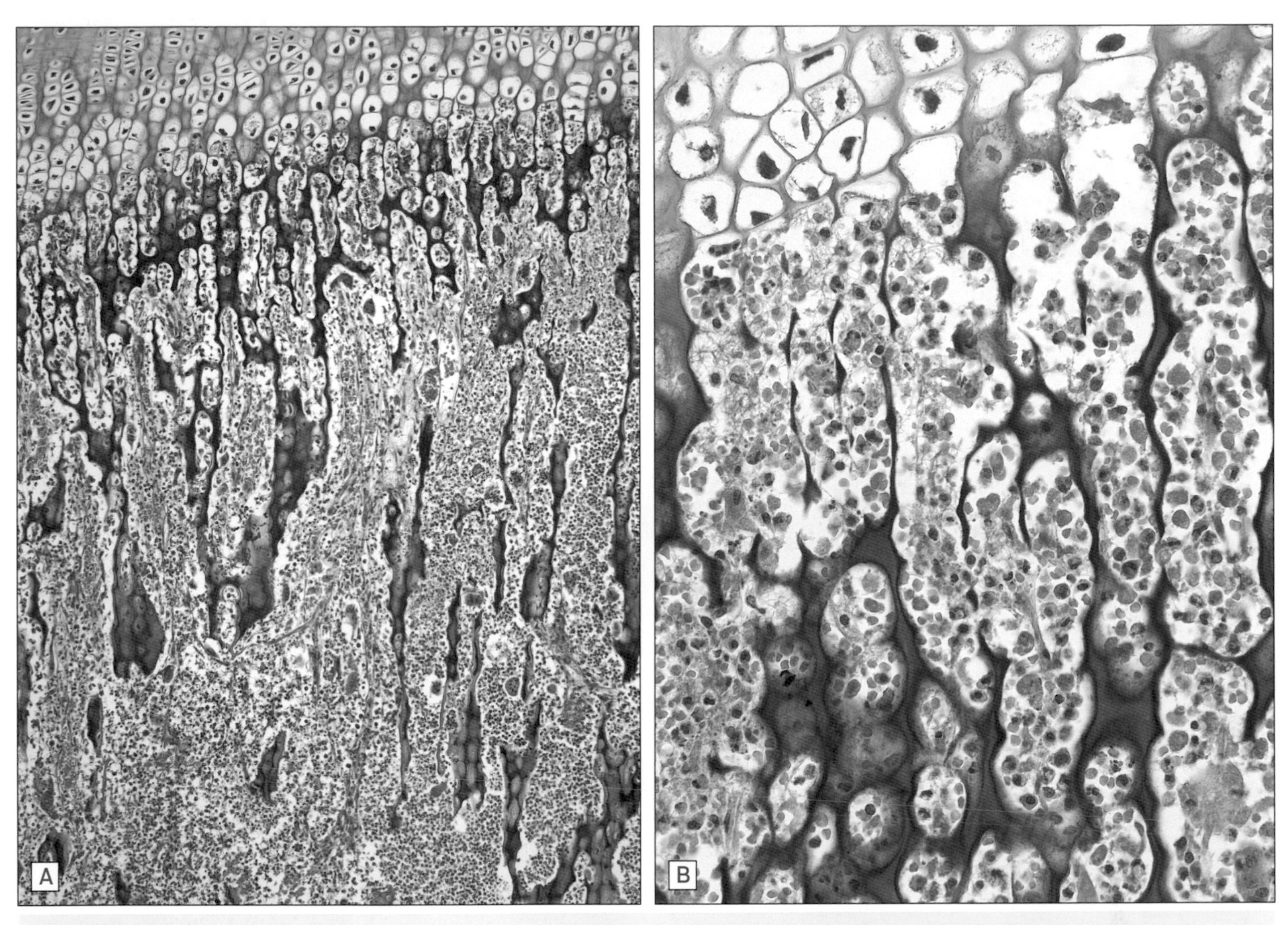

Figure 1.98 Metaphyseal osteopathy, dog. **A.** Acute disease showing normal physis and intense inflammatory reaction between trabeculae in the primary and secondary spongiosa. Trabeculae are delicate and consist largely of calcified cartilage with little, if any, osteoid. **B.** Higher-power view of primary spongiosa from the same animal. Calcified cartilage spicules devoid of an osteoid layer are separated by neutrophils and necrotic cellular debris. No osteoblasts are apparent.

time there is proliferation of mesenchymal tissue in the marrow spaces, replacing the suppurative exudate and providing precursor cells for the reconstruction of the damaged tissues. In those animals that have recurrences of the disease, acute inflammatory changes are superimposed on the osteogenic fibrous tissue in marrow spaces. Radiologically, the collar of periosteal bone may obscure metaphyseal lesions.

Although there have been numerous proposed causes for metaphyseal osteopathy, none has been proven. Initial reports suggested vitamin C deficiency as a likely cause because of the radiographic similarity between this disease and scurvy of children, but the histological changes are quite different and, in cases of metaphyseal osteopathy where liver levels of ascorbic acid were measured, they were normal. Hypervitaminosis D and "overnutrition" have also been incriminated, but neither of these, nor imbalances of other nutrients such as calcium, phosphorus, or vitamin A would be expected to produce the inflammatory lesions typical of metaphyseal osteopathy. Arguments in support of a nutritional cause are unconvincing. Based on clinical signs, the suppurative nature of the early lesions, and their predilection for osteochondral complexes of metaphyses and epiphyses, *an infectious etiology, probably bacterial, seems likely*. This possibility was suggested in an excellent description of metaphyseal osteopathy in a litter of Weimaraner pups, which also had suppurative lesions in soft tissues (see Woodard 1982). Although hematogenous osteomyelitis is considered uncommon in dogs, it is a consistent feature of Border Collie puppies with an inherited form of persistent neutropenia, and occurs in some puppies that survive canine parvovirus infection, probably following bacteremia established during a period of neutropenia. The lesions in affected animals are indistinguishable from those of metaphyseal osteopathy (Fig. 1.99). Further support for an infectious etiology in metaphyseal osteopathy is provided by the demonstration of *E. coli* bacteremia in a dog with characteristic radiographic lesions.

A possible link has been suggested between metaphyseal osteopathy and canine distemper vaccination, at least in Weimaraner puppies, but radiographic evidence has not been supported by histopathology. Canine distemper virus mRNA has been detected in osteoblasts and osteoclasts from metaphyseal bone of dogs with metaphyseal osteopathy, but viral mRNA can also be detected in the metaphysis of distemper-infected dogs without metaphyseal osteopathy. Canine distemper virus is known to induce metaphyseal sclerosis secondary to its action on osteoclasts (see above), but this change does not resemble the suppurative, inflammatory lesion of metaphyseal osteopathy.

Based on the clinical and histological evidence available, the concept of an infectious, probably bacterial, etiology for metaphyseal osteopathy is the most appealing. This does not however imply the involvement of a specific agent. Several bacteria are known to cause hematogenous osteomyelitis in other species, and a similar range of organisms may be involved in dogs. Proof of bacterial infection in metaphyseal osteopathy is difficult as most affected animals survive, and those that are subjected to postmortem examination are usually either at an advanced stage of the disease or have been treated with antibiotics prior to death or euthanasia. In reality, many cases of metaphyseal osteopathy caused by bone infection in dogs could remain undetected, especially in dogs that are able to re-establish an effective immune response and eliminate the infection. Perhaps clinical disease is confined to animals with defective immunity or those that receive an overwhelming infection during a period when their defense mechanisms are reduced by an immunosuppressive viral infection.

Bibliography

Harrus S, et al. Development of hypertrophic osteodystrophy and antibody response in a litter of vaccinated Weimaraner puppies. J Small Anim Pract 2002;43:27–31.

Malik R, et al. Concurrent juvenile cellulitis and metaphyseal osteopathy: an atypical canine distemper virus syndrome. Aust Vet Pract 1995;25:62–67.

Mee AP, et al. Canine distemper virus transcripts detected in the bone cells of dogs with metaphyseal osteopathy. Bone 1993;14:59–67.

Schulz KS, et al. *Escherichia coli* bacteremia associated with hypertrophic osteodystrophy in a dog. J Am Vet Med Assoc 1991;199:1170–1173.

Teare JA, et al. Ascorbic acid deficiency and hypertrophic osteodystrophy in the dog: A rebuttal. Cornell Vet 1979;69:384–401.

Woodard JC. Canine hypertrophic osteodystrophy, a study of the spontaneous disease in littermates. Vet Pathol 1982;19:337–354.

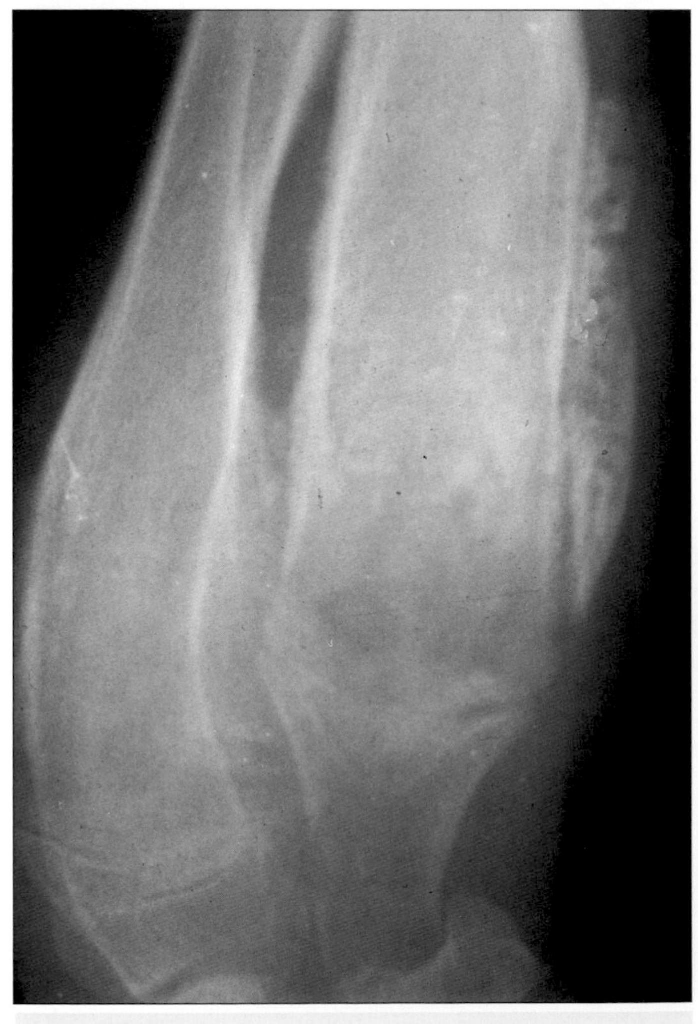

Figure 1.99 Periosteal new bone forming a collar around the metaphysis of the distal radius and ulna in a 5-month-old pup that had survived infection by *Canine parvovirus*. The lesions were bilateral and radiographically, were indistinguishable from chronic metaphyseal osteopathy.

Canine panosteitis

Canine panosteitis (panostosis, juvenile osteomyelitis, enostosis, eosinophilic panosteitis) is a disease of unknown cause that, like metaphyseal osteopathy, usually affects dogs of the large and giant breeds between 5–12 months of age. Occasionally, small dogs such as Miniature Schnauzer and Scottish Terrier are affected and the age range extends from 2 months

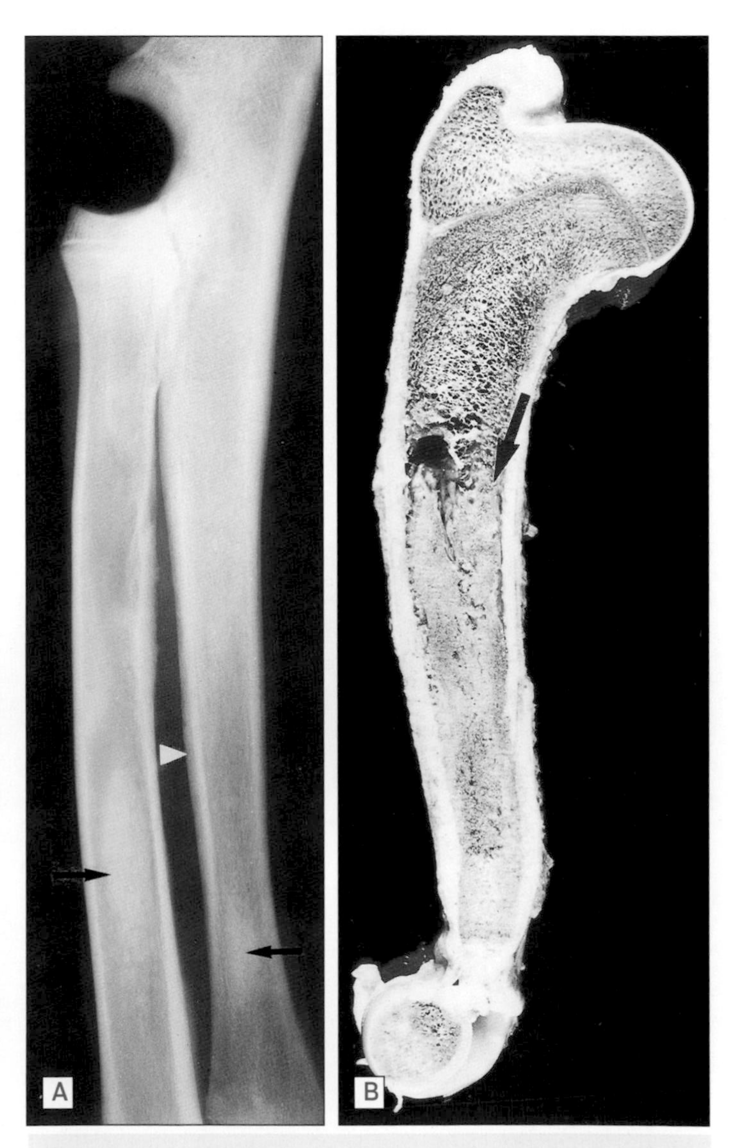

Figure 1.100 Panosteitis, dog. **A.** Radius and ulna showing focal and diffuse medullary densities (arrows) and periosteal reaction (arrowhead). (Courtesy of DC Van Sickle.) **B.** Humeral marrow distal to arrow is filled with woven bone.

to 5 years. The disease was first described as eosinophilic panosteitis of German Shepherds and 75% of reported cases involve this breed. More than two-thirds of affected dogs are males. Although an inflammatory origin for panosteitis is not convincing, the disease is included here for convenience.

Clinical signs vary from *mild to severe lameness*, which may shift from one bone to another. The disease is prone to remission and exacerbation, and is *usually self-limiting* after one to several months. The lameness is associated with abnormalities in the diaphysis of a long bone, usually in the foreleg. Multiple bone involvement occurs in about 50% of cases and rarely, other bones such as ilium and metatarsals are affected.

Because the disease is self-limiting and is well recognized by radiologists, pathologic studies are few and the lesions are defined in terms of their radiographic appearance. At the time when clinical signs begin, no lesions may be visible. About 10 days later, initial involvement of the long bone is seen as an increased density or densities of the medulla in the region of the nutrient foramen. The density may increase in size, sometimes filling the entire medullary cavity, or may remain localized (Fig. 1.100A, B). If the reaction extends to the cortex, marked cortical thickening may result due to periosteal proliferation. When the animal recovers, the increased density disappears over a period of weeks to months.

The initial increased radiodensity is due to expanding areas of fibrovascular tissue in the bone marrow, which are rapidly replaced by woven bone (Fig. 1.101A). This bone is subject to consecutive episodes of formation and resorption, thus reversal and resting lines are often present in the same trabeculae, and osteoclasts and osteoblasts are active in the same microscopic field. Cartilage is sometimes formed in the fibrovascular tissue. Periosteal woven bone formation may be stimulated and this, like the medullary bone, is replaced by lamellar bone before being replaced over the ensuing months (Fig. 1.101B). The older, more mature bone in the center of the medullary lesions is removed first.

In most dogs, there is no evidence of inflammatory infiltrates in the lesions, but sometimes plasma cells and histiocytes are present. Eosinophilia is an inconstant feature of the hemogram and serum chemistry is unremarkable. Abnormalities in clotting times are inconstant findings.

The cause of canine panosteitis is not known. Genetic and allergic factors, hyperestrogenism, filterable agents, and various bacteria have been proposed, but the evidence is inconclusive. A viral etiology, particularly *Canine distemper virus*, has also been suggested because of the pyrexia, tonsillitis, and leukocytosis that occur in some cases. In females, the onset of signs is sometimes associated with estrus and it is thought that other physiological stress may precipitate the disease. The occurrence of panosteitis in dogs with hemophilia A suggests that sometimes the disease might be a sequel to intraosseous hemorrhage.

Bibliography

Grondalen J, et al. Enostosis (panosteitis) in three dogs suffering from hemophilia A. Canine Pract 1991;16:10–14.

Muir PM, et al. Panosteitis. Compend Contin Educ Pract Vet 1996;18:29–33.

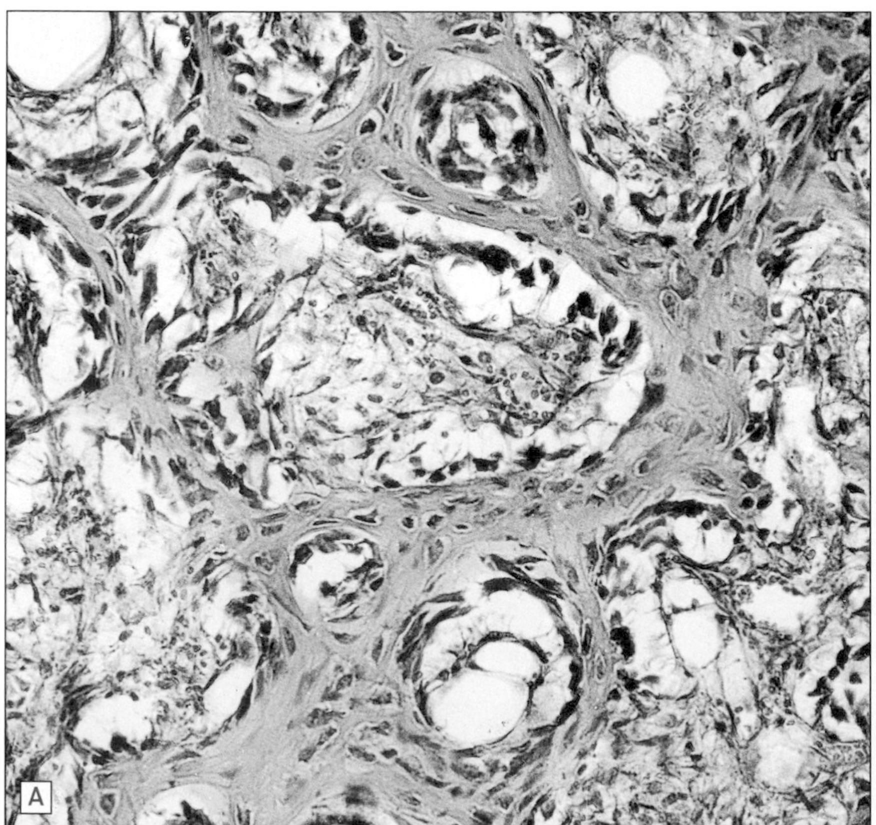

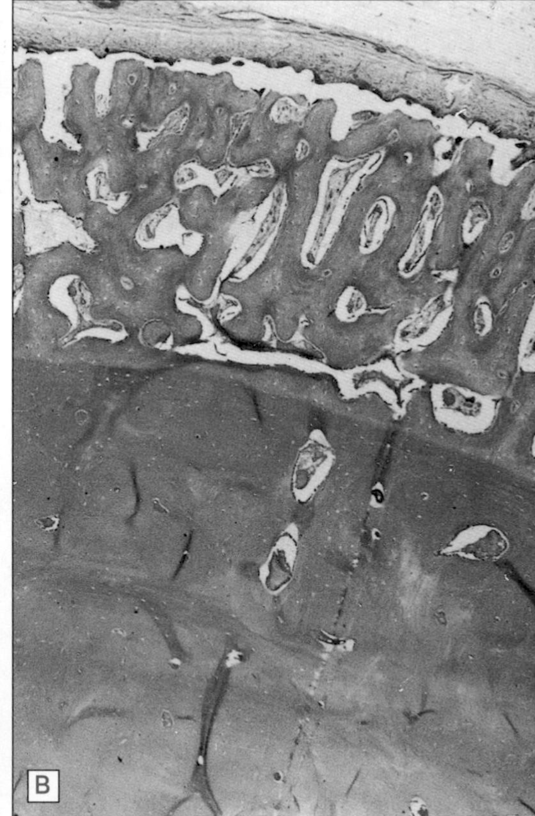

Figure 1.101 Panosteitis, dog. **A.** Rapidly developing trabeculae of woven bone in the marrow cavity. (Courtesy of DC Van Sickle.) **B.** New bone formation beneath the periosteum. (Courtesy of KA Johnson.)

HYPEROSTOTIC DISEASES

Excessive bone formation or hyperostosis occurs as a nonspecific response to various forms of bone injury, including trauma, infection, metabolic disturbances, mineral and vitamin imbalances, subperiosteal hemorrhage, and neoplasia. Many of these have been discussed already in this chapter. The periarticular exostoses or osteophytes that develop in association with degenerative joint disease further illustrate this predictable response of bone to injury or inflammation in adjacent tissues. This section includes a group of poorly understood diseases of humans and animals, characterized by marked hyperostosis in the absence of any apparent cause.

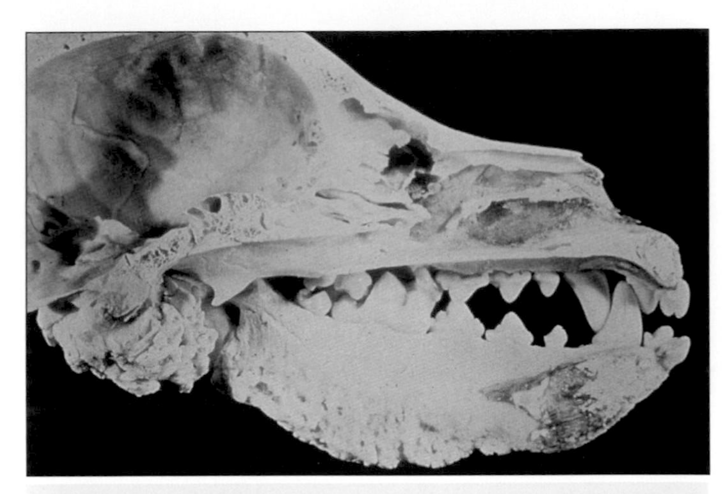

Figure 1.102 Craniomandibular osteopathy, dog. Macerated specimen showing extensive new bone formation along the mandible and around the tympanic bulla.

Craniomandibular osteopathy

Craniomandibular osteopathy, also known as *"lion jaw", is a proliferative disorder usually confined to the bones of the skull, in particular the mandibles, occipital, and temporal bones.* The tympanic bullae are often severely affected. Lesions are bilateral but irregular and may also involve the parietal, frontal, and maxillary bones. Occasionally, there is subperiosteal and extraperiosteal proliferation of new bone associated with long bones. The disease is most common in West Highland White Terriers, but is also described in several other breeds, including Scottish Terriers, Labrador Retrievers, Great Danes, Doberman Pinschers, Cairn Terriers, German Wirehaired Pointers, Pyrenean Mountain Dogs, and in a Boxer, a Boston Terrier and an English Bulldog.

The disease is usually recognized at approximately 4–7 months of age because of either discomfort while chewing or inability to open the mouth to eat. Proliferative changes may be palpable or grossly visible, and pain is elicited when attempting to open the mouth. Radiographic findings are characterized by more or less symmetrical enlargement of the mandibles and tympanic bullae, although the lesions may occur independently. Ossification of soft tissues, especially near the angular processes of the mandibles, may result in fusion of the processes to the bullae and ankylosis. The disease has an intermittent, progressive course lasting several weeks to a few months. It is often self-limiting and nonfatal, although some dogs are killed because they cannot eat. During clinical exacerbations, which tend to recur every 2–3 weeks, fever is present but laboratory data are normal.

At the height of the disease, atrophy of the muscles of mastication and increased fibrous and osseous tissue of the head are obvious. The full extent of the bone changes is best demonstrated in radiographs and macerated specimens (Fig. 1.102). In the mandible, new bone deposition is usually most prominent in the region of the angle, involving medial, ventral, and lateral aspects but tending to avoid the alveolar bone. The tympanic bullae are often enlarged two to three times and filled with new bone.

Histologic changes in the mandible involve the endosteum, periosteum, and trabecular bone and present a complex pattern of intermittent and concurrent formation and resorption. The mosaic of reversal and resting lines resulting from this cellular activity (Fig. 1.103) bears some resemblance to the changes seen in Paget's disease of man, but further comparison is unjustified. The significance of this mosaic pattern is easily overemphasized since the mandible of growing dogs is a site of intense bone modeling as teeth mature, erupt, and drift during normal development. Bone resorption in craniomandibular osteopathy appears to be random and disoriented, involving both pre-existing lamellar trabeculae and newly formed woven bone. Similarly, bone formation occurs simultaneously in many areas, evolving from fibrous tissue, which frequently fills the marrow

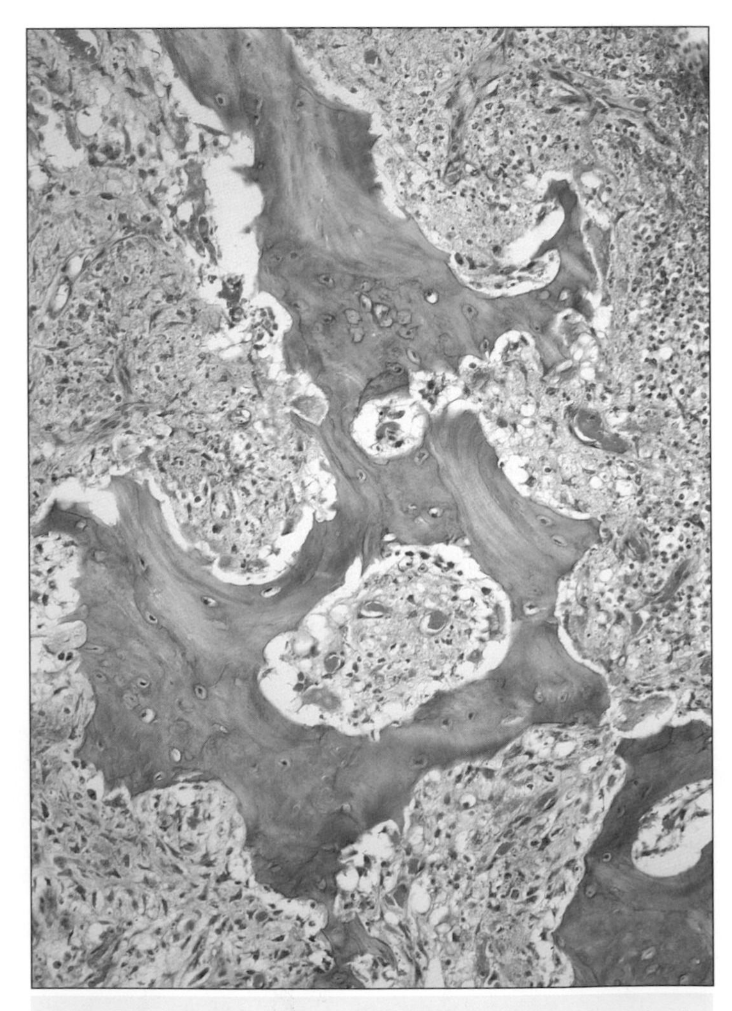

Figure 1.103 Craniomandibular osteopathy, dog. Ragged bone trabeculae with scalloped margin indicating active osteoclastic resorption. The trabeculae contain a mosaic of woven and mature lamellar bone demarcated by cementing lines.

spaces and thickens the periosteum. Lymphocytes, plasma cells, and neutrophils are sometimes present in areas of active osteogenesis.

As the disease subsides, formation of woven bone may be superseded by lamellar bone production, and existing woven trabeculae are replaced by lamellar bone, which is then gradually resorbed. In some cases, especially where fusion of mandibles to tympanic bullae is present, resorption is insufficient to allow restitution of normal function.

The cause of craniomandibular osteopathy is not known. The presence of inflammatory infiltrates raises the possibility of an infectious agent, but none has been demonstrated. In West Highland White and Scottish Terriers, there is evidence of a genetic etiology with autosomal recessive inheritance. However, the occurrence of the syndrome in diverse breeds suggests that there may be more than one cause of the condition. Alternatively, there may be an inherited predisposition in several breeds but the presence of an additional factor, perhaps an infectious agent, is required for the disease to be expressed. The etiology and pathogenesis of a similar condition in children, infantile cortical hyperostosis, are also unknown.

Bibliography

Padgett GA, Mostosky UV. The mode of inheritance of craniomandibular osteopathy in West Highland white Terrier dogs. Amer J Med Genet 1986;25:9–13.

Watson ADJ, et al. Craniomandibular osteopathy in dogs. Compend Contin Educ Pract Vet 1995;17:911–922.

Hypertrophic osteopathy

This syndrome, which is also known as "Marie's disease" or hypertrophic pulmonary osteopathy, is characterized by diffuse, periosteal new bone formation along the diaphyses and metaphyses of certain limb bones in association with a chronic inflammatory or neoplastic lesion, usually in the thoracic cavity. It occurs in humans, and is reported in several domestic animal species, most often dogs. Occasionally, hypertrophic osteopathy occurs in association with nonthoracic lesions, such as botryoid rhabdomyosarcoma of the urinary bladder in dogs and ovarian tumors in horses. Rarely, the disease occurs in animals with no detectable visceral lesions.

The thoracic lesions associated with hypertrophic osteopathy are diverse. In dogs, it occurs most often with primary or secondary pulmonary neoplasms, but also with granulomatous pleuritis, granulomatous lymphadenitis of bronchial or mediastinal nodes, chronic bronchitis, *Dirofilaria immitis* infection, esophageal granulomas, and tumors provoked by *Spirocerca sanguinolenta,* and with neoplastic disease of the thoracic wall. In horses, it is more often associated with granulomatous inflammatory diseases involving the thoracic cavity. Hypertrophic osteopathy is present only in a minority of animals with thoracic lesions, but the incidence is much higher in some types than in others. For example, dogs with pulmonary metastases from osteosarcoma are much more likely to develop the syndrome than are dogs with metastatic carcinoma. It is also possible that many mild cases of hypertrophic osteopathy are missed both clinically and through incomplete examination of the limb bones at necropsy.

The *periosteal new bone formation in hypertrophic osteopathy is usually confined to the limbs,* and in the dog, involves particularly the radius, ulna, tibia, metacarpals, and metatarsals, with relative sparing of the bones of the upper limbs and phalanges (Fig. 1.104). The more distal limb bones are generally affected first, the lesions then extending proximally. The extent of the osteophytes is best demonstrated in radiographs and macerated specimens where, in florid cases, they appear as wart or cauliflower-like accretions extending along the whole length of the bone (Fig. 1.105). Cross-sections of bone demonstrate the asymmetric development of these accretions, which tend to occur initially and most severely where the periosteum is free of tendinous insertions or adjacent bones. Occasionally, osteophytes occur on the vertebrae and skull, and minor endosteal lesions occur infrequently. *Articular surfaces are not involved in animals but are often affected in human cases,* hence the frequent use of the term hypertrophic osteoarthropathy for the human disease. Although the lesions of hypertrophic osteopathy are progressive, they regress if the primary thoracic lesion is removed.

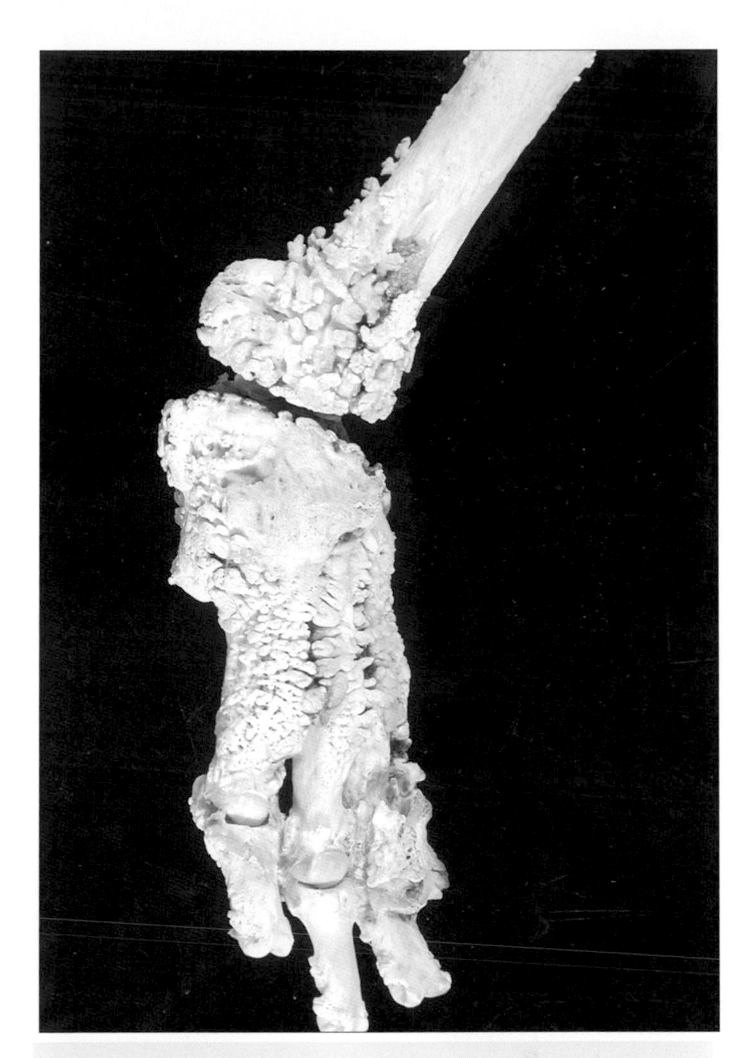

Figure 1.104 Hypertrophic osteopathy, dog. Periosteal new bone involving the metacarpals and radius-ulna, but with relative sparing of the phalanges.

Histologically, the earliest changes are hyperemia and edema, with proliferation of highly vascular connective tissue in the periosteum, in some cases leading to extensive hemorrhage. These changes are associated with a rapid increase in peripheral blood flow in the distal half of the limbs and may be accompanied by a light infiltrate of lymphocytes and plasma cells. Shortly thereafter, osteoblasts deposit osteoid on the existing cortical bone and then, if the disturbance is severe, begin to lay down new trabeculae perpendicular to the original cortex. The new bone may be deposited with extraordinary rapidity, and the width of the cortex may be doubled in a few weeks. In the early and active stages of the disease, the new bone is clearly distinguishable from the original cortex because the former is trabecular and the latter compact. Later, the distinction may be less distinct because the original cortex is converted to spongy bone by resorption from within the vascular canals and the endosteal surface.

The *pathogenesis of hypertrophic osteopathy is obscure* but increased blood flow to the limbs is a consistent early change. Several hypotheses have been proposed, including hypoxia, arteriovenous shunting, neurogenic and humoral mechanisms, but none consistently fits the clinical and experimental observations. According to the *neurogenic theory*, impulses originating in the thoracic lesion travel via the vagus nerve to the brainstem and initiate reflex vasodilation in the limbs, either by humoral or neural means. Limited support for this theory is provided by the regression of bone lesions in some, but not all, human and canine cases treated by vagotomy. The *humoral hypothesis* proposes either that the primary lesion produces a hormone or hormone-like substance or that arteriovenous anastomoses in the primary lesion prevent catabolism of such a substance in the lung. The hormone then produces the secondary skeletal lesions. Support for this hypothesis is derived from the production of typical skeletal lesions following experimental venoarterial shunts in dogs, but there is no evidence of such shunts in most spontaneous cases. In a very limited number of cases, Marie's disease has been restricted to one limb, and vascular abnormalities are generally found in those cases. It has also been suggested that reduced oxygenation of peripheral blood, resulting from congenital or acquired arteriovenous shunts, stimulates periosteal osteophyte production. More recently, it has been proposed that the primary lesion in hypertrophic osteopathy might cause inappropriate stimulation of an extra-renal volume receptor system controlled by innervation of blood vessels by branches of the vagus and glossopharyngeal nerves. It is suggested that stimulation of this system as a result of blood flow in anomalous vascular channels associated with the primary thoracic lesion, may activate the cerebral salt center leading to retention of extracellular sodium, fluid retention, and increased blood supply to the limbs. This does not however explain the occurrence of hypertrophic osteopathy in animals in association with tumors of the urinary bladder or ovary.

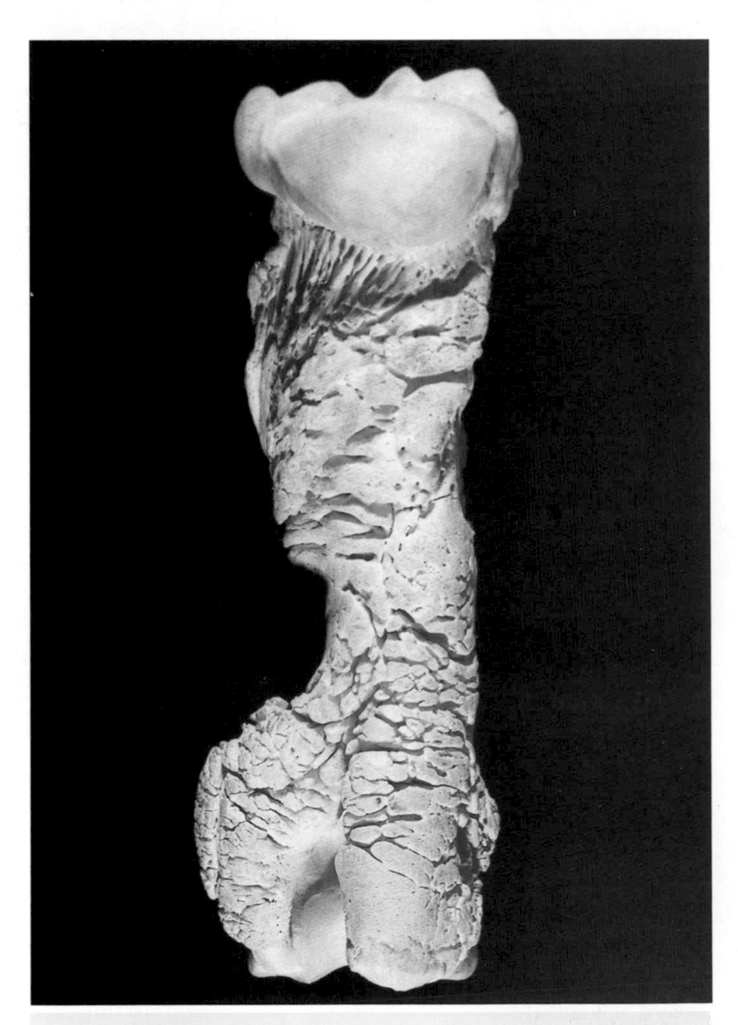

Figure 1.105 Hypertrophic osteopathy, horse. Florid periosteal reaction along the shaft of the humerus.

Bibliography

Doyle L. Pathogenesis of secondary hypertrophic osteoarthropathy: a hypothesis. Eur Respir J 1989;2:105–106.

Hesselink JW, van den Tweel JG. Hypertrophic osteopathy in a dog with a chronic lung abscess. J Am Vet Med Assoc 1990;196:760–762.

Mair TS, et al. Hypertrophic osteopathy (Marie's disease) in Equidae: a review of twenty four cases. Equine Vet J 1996;28:256–263.

Canine diffuse idiopathic skeletal hyperostosis

Diffuse idiopathic skeletal hyperostosis is a hyperostotic disorder of man that appears to have a counterpart in dogs, particularly large and giant breeds such as Labrador Retrievers and Great Danes. *The disease in dogs is characterized by progressive new bone formation along vertebral bodies, sometimes leading to fusion; progressive osseous fusion of the ilium, pubis, femur, and ischium; and development of para-articular bony lesions around certain joints of the appendicular skeleton.*

The vertebral exostoses tend to occur at ligamentous insertions (enthesiophytes) and appear to vary in their distribution between different regions of the spine. The lesions are more extensive than those of ankylosing spondylosis, involving the ventral and lateral aspects of three or more contiguous vertebral bodies, and are not accompanied by evidence of disk degeneration. Furthermore, the new bone formation also occurs on vertebral arches, dorsal spinous processes, and articular processes, where it is very unlikely to be associated with degenerative disk disease. The initial para-articular lesions in the appendicular skeleton are fibrocartilaginous, but undergo endochondral ossification to produce bony lesions, which may progress to result in joint fusion. Intra-articular structures are not affected.

There are several other hyperostotic diseases in dogs that must be differentiated from diffuse idiopathic skeletal hyperostosis. These include ankylosing spondylosis, spondylosis deformans, spinal osteoarthrosis, vitamin A toxicity, and hepatozoonosis, all of which are discussed elsewhere in this chapter. *Radiographic criteria* that might suggest a diagnosis of diffuse idiopathic skeletal hyperostosis in dogs include the following:

- flowing calcification and ossification along ventral and lateral aspects of three contiguous vertebral bodies leading to bony ankylosis;
- preservation of normal disk width in affected areas and absence of significant degenerative disk disease, such as end-plate sclerosis, nuclear calcification and localized spondylosis deformans;
- osteophytes around vertebral articular facets;

- formation of pseudoarthroses between the bases of spinous processes;
- periarticular osteophytes in addition to calcification and ossification of soft-tissue attachments (enthesiophytes) in the axial and appendicular skeleton;
- periarticular osteophytes, sclerosis and ankylosis of sacroiliac joints; and
- bony ankylosis of the symphysis pubis.

The presence of any four of the first five criteria is considered sufficient to support the diagnosis.

The *etiology of diffuse idiopathic skeletal hyperostosis is unknown*, but it appears to represent an exaggerated response to stimuli that would normally induce little, if any new bone formation. For this reason, *the disease has been referred to as an ossifying diathesis*. In human patients with diffuse idiopathic skeletal hyperostosis, excessive heterotopic ossification occurs after hip surgery, and in dogs, the formation of periarticular osteophytes is out of proportion to any degenerative changes in the associated joint. No predisposing cause can be found for most of the skeletal lesions in this syndrome but their close association with joints, and insertion sites for ligaments, tendons, and muscles cannot be ignored. Perhaps minor traumatic episodes at these sites result in excessive local production of specific growth factors, (e.g., TGF-β, FGFs, and BMPs) in susceptible individuals.

Bibliography

Morgan JP, Stavenborn M. Disseminated idiopathic skeletal hyperostosis (DISH) in a dog. Vet Radiol 1991;32:65–70.

Woodard JC, et al. Canine diffuse idiopathic skeletal hyperostosis. Vet Pathol 1985;22:317–326.

Canine hepatozoonosis

Periosteal new bone formation, similar to that occurring in hypertrophic osteopathy, is a feature of canine hepatozoonosis caused by *Hepatozoon americanum* infection of dogs in the southern USA. The osseous lesions also consistently develop in experimentally infected dogs and coyotes. *The periosteal reaction occurs primarily on the diaphyseal regions of the more proximal limb bones* (Fig. 1.106A), but also may involve bones of the axial skeleton, including the ilium (Fig. 1.106B) and vertebrae, the lesions differing in distribution to those of hypertrophic osteopathy. In early reports of canine hepatozoonosis, it was suggested that the periosteal new bone formation was secondary to local irritation caused by the presence of *Hepatozoon americanum* cysts in adjacent muscle fibers. The absence of microscopic evidence to support this hypothesis, and the widespread, often symmetrical, distribution of lesions *suggests that humoral rather than local factors are involved in the pathogenesis of the bony lesions*.

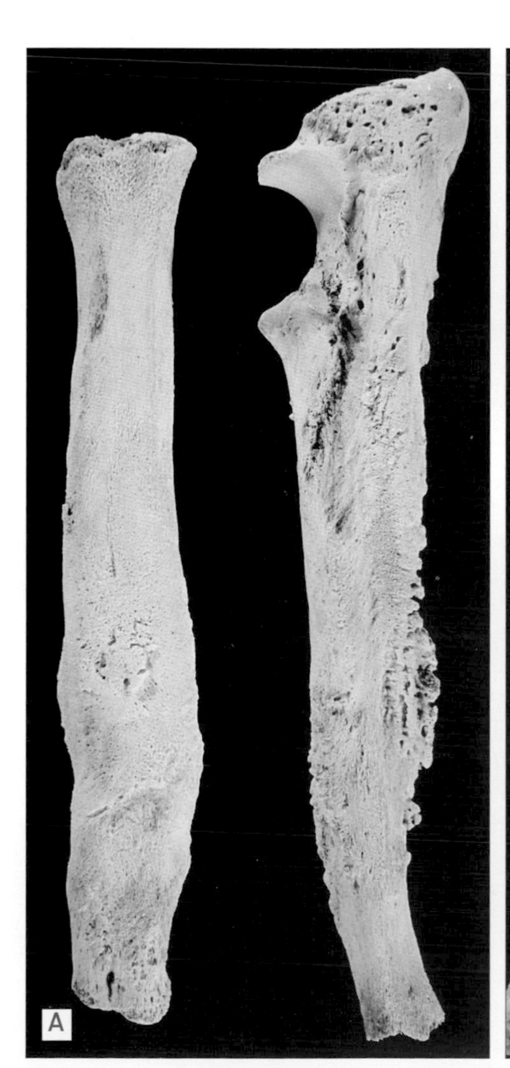

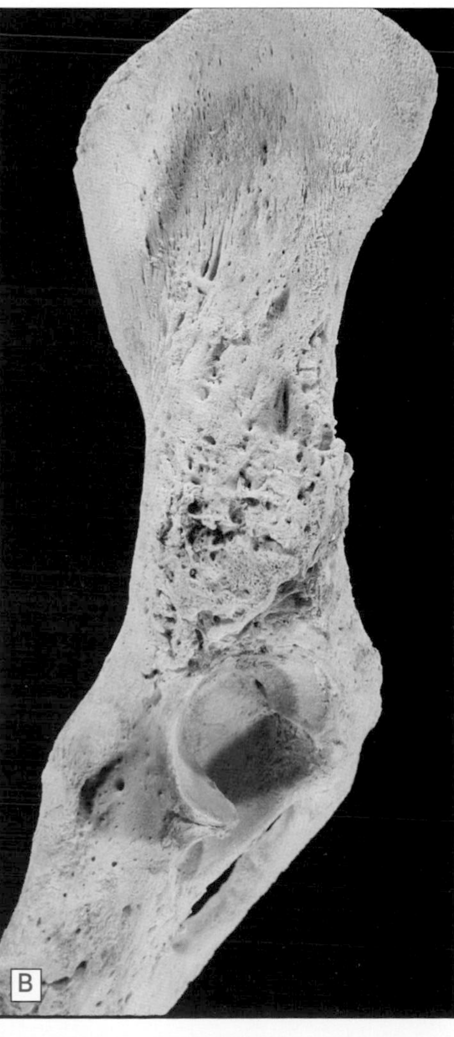

Figure 1.106 Canine hepatozoonosis. A. Periosteal reaction along the diaphyses of the radius and ulna of a 1-year-old dog that had been infected with *Hepatozoon americanum* for approximately 9 months. **B.** Ilium from the same dog, showing prominent periosteal reaction.

Clinical signs of canine hepatozoonosis include pyrexia, depression, weakness, muscle atrophy, and gait abnormalities ranging from stiffness to recumbency. Leukocytosis due to mature neutrophilia, and sometimes a left shift, is a consistent laboratory finding. The disease leads to *chronic debilitation and eventual death*. Different stages of this protozoon agent may be found in skeletal muscles throughout the body, often inducing a pyogranulomatous inflammatory response. The parasite is not present in bone, but may be detected in muscle fibers close to the periosteal surface. Except for a single report from Japan, periosteal new bone formation has not been described in association with *Hepatozoon canis* infection, which occurs in the Old World. The agent of canine hepatozoonosis in North America was initially considered a more virulent strain of *Hepatozoon canis*, but differences in the nature and distribution of lesions, in addition to morphologic differences in gamonts, led to its classification as a separate species.

Bibliography

Craig TM, et al. *Hepatozoon canis* infection in dogs: clinical, radiographic and hematologic findings. J Am Vet Med Assoc 1978;173:967–972.

Macintire DK, et al. Hepatozoonosis in dogs: 22 cases (1989–1994). J Am Vet Med Assoc 1997;210:916–922.

Panciera RJ, et al. Skeletal lesions of canine hepatozoonosis caused by *Hepatozoon americanum*. Vet Pathol 2000;37:225–230.

TUMORS AND TUMOR-LIKE LESIONS OF BONES

Primary tumors of bones are common in dogs and to a lesser extent in cats, but occur infrequently or rarely in other domestic animals. They may arise from any of the mesenchymal tissues present in bones, including precursors of bone, cartilage, fibrous tissue, adipose tissue, and vascular tissue, but *tumors of bone and cartilage-forming cell lines are the most common*. In humans, most primary tumors of bones are benign but this does not apply to all animal species. In dogs, most tumors of bones are malignant. Benign and malignant tumors of bones occur with approximately equal frequency in cats, but in horses, cattle, and other domestic animals, benign tumors of bones are much more common than malignant ones. Secondary tumors of bones, in particular metastatic carcinomas, are very common in humans but are seldom diagnosed in animals. The prevalence of secondary bone tumors in animals is no doubt underestimated as the skeleton is seldom examined in detail either radiographically or at necropsy, but it is almost certainly much lower than in humans. Several comprehensive surveys and reviews of bone tumors have been published and are included in the bibliography at the end of this section.

The classification of primary tumors and tumor-like lesions of bones in domestic animals is generally similar to that developed for humans, but there are too many differences in morphology and prognosis to allow direct extrapolation. The system used in this chapter is based on that proposed in the most recent World Health Organization fascicle on *Histological Classification of Bone and Joint Tumors of Domestic Animals* (Table 1.3). Rather than discuss benign and malignant tumors separately, as in the WHO system, the most important of these tumors will be grouped according to the nature of the predominant matrix that they produce. This reflects the manner in which a pathologist is likely to approach the diagnosis of a bone tumor.

Table 1.3 Histological classification of tumors and tumor-like lesions of bones*

Benign tumors
- Chondroma
- Feline osteochondromatosis
- Hemangioma
- Myxoma of the jaw
- Ossifying fibroma
- Osteoma
- Osteochondroma

Malignant tumors
- Central
  1. Chondrosarcoma
  2. Fibrosarcoma
  3. Giant cell tumor of bone
  4. Hemangiosarcoma
  5. Liposarcoma
  6. Multilobular tumor of bone
  7. Osteosarcoma
     a. poorly differentiated
     b. osteoblastic
        — nonproductive
        — productive
     c. chondroblastic
     d. fibroblastic
     e. telangiectatic
     f. giant cell type
- Peripheral
  1. Maxillary fibrosarcoma (dogs)
  2. Parosteal osteosarcoma
  3. Periosteal chondrosarcoma
  4. Periosteal fibrosarcoma
  5. Periosteal osteosarcoma
- Tumors of bone marrow
  1. Malignant lymphoma
  2. Plasma cell myeloma

Tumor-like lesions
- Aneurysmal bone cyst
- Epidermoid cyst of the phalanx
- Exuberant fracture callus
- Fibrous dysplasia
- Solitary (unicameral) bone cyst
- Subchondral (juxtacortical) bone cyst

Based on World Health Organization International Histological Classification of Tumors of Domestic Animals.

It is often difficult to classify a bone tumor into one category or another with confidence, as the predominant matrix may vary throughout the tumor and poorly differentiated sarcomas may reveal little evidence of their lineage. Since the prognosis of different bone tumors varies markedly, accurate classification by the pathologist will greatly assist the clinician or surgeon and should be attempted, but only in cases where sufficient tissue and information is provided. The pathologist must not feel pressured into making a definitive diagnosis in cases where either the specimen or the history is inadequate. There are many benign lesions of bones that may resemble malignant bone tumors and the consequences of an incorrect diagnosis can be substantial.

The clinical history and radiographic appearance are often crucial to an accurate diagnosis of a bone lesion and the pathologist should not rely on microscopic features alone. In addition to knowledge of the species, breed, and age of the animal, it is important to be aware of the location of the lesion and its duration. Certain bone tumors in man and animals occur with increased frequency at specific sites, hence the value of knowing the exact location of the lesion. It is also important to know if there has been a previous fracture or infection at the site, or whether the animal has recently suffered from a systemic disease or soft tissue tumor, which may have spread to the bone. Radiographs provide valuable additional information on the extent, nature, and behavior of a bone tumor. They can also be of considerable value to the surgeon or pathologist in establishing a list of likely differential diagnoses, and selecting sites for histological or cytological examination. Radiographs of a bone lesion at necropsy will often provide more information of diagnostic relevance than gross examination of the affected bone, but the radiographic appearance can seldom allow reliable differentiation of primary tumors, secondary tumors, and inflammatory lesions of bones.

Proliferation of new, woven bone is a common response to various forms of bone injury and should not be misinterpreted as osteosarcoma. This reactive bone may be deposited beneath an elevated periosteum and form the so-called *Codman's triangle* (see Fig. 1.16), which often occurs in osteosarcoma but also in other lesions where the periosteum is separated from the underlying bone. When the periosteum is breached, the radiating spicules of reactive bone expanding out from the original lesion may create a "sunburst" effect in radiographs. Reactive bone is not confined to the periosteal surface. Many primary and secondary tumors growing within the bone marrow stimulate endosteal new bone formation, as do many inflammatory lesions. In the early stages of formation, reactive bone consists of rapidly proliferating, immature mesenchymal cells producing spicules of unmineralized osteoid. These spicules usually merge with broader trabeculae of woven bone lined by a single layer of plump osteoblasts (Fig. 1.107), unlike osteosarcoma, where the spaces between spicules or islands of tumor bone are generally filled with malignant osteoblasts (see Fig. 1.109B). However, in small biopsy samples, differentiation of early reactive bone from osteosarcoma may be extremely difficult, if not impossible.

In addition to new bone formation, *osteolysis is also a feature of many bone tumors* and osteoclasts can often be seen resorbing mature bone as the advancing tumor permeates the marrow cavity or invades the cortex. The gross and radiographic appearance of a bone tumor reflects the balance between bone resorption and new bone formation. *Biopsy samples, or samples collected for histology or cytology from a suspected bone tumor during necropsy, should always include areas of lysis, as these areas are most likely to contain cells of diagnostic significance.* Too often, samples submitted to the pathologist for examination consist entirely of reactive bone and no diagnosis is possible. In such cases, it is important that the pathologist does not exclude the possibility of an underlying tumor and if the history and radiographic appearance suggest neoplasia, examination of further biopsies, including areas of lysis, is recommended.

Bone-forming tumors

Osteoma, ossifying fibroma, and fibrous dysplasia

These benign tumors are uncommon in domestic animals and there is considerable confusion over their classification and diagnosis. All three arise primarily from the bones of the skull, particularly those bones that develop by intramembranous ossification. Fibrous dysplasia is not a true neoplasm of bones but is included in this group because of the need to differentiate it from osteoma and ossifying

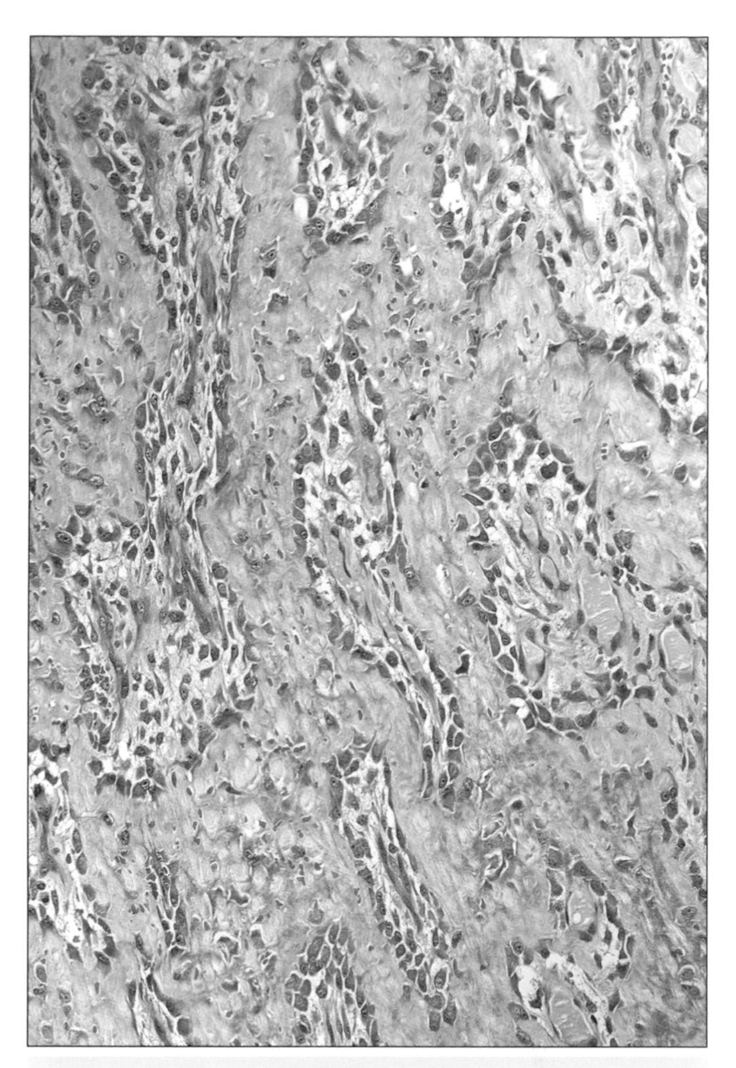

Figure 1.107 Trabeculae of **reactive, woven bone** lined by a single layer of plump osteoblasts.

fibroma. Furthermore, some authors have suggested that osteomas are hamartomas rather than true tumors, while others claim that they represent the sclerotic end stage of fibrous dysplasia.

An **osteoma** is a *dense, smoothly contoured, protruding mass of well-differentiated bone* originating from a periosteal surface and merging with the underlying bone. Exostoses induced by localized periosteal damage may closely resemble osteomas, but osteomas generally show *slow, progressive enlargement* and sometimes achieve a very large size. They are found most often in the mandible, maxilla, nasal sinuses, and bones of the face and cranium in horses and cattle, but also occur in other species. Osteomas occasionally arise from bones of the pelvis, or tubular bones of the limbs, and *must be differentiated from osteochondromas*. In osteochondroma, the bone forms by endochondral ossification beneath a cap of hyaline cartilage and there is continuity between the intertrabecular spaces of the tumor and the marrow cavity of the bone.

Osteomas are often extremely hard, especially if they have been growing for some time, and must be cut with a saw. Clinical signs, other than disfigurement, may be nonexistent or may relate to compression of adjacent structures.

Histologically, osteomas consist of trabecular bone formed by osteoblasts, remodeled by osteoclasts and ultimately converted almost entirely to *lamellar bone*. The trabeculae are gradually thickened by appositional growth so that ultimately the spaces between them are relatively inconspicuous, and the density of the tumor mass approaches that of mature cortex. Such tumors are virtually indistinguishable from exostoses; location and clinical history should be considered in differentiating the two. Actively expanding osteomas have a border of connective tissue resembling periosteum and the slender trabeculae forming beneath this layer are arranged approximately perpendicular to the surface. The superficial trabeculae of an osteoma may consist of woven bone while those in deeper regions are broader and consist largely or completely of lamellar bone.

Osteoid osteoma, a distinct form of osteoma in humans, has also been reported in a cat. This tumor is characterized by a discrete, intra-osseous nidus of active bone formation in which disorganized trabeculae are surrounded by a rim of sclerotic bone. The trabeculae of immature bone are lined by plump osteoblasts but show no evidence of malignancy.

Ossifying fibroma is a rare fibro-osseous tumor of the head, occurring most frequently in young horses less than a year of age, and primarily involving the rostral mandible. There are occasional reports of the tumor in cats, dogs, and sheep. Typically, ossifying fibroma is a sharply demarcated, expansile mass, which distorts the normal contours of the affected bone. The tumor *consists of spindle-shaped fibroblasts, which appear to transform into osteoblasts and form irregular spicules of woven bone*, which are lined by plump osteoblasts. Lamellar bone is extremely rare in ossifying fibroma, but may be formed where woven bone trabeculae are resorbed and replaced.

There are several lesions from which ossifying fibroma must be distinguished, including osteoma, fibrous dysplasia, osteosarcoma, and perhaps even fibrous osteodystrophy, especially in horses. In osteomas, the spaces between trabeculae may contain marrow rather than fibrous connective tissue, and the trabeculae are larger and denser with a much greater proportion of lamellar bone. The bone spicules of fibrous dysplasia are usually more uniform and are not rimmed by osteoblasts. The connective tissue cells of ossifying fibroma lack the pleomorphism and high mitotic index of osteosarcoma and the bone is formed in a more regular and uniform manner. Confusion with fibrous osteodystrophy is unlikely as long as an adequate history accompanies a small bone biopsy. The lesions of fibrous osteodystrophy are bilaterally symmetrical and large osteoclasts are often present amongst the loose connective tissue surrounding trabeculae of woven bone.

The biologic behavior of ossifying fibroma is obscure but *malignant transformation is not known to occur*. Bone is not an inert tissue and it seems reasonable that remodeling of woven trabeculae and replacement by lamellar bone within the tumor could occur. If so, then a maturing ossifying fibroma might eventually resemble an osteoma with hematopoietic cells colonizing spaces between trabeculae of lamellar bone.

Fibrous dysplasia is a rare, fibro-osseous lesion of bone that is thought to be a *developmental abnormality of bone-forming mesenchyme rather than a neoplasm*. It is characterized by smoothly contoured, expanding fibro-osseous lesions involving one or several bones. Although well documented in humans, there are few reliable reports of fibrous dysplasia in animals, but there seems little doubt that the condition does occur in several animal species, including horses, dogs, and domestic cats. As in humans, young animals are most commonly affected.

Some published reports of fibrous dysplasia in animals are questionable, the lesions in some cases appearing more consistent with ossifying fibroma. Furthermore, a description of familial canine polyostotic fibrous dysplasia in three Doberman Pinscher pups most likely represents a polyostotic form of unicameral bone cysts. It is also possible that some cases of fibrous dysplasia have been misdiagnosed as various tumors of bones.

Osteosarcoma

This malignant tumor is the most common primary neoplasm of the appendicular skeleton in dogs and cats. In general, it is a rapidly progressive tumor with early metastasis to the lungs leading to early mortality. Most osteosarcomas arise from within bones, particularly in the metaphyseal regions of long bones, and are referred to as **central osteosarcomas**. Less commonly, osteosarcomas arise in the periosteum or even in extraskeletal tissues. Two types of **peripheral osteosarcoma** may arise in the periosteum. One is referred to as **periosteal osteosarcoma** and may show similar biologic behavior to central osteosarcoma; the other is **parosteal (juxtacortical) osteosarcoma**, which shows greater differentiation, slower growth, and a much better prognosis than central osteosarcoma.

Osteosarcoma accounts for approximately 80% of primary bone tumors in dogs and 70% in cats. In **dogs**, the mean age of occurrence is around 7.5–8 years, but the range is broad and animals less than 2 years of age are sometimes affected. The tumor occurs predominantly in large and medium-sized breeds and has a strong site preference. The appendicular skeleton is affected three to four times as often as the axial skeleton and the forelimbs 1.6–1.8 times as often as the hindlimbs. Most osteosarcomas in the forelimbs involve the *metaphyses of either the distal radius or proximal humerus* (Fig. 1.108A). The *distal femur and proximal tibia* (Fig. 1.108B) are favored sites in the hindlimb. Approximately 50% of osteosarcomas of the axial skeleton occur in bones of the head and 50% in the ribs, vertebrae, and pelvis. Osteosarcomas of the appendicular skeleton occur more often in male dogs than in females, but this sex difference does not appear to apply to tumors of the axial skeleton. In addition to the sites mentioned above, osteosarcomas occasionally occur at sites of chronic irritation and repair, such as those associated with osteomyelitis, bone infarcts, or the presence of an internal fixation device. In such cases, the tumor may originate from the diaphyseal region of long bones, or other locations not normally considered predilection sites for osteosarcoma.

The mean age of osteosarcoma in **cats** is 10.5 years (range 3–18 years) and there is no apparent breed predisposition. Most studies of osteosarcoma in cats involve fewer cases than in dogs and information on predilection sites is less precise. Although the appendicular skeleton appears to be involved more frequently than the axial skeleton, the ratio is less than in dogs and there is no apparent predilection for the forelimbs. Unlike dogs, most osteosarcomas in cats arise in the diaphyses of long bones, rather than the metaphyses.

Osteosarcomas are rare in domestic animals other than dogs and cats, but are reported occasionally in horses, cattle and sheep. In these species, the tumor generally involves bones of the head, particularly the mandible.

The *gross and radiographic appearance of central osteosarcoma varies markedly*, depending on the behavior of the tumor cells and the matrix they produce. Some subtypes are predominantly lytic, some

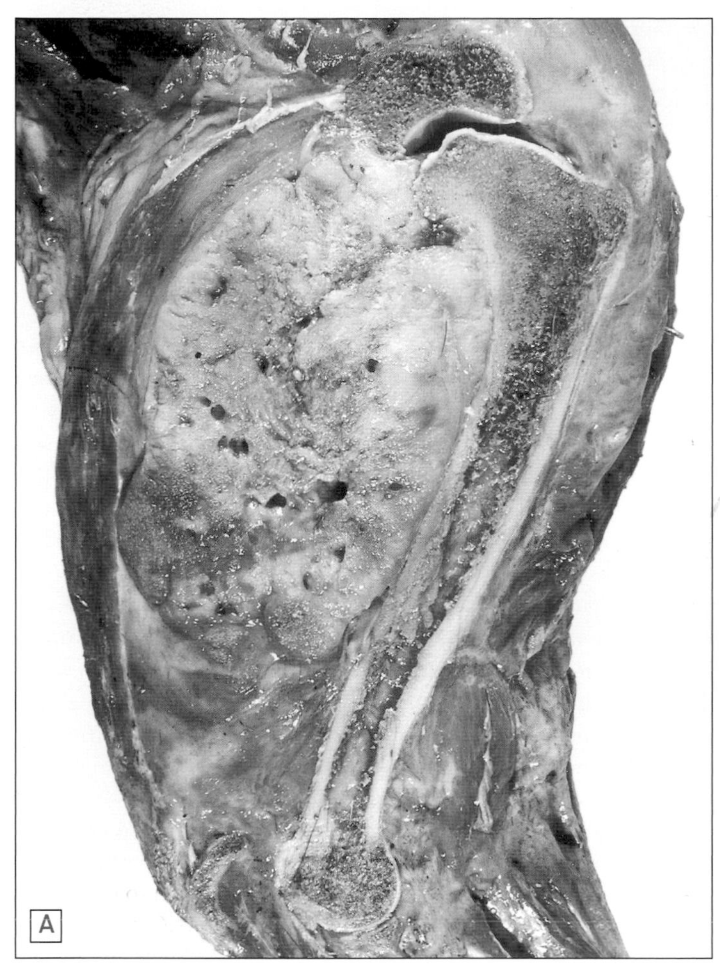

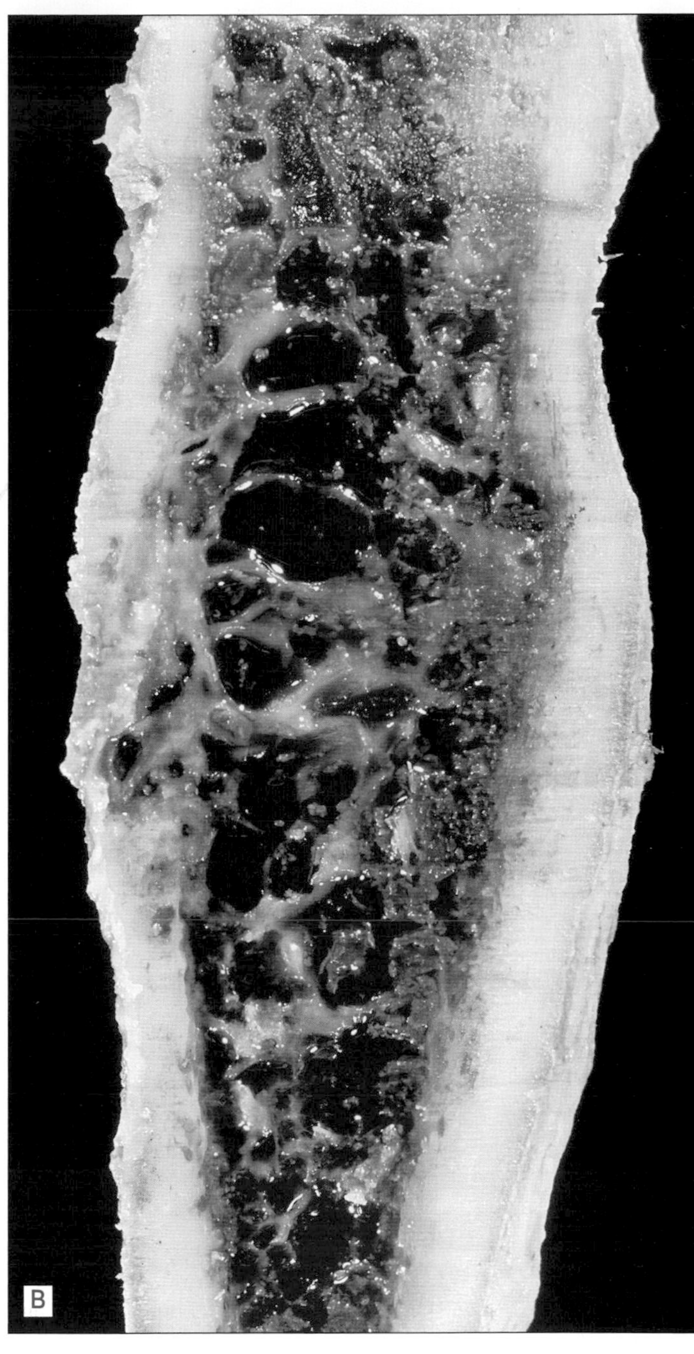

Figure 1.108 A. Compound osteosarcoma originating in the proximal humerus of a dog. **B. Telangiectatic osteosarcoma** in the proximal tibia. Multiple, blood-filled spaces resembling hemangiosarcoma.

are productive, while others comprise a mixture of both destructive and proliferative elements. Assessment of the gross features is greatly enhanced by radiographs of dissected and bisected specimens. Radiolucent or osteolytic tumors are usually hemorrhagic and soft, and often contain light yellow areas of necrosis. Pathological fractures may accompany erosion of cortical bone and osteolytic tumors tend to invade the adjacent soft tissues early in their course. Radiodense tumors are various shades of gray on gross examination and areas of tumor bone and tumor cartilage give a stippled appearance to radiographs and a gritty texture when cut. In compound osteosarcomas, tumor cartilage is sometimes recognizable by its texture and color, and tends to be located at the periphery of the neoplasm. Productive tumors frequently provoke a more marked periosteal reaction than the osteolytic tumors. Osteosarcomas of long bones commonly, perhaps invariably, erode cortical bone but although they tend to invade the epiphysis rather than the diaphysis, they rarely penetrate the adjacent articular cartilage. Telangiectatic osteosarcomas are soft and dark red, and closely resemble hemangiosarcomas grossly.

The *histologic appearance of osteosarcomas varies markedly,* but the production of osteoid and/or tumor bone by malignant osteoblasts is a common factor. The tumor matrix may also contain variable quantities of cartilage and collagen, but *if tumor osteoid is present then the tumor is classified as osteosarcoma.* This reflects the greater malignant potential of malignant osteoblasts than either chondroblasts or fibroblasts. Bone formation also occurs in some chondrosarcomas, but indirectly through endochondral ossification of tumor cartilage, and should not be misinterpreted as tumor bone. Similarly, osseous metaplasia of multipotential mesenchymal cells in tumors of nonosseous origin, such as mammary carcinomas, may create confusion.

Malignant osteoblasts may be spindle-shaped cells resembling fibroblasts or plump, oval or rounded cells with basophilic cytoplasm and eccentric, hyperchromatic nuclei, more closely resembling non-neoplastic osteoblasts. Mitotic figures are often very common. The nature and amount of osteoid is highly variable. In some cases, it consists of hyaline, eosinophilic material arranged in thin strands or narrow ribbons amongst the malignant cells, producing a lace-like pattern (Fig. 1.109A). In others, the osteoid is present as irregular islands or spicules separated by malignant osteoblasts (Fig. 1.109B). Thin strands of osteoid may closely resemble collagenous fibrous tissue and distinguishing the two forms of matrix may be impossible. Both are birefringent, reflecting their collagen content, and reliable differentiation is not possible using histochemical stains. Fibrin in areas of hemorrhage may also be mistaken for osteoid, but is not birefringent. In general, osteoid is less fibrillar than collagen, more amorphous, and often partly or completely surrounds the tumor cells, entrapping them in lacunar spaces.

Formation of endosteal and periosteal new bone is a feature of a variety of inflammatory and neoplastic bone lesions, not just osteosarcoma, and must be differentiated from tumor bone. This may be difficult in small biopsy samples. Distinguishing between osteosarcoma and an early fracture callus presents an even greater challenge. Rapidly proliferating, plump mesenchymal cells surrounding themselves with osteoid are a feature of fracture repair (see Fig. 1.19), especially during the first few days, and may easily be confused with osteosarcoma. Evidence of maturation within the callus is a useful differentiating feature, and the cell population would be expected to show less atypia than most osteosarcomas. Not surprisingly, the histologic appearance may be extremely difficult to interpret in cases where pathological fracture has occurred in association with an osteosarcoma. *Knowledge of the clinical history and radiographic findings are particularly important adjuncts to histology in such cases.*

Multinucleate giant cells with features of osteoclasts are often scattered throughout osteosarcomas, sometimes in sufficient numbers to suggest a diagnosis of giant cell tumor, but demonstration of osteoid production by the tumor cells allows exclusion of the latter option. In rapidly growing osteosarcomas, large areas of coagulation necrosis and hemorrhage are often present, probably due to localized ischemia.

As shown in Table 1.3, osteosarcomas may be subclassified according to the predominant histologic pattern. This scheme is an adaptation of a system developed for use in human medicine and is now well accepted by veterinary pathologists. *Subclassification of osteosarcomas can be justified in that it may lead to the identification of correlations of osteosarcoma subtype with prognosis, and susceptibility to therapy.* For example, fibroblastic osteosarcomas in dogs and human patients have been shown to possess a relatively favorable prognosis, while the prognosis for the telangiectatic form is very poor. However, the exercise is not always straightforward because of the inherent variability present within many osteosarcomas, and the fact that a subdominant pattern may appear to be the most malignant. *Classification into one of the six categories is determined by the predominant pattern in representative sections from the tumor,* but if no single pattern is dominant, the tumor is best categorized as a *combined type osteosarcoma.* In cases where only small fragments of tissue are received for examination, the main aim should be to determine whether the tumor is an osteosarcoma, rather than what subtype it belongs to.

- In **poorly differentiated osteosarcoma**, the tumor cells vary from small cells resembling those of bone marrow stroma, to large, pleomorphic cells of an undifferentiated sarcoma. The only clue that the tumor is an osteosarcoma is the presence of small quantities of *unequivocal tumor osteoid.* These tumors are generally highly aggressive, forming lytic bone lesions, and often are associated with pathological fractures.
- **Osteoblastic osteosarcomas** are recognizable by the presence *of cells with features of anaplastic osteoblasts* throughout much of the tumor (Fig. 1.109C). The tumor cells have hyperchromatic, often eccentric nuclei and variable quantities of basophilic cytoplasm. The cell borders are often angular and there may be a pale Golgi zone adjacent to the nucleus. Osteoblastic osteosarcomas may be *further subclassified into nonproductive and productive osteosarcomas* depending on the quantity of tumor bone produced. Moderately productive osteoblastic osteosarcoma (Fig. 1.109A, B) is the most common subtype of osteosarcoma in dogs. Radiographically, there is a mixed pattern of destruction and production. In some cases with abundant tumor bone formation, differentiation of tumor bone from reactive bone may be difficult or impossible.
- In **chondroblastic osteosarcomas**, *the malignant mesenchymal cells directly produce both osteoid and chondroid matrices.* Although the two components are usually intermixed, they remain separate in some tumors and small biopsy specimens may lead to an incorrect diagnosis of chondrosarcoma.
- **Fibroblastic osteosarcomas** consist of a population of *spindle cells* similar to those of fibrosarcoma, within which there is evidence of *osteoid or bone formation by tumor cells.* The spicules of bone may be sparse, especially in early lesions, and it is not uncommon for such tumors to initially be diagnosed as fibrosarcomas then later reclassified as osteosarcoma following examination of further biopsies. In one study, the prognosis for dogs with fibroblastic osteosarcoma was more favorable than for other subtypes.
- **Telangiectatic osteosarcoma** is an *aggressive, osteolytic tumor* consisting of a mixture of solid areas and blood-filled spaces, grossly and radiographically resembling hemangiosarcoma (Fig. 1.108B). Histologically, telangiectatic osteosarcoma can be *differentiated from hemangiosarcoma by the presence of occasional spicules of osteoid among pleomorphic, malignant mesenchymal cells* (Fig. 1.110), although a careful search is often required in order to detect osteoid. Furthermore, the blood-filled spaces present throughout the tumor are lined by tumor cells, not endothelium. Metastases of telangiectatic osteosarcomas generally resemble the primary tumor, containing many cystic spaces filled with blood. In human patients and dogs, *this subtype is associated with a less favorable prognosis than all other forms of osteosarcoma.*
- **Giant cell osteosarcomas** resemble nonproductive osteoblastic osteosarcoma histologically, but possess areas in which tumor giant cells predominate and must be differentiated from malignant giant cell tumors of bone.

Although cytology is usually less reliable than histology in the diagnosis of mesenchymal tumors, central osteosarcomas can often be diagnosed with confidence on examination of *fine-needle aspiration biopsies or imprints* prepared from tissue biopsy samples. Cytological preparations from osteosarcomas are usually more cellular than aspirates or imprints from soft tissue sarcomas, and the cells may have characteristic features of malignant osteoblasts. In many cases,

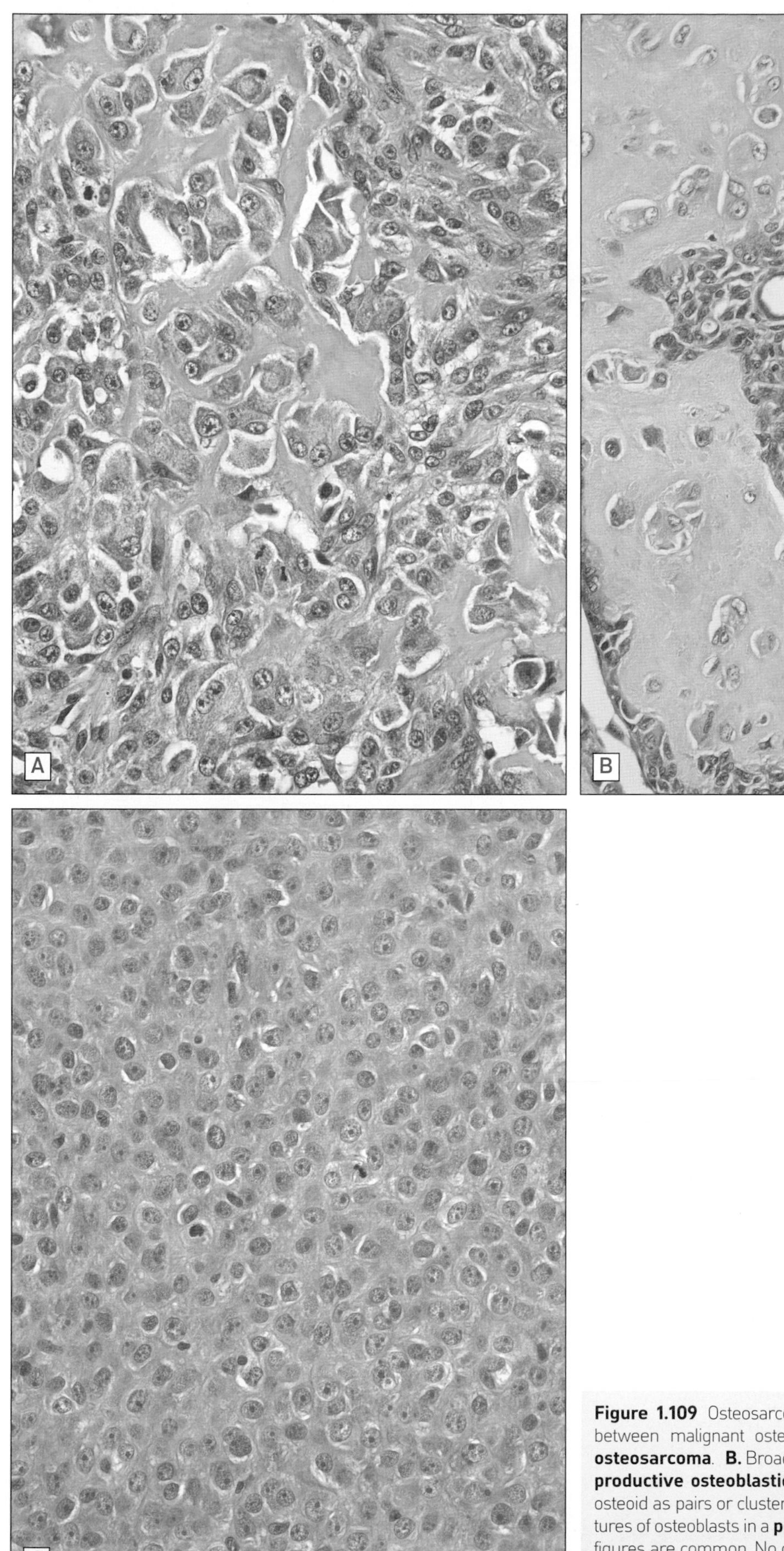

Figure 1.109 Osteosarcoma, histological patterns. **A.** Lacy strands of osteoid between malignant osteoblasts in a **moderately productive osteoblastic osteosarcoma**. **B.** Broad lakes of osteoid separated by malignant osteoblasts in a **productive osteoblastic osteosarcoma**. Many tumor cells are trapped in the osteoid as pairs or clusters. **C.** Sheets of anaplastic mesenchymal cells with features of osteoblasts in a **poorly productive osteoblastic osteosarcoma**. Mitotic figures are common. No osteoid is apparent in this field but small quantities were detected elsewhere in the tumor.

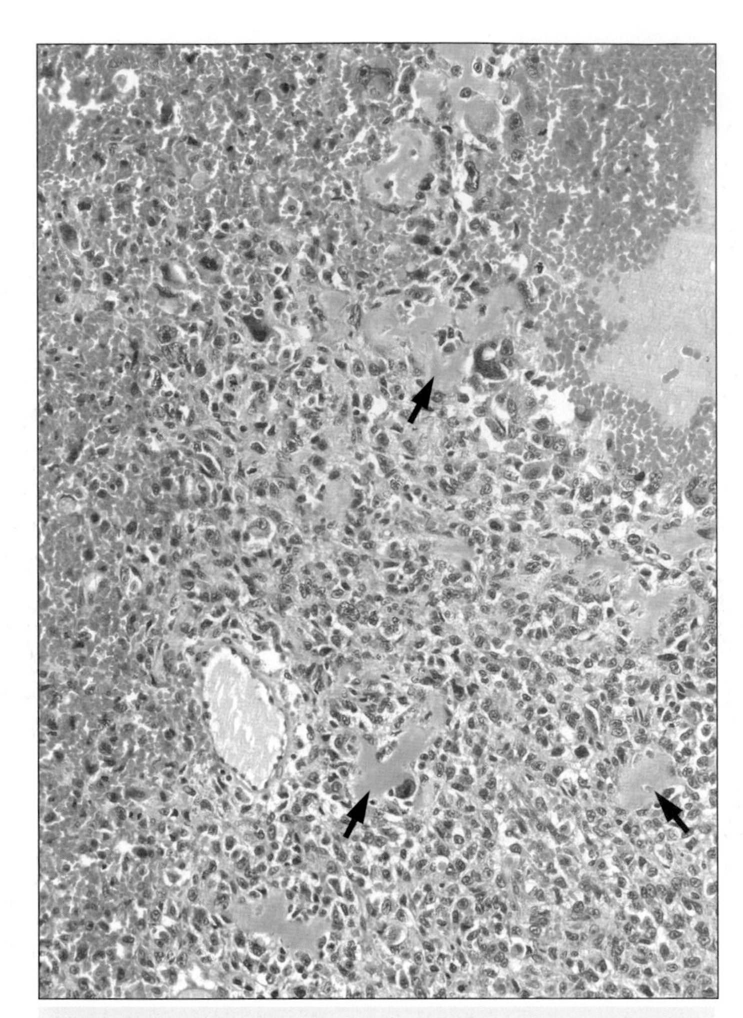

Figure 1.110 Telangiectatic osteosarcoma, dog. Malignant mesenchymal cells forming spicules of matrix resembling osteoid (arrows) and closely associated with large, blood-filled spaces.

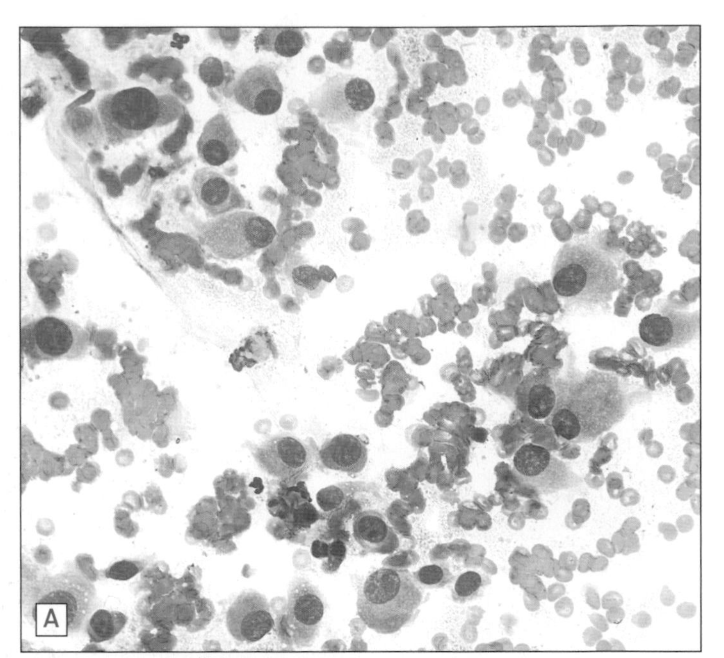

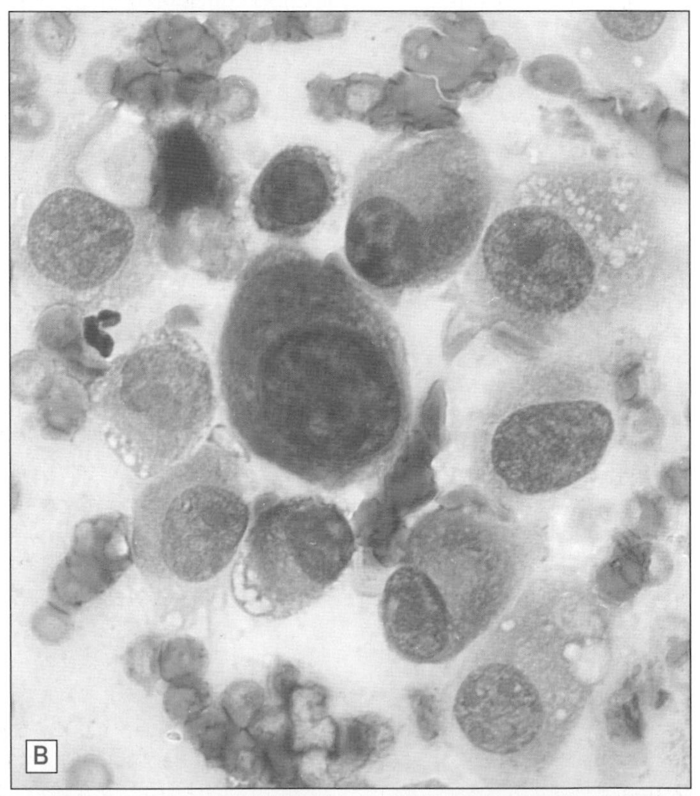

Figure 1.111 Cytological appearance of **osteosarcoma**. **A.** Moderate numbers of oval to pyriform-shaped cells with eccentric nuclei, basophilic cytoplasm and pale Golgi zone adjacent to the nucleus of some cells. There is moderate variation in nuclear size and N:C ratio. **B.** Higher-power view of malignant osteoblasts including one cell with a very large, hyperchromatic nucleus and deeply basophilic cytoplasm.

the cytological characteristics, together with clinical history and radiography, will be sufficient to allow a definitive diagnosis of osteosarcoma, but malignancy cannot be excluded on the basis of cytology as the sample may not be sufficiently representative of the lesion. Since most osteosarcomas originate from within the medullary cavity, shallow aspirates may be largely acellular or, at best, just contain a small number of reactive osteoblasts (see Fig. 1.2). Furthermore, some productive subtypes of osteosarcoma with extensive tumor bone formation may not yield significant numbers of tumor cells to cytological preparations and aspirates from telangiectatic osteosarcomas may be too heavily contaminated with blood to be of value. Even in cases where a cytological diagnosis of osteosarcoma can be made, classification of the tumor into one of the subtypes listed above is not possible.

Malignant osteoblasts may be present individually or in clusters in cytological preparations and are sometimes closely associated with brightly eosinophilic strands or islands of *osteoid*. They vary from round or oval to plump, fusiform cells, often with an eccentric nucleus and deeply basophilic cytoplasm (Fig. 1.111A, B). The cytoplasm may have a pale Golgi zone adjacent to the nucleus and, in some cases, there are variable numbers of *small, clear, intracytoplasmic vacuoles and/or fine pink granules*. Similar pink granules may also be present in tumor cells from chondrosarcomas or occasionally fibrosarcomas. In anaplastic osteosarcomas, there may be marked anisokaryosis, multiple large, irregular-shaped nucleoli and variable nuclear to cytoplasmic ratio. Mitotic figures are common and may be abnormal. In contrast, well-differentiated osteosarcomas may consist largely of relatively uniform-sized cells with many features of reactive

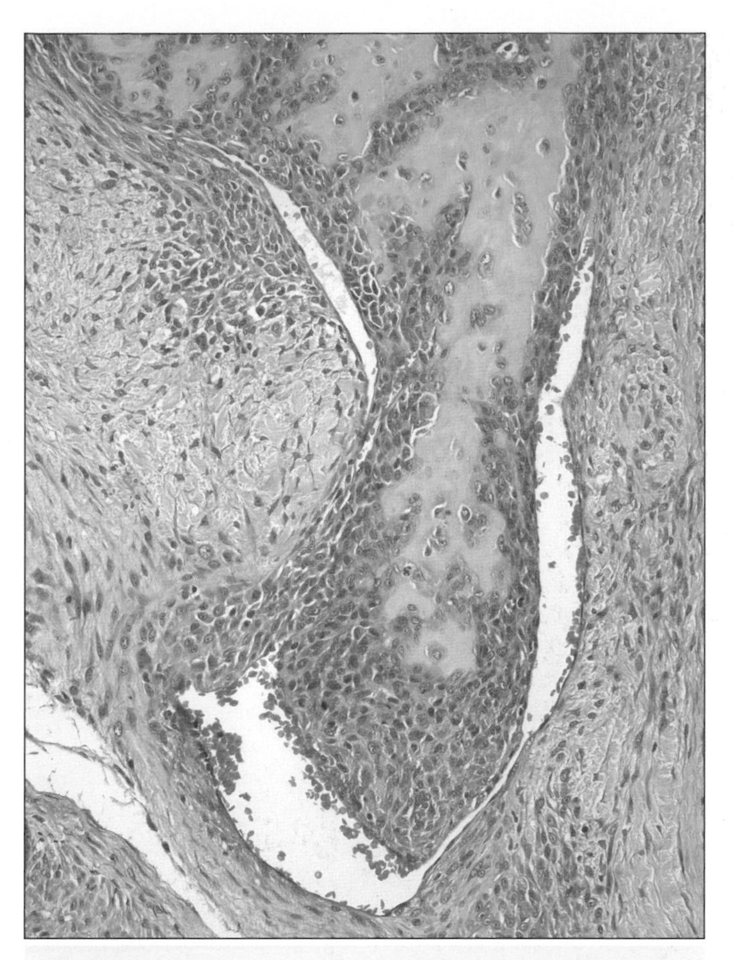

Figure 1.112 Tumor tissue containing osteoid invading a large vein at the margin of an **osteosarcoma**.

osteoblasts. A similar population of reactive osteoblasts associated with strands of osteoid may be harvested from an early fracture callus, highlighting the importance of clinical history and knowledge of the radiographic appearance of the lesion. *Unless the characteristics of malignancy are unequivocal, histological examination is recommended.*

Central osteosarcoma is perhaps the most malignant group of tumors of animals, at least in dogs. *The prognosis for all subtypes is very poor.* Hematogenous metastasis to the lungs commonly occurs early in the disease. Vascular invasion can sometimes be detected at the tumor margins (Fig. 1.112). Pulmonary metastases are detected radiographically in approximately 10% of canine appendicular and axial osteosarcomas at the time of initial diagnosis and it is likely that most dogs with osteosarcoma will eventually develop metastases if their lives are prolonged by surgery or other forms of treatment. In one study, dogs with telangiectatic osteosarcoma had a 100% metastatic rate. Hematogenous metastasis to other organs, including the skeleton, also occurs but osteosarcomas seldom spread to regional lymph nodes. The median survival time for dogs with appendicular skeletal osteosarcomas is only 14–19 weeks. Survival time is only marginally better (22 weeks) in dogs with osteosarcomas of the axial skeleton, although osteosarcomas of the mandible, and those with osteoblastic tumors of paranasal sinuses and calvaria generally have a better prognosis.

The incidence of *metastasis in cats* with central osteosarcoma is considerably less than in dogs and the prognosis is therefore more favorable. A median survival time of 49.2 months has been observed in cats with appendicular osteosarcoma following treatment by amputation, but the number of animals in most studies of feline osteosarcoma has been small.

Periosteal and parosteal (juxtacortical) osteosarcoma are referred to as **peripheral osteosarcomas** because of their origin on or near the surface of bones. Two types of **periosteal osteosarcoma** have been recognized in dogs. One is a highly aggressive tumor with similar histologic features and biologic behavior as central osteosarcoma, the other being more differentiated and with a more favorable prognosis. Too few cases of periosteal osteosarcomas have been reported in dogs and other domestic animals to provide reliable data on the age, sex, and site incidence. It is possible that the more aggressive forms of periosteal osteosarcoma in dogs are actually central osteosarcomas arising from the outer metaphyseal regions of a long bone and adopting an eccentric growth pattern.

Parosteal osteosarcomas also arise in the periosteal connective tissue but have a characteristic clinical behavior and histologic pattern. These tumors are reported in dogs, cats, and a horse and follow a longer clinical course than central osteosarcomas. Most cases are presented as a firm, slowly enlarging mass on the surface of a bone. Radiographically, the tumor has an evenly contoured margin and the underlying cortex is generally intact. This is in contrast to osteochondroma, where the marrow cavity of the tumor is continuous with that of the adjacent bone. In histological sections, parosteal osteosarcoma consists of *broad trabeculae of well-differentiated bone separated by moderately cellular fibrous connective tissue showing some pleomorphism, but no convincing evidence of malignancy* (Fig. 1.113). Differentiation from reactive bone may present a significant challenge. Metastasis of parosteal osteosarcoma to the lungs occurs late, if at all.

Osteosarcomas occasionally arise in soft tissues of dogs and cats, in the absence of a primary bone lesion. These **extraskeletal osteosarcomas** occur most often in the *mammary gland*, but may also arise in the gastrointestinal tract, subcutaneous tissues, spleen, urinary tract, liver, skin, muscle, eye, and thyroid gland. They also arise in the esophagus in association with *Spirocerca lupi* infestation. In general, extraskeletal osteosarcomas occur in older dogs than skeletal osteosarcomas (mean age 10.6–11.5 years) and show no apparent predilection for large breeds. Although distant metastases are common, the lungs are involved less often than in skeletal osteosarcomas, and death is usually due to either local recurrence or euthanasia at the time of diagnosis. The mean survival time is reported to be lower than for skeletal osteosarcomas, in part due to the later detection of intra-abdominal tumors and limited surgical options for tumors at some sites. Osteosarcoma of the mammary gland of bitches should not be confused with the *more common, nonneoplastic, osseous metaplasia* that occurs in association with mammary carcinomas.

Extraskeletal osteosarcoma appears to be less common in cats than in dogs, but has been reported in the eye following ocular trauma, and in the mammary area of a 12-year-old cat. In the latter case, the tumor recurred following surgical removal and widespread lung metastases were detected at necropsy.

Bibliography

Bitetto WV, et al. Osteosarcoma in cats: 22 cases (1974–1984). J Am Vet Med Assoc 1987;190:91–93.

Dubielzig RR, et al. Bone sarcomas associated with multifocal medullary bone infarction in dogs. J Am Vet Med Assoc 1981;179:64–68.

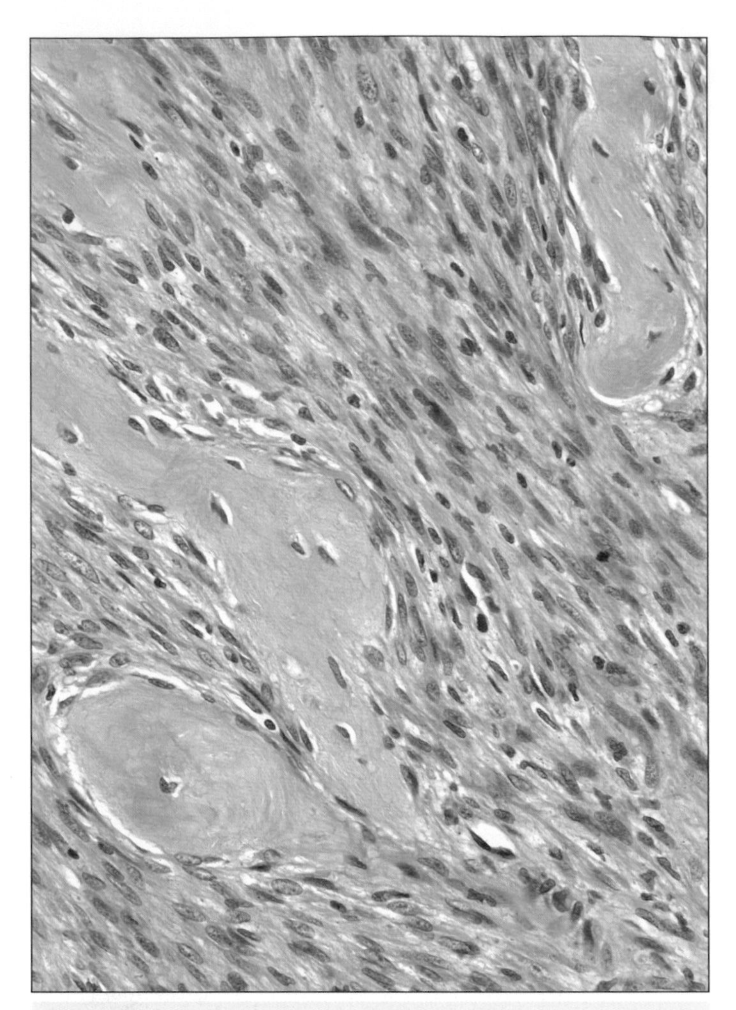

Figure 1.113 Parosteal osteosarcoma, dog. Broad, disoriented, bony trabeculae separated by uniformly cellular tissue resembling immature fibrous tissue.

Easton CB. Extraskeletal osteosarcoma in a cat. J Am Anim Hosp Assoc 1994;30:59–61.

Gleiser CA, et al. Telangiectatic osteosarcoma in the dog. Vet Pathol 1981;18:396–398.

Hammer AS, et al. Prognostic factors in dogs with osteosarcomas of the flat or irregular bones. J Am Anim Hosp Assoc 1995;31:321–326.

Kuntz CA, et al. Extraskeletal osteosarcomas in dogs: 14 cases. J Am Anim Hosp Assoc 1998;34:26–30.

Lagenbach A, et al. Extraskeletal osteosarcoma in dogs: a retrospective study of 169 cases (1986–1996). J Am Anim Hosp Assoc 1998;34:113–120.

Livesey MA, et al. Epistaxis in a thoroughbred weanling caused by fibrous dysplasia. Equine Vet J 1984;16:144–146.

Miller WW, Boosinger TR. Intraocular osteosarcoma in a cat. J Am Anim Hosp Assoc 1987;23:317–320.

Morse CC, et al. Equine juvenile mandibular ossifying fibroma. Vet Pathol 1988;24:415–421.

Richardson DW, et al. Rostral mandibulectomy in five horses. J Am Vet Med Assoc 1991;199:1179–1182.

Rosendal S. Osteoma in the oral cavity in a pig (*Sus scrofa*). Vet Pathol 1979;16:488–490.

Slayter MV, et al. Histological Classification of Bone and Joint Tumors of Domestic Animals. W.H.O. Second Series vol 1. Armed Forces Institute of Pathology, American Registry of Pathology: Washington DC, 1994.

Spodnick GJ, et al. Prognosis for dogs with appendicular osteosarcoma treated by amputation alone: 162 cases (1978–1988). J Am Vet Med Assoc 1992;200:995–999.

Stevenson S, et al. Fracture-associated sarcoma in the dog. J Am Vet Med Assoc 1982;180: 1189–1196.

Thompson KG, Pool RR. Tumors of bones. In: Meuten DJ, ed. Tumors in Domestic Animals. 5th ed. Ch 5. Ames, IA: Iowa State University Press, 2002:245–317.

Wilson RB. Monostotic fibrous dysplasia in a dog. Vet Pathol 1989;26:449–450.

Cartilage-forming tumors

Tumors consisting entirely or predominantly of cartilage are *uncommon* in the skeleton of domestic animals. They are diagnosed most frequently in dogs, where approximately 10% of skeletal tumors are cartilaginous, and in sheep, where chondromas comprise a relatively high proportion of skeletal tumors. Cartilaginous tumors often contain areas of bone formed by endochondral ossification of tumor cartilage. This should not be mistaken for the tumor bone formed directly from neoplastic mesenchymal cells in osteosarcoma. Repairing fractures also contain cartilage and bone in various proportions at different stages of maturity and could be confused with cartilage- or bone-forming tumors.

Extra-skeletal tumors containing cartilage also occur, particularly those arising as a component of lipomatous soft tissue masses (chondrolipomas). Cartilaginous tissue is also present and may become dominant in mixed tumors of mammary and salivary gland origin.

Chondroma

A chondroma is a benign neoplasm of cartilage but, in veterinary medicine, the term has often been used loosely to include benign proliferations of cartilage in several extraskeletal tissues. Primary chondromas of bone are separable into *enchondromas*, which originate within the medullary cavity of a bone and *ecchondromas*, which arise from cartilage elsewhere in the skeleton. Both forms are rare in animals. Enchondromas are sometimes polyostotic, in which case the syndrome is referred to as *enchondromatosis*. It is likely that many tumors diagnosed as chondromas in animals are in fact osteochondromas or low-grade chondrosarcomas, especially in cases where the pathologist is not provided with an adequate history or access to radiographs of the lesion.

Chondromas occur rarely in dogs, cats, and cattle, and although considered to be more common than other skeletal tumors in sheep, they are infrequently diagnosed in this species. The tumors are typically firm to hard, smooth or nodular, roughly spherical masses with a relatively thin fibrous capsule. They involve flat bones and ribs more commonly than long bones. On cut surface, a lobular pattern may be evident due to dissection of the blue-white cartilage by fibrous septa. Areas of mineralization or ossification appear as chalk-white stippling. Myxomatous tissue, which occurs in some chondromas, has a gelatinous texture grossly and seems prone to hemorrhage and necrosis.

Histologically these benign tumors consist of irregular lobules of hyaline cartilage with cells that are, by definition, quite regular in size and appearance and typically chondrocytic. This is especially true of enchondromas. The matrix is usually more fibrous than that of normal hyaline cartilage. Foci of endochondral ossification and mineralization may be present, and lobules of myxomatous tissue sometimes develop. Differentiation between chondroma and low-grade chondrosarcoma is difficult on the basis of histopathology and may require the assessment of biological behavior in sequential radiographs.

Chondromas expand slowly, and a rapid change in size may indicate malignant transformation. Expanding tumors within the medullary cavity cause bone deformation and may predispose to fracture.

Osteochondroma

An osteochondroma is a benign, cartilage-capped tumor-like exostosis arising from the surface of an endochondral bone adjacent to a physis or subarticular growth cartilage. The tumor may be monostotic or polyostotic, in which case the terms **multiple cartilaginous exostosis** or **osteochondromatosis** are often used. In **humans, dogs**, and **horses**, the disease is inherited as an autosomal dominant trait and would be more appropriately classified as a *skeletal dysplasia* than a neoplasm, but is included here for convenience.

In dogs, the lesions usually are not present at birth but arise in young animals and continue to enlarge until the skeleton matures. In affected horses, the lesions are often present at birth and tend to be bilaterally symmetrical. During the phase of expansion, the outgrowths consist of a thin outer cap of hyaline cartilage resembling poorly organized growth plate, adjacent to the epiphyseal plate, which undergoes endochondral ossification from its deep surface (Fig. 1.114A). *Trabecular bone and bone marrow within the mass are continuous with the marrow cavity of the parent bone. This is a useful diagnostic feature in the differentiation of osteochondromas from some other hyperplastic or neoplastic bony masses.* Once bone growth ceases, the cartilage cap is replaced by bone. The trabecular bone in osteochondromas is not remodeled and the mineralized cartilage cores persist. *The nature of the genetic defect in osteochondroma is not known but is suspected to involve the perichondrial ring.* Peripheral nodules of physeal cartilage are pinched off and grow laterally, the lesions eventually finishing up in the metaphyseal region some distance from the original growth plate.

The lesions of osteochondroma are variable in their location but common sites in dogs and horses are the metaphyses of long bones, the pelvis, ribs, scapula, and vertebrae. Although many cases are merely of esthetic rather than clinical significance, lesions in some locations interfere with the action of ligaments or tendons and exostoses derived from vertebrae sometimes protrude into the spinal canal, resulting in spinal cord compression (Fig. 1.114B). Furthermore, *they may undergo malignant transformation into chondrosarcoma or osteosarcoma.* From 5 to 25% of human patients with the syndrome eventually develop chondrosarcoma, and similar cases have occurred in dogs and horses. In one series of eight cases of multiple cartilaginous exostoses in dogs, three developed chondrosarcoma, suggesting that the risk of malignant transformation in affected dogs is relatively high.

Osteochondromatosis in **cats** occurs in mature animals and tends to involve flat bones, including bones derived from intramembranous ossification. Long bones are seldom affected. The lesions in cats appear to arise as *multifocal areas of osteocartilaginous hyperplasia in the periosteum and undergo progressive enlargement.* Their behavior is therefore more consistent with that of a true tumor, unlike that of osteochondromas in dogs and horses. Furthermore, the lesions in cats are usually not continuous with the marrow cavity of the adjacent bone. It seems likely that this syndrome in cats is not analogous to that in the other species and a link with *Feline leukemia virus* has been made, and virus particles identified within lesions. Malignant transformation of feline osteochondroma is also reported.

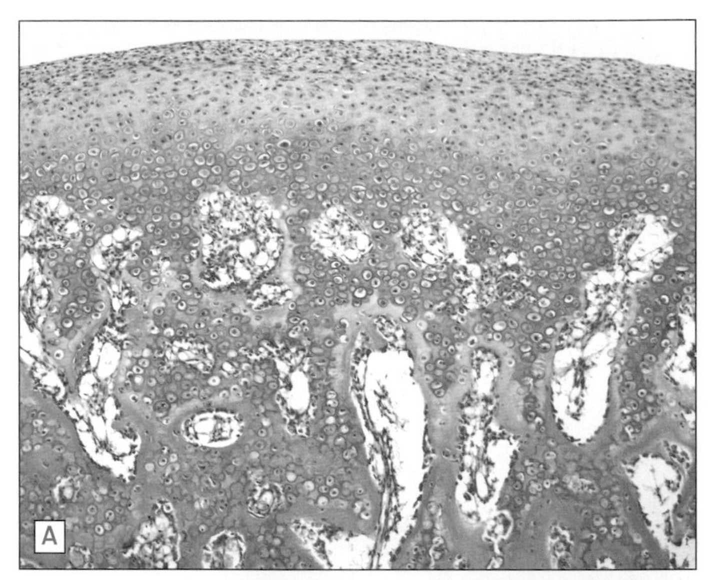

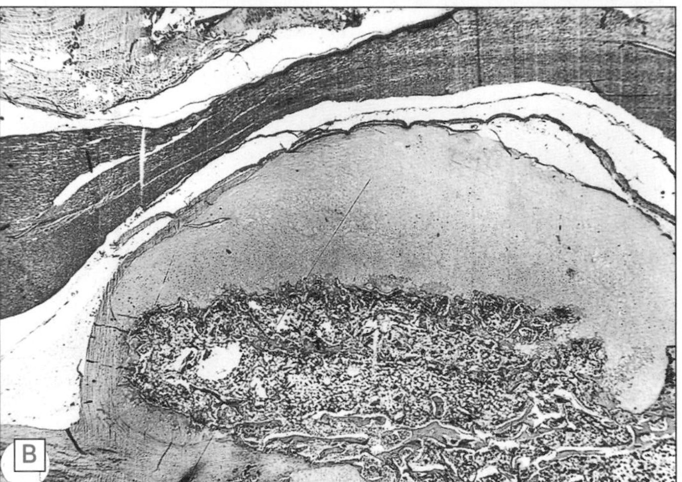

Figure 1.114 Osteochondroma, dog. **A.** Outer layer of proliferating chondrocytes differentiating into disorganized hyaline cartilage with randomly distributed hypertrophic chondrocytes. Endochondral ossification is occurring at the deep surface of the cartilage cap. **B.** Compression of spinal cord by osteochondroma originating from vertebra.

Multilobular tumor of bone

Multilobular tumor of bone is a slow-growing but locally aggressive and potentially malignant tumor, occurring most often in the skull of dogs, but occasionally in the cat and horse. Many alternative terms have been proposed for the tumor, including chondroma rodens, cartilage analogue of fibromatosis, calcifying aponeurotic fibroma, multilobular chondroma or osteoma, and multilobular osteochondrosarcoma. In dogs, it is primarily a disease of middle-aged to older animals, occurring most often in medium or large breeds, but rarely in giant breeds. In one study of 39 cases, the median age was 8 years (range 4–17 years) and the median weight was 29 kg, although four dogs weighed less than 25 kg. Three cases have been recorded in cats, varying in age from 9 months to 8 years, and there is one report in a 12-year-old Thoroughbred mare.

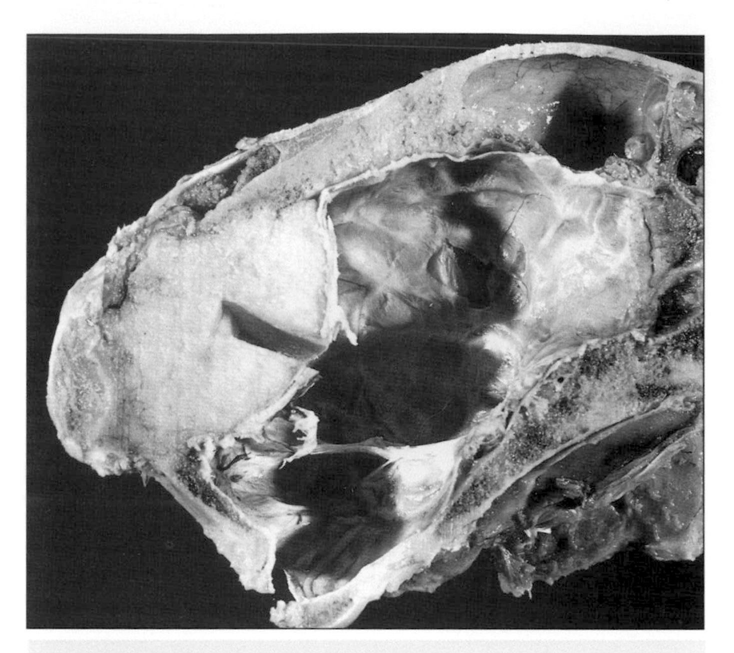

Figure 1.115 Multilobular tumor of bone impinging on the brain of a dog.

The tumor is usually present as a *firm, immovable mass on the surface of skull bones* and clinical signs relate to the compression and disturbance of function in adjacent structures. The swelling apparent from the skull surface may provide little indication of the degree to which the tumor impinges on adjacent organs, such as the brain (Fig. 1.115). Multiple small gritty foci are usually evident grossly on cut surface and a stippled appearance may be observed in radiographs of the tumor.

Histologically, the multilobular tumor of bone has a characteristic pattern consisting of multiple circular, oval or irregular-shaped nodules of cartilaginous, osseous, or osteocartilaginous tissue separated by narrow fibrovascular septa (Fig. 1.116A, B). In certain areas of some tumors, broad, ill-defined zones of mesenchymal tissue merge with the nodules. The cartilaginous nodules usually are surrounded by spindle-shaped septal cells, contiguous with the plump oval nuclei of the neoplastic chondrocytes in the center of each lobule. The tumor cells produce a pale, eosinophilic or faintly basophilic matrix, which mineralizes at the center of the lobule. Resorption of mineralized cartilage and endochondral bone formation sometimes occurs and occasionally, osteoclastic remodeling of bone develops. In these nodules, the matrix-producing cells are unequivocally chondrocytic in appearance. In bony nodules, the mesenchymal cells produce a matrix that

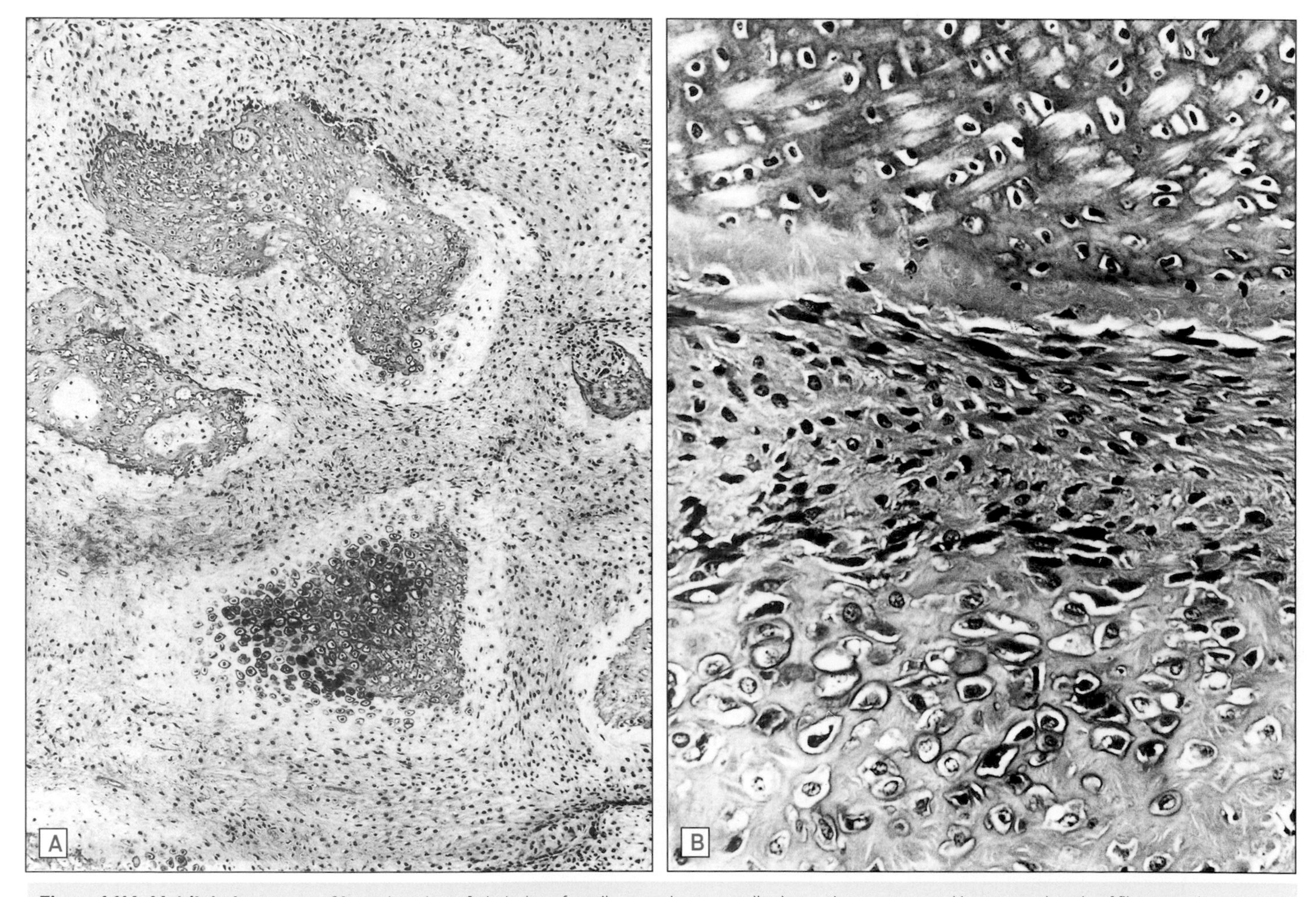

Figure 1.116 Multilobular tumor of bone in a dog. **A.** Lobules of cartilage and osteocartilaginous tissue separated by narrow bands of fibrovascular stroma. **B.** Higher-power view showing adjacent lobules of neoplastic chondroid tissue and intermediate stroma.

ossifies rather than mineralizes. In some tumors, the bone is produced by angular osteoblasts with abundant basophilic cytoplasm but in others, oval cells of indeterminate type produce a tissue reminiscent of chondroid bone. The mineralization process tends to progress centrifugally to involve the entire nodule, and the septal tissue then consists of dense collagen. In these areas, the tumor is extremely hard. Osseous and cartilaginous tissue may be present in the same nodule and some tumors contain both osseous and cartilaginous nodules. Although the nodular pattern predominates, resorption of the hard tissues does occur and nodules may be replaced by dense connective tissue containing areas of cartilaginous metaplasia.

Surgical removal is often difficult because of the location of these tumors and local recurrence occurs in about 50% of cases. Malignant transformation often occurs in tumors that are long-standing or recurrent. Indicators of malignancy include mitotic activity, loss of the orderly lobular architecture, necrosis, hemorrhage, and overgrowth of one of the mesenchymal elements. The characteristic appearance of multilobular tumors is retained in metastases.

Chondrosarcoma

Chondrosarcomas are malignant mesenchymal tumors in which the neoplastic cells produce variable quantities of cartilaginous or fibrillar matrix, but not osteoid. Although bone may be present in chondrosarcomas, it forms by endochondral ossification of tumor cartilage, rather than being produced directly by malignant mesenchymal cells.

Primary chondrosarcomas are those that arise from either within a bone (central or medullary chondrosarcoma) or from the periosteal surface (peripheral chondrosarcoma), the former being the most common in animals. The term *secondary chondrosarcoma* refers to those that develop by malignant transformation of cartilage in an osteochondroma.

Chondrosarcoma is *reported most frequently in the dog*, where it accounts for approximately 10% of primary tumors of bones and is second only to osteosarcoma in incidence. In most other domestic species, chondrosarcoma is a relatively rare tumor and too few cases are reported to provide reliable information on its clinicopathological features. In sheep, chondrosarcoma is considered to occur more frequently than osteosarcoma, but it remains a rare tumor in this species.

In dogs, chondrosarcoma occurs most often in medium to large breeds, particularly Boxers, German Shepherds, Golden Retrievers and various mixed breeds, but is rare in small and giant breeds. Although a broad age range is reported, the tumor is *most common in middle-aged to older dogs*, the mean age of affected animals varying from 5.9 to 8.7 years. No sex predilection is recognized. There are fewer data on the age incidence of chondrosarcoma in cats, but in one review, a mean age of 8.8 years was reported.

In all species, chondrosarcomas *involve flat bones more often than long bones*. The ribs, turbinates, and pelvis are common sites in dogs, although nasal chondrosarcomas are rare in Boxers. Chondrosarcomas may also occur in the appendicular skeleton of dogs, including, but not restricted to, sites of predilection for osteosarcomas. In cats, chondrosarcomas are reported in both flat bones (especially the scapula) and long bones, but in this species, the published data are inadequate to draw reliable conclusions regarding site predilection. In sheep, the cartilages of the sternocostal complex were the most common site for chondrosarcoma in one survey, followed by the scapula and tuber coxae. In cattle and horses, chondrosarcomas are found most often on flat bones, but long bones are occasionally affected.

Grossly, central chondrosarcomas are firm or hard and may consist of either several large lobules resembling hyaline cartilage or multiple small, contiguous nodules of translucent, blue-white or pink tissue. In some tumors, especially those in the nasal cavity, there are soft, mucoid areas, and in others, there are chalky white foci of mineralization or ossification. Chondrosarcomas *tend to grow expansively* and have a smooth surface and a capsule that merges with surrounding fibrous tissue. The more highly malignant tumors may contain areas of necrosis and hemorrhage. Nasal chondrosarcomas tend to destroy turbinates, fill the nasal cavity (Fig. 1.117A, B) and may either spread into adjacent sinuses or penetrate overlying bone and infiltrate adjacent soft tissues. When in long bones, chondrosarcomas may produce lytic lesions similar to osteosarcomas. Periosteal chondrosarcomas are less common in animals than central chondrosarcomas and usually occur as slow-growing, nodular masses on the surface of flat bones in older dogs and cats.

Histologically, well-differentiated chondrosarcomas show few indications of malignancy and closely resemble benign tumors of cartilage (Fig. 1.118A). Endochondral ossification of tumor cartilage may be present and should not be mistaken for the formation of tumor bone. *Knowledge of the clinical and radiographic features is often essential to accurate classification of cartilaginous tumors.* Fortunately for the veterinary pathologist, most chondrosarcomas in animals are well advanced before the owner seeks veterinary advice and biopsy samples are collected. In fact, the challenge may be to decide whether a malignant mesenchymal tumor involving bone is a chondrosarcoma, osteosarcoma, or some other sarcoma of bone. Such a decision is important, bearing in mind the differences in prognosis. In some chondrosarcomas, the matrix becomes fibrillar and hyalinized, resembling osteoid, and differentiation from osteosarcoma may be very difficult, especially in small biopsy samples. Chondrosarcomas in the sinonasal region of dogs are often characterized by nodules of variously differentiated chondroid tissue forming within poorly differentiated mesenchymal elements (Fig. 1.117C, D).

Microscopic features of malignancy in central chondrosarcomas include the presence of many tumor cells with plump nuclei and prominent nucleoli, binucleate tumor cells, and large chondrocytes with single or multiple nuclei (Fig. 1.118A, B). Mitotic figures are seldom present in well-differentiated chondrosarcomas and even a single mitotic figure strongly supports a diagnosis of malignancy in this tumor. In poorly differentiated, more malignant chondrosarcomas, mitotic figures may be relatively common (Fig. 1.119).

Fine-needle aspiration biopsies from chondrosarcomas usually contain fewer cells than osteosarcomas but, on low-power examination, *lakes of bright pink chondroid matrix* may be evident (Fig. 1.120). The tumor cells are similar to those from osteosarcomas, varying from round to fusiform, possessing large, hyperchromatic nuclei and basophilic cytoplasm, which sometimes contains fine pink granules. Anisokaryosis is generally a prominent feature and there may be multinucleate tumor cells. Although a presumptive diagnosis of chondrosarcoma may be possible in cytologic specimens, *confirmation requires histopathology*. Malignant chondroblasts and osteoblasts have too many features in common to allow reliable differentiation cytologically, and some osteosarcomas have extensive chondroid matrix.

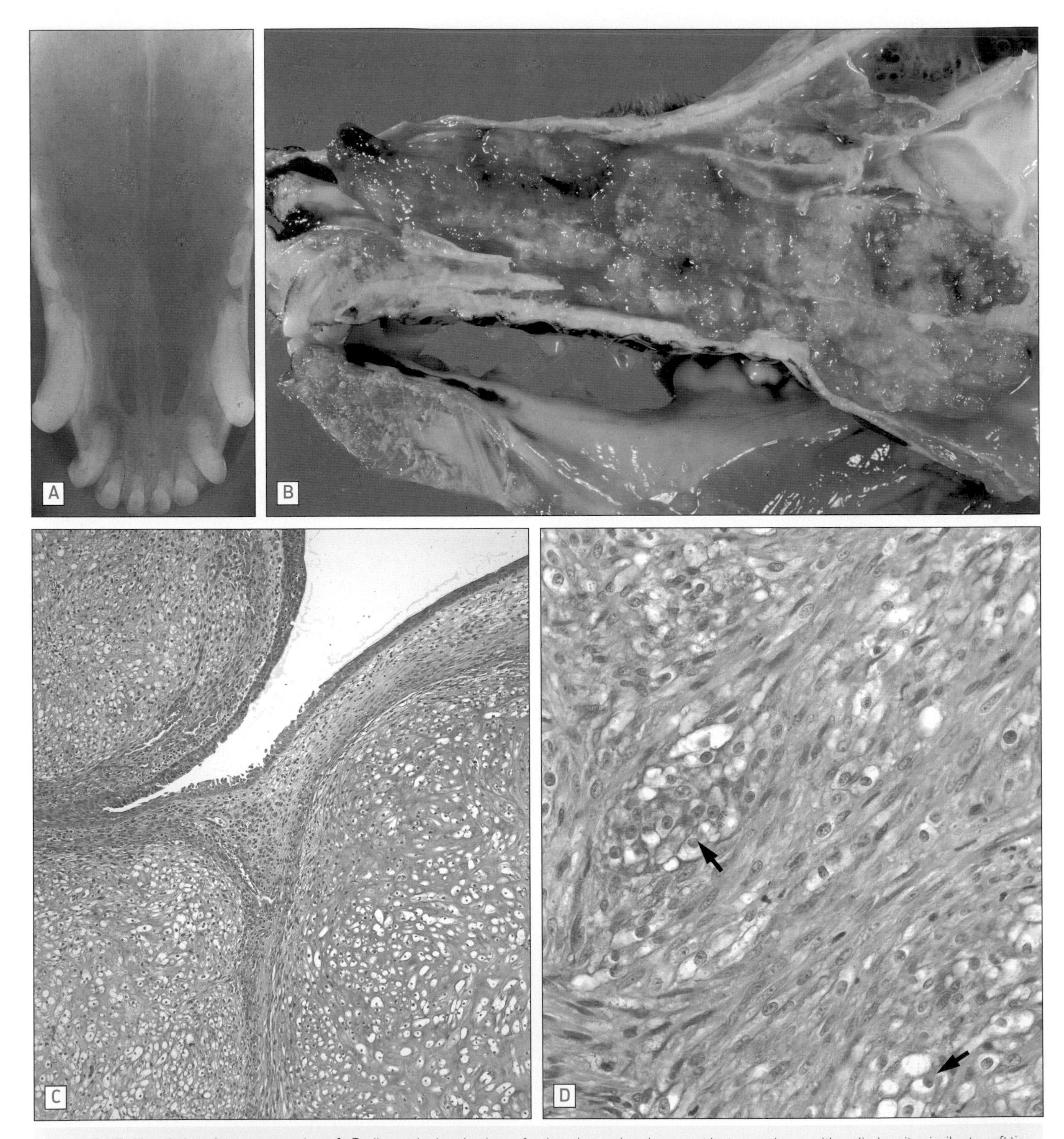

Figure 1.117 Nasal chondrosarcoma, dog. **A.** Radiograph showing loss of trabeculae and replacement by tumor tissue with radiodensity similar to soft tissue. **B.** Sagittal section through the skull of the same dog. Nodules of tumor tissue resembling hyaline cartilage fill the nasal cavity and extend into the nasopharynx. The tumor is eroding into the presphenoid bone, cribriform plate, and hard palate. **C.** Nodules of relatively well-differentiated hyaline cartilage beneath the nasal mucosa bulge into the attenuated lumen of the nasal cavity. **D.** Higher-power view of the same tumor, showing areas of chondroid differentiation (arrows) closely associated with poorly differentiated mesenchymal elements.

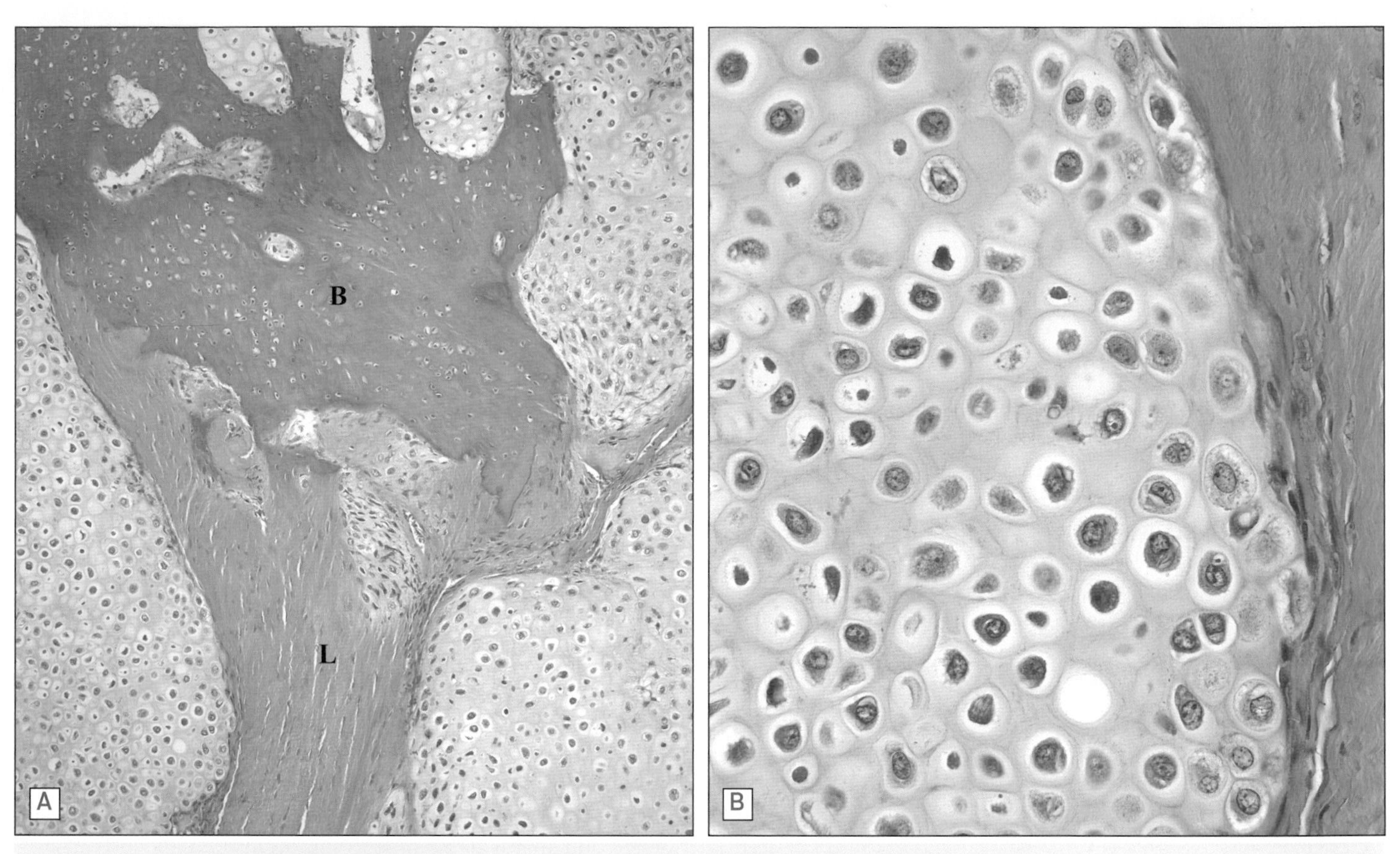

Figure 1.118 Chondrosarcoma, dog. Distal radius. **A.** Nodules of well-differentiated hyaline cartilage surrounding a ligament (L) at its insertion site and invading the adjacent bone (B). **B.** Higher-power view showing the plump, neoplastic chondrocytes compressing the ligament. Most of the tumor cells have large, variably sized nuclei and prominent nucleoli. Some lacunae contain more than one cell.

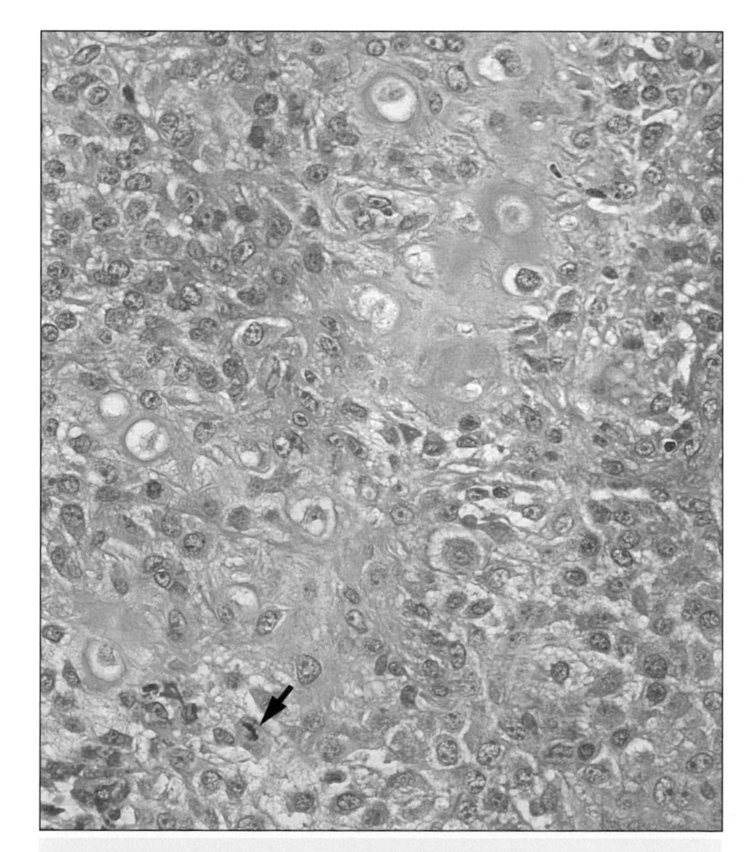

Figure 1.119 Poorly differentiated chondrosarcoma, dog. Anaplastic mesenchymal cells showing evidence of chondroid differentiation in some areas. Note the mitotic figure (arrow).

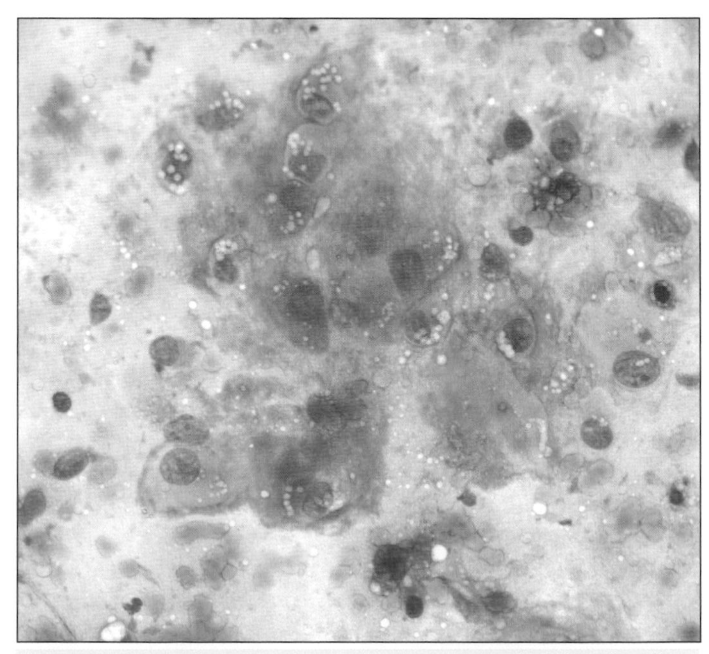

Figure 1.120 Cytological preparation from a **chondrosarcoma** in a dog. Several oval to fusiform cells, often with eccentric nuclei, prominent nucleoli, and basophilic cytoplasm, are closely associated with a background of brightly eosinophilic matrix.

Chondrosarcomas tend to grow more slowly and metastasize later than osteosarcomas, and typically follow a longer clinical course. Local invasion is common, as is recurrence following surgical removal, but the chance of successful removal from accessible sites is much greater than for osteosarcoma. Metastasis is usually to the lungs, but other visceral organs such as the kidney, liver, heart, and skeleton are sometimes involved.

Bibliography

Brown RJ, et al. Multiple osteochondroma in a Siamese cat. J Am Vet Med Assoc 1972;160:433–435.

Dernell WS, et al. Multilobular osteochondrosarcoma in 39 dogs: 1979–1993. J Am Anim Hosp Assoc 1998;34:11–18.

Diamond SS, et al. Multilobular osteosarcoma in the dog. Vet Pathol 1980; 17:759–763.

Doige CE. Multiple cartilaginous exostoses in dogs. Vet Pathol 1987;24:276–278.

Doige CE. Multiple ostechondromas with evidence of malignant transformation in a cat. Vet Pathol 1987;24:457–459.

Jacobson LS, Kirberger RM. Canine multiple cartilaginous exostosis: unusual manifestations and a review of the literature. J Am Anim Hosp Assoc 1996;32:45–51.

McCalla TL, et al. Multilobular osteosarcoma of the mandible and orbit in a dog. Vet Pathol 1989;92–94.

Morton D. Chondrosarcoma arising in a multilobular chondroma in a cat. J Am Vet Med Assoc 1985;186:804–806.

Patnaik AK, et al. Canine sinonasal skeletal neoplasms: chondrosarcomas and osteosarcomas. Vet Pathol 1984;21:475–482.

Pool RR, Carrig CB. Multiple cartilaginous exostoses in a cat. Vet Pathol 1972;9:350–359.

Popovitch CA, et al. Chondrosarcoma: a retrospective study of 97 dogs (1987–1990). J Am Anim Hosp Assoc 1994;30:81–85.

Richardson DW, Acland HM. Multilobular osteoma (chondroma rodens) in a horse. J Am Vet Med Assoc 1983;182:289–291.

Riddle WE, Leighton R. L. Osteochondromatosis in a cat. J Am Vet Med Assoc 1970;156:1428-1430.

Shupe JL, et al. Hereditary multiple exostoses: clinicopathologic features of a comparative study in horses and man. Am J Vet Res 1979;40:751–757.

Sylvestre AM, et al. A case series of 25 dogs with chondrosarcoma. J Vet Comp Orthop Traum 1992;4:13–17.

Fibrous tumors of bones

Fibrous tumors of bones are less common in domestic animals than tumors forming bone or cartilage. Ossifying fibroma and fibrous dysplasia are discussed above with osteoma, because of the similarities between these three benign tumors. Skeletal **fibromas** are extremely rare in animals, unlike humans where nonossifying fibromas are relatively common.

Skeletal **fibrosarcomas** arise from connective tissue stroma in either the medullary cavity or periosteum. Their histologic and gross appearances are essentially the same as that of fibrosarcomas elsewhere, although their innocuous microscopic appearance often belies their invasive tendencies. Central (medullary) fibrosarcomas are less common than those originating from the periosteum. They probably comprise about *5% of primary skeletal tumors in dogs* and occur predominantly in mature male dogs of large and medium breeds, but are rarely reported in other species.

In dogs, **central fibrosarcomas** arise most often in *metaphyses of long bones* and cause lytic lesions that must be differentiated from fibroblastic osteosarcomas. They are also reported in the mandible and vertebral column of dogs. It is likely however, that the prevalence of skeletal fibrosarcoma is overestimated. In one study, six of 11 tumors originally diagnosed as skeletal fibrosarcoma were reclassified as osteosarcoma following re-examination and identification of areas of osteoid production by tumor cells. Because of the poorer prognosis of osteosarcoma, an accurate diagnosis carries considerable clinical relevance. The pathologist should not be tempted to diagnose skeletal fibrosarcoma if the quantity of tissue available for examination is inadequate. Sequential radiographs of the lesion may be of diagnostic value because *fibrosarcomas of bone, although they are primarily destructive, usually progress more slowly than osteosarcomas or other highly malignant bone tumors.*

Periosteal fibrosarcomas occur in most species and *tend to involve flat bones* especially those of the head, but also occur on the scapula and occasionally on long bones. They enlarge slowly, causing disfigurement of the involved bone and are intimately attached to the bone surface. Erosion of the adjacent bone cortex may eventually predispose to pathological fracture.

Maxillary fibrosarcoma of the dog is technically a periosteal fibrosarcoma but it is classified separately from other tumors of this type because of its more frequent occurrence, and evidence that *it responds to combined radiation–hyperthermia therapy*. Maxillary fibrosarcomas occur primarily in middle-aged dogs, usually around 7 years of age, and appear to be most common in the Golden Retriever, Doberman Pinscher and German Shepherd breeds. In one large survey of canine bone tumors, ten of 31 fibrosarcomas involved the maxilla. Typically, the mass is broadly adherent to the periosteal surface of the maxilla (Fig. 1.121A, B).

Classification of periosteal fibrosarcomas as low-grade fibrosarcomas is based more on their invasive behavior than their histological appearance, which is often deceptively benign. They are less cellular than fibrosarcomas in other sites, lack the characteristic pattern of interwoven bundles and often contain a highly collagenous stroma with minimal pleomorphism of tumor cells (Fig. 1.121C). Biopsy samples from such tumors will often be misinterpreted as fibroma or fibrous repair tissue, especially if the pathologist is unaware of the clinical history or radiographic findings.

Although periosteal fibrosarcomas can often be dissected free from the underlying bone, *they often recur*. Metastasis to the lungs rarely occurs.

Vascular tumors of bones

Although tumors of vascular tissue are described with the circulatory system, *they can occur as primary bone tumors* and will therefore be mentioned briefly here. Intraosseous **hemangioma** is extremely rare in domestic animals. **Hemangiosarcoma** occurs occasionally as a primary bone tumor, especially in dogs, and is considered slightly less common than primary fibrosarcoma of bone. In one survey of 152 primary bone sarcomas in dogs, four were hemangiosarcomas. The tumor is found mainly in large and medium-sized breeds, with Boxers, German Shepherds and Great Danes over-represented. The *proximal and distal ends of long bones are most often affected* but tumors are also reported in the pelvic bones, sternum, ribs, maxilla, and vertebrae.

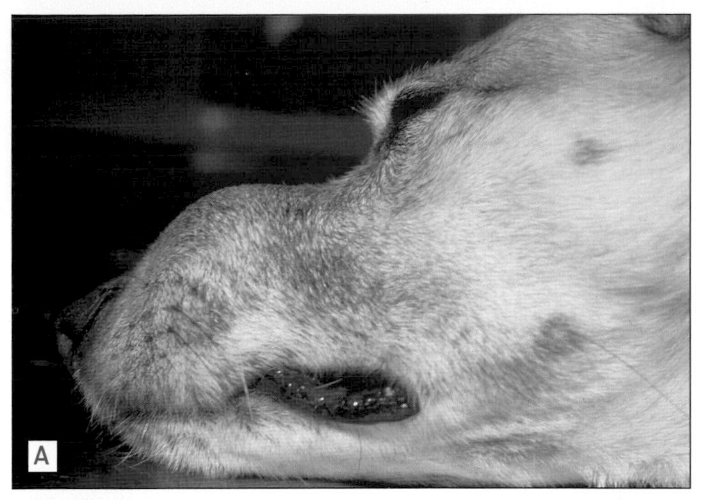

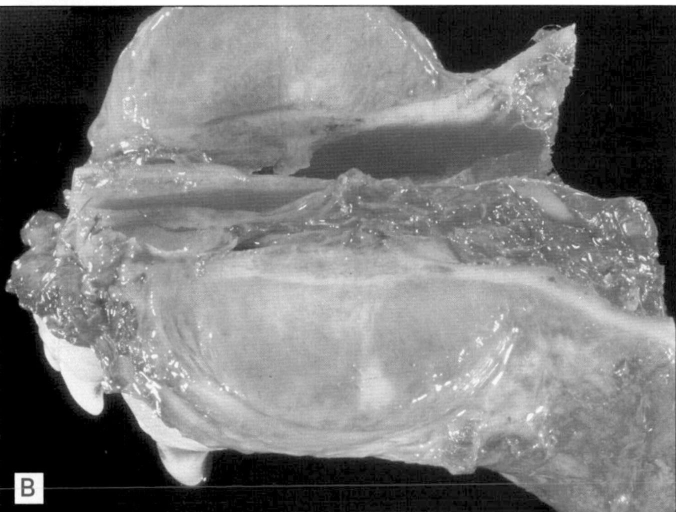

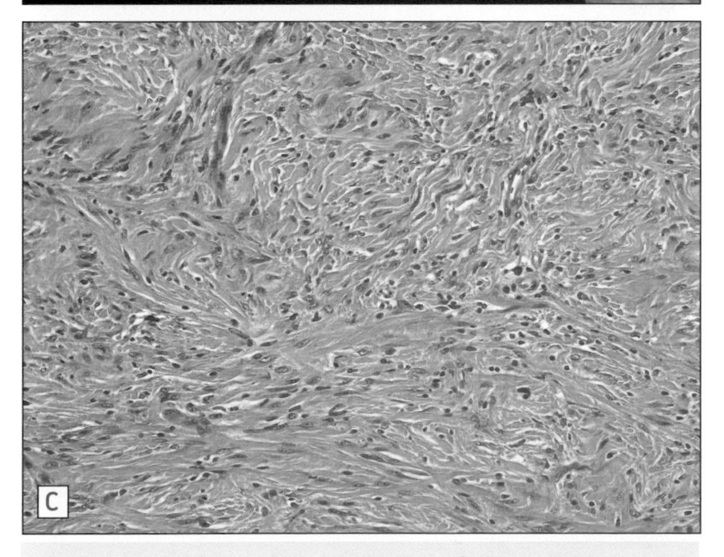

Figure 1.121 Maxillary fibrosarcoma, dog. **A.** Firm swelling over the rostral maxilla. **B.** Sagittal section through the nasal cavity of the same dog. The mass is firmly adherent to the outer surface of the maxillary bone and partly surrounding it. **C.** Interwoven bundles of well-differentiated fibrous tissue showing little microscopic evidence of malignancy.

Skeletal hemangiosarcoma is an aggressive tumor causing bone destruction and often predisposing to pathological fracture. The tumor tends to remain within the medullary cavity rather than invade adjacent soft tissues, but erodes and weakens the cortex. *Grossly*, the tumor resembles hemangiosarcomas of other organs, consisting of spongy, dark red tissue, and *cannot be reliably differentiated from telangiectatic osteosarcoma and aneurysmal bone cysts. Diagnosis is based on the demonstration in microscopic sections of malignant endothelial cells forming vascular channels*, at least in some areas of the tumor. The supporting stroma may become impregnated with plasma proteins, forming a hyaline material resembling osteoid and leading to an incorrect diagnosis of telangiectatic osteosarcoma. *In telangiectatic osteosarcoma, malignant osteoblasts rather than endothelial cells line the blood-filled spaces*, but the distinction is often difficult, especially in small biopsy samples or at sites of pathological fracture. Hemangiosarcomas occasionally metastasize to bones from other tissues and thorough postmortem examination of an affected animal is required before the tumor can be considered to be of bone origin.

Other primary tumors of bones

Giant cell tumor of bone is a recognized entity in humans but is rare in domestic animals with only isolated reports in **dogs** and **cats**. Some reported cases in animals are not convincing and may represent other tumors in which osteoclasts are prominent. Giant cell tumors of humans and animals *typically cause expansile osteolytic masses in the ends of long bones*, often involving much of the subchondral epiphyseal bone. Involvement of metacarpal bones and of the axial skeleton is also recorded in dogs and cats. As the mass expands, it destroys cortex but tends to remain at least partly circumscribed by a thin shell of bone. The osteolytic nature of the tumor combined with its bony shell creates a characteristic "soap-bubble" appearance in clinical radiographs.

The tumor is characterized *histologically* by the presence of *large numbers of multinucleated giant cells closely associated with neoplastic mononuclear cells*. The giant cells, which resemble osteoclasts, are often very large and are scattered uniformly throughout the tumor (Fig. 1.122). Their nuclei resemble those of the mononuclear cells. In some tumors there may be areas of collagen and/or osteoid formation, but this is not a prominent feature and the matrix may be produced by reactive fibroblasts and/or osteoblasts respectively, rather than by the tumor cells. The tumor is highly vascular and may contain cavernous spaces and areas of hemorrhage, leading to possible confusion with aneurysmal bone cyst, which also contains variable numbers of multinucleated giant cells. Osteosarcomas may also contain many osteoclasts in some areas and be mistakenly diagnosed as giant cell tumors.

In cytological preparations, the presence of a large percentage of multinucleated giant cells among many plump, spindle-shaped, or ovoid mesenchymal cells, suggests the possibility of giant cell tumor. Giant cells may also be present in aspirates from other bone lesions, particularly osteosarcoma, but the percentage in giant cell tumors is likely to be much higher. In one report of this tumor in a dog, 25% of all cells obtained by fine-needle aspiration biopsy were multinucleated giant cells. However, definitive diagnosis still requires histological examination of sections from representative areas of the mass. The histogenesis of giant cell tumor is uncertain, but immunochemical staining suggests that the mononuclear tumor cells are of histiocytic origin and that the giant cells arise from their fusion. C-type viral particles were found to be budding from tumor cells in one feline giant cell tumor but their significance is unknown.

Because there are so few documented cases of giant cell tumor in animals, there is inadequate information to provide an indication of their biological behavior. Benign and malignant forms are also reported in animals, the former being most common. In humans, most giant cell tumors are benign, but they commonly recur following surgery and approximately 5–10% are malignant, metastasizing predominantly to the lungs.

Because of the marked differences in prognosis between giant cell tumor and osteosarcoma, both of which may contain many multinucleated giant cells, *a diagnosis of giant cell tumor should never be made from small biopsy samples that are not representative of the lesion.*

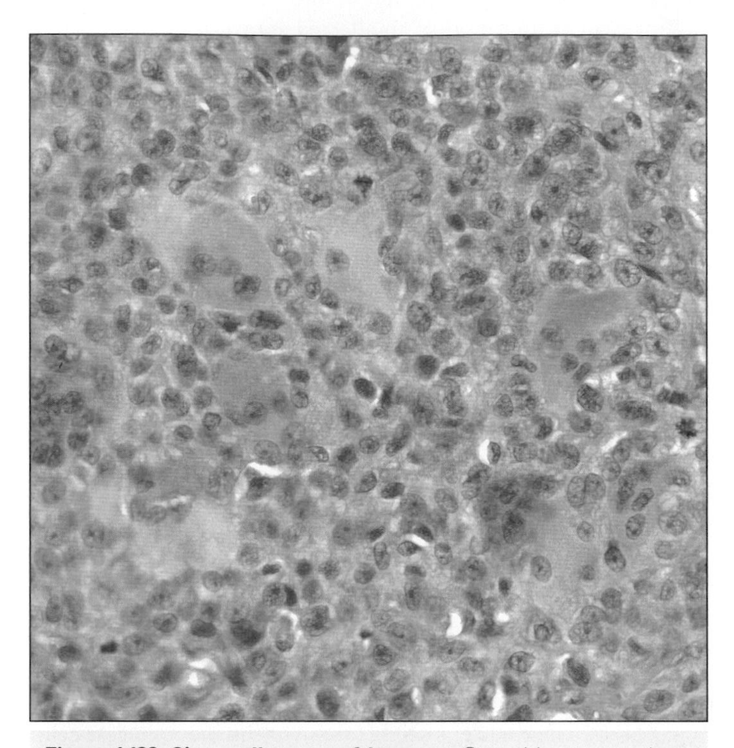

Figure 1.122 Giant cell tumor of bone, cat. Several large, sometimes abnormally shaped, multinucleated giant cells resembling osteoclasts scattered amongst a population of mononuclear cells.

Liposarcoma is a rare primary bone tumor in animals, resembling its soft-tissue counterpart but forming osteolytic bone lesions. The tumor cells typically contain variable numbers of intracytoplasmic vesicles, often with an eccentrically positioned nucleus but, in some areas, may consist of less well-differentiated spindle cells. **Osteoliposarcoma**, a form of **malignant mesenchymoma**, is a malignant neoplasm containing liposarcomatous and osteosarcomatous tissue and is recorded in the dog.

Plasma cell myeloma, a malignant tumor of plasma cells within the bone marrow, typically produces discrete, multicentric, lytic lesions in bones, especially those involved in active hematopoiesis. The disease occurs most often in **dogs** but is also reported occasionally in **cats** and **horses**. The mean age of affected dogs is approximately 9.5 years (range 2.5 to 16 years) and males are affected more frequently than females. In cats, like dogs, there is a higher incidence in males but no sex predilection is recognized in the small number of cases reported in horses.

A feature of plasma cell myeloma in all species is the *production of a homogeneous immunoglobulin or immunoglobulin fragment (paraprotein or M-component),* which appears as a monoclonal spike on serum protein electrophoresis. The disease may also be accompanied by Bence–Jones proteinuria, hyperviscosity syndrome, and hypercalcemia. Involvement of vertebral bodies may result in paraplegia due to protrusion of tumor masses into the spinal canal, or secondary to pathological fractures of vertebral bodies. Discrete, "punched-out" foci of osteolysis (Fig. 1.123A), of various sizes, and often involving multiple bones, are present in approximately two-thirds of dogs with plasma cell myeloma, but appear to be less common in affected horses. In dogs, the principal sites of bone involvement are vertebrae, especially in the thoraco-lumbar region, femur, pelvis, humerus, and ribs. Bones of the distal limb are seldom involved in dogs, unlike cats where they appear to be involved as often as proximal bones of the limb.

Grossly, the lytic foci consist of soft, fleshy or gelatinous, dark red nodules, replacing trabecular bone. The lesions are often multiple and may be associated with a pathological fracture. Histological or cytological examination reveals a relatively pure, dense population

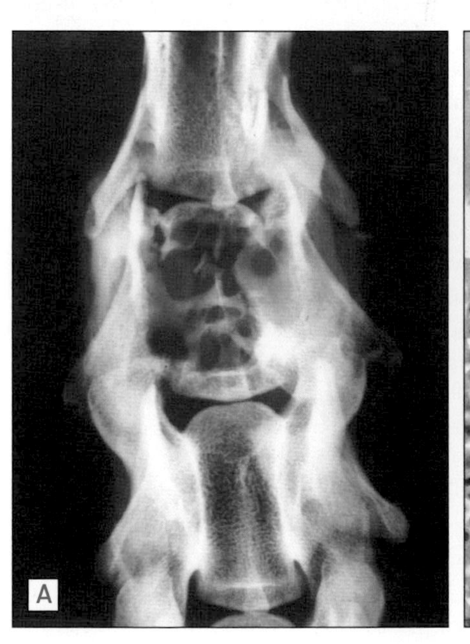

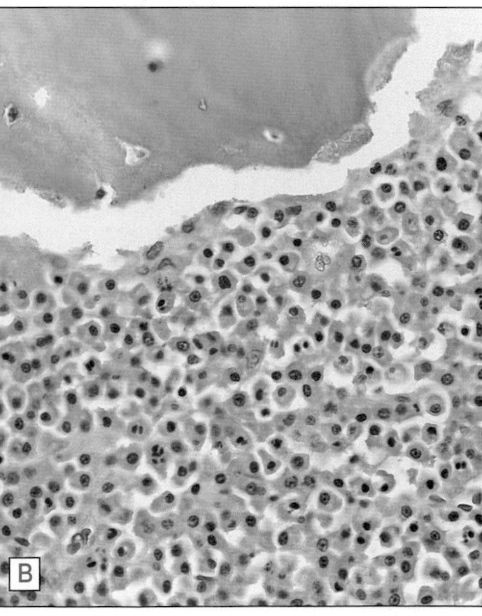

Figure 1.123 Plasma cell myeloma, dog. **A.** Discrete, "punched out" osteolytic foci in a cervical vertebra. **B.** Monomorphic population of plasma cells replacing normal marrow architecture.

of plasma cells (Fig. 1.123B), which may be either well-differentiated or large, anaplastic round cells with a high mitotic index.

Malignant lymphoma may also occur as a primary tumor of bone in humans and animals but, more frequently, bone involvement occurs in association with multicentric lymphoma. There are few reported cases of primary skeletal lymphoma in **dogs**, but most have occurred in animals less than 1 year of age. The lesions in dogs are typically lytic and multiple, and cannot be distinguished radiographically or grossly from plasma cell myeloma. Pathological fractures and hypercalcemia are reported, but hypercalcemia is not a consistent feature of the disease, even when the bone lesions are extensive. Microscopically, sheets of monomorphic lymphocytes replace bone trabeculae and the contents of the marrow cavity in areas of lysis.

Infiltration of bone marrow, together with *multifocal to locally extensive bone infarction*, is reported in **calves** with the juvenile, sporadic form of malignant lymphoma. Affected calves also have generalized lymph node enlargement and variable involvement of other organs, including liver, kidney, and spleen. The bone infarcts are readily visible grossly as discrete, pale areas (Fig. 1.124A), but are not detected unless the bones are sectioned during postmortem examination. The mechanism of the tumor-associated bone marrow necrosis is not clear, but ischemia secondary to infiltration of the marrow with malignant cells is the most likely explanation. Histologically, the infarcted areas may include either neoplastic or nonneoplastic tissue and are often bordered by a zone of edematous connective tissue (Fig. 1.124B).

Bibliography

Bingel SA, et al. Haemangiosarcoma of bone in the dog. J Small Anim Pract 1974;15:303–322.

Brewer WG, Turrel JM. Radiotherapy and hyperthermia in the treatment of fibrosarcoma in the dog. J Am Vet Med Assoc 1982;181:146–150.

Brodey RS, Riser WH. Liposarcoma of bone in a dog: A case report. J Am Vet Radiol Soc 1966;7:27–33.

Edwards DF, et al. Plasma cell myeloma in the horse. A case review and literature review. J Vet Int Med 1993;7:169–176.

LeCouteur RA, et al. A case of giant cell tumor of bone (osteoclastoma) in a dog. J Am Anim Hosp Assoc 1978;14:356–362.

Misdorp W, van der Heul RO. An osteo-(chondro-) liposarcoma ("malignant mesenchymoma") of the radius in a dog, with two types of metastases. Zbl Veterinaermed [A] 1975;22:187–192.

Osborne CA, et al. Multiple myeloma in the dog. J Am Vet Med Assoc 1968;153:1300–1319.

Sheafor SE, et al. Hypercalcaemia in two cats with multiple myeloma. J Am Anim Hosp Assoc 1996;32:503–508.

Thompson KG, Pool RR. Tumors of bones. In: Meuten DJ, ed. Tumors in Domestic Animals. 5th ed. Ames, IA: Iowa State University Press, 2002:245–317.

Thornberg LP. Giant cell tumor of bone in a cat. Vet Pathol 1979;16:255–257.

van Bree H, et al. Cervical cord compression as a complication in an IgG multiple myeloma in a dog. J Am Vet Med Assoc 1983;19:317–323.

Weber NA, Tebeau CS. An unusual presentation of multiple myeloma in two cats. J Am Anim Hosp Assoc 1998;34:477–483.

Wesselhoeft Ablin L, et al. Fibrosarcoma of the canine appendicular skeleton. J Am Anim Hosp Assoc 1991;27:303–309.

Zachary JF, et al. Multicentric osseous hemangiosarcoma in a Chianina-Angus steer. Vet Pathol 1981;18:266–270.

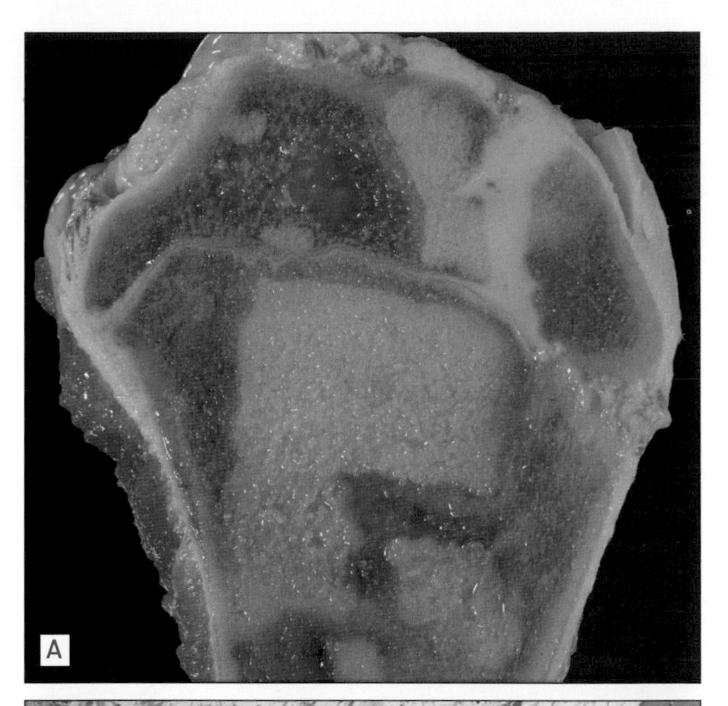

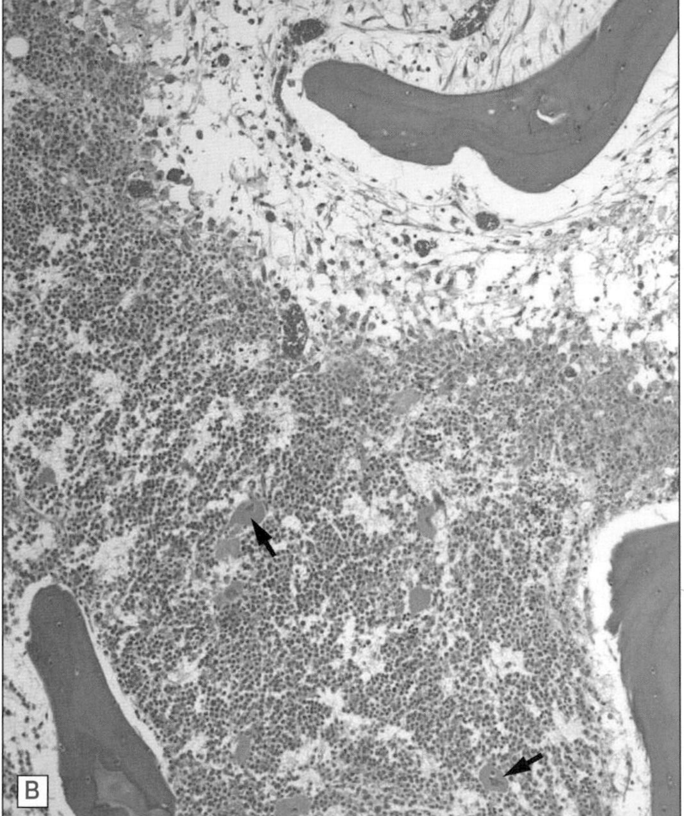

Figure 1.124 Malignant lymphoma, 6-month-old calf. **A.** Multiple, irregular-shaped, pale foci representing medullary infarcts throughout the epiphysis and metaphysis of the proximal tibia. Similar lesions were detected in most other long bones. **B.** Sheets of necrotic tumor cells in an infarcted area, bordered by a zone of edematous connective tissue. Several necrotic megakaryocytes (arrows) are scattered amongst the tumor cells.

Secondary tumors of bones

Malignant neoplasms originating in soft tissues or in the skeleton may involve bone secondarily either by hematogenous metastasis or direct

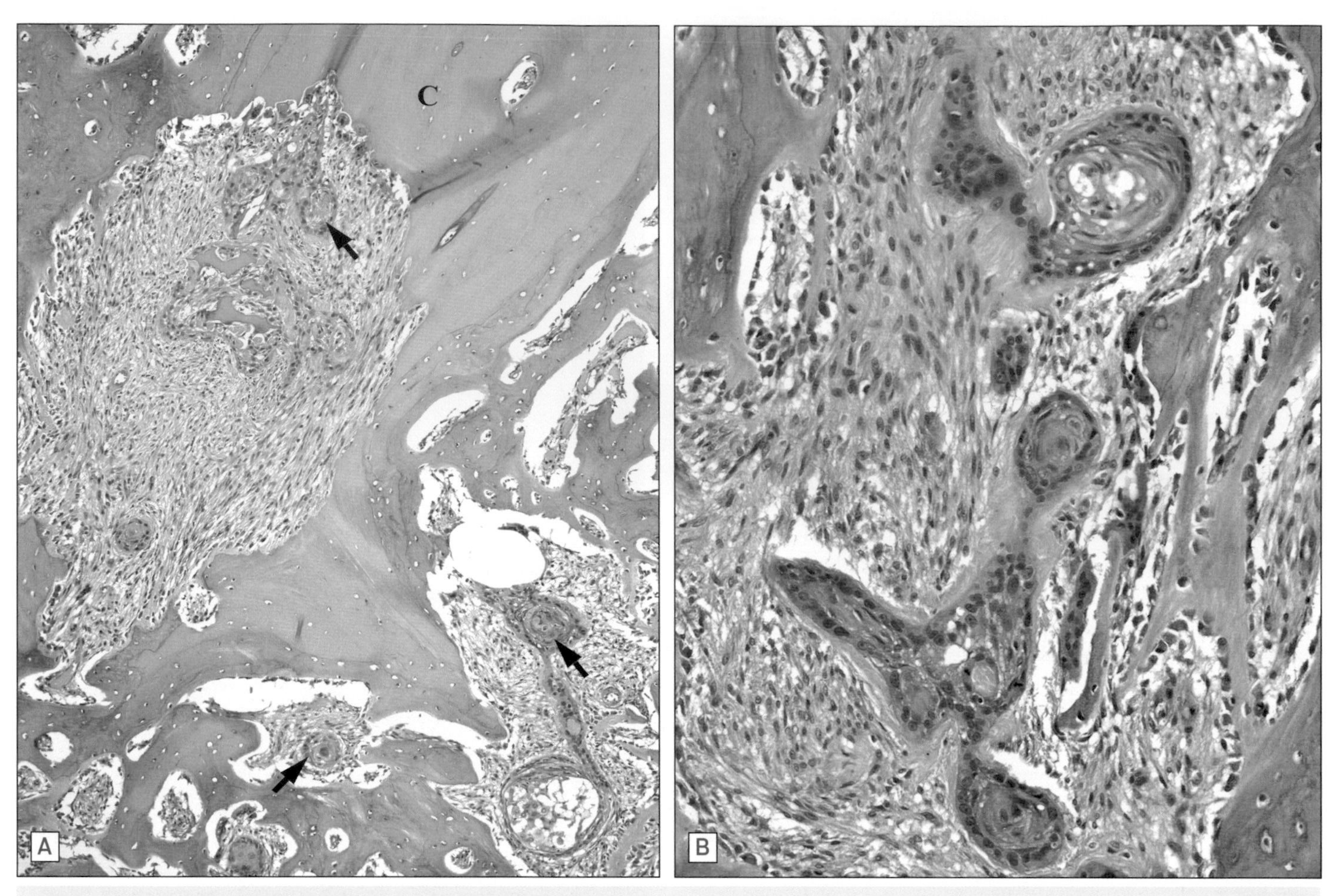

Figure 1.125 Squamous cell carcinoma, cat. Mandible. **A.** Cords of epithelial cells (arrows) surrounded by a marked fibroblastic response invading the dense cortical bone (C) and adjacent reactive bone. **B.** Closer view of tumor cells showing evidence of squamous differentiation.

extension. **Metastatic bone disease** is very common in humans but is *generally considered rare in domestic animals*. Several explanations for this discrepancy have been proposed. The life span of most farm animals is abbreviated by slaughter, and that of many pets by euthanasia, thus limiting the time for tumors to develop, metastasize and, perhaps most importantly, produce signs of metastatic disease.

While there appears to be a genuine difference between the frequency of skeletal metastases in humans and domestic animals, *metastatic bone disease in animals is likely to be much more common than is realized*. The skeleton of animals with malignancies at other sites is seldom examined in detail, either radiographically or during necropsy, and skeletal metastases could easily be missed. In one survey, skeletal metastases were identified in 5.8% of dogs with metastatic carcinoma, but since fewer than 20% of the dogs underwent bone scan, skeletal radiography, or necropsy, the true prevalence was probably much greater. In another study, 98 dogs with a variety of carcinomas were subjected to thorough examination of the skeleton at necropsy. The spine, pelvis, and long bones were sectioned longitudinally and the ribs inspected visually. Macroscopic metastases were detected in 21 (21.4%) of the 98 dogs. The prevalence of metastases would almost certainly have been even higher had the bones been scanned or radiographed, or if the skeleton had been subjected to detailed microscopic examination.

Carcinomas metastasize to the skeleton of dogs much more commonly than sarcomas and the most common tissues of origin are the mammary gland, thyroid, prostate, ovary, and lung. The ribs, vertebrae, and proximal long bones are the favored locations for skeletal metastases in dogs.

Information on the prevalence of skeletal metastases in cats is scarce, but there are occasional reports of pulmonary and mammary carcinomas metastasizing to the bones in this species. Interestingly, metastatic carcinomas in the skeleton of cats more frequently involve bones of the distal limb (acrometastases), unlike humans and dogs where skeletal metastases are uncommon in bones distal to the elbow or stifle.

Secondary bone tumors generally produce osteolytic lesions that are difficult, if not impossible, to distinguish radiographically from primary bone tumors. This may contribute to the underdiagnosis of secondary bone tumors in cases where the radiographic diagnosis is not confirmed by histological or cytological examination of biopsy specimens. For example, in a report of 20 metastatic bone tumors in dogs, the radiographic diagnosis was primary bone tumor in all but one case.

In general, dogs with skeletal metastases are older than dogs with primary tumors of bones (median age 8.5–10 years), and there is no obvious breed or size predilection. Unlike primary bone sarcomas, metastatic skeletal carcinomas are found most commonly in dogs weighing less than 25 kg and approximately 30% of such tumors are found in small dogs weighing less than 15 kg.

A definitive diagnosis of metastatic bone tumor is based on either cytological or histological examination of fine-needle aspirates or tissue biopsies respectively but, in most cases, the tumor cells provide few indications as to the tissue of origin. Even after thorough postmortem examination, the primary site of a metastatic skeletal carcinoma may not be apparent, although malignant epithelial cells within a skeletal lesion can only be derived from an extraskeletal carcinoma. Osteosarcomas sometimes metastasize from the bone of origin to other skeletal sites, in which case the secondary lesions may be in atypical locations and may appear to have been present for different lengths of time. For some sarcomas, such as hemangiosarcoma, which may originate in bone or other tissues, it may be impossible to determine whether skeletal involvement is primary or secondary but if the tumor is present in several skeletal sites then metastasis is more likely.

Malignant tumors in soft tissues adjacent to a bone may penetrate the bone by direct extension and can be referred to as **invasive tumors of bones**. *This is a feature of some types of tumor, in particular squamous cell carcinoma of the digits and oral cavity in dogs and cats.* These aggressive tumors frequently invade the periosteum of the underlying bone, erode the cortex, and penetrate the medullary cavity. In dogs, bone invasion is reported to occur in 77% of oral squamous cell carcinomas. Microscopically, cords of anaplastic epithelial cells, showing evidence of squamous differentiation, permeate the osseous and extra-osseous tissues, and are accompanied either by an osteoblastic reaction or a prominent fibroblastic response with osteoclastic resorption of adjacent bone (Fig. 1.125A, B). Squamous cell carcinomas of the canine digit not only invade bone but also metastasize to local lymph nodes, and eventually to the lungs.

Other tumors that appear to have an affinity for bone invasion are *malignant melanomas of the oral cavity in dogs* and *fibrosarcomas of the canine skull and long bones*. Tumors of dental origin, including acanthomatous epulis, ameloblastoma, and fibroameloblastoma, may also extend into the maxilla or mandible of dogs and cats.

Bibliography

Cooley DM, Waters DJ. Skeletal metastasis as the initial clinical manifestation of metastatic carcinoma in 19 dogs. J Vet Intern Med 1998;12:288–293.

May C, Newsholme SJ. Metastasis of feline pulmonary carcinoma presenting as multiple digital swelling. J Small Anim Pract 1989;30:302–310.

Russell RG, Walker M. Metastatic and invasive tumors of bone in dogs and cats. Vet Clin North Am Small Anim Clin 1983;13:163–180.

Waters DJ, et al. Skeletal metastases in feline mammary carcinoma: case report and literature review. J Am Anim Hosp Assoc 1998;34:103–108.

Tumor-like lesions of bones

Several nonneoplastic lesions of bones occur in humans and domestic animals and must be differentiated from primary and secondary bone tumors. Included amongst these are various forms of **bone cysts**, some of which are not true cysts as defined by pathologists but appear "cystic" radiographically.

Solitary or **unicameral bone cysts** are reported in the *metaphyses of long bones in children and young dogs*, a breed predisposition having been suggested in Doberman Pinschers. The lesions may be monostotic or polyostotic and are generally lytic and expansile, with erosion of the cortex and little or no periosteal new bone formation. In radiographs, shelves of bone often project from the cyst wall, but in most cases, these are incomplete and the cysts are unicameral. Pathological fracture may occur due to the localized bone destruction. *The cyst cavity is filled with clear or sanguineous fluid and lined by a connective tissue membrane of variable thickness, with scattered multinucleate giant cells and hemosiderin-containing macrophages.* The pathogenesis of unicameral bone cysts is uncertain but they may be the result of impaired venous drainage from sites of active endochondral ossification. Recurrence following surgical drainage and curettage is uncommon.

Aneurysmal bone cysts have been reported rarely in dogs, cats, horses, and cattle. Radiographically, they appear as *expansile, osteolytic lesions* (Fig. 1.126A) *contained by a thin, "ballooned" periosteum and with an internal "soap-bubble" appearance* and must be differentiated from osteosarcoma, hemangiosarcoma, fibrosarcoma, and plasma cell myeloma. Too few cases are reported in animals to establish age or site prevalence, although lesions are described in bones of both the axial and appendicular skeleton. The gross appearance of aneurysmal bone cysts closely resembles telangiectatic osteosarcoma and hemangiosarcoma, typically exuding blood from the cut surface, and may contain solid areas in addition to multiple blood-filled cysts. Pathological fracture may be present.

Fine-needle aspiration biopsies are unlikely to be useful in the diagnosis of either aneurysmal or unicameral bone cysts as the preparations are likely to be heavily contaminated with blood. Confirmation of the diagnosis requires histopathological examination of biopsy specimens. *The lesion consists of cavernous blood-filled spaces* (Fig. 1.126B) *separated by septa of loosely arranged spindle cells with scattered multinucleate giant cells and hemosiderin-containing macrophages*, similar to the lining of unicameral bone cysts. Osteoid or spicules of reactive bone may be present in the surrounding connective tissue (Fig. 1.126C) and should not be mistaken for tumor bone. The pathogenesis of these lesions is not known, but altered blood flow, perhaps secondary to trauma or some other bone disease, such as malignancy, is believed to play a role.

Subchondral (juxtacortical) bone cysts occur in young horses, pigs, and occasionally in other species, as a manifestation of osteochondrosis. The lesions are typically 5–10 mm in diameter and may be multilocular. In horses, subchondral cysts are found most frequently beneath the articular surfaces of phalanges, but also occur in femoral condyles and a range of other bones. *The cysts may develop either from residual nodules of epiphyseal cartilage or within foci of subarticular hemorrhage.* Histologically, the lesions are not always cystic, instead consisting of fibrous tissue with extensive myxoid matrix or, in some cases, degenerate cartilage. Cystic spaces lined by fibrous tissue and containing fluid, possibly of synovial origin, are present within some lesions. In humans, subchondral cysts occur in association with degenerative joint disease and are thought to be secondary to either synovial fluid intrusion or bony contusion.

Intraosseous epidermoid cysts *are reported rarely in dogs as a cause of lytic lesions in the distal phalanx.* At this site, they must be differentiated from nail-bed carcinomas, malignant melanomas, and osteomyelitis. One reported case involved the tenth thoracic vertebral body of a dog. Similar lesions occur in the distal phalanx and skull of humans. Radiographically, there may be a sclerotic reaction around one or more lytic foci and extensive periosteal new bone formation. Grossly, the lesion consists of multilocular cysts containing pale cream, crumbly material. Microscopically, *the cysts are lined by well-differentiated, stratified squamous, keratinizing epithelium and filled with layers of keratinized squames.* The squamous epithelium may show marked pseudoepitheliomatous hyperplasia and could be mistaken

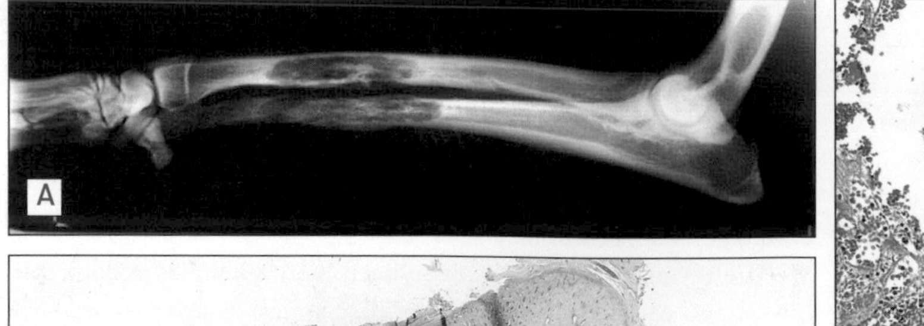

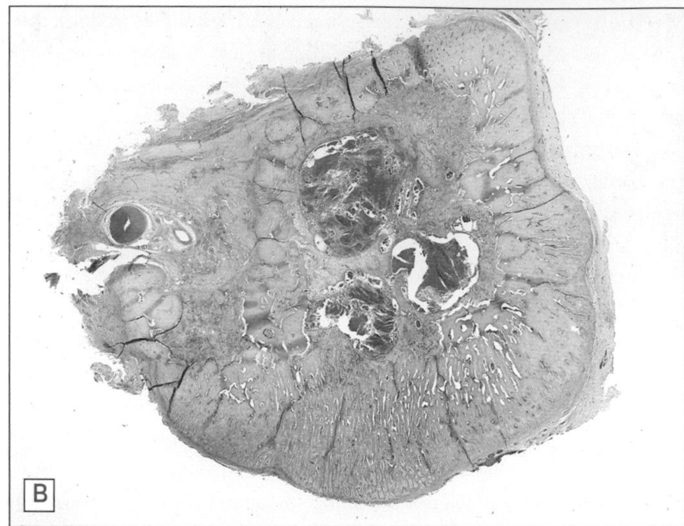

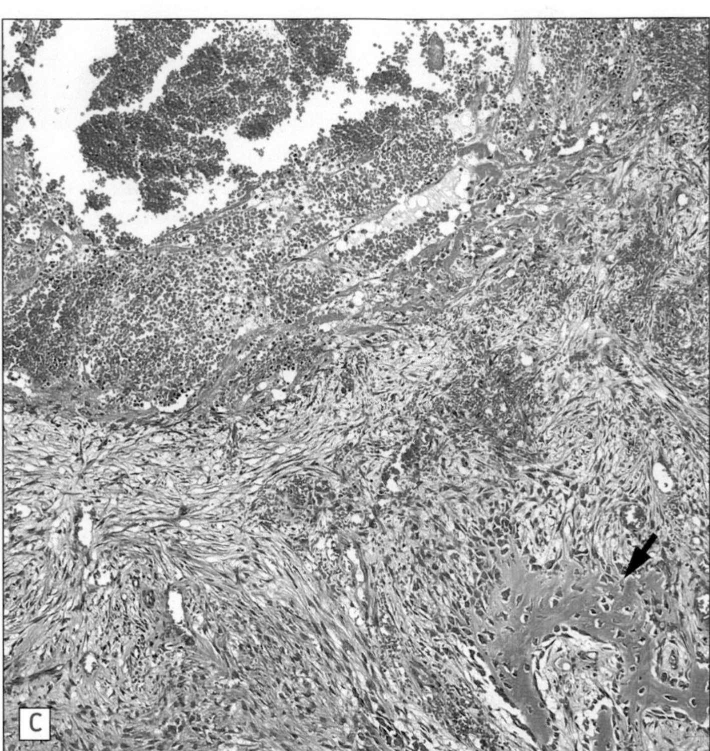

Figure 1.126 Aneurysmal bone cyst, 1-year-old dog. Radius and ulna. **A.** Radiograph showing expansile, osteolytic lesions in the distal diaphyseal regions of the radius and ulna. **B.** Subgross, transverse section of ulna showing cavernous, blood-filled spaces surrounded by loose connective tissue, reactive bone, and remnants of cortical bone. **C.** Reactive bone (arrow) forming in the connective tissue near a blood-filled space.

for squamous cell carcinoma, especially if a biopsy sample is inadequate. The cysts are generally supported by a dense fibrous stroma and surrounded by thickened bone trabeculae. The pathogenesis of intra-osseous epidermoid cysts is uncertain, but the digital lesions are believed to be *secondary to a penetrating wound*, with traumatic implantation of epidermal fragments into the underlying bone. Cysts involving the skull of humans, and vertebral body of a dog, may represent *rests of heterotopic ectoderm* that have become sequestered along lines of closure during embryonic development.

An **exuberant fracture callus** containing extensive areas of disorganized and primitive bone, cartilage, and fibrous tissue *may also resemble a primary bone tumor*. Even in cytological and histological preparations, differentiation of an early callus from osteosarcoma and chondrosarcoma can present a significant challenge, especially in cases where the clinical and radiographic history is inadequate.

Bibliography

Belknap EB, et al. Aneurysmal bone cyst in a Holstein bull. J Am Vet Med Assoc 1992;201:1413–1415.

Biller DS, et al. Aneurysmal bone cyst in the rib of a cat. J Am Vet Med Assoc 1987;190:1193–1195.

Bowles MHY, Freeman K. Aneurysmal bone cyst in the ischia and pubes of a dog: A case report and literature review. J Am Anim Hosp Assoc 1986;23:423–427.

Carrig CB, Seawright AA. A familial canine polyostotic fibrous dysplasia with subperiosteal cortical defects. J Small Anim Pract 19609;10:397–405.

Homer BH, et al. Intraosseous epidermoid cysts in the distal phalanx of two dogs. Vet Radiol Ultr 1992;33:133–137.

McIlwraith CW. Subchondral cystic lesions (osteochondrosis) in the horse. Compend Cont Educ Pract Vet 1982;4:S282–S291.

Momiyama N, et al. Aneurysmal bone cyst in a colt. Equine Vet J 1999;11:243–246.

Pernell R, et al. Aneurysmal bone cyst in a 6-month-old dog. J Am Vet Med Assoc 1992;201:1897–1899.

Schrader SC, et al. Bone cysts in two dogs and a review of similar cystic lesions in the dog. J Am Vet Med Assoc 1983;182:490–495.

Shiroma JT, et al. Pathological fracture of an aneurysmal bone cyst in a lumbar vertebra of a dog. J Am Anim Hosp Assoc 1993;29:434–437.

Diseases of joints

GENERAL CONSIDERATIONS

Three main types of joints or articulations unite adjacent bones and/or cartilaginous structures throughout the skeleton. These are classified on the basis of their morphology and tissue composition as *fibrous, cartilaginous, or synovial joints*. This method of classification has limitations as some joints contain a mixture of the different tissue types, while others change their composition during maturation. Furthermore, even within each category, there is considerable variation in the amount of movement between adjacent skeletal structures.

In spite of these limitations, the system is widely accepted in the medical and veterinary literature and is used throughout this chapter.

Fibrous joints

In these joints the *bones are united by fibrous tissue*, which allows little movement between them. Fibrous joints are *subdivided into sutures, syndesmoses, and gomphoses*.

Sutures are limited to the *skull*, where they allow continued growth of cranial bones by intramembranous ossification as the brain matures. Osteogenic cells form a cambial layer adjacent to the bone-forming surfaces and are separated by intervening layers of fibrous tissue, which vary in thickness depending on their location. Broader sheets of fibrous tissue often occur at the junctions of three adjacent skull bones and are referred to as **fontanelles**. A bony union or **synostosis** replaces the fibrous tissue of many sutures once growth ceases.

A **syndesmosis** is a fibrous joint in which *adjacent bones are united by an interosseous ligament or membrane*, such as occurs in some species between the shafts of the tibia and fibula and between the radius and ulna. Syndesmoses contain fibrous and elastic connective tissue in variable proportions. Consequently, minor movement may occur between the bones due to stretching of the ligament or membrane.

Gomphoses are specialized fibrous *joints between the teeth and either the mandible or maxilla*. The membrane between tooth and bone is termed the **periodontal ligament**, and although it contains no elastic fibers, it allows slight movement of the tooth.

Cartilaginous joints

These are joints in which the *union consists of either hyaline or fibrocartilage*, or a combination of the two. There are two types of cartilaginous joints, *synchondroses and symphyses*.

Synchondroses are *temporary joints* that exist only while the skeleton is growing and are replaced by bone once the skeleton matures. *Physeal growth plates*, which unite the separate centers of ossification in long bones, are synchondroses consisting of well-organized hyaline cartilage. Synchondroses also exist between bones forming by endochondral ossification in the basicranium.

Symphyses are located in the *mid-sagittal plane of the body and are permanent joints*, unlike synchondroses. The adjacent bones are capped by a thin layer of hyaline cartilage, which blends with fibrocartilage, forming a joint with great strength while still allowing a limited amount of movement. Examples are the *pubic symphysis and intervertebral disks*. Intervertebral disks unite each pair of vertebrae in the vertebral column, with the exception of the atlas and axis.

Diseases of **intervertebral disks** are very common in humans and certain domestic animals. For this reason, a brief discussion of the unique structure and function of these joints is appropriate. Each disk contains *a central core, the* **nucleus pulposus**, which is a remnant of the notochord. In young animals, the nucleus pulposus is gelatinous and translucent (Fig. 1.127). The matrix consists of glycosaminoglycans, particularly chondroitin-6-sulfate, keratan sulfate, and hyaluronan (hyaluronic acid), collagen (mainly type II) and a large amount of water. The cellular concentration is relatively sparse and consists predominantly of *chondrocytes*, which are often arranged in small clusters, and fibrocytes. The nucleus pulposus of immature animals may also contain clusters of notochordal or physaliferous cells, which have abundant finely vacuolated cytoplasm filled with glycogen. With aging, the glycosaminoglycan and water concentration of intervertebral disks declines and the number of fibrocytes increases. *The nucleus pulposus is surrounded by the* **annulus fibrosus**, which is broader ventrally than dorsally and consists of concentric layers of fibrocartilage. The direction of the collagen fibers alternates between each layer. The matrix of the annulus fibrosus consists predominantly of type I collagen, with lesser quantities of glycosaminoglycans. *Fibrocytes* are the predominant cell type. Fine nerve endings are present in the outer third of the annulus fibrosus. *The cranial and caudal boundaries of intervertebral disks are occupied by* **cartilaginous end plates**, which consist of hyaline cartilage and are in direct apposition to the vertebral bodies on either side of the joint. Collagen fibers from the annulus fibrosus merge with those of the cartilaginous end plates and become embedded in the bony trabeculae of the vertebral body, forming a strong, stable union.

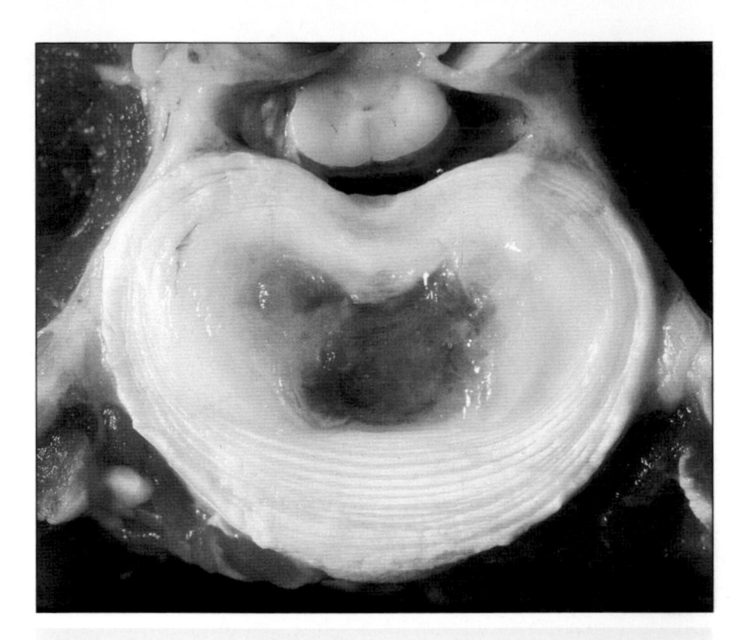

Figure 1.127 Intervertebral disk of a young dog. The gelatinous nucleus pulposus is surrounded by the annulus fibrosus, which consists of concentric layers of fibrocartilage.

Dorsally and ventrally, the intervertebral disks merge with the **dorsal and ventral longitudinal ligaments**, which run the length of the spinal column. The dorsal longitudinal ligament lies in the floor of the vertebral canal, merging with each disk as it passes, except between the second and tenth thoracic vertebrae. In this region, *conjugal ligaments* connecting the heads of the corresponding ribs cross the floor of the canal between the dorsal longitudinal ligament and the dorsal portion of the annulus fibrosus. The extra support provided by the conjugal ligaments is no doubt responsible for the low incidence of disk protrusions between the second and tenth thoracic vertebrae in dogs.

Intervertebral disks are designed to allow limited movement between adjacent vertebral bodies when the vertebral column is subjected to a wide variety of different loading conditions, including compression, tension, bending, shear forces, and torsion. Degenerative changes occurring in the nucleus pulposus and/or annulus fibrosus as part of the aging process or in disease states can markedly alter the ability of intervertebral disks to withstand such forces.

Synovial joints

Synovial or **diarthrodial** joints are found predominantly in the appendicular skeleton and allow considerable movement between adjacent bones. The bone ends in these specialized joints are covered by *hyaline articular cartilage* and an *articular capsule* surrounds a central cavity filled with *synovial fluid*. Some synovial joints are supported by ligaments, while others, such as the femorotibial joint, contain fibrocartilaginous menisci. Because of the importance of these joints, and the frequency with which they are involved in disease processes, the individual components of synovial joints will be discussed in more detail.

Articular cartilage is the key component of synovial joints, being required to withstand the compressive forces associated with weight bearing in addition to the shear forces that occur during motion. Grossly, it is smooth, bluish-white, and turgid in young animals but, with advancing age, it becomes yellow, opaque, and less elastic. The thickness of articular cartilage varies between and within joints, tending to be thickest at points of maximum weight bearing.

The matrix of articular cartilage is approximately 70–80% water. *The organic component consists largely of proteoglycans, type II collagen, and lesser quantities of types V, VI, IX, X, and XI.* Although not apparent in routine histologic preparations, the type II collagen fibrils are arranged in loops with either end firmly embedded in the calcified zone. Therefore, the fibrils located in the superficial zone are oriented parallel to the articular surface, while those in the radial zone are more vertical. This arrangement presumably enhances the ability of articular cartilage to withstand the range of shear and compressive forces to which it is exposed. In addition to covalent cross-links between chains of type II collagen in articular cartilage, there are intermolecular links between type II and type IX collagen. Type IX collagen is a small, nonfibrillar molecule, comprising only 1–2% of articular cartilage, but appears to be important in anchoring proteoglycan molecules to collagen and stabilizing the network of collagen fibers within the matrix.

The *proteoglycan subunits of articular cartilage* consist of a core protein with the glycosaminoglycan molecules chondroitin-6-sulfate, chondroitin-4-sulfate, and keratan sulfate attached. A small peptide referred to as *link protein* links the amino-terminal end of the core protein in proteoglycan subunits to hyaluronan (hyaluronic acid) filaments, thus forming massive, stable proteoglycan aggregates. The term *aggrecan* is applied to the proteoglycan monomers that link with hyaluronan, and the complex is referred to as an aggrecan aggregate. The glycosaminoglycan molecules in these aggregates are negatively charged because of the presence of many carboxyl and sulfate groups and therefore remain separated when attached to the core protein. Water molecules are trapped and immobilized by the negative charges and the meshwork of large, hydrophilic molecules, resulting in the *formation of a gel* supported by a delicate reticular arrangement of collagen fibrils. Water can move only slowly within this meshwork, thus allowing articular cartilage to maintain its turgidity when subjected to a compressive load. This flow of water during movement is important in promoting the transport of nutrients to chondrocytes within the articular cartilage and providing lubricant for the joint. Small quantities of nonaggregating proteoglycan monomers, including decorin and biglycan, are also found in articular cartilage. The role of these proteoglycans, which consist of chondroitin sulfate and dermatan sulfate, is not clear.

Histologically, the cellular concentration of articular cartilage is low, especially in adults, and the chondrocytes are not distributed randomly. In the *superficial or gliding zone*, the chondrocytes are relatively small and flattened, with their long axis parallel to the articular surface. Beneath this layer, is an *intermediate (transitional) zone* in which the chondrocytes are round or ovoid, then a *radial zone*, in which large, round chondrocytes line up vertically in short columns reminiscent of those in the physis. The proteoglycan content of the transitional and radial zones is greater than that of the superficial zone. The fourth recognizable zone in mature articular cartilage is the *calcified zone*, which is separated from the radial zone by an irregular basophilic line, referred to as the "*tidemark*." Although collagen fibrils do not cross from the calcified zone of articular cartilage into subchondral bone, the undulating nature of this osteochondral interface provides a strong attachment with considerable resistance to shearing forces. In immature animals, endochondral ossification beneath the articular cartilage contributes to the growth in size of the epiphysis. The metachromasia of cartilage matrix with stains such as toluidine blue is due to its glycosaminoglycan content. When proteoglycans are lost, metachromasia is reduced, the intercellular substance stains positively by the periodic acid-Schiff (PAS) method, and collagen fibers are more prominent.

Although the collagen component of articular cartilage is relatively stable, the *proteoglycan macromolecules are constantly being degraded and replaced*, perhaps as part of an internal remodeling system mediated by autodegradative enzymes. Various zinc-dependent metalloproteinases are secreted by the chondrocytes and cleave the core protein, link protein, and hyaluronan molecules at specific locations. The fragments diffuse into the synovial fluid then into the synovial membrane, where they are removed by lymphatics. Overactivity of these proteases may be responsible for cartilage degradation in degenerative joint disease and immune-mediated arthritis. Chondrocytes in articular cartilage must continually synthesize new matrix components in order to replace those that are degraded and lost. They respond to various soluble mediators, including synovial cytokines, such as tumor necrosis factor and interleukin-1, in addition to mechanical loading, changes in hydrostatic pressure and even to electric fields. A serine proteinase inhibitor and various collagenase inhibitors have been isolated from human and bovine articular cartilage. These are probably important in the regulation of extracellular matrix degradation.

Articular cartilage is devoid of blood vessels and nerves. The chondrocytes within articular cartilage therefore depend on diffusion of nutrients from synovial fluid through the extracellular matrix, except in immature animals where a proportion of the nutrients entering articular cartilage may diffuse through the relatively permeable subchondral bone. Because of the absence of nerve endings, damage to articular cartilage does not cause pain unless there is concomitant injury to the subchondral bone and/or joint capsule, both of which are well supplied with nerves. The surface of the cartilage appears to be porous, at least in macromolecular dimensions, and the diffusion of nutrients into cartilage is aided by the massaging effect of normal movement. It appears that the integrity of the cartilage is preserved only if joint movements are physiological in their range and pressure. *Sustained excesses of pressure and prolonged disuse accelerate degeneration.* The latter is of particular relevance in animals with limb fractures, where one or more joints may be immobilized by casting or external fixation. Such fixators should be left in place for the shortest time possible and, ideally, allow up to 10 degrees of joint motion.

The chemical composition of articular cartilage alters with advancing age. Although the collagen content remains relatively stable throughout life, the proteoglycan content slowly decreases from birth. The protein core and glycosaminoglycan chains are longer in immature animals than in adults and there is a rapid decline in the concentration of chondroitin-4 sulfate with aging. This is accompanied by a corresponding increase in the concentration of keratan sulfate.

The thin plate of **subchondral bone**, to which the articular cartilage is attached, is approximately *ten times more deformable than cortical bone*. This is important in allowing more even distribution of the load between the articular cartilage and the bone at times of peak loading. In chronic degenerative joint diseases, the subchondral bone may become denser. In such cases, the articular cartilage is required to bear an increased proportion of the burden and the degenerative process is accelerated. There is some debate as to whether thickening of the subchondral bone precedes degeneration of the articular cartilage in degenerative joint diseases, or occurs as a sequel, but it is likely that the two processes occur concurrently.

In some joints of cattle, horses, and pigs, nonarticulating depressions known as **synovial fossae** (Fig. 1.128) are present near the midline. These normal structures are bilaterally symmetrical and are acquired during the first months of postnatal life as a consequence of joint modeling. During skeletal growth, acquired incongruities in central areas of certain joints cause progressive loss of contact between apposing articular surfaces. While the superficial or gliding layer of the articular cartilage in these areas persists, chondrocytes in the deeper zones of the subarticular growth cartilage are not maintained and gradually disappear. Gradually, synovial fossae appear as central depressions having distinct borders and a smooth, blue to pink surface, reflecting the proximity of the subchondral capillary bed. A study in 50 swine found that synovial fossae were not present at birth, but were present commonly after 4–5 months of age on the articular surfaces of the scapula, distal humerus, proximal radius, distal radius, and distal surface of the intermediate carpal bone. *It is important that synovial fossae are not mistaken for lesions in the articular cartilage or as indicators of collapsed subchondral bone*. In general, they are of no significance, although in horses they may be structural points of weakness where infection can be passed between the joint cavity and the subchondral bone. In diseased joints, synovial fossae may become more prominent due to hyperemia of the synovium or the underlying epiphyseal bone.

An **articular capsule** surrounds each synovial joint and consists of an outer fibrous capsule and an inner synovial membrane. The **fibrous capsule** consists of parallel bundles of dense, fibrous connective tissue and merges with the periosteum of the bones on either side of the joint. This strong capsule restricts the range of movement possible between articulating bone ends and is supported in some areas by focal thickenings or **ligaments**. Intra-articular ligaments, such as the cruciate ligaments of the stifle, add further support in some joints. **Tendons** may also attach to the articular capsule, adding strength to areas that require it. Collagen fibers from ligaments and tendons may be attached to the fibrous capsule or may attach to bone at sites referred to as **entheses**. At these sites, collagen fibers from the tendon merge with zones of unmineralized then

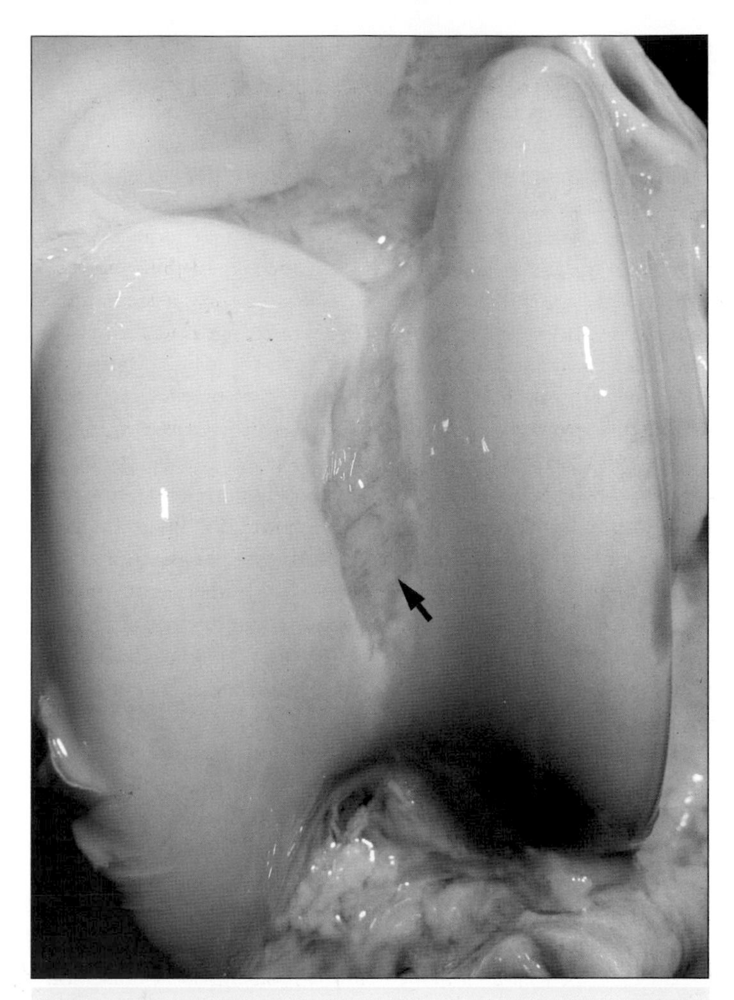

Figure 1.128 Synovial fossa (arrow) in the groove between articular condyles of the talus in a horse.

mineralized fibrocartilage, before becoming incorporated into bone as **Sharpey's fibers**. Entheses are well served by anastomosing blood vessels originating within the peritenon, perichondrium, and periosteum, and have a prominent nerve supply. Excessive tension on ligaments may lead to rupture of the ligament, or to an avulsion fracture, where a fragment of bone is detached with the enthesis intact. The latter is not uncommon in animals with rickets or fibrous osteodystrophy. The fibrous capsule is well supplied with blood vessels, lymphatics, proprioceptive nerves, and pain receptors. Thickening of the fibrous capsule in animals with chronic joint diseases leads to reduced motion or stiff joints but may be difficult to appreciate clinically or at necropsy.

In the *femorotibial joints* of domestic animals, *semilunar fibrocartilaginous disks, or* **menisci**, provide additional stability. These structures are firmly attached to ligaments, or to the fibrous layer of the joint capsule, and extend into the joint space between the articulating bone surfaces. Menisci are not lined by a synovial membrane but are innervated and have a blood supply. Similar, but more circular or oval structures, referred to as **articular disks**, *are present in the temporomandibular joint*. Articular disks may possess a central perforation. Intrameniscal calcification and ossification in the stifle joint occurs uncommonly in humans and has been reported in cats. Such lesions must be differentiated from intra-articular avulsion fractures or loose bodies in clinical radiographs.

The **synovial membrane** is a smooth, glistening, highly vascular layer that lines the inner surface of the fibrous capsule. It also covers any intra-articular ligaments or tendons and is reflected on intra-articular bone where it merges with the periosteum or the perichondrium, as the case may be. In the transition zone, it merges with the articular margins and spreads for a short distance over the non-weight-bearing articular cartilage. In some areas, particularly in recesses of the joint, the synovial membrane has many *small, villus projections,* which presumably permit expansion of the synovial membrane in association with joint movement or changes in intra-articular pressure. These synovial villi are not easily discerned macroscopically in normal joints but may become enlarged, hyperemic, and more numerous in some chronic inflammatory or degenerative diseases of joints. In addition, thickened folds of synovial membrane, often containing adipose tissue, extend into the joint cavity. These *fat pads* generally occupy depressions on the articular surface and are displaced during motion. Synovial membranes lining tendon sheaths and bursae are structurally similar to those lining diarthrodial joints.

The *synovial membrane generally consists of two layers,* a thin, cellular **intima** on the inner surface and a **subintima**, which contains variable quantities of areolar, adipose, and fibrous tissue. The loose fibrous connective tissue of the subintima merges with the dense fibrous capsule. The subintima is richly vascular, and contains many lymphatics and nerves, together with a small number of histiocytes. Dendritic cells similar to the antigen-processing Langerhans cells of skin have been identified in the synovium and have been shown to interdigitate with T-lymphocytes. Specialized post-capillary venules with cuboidal endothelial cells, referred to as *high endothelial venules,* allow lymphocytes to migrate easily from the blood into the subintima of the synovial membrane in certain inflammatory conditions. In areas where the synovial membrane lines intra-articular ligaments or tendons, the subintimal layer is usually attenuated or inapparent.

The synovial intima consists of *synoviocytes* forming an ill-defined layer, one to three cells deep. The cells vary in shape from fusiform to polygonal. No basement membrane exists between the synovial intima and subintima and the *synoviocytes are of mesenchymal rather than epithelial origin.* In some areas, the synoviocytes are closely packed, while elsewhere they are relatively sparse and the subintimal layer may be directly apposed to the joint cavity. Two types of synoviocytes, referred to as type A (macrophage-like) and type B (fibroblast-like) cells, are recognized on the basis of their morphology, function, and immunochemical staining. *Type A synoviocytes originate from the bone marrow and have phagocytic and antigen-processing functions.* Ultrastructurally, they resemble tissue macrophages, possessing a dense, heterochromatin-rich nucleus, many cytoplasmic vacuoles and poorly developed rough endoplasmic reticulum. They are primarily responsible for removing and degrading particulate matter from the joint cavity and possess antigen-processing properties. *Type B synoviocytes are probably of fibroblastic origin.* They have a well-developed Golgi apparatus, prominent rough endoplasmic reticulum and are responsible for the synthesis of hyaluronan in addition to matrix components, including collagen. They are also equipped with various enzymes capable of degrading cartilage and bone. Both cell types produce cytokines and other mediators. Cells with ultrastructural characteristics intermediate between types A and B synoviocytes, so-called *intermediate or type C cells,* have also been described.

The synovial membrane is freely permeable in either direction to molecules of small dimension, which may be removed by the capillaries and lymphatics. Larger particles are phagocytosed by type A synoviocytes. The removal of particulate matter from the joint and its deposition in the subintimal layer is a continuous process. Because of the long life span of type A synoviocytes, estimated to be from 3–6 months, phagocytosed particulate matter may persist in the synovium for long periods. When the volume is large, as may occur in diseased joints, its presence in the synovial membrane stimulates fibrosis of the capsule, contributing to the swelling and fixation of diseased joints. *The synovial membrane proliferates markedly in certain disease states,* and has considerable powers of regeneration following injury or synoviectomy. *In chronic synovitis, lymphocytes and plasma cells diffusely infiltrate the synovial membrane, and may accumulate in hypertrophic synovial villi.* The lymphocytes are sometimes arranged in follicles.

The transitional zone of the synovial membrane is characterized by a gradual merging of the synovial membrane with the periosteum and cartilage margin. The intima is well vascularized where it extends onto the cartilage surface and it is in this area that erosion, or alternatively lipping and osteophyte formation, often occurs in chronic arthritis and degenerative arthropathy. The transitional zone of the synovial membrane is also the initial site of synovial proliferation and development of the *vascular granulation tissue or* **pannus,** which sometimes spreads across the articular cartilage in chronically inflamed joints. Pannus may also develop from the marrow spaces of subchondral bone and extend onto the articular surface through defects in the cartilage. *This layer of granulation tissue interferes with the normal nutrition of articular cartilage and is capable of eroding and destroying cartilage through the activity of cytokines and collagenases.* Collagenases may be synthesized by cells in diseased synovial membranes, by granulation tissue, and by neutrophils in the synovial fluid. The collagens of the synovial membrane itself are generally resistant to these collagenases because of their cross-linking. Adhesion of pannus to opposing articular surfaces *may cause fibrous ankylosis* and, if bone is formed in the connective tissue, bony ankylosis results. Few animals are permitted to survive to the stage of bony ankylosis, but fibrous ankylosis occurs occasionally in pigs with mycoplasma arthritis and in other chronic arthritides. Bony ankylosis sometimes involves the intercarpal joints of racing horses.

Synovial chondromatosis (osteochondromatosis) is a syndrome characterized by the presence of *many nodules of hyaline cartilage, some of which may undergo ossification, in the synovial membrane* (Fig. 1.129). It is widely believed that these nodules develop by metaplasia, or even benign neoplasia, of mesenchymal elements in the synovium. An alternative hypothesis is that, at least in some cases, they are derived from fragments of cartilage eroded from a damaged articular surface as part of a pre-existing joint disease. Such fragments are capable of surviving, and growing, in the synovial fluid, which provides a nutritious culture medium. Some may attach and become embedded in the synovial membrane, where survival and proliferation of chondrocytes within fragments would also be expected. Some of these bodies then become vascularized and undergo endochondral ossification. Some human patients and animals with synovial chondromatosis also have either few or multiple loose bodies free within the synovial fluid. These could represent nodules that have developed within the synovial membrane and become detached, but it seems more likely that they are of articular cartilage origin and have grown within the joint space, as occurs in some animals with osteochondrosis. However, synovial

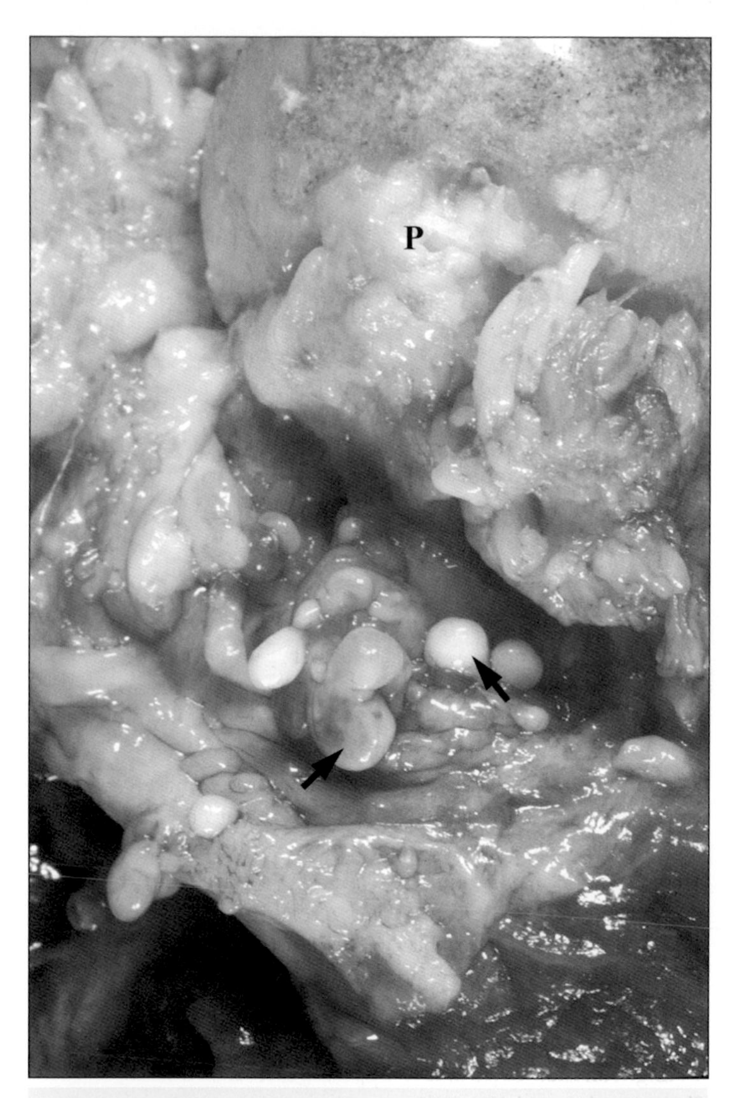

Figure 1.129 Synovial chondromatosis associated with degenerative joint disease in the hip of a dog. Several smooth, oval, cartilaginous nodules (arrows) are present within or attached to the synovium. Also note the villus hypertrophy, pannus formation (P), and eburnation of the femoral head. (Courtesy of RA Fairley.)

chondromatosis sometimes occurs in the absence of an underlying articular disease, or involves extra-articular structures such as bursae or tendon sheaths. Such cases, referred to as **primary synovial chondromatosis**, are more likely to be due to chondroid metaplasia of subsynovial fibroblasts, although the possibility that they are seeded by microscopic fragments of cartilage released from mildly damaged articular surfaces should be considered.

Synovial fluid is a viscous, clear, colorless or slightly yellow fluid, and is the main source of nutrients for articular cartilage. Essentially, *it is a dialysate of plasma, modified by the addition of hyaluronan, glycoprotein, and various other macromolecules by synoviocytes and other cells in the synovial membrane*. Electrolytes and small molecules such as glucose, lactate, and some small plasma proteins are able to move freely into and out of the synovial fluid through the synovial membrane, but large proteins such as fibrinogen are excluded. The viscous nature of synovial fluid reflects its high concentration of hyaluronan and varies between joints, as does the volume of fluid.

Hyaluronan is believed to function as a lubricant for the synovial membrane and periarticular tissues, but it probably plays little, if any part, in lubricating the motion between opposing cartilage surfaces. Lubrication of synovial joints under relatively light loading relies on the presence of the glycoprotein **lubricin**, which adheres to the surface of articular cartilage and binds a highly insoluble, **surface-active phospholipid** with strong lubricating properties. Recent studies have demonstrated that *it is the surface-active phospholipid, rather than lubricin, that actually lubricates the joint*. This is referred to as boundary lubrication. *Lubrication of articular surfaces under heavier loads depends on hydrostatic (weeping) lubrication*, which involves the seepage of water from the matrix when the cartilage is compressed. The water is squeezed onto the articular surface just ahead of the contact area and accumulates in the many minute depressions that are normally present. Once the compressive force is removed, the fixed charges within the cartilage attract the water and small solutes back into the matrix, and the cartilage returns to its original shape.

Normal diarthrodial joints contain only a very small volume of synovial fluid but the volume generally increases greatly in response to injury or inflammation. This is most likely due in part to increased vascular permeability in the synovial membrane following the release of inflammatory mediators such as prostaglandins and cytokines. The resulting increase in protein concentration of synovial fluid alters the normal oncotic balance and therefore fluid volume. In damaged joints, increased lymphatic drainage accelerates the clearance of proteins and cartilage breakdown products from synovial fluid.

Synovial fluid normally contains a small number of mononuclear cells and occasional free synoviocytes. Neutrophils and erythrocytes are uncommon unless the joint has been damaged, the synovial membrane is inflamed, or the sample has been contaminated with blood during collection. *The number of neutrophils increases markedly in both septic and nonseptic inflammatory diseases of the joint*. The synovial fluid may become turbid and less viscous depending on the number of neutrophils that are present.

Response of articular cartilage to injury

Because of its avascular nature and the absence of undifferentiated cells with the ability to respond to injury, *articular cartilage has only limited powers of regeneration*. The chondrocytes of mature articular cartilage show little if any sign of mitotic activity and have limited capacity for increasing matrix synthesis. Furthermore, their encasement in lacunae restricts their capacity to migrate to areas of damage. The regenerative potential of articular cartilage decreases even further with advancing age as the number of chondrocytes declines and the size of matrix proteoglycans decreases.

The response of articular cartilage to injury varies with the nature of the insult and with the depth of the lesion. *Superficial lacerations that do not penetrate the tidemark, and therefore fail to cause hemorrhage or inflammation, do not heal*. Chondrocytes adjacent to the lesion may proliferate, forming small clusters (*chondrones*), and may produce new matrix, but they do not migrate into the lesion. Within a few weeks of injury the chondrocyte response subsides, the lesion persisting for long periods but without progressing to chondromalacia or degenerative joint disease.

The repair of injuries that involve the full depth of the articular cartilage and penetrate subchondral bone differs markedly from the repair of superficial lesions. Hemorrhage occurs from blood vessels in the subchondral bone and the lesion becomes filled with a hematoma. Inflammatory cells and primitive mesenchymal cells invade the hematoma, probably under the influence of local growth factors, such as PDGF and TGF-β, derived from platelets and from the damaged bone. Within approximately 2 weeks of injury, some of the mesenchymal cells in the lesion have features of chondrocytes and begin to produce a matrix rich in proteoglycans, but also containing type II collagen. By 6–8 weeks, the defect is filled with fibrocartilage, which is firmly bonded to the adjacent hyaline articular cartilage. New bone formation occurs at the base of the lesion, restoring the subchondral bone plate, but the new bone does not extend into the area previously occupied by articular cartilage, remaining well below the articulating surface. The fibrocartilage repair tissue is analogous to the fibrous scar that repairs most other tissues and although it is an adequate replacement for articular cartilage at sites of deep injury, it does not perform as well when subjected to mechanical loading. In general, *most large defects in articular cartilage will eventually progress to degeneration after being filled with fibrocartilaginous repair tissue*. Early signs of degeneration may be present within a year of injury, although in some situations the repair tissue appears to function satisfactorily for a prolonged period and may become remodeled to more closely resemble normal articular cartilage. Interestingly, continuous passive motion of articular surfaces subjected to full-thickness injury has been shown to stimulate more rapid and successful healing of the articular cartilage than either complete immobilization or intermittent active motion.

Subchondral cystic lesions in horses are considered a manifestation of osteochondrosis, but in a recent study, similar lesions were induced experimentally by creating full-thickness defects in the articular cartilage and extending them 4 mm into the subchondral bone. Histologically, the lesions consisted of variable quantities of fibrous connective tissue, fibrocartilage, and bone. This study suggests that *trauma to weight-bearing surfaces, in addition to osteochondrosis, may predispose to subchondral cystic lesions in horses.*

Bibliography

Barrie HJ. Intra-articular loose bodies regarded as organ cultures in vivo. J Pathol 1978;125:163–169.

Behrens F, et al. Biochemical changes in articular cartilage after joint immobilization by casting or external fixation. J Orthop Res 1989;7:335–343.

Desjardins MR, Hurtig MB. Cartilage healing with emphasis on the equine model. Can Vet J 1990;31:565–572.

Doige C, Horowitz A. A study of articular surfaces and synovial fossae of the pectoral limb of swine. Can J Comp Med 1975;39:7–16.

Edwards JC. The origin of type A synovial lining cells. Immunobiology 1982;161:227–231.

Hamerman D. The biology of osteoarthritis. N Engl J Med 1989;320:1322–1330.

Johnston SA. Osteoarthritis: joint anatomy, physiology and pathobiology. Vet Clin North Am: Small Anim Pract 1997;27:699–723.

Morris NP, Keene DR, Horton WA. Morphology and chemical composition of connective tissue: cartilage. In: Royce PM, Steinmann B, eds. Connective Tissue and its Heritable Disorders. Molecular, Genetic and Medical Aspects. 2nd ed. New York: Wiley-Liss, 2002:41–65.

Muller-Ladner U, et al. Structure and function of synoviocytes. In: Koopman WJ, ed. Arthritis and Allied Conditions. 13th ed. vol 1. Baltimore, MD: Williams & Wilkins, 1996:243–254.

Poole AR. Cartilage in health and disease. In: Koopman WJ, ed. Arthritis and Allied Conditions. 13th ed. vol 1. Baltimore, MD: Williams & Wilkins, 1996:255–308.

Ralphs JR, Benjamin M. The joint capsule: Structure, composition, aging and disease. J Anat 1994;184:503–509.

Ray CS, et al. Development of subchondral cystic lesions after articular cartilage and subchondral bone damage in horses. Equine Vet J 1996;28:225–232.

Salter RB, et al. The biologic effect of continuous passive motion on the healing of full-thickness defects in articular cartilage. An experimental investigation in the rabbit. J Bone Joint Surg 1980;62-A:1232–1251.

Sandy JD, et al. Structure, function and metabolism of cartilage proteoglycans. In: Koopman WJ, ed. Arthritis and Allied Conditions. 13th ed. vol 1. Baltimore, MD: Williams & Wilkins, 1996:229–242.

Schwartz IM, Hills BA. Surface-active phospholipid as the lubricating component of lubricin. Br J Rheumatol 1998;37:21–26.

Whiting PG, Pool RR. Intrameniscal calcification and ossification in the stifle joint of three cats. J Am Anim Hosp Assoc 1985;21:579–584.

DEVELOPMENTAL DISEASES OF JOINTS

Osteochondrosis

Osteochondrosis is a common and important disease of pigs, horses, and large breeds of dog, but also occurs in cattle, sheep, and farmed deer. Young, fast-growing animals are most susceptible to osteochondrosis, especially breeds selected for rapid growth. The disease is most likely analogous to human osteochondrosis and to tibial dyschondroplasia in chickens and turkeys. It is characterized by multifocal abnormalities in endochondral ossification involving articular–epiphyseal cartilage complexes (the immature cartilage covering the ends of growing long bones) and growth plates. As such, osteochondrosis is not strictly a disease of joints, but since the clinical and pathological manifestations relate primarily to lesions in articular cartilage, it is included in this section. **Dyschondroplasia** is a more appropriate name for this disease as the initial lesion is in the growing cartilage, but the term osteochondrosis has become entrenched in the literature and a change in nomenclature is now unlikely to gain widespread acceptance. Other synonyms for the disease are **osteochondrosis dissecans** and **osteochondritis dissecans**. Such differences in terminology are due, at least in part, to the variation in lesions when examined at different stages. Severe degenerative joint disease is a common sequel to osteochondrosis and is one of the most common causes of lameness in domestic animals, especially in swine, horses, and certain large breeds of dog.

The *etiology and pathogenesis of osteochondrosis are poorly understood* and have been the subject of considerable recent debate, but valuable clues have emerged from studies in swine, horses, and dogs. The etiology is multifactorial, but most likely involves the effect of trauma or biomechanical factors on cartilage that has been weakened by nutritional or hormonal imbalances, vascular disruption, or genetic factors. Whatever the cause, the initial lesion in the articular–epiphyseal cartilage complex of each species where detailed studies have been performed are remarkably similar, *suggesting a common pathogenesis, most likely involving ischemic damage to the growing cartilage.*

In adult animals articular cartilage is avascular, relying on diffusion of nutrients from synovial fluid, but the articular–epiphyseal cartilage complex of immature animals depends on the presence of viable blood vessels within cartilage canals, at least for the first few months of life. These vessels, which appear to arise from the perichondrium, gradually disappear as the lumens of cartilage canals become filled with hyaline cartilage in a process referred to as *chondrification*. Investigation of the vascular supply to the femoral condyles of swine

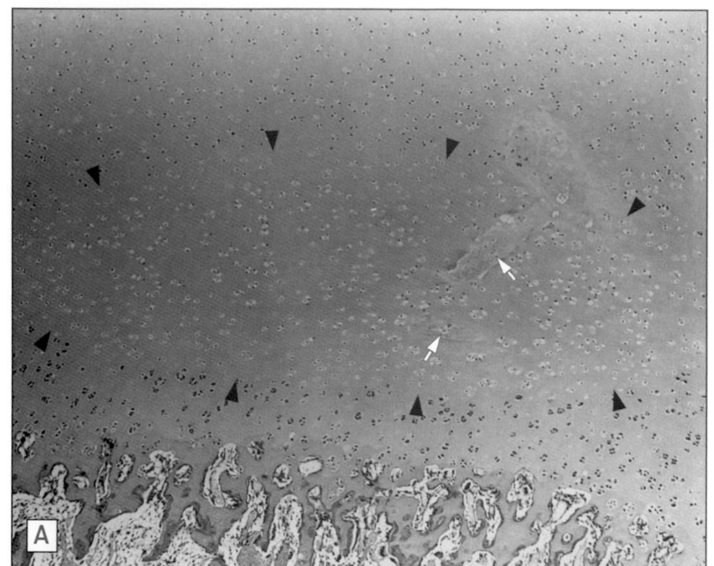

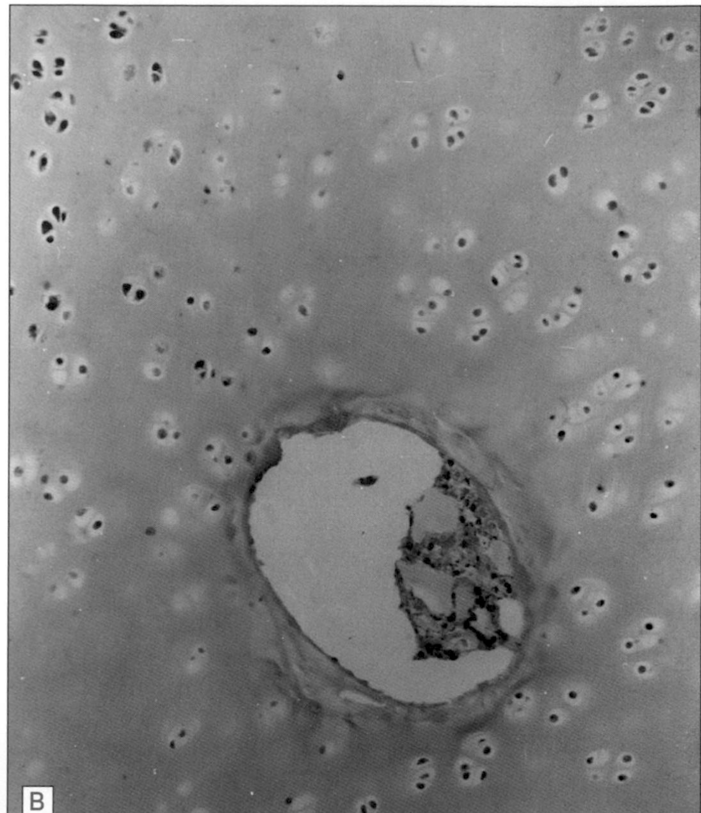

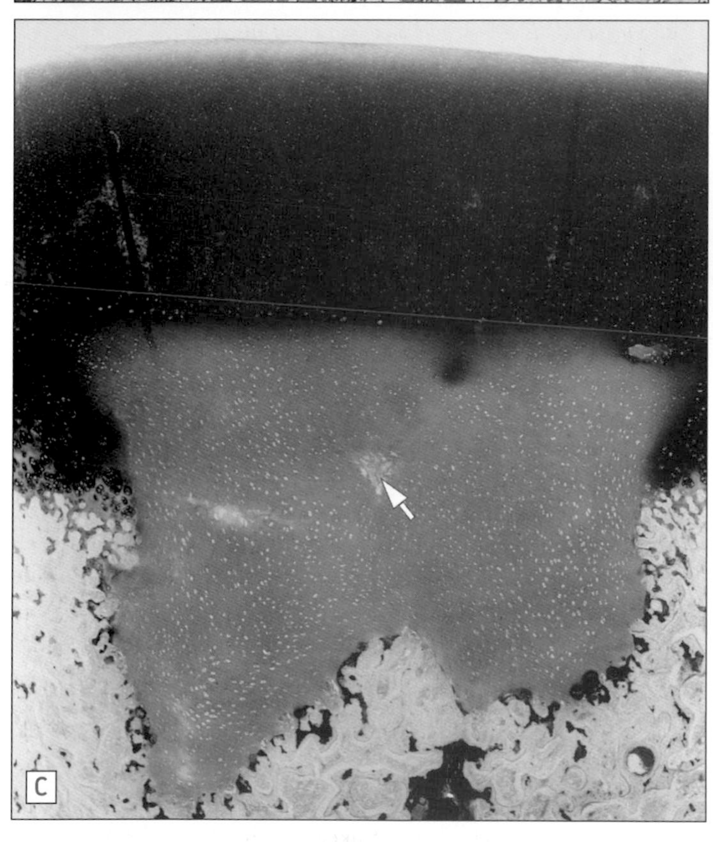

Figure 1.130 Osteochondrosis, pig. (Courtesy of CS Carlson.) **A.** Earliest lesion showing area of chondronecrosis (bounded by arrowheads) in epiphyseal cartilage immediately above the chondro-osseous junction. Necrotic cartilage canal vessels (arrows) are present in the necrotic zone. **B.** Closer view of necrotic cartilage canal vessel surrounded by necrotic cartilage. **C.** Focal area of necrotic cartilage and impaired endochondral ossification in the lateral femoral condyle of a young pig. Note the necrotic cartilage canal vessel (arrow). Section stained with alcian blue.

revealed that the cartilage of both condyles is fully vascularized at 2 weeks of age but that the blood supply recedes with maturity. By the time the pigs are 4–5 months of age the condyles are virtually avascular. In horses, cartilage canal blood vessels have disappeared from the articular–epiphyseal cartilage complex of the distal tibia by 3 months of age, and from the femoral condyles by 5 months.

Surgical interruption of the cartilage canal vascular supply in growing pigs at approximately 2 months of age results in necrosis of subarticular epiphyseal cartilage, but not of the overlying articular cartilage. This closely resembles the earliest lesion of osteochondrosis identified in the articular–epiphyseal cartilage complex of pigs and horses, wherein focal areas of cartilage necrosis and chondrolysis associated with necrotic cartilage canal blood vessels are confined to the epiphyseal cartilage and do not involve either the overlying articular cartilage or the subchondral bone (Fig. 1.130A, B). Similar early lesions have also been recognized in dogs and calves. These observations suggest that there is a risk period during which the epiphyseal cartilage of the articular–epiphyseal cartilage complex is dependent on the blood supply delivered by cartilage canal vessels. Disruption of the blood supply during this period in a young, rapidly growing animal may be the initial event in osteochondrosis. Local ischemia to this zone of developing cartilage would lead to necrosis, delayed endochondral ossification, and an extension of necrotic cartilage into the subchondral bone. Such lesions would not be expected to occur once the cartilage canals have closed and the cartilage is deriving its nutrients by diffusion from synovial fluid.

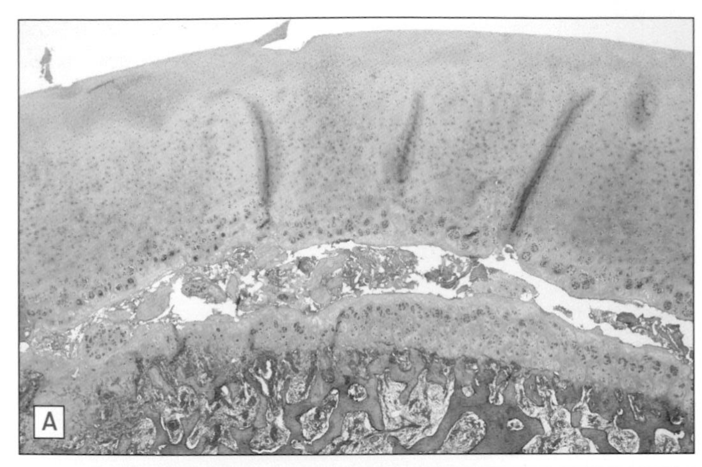

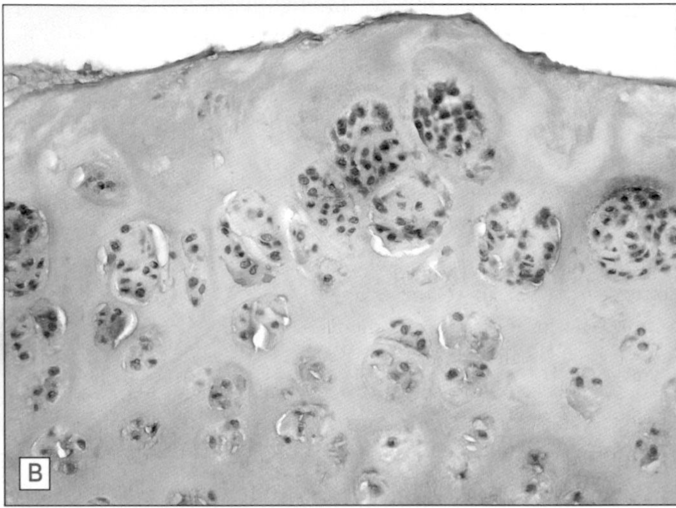

Figure 1.131 Osteochondrosis, foal. **A.** Horizontal cleft in deep layer of necrotic cartilage. **B.** Higher power of cartilage lining the cleft, showing acellular areas of chondronecrosis and many clusters of proliferating chondrocytes (chondrones) indicating a response to injury.

The presence of necrotic cartilage in the articular–epiphyseal cartilage complex induces *localized failure of endochondral ossification*. The necrotic cartilage does not mineralize or become invaded by blood vessels from the epiphyseal bone, and extends into the subchondral bone as ossification continues in adjacent, unaffected areas of cartilage (Fig. 1.130C). Small defects are unlikely to cause problems and no doubt heal spontaneously. Islands of necrotic cartilage left behind in the subchondral bone of the epiphysis are often found incidentally in various stages of repair. If the lesion is sufficiently large, clefts form in the deep layers of necrotic cartilage (Fig. 1.131A, B), presumably due to the trauma of weight bearing. The cleft may cause extensive underrunning of the articular cartilage and eventually join with the articular surface, creating a flap, which either remains attached or becomes separated, *forming a loose body or "joint mouse."* Loose bodies may survive and enlarge within the joint space, deriving their nutrients from the synovial fluid, and may even undergo endochondral ossification. Some become attached to the synovial membrane. At this advanced stage, the lesion is accompanied by inflammatory changes in the synovium and is often referred to as osteochondritis dissecans.

Another potential sequel of osteochondrosis involving the articular–epiphyseal cartilage complex is the *formation of subchondral cystic lesions* consisting initially of degenerate or necrotic cartilage, which is eventually replaced with fibrous tissue. This lesion, which appears to be most common in horses, will be discussed in more detail later in this section.

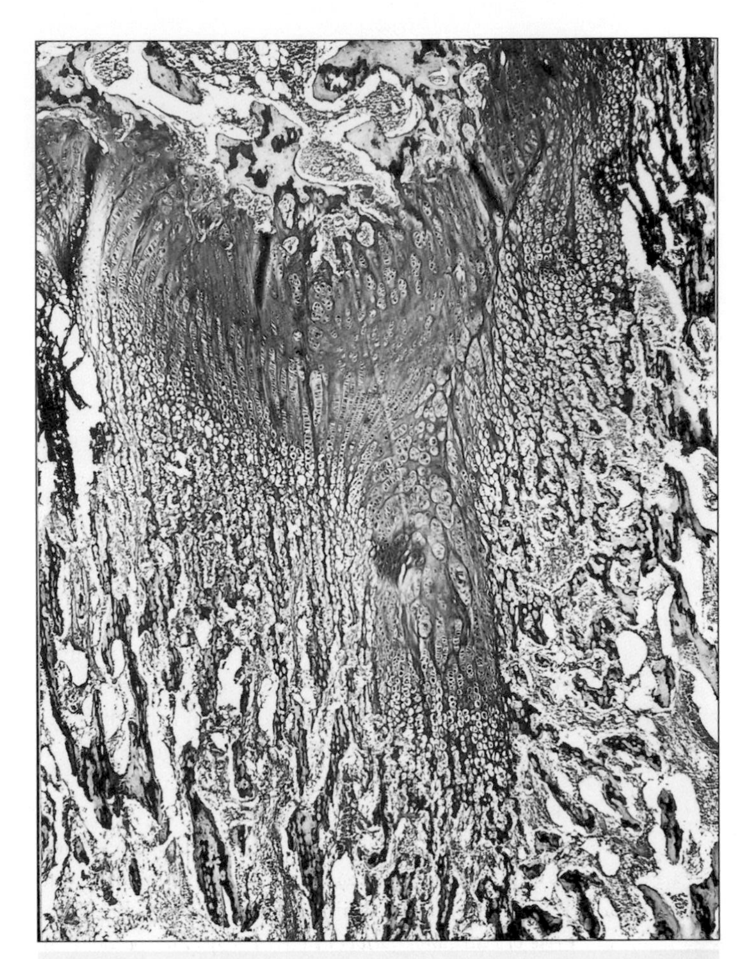

Figure 1.132 Focal retention of physeal cartilage (**metaphyseal dysplasia**) in osteochondrosis in a pig.

The physeal lesions of osteochondrosis differ morphologically from those involving the articular–epiphyseal cartilage complex, suggesting the possibility of a different pathogenesis. *Early lesions in the growth plate consist of cone-shaped foci of retained cartilage extending into the metaphysis* (Fig. 1.132), but rather than containing necrotic cartilage, these foci of metaphyseal dysplasia consist of viable hypertrophic chondrocytes. This does not exclude the possibility of an ischemic origin as experimental vascular disruption has been shown to induce similar changes in the growth plate of young pigs and lesions identical to tibial dyschondroplasia in chickens. It has also been suggested that these retained wedges of hypertrophic cartilage may be secondary to the development of trabecular microfractures in the primary spongiosa near the chondro–osseous interface. Such fractures would interfere with vascular invasion of the mineralized cartilage during endochondral ossification leading to persistence of hypertrophic zone chondrocytes. A similar mechanism has been proposed for the multifocal physeal thickening observed in Alaskan Malamute dogs with chondrodysplasia.

Although several possible causative factors have been incriminated in osteochondrosis, *there seems little doubt that the etiology is multifactorial*, and it is likely that differences between species exist. A *genetic predisposition* to osteochondrosis appears to exist in most species. This is at least partly related to the *predisposition for rapid growth*, as the prevalence is greatest in species and breeds where this attribute has been emphasized. Furthermore, in species other than pigs, the prevalence is higher in males than females, presumably due to their more rapid growth. The occurrence of many familial cases of osteochondrosis in humans, and the apparent increase in prevalence within certain genetic lines in animals, suggests that there is *also a direct genetic component to the disease*, at least in some cases. A heritability coefficient of 0.24–0.27 has been estimated from a study of Standardbred horses in Sweden.

Trauma almost certainly plays an important role, as supported by the increased prevalence of articular lesions at sites of greatest weight-bearing force. Furthermore, pigs housed on hard surfaces appear to have increased incidence and severity of the disease. Whether trauma alone is capable of causing osteochondrosis is questionable, but the forces associated with weight bearing and motion, when inflicted on large foci of degenerate or necrotic cartilage, would be expected to predispose to cleft formation and separation of cartilage flaps from subchondral bone. The role of trauma in the etiology of physeal lesions is difficult to determine, but compressive forces acting vertically on articular surfaces inevitably are transmitted through epiphyseal bones to the growth plate. This could damage the vascular supply to the physis, especially in young animals still dependent on transphyseal blood vessels within cartilage canals.

Rapid growth and optimal nutrition are considered necessary for the development of osteochondrosis in most animal species, but contradictory evidence has been obtained from experimental studies and *the exact role of nutritional factors in the etiology of osteochondrosis remains to be determined*. A comparison of weanling swine fed either 12% or 16% protein in their ration demonstrated a reduced growth rate in the former group but no reduction in the incidence of osteochondrosis. This does not however exclude the possibility that further reduction in growth rate may have been beneficial, as in this study all pigs in both groups developed lesions. In another study, swine fed a balanced ration at 70% of that of controls grew more slowly, and had less severe lesions of osteochondrosis than controls when slaughtered at the same weight (90 kg). However, a comparison of lesions in pigs from both groups when they were slaughtered at the same age (208 days) revealed that the lesion score was highest in pigs on the restricted ration. These data suggest that although restricted growth rate did not reduce the severity of osteochondrosis, there was some resolution of the lesions in pigs on the restricted ration by the time they reached slaughter weight.

Experimental prolonged excess of dietary calcium is reported to increase the prevalence and severity of osteochondrosis in susceptible breeds of dog but does not appear to influence the disease in pigs and its relevance to the naturally occurring disease is questionable. Increased dietary calcium is believed to result in hypercalcemia and hypergastrinemia, both of which would be expected to induce hypercalcitoninemia and impaired bone resorption, but suggestions that osteochondrosis results from this mechanism are speculative and unproven. Of more significance is the apparent link between primary or secondary copper deficiency and osteochondrosis in horses, pigs, and deer. *Low dietary copper or high dietary levels of copper antagonists, including zinc and molybdenum, have been associated with both experimental and natural osteochondrosis*. Calcium is also a copper antagonist thus providing a possible explanation for the reported effect of high dietary calcium on osteochondrosis in dogs. As a component of the enzyme lysyl oxidase, copper is involved in strengthening collagen molecules in articular cartilage, and other connective tissues, by the formation of intermolecular cross-links. Copper deficiency could therefore weaken articular cartilage and the walls of small blood vessels in cartilage canals, rendering them more susceptible to the forces of weight bearing or other trauma.

Various hormones have been implicated in the etiology of osteochondrosis. Growth hormone and somatomedins stimulate the activity of chondrocytes both in vitro and in vivo and have been shown experimentally to increase the severity of osteochondrosis lesions in the articular–epiphyseal cartilage complex of pigs. Furthermore, high levels of growth hormone are present in young dogs of large breeds at the stage where they are most susceptible to the development of osteochondrosis. Insulin and insulin-like growth factors I and II are also mitogenic for chondrocytes and may provide an explanation for the apparent link between osteochondrosis and the feeding of high-energy diets, which would be expected to induce hyperinsulinemia. Lesions resembling osteochondrosis with extensive underrunning of cartilage have occurred in horses following the administration of glucocorticoids. A possible link between copper and hormone levels has been suggested and warrants further investigation. Several hormones, including glucocorticoids, insulin, insulin-like growth factor-I, interleukin-1, estrogen, and progesterone have been shown to alter metallothionein synthesis and are therefore capable of altering copper metabolism. Furthermore, growth hormone has been shown to reduce copper retention in pigs. This may help to explain the increased incidence of osteochondrosis in rapidly growing young animals.

Thrombosis of small blood vessels within cartilage canals has been suggested as a possible cause of ischemia to the articular–epiphyseal cartilage complex and to physeal cartilage. Lipid emboli were observed in the lumen of these vessels in one study, but their origin and significance is not known. Fibrin thrombi occurring in association with bacteremia or septicemia could also cause thrombosis of cartilage canal vessels. It is unlikely however that the majority of cases of osteochondrosis occur by this mechanism.

Because of differences between species in the nature and distribution of lesions, and their sequelae, it is appropriate to consider each species separately.

1. **Swine** As in other species, *microscopic lesions of osteochondrosis in swine are far more common than clinical signs or gross examination at necropsy would suggest*. In some studies, up to 100% of rapidly growing young pigs had microscopic changes of osteochondrosis in their growth plates or articular–epiphyseal cartilage complexes. Clearly, the vast majority of such lesions heal uneventfully and only those that are sufficiently large, or subjected to excessive trauma, progress to become clinically significant. At this stage, gross lesions are likely to be present in one or several joints. *Predilection sites in pigs* are the joint surfaces of the medial humeral and femoral condyles, anconeal process, lumbar vertebrae, mediodistal part of the talus, humeral head, glenoid cavity of the scapula, distal ulna, and dorsal acetabulum. *Physeal lesions* occur most commonly in the distal ulna, distal femur, costochondral junctions, femoral and humeral heads, thoracolumbar vertebrae, and the ischial tuberosity.

   The articular lesions of osteochondrosis are often bilateral, and may be symmetrical. It is important to distinguish them from synovial fossae, which are present as normal structures in some joints. *Early articular lesions* appear as thickened, white or cream foci of articular cartilage, which are sharply demarcated from adjacent normal areas of cartilage. In some cases the articular cartilage, which is not directly affected in osteochondrosis, will be depressed or wrinkled due to collapse of necrotic cartilage in the underlying articular–epiphyseal cartilage complex. *In more advanced lesions, the affected cartilage usually shows evidence of separation and underrunning* (Fig. 1.133), and there may be nodules of cartilage reflecting attempts at repair. In other cases, *underrun segments of articular cartilage may be detached completely, leaving a deep ulcer with exposure of subchondral bone* (Fig. 1.134). Lesions of this type are referred to as **osteochondritis dissecans** and occur most frequently on weight-bearing surfaces of the medial condyles of the humerus and femur in pigs of 5–7 months of age. In such cases, large fragments of articular cartilage may be present within the joint space. Since these so-called loose bodies or joint mice obtain nutrients by diffusion from synovial fluid, they can survive and grow within the joint, and may be larger than the defect from which they originated. The dissecting lesion does not involve bone but sometimes flaps of cartilage contain osseous tissue. This probably develops by endochondral ossification following invasion of vessels and cells from the area of attachment. The defect in the articular surface is initially filled with vascular connective tissue, which eventually is converted to fibrocartilage. Even if a dissecting lesion does not result, hemorrhage and fibrosis may occur in the subchondral bone and the resulting localized radiolucent area may be the basis for one type of "bone cyst" in osteochondrosis. *Degenerative arthropathy is common in the late stages of the disease*, but evidence that osteochondrosis was involved may no longer be apparent grossly. Even histologically, the changes may be too altered by secondary changes to reflect the initial lesion. Synovial villi may be enlarged and mild lymphoplasmacytic inflammation with scant fibrinous exudate may be present in the synovium, but these changes are nonspecific.

Severe **growth plate lesions** associated with osteochondrosis may appear grossly as thickened foci. *Microscopically these foci, which are sometimes referred to as metaphyseal dysplasia, consist of persistent hypertrophic chondrocytes* (Fig. 1.132) and are associated with delayed mineralization. *Such lesions are similar to those of rickets* and may present a diagnostic challenge to the pathologist, especially since trabecular microfractures in the primary spongiosa may also occur in osteochondrosis and imply an underlying metabolic bone disease. In osteochondrosis, the mineralization failure is transient

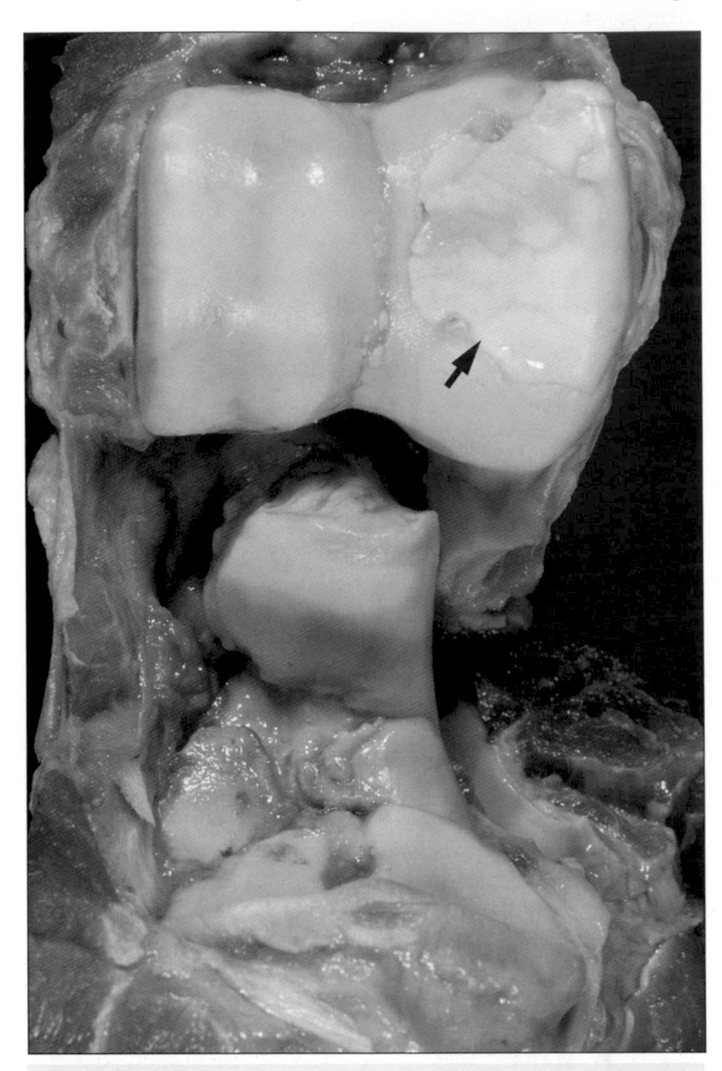

Figure 1.133 Osteochondrosis, pig. Elbow joint. Large area of thickened, underrun articular cartilage (arrow) on the medial humeral condyle, sharply demarcated from adjacent normal cartilage. (Courtesy of RA Fairley.)

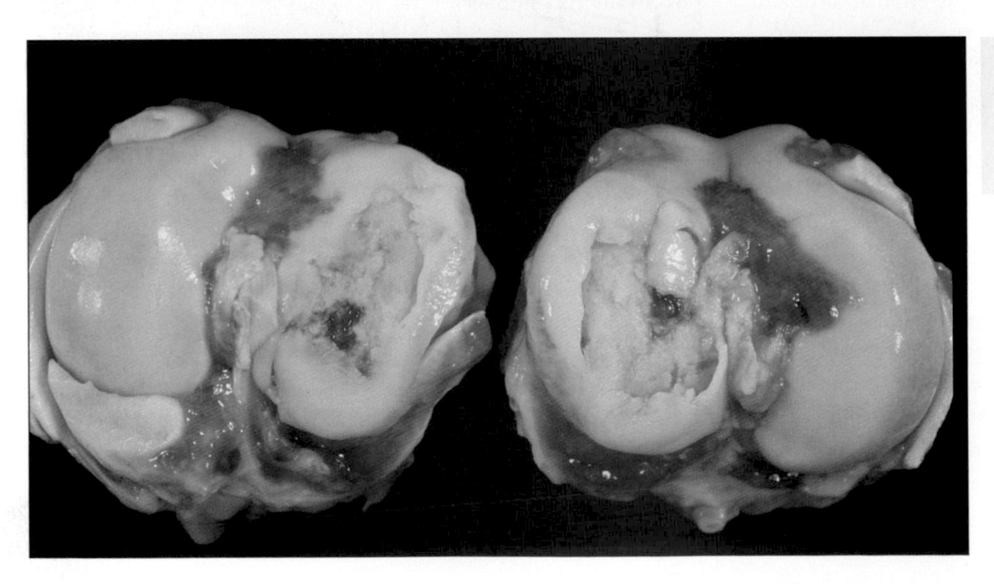

Figure 1.134 Osteochondrosis, pig. Bilateral detachment of articular cartilage on medial femoral condyles with exposure of subchondral bone. Lesions of this type are referred to as **osteochondritis dissecans**. (Courtesy of RA Fairley.)

and focal, and there is no evidence of delayed mineralization of osteoid, as occurs in rickets. The fate of these metaphyseal lesions is varied. Some undergo relatively normal ossification, others persist as nodules of cartilage in the metaphysis, while many degenerate and are replaced by fibrous tissue in which woven bone or fibrocartilage develops.

Irregular eosinophilic streaks, associated with areas of disorganized growth plate architecture, also occur in osteochondrosis (Fig. 1.135A). These may reflect either vestiges of cartilage canals or infraction lines occurring as a sequel to growth plate trauma. Similar eosinophilic streaks are normally present in the growth plates of young animals but are usually parallel to cartilage columns. In osteochondrosis they are often stellate and may subdivide the physeal cartilage into disorganized, sometimes degenerate, lobules. *Bony bridges*, uniting the epiphysis and metaphysis and effectively closing the growth plate at that location, may develop at sites of physeal degeneration (Fig. 1.135B). *Angular limb deformity* resulting from premature closure of a growth plate on one side and continued growth on the other is a potential sequel to this lesion but appears to be less common in pigs than in other species.

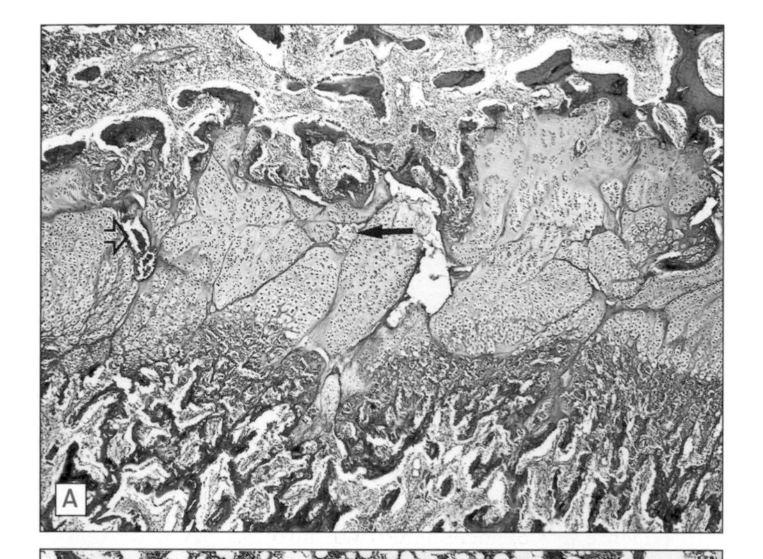

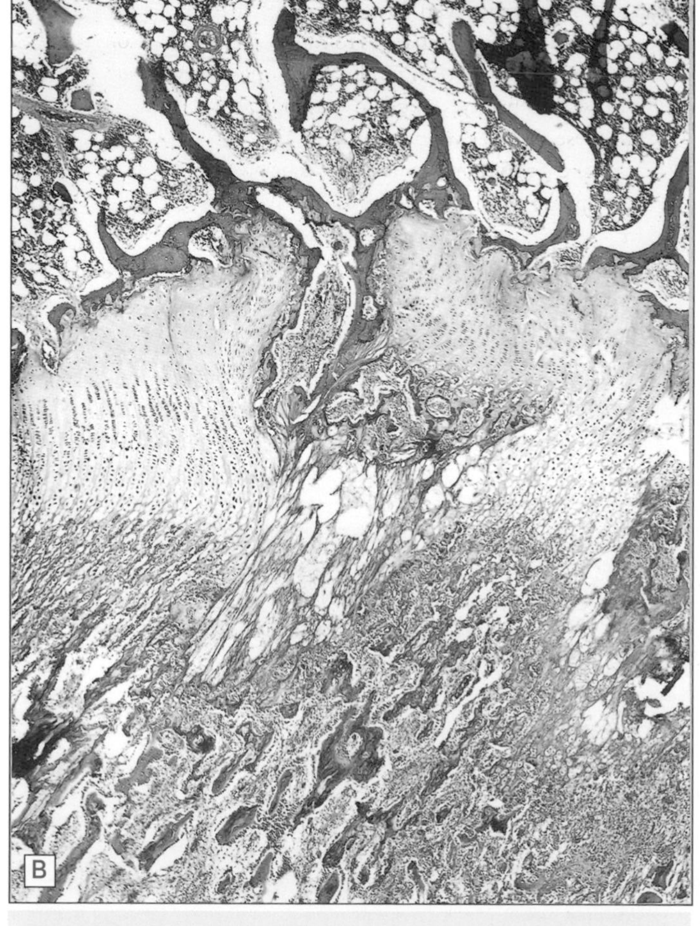

Figure 1.135 Osteochondrosis, pig. **A.** Eosinophilic streaks and focal cavitation (arrow) in a disorganized physis. **B.** Focal degeneration of the physis with formation of a bony bridge between the epiphysis and metaphysis.

Another manifestation of osteochondrosis in swine is **epiphysiolysis**, *the separation of an epiphysis from metaphyseal bone.* This is a traumatic lesion, predisposed to by a defect in growth cartilage of the physis, and probably develops either from an extended eosinophilic streak or from areas of necrosis in the growth cartilage, rather than from foci of metaphyseal dysplasia. *The common sites for epiphysiolysis are femoral head* (Fig. 1.136*), ischiatic tuberosity of females, and lumbar vertebrae.* The distal epiphysis of the ulna and the anconeal process may also be involved, although strictly speaking the lesion involving the latter should not be called epiphysiolysis. In pigs, unlike dogs, the anconeal process does not develop from a separate ossification center, so **apophysiolysis** is a more appropriate term. Separation may be complete, as is often the case with the ischiatic tuberosity, or partial, as occurs in the head of the femur, which sometimes remains attached at its lateral margin. Separation probably occurs when the process of endochondral ossification reaches or approaches the cartilage defect. The resulting fracture may extend in a jagged crack through primary and secondary spongiosa.

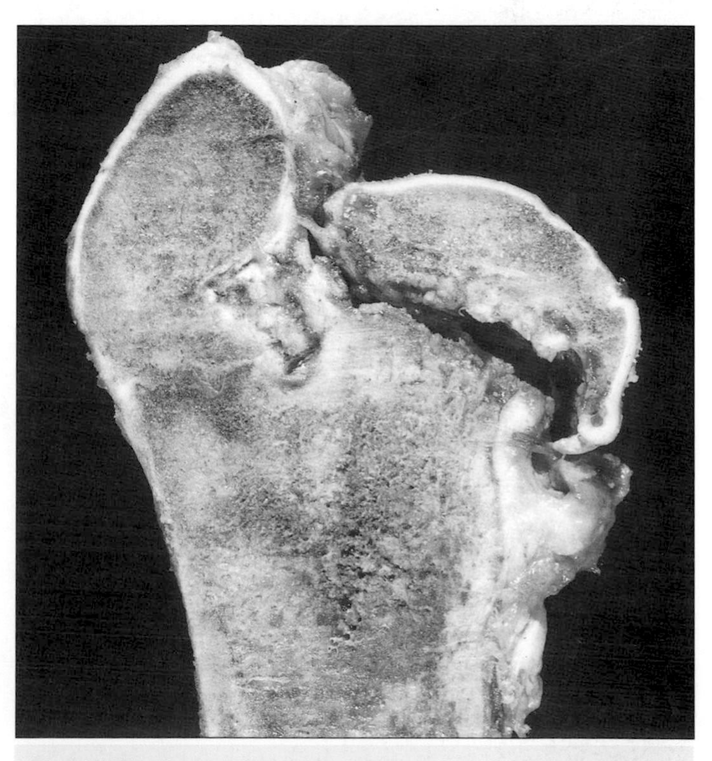

Figure 1.136 Osteochondrosis, pig. Epiphysiolysis of the femoral head.

2. **Dogs** *Osteochondrosis in dogs includes several orthopedic diseases, usually occurring in young fast-growing males of large and giant breeds.* Osteochondritis dissecans of the shoulder joint is the classic presentation of the disease, but similar lesions may also occur in other major joints. In addition, *ununited anconeal process and fragmented coronoid process* are believed to be manifestations of osteochondrosis in dogs.

The major predilection site for **osteochondritis dissecans** *in dogs is the caudal aspect of the humeral head.* In susceptible breeds, lesions are common between 4 and 8 months of age and are bilateral in approximately 70% of cases. Many lesions resolve spontaneously but others progress to cause severe lameness due to degenerative joint disease. As in pigs, *early lesions* are visible grossly as discrete gray/white or cream foci in the articular surface representing areas of thickened or underrun cartilage (Fig. 1.137A, B, C). Flaps of cartilage often detach from these sites and form loose bodies, leaving large ulcers that are gradually filled with fibrocartilage. Healing of such defects is never perfect and partly healed lesions of osteochondritis dissecans are often detected several months, or even years, later in the shoulder joints of dogs with chronic degenerative joint disease (Fig. 1.138). Such lesions may also be found incidentally, reflecting their high prevalence in certain breeds and the fact that they are not always symptomatic.

Osteochondritis dissecans also occurs in several other locations in dogs, including the medial aspect of the humeral condyle, the lateral, and less frequently the medial, condyle of the femur, and the medial trochlear ridge of the tibial tarsal bone. Lesions at these sites can be bilateral and may either cause lameness at a young age when the lesion are active, or predispose to degenerative joint disease.

Lesions in the humeral condyle form part of the **elbow dysplasia syndrome**, *which also includes ununited anconeal process and fragmented (ununited) medial coronoid process of the ulna.* The latter two conditions may also occur separately (see below), or in other combinations. Together the three lesions, which are often bilateral, cause foreleg lameness in young, usually large, growing dogs and often lead to arthropathy associated with periarticular osteophytes. The elbow dysplasia syndrome is characterized by incongruity of the joint caused by a step between the cranial margin of the proximal ulna and the caudal margin of the proximal radius. An increase in length of the proximal ulna is responsible for the incongruity and results in disruption of the normal continuous curve made by the profile of the trochlear notch of the ulna and the articular cartilage of the radius. Trauma from normal use most likely precipitates lesions.

Ununited anconeal process, which develops as an *epiphysiolysis*, is most common in the German Shepherd, but also occurs in other large and giant breeds. The ossification center of the anconeal process develops at about 11–13 weeks and expands for about 6 weeks until osseous union with the ulna is achieved by 4–5 months. If extensive fissures develop in the bipolar growth cartilage between the process and the ulnar diaphysis, normal plate closure does not occur and a fibrocartilaginous or fibrous union results.

Ununited (or fragmented) medial coronoid process of the ulna is less well known, but apparently more common, than ununited anconeal process. The coronoid process does not develop from a separate ossification center and is not easily seen in radiographs. Usually the first indications of disease are osteophytes around the anconeal process and the medial epicondyle of the humerus. Golden and Labrador Retrievers and Rottweilers are particularly prone to this condition. *In affected dogs, the medial coronoid process consists of one or several fragments, which may be in their normal position or completely separated from the articular surface of the proximal ulna as joint mice.* Lesions begin as vertical fissures in the proximal face of the articular cartilage and extend into the subchondral bone. They may reach the vertical joint surface or the area of insertion of the annular ligament.

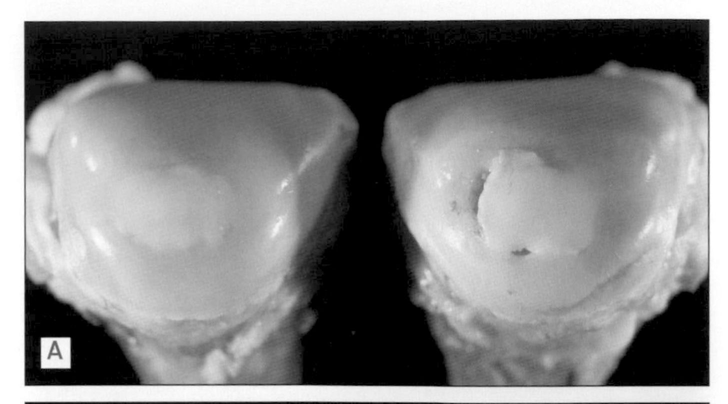

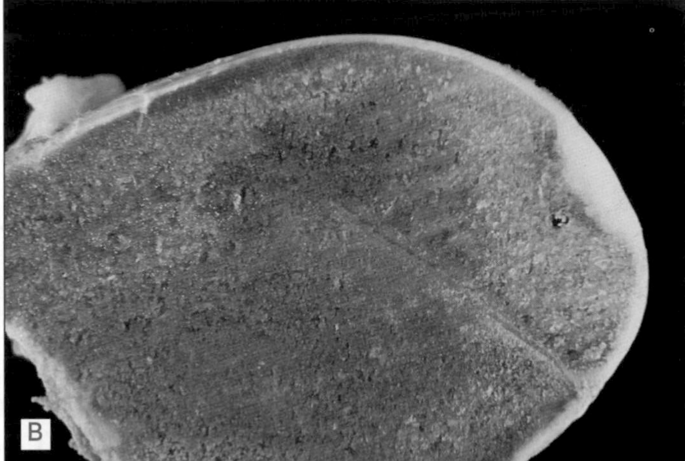

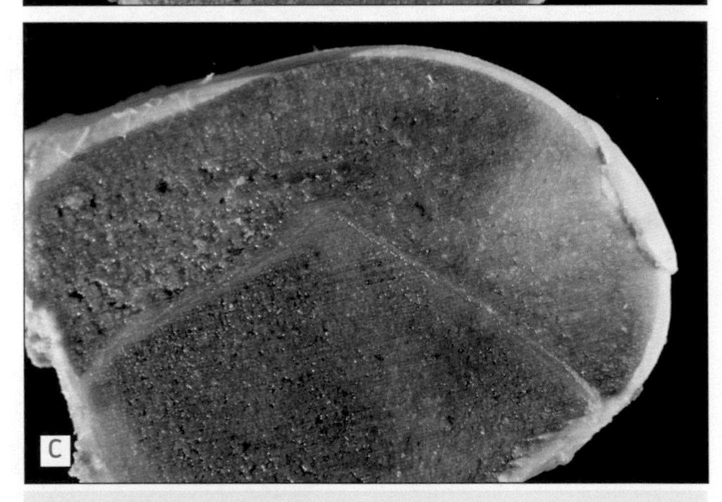

Figure 1.137 Osteochondrosis, dog. **A.** Early, bilateral lesions involving the caudal aspect of the humeral head in a 5-month-old Irish Wolfhound. **B, C.** Sagittal sections of the lesions shown in (**A**). In (**B**) the articular cartilage is thickened, while in (**C**) the thickened cartilage has become detached from the subchondral bone.

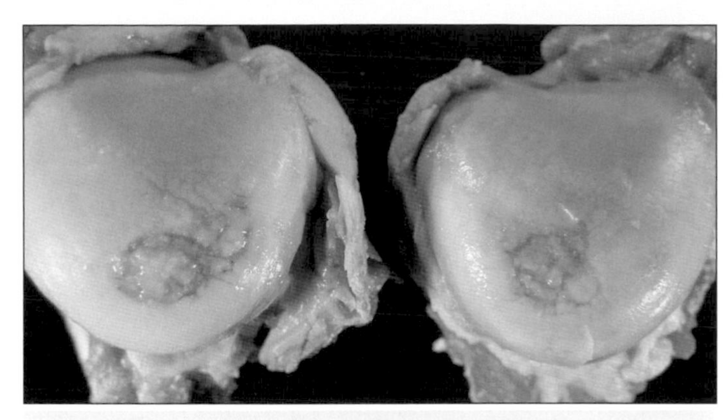

Figure 1.138 Partly healed lesions of **osteochondritis dissecans** in both humeral heads of a 4-year-old Great Dane with degenerative joint disease of both shoulder joints.

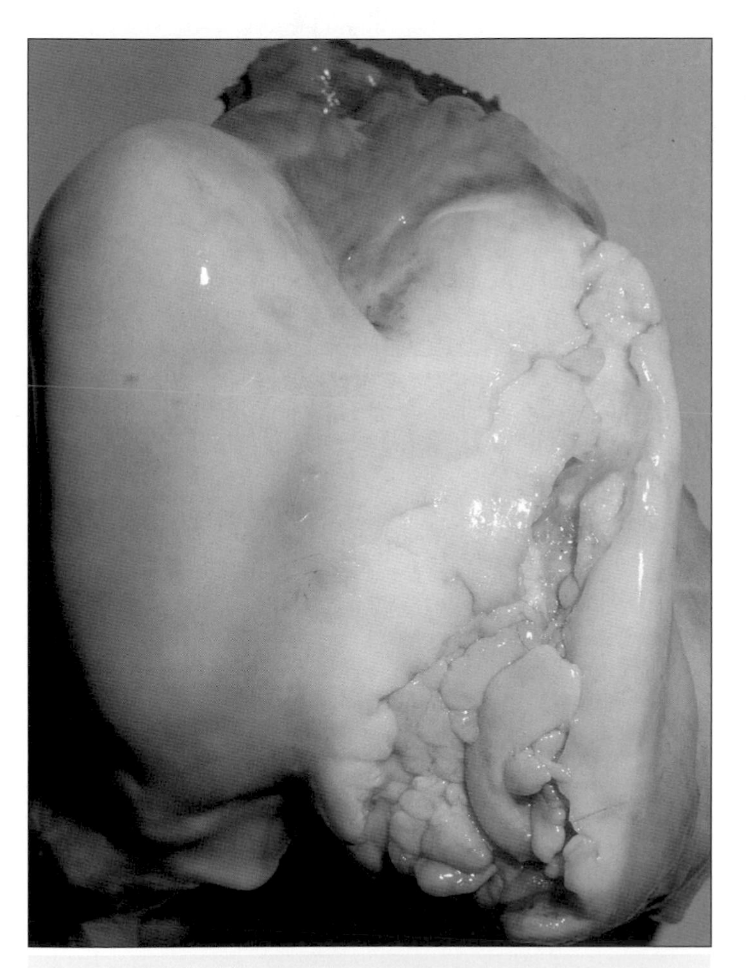

Figure 1.139 Osteochondrosis, horse. Extensive underrunning and displacement of articular cartilage on the lateral trochlear ridge of a 6-month-old foal. The many small cartilage nodules represent attempts at repair.

When complete separation of the fragment or fragments does not occur, the walls of the fissure become lined by fibrocartilage.

Other conditions in dogs, which are probably manifestations of osteochondrosis, include *retained cartilage core of the distal ulna* (Fig. 1.55A, B), and *slipped capital femoral epiphysis*. Retained cartilage cores also develop in the other long-bone metaphyses and may lead to growth deformities of the distal femur and proximal tibia. Canine hip dysplasia has been suggested as a possible manifestation of osteochondrosis but because of doubts over this classification, the disease is considered separately.

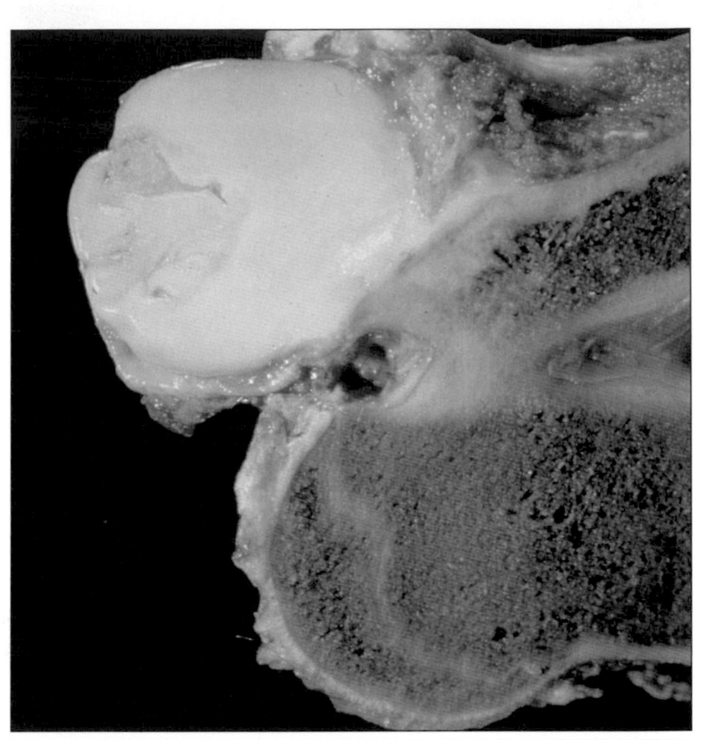

Figure 1.140 Osteochondrosis, horse. Flaps of detached cartilage on an articular facet of a cervical vertebra in a foal.

3. **Horses** Osteochondrosis is an important skeletal disease in horses of several breeds, and its incidence worldwide appears to be increasing. The term **developmental orthopedic disease** has been used to group osteochondrosis with several other skeletal diseases of young horses, some of which may occur as a sequel to, or as different manifestations of osteochondrosis. *These include osteochondritis dissecans, physitis, subchondral bone cysts, angular limb deformities, and wobbler syndrome.*

Although the lesions of osteochondrosis in horses may be widespread, there are several *predilection sites*, including the lateral trochlear ridge (Fig. 1.139) and medial condyle of the femur, the patella, the dorsal edge of the sagittal ridge of the distal tibia, and various sites in the tarsal and fetlock joints. In these locations, the pathogenesis of lesions is probably similar to that described earlier. Ossification of attached cartilage flaps seems to be more common in the horse than in other species. Lesions of osteochondrosis may also involve articular processes of cervical vertebrae (Fig. 1.140). Healing of such lesions may be characterized by formation of exostoses, which encroach on the spinal canal, or create asymmetry of articular facets, thus predisposing to wobbler syndrome.

Osteochondrosis in horses has been incriminated as a *predisposing lesion in the development of* **subchondral cystic lesions**, which are most common on the distal aspect of the medial femoral condyle (Fig. 1.141), distal aspect of the metacarpus, in addition to the carpus, elbow, and phalanges. It is suggested that subchondral cysts may develop from invaginations of articular cartilage, remnants of necrotic cartilage derived from the articular–epiphyseal cartilage complex, or in response to leakage of synovial fluid into subchondral bone through defects in articular cartilage. Such

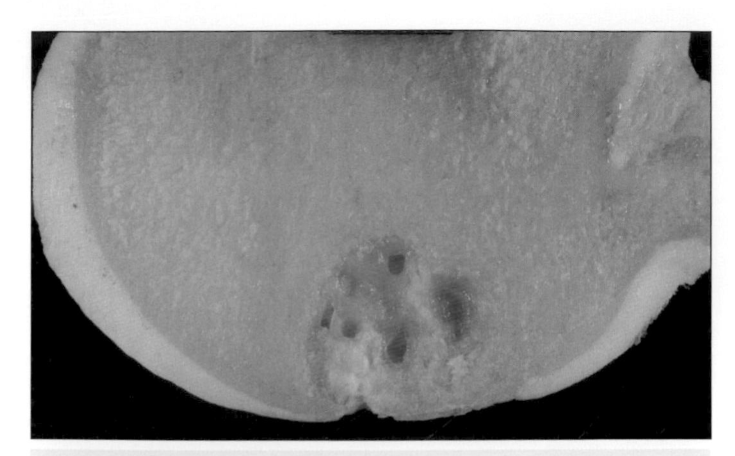

Figure 1.141 Osteochondrosis, horse. Subchondral cystic lesion in the medial femoral condyle. (Courtesy of NC State University.)

lesions have also been reproduced experimentally in young horses following traumatic damage to the articular cartilage and its supporting subchondral bone, suggesting that not all subchondral cysts are related to osteochondrosis. Histologically, the cysts usually consist of variable quantities of fibrous tissue and fibrocartilage, and are surrounded by sclerotic bone trabeculae.

Focal thickening of the growth plate, similar to metaphyseal dysplasia of pigs, is recognized as a manifestation of osteochondrosis in young foals. **"Physitis"** *or* **"epiphysitis"** *are commonly used clinical terms to describe these lesions, but both are misleading as the lesions are not inflammatory in origin.* The latter term is particularly inappropriate since the epiphysis is not involved. The lesions are thought to predispose to premature closure of growth plates and therefore *may induce angular limb deformity*. Epiphysiolysis is seldom reported in horses as a manifestation of osteochondrosis but has been described recently involving the physes of all cervical vertebrae from C3 to C7 in a 16-month-old filly.

Foals with congenital and neonatal angular limb deformities sometimes have concomitant hypoplasia of carpal bones and osteochondritis dissecans. These early lesions may both be manifestations of defective growth and maturation of cartilage. Lesions consistent with osteochondrosis were found at necropsy in the tarsal joints of 36 of 50 young horses with *spavin*, suggesting that osteochondrosis may be an important cause of this condition, at least in young animals.

Lesions of the palmar surface of the distal end of the metacarpal in adult racing Thoroughbreds are often discussed with the osteochondroses. These defects develop on the articular surface in contact with the proximal sesamoids. The *initial lesion* consists of fracture and necrosis of the subchondral bone, probably secondary to the trauma of hard running. With rest, *the fracture may heal* since articular cartilage above the fracture, nourished by synovial fluid, remains viable and probably holds the bone fragment in place. Collapse of subchondral tissues causes depression of the intact articular cartilage, but revascularization and healing may occur. On occasion, the complete fragment breaks free and this type of osteochondritis dissecans is analogous to some of the lesions described in man. The fact that horses so affected are adults, and are athletes in hard training, suggests that these lesions of the palmar surfaces of metacarpals *should be classified with stress fractures* rather than with osteochondrosis.

The relationship between copper deficiency and osteochondrosis in horses is compelling. Lesions indistinguishable from naturally occurring osteochondritis dissecans were reproduced experimentally in foals weaned from their dams at birth and fed on copper-deficient milk. Furthermore, there are several reports of similar lesions occurring in different parts of the world in foals grazing either copper-deficient pasture or pasture contaminated with the copper antagonists zinc and cadmium. Neonatal foals obtain copper primarily from milk, and yet mare's milk normally contains low copper concentrations and does not respond to supplementation. Foals born with inadequate hepatic copper reserves may therefore develop copper deficiency at an early age unless supplemented. Interestingly, supplementation of mares during late pregnancy and of their foals from 90 to 180 days of age appeared to reduce the prevalence and severity of osteochondrosis, even though unsupplemented control animals were fed at a level slightly above National Research Council recommended levels. There are also claims that copper supplementation has a palliative effect on established lesions of osteochondrosis. Possible mechanisms by which copper deficiency might predispose to osteochondrosis were discussed earlier in this section. Clearly, further work is needed in order to determine the precise role of copper in the etiology of osteochondrosis in horses and other species.

4. **Cattle** There are only occasional reports of osteochondrosis in cattle, but *the disease is likely to be much more common in this species than is currently recognized.* Due to financial constraints and difficulties in detailed radiologic examination, many lame cattle are sent for slaughter without definitive diagnosis. In a survey of middle-aged bulls slaughtered for nonmedical reasons, lesions of osteochondrosis were detected in the stifle joint of three of 25 animals in the absence of clinical lameness. Degenerative joint disease was detected in the stifle of 14 of the 25 bulls and although these lesion were too advanced to accurately determine their origin, the fact that the lesions identified as osteochondrosis, and those of degenerative joint disease both had a predilection for the lateral trochlear ridge, suggested that at least some cases of degenerative joint disease in this population of bulls were secondary to osteochondrosis. Other predilection sites for osteochondrosis in cattle are the humeral head, distal radius, elbow joint, and the tibial tarsal and occipital condyles.

Lesions characterized by focal thickening and chondrolysis are described in the growth cartilage of the articular–epiphyseal cartilage complex in young calves, *suggesting that the pathogenesis of the articular lesions in cattle is the same as in other species.* An association has been made between high-energy concentrate feeding and osteochondrosis in cattle, but the syndrome has also been reported in unsupplemented beef cattle grazing pasture. A possible genetic predisposition was suggested in the latter report.

Physeal lesions similar to those in pigs with osteochondrosis are described in the metacarpal and metatarsal bones of fast-growing, grain-fed, housed calves. In many cases, radiographic lesions characterized by focal thickening of the growth plate are accompanied by lameness and postmortem examination has revealed eosinophilic streaks and focal persistence of the hypertrophic zone. Disruption of the growth plate with bony bridging between the metaphysis and epiphysis is also recorded in affected calves. Hard floors apparently increase the number and severity of lesions, supporting the role of trauma in susceptible animals.

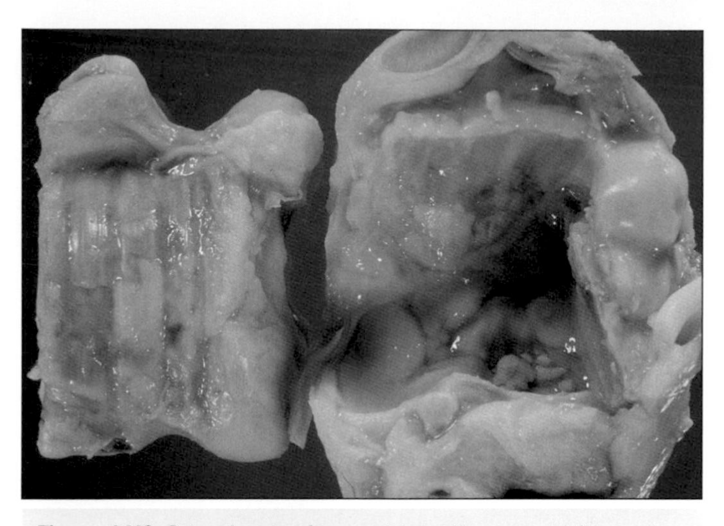

Figure 1.142 Osteochondrosis associated with copper deficiency in a farmed red deer. Extensive erosion of articular cartilage on the plantar surface of the talus and its opposing articular surface. Only small islands of cartilage remain and there are deep linear grooves in the exposed subchondral bone.

5. **Deer** *A strong association is recognized between osteochondrosis and copper deficiency in farmed red deer and wapiti x red deer hybrids in New Zealand.* On some farms, more than 30% of the fawns are affected. Lameness may be noticed as early as 1 month of age, but more commonly, the problem is not noticed until weaning at around 4 months of age. *Epiphysiolysis of the femoral head* is a common manifestation of the disease and may be bilateral. Animals with this lesion are severely lame and may adopt a "bunny-hopping" gait or "cow-hocked" stance. Other predilection sites are the carpal, hock (Fig. 1.142), and stifle joints. The lesions are usually bilateral. Affected deer invariably have low serum and/or liver copper concentrations and the disease can be prevented by copper supplementation of pregnant hinds.
6. **Sheep** Osteochondrosis appears to be *rare* in sheep, but has been reported as a cause of lameness in young, rapidly growing, Suffolk ram lambs. It is likely that the incidence of osteochondrosis in sheep will increase with continued selection for rapid growth. Microscopic lesions are common in growth plates of fast-growing lambs, but few of these progress to gross lesions. Valgus and varus limb deformities are common in ram lambs in feedlots and test stations in the USA and also occur in other countries. Grossly, some affected rams have thickening of the distal radial physis, similar to the growth plate lesions of osteochondrosis but joint changes are absent. Vascular and growth plate lesions mimicking osteochondrosis can be produced experimentally in lambs by procedures that increase weight bearing. Epiphysiolysis of the distal radial growth plate, associated with deformity of the forelimbs, is reported in 3-month-old lambs, supporting the concept that the physeal lesions of osteochondrosis may be one cause of angular limb deformity in sheep.

Bibliography

Caperna TJ, et al. Interrelationships of exogenous porcine growth hormone administration and feed intake level affecting various tissue levels of iron, copper, zinc and bone calcium of growing pigs. J Anim Sci 1989;67: 654–662.

Carlson CS, et al. Osteochondrosis of the articular-epiphyseal cartilage complex in young horses: evidence for a defect in cartilage canal blood supply. Vet Pathol 1995;32:641–647.

Carlson CS, et al. Ischemic necrosis of cartilage in spontaneous and experimental lesions of osteochondrosis. J Orthop Res 1991;9:317–329.

Cymbaluk NF, Smart ME. A review of possible metabolic relationships of copper to equine bone disease. Equine Vet J 1993;Suppl 16:19–26.

Duff SRI. Histopathology of growth plate changes in induced abnormal bone growth in lambs. J Comp Pathol 1986;96:15–24.

Ekman S, Carlson CS. The pathophysiology of osteochondrosis. Vet Clin North Am 1998;28(1): 17–32.

Farnum CE, Wilsman NJ. Ultrastructural histochemical evaluation of growth plate cartilage matrix from healthy and osteochondritic swine. Am J Vet Res 1986;47:1105–1115.

Firth EC, Poulos FW. Retained cartilage in the distal radial physis of foals. Vet Pathol 1984;21:10–17.

Girard C, et al. Multiple vertebral osteochondrosis in a foal. J Vet Diagn Invest 1997;9:436–438.

Goedegebuure SA, Hazewinkel HAW. Morphological findings in young dogs chronically fed a diet containing excess calcium. Vet Pathol 1986;23:594–605.

Gunson DE, et al. Environmental zinc and cadmium pollution associated with generalized osteochondrosis, osteoporosis and nephrocalcinosis in horses. J Am Vet Med Assoc 1982;180:295–299.

Hill BD, et al. Investigation of osteochondrosis in grazing beef cattle. Aust Vet J 1998;76:171–175.

Hill MA. Causes of degenerative joint disease (osteoarthrosis) and dyschondroplasia (osteochondrosis) in pigs. J Am Vet Med Assoc 1990;197:107–113.

Hurtig M, et al. Correlative study of defective cartilage and bone growth in foals fed a low-copper diet. Equine Vet J Suppl 1993;16:66–73.

Jensen R, et al. Osteochondrosis in feedlot cattle. Vet Pathol 1981;18:529–535.

Keller GG, et al. Correlation of radiographic, necropsy and histologic findings in 8 dogs with elbow dysplasia. Vet Radiol Ultr 1997;38:272–276.

McLaughlin BG, et al. Carpal bone lesions associated with angular limb deformity in foals. J Am Vet Med Assoc 1981;178:224–230.

Nakano T, et al. Leg weakness and osteochondrosis in swine: A review. Can J Anim Sci 1987;67:883–901.

Ray CS, et al. Development of subchondral cystic lesions after articular cartilage and subchondral bone damage in young horses. Equine Vet J 1996;28:225–232.

Scott CA, et al. Osteochondrosis as a cause of lameness in purebred Suffolk lambs. Vet Rec 1996;139:165–167.

Thompson KG, et al. Osteochondrosis associated with copper deficiency in young farmed red deer and wapiti x red deer hybrids. NZ Vet J 1994;42:137–143.

Uhthoff HK, et al. Epiphysiolysis, a possible cause of limb deformities in lambs. Ann Rech Vet 1982;13:237–244.

Visco DM, et al. Cartilage canals and lesions typical of osteochondrosis in growth cartilages from the distal part of the humerus of newborn pigs. Vet Rec 1991;128:221–228.

Watrous BJ, et al. Osteochondrosis and juvenile spavin in equids. Am J Vet Res 1991;52:607–612.

Wegener KM, Heje NI. Dyschondroplasia (osteochondrosis) in articular-epiphyseal cartilage complexes of three calves from 24 to 103 days of age. Vet Pathol 1992;29:562–563.

Weisbrode SE, et al. Osteochondrosis, degenerative joint disease, and vertebral osteophytosis in middle-aged bulls. J Am Vet Med Assoc 1982;181: 700–705.

Weiss S, Loeffler K. Histology of cartilage channels in the epiphyseal cartilage with reference to localization of osteochondrosis dissecans in young dogs. Duetsche Tier Woch 1996;103:164–169.

White SL, et al. Radiographic, macroscopic and microscopic changes in growth plates of calves raised on hard flooring. Am J Vet Res 1984;45:633–639.

Hip dysplasia

Hip dysplasia is the most common skeletal disease of large and giant breeds of dogs, but may occur in all dog breeds and is occasionally reported in cats, cattle, and horses. *The disease is characterized by a lack of conformity between the femoral head and acetabulum, resulting in subluxation and, invariably, degenerative joint disease.* A polygenic mode of inheritance is postulated in dogs, and estimates of heritability have varied from 0.2 to 0.6. Environmental effects are believed to play a significant role in the severity of lesions. In particular, growth rate during the first few weeks of life appears to be important; faster-growing dogs having more severe lesions. Overfeeding young pups of susceptible breeds has been shown to shorten the time to first appearance of hip dysplasia and increase its severity. In another study, limiting the food consumed by Labrador Retrievers between 6 weeks and 1 year of age reduced both the incidence and severity of the disease.

1. **Dogs** Increased joint laxity is a common feature in dogs with hip dysplasia and appears to have a hereditary basis. *Although the cause of joint laxity is not clear, it is well established that dogs with hip dysplasia generally have low pelvic muscle mass.* The hip joint, probably more than any other joint, depends on muscle action to maintain the relationships between articulating surfaces during weight bearing and motion. Breeds such as Greyhounds, which do not get hip dysplasia, have a much greater muscle mass than German Shepherd Dogs, in which the disease is common. Hypotrophy of pectineal muscles, due to a developmental neuropathy, has also been suggested as a predisposing cause of hip dysplasia in dogs. Spasm or shortening of the pectineal muscle would be expected to create an upward force by the femoral head on the dorsal rim of the acetabulum. Such a force during early postnatal development of the hip joint could result in abnormal modeling and a dysplastic joint.

   It is possible that the basic defect in hip dysplasia is intrinsic to the hip joint, rather than to its supporting structures. It has been suggested that hip dysplasia is a manifestation of osteochondrosis but this hypothesis does not appear to be widely supported.

   Radiographic evidence of hip dysplasia in affected pups is usually not apparent until about 6 months of age, but may be detected earlier in severe cases or much later in dogs with mild lesions. *A radiographic diagnosis of hip dysplasia is based on the presence of subluxation of the joint or evidence of degenerative joint disease, or both.*

   The *gross lesions* of canine hip dysplasia vary with the stage of the disease. In the early stages, acetabula appear shallow, there is subluxation of the femoral head, and the articular cartilage may be dull or roughened. *The lesions are most prominent in weight-bearing areas of the femoral head and the dorsal rim of the acetabulum.* As the disease progresses, the articular cartilage becomes yellow or gray and erosion leads to fibrillation, then eburnation, with sclerosis of the subchondral bone. Osteophytes may develop at chondro-osseous margins. The shape of the femoral head may be altered due to the abnormal forces associated with subluxation and the femoral neck may become thickened as enthesiophytes develop at the attachment of the joint capsule. The joint capsule may be thickened with fibrous connective tissue and granulation tissue developing within the synovial membrane may extend over part of the articular surface as a pannus. In advanced stages, evidence of hip dysplasia may be masked by the manifestations of severe, degenerative joint disease. In some cases, the formation of osteophytes around the acetabular rim may disguise its original shallowness. In dogs with severely dysplastic joints, advanced changes of degenerative joint disease may be present by one year of age.

   Microscopic changes in hip dysplasia are those of degenerative joint disease (see below) and contribute nothing specific to the diagnosis. Early lesions include edema and tearing of collagen fibers in the ligament of the head of the femur and hypertrophy and hyperplasia of synoviocytes in the synovial membrane. Later in the disease, synovial villi may be infiltrated with mononuclear cells, the joint capsule is thickened with fibrous tissue, and the eroded articular cartilage contains clusters of proliferating chondrocytes.

2. **Cats** *Hip dysplasia is much less common in cats than in dogs*, but its frequency in the general cat population is probably underestimated. Many cats with radiographic evidence of hip dysplasia are asymptomatic and *the diagnosis is often incidental.* In a survey of 648 cats representing 12 breeds, the overall frequency of hip dysplasia was about 6.6%. Persians and Himalayans had a higher prevalence rate (15.8% and 25.0%, respectively) but only small numbers of these purebreds were included in the study and the results may be misleading. Other studies have indicated a very high prevalence of hip dysplasia in the Maine Coon breed of cat, which, like the Persian and Himalayan breeds, has a larger body size and a relatively small gene pool. As in dogs, no sex predilection is apparent in cats.

   The role of joint laxity in the pathogenesis of feline hip dysplasia is uncertain and requires further investigation. A consistent observation in cats with hip dysplasia is an *abnormally shallow acetabulum*, rather than subluxation of the joint, which is a feature of the disease in dogs. The shallow acetabulum predisposes to degenerative joint disease but the distribution of lesions in cats differs from that in dogs. The most extensive remodeling and proliferative changes in affected cats involve the craniodorsal acetabular margin, whereas in dogs the dorsal rim of the acetabulum is most severely affected. A further difference is the lack of remodeling of the femoral neck in cats with hip dysplasia.

3. **Cattle** *Hip dysplasia in cattle is best known in Herefords* but also occurs in the Aberdeen Angus, Galloway, and Charolais breeds. An inherited component is suspected but too few cases are reported to allow confirmation or characterization of the mode of inheritance. The disease is largely confined to males. Although some calves may be affected at birth, clinical lameness usually commences from 3 months to 2 years of age. Since lame bulls are more often sent for slaughter than subjected to postmortem examination, the true prevalence of hip dysplasia in cattle may be much higher than is realized. The lesions are generally bilateral and are characterized by shallow acetabula and degenerative arthropathy involving both the femoral head and acetabulum. *Rapid growth and mineral deficiencies appear to exacerbate the condition*, and it is likely that at least some cases of hip dysplasia in cattle represent manifestations of osteochondrosis.

Luxations and subluxations

Congenital luxations are rare in animals but **atlanto-axial subluxations** are reported in dogs, goats, cattle, and horses. In dogs, miniature and toy breeds are usually affected. *The underlying lesion appears to be failure of fusion of the odontoid process to the body of the axis.* Clinical signs vary from neck pain to tetraplegia, with age of onset varying from a few months to several years. *Absence or hypoplasia of the odontoid process occurs in calves*, often in conjunction with atlanto-occipital fusion. Tetraplegia may be present at birth or develop at several months of age. In both dogs and calves, *fusion of the odontoid process with the axis* normally occurs in the early months of life and it is possible that in some cases postnatal influences are responsible for the condition.

Atlanto-axial subluxations occur in some *Arabian foals* with a familial, probably inherited, syndrome involving occipitalization of the atlas and atlantalization of the axis. Affected foals may be dead or tetraparetic at birth, or develop progressive ataxia within a few months. They have atlanto-occipital fusion and atlantal condyles that articulate with a malformed axis, thereby displacing the cranio-vertebral articulation caudally. *Congenital atlanto-occipital fusion with a wedge-shaped vertebral piece and cervical scoliosis* also occurs in horses as a sporadic defect unrelated to the Arabian condition. Subluxations of cervical vertebrae in horses and dogs are discussed with cervical vertebral stenotic myelopathy ("wobbler syndrome") earlier in this chapter.

Temporomandibular subluxation is reported in Basset Hounds and Irish Setters. Clinically, open-mouth locking of jaws occurs when the zygomatic arch interferes with the normal movement of the coronoid process of the mandible. Developmental abnormalities in the condyloid process of the mandible and the mandibular fossa of the temporal bone are responsible for subluxation but the *cause of the dysplasia is unknown*. The lesions are bilateral. A similar condition in American Cocker Spaniels may be bilateral or unilateral. In these animals, temporomandibular subluxation may be elicited by manipulation but is not associated with spontaneous clinical signs. Dysplasia of the mandibular fossa and hypoplasia or aplasia of the retroglenoid process are responsible for the excess joint mobility.

Subluxation of the carpus is reported as a sex-linked recessive trait in a colony of dogs in which hemophilia A also existed, although the two disorders do not occur in the same animals. Signs of carpal subluxation first appear when the animals begin to walk. Most carpal subluxations and luxations are secondary to trauma.

Patellar luxations and **subluxations** are common in dogs, less so in horses, and rare in other species. In **dogs**, most are associated with anatomical defects and are probably inherited as polygenic traits. Females are affected 1.5 times as often as males. The condition may be unilateral or bilateral and luxations of variable severity may occur either medially or laterally. Occasionally they occur in both directions. Medial luxations account for about three-quarters of the cases and are *most common in small dogs*, especially Pomeranians, Yorkshire Terriers, Chihuahuas, Miniature and Toy Poodles and Boston Terriers. Lateral luxations tend to occur in larger dogs including some giant breeds, such as Great Dane, St. Bernard, and Irish Wolfhound. Clinical signs commonly develop within the first few months of life, but may be present at birth. Various anatomical defects involving the femorotibial joint, and sometimes the entire limb, are present in affected dogs and may be adaptational deformities. Patellar luxation in **horses** almost always occurs in a lateral direction and is associated with hypoplasia of the lateral ridge of the femoral trochlea. It is sometimes congenital and bilateral in both foals and calves. The condition probably is inherited in ponies, and perhaps also in horses. Patellar luxation is rarely reported in **cats** and most cases appear to have a traumatic origin. A genetic predisposition has however been suggested in the Abyssinian and Devon Rex breeds.

The *consequences of luxations and subluxations* vary with the species of animal and the joint involved. In general, subluxations, whether they are genetic or traumatic in origin, *predispose to degenerative joint disease* due to instability of the joint. Luxations are more likely to damage periarticular soft tissues and, if the articular cartilage remains in persistent contact with soft tissues, it degenerates and is replaced by fibrous tissue and bone. If movement is minimal, a *fibrous or bony fixation* may develop, but continued movement may result in the formation of a new joint. Fibrous tissue about the dislocated bone ends sometimes becomes organized into an articular capsule with a synovial lining, but the articular surfaces are covered with fibrous tissue rather than articular cartilage.

Abnormal positioning of joints in terms of overextension or overflexion occurs in animals with **arthrogryposis**, but only in the most severe cases are the articular surfaces deformed. The primary lesion is in the central nervous system, where the congenital absence of motor neurons supplying selected muscles results in muscular atrophy and overextension or overflexion of the opposing unaffected muscle groups. **Congenital torticollis**, whether or not it is associated with a branchiocephalic fold, is associated with articular abnormalities of the cervical vertebrae in sympathy with the concertina-like compression that occurs on the concave side of the deviation.

Bibliography

Cardinet GH, et al. Association between pelvic muscle mass and canine hip dysplasia. J Am Vet Med Assoc 1997;210:1466–1473.

Carnahan DL, et al. Hip dysplasia in Hereford cattle. J Am Vet Med Assoc 1968;152:1150–1157.

Geary JC, et al. Atlanto axial subluxation in the canine. J Small Anim Pract 1967;8:577–582.

Hoppe F, Svalastoga E. Temporomandibular dysplasia in American Cocker Spaniels. J Small Anim Pract 1980;21:675–678.

Howlett CR. Pathology of coxofemoral arthropathy in young beef bulls. Pathology 1973;5:135–144.

Johnson KA. Temporomandibular joint dysplasia in an Irish setter. J Small Anim Pract 1979;20: 209–218.

Keller GG, et al. Hip dysplasia: a feline population study. Vet Radiol Ultras 1999;40:460–464.

Ladds P, et al. Congenital odontoid process separation in two dogs. J Small Anim Pract 1970;12:463–471.

Leighton EA. Genetics of canine hip dysplasia. J Am Vet Med Assoc 1997;210:1474–1479.

Lust G, et al. Joint laxity and its association with hip dysplasia in Labrador Retrievers. Am J Vet Res 1993;54:1990–1999.

Lust G. An overview of the pathogenesis of canine hip dysplasia. J Am Vet Med Assoc 1997;210:1443–1445.

Mayhew IG, et al. Congenital occipito-atlantoaxial malformations in the horse. Equine Vet J 1978;10:103–113.

Meagher DM. Bilateral patellar luxation in calves. Can Vet J 1974;15:201–202.

Morgan SJ. Pathologic alterations in canine hip dysplasia. J Am Vet Med Assoc 1997;210:1446–1450.

Pick JR, et al. Subluxation of the carpus in dogs. An X chromosomal defect closely linked with the locus for hemophilia A. Lab Invest 1967;17:243–248.
Priester WA. Sex, size, and breed as risk factors in canine patellar dislocation. J Am Vet Med Assoc 1972;160:740–742.
Robinson WF, et al. Atlanto-axial malarticulation in Angora goats. Aust Vet J 1982;58:105–107.
Smith GK, et al. Evaluation of the association between medial patellar luxation and hip dysplasia in cats. J Am Vet Med Assoc 1999;215:40–45.
Weaver AD. Hip dysplasia in beef cattle. Vet Rec 1978;102:54–55.
White ME, et al. Atlanto-axial subluxation in five young cattle. Can Vet J 1978;19:79–82.

DEGENERATIVE DISEASES OF JOINTS

Synovial joints

Degenerative diseases involving the major weight-bearing joints of the limbs are very common in humans and domestic animals. In human medicine, the term **"osteoarthritis"** is preferred for this group of diseases although it incorrectly implies an inflammatory origin. **Degenerative joint disease** is a more appropriate term, based on the putative pathogenesis, and will be used in this chapter. Other commonly used *synonyms include osteoarthrosis and degenerative arthropathy*.

Degenerative joint disease is not a specific entity, but a common sequel to various forms of joint injury and involves an interaction between biologic and mechanical factors on the articular cartilage, subchondral bone, and synovium. It can be either *monoarticular or polyarticular* and may be classified as either *primary or secondary*. **Primary** *degenerative joint disease refers to those cases where there is no apparent predisposing cause and generally occurs in older animals*. Such cases may reflect an acceleration of the normal aging changes that occur in joints. Mild degenerative changes in weight-bearing articular surfaces, including yellowing and fibrillation of cartilage, are common incidental findings in adult dogs at necropsy. In the absence of clinical signs of lameness it is difficult to justify a diagnosis of degenerative joint disease in such cases, but it is likely that these represent the early manifestations of the disease and probably account for the mild lameness and stiffness seen in many old dogs.

Secondary *degenerative joint disease is associated with an underlying abnormality in the joint or its supporting structures, predisposing to premature degeneration of the cartilage. Any condition that causes direct damage to the articular cartilage, creates instability, or results in abnormal directional forces can predispose to degenerative joint disease*. For example, secondary degenerative joint disease is an inevitable consequence of the joint laxity in dogs with hip dysplasia, due to the effect of abnormal mechanical forces on articular cartilage. Traumatic injuries to ligaments may also create joint instability leading to degenerative joint disease. Incongruity of opposing articular surfaces, as occurs in many animals with osteochondrosis, is a common cause of degenerative joint disease involving the shoulder, elbow, stifle, and hock joints of dogs and other species. Other disorders that may predispose to secondary degenerative joint disease include malaligned limb fractures, angular limb deformities, aseptic necrosis, or metabolic bone diseases with collapse of subchondral bone, inherited defects in cartilage or collagen formation, septic arthritis, and hemarthrosis. Persistent hemarthrosis, as occurs in animals with hemophilia or other coagulopathies, may lead to chronic, proliferative synovitis with accumulation of hemosiderin-containing macrophages in the synovium. Invasive pannus may develop from the hyperplastic synovial tissue and spread out over the articular surface.

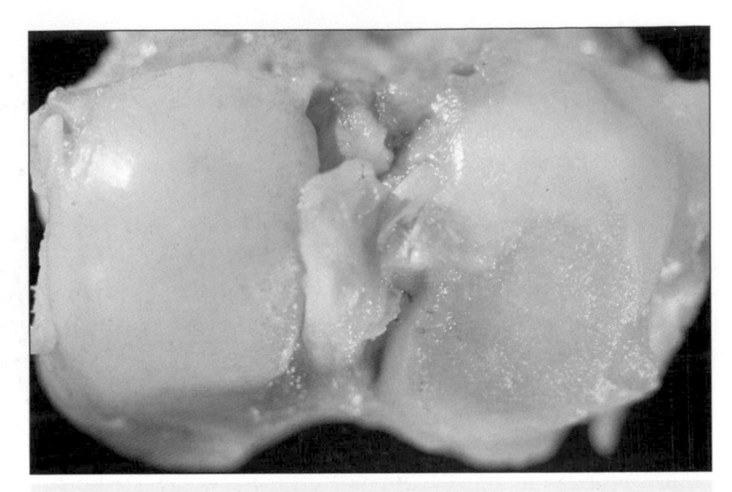

Figure 1.143 Degenerative joint disease, dog. Fibrillation of articular cartilage on the femoral condyle.

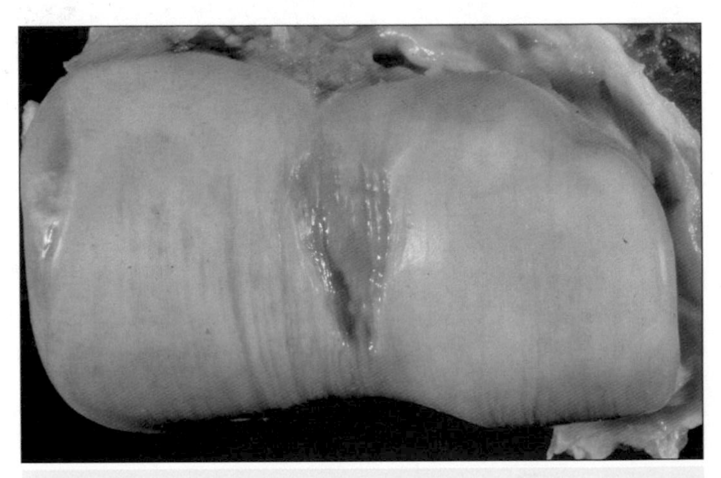

Figure 1.144 Degenerative joint disease, horse. Linear grooves (wear lines) in the articular cartilage of the distal humerus. The depressed area between the condyles is a developing synovial fossa. (Courtesy of SE Weisbrode.)

The *gross lesions* of degenerative joint disease are similar whether the disease is primary or secondary in origin, although the lesions of secondary degenerative joint disease are generally more severe by the time an affected animal comes to necropsy. *The earliest gross lesion is roughening of the articular cartilage in areas of weight bearing* (Fig. 1.143) due to loss of proteoglycans from the matrix and unmasking of the collagen fibrils. This is referred to as **fibrillation**. Initially, only the superficial layers are involved but, with continued abrasion of the degenerate cartilage, vertical fissures develop in deeper layers in the direction of collagen fibril alignment and may extend to the subchondral bone. In hinge-type joints, such as the hock, fetlock, and elbow, *linear grooves (wear lines)* may be present in the cartilage in the direction of joint movement (Fig. 1.144). These are found relatively commonly in the joints of adult horses. Their cause is uncertain and they are not necessarily associated with progressive lesions. Progressive erosion of fibrillated cartilage is accompanied by sclerosis of the subchondral bone. In advanced lesions, *the articular cartilage may be*

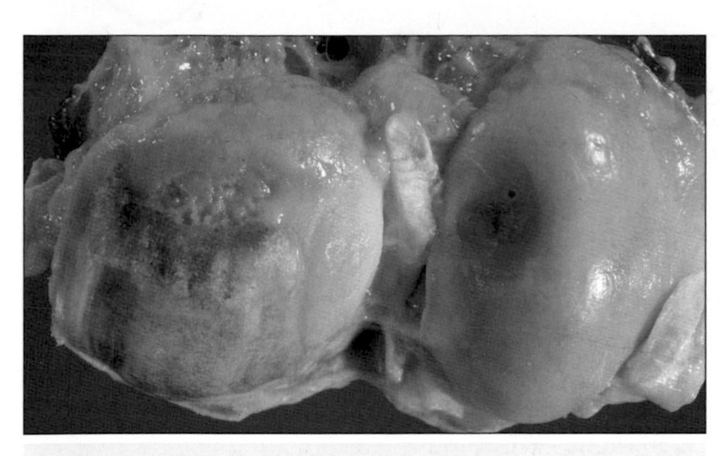

Figure 1.145 Chronic degenerative joint disease of the stifle joint in a cow. Loss of articular cartilage on the medial condyle with eburnation of the exposed subchondral bone. A smaller lesion is present on the lateral condyle.

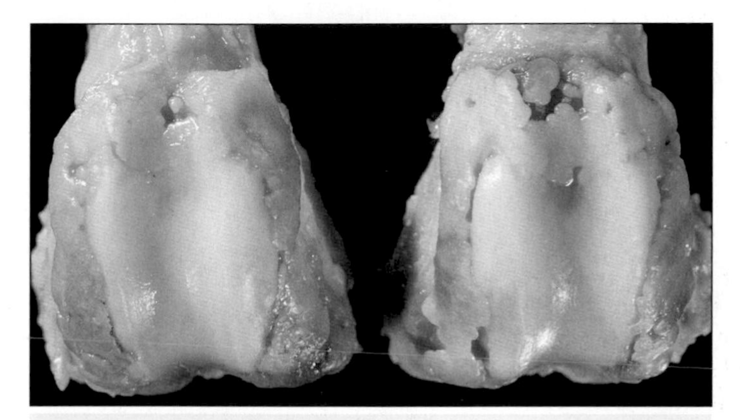

Figure 1.146 Degenerative joint disease, dog. Extensive osteophyte formation along the chondro-osseous margins of both stifles.

completely ulcerated in areas of maximum weight bearing and the exposed bone worn smooth, a process referred to as **eburnation** (Fig. 1.145). Increased stiffness of the sclerotic subchondral bone may accelerate the loss of the overlying cartilage due to reduced flexibility during weight bearing. In fact, some investigators have proposed that sclerosis of subchondral bone may be the initial lesion in degenerative joint disease. More likely, this is just one of a combination of factors involved in progression of the disease. Cystic lesions are often present beneath eburnated surfaces in human patients with degenerative joint disease but are seldom seen in domestic animals. *Another consistent gross feature of degenerative joint disease is the formation of* **osteophytes** *at the margin of articular cartilage and bone* (Fig. 1.146). These small, nodular, outgrowths of bone, covered by a thin layer of hyaline cartilage may surround the articular surface and either distort its shape or obscure the boundary between the articular surface and the supporting bone. Osteophytes develop rapidly following joint injury and can be detected as early as 7 days after a joint has been unstable experimentally. Changes also occur in the synovium and joint capsule of animals with degenerative joint disease. The joint capsule is thickened with fibrous connective tissue and there is likely to be hypertrophy of synovial villi.

A variety of *histologic changes* have been reported in the articular cartilage of animals and humans with degenerative joint disease. *Reduction in metachromatic staining of the superficial cartilage matrix,* presumably associated with the loss of proteoglycan, is a common early change and may be accompanied by necrosis of chondrocytes in the tangential layer. *Clusters of proliferative chondrocytes (brood capsules or chondrones) may be present*, especially adjacent to fissures in areas of fibrillation (Fig. 1.147A). Elsewhere, the density of chondrocytes is

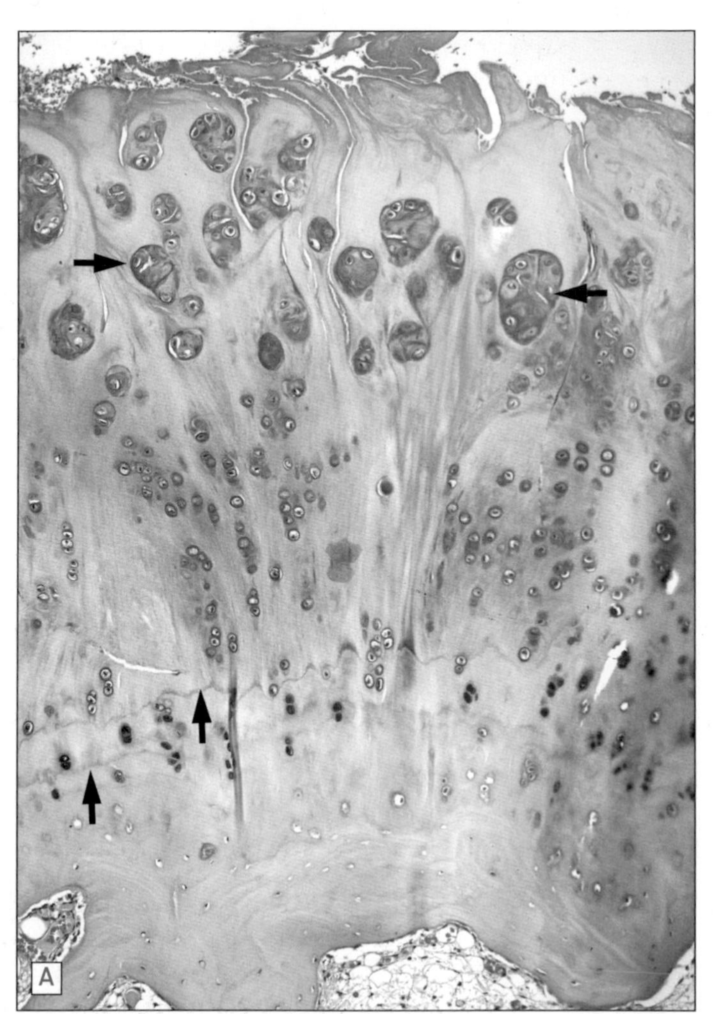

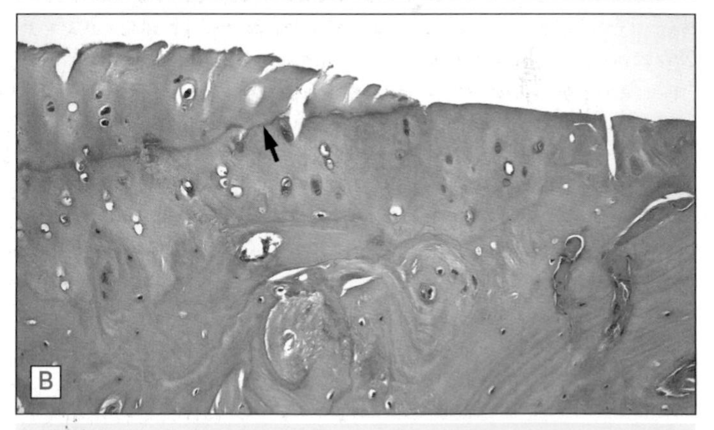

Figure 1.147 Degenerative joint disease, dog. **A.** Fibrillated articular cartilage with irregular surface, eosinophilic matrix and disorganization of chondrocytes. Several chondrones (horizontal arrows) are adjacent to clefts in superficial layers. The tidemark is duplicated in some areas (vertical arrows). **B.** Junction between areas of fibrillation and eburnation. The frayed cartilage becomes eroded to the level of the tidemark (arrow) at which stage it is replaced by an articular surface comprised of mineralized cartilage then sclerotic bone.

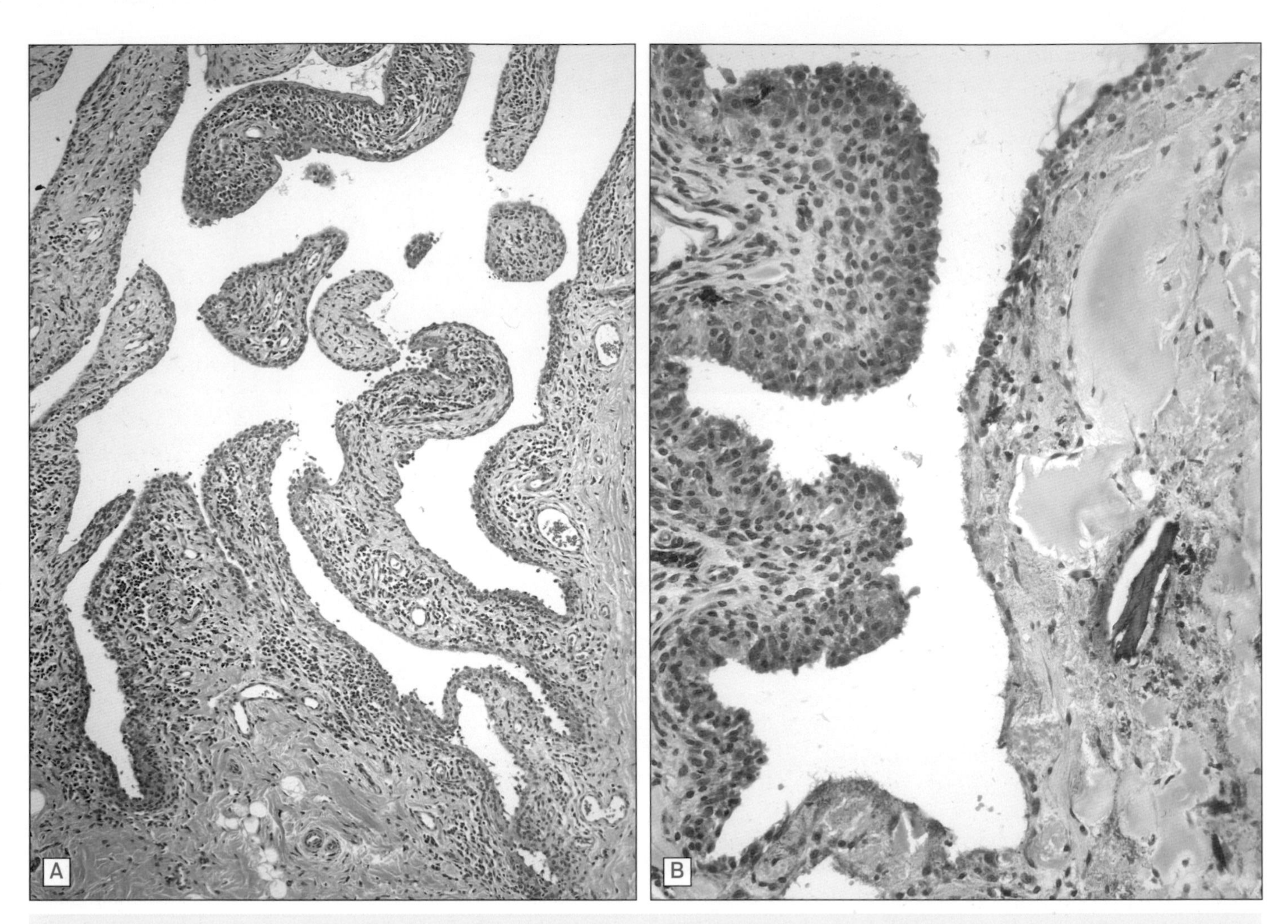

Figure 1.148 Chronic degenerative joint disease. **A.** Hypertrophic villi lined by plump synoviocytes and infiltrated with mononuclear inflammatory cells. **B.** Fragments of degenerate cartilage and occasional spicules of bone, most likely derived from the eroded articular surface, embedded in the synovium. The adjacent villi are lined by hyperplastic synoviocytes.

often reduced but remnants of degenerate cells may still be apparent. In advanced lesions, *the overall thickness of the degenerate cartilage may be markedly reduced*, the surface is irregular, and deep clefts may be present. Collagen fibrils within the matrix appear more prominent. The tidemark is often duplicated or disrupted, and may be penetrated by blood vessels. *Fibrillated cartilage merges with areas of eburnation* (Fig. 1.147B), where the articular cartilage is absent and the trabeculae of subchondral bone show variable degrees of thickening and/or remodeling. In chronic degenerative joint disease, *synovial villi are hypertrophic*, sometimes branching and are lined by plump, hyperplastic synoviocytes (Fig. 1.148A). Small to moderate numbers of *mononuclear inflammatory cells*, predominantly lymphocytes, in addition to hemosiderin-containing macrophages are often present. *Fragments of degenerate cartilage*, presumably derived from the eroded articular surface, may be embedded in the synovium or attached to its surface (Fig. 1.148B). Such fragments may enlarge through proliferation of surviving chondrocytes and may be an early stage of secondary osteochondromatosis (see p. 134).

The *pathogenesis of degenerative joint disease is complex* and continues to be debated in human medicine, even after many decades of research and observation. Although there are differing hypotheses on the exact sequence of events, most investigators conform to the view that the disease is *primarily degenerative in nature and that the accompanying inflammatory changes are secondary*. It must be recognized however, that lesions of degenerative joint disease will also develop as a sequel to chronic inflammation in many primary inflammatory conditions of man and domestic animals. There is convincing evidence that the *chondrocytes* of articular cartilage play an important role in the early stages of disease development. These post-mitotic cells normally survive throughout the life of the individual and maintain a balance between degradation and repair of the cartilage matrix under the influence of cytokines, growth factors, and direct physical stimuli. Disruption of this balance in favor of matrix catabolism occurs in the early stages of degenerative joint disease and is reflected by depletion of the proteoglycan aggregates, aggrecan, which are a major component of cartilage matrix. Continued reduction in the proteoglycan content of the matrix, together with damage to collagen fibrils, interferes with the viscoelastic properties of articular cartilage. As a result, progressive loss of cartilage occurs under the influence of normal biomechanical forces.

The early loss of matrix components in degenerative joint disease is mediated by degradative enzymes, including metalloproteinases, serine proteinases, cysteine proteinases, and aggrecanase. Many of these enzymes are derived from chondrocytes, but synoviocytes and inflammatory cells may also produce them. Natural inhibitors of these enzymes are normally present in articular cartilage but are deficient in degenerative joint disease. Several zinc-dependent metalloproteinases are recognized but the collagenases, stromelysins, and gelatinases appear to be the most important in cartilage degradation. Collagenase and stromelysin are synthesized as latent enzymes in cartilage and can be activated by plasmin and plasminogen activator or inhibited by plasminogen activator inhibitor-1. Collagenase breaks down the scaffolding of type-II collagen, while stromelysin cleaves aggrecan in addition to some types of collagen. Degradation products of aggrecan and type-II collagen may remain in the cartilage matrix or diffuse into the synovial fluid, where they can be detected. Proteoglycan fragments in synovial fluid may be either phagocytosed by synovial cells or enter lymphatics in the synovium.

Various cytokines and growth factors are also believed to be involved in the pathogenesis of degenerative joint disease, particularly in the generation of the inflammatory response. Most attention has focused on the role of the cytokines interleukin-1, interleukin-6, and tumor necrosis factor-α. Interleukin-1 and tumor necrosis factor-α have been shown to increase the synthesis of metalloproteinases and plasminogen activators, and to induce the resorption of cartilage both in vitro and in vivo. Interleukin-1 also stimulates fibroblasts to synthesize collagen type I and type II, and may therefore contribute to fibrous thickening of the joint capsule in degenerative joint disease. The role of interleukin-6 is less clear but it is released in vitro by chondrocytes from normal and degenerate cartilage and may be involved in autocrine stimulation of chondrocyte proliferation. It has also been detected in the synovial fluid of human patients with various arthropathies and may be an important intermediate signal for the activities of interleukin-1 and tumor necrosis factor-α. Growth factors, such as insulin-like growth factor-1 and transforming growth factor-β, have an anabolic effect on connective tissues and have been shown to stimulate proteoglycan and collagen synthesis. They can also inhibit or reverse some of the catabolic effects of interleukin-1. Similarly, the cytokine γ-interferon inhibits the action of interleukin-1 on metalloproteinase production and proteoglycan depletion from cartilage. These observations support the concept of a complex interaction between cytokines and growth factors in the pathogenesis of degenerative joint disease.

Inflammatory changes in the synovium of humans and animals with degenerative joint disease are most likely secondary to the stimulation of interleukin-1 and tumor necrosis factor-α by synoviocytes following the release of degraded collagen and proteoglycan fragments from degenerate cartilage. The neuropeptide, substance P, may also be involved. This peptide has been detected in the synovial membrane and fluid of human patients with degenerative joint disease and has been shown to activate both inflammatory cells and synoviocytes, in addition to stimulating the secretion and action of interleukin-1.

Primary and secondary degenerative joint diseases are common in most domestic animal species, but in dogs, horses, and cattle, certain types are either sufficiently common or important to warrant discussion as separate entities.

Degenerative joint diseases of horses

Although degenerative joint diseases may affect a wide range of synovial joints in horses, those involving the *interphalangeal, metacarpophalangeal, and hock joints* are of particular importance. *These joints are subjected to considerable biomechanical loading during motion*, especially in performance horses, and are therefore predisposed to traumatic injury to the articular cartilage, subchondral bone, or supporting structures. *In joints subjected to considerable motion, such as the metacarpophalangeal joints, the changes of degenerative joint disease are usually characterized by gradual erosion of articular cartilage, sclerosis of subchondral bone, chronic synovitis, and gradual stiffening of the joint due to fibrous thickening of the joint capsule.* In low-motion joints, such as the proximal and distal interphalangeal, distal intertarsal, and tarsometatarsal joints, maximum loading during motion is focused on a restricted area. In these joints, the lesion typically is characterized by full-thickness necrosis of the articular cartilage with limited wearing, focal damage to subchondral bone, and bony ankylosis. Degenerative changes involving the navicular bone and the adjacent deep digital flexor tendon, referred to as *navicular syndrome*, probably have a similar pathogenesis and will be discussed here, although they are more appropriately classified as a form of bursitis rather than with degenerative joint diseases.

Metacarpophalangeal (fetlock) joints

Traumatic and degenerative diseases of the metacarpophalangeal (fetlock) joints of the foreleg are *more common than similar lesions affecting any of the other limb joints*. This susceptibility to injury presumably reflects the relatively small surface area of this joint in comparison to most others and the considerable range of motion expressed by the joint. Furthermore, during racing, the entire weight of the animal is transmitted to the ground through this joint during one phase of the stride. *Poor conformation and excessive training of horses at a young age no doubt contribute to the development of lesions in this and other joints.* **Traumatic synovitis** of the dorsal joint capsule often results from repeated overextension of the fetlock joint in the racehorse. At the point of maximum extension, the *proximodorsal margin of the proximal phalanx traumatizes the fibrous synovial pad* covering the dorsal surface of the distal end of the cannon bone. In response to constant trauma, the fibrous pad becomes enlarged due to hyperemia, edema, and fibroplasia, and extends across the adjacent dorsal articular margin of the cannon bone. Degeneration of the underlying articular cartilage occurs as a result of impaired access to synovial fluid and release of inflammatory mediators from the inflamed synovium. In cases where the inflammation resolves and the synovial pad retracts, the degenerate, pitted articular surface remains as evidence. In other cases, hemorrhage from the traumatized synovial pad and the insertion line of the joint capsule results in the formation of an organizing hematoma. *The firm yellow/brown lesion on the dorsal surface of the distal cannon bone is referred to as* **villonodular synovitis**. The histological features of these lesions vary with their duration. In the subacute stages, they include a mixture of hemosiderin-containing macrophages and well-ordered granulation tissue. Chronic lesions consist of dense, poorly vascularized fibrous tissue infiltrated by mononuclear inflammatory cells and covered by a layer of synoviocytes.

Another common change involving the metacarpophalangeal joint in performance horses is the *formation of a periarticular lip along the dorsal articular margin of the proximal phalanx*. Initially, the lip consists of an overgrowth of articular cartilage, but its deeper layers undergo endochondral ossification, creating an *osteophyte* that can be detected radiographically. With repeated trauma, microscopic or macroscopic chip fractures may develop in the bony support of the lip. The repair of such fractures is often compromised by the continued trauma of racing or training, and loosened chip fractures, attached to the adjacent bone by granulation tissue, may cause synovitis and acute clinical signs.

Traumatic osteochondrosis

Small, ovoid, "bruised" defects about 2–4 mm in diameter are relatively common incidental findings in the palmar articular surface of the condyle of the cannon bone in racehorses at necropsy. More severe lesions of this type are symptomatic and are characterized by apparent collapse of the articular cartilage into a defect in the subchondral bone. These lesions are referred to as traumatic osteochondrosis. They typically occur in highly trained, mature racehorses and are believed to result from focal sclerosis of subchondral bone, leading to microfractures and bone necrosis. During the repair process, the lesion is susceptible to displacement or collapse, particularly if strenuous exercise persists during this period.

Transverse ridge arthrosis

This is a degenerative lesion involving the transverse ridge of the condyle of the cannon bone, particularly in the foreleg. The lesions vary from mild fibrillation to the development of deep ulcers extending into the underlying bone. The transverse ridge develops between the dorsal articular surface of the condyle, which articulates with the proximal phalanx, and the palmar surface of the condyle, which articulates with the proximal sesamoid bones. If the fetlock joint is overextended during racing, the base of the proximal sesamoid bone overrides the transverse ridge, exposing it to shearing forces and eventually leading to degeneration.

Instability of the metacarpophalangeal joint created by experimental transection of the medial collateral and the lateral collateral sesamoidean ligaments in horses has been used to induce lesions similar to those of naturally occurring degenerative joint disease. The lesions included scoring lines (linear erosions) in the articular cartilage and osteophyte formation along the lateral articular margin of the sesamoid bone and lateral aspect of the proximal phalanx.

Ringbone

Degenerative diseases of **interphalangeal joints** are commonly referred to as *ringbone*. *High* or *low* ringbone refers to involvement of the *proximal or distal interphalangeal joints* respectively. *The lesions are typically bilateral and primarily involve the forelimbs.* In young horses, subchondral cystic lesions associated with osteochondrosis are considered an important predisposing factor in high ringbone, although similar subchondral lesions can also be induced by trauma to the articular surface of young animals. In older horses, instability of the joint secondary to traumatic injuries to the joint capsule, ligaments, or tendons supporting the joint may be involved. Alternatively, repeated episodes of minor trauma from athletic activity, or mechanical stresses associated with faulty conformation, may place excessive strain on the insertion lines of the dorsal joint capsule. Degenerative disease of the proximal interphalangeal joint also occurs secondary to subluxation of the joint following fractures of the palmar or plantar eminences of the middle phalanx. High ringbone is found most often in adult horses used for western events or polo, where horses running at high speed make abrupt stops, turns, and twisting motions.

The severity of the articular and periarticular lesions of high ringbone varies markedly between individuals. In the *early stages of the disease*, affected joints may be partly immobilized by fibrous thickening of the dorsal joint capsule and there may be early cartilage degeneration of one or both condyles of the distal first phalanx and the apposing glenoid cavity of the proximal second phalanx. Joint fluid is normal and the synovium is not congested. The periarticular response, which includes fibrous thickening of the dorsal joint capsule and bone formation beginning in the joint capsule insertion line, is a much more prominent feature than the cartilaginous changes. *The periarticular bony response on the dorsal surface of the joint gives the lesion its name*. In *advanced lesions*, full-thickness necrosis of the articular cartilage, followed by erosions in the subchondral bony plate, may lead to *ankylosis*. In cases where there is residual joint motion, there is eburnation of the ulcerated articular surfaces, thickening of the subchondral bony plates and inhibition of ankylosis.

Degenerative disease of the distal interphalangeal (coffin) joint

This occurs most often in racehorses, probably as a result of repeated minor trauma. *The Quarter Horse breed appears predisposed to problems of this joint*, possibly because their relatively small hoof diameter, short, upright pasterns, and large body size place greater stress on the joint during racing at high speeds. Periarticular osteophytes and enthesiophytes involving the distal aspect of the middle phalanx or the extensor process of the distal phalanx, characteristic of low ringbone, are present in some, but not all cases of degenerative joint disease of the coffin joint. In other cases the disease is less obvious clinically and radiographically and may be confused with navicular syndrome.

Bone spavin

This is a degenerative disease of the tarsus of the horse and occasionally the ox. Structural changes in this disorder are essentially the same as those occurring in high ringbone and presumably have a similar pathogenesis, initiated by sustained loading and joint immobilization. The *major lesions develop on the medial side of the tarsus*, primarily involving the distal intertarsal joint and, less commonly, the tarsometatarsal and proximal intertarsal joints. Examination of early cases of bone spavin, centered in the distal intertarsal joint, indicates that periarticular fibrosis initially immobilizes the dorsomedial side of the joint. "Kissing lesions" subsequently develop in articular cartilage adjacent to the dorsomedial margins of the apposing articular surfaces of the central and third tarsal bones. *Early lesions* show full-thickness necrosis of the apposed cartilage surfaces and intense bone remodeling within the thickened subchondral bony plate. *Intermediate lesions* show penetration of the necrotic cartilage by granulation tissue from the areas of intense subchondral bone remodeling. As the *lesion progresses*, granulation tissue extends across the joint space through areas of necrotic cartilage and establishes a *fibrous ankylosis*, which later gives way to a more stable *bony ankylosis*.

Navicular syndrome (navicular disease)

This is a degenerative disorder involving the distal half of the flexor surface of the navicular bones of the forelegs of mature horses. Various theories for its etiology have been proposed, but a biomechanical origin, associated with the combined effect of abnormal forces and poor conformation, is currently favored. An alternative hypothesis, whereby thrombosis of arterioles supplying the distal region of the navicular bone leads to ischemic necrosis of the bone, has failed to gain support.

Horses having *abnormal foot conformation*, i.e., bone and joint alignments at either end of the spectrum for the breed, are predisposed to navicular syndrome. At one end of this spectrum are *racing Thoroughbreds with very long toes and low heels*. In horses with this conformation, the deep digital flexor tendon places sustained pressure against the distal border of the flexor surface of the navicular bone. At the other end of the spectrum are those American Quarter Horses with an *extremely upright foot conformation*. In such animals, the deep digital flexor tendon exerts repetitive concussive forces on the distal border of the flexor surface of the navicular bone during exercise. Either sustained pressure or repetitive concussion can activate the remodeling processes in the subchondral region of the navicular bone in an attempt to adapt the flexor cortex to these biomechanical stresses. If pressure or concussive forces are of low intensity and of limited duration, the subchondral bone and spongiosa thicken sufficiently to absorb, diffuse, and redistribute the load. In such horses, the navicular bones are sclerotic and the fibrocartilage of the flexor surface of these horses often shows degenerative changes, but there is no clinical lameness.

When the sustained load or concussive forces acting on the distal border of the flexor surface of the navicular bone exceeds the physiologic limit, an exaggerated bone remodeling response is initiated. This eventually creates *lytic lesions in the subchondral bone beneath the flexor surface of the navicular bone*. Granulation tissue arises within these sites of intense bone remodeling in the same manner as it does in high ringbone and bone spavin. The granulation tissue eventually penetrates the overlying layer of degenerate fibrocartilage and forms fibrous adhesions to the apposing dorsal surface of the deep digital flexor tendon.

Bone marrow fibrosis and distended veins can be demonstrated in the marrow spaces of the subchondral bone and spongiosa located in the distal halves of the navicular bones of horses with navicular syndrome. It appears that vessels participating in the intense bone remodeling response leak edema fluid into the marrow spaces of the subchondral spongiosa supporting the flexor surface of the bone. This fluid is organized by fibrous tissue, which forms at the drainage angle in the medullary cavity of the distal border of the navicular bone. Blood vessels in this area are entrapped in the fibrous tissue, which retards venous drainage, resulting in distended veins, venous hypertension, and pain.

Enlarged vascular channels can often be seen radiographically in horses with navicular syndrome. As the tiny nutrient arteries enter along the floor of the synovial fossae, which are located on the distal border of the navicular bone, each main artery sends off small branches to the synovial lining of each of the respective synovial fossae. As part of the hyperemia associated with the remodeling process, the synovial lining of the fossae also undergoes active hyperemia. Osteoclasts are attracted to the site and activated to resorb bone, thus enlarging the synovial fossae and eventually eroding into the navicular bone. The *resorptive process* follows the pathway of the nutrient artery into the medullary cavity of the distal border of the navicular bone, creating deep synovial invaginations that are recognized on radiographs as enlarged vascular channels.

Degenerative joint diseases of dogs

Primary and secondary degenerative joint diseases are relatively common in adult dogs, particularly medium and large breeds, and usually involving the major weight-bearing joints. Secondary degenerative joint disease in dogs most often occurs as a sequel to joint instability or incongruity following dysplastic diseases of the hip or elbow or to the various manifestations of osteochondrosis. These are discussed in more detail elsewhere in this chapter.

Primary degenerative joint disease is sufficiently common in aged dogs to be regarded by many as an *inevitable consequence of aging*. Gross lesions are often found incidentally at necropsy in animals that had shown no clinical evidence of lameness. In one study, 31 (21%) of 150 randomly selected dogs had degenerative lesions in the *stifle joint* at necropsy. In 23 of these dogs, the lesions were bilateral. Degenerative joint disease of the shoulder and hip joints are also common in middle-aged and old dogs. The lesions are usually bilateral and develop slowly, starting at around 5–6 years of age as areas of softening and yellow discoloration on regions of articular cartilage subjected to maximum weight-bearing stress, then progress to fibrillation (see Fig. 1.143) and sometimes eburnation. Osteophytes frequently line the chondro–osseous junction (see Fig. 1.146) and may encircle the articular surface. In severe cases, the joint capsule is thickened and synovial villi are hypertrophic.

Degenerative joint disease of the *shoulder joint* may be related to joint laxity. Like the hip joint, the shoulder relies on muscular strength for stability. Atrophy of muscles with aging could therefore permit excessive joint mobility and persistent mild trauma to the articular cartilage. The fact that the dog bears 65–70% of its body weight on its forelegs may account for the development of lesions in shoulders more frequently than in hips. The shoulder lesions of primary degenerative joint disease may be difficult to distinguish from the degenerative lesions that occur as a sequel to osteochondrosis, especially in the advanced stages. Both typically affect the caudal aspect of the humeral head, and both are generally bilateral. However, as described earlier in this chapter, osteochondrosis develops at a much earlier age than primary degenerative joint disease and although healed lesions of osteochondrosis may be found incidentally in older dogs, they represent the repair of a cartilage defect, rather than progressive degeneration of articular cartilage from its superficial layers.

Degenerative joint diseases of cattle

Degenerative joint disease of the *stifle joint* occurs in mature dairy cows and is reported as a *possible inherited trait in Holsteins and Jerseys*. Clinical signs include lameness and muscle atrophy. The lesions are bilateral, and appear to develop in the conventional manner. Cartilage degeneration, erosion, eburnation, and osteophyte formation occur on the distal femur and are most severe on the medial aspect (see Fig. 1.145). Complementary lesions are present in the proximal tibia and shredding of the medial meniscus is common (Fig. 1.149).

Stifle arthropathy also occurs in stud dairy and beef bulls and may be secondary to poor conformation, ligament damage, or ruptured meniscus during fighting, or as a consequence of osteochondrosis. The latter may be an important cause of wastage of well-grown beef bulls that have been fed for optimal growth prior to sale or showing.

Degenerative joint disease of the *hock joints (spavin)* has been described as a problem in *tied Swedish dairy cows*. In one study, 37%

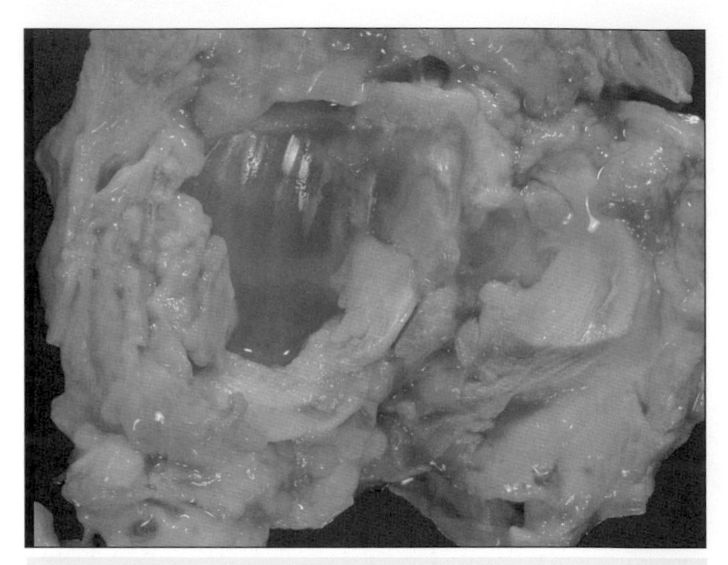

Figure 1.149 Degenerative joint disease, cow. Proximal tibia of same stifle joint as shown in Fig. 1.145. Shredding of medial meniscus, eburnation of medial articular surface (corresponding to medial condylar lesion), and marked fibrous thickening of joint capsule.

of animals were affected. The changes developed before the cows were 2 years old and increased in severity with age, sometimes progressing to ankylosis.

A lethal syndrome characterized by generalized degenerative joint disease and brachygnathia superior is reported in Angus calves. Affected calves have facial abnormalities, including reduced length of maxillary and palatine bones, together with abnormalities in all major joints. Macroscopic changes vary from reduced luster of articular cartilage to erosions and deep ulcers, eburnation of exposed subchondral bone, and thickening of joint capsules. Histologic lesions include degeneration of the articular cartilage matrix and necrosis of chondrocytes, in addition to fibrillation, chondrone formation, and chronic synovitis. Physeal abnormalities are also described. A genetic defect in the composition of cartilage matrix is suspected but the mode of inheritance is uncertain.

Bibliography

Holmberg T, Reiland S. The influence of age, breed, rearing intensity and exercise on the incidence of spavin in Swedish dairy cattle. Acta Vet Scand 1984;25:113–127.

Jayo M, et al. Brachygnathia superior and degenerative joint disease: a new lethal syndrome in Angus calves. Vet Pathol 1987;24:148–155.

McDevitt C, et al. An experimental model of osteoarthritis; early morphological and biochemical changes. J Bone Joint Surg [Br] 1977;59B:24–35.

McIlwraith CW, Goodman NL. Conditions of the interphalangeal joints. Vet Clin North Am: Equine Pract 1989;5:161–178.

McIlwraith CW, van Stickle DC. Experimentally induced arthritis of the equine carpus: histologic and histochemical changes. Am J Vet Res 1981;42:209–217.

Nickels FA, et al. Villonodular synovitis of the equine metacarpophalangeal joint. J Am Vet Med Assoc 1976;168:1043–1046.

Pedersen NC, Pool RR. Canine joint disease. Vet Clin North Am: Small Anim Pract 1978;8:465–493.

Pelletier J-P, et al. Etiopathogenesis of osteoarthritis. In: Koopman WJ, ed. Arthritis and Allied Conditions. 13th ed. vol 2. Baltimore, MD: Williams & Wilkins, 1996:1969–1984.

Pool RR. Pathologic manifestations of joint disease in the athletic horse. In: McIlwraith CW, Trotter GW, eds. Joint Disease in the Horse. Philadelphia, PA: W. B. Saunders Co., 1996:87–104.

Pool RR, Meagher DM. Pathologic findings and pathogenesis of racetrack injuries. Vet Clin North Am: Equine Pract 1990;6:1–30.

Pool RR, et al. Pathophysiology of navicular syndrome. Vet Clin North Am: Equine Pract 1989;5:109–129.

Poole AR. Cartilage in health and disease. In: Koopman WJ, ed. Arthritis and Allied Conditions. 13th ed. vol 1. Baltimore, MD: Williams & Wilkins, 1996:255–308.

Simmons EJ, et al. Instability-induced osteoarthritis in the metacarpophalangeal joint of horses. Am J Vet Res 1999;60:7–13.

Tirgari M, Vaughan LC. Arthritis of the canine stifle joint. Vet Rec 1975;96:394–399.

Trotter GW, et al. Degenerative joint disease with osteochondrosis of the proximal interphalangeal joint in young horses. J Am Vet Med Assoc 1982;180:1312–1318.

Vaughan LC. Orthopaedic problems in old dogs. Vet Rec 1990;126:379–388.

Cartilaginous joints

The most important degenerative diseases of cartilaginous joints are those affecting *intervertebral disks*. Such diseases are of particular importance in humans and dogs, but are rare in other species, as are degenerative diseases of other cartilaginous joints. **Degeneration of intervertebral disks** occurs in all dog breeds as part of the aging process, but there are significant differences between chondrodystrophic and nonchondrodystrophic breeds in the nature of the degeneration, and the age at which it occurs.

In **chondrodystrophic breeds**, such as the Dachshund, Pekingese, Poodle, Beagle and Cocker Spaniel, *the nucleus pulposus starts to degenerate early in life* and by one year of age, it has become largely replaced by dry, gray/white or yellow, cartilaginous material (Fig. 1.150A). The initial microscopic change is thickening of the delicate fibrocartilaginous septa between cellular clusters, dividing the nucleus pulposus into lobules. Chondrocyte proliferation within the nucleus leads to *replacement of the original structure with chondroid tissue* within the first year of life. No lesions are apparent in the annulus fibrosus at this stage. The change in the nucleus pulposus in chondrodystrophic dogs *occurs in all disks* throughout the length of the vertebral column and is accompanied by a decline in the glycosaminoglycan and water content, and an increase in the collagen content of the matrix. Beginning at the periphery, *the chondroid tissue in the nucleus pulposus degenerates and mineralizes*, eventually becoming a crumbly mass (Fig. 1.150B). At this stage, there is *degeneration of the inner lamellae of the annulus fibrosus*, probably due to the altered viscoelastic properties of the degenerate nucleus pulposus. Individual lamellae may tear and allow degenerate nuclear material to escape into the annulus. Meanwhile, degeneration of the annulus fibrosus continues until the outer lamellae are also involved.

In **nonchondrodystrophic dogs**, *the normal mucoid nature of the nucleus pulposus persists, at least until middle age*, and although it may become dry and more fibrous with advancing age, it seldom mineralizes. Occasionally, fibrous metaplasia of the nucleus pulposus occurs in relatively young dogs of nonchondrodystrophic breeds, but such changes are believed to be secondary to *focal disruption of lamellae in the annulus fibrosus*, presumably as a result of trauma. In support of this belief is the observation that these lesions are *generally confined to a single disk*, unlike the generalized changes that occur in the nucleus pulposus of chondrodystrophic dogs. Traumatic damage to the annulus fibrosus would be expected to alter the biomechanical properties of

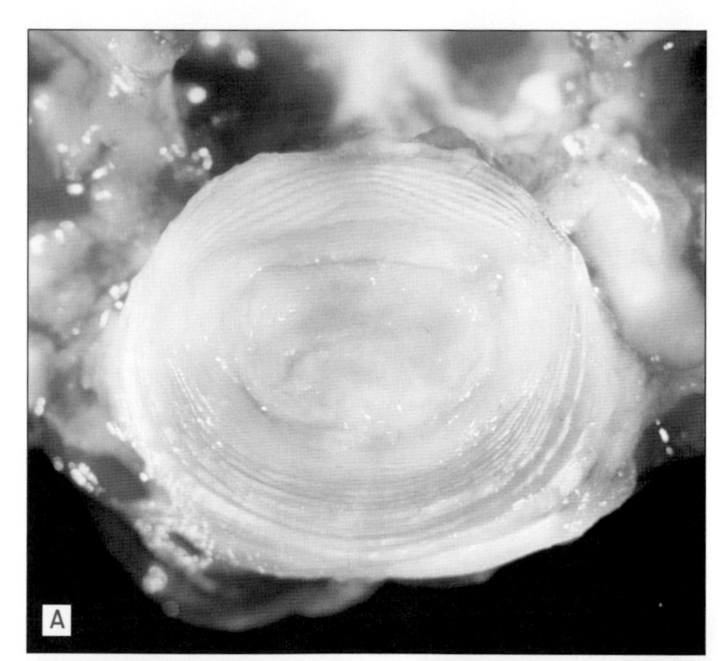

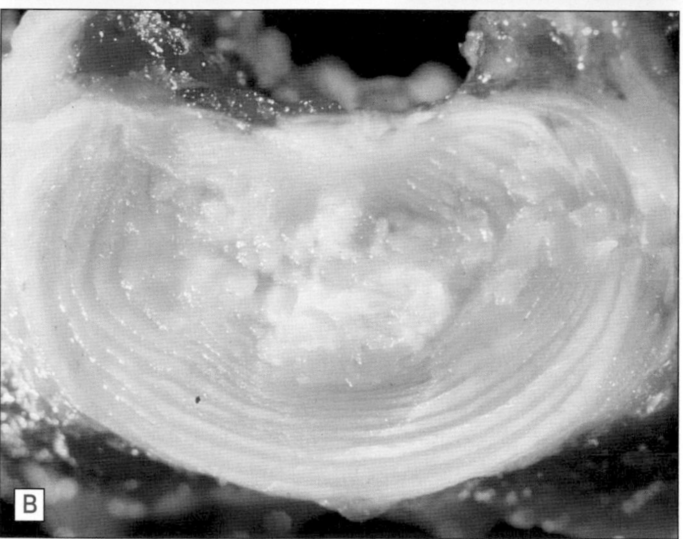

Figure 1.150 Intervertebral disk degeneration. **A.** Dry, gray/white nucleus pulposus (compare with Fig. 1.127) **B.** Chalky white foci of mineralization in the nucleus pulposus of a chondrodystrophic dog. Inner layers of annulus fibrosus are also degenerate.

the entire disk, leading to adaptive, and eventually degenerative, changes in the nucleus pulposus. Presumably, this same mechanism of intervertebral disk degeneration can occur in chondrodystrophic breeds, but the changes would be difficult to differentiate from the more severe, and more common, lesions outlined above.

Not surprisingly, *significant differences exist between chondrodystrophic and nonchondrodystrophic breeds of dog in the biochemical composition of their intervertebral disks.* At birth, the nucleus pulposus of chondrodystrophic disks contains up to 12 times more collagen than proteoglycan. The collagen composition increases rapidly with maturity, and by 11 months of age averages 25%. In nonchondrodystrophic breeds the collagen content of intervertebral disks remains below 5% for most of the animal's life. At all ages, the proteoglycan content of the intervertebral disk in chondrodystrophic breeds is significantly less than that of nonchondrodystrophic breeds.

The nucleus pulposus of *equine intervertebral disks* is more fibrous than that of dogs and its demarcation from the annulus fibrosus is less distinct. Although the nucleus pulposus of horses becomes less cellular with age, no chondroid or fibrous metaplasia occurs. In *cats*, macroscopic signs of intervertebral disk degeneration are not apparent until the animal is almost senile. Degenerative changes similar to those occurring in nonchondrodystrophic dogs are described in *adult sows and boars*, but dorsal herniation of the nucleus pulposus into the spinal canal has not been reported in this species. *Although disk protrusions are reported occasionally in cats and horses, discussion in the following section will concentrate on the syndrome in dogs*, for which there is a considerable volume of information.

Herniation of intervertebral disks

Because of their altered biomechanical properties, and their inability to withstand the normal range of forces associated with motion, *degenerate intervertebral disks are predisposed to complete or partial herniation or protrusion of nucleus pulposus material through the annulus fibrosus.* Many herniations are asymptomatic, but damage to adjacent structures, such as the spinal cord or peripheral nerve roots, is common and will be reflected by the clinical signs. Because of the eccentric location of the nucleus pulposus within the annulus fibrosus, most herniations occur through the narrower dorsal or dorsolateral regions of the annulus. In fact, *dorsal herniation of disk material into the spinal canal is considered the most common cause of paresis or paralysis in dogs.* Ventral herniation also occurs and may predispose to spondylosis (see below) and, on rare occasions, *nuclear material may herniate through the cranial or caudal cartilaginous end plate into a vertebral body, forming a so-called "Schmorl's node."*

Two types of dorsal herniation (types I and II) were recognized in classical descriptions of the disease in dogs by Hansen. **Type I herniations** *are characterized by a massive extrusion of degenerate nuclear material through the annulus fibrosus and dorsal longitudinal ligament into the spinal canal* (Fig. 1.151A). The sudden compression of the spinal cord, and/or peripheral nerve roots, typically causes *acute pain, paresis, or paralysis*, depending on the volume of extruded material and its location. Extradural hemorrhage may accompany laceration of longitudinal venous sinuses in the spinal canal. In some cases, severe damage to the spinal cord, or its vascular supply, results in *extensive hemorrhagic myelomalacia and ascending syndrome.* More commonly, the myelomalacia remains localized to a few cord segments. *The irritant nuclear material induces an inflammatory reaction* within the spinal canal and may become adhered to the dura.

Type II herniations generally develop slowly and are characterized by *partial herniation of the nucleus pulposus through ruptured annular fibers*, eventually resulting in bulging of outer lamellae and the intact dorsal longitudinal ligament into the spinal canal (Fig. 1.151B). Damage to the cord or peripheral nerve roots is much less than in type I herniations and clinical signs are generally mild.

Type I herniations of intervertebral disks are largely confined to chondrodystrophic dogs, particularly Dachshunds, and generally occur between 3 and 7 years of age. *Type II herniations are usually seen in nonchondrodystrophic dogs* between 6 and 8 years of age but can occur in any breed, as well as in humans, cats, and occasionally other species. Type I herniations are seldom reported in nonchondrodystrophic dogs.

Disk protrusions occur most frequently at sites of greatest vertebral mobility. In dogs, 70% of clinical cases of intervertebral disk disease are the

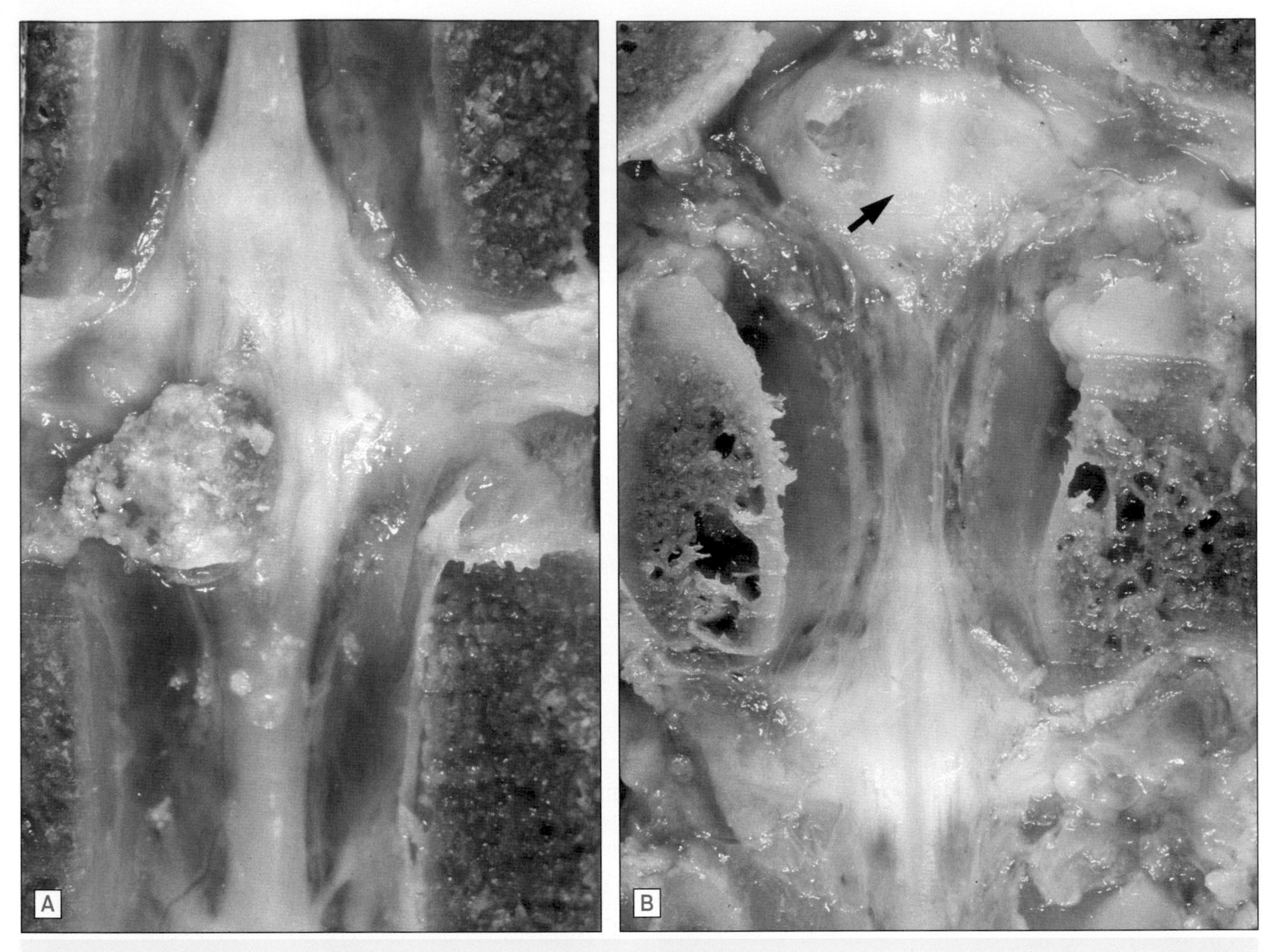

Figure 1.151 Degeneration and herniation of canine intervertebral disks. **A.** Herniation of a crumbly mass of degenerate disk material into the spinal canal through a tear in the dorsal longitudinal ligament (type I herniation). (Courtesy of RA Fairley.) **B.** Partial herniation of degenerate disk material (type II herniation) causing dorsal longitudinal ligament to bulge into the spinal canal (arrow). The adjacent disk is normal. (Courtesy of RA Fairley.)

result of herniations between the 12th thoracic and 2nd lumbar vertebrae. Approximately 15% of cases occur in the cervical region. Neurological signs associated with cervical disk protrusions are usually less severe than those involving the thoracolumbar region as the cervical cord occupies comparatively less space in the spinal canal, allowing more room for displacement before compressive damage occurs.

Herniations of intervertebral disks are *rare in horses* but occasionally are reported in the *cervical region*. Furthermore, in one study of cervical intervertebral disks in 17 clinically normal horses, partial extrusion of nuclear material through the annulus fibrosus, similar to type II lesions in dogs, was detected histologically in five horses. No intervertebral disk herniations have been reported in the thoracolumbar region of horses, probably because of the relative inflexibility of the equine spine in comparison to dogs and humans, and the strong longitudinal ligaments supporting the spine in this species. The mechanism of the cervical herniations in horses is not clear, but traumatic damage to the disk or adjacent vertebrae is a likely possibility, at least in some cases.

Ischemic myelopathy caused by **fibrocartilaginous embolism** *of spinal blood vessels is recognized as a possible sequel to degenerative disk disease in dogs*. Clinical signs relate to acute, severe, spinal cord damage similar to that associated with type I herniations of intervertebral disks, but the syndrome is *generally associated with type II herniations and is most common in nonchondrodystrophic dogs of large and giant breeds*. The spinal lesions may involve several vertebral segments and appear grossly as areas of swelling, malacia, and hemorrhage. Microscopically, fibrocartilaginous material, similar to that found in the degenerate nucleus pulposus, can usually be detected in the lumen of venules or arterioles (sometimes both) in areas of malacia. The mechanism by which embolic nuclear material enters the spinal vasculature is not clear. Venous emboli are probably caused by herniation of nuclear material directly into the overlying venous sinus, but arterial emboli are more difficult to explain. One suggestion is that they pass through arteriovenous communications from the venous circulation. Alternatively, they may directly penetrate arterioles in the degenerate annulus fibrosus and be extruded up to the radicular artery, from where they could gain access to the spinal cord. The possibility that such emboli develop following prolapse of the nucleus pulposus into the marrow cavity of an adjacent vertebral body has also been suggested, and is supported by experimental evidence. Demonstration of

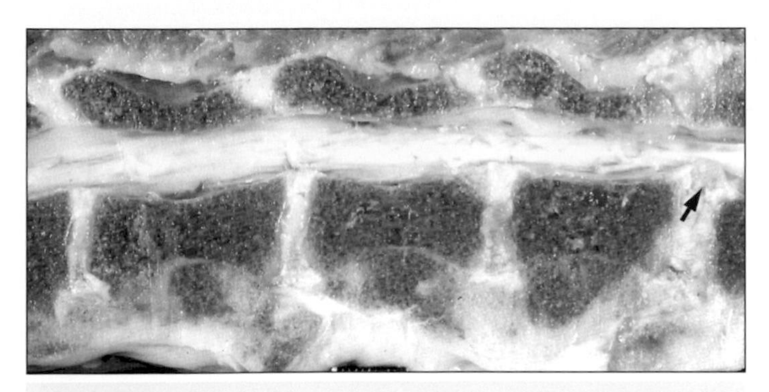

Figure 1.152 Ankylosing spondylosis, dog. Adjacent vertebral bodies united by thick, bony bridges along their ventral aspect. Also notice the type II disk herniation (arrow). (Courtesy of R. A. Fairley.)

Schmorl's nodes in vertebral bodies in the vicinity of spinal lesions would add further support to this hypothesis.

Fibrocartilaginous embolism has also been reported occasionally in pigs, cats, horses, and sheep. Of these species, pigs appear to be affected most frequently. The syndrome has occurred in weaner pigs as young as 45 days of age and, on one property, occurred in up to 25 of 1800 finishing pigs that had been sorted for slaughter at a weight of 126 kg. No degenerative changes in intervertebral disks, or other apparent predisposing factors, have been recognized in affected pigs. It is suggested that a *combination of heavy muscling and abrupt activity or excitement* may create increased pressure within intervertebral disks of young pigs and predispose to herniation of nuclear material into adjacent vertebrae or blood vessels. However, detailed dissection of disks and vertebrae in the vicinity of spinal lesions does not appear to have been performed.

Spondylosis

Spondylosis (spondylosis deformans, ankylosing spondylosis) is a common degenerative disease of the vertebral column characterized by the formation of osteophytes at the ventral and lateral margins of vertebral bodies adjacent to intervertebral spaces. The osteophytes may appear as spurs growing towards the adjacent vertebral body or as complete bony bridges with fusion of vertebrae (Fig. 1.152). Osteophytes also may be found dorsolaterally, projecting into the vertebral canal, but these are small and uncommon. In some cases, spondylosis is accompanied by degeneration of the synovial joints of the articular facets, and the reactive osteophytes may produce concurrent ankylosis of these articulations.

The *pathogenesis* of spondylosis is believed to involve an *initial degenerative change in the ventral annulus fibrosus*, probably secondary to trauma. Separation or tearing of the collagenous attachment of the annulus fibrosus from the adjacent vertebral body predisposes to mild ventral displacement of the annulus fibrosus and stretching of the ventral longitudinal ligament. This induces formation of bony outgrowths or spurs at the ventral margin of the intervertebral disk. As the disease progresses, further displacement of the annulus fibrosus and stretching of the ventral longitudinal ligament leads to more extensive osteophyte formation and eventually to bony bridging of the intervertebral space.

Spondylosis occurs most frequently in bulls, pigs, and dogs, and is seen less often in other domestic animal species. It is important in bulls kept in artificial breeding centers where it is presumably related to repeated traumatic damage to intervertebral disks during semen collection; *lesions are found in almost any bull past middle age.* Osteophytes develop mainly on the caudal end of thoracic vertebrae and the cranial end of lumbar vertebrae, and their incidence and size tends to decrease in either direction from the thoracolumbar junction. The greatest number and size of osteophytes is therefore in the area of greatest spinal curvature where maximum pressure on the disks during the thrust of service would be expected. The sequence of osteophyte development begins with severe degeneration of the annulus fibrosus, which may be present in bulls as young as 2 years of age. The osteophytes develop first in the outer annulus fibrosus and at its insertion to the rim of the vertebra. Growth is also in part by periosteal apposition and osseous metaplasia of ligaments. The trabecular bone of the osteophytes becomes continuous with that of the vertebral body and eventually is densely sclerotic. A thick layer of bone may be deposited along the ventral and ventrolateral aspects of the vertebral bodies (Fig. 1.153). In late stages, the heads of many ribs and the articular processes of the vertebrae bear large irregular osteophytes, which frequently cause ankylosis of the corresponding joint.

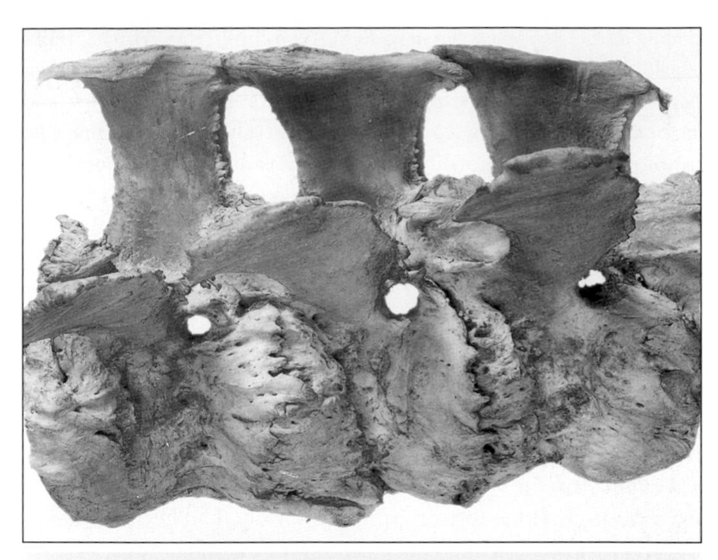

Figure 1.153 Ankylosing spondylosis, bull. Fusion of adjacent vertebral bodies by new bone deposited on ventral and ventrolateral surfaces.

Although spondylosis is a *common incidental finding in breeding bulls, the disease is sometimes associated with mild or severe clinical signs.* Affected bulls may show caudal weakness and ataxia, or even paralysis, after dismounting from service. They may continue to be mildly ataxic or recover, only to be affected again later. The onset of signs is usually associated with fracture of the vertebral bodies and of the ankylosing new bone, which is dense, but tends to be brittle. The line of fracture tends to follow a large penetrating vessel to the intervertebral disk, which is frequently separated, and then to diverge across the dorsal corner of one or other vertebra. There is little displacement of the fractured ends in most cases, which accounts for the incomplete spinal syndrome. Trauma to the spinal cord is usually mild and paralysis is usually secondary to either hemorrhage or repeated trauma.

In *dogs*, the incidence of spondylosis increases with age after about the fifth year, and *vertebral osteophytes are a common incidental finding during radiography or at necropsy*. As in bulls, the primary morphologic change in dogs and cats with spondylosis is in the *annulus fibrosus*. In dogs, most lesions occur in the region of the first and second lumbar vertebrae, an area of relatively high mobility. The lumbosacral articulation is also often involved. The link between spondylosis and clinical signs in dogs is questionable, but it seems likely that severe lesions are responsible for spinal stiffness and pain, and reduced enthusiasm for physical activity.

Ankylosing spondylosis is a relatively common incidental finding in adult sows and boars. Although no specific predisposing factors have been identified, degenerate intervertebral disks or narrow disk spaces are often associated with the lesions. The osteophytes most commonly involve *lumbar vertebrae*, especially those in the lumbosacral region. Ankylosis, if present, may be confined to the ventral aspect of the vertebral bodies, but in some cases there is extensive new-bone formation in the vertebral arches, thus fusing the articular processes and encroaching on the spinal canal.

Spondylosis in *horses* is comparable to that in other species, but the evolution of the osteophytes has not been studied in detail. Vertebral ankylosis in *cats* with chronic vitamin A toxicity is discussed elsewhere.

Bibliography

Benson JE, Schwartz KJ. Ischemic myelomalacia associated with fibrocartilaginous embolism in multiple finishing swine. J Vet Diagn Invest 1998;10:274–277.

Bray JP, Burbidge HM. The canine intervertebral disk. Part one: structure and function. J Am Anim Hosp Assoc 1998;34:55–63.

Bray JP, Burbidge HM. The canine intervertebral disk. Part two: Degenerative changes – nonchondrodystrophoid versus chondrodystrophoid disks. J Am Anim Hosp Assoc 1998;34:135–144.

Cauzinille L, Kornegay N. Fibrocartilaginous embolism of the spinal cord in dogs: review of 36 histologically confirmed cases and retrospective study of 26 suspected cases. J Vet Intern Med 1996;10:241-245.

Doige CE. Pathological changes in the lumbar spine of boars. Can J Comp Med 1980;44:382–389.

Furr MO, et al. Intervertebral disk prolapse and diskospondylitis in a horse. J Am Vet Med Assoc 1991;198:2095–2096.

Gaschen L, et al. Intervertebral disk herniation (Schmorl's node) in five dogs. Vet Radiol Ultr 1995;36:509–516.

Morgan JP, et al. Spondylosis deformans (vertebral osteophytosis) in the dog. J Small Anim Pract 1967;8:57–66.

Scott HW, O'Leary MT. Fibrocartilaginous embolism in a cat. J Small Anim Pract 1996;37:228–231.

Thomson RG. Vertebral body osteophytes in bulls. Pathol Vet 1969;[Suppl]6:1–46.

Tosi L, et al. Fibrocartilaginous embolism of the spinal cord: a clinical and pathogenic reconsideration. J Neurol Neurosurg Psych 1996;60:55–60.

Yovich JV, et al. Morphologic features of the cervical intervertebral disks and adjacent vertebral bodies of horses. Am J Vet Res 1985;46:2372–2377.

INFLAMMATORY DISEASES OF JOINTS

Inflammatory diseases of joints are generally referred to as either **arthritis** or **synovitis**. Although these terms are sometimes used interchangeably, they have slightly different meanings. *Synovitis refers to inflammation of a synovial membrane, whereas arthritis implies inflammation of other joint components in addition to the synovial membrane.* Inflammation of *tendon sheaths* often accompanies inflammation of an adjacent synovial joint and is referred to as **tenosynovitis** (synonyms: tendosynovitis or tendovaginitis). Secondary inflammatory changes are a feature of many chronic degenerative joint diseases, hence the commonly used term *osteoarthritis*, but in this section discussion will be confined to joint diseases that are primarily inflammatory in origin.

Arthritis may be either *infectious or noninfectious*, depending on the etiology. *Infectious arthritis occurs most frequently in farmed livestock and horses*, especially in young animals where it is a common sequel to neonatal bacteremia. *Most cases of noninfectious arthritis occur in dogs or cats and are immune-mediated*. Further classification is based on the duration of the lesion, the nature of the exudate, and the host response.

Fibrinous arthritis

This is typical of many *acute inflammatory diseases* of synovial joints, particularly those caused by *bacterial infections*. The presence of fibrin within synovial fluid indicates increased permeability of blood vessels in the synovial membrane, as fibrinogen and other large molecules are normally excluded. *Fibrin clots* may be floating free within the joint fluid, attached to the synovial membrane or lodged within recesses of the joint (Fig. 1.154A). In some cases, *sheets of yellow fibrin* partially or completely cover the synovial membrane, which is often edematous and hyperemic or may be studded with petechiae (Figs 1.154B, 1.155). *Synovial villi*, which are barely noticeable in normal joints, may become prominent macroscopically due to the edema and hyperemia. The synovial fluid is increased in volume and is usually slightly *turbid and mucinous*. When the inflammatory reaction is severe, there may be *gross edema of the periarticular tissues*. At this early stage, microscopic changes in the synovial membrane consist of edema and vascular engorgement, with few inflammatory cells. *Serous fluid or serofibrinous exudate* often infiltrates the fibrous layer of the articular capsule and the adjacent periarticular tissue.

In arthritis of longer duration, edema of synovial tissues is less apparent but the joint capsule and synovial membrane are thickened due *to proliferation of stromal cells and synoviocytes*, the latter often becoming several layers thick. *Sheets of fibrin containing variable numbers of neutrophils and fibroblasts may be attached to the surface* (Fig. 1.156). Villi continue to enlarge as a result of the cellular proliferation and may become extensively branched, with increasing numbers of lymphocytes and plasma cells, but few neutrophils (Fig. 1.157). Extravasated neutrophils pass quickly into the synovial fluid but seldom in sufficient numbers to give the fluid a purulent character. *Hypertrophy of villi* is greatest in the transition zone, and the proliferating fibrous stroma is joined by proliferating perichondrium to produce a fringe of granulation tissue, which spreads across the articular cartilage as a pannus and causes degeneration of the underlying cartilage.

Early resolution of the infection in animals with fibrinous arthritis is common, especially in smaller joints. However, the extensive deposits of fibrin in severe cases cannot be effectively removed by fibrinolytic mechanisms. Instead, the fibrin, which is deposited on the synovial membrane and within the layers of the articular capsule and periarticular tissue, is progressively invaded by fibrous tissue, leading to enlargement and restricted movement of affected joints.

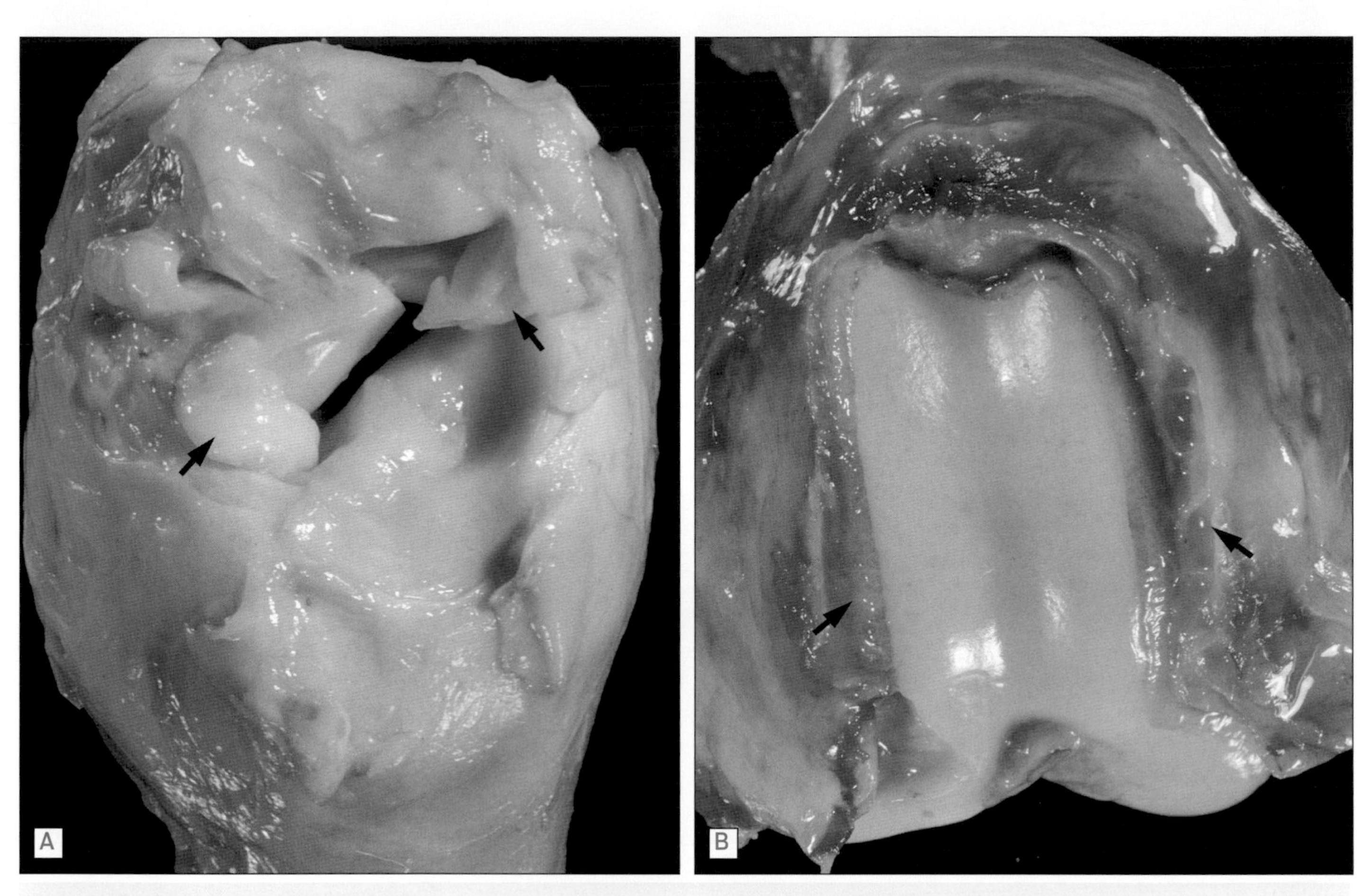

Figure 1.154 Fibrinous polyarthritis, calf. **A.** Large fibrin clots in the carpal joint (arrows). **B.** Stifle joint from the same calf showing an edematous, hyperemic synovial membrane covered by fibrin (arrows). The calf also had suppurative osteomyelitis (see Fig. 1.89A).

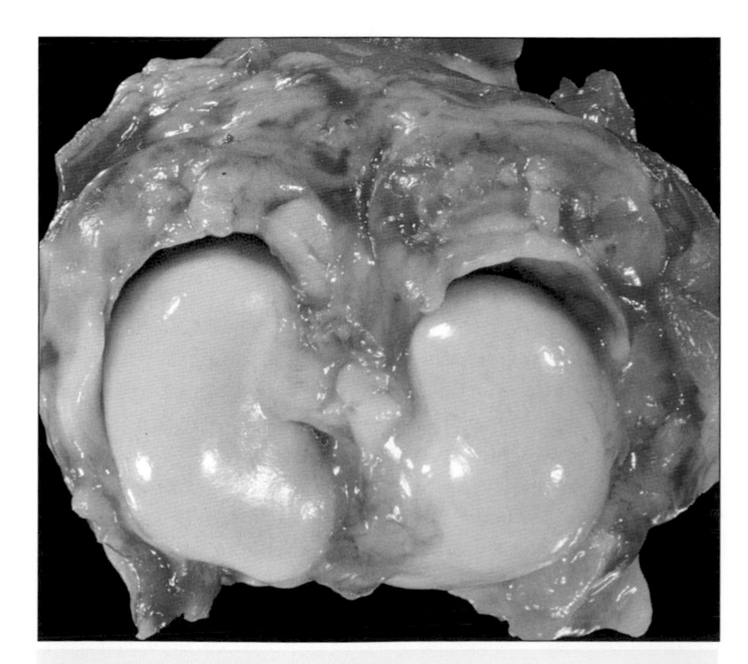

Figure 1.155 Fibrinous arthritis, pig. *Staphylococcus aureus* infection. The synovial membrane surrounding the femoral condyles is markedly thickened due to edema and an adherent layer of fibrin. Many petechiae are present in some areas.

The synovial lining is repaired by proliferation of synoviocytes. *Articular cartilage generally remains intact* in fibrinous arthritis, except in areas where it is covered by pannus. Pannus formation in joints with restricted movement may result in adhesions between apposed articular surfaces, leading to ankylosis.

Low-grade inflammation, with intense lymphocytosis, may persist in the synovial membrane, even in cases where the infection has apparently resolved. This may be due either to the persistence of an infectious agent that cannot be cultured or to ineffective removal by macrophages of the peptidoglycan components of microbial cell walls. For example, the cell wall of group A streptococci is relatively resistant to degradation by mammalian lysosomal enzymes, and is capable of provoking *persistent inflammation* in synovial tissues. Cell wall peptidoglycans from various other organisms, including *Erysipelothrix rhusiopathiae* also have this ability. All bacterial cell walls contain peptidoglycans, but there is considerable structural heterogeneity between bacterial species, and the types of side chain on the molecules probably determine their arthritogenic potential.

Purulent (suppurative) arthritis

This is characterized by the presence of *significant numbers of neutrophils in the synovial fluid, synovial membrane, and sometimes in adjacent structures*. When caused by bacterial infection, the neutrophils are usually abundant and may show *degenerative changes* in cytologic preparations of joint fluid. This is often referred to as **septic**

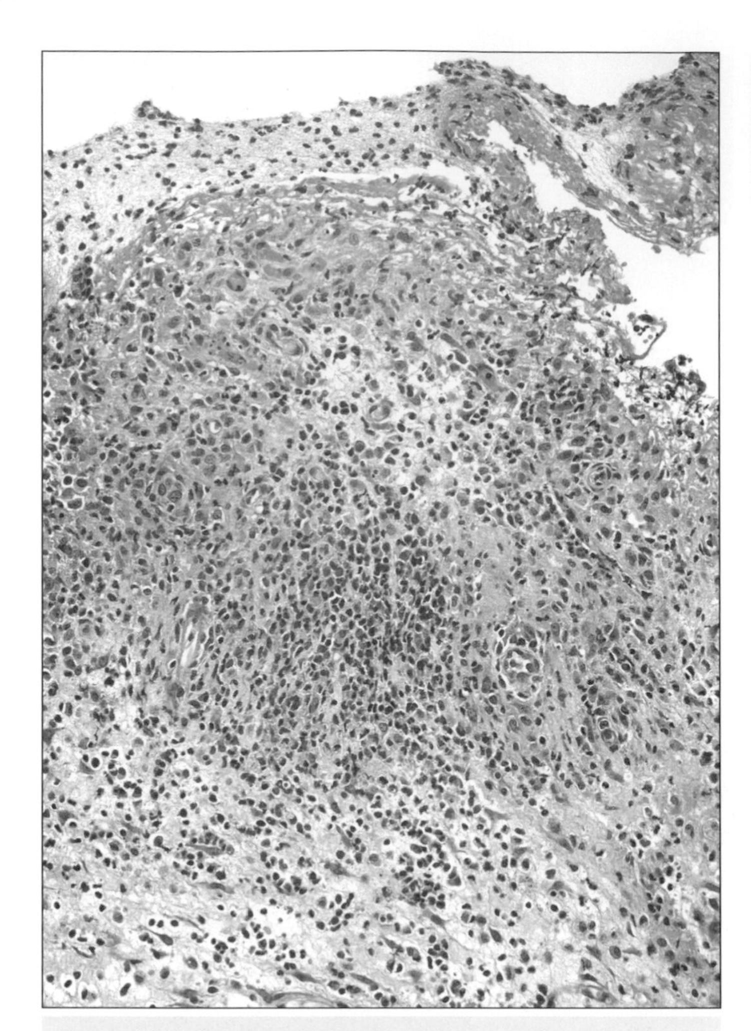

Figure 1.156 Subacute fibrinous arthritis, pig. *Streptococcus suis* type 1 infection. Edema, early proliferation of stromal cells and mixed cellular infiltration of synovial membrane. Fibrinous exudate containing moderate numbers of neutrophils is attached to the surface.

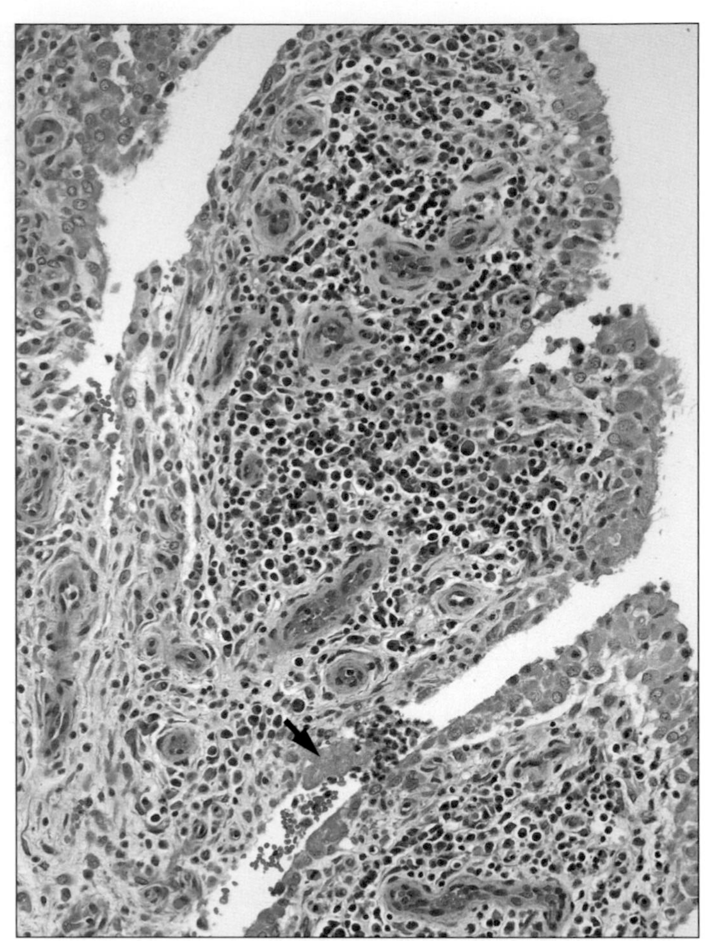

Figure 1.157 Chronic fibrinous arthritis, pig. *Streptococcus suis* type 2 infection. Hypertrophic villi infiltrated with mononuclear cells and lined by hypertrophic synoviocytes. A small fibrin tag and a cluster of neutrophils are trapped between two villi (arrow).

arthritis. Neutrophilic inflammation is a feature of arthritis caused by *Mycoplasma* spp., *Borrelia burgdorferi*, and certain viruses, but in these infections the neutrophils in synovial fluid are *nondegenerate*. Noninfectious, *immune-mediated arthritis* is also characterized by the presence of nondegenerate neutrophils in synovial fluid and differentiation from infectious arthritis is often difficult. *Bacteria are seldom observed in synovial fluid in animals with septic arthritis and false negatives on bacterial culture are common.*

Septic arthritis is often monoarticular and is *potentially a much more destructive process than fibrinous arthritis*. The synovial fluid is initially thin and cloudy but may resemble frank pus after a few days. *Destruction of articular cartilage* is much more likely to occur in septic arthritis than in fibrinous arthritis. *Lysosomal enzymes*, particularly collagenase, released from degenerating neutrophils probably play an important role in the cartilage destruction. Cytokines of macrophage origin, such as interleukin-1 and tumor necrosis factor-α, have also been shown to induce the resorption of cartilage both in vitro and in vivo and are most likely involved in chondrocyte-mediated cartilage degradation by stimulating the synthesis of metalloproteinases and plasminogen activators.

Complete resolution of septic arthritis is possible if the infection is eliminated spontaneously or by antibiotic therapy before erosion of cartilage occurs, but if the inflammatory process persists, the joint and adjacent structures will be severely altered. Cartilage degeneration occurs mainly at sites of weight bearing or at the articular margins, the latter in association with pannus formation. *Erosion of the degenerate cartilage may allow infection to enter the subchondral bone, resulting in purulent osteomyelitis* with extensive underrunning and separation of the articular cartilage. In such cases, it may be difficult to determine whether the arthritis preceded the osteomyelitis or vice versa, or whether the infectious agent gained access to both sites independently. Granulation tissue originating in the subchondral bone may grow out over the degenerate articular surface and predispose to ankylosis.

The suppurative process may extend to *involve adjacent tendon sheaths* and outwards from the synovial membrane of the articular capsule to *produce cellulitis in periarticular tissues*. The articular region is then greatly enlarged and the proliferation of fibrous tissue in response to inflammation, or during the healing process, results in permanent joint stiffness. In some cases, localization of the cellulitis into a periarticular abscess may be followed by *fistulation to the skin*. Fistulation to the skin surface may also result directly from empyema of the joint. Adhesions between tendons and tendon sheaths frequently occur in cases where tenosynovitis has developed in association with septic arthritis.

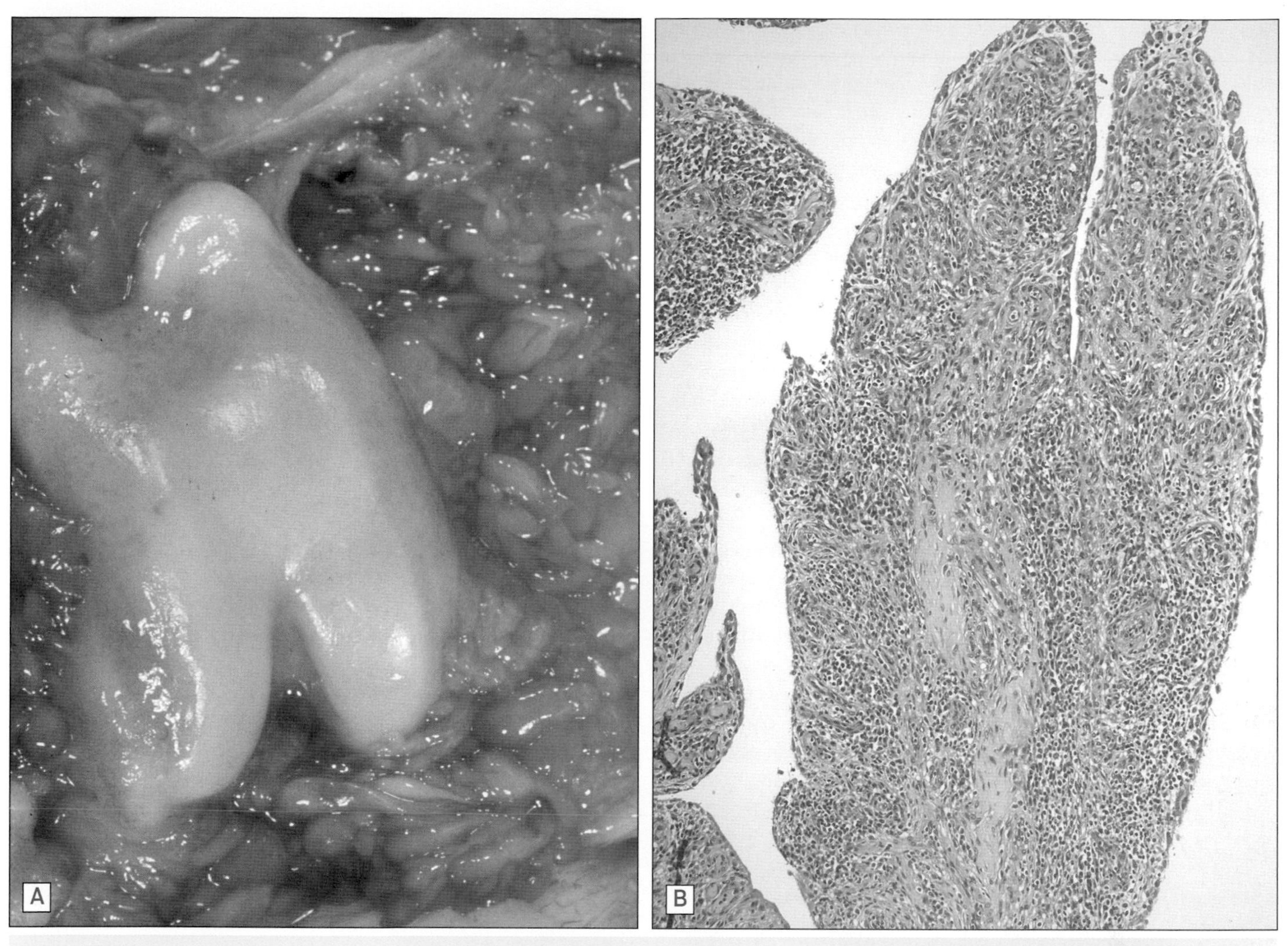

Figure 1.158 Proliferative arthritis, pig. **A.** Marked hypertrophy and hyperplasia of synovial villi in the stifle joint. (Courtesy of RA Fairley.) **B.** Hypertrophic villus in a pig with chronic *Erysipelothrix rhusiopathiae* infection. Note the stromal cell proliferation, mononuclear infiltration, and prominent synoviocyte layer.

Fibrinopurulent arthritis

Although it is convenient to classify inflammatory diseases of joints as fibrinous or purulent on the nature of the exudate, in reality, *many diseases would be better classified as* **fibrinopurulent arthritis**, *because the exudate consists of both fibrin and neutrophils*. In the chronic stages of many infectious and noninfectious forms of arthritis, lymphocytes and/or plasma cells are the major cell types infiltrating the synovial membrane (see Figs 1.148; 1.157). In such cases, **lymphocytic/plasmacytic synovitis** is a more appropriate morphological diagnosis. The term **proliferative arthritis** is often used to describe *chronic inflammatory diseases of joints where hypertrophy and hyperplasia of synovial villi is a prominent feature* (Fig. 1.158A, B).

An accurate etiologic diagnosis in animals with inflammatory diseases of joints may be crucial to a successful clinical outcome. In particular, failure to differentiate infectious and noninfectious causes of purulent arthritis can lead to inappropriate treatment and significantly alter the prognosis. *It is also important for septic arthritis to be recognized early and treated with an appropriate antibiotic in order to prevent degeneration of articular cartilage*. In addition to clinical history, analysis of synovial fluid often provides useful information but seldom allows a definitive diagnosis. As mentioned elsewhere in this section, many infectious and noninfectious forms of arthritis are characterized by increased numbers of neutrophils in synovial fluid. The neutrophils may show degenerative changes in bacterial infections but this is often difficult to appreciate in synovial fluid where the high concentration of hyaluronan prevents the cells from flattening out on the slide. Furthermore, not all bacteria induce such changes in neutrophils. Culture of bacteria or other agents from an inflamed joint allows a definitive diagnosis but false negatives are common. Culture of synovial membrane has been considered more sensitive but, in one study, *incubation of synovial fluid in a blood culture medium prior to culture yielded better results than either direct culture of the synovial fluid or culture of synovial membrane biopsies*. Microscopic examination of *synovial membrane biopsies* provides information on the nature of the inflammatory response and may be useful in differentiating chronic inflammatory and degenerative diseases of joints. Further information on diagnostic methods and details of laboratory results in specific diseases are discussed below.

Infectious arthritis

A variety of infectious agents, including *bacteria, viruses, and fungi*, are capable of infecting diarthrodial joints in humans and domestic animals. *In many, if not most situations, the arthritis is but one manifestation of a systemic infection*, with inflammatory lesions involving several tissues. In other cases, the infection may appear to be confined to one or more joints, suggesting either an affinity for synovial membranes or persistence of the infection in joints after being cleared from other sites. *Certain infectious agents may initiate a sterile synovitis in response to primary inflammatory lesions at sites distant from joints*. The mechanism of this form of arthritis is not clear, but it most likely involves an *immune-mediated reaction to nonviable bacterial components*, such as the bacterial wall antigen peptidoglycan, deposited in the synovial membrane, rather than direct infection of the joint by the agent. These forms of arthritis are discussed later under the heading Noninfectious (immune-mediated) arthritis.

A list of microorganisms that are commonly associated with infectious arthritis in domestic animals is presented in Table 1.4. Many agents other than those included in the list are capable of causing arthritis, but usually in isolated cases. Cats are not included in the list as infectious arthritis in this species is rare.

Some generalizations may be made about the prevalence of these infections relative to age. In *sheep*, with the exception of infection by *Mycoplasma* spp., infectious arthritis is primarily a disease of lambs. In *cattle*, streptococcal and coliform polyarthritis are neonatal, whereas infections due to *A. pyogenes* and *Salmonella* spp. may occur at any age. Streptococcal polyarthritis in *swine* is often a neonatal disease but the other infections are usually observed in weaned pigs. In *horses*, the organisms listed, other than *Salmonella* spp., generally cause intrauterine or neonatal infections.

Table 1.4 Common causes of infectious arthritis in domestic animals

Sheep
- *Chlamydophila pecorum*
- *Erysipelothrix rhusiopathiae*
- *Escherichia coli*
- *Histophilus somni*
- *Mycoplasma* spp.
- *Staphylococcus* spp.
- *Streptococcus* spp. (including types 1 & 2)

Goats
- *Mycoplasma* spp.
- Retrovirus

Swine
- *Actinobacillus suis*
- *Arcanobacterium pyogenes*
- *Brucella suis*
- *Erysipelothrix rhusiopathiae*
- *Escherichia coli*
- *Haemophilus parasuis*
- *Mycoplasma* spp.
- *Salmonella* spp.
- *Staphylococcus aureus*
- *Staphylococcus hyicus* ssp. *hyicus*
- *Streptococcus* spp. (including groups C & L)
- *Streptococcus suis* (types 1 & 2)

Cattle
- *Arcanobacterium pyogenes*
- *Escherichia coli*
- *Histophilus somni*
- *Mycoplasma bovis*
- *Salmonella* spp.
- *Streptococcus* spp.

Horses
- *Actinobacillus equuli*
- *Escherichia coli*
- *Klebsiella* spp.
- *Rhodococcus equi*
- *Salmonella* spp.
- *Streptococcus* (Group C)

Dogs
- *Blastomyces dermatitidis*
- *Borrelia burgdorferi*
- *Ehrlichia ewingii*
- *Escherichia coli*
- *Staphylococcus* spp.
- *Streptococcus* spp.

Bacteria

Bacterial arthritis is common in horses and food animals, usually as a sequel to neonatal bacteremia following omphalophlebitis ("navel ill"), or infections of the gastrointestinal tract or lungs. In many cases, the origin of the infection is not apparent either clinically or at necropsy, but inadequate transfer of colostral immunoglobulins is a common predisposing factor. The richly vascular synovial membrane appears to be a favored site for localization of bloodborne bacteria. Experimental studies have shown that viable bacteria injected intravenously lodge in the synovial membrane and gain access to synovial fluid more readily than to spinal fluid, aqueous humor, and urine.

Hematogenous bacterial infections in neonatal animals typically cause *polyarthritis*. Infected joints are generally hot, painful, and swollen due to the hyperemia and edema of the synovial membrane and joint capsule, and the increased quantity of synovial fluid. Although the infection may resolve in some joints, it often persists in others, particularly the large joints of the limbs, causing severe septic arthritis with destruction of articular cartilage. *Many, if not most young animals with septic arthritis of hematogenous origin also have osteomyelitis in the epiphyses or metaphyses of adjacent bones* (Figs 1.89A, 1.154A, B). This may be due to concurrent localization of the organism in the bone and synovial membrane, or may reflect the close vascular relationship between the epiphyseal bone and synovial membrane in young animals, with spread of infection from one site to the other. Foci of osteomyelitis originating at sites of endochondral ossification in the epiphysis, immediately beneath the articular cartilage, may underrun and penetrate the cartilage, spreading the infection directly into the synovial fluid. In joints where the capsule attaches distal to the physis, inflammatory foci in the metaphysis may contaminate the synovial fluid by penetrating the cortex near the physeal margin. This region is relatively porous in young animals because of the intense structural modeling that occurs in the metaphyseal cortex during rapid growth. The prevalence of concurrent bone involvement should always be considered in animals with bacterial arthritis as even if the arthritis can be successfully treated, the animal may eventually succumb to the effects of chronic osteomyelitis.

The reason why certain organisms are more likely to localize in the synovial membrane than others during bacteremia is not clear, but experimental evidence suggests that it is not purely due to chance. Studies in mice have indicated that *adherence* of *Staphylococcus aureus* to collagen is likely to be involved in the pathogenesis of septic arthritis and osteomyelitis. Other organisms causing arthritis have also been shown to possess *collagen-binding components*.

Spread of infection to joints from adjacent soft tissues is uncommon as the dense, fibrous layer of the joint capsule provides an effective barrier, but it may occur in necrotizing disorders such as necrobacillosis and footrot in cattle.

Direct implantation of bacteria into a synovial joint may occur as a sequel to a *penetrating wound* from the skin surface. This is the most common cause of bacterial arthritis in *dogs and cats*, where the disease occurs more often in adolescent and adult animals than in neonates. The arthritis is *monoarticular* and a mixed population of opportunistic bacteria is likely to be involved, often resulting in a highly destructive inflammatory response. *Arthroscopic surgery* and collection of synovial fluid by *fine-needle aspiration* may also introduce bacteria to a joint.

Although many different bacteria have been associated with arthritis in domestic animals, some specific types of bacterial arthritis are sufficiently important to warrant discussion in more detail.

Erysipelas

Erysipelothrix rhusiopathiae, *the cause of porcine erysipelas and erysipeloid in man, is a gram-positive bacillus with a wide geographic distribution and host range.* It causes outbreaks of disease in *pigs, lambs, and birds*, and sporadic disease in the other domestic species. The organism is widespread in nature and is capable of survival, and perhaps growth, in decaying material of animal origin. It may be present in the soil of pig pens and in pit slurry, and survives for 2–3 weeks on pasture spread with slurry. It is resistant to many disinfectants and is capable of infecting many species, some of them in epidemic proportions. In spite of these epidemiological features, *pigs are probably the principal source of infection for other pigs. Erysipelothrix rhusiopathiae* can persist for many months in the lesions of diseased pigs, and it is often carried in the tonsils, intestine, bone marrow, and gallbladder of healthy swine.

Porcine erysipelas occurs in pigs of all ages, but the most susceptible are those from 2 months to 1 year of age, and pregnant sows. The latter may abort or give birth to stillborn young, from which the organism can be cultured. The disease can be produced by ingestion of the organism, contamination of cutaneous wounds, or as a result of bites of infected flies. The manifestations of erysipelas in pigs vary from an *acute septicemic form*, which is usually fatal, to *mild and chronic forms* characterized by necrosis of the skin, endocarditis, and polyarthritis. *In epidemics, the septicemic form predominates, whereas in endemic areas the disease tends to be sporadic, with cases of septicemia, polyarthritis, or endocarditis occurring in varying proportions.*

The **acute disease** is a *febrile septicemia*, which usually develops within 24 h of exposure to virulent organisms and produces *disseminated intravascular coagulation*. Endothelial cells of capillaries and venules throughout the body swell, monocytes adhere to them, and by 2–3 days microthrombi are widespread. By 4 days, accumulation of fibrin within and around vessels, bacterial invasion of endothelium and diapedesis of erythrocytes are prominent. Perivascular fibrin incites connective tissue proliferation in sites such as synovial membranes. *Grossly*, there is *purple discoloration of the skin* due to congestion and, in some cases, thrombosis of dermal capillaries and venules. Lesions may not be specific in pigs that die at this stage. *Petechiae or ecchymoses* may be present on serous membranes, the *spleen is almost always swollen and red,* and there may be *congestion and infarction in the gastric mucosa.* The latter lesion occurs in many acute infections in pigs. Subsidence of the acute disease, or a milder initial course, often leads to swelling of joints, lameness, and characteristic erythematous lesions in the skin.

The *cutaneous lesions* of porcine erysipelas are *roughly rhomboidal* and slightly raised. They are readily visible in light-skinned pigs and palpable when not visible in dark-skinned pigs. The skin within the rhomboid may be uniformly *bright red or purple*, but in some lesions only the margins and center are discolored. The latter lesions may progress to complete discoloration, or may return to normal within a few days. The uniform, bright red lesions may also resolve, leaving only an area of scurfiness as a residue. The dark red or purple lesions undergo dry necrosis and may eventually peel off or, if forcibly detached, expose a raw base. Occasionally, the skin lesions coalesce over large areas and lead to extensive cutaneous necrosis. The *tip of the tail and ears* may also become dark, shrunken, and leathery due to *ischemic necrosis*. Microscopically, there is neutrophilic infiltration of the walls of small dermal arterioles, many of which contain *cellular thrombi*. Suppurative inflammation of sweat glands is also a consistent microscopic finding, but otherwise the reaction is most severe at the junction of dermis and subcutis. *Similar cutaneous infarcts occasionally occur in other septicemic bacterial diseases* and the lesions should not therefore be considered pathognomonic for erysipelas. Confirmation requires culture of the organism from the undersurface of skin lesions or from other tissues.

By the time the cutaneous lesions of porcine erysipelas develop, lesions also may be found in *visceral organs*. In addition to *splenic enlargement*, numerous *petechiae may be visible in the renal cortices* and there is sometimes intense interstitial hemorrhage in the medulla. The renal cortical petechiae arise in part from small venules, but mainly from glomeruli. The *characteristic glomerular lesion of erysipelas is focal fibrinoid necrosis of the tufts, with intracapsular hemorrhage.* Less specific changes that might also be present include diffuse glomerulitis, characterized by swelling or proliferation of the glomerular endothelium, and segmental sludging of erythrocytes in some glomerular tufts. The latter lesion probably precedes fibrinoid necrosis and intratubular hemorrhage. Occasionally, gram-positive bacterial colonies are found in the necrotic tufts or in intertubular capillaries, where they are associated with tiny, intense foci of neutrophils.

The articular lesions of acute erysipelas are typically those of *fibrinous polyarthritis* (see above). The volume of synovial fluid is increased and the synovial membrane is hyperemic. In some cases, the synovial arterioles show necrotizing inflammation and extensive plugging by cellular thrombi.

Lesions in other tissues are not specific. There is leukocytosis with many mononuclear cells in hepatic sinusoids. The *lungs show typical lesions of bacteremia*, with organisms sequestered in the pulmonary capillaries, but without the focal localization of embolic pneumonia. The alveolar capillaries are intensely hyperemic and contain numerous sequestered leukocytes. Later, the alveolar walls tend to thicken as a result of cellular infiltration, mononuclear cells predominating, and this is accompanied by alveolar flooding and increased alveolar macrophages. The *skeletal musculature often shows extensive degeneration*, although it may be too recent to be visible grossly. Whether the muscular degeneration is an example of the classic change described as Zenker's degeneration or is mainly due to peripheral arteriolitis is difficult to determine. Of the remaining tissues, the *brain and eyes* appear to harbor lesions most consistently. The organisms localize in the choroid and the ciliary process and provoke an intense neutrophilic inflammatory response. In the brain, there is cerebral leukocytosis and degeneration of blood vessels in the cerebral white matter. Embolic bacterial colonies, together with a tiny surrounding zone of neutrophils and a few eosinophils, may be found in small vessels of the brain and spinal cord. Such foci of inflammation are quite common and are not always associated with visible organisms. The neural lesions do not produce neurological signs.

Chronic erysipelas in swine is characterized by *vegetative valvular endocarditis and/or arthritis*. Localization of the organism in heart valves and joints occurs as a sequel to either acute, nonfatal septicemia or mild, perhaps inapparent, systemic disease. The *mitral valves* are most often involved and pigs that die of endocarditis have congestive heart failure and embolism. *Large infarcts in the spleen and kidneys* are particularly common. The valvular lesions may be very large, consisting of layers of fibrin with variable numbers of trapped inflammatory cells. During the active stage, masses of gram-positive bacteria can be found near the surfaces of the thrombi. In older lesions, the bacterial colonies are buried more deeply in the thrombi and usually cannot be cultured.

Arthritis is a common expression of chronic erysipelas in pigs and may be unassociated with earlier acute or subacute signs of infection. It can be reproduced experimentally by injections of the organism, and also occurs in vaccinated swine. *Although vaccination seems useful in preventing the acute syndrome and mortality, it appears to enhance susceptibility to polyarthritis.* The number of joints affected following experimental inoculation of susceptible pigs depends on the number of organisms used and the strain of organism. In pigs with acute arthritis, organisms may be isolated from grossly normal as well as inflamed joints, but isolation from affected joints may be difficult in the chronic disease. Persistence of the inflammation in such cases may be due to the presence in synovial tissues of bacterial antigens, rather than intact organisms. Antigens persist for up to 18 months in arthritic joints and specific antibodies found in synovial fluid may be produced by plasma cells in the synovial membrane. Culture of the sediment from centrifuged synovial fluid however, usually yields a few organisms, even in very chronic erysipelas.

The *lesions in chronic erysipelas arthritis* vary in severity. In mild cases, there is excess synovial fluid and villus hypertrophy, but the articular capsule may appear normal. In severe cases, there is extensive villus hyperplasia and hypertrophy over much of the synovial membrane (Fig. 1.158A), together with pannus formation and cartilage degeneration. The hypertrophic villi are hyperemic and infiltrated with mononuclear cells, including plasma cells (Fig. 1.158B). *Diskospondylitis* is also a feature of chronic erysipelas.

Acute and chronic arthritis, similar to that caused by *Erysipelothrix rhusiopathiae* infection, also occur in pigs in association with certain other bacterial and mycoplasmal infections and *in many cases, the etiology remains undetermined.* The development of molecular biological techniques capable of demonstrating the presence of small quantities of persistent antigen may improve our diagnostic success with such cases in the future.

Erysipelas in sheep is usually the result of *percutaneous infection*, entry being gained through the *umbilicus, docking and castration wounds, shear wounds, and cuts or abrasions acquired during dipping.* The lesion in sheep may be confined to the skin and subcutis at the point of entry, or there may be bacteremia with localization in joints. Rarely, death may occur from septicemia.

Fibrinopurulent polyarthritis, and osteomyelitis, is the usual form of erysipelas seen in young lambs after docking or castration, and sometimes following umbilical infections. The arthritis is subacute or chronic and the morbidity may be as high as 50%. Mortality is low, and is a consequence of severe lameness rather than a direct result of the infection. The main limb joints are involved. In the early stages, there is synovitis with an increased volume of turbid synovial fluid. Later, the fibrinous exudate may coagulate into firm pads. Articular cartilage is initially unaffected, but foci of osteomyelitis in the subchondral epiphyseal bone may lead to collapse of the overlying articular surface and formation of irregular pits or ulcers with a base of granulation tissue. In the chronic stages, the joints are stiffened and deformed by periarticular fibrosis and by periosteal and perichondral osteophytes.

Cutaneous infections following dipping are associated with contamination of nonbactericidal dips with *E. rhusiopathiae*. Lesions occur most often about the *fetlocks* but invasion may occur wherever the skin is injured and contaminated. Post-dipping infections, which mimic cutaneous erysipelas, are occasionally caused by both *Arcanobacterium pyogenes* and *Corynebacterium pseudotuberculosis*. Cutaneous erysipelas may also occur when sheep are confined in wet, contaminated pens.

Lameness is severe and out of proportion to the gross changes in affected feet. The disease is febrile in some animals and associated with rapid wasting, but recovery occurs in 2–3 weeks. The affected pasterns are hot and painful, and there is regional lymphadenitis. The coronary band may be swollen and the swelling, which is always slight, may extend to the metacarpal or metatarsal regions. The affected areas are progressively depilated. Incision reveals moderate erythema and slight edema of the subcutis.

Histologically, there is acute inflammation very similar to that seen in the cutaneous lesions of porcine erysipelas. There are superficial pustules in the epidermis. In the outer layers of the dermis, there is perivascular edema, accumulation of neutrophils and cellular thrombi within vessels. The reaction is more severe in the deeper layers of the dermis and is characterized by suppurative hydradenitis, necrotizing vasculitis, and vascular thrombosis. Similar changes occur in the *sensory laminae of the foot* and are responsible for the severe lameness. In the course of 2–3 weeks, the inflammatory reaction resolves completely, except for residual lesions in the larger blood vessels.

Streptococcal septicemia and polyarthritis

Streptococci cause a variety of infections in domestic animals, including *septicemia, meningitis, polyarthritis, bronchopneumonia, and endocarditis*. In **swine**, there are well-defined syndromes of streptococcal septicemia, with localization in synovial structures, meninges, and elsewhere, caused by ***Streptococcus suis***. This organism shares cell-wall antigens with streptococci of Lancefield's group D but is not genetically related to them. Over 30 serotypes have now been recognized but those most frequently associated with arthritis are types 1, 2, 7, and 14. *In general,* Streptococcus suis *serotype 1 infects suckling pigs and is not pathogenic for other species, whereas serotype 2 tends to cause disease in weaner and feeder pigs and also cause meningitis and septicemia in man.* Serotype 7 may also have zoonotic significance. Interestingly, some serotype 2 strains cause only nonfatal pneumonia in gnotobiotic pigs, even following dexamethasone treatment. Increased virulence may depend on certain high-molecular-weight, cell-wall proteins that are released by muramidase.

***Streptococcus suis* type 1** may cause disease in piglets from 2 to 10 weeks of age, but most cases occur in the *2–3-week age group*. The disease may occur in one or all pigs in a litter, and a number of litters may succumb over a period of weeks. The infection is initially *bacteremic or septicemic* and death may occur at this stage with little evidence of localization in visceral organs. The spleen is slightly enlarged and purple, petechiae may be present in the renal cortex, and the lungs are hyperemic with small pleural hemorrhages. There may be a slight excess of fluid in serous cavities. When the course of the disease is slightly longer, there are signs of *arthritis and meningitis*. All joints may be affected but the lesions are most obvious in the large limb joints. The synovial fluid is increased in volume, slightly mucinous, and turbid due to the presence of neutrophils. Occasional gram-positive cocci may be seen in smears. The meningitis is fibrinopurulent and affects mainly the basal meninges. Clumps of fibrin may be found floating free in lateral ventricles or attached to choroid plexuses. The cerebral aqueduct and/or foramina of Luschka may be occluded by exudate or by ependymal reaction, leading to internal hydrocephalus.

Streptococcus suis type 1 is most likely *carried in the nasopharynx of sows* and transferred to their offspring shortly after birth. The portal of entry is the palatine tonsil. Piglets infected experimentally may have bacteremia for 2–3 weeks, after which time, the developing immunity eliminates infection from the blood and internal organs. The organism is relatively harmless unless it becomes established in joints or meninges.

Disease caused by ***Streptococcus suis*** **type 2** may be clinically and pathologically similar, but often the range of lesions is greater. The organism is *carried in the palatine tonsils of pigs*, and *infection is probably by the respiratory route*. In infected herds, it is isolated from up to 80% of clinically normal pigs and is commonly found in nasal turbinates and pneumonic lungs, where it is probably a secondary invader. Limited outbreaks do occur but *sporadic, isolated disease is more common*. The incubation period varies from 1 to 14 days and the clinical course from 4 to 48 h. Affected pigs are usually about 10–14 weeks of age and the most significant lesion is *purulent meningitis*, which, along with *polyserositis*, is visible grossly in about 50% of pigs. The bacteria probably enter the cerebrospinal fluid within monocytes via the choroid plexuses. *Purulent arthritis* occurs in a few animals, usually those at the lower end of the age range. *Fibrinopurulent pericarditis, endocarditis, or hemorrhagic, necrotizing myocarditis* occur in some pigs. Endocarditis most often affects the mitral valve. The myocarditis grossly may resemble mulberry heart disease but *the histologic lesions of necrotizing vasculitis and diffuse inflammation associated with bacteria are distinctive*.

Occasionally, *Streptococcus suis* type 2 causes *septicemia in newborn piglets*. Pigs dying acutely may show few lesions other than marked congestion of lungs and meninges with perhaps a few strands of fibrin adherent to the pleura, but purple discoloration of the skin and other signs of septicemia are usually present. *Streptococcus suis* is occasionally isolated from suppurative lesions in ruminants.

Streptococcus equisimilis also has been isolated from the joints of pigs with purulent arthritis. In experimental infections, other streptococci, such as *Streptococcus pyogenes* (Lancefield's group A) and group C streptococci produce arthritis and osteomyelitis, in swine.

Streptococci also cause *polyarthritis and meningitis* in **calves**. Metastatic iridocyclitis occurs in many bacterial infections in which polyarthritis occurs, but in none is it so consistent or prominent as in the *streptococcal disease of neonatal calves*. The disease is probably secondary to *umbilical infection* in most cases but, because ocular lesions may be visible grossly by 24 hours of life, there is a possibility that some infections are intrauterine. The clinical signs are of *hypopyon, corneal opacity and meningitis* and because of the strong affinity of the organisms for the meninges and eyes, the disease is without a chronic phase. The arthritis is acute and there is no obvious joint swelling.

In **lambs**, *Streptococcus* spp. are probably second only to *Erysipelothrix rhusiopathiae* as a cause of polyarthritis, although in a UK study, *Streptococcus dysgalactiae* was easily the most common isolate from the joints of arthritic lambs. The *umbilicus* is accepted as the likely route of entry in most cases and this is supported by the high prevalence of the disease in sucklings. There is some variation in the combination of lesions seen at necropsy, probably due to differences in the species and strains of organisms involved. Specific typing of *Streptococcus* spp. is not a routine procedure.

Localization of *Streptococcus* spp. in the joints and other organs of lambs is a sequel to bacteremia. Some lambs die acutely of septicemia and show few gross lesions. *Localization* in various tissues occurs in the course of 1–2 days and may involve any one or a combination of sites, including *the uvea, cerebrospinal meninges, valvular endocardium, myocardium, kidneys, and joints*. Meningeal localization seldom occurs in the absence of polyarthritis, but the latter may not be clinically evident in cases with a short clinical course. Polyarthritis may however occur alone. The infection may subside in many joints, persisting only in the larger limb joints and causing chronic lesions of purulent arthritis. In approximately 20% of lambs with subacute or chronic polyarthritis, there is coincident valvular endocarditis.

Coliform polyarthritis

Escherichia coli *often localizes in the joints or meninges (or both) in farm animals, but is a rare cause of arthritis in dogs*. In septicemic colibacillosis of neonatal **calves**, polyarthritis and tenosynovitis are common, but are easily overlooked or overshadowed by other manifestations of acute septicemia, including meningitis and polyserositis. The organism may enter the blood from the gut, oropharynx, or umbilicus. The lesions in calves are similar to those of streptococcal infection although iridocyclitis, with grossly visible hypopyon, occurs less frequently in association with coliform polyarthritis. In some cases, the polyarthritis is chronic, with lesions restricted to one or two of the larger limb joints and tending to be symmetrical. Chronic coliform arthritis in calves is often coincident with interstitial nephritis (white-spotted kidney), which may develop into descending pyelonephritis.

Polyarthritis caused by *Escherichia coli* also occurs commonly in **horses** and **pigs**, but does not appear to be a common isolate from the joints of lambs with polyarthritis.

Staphylococcal arthritis

Staphylococcus aureus *is a relatively common cause of polyarthritis in farm animals and monoarticular arthritis in dogs*. In lambs, *Staphylococcus aureus* may occur as a sporadic infection or as a complication of tick pyemia. In the UK, the latter syndrome occurs in lambs born onto tick-infested ground, particularly during the spring when tick activity is at a peak. The agent gains entry to the blood through bites of the blood-sucking nymphal stage of the tick *Ixodes ricinus*, then localizes in the synovial membrane and various internal organs. Vertebral osteomyelitis is a frequent complication of *Staphylococcus aureus* septicemia in affected lambs, often leading to ataxia or paralysis following collapse of necrotic bone into the spinal canal.

In one study, ***Staphylococcus hyicus*** subspecies *hyicus* was an important cause of fibrinopurulent arthritis in **pigs** up to 12 weeks of age. Lesions were most common in the *elbow and tarsal joints*. The palatine tonsil is considered an important site of entry for this organism in pigs. *Staphylococcus hyicus* subspecies *hyicus* produces *protein A*, which aids in attachment of the bacteria, and *exfoliative factors*, which may promote epithelial erosion and assist in the invasive process. The altered epithelial environment created by *Staphylococcus hyicus* subspecies *hyicus* in tonsillar crypts may also facilitate the entry of other bacteria to the blood or lymph of young pigs.

Staphylococcus spp. were the most common bacteria isolated from the synovial fluid in a study of 19 cases of *septic arthritis* in **dogs**. Interestingly, although all dogs included in the study had increased numbers of neutrophils in their synovial fluid, the *neutrophils were nondegenerate* in all but one case. This reinforces the point that detection of toxic neutrophils in synovial fluid is not a reliable means of differentiating septic arthritis from noninfectious, immune-mediated arthritis in dogs.

Haemophilus and *Histophilus* septicemia and arthritis

Glasser's disease *is a fibrinous meningitis, polyserositis, and/or polyarthritis of* ***pigs****, caused by* ***Haemophilus parasuis***. The organism is part of the normal flora of the upper respiratory tract of conventional pigs but is often isolated from pneumonic lungs and regarded as a secondary invader. It is acquired from the dam shortly after birth but colostral antibodies usually protect young piglets against disease. Active immunity develops by 7–8 weeks. *Haemophilus parasuis* occasionally produces severe outbreaks of disease in animals aged around 5–12 weeks, usually following transportation or other management stress. Cesarian-derived pigs are susceptible at any age and often develop Glasser's disease after introduction to a boar test-station or a conventional herd.

Glasser's disease is defined on an etiological basis, as there are other organisms, such as *Streptococcus suis*, which produce similar lesions and similar diseases. *Mycoplasma* spp. also produce serositis and arthritis in swine but the diseases are more chronic, and meningitis is either absent or lymphocytic, depending on the species of mycoplasma involved.

Glasser's disease is peracute, with high fever, lameness, and neurological disturbances, including paresis, stupor, and hyperesthesia. As in other septicemic diseases of pigs, the skin may show purple discoloration. The course is 1–2 days and without treatment, the mortality rate is very high. Usually, *serofibrinous meningitis, pericarditis, pleuritis, peritonitis, and synovitis of many joints* characterize the morbid picture. In individual cases, all these tissues, or any combination of them, may be inflamed. Occasionally the lesions occur in only one site and, in some pigs or some outbreaks, gross lesions are absent. *Predilection sites* for lesions of Glasser's disease are *meninges, joints, peritoneum, pleura, and pericardium in descending order*. Meningitis, which is more severe in the cranial than the spinal meninges, occurs in more than 80% of affected pigs. *Polyarthritis is most severe in the atlanto-occipital and large limb joints*. The synovial fluid is increased in volume and turbid due to increased numbers of neutrophils. The *synovitis* is characterized by the presence of gray-yellow fibrin, which covers the membrane or accumulates as a meniscus-like pad between articular surfaces. The *gastric fundic mucosa* is often intensely reddened due to venous infarction, a change that accompanies septicemia of several causes in pigs.

The *microscopic lesions* of *Haemophilus parasuis* infection in pigs are those of septicemia and fibrinous inflammation. Thrombosis of vessels in the skin, meninges, and renal glomeruli is often prominent. The organism can best be cultured from visceral pleura, providing the interval from death to postmortem examination is relatively short. It is seldom isolated from other sites.

Histophilus somni, previously known as ***Haemophilus agni***, ***Histophilus ovis***, or ***Haemophilus somnus***, produces an acute, fulminating, septicemic disease in **lambs** and a more chronic disease in older sheep. The disease appears to be associated with high levels of feeding but the reason for this association is unclear. Little is known of the biology of the organism, or the pathogenesis of the infection, but *H. somni* is a commensal of the genital tract of sheep and could be transmitted to newborn lambs during parturition.

Lambs with *H. somni* septicemia are usually *found dead*, the course of the disease being less than 12 h. Clinically, there is fever, depression, and extreme reluctance to move. Animals that survive for more than 24 h develop *fibrinopurulent arthritis, choroiditis, and basilar meningitis*. The disease tends to remain enzootic in a flock and losses may continue for several months. *The most constant postmortem findings are multiple hemorrhages throughout the carcass*. The hemorrhages vary in severity, but are usually most obvious in lambs dying acutely. The intermuscular connective tissue is wet and slightly stained with blood. The large blotchy hemorrhages of the serosa lack specificity, but *tiny streaks of hemorrhage that are quite diagnostic can usually be seen in the muscles*. They are best appreciated by viewing the intact muscle through the perimysium, and are usually most common near the tendinous attachments. In all cases except the most acute, small foci of necrosis, surrounded by a red halo, are present in the liver. The spleen is enlarged, the pulp soft and juicy. The *absence of pulmonary lesions* usually allows differentiation of this infection from *Mannheimia haemolytica* septicemia, which produces similar hepatic lesions. In *mature animals*, a more extended course is usual and lesions include myocarditis, embolic nephritis, and meningoencephalitis, similar to the lesions of *H. somni* infection in cattle.

Histologically, there is evidence of *overwhelming intravascular bacterial multiplication*. Blood vessels in many tissues are plugged with bacteria and some of the emboli give rise to *acute vasculitis and secondary infarctions*. All tissues share to some extent in this reaction, but there is preferential involvement of liver and muscle. In these organs, there is often severe inflammation in the parenchyma adjacent to the damaged vessels.

In spite of the fact that the tissues often teem with the organisms, bacteriological confirmation may not be obtained unless samples are taken very soon after death and cultured in media enriched with blood or tissue fragments, and preferably in an atmosphere of 10% carbon dioxide. Even so, previous antibiotic treatment significantly impairs isolation of this organism.

Acute serofibrinous arthritis involving one or two joints, usually including the atlanto-occipital joint, occurs regularly in **cattle** with meningoencephalitis caused by ***H. somni***. These animals die suddenly, usually have hemorrhagic necrosis in the brain, and yield *H. somni* on culture (see Vol. 1, Nervous system).

Borreliosis

Borrelia burgdorferi was first recognized in 1975 as a cause of a multisystemic disease (*Lyme disease, Lyme borreliosis*) in man. More recently, it has been associated with disease in domestic animals, including *dogs, horses, cattle, and cats.* In all species, *infection is far more common than disease,* but the host–bacterium interactions responsible are not well defined. *Arthritis is a common feature of disease in animals and human patients with borreliosis.* Other lesions include *myocarditis and nephritis in dogs, ocular disease and probably encephalitis in horses, and abortion in cattle.*

In North America, the three-host tick *Ixodes dammini* is the primary vector for *B. burgdorferi.* Tick eggs are deposited by engorged females in summer and hatch in about 1 month. Larvae engorge for a few days in the period May–September and about 2 months later molt to the nymphal stage. In the following spring–summer period they feed, drop off and molt to the adult stage. This 2-year cycle may be extended to 4 years since unfed larvae and nymphs may overwinter. Larvae and nymphs feed mainly on birds and small mammals in North America, *Peromyscus* spp. (white-footed mouse and deer mouse) are the main mammalian hosts. The adults attach mainly to large mammals, particularly *Odocoileus virginianus,* the white-tailed deer, but raccoons, dogs, horses, cattle, and people are among the potential victims. *Borrelia infection in the principal wildlife hosts is essentially asymptomatic.* Similar epidemiological patterns involving ticks of the *Ixodes ricinus* group and various animal hosts exist in other parts of the world. In North America, *B. burgdorferi* has been isolated from deer flies and horse flies, which are potentially effective mechanical vectors, and from mosquitoes, which are likely less important. Such vectors are significant only in areas where efficient tick vectors maintain infection among wildlife populations.

Both transovarial and trans-stadial transmission of *B. burgdorferi* occur, but only the latter is epizootiologically important. Intrastadial and interstadial transmission, which occur when several larvae and nymphs feed on an infected host, is of greatest significance in the spread of infection. *Transmission of infection to large mammals is usually by the bite of an adult tick and requires attachment for about 24 h.* The organism may be present in the urine of *Peromyscus* spp. and cattle, but the prevalence of infection by direct contact is not known.

The most common clinical signs in **dogs** with borreliosis are anorexia, lethargy, and lameness in association with fever and lymphadenopathy. Severe depression occurs in some cases and may be due to meningitis. The *arthritis is typically intermittent and involves one or more joints,* often including the carpus. Detailed pathologic descriptions are unavailable since antibiotic treatment appears to be successful and experimental reproduction of disease in dogs is not. In people, the arthritis may be recurrent, leading eventually to ulceration of cartilage. In experimentally infected Lewis rats, acute exudative arthritis, tendonitis and bursitis occur by 30 days post-infection, then regress, but exacerbations develop in some animals. Synovial, but not cartilaginous, ulceration occurs in rats, and there is villus hyperplasia with lymphoplasmacytic and macrophage infiltrates in the synovial membranes. Lymphoplasmacytic myocarditis also occurs in rats, and nonsuppurative myocarditis develops in a small proportion of affected dogs. Clinical evidence of renal disease is also seen in a few dogs and organisms can be demonstrated in the kidney, but the lesions are poorly defined.

In **horses**, signs of borreliosis include lethargy, low-grade fever, painful, swollen joints, and reluctance to move. Laminitis and panuveitis may also occur but are less common. The organism has been demonstrated in anterior chamber fluid and a probable case of encephalitis caused by *B. burgdorferi* is recorded in a horse. Few necropsies on affected horses are reported but it appears that arthritis is present and resembles that seen in dogs, with the addition of marked thickening and hyalinization of arterioles in synovial tissues.

Although there are few reports in **cattle,** it appears that the disease in this species is associated with *abortion,* and may develop into a chronic illness with relapses following treatment, eventually leading to emaciation. In other respects, the disease resembles that seen in dogs and horses. *Arthritis is common and there is limited evidence of myocarditis and nephritis.* In people, a characteristic skin lesion, *erythema chronicum migrans,* may develop at the site of the tick bite, and represents the first stage of Lyme disease. Similar areas of discoloration have been described on bovine mammary skin.

Borrelia burgdorferi has been isolated from blood, urine, colostrum, and synovial fluid of cows, and the blood of a newborn calf. Antibodies in the blood of an aborted fetus suggest that the organism may cross the placenta. Diagnosis of borreliosis is made to some extent by exclusion. *Borrelia burgdorferi* may be demonstrable by *dark-field or phase-contrast microscopy in urine or synovial fluid* and by *silver, immunoperoxidase or immunofluorescent stains in synovial membranes or other tissues.* Isolation of the organism may be possible by using special media. Often the diagnosis is based on typical signs in an animal with a high titer and potential or known exposure to the organism. There is serological cross-reactivity between *B. burgdorferi* and some other spirochetes, but apparently not with leptospires.

Rickettsial polyarthritis

Ehrlichiosis has occasionally been associated with polyarthritis in **dogs**. The syndrome is characterized by acute-onset fever with pain and swelling in one or more joints of the limbs. The synovial fluid has an increased protein concentration and a high cell count, of which 60–80% are neutrophils. *Morulae are occasionally observed within the cytoplasm of neutrophils, eosinophils, or monocytes in synovial fluid, and in circulation.* This differs from *Ehrlichia canis* infection, in which morulae typically are found in monocytes and lymphocytes. Although *Ehrlichia canis* titers are generally positive in affected dogs, the strain of the organism involved in *canine polyarthritis* has been tentatively named ***Ehrlichia ewingii***.

Chlamydial polyarthritis

The genera ***Chlamydia*** and ***Chlamydophila*** contain several species of obligate intracellular gram-negative bacteria characterized by the absence of cell-wall peptidoglycans. The former *Chlamydia psittaci* has been redefined as the *Chlamydophila* species: *C. abortus* (mammals), *C. psittaci* (birds), *C. felis* (cats), and *C. caviae* (guinea pigs). *Chlamydia pecorum* is renamed *Chlamydophila pecorum.* The former *Chlamydia trachomatis* has been subdivided to include the *Chlamydia* species: *C. trachomatis,* which infects humans, and *C. suis,* which infects swine.

- ***Chlamydophila abortus*** is an important cause of abortion in several species, including goats, cattle, and sheep, in which it is responsible for *"enzootic" abortion of ewes* in the United Kingdom.
- ***Chlamydophila psittaci*** is well recognized as an infectious agent of birds with zoonotic potential.
- ***Chlamydophila felis*** causes conjunctivitis and rhinitis in cats.
- Only ***Chlamydophila pecorum*** is currently recognized as a cause of arthritis in domestic animals.

Sporadic or epidemic C. pecorum polyarthritis occurs in calves and lambs, and occasionally in other animals. The natural habitat of chlamydiae is the intestinal tract, where the organism multiplies in the mucosal epithelium before entering the lamina propria. Nonvirulent strains rarely progress beyond the mesenteric nodes. Following oral exposure of calves to virulent strains, the chlamydiae spread to the liver and mesenteric nodes via blood vessels and lymphatics of the lower small intestine. Multiplication in these sites is followed by a primary, low-level chlamydemia with localization and multiplication in spleen, liver, lungs, and kidneys. The joints are infected during a secondary chlamydemia, and arthritogenic strains produce their most severe effects in synovial membranes, with clinical arthritis developing about 10 days after oral inoculation. Severe watery or bloody diarrhea often occurs a few days prior to the development of arthritis.

The disease in calves is severe, causing a high mortality rate both naturally and experimentally. Affected calves may be weak at birth, suggesting intrauterine infection. In these animals, fever, anorexia, reluctance to stand or move, and swelling of joints develop in 2–3 days and death occurs 2 days to 2 weeks after the onset of signs. *All or many joints are affected*, those of the limbs most severely. The subcutaneous and adjacent periarticular tissues are edematous with clear fluid, which also extends around tendon sheaths. Surrounding muscles are hyperemic and edematous with petechiae in the fascia. Joint cavities are distended with turbid yellow-gray fluid, and strands or wads of fibrin adhere to the synovium. Viscera may show changes attributable to systemic infection.

The ovine syndrome is less severe, being characterized by high morbidity but negligible mortality, even though the infection is systemic. Affected lambs show conjunctivitis, depression, anorexia, reluctance to move, joint stiffness that disappears with exercise, and loss of weight. Most lambs recover, but a few are permanently lame. *The articular lesions are similar to those in calves although modified by the milder reaction*, the longer course allowing fibrotic thickening of tendon sheaths and articular capsules and hyperplasia of synovial villi. In soft tissues, including the central nervous system, histologic traces of inflammation are present. The organism is sometimes demonstrable in the cytoplasm of synovial cells stained by the Giemsa, Gimenez, or modified Stamp methods.

Bibliography

Anderson BE, et al. *Ehrlichia ewingii* sp. nov., the etiologic agent of canine granulocytic ehrlichiosis. Intl J Syst Bacteriol 1992;42:299–302.

Appel MJG. Lyme disease in dogs and cats. Compend Contin Educ Pract Vet 1990;12:617–625.

Bellah JR, et al. *Ehrlichia canis*-related polyarthritis in a dog. J Am Vet Med Assoc 1986;189:922–923.

Bennett D, Taylor DJ. Bacterial infective arthritis in the dog. J Small Anim Pract 1988;29:207–230.

Burgess EC, et al. Arthritis and systemic disease caused by *Borrelia burgdorferi* infection in a cow. J Am Vet Med Assoc 1987;191:1468–1470.

Cohen ND, Cohen D. Borreliosis in horses: A comparative review. Compend Contin Educ Pract Vet 1990;12:1449–1458.

Cutlip RC, Ramsey FK. Ovine chlamydial polyarthritis: sequential development of articular lesions in lambs after intra-articular exposure. Am J Vet Res 1973;34:71–75.

Eamens GJ, Nicholls PJ. Comparison of inoculation regimes for the experimental production of swine erysipelas arthritis. I Clinical, pathological and bacteriological findings. Aust Vet J 1989;66:212–216.

Firth EC. Current concepts of infectious polyarthritis in foals. Equine Vet J 1983;15:5–9.

Fukushi H, Hirai K. Proposal of *Chlamydia pecorum* sp. nov. for *Chlamydia* strains derived from ruminants. Int J Syst Bact 1992;42:306–308.

Gogolewski RP, et al. *Streptococcus suis* serotypes associated with disease in weaned pigs. Aust Vet J 1990;67:202 –204.

Hariharan H, et al. An investigation of bacterial causes of arthritis in slaughter hogs. J Vet Diagn Invest 1992;4:28–30.

Higgins R, et al. Isolation of *Streptococcus suis* from cattle. Can Vet J 1990;31:529.

Hill BD, et al. Importance of *Staphylococcus hyicus* ssp *hyicus* as a cause of arthritis in pigs up to 12 weeks of age. Aust Vet J 1996;73:179–181.

Johnston KM, et al. An evaluation of nonsuppurative joint disease in slaughter pigs. Can Vet J 1987;28:174–180.

Luque I, et al. *Streptococcus suis* serotypes associated with different disease conditions in pigs. Vet Rec 1998;142:726–727.

Marchevsky AM, Read RA. Bacterial septic arthritis in 19 dogs. Aust Vet J 1999;77:233–237.

Montgomery RD, et al. Comparison of aerobic culturette, synovial membrane biopsy, and blood culture medium in detection of canine bacterial arthritis. Vet Surg 1989;18:300–303.

Nietfeld JC. Chlamydial infections in small ruminants. Vet Clin North Am Food Anim Pract 2001;17:301–314.

Shewen PE. Chlamydial infection in animals: a review. Can Vet J 1980;21:2–11.

Smart NL, et al. Glasser's disease and prevalence of subclinical infection with *Haemophilus parasuis* in swine in southern Ontario. Can Vet J 1989;30:339–343.

Watkins GH, Sharp MW. Bacteria isolated from arthritic and omphalatic lesions in lambs in England and Wales. Vet J 1998;155:235–238.

Waxler GL, Britt AL. Polyserositis and arthritis due to *Escherichia coli* in gnotobiotic pigs. Can J Comp Med 1972;36:226–233.

Wood RL. Swine erysipelas – a review of prevalence and research. J Am Vet Med Assoc 1984;184:944–949.

Wood RL, et al. Osteomyelitis and arthritis induced in swine by Lancefield's Group A streptococci (*Streptococcus pyogenes*). Cornell Vet 1971;61:457–470.

Mycoplasmal arthritis

Mycoplasmas are ubiquitous organisms, which are difficult to isolate, propagate, and identify, and often difficult to associate with specific diseases. Polyserositis and polyarthritis produced by these organisms are problems of considerable magnitude in farm animals, and often complicate mycoplasma ("enzootic") pneumonia or other disease syndromes. The diseases are seldom fatal, but produce a lingering debility from which animals never completely recover. Because of the difficulty in isolating mycoplasmas from routine diagnostic specimens, the prevalence of diseases caused by these agents is probably underestimated.

Swine

Three *Mycoplasma* species are pathogenic for swine:

- *Mycoplasma hyopneumoniae (suipneumoniae)* causes enzootic pneumonia;
- *Mycoplasma hyorhinis* causes polyserositis and *polyarthritis*, usually in animals about 3–10 weeks of age;
- *Mycoplasma hyosynoviae* also causes *polyarthritis*, but not polyserositis, and usually in pigs over 10 weeks of age.

Other mycoplasmas are sometimes associated with various diseases of swine but they are not primary pathogens.

Mycoplasma hyorhinis *is a commensal or parasite of the nasal passages in most pigs*, but often colonizes pneumonic lesions, especially those of mycoplasmal pneumonia. Although it does not noticeably alter the lung lesion, infected lungs might be the primary site for entry of the agent into the blood. The pathogenicity of *M. hyorhinis* is enhanced by intercurrent disease and various forms of stress. After an incubation period of 3–4 days, the infection produces an erratic febrile reaction, anorexia, depression, and loss of body weight. Growth rate remains retarded, although after a month or so there may be signs of recovery. The infection is more likely to be fatal in suckling piglets or those with intercurrent pneumonia.

Mycoplasma hyorhinis has a predilection for collagen-containing structures, including serous and synovial membranes and cartilage, but evidence of meningitis is either absent or mild. When present, the meningitis is lymphocytic in nature. The systemic infection persists for at least 2 months after experimental inoculation. *The serosal lesions may vary and any combination of epicarditis, pleuritis, and/or peritonitis is possible.* The serosal reaction is serofibrinous, and the cellular component is mononuclear with focal accumulations of neutrophils. The epicardium is uniformly affected, whereas pleuritis may be confined to the ventral margin of the lung and the pleura between lobes, and may extend to the outer surface of the pericardial sac. The peritoneal exudate is patchy and may be concentrated in the anterior abdomen, especially between the liver and diaphragm, but often involves loops of intestine and the coiled colon. Progressive organization of exudates produces tough adhesions, but even after many weeks there is still histologic evidence of active inflammation, which is consistent with the persistence of the organism.

While the effects of polyserositis predominate early in the disease, signs of *polyarthritis* become evident once villus hypertrophy, synovial thickening, and organization of fibrinous exudate replace the initial synovial edema and hyperemia. In the chronic disease, thickening and brown discoloration of joint capsules, erosion and discoloration of articular cartilages, and pannus formation are observed. Discoloration of joint structures is probably a sequel to synovial hemorrhage.

Early *microscopic changes* consist of hyperemia, diffuse lymphocyte and macrophage infiltration, and mild villus hypertrophy, followed by ulceration of synovial membranes. Fibrinopurulent exudate is consistently present in virtually all joints, and is most abundant in the recesses where the synovial membrane is reflected from the articular cartilage. Later, perivascular lymphoplasmacytic accumulations and more pronounced villus hypertrophy become evident and fibrinous exudate is less prominent. Early in experimental infections, mycoplasmas invade the lacunae of superficial chondrocytes, and degeneration of chondrocytes combined with the enzymatic activity of adherent neutrophils produces erosions of articular cartilage.

In chronic *Mycoplasma hyorhinis* synovitis, there is marked villus hypertrophy and proliferation of synovial cells. Perivascular cuffs are less prominent, but *lymphoid follicles*, often surrounded by lymphatics, occur frequently in the villi. Dense fibrosis of some villi is evident. Erosions, developing first at the periphery of the articular cartilages, later occur centrally, and *erosion of cartilage and subarticular bone by pannus* is not unusual in advanced cases. Joint contractures are associated with the chronic arthritis and thickened joint capsules. Chronic lesions remain active for many months, and the organism can often be cultured from surface exudate in these joints.

Mycoplasma hyosynoviae is carried persistently in the pharynx and tonsils of many sows and may be transmitted to their offspring. Infection of pigs less than 6 weeks of age is uncommon and separation of piglets from their dams by 5 weeks of age usually prevents transmission. Clinical disease often develops following management stress and is more frequent, and more severe, in pigs with poor conformation and gait.

Following experimental infection with *Mycoplasma hyosynoviae*, there is an incubation period of 5–10 days. Lameness, lasting 3–10 days, occurs in many pigs and may involve one joint or several. *Many pigs recover completely but lameness due to chronic arthritis persists in 5–15% of infected swine.* The early pathologic changes resemble those caused by *Mycoplasma hyorhinis*. Chronic lesions are not fully described but are also likely to be qualitatively similar to those of *Mycoplasma hyorhinis*.

Failure to isolate organisms from the joints of many pigs with *chronic mycoplasma arthritis* may be due to difficulties in culturing the organism. Alternatively, the continued inflammatory reaction may be due to an immune response to persisting mycoplasma antigen, rather than a viable agent. Support for this view is derived from the observation that rabbits sensitized to *Mycoplasma arthritidis*, either by infection or hyperimmunization, develop chronic arthritis when challenged with nonviable *Mycoplasma arthritidis* antigen. Antibody in the synovial fluid of sensitized animals could retain antigen in immune complexes. These complexes may become deposited in synovial tissues and articular cartilage and stimulate a cell-mediated immune response with generation of cytokines capable of inducing tissue damage. The nature of the putative antigens is undetermined. Since mycoplasmas lack a cell wall and cannot synthesize peptidoglycans, the antigen must differ from the antigens responsible for inducing chronicity in some bacterial arthritides. Whether this hypothesis is correct, or relevant to the natural disease, is undetermined.

Goats

Mycoplasma spp. cause several important disease syndromes in goats, including contagious caprine pleuropneumonia (see Vol. 2, Respiratory system) and contagious agalactia (see Vol. 3, Male genital system). A **septicemia-arthritis** syndrome caused by either ***Mycoplasma mycoides*** **subsp.** ***mycoides*** or ***Mycoplasma capricolum*** **subsp.** ***capricolum*** occurs in goats. *Mycoplasma mycoides* subsp. *mycoides* is separable into two groups on the basis of colony type (large and small). *Mycoplasma mycoides* subsp. *mycoides* (small colony) type is the etiologic agent of contagious bovine pleuropneumonia and should not be confused with *Mycoplasma mycoides* subsp. *mycoides* (large colony) type, which is a common infection of goats in several countries.

Mycoplasma putrifaciens occasionally causes polyarthritis and mastitis in goats. *Mycoplasma agalactiae*, the cause of contagious agalactia, also may be associated with arthritis following extension of infection from periarticular connective tissues.

The **septicemia-arthritis syndrome in goats** is acutely febrile and associated with a drop in milk yield due to *mastitis*. In the course of about 2 days, affected animals develop *acute polyarthritis*, but in suckling kids, the disease is peracute and localization in joints is less obvious. During the *systemic phase of the infection*, there is a generalized acute lymphadenitis, splenitis, histiocytic meningitis, glomerulitis, renal tubular degeneration, and focal coagulative necrosis in the liver. Fibrinous peritonitis and pleuritis are sometimes present. Capillaries in many organs may contain thrombi, probably reflecting disseminated intravascular coagulation. Diffuse interstitial pneumonia characterized by infiltration of alveolar walls with neutrophils or monocytes, and leakage of protein-rich fluid into alveoli, develops in kids. In adults, the pneumonia tends to be less diffuse and more chronic. *The articular lesion is a severe fibrinopurulent inflammation, usually involving many synovial structures.*

The epidemiology of the septicemia-arthritis syndrome is incompletely understood. Some do probably acquire *Mycoplasma capricolum* subsp. *capricolum* via the teat canal and infection can spread to the opposite gland. Some kids are probably infected via milk but horizontal transmission of both *Mycoplasma capricolum* subsp. *capricolum* and *Mycoplasma mycoides* subsp. *mycoides* (large colony) type occurs among young kids housed together. An outbreak of septicemia and fibrinous polyarthritis caused by *Mycoplasma mycoides* subsp. *mycoides* (large colony type) occurred in New Zealand in 3–20 day old dairy goat kids fed pooled colostrum contaminated with organisms by a doe with mastitis. In total, 34 of 64 kids were affected and 3 died.

Sheep

Septicemia and arthritis caused by *Mycoplasma capricolum* subsp. *capricolum*, or a closely related organism, is reported in **lambs** exposed to goats' milk. The disease was similar to that described in kids.

Cattle

Mycoplasma mycoides subsp. *mycoides* (small colony) type, the agent of **contagious bovine pleuropneumonia**, causes *polyarthritis and endocarditis* in a proportion of **calves** in which it is used as a vaccine. Sporadic outbreaks of polyarthritis in cattle, not associated with *Mycoplasma mycoides* subsp. *mycoides* vaccination also occur in North America and Australia and are probably caused by *Mycoplasma bovis*. This organism also causes mastitis, with or without arthritis, and is often isolated from bovine fibrinous pneumonia where its significance is poorly understood. *Mycoplasma alkalescens, Mycoplasma californicum,* and *Mycoplasma canadense* have all been associated with arthritis and mastitis in cattle. Although *Mycoplasma mycoides* subsp. *mycoides* (large colony) type is not considered to be pathogenic for cattle, an outbreak of arthritis caused by this agent was recently reported in artificially reared dairy calves in New Zealand. This was the result of feeding contaminated goats' milk from a dairy goat farm where an outbreak of arthritis was also occurring in goat kids. No lateral spread of infection occurred amongst the calves.

Mycoplasma bovis probably enters the circulation *from the lungs* and localizes in synovial membranes. Oral infection of calves from the milk of a mastitic dam may also occur. Outbreaks of disease usually occur in *feedlots* and are often preceded by management stress. Usually 15% of animals show signs of lameness, followed within 1 or 2 days by severe swellings around joints. The *stifle, shoulder, hock, and elbow joints are most often affected*, but severe lesions usually develop in only one limb.

In *acute disease*, the joints are distended by opaque cream-colored fluid containing flakes of fibrin. Synovial membranes are red and swollen. Microscopic changes include light to diffuse infiltrations of lymphocytes, macrophages, and plasma cells in addition to hyperplasia of synovial cells and synovial villi. Focal perivascular necrosis and ulceration of the synovial membrane may be present and attract numerous neutrophils, which accumulate in joint spaces.

Most affected animals recover in 1–2 months but a few develop *chronic arthritis* and are culled. These animals have a *proliferative and erosive arthritis with well-vascularized pannus* extending from the thickened synovial membrane across the articular cartilage. Spread of inflammation to the subchondral bone with development of *osteomyelitis* occurs in some animals. The predominant cells in the chronic synovial lesions are lymphocytes and plasmacytes, with fewer neutrophils and macrophages. Isolation of mycoplasmas is relatively easy in the acute disease but is often more difficult in chronic stages.

Cats and dogs

Occasionally, mycoplasma arthritis occurs in cats and dogs. ***Mycoplasma gateae*** is reported as a cause of polyarthritis and tenosynovitis in cats, and ***Mycoplasma felis*** was recovered from the joint of a cat with suspected immune deficiency. ***Mycoplasma spumans*** was isolated from a Greyhound with polyarthritis and is considered a possible cause of the infectious arthritis seen in that breed in Australia.

Bibliography

Adegboye DS, et al. *Mycoplasma bovis*-associated pneumonia and arthritis complicated with pyogranulomatous tenosynovitis in calves. J Am Vet Med Assoc 1996;209:647–649.

Barton MD, et al. Isolation of *Mycoplasma spumans* from polyarthritis in a Greyhound. Aust Vet J 1985;62:206.

DaMassa AJ, et al. Comparison of caprine mycoplasmosis caused by *Mycoplasma capricolum*, *Mycoplasma mycoides* subsp *mycoides*, and *Mycoplasma putrefaciens*. Israel J Med Sci 1987;23:636–640.

Hagedorn-Olsen T, et al. Gross and histopathological findings in synovial membranes of pigs with experimentally induced *Mycoplasma hyosynoviae* arthritis. APMIS 1999;107:201–210.

Henderson JP, Ball HJ. Polyarthritis due to *Mycoplasma bovis* infection in adult dairy cattle in Northern Ireland. Vet Rec 1999;145:374–376.

Hooper PT, et al. Mycoplasma polyarthritis in a cat with probable severe immune deficiency. Aust Vet J 1985;62:352.

Jackson R, King C. *Mycoplasma mycoides* subspecies *mycoides* (large colony) infection in goats – a review with special reference to occurrence in New Zealand. Surveillance 2002;29:8–12.

Moise NS, et al. *Mycoplasma gateae* arthritis and tenosynovitis in cats: case report and experimental reproduction of the disease. Am J Vet Res 1983;44:16–21.

Pfutzner H, Sachse K. *Mycoplasma bovis* as an agent of mastitis, pneumonia, arthritis and genital disorders in cattle. Rev Sci Tech Off Int Epiz 1996;15:1477–1494.

Roberts ED, et al. The pathology of *Mycoplasma hyorhinis* arthritis produced experimentally in swine. Am J Vet Res 1963;24:19–31.

Rosendal S, et al. *Mycoplasma mycoides* subspecies *mycoides* as a cause of polyarthritis in goats. J Am Vet Med Assoc 1979;175:378–380.

Ruhnke HL, et al. Isolation of *Mycoplasma mycoides* subspecies *mycoides* from polyarthritis and mastitis of goats in Canada. Can Vet J 1983;24:54–56.

Stokka GL, et al. Lameness in feedlot cattle. Vet Clin North Am Food Anim Pract 2001;17:189–207.

Swanepoel R, et al. *Mycoplasma capricolum* associated with arthritis in sheep. Vet Rec 1977;101:446–447.

Other infectious agents

Viral arthritis

Few viral agents have been incriminated either directly or indirectly with arthritis in domestic animals.

Goats

The best-characterized example of viral arthritis in animals is **caprine arthritis-encephalitis**. This syndrome is caused by persistent infection with a *nononcogenic retrovirus (lentivirus)*. The neurologic, mammary, respiratory and systemic features are described in Vol. 1,

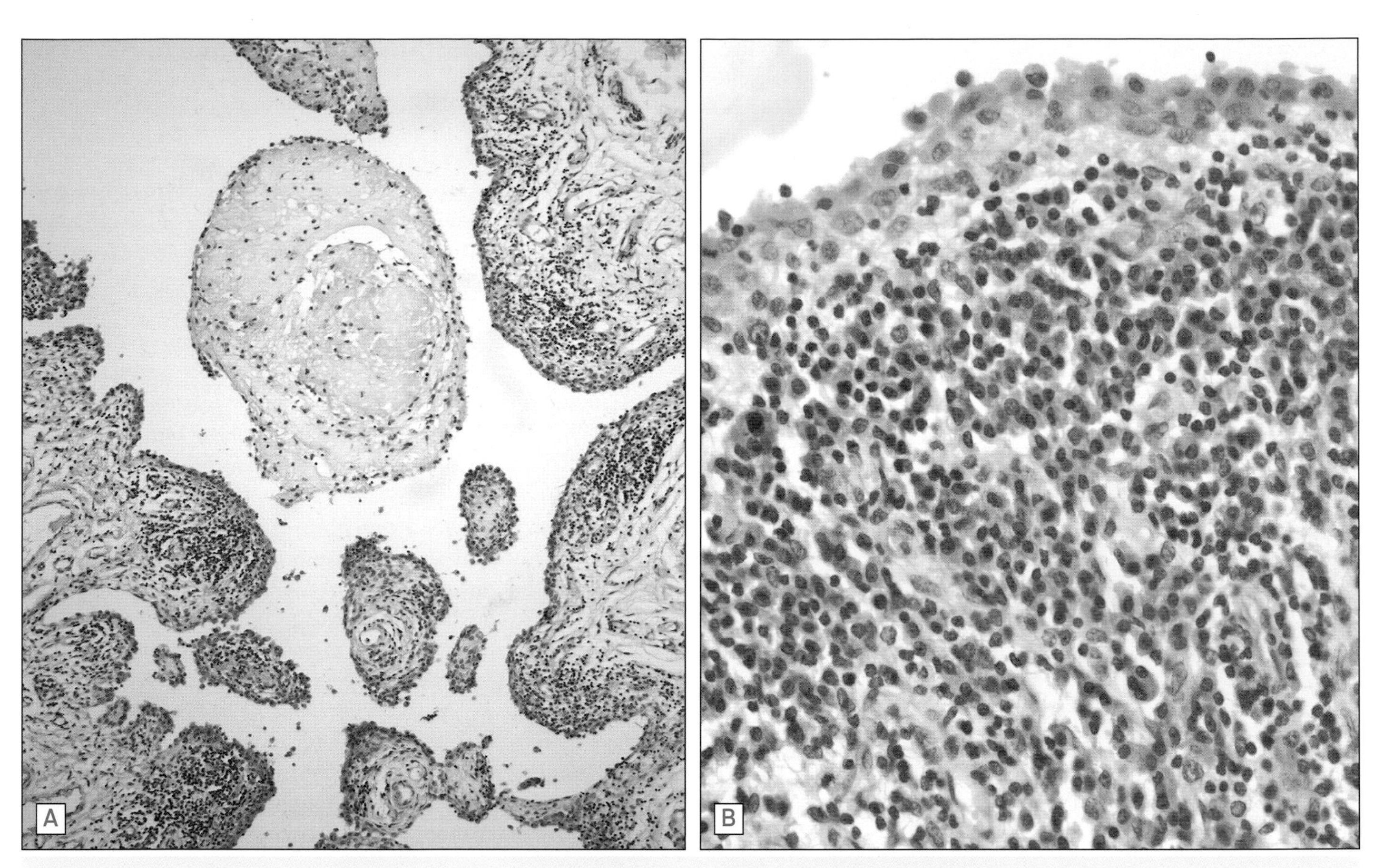

Figure 1.159 Caprine arthritis-encephalitis. **A.** Hypertrophic, edematous synovial villi containing aggregates of mononuclear cells. **B.** Closer view showing intense plasmacytic infiltration of the synovium and hypertrophy of synoviocytes on the surface.

Nervous system. *In many herds, arthritis is the major or only clinical manifestation of infection*, with signs of lameness often associated with carpal hygromas, weight loss, and reduced milk production. The prevalence of infection in a herd may reach 100%, but expression of disease is variable and rarely exceeds 25–30%.

A high prevalence of unilateral or bilateral carpal hygromas is a characteristic clinical feature of caprine arthritis-encephalitis. The hygromas are chronic lesions that appear as flattened, cystic, subcutaneous distensions over the cranial carpus, and are filled with yellow or bloody fluid, often containing fibrinous or gelatinous masses. Usually, there is no communication with the carpal joint or tendon sheaths. The tendon sheaths and joint capsule are thickened by fibrous tissue, in which collagen degeneration and mineralization may occur. In many cases, the major joints, especially carpus and stifle, are distended with clear yellow fluid. Other gross changes, which are also seen most often in the carpus and stifle, include hypertrophy of synovial villi, fibrillation and erosion of cartilage, and destruction of joint structures by pannus. Lymphocytic/plasmacytic arthritis is demonstrable microscopically in many joints.

Caprine arthritis encephalitis virus is readily transmitted to kids in colostrum and milk, and horizontal transmission probably occurs. Although the colostrum may contain antibody this does not influence viral transmission. In blood, the virus is present in monocytes and is activated when they mature into macrophages. Following infection, there is vascular injury to synovial structures, with exudation of plasma proteins into synovial fluid. Synovial villi hypertrophy, become edematous and accumulate focal and diffuse infiltrations of plasma cells and lymphocytes (Fig. 1.159A, B) and scattered macrophages, which are sometimes multinucleated. Some villi may be fibrosed, and there is hyperplasia of synoviocytes on their surfaces. Hyalinized masses of fibrin also form villus-like structures in inflamed joints, and layers of fibrin may cover the synovial membrane in some areas.

Sheep

A related lentivirus of sheep, the ***Visna/maedi virus***, causes *chronic, non-suppurative arthritis* in this species, and also produces arthritis in goat kids experimentally. Similarly, the *Caprine arthritis encephalitis virus* induces arthritis experimentally in lambs but natural cross infections are not known to occur.

In *lentivirus arthritis*, macrophages and lymphocytes are the predominant cells in synovial fluid. A small number of the macrophages are infected with the virus but there is a reduction in virus gene expression, possibly due to the presence of interferon in the synovial fluid. Plasma cells in the inflamed synovia produce immunoglobulin G_1, presumably in response to persistent infection, and the concentration in synovia is higher than that in serum. The relevance of this to lesion development is unclear since the predominant lymphocytes in the synovia are T cells and there is some suggestion that interaction between these cells and macrophages may be responsible for the chronic inflammatory response.

Cats

Lameness caused by acute arthritis is reported in cats in association with ***Feline calicivirus*** infection, or 5–7 days after live-virus vaccination. In one study, intra-articular inoculation or contact exposure of cats to a field strain of *Feline calicivirus* resulted in acute arthritis in addition to oral and nasal ulceration, conjunctivitis, and ocular discharge, which are more typical of the infection. Only mild lameness was induced by the vaccine strain. The gross and microscopic changes have not been well characterized, at least in natural infections, although viral antigen has been demonstrated in the supporting and lining cells of the synovial membrane by immunostaining.

Fungal arthritis

Arthritis involving one or more joints occurs in some dogs with systemic fungal infections. In some cases, the arthritis is probably *immune-mediated*, following the deposition of immune complexes in the synovial membrane, but *hematogenous localization* of fungal agents in joints, or *direct spread from osteomyelitic lesions* in adjacent bones also occurs. Fungi identified in arthritic joints of dogs have included *Blastomyces, Histoplasma*, *Coccidioides*, *Cryptococcus*, and *Sporothrix* species. Radiography may reveal a destructive process in a bone or bones adjacent to the joint and erosive changes in articular cartilage. The causative agent is sometimes evident on cytological examination of synovial fluid obtained by arthrocentesis. Histologically, the synovial inflammation is usually *pyogranulomatous*.

Protozoal arthritis

Proliferative synovitis may be associated with *visceral leishmaniasis* caused by the protozoal agent *Leishmania donovani*. Synovial villi in affected joints are hypertrophic and infiltrated with plasma cells and macrophages, some of which may contain the organism. The agent is occasionally demonstrated in macrophages collected from synovial fluid.

Bibliography

Bloomberg MS, et al. Cryptococcal arthritis and osteomyelitis in a dog. Compend Contin Educ Pract Vet 1983;5:609–617.

Bulgin MS. Ovine progressive pneumonia, caprine arthritis-encephalitis, and related lentiviral diseases of sheep and goats. Vet Clin North Am Food Anim Pract 1990;6:691–704.

Cutlip RC, et al. Arthritis associated with ovine progressive pneumonia. Am J Vet Res 1985;46:65–68.

Dawson S, et al. Acute arthritis of cats associated with feline calicivirus infection. Res Vet Sc 1994;56:133–143.

Goad DL, Pecquet Goad ME. Osteoarticular sporotrichosis in a dog. J Am Vet Med Assoc 1986;189:1326–1328.

Huss BT, et al. Polyarthropathy and chorioretinitis with retinal detachment in a dog with systemic histoplasmosis. J Am Anim Hosp Assoc 1994;30:217–224.

Scott-Adams D, et al. A pathogenetic study of the early connective tissue lesions of viral caprine arthritis-encephalitis. Am J Pathol 1980;99:257–278.

von Bodungen U, et al. Immunohistology of the early course of lentivirus-induced arthritis. Clin Exp Immunol 1998;111:384–390.

Woodard JC, et al. Caprine arthritis-encephalitis: clinicopathologic study. Am J Vet Res 1982;43:2085–2096.

Yamaguchi RA, et al. *Leishmania donovani* in the synovial fluid of a dog with visceral leishmaniasis. J Am Anim Hosp Assoc 1983;19:723–726.

Miscellaneous inflammatory lesions of joint structures

Bursitis

Bursitis often occurs as part of the synovial localization of *hematogenous* infections. In addition, there are *isolated forms* of bursitis, especially in horses, that appear to be initiated by *trauma* and are characterized by accumulation of excess serous fluid and variable degrees of synovial hypertrophy. They represent loci of lowered resistance and are predisposed to the localization of organisms, which may alter the nature of the inflammatory reaction while contributing to its progression. *The bursae that cover bony prominences are especially liable to traumatic injury*. Capped elbow and capped hock are examples of *serous bursitis*. Carpal bursitis is also known as *hygroma* and is not uncommon in cattle and sheep. The distended bursae are sometimes filled with fibrin concretions (Fig. 1.160). In cattle, large hygromas should be suspected of being secondarily infected with *Brucella abortus*. Carpal hygromas are also common in adult goats infected with *Caprine arthritis encephalitis virus*.

"Fistulous withers" and "poll evil" are the most serious forms of bursitis in horses and mules, affecting the supraspinous and atlantal bursae respectively. The affected bursae are those between the nuchal ligament and the second, or less often, the third, fourth, or fifth, thoracic spine in the case of "fistulous withers," and between the nuchal ligament and the dorsal arch of the atlas in the case of "poll evil." In both syndromes, the inflammation is *suppurative and granulomatous*, and there

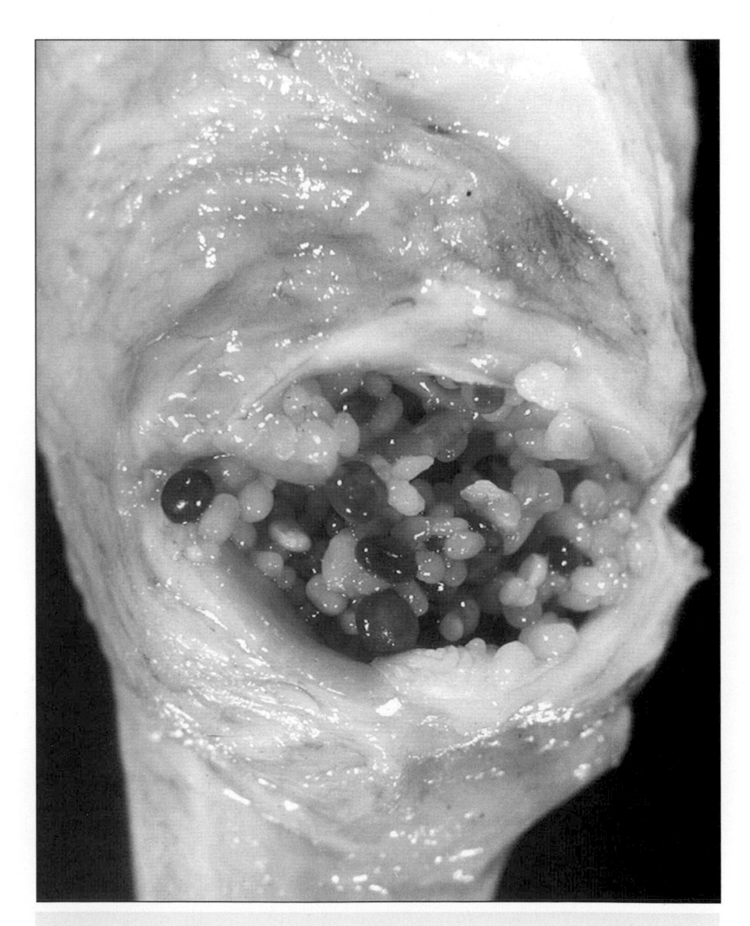

Figure 1.160 Chronic carpal bursitis in a sheep. Thickened fibrous wall surrounding numerous fibrin concretions.

is a tendency to fistulate to the skin surface. Less commonly, the inflammation extends into adjacent fibrous connective tissues as a cellulitis, or induces destructive osteitis of adjacent bones. Inflammation of the navicular bursa is discussed with navicular syndrome.

The primary lesions of "fistulous withers" and "poll evil" may be either *traumatic or inflammatory*. The trauma may be caused by a penetrating wound, with introduction of infection, or blunt injury, producing contusions in which organisms localize hematogenously. Inflammatory lesions are associated with a variety of organisms, including the nematode *Onchocerca cervicalis,* which localizes in the nuchal ligament and environs, provoking mineralized granulomas when it dies. However, in areas where the prevalence of *O. cervicalis* infection is high, the prevalence of bursitis is not, and *the etiologic role of the parasite is questionable*. In brucellosis-endemic areas, *Brucella abortus* is often isolated from closed lesions of bursitis, and vaccination is considered a useful method of treatment. *Actinomyces bovis*, a common component of the normal bovine oral flora, sometimes can be cultured from closed lesions in horses, and exposure to cattle is considered a predisposing factor. In North America, and other locations where the incidence of brucellosis and the exposure of horses to cattle are declining, isolation of *Brucella abortus* and *Actinomyces bovis* from equine bursitis has also waned. *Streptococcus zooepidemicus* is now the most common isolate from closed lesions but several other bacteria have also been implicated. The infections are *probably hematogenous*, but it is not clear whether a predisposing bursal lesion is required. *Actinomyces bovis,* in particular, is an unlikely primary pathogen, since in its own niche it is an uncommon opportunistic invader of traumatized oral mucosa. Furthermore, it does not establish itself in regional lymph nodes draining the lesions of osteomyelitis in which it flourishes.

Adventitious bursitis of the hock is common in finishing pigs, particularly those kept on slatted floors. A study conducted on 21 properties in south-west England revealed an overall prevalence of 51.0% with a range of 10.1 to 84.0%. The bursae are typically found immediately distal to the hock on the lateroplantar, plantar, and medial aspects of the joint. The lesions are thought to arise through traumatic injury to lymphatic vessels and capillaries, followed by the accumulation of fibrinous exudate within affected bursae.

Diskospondylitis

Diskospondylitis is inflammation of an intervertebral disk leading to osteomyelitis of contiguous vertebrae. It occurs occasionally in dogs and pigs, and less often in cats, horses, cattle, and sheep. Most cases are caused by bacteria, usually as a result of primary bacteremia, but also secondary to a chronic infection elsewhere in the body. Fungi, such as *Aspergillus terreus*, are occasionally involved in dogs.

In **dogs**, diskospondylitis occurs most often in *large males* and usually involves the *lumbosacral spine*, causing hyperesthesia, stilted gait, and/or pelvic limb lameness. *Staphylococcus aureus* is the most common cause, although several other bacteria have been incriminated and *Brucella canis* should be considered in countries or regions where it is known to occur. Often, there is concurrent disease, such as a urogenital infection. Diskospondylitis and osteomyelitis of lumbar vertebrae has been associated with migrating grass seeds in dogs. It is suggested that ingested seeds occasionally penetrate the intestinal wall at the caudal duodenal flexure and ascend in the mesoduodenum to the lumbar vertebrae, carrying bacteria with them.

In **pigs**, most lesions occur in the *upper thoracic and upper lumbar spine* following *hematogenous* localization of bacteria. *Erysipelothrix rhusiopathiae, Arcanobacterium pyogenes,* and *Staphylococcus aureus* are the most common agents involved but, in some geographic areas, *Brucella suis* may be an important cause of the disease. Diskospondylitis in **horses** most often involves the cervical vertebrae, inducing signs of neck pain. In some cases, there is a history of a penetrating wound to the neck. Medical or surgical therapy is often successful in dogs but seldom in horses.

Organisms causing diskospondylitis probably localize initially in the outer part of the annulus fibrosus, where they stimulate an inflammatory reaction. Alternatively, localization in the vertebral body with extension to the disk may occur. Early radiographic changes are reduction of the intervertebral disk space and loss of density in the vertebral endplates. Gross lesions appear as soft, gray areas of discoloration and disruption in the disk, often extending into adjacent vertebrae through disrupted end plates (Fig. 1.161). *Complete destruction of disks, with fibrous replacement and formation of vertebral osteophytes, occurs late in the disease*. Such lesions are easily confused with spondylosis due to primary degeneration of the annulus fibrosus. The inflammatory reaction may extend dorsally into the spinal canal causing meningomyelitis, or laterally, causing paravertebral abscessation. *Microscopic lesions* of diskospondylitis vary with the stage of the disease and the nature of the causative organism. Early bacterial infections are characterized by suppurative inflammation, hemorrhage, and necrosis of intradiskal structures and adjacent bones. In chronic lesions, vascular connective tissue, infiltrated with mononuclear or mixed inflammatory cells, predominates.

Calcium crystal-associated arthropathy (pseudogout)

A syndrome characterized by the deposition of *calcium pyrophosphate dihydrate* ($Ca_2P_2O_7{\cdot}2H_2O$) *crystals* in articular and para-articular tissues is well recognized in humans and is reported occasionally in *aged dogs*. The lesions may occur as single, tumor-like, periarticular masses (Fig. 1.162) developing over a period of several months or even years. The lateral and dorsal aspects of the metatarsophalangeal joint of the 5th digit were involved in a 13-year-old female Golden Retriever. A similar mass involving the carpal joint was diagnosed in a 15-year-old male English Pointer. Mild, progressive lameness was reported in

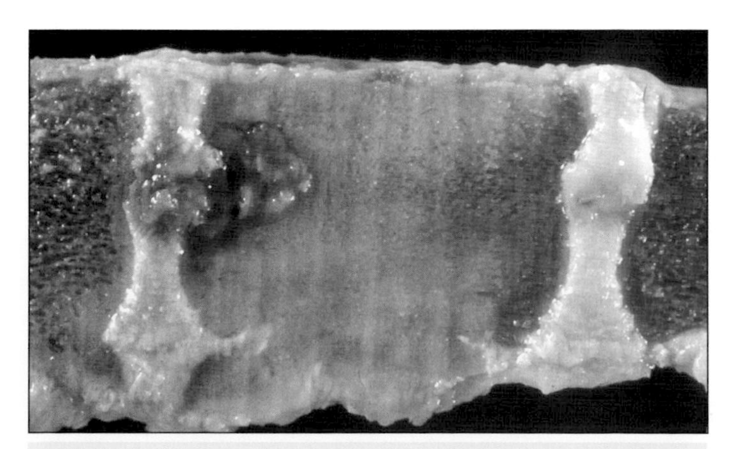

Figure 1.161 Diskospondylitis, dog. Inflammation of intervertebral disk and extension into adjacent vertebral body, causing local bone lysis. The remainder of the vertebral body is sclerotic.

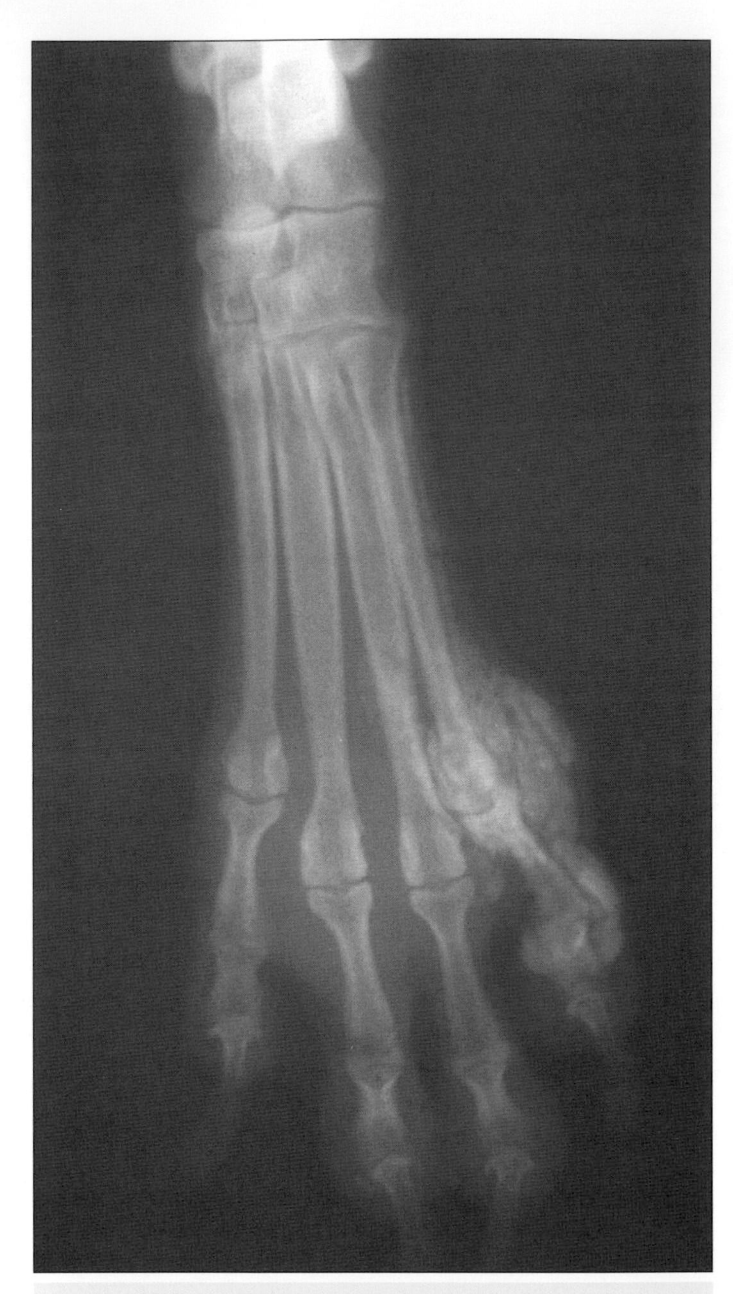

Figure 1.162 Calcium pyrophosphate dihydrate crystal deposition disease (**pseudogout**), dog. Radiodense mass adjacent to the metatarsophalangeal joint of the 5th digit and extending along the 1st phalanx.

the latter dog. In both cases, the lesions consisted of *multiple, hard, chalky white nodules separated by fibrous septa*. Although the masses were adherent to the joint capsule, they did not involve joint cavities or articular surfaces. Microscopically, the chalky nodules consisted of variable-sized deposits of pale brown crystalline material and were separated by bands or islands of fibrous or cartilaginous connective tissue. A *granulomatous inflammatory reaction*, which included many large, multinucleated giant cells, was closely associated with the crystalline deposits. The crystals were weakly birefringent, rhomboidal or rectangular, and stained positively with Alizarin red.

A more acute form of the disease characterized by nonweight-bearing lameness in both forelimbs and the left hindlimb was diagnosed in a 13-year-old Keeshond. Cytological examination of synovial fluid from both carpal joints revealed 60% mononuclear cells and 40% neutrophils. Weakly birefringent rectangular and rhomboid crystals, which stained positively with Alizarin red, were present extracellularly and within neutrophils, monocytes, and synovial lining cells. Clinically, *this acute form of pseudogout closely resembles septic arthritis*.

The pathogenesis of this syndrome, now referred to as calcium pyrophosphate dihydrate crystal deposition disease, is unknown, but acute episodes in human patients may follow surgery, trauma, or severe medical conditions, such as myocardial infarction.

True gout, which is associated with the deposition of urate crystals within joint structures occurs commonly in humans, but does not occur in mammalian species possessing the enzyme uricase. *There are no convincing reports of gout in either dogs or cats, and even Dalmatian dogs, with their high serum uric acid concentrations, do not appear to develop the disease.*

Bibliography

Cohen ND, et al. Fistulous withers in horses: 24 cases (1984–1990). J Am Vet Med Assoc 1992;201:121–124.

Colbourne CM, et al. Cervical diskospondylitis in two horses. Aust Vet J 1997;75:477–479.

de Haan JJ, Andreasen CB. Calcium crystal-associated arthropathy (pseudogout) in a dog. J Am Vet Med Assoc 1992;200:943–946.

Doige CE. Diskospondylitis in swine. Can J Comp Med 1980;44:121–128.

Kerwin SC, et al. Diskospondylitis associated with *Brucella canis* infection in dogs: 14 cases (1980–1991). J Am Vet Med Assoc 1992;201:1253–1257.

Malik R, et al. Bacterial diskospondylitis in a cat. J Small Anim Pract 1990;31: 404–406.

Mouttotou N, et al. Adventitious bursitis of the hock in finishing pigs: prevalence, distribution and association with floor type and foot lesions. Vet Rec 1998;142:109–114.

Thomas WB. Diskospondylitis and other vertebral infections. Vet Clin North Am Small Anim Pract 2000;30:169–182.

Turnwald GH, et al. Diskospondylitis in a kennel of dogs: Clinico-pathologic findings. J Am Vet Med Assoc 1986;188:178–183.

Watt PR, et al. Disseminated opportunistic fungal disease in dogs: 10 cases (1982–1990). J Am Vet Med Assoc 1995;207:67–70.

Noninfectious (immune-mediated) arthritis

The term **immune-mediated arthritis** is used to classify a group of *inflammatory but noninfectious diseases of joints*. The inflammation is in response either to persistence of antigenic material in the synovium of affected joints, possibly as a sequel to previous infection, or to deposition in the synovium of immune complexes derived from inflammatory lesions elsewhere in the body. The *lesions may resemble those of infectious arthritis*, which is not surprising, as the mediators produced during the inflammatory process are quantitatively and qualitatively similar. Furthermore, *synovial fluid from both forms of arthritis is characterized by the presence of increased numbers of neutrophils. Demonstration of toxic change in the neutrophils is often mentioned as a means of differentiating infectious from immune-mediated arthritis, but this is unreliable*. First, not all bacteria induce significant toxic change in synovial neutrophils. Second, unless the viscosity of the synovial fluid is reduced by the lytic action of lysosomal enzymes on hyaluronan, the neutrophils may not "flatten out" sufficiently in direct smears for signs of nuclear degeneration to be apparent.

Immune-mediated arthritis is typically a *polyarthritis* and occurs most often in *dogs and cats*. Erosive and nonerosive forms of the disease are recognized.

- In the *erosive form*, the immunologic process is centered in the joint and stimulates pannus formation, which may result in erosion of the margins of articular cartilage, instability or luxation of joints, or fusion of low-motion joints. The erosive pattern of immune-mediated arthritis is a feature of *rheumatoid-like arthritis of dogs, polyarthritis of Greyhounds, and feline chronic progressive polyarthritis.*
- In the *nonerosive form*, the primary disease is located elsewhere in the body and the products of the immune process are transported to the capillary bed of the synovium of affected joints. Since the primary disease may be transient, cyclic, or responsive to treatment, and is not centered in the joint, products of the immune response that initiate the synovitis can be cleared periodically or permanently from the joint. Consequently, there is no chronic stimulation of pannus or destruction of articular surfaces. Nonerosive immune-mediated arthritis is seen in *idiopathic polyarthritis of dogs, drug-induced arthritis, polyarthritis/myositis syndrome of dogs, lymphocytic/plasmacytic arthritis, and systemic lupus erythematosus*. It is also seen in some animals with chronic enteropathies and other chronic infections.

Erosive athritis

Rheumatoid arthritis

This potentially deforming and crippling disorder is well described in humans, where it is defined by a combination of clinical, pathological, and laboratory criteria. The American Rheumatism Association lists 11 features of the disease, at least seven of which must be present to establish the diagnosis. Furthermore, certain diseases, such as bacterial arthritis, bacterial endocarditis, and systemic lupus erythematosus, must be excluded in order to permit the diagnosis. *The cause of rheumatoid arthritis in humans is not known*, although many aspects of its pathogenesis are understood.

A disease resembling human rheumatoid arthritis is recognized uncommonly in **dogs** and rarely in **cats**. In dogs, it typically affects small and toy breeds, but there is no sex or age predilection. Affected animals initially have episodes of anorexia, depression, and fever, with generalized or shifting lameness associated with swelling around one or more joints. The clinical course is progressive and in the advanced stages of the disease, multiple joints, particularly carpal, tarsal, and phalangeal joints, are persistently swollen, painful, and may be unstable due to weakening of periarticular soft tissues and destruction of articular cartilage and subchondral bone.

Radiographic changes in the early stages of rheumatoid arthritis may be confined to soft tissue swellings, with no apparent alterations to the joint space. As the disease progresses, there is loss of bone density around the joint, collapse of the joint space, and focal radiolucent areas may develop in the subchondral bone (Fig. 1.163A). Other changes may include periarticular osteophytosis, subluxation, or luxation of the joint and fibrous or bony ankylosis, especially in the advanced stages of the disease.

The prominent gross features of early rheumatoid arthritis are thickening and brown discoloration of the joint capsule, with hypertrophy and hyperplasia of synovial villi (Fig. 1.163B, C). Fibrin may be attached to the synovial membrane. Histologically, the enlarged villi are infiltrated with large numbers of lymphocytes and plasma cells and are lined by hypertrophic synoviocytes. Extravasated erythrocytes are often seen within the synovium, as are hemosiderin-laden macrophages, which account for the brown discoloration seen grossly. Degeneration of articular cartilage commences at the margins of the joint where *granulation tissue from the inflamed synovium either spreads across the articular cartilage as a pannus* (Fig. 1.164A) or invades the epiphysis, destroying subchondral bone, and undermining the articular cartilage (Fig. 1.164B). Erosion of central regions of articular cartilage (Fig. 1.163B, C) occurs later in the disease process, probably as a consequence of joint instability and the action of enzymes and mediators released as part of the chronic synovitis. Periosteal new bone sometimes develops at the attachment of thickened joint capsules, but productive osseous changes are always minimal.

Various infectious agents have been implicated as etiologic factors in rheumatoid arthritis of humans and animals. Although none has been shown to be directly involved, indirect involvement through the generation of immune complexes or induction of autoimmunity by molecular mimicry, are possible mechanisms. *Whether the disease is triggered by an infectious agent, or is a manifestation of autoimmunity, there seems little doubt that deposition of immune complexes in articular structures is central to the pathogenesis of rheumatoid arthritis.* Local activation of the complement cascade by these immune complexes leads to generation of proinflammatory peptides such as C3a and C5a, which are chemotactic for neutrophils and induce their degranulation. Type A synoviocytes are efficient antigen-presenting cells and are capable of secreting cytokines that modulate the immune response. Furthermore, high concentrations of granulocyte-monocyte colony stimulating factors in rheumatoid joints can induce monocyte precursors to differentiate into dendritic cells, which are also highly effective at antigen presentation. *Rheumatoid factors*, autoantibodies of the IgM, IgG, or IgA subclasses directed against altered host IgG, are found in synovial fluid, and sometimes in the serum, of dogs with rheumatoid arthritis. *Anti-type II collagen autoantibodies* have also been demonstrated in the synovial fluid of dogs with rheumatoid arthritis. About 25% of dogs with rheumatoid arthritis have rheumatoid factor of the IgM type in their serum. The IgG rheumatoid factor may be more important in dogs but its prevalence in the serum of affected dogs is not known. Rheumatoid factors also are found in a small proportion of dogs and people that do not have joint disease.

Canine distemper virus antigens have been demonstrated in immune complexes precipitated from synovial fluids of dogs with rheumatoid arthritis, suggesting the possibility of a causal role for this virus either following natural infection or vaccination. This would not be surprising since several viral agents have been implicated in human rheumatoid arthritis and the disease in humans often follows viral infection or vaccination.

The joint lesions of *chronic erysipelas and mycoplasmal infections in swine* have features of rheumatoid arthritis and the difficulty in isolating infectious organisms from such joints suggests that an immune mechanism may be involved. In fact, these diseases have been suggested as models for human rheumatoid arthritis.

Polyarthritis of Greyhounds

An *erosive polyarthritis*, which does not appear to have an immune basis, is described in young Greyhounds in Australia, the UK, and the

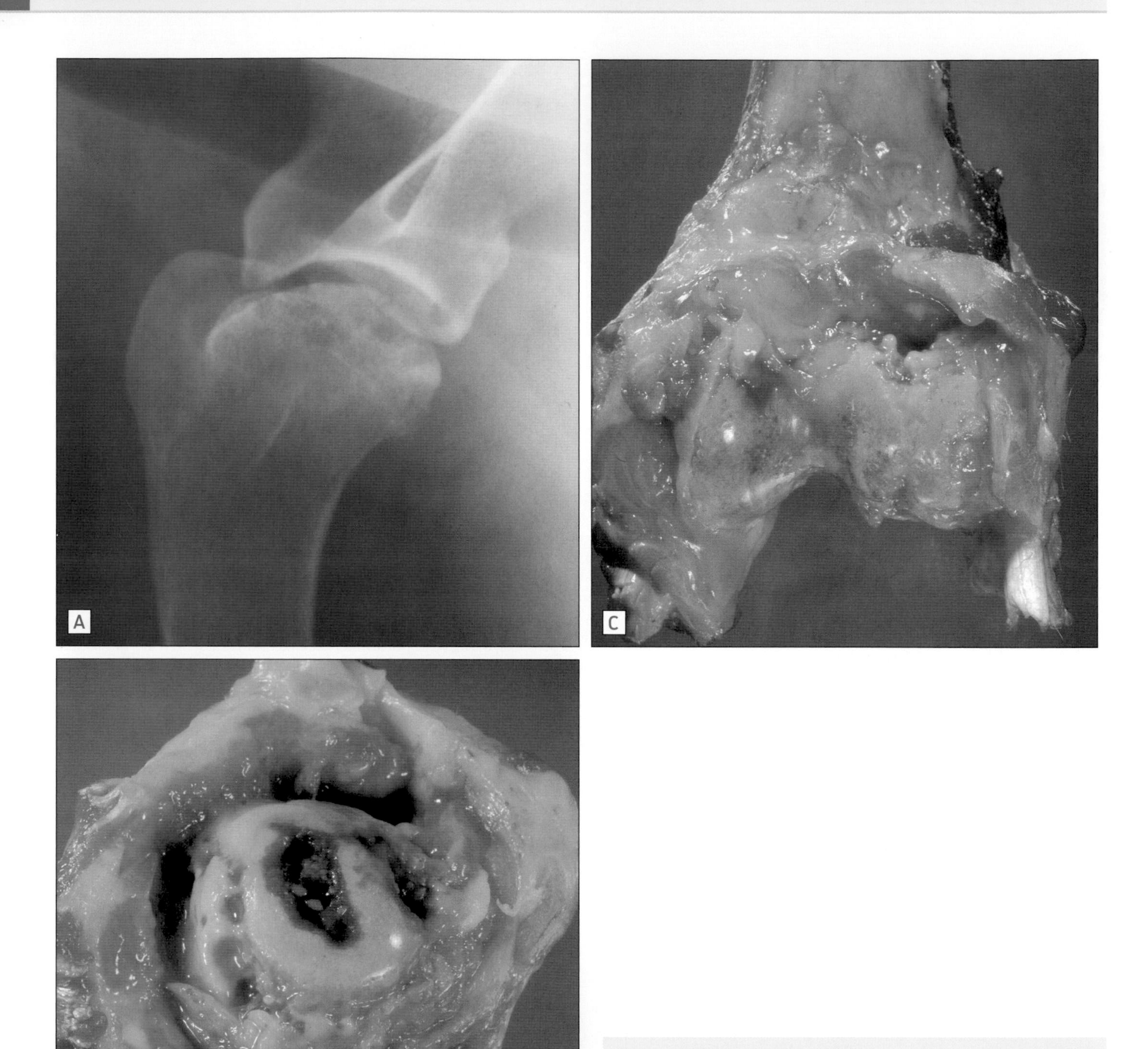

Figure 1.163 Rheumatoid arthritis, dog. **A.** Multifocal, subchondral radiolucent areas in the humeral epiphysis and scapula. **B.** Humeral head from the same dog. Note the deep pits in the eburnated articular surface and the thick joint capsule. The synovial membrane is discolored tan due to the presence of hemosiderin-containing macrophages. **C.** Eburnation and pitting of the condyles of the distal humerus from the same dog.

US. The disease affects dogs of both sexes and usually begins insidiously between 3 and 30 months of age. Mild to severe lameness and joint swellings, involving limb joints distal to, and including, elbows and stifles are observed clinically. Superficial lymph nodes are enlarged. Despite considerable effort, *no infectious agent has yet been identified and the syndrome does not appear to be related to athletic activity*.

Gross findings in affected joints include an excess of turbid synovial fluid, with fibrin clots in severe cases, yellow/brown discoloration, and thickening of synovial membranes, sometimes with adherent fibrin plaques, ecchymotic hemorrhages in the synovial membrane and erosions of articular cartilage. *Lesions are common in the first and second phalangeal joints, and in carpal, tarsal, elbow, and stifle joints*. Occasionally, shoulder, hip, and atlanto-occipital joints are involved.

Microscopic lesions include *necrosis of articular cartilage and proliferative synovitis*. The articular cartilage shows either full-thickness necrosis or necrosis of deep layers with relative sparing of superficial zones. Cartilage erosion sometimes extends to the subchondral bone. Typical changes in the synovium include villus hypertrophy, proliferation of synovial cells, and infiltration by lymphocytes, plasma cells, and neutrophils. In some areas, the lymphocytic infiltrates are

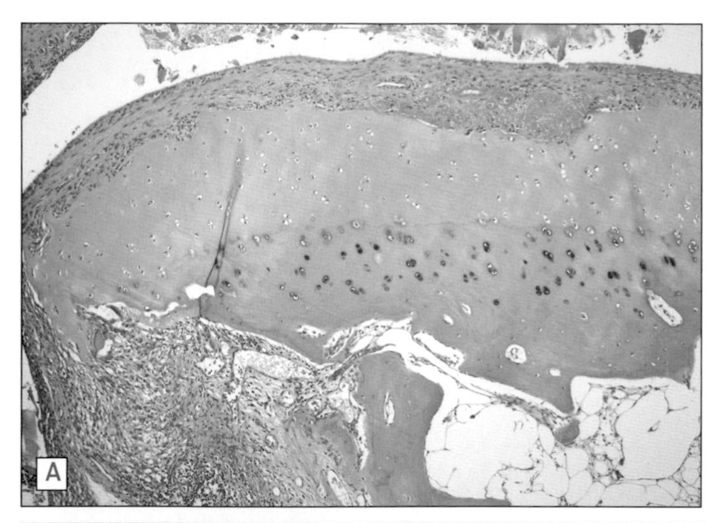

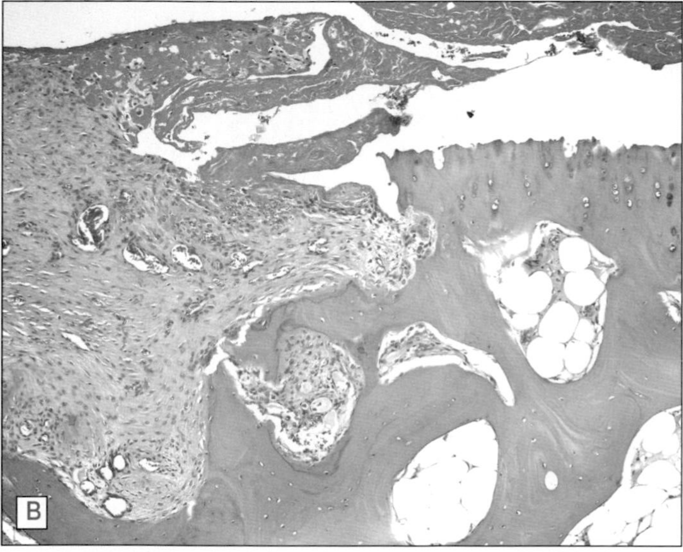

Figure 1.164 Rheumatoid arthritis, dog. **A.** Pannus spreading across articular cartilage from the joint margin. The cartilage beneath the pannus is degenerate. **B.** Granulation tissue invading the epiphysis and encroaching on the eroded articular surface. Note the osteoclasts resorbing bone in front of the advancing granulation tissue. Fibrin is adherent to the surface.

intense and may form follicles. There is no evidence of vasculitis. Pannus formation is often present, but never extensive, and changes in subchondral bone are usually minimal.

Feline chronic progressive polyarthritis

Two forms of this disease are recognized; an *erosive form*, which resembles rheumatoid arthritis of dogs and humans, and a more common form characterized by *periosteal proliferation*.

The **erosive form** occurs in older cats and can affect either sex. It has an *insidious onset, chronic progression,* and clinical signs are largely restricted to symmetrical deformities of the *carpus, tarsus, and digits* due to loss of joint margins, subluxation, collapse of joint space, and ankylosis. The synovial fluid contains low to moderate numbers of neutrophils and lymphocytes. Synovial membranes are heavily infiltrated with lymphocytes and plasma cells and enlarged synovial villi often contain prominent lymphoid follicles with germinal centers. Rheumatoid factor is absent. Infection with *Feline leukemia virus* is present in about 50% of affected cats.

The **periosteal proliferative form** occurs only in relatively *young, intact or neutered male cats,* usually between 18 months and 5 years of age. The disease is etiologically *linked to infection with Feline syncytia-forming virus and Feline leukemia virus.* Evidence of *Feline syncytia-forming virus* infection is present in all affected cats and 60% also have evidence of *Feline leukemia virus* infection, but the disease cannot be reproduced by experimental infection with either of the two agents, or with cell-free synovial tissue from affected cats. Because many cats are infected with both viruses without ever becoming ill, it is thought that the periosteal proliferative form of feline chronic progressive polyarthritis is an *unusual manifestation of Feline syncytia-forming virus infection in cats that are somehow predisposed.* The role of *Feline leukemia virus* is unclear, but it may potentiate the activity of the other viral agent. A similar syndrome has been reported in a 4-year-old cat that was seropositive for both *Feline syncytia-forming virus* and *Feline immunodeficiency virus.*

The disease is characterized by sudden onset of high fever, severe pain in joints and tendon sheaths, and lymphadenopathy associated with affected joints. Synovitis is initially characterized by the presence of *fibrinopurulent synovitis but later, plasma cells and lymphocytes predominate.* Rheumatoid factor is absent. Synovial lining cells are hyperplastic throughout the course of the disease, but villus hypertrophy and pannus formation are uncommon until late in the disease. Swollen lymph nodes biopsied early in the disease have exuberant lymphoid hyperplasia, including marked extracapsular extension, and could be mistaken for lymphosarcoma.

The skeletal lesions are bilateral and *most frequently involve the tarsometatarsal and carpometacarpal joints,* but the elbow and stifle joints, and the articular facets of the thoracic and lumbar spine, may also be affected. The periosteal new bone consists of trabeculae of woven bone and the intertrabecular spaces often are infiltrated with lymphocytes and plasma cells. Pannus formation usually occurs late in the disease and leads to periarticular erosions of joint margins, collapse of joint spaces, and fibrous ankylosis, but subluxation is not a feature. This pattern of disease is similar to Reiter's arthritis of humans.

Nonerosive arthritis

There are several diverse causes of noninfectious, nonerosive arthritis in dogs and cats, but the mechanism in each syndrome appears to be immune mediated and the presenting signs are similar. Clinically, the joint disease tends to be intermittent, and periods of remission may occur. One or several joints of the distal limbs may be involved, particularly the smaller joints of the manus and pes. There are essentially no radiographic changes except for joint distension and soft tissue swelling, although signs may have been present for months. Occasionally, slight narrowing of the joint space is evident, and distension of the joint cavity is demonstrable by contrast arthrography. Gross lesions in affected joints are minimal. Histologically, there is edematous thickening and inflammation of the synovial membrane. Neutrophils are concentrated at the intimal layer of the synovium and may be quite numerous, depending upon the stage of the disease. Sparse accumulations of plasma cells and lymphocytes are present in the deeper layers of the synovium and fibrous joint capsule. Villus hyperplasia and pannus are not seen.

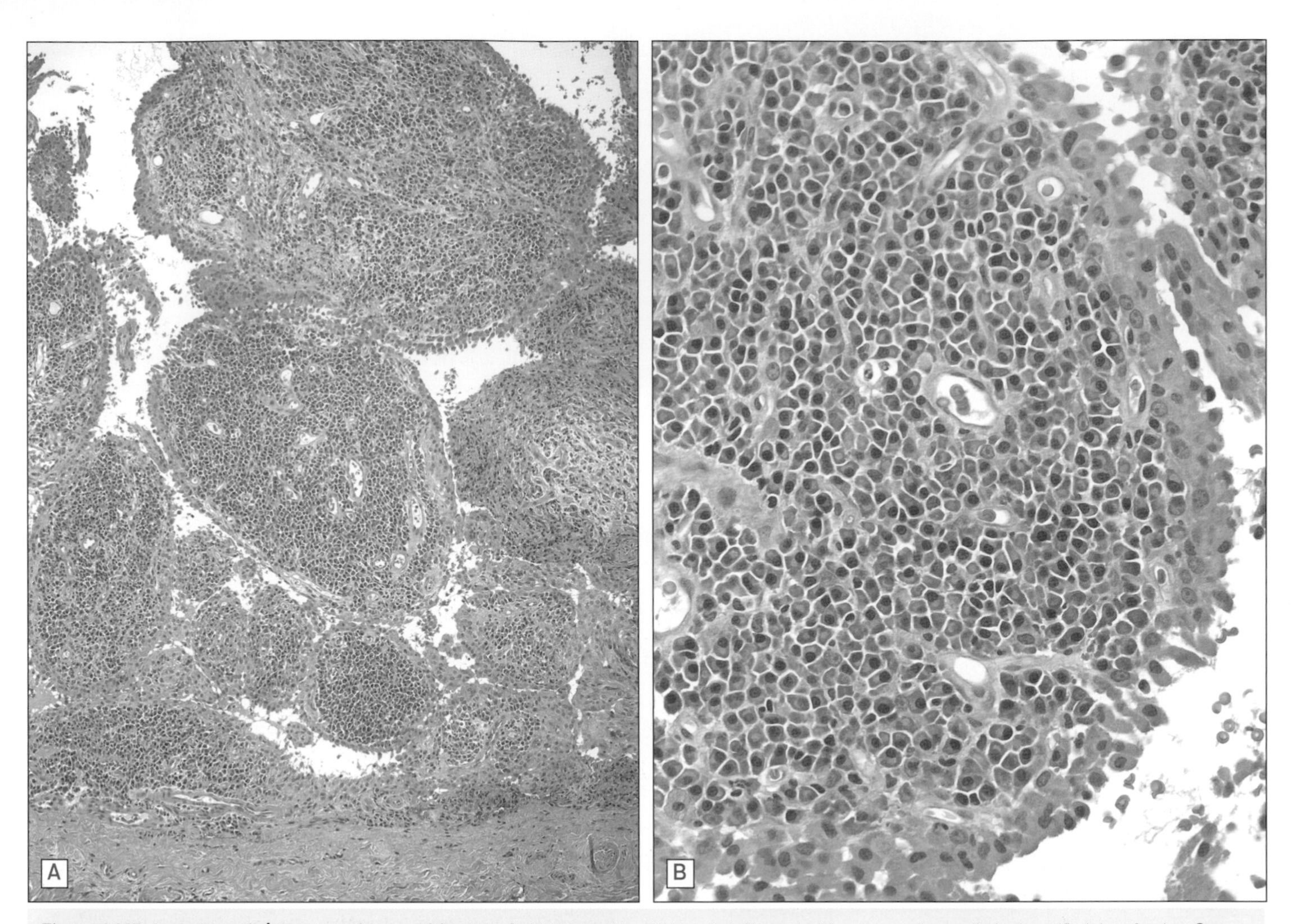

Figure 1.165 Lymphocytic/plasmacytic synovitis, dog. **A.** Hypertrophic villi heavily infiltrated with mononuclear cells in the stifle joint of a dog, 2 years after surgery for correction of patellar luxation. **B.** High-power view of a villus from the same dog. The villus is infiltrated with an almost pure population of plasma cells. Note the hypertrophy and hyperplasia of synovial cells.

Synovial fluid cytology is useful in the diagnosis of noninfectious, nonerosive arthritis, but is not specific and often does not allow differentiation from infectious arthritis or from erosive forms of noninfectious arthritis. The characteristic feature is a mild to moderate increase in cellularity, most cells of which are nondegenerate neutrophils.

Idiopathic polyarthritis is considered the most common form of nonerosive, immune-mediated arthritis in dogs, but is diagnosed only when other types of inflammatory joint disease have been excluded. Arthritis is the only manifestation, but pyrexia, inappetance, and lethargy generally accompany the lameness. The polyarthritis associated with **systemic lupus erythematosus** of dogs and cats is similar to that of idiopathic polyarthritis, but may be accompanied by evidence of disease in other organs systems, such as the skin, kidney, bone marrow, or neuromuscular system. *In many cases, only the presence of antinuclear antibody in serum distinguishes the two syndromes.* Neutrophils containing phagocytosed, partially degraded nuclear material, referred to as lupus erythematosus cells (LE cells), are rarely detected in the synovial fluid of animals with systemic lupus erythematosus. The phagocytosed nuclear material in LE cells is dense, diffusely pink or purple, and displaces the nucleus to the periphery of the cell. Leukophagocytic macrophages and neutrophils containing more granular nuclear remnants are common in the synovial fluid of acutely inflamed joints and should not be misinterpreted as LE cells.

Nonerosive polyarthritis has been recognized in animals and humans in association with a **variety of chronic diseases**, such as bacterial endocarditis, urinary tract infections, diskospondylitis, periodontitis, chronic otitis media or interna, pyometra, dirofilariasis, and fungal infections. **Inflammatory bowel disease** has also been associated with polyarthritis in canine and human patients. Although the possibility that infection may be involved in some of these nonerosive forms of polyarthritis is virtually impossible to exclude, the weight of evidence suggests that the synovitis is secondary to deposition of circulating immune complexes in the synovial capillary bed. In those cases associated with inflammatory processes at other sites, the inflammation presumably does not persist long enough, or is not severe enough, to initiate pannus formation or induce cartilage erosion. In the most common primary or idiopathic form, the origin and nature of the antigen responsible for initiating the disease is unknown.

Drug-induced polyarthritis, thought to be immune-mediated, develops in a small proportion of dogs, particularly Dobermans, treated with *sulfonamides*. Combination drugs containing sulfadiazine are usually responsible but sulfamethoxazole is also incriminated. The drug may act directly as *an antigen or as a hapten* in combination with host proteins. Signs of polyarthritis and fever, sometimes with lymphadenopathy, anemia, leukopenia, and thrombocytopenia, develop after 8–20 days of treatment. Clinical signs regress within 2–5 days of drug withdrawal and, in one report, recurred within 2 hours to 5 days in six of six dogs that were re-exposed.

A syndrome characterized by nonerosive **polyarthritis** and **polymyositis** has been reported in six young adult dogs, five of which were Spaniels. Clinical signs included stiffness, pain and swelling of multiple joints, muscle pain, muscle atrophy, and pyrexia. Affected dogs have no circulating antinuclear antibodies or rheumatoid factors but show chronic active inflammatory changes in muscle and synovial membrane biopsies.

Plasmacytic/lymphocytic synovitis is an insidious, nonerosive arthritis involving primarily the *stifle joint of small and medium-sized breeds of dog*. The syndrome may be accompanied by joint laxity and partial or complete rupture of the cranial cruciate ligament but it is seldom possible to determine which lesion came first. It is possible that the synovitis in these animals reflects an exaggerated immune response to mediators or antigens released following ligament damage, surgical correction, or as a result of an ensuing degenerative joint disease. Radiographic evidence of degenerative joint disease may be present in some cases. The synovial membrane is thickened, edematous, and red/yellow on gross examination. Microscopic examination reveals a *marked diffuse and/or nodular plasmacytic/lymphocytic infiltration of the synovium and hypertrophy of synovial cells* (Fig. 1.165A, B). Villus hypertrophy may also be a feature. Unlike other forms of immune-mediated arthritis, the increase in cellularity of the synovial fluid is due predominantly to small mononuclear cells rather than neutrophils, the latter comprising only 10–40% of the cell population.

Bibliography

Becker KM, et al. Polyarthropathy in a cat seropositive for feline syncytial-forming virus and feline immunodeficiency virus. J Am Anim Hosp Assoc 1994;30:225–232.

Bell SC, et al. Canine distemper viral antigen and antibodies in dogs with rheumatoid arthritis. Res Vet Sci 1991;50:64–68.

Bennett D. Immune-based erosive inflammatory joint disease of the dog: canine rheumatoid arthritis. 2. Pathological investigations. J Small Anim Pract 1987;28:799–819.

Bennett D. Immune-based nonerosive inflammatory joint disease of the dog. 1. Canine systemic lupus erythematosus. J Small Anim Pract 1987;28:871–889.

Bennett D. Immune-based nonerosive inflammatory joint disease of the dog. 3. Canine idiopathic polyarthritis. J Small Anim Pract 1987;28:909–928.

Bennett D, Kelly DF. Immune-based nonerosive inflammatory joint disease of the dog. 2. Polyarthritis/polymyositis syndrome. J Small Anim Pract 1987;28:891–908.

Bennett D, et al. Bacterial endocarditis with polyarthritis in two dogs associated with circulating auto-antibodies. J Small Anim Pract 1978;19:185–196.

Carter SD, et al. Canine rheumatoid arthritis and inflammatory cytokines. Vet Immunol Immunopathol 1999;69:201–214.

Cribb AE. Idiosyncratic reactions to sulfonamides in dogs. J Am Vet Med Assoc 1989;195:1612–1614.

Fournel C, et al. Canine systemic lupus erythematosus. I: A study of 75 cases. Lupus 1992;1:133–139.

Galloway RH, Lester SJ. Histopathological evaluation of the stifle joint synovial membrane collected at the time of repair of cranial cruciate ligament rupture. J Am Anim Hosp Assoc 1995;31:289–294.

Huxtable CR, Davis PE. The pathology of polyarthritis in young Greyhounds. J Comp Pathol 1976;86:11–21.

Krum SH, et al. Polymyositis and polyarthritis associated with systemic lupus erythematosus in a dog. J Am Vet Med Assoc 1977;170:61–64.

Little DJL, Carmichael S. Trimethoprim sulphonamide hypersensitivity in dogs. Vet Rec 1990;127:459–460.

Pedersen NC, et al. Noninfectious canine arthritis: rheumatoid arthritis. J Am Vet Med Assoc 1976;169:295–303.

Pedersen NC, et al. Feline chronic progressive polyarthritis. Am J Vet Res 1980;41:522–535.

Schumacher HR, et al. Synovial pathologic changes in spontaneous canine rheumatoid-like arthritis. Arthritis Rheum 1980;23:412–423.

Woodard JC, et al. Erosive polyarthritis in two Greyhounds. J Am Vet Med Assoc 1991;198: 873–876.

TUMORS AND TUMOR-LIKE LESIONS OF JOINTS

A range of neoplastic and non-neoplastic lesions occurs in domestic animals in the vicinity of joints, but most are rare and poorly characterized. The most recent World Health Bulletin on the histological classification of bone and joint tumors lists only synovial sarcoma and villonodular synovitis as tumors and tumor-like lesions of joints and related tissues. Although veterinary pathologists recognize many lesions other than these two, only the most common are included here. For further information, the reader is referred to the bibliography at the end of this section.

Tumors in the region of joints may be either *benign or malignant* and *arise from synovioblastic cells* in the synovial membrane *or from a range of supporting structures*, including fibroblastic, vascular, and nervous tissue. Because of the similarity between synovial tumors and other mesenchymal tumors, the potential for misdiagnosis is high, especially when these lesions occur so infrequently and diagnostic criteria are largely extrapolated from the human medical literature.

As with tumors of bones, the availability of a detailed clinical history and knowledge of the radiographic and gross findings prior to microscopic examination of the lesion are likely to enhance the accuracy of the diagnosis. In particular, radiography will usually indicate whether the lesion is centered on a joint or tendon sheath, the presence of mineralization, and any bone involvement. Cytological evaluation of fine-needle aspirates or scrapings prepared from tissue biopsies may provide useful information on the nature of the tumor cells, but in most cases, histologic examination is required.

Benign tumors and tumor-like lesions of joints

Although several benign proliferative lesions of the synovium have been described in man and animals, most are rare and, for many of them, there is debate over whether they are neoplastic or inflammatory.

Pigmented villonodular synovitis is recognized occasionally in the *major weight-bearing limb joints, particularly the stifle and hip, of* *adult dogs*. Grossly, the synovial membrane in affected joints is thickened with plump, tan or dark brown villi and articular surfaces show features of mild degenerative joint disease. Histologically, the thickened synovial membrane consists of *closely packed villi of various sizes and shapes, and slit-like spaces lined by synovial cells*. The spaces may represent tangential sections through gaps between adjacent villi. Hyperplastic synovial cells are present throughout much of the thickened synovium but do not invade the joint capsule and although binucleate forms are often present, they show no cytologic features of malignancy. Multinucleated giant cells are sometimes present, together with hemosiderin-containing macrophages. *The lesion may be difficult to differentiate from chronic infectious synovitis, or a chronic synovial response to either hemarthrosis or degenerative joint disease.*

Villonodular synovitis of the *equine metacarpophalangeal or metatarsophalangeal joints* is a chronic inflammatory condition characterized by the formation of a nodular mass involving the synovium near the dorsoproximal attachment of the joint capsule. As mentioned earlier in this chapter, this lesion is considered *secondary to persistent trauma* and has features of a resolving hematoma.

Localized nodular tenosynovitis is another benign lesion of questionable origin and with a variety of synonyms in the human literature, including benign synovioma; a term that is no longer advocated for use in either humans or animals. The lesion has been reported only occasionally in *dogs*, although nodular lesions of tendons previously diagnosed as benign synovioma probably constitute additional examples of localized nodular tenosynovitis. The most common sites for these firm, solitary lesions are the *tendons and tendon sheaths of the extensors and flexors of the feet, particularly in the region of the metacarpus and metatarsus*. The microscopic appearance varies between and within lesions, but usually includes cellular areas containing proliferating synoviocytes, hemosiderin-containing macrophages, multinucleated giant cells and mononuclear inflammatory cells. Cleft-like spaces lined by synoviocytes are often present in some areas. There are *similarities between this lesion and benign giant cell tumor of tendons and tendon sheaths*, and it is possible that these are variants of the same disease process.

Benign giant cell tumors of tendons and tendon sheaths appear to arise from synovioblastic cells surrounding tendons and tendon sheaths and are relatively common in animals. Microscopically, the lesion is characterized by the presence of *numerous multinucleated giant cells, which are thought to develop from proliferating synovioblasts*. Some lesions are predominantly solid while others contain many cleft-like spaces. The tumor cells show no convincing features of malignancy but, although they do not metastasize, recurrence following surgical removal is likely.

Benign vascular lesions referred to as either **synovial hemangiomas** or **vascular hamartomas** have been reported in the *carpal and digital sheaths of the forelegs in young horses*. The lesions may be apparent from an early age and enlarge slowly, or may become acutely apparent following rupture and formation of hematomas. Microscopically, the lesions consist of *multiple nodules of well-differentiated capillaries separated by septa of fibrous tissue*. Apparent invasion of adjacent structures, including tendons, occurs in some cases, but the endothelial cells lining capillaries show no features of anaplasia, and metastasis is not reported. Reports of hemangiosarcomas involving the tendon sheaths of young horses are most likely further examples of benign vascular tumors that would be more appropriately classified as vascular hamartomas.

Synovial chondromatosis (osteochondromatosis) is a tumor-like lesion characterized by the presence of *multiple nodules of hyaline cartilage, some of which may undergo ossification, in the synovial membrane*. Although synovial chondromas are widely considered to arise by metaplasia of synovial cells within the synovial membrane, an alternative hypothesis suggests that the cartilage nodules may in fact be derived from fragments of cartilage from the articular surface. Such fragments released into the joint space may continue to enlarge within the joint as they derive their nutrients from the synovial fluid. Some may become incorporated into the synovial membrane, where they could also survive and grow within the richly vascular synovial membrane and, in some cases, become ossified following vascular invasion. This mechanism is most likely in cases where there is an associated degenerative joint disease, but the syndrome sometimes occurs in the synovial membrane of apparently normal joints or bursae. In such cases, chondroid metaplasia of synovial mesenchymal cells is a more attractive pathogenesis.

Various other benign, tumor-like lesions occurring in the vicinity of joints, including **tumoral calcinosis** and **fibrodysplasia ossificans progressiva** are discussed earlier in this chapter under the heading Ectopic mineralization and ossification.

Malignant tumors of joints

Because of the infrequent occurrence of these tumors in animals, their classification has largely been based on extrapolation from the medical literature. This has not been straightforward, as the classification of certain malignant periarticular tumors of humans is confusing. For example, there is evidence that tumors classified as synovial sarcoma in human patients are not of synovial origin at all. Furthermore, there is debate over the use of such terms as malignant fibrous histiocytoma and malignant giant cell tumors of soft parts, both in animals and humans. The use of such categories in this section is more in recognition that they are well established in the veterinary literature than an endorsement of their validity. *A more precise and widely accepted classification system for malignancies of joints will necessitate the use of immunochemical or molecular techniques to better determine the histogenesis of the tumor cells.*

Synovial sarcoma in humans is characterized by a biphasic pattern, comprising both *mesenchymal and epithelial elements*. In some tumors, a "pseudoglandular" appearance is created by epithelial elements, which often form irregular cleft-like spaces surrounded by neoplastic mesenchymal cells. In other cases, the mesenchymal elements predominate and the tumor may be difficult to differentiate from other sarcomas, particularly fibrosarcoma. The neoplastic epithelial cells in these tumors possess tight junctions and are arranged on a basal lamina. In addition, they stain positively with the epithelial markers cytokeratin and epithelial membrane antigen. *Synovial cells are of mesenchymal, rather than epithelial, origin* and are not arranged on a basal lamina. The fact that these tumors in human patients frequently occur at sites distant from joints creates further doubt over their synovial origin and suggests that extrapolation to animals is inappropriate.

Synovial sarcoma is rare in animals, but has been reported in dogs and occasionally in cats and cattle. In **dogs**, synovial sarcoma is reported mainly *in large but not giant breeds* and although it is most common around middle age, the *age range is broad* (1–15 years). The tumor is found most often near one of the *major weight-bearing joints*, the *stifle* being the most common and followed in decreasing order by the elbow, shoulder, tarsus, carpus, and hip. Occasionally, joints of the axial skeleton are involved. Synovial sarcoma may also originate from the region of *tendons or tendon sheaths*, usually the flexor or extensor tendons of the limbs proximal to the carpus and tarsus. Grossly, *the tumor has indistinct borders* and may infiltrate along fascial planes leading away from the affected joint. Some synovial sarcomas contain cystic spaces filled with mucinous material. The synovial membrane may be largely replaced by tumor tissue and invasion of epiphyseal bone may occur at the insertion of the joint capsule.

Histologic descriptions of synovial sarcoma in animals frequently imply the presence of two distinct cell populations by reference to a synovioblastic or "epithelioid" cell type and a fibroblastic cell type. This no doubt reflects extrapolation from synovial sarcoma in humans, although *there is some doubt that these biphasic tumors actually occur in animals*. The tumor cells in synovial sarcomas of animals may vary in shape from polygonal to spindle-shaped, the relative proportion of each type varying between tumors, and even within the same tumor. *In cases with a predominance of spindle cells, the tumor may be virtually indistinguishable from fibrosarcoma, but other tumors may consist predominantly of sheets of synovioblastic cells more closely resembling normal synoviocytes.* Cavities or slit-like spaces containing *proteinaceous fluid or mucoid material* and lined by a poorly defined layer of malignant synovioblasts may form within sheets of tumor cells (Figs 1.166A, B, 1.167A). The malignant synovioblastic cells of synovial sarcoma often have eccentric circular to oval nuclei, which vary in size and may contain one or more prominent nucleoli. The mitotic rate is highly variable, as is the frequency of binucleate and multinucleate giant cells. Individual cells may be surrounded by an eosinophilic matrix resembling osteoid (Fig. 1.167B), sometimes leading to an incorrect diagnosis of osteosarcoma. In some canine synovial sarcomas, especially those involving tendons or tendon sheaths, *nodules of myxomatous tumor tissue* are scattered among areas that are more solid. The myxoid matrix may surround individual stellate tumor cells, clusters of tumor cells, or fill multiple spaces within the tumor. Synovial sarcomas with abundant myxoid change are difficult to differentiate from myxosarcoma or malignant peripheral nerve sheath tumors. The perivascular orientation of synovioblastic or fibroblastic tumor cells in some tumors might also cause confusion with hemangiopericytoma, especially in lesions where there is infiltration of the skin adjacent to the joint or tendon sheath.

In cytologic preparations, synovial sarcoma may yield a population of plump, malignant mesenchymal cells with eccentric nuclei and basophilic cytoplasm, together with variable numbers of spindle cells and multinucleated giant cells, but histopathology is required to reliably differentiate the tumor from osteosarcoma and various other sarcomas.

Canine synovial sarcomas *commonly recur following surgical excision* and, in one study, *20 of 37 cases (54%) metastasized*. Metastases were found most often in the lungs and regional lymph nodes. The clinical course may vary from less than a month to greater than a year.

Only isolated cases of synovial sarcoma are reported in species other than dogs, and the diagnosis is not always conclusive.

Histiocytic sarcoma is recognized as a *rapidly growing, locally aggressive tumor* often occurring in *close proximity to a joint in dogs*, particularly flat-coated Retrievers, Golden Retrievers, Labrador Retrievers, Bull Mastiffs and Rottweilers. The tumor has been recognized in dogs of both sexes from 4 to 13 years of age. Similar tumors also arise from the skin or subcutaneous tissue and infiltrate underlying tissues. It is likely that many histiocytic sarcomas originating in the joint capsule are incorrectly diagnosed as synovial sarcoma.

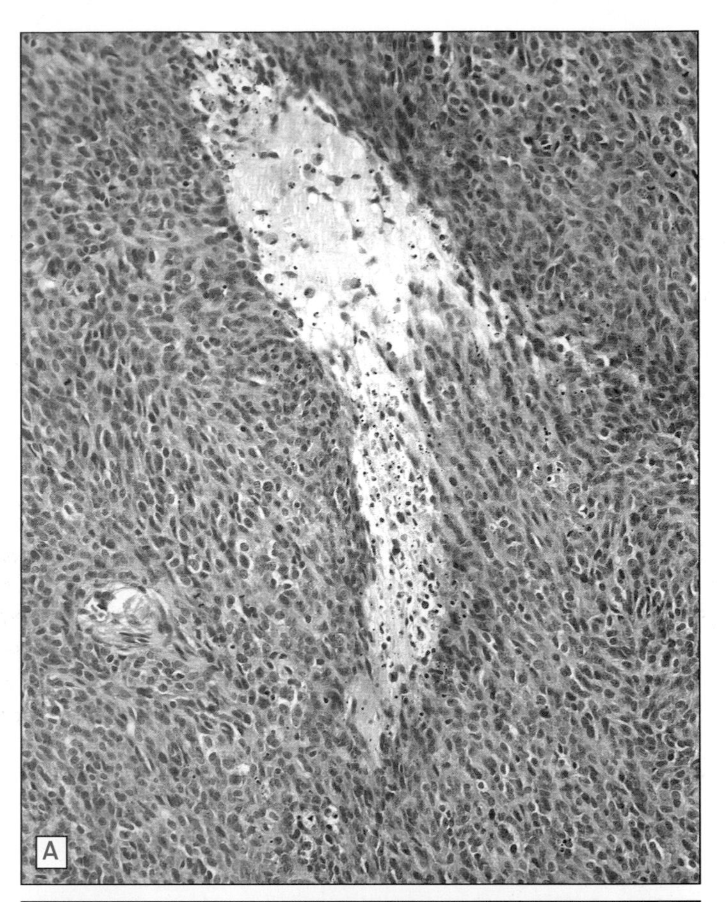

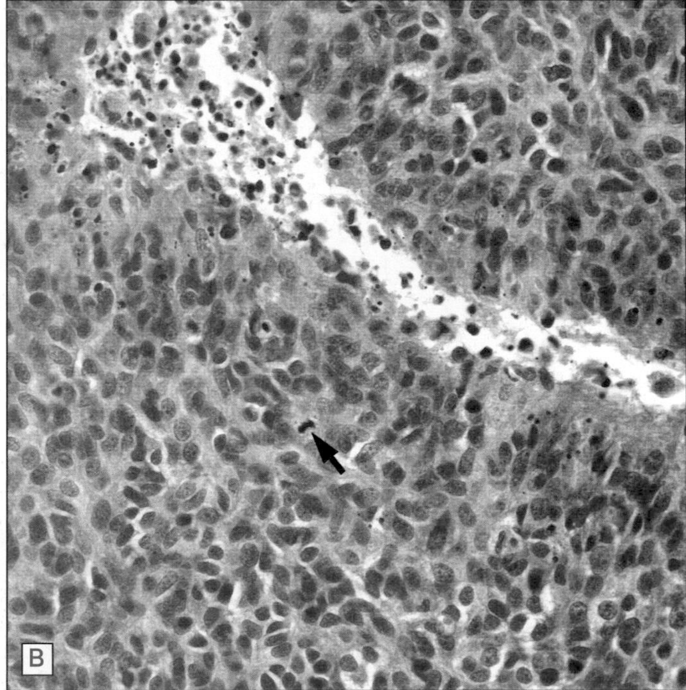

Figure 1.166 Synovial sarcoma, dog. **A.** Sheets of disorganized spindle cells surrounding and lining a poorly defined cavity. **B.** Higher-power view of the same tumor showing a narrow cleft surrounded by tumor cells. Occasional mitotic figures are present (arrow).

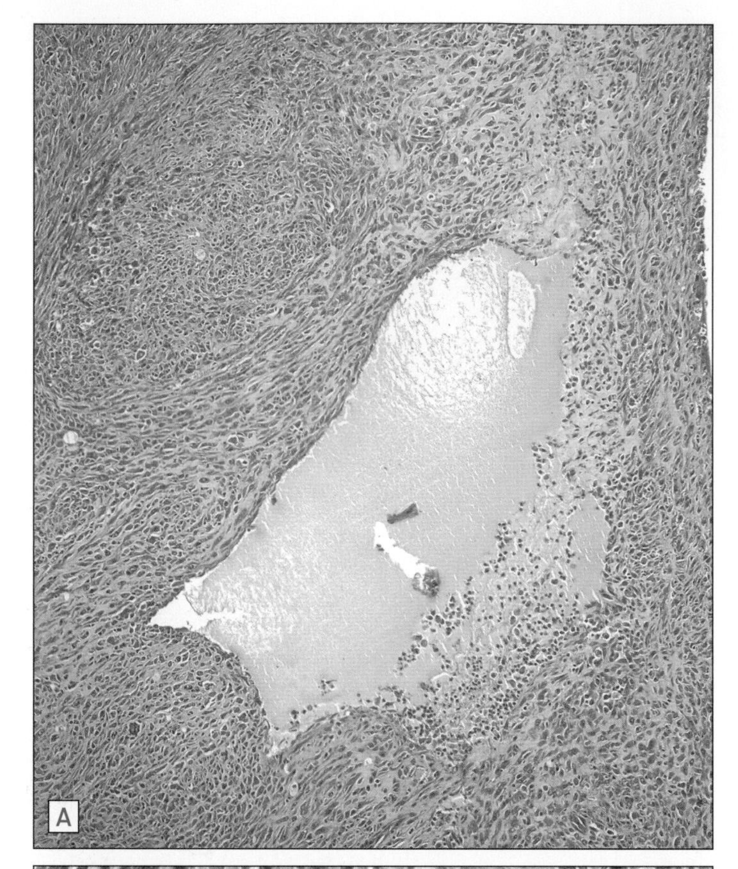

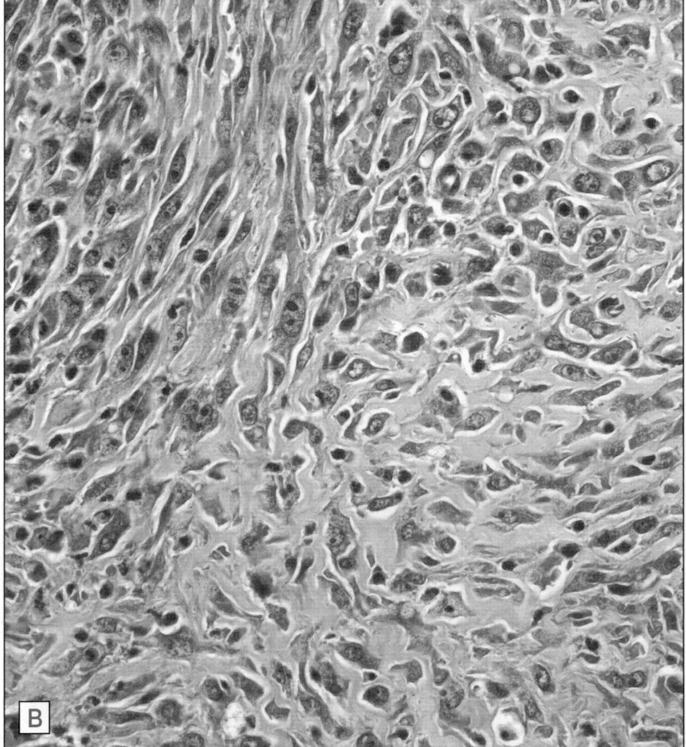

Figure 1.167 Synovial sarcoma, dog. **A.** Large cavity surrounded by malignant synovioblastic cells and containing proteinaceous fluid. **B.** Same tumor at higher power showing fusiform to polygonal tumor cells, many of which are surrounded by eosinophilic matrix similar to osteoid.

A recent retrospective study of 35 canine synovial tumors, using immunochemical staining for antibodies to cytokeratin and CD18, found that 51% of them were histiocytic sarcomas.

Dendritic (Langerhans) cells, which are known to occur in the synovial membrane, are considered the cell of origin of histiocytic sarcomas in the region of joints, although precise classification of the tumor requires the development of specific immunochemical stains.

Clinically, the tumor produces soft tissue swellings around or in the vicinity of major limb joints and may be accompanied by lytic lesions in the epiphyses or metaphyses of adjacent bones. On gross examination, the synovial membrane and joint capsule may show marked nodular or diffuse thickening with gray/pink, fleshy tumor tissue (Fig. 1.168A), which may extend into adjacent soft tissues. Histologically, *the synovial membrane and joint capsule are infiltrated with malignant histiocytic cells*, sometimes forming nodules protruding into the joint space (Fig. 1.168B) or causing marked thickening of synovial villi. The nuclei of tumor cells vary considerably in size and shape, and often contain large, irregularly shaped nucleoli (Fig. 1.168C). The cells have a moderate to large quantity of eosinophilic cytoplasm, which sometimes contains many small vacuoles. Multinucleated giant cells with variable-sized nuclei are common and the mitotic rate is usually high. Neutrophils, eosinophils, lymphocytes, and plasma cells may be present in variable numbers throughout the tumor. Similar tumor cells may be present between bone trabeculae in adjacent bones, presumably due to direct invasion from the attachment of the joint capsule or the adjacent muscle. *Cytological preparations* generally reveal a monomorphic population of large round cells with circular to oval or indented nuclei and abundant cytoplasm, which may contain many discrete vacuoles (Fig. 1.169A, B). Multinucleated giant cells containing nuclei of various sizes are common, as are abnormal mitotic figures.

Canine histiocytic sarcoma is not only locally aggressive, but *frequently metastasizes* to regional lymph nodes and occasionally to the lungs and other visceral organs. In the retrospective study referred to above, 91% of histiocytic sarcomas metastasized, and the average survival time was 5.3 months. The prognosis is therefore poor, and early diagnosis followed by amputation of the affected limb offers the best chance of survival.

Bibliography

Affolter VK, Moore PF. Histiocytosis. Pisa, Italy: Proc Eur Soc Vet Derm 14th Annual Congress, 5–7 Sept, 1997:101–104.

Carb A, Halliwell WH. Nodular tenosynovitis of the flexor tendon in two dogs. J Am Anim Hosp Assoc 1982;18:867–871.

Colbourne CM, et al. Vascular hamartomas of the dorsal carpal region in three young thoroughbred horses. Aust Vet J 1997;75:20–23.

Craig LE, et al. The diagnosis and prognosis of synovial tumors in dogs: 35 cases. Vet Pathol 2002;39:66–73.

Dickersin GR. Synovial sarcoma: a review and update with emphasis on the ultrastructural characterization of the nonglandular component. Ultrastr Pathol 1991;15:379–402.

Griffith JW, et al. Synovial sarcoma of the jaw in a dog. J Comp Path 1987;97:361–364.

Johnstone AC. Congenital vascular tumors in the skin of horses. J Comp Path 1987;97:365–368.

Kay PR, et al. The etiology of multiple loose bodies. Snow storm knee. J Bone Joint Surg 1989;71:501–504.

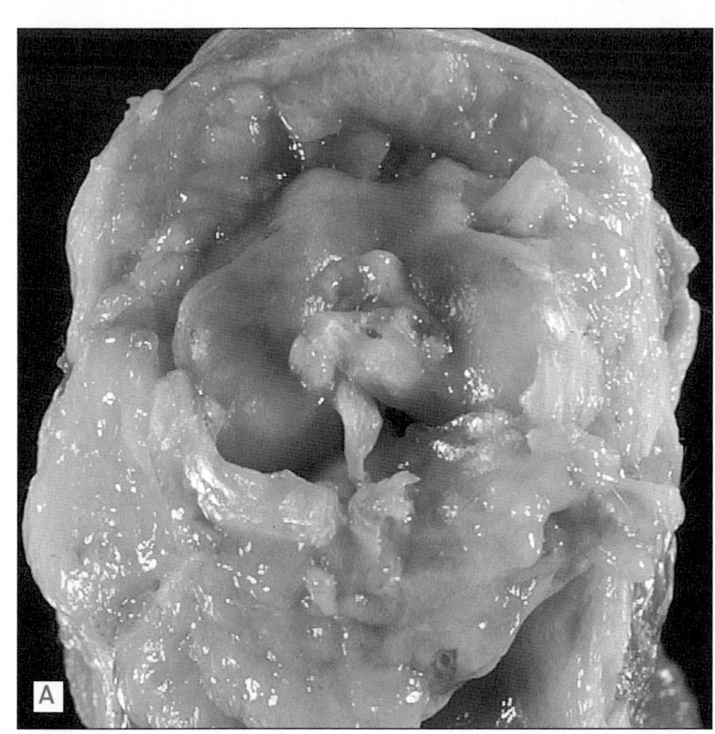

Figure 1.168 Histiocytic sarcoma, dog. Stifle joint. **A.** Massive thickening of joint capsule with fleshy tumor tissue. **B.** Nodular infiltration of synovial membrane with malignant histiocytic cells. **C.** Closer view of tumor cells showing marked anisokaryosis and anisonucleoliosis in addition to multinucleated cells and abnormal mitotic figures (arrows).

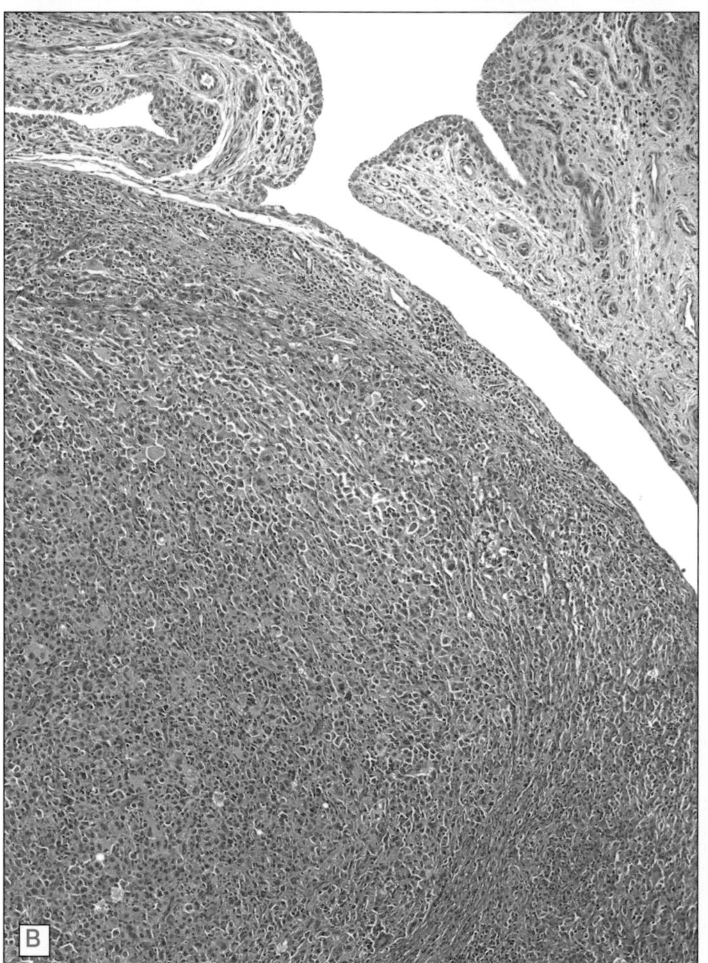

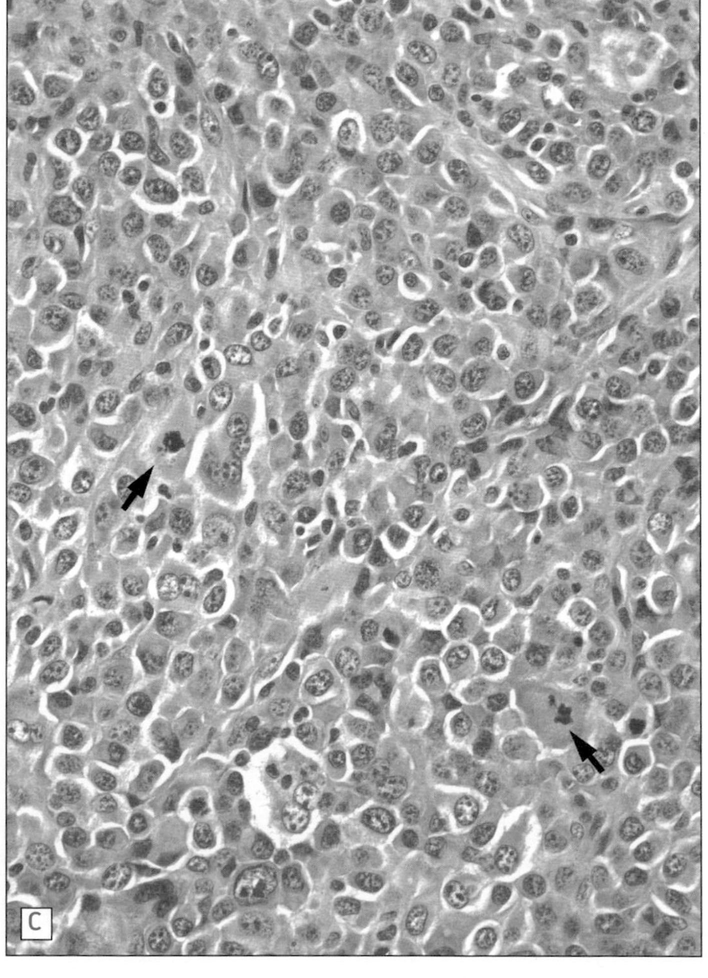

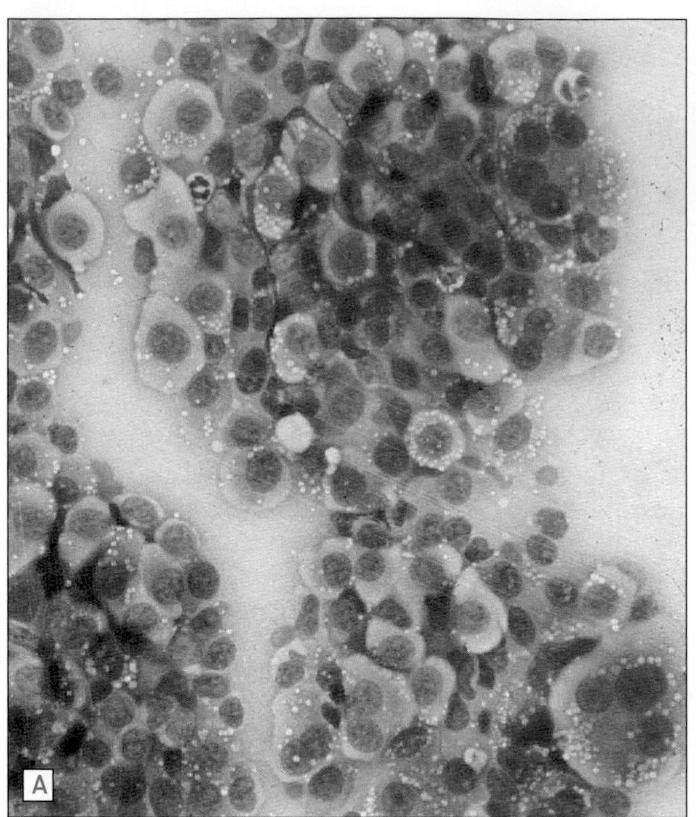

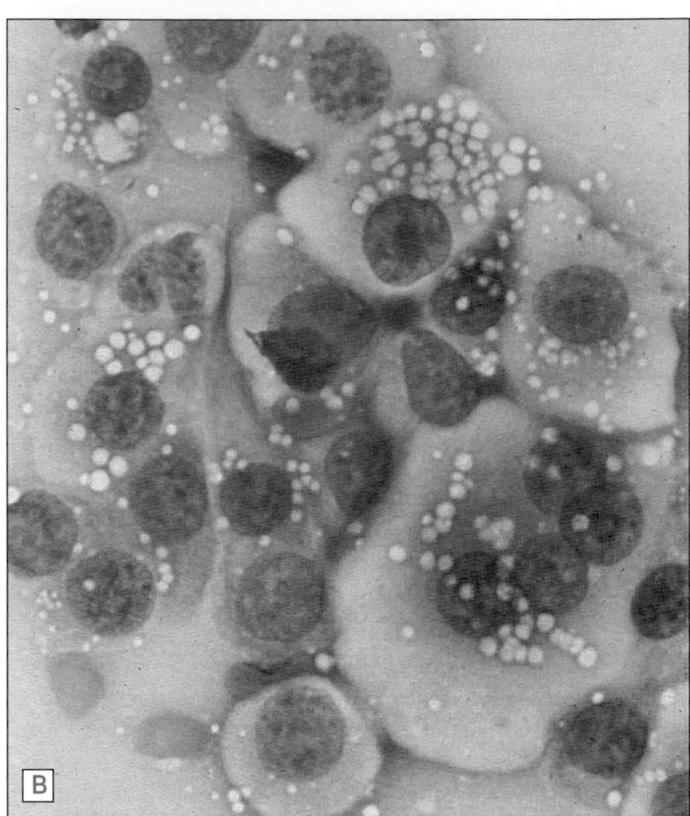

Figure 1.169 Histiocytic sarcoma, dog. **A.** Cytological preparation (scraping) of tumor involving the shoulder joint of a Retriever. The tumor cells are sometimes binucleate or multinucleate and many contain discrete intracytoplasmic vacuoles. **B.** Closer view showing large histiocytic cells, including a multinucleate form.

Marti JM. Bilateral pigmented villonodular synovitis in a dog. J Small Anim Pract 1997;38:256–260.

McGlennon NJ, et al. Synovial sarcoma in the dog – a review. J Small Anim Pract 1988;29:139–152.

Miettinen M, Virtanen I. Synovial sarcoma – a misnomer. Am J Pathol 1984;117:18–25.

Pool RR, Thompson KG. Tumors of joints. In: Meuten DJ, ed. Tumors in Domestic Animals. 4th ed. Ames, IA: Iowa State University Press, 2002:Ch 4.

Salisbury JR, Isaacson PG. Synovial sarcoma: an immunohistochemical study. J Pathol 1985;147:49–57.

Silva-Krott IU, et al. Synovial sarcoma in a cat. J Am Vet Med Assoc 1993;203:1430–1431.

Slayter MV, et al. In: Histological Classification of Bone and Joint Tumors of Domestic Animals. W.H.O. Second Series, vol 1. Washington DC: Armed Forces Institute of Pathology, American Registry of Pathology, 1994.

Somer T, et al. Pigmented villonodular synovitis and plasmacytoid lymphoma in a dog. J Am Vet Med Assoc 1990;197:877–879.

Van Pelt RW, et al. Multiple hemangiosarcomas in the tarsal synovial sheath of a horse. J Am Vet Med Assoc 1972;161:49–52.

2 Muscle and tendon

John F. Van Vleet and Beth A. Valentine

Muscles

ACKNOWLEDGMENTS

Dr. Thomas J. Hulland (University of Guelph), author of this chapter in the 2nd, 3rd, and 4th editions, is fully acknowledged for his great contribution to the original text and illustrations. Dr. M. Donald McGavin (University of Tennessee) generously gave his time and energy to review this chapter and assist with photomicroscopy. We also appreciate the manuscript review and comments of Dr. Brad Hanna (University of Guelph).

Muscles

DEVELOPMENT AND STRUCTURE

Development

Development of striated muscle in the embryo is from *mesodermal somites,* which give rise to *myotomes*. Within each myotome, which corresponds roughly to a vertebral body segment, with its spinal nerve, the individual muscles develop by a process of aggregation and migration of presumptive myoblastic cells. It is very likely that the undifferentiated mesodermal cells will be committed to a muscle destiny some time before significant structural change is visible, and the earliest detectable modification to presumptive myoblasts is a cross-sectional rounding of the spindle-shaped cells. By this time as well, there may be subtle distinctions between those cells that will become myofibers and those that will become satellite cells.

The first clear sign of differentiation is the *migration of presumptive myoblasts*, destined to become myofibers, into the regions where future muscles will appear; this occurs before any nerve influence is exerted. The direct connection of the nerve to the myotome determines the subsequent route of innervation, but because migration has occurred, the muscle may receive nerve sprouts (as it has received myoblast group components) from more than one myotome.

The second phase of muscle development is incompletely separated from the first and subsequent phases. It begins with the *early development of sarcoplasmic components,* such as myofibrils, which identify the cells as muscle. The commitment to myogenesis is mutually exclusive with cell replication, and, with possible rare exceptions, committed myoblasts are post-mitotic. Myoblasts begin to fuse into elongated multinucleated cells about the time myogenesis begins.

Subsequent development of the myotube allows it to become a well-developed muscle fiber and consists of stepwise construction of *actin and myosin filaments*, the formation of the *Z band* into which the thin actin filaments insert, and the evolution of the *tubular systems*. The last of these steps, the invagination of the T tubular system from caveolae or other small, regular recesses on the outer sarcoplasmic membrane, provides an elaborate system of tubules that run parallel to the Z bands and make contact with all developing myofibrillar units.

The fourth phase of development is one in which the evolving fiber grows, increases the number of myofibrils and nuclei, and moves the latter to the subsarcolemmal position. During the final phase of development, the development of a basal lamina and an additional sheath of collagen, fibroblasts and capillaries invest each developing myotube as orientation of the fiber into its final position of tension takes place. Development of fibers up to this point, just after the end of the first trimester, is independent of any neural connection, but subsequent fiber enlargement and the considerable increase in the number of fibers that occurs during the immediate prenatal and postnatal periods, is dependent on a functional neural connection. The terminal differentiation of skeletal muscle is therefore largely determined by the characteristics of the neural connections although locally acting myogenic factors also contribute.

The genetic and molecular events in muscle development, and also in muscle regeneration, are rapidly becoming known. As might be expected, the organization and control of gene and protein expression during muscle cell specification and differentiation is complex. *Myogenic regulatory factors* (MRF) are centrally involved in transcription regulation in muscle and include MyoD, myogenin, Myf5, and MRF4. These muscle-specific proteins and a variety of growth factors influence gene and protein expression during the development of skeletal muscle.

The muscle fiber increase in late gestation in domestic animals is probably comparable in all species, but it has been particularly well studied in the pig and is more orderly in that species than in others. Within what will become a primary bundle of muscle fibers, *1–6 primary or template myofibers become the focal point of the proliferation* that, by early postnatal life, has produced one or more sublobular clusters of fibers within each primary bundle. It is not clear whether new fibers are produced next to the template fiber by a process of template fiber budding, or by incomplete or complete longitudinal division. Alternatively they may be derived from local myoblastic or satellite cells that begin development within the basal lamina of the primary fiber and then separate and develop their own completely investing basal lamina. What is clear is that they are produced in waves, with subsequent fibers pushing those formed earlier to the periphery of the sublobule. Template fibers are always histochemically type 1, but the newly formed fibers are type 2 until near the time of birth when a proportion of them (few or several depending on the muscle and the species) which lie closest to the template fiber will begin to modify to become type 1 fibers (Fig. 2.1A, B). The latter process may continue for 6 months or more after birth, and it may be that the process reverses again in early postnatal life in some muscles of the body.

During the period when templating is occurring, new fibers rapidly become innervated and, it seems, do not later change neural connections. In view of the described changes of fiber type, thought to be associated with exercise, it is difficult to reconcile other evidence that suggests that a single motor nerve axon can serve only one histochemical type of muscle fiber. The paradox may be resolved if it is accepted that some fibers have, or develop, different kinds of energy metabolism that they use selectively depending on work demands. Alternatively, a change in the activity of the nerve may induce biochemical changes in the muscle fiber clusters, and hence a change in fiber type identity. This explanation is consistent with the fact that the functional capacity of a muscle fiber is limited by its nerve connection and its cytoplasmic components and of these probably only the latter can be modified.

Gross anatomy

Muscle structure is arranged around *muscle fibers*. Muscle fibers are variable in size depending on age, exercise, nutritional status, position and function of the muscle in question, and on species, although the fibers of a mouse are only a little smaller than those of a horse. Muscle fibers in the extrinsic muscles of the eye are consistently small (10–30 μm in diameter) and round; those of the major limb muscles vary from an average least diameter of 40–65 μm and, although rounded in the fresh state, often appear polygonal when

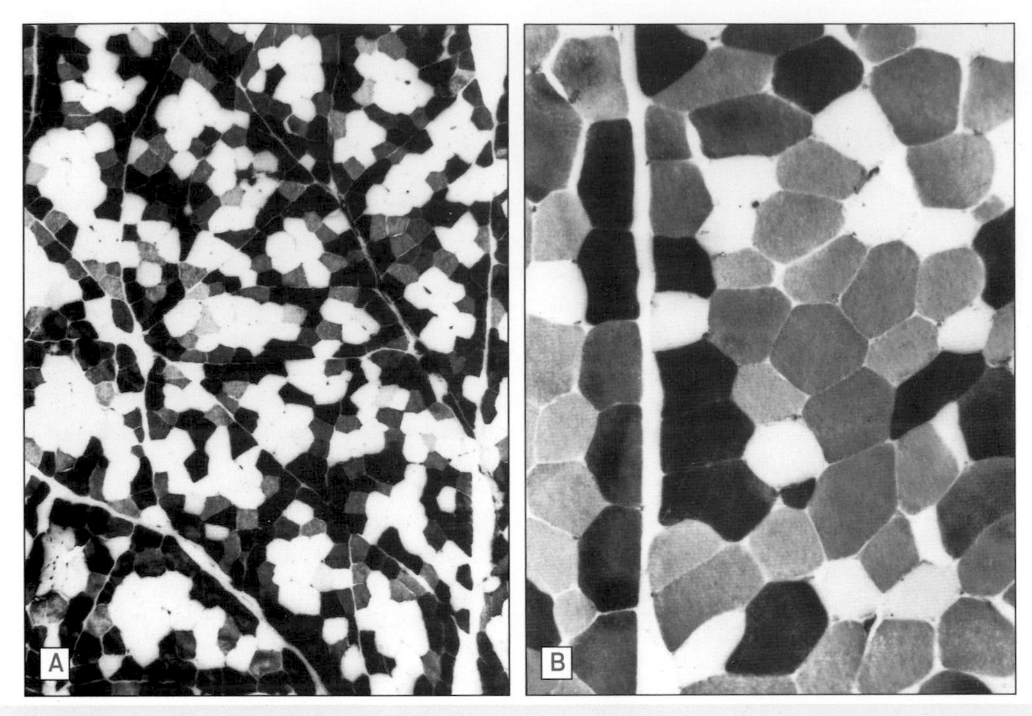

Figure 2.1 A. ATPase (alkaline) histochemical preparation of normal calf muscle to show light type 1 sublobular "**template clusters**." **B. Dark type 2 fibers** clustered along edges of primary bundles. (Courtesy of TJ Hulland.)

fixed. The size of fibers increases with age until puberty, at which time males have slightly larger fibers than females. In old age, with certainty, but perhaps beginning in early maturity, the fiber diameter slowly decreases. In those domestic animals that have been studied, the size distribution of muscle fibers conforms more or less to a biological distribution curve, although in most postural muscles the curve is skewed by a small population of large fibers extending upwards from the expected upper size limit. In most instances, these large fibers are from the type 1 fiber population, but in some muscles in some species they may be from the type 2 group. A distinctly bimodal curve readily develops in a muscle when disease, pregnancy, or nutritional status prompts withdrawal of muscle protein for general maintenance. This also increases the likelihood that large fibers will be round rather than polygonal in routine preparations.

Microscopic structure

The **structure of the muscle cell** or muscle fiber is quite well defined (Fig. 2.2). The outer component is a thin amorphous, but apparently quite tough, *basal lamina* consisting of three layers which, on most muscle cell surfaces, seems to be thrown into gentle folds. Atrophy of the fiber leads to much more obvious accordion-like folds of the basal lamina. *Within this basal lamina are two separate cell populations with very similar nuclei: the multinucleate myofiber, and the small, more numerous satellite cells,* which play an important role in fiber repair and regeneration (Fig. 2.3A, B). The nuclei of both cell types are oriented to the long axis of the muscle fiber and are distributed regularly in a spiral manner. In normal muscle, less than 3% of the nuclei of the multinucleate myofiber cell are displaced internally, but

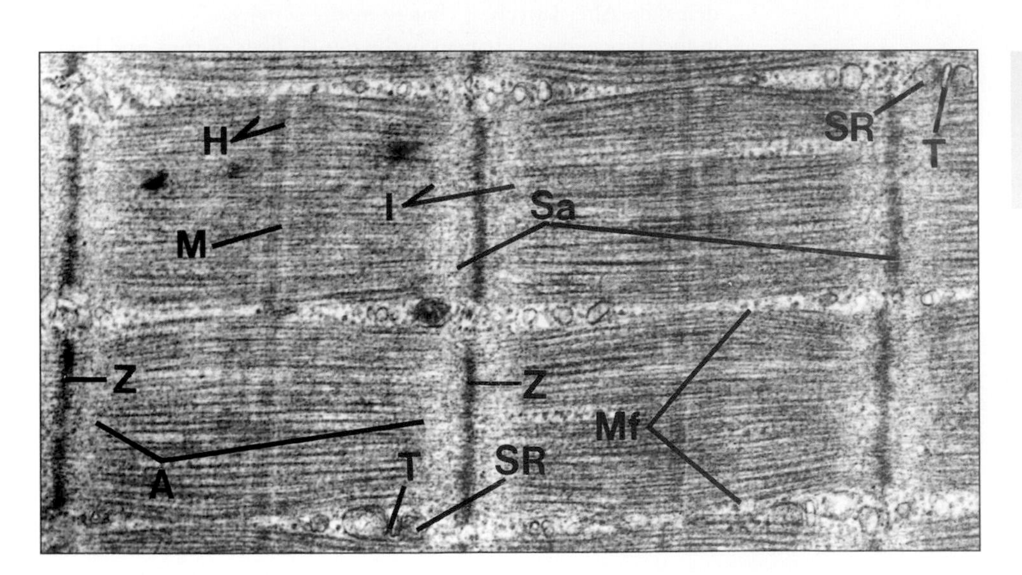

Figure 2.2 Normal horse muscle. Anisotropic band (A), H band (H), isotropic band (I), M line (M), myofibril (Mf), one sarcomere (Sa), sarcoplasmic reticulum (SR), T-tubule (T), Z band (Z). (Courtesy of TJ Hulland.)

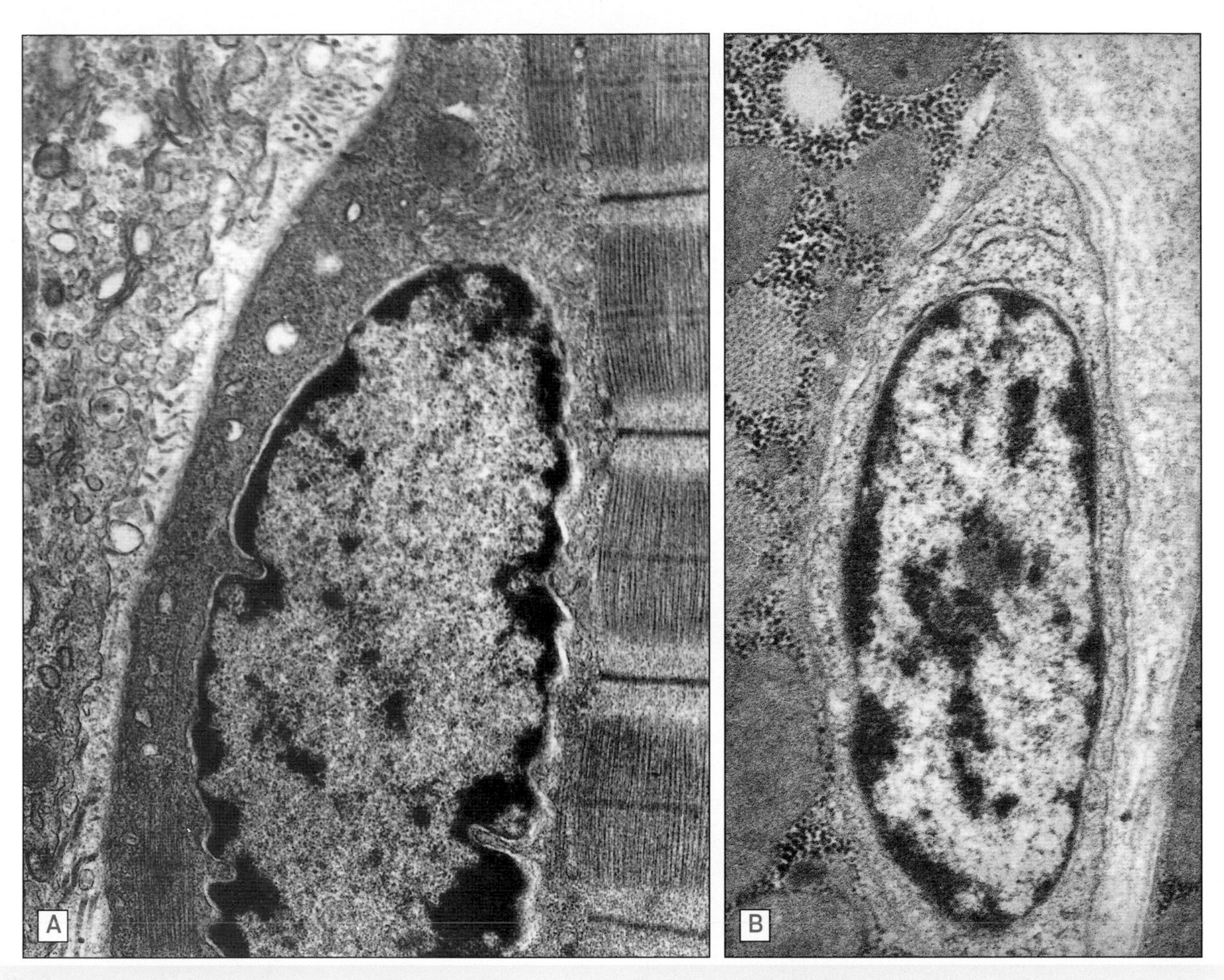

Figure 2.3 **A.** Myofiber nucleus and adjacent myofibril. **B.** Satellite cell nucleus. (Courtesy of TJ Hulland.)

the number tends to be higher adjacent to points where muscle and tendon interdigitate, or where muscle and bone meet through a short ligament or tendon. Nuclei are slender, oval, have evenly distributed chromatin and single, small nucleoli. The **satellite cells**, initially described by Mauro in 1961, consist of a simple cell membrane around a nucleus, a minimum of cytoplasm with mitochondria and a scant tubular system, all of which lie in a shallow indentation on the myofiber surface within the basal lamina. Satellite cells constitute 1–30% of the visible nuclei associated with a muscle fiber; the higher figure describes the neonatal state, the lower, old age. In mature muscle, 3–5% of the nuclei are satellite cells; a modest concentration of them occurs adjacent to motor end plates.

Satellite nuclei have been thought to be the only ones in muscle capable of mitotic division in postnatal life, and each time these cells divide in a growing muscle they contribute one myocytic nucleus and a minute amount of cytoplasm to the growing pool of nuclei in the enlarging multinucleate, myofiber cell. The other daughter cell remains as part of the satellite cell pool outside the myocyte and retains mitotic capability. It is clear that this mechanism will make the satellite cells a progressively smaller proportion of the total nuclear population within the basal lamina since their number remains constant from birth while the nonreplicating postmitotic myofiber nuclei increase in number cumulatively.

New concepts are emerging on the exclusive role of satellite cells in postnatal growth, repair and maintenance of skeletal muscle. Recent studies in mice have demonstrated that *hematopoietic stem cells from bone marrow may participate in regeneration of skeletal muscle.* However, the contribution of bone marrow-derived myogenic progenitor cells in the overall process of muscle cell regeneration, a process previously thought to exclusively involve satellite cells producing myogenic precursor cells, is still unclear. The potential may now exist for therapy by delivery of bone marrow-derived stem cells, via injection into the circulation, to damaged muscle cells to augment regeneration in diseases such as muscular dystrophy where the satellite cell population has become depleted and/or ineffective.

Ultrastructure

The most distinctive characteristic of skeletal muscle cells is the presence of **striated myofibrils**, approximately 0.5–1.0 μm in diameter, consisting, in cross-section, of thousands of regularly sized and regularly oriented **myofilaments** (Fig. 2.2). In longitudinal section, *contractile units or sarcomeres* about 20 μm long extend from one Z band to the next, and consist of bands and lines created by the stacking of thick and thin filaments with protein aggregates at certain places. The *thin filaments* (6 nm wide; actin, tropomyosin, and troponin) are fixed into the electron-dense *Z band* of noncontractile protein and incompletely overlap the *thick filaments* (16 nm wide; myosin). The zone of no overlap adjacent to the Z band is referred to as the *I band*. The central zone between the ends of the thin filaments in which only thick filaments are visible is the *H band*, and this is divided by a *thin dense line of M substance* on each filament, and collectively these create the *M line*. The *A band* is the wide central zone which extends from one end of the thick filaments to the other and alternates with the I band. *In sarcomere contraction, Z bands move closer together reducing I and H band widths.* In cross section at a central point where thick and thin filaments are present, one myosin filament is surrounded at regular intervals by six thin filaments, or 12 when the sarcomere is in strong contraction.

Myofibrils are surrounded by *sarcoplasm*, which makes up 30–40% of the fiber volume, and in it are elements of the T-tubular system, the sarcoplasmic reticulum, mitochondria, lysosomes, glycogen granules, and often, fat droplets. The endoplasmic tubular systems in the muscle fibers of all mammals regularly come together to surround myofibrils and meet in triads with the T tubule between two tubular segments of sarcoplasmic reticulum at frequent regular intervals. In many animals these triads can be found at each end of each sarcomere, an arrangement which ensures very extensive direct surface membrane contact between the cell surface, the sarcomeres and the endoplasmic reticulum. Sarcoplasm between the myofibrils and the outer cell membrane is often rich in mitochondria and glycogen granules.

Quite apart from their ability to shorten in active contraction, *myofibrils are capable of easy and rapid length adjustment accomplished by shedding or adding one or more sarcomeres.* Under ideal experimental circumstances, up to 25% of the sarcomeres may be lost in a 24-hour period, a statistic which emphasizes that, even in the healthy animal, there is potential for a considerable flux of muscle protein to allow for rapid dismantling and reconstruction of myofibrils. Muscle has a high requirement for arginine, glucogenic amino acids, and energy, reflected in part by the high turnover of glycogen in normal muscle. The breadth of myofibrils increases or decreases equally rapidly by building or discarding myofilaments. When new myofibrils are required, an existing large myofibril splits longitudinally, but when atrophy reduces the need for some myofibrils they are simply dismantled sarcomere by sarcomere or reduced in size by destruction of the most peripheral myofilaments.

Outside the muscle fibers and their satellite cells are *three magnitudes of connective tissue framework.* Intimately applied to the basement membrane of each muscle fiber is the net-like **endomysium**, which carries the capillary network with its longitudinal orientation. Around each primary bundle of 40–150 fibers is the thicker **perimysium** in which run larger vessels, nerve trunks, and sensory neuromuscular spindles. Around the outside of the muscle, or a major head of a muscle, lies the **epimysium,** which carries tendon organ sensory endings and sometimes prominent tendinous bands.

Histochemical fiber types

Types of muscle fibers may be distinguished by many histochemical and immunohistochemical techniques available for studying the enzyme components; each new technique demonstrates an ever-expanding heterogeneity of muscle fibers. Many of these techniques subdivide the muscle fiber population in the same ways, and in many instances the subdivisions seem to bear little relationship to the biological response created by disease. The two techniques that seem best to identify different biological activities are the *alkaline- and acid-resistant adenosine triphosphatase procedures* and the *nicotinic acid dehydrogenase tetrazolium reductase (NADH-TR) test* for oxidative enzyme activity. These allow the division of the muscle population into two major groups and several subgroups (Fig. 2.1A, B):

- **type 1 fibers** rich in oxidative enzymes and showing slow-twitch, red color characteristics (myoglobin); generally assumed to be fibers with a predominantly oxidative energy source appropriate for sustained activity;
- **type 2 fibers** rich in glycogen showing a fast-twitch response and paler color; generally assumed to be fibers with a predominantly glycolytic energy source appropriate for short-term, strong activity.

Both types of fiber contain a broad spectrum of enzymes, which makes them capable of a wide range of biochemical activity and, in certain circumstances, an interconversion of working types.

Some species, particularly the pig and the horse, have fibers apparently rich in both oxidative and glycolytic ingredients, and *many domestic animals have fibers that lack the clear-cut divisions that seem evident in the muscles of man and laboratory animals.* The type 2 fibers can be histochemically subdivided by ATPase response into subtypes but, for purposes of predicting biological activity and identifying diseases, the two main types seem to have the greatest relevance. A special subgroup of the glycolytic, type 2 group found in the masticatory muscles of the dog represent an exception to this because they display antigenic differences from other muscles and this makes them vulnerable to a unique disease process. Examination of a muscle in which about equal numbers of type 1 and type 2 fibers are present might suggest a random checkerboard distribution of the types; however, *type 2 fibers are disproportionately found on the periphery of primary bundles, and type 1 fibers are disproportionately at the center of nests of fibers within the primary bundle* (Fig. 2.1A, B). These observations are consistent with knowledge of the late fetal fiber evolution.

Muscles used repetitively but slowly and persistently should have high levels of type 1 fibers while those used for short bursts of activity should have high levels of type 2 fibers. This is often the case; for example the diaphragm of cattle often has 80–95% of type 1 fibers while most other skeletal muscles have 10–60% type 1 fibers. On the other end of the scale, the longissimus and semitendinosus muscles, the two muscles which are most enlarged in racing Greyhounds and Thoroughbred horses, have ~80–95% type 2 fiber content. Obligatory postural muscles, such as the supraspinatus, tend to have a 40–50% type 1 component, but so do muscles which are used relatively sparingly. Individual variation in fiber proportions is quite wide, and this is magnified by breed, muscle region, and species differences. The anatomic position and the function of a muscle in an animal can provide only a general indication of its fiber composition. In the horse, the proportion of type 1 fibers increases in deeper levels of large muscle masses, and the very deep postural muscles of the limbs, such as the medial head of the triceps and the vastus intermedius, are almost entirely type 1 fibers.

Specialized structures

Sensory muscle spindles *are found in all skeletal muscles in and anchored to the perimysial connective tissue and associated with a small nerve radicle, which contains 6–20 large sensory fibers.* They are more numerous in some muscles than others and are generally difficult to find in the larger muscles of mature animals. Spindles are about 0.5–3.0 mm long and 200–500 μm wide (Fig. 2.4). The intrafusal (central) space

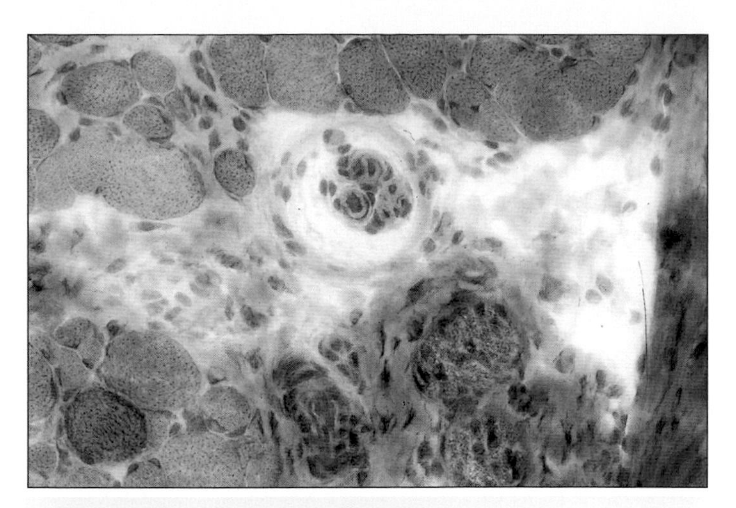

Figure 2.4 Sensory muscle spindle in cross-sectioned normal muscle. Frozen section, modified Gomori's trichrome.

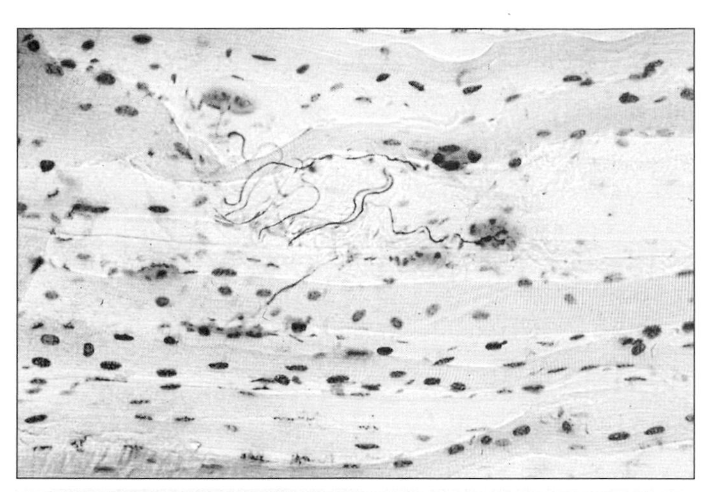

Figure 2.5 Motor end-plate in longitudinal section of canine muscle. Silver stain. (Courtesy of BJ Cooper.)

enclosed within the fibrous, multilayered outer sheath is continuous with lymphatic space and contains 2–20 specialized *small intrafusal muscle fibers*. The intrafusal fibers are histochemically different from the extrafusal fibers but share the same motor nerve. However, intrafusal fibers are innervated by a different, smaller group of motor neurons than those innervating extrafusal fibers. The intrafusal fibers have a high content of nuclei often contained in a central "nuclear bag" region, or linearly distributed up the middle of the small round fibers. Abundant sensory axons entering the spindle have "flower-spray," "grape-cluster," or spiral endings on the intrafusal fibers, and these structures collectively give rise to impulses, which record muscle stretch and contribute to proprioception. *Complex spindles* consisting of 2–10 spindles, incompletely overlapping end on end, are sometimes found in skeletal muscles and may be an expression of anomalous development. Intrafusal fibers generally do not participate in the pathologic processes, which involve extrafusal fibers, with the possible exception of nutritional myopathy. Intrafusal fibers are also resistant to atrophy.

Motor end-plates *are the sites of synaptic transmission of acetylcholine from nerve ends to muscle receptors at which sites a surface-membrane-conducted, polarizing impulse is initiated.* The interface takes the form of a complex, pretzel-shaped neural termination, which is pressed into a shallow but convoluted, cholinesterase-laden, synaptic gutter of matching shape on the myofiber surface. The end plate is contained within the endomysium, and extensions of the endomysial connective tissue ensheath the bare terminal axon for a short distance until its myelin sheath is reached (Fig. 2.5). A little more than one end-plate for each muscle fiber exists in skeletal muscle, and although supernumerary endings (subterminal sprouts) can develop, such structures are rarely found in normal muscle. One motor neuron gives rise to an extremely variable number of terminal axons with one end-plate each, the number being inversely proportional to the fineness of motor movement required of the muscle, and directly proportional to the relative diameter of the muscle fibers. Thus, in the extrinsic ocular muscle the axon:end-plate ratio may be as low as 1:10 on small round muscle fibers, whereas in the gastrocnemius or gluteus muscles the ratio may be 1:2000 on muscle fibers near the upper size limits. Terminal axons are given off at nodes of Ranvier in clusters of 5–30 per node to make muscle end-plate contact locally via a short, fine terminal axon. Although a low neural impulse level to skeletal muscle is translated into contraction of only a proportion of the muscle fibers, this is clearly not a form of muscle regulation that can lead to finely controlled movement and consequently fine movement must be controlled by a low neural ratio.

Bibliography

Armstrong RB. Distribution of fiber types in locomotory muscles of dogs. Am J Anat 1982;163:87–98.

Baker JH, Hall-Craggs ECB. Changes in length of sarcomeres following tenotomy of the rat soleus muscle. Anat Rec 1978;192:55–58.

Blot S. Myopathies in domestic carnivores. Part 1. The skeletal striated muscle: structure, function, and symptomatology. Eur J Compan An Pract 1996;6:42–55.

Brown SC, et al. The molecular and cellular biology of muscle. In: Karpati G, Hilton-Jones D, Griggs RC, eds. Disorders of Voluntary Muscle. 7th ed. New York: Cambridge University Press, 2001:42–59.

Campion DR. The muscle satellite cell: a review. Int Rev Cytol 1984;87:225–251.

Cardinet GH, III. Skeletal muscle function. In: Kaneko JJ, Harvey JW, Bruss ML, eds. Clinical Biochemistry of Domestic Animals. 5th ed. San Diego, CA: Academic Press, 1997:407–440.

Ferrari G, et al. Muscle regeneration by bone marrow-derived myogenic progenitors. Science 1998;279:1528–1530.

Franzini-Armstrong C, Fischman DA. Morphogenesis of skeletal muscle fibers. In: Engel AG, Franzini-Armstrong C., eds. Myology, Basic and Clinical. 2nd ed. New York: McGraw-Hill, 1994:74–96.

Gauthier GF. The muscular tissue. In: Weiss L, ed. Histology: Cell and Tissue Biology. 5th ed. New York: Elsevier Biomedical, 1983:256–281.

Hadlow WJ. Diseases of skeletal muscle. In: Innes JRM, Saunders LS, eds. Comparative Neuropathology. New York: Academic Press, 1962:147–243.

Horwitz AF, et al. The plasma membrane of the muscle fiber: composition and structure. In: Engel AG, Franzini-Armstrong C., eds. Myology, Basic and Clinical. 2nd ed. New York: McGraw-Hill, 1994:200–222.

Kelly AM, Rubinstein NA. Development of neuromuscular specialization. Med Sci Sport Exerc 1986;18:292–298.

Mauro A. Satellite cell of skeletal muscle fibers. J Biophy Biochem Cytol 1961; 9:493–495.

Miller JB. Developmental biology of skeletal muscle. In: Karpati G, Hilton-Jones D, Griggs RC, eds. Disorders of Voluntary Muscle. 7th ed. New York: Cambridge University Press, 2001:26–41.

Sabourin LA, Rudnicki MA. The molecular regulation of myogenesis. Clin Genet 2000;57:16–25.
Schmalbruch H. Skeletal Muscle. New York: Springer-Verlag, 1985.
Schultz E, McCormick KM. Skeletal muscle satellite cells. Rev Physiol Biochem Pharmacol 1994;123:213–257.
Seale P, Rudnicki MA. A new look at the origin, function, and "stem cell" status of muscle satellite cells. Dev Biol 2000;218:115–124.
Valberg SJ. Muscular causes of exercise intolerance in horses. Vet Clin N Am: Eq Pract 1996;12:495–515.

DISTURBANCES OF GROWTH AND POSTMORTEM ALTERATIONS

As with many tissues, muscle has a fairly limited repertoire of changes. Many of the same histopathologic features are seen in different muscle disorders. Determination of possible causes for muscle changes often requires careful evaluation of the signalment, clinical history, and clinicopathologic findings as well as gross and histopathologic findings. *Muscle atrophy, hypertrophy*, and *postmortem changes* are commonly encountered in pathologic specimens and are the focus of this section. Degenerative and regenerative reactions are discussed in the next section.

Atrophy

Muscle atrophy *can refer to reduction in overall muscle mass.* Reduction in mass most often reflects *decreased myofiber diameter* that can involve all fibers uniformly or that can selectively involve muscle fiber types. Histochemical evaluation of fiber types is often necessary to clearly distinguish the type of atrophy present. In many circumstances, type 2 glycolytic fibers are more sensitive to atrophy than are type 1 oxidative fibers. Morphometric analysis of overall fiber diameter may be necessary to confirm a decrease in muscle mass due to mild overall reduction of myofiber diameter.

All fibers undergoing a reduction in size *lose myofilaments and myofibrils* by a process of more or less simultaneous disaggregation of actin and myosin filaments and disintegration of the protein of Z bands. Briefly, in the sequence, a slight sarcoplasmic space appears between the shrinking myofibrillar mass and the plasma membrane, but the membrane (and the basal lamina) soon begins to wrinkle and condense to accommodate the new slimmer lines. After a brief lag, mitochondria, glycogen granules, and lysosomes are reduced in number and size. After a slightly longer lag phase, the tubular systems are reduced in volume. Removal of cytoskeletal proteins, organelles, and glycogen is by autophagy. Atrophy does not involve sarcolemmal damage and therefore is not associated with increased serum activity of CK or AST. Provided that the time interval is relatively short, the influences inducing atrophy are removed, and the muscle environment is returned to normal, *the sequence can be reversed* and fibers can be restored to normal size.

Denervation atrophy

Myofibers that have lost connection with peripheral nerves due to neuropathy or neuronopathy undergo rapid and severe atrophy due to denervation. This form of atrophy has also been referred to in the somewhat contradictory terms "neurogenic atrophy." Denervation atrophy is characterized histologically by *severe fiber atrophy involving type 1 and type 2 fibers*. Mild denervation will result in scattered single or small contiguous groups (*small group atrophy*) of severely atrophied fibers compressed into angular shapes (*angular atrophy*) by adjacent innervated fibers (Fig. 2.6). More extensive denervation will result in large groups of small rounded fibers (*large group atrophy*), as there are no innervated fibers in the area to cause angular change in the denervated fibers (Fig. 2.7). Even in the absence of histochemical preparations, muscle containing extensive small and large group atrophy is most likely to be denervated, and a careful examination of intramuscular nerves (Fig. 2.8), peripheral nerve trunks, ventral nerve roots, and motor neurons is indicated. In addition to those features of atrophy described above, the rapid and severe atrophy due to denervation often results in clustering of myonuclei (nuclear clumping).

Denervation atrophy is relatively common in animals. It is part of many congenital dysplasias involving skeletal muscle that cause contracture or arthrogryposis. Denervation atrophy is always accompanied by muscle weakness or paralysis, but the clinical signs may be mild if the nerve is small or the damage is mild. Some of the best-known examples of denervation atrophy in animals are *laryngeal hemiplegia in horses* caused by axonal degeneration of the left recurrent laryngeal nerve, injury to the supraspinatus nerve by trauma or the pressure of a poorly fitting collar in a work horse ("*sweeney*"), symmetrical (such as due to equine motor neuron disease), or

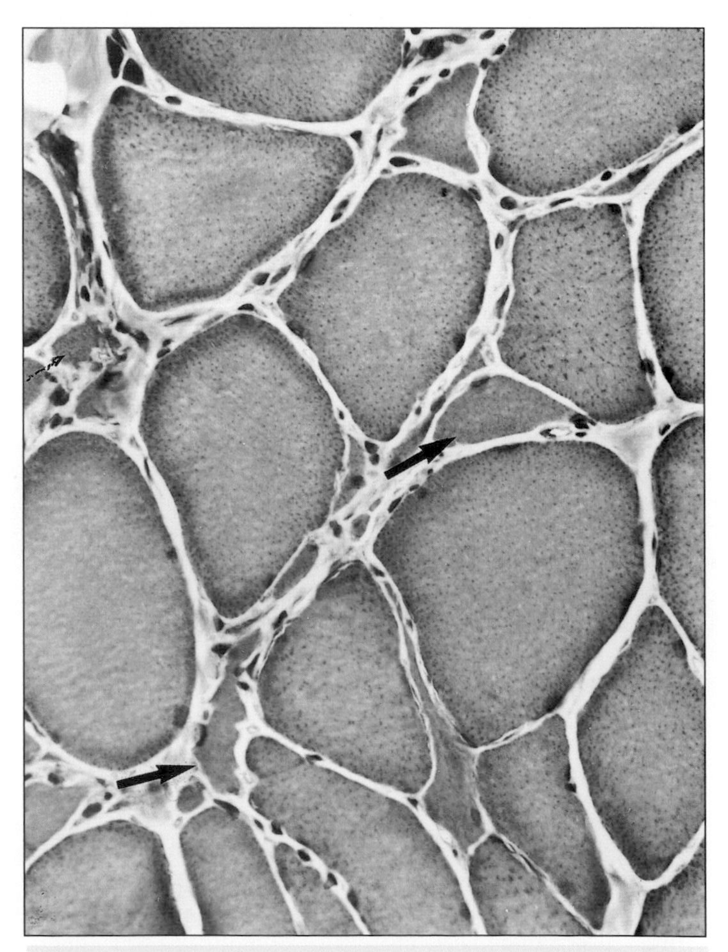

Figure 2.6 Severe angular atrophy (arrows) of small continguous groups of fibers (small group atrophy) due to denervation in a dog. (Courtesy of TJ Hulland.)

asymmetrical (the hallmark of equine protozoal myeloencephalitis) *gluteal atrophy in the horse*, and *radial or brachial paralysis in dogs and horses* due to trauma. Lesions involving the ventral gray matter of the spinal cord or the ventral roots emerging from the spinal canal, and inherited or acquired peripheral neuropathies, are also common causes of denervation atrophy.

Denervation atrophy is rapid and severe. It is accompanied by abnormal spontaneous activity (fibrillations, positive sharp waves, and sometimes myotonic bursts) detectable with concentric needle electromyography. *Within 2–3 weeks, two-thirds of the muscle mass can be lost.* This reduction in mass may be readily observed or may require careful palpation of muscle mass for detection. Given the variable muscling of different breeds of dogs and horses, a diagnosis of symmetric muscle atrophy can be difficult.

As stated above, *the hallmark of denervation atrophy is involvement of both type 1 and type 2 fibers.* Type 2 fibers can, however, be preferentially atrophied, especially early on in the denervation process. The denervation of equine motor neuron disease is somewhat unique, in that there is preferential atrophy of type 1 fibers, presumably due to oxidative injury to type 1 motor neurons due to vitamin E deficiency (Fig. 2.9). The fiber type of the muscle is determined by the electrical activity of the nerve fiber supplying that motor unit. If a denervated motor unit is reinnervated by terminal nerve sprouts from an adjacent intact nerve, the fiber type will be converted to that of the newly innervating nerve, and the reinnervated myofibers will rapidly regain normal diameter. Thus, alteration of the normal mosaic distribution of fiber types to one of clusters of type 1 and type 2 fibers (*fiber type grouping*), which can only be demonstrated on histochemical preparations, is characteristic of denervation followed by reinnervation (Fig. 2.10). If there is subsequent degeneration of the reinnervating nerve this will result in denervation atrophy of a group of fibers all of the same fiber type (*type-specific group atrophy*). This finding is indicative of on ongoing denervating process. Although such disorders occur, it is curious that type-specific group atrophy is rarely seen in animals.

Severe and chronic denervation will be accompanied by a variable degree of endomysial fibrosis. Admixed innervated fibers often undergo

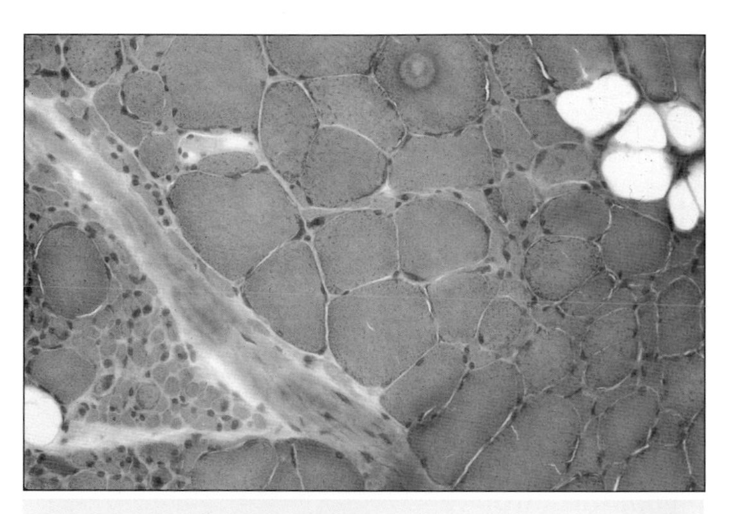

Figure 2.7 Small and large group atrophy in the vastus intermedius muscle of a horse with denervation due to equine motor neuron disease. Denervated fibers are admixed with moderately hypertrophied fibers. Frozen section, modified Gomori's trichrome. (From McGavin MD, Zachary JF. Pathologic Basis of Veterinary Disease, 2006, with permission of Elsevier Ltd.)

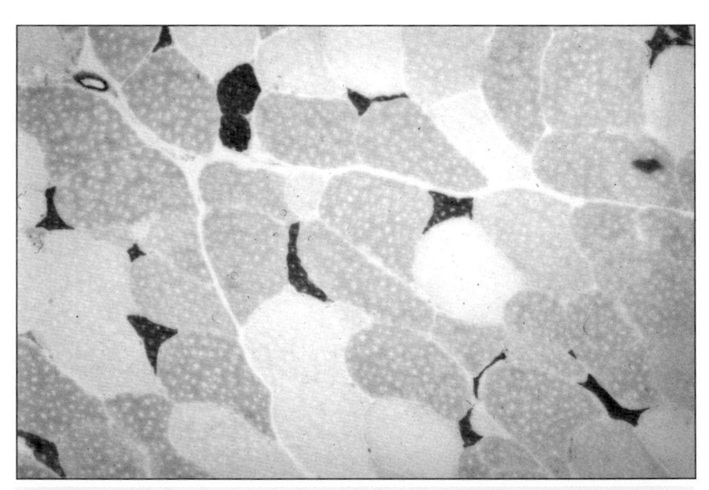

Figure 2.9 Selective angular atrophy of type 1 (dark staining) fibers in a horse with equine motor neuron disease. Frozen section, ATPase, acid preincubation.

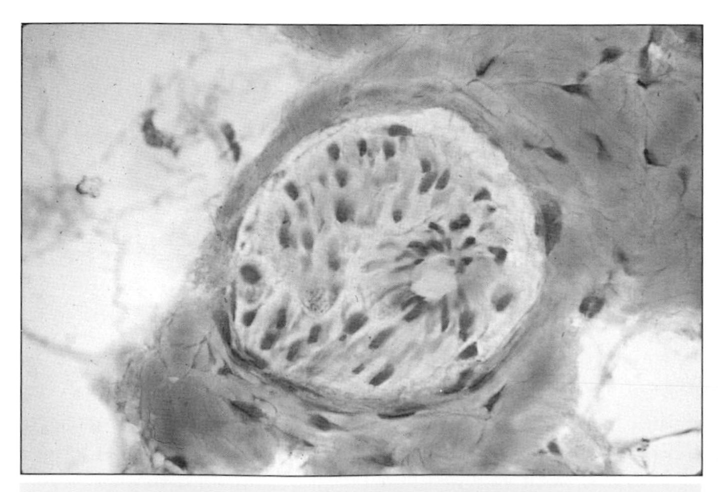

Figure 2.8 Intramuscular nerve from a horse with equine motor neuron disease. There is marked **loss of myelinated fibers** (only 1 remains), with endoneurial fibrosis. Frozen section, modified Gomori's trichrome.

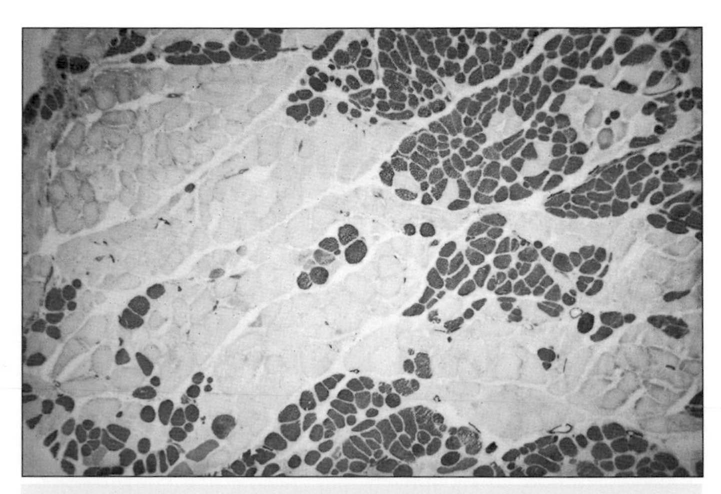

Figure 2.10 Fiber type grouping of type 1 (dark staining) and type 2 (light staining) fibers due to denervation and reinnervation in the laryngeal muscle of a horse. Frozen section, ATPase, acid preincubation.

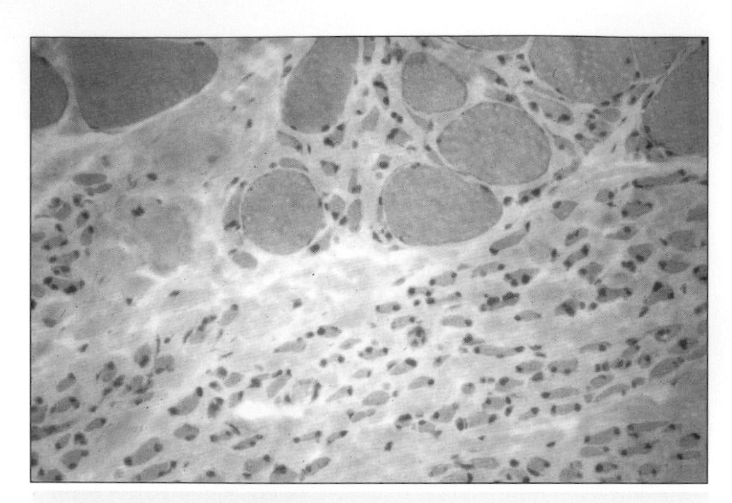

Figure 2.11 Severe large group atrophy with marked endomysial fibrosis due to chronic denervation in the medial head of the triceps of a horse with chronic equine motor neuron disease. There is severe compensatory hypertrophy of other fibers. Frozen section, modified Gomori's trichrome.

compensatory hypertrophy (see below; Figs 2.7, 2.11). Although both type 1 and type 2 fibers will undergo hypertrophy, type 1 muscle fibers appear to be somewhat resistant to denervation atrophy in many circumstances, and may be the predominant hypertrophied fiber type seen. Even without histochemical preparations to determine fiber types, *a pattern of large-diameter fibers admixed with severely atrophied fibers is very characteristic of severe and chronic denervation*. In very severe cases, there can be eventual loss of denervated myofibers, with replacement of muscle by fibrous connective tissue and often also by fat. Determining the cause of the severe atrophy in such "end-stage muscles" can be very difficult, as both severe chronic neuropathic processes and severe chronic myopathic processes are possible.

Disuse atrophy

Disuse atrophy *occurs due to decreased contractile activity of innervated muscle*. Decreased muscular activity due to painful lameness, bone fracture or disease, or limb immobilization are most common. Disuse atrophy in humans and experimental animals *classically involves predominantly type 2 fibers*, although this pattern is not seen in all muscles in people with disuse atrophy. Although a type 2 predominant atrophy is seen in some cases of disuse atrophy in domestic animals, in many cases there is overall atrophy of all fiber types with no clear preferential pattern. As no workload is imposed on muscle fibers undergoing disuse atrophy, there will be no compensatory hypertrophy of fibers.

Atrophy of cachexia

Atrophy of cachexia and malnutrition *occurs when an animal is unable to supply enough dietary nutrients to maintain muscle; muscle proteins become the source of nutrients for the rest of the body*. One to five per cent of the contractile muscle substance is dismantled each day, and in normal animals an equal or greater amount is reconstructed. In view of the large bulk of the body muscle, this represents a very large amount of protein that can be borrowed on a daily basis. Net loss of muscle protein probably starts hours after negative nitrogen balance has been reached. The muscle atrophy of cachexia associated with chronic illness and neoplasia is hastened by circulating cytokines such as *tumor necrosis factor* ("*cachectin*"), which act systemically to increase catabolism, including catabolism of myofibers. The atrophy of cachexia is gradual, and the process may take years if the net withdrawal of muscle protein is subject to fluctuations, or is irregular or slight.

In the dog, *atrophy of temporal muscles* is often prominent and can occur fairly rapidly in animals ill for any reason. The *back and thigh muscles* are also susceptible to severe atrophy due to cachexia. Histochemically, *type 2 fibers are depleted preferentially in cachexia* (Fig. 2.12A, B). Similar to the case in denervation atrophy and some cases of disuse atrophy, type 1 muscle fibers are resistant to atrophy due to cachexia. In most cases, the degree of atrophy achieved through cachexia is not as severe as that seen in denervation atrophy, and the history will provide clinical features and a time frame for the atrophy that should enable differentiation of cachexia from disuse and denervation atrophy.

Atrophy of endocrine disease

Neuromuscular weakness and muscle atrophy can accompany hypothyroidism and hypoadrenocorticism in the dog. In both disorders, *selective atrophy of type 2 fibers* is seen (Fig. 2.13). No compensatory type 1 hypertrophy occurs. The finding of contiguous groups of mildly angular atrophied fibers can suggest denervation atrophy, and histochemical preparations to reveal the selective type 2 involvement may be necessary. In general, the atrophy of type 2 fibers in endocrine myopathy is not as severe as the atrophy of denervation. *Selective type 2 fiber atrophy due to endocrine disease must be differentiated from that of cachexia or disuse*.

Myopathic atrophy

Atrophy of fibers commonly occurs in myopathic conditions, and contributes to the nonspecific myopathic change of increased fiber size variation. Selective type 1 fiber atrophy is seen in many congenital myopathies in humans, and also occurs in cats with nemaline myopathy (Fig. 2.14). In such cases, *the use of histochemical procedures is essential to distinguish the selective type 1 atrophy that is suggestive of primary myopathy*. Other myopathies result in mild rounded atrophy of both fiber types, usually occurring randomly throughout the sections. Chronic myopathic change often involves hypertrophy (see below) as well as atrophy. Hypertrophied fibers are prone to fiber splitting, and some of the rounded small-diameter fibers interpreted as atrophic in chronic myopathic conditions may represent fiber splitting.

Hypertrophy

As with atrophy, **hypertrophy** *can refer to the muscle as a whole or to increased diameter of myofibers*. Overall muscular hypertrophy occurs in cattle as an inherited defect in myostatin, resulting in an increased number of otherwise relatively normal-diameter fibers ("*double muscling*"). Overall muscular hypertrophy occurs due to physiologic increase in myofiber diameter due to *exercise conditioning*. The muscles of animals with myotonic myopathy often appear enlarged, which may be due to prolonged muscle contraction as well as to myofiber

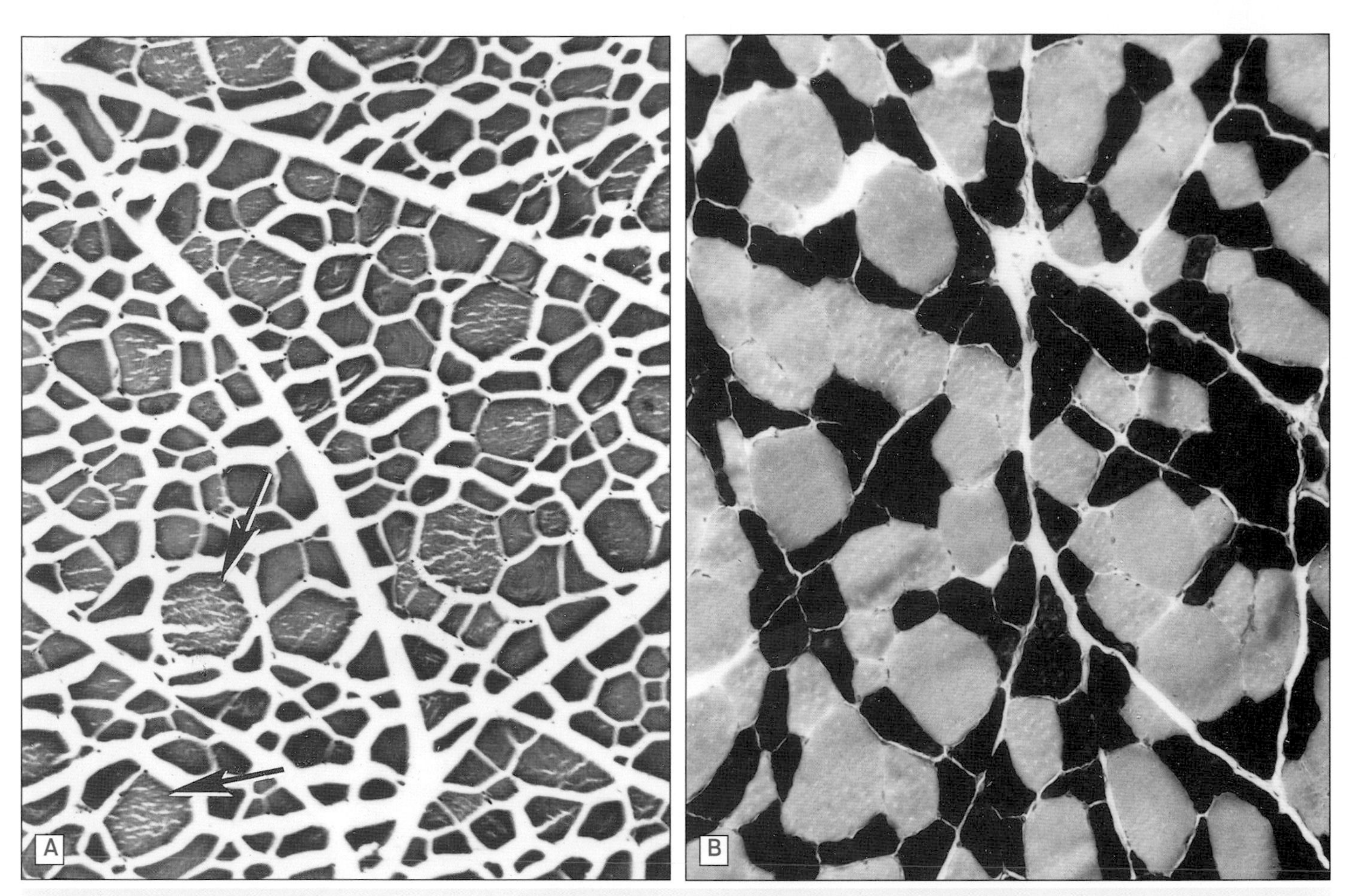

Figure 2.12 Atrophy of cachexia. **A.** Atrophy-resistant type 1 fibers are prominent (arrows) in formalin-fixed muscle from a calf; H&E stain. **B.** Preferential atrophy of type 2 (dark-staining) fibers in an emaciated sheep; frozen section, ATPase, alkaline preincubation. (Courtesy of TJ Hulland.)

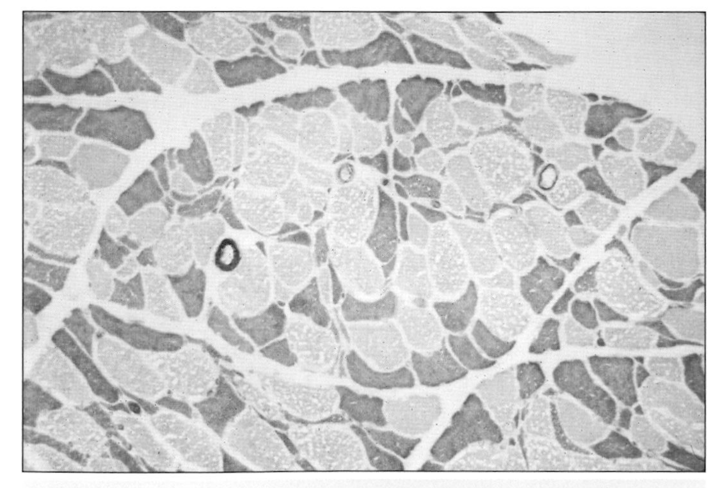

Figure 2.13 Preferential atrophy of type 2 (dark staining) fibers in a dog with **hypothyroid myopathy**. Frozen section, ATPase, alkaline preincubation.

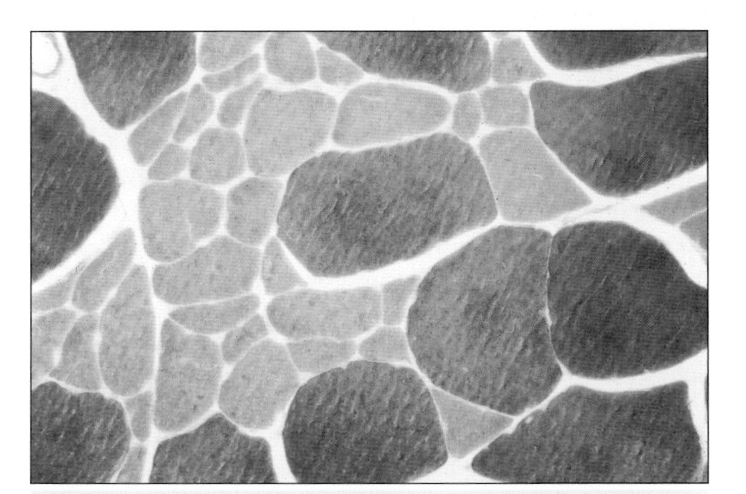

Figure 2.14 Selective atrophy of type 1 (light staining) fibers in a cat with congenital **nemaline myopathy**. Frozen section, ATPase, alkaline preincubation.

hypertrophy. Muscular hypertrophy is a characteristic feature of Duchenne-type X-linked muscular dystrophy in the cat, and occurs to a lesser degree in dystrophic dogs. Individual myofiber hypertrophy is often seen histologically in myopathic and neuropathic conditions in which there is overall reduction in muscle mass due to concurrent myofiber atrophy or loss. Lastly, muscle may appear enlarged due to pseudohypertrophy, as in chronically damaged muscles replaced by masses of fibrous tissue and/or fat, or due to fascial thickening in cats with fibrodysplasia ossificans progressiva.

Physiologic hypertrophy

Myofiber hypertrophy is considered physiologic when it occurs due to increased workload. This is a desirable process in athletes, and is accomplished through exercise conditioning. This process of physiologic hypertrophy of fibers is *accomplished by adding sarcomeres, by adding myofilaments to the periphery of myofibrils, and by adding new myofibrils to the existing ones by a process of longitudinal splitting*. There are sharp upper limits for this type of hypertrophy, and for animals it lies somewhere between 80 and 100 μm in diameter.

Compensatory hypertrophy

Compensatory myofiber hypertrophy occurs in muscle in which some myofibers are weak or dysfunctional due to myopathic or neuropathic disorders. In a sense, *this is a type of workload-increased hypertrophy* imposed on fibers less severely affected or unaffected by the myopathic or neuropathic condition. In such cases, fibers of 150–200 μm diameter can develop. Hypertrophied fibers in myopathic and neuropathic conditions are often abnormal, and may contain one or more internal nuclei, may undergo longitudinal splitting, or can develop bizarre cytoarchitectural disarray such as the formation of ring fibers and whorled fibers (Fig. 2.15). Longitudinal splitting allows one or more capillaries to be located near the center of the muscle fiber (Figs 2.16A, B, 2.17). When division is more or less complete, two or often more fibers become arranged in an "orange section" array (Fig. 2.16B) and appear as a cluster of the same fiber type that should not be mistaken for fiber type grouping.

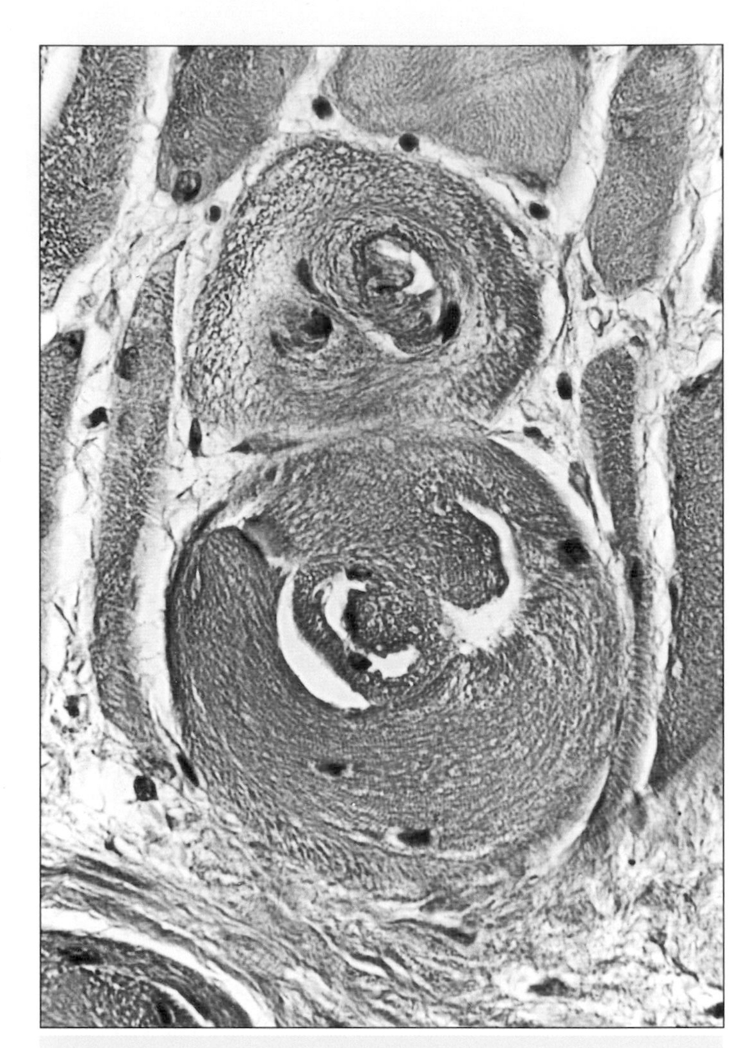

Figure 2.15 Bizarre cytoarchitectural alterations (clefting, whorling and internal nuclei) of **hypertrophied fibers in a denervated muscle**. (Courtesy of TJ Hulland.)

Postmortem changes

It is an unfortunate fact that veterinary pathologists are often involved in the postmortem examination of animals that have not recently expired. *Postmortem changes in muscle are common but variable*, making interpretation of the gross appearance of muscle difficult. In a well-fed animal that dies suddenly, the muscles can become very pale. Pallor may be caused by the accumulation of lactic acid in ischemic muscle. In other animals, particularly those whose glycogen stores have been depleted by chronic disease or malnutrition, the muscles become unusually dark after death. A wide range of differences in color and consistency of muscle normally exists among various species. Pallor of muscles also is present in animals that are anemic from copper or iron deficiency or blood loss, and is often normal in neonatal animals. Dark-red staining of muscle can be indicative of antemortem rhabdomyolysis, or can occur during putrefaction. Given the difficulty in interpretation of gross changes, it behooves the pathologist to take multiple muscle samples for histologic evaluation.

Rigor mortis *is contracture of the skeletal muscle that develops after death*. Rigor mortis is characterized by stiffening of the muscles and immobilization of the joints. It proceeds in orderly fashion from the muscles of the jaw to those of the trunk and then to those of the extremities, and it passes off in the same order. The time of onset, in average circumstances, is 2–4 h after death; maximum rigor is achieved in 24–48 h, after which it disappears. The intensity of rigor varies considerably as does the time of onset. *The factors influencing the time of onset and degree of rigor are the glycogen reserves, the pH of the muscles at the time of death, and the environmental temperature*. Rigor is slight or absent in cachectic or chronically debilitated animals. Rigor occurs with extraordinary rapidity in animals that die during or shortly after intense muscular activity, when muscle pH and glycogen stores are low. Onset of rigor can be delayed in well-rested, well-fed animals. It is hastened in onset and disappearance in a warm environment, and retarded in a cold environment. The chemical events in rigor are a modification of those occurring in normal contraction. Immediately after death, glycogen is converted to lactic acid by anaerobic glycolysis and creatine phosphate is broken down to produce creatine. These are both mechanisms for the resynthesis of adenosine triphosphate from adenosine diphosphate. Rigor will occur when the rate of adenosine triphosphate degradation exceeds its rate of synthesis. Muscle does not require energy to contract, but contraction is dependent on the presence of free calcium ions. Sequestration of calcium requires energy and is necessary for muscle relaxation. *Rigor develops because muscles deprived of energy are unable to maintain calcium in sequestered stores*. The eventual disappearance of rigor, and its failure to develop in cachectic animals, may be due to complete exhaustion of the chemical systems that produce energy and/or myofibrillar protein loss or breakdown.

Skeletal muscle is also prone to various *artifactual changes* that interfere with accurate histologic evaluation. Muscle collected from freshly dead animals, especially horses, is often still capable of vigorous

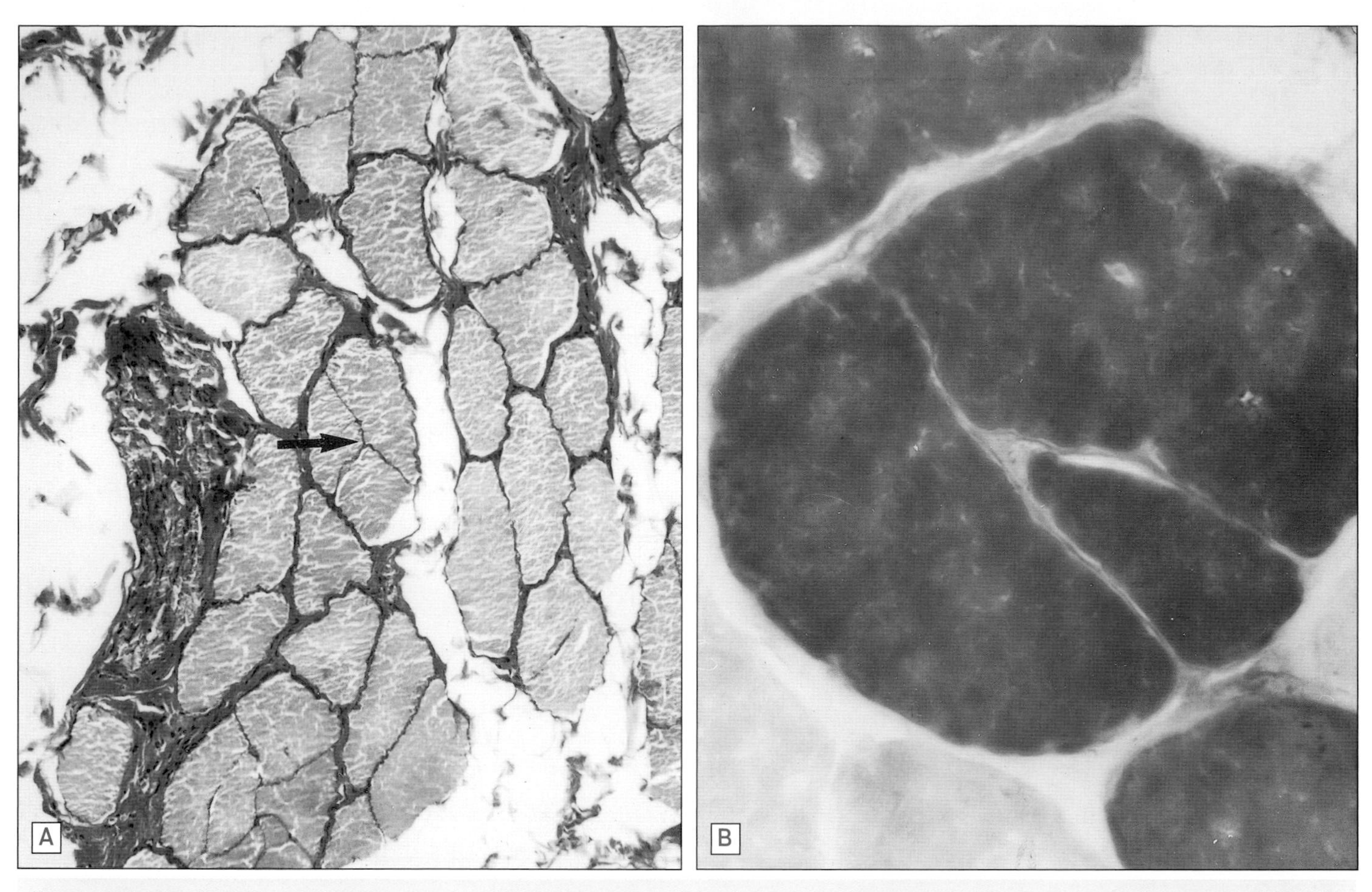

Figure 2.16 Fiber splitting. A. Fiber hypertrophy with fiber subdivisions (arrow). **B.** Hypertrophied fiber with early subdivision ("orange section" array). (Courtesy of TJ Hulland.)

contraction when myofiber ends are cut, allowing calcium-rich extracellular fluid to enter the myofiber and trigger the contractile apparatus. Exposure to formalin can also trigger contraction in fresh muscle samples. Various procedures have been advocated for elimination of the resultant contraction band artifact in muscle. It has been suggested that delayed sampling, following "curing" of the carcass, will result in better histologic preparations. Although the myofilamentous elements of myofibers are somewhat resistant to autolysis, and overall architecture of muscle will be better preserved postmortem than that of nervous tissue or gastrointestinal mucosa, this type of processing must still be considered less than ideal. Rapid postmortem loss of glycogen will often result in inability to diagnose a glycogen storage myopathy, and postmortem alterations in mitochondria and other organelles will interfere with ultrastructural evaluation. Histochemical procedures are also affected by postmortem autolysis, with resultant loss of fiber typing ability.

An extremely valuable procedure for collection of fresh muscle samples at necropsy, but also by biopsy, is *collection of muscle strips in a specially designed muscle clamp*. Samples are clamped in situ, following careful undermining of a strip of longitudinally arranged muscle fibers. The clamp ensures that the calcium influx occurring when fibers are cut transversely does not result in fiber contraction. It is recognized, however, that not all veterinary pathologists will have access to these muscle clamps. Utilization of a similar sampling technique, i.e., the isolation of a longitudinal strip of muscle approximately 2–3 cm long and 1 cm diameter and undermining the strip prior to cutting transversely across myofibers, will minimize artifact during sampling if followed by *pinning the strip to a rigid surface such as a piece of wooden tongue depressor*. This procedure will mimic the action of a muscle clamp and will provide good pathologic specimens for routine pathologic evaluation. Fixation in formalin cooled to refrigerator temperature can aid in preservation of glycogen.

When evaluating skeletal muscle samples, *it is essential to prepare both transverse and longitudinal sections*, and the sampling method described above will help to ensure that such sections are obtained. *Transverse sections* are needed in order to evaluate fiber diameter and presence of internal nuclei, as well as for detection of various cytoarchitectural changes. *Longitudinal sections* are often useful to confirm acute myonecrosis and regeneration as well as to determine the length of segment involved. Intramuscular nerves are often easier to find and to examine in longitudinal muscle sections. The use of *special staining techniques*, such as Masson trichrome stain, reticulin stain, phosphotungstic acid hematoxylin, and periodic acid-Schiff (PAS) stain for glycogen can be particularly useful when evaluating muscle samples fixed in formalin. Interpretation of early degenerative change and its distinction from artifactual or autolytic change sometimes requires all available information about time and circumstances of death as well as clinical signs and biochemical changes shown prior to death.

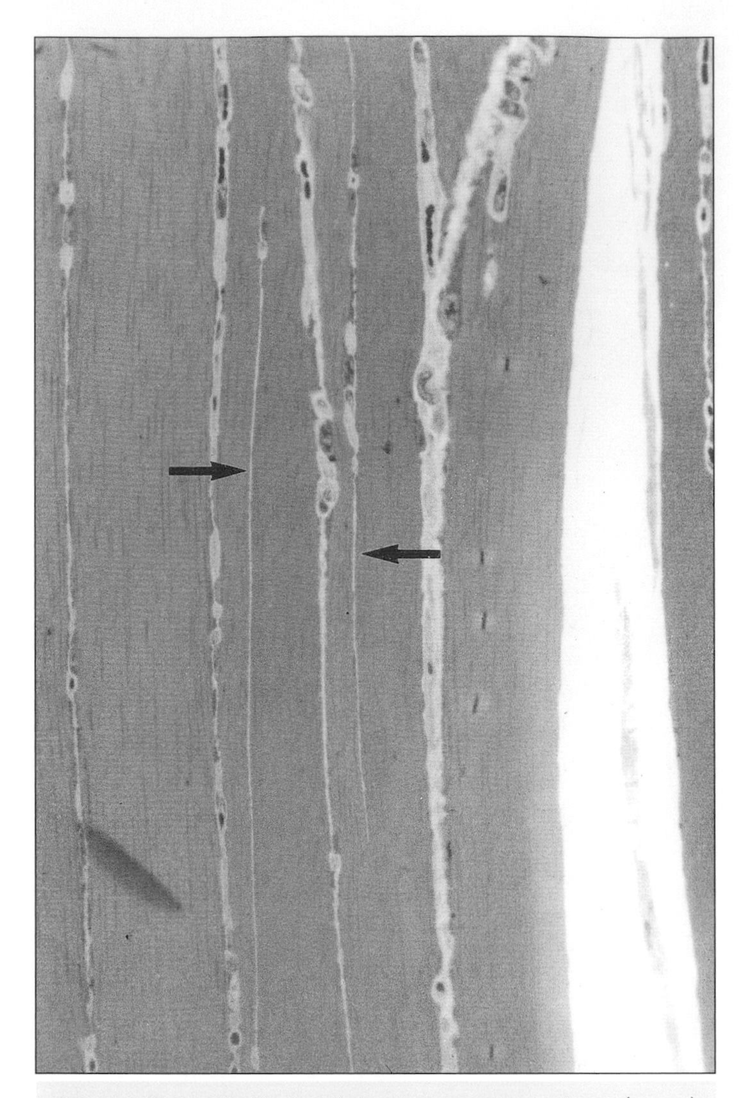

Figure 2.17 Longitudinal splitting in two adjacent fibers (arrows). (Courtesy of TJ Hulland.)

Bibliography

Anderson LVB. The molecular basis of muscle disease. In: Karpati G, Hilton-Jones D, Griggs RC, eds. Disorders of Voluntary Muscle. 7th ed. New York: Cambridge University Press, 2001:60–79.

Banker BQ, Engel AG. Basic reactions of muscle. In: Engel AG, Franzini-Armstrong C., eds. Myology, Basic and Clinical. 3rd ed. New York: McGraw-Hill. 2004:691–748.

Bradley R. Skeletal muscle biopsy techniques in animals for histochemical and ultrastructural examination and especially for the diagnosis of myodegeneration in cattle. Br Vet J 1978;134:434–444.

Cardinet GH, Holiday TA. Neuromuscular diseases of the domestic animals: a summary of muscle biopsies from 159 cases. Ann NY Acad Sci 1979;317:290–313.

Carpenter S. Electron microscopy in the study of normal and diseased muscle. In: Karpati G, et al., eds. Disorders of Voluntary Muscle. 7th ed. New York: Cambridge University Press, 2001:296–318.

Cooper BJ. Animal models of human muscle disease. In: Karpati G, et al., eds. Disorders of Voluntary Muscle. 7th ed. New York: Cambridge University Press, 2001:187–215.

Cullen MJ, Mastaglia FL. Pathological reactions of skeletal muscle. In: Mastaglia FL, Walton J, eds. Skeletal Muscle Pathology. Edinburgh: Churchill-Livingstone, 1982:88–95 and 102–105.

Dickinson PJ, Le Couteur RA. Muscle and nerve biopsy. Vet Clin North Am Small Anim Pract 2002;32:63–102.

Dubowitz V. Definition of pathological changes seen in muscle biopsies. In: Dubowitz V, ed. Muscle Biopsy, A Practical Approach. 2nd ed. London: Bailliére Tindall, 1985:82–103.

Dyer KR, et al. Peripheral neuropathy in two dogs: correlation between clinical, electrophysiological and pathological findings. J Small Anim Pract 1986;27:133–146.

Edström L, Grimby L. Effect of exercise on the motor unit. Musc Nerv 1986;9:104–126.

Essén-Gustavsson B, et al. Muscular adaptation of horses during intensive training and detraining. Equine Vet J 1989;21:27–33.

Fjelkner-Modig S, Ruderus H. Part I. The influence of exhaustion and electrical stimulation on the meat quality of young bulls: Postmortem pH and temperature. Meat Sci 1983;8:185–201.

Fjelkner-Modig S, Ruderus H. Part II. The influence of exhaustion and electrical stimulation on the meat quality of young bulls: physical and sensory properties. Meat Sci 1983;8:203–220.

Honikel KO, et al. The influence of temperature on shortening and rigor onset in beef muscle. Meat Sci 1983;8:221–241.

Hulland TJ. Histochemical and morphometric evaluation of skeletal muscle of cachectic sheep. Vet Pathol 1981;18:279–298.

Kakulas BA, Cooper BJ. Experimental and animal models of human neuromuscular disease. In: Walton J, et al., eds. Disorders of Voluntary Muscle. New York: Churchill Livingstone, 1994:437–496.

Lexell J, et al. What is the cause of the ageing atrophy? J Neurol Sci 1988;84:275–294.

McGavin MD. Muscle biopsy in veterinary practice. Vet Clin North Am Small Anim Pract 1983;13:135–144.

McGavin MD, Valentine BA. Muscle. In: McGavin MD, et al., eds. Thomson's Special Veterinary Pathology. 3rd ed. St. Louis, MO: Mosby, 2001:461–473.

Riley DA, Allin EF. The effects of inactivity, programmed stimulation and denervation on the histochemistry of skeletal muscle fiber types. Exp Neurol 1973;40:391–413.

Sewry CA. Electron microscopy. In: Lane RJM, ed. Handbook of Muscle Disease. New York: Marcel Dekker, 1996:81–93.

Sivachelvan MN, Davies AS. Induction of relative growth changes in the musculoskeletal system of the sheep by limb immobilization. Res Vet Sci 1986;40:173–182.

DEGENERATION AND REPAIR OF MUSCLE

Degeneration may involve parts or all of the cellular structures and often occurs segmentally along the length of the myofibers. The myofibrils alone, or myofibrils and sarcoplasm may undergo degenerative change leaving the sarcolemmal basal lamina, myonuclei, and satellite cells viable and intact. The next level of segmental degeneration leaves only the satellite cell nuclei and the basal lamina in place, and the third level destroys the satellite cells. The fourth level of segmental destruction destroys endomysial connective tissue cells and capillaries as well. *Regenerative responses* differ at each of these levels. Because the myofibers are so long, it is quite possible for a segment or several segments of a fiber to be destroyed without all of the cells being adversely affected although subsequent reparative events sometimes fail to reconstruct the original fiber completely. On the other hand, it is distinctly possible for a fiber to suffer repeated segmental destruction throughout its life span, and to be restored each time to completeness.

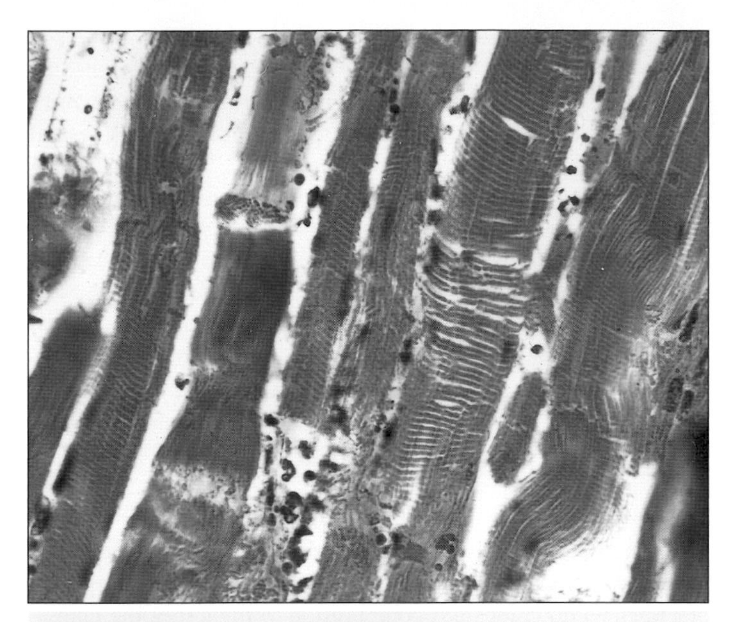

Figure 2.18 Hypercontracted fibers in a downer cow. (Courtesy of TJ Hulland.)

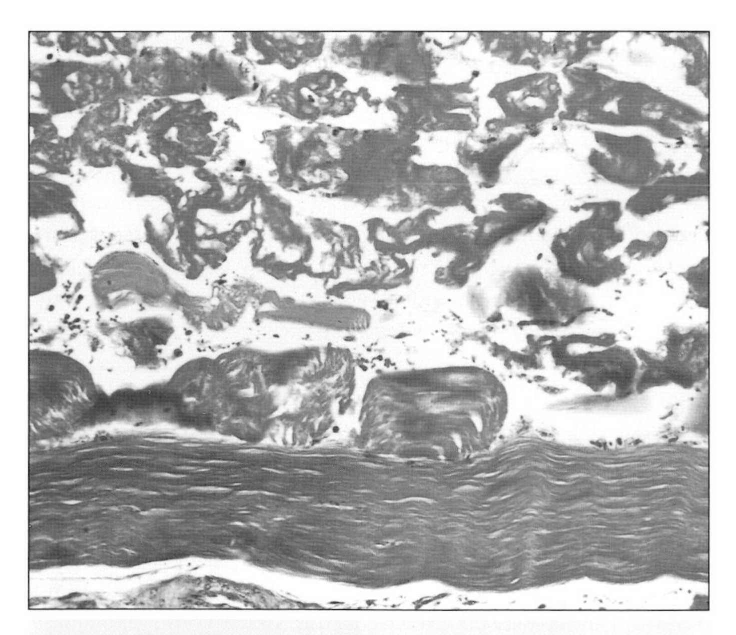

Figure 2.19 Hyaline degeneration in nutritional myopathy in a cow. (Courtesy of TJ Hulland.)

Thus, complete muscle cell death is an exceptional event even in extensive lesions, but destructive events usually have some lasting effect on the shape or number of fibers (see Regeneration and repair of muscle).

Histopathologic evidence of segmental degeneration of muscle fibers along with the events of regeneration and repair are the common expression of many muscle diseases in animals. Kakulas developed a classification for the degenerative lesions of muscle based on spatial distribution and temporal patterns that is often useful to identify broad etiologic categories of muscle disease. *Four categories of muscle injury reactions were established as follows: (1) focal monophasic, (2) multifocal monophasic, (3) focal polyphasic, and (4) multifocal polyphasic* (Kakulas, 1981).

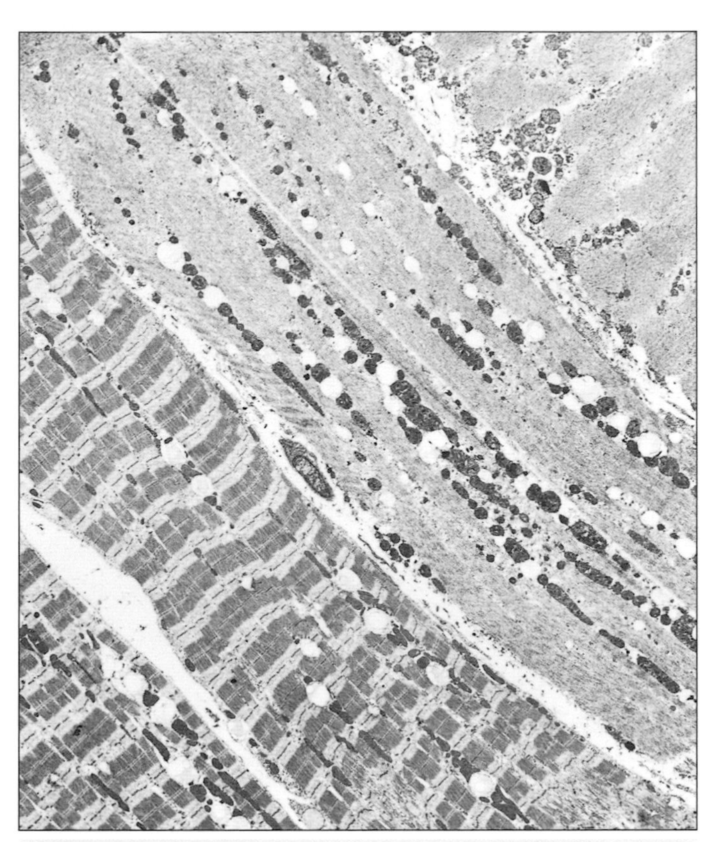

Figure 2.20 Coagulative necrosis (top) and areas of myofibrillar lysis (bottom) in a foal. (Courtesy of TJ Hulland.)

- *Focal monophasic reactions* result from an isolated single mechanical injury, such as external trauma or needle insertion.
- In *multifocal monophasic reactions*, a single insult – such as exposure to various myotoxic drugs, chemicals, or metabolic disorders – may initiate widespread muscle lesions, but all the alterations are in the same phase of injury.
- *Focal polyphasic reactions* result from repeated mechanical injury in the same site.
- *Multifocal polyphasic reactions* are frequent in muscular diseases of animals, and result from continued insults applied over a prolonged time, such as from nutritional deficiencies and genetic disorders (as in muscular dystrophies). The lesions are widespread in the musculature and various pathological reactions – including degeneration, leukocytic invasion during resolution, and regeneration – will occur concurrently.

Muscle fiber degeneration is frequently associated with alterations of cellular membranes, and membrane failure takes the form of segmental myofiber degeneration. Initiation of events that lead to contraction is by nerve-triggered activation of skeletal muscle ion channels resulting in a muscle action potential. Muscle contraction is initiated by passive release of calcium ions from the sarcoplasmic reticulum, but energy is required to recapture calcium ions to allow muscle fiber relaxation. Exhaustion of phosphate-bonded energy reserves often leaves the muscle fiber in a state of calcium-abundant contraction or hypercontraction which soon reduces the complex myofilaments to a coagulum of contractile proteins (Figs 2.18–2.21). *There appears to be a final common destructive pathway of* **mitochondrial calcium overload,** *which begins with many different causes of*

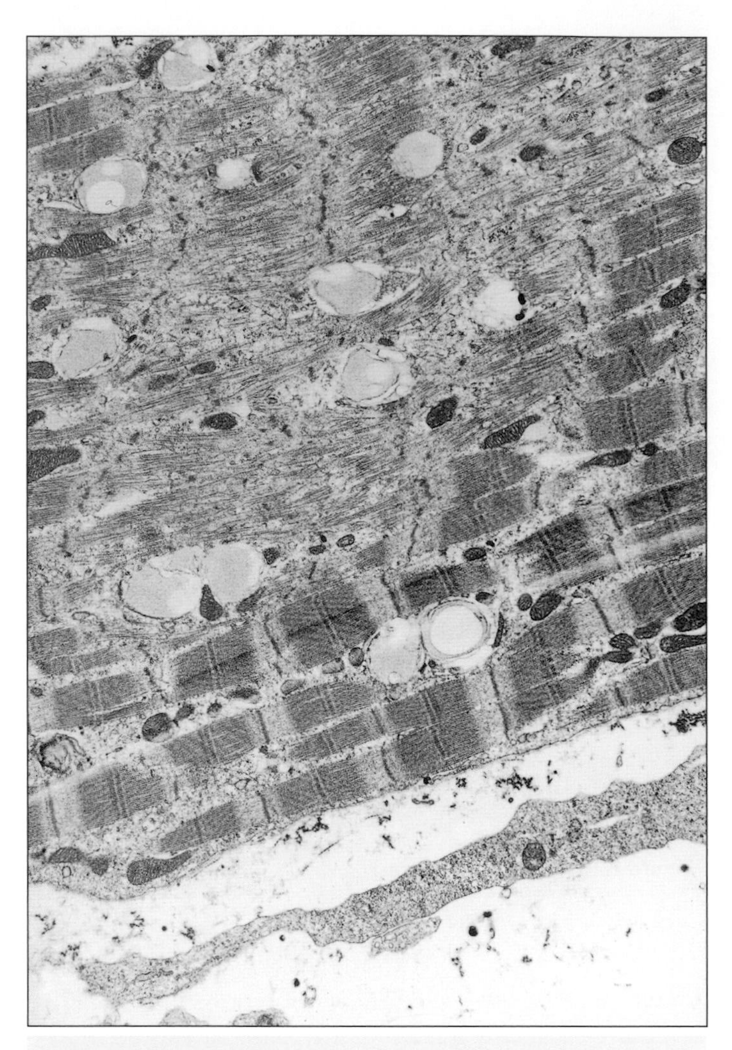

Figure 2.21 Myofibrillar lysis and lipid droplet accumulation in a foal. (Courtesy of TJ Hulland.)

membrane or energy failure and ends with hypercontraction and coagulation of the contractile proteins. Most animal myopathies seem to fit well into this sequence of events, particularly the nutritional myopathies. Grossly visible mineralization occurs several hours after the onset of protein coagulation during which striations are lost (*hyaline degeneration*). Calcium is released belatedly in degenerated myofibrils from calcium-saturated mitochondria as they disintegrate. Although the almost chalky mineralization seen grossly in many cases of nutritional myopathy is usually referred to as dystrophic, it is not at all certain that such accumulations can occur as a result of a purely passive collection of mineral from the blood on dead tissue protein. At the very least, it seems to require that mitochondria become overloaded with calcium early in the degenerative process.

Some cases of nutritional myopathy and toxic myopathy may have very similar microscopic degenerative changes not characterized by mineralization to any appreciable extent, even though the lesions are as extensive as those in typical "white muscle disease." Degenerate muscle may be very difficult to detect on gross examination when it is unmineralized, and consequently is likely to escape detection. The event that determines whether mineralization occurs in addition to the variable of the amount of blood calcium available may well be the period after hypercontraction, during which cellular membranes allow calcium into the cell and mitochondria continue to collect calcium from the cytosol. Eventually such activity will be ended by membrane disintegration and a release of calcium to the cytosol again, but calcium gathering could continue for a period of several hours.

The hypercontracted eosinophilic coagulum in segmental hyaline degeneration is readily removed by macrophages both in its earlier, premineralized state and in the later mineralized stage of granular degeneration. *The early pale, hyaline stage develops into typical* **Zenker's degeneration**, *which is a highly eosinophilic, homogeneous mass.* It sometimes retains faintly visible, tightly contracted striations, although these are eventually lost.

Regeneration and repair of muscle

The ability of muscle to repair itself is remarkable considering its high specialization and the great length and great vulnerability of individual fibers. The ability to rapidly repair the damaged segment of a fiber, without apparent complication to the rest of the fiber, is without parallel in other cells of the body. A muscle cell consists of a single large multinucleate myofiber adjacent to which is a large population of uninuclear satellite cells, outside the plasma membrane but within the tough basal lamina. *The major participants in the regenerative sequence are macrophages from the blood, the satellite cells, because only they, within the muscle, have retained the capability for mitotic division, and the basal lamina, which acts as a very efficient scaffold.* The integrity of the basal lamina determines from the very beginning how effective regeneration will be and whether the outcome will be regeneration of myofibers, fibrous replacement, or a mixture of the two. An intact basal lamina effectively keeps myonuclei, satellite nuclei, and myoblastic cells inside. It is equally efficient in keeping fibroblastic cells out, but allows phagocytic cells easy entry and exit.

If damage to the fiber is *segmental* and such that only the myofibrils and the sarcoplasm along with its subcellular components have been injured, the first visible event of regeneration is an early rounding-up of satellite cells as they prepare to undergo mitotic division. The proliferated satellite cells become apparent in hours as they leave their former sublaminal site. After about 12 hours, macrophages appear and they may or may not be accompanied by a short-lived wave of neutrophils and eosinophils. These inflammatory cells are rich sources of growth factors and cytokines such as insulin-like growth factor (IGF)-1, platelet-derived growth factor (PDGF), and interleukin (IL)-6 that promote satellite cell and myoblast proliferation and differentiation. These cell types freely enter the mineralized damaged fiber. Macrophages dissolve and remove the debris (Fig. 2.22); neutrophils disappear unless infection complicates the process. Removal of sarcoplasmic debris leaves some space enclosed within the collapsing sarcolemma; and proliferating satellite cells are seen in the sarcolemmal tube. These cells are now termed myoblasts.

Myoblasts increase in number until a critical myoblastic mass is reached. Only then do myoblasts begin to fuse, and this triggers the next sequence of events. Five or six days after degeneration occurred, fusion of myoblasts has produced *unpolarized myotube giant cells* that begin to send out cytoplasmic processes as their nuclei divide (Fig. 2.23). Guided by the basal lamina, some processes make contact with remaining viable segments of the original fiber. They make effective union by dissolving cell membranes and uniting the cytosols into a single myofiber. The free pole of the myotube giant cell then

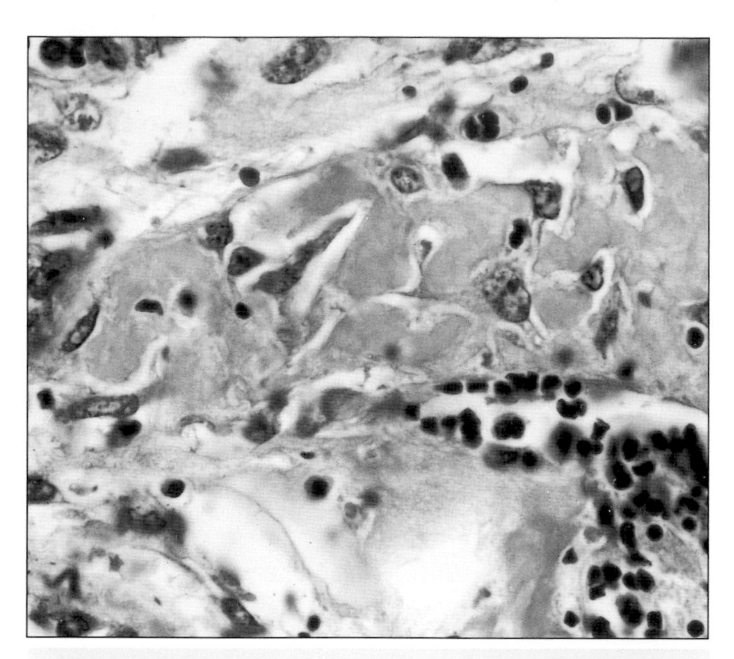

Figure 2.22 Necrotic myofiber with surviving satellite cells and invading macrophages. (Courtesy of TJ Hulland.)

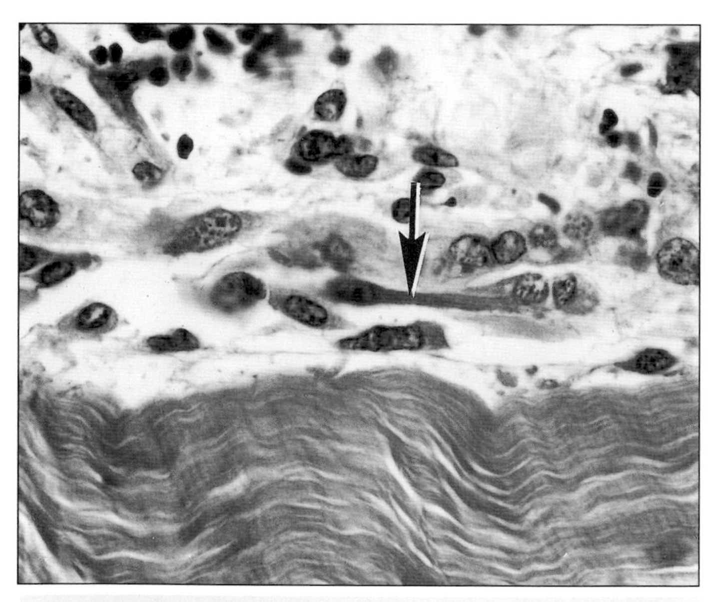

Figure 2.23 Regeneration, with elongating myoblasts (arrow). (Courtesy of TJ Hulland.)

becomes a *polarized regenerative probe,* which grows within the cleared space of the collapsed sarcolemmal sheath. Other myotube cells in the regenerating myofiber may not make contact with other myotubes for some time, and remain as unpolarized giant cells until an adjacent myotube's process contacts them. *A growing myotube characterized by its basophilic cytoplasm and central row of nuclei can grow for relatively long distances as long as the basal lamina is intact and no fibrous tissue intrudes and obstructs* (Fig. 2.24). If the basal lamina sheath is ruptured, the myotube protrudes from the ruptured sarcolemmal tube as a syncytial giant cell and can grow into the proliferating fibrous tissue for only 2–5 mm.

When a myotube has made contact with the next viable segment of the original fiber, at about 10–14 days, the next stage

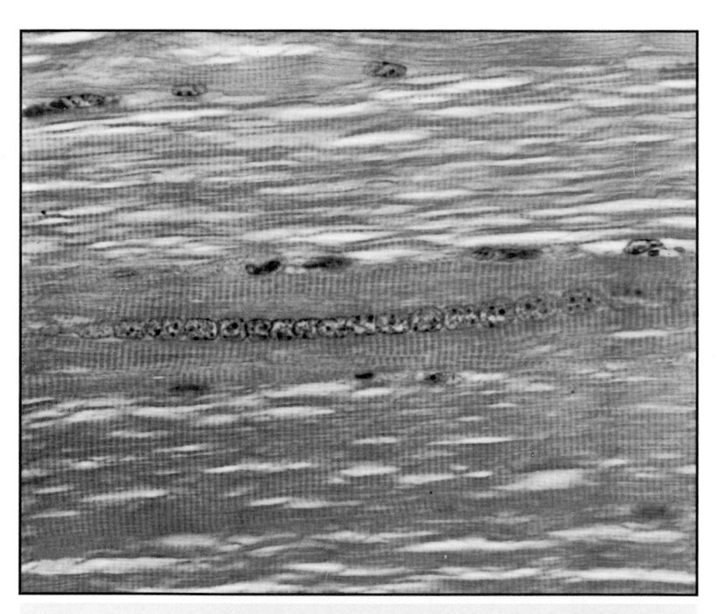

Figure 2.24 Regeneration, with a fiber with a row of central nuclei. (Courtesy of TJ Hulland.)

consists mostly of *production of new sarcomeres in the enlarging fiber.* The new fiber has to find growing space between existing fibers but seems able to do this efficiently. As myofibrils, sarcoplasm, and other organelles are added, the fiber becomes less basophilic, and from 7–21 days the nuclei migrate from their central or internal position to lie just under the new cell membrane – the normal position in a mature myofiber. Only in the most ideal of circumstances are all the parts restored to the predegeneration state by the efficient regeneration process described above. At the very least, two basal laminae, one inside the other, persist; later they may fuse. Any proliferating satellite cell/myoblasts, which do not enter the original cell, or any myotube processes which escape from it, may produce muscle giant cells that reflect abortive attempts at myofiber regeneration.

Considering the possibility of breaks in the sarcolemmal tubes, the potential for myoblast formation, which may be inside or outside the original myofiber and the potential for distortion of development by fibrous tissue invasion, it is easy to understand that the final result may not be perfect. *The longer and more numerous the gaps in sarcolemmal tubes are, the more potential there is for aberrations in repair.* The most important factors in preventing such aberrations seem to be the viability of nuclei and the wholeness of the basal lamina. Although sometimes extensively destructive, *nutritional, exertional and most toxic myopathies are likely to repair very well with minimal fibrosis. Primary dystrophies repair well but degenerate again* and eventually residual lesions of fibrosis will become prominent. *Ischemic damage repairs badly or not at all* because satellite nuclei and endomysial cells may have been killed. Fibrous replacement will be the end result. Ischemia with early reflow permits some regenerative repair, particularly around the outside of primary bundles where blood flow returns first but central fibrous replacement will occur. *Fibrosis may be the dominant feature in healed lesions of myositis and physical injury.*

The reduced regenerative capability that develops with maturity may be related to low numbers of potential myoblasts as the proportion of satellite cells to the total nuclear population in the fiber drops with age.

Other types of degeneration

Vacuolar degeneration, an infrequent alteration in muscle fibers (Fig. 2.25) is associated with *electrolyte abnormalities,* such as hyperkalemia in horses with hyperkalemic periodic paralysis, and in the diaphragm of rodents given intraperitoneal injections of doxorubicin. **Fatty degeneration** with small fat vacuoles is a very common finding in *emaciated or anorectic animals* because muscle is able to use triglycerides directly as a source of energy. Rows of minute droplets are held in considerable quantity by type 1 (oxidative) fibers, but type 2 fibers often contain neutral fat also (see Fig. 2.21). The presence of these fat droplets may be more evident in those myofibrils remaining in advanced cachectic atrophy, but it apparently implies no pathologic change in muscle as even well-nourished animals carry some droplets in their muscles. Quite separate from these aggregations of minute fat droplets, larger fat droplets may be seen in muscle fibers in the dog and horse. Their cause is not known.

So-called **discoid degeneration** represents the phenomenon of *hypercontraction*. It develops when hypoxia plays a major part in the production of muscle lesions. The muscle striations, but not all of their fine features, are preserved and the fiber begins to separate at the Z bands (see Fig. 2.18).

Xanthomatosis (lipofuscinosis) is the term used to describe the *accumulation of abnormal amounts of yellow-brown to bronze pigment in some skeletal muscles and myocardium, and often also in adrenal cortex and distal convoluted tubules of the kidney*. Black hair coats may become brown, and white skin may become yellow, but the presence of the pigment appears not to be detrimental to the health of the animal. The build-up of "wear-and-tear pigments" in old animals, particularly high-producing dairy cows is indistinguishable morphologically from xanthomatosis but it is sometimes associated with myocardial failure. There appears to be a disproportionately high incidence of xanthomatosis in Ayrshire cows and among old cows of all breeds slaughtered for human consumption; in one study the incidence was about 0.1–0.5% overall compared to 10–25% for Ayrshires.

Skeletal muscles most frequently or most extensively involved are the *masseter muscles* and the *diaphragm*. Muscle fibers are of normal diameter or smaller, but may be dark brown or even black-brown. Pigment granules, some of which stain positively with lipid and PAS stains, tend to be located within lysosomes found perinuclearly under the sarcolemma or centrally in the fiber. Particles are irregular in size and shape and on electron microscopic examination show a wide variation in shape and organization. All are electron-dense and some are membrane-bound and it is presumed that they represent degraded lipid substances that have accumulated in phagolysosomes.

Other myofiber alterations

A variety of inclusion-like structures or focally abundant or altered structural components occur in the myopathies of animals and are termed **cytoarchitectural changes** (Figs 2.26, 2.27). Similar alterations in the muscles of humans sometimes are associated with specific diseases but such relationships have not been established in most animal diseases. **Nemaline rods** have been found in a myopathy of cats and in occasional cases in dogs, with or without hypothyroidism. The rods represent accumulations of Z band material as confirmed by electron microscopy (see Congenital and inherited defects). **Targetoid fibers** (central zones of myofibrillar disruption)

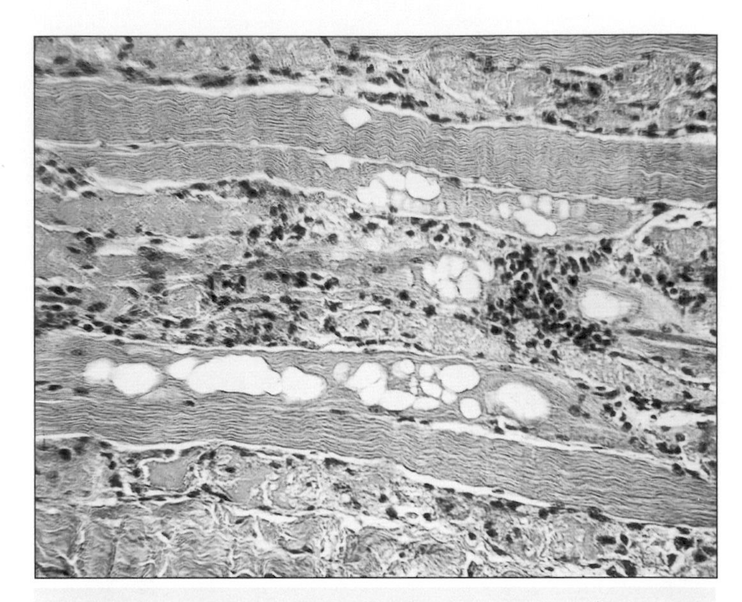

Figure 2.25 Vacuolar degeneration of muscle in a cow. (Courtesy of W Hadlow.)

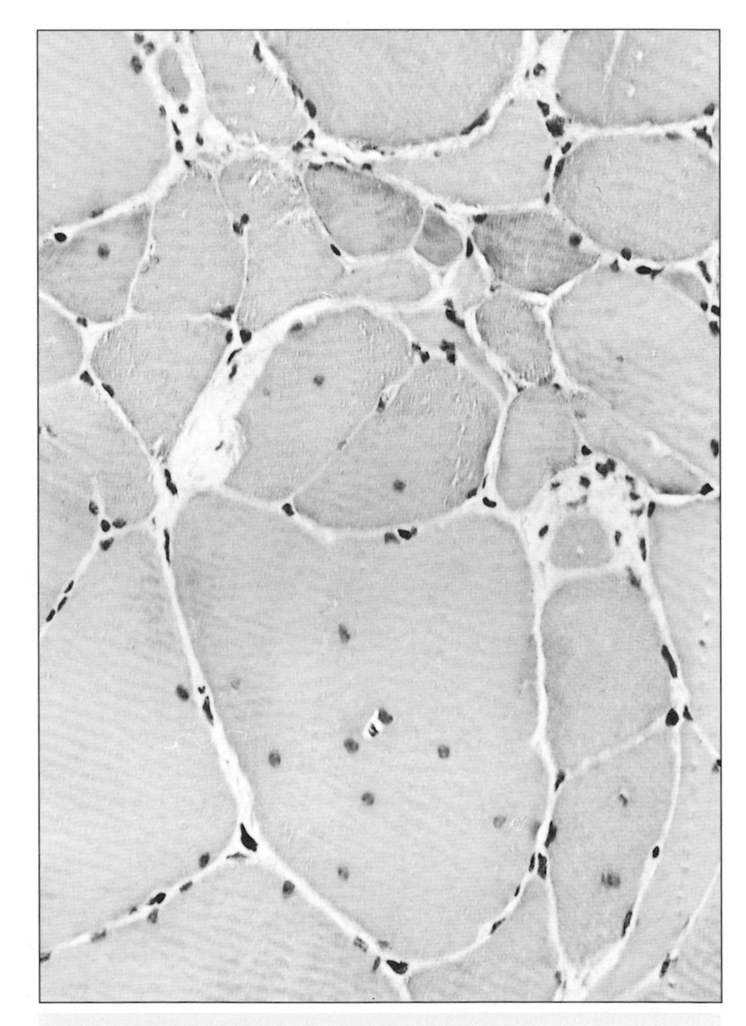

Figure 2.26 Myopathic alterations of internal nuclei and variation in fiber size in a horse. (Courtesy of TJ Hulland.)

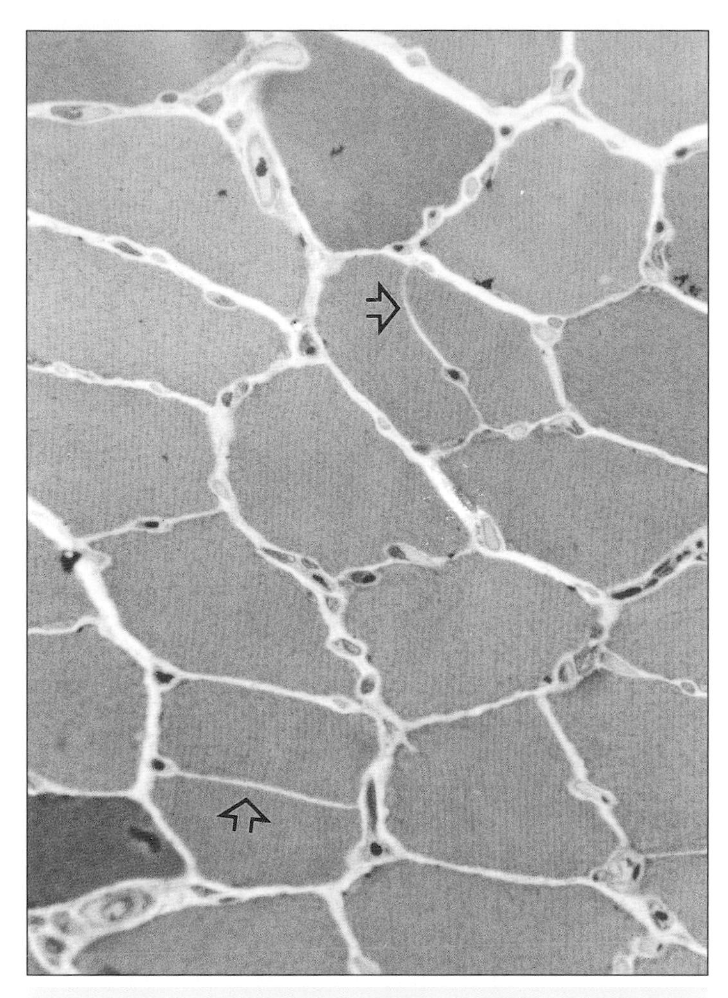

Figure 2.27 Myopathic alteration of **fiber splitting** (arrows) in a horse. (Courtesy of TJ Hulland.)

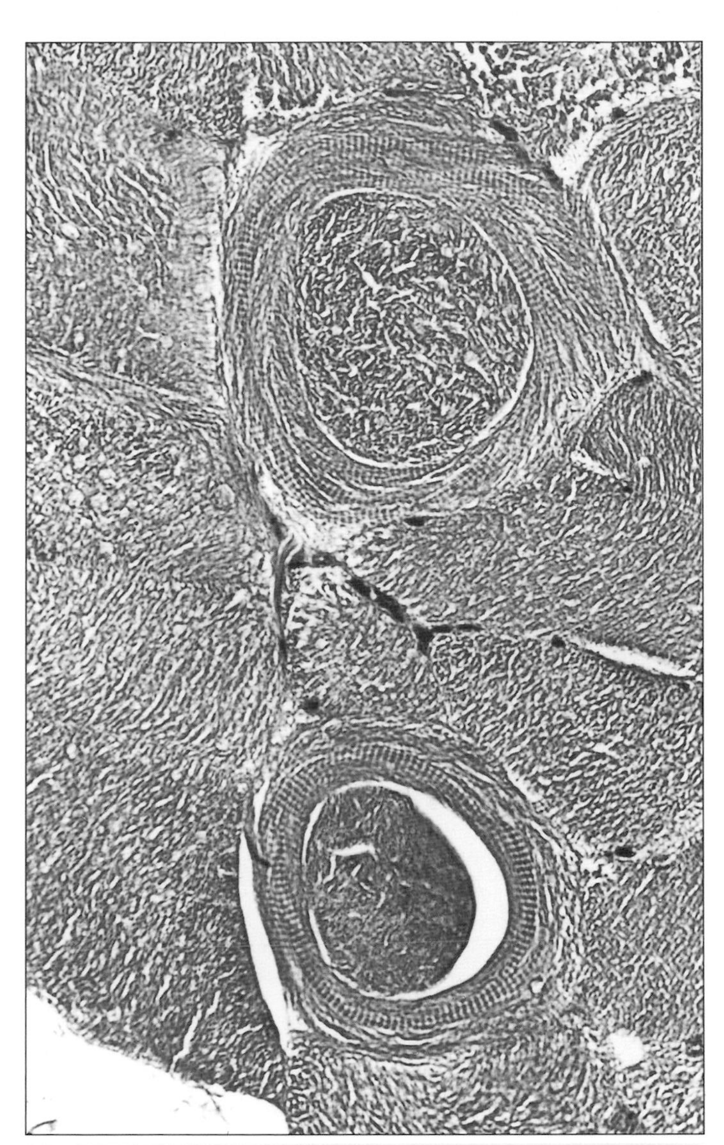

Figure 2.28 Two fibers with **ringbinden** in a horse. (Courtesy of TJ Hulland.)

and **ragged red fibers** (mitochondrial-laden) have been seen in myotonic muscle disease in dogs, and **peripheral and central sarcoplasmic masses** have been observed in the muscles of sheep and cattle in dystrophy. Abnormal **glycogen accumulations** may develop in the muscles of dogs, sheep, cattle, cats, and horses (see also Congenital and inherited defects). In all species, these are generally nonmembrane-bound collections. The deposits are PAS positive and digested by diastase and are usually just under the sarcolemma.

Ringbinden (ring fibers) is one of the unusual findings that may be left behind when denervation or tenotomy is combined with atrophy and regeneration. *It is a formation of disoriented peripheral myofibrils, which wrap themselves around a muscle fiber in a tight spiral fashion* (Fig. 2.28). Satellite cell nuclei can migrate and they sometimes orient their long axes transversely rather than longitudinally. Circular myofibrils accompanied by a mass of disrupted subsarcolemmal contractile elements presumably represent a true, but nonspecific, degeneration of myofibers. Ring fibers most often occur naturally in animals showing evidence of denervation atrophy, with or without evidence of ischemic muscle damage. Horses cast and anesthetized for several hours may also develop these lesions.

The role of **apoptosis** in skeletal muscle disease is still unclear. Although apoptosis represents an important activity in myoblasts during normal differentiation and development, its *role in postmitotic mature myofibers is uncertain*, but activated satellite cells may undergo apoptosis. Multinucleated skeletal muscle myotubes in cell culture exposed to staurosporine, a protein kinase inhibitor known to induce apoptosis in a variety of cell types, underwent the morphologic and biochemical features of apoptosis. In several models of muscle disease (X-linked muscular dystrophy in mouse, bupivacaine injury of immature rat muscle), apoptosis precedes the development of necrosis. Further studies are needed to establish the role and the importance of apoptosis in muscle diseases of animals and human beings.

Bibliography

Allbrook D. Skeletal muscle regeneration. Musc Nerv 1981;4:234–245.

Best TM, Hunter KD. Muscle injury and repair. Phys Med Rehabil Clin North Am 2000;11:251–266.

Bornemann A, et al. Satellite cells as players and targets in normal and diseased muscle. Neuropediatrics 1999;30:167–175.

Cardinet GH. Part III. Skeletal muscle function. In: Kaneko JJ, et al., eds. Clinical Biochemistry of Domestic Animals. 5th ed. New York: Academic Press, 1997:407–440.

Carlson BM, Faulkner JA. The regeneration of skeletal muscle fibers following injury: a review. Med Sci Sport Exerc 1983;15:187–198.

Carpenter S. Electron microscopy in the study of normal and diseased muscle. In: Karpati G, et al., eds. Disorders of Voluntary Muscle. 7th ed. New York: Cambridge University Press, 2001:296–318.

Chargé SBP, Rudnicki MA. Cellular and molecular regulation of muscle regeneration. Physiol Rev 2004;84:209–238.

Cooper BJ. Animal models of human muscle disease. In: Karpati G, et al., eds. Disorders of Voluntary Muscle. 7th ed. New York: Cambridge University Press, 2001: 187–215.

Duncan CJ, Jackson MJ. Different mechanisms mediate structural changes and intracellular enzyme efflux following damage to skeletal muscle. J Cell Sci 1987;87:183–188.

Grounds MD. Towards understanding skeletal muscle regeneration. Pathol Res Pract 1991;187:1–22.

Hadlow WJ. Diseases of skeletal muscle. In: Innes JRM, Saunders LZ, eds. Comparative Neuropathology. New York: Academic Press, 1962:147–243.

Husmann I, et al. Growth factors in skeletal muscle regeneration. Cytokine Growth Factor Rev 1996;7:249–258.

Kakulas BA. Experimental myopathies. In: Walton J, ed. Disorders of Voluntary Muscle. 4th ed. New York: Churchill-Livingstone, 1981:389–416.

Karpati G, et al. Disorders of Voluntary Muscle. 7th ed. New York: Cambridge University Press, 2001.

Lane RJ, ed. Handbook of Muscle Disease. New York: Marcel Dekker, 1996.

Lescaudron L, et al. Blood-borne macrophages are essential for the triggering of muscle regeneration following muscle transplant. Neuromuscul Disord 1999;9:72–80.

McArdle A, et al. Apoptosis in multinucleated skeletal muscle myotubes. Lab Invest 1999;79:1069–1076.

McGavin MD, Valentine B. Muscle. In: McGavin MD, et al., eds. Thomson's Special Veterinary Pathology. 3rd ed. Philadelphia, PA: Mosby, 2001:461–498.

Shelton GD, Cardinet GH. Part III. Pathophysiologic basis of canine muscle disorders. J Vet Inter Med 1987;1(1):36–44.

Van Vleet JF. Pathological reactions of skeletal muscle to injury. In: Jones TC, et al., eds. ILSI Monographs on Pathology of Laboratory Animals: Cardiovascular and Musculoskeletal Systems. New York: Springer Verlag, 1991:109–126.

Van Vleet JF. Skeletal muscle. In: Jones TC, et al., eds. Veterinary Pathology. 6th ed. Philadelphia, PA: Williams & Wilkins, 1997:873–897.

Wrogemann K, Pena SDJ. Mitochondrial calcium overload: a general mechanism for cell-necrosis in muscle diseases. Lancet 1976;1:672–673.

CONGENITAL AND INHERITED DEFECTS

There are numerous conditions affecting skeletal muscle development, integrity, and function in animals. Congenital myopathic and neuropathic conditions are apparent at birth or soon thereafter, usually within the first year of life, and may or may not be inherited. *Pedigree analysis and breeding studies often help to distinguish those congenital disorders that are also inherited.* Inherited disorders affecting skeletal muscle in animals in which the gene defect is known are listed in Table 2.1. Gene mutations leading to skeletal muscle dysfunction are most often *point mutations*, e.g., hyperkalemic periodic paralysis (HYPP) in horses, phosphofructokinase (PFK) deficiency in dogs, and myophosphorylase deficiency in cattle. Some disorders, e.g., canine X-linked muscular dystrophy, can occur due to either point mutations or deletions, and the genetically characterized cases of feline X-linked muscular dystrophy have been due to a gene deletion.

Following tradition, congenital and inherited defects of skeletal muscle are discussed separately from the congenital and inherited myopathies, although it is recognized that the distinction between these two groups is not always clear. Numerous disorders are difficult to classify using traditional classification schemes, and diseases or syndromes can change their status as a result of investigation and new information.

Abnormal development of neuroectoderm that involves the lower motor neuron portion of the nervous system will also affect skeletal muscle. Although the primary defect is in the nervous system, the profound effect these disorders can have on skeletal muscle development and function warrant a brief discussion here.

Primary CNS conditions

Neuroectodermal defects affecting the innervation of individual myotomes and the muscles that form from them can result in abnormal muscle development. Given the complex interaction of myogenic and neurogenic cells during development, it is often difficult to define the exact nature of the defect. Neuroectodermal defects can result in abnormal muscle development or structure due to lack of innervation, to loss of innervation, or to abnormal motor neuron activity.

For proper in utero development, muscles require normal innervation. Without it they atrophy or fail to develop normally (hypotrophy) and are more or less replaced by fibrous tissue and fat. Associated with each embryonic spinal cord segment is a myotome, a collection of cells with myoblastic potential, which migrate as the fetus develops and that ultimately form muscle. Committed myoblastic cells from one myotome may contribute to several muscles. Later, nerves from the same spinal segment follow the route of the myoblastic cells and innervate the same muscles. Most developing muscles are formed from myoblastic cells and nerves from two to six cord segments, but a few small muscles of the distal limbs receive contributions from only one. This explains why some muscles innervated from only one segment are vulnerable to denervation or lack of innervation resulting from a cord lesion involving a single segment, while a cord lesion of similar extent contributing innervation to muscles receiving cells and nerves from multiple segments can be associated with apparently normal muscle and nerve development. In the latter case, collateral innervation from nerves arising in normal cord segments can develop.

Developing skeletal muscle motor units are innervated by more than one nerve and, in some species such as the dog, this polyinnervation is still present at birth. With maturation of the neuromuscular unit the innervation pattern is simplified to one of one nerve fiber per motor unit. This pattern of polyinnervation can further complicate the pathologic findings in muscle from animals with neuroectodermal defects.

Arthrogryposis and dysraphism

Arthrogryposis *literally means crooked joint.* The terms *congenital articular rigidity* and *arthrogryposis multiplex congenita* are also used to describe this syndrome. Arthrogryposis can involve one or more limbs, depending on the underlying neuroectodermal defect. Severely affected animals may also have scoliosis, kyphosis, and torticollis, and the limbs or parts of limbs may be rotated, abducted, or curled backwards or forwards in grotesque positions (Fig. 2.29). Newborn animals afflicted with arthrogryposis are sometimes stillborn and may show autolysis indicative of in utero death 2–4 days earlier. Hydramnios is disproportionately associated with these, as is dystocia. Many, perhaps most, are of normal skeletal size although some are

Table 2.1 Animal myopathies in which the gene defect is known

Disorder	Gene affected	Type of disease	Species/breed affected
X-linked muscular dystrophy	Dystrophin	Muscular dystrophy	Various dog breeds; DSH cats
Double muscling	Myostatin	Muscular hyperplasia	Various beef breeds
Porcine stress syndrome	Ryanodine receptor	Malignant hyperthermia	Various pig breeds
Phosphofructokinase (PFK) deficiency	PFK, muscle isozyme	Carbohydrate metabolic defect	English Springer Spaniels, American Cocker Spaniels
Hyperkalemic periodic paralysis (HYPP)	Skeletal muscle sodium channel	Channelopathy leading to myotonia and paralysis	Impressive line of Quarter Horses
Glycogen storage disease	Myophosphorylase	Carbohydrate metabolic defect	Charolais cattle
Canine myotonia	Skeletal muscle chloride channel – ClC-1	Channelopathy leading to myotonia	Miniature Schnauzer

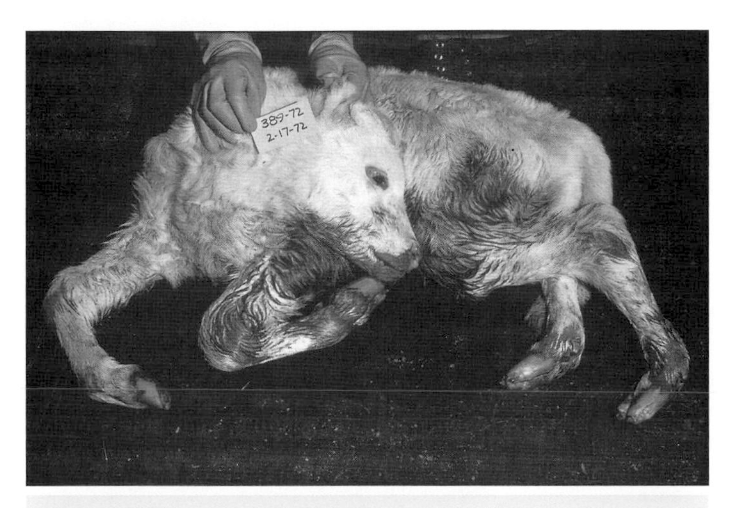

Figure 2.29 Newborn calf with **arthrogryposis**. (Courtesy of S Snyder.)

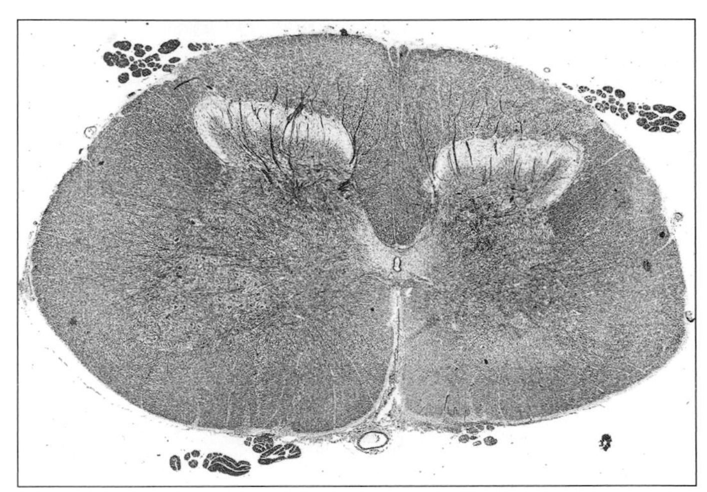

Figure 2.30 Failure of development of the right ventral horn in a calf with **myelodysplasia**. (Courtesy of TJ Hulland.)

considerably smaller than normal or smaller than littermates. In the rare cases in which the limb involvement is unilateral, the animal is likely to be born alive.

The causes of arthrogryposis are often not clear, although the underlying cause is generally agreed to be decreased limb movement in utero. Both myogenic and neurogenic disorders can result in decreased limb movement and arthrogryposis, but *denervation is by far the most common cause.* Arthrogrypotic fixation of the joints of lambs, calves, piglets, and foals, and less frequently of kittens and puppies, occurs with some regularity, and sometimes in epidemics. In cases of epidemic incidence, viral infections or toxins affecting the nervous system (see below) are most likely.

Unequivocal links exist between arthrogryposis and *the recognizable lesions caused by arrest or delay of neural tube closure* (**dysraphism**). These include, in the extreme, spina bifida and cord agenesis, but also anomalies of the dorsal septum, anomalies of the central canal such as hydromyelia and syringomyelia, anomalies of the dorsal, central or ventral gray matter (Fig. 2.30), and anomalies of the ventral median fissure (see Vol. 1, Nervous system). Dysraphism does not always lead to arthrogryposis; segmental lesions are sometimes found in clinically normal animals.

Obvious spinal cord and/or peripheral nerve abnormalities are present in a proportion, perhaps a majority, of arthrogrypotic domestic animals. In the rest, although an absence of primary myogenic or osteogenic lesions seems to point to a neurologic cause, the identity of the failed neural component is not obvious on routine investigation. Several careful studies of unilateral arthrogryposis in animals and children have indicated that the neural changes can be subtle and varied. The number of motor neurons in an apparently normal cord may be segmentally reduced, particularly in the caudal portion of the thoracic and lumbar eminences; or the number of motor neurons may be increased, or the neurons may be disoriented. Beyond this, conjecturally, there could be failure of neural direction, or connection, or of end-plate development.

Affected animals may have obvious reduction in mass of affected muscle due to atrophy or hypotrophy. Muscle mass can, however, appear superficially normal if there is replacement of the lost muscle mass by local masses of neonatal fat (Fig. 2.31). Dissection of major nerve trunks and muscle often is very difficult. Nerve trunks often appear to be normal on gross examination. Where comparisons are possible, peripheral nerve trunks in affected limbs may be demonstrably smaller and lacking some fascicles, although individual axons are normal.

Histologically, marked fiber size variation due to irregularity of muscle development may be evident. Groups of normal muscle can occur admixed with, or adjacent to, groups of small round muscle fibers (Fig. 2.32). Rarely, a typical denervation pattern of clusters of large

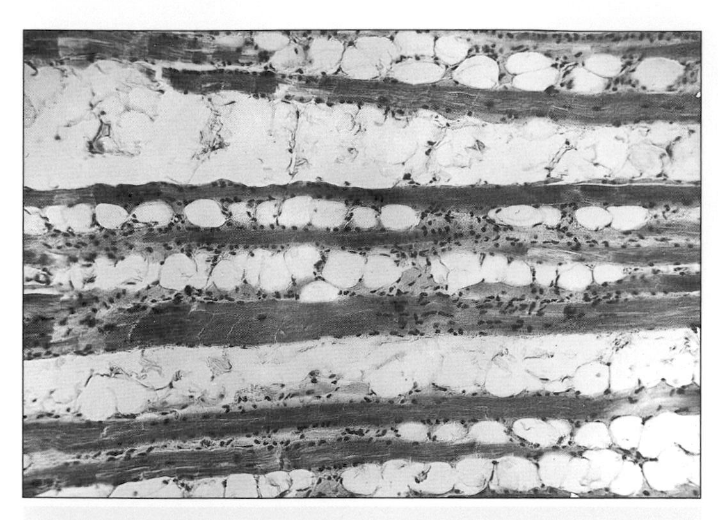

Figure 2.31 Muscle hypotrophy and fat replacement in a calf with arthrogryposis due to myelodysplasia. (Courtesy of TJ Hulland.)

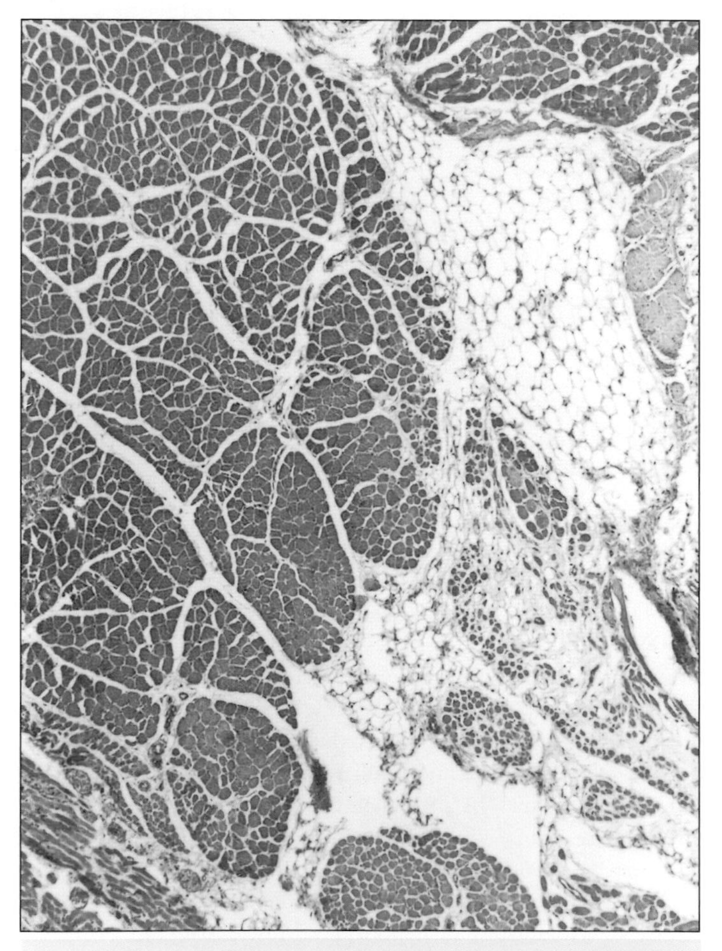

Figure 2.32 Admixed fascicles composed of myofibers of varied diameter, often with admixed fat infiltration, indicative of **asynchronous myofiber development** in an animal with arthrogryposis. (Courtesy of TJ Hulland.)

and clusters of small fibers can be seen. Abnormalities resulting in denervation and reinnervation will result in fiber type grouping. Other alterations in the fiber type pattern, such as type 1 fiber predominance (Fig. 2.33), are more difficult to explain but may reflect abnormal innervation or neural activity. Variable portions of muscle may be composed of adipose tissue.

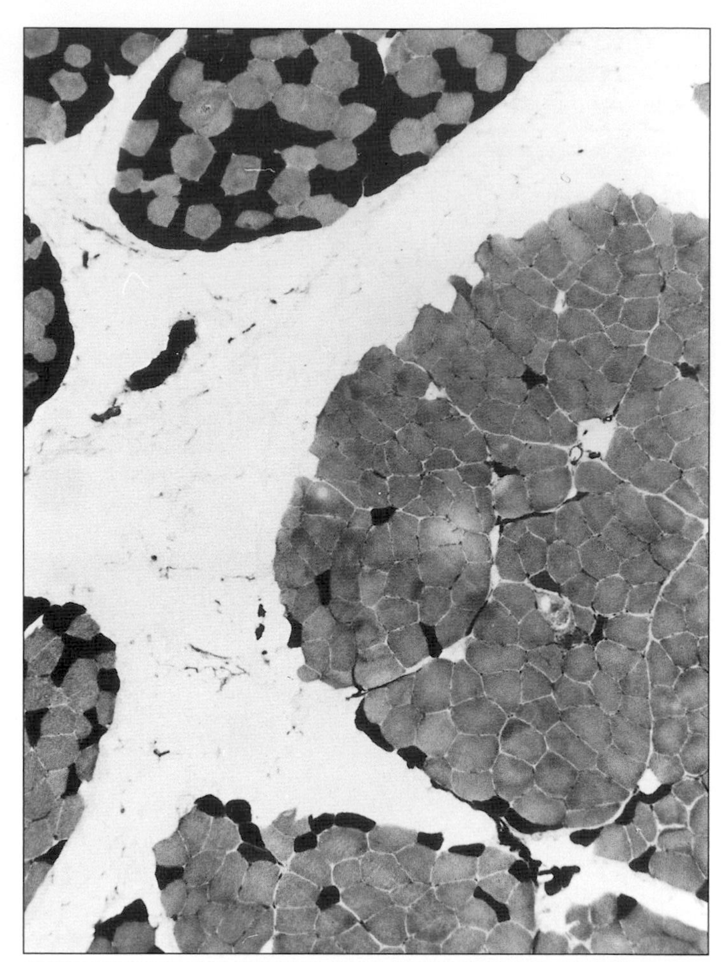

Figure 2.33 Fascicles exhibiting **type 1** (pale staining) **fiber predominance** in a lamb with arthrogryposis. Frozen section, ATPase, alkaline pre-incubation. (Courtesy of TJ Hulland.)

As noted above, it is often impossible to relate lesions to a specific cause. The critical event must occur early in pregnancy. *Genetic causes* are postulated in calves, sheep, and pigs, but the establishment of such a relationship does not require a different pathogenetic mechanism since the gene effect would apparently be directed at the neural component. Syndromes in the Charolais, Friesian, Swedish, and Red Danish breeds of cattle, sometimes associated with cleft palate, are consistent with that of a simple recessive or modified recessive characteristic. *Environmental toxins or viruses* may result in a similar disease pattern. The viruses of Akabane disease, Cache Valley fever, bluetongue, and border disease cause outbreaks of arthrogryposis in cattle and/or sheep. *Lupinus laxiflorus* (wild lupine), and other plant toxins, also cause deformities in fetuses when they are ingested by the dam during early pregnancy (see Vol. 1, Bones and joints).

Congenital flexures

Pastern contracture and immobility by itself can sometimes be part of arthrogryposis. If the flexure is combined with some degree of distal limb rotation, the pathogenesis is likely to be associated with neural and muscle changes as a minor expression of arthrogryposis. Many lambs, foals, and calves are born with an apparent inability to straighten the fetlock and sometimes other distal joints, yet deformities are minimal and muscle loss is not apparent. The problem in these cases seems to relate to the holding of the affected joint or joints in flexion without relief during a period of time in late gestation. The affected muscles appear to have reacted as they would following tenotomy by losing sarcomeres from the ends of myofibrils. This makes the joint initially incapable of extension, but under more or less constant tension the lost sarcomeres are quickly returned in hours or days. Such an explanation seems applicable because many affected foals and lambs recover completely within a few days to weeks. The original joint-fixing event can only be guessed at, but it would be easy to understand how it might happen in species in which the fetal size and limb length are high in relation to dam size.

Bibliography

Abbott LC, et al. Crooked calf disease: a histological and histochemical examination of eight affected calves. Vet Pathol 1986;23:734–740.

Banker BQ. Arthrogryposis multiplex congenita: spectrum of pathologic changes. Human Pathol 1986;17:656–672.

Cho DY, Leipold HW. Congenital defects of the bovine central nervous system. Vet Bull 1977;47:489–504.

Edwards JF, et al. Ovine arthrogryposis and central nervous system malformations associated with in utero Cache Valley virus infection: spontaneous disease. Vet Pathol 1989;26:33–39.

Gardner-Medwin D. Neuromuscular disorders in infancy and childhood. In: Walton G, Karpati G, et al., eds. Disorders of Voluntary Muscle. 6th ed. New York: Churchill-Livingstone, 1994:809-811.

Hartley WJ, et al. Serological evidence for the association of Akabane virus with epizootic bovine congenital arthrogryposis and hydranencephaly syndromes in New South Wales. Aust Vet J 1975;51:103.

Haughey KG, et al. Akabane disease in sheep. Aust Vet J 1988;65:136–140.

Mayhew IG. Neuromuscular arthrogryposis multiplex congenita in a thoroughbred foal. Vet Pathol 1984;21:187–192.

Nawrot PS, et al., Arthrogryposis: an inherited defect in newborn calves. Aust Vet J 1980;56:359–364.

Nes N, et al., Hereditary lethal arthrogryposis ("muscle contracture") in horses. Nord Vet-Med 1982;34:425–430.

Russell RG, et al. Variability in limb malformations and possible significance in the pathogenesis of an inherited congenital neuromuscular disease of Charolais cattle (syndrome of arthrogryposis and palatoschisis). Vet Pathol 1985;22:2–12.

Muscular defects

Defects in the form and disposition of muscles associated with neuraxial deformities are quite common but there are four syndromes of importance affecting muscle that are not associated with lesions in nervous tissue.

"Splayleg" (myofibrillar hypoplasia) in piglets

Splayleg, *also called spraddle-leg, is a disease of neonatal piglets.* It occurs in all countries with a well-developed pig-rearing industry. The incidence of the disease fluctuates inexplicably but frequently appears as a farm or regional outbreak. The disease incidence within litters is variable and a sow may produce consecutive litters with the disease. Genetic predisposition and infectious or nutritional causes are postulated but not proven.

Piglets with splayleg assume a posture with the hindlegs or all four legs laterally extended (Fig. 2.34). They are apparently unable to adduct them or retrieve them from a forward or backward position. Mobility is reduced and affected pigs are susceptible to accidents or may starve due to an inability to compete to suckle. *The locomotor defect is transient and within a week, or at most two, survivors appear normal.*

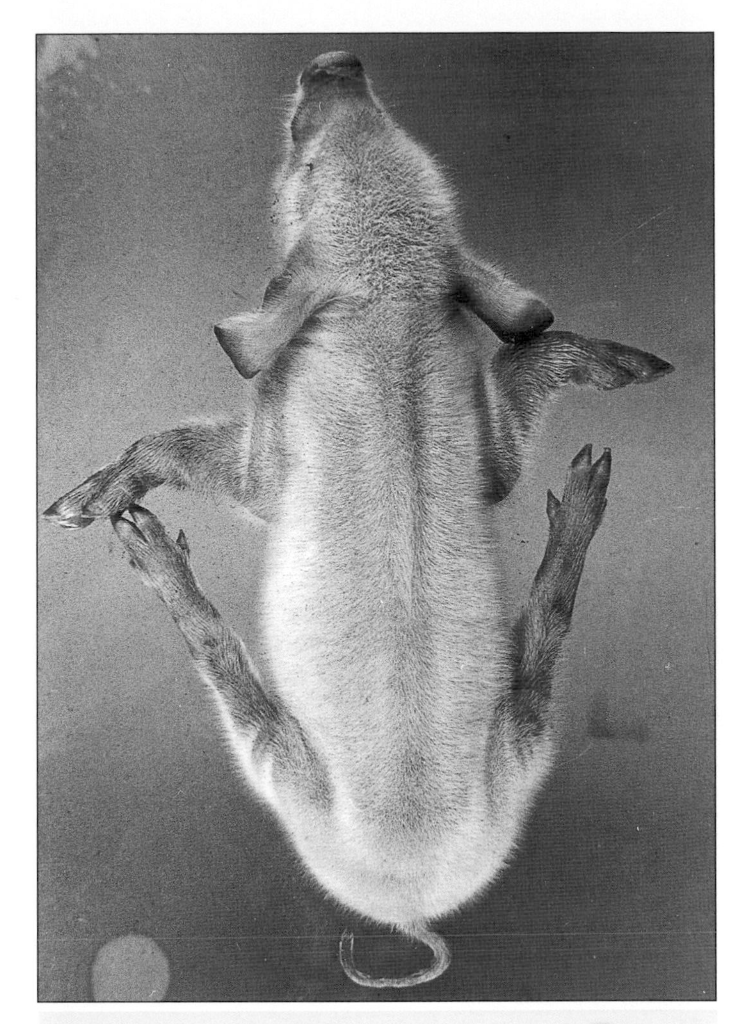

Figure 2.34 Piglet with **splayleg**. (Courtesy of TJ Hulland.)

The clinical signs of splayleg reflect muscle weakness. Not all piglets suffering from splayleg have primary muscle disease; other conditions cause similar signs, but much less frequently. Developmental abnormalities of spinal closure may be responsible (see Arthrogryposis and dysraphism) and myopathy induced by the injection of saccharated iron may produce a similar syndrome in one or more litters. The splayleg syndrome described here is unrelated to either of the above causes. The most common finding in skeletal muscle of affected pigs is *reduced diameter of myofibers with an abnormally small mass of myofibrils within individual muscle fibers* (Fig. 2.35A, B), and increased cytoplasmic glycogen filling the large extramyofibrillar spaces. It is also possible, however, to find the same histologic picture of apparent myofiber immaturity in clinically normal neonatal piglets. It may be that subtle differences in the degree of myofiber immaturity is the explanation for the variable clinical expression.

In the late intrauterine development of skeletal muscles in pigs, the muscle mass is increased by the *"stem line-template" method of new muscle fiber production.* A large type 1 muscle fiber centrally located within a sublobule (a segment of a primary bundle) of developing

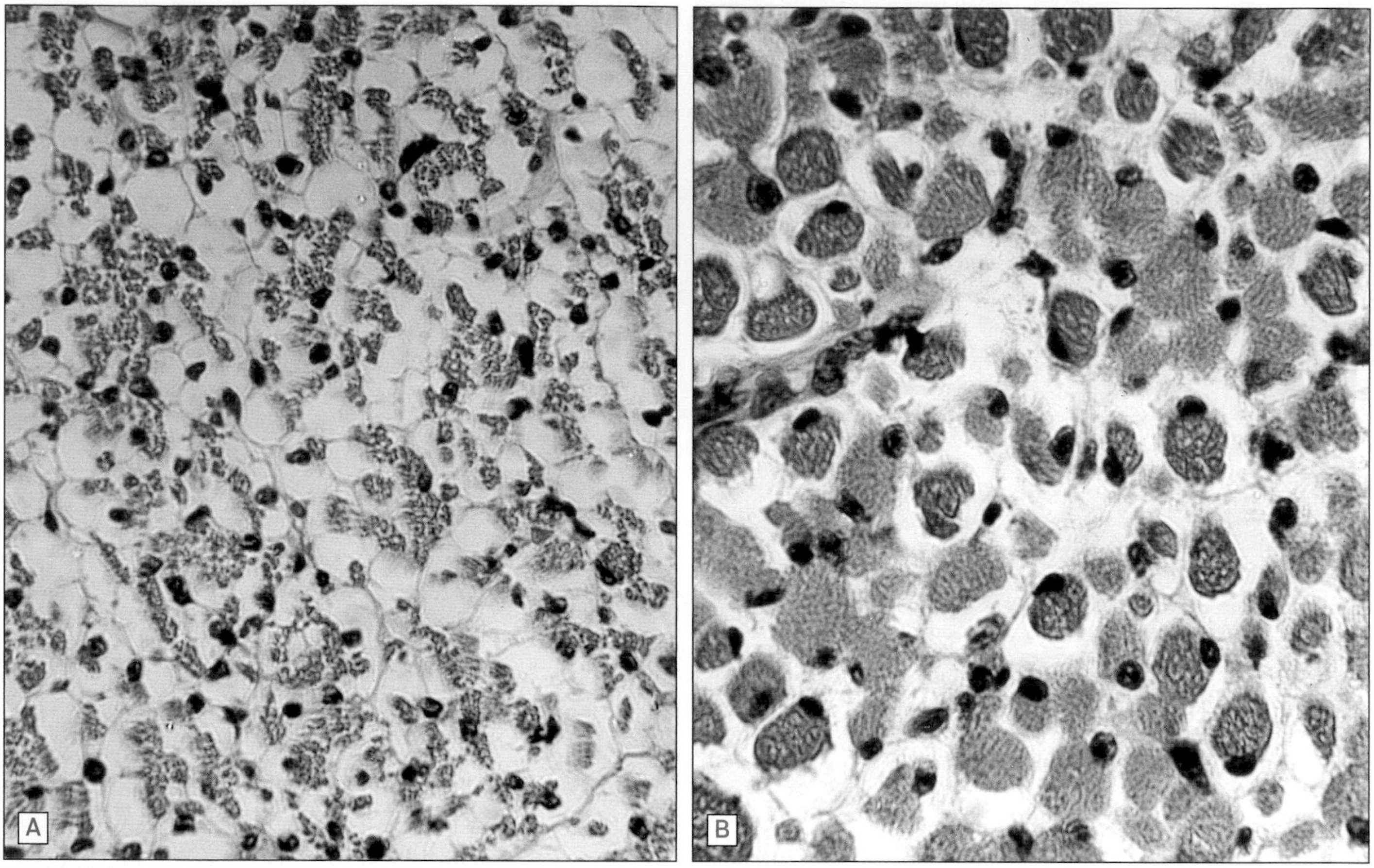

Figure 2.35 **A.** Reduced diameter of myofibers in a neonatal piglet with **splayleg**. (Courtesy of W Hadlow.) **B. Normal** neonatal piglet muscle. (Courtesy of W Hadlow.)

muscle apparently divides longitudinally to create a smaller daughter fiber, or acts as a template beside which a new fiber evolves from myoblasts. The new fiber has characteristics of a type 2 fiber. The central template fiber continues to spawn new fibers, gradually pushing those formed earlier to the periphery and thereby creating a sublobule of 10–20 fibers. Beginning at about the time of birth, a few of the most recently formed type 2 fibers adjacent to the primary or template fiber take on the characteristics of the central type 1 fiber. This early postnatal period also seems to mark the end of vigorous new fiber production, although some increase may continue in some circumstances. In the critical period just before and just after birth, splayleg pigs show an irregularity or retardation in the transition of type 2 fibers to type 1 fibers in the central sublobular region. *These findings in pigs with splayleg suggest delayed maturation of muscle in utero.* Examination of muscle from recovered piglets indicates that postnatal maturation continues, and the muscles from such pigs are indistinguishable from control piglets.

The characteristic lesions of myofibrillar hypoplasia are only partly revealed by light microscopy. Affected muscles, chiefly the longissimus, semitendinosus, and triceps, are incompletely or irregularly involved, and *the most obvious change is lightness of staining with eosin due to the low volume of myofibrils within outer cell membranes of normal volume.* The remainder of the fiber sheath appears to be empty but sometimes contains a nucleus or thin pink proteinaceous fluid. In longitudinal section, myofibrils appear to be diluted by watery fluid or clear strips of space. PAS staining reveals *marked accumulation of cytoplasmic glycogen.*

Electron microscopic examination of muscle from pigs with splayleg reveals segmental Z-line distortion with dispersal of the electron-dense material (Z-line streaming), loss of register and alignment of sarcomeres, reduced volume of myofilaments, and myofilament splitting and disarray. Glycogen granules are abundant, and there are increased numbers of ribosomes. Although degenerative changes, including increased phagolysosomes and lysis of myofilaments, have been described, this is not a consistent finding.

Myofibrillar hypoplasia has been reported as an isolated case in a *6-week-old calf.* Lesions very similar to those in splayleg pigs were seen. A clinical syndrome similar to splayleg occurs in puppies, and affected pups are known as "*swimmer pups*." Affected pups may have underlying myopathy or neuropathy, but more often this syndrome is seen in rapidly growing, overnourished pups. Dorsoventral flattening of the sternum often occurs. Affected pups often recover completely if measures such as use of a type of harness to help keep legs under the body and assisted exercise are employed.

"Double muscling" (muscular hyperplasia) in cattle

Economic pressure to produce beef cattle with increased muscling has undoubtedly led to perpetuation of multiple genetic defects involving muscle development. The best characterized of these is the defect known as double muscling. This disorder occurs within several beef breeds, including Charolais, Santa Gertrudis, South Devon, Angus, Belgian Blue, Belgian White, and Piedmontese cattle.

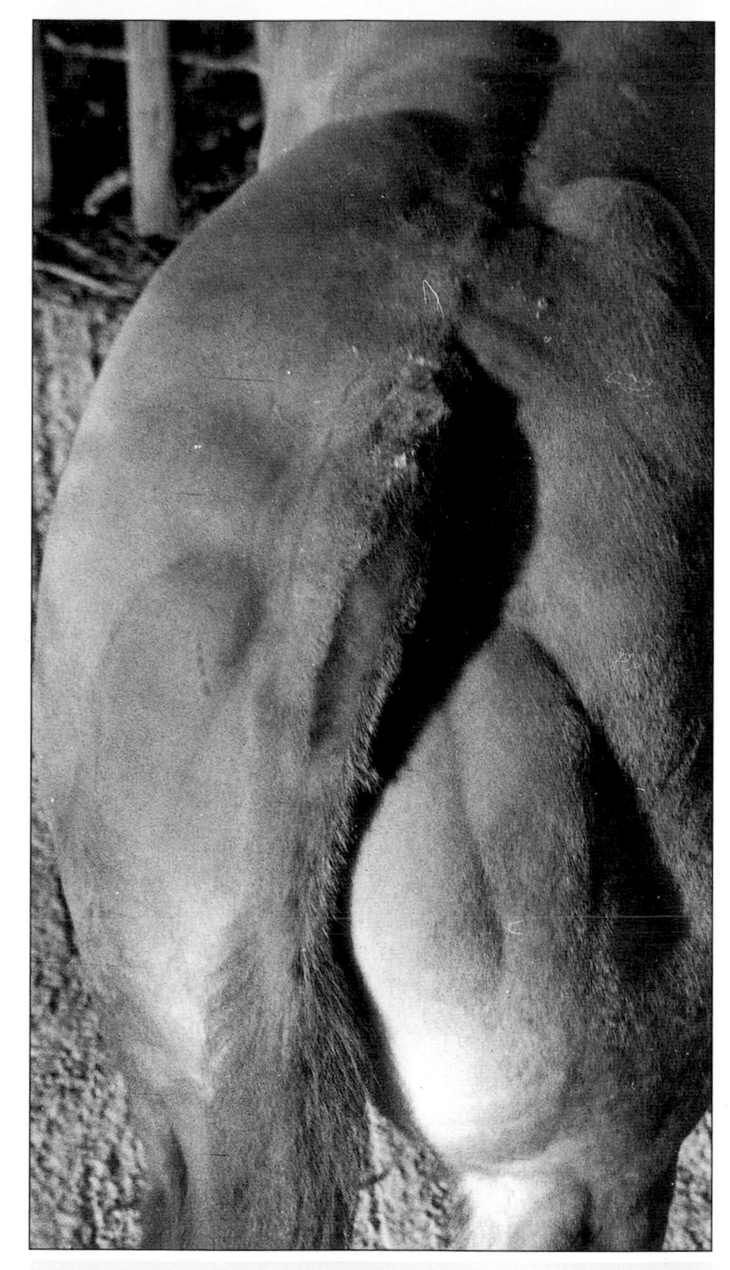

Figure 2.36 Congenital muscular hyperplasia in a calf. (Courtesy of JC MacKellar.)

It is characterized by an *increase in the number of fibers in affected muscles. The individual fibers are of normal size and structure.* This is in contrast to findings in other cattle with increased muscle bulk that are not double-muscled, in which a normal number of hypertrophied muscle fibers is found. In double-muscled homozygotes showing the full effect of the hyperplasia, the increase in gross muscle size is substantial, although not twice normal as the common name "double muscle" might suggest. In fact, the contours of the large muscles are regular and normal except for rather prominent topographical clefts between muscles which are associated with large individual muscle size, reduced body fat proportion and thin skin (Fig. 2.36). Bones may be lighter than normal and are often marginally shorter. Probably all striated muscles of the body are affected to some degree but *the muscles showing the most obvious change are those of the thighs, rump, loin, and shoulder* giving the calf a very athletic appearance and predisposing to dystocia. Some fiber increase is manifested by heterozygotes but the level of heritability seems to be low and subject to capricious variability of penetrance or expression. A higher proportion of type 2B glycolytic fibers and a decreased capillary density are found in muscle from doubled-muscled cattle.

This disorder has been found to be due to *genetic defects in the myostatin gene*, which normally functions to limit skeletal muscle growth. Other genes are likely to be involved in the development of double muscling, as the degree of double muscling in Belgian Blue cattle is significantly greater than in double-muscled Piedmontese cattle, despite the fact that both breeds have genetic defects that apparently result in inactivation of myostatin.

Muscular hyperplasia is also well documented in the *Callipyge phenotype in sheep* – the disease is only seen in heterozygote males and the molecular basis of the defect is associated with a mutation on chromosome 18. The condition is associated with hyperplasia of hindquarters and hindlimb musculature.

Muscular steatosis

Muscular steatosis *is a disease characterized by too much fat deposited within muscles.* It carries an inference that the fat is where muscle once was or ought to have been; effectively, *fat replacement of muscle fibers*. Fat infiltration of muscle is a *common nonspecific finding in chronic myopathic and neuropathic disorders that affect muscle.* The adipocytes that infiltrate muscle are derived from intramuscular mesenchymal cells. Fat infiltration may be accompanied by variable degrees of fibrosis. Steatosis of muscle is *best considered a reaction of chronically damaged or denervated muscle*, rather than a true developmental muscular defect.

The syndrome known as muscular steatosis in livestock is not typically associated with fibrosis. *It appears in clinically healthy animals, and it is usually a problem only in meat inspection.* Although previous damage due to neural lesions, nutritional myopathy, exertional myopathy, ischemia, or trauma are possible underlying causes, in most cases an exact cause is not determined. Studies on steatosis in normal market pig carcasses indicate that about 1–5% of pigs have small steatotic lesions and that a smaller proportion have extensive lesions of the anterior thigh or loin muscles (Fig. 2.37).

Sometimes the steatosis affects several muscles of one limb, but more often it affects only one or several muscles in one region. It may be bilaterally symmetrical or asymmetrical. Rarely does it affect all of one muscle and the dividing line between normal and fatty muscle is not sharp. Surviving muscle fibers in the marginal areas may be normal or smaller than normal but are often angular in fixed tissue as a result of adjacent pressure from turgid lipocytes.

Congenital clefts of the diaphragm

The embryologic development of the diaphragm is complex, with contributions from several different tissues. The septum transversum forms the central tendon, the dorsal aspect of the caudal mediastinum (the dorsal mesoesophagus) forms the diaphragm surrounding the esophagus and aorta, and the right and left pleuroperitoneal membranes fuse to close the pleuroperitoneal canals and form the final complete diaphragm.

Congenital diaphragmatic clefts affect all species either alone or as part of a more generalized malformation. *The most common defect involves the left dorsolateral and central portions of the diaphragm, indicative of failure of closure of the left pleuroperitoneal canal.* The clefts may permit

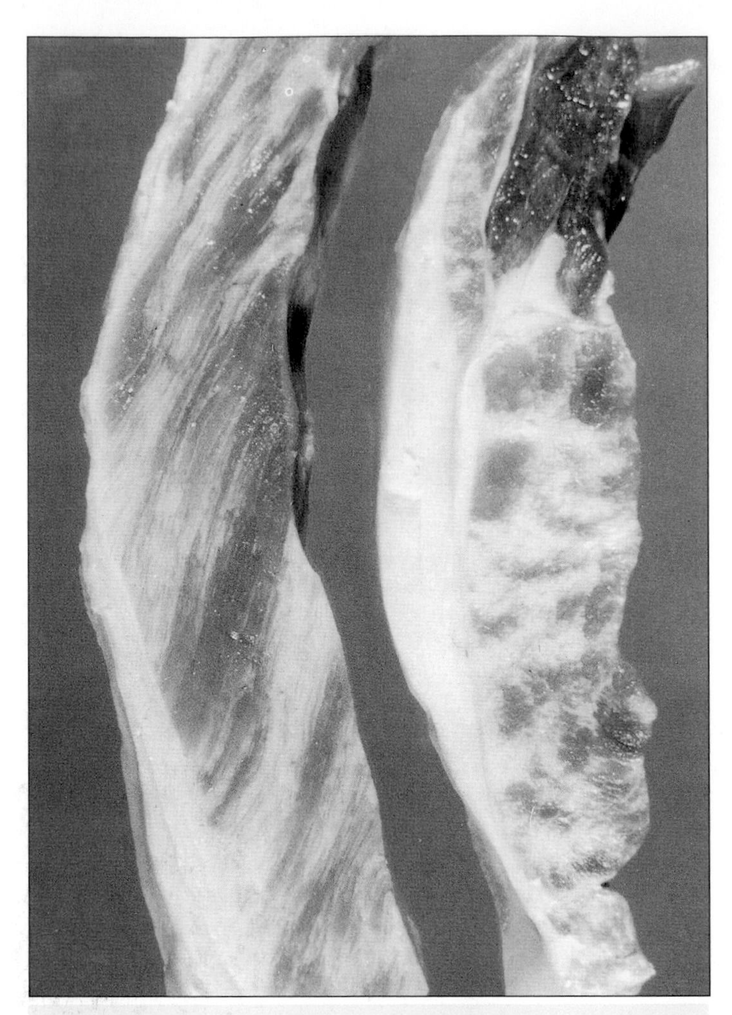

Figure 2.37 Steatosis of the loin muscle of a clinically normal pig. (Courtesy of TJ Hulland.)

the herniation of tissues ranging in size from a small button of liver to extensive displacement of viscera. In very large congenital clefts, the diaphragm may be represented by only a narrow rim of muscle that does little more than mark the diaphragmatic origin. Congenital clefts must be differentiated from acquired but healed lacerations of the diaphragm. The occurrence of congenital diaphragmatic hernia is best documented in the *dog* and in the *rabbit*. In the dog, incomplete closure of the left pleuroperitoneal canal is most common. In the rabbit, both defective closure of the left pleuroperitoneal membrane and absence of the major portion of the left diaphragm have been reported. Autosomal recessive inheritance has been proposed in both dogs and rabbits. The occurrence of congenital diaphragmatic hernias in five of 27 puppies from three father–daughter matings would support this form of inheritance, however further inbreeding of this particular colony of dogs failed to produce any subsequent pups with diaphragmatic hernias, suggesting that the genetic defect is likely to involve multiple genes.

Bibliography

Bidwell CA, et al. Differential expression of the GTL2 gene within the callipyge region of ovine chromosome 18. Anim Genet 2001;32:248–256.

Bradley R, et al. The ultrastructural morphology of the skeletal muscles of normal pigs and pigs with splayleg from birth to one week of age. J Comp Pathol 1980;90:433–446.

Butterfield RM. Muscular hypertrophy of cattle. Aust Vet J 1966;42:37–39.

Carpenter CE, et al. Histology and composition of muscles from normal and callipyge lambs. J Anim Sci 1996;74:388–393.

Dickman S. Gene mutation provides more meat on the hoof. Science 1997; 277:1922–1923.

Ducatelle R, et al. Spontaneous and experimental myofibrillar hypoplasia and its relation to splayleg in newborn pigs. J Comp Pathol 1986;96:433–445.

Geesink GH, Koohmaraie M. Postmortem proteolysis and calpain/palpstatin activity in callipyge and normal lamb biceps femoris during extended post mortem storage. J Anim Sci 1999;77: 1490–1501.

Grobet L, et al. A deletion in the bovine myostatin gene causes the double-muscled phenotype in cattle. Nat Genet 1997;17:71–74.

Ott RS. Muscular hypertrophy in beef cattle: déjà vu. J Am Vet Med Assoc 1990;196:413–415.

Stavaux D, et al. Muscle fibre type and size, and muscle capillary density in young double-muscled blue Belgian cattle. Zentralbl Veterinarmed [A] 1994;41:229–236.

Swatland HJ. Developmental disorders of skeletal muscle in cattle, pigs and sheep. Vet Bull 1974;44:179–202.

Szalay F, et al. Retarded myelination in the lumbar spinal cord of piglets born with spread-leg syndrome. Anat Embryol 2001;203:53–59.

Valentine BA, et al. Canine congenital diaphragmatic hernia. J Vet Int Med 1988;2:109–112.

Muscular dystrophy

The muscular dystrophies of humans are defined as inherited progressive myopathies characterized histologically by ongoing muscle fiber degeneration and regeneration. Peripheral nerves and neuromuscular junctions are normal, although a recent study in humans and mice found cognitive disorders and increased susceptibility of the CNS to injury in individuals with Duchenne dystrophy. The advent of molecular genetics has begun to further designate these disorders according to their genetic basis and has aided in validating several animal disorders as true animal models of human disease. Given the high conservation of genes on the mammalian X chromosome, it was suspected that progressive degenerative myopathies inherited as an X-linked recessive trait in animals were likely to be homologs of the X-linked Duchenne and Becker muscular dystrophies of humans. Molecular genetic analysis has proven this to be the case. **True muscular dystrophy**, *homologous to Duchenne and Becker muscular dystrophy of humans, occurs in the dog, cat, and mouse.* Duchenne and Becker muscular dystrophy are X-linked recessive disorders of humans caused by defects in the gene coding for dystrophin, a sarcolemmal-associated cytoskeletal protein. Immunostaining of frozen sections of muscle and Western blot analysis for dystrophin in snap-frozen muscle samples are necessary for confirmation of dystrophin-deficient muscular dystrophy. It is interesting that dystrophin deficiency results in progressive muscle atrophy in most breeds of dogs, but causes marked muscular hypertrophy in the mouse, cat, and Rat Terrier dog. Muscle fiber hypertrophy occurs, especially in early stages of the disorder, but extensive fiber necrosis leads to overall muscle atrophy in most cases. At this time there is no explanation for this phenomenon, although it would appear that muscle hypertrophy is more apparent in animals of small stature.

In animals, a number of muscle disorders have been erroneously designated as "muscular dystrophy," most notably those degenerative myopathies occurring secondary to nutritional deficiency. An inherited progressive myopathy in sheep has been described as a muscular dystrophy and is included in this section, although this disorder might be better classified as a congenital progressive myopathy because cytoarchitectural alterations are the hallmarks of this disorder, and on-going fiber degeneration and regeneration are not typical features. Other inherited myopathies in dogs and cattle, many of which have been described as muscular dystrophies, are considered to be less likely candidates for true muscular dystrophy and are described in the Congenital myopathy section.

Canine X-linked muscular dystrophy

Sporadic reports from around the world of a severe progressive degenerative myopathy affecting young male dogs led to the establishment of a breeding colony of affected Golden Retriever dogs. Although a similar disorder has now been identified in many breeds, including Irish Terrier, Samoyed, Rottweiler, Dalmatian, Shetland Sheepdog, Labrador Retriever, German Shorthaired Pointer, Brittany Spaniel, Rat Terrier, Belgian Groenendael Shepherd, and Schnauzer, *the disease is best characterized in the Golden Retriever.*

Affected pups may be normal or slightly small at birth. Some affected pups may show severe progressive weakness leading to death within the first few weeks of life. This may be particularly true of affected pups in large litters that include normal and carrier pups, and may in part be due to inability to compete for food. Other pups show no signs of disease until approximately 8 weeks of age, when reduced jaw mobility, exercise intolerance, and a stiff-legged gait become apparent. Serum activities of creatine kinase (CK) and aspartate aminotransferase (AST) are, however, markedly increased, indicative of severe myodegeneration, even in neonates with inapparent disease, and levels of CK and AST continue to rise until peaking at about 6 months of age. Serum CK and AST levels in older dogs are always high, but tend to be decreased as compared to younger dystrophic dogs. Serum activities of CK and AST are highest if blood is drawn 4–6 hours after exercise. *Clinical signs of neuromuscular weakness are progressive until approximately 8–12 months of age, when the disease tends to stabilize.* The severity of the disorder is variable, with some dogs developing severe muscle atrophy and contractures by 6 months of age (Fig. 2.38) and others remaining stiff, muscle wasted, and exercise intolerant but without severe impairment of joint mobility. Dystrophic dogs have a characteristic stiff-legged shuffling gait and a thickening of the muscles of the base of the tongue and under the jaw, tend to drool excessively, and develop abdominal breathing and often deformation of the ribcage due to diaphragmatic contracture. Esophageal dysfunction is common, and dystrophic dogs may develop aspiration pneumonia due to regurgitation. The severity of the disease varies among breeds. Although muscle atrophy is more obvious than hypertrophy in the Golden Retriever and Rottweiler, in other breeds such as the Rat Terrier there is progressive development of muscular hypertrophy resulting in obvious increased bulk, particularly involving muscles of the thigh, neck, and shoulder girdle. Breed size may have some role in the type and severity of changes, with larger breeds being most severely affected. Female carriers are clinically normal, although higher than normal levels of serum CK and AST are apparent, particularly in carriers under 6 months of age.

Concentric needle electromyography reveals marked spontaneous activity in the muscles of dystrophic dogs. Although the complex repetitive activity generated by canine dystrophic muscle was initially interpreted as a myotonia, resulting in characterization of this disorder as a myotonic myopathy, careful analysis of the electrical activity indicates that these bursts do not wax and wane but rather start and

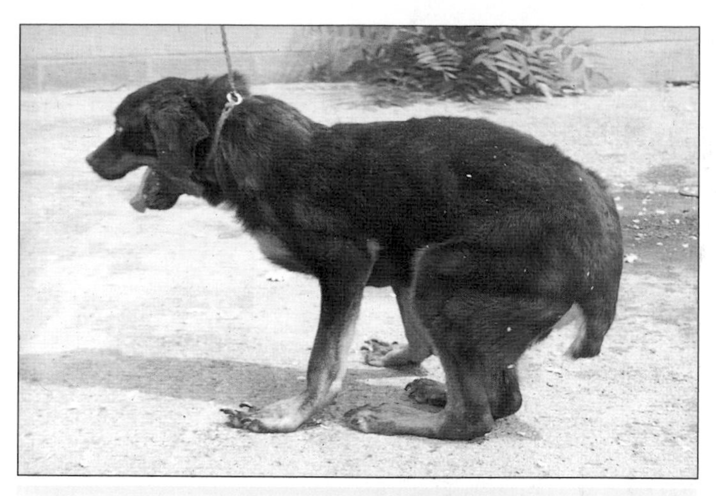

Figure 2.38 One-year-old male Rottweiler dog with severe **X-linked muscular dystrophy**.

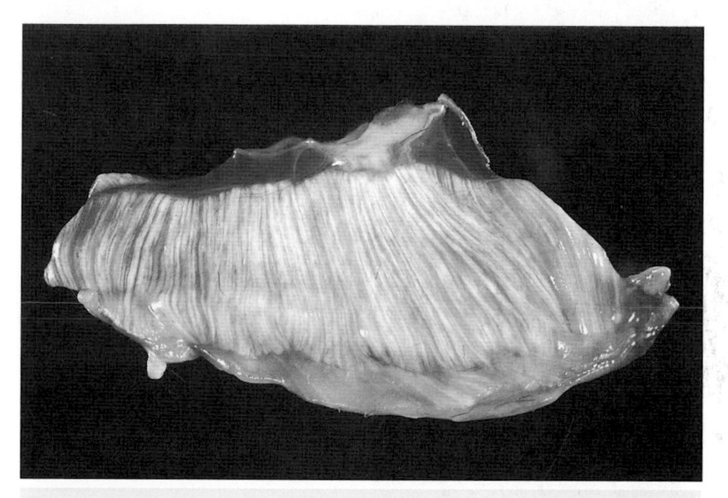

Figure 2.39 Pale streaking of diaphragm muscle due to **massive necrosis** in a neonatal pup with fulminant X-linked muscular dystrophy. (From McGavin MD, Zachary JF. Pathologic Basis of Veterinary Disease, 2006, with permission of Elsevier Ltd.)

stop abruptly and are *characteristic of pseudomyotonia.* Although the exact cause of this electrical activity is not known, membrane instability associated with clusters of degenerating and regenerating fibers is suspected.

Pups dying with fulminant neonatal disease have characteristic gross pathologic findings of severe degeneration of the diaphragm and strap muscles, including the trapezius and sartorius muscles of the limbs, characterized by pale white streaks within affected muscles (Fig. 2.39). Histologic evaluation reveals massive acute muscle fiber necrosis and mineralization, and similar findings are present in tongue muscle. This selective involvement of muscles in neonatal pups may reflect exercise-induced injury in muscles used for breathing, crawling, and suckling and may also involve the susceptibility to injury of more mature, larger-diameter fibers.

Gross pathologic examination of affected dogs that survive the neonatal period typically reveals pale musculature that may be slightly firm, especially true of the sartorius muscles of the hindlimbs. The diaphragm often exhibits the most striking changes, with thickening, contracture, and fibrosis evident (Fig. 2.40). On histologic examination, muscle samples exhibit the characteristic findings of muscular dystrophy. *Numerous swollen and dark staining fibers (so-called large dark*

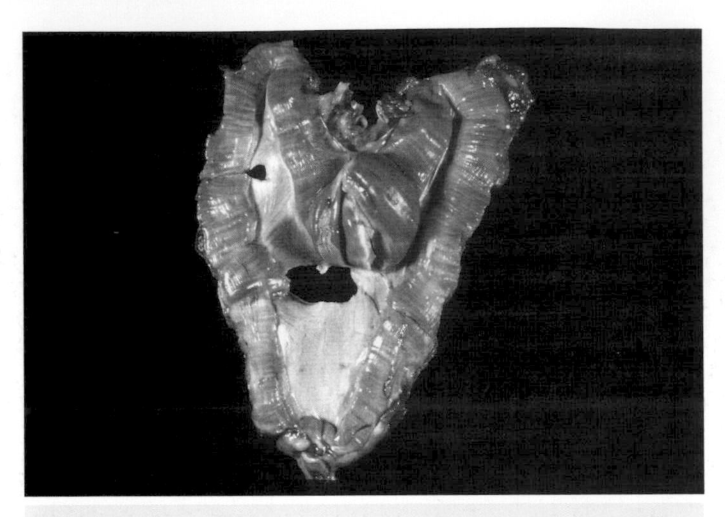

Figure 2.40 Severe diaphragmatic **muscular fibrosis and contraction** in a young adult dog with X-linked muscular dystrophy.

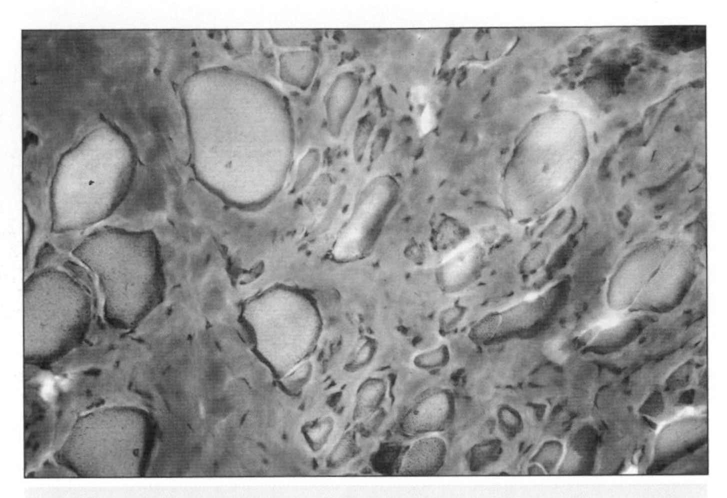

Figure 2.42 **Marked endomysial fibrosis** in the sartorius muscle of a dog with X-linked muscular dystrophy. Remaining fibers have variable diameter and frequently contain internal nuclei. Frozen section, modified Gomori's trichrome.

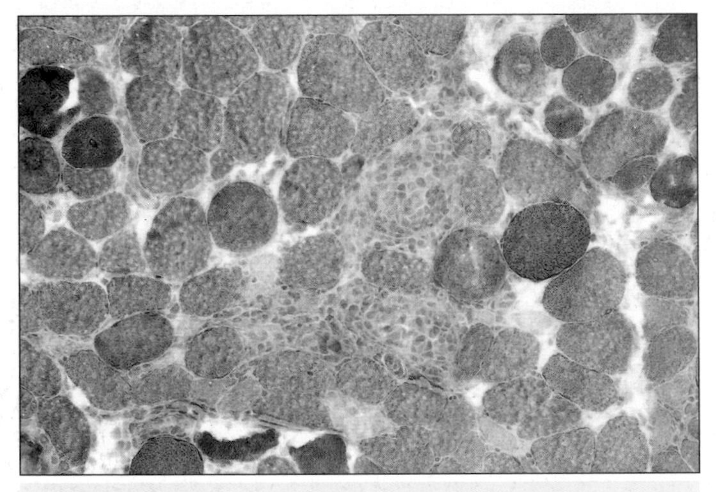

Figure 2.41 Characteristic **multifocal, polyphasic necrosis** in muscle from a dog with X-linked muscular dystrophy. There are characteristic large dark fibers as well as clusters of overtly necrotic fibers with macrophage infiltration. Frozen section, modified Gomori's trichrome. (Courtesy of BJ Cooper.)

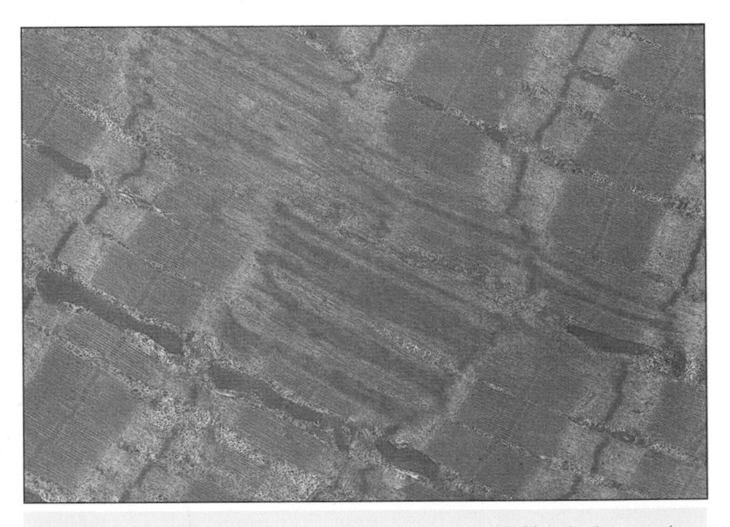

Figure 2.43 **Streaming of Z bands** in a pup with X-linked muscular dystrophy.

fibers) are seen throughout the sections and are considered to be the earliest stage of muscle fiber degeneration. Small clusters of overtly *necrotic fibers*, either in a coagulative state or macrophage-infiltrated, and of *regenerate fibers* are seen (multifocal, polyphasic necrosis; Fig. 2.41). Scattered *mineralized fibers* are common. The basal lamina of necrotic fiber segments is preserved, resulting in the presence of "empty sarcolemmal tubes" and in the ability to fully regenerate affected fiber segments. Muscle spindles are unaffected. With increasing age the degree of overt fiber necrosis and regeneration decreases. In *older dystrophic dogs*, marked fiber size variation, with internal nuclei, cytoarchitectural changes including nemaline rods, and a type 1 fiber predominance may be seen. Endomysial fibrosis and fat infiltration, the hallmark of advanced Duchenne dystrophy in boys, occurs in some muscles (Fig. 2.42), but is variable and typically less apparent in the dog.

In addition to evidence of fiber necrosis and regeneration, ultrastructural studies of muscle from dystrophic dogs have found small areas of apparent sarcolemmal defects in otherwise normal-appearing fibers. *Non-specific cytoarchitectural changes*, including increased mitochondrial content and Z-line streaming are also seen (Fig. 2.43). Alizarin red staining of frozen sections has confirmed that influx of calcium, probably through defects in the sarcolemma, is an early event leading to muscle fiber necrosis in dystrophic muscle (Fig. 2.44). Although considered to be an essential cytoskeletal protein and known to be part of a membrane-associated complex, *the exact function of dystrophin and the cause of muscle fiber necrosis in dystrophin-deficient muscle is still not clear.*

Cardiac muscle of dystrophic dogs 6 months or older exhibits myofiber necrosis, mineralization, and fibrosis of the myocardium in a subepicardial pattern. The left ventricular wall and right side of the interventricular septum are most severely affected (Fig. 2.45). The development of *progressive degenerative cardiomyopathy* is a hallmark of Duchenne and Becker muscular dystrophy in man, and often eventually results in congestive heart failure in older dystrophic dogs.

Immunostaining of frozen sections for dystrophin typically reveals complete absence of this sarcolemmal-associated protein (Fig. 2.46A, B), although partial expression may be present in Becker-type mutations or in so-called revertant fibers, which are fibers that have undergone genetic mutation allowing dystrophin expression. Cardiac muscle in dystrophic dogs completely lacks dystrophin. Although dystrophin expression has been absent or nearly absent in the dystrophic dogs

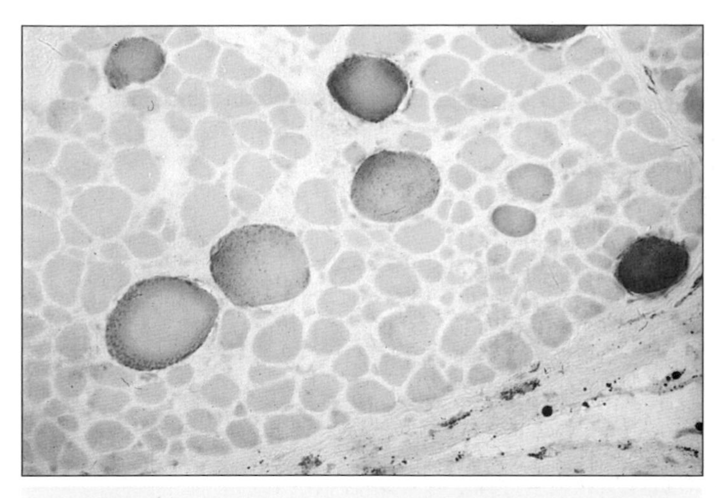

Figure 2.44 Numerous large apparently intact fibers with dark staining due to **calcium influx** indicative of sarcolemmal damage in a dog with X-linked muscular dystrophy. Frozen section, alizarin red S.

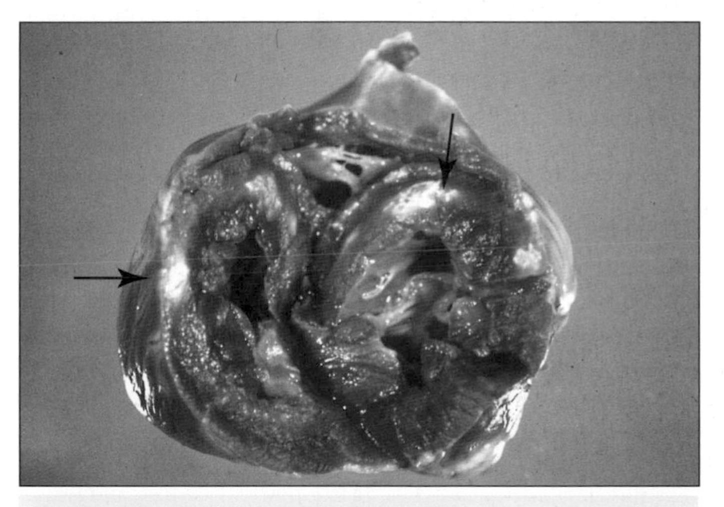

Figure 2.45 Multifocal pale zones of **myocardial necrosis and mineralization** (arrows) within the left ventricular wall and interventricular septum of a dog with X-linked muscular dystrophy. (Courtesy of BJ Cooper.)

studied to date, it is possible that animals expressing an abnormal truncated or elongated dystrophin will be found.

Muscle from young female carriers often contains numerous large dark fibers and scattered necrotic and regenerating fibers. The degree of overt necrosis and regeneration appears to be less than the proportion of large dark fibers seen, suggesting that membrane repair in some large dark fibers is possible. By about 6 months of age, evidence of degeneration or regeneration is rare. This reflects the mosaic pattern of dystrophin expression in carrier muscle. This mosaic pattern is most apparent in neonatal carriers, with loss of skeletal muscle mosaicism by about 6 months of age. This phenomenon is thought to reflect up-regulation or translocation of dystrophin throughout the mosaic muscle fiber. Cardiac muscle, composed of uninucleate cells incapable of regeneration, maintains a striking mosaicism for dystrophin for the life of the animal, and carrier females also develop cardiac muscle necrosis and progressive fibrosis in a pattern similar to that seen in dystrophic males. Curiously, although the fibrosis of cardiac muscle in older female carriers is quite striking, overt cardiac failure does not occur.

Feline X-linked muscular dystrophy

As in studies of canine muscular dystrophy, the recognition of a severe progressive degenerative myopathy in young male cats led to breeding studies of affected cats. To date, this disorder has only been reported in cats of mixed breeding. Its occurrence in Europe as well as North America suggests that, similar to canine X-linked muscular dystrophy, the feline dystrophin gene is prone to spontaneous mutation.

Affected cats develop marked muscle hypertrophy, stiff gait, "bunny-hopping" in the rear limbs, reduced activity and difficulty jumping up onto furniture and other objects. Clinical signs may be recognized as early as 5 months or as late as 2 years of age. Thickening of tongue muscle may result in difficulties prehending food and in drooling. Regurgitation due to esophageal dysfunction may also be evident. Given the fairly subtle signs, it is likely that affected cats may not be recognized by owners as being abnormal. Muscular hypertrophy is most evident in the muscles of the neck and proximal limbs (Fig. 2.47). Dystrophic cats are prone to development of a *malignant hyperthermia-like syndrome* associated with restraint or general anesthesia. Serum activities

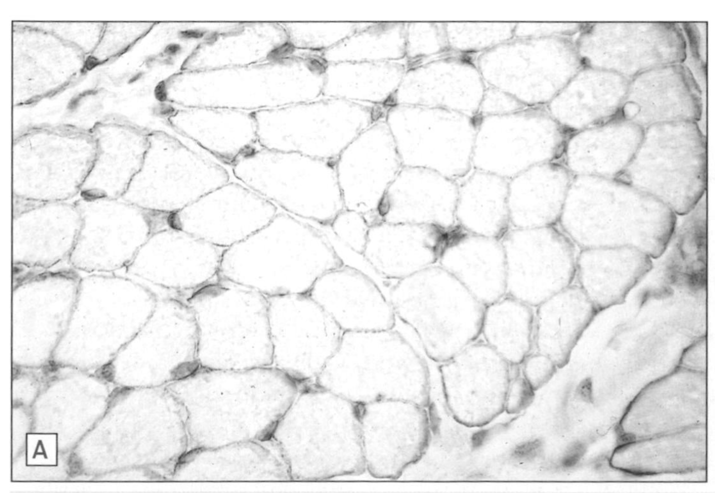

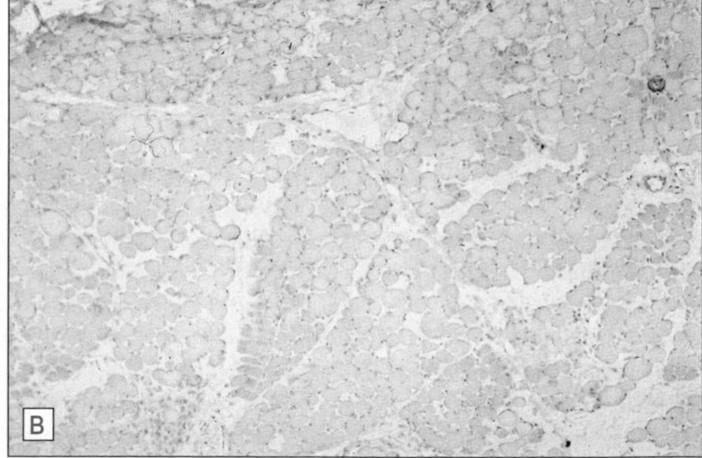

Figure 2.46 **A. Dystrophin** immunostaining of **normal** canine muscle, showing diffuse sarcolemmal staining. Frozen section, immunoperoxidase. (Courtesy of BJ Cooper.) **B. Dystrophin is completely absent** in muscle from a dog with X-linked muscular dystrophy. Frozen section, immunoperoxidase. (Courtesy of BJ Cooper.)

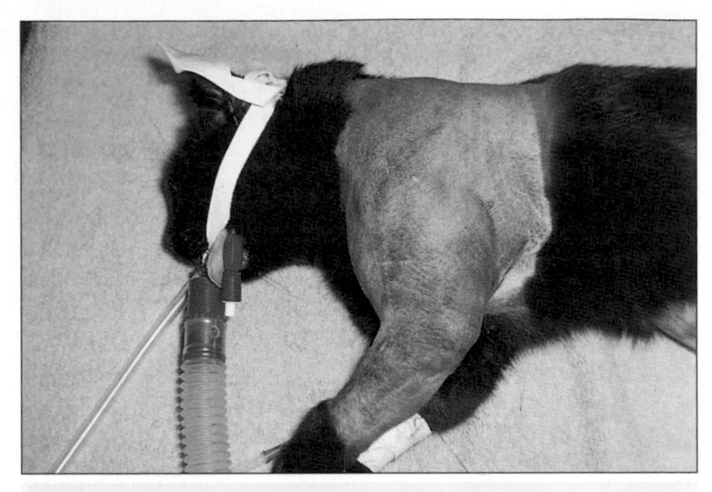

Figure 2.47 Marked hypertrophy of cervical and proximal forelimb muscles in a **cat with X-linked muscular dystrophy**. (Courtesy of BJ Cooper.)

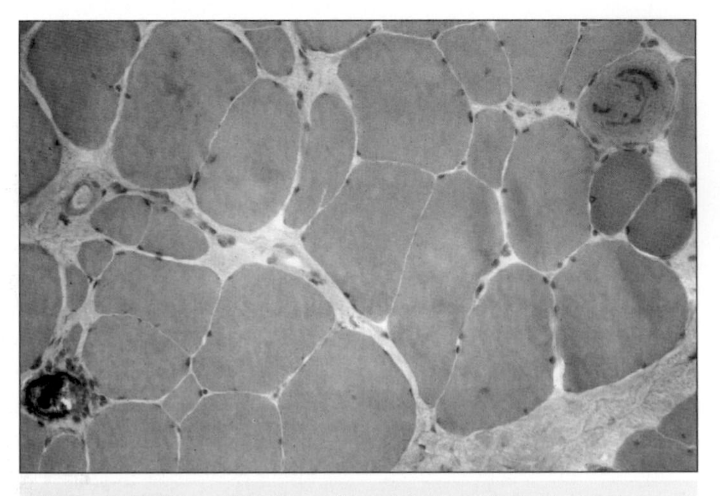

Figure 2.48 Excessive fiber size variation with both atrophy and hypertrophy, internal nuclei, and with scattered mineralized and bizarre fibers, in a cat with X-linked muscular dystrophy. Frozen section H&E. (Courtesy of BJ Cooper.)

of CK and AST are typically very high, and increases can be detected in kittens as young as 3 weeks of age. Electromyographic studies of affected cats reveal bizarre complex repetitive activity similar to that seen in the dystrophic dog.

At necropsy, affected cats have thickening of the muscular wall of the esophagus as well as marked thickening and contraction of the diaphragm. Skeletal muscle is often diffusely pale as well as displaying various degrees of hypertrophy. Pale streaks are often visible in the left ventricular wall and interventricular septum.

Histologic evaluation reveals *marked fiber size variation with numerous hypertrophied fibers often containing multiple internal nuclei.* Scattered clusters of necrotic and regenerating fibers with scattered mineralized myofibers are seen, and fibers with bizarre cytoarchitecture can occur (Fig. 2.48). The degree of myofiber degeneration and regeneration is often less than that seen in dystrophic dogs. Endomysial fibrosis occurs, but is minimal.

Foci of necrosis and mineralization of cardiac myofibers, followed by progressive fibrosis, can be seen in the left ventricular wall and interventricular septum of affected cats in a pattern similar to that seen in dystrophic dogs and in Duchenne and Becker muscular dystrophy. Cardiac lesions are not, however, a consistent finding in dystrophic cats, and clinical signs of cardiac insufficiency have not been reported, although experimental studies using inbred cats demonstrated left ventricular hypertrophy in all affected animals.

Muscular dystrophy, not X-linked, has also been described in cats associated with laminin deficiency. Affected cats developed progressive muscle weakness and atrophy, and also had peripheral neuropathies. In cases that survive for extended periods, fibrous replacement of atrophic muscle is severe.

Ovine muscular dystrophy

Muscular dystrophy of Merino sheep is an autosomal recessive disorder that occurs in widely separated flocks in Australia. This disorder affects about 1–2% of the progeny each year. The sexes are equally affected and *skeletal muscle of affected sheep expresses dystrophin in a normal manner, consistent with the non-X-linked nature of this disorder.* Although similarities to myotonic dystrophy of man have been proposed, there is no compelling evidence that this is the case.

Initial signs are *lack of normal growth and reduced flexion of the hindlimbs* that lead to aberrations of gait or, in mild cases, just stiffness. Subtle clinical signs may be detected in lambs at 3–4 weeks of age. The rate of progression of this disorder is extremely variable but the majority of cases have clear-cut signs of hindlimb gait abnormalities by 6–12 months of age and are severely affected by 2–3 years of age. Under field conditions, the animals often die of inanition at 6–18 months of age. With care, some animals can be maintained for up to 5 years, during which time the clinical disease is slowly progressive. Serum activity of CK is increased at rest in animals with unequivocal clinical signs of muscle dysfunction and is increased further following exercise. No electromyographic abnormalities are found.

On postmortem examination, apart from emaciation, the prominent changes are in the vastus intermedius, soleus, anconeus, and medial head of the triceps, where normal muscle may be replaced by mature adipose tissue. The muscles in advanced cases appear gray, and are hard and atonic. Involvement of other muscles, most often the extensors of the hip, stifle, and hock joints and flexors of the shoulder, carpus, and digits, is limited to microscopic changes only, although these muscles may exhibit some degree of pallor. Affected muscles have a high proportion of type 1 fibers, and it appears that this accounts for the distribution of lesions, as this disorder affects only type 1 fibers.

The initial stages of the dystrophic lesion are heralded by a general hypertrophy of type 1 fibers followed by loss of myofibrils and formation of characteristic sarcoplasmic masses at the periphery or in the central portion of the cell (Fig. 2.49A, B). This is followed by an irregular atrophy of fibers. Fiber proportions remain normal. Compensatory hypertrophy of fibers is often accompanied by fiber splitting, resulting in fiber nesting ("orange section" clusters). A few fibers develop peripheral annular fibrils ("ring fibers," or "ringbinden"). Many fibers acquire internally located nuclei. Hypercontracted fiber segments are observed only sporadically, and regenerative fibers are rare or nonexistent. Muscles undergo progressive loss of fibers which may reach 80–100% in animals over 2 years of age, and undergo progressive fat infiltration and/or endomysial fibrosis (Fig. 2.50A, B, C). In advanced muscle lesions, aggregates of lymphoid and histiocytic cells occur but these seem to be unimportant in the genesis of lesions.

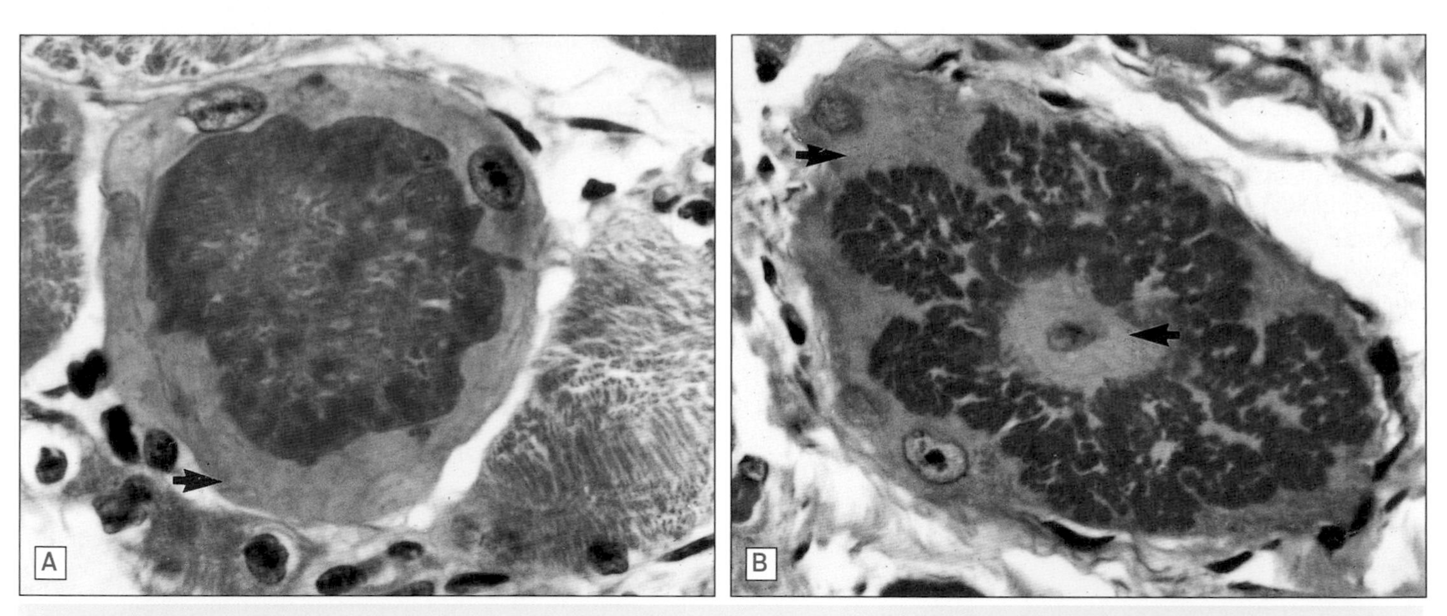

Figure 2.49 Myofibers in the vastus intermedius muscle of a **sheep with muscular dystrophy**. **A.** Myofiber with pale peripheral sarcoplasmic masses (arrow) and large vesicular nuclei. **B.** Myofiber with central and peripheral pale sarcoplasmic masses (arrows) and large vesicular nuclei. (Courtesy of MD McGavin.)

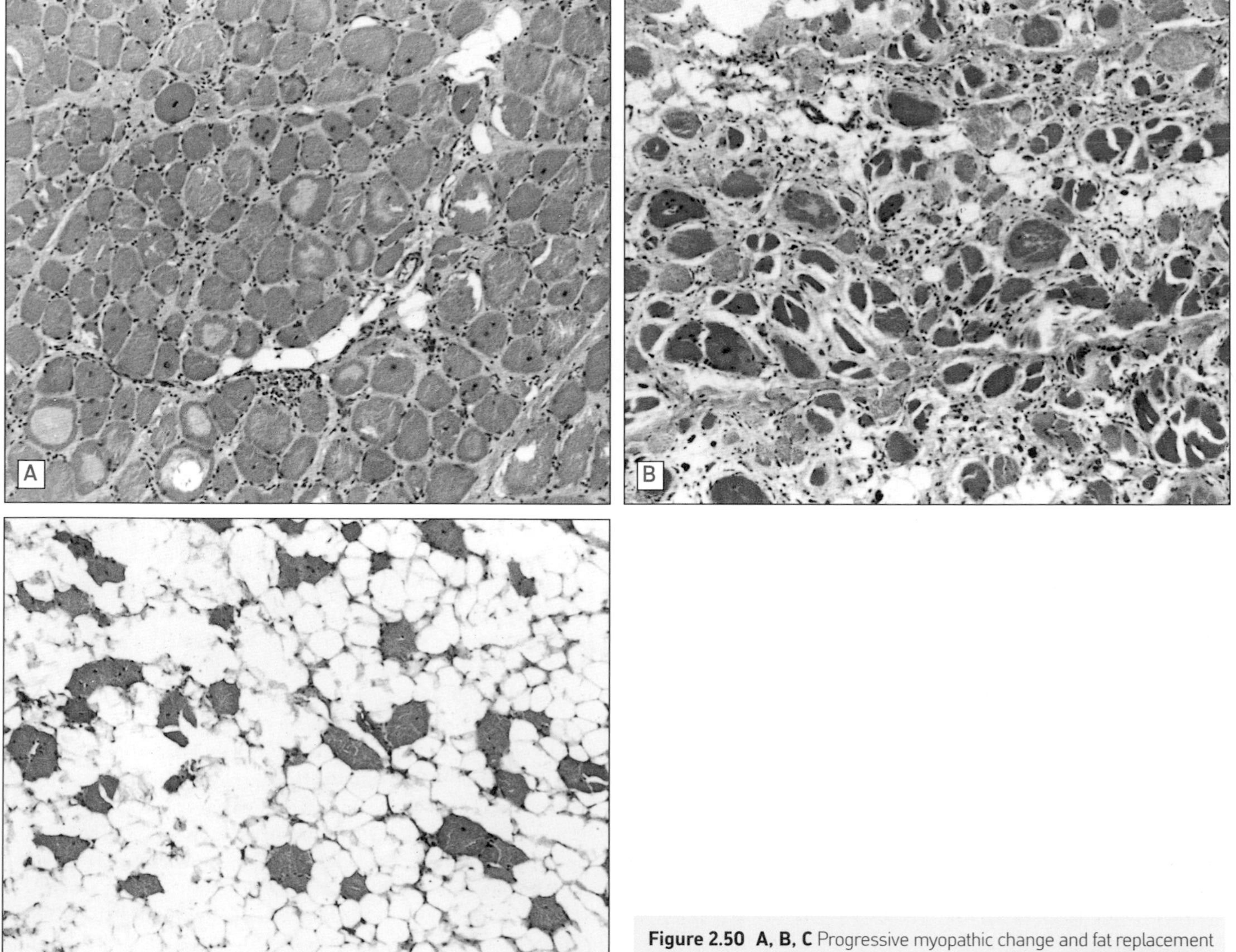

Figure 2.50 A, B, C Progressive myopathic change and fat replacement in the vastus intermedius muscle of a **sheep with muscular dystrophy**. (Courtesy of MD McGavin.)

Ultrastructural findings include *focal myofibril degeneration and Z-line abnormalities, including nemaline rods*. The distinctive sarcoplasmic masses are found to contain a mixture of normal organelles and tubular and fibrillar structures, including abnormal Z-line material. Immunocytochemical studies indicate profound alterations in cytoskeletal elements, including *loss of alpha actinin and proliferation of desmin*. Desmin forms the major constituent of the sarcoplasmic masses. Similar abnormal expression of desmin has been demonstrated in a growing number of myopathies affecting people and animals, and the term "myofibrillar myopathy" has been proposed for such disorders.

Bibliography

Al-Shehab A, et al. Immunocytochemical studies of the cytoskeleton in congenital progressive ovine muscular dystrophy (OD). Acta Cardiomiologica 1994;6:45–57.

Anderson JL, et al. Brain function in Duchenne muscular dystrophy. Brain 2002;125:4–13.

Carpenter JL, et al. Feline muscular dystrophy with dystrophin deficiency. Am J Pathol 1989;135:909–919.

Cooper BJ. Animal models of human muscle disease. In: Karpati G, et al., eds. Disorders of Voluntary Muscle. 7th ed. New York: Cambridge University Press, 2001:187–215.

Cooper BJ, et al. Mosaic expression of dystrophin in carriers of canine X-linked muscular dystrophy. Lab Invest 1990;62:171–178.

Cozzi F, et al. Development of muscle pathology in canine X-linked muscular dystrophy. II. Quantitation characterization of histopathologic progression during postnatal skeletal muscle development. Acta Neuropathol 2001;101:469–478.

De Blecker JL, et al. Part II. Myofibrillar myopathy with abnormal foci of desmin positivity. Immunocytochemical analysis reveals accumulation of multiple other proteins. J Neuropathol Exp Neurol 1996;55:563–577.

Dent AC, et al. Congenital progressive ovine muscular dystrophy in Western Australia. Aust Vet J 1979;55:297.

Gaschen F, et al. Lethal peracute rhabdomyolysis associated with stress and general anesthesia in three dystrophin-deficient cats. Vet Pathol 1998; 35:117–123.

Gaschen F, Burgunder JM. Changes in skeletal muscle in young dystrophin-deficient cats: a morphological and morphometric study. Acta Neuropathol 2001;101:591–600.

Gaschen L, et al. Cardiomyopathy in dystrophin-deficient hypertrophic feline muscular dystrophy. J Vet Int Med 1999;13:346–356.

Kornegay JN, et al. Muscular dystrophy in a litter of golden retriever dogs. Muscle Nerve 1988;11:1056–1064.

Nakada H, et al. Positive immunostaining of ovine congenital progressive muscular dystrophy with antibody against N- and C-terminal dystrophin. Aust Vet J 1990;67:271–272.

O'Brien DP, et al. Laminin alpha 2 (merosin)–deficient muscular dystrophy and demyelinating neuropathy in two cats. J Neurol Sci 2001;189:37–43.

Richards RB, Passmore IK. Ultrastructural changes in skeletal muscle in ovine muscular dystrophy. Acta Neuropathol 1989;79:168–175.

Richards RB, et al. Skeletal muscle pathology in ovine congenital progressive muscular dystrophy. Part I. Histopathology and histochemistry. Acta Neuropathol 1988;77:95–99 and 161–167.

Shelton GD, Engvall E. Muscular dystrophies and other inherited myopathies. Vet Clin N Am Small Anim Pract 2002;32:103–124.

Shelton GD, et al. Muscular dystrophy in female dogs. J Vet Intern Med 2001; 15:240–244.

Valentine BA, Cooper BJ. Canine X-linked muscular dystrophy: selective involvement of muscles in neonatal dogs. Neuromusc Dis 1991;1:31–38.

Valentine BA, et al. Development of Duchenne-type cardiomyopathy. Am J Pathol 1989;135:671–678.

Valentine BA, et al. Canine X-linked muscular dystrophy: morphologic lesions. J Neurol Sci 1990;97:1–23.

Valentine BA, et al. Canine X-linked muscular dystrophy as an animal model of Duchenne muscular dystrophy: a review. Am J Med Genet 1992;42:352–356.

Vos JH, et al. Dystrophy-like myopathy in the cat. J Comp Pathol 1986;96:335–341.

Wentink GH, et al. Myopathy with a possible recessive X-linked inheritance in a litter of Irish terriers. Vet Pathol 1972;9:328–349.

Wetterman CA, et al. Hypertrophic muscular dystrophy in a young dog. J Am Vet Med Assoc 2000;216:878–881.

Inherited and congenital myopathies

Many animal disorders have been compared to similar disorders in humans, but such comparisons are rarely validated. Several disorders are included in this section that have previously been designated as muscular dystrophies; the myopathy of sheep included in the muscular dystrophy section might be better classified as an inherited progressive myopathy. Inherited metabolic disorders are described in the Metabolic myopathies section. *The classification of myopathies in animals, similar to those in people, is subject to modification based on findings of on-going genetic and pathogenetic studies as well as on changes in disease definitions.*

Breed-associated myopathies in the dog

Several myopathic disorders are recognized in dogs that are breed-specific and it is likely that many more will be identified in the future. An inherited basis is suspected, if not confirmed, in most cases of breed-associated myopathies.

Myopathy of Labrador Retrievers

An inherited myopathy in Labrador Retrievers has been reported from Europe, North America, and Australia. The disorder occurs in working dog lines and not in show lines and is inherited as an *autosomal recessive disorder*. Both yellow and black Labrador Retrievers are affected.

Clinical severity is quite variable. Evidence of *stunting, reduced exercise tolerance, and a stiff "bunny hopping" gait* may be apparent soon after birth or may not occur until about 6 months of age. Affected dogs may always have a slightly stiff gait and low head carriage, or may be apparently normal at rest. Exercise in affected dogs leads to increasing signs of weakness and collapse. Clinical signs are exacerbated by cold ambient temperature. Muscle atrophy may or may not be apparent. *The temporalis muscles appear to be particularly prone to atrophy*. Decreased or absent patellar reflexes are a consistent finding in affected dogs. Megaesophagus leading to regurgitation may occur, but is uncommon. This disorder may progress, but often stabilizes by 6 months to 1 year of age, and affected dogs may show some degree of improvement with age. Electromyography reveals bizarre spontaneous, high-frequency activity. Serum activities of CK and AST are normal or only slightly increased.

Gross pathologic examination may indicate normal or slightly reduced muscling. On histological examination, *affected muscles exhibit a marked increase in fiber size variation that is most severe in older dogs*. Although initial reports indicated a type 2 fiber deficiency,

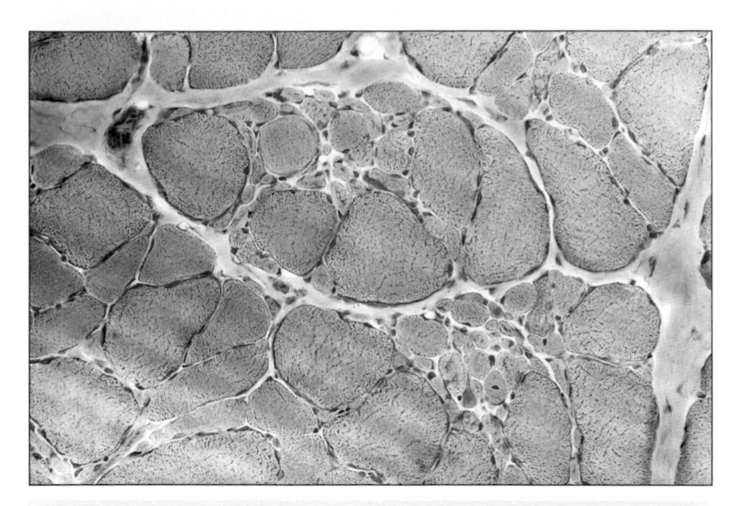

Figure 2.51 Increased variation in fiber diameter with groups of angular atrophied fibers and groups of fibers with rounded atrophy (mimicking denervation atrophy) in a Labrador Retriever with **congenital myopathy**. Frozen section, modified Gomori's trichrome.

subsequent studies indicate that, although alterations in fiber type are typical, atrophy or deficiency of type 2 fibers is variable. Scattered angular atrophied fibers may be seen. Fiber type grouping and small and large group atrophy are common (Fig. 2.51). Alterations in mitochondrial distribution are often striking, with peripheral mitochondrial aggregates and cytoplasmic zones devoid of mitochondria. Fibers with internal nuclei, whorled fibers, and split fibers are seen. There are scattered necrotic and regenerate fiber segments. Endomysial fibrosis is minimal. Despite the angular atrophy and fiber type grouping suggestive of denervation, motor nerve conduction velocities are normal and no abnormalities have been found in the peripheral or central nervous systems.

Myopathy of Bouvier des Flandres dogs

A *degenerative polymyopathy* occurs in the Bouvier des Flandres dog. Although the inheritance is not known, both sexes are affected. *Esophageal and swallowing muscles appear to be preferentially involved*, although generalized weakness occurs and histopathologic changes are seen in multiple muscles.

Affected dogs may not be recognized until 1–2 years of age when regurgitation due to megaesophagus becomes apparent. Clinical severity is variable, however, and affected pups may be slightly stunted and display locomotor and swallowing difficulties as early as 7 weeks of age. Generalized muscle atrophy, weakness, and a peculiar paddling gait are characteristic. Serum activities of CK and AST are typically moderately increased. Bizarre high-frequency activity is seen with concentric needle electromyography.

Gross pathologic findings are *generalized muscle atrophy and pallor and megaesophagus*. Histopathologic changes include moderate to severe increase in fiber size variation with rounded atrophy and hypertrophy of both fiber types. Severe cytoarchitectural changes are seen, including whorled fibers, split fibers, and fibers with internal nuclei. Multifocal myofiber necrosis and regeneration occurs, but is generally not striking. Endomysial and perimysial fibrosis occurs, but is relatively mild. Cardiac myofiber degeneration and fibrosis may also be present.

Canine dermatomyositis

A syndrome of crusting and alopecic skin lesions and associated myositis has been described in *Shetland Sheepdogs, Collies* and in a Pembroke Welsh Corgi dog. Canine dermatomyositis is thought to be inherited as an *autosomal dominant disorder* based on genetic studies in the Collie dog. This disorder has been likened to human dermatomyositis, which is thought to involve autoimmune mechanisms. In people, characteristic findings are a skin rash of the face, upper chest, and skin overlying joints, and muscle weakness with perifascicular atrophy and immune complex deposition and damage in skeletal muscle capillaries. Dogs with dermatomyositis develop distinctive skin lesions with basal cell degeneration and subepidermal cleft formation, but muscle lesions are not consistently found. Serum activities of CK and AST are normal. Nonsuppurative inflammation and atrophy of temporal and masseter muscles have been seen in affected dogs, however *electrodiagnostic and histologic studies of a group of affected Shetland Sheepdogs did not reveal convincing evidence of a primary myositis*. Muscle inflammation, when present, appeared to represent extension of inflammation from overlying ulcerated and inflamed skin lesions.

Other canine myopathies

A juvenile-onset distal myopathy occurs in Rottweiler dogs. Both males and females are affected, and clinical signs of muscle weakness and plantigrade and palmigrade stance are evident at about 2 months of age. The disorder is progressive, and is characterized histopathologically by *marked myofiber atrophy and fat infiltration with mild myonecrosis and endomysial fibrosis.* Serum activities of CK and AST are normal or only slightly increased. Electromyographic studies reveal rare fibrillations and positive sharp waves. The finding of decreased serum and muscle carnitine levels and improvement following carnitine supplementation suggest that *this may be a form of metabolic myopathy involving lipid metabolism*.

A *polymyopathy* with involvement of esophageal musculature occurs in association with dyserythropoiesis and cardiomegaly in *English Springer Spaniel dogs*. Findings in affected skeletal muscle include marked increase in fiber size variation with both rounded atrophy and hypertrophy and many fibers with internal nuclei. Central linear or irregular granular inclusions within myofibers that are visible on H&E and Gomori trichrome-stained frozen sections are characteristic. Inclusions are often associated with fiber splitting.

A myopathy with scattered degenerate and regenerate fibers and intramyofiber core-like structures has been seen in a young adult *Great Dane dog* with muscle weakness and atrophy. Ultrastructural evaluation revealed that the cores consist of disarrayed myofilaments and thickened Z-lines similar to nemaline rods.

Nemaline rods within myofibers occur as a nonspecific change in various canine myopathic conditions, and have been described in dogs with *X-linked muscular dystrophy*, hypothyroidism, and Cushing's syndrome. *Nemaline rods are formed by expanded Z-lines and are visible only in frozen sections stained with Gomori's trichrome stain or on ultrastructural evaluation*. Ultrastructurally, nemaline rods are electron-dense structures with periodicity similar to the Z-band material from which these structures arise. Congenital nemaline myopathy has been described in a 10-month-old Border Collie dog and adult-onset nemaline myopathy occurred in an 11-year-old Schipperke dog. Affected dogs displayed exercise intolerance and muscle weakness.

Endocrine myopathies are well recognized in humans, but in dogs are uncommon conditions sporadically associated with hypothyroidism, hyperadrenocorticism, and diabetes mellitus.

Inherited and congenital myopathies of cats

Primary congenital myopathies are less commonly described in cat than in dogs. Some are better characterized than others. It is possible that, given the relatively sedentary life of most house cats, a subtle neuromuscular dysfunction could be overlooked.

Nemaline myopathy of cats

An apparently inherited congenital myopathy characterized by intramyofiber nemaline rods occurs in mixed-breed cats. Both males and females are affected. This congenital myopathy is similar to congenital nemaline rod myopathy of people.

Affected cats exhibit signs of *progressive neuromuscular dysfunction* characterized by reluctance to move, a crouched "jerky" and hypermetric gait, muscle twitching, muscle atrophy, and hyporeflexia. Serum activities of CK and lactic dehydrogenase are mildly increased. No abnormalities are detected on electromyographic studies.

Muscle atrophy most severe in the proximal limb muscles and muscles of mastication is seen on gross examination. Characteristic histopathologic findings are seen with frozen section histochemistry, and include *atrophy of type 1 and type 2A fibers and presence of nemaline rods.* Nemaline rods are only visible with Gomori's trichrome stain (Fig. 2.52) and occur primarily within atrophied type 1 and 2A fibers and only rarely in type 2B fibers. Nemaline rods are also seen in toluidine blue-stained Epon-Araldite embedded sections and in sections examined by electron microscopy (Fig. 2.53). Fiber size variation and marked fiber splitting are also seen. Fiber typing is often indistinct in areas in which myofibers exhibit extensive fiber splitting. Fiber necrosis and regeneration are uncommon but may be seen, especially in younger cats.

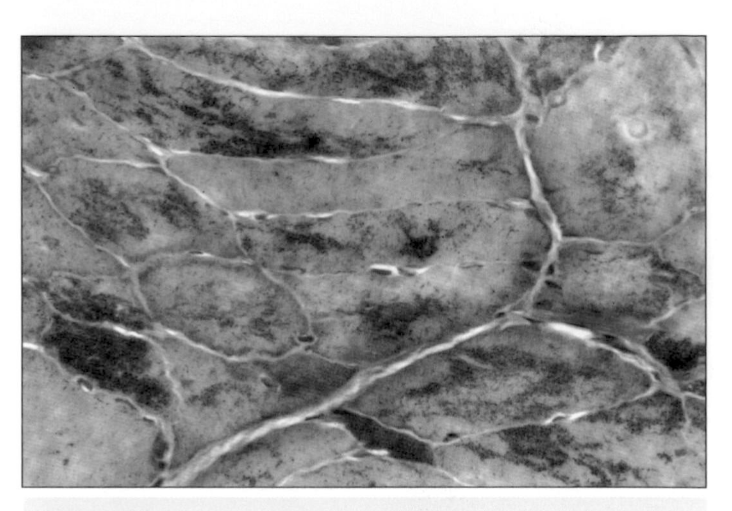

Figure 2.52 Numerous aggregates of dark staining nemaline rods in muscle from a cat with **congenital nemaline myopathy**. Frozen section, modified Gomori's trichrome.

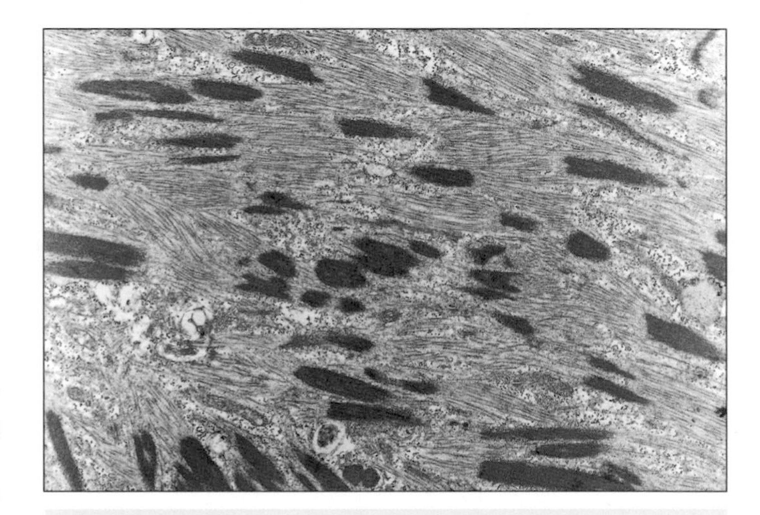

Figure 2.53 Dense staining elongate bodies composed of Z-disk material with associated myofilaments characteristic of nemaline rods in a cat with **congenital nemaline myopathy**. (Courtesy of BJ Cooper.)

Other feline myopathies

A syndrome of *feline hyperesthesia* has been recognized for many years. Detailed studies of frozen section muscle biopsies of epaxial muscle from affected cats have found numerous rimmed vacuoles. The contents of these vacuoles stain with monoclonal antibodies to paired helical filaments and beta amyloid, and this disorder has been likened to *human inclusion-body myositis.*

A myopathy causing spasticity has been reported in Devon Rex cats. Autosomal recessive inheritance is suspected. Affected cats exhibit neuromuscular dysfunction from an early age, typically from 3 to 23 weeks of age. Ventroflexion of the neck, exercise intolerance, megaesophagus, a hypermetric forelimb gait, muscle tremors, and collapse with exercise are characteristic. Serum activities of CK and AST are normal. Electromyographic studies indicate that abnormal spontaneous activity is rare and motor nerve conduction and repetitive nerve stimulation studies are normal. Sudden death due to laryngospasm is common. Histopathologic findings are consistent with a primary myopathy and are characterized by excessive fiber size variation due to rounded and angular atrophy and marked hypertrophy, internal nuclei, fiber splitting, and scattered necrotic and regenerate fibers. Endomysial fibrosis occurs in older affected cats.

Inherited and congenital myopathies of cattle

Congenital and inherited myopathies have been described in beef and dairy breeds. Double muscling in beef breeds, a genetic defect in the myostatin gene, is discussed under the heading Congenital and inherited defects. Myopathy due to glycogen storage disease is described in the Metabolic myopathy section.

Myopathy of the diaphragmatic muscle (diaphragmatic dystrophy)

An inherited myopathy affecting primarily diaphragmatic and intercostal muscles has been described in *Meuse-Rhine-Yssel cattle in The Netherlands and in Holstein-Friesian cattle in Japan.* The disorder in these two breeds appears to be identical. The disorder affects males and females, and is suspected to be transmitted as an autosomal recessive trait.

Clinical signs in affected cattle occur in adults from 2 to 10 years of age and include *loss of appetite and condition, decreased rumen activity, and recurrent bloat.* Serum activities of CK, AST, and LDH are normal.

Abnormal spontaneous activity was not seen in an electromyographic study of the diaphragm of affected Meuse-Rhine-Yssel cattle, although subtle changes in motor unit potentials were found.

The most severe gross pathologic changes are found in the *diaphragm, which is swollen, pale, and inflexible*. Similar changes are seen in intercostal muscles. Microscopic changes of myopathy occur in many other muscles and become more obvious as the disease progresses. Affected fibers exhibit marked cytoarchitectural alterations including vacuolar change, sarcoplasmic masses, atrophy and hypertrophy of fibers, numerous internal nuclei, marked fiber splitting, and central core-like lesions. *These core-like lesions are the most distinctive finding in this disorder*. Frozen section histochemistry studies demonstrate lack of mitochondrial enzyme staining within the cores, but strong staining at the periphery, similar to the cores and rimmed vacuoles described in several human myopathies. Scattered necrotic fiber segments are seen, often with macrophage infiltration. Endomysial fibrosis occurs and appears to be progressive. *Myocardial fibers contain distinctive centrally located inclusions* that are intensely acidophilic on H&E stain and dark green with Gomori's trichrome stain. On ultrastructural examination, the core-like lesions in skeletal muscle and the inclusions within cardiac myocytes consist of *disordered myofilaments with streaming of Z-line material*. Immunohistochemical studies of affected Holstein-Friesian cattle demonstrate that the core-like lesions in skeletal muscle contain actin and ubiquitin, but lack alpha actinin, desmin, and vimentin. Similar studies of myocardial fibers found variable ubiquitin reactivity of cardiac inclusions, and increased desmin reactivity on the periphery of the inclusions. It is proposed that this bovine disorder *may be a form of myofibrillar myopathy*.

Other bovine myopathies

Congenital myopathy occurs in *Braunvieh × Brown Swiss calves*. Both males and females are affected. These calves are abnormal at or soon after birth, with rapidly progressive muscle weakness and recumbency developing within 2 weeks of birth. Histological findings are marked fiber size variation due to fiber atrophy and hypertrophy, fiber splitting of hypertrophied fibers, disorganization of myofibrils, nemaline rods, internal nuclei, and peripheral eosinophilic inclusions. Fiber necrosis, regeneration, and endomysial fibrosis are not seen. Ultrastructural evaluation reveals that peripheral inclusions consist of tightly packed filamentous structures. Myofibrillar and mitochondrial disarray are also seen.

A congenital myopathy has been reported in a single Friesian calf that showed progressive weakness from birth. Muscle fibers were poorly developed and often exhibited lack of adequate myofibrils similar to myofibrillar hypoplasia of piglets. The most striking abnormality was the absence of Z-lines and presence of intracytoplasmic electron dense inclusions.

A degenerative myopathy characterized by necrotizing vasculopathy within skeletal muscle occurs in *young Gelbvieh cattle* (Fig. 2.54). The cause of this disorder is not known, although both immune-mediated and vitamin E deficiency-associated vasculopathy have been proposed.

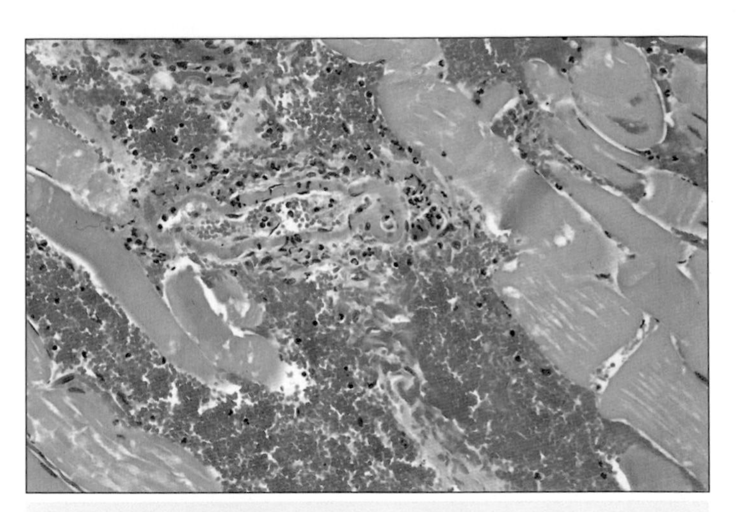

Figure 2.54 Necrotizing vasculitis and hemorrhagic necrosis of muscle in a Gelbvieh steer. (Courtesy of BJ Cooper.)

Inherited and congenital myopathies of sheep

The progressive inherited myopathy of *Merino sheep* in Australia has been described in the Muscular dystrophy section. A suspected autosomal recessive congenital myopathy has been described in *Border Leicester sheep*. At birth, affected lambs have clinical signs similar to lambs with cerebellar cortical atrophy ("daft lambs") but central nervous system lesions are absent. Clinical signs consist of difficulty or inability to rise and a peculiar arching of the neck with the head pressed back in an opisthotonos-like position. Pathologic findings in muscle are primarily within the cervical muscle and consist of abnormal fiber size variation due to fiber atrophy and hypertrophy. It has been proposed that small-diameter fibers represent delayed myofiber differentiation and maturation rather than atrophy. Ultrastructural abnormalities, including electron-dense bodies within axons of intramuscular nerves, suggest that myofiber lesions may reflect functional deficits of peripheral nerves rather than a primary myopathic process.

Bibliography

Bradley R. Hereditary "daft lamb" disease of border Leicester sheep: the ultrastructural pathology of the skeletal muscles. J Pathol 1978;125:205–212.

Bradley R. A primary bovine skeletal myopathy with absence of Z discs, sarcoplasmic inclusions, myofibrillar hypoplasia and nuclear abnormality. J Comp Pathol 1979;89:381–388.

Braund KG, et al. Investigating a degenerative polymyopathy in four related Bouvier des Flandres dogs. Vet Med Small Anim Clinician 1990;85:558–570.

Cooper BJ, et al. Nemaline myopathy of cats. Muscle Nerve 1986;9:618–625.

Delauche AJ, et al. Nemaline rods in canine myopathies: 4 case reports and literature review. J Vet Int Med 1998;12:424–430.

Furuoka H, et al. Immunohistochemical and electron microscopical studies of myocardial inclusions in hereditary myopathy of the diaphragmatic muscles in Holstein-Friesian cattle. Acta Neuropathol 1999;97:185–191.

Furuoka H, et al. Immunohistochemical study of some cytoskeletal proteins in hereditary myopathy of the diaphragmatic muscles in Holstein-Friesian cattle. Acta Neuropathol 1999;97:177–184.

Goedegebuure SA, et al. Dystrophy of the diaphragmatic muscles in adult Meuse-Rhine-Yssel cattle: electromyographical and histological findings. Vet Pathol 1983;20:32–48.

Hafner A, et al. Congenital myopathy in Braunveih x brown Swiss calves. J Comp Pathol 1996;115:23–24.

Hanson SM, et al. Juvenile-onset distal myopathy in Rottweiler dogs. J Vet Int Med 1998;12:103–108.

Hargis AM, et al. A skin disorder in three Shetland sheepdogs: comparison with familial canine dermatomyositis of collies. Comp Cont Educ Pract Vet 1985; 7:306–318.

Hargis AM, et al. Post-mortem findings in a Shetland sheepdog with dermatomyositis. Vet Pathol 1986;23:509–511.

Haupt KH, et al. Familial canine dermatomyositis: clinical, electrodiagnostic, and genetic studies. Am J Vet Res 1985;46:1861–1869.

Holland CT, et al. Dyserythropoiesis, polymyopathy, and cardiac disease in three related English Springer spaniels. J Vet Int Med 1991;5:151–159.

Kramer JW, et al. Inheritance of a neuromuscular disorder of Labrador Retriever dogs. J Am Vet Med Assoc 1981;179:380–381.

Malik R, et al. Hereditary myopathy of Devon rex cats. J Small Anim Pract 1993;34:539–546.

March PA, et al. Electromyographic and histological abnormalities in epaxial muscles of cats with feline hyperesthesia syndrome. J Vet Int Med 1999;13:2389.

McKerrell RE, Braund KG. Hereditary myopathy in Labrador Retrievers: a morphologic study. Vet Pathol 1986;23:411–417.

Nakamura N. Dystrophy of the diaphragmatic muscles in Holstein-Friesian steers. J Vet Med Sci 1996;58:79–80.

Newsholme SJ, Gaskell CJ. Myopathy with core-like structures in a dog. J Comp Pathol 1987;97:597–600.

Peeters ME, Ubbink GJ. Dysphagia-associated muscular dystrophy: a familial trait in the Bouvier des Flandres. Vet Rec 1994;134:444–446.

Robinson R. 'Spasticity' in the Devon rex cat. Vet Rec 1992;130:302.

Vite CH. Myotonia and disorders of altered muscle cell membrane excitability. Vet Clin N Am Small Anim Pract 2002;32:169–187.

Watson ADJ, et al. Myopathy in a Labrador retriever. Aust Vet J 1988;65:226–227.

White SD, et al. Dermatomyositis in an adult Pembroke Welsh corgi. J Am An Hosp Assoc 1992;28:398–401.

Myotonic and spastic syndromes

Myotonia *is defined clinically as a temporary inability of skeletal muscle fibers to relax, resulting in transient uncontrollable muscle tension as a result of voluntary muscle contraction, and is manifested clinically as muscle stiffness.* Electromyographically, myotonia is characterized by waxing and waning spontaneous electrical activity ("dive bomber" sounds) evident following needle insertion or muscle percussion during concentric needle electromyography. In many, but not all, myotonic syndromes, prolonged focal muscle contraction may be elicited by muscle percussion, a phenomenon known as "*dimpling*" (Fig. 2.55). Myotonia may be inherited or acquired. Myotonia is most obvious on initiation of muscle contraction and often improves with continued exercise. Affected individuals may be normal between episodes or have persistent muscle stiffness resulting in a stiff gait. Myotonic syndromes reflect muscle membrane electrical abnormalities, most often associated with *ion channel defects*. Ion channel disorders are a diverse group of disorders, collectively termed the *channelopathies*, and many involve the abnormal regulation of chloride and sodium ions.

In animals, confirmed or suspected inherited myotonias are most common. Drug- or toxin-induced myotonia occurs in humans, and a report of transient myotonia in a dog following ingestion of a phenoxy herbicide indicates that such induced forms of myotonia are possible in animals. Hypercortisolism due to endogenous or exogenous corticosteroids can induce a myotonia-like syndrome in dogs, although this disorder is best classified as a *pseudomyotonia*. Pseudomyotonic electrical discharges are also a feature of X-linked Duchenne-type muscular dystrophy in the dog and cat, and the canine disorder has been erroneously described as a myotonic myopathy.

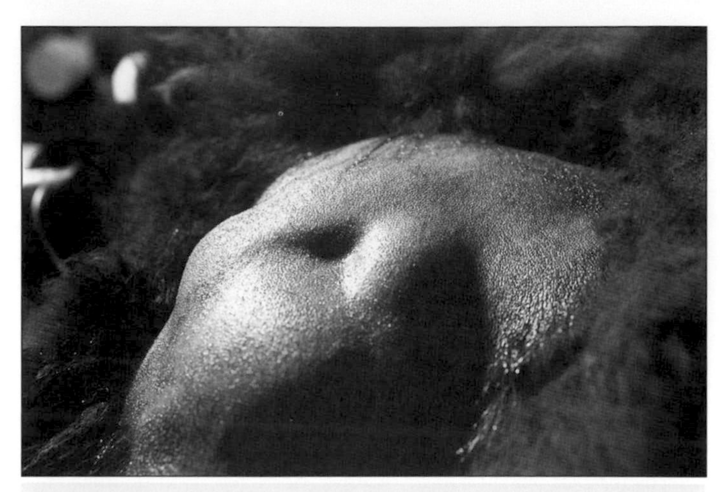

Figure 2.55 Dimpling following percussion in a Chow Chow dog with **congenital myotonia**. (Courtesy of L Fuhrer.)

Several syndromes involving *episodic spasticity of limb movements* are recognized in animals. The cause of these spastic syndromes is poorly understood, although an inherited basis is often suspected. Although primary myopathy is suspected in some cases, it is also possible for abnormal peripheral or central nervous system activity to result in episodic spasticity.

Myotonia in the dog

A *congenital myotonic syndrome* has been described in several breeds of dog, including Chow Chow, Staffordshire Terrier, and Miniature Schnauzer dogs. A suspected *adult-onset myotonic syndrome* has been described in the Rhodesian Ridgeback and Boxer dog. Clinical signs in myotonic dogs are often misinterpreted as a shifting leg lameness. Myotonia has been best characterized in the Chow Chow and Miniature Schnauzer dog.

Myotonia in the Chow Chow

This disorder occurs in Chow Chow dogs worldwide, including North America, Europe, Australia, and New Zealand. It may be that breeding for heavy muscling has concentrated the trait in this breed. Myotonia in Chow Chows affects both sexes, and is likely to be an *autosomal recessive trait*. Mildly affected animals, however, may go undetected. The specific muscle defect leading to myotonia in the Chow Chow is still not known.

Clinical signs of stiff gait and muscular spasm on initiation of movement may be apparent as early as 6 weeks of age. Electromyographic evidence of myotonia precedes obvious clinical signs and persists for the life of the animal. Laryngospasm is common, causing episodic collapse or cyanosis, and affected dogs often have a weak or hoarse bark. Muscular contraction occurring when affected dogs attempt to rise often results in transient splaying of the forelimbs followed by sufficient relaxation to allow the dog to stand and ambulate, although affected Chow Chows often have a persistent stiffness of gait. Affected dogs may have a stiff "bunny hopping" gait in the pelvic limbs, and muscular hypertrophy is evident in early stages. Percussion of limb or tongue musculature results in dimpling (Fig. 2.55). Serum activity of creatine kinase may be mildly increased. Muscle atrophy may develop in older animals.

In young myotonic dogs, the muscles may appear hypertrophied. In older affected dogs, muscle atrophy may be more obvious, and muscles may appear slightly pale. Histopathologic findings in affected muscle are minimal in early stages of the disorder. Only rare necrotic fibers are seen. With time, *progressive myopathic changes*, including excessive fiber size variation due to both hypertrophy and atrophy, internal nuclei, and mild endomysial fibrosis may be apparent. *Chronic myopathic changes, in particular numerous fibers with one or more internal nuclei, are the most consistent finding in muscle from older myotonic Chow Chows.*

Myotonia in the Miniature Schnauzer

Myotonia in the Miniature Schnauzer, reported as "myotonic myopathy," is also suspected to be due to *autosomal recessive inheritance* and appears to be clinically and histopathologically similar to myotonia in the Chow Chow. Abnormal muscle membrane chloride conductance in the Miniature Schnauzer is due to mutations in a skeletal muscle voltage-dependent chloride channel, CIC-1.

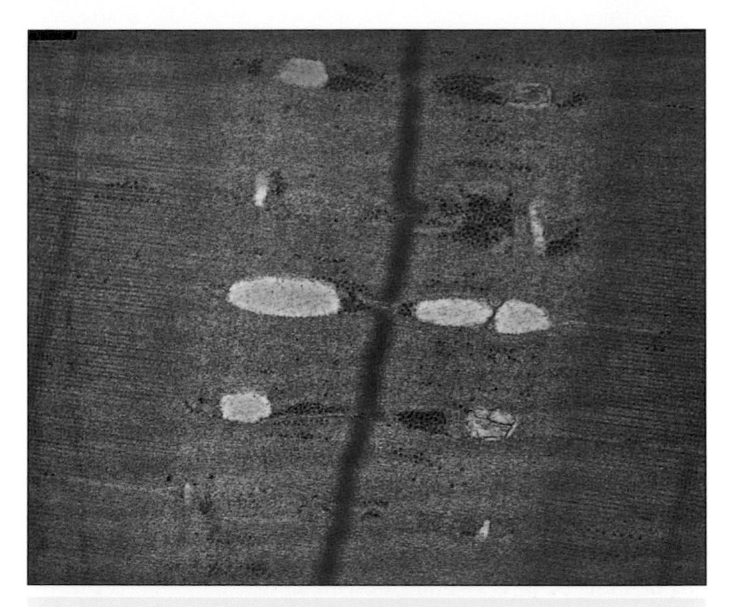

Figure 2.56 Dilated sarcotubular elements in muscle from a cat with **congenital myotonia**. (Courtesy of JF Cummings.)

Myotonia in the cat

A suspected inherited congenital myotonia occurs in mixed breed cats. Clinical signs include a *crouched and stiff hindlimb gait and marked hypertrophy of proximal appendicular muscle evident at about 4 months of age*. These clinical signs of myotonia resemble those of male cats with muscular dystrophy, however serum activities of CK and AST in myotonic cats are normal. Vocalization is weak, facial muscle spasms may be seen, and transient laryngospasm may occur. Electromyography reveals characteristic waxing and waning myotonic activity. Muscle percussion induces "dimpling." *Increased variation in fiber size due to prominent fiber hypertrophy is the primary histopathologic finding.* Fibers with multiple tiny clear cytoplasmic vacuoles may be seen, especially in plastic-embedded sections. Ultrastructural evaluation reveals mild dilation of T-tubules and terminal cisternae of the sarcoplasmic reticulum (Fig. 2.56). Clinical signs are apparently not progressive. Both males and females are affected, and the underlying defect is as yet unknown.

Myotonia in the goat

Congenital myotonia in the goat has been recognized for many years. *The myotonic goat is said to be the oldest recognized animal model of an inherited human skeletal muscle disease.* In fact, these so-called *"fainting goats"* are prized by certain breeders. If nothing else, the advantages of keeping such goats include the difficulty myotonic goats have in jumping fences due to muscle spasms associated with initiation of muscle contraction.

Myotonia in goats is inherited as *an autosomal dominant trait, with probable incomplete penetrance*. This disorder has been shown to be due to mutation in a skeletal muscle voltage-dependent chloride channel, CIC-1, which causes decreased skeletal muscle chloride channel conductance. This condition is very similar to congenital myotonia (Thomsen's disease) in humans.

Affected goats show clinical signs of myotonia within 2 weeks of birth. Attacks are most often initiated by startling an affected goat. Affected goats assume a "sawhorse" stance and often fall over. Myotonic episodes are transient and affected goats are normal in between episodes. Percussion induces a prolonged muscle "dimpling," and concentric needle electromyography reveals characteristic waxing and waning myotonic potentials. Serum activities of CK and AST are normal.

There are no gross abnormalities in myotonic goats, and affected goats do not appear to be heavily muscled. Histopathologic changes in muscle examined by light microscopy are minimal, with only mild increase in fiber size variation due primarily to fiber hypertrophy and, in some cases, increased internal nuclei. On ultrastructural examination, dilated and proliferated sarcoplasmic reticulum and T-tubules are evident.

Periodic paralyses

The periodic paralyses are a group of inherited muscle disorders. In humans, hypokalemic, normokalemic, and hyperkalemic periodic paralyses are recognized. Although electrical myotonia and pseudomyotonia is a feature of many of the periodic paralyses, the transient attacks of paralysis are associated with muscle hypotonia rather than hypertonicity. These disorders are *sometimes referred to as paramyotonias* rather than true myotonic syndromes. The periodic paralyses are *due to ion channel defects that affect muscle sodium channel activity* and alter the muscle membrane potential. To date, only hyperkalemic periodic paralysis has been recognized in animals. The most common and the best-characterized syndrome occurs in horses. A similar disorder has been seen in a young American Pit Bull dog.

Hyperkalemic periodic paralysis in horses

Hyperkalemic periodic paralysis (HYPP) occurs in horses related to the Quarter Horse stallion "Impressive" and is inherited as an autosomal dominant trait. Homozygotes exhibit more severe signs of muscle dysfunction than do heterozygotes. The diagnosis of HYPP in horses can be confirmed by DNA testing.

Foals homozygous for HYPP often exhibit a peculiar respiratory noise due to *laryngospasm*, and may develop dysphagia and emaciation during the first 2 years of life. Laryngospasm and pharyngeal collapse associated with exercise is common. Such horses must be considered nonviable as performance animals. Heterozygotes may appear to be clinically normal, but are prone to transient attacks of paralysis. Initial signs include muscle fasciculations, flashing of the third eyelid, muscle spasm, and inspiratory stridor. In severe attacks, these signs will be followed by collapse to sternal or lateral recumbency associated with limb hypotonia. Attacks typically last from a few minutes to a few hours. Electromyography performed when animals are apparently normal reveals myotonic discharges and complex repetitive activity (pseudomyotonia).

Serum chemistry analysis often reveals higher than normal potassium levels in affected horses, particularly during attacks of weakness, but this finding is variable. Serum activities of CK and AST are normal or only very slightly increased. Clinical signs of weakness can be induced in HYPP horses with an oral potassium challenge test, high potassium feeds such as alfalfa or molasses-containing feeds, stress, or cold weather. *Sudden death* may occur in HYPP horses, perhaps due to effects of increased blood potassium on cardiac function. Attacks may also be precipitated by inhalant anesthetic agents, and may resemble malignant hyperthermia.

The underlying defect in HYPP in horses, as in man, is a mutation in the muscle sodium channel leading to increased open time. The increased influx of sodium through defective channels results in compensatory loss of muscle potassium, hence the hyperkalemia. Increased concentration of potassium ions outside the cell may further activate the abnormal sodium channels. The alteration in resting muscle membrane potential can lead to increased muscle action potentials and muscle fasciculations and spasms as well as to complete depolarization with inactivation of sodium channel activity and collapse.

There are no gross findings in horses with HYPP, other than frequent heavy and well-defined muscling. Although a vacuolar myopathy similar to humans with hyperkalemic periodic paralysis has been reported, in most cases of equine HYPP, *abnormalities are not found on light microscopy*. Ultrastructural findings of dilated sarcotubular elements are characteristic of HYPP, and are similar to those seen in myotonia in the cat and goat. DNA testing is now available on cells obtained from mane hairs rather than on blood, which is a boon for the pathologist who can now obtain the appropriate sample for testing in cases of otherwise unexplained death in Quarter-Horse-related breeds.

Myotonic dystrophy-like disorders in dogs and horses

Myotonic dystrophy is the most common inherited myotonic disorder in humans, affecting approximately 5 per 100 000 people, and is inherited as an autosomal dominant condition. Onset of obvious clinical signs is most often in late childhood, although this is quite variable, and a congenital form is also recognized. Myotonic dystrophy is a multisystem disorder associated with a constellation of signs, including cataracts and testicular atrophy. Muscle dysfunction is progressive, although the clinical signs of muscle dysfunction remain relatively mild. Findings in muscle biopsies include selective atrophy of type 1 fibers, hypertrophy of type 2 fibers, internal nuclei, ring fibers, and sarcoplasmic masses. However, these histopathologic findings are not specific for myotonic dystrophy. Attempts have been made to classify a group of animal disorders as animal models of myotonic dystrophy based on some similarities in clinical and pathologic findings, but the evidence for this is unconvincing. In particular, the involvement of other organ systems is generally lacking. The genetic defect in human myotonic dystrophy has been shown to be an abnormal expansion of a trinucleotide (CTG) repeat in a gene coding for a serine-threonine protein kinase. Similar molecular studies are lacking in animals. Myotonic dystrophy-like disease has been reported in a Rhodesian Ridgeback dog and in a Boxer dog. The best characterized of the myotonic dystrophy-like disorders occurs in the horse.

Myotonic dystrophy-like disease in the horse

A progressive early-onset myopathy associated with clinical and electrical myotonia and profound cytoarchitectural alterations in muscle occurs sporadically in horses. Breeds affected include Quarter Horse, Thoroughbred, and Standardbred, and both males and females appear to be equally represented. Although the early onset of clinical signs suggests that this disorder is congenital, to date there is no proof that it is inherited, and affected foals appear to occur only sporadically.

Affected foals may have difficulty standing at birth or, more commonly, develop a *progressive stiff gait with marked prominence of proximal limb muscles*, especially the gluteal muscle, evident at about 1 month of age. Percussion of muscle induces prolonged muscle dimpling. Affected foals become progressively weaker and have difficulty rising, with later development of muscle atrophy. Serum activities of CK and AST may be mildly increased. Concentric needle electromyography reveals characteristic myotonic and pseudomyotonic discharges.

At necropsy, affected muscles are often hypertrophied (Fig. 2.57) and may contain fibrous tissue and linear streaks due to fat

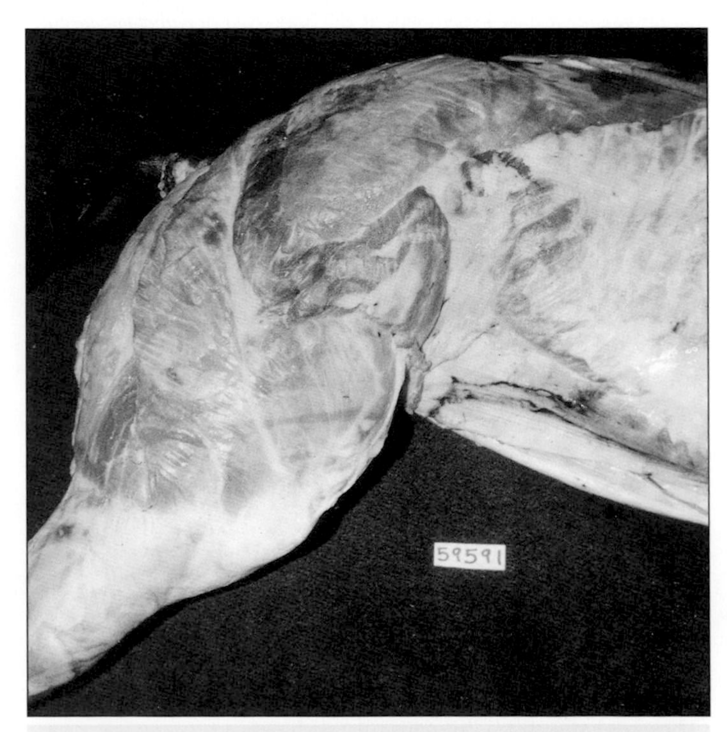

Figure 2.57 Muscular hypertrophy of the hindquarters in a foal with **myotonic dystrophy-like disease**. (Courtesy of TJ Hulland.)

infiltration. Severe lesions are pale and yellow-white. Atrophy of affected muscles may also be seen. There is a selective involvement of muscle, with *the most severe lesions found in the longissimus, iliopsoas, medial gluteal, biceps femoris, semitendinosus, semimembranosus, and sartorius muscles*. The triceps brachii and rectus femoris are less severely affected.

Histopathologic findings are a marked increase in fiber size variation with fiber hypertrophy as well as rounded atrophy and severe cytoarchitectural changes including pale-staining peripheral sarcoplasmic masses, internal nuclei, and small clear vacuoles (Fig. 2.58). Ring fibers and fiber splitting can also be seen. Only scattered necrotic and regenerate fibers are seen. Alterations in fiber type distribution in affected muscles include type 1 fiber predominance and fiber type grouping. Peripheral and intramuscular nerves, however, are histologically normal. Endomysial and perimysial fibrosis occurs, but is variable.

On ultrastructural examination, sarcoplasmic masses are composed of ribosomes, mitochondria, and disarrayed myofibrils.

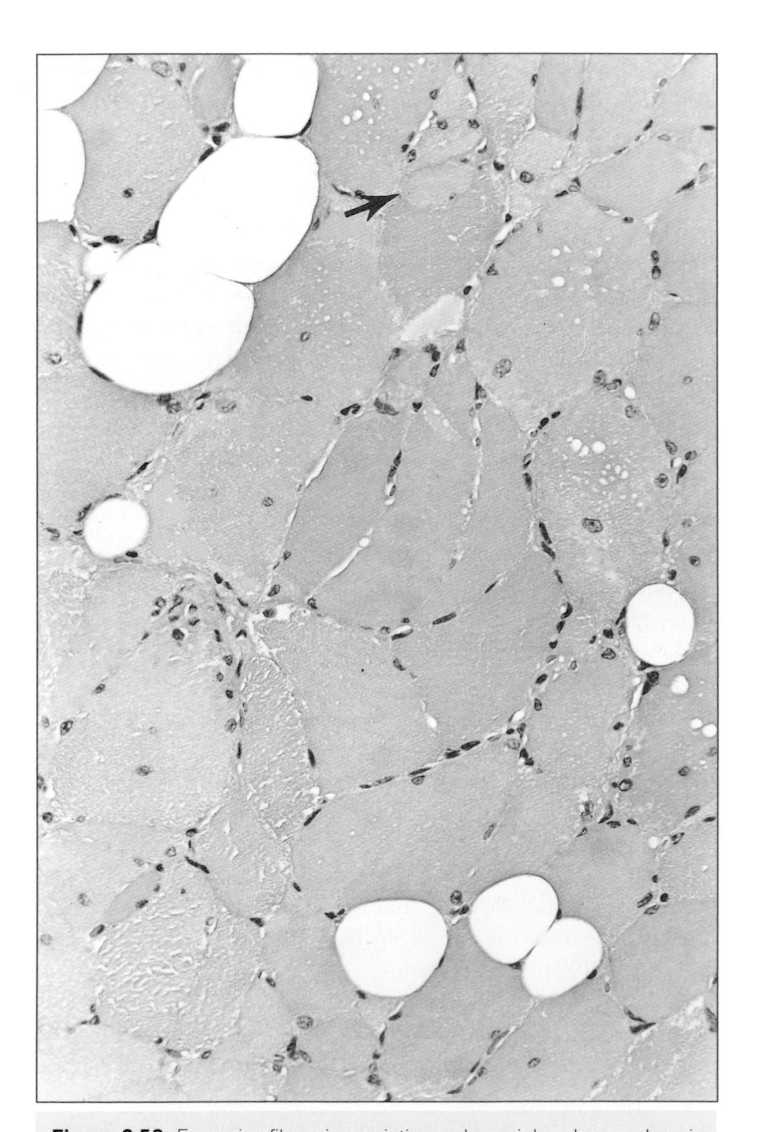

Figure 2.58 Excessive fiber size variation, pale peripheral sarcoplasmic masses (arrow), internal nuclei, fine cytoplasmic vacuoles, and fat infiltration in muscle from a **foal with myotonic dystrophy-like disease**.

Other myotonic-like disorders in the horse

A syndrome resembling *stiff-man syndrome* occurs in the horse. *Affected horses exhibit periodic muscle stiffness and spasms*. Muscle spasms are initiated by voluntary movement. Muscle hypertrophy may be evident. Electromyography reveals persistent motor unit activity, but no abnormal primary spontaneous activity of muscle is seen. Muscle biopsy samples are reported to be normal. A disorder involving *autoantibodies to glutamic acid decarboxylase*, resulting in a neuromyotonic syndrome similar to that occurring in humans, is proposed.

A syndrome of episodic painful muscle spasms associated with prolapse of the third eyelid has been described in horses with ear tick (Otobius megnini) infestation. Percussion of affected muscle groups results in muscle dimpling. Serum activities of CK and AST are often moderately to markedly increased. Electromyographic studies are normal unless muscle contracture occurs secondary to needle placement. No abnormalities have been reported in muscle biopsy samples. Clinical signs resolve following removal or insecticidal treatment of the ear ticks.

Spastic syndromes

"Scotty cramp" is an episodic motor disease, primarily of Scottish Terrier dogs. This disorder most often begins at 2–6 months of age, but adult onset is also possible. It is characterized by *hindlimb and pelvic muscle hypertonicity* along with upward arching of the back for periods of 1–30 minutes, and is precipitated by exercise or excitement. No consistent gross or histologic abnormalities are found in the central nervous system, peripheral nerves or skeletal muscles.

Muscle hypertonicity precipitated by exercise or excitement has been described in several *Cavalier King Charles Spaniels*. Vacuolation of scattered muscle fibers and several minor ultrastructural changes occur, but there is no clear indication of the cause.

"Dancing Doberman" disease has been described as a spastic disease of *one or both hocks* in Doberman Pinschers of any age. The animals are reluctant to bear weight continuously and exhibit a peculiar shifting hindleg action resembling dancing. This appears to be a nonspecific sign, since some of these dogs apparently have a localized myopathy and others have evidence of a neuropathy.

A congenital myopathy in *Devon Rex cats* results in spasticity and is described in the section on Inherited and congenital myopathies.

Spastic paresis of cattle affecting one or both hindlegs is usually seen in calves 3–7 months of age, although onset of signs can occur in adults. The disease appears first as an exaggerated straightness of the hock that increases to the point of *inability to flex the hock*. In the later stages, in animals with unilateral involvement, the affected limb may swing stiffly like a pendulum or be held out in an abnormal cranial or caudal position. The disease, also called *"contraction of the Achilles tendon," "straight hock," or "Elso heel"* (the latter derived from the name of the Friesian bull, some of whose progeny, had the disease), is worldwide in distribution. It affects primarily Holstein-Friesian cattle but has been found in several other dairy and beef breeds, and has a distinct familial pattern. Deafferentation (cutting of the sensory nerve root) of the gastrocnemius muscle relieves the effect, suggesting that the defect is an *unmodulated or uncontrollable sensory-motor reflex loop*.

A related syndrome, referred to as *"spastic syndrome," "crampy spasticity," or "stretches"* affects mature animals, usually *bulls*, and causes periodic and sudden extension and stiffening of both hindlegs. During episodes the back is arched and the neck is extended. Episodes last for a period of seconds to minutes. The disease is progressive and it is reportedly associated with straight hocks and a variety of other abnormalities of bone, joints, or spinal column.

Bibliography

Amann JF, et al. Myotonia in a chow chow. J Am Vet Med Assoc 1985;187:415–417.

Atkinson JB, et al. Myotonia congenita. A histochemical and ultrastructural study in the goat: comparison with abnormalities found in human myotonia dystrophica. Am J Pathol 1981;102:324–335.

Bailey JE, et al. Hyperkalemic periodic paralysis episode during halothane anesthesia in a horse. J Am Vet Med Assoc 1996;208:1859–1865.

Berchtold MW, et al. Calcium ion in skeletal muscle: its crucial role for muscle function, plasticity, and disease. Physiol Rev 2000;80:1215–1265.

Bijlevald K, Hartman W. Electromyographic studies in calves with spastic paresis. Tijdschr Diergeneesk 1976;101:805–808.

Bradley R, Wijeratne WVS. A locomotor disorder clinically similar to spastic paresis in an adult Friesian bull. Vet Pathol 1980;17:305–315.

Bryant SH. Myotonia in the goat. Ann NY Acad Sci 1979;317:315–325.

Carr EA, et al. Laryngeal and pharyngeal dysfunction in horses homozygous for hyperkalemic periodic paralysis. J Am Vet Med Assoc 1996;209:798–803.

Chrisman CL. Dancing Doberman disease: clinical findings and prognosis. Prog Vet Neurol 1990;1:83–90.

De Ley G, De Moor A. Bovine spastic paralysis: Results of surgical deafferentation of the gastrocnemius muscle by means of spinal dorsal root resection. Am J Vet Res 1977;38:1899–1900.

Duncan ID, Griffiths IR. A myopathy associated with myotonia in the dog. Acta Neuropath 1975;31:297–303.

Harper PS. Myotonic dystrophy. In: Karpati G, Hilton-Jones D, Griggs RC, eds. Disorders of Voluntary Muscle. 7th ed. New York: Cambridge University Press, 2001:541–559.

Harrington ML, et al. Suspected herbicide toxicosis in a dog. J Am Vet Med Assoc 1996;209:2085–2087.

Hegreberg GA, Reed SM. Skeletal muscle changes associated with equine myotonic dystrophy. Acta Neuropathol 1990;80:426–431.

Jezyk PF. Hyperkalemic periodic paralysis in a dog. J Am Anim Hosp Assoc 1982:18:977–980.

Kortz G. Canine myotonia. Sem Vet Med Surg (Small Animal) 1989;4:141–145.

Lehmann-Horn F, et al. Periodic paralysis: understanding channelopathies. Curr Neurol Neurosci Rep 2002;2:61–69.

Madigan JE, et al. Muscle spasms associated with ear tick (Otobius megnini) infestations in five horses. J Am Vet Med Assoc 1995;207:74–76.

Meyers KM, et al. Muscular hypertonicity: Episodes in Scottish Terrier dogs. Arch Neurol 1971;25:61–68.

Naylor JM. Hyperkalemic periodic paralysis. Vet Clinic N Am: Eq Pract 1997;13:129–144.

Nollet H, et al. Suspected case of stiff-horse syndrome. Vet Rec 2000;146:282–284.

Reed SM, et al. Progressive myotonia in foals resembling human dystrophia myotonica. Muscle Nerve 1988;11:291–296.

Rhodes TH, et al. A missense mutation in canine ClC-1 causes recessive myotonia congenita in the dog. FEBS Lett 1999;456:54–58.

Sarli G, et al. Dystrophy-like myopathy in a foal. Vet Rec 1994;135:156–160.

Shirakawa T, et al. Muscular dystrophy-like disease in a thoroughbred foal. J Comp Pathol 1989;100:287–294.

Shires PK, et al. Myotonia in a Staffordshire terrier. J Am Vet Med Assoc 1983;183:229–232.

Shores A, et al. Myotonia congenita in a Chow Chow pup. J Am Vet Med Assoc 1986;188:532–533.

Simpson ST, Braund KG. Myotonic dystrophy-like disease in a dog. J Am Vet Med Assoc 1985;186:495–498.

Smith BR, et al. Possible adult onset myotonic dystrophy in a boxer. J Vet Intern Med 1998;12:120.

Spier SJ, et al. Hyperkalemic periodic paralysis in horses. J Am Vet Med Assoc 1990;197:1009–1017.

Toll J, et al. Congenital myotonia in 2 domestic cats. J Vet Int Med 1998;12:116–119.

Vite CH, et al. Myotonic myopathy in a miniature schnauzer: case report and data suggesting abnormal chloride conductance across the muscle membrane. J Vet Intern Med 1998;12:394–397.

Metabolic myopathies

Abnormal skeletal muscle metabolism leading to neuromuscular dysfunction is most often due to inborn errors of metabolism, but can occur due to acquired metabolic defects. In some disorders, a metabolic defect is suspected based on clinical and pathologic findings but an exact cause remains elusive. Metabolic defects can affect multiple organ systems, with metabolically active organs such as skeletal muscle, cardiac muscle, nervous tissue, and liver being most severely compromised. Muscle dysfunction can, however, be the primary or the only clinical sign. In some such cases, the occurrence of tissue-specific isozymes of enzymes involved in metabolism can explain selective organ dysfunction, and in other cases the cause is not clear.

In *humans*, metabolic myopathies are broadly classified into four groups according to the type of metabolism affected:

- carbohydrate metabolic disorders,
- disorders of lipid metabolism,
- disorders of mitochondrial metabolism ("mitochondrial myopathies"),
- disorders of adenine nucleotide metabolism (myoadenylate deaminase deficiency).

Clinical signs of progressive muscle weakness, or of exercise-induced muscle cramping, contracture, and rhabdomyolysis are most common. Skeletal muscle dysfunction may occur due to inadequate energy production, to disruption of myofibrillar structure due to storage of carbohydrate or lipid, or to a combination of these factors. To date, the confirmed or suspected metabolic myopathies in animals that have been identified include disorders of carbohydrate metabolism, mitochondrial function, and lipid metabolism.

It should be noted that the terminology regarding *periodic acid-Schiff (PAS) positive, amylase-resistant inclusions* that occur within myofibers in some metabolic disorders is confusing. Terms such as *amylopectin, amylopectin-like, polyglucosan bodies, Lafora bodies, and complex polysaccharide have all been applied to this material.* Until detailed biochemical analysis of this type of stored material is available it is safe to say that *all these terms describe a similar type of material.*

Metabolic myopathies of the dog

Glycogen storage disease type II in Lapland dogs

A canine model of Pompe's disease due to acid maltase (acid α-glucosidase) deficiency has been recognized in the Lapland dog. Massive glycogen storage occurs in multiple organs, but skeletal, myocardial, and smooth muscle are most severely involved. The disorder is inherited as an autosomal recessive trait.

Clinical signs of progressive weakness and regurgitation due to megaesophagus are present from about 6 months of age. Myocardial dysfunction is also a feature. Affected dogs typically die at 10–18 months of age.

Overall muscle atrophy and megaesophagus are found on gross pathologic examination. Histologic examination reveals massive glycogen storage in multiple organs. Stored material is visible in routine preparations as clear vacuoles. This material stains positively with PAS stain and is digested by amylase (diastase), consistent with glycogen. Ultrastructural studies indicate that *the stored glycogen is membrane-bound within lysosomes.*

Phosphofructokinase deficiency (glycogenosis type VII) in English Springer Spaniels and American Cocker Spaniels

Phosphofructokinase (PFK) is a rate-controlling glycolytic enzyme. Quantitative and qualitative alterations in PFK activity can significantly alter energy metabolism in cells such as erythrocytes and skeletal muscle cells that rely heavily on glucose metabolism for energy. PFK is a tetramer composed of liver, muscle, and platelet type subunits in tissue-specific patterns. *The genetic mutation is a point mutation in the muscle isozyme of PFK, and a PCR-based test can detect affected and carrier animals.*

In English Springer Spaniels and American Cocker Spaniels, deficiency of the muscle isozyme of PFK results in *recurrent hemolytic episodes due to defective erythrocyte carbohydrate metabolism.* Variable hematocrit and persistent high reticulocyte counts are typical findings. Episodes are most often initiated by exercise or excitement, as PFK-deficient erythrocytes are particularly sensitive to lysis associated with a mildly increased pH of blood (alkalemia) resulting from hyperventilation. Skeletal muscle cells are apparently protected to some degree by up-regulation of the liver isozyme of PFK. Exercise intolerance, exercise-induced muscle cramps, and progressive muscular atrophy and weakness can occur, however, particularly in older PFK-deficient dogs. Erythrocyte PFK activity is markedly reduced in affected dogs, and moderately decreased in heterozygotes.

In humans with PFK deficiency, clinical signs are entirely due to muscular dysfunction, with exercise-induced cramps and myoglobinuria being most common. Late-onset progressive muscle weakness may also occur. The differences in clinical signs in affected dogs reflect the sensitivity of canine erythrocytes to alkalosis-induced lysis and possibly also to the high reliance of canine muscle on oxidative metabolism and less reliance on anaerobic glycolysis.

In older PFK-deficient dogs, examination of skeletal muscle may reveal *chronic myopathic changes including excessive fiber size variation and intramyofiber vacuoles and inclusions of material* that is stained lightly by hematoxylin in H&E-stained sections. This material is *intensely PAS-positive* and resists digestion by amylase (diastase), consistent with an amylopectin-like complex polysaccharide. Accumulation of this material appears to be a function of age. Ultrastructural studies indicate that this material is composed of nonmembrane-bound granular filamentous and amorphous material. Other findings at necropsy include marked extramedullary hematopoiesis and hemosiderosis due to recurrent hemolysis.

Other canine metabolic myopathies

- *Mitochondrial myopathy* causing episodic weakness and exercise-induced lactic acidosis has been described in a litter of Old English Sheepdogs.
- *Familial myoclonic epilepsy* with polyglucosan bodies in skeletal muscle occurs in miniature wire-haired Dachshunds.
- Neuromuscular weakness associated with *increased lipid accumulation and decreased carnitine activity* within skeletal muscle has been described as an acquired disorder in a variety of dog breeds.
- *Lipid storage myopathy* is thought to reflect abnormal lipid metabolism. It should be noted that increased intramyofiber lipid is normal in pups up to about 2 months of age and should not be interpreted as a lipid storage myopathy.

Metabolic myopathy of the cat

Metabolic myopathy in Norwegian Forest cats

A glycogen storage disease type IV due to deficiency of glycogen branching enzyme occurs as an autosomal recessive trait in Norwegian Forest cats. Although glycogen storage occurs in multiple organ systems in the cat, it is dysfunction of skeletal muscle, cardiac muscle, and nervous tissue that characterizes the feline disorder. In contrast, glycogen storage type IV of humans typically results in early-onset and progressive hepatic cirrhosis and liver failure. The molecular basis for this difference between cats and humans is as yet unknown.

Two clinical syndromes have been identified. The most common is the birth of fully developed kittens that are either stillborn or that die within a few hours of birth. Affected kittens that survive the neonatal period develop *progressive neuromuscular weakness, muscle atrophy, and cardiac dysfunction* beginning at about 5–7 months of age. Affected cats are often mildly febrile, exhibit generalized muscle tremors and a "bunny hopping" pelvic limb gait. *Progression to tetraplegia is rapid*, occurring within about 2 months following onset of clinical signs. Electromyography reveals abnormal spontaneous activity in multiple muscles. Cardiologic abnormalities include concentric left ventricular hypertrophy, left atrial dilation, decreased relaxation of the left ventricular wall during diastole, and focal hyperechoic areas in the subendocardial region of the left ventricular wall. Serum activities of CK and ALT are often increased. Glycogen branching enzyme activity in muscle, liver, and leukocytes is markedly reduced in affected cats, and moderately to severely reduced in clinically normal parents of affected cats.

Gross pathologic findings are absent in stillborn kittens or kittens dying soon after birth. In older affected animals, *severe generalized skeletal muscle atrophy* is evident. Fibrous replacement of muscle may be seen. *Left ventricular hypertrophy and left atrial dilation* are typical, and foci of fibrosis may be evident within the left ventricular myocardium.

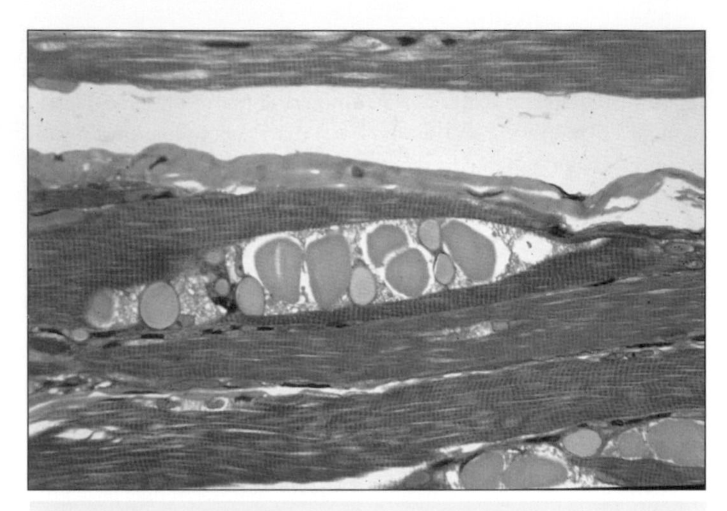

Figure 2.59 Multiple spherical to ovoid pale hyaline inclusions of complex polysaccharide in muscle from a Norwegian Forest cat with **glycogen branching enzyme deficiency** (glycogenosis type IV). (Courtesy of TJ Van Winkle.)

Characteristic histopathologic findings are nonmembrane-bound inclusions of *pale blue material within cells of many organs* (Fig. 2.59). This material is PAS-positive and amylase-resistant. Skeletal muscle, cardiac muscle, and central and peripheral nervous tissue are most severely affected and accumulation of stored material in these organs is accompanied by severe degenerative changes.

Metabolic myopathies of the horse

Equine polysaccharide storage myopathy

A glycogen storage myopathy occurs in many breeds of horses. This disorder has been recognized sporadically for many years. Only recently have studies begun to reveal the variety of clinical disorders associated with polysaccharide storage myopathy in horses as well as the wide range of breeds affected.

Equine polysaccharide storage myopathy is most common in draft, warmblood, and Quarter-Horse-related breeds. In draft-related breeds, a prevalence of over 50% has been reported. This disorder has also been recognized in virtually all other breeds, including ponies and miniature horses. Clinical signs range from recurrent exertional rhabdomyolysis, to progressive weakness that may or may not be accompanied by overt muscle atrophy, to mechanical lameness of the pelvic limbs. Subclinical cases are common. Serum activities of CK and AST may or may not be increased in affected horses. Although *an inherited basis is suspected*, the nature of the inheritance is still unclear.

Gross pathologic findings vary from no significant findings to obvious pale streaks within affected muscle. Muscle atrophy may or may not be evident. Red staining of muscle due to myoglobin release may be seen at postmortem examination of horses dying due to rhabdomyolysis. Careful evaluation of the diaphragm is indicated in animals dying with respiratory failure following clinical rhabdomyolysis, as *severe diaphragmatic necrosis can occur.*

Histopathologic findings are variable. In the most severe cases numerous round to irregularly shaped *blue-gray inclusions are seen within skeletal muscle fibers* on H&E-stained sections (Fig. 2.60). *Inclusions may be single or multiple and are segmental, replacing up to 90% or more of the cross-sectional area of affected fiber segments* (Fig. 2.61). These

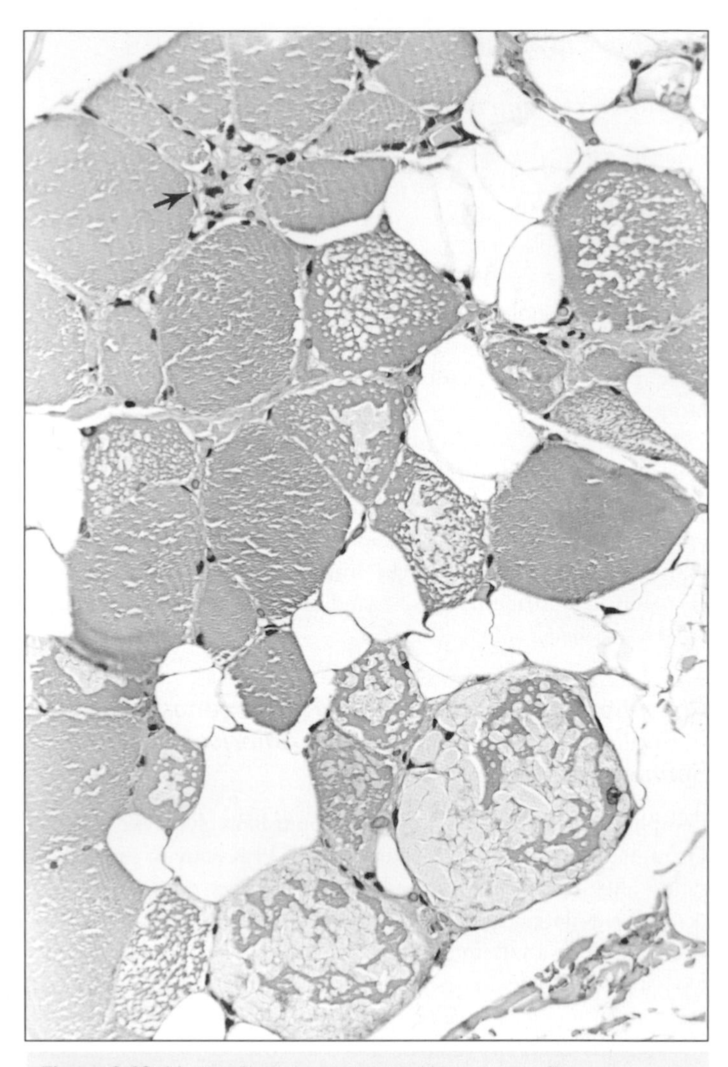

Figure 2.60 Marked fiber size variation with numerous fibers containing multiple vacuoles and inclusions of pale complex polysaccharide in a draft horse with severe chronic **polysaccharide storage myopathy**. A focus of interstitial macrophages (arrow) is indicative of previous segmental necrosis.

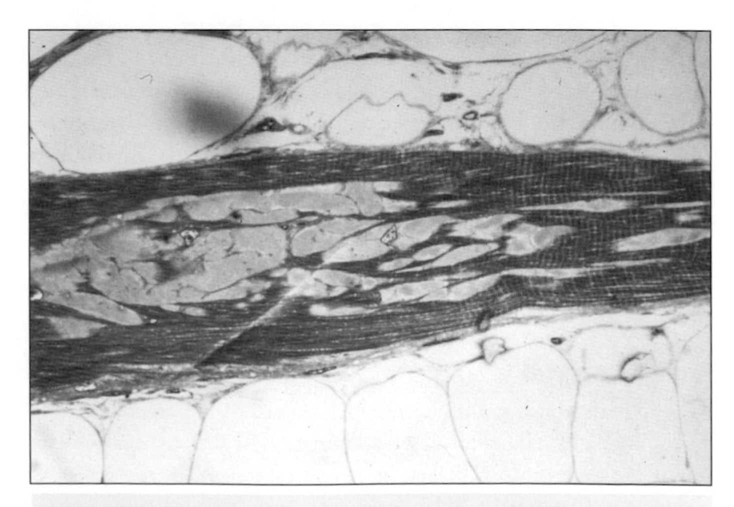

Figure 2.61 Multiple pale inclusions of complex polysaccharide replace large portions of fiber segments in a horse with **polysaccharide storage myopathy**. (Courtesy of JF Cummings.)

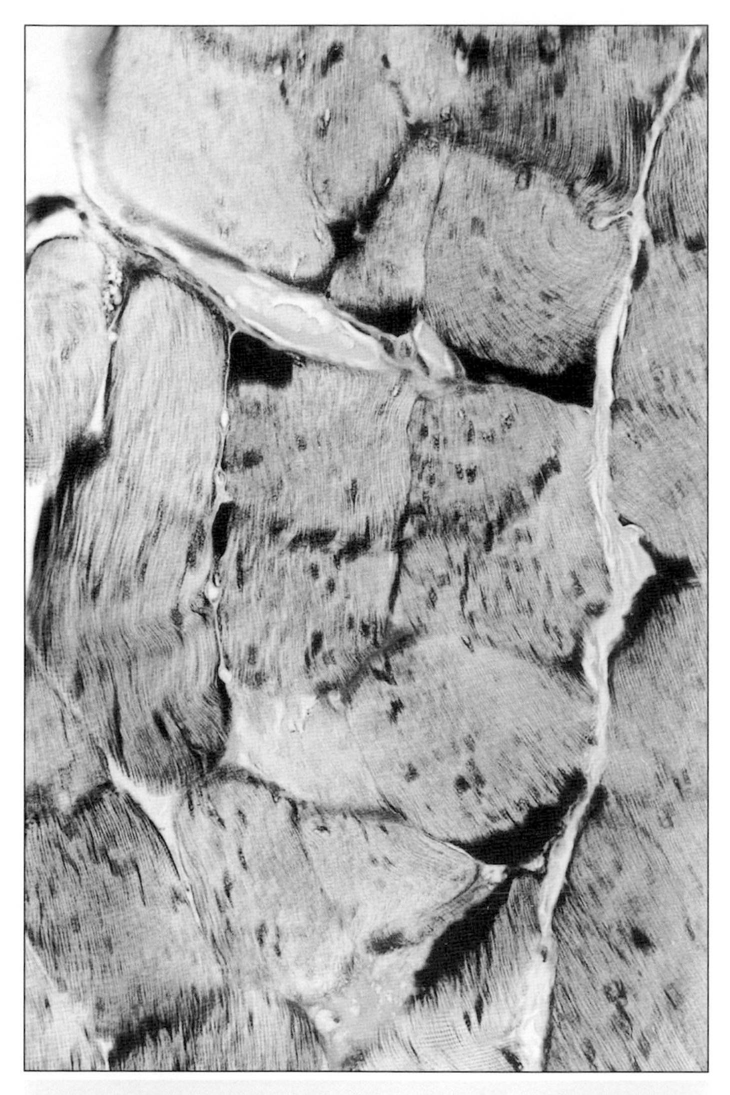

Figure 2.62 Multiple fibers with peripheral aggregates of densely stained glycogen in muscle from an Arabian horse with **polysaccharide storage myopathy**. Fibers also contain increased coarse granular glycogen. Periodic acid-Schiff.

inclusions are PAS-positive and amylase-resistant, consistent with a form of *complex polysaccharide. Inclusions occur only in type 2B glycolytic and 2A oxidative-glycolytic fibers*. Muscles that are strongly type 2 in composition, including semimembranosus, semitendinosus, gluteal, longissimus, and pectoral muscles, are most severely affected. In all cases in which inclusions of complex polysaccharide are seen, other fibers contain subsarcolemmal rounded vacuoles that are either clear or that contain pale pink hyaline material on H&E-stained sections. This material is PAS-positive and amylase-sensitive, consistent with *glycogen*. Fibers with complex polysaccharide or glycogen inclusions often occur in clusters, particularly at the periphery of fascicles. A more subtle pathologic change, involving only subsarcolemmal inclusions of glycogen, is seen in horses believed to have a form of the same disorder (Fig. 2.62). Numerous clear vacuoles within the fiber interior as well as in a subsarcolemmal location can also be seen. Aggregates of glycogen and of amylase-resistant material often contain ubiquitin. *Chronic myopathic changes* are often found, especially in older affected horses, and include excessive fiber size variation due to fiber atrophy and/or hypertrophy and increase in internal nuclei

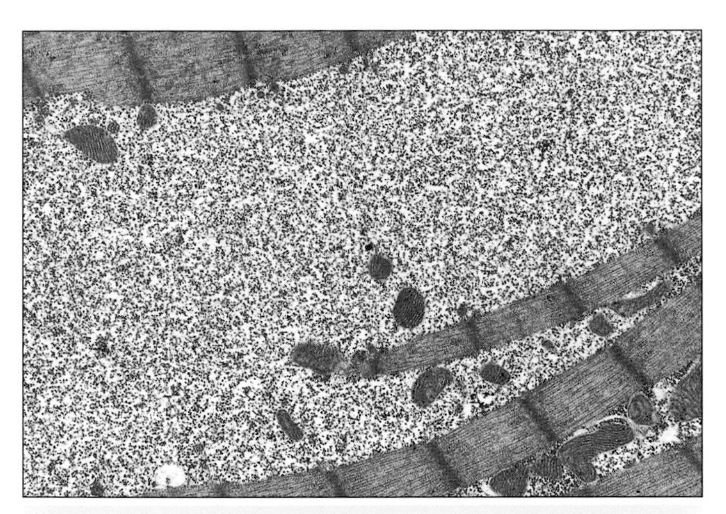

Figure 2.63 Aggregates of granular glycogen with attenuation of myofibrils in a horse with **polysaccharide storage myopathy**. (Courtesy of JF Cummings.)

within myofibers. Scattered myofiber necrosis or regeneration may or may not be seen. Macrophages within necrotic fiber segments or found as small clusters within the interstitium often contain PAS-positive, amylase-resistant complex polysaccharide. In very severe cases, to date only documented in draft-related horses with apparent sudden onset of inability to rise, massive replacement of skeletal muscle by infiltrating adipose tissue can be seen. Other organs, with the exception of rare cases with inclusions of complex polysaccharide within cardiac myofibers, are unaffected.

Ultrastructural examination of affected muscle indicates that *glycogen storage is not intralysosomal but rather is dispersed within the cytoplasm*. Loss or attenuation of myofibrils occurs (Fig. 2.63). Organized inclusions of PAS-positive, amylase-resistant material are composed of tangled fibrillar material studded with glycogen particles.

Despite the clinical and pathologic similarities to myopathies due to carbohydrate metabolic defects in people, dogs, and cats, extensive studies have failed to document a defect in either glycolytic or glycogenolytic pathways in muscle from affected horses. However, diets designed to minimize starch and sugar intake and maximize fat intake have proven to be extremely successful in controlling clinical signs of skeletal muscle dysfunction, *suggesting that this equine disorder involves an as-yet unknown abnormality in carbohydrate metabolism*. Curiously, studies of a small number of horses indicate that pathologic findings are not obviously altered by dietary therapy.

Other metabolic myopathies of horses

A *mitochondrial myopathy* due to deficiency of complex 1 respiratory chain enzyme has been described in an Arabian. Profound exercise intolerance and exercise-induced lactic acidosis without evidence of exercise-induced muscle necrosis were seen.

Glycogen brancher enzyme deficiency occurs in Quarter Horse foals. Affected foals may be aborted or stillborn, or develop weakness and die of cardiac failure in the first few months of life. Characteristic spherical or ovoid inclusions of PAS-positive amylase-resistant amylopectin are seen within skeletal and myocardial fibers, particularly Purkinje fibers (Fig. 2.64). Similar material is seen to a lesser degree in many other organs.

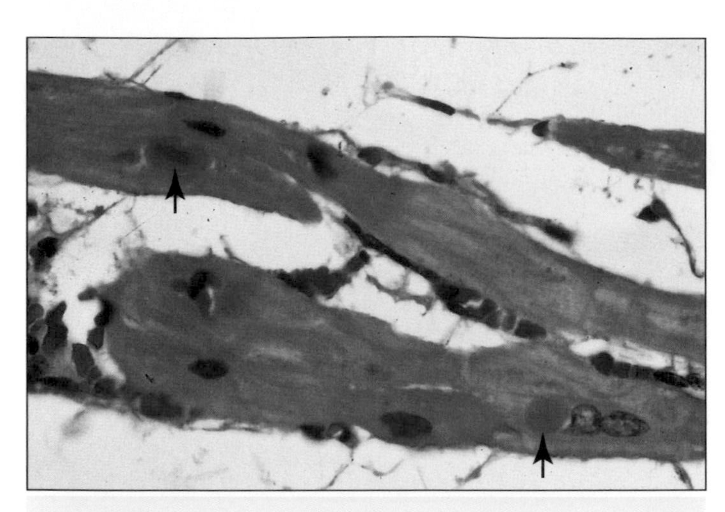

Figure 2.64 Spherical-to-ovoid bodies of complex polysaccharide within Purkinje fibers and cardiac myocytes in a Quarter Horse foal with **glycogen branching enzyme deficiency**. (Courtesy of BJ Cooper.)

Metabolic myopathies of cattle and sheep

Biochemical abnormalities leading to abnormal glycogen storage within skeletal muscle occur in sheep and cattle. In some cases, the disorder is generalized and in others it is confined to skeletal muscle. *Clinical signs of neuromuscular weakness in young sheep and cattle due to metabolic myopathy must be distinguished from the more common nutritional myopathies.*

Bovine metabolic myopathy due to myophosphorylase deficiency

Glycogen phosphorylase is an essential glycolytic enzyme. Tissue-specific isoforms exist, and the skeletal muscle isoform is known as myophosphorylase. *An autosomal recessive defect in the myophosphorylase gene similar to McArdle's disease in people occurs in Charolais cattle, and results in metabolic dysfunction confined to skeletal muscle.* Clinical signs of exercise intolerance and exercise-induced collapse can be seen in affected cattle as young as 7 weeks of age. Increased serum activities of CK and AST are characteristic. Subsarcolemmal vacuoles due to glycogen storage within myofibers are characteristic, and biochemical and histochemical studies reveal a *complete lack of myophosphorylase activity.* Testing of DNA from peripheral white blood cells will detect homozygotes and heterozygotes.

Glycogenosis type II (Pompe's disease) in cattle

Glycogen storage disease due to acid maltase (acid α-glucosidase) deficiency occurs as an autosomal recessive trait in Shorthorn and Brahman cattle. Two clinical syndromes are reported in Shorthorn cattle. An *early-onset form* results in intralysosomal glycogen storage within skeletal, cardiac, and smooth muscle, and in neurons of the central and autonomic nervous systems. Clinical signs of cardiac dysfunction predominate, leading to death due to cardiac failure. A *late-onset form* develops clinical signs predominantly of muscle weakness. Serum activity of CK is often increased, sometimes markedly. In Brahman cattle, glycogenosis type II results in early-onset signs of poor growth and neurologic dysfunction.

Glycogen storage diseases of sheep

A *generalized form* of glycogen storage disease occurs in sheep. Glycogen storage confined to skeletal muscle due to *myophosphorylase deficiency* also occurs, and is similar to the disease in cattle.

Metabolic myopathies of other species

Acid maltase deficiency (glycogenosis type II) resulting in generalized glycogen storage occurs in *Japanese quail*. These birds have been studied as an animal model of acid maltase deficiency of people. Clinical signs of muscle dysfunction predominate, and include inability to right themselves following placement in dorsal or lateral recumbency, and poor wing movements. Weakness is progressive. Abnormal accumulation of membrane-bound glycogen particles occurs as early as day 16 of embryonal development. Progressive glycogen storage resulting in *vacuolar myopathy*, with formation of autophagic vacuoles followed by fiber loss and fatty replacement, are characteristic. Abnormal glycogen storage also occurs in cardiac and smooth muscle as well as in neurons in the brain and spinal cord.

Bibliography

Angelos SM, et al. Myophosphorylase deficiency associated with rhabdomyolysis and exercise intolerance in 6 related Charolais cattle. Muscle Nerve 1995;18:736–740.

Bilstrom JA, et al. Genetic test for myophosphorylase deficiency in Charolais cattle. Am J Vet Res 1998;59:267–270.

Breitschwerdt EB, et al. Episodic weakness associated with exertional lactic acidosis and myopathy in Old English sheepdog littermates. J Am Vet Med Assoc 1992;201:731–736.

Carpenter S, Karpati G. Lysosomal storage in human skeletal muscle. Hum Pathol 1986;17:683–703.

Cooper BJ. Animal models of human muscle disease. In: Karpati G, et al., eds. Disorders of Voluntary Muscle. 7th ed. New York: Cambridge University Press, 2001: 187–215.

DiMauro S, et al. Metabolic myopathies. Am J Med Genet 1986;25:635–651.

Edwards JR, Richards RB. Bovine generalized glycogenosis type II: A clinicopathological study. Br Vet J 1979;135:338–348.

Fitzmaurice SN, et al. Familial myoclonic epilepsy with skeletal muscle polyglucosan bodies in the miniature wire-haired dachshund. J Vet Int Med 1999;13:239.

Fyfe JC, et al. Glycogen storage disease type IV: Inherited deficiency of branching enzyme deficiency in cats. Pediatr Res 1992;32:719–725.

Giger U, et al. Inherited Phosphofructokinase deficiency in an American cocker spaniel. J Am Vet Med Assoc 1992;201:1569–1571.

Gullotta F. Metabolic myopathies. Path Res Pract 1985;180:10–18.

Harvey JW, Giger U. Animal model: muscle-type phosphofructokinase deficiency (glycogen storage disease type VII). Comp Pathol Bull 1991;23:3–4.

Higuchi I, et al. Acid maltase deficiency in the Japanese quail; early morphological event in skeletal muscle. Acta Neuropathol (Berl) 1987;73:32–37.

Howell J.McC, et al. Infantile and late onset form of generalized glycogenosis type II in cattle. J Pathol 1981;134:266–277.

Jolly RD, et al. Generalized glycogenosis in shorthorn cattle - heterozygote detection. Aust J Exp Biol Med Sci 1977;55:141.

O'Sullivan BM, et al. Generalized glycogenosis in Brahman cattle. Aust Vet J 1981;57:227–229.

Pleasure D, Bonilla E. Skeletal muscle storage diseases: myopathies resulting from errors in carbohydrate and fatty acid metabolism. In: Mastaglia FL, Walton J, eds. Skeletal Muscle Pathology. Edinburgh: Churchill-Livingstone, 1982:340–359.
Rafiquzzaman M, et al. Glycogenosis in the dog. Acta Vet Scand 1976;17:196.
Render JA, et al. Amylopectinosis in fetal and neonatal Quarter horses. Vet Pathol 1999;36:157–160.
Shelton GD, et al. Lactic acidemia, hyperalanemia and carnitine abnormalities in dogs with lipid storage myopathy. J Neuropathol Exp Neurol 1995;54:457.
Thompson AJ, et al. Polysaccharide storage myopathy. Muscle Nerve 1988;11:349–355.
Valberg SJ, et al. Polysaccharide storage myopathy associated with recurrent exertional rhabdomyolysis in horses. Neuromusc Dis 1992;2:351–359.
Valberg SJ, et al. Skeletal muscle mitochondrial myopathy as a cause of exercise intolerance in a horse. Muscle Nerve 1994;17:305–312.
Valberg SJ, Hodgson DR. Diseases of muscle. In: Smith BP, ed. Large Animal Internal Medicine. 3rd ed. St. Louis, MO: Mosby, 2002:1266–1291.
Valberg SJ, et al. Skeletal muscle glycolytic capacity and phosphofructokinase regulation in horses with polysaccharide storage myopathy. Am J Vet Res 1998;59:782–785.
Valentine BA, et al. Muscle glycogen, myopathy, and diet. World Eq Vet Rev 1997;2:27–31.
Valentine BA, et al. Muscle biopsy diagnosis of equine motor neuron disease and equine polysaccharide storage myopathy. Eq Vet Educ 1998;10:42–50.
Valentine BA, et al. Polysaccharide storage myopathy in Morgan, Arabian, and Standardbred related horses and Welsh-cross ponies. Vet Pathol 2000;37:193–196.
Valentine BA, et al. Incidence of polysaccharide storage myopathy in draft horse-related breeds: a necropsy study of 37 horses and a mule. J Vet Diagn Invest 2001;13:63–68.
Valentine BA, et al. Role of dietary carbohydrate and fat in horses with equine polysaccharide storage myopathy. J Am Vet Med Assoc 2001;219:1537–1544. Erratum in: J Am Vet Med Assoc 2002;220:211.
Walvoort HC. Glycogen storage disease type II in the Lapland dog. Vet Quarterly 1985;7:187–190.

Congenital myasthenia gravis

Two clearly defined types of myasthenia gravis occur in humans and animals; both congenital and acquired myasthenia gravis have been described in dogs and cats.

- The *congenital disease* is due to an inherent defect in acetylcholine end-plate receptors.
- The more common *acquired disease* is an immune-mediated disorder due to circulating anticholinesterase receptor antibodies and is discussed in the section on Immune-mediated conditions.

Canine congenital myasthenia

In the dog, congenital myasthenia gravis has been described in Jack Russell Terriers, Springer Spaniels, Smooth Fox Terriers, and the Gammel Dansk Hønsehund. The disorder is inherited as an *autosomal recessive trait*. Affected dogs are clinically normal at birth but develop clinical signs of *exercise-induced weakness and collapse* at an early age. Clinical signs are apparent at about 5–8 weeks of age in affected Springer Spaniels and Jack Russell Terriers, and at about 12–16 weeks of age in the Gammel Dansk Hønsehund. Clinical signs are progressive in growing Jack Russell Terriers and Springer Spaniels, often leading to recumbency. The disorder is not progressive in the Gammel Dansk Hønsehund. Esophageal dysfunction leading to megaesophagus may occur in the Springer Spaniel and Smooth Fox Terrier. A decremental response occurs with repetitive nerve stimulation studies. Circulating antibodies to acetylcholine receptors are not found, but affected dogs improve with anticholinesterase therapy.

No abnormalities are seen in the motor end plate by light microscopy. Ultrastructural evaluation reveals *decreased density of postsynaptic acetylcholine receptors and shallow secondary clefts in the end-plate synaptic gutters*. Studies in the Jack Russell Terrier have shown a decreased rate of insertion of acetylcholine receptors into the post-synaptic membrane. Young animals are apparently able to function normally, but with growth this reduced acetylcholine receptor density results in neuromuscular weakness.

Feline congenital myasthenia

Myasthenia gravis is less commonly described in cats. This disorder has been described in Siamese and in domestic shorthaired cats. Mode of inheritance is not known. Clinical signs of *episodic weakness* are first noted at about 4–5 months of age. Affected cats may have a weak voice and the disorder may progress to tetraplegia. Megaesophagus has not been reported. A decremental response is seen with repetitive nerve stimulation, and circulating antibodies to acetylcholine receptors are not found. Clinical improvement can be seen with oral or intravenous anticholinesterase therapy. Acetylcholine receptor density was found to be 66% of normal in one cat studied.

Bibliography

Flagstad A, et al. Congenital myasthenic syndrome in the dog breed Gammel Dansk Hønsehund: clinical, electrophysiological, pharmacological and immunological comparison with acquired myasthenia gravis. Acta Vet Scand 1989;30:89–102.
Johnson RP, et al. Myasthenia in Springer spaniel littermates. J Small Anim Pract 1975;16:641–647.
Joseph RJ, et al. Myasthenia gravis in the cat. J Vet Int Med 1988;2:75–79.
Lennon VA, et al. Acquired and congenital myasthenia gravis in dogs – a study of 20 cases. In: Satoyoshi E, ed. Myasthenia Gravis – Pathogenesis and Treatment. Tokyo: University of Tokyo Press, 1981:41–54.
Miller LM, et al. Congenital myasthenia gravis in 13 smooth fox terriers. J Am Vet Med Assoc 1983;182:694–697.
Odo K, et al. Congenital canine myasthenia gravis: I. Deficient junctional acetylcholine receptors. Muscle Nerve 1984;7:705–716.
Odo K, et al. Congenital canine myasthenia gravis: II. Acetylcholine receptor metabolism. Muscle Nerve 1984;7:717–724.
Palmer AC, et al. Autoimmune form of myasthenia gravis in a juvenile Yorkshire terrier x Jack Russell terrier hybrid contrasted with congenital (non-autoimmune) myasthenia gravis of the Jack Russell. J Small Anim Pract 1980;21:359–364.
Trojaborg W, Flagstad A. A hereditary neuromuscular disorder in dogs. Muscle Nerve 1982;5:S30–S38.
Wilkes MK, et al. Ultrastructure of motor endplates in canine congenital myasthenia gravis. J Comp Pathol 1987;97:247–256.

Malignant hyperthermia

Malignant hyperthermia (MH) *is a condition that results in a sudden increase in myoplasmic calcium concentration leading to prolonged myofiber contraction and muscle rigidity, hypermetabolism, tachycardia, dyspnea, metabolic acidosis, and life-threatening hyperthermia. Severe acute rhabdomyolysis is the primary histopathologic finding*. Episodes are triggered by a variety of circumstances, including stress and pharmacologic agents such as halothane anesthesia. Malignant hyperthermia is an inherited disorder in humans, pigs, and some dogs. *The defect is in the ryanodine receptor*, a calcium-release channel of the sarcoplasmic reticulum that serves a critical role in triggering release of calcium from the sarcoplasmic reticulum during excitation–contraction coupling. Malignant hyperthermia in humans may be due to more than one genetic defect involving the ryanodine receptor. Other myopathic disorders leading to susceptibility to MH occur, and therefore *MH is best regarded as a syndrome rather than a single entity*. Susceptible individuals may have mildly increased serum CK activities and increased erythrocyte fragility. Testing for MH susceptibility classically involves in vitro exposure of muscle biopsy samples to various concentrations of caffeine and halothane. Muscle from MH-susceptible individuals exhibits contraction at relatively low concentrations of these pharmacologic agents as opposed to normal individuals.

Malignant hyperthermia-like episodes also occur in *anesthetized horses*, although an inherited basis has not been documented in the horse. Ryanodine receptor defects have been documented in a small number of cases. It may also be triggered in horses by injection of succinylcholine. Malignant hyperthermia-like episodes may also occur in people or animals with other underlying myopathies. This is certainly the case in cats with X-linked muscular dystrophy, in which anesthesia or the stress of restraint can trigger episodes of fatal hyperthermia. Underlying HYPP has been associated with malignant hyperthermia-like episodes associated with anesthesia in horses, and it is possible that other myopathic conditions may predispose horses to this disorder.

Malignant hyperthermia in pigs (porcine stress syndrome)

Malignant hyperthermia in pigs renders them susceptible to episodes associated with stresses such as handling, transportation, or fighting, and *may result in sudden death*. The meat of affected pigs is usually *pale, soft, and exudative (PSE pork)*. Porcine stress syndrome has been recognized in Europe and North America for a long time as "*herztod*" or *back muscle necrosis* of pigs. *Susceptible pigs exhibit intense, immobilizing limb and torso muscle rigidity, respiratory difficulty, tachycardia, acidosis and, often, rapid death*. Heavy-muscled pigs seem to be most susceptible to the clinical disease. Prior to identification of the ryanodine receptor gene defect, a large body of literature accumulated regarding various biochemical abnormalities detected in affected muscle and in affected animals. Recently, *a single point mutation in the skeletal muscle ryanodine receptor (ryr1) at locus HAL-1843 leading to increased channel open time has been shown to be the cause of MH* in domestic pigs, including Pietrain, Yorkshire, Poland China, Duroc, and Landrace breeds. DNA testing of peripheral blood for the HAL-1843 gene defect is available commercially. Genetic studies point to a single affected founder pig followed by widespread dissemination of the gene, and it has been suggested that these pigs have been selected for based on their heavy muscling and decreased body fat. Malignant hyperthermia occurs in all pork-producing countries of the world. It has been estimated that 2–30% of purebred breeding pigs are susceptible to malignant hyperthermia. A similar syndrome of MH appears to occur in *Vietnamese pot-bellied pigs*. In one case of a pot-bellied pig dying due to anesthesia-induced hyperthermia, a gene defect at HAL-1843 was detected. Testing of parents of another pot-bellied pig with suspect malignant hyperthermia, however, did not reveal HAL-1843 defects, suggesting that in pigs, as in humans, *more than one gene defect may lead to MH*.

Postmortem examination of the muscles of susceptible pigs that have not endured an episode of hyperthermia recently reveals normal muscles. *Pigs dying of hyperthermia have pale muscles that are wet and apparently swollen*. *Rigor mortis develops unusually rapidly*. In addition to lesions of skeletal muscle, *lesions of acute heart failure*, such as pulmonary edema and congestion, hydropericardium, hydrothorax, and hepatic congestion, often are present. The muscles most likely to be affected are those of the *back, loin, thigh, and shoulder*. Although both type 1 and type 2 myofibers undergo necrosis, muscles with a high proportion of type 2 fibers such as longissimus, psoas, and semitendinosus are most extensively and most frequently affected, and these should be examined histologically. Hemorrhages sometimes are present in muscles, and in the warm carcass a marked lowering of muscle pH to 5.8 or lower can be detected. On cooling, the pH rises rapidly towards neutrality. Myocardial pallor involving the ventricular muscles sometimes occurs but the clinical signs of tachycardia are probably related to acidosis.

Microscopic examination of malignant hyperthermia susceptible animals not recently affected by hyperthermic episodes reveals normal muscle fibers, or there may be a few degenerate fibers. *There is nothing distinctive about the appearance of the degenerate fibers*. In pigs dying acutely of malignant hyperthermia, *muscle fibers are separated by edema fluid*. This is evident in rapidly fixed specimens only and may be lost in processing. Changes in muscle fibers are widespread and are typically characterized as *multifocal monophasic injury*. It is possible, however, to find polyphasic injury in pigs with recent nonfatal episodes of MH, and underlying chronic myopathic changes may also be observed. Degenerative changes vary from segmental hypercontraction (Fig. 2.65) to overt coagulative necrosis. *Hypercontraction* is the most common lesion in skeletal muscle. Myocardial lesions include multifocal granular degeneration of myocytes, contraction band necrosis, and myocytolysis.

Malignant hyperthermia in dogs

There are sporadic reports of *MH-like episodes* in various breeds of dogs. *Exercise-induced hyperthermia* has been seen in English Springer Spaniels and in Labrador Retrievers. *Ingestion of hops* can trigger a MH-like episode in susceptible dogs, and this condition has been most commonly seen in Greyhounds. Studies of a breeding colony of mixed-breed dogs susceptible to anesthesia-induced MH determined that the disorder was inherited as a dominant trait with variable severity. A genetic defect has yet to be identified in MH-susceptible dogs and *it is possible that MH in dogs is a heterogeneous disorder*. Chronic myopathic changes including internal nuclei, increased fiber size variation, and fiber hypertrophy may be seen in muscle from MH-susceptible dogs. Histologic lesions in dogs dying due to

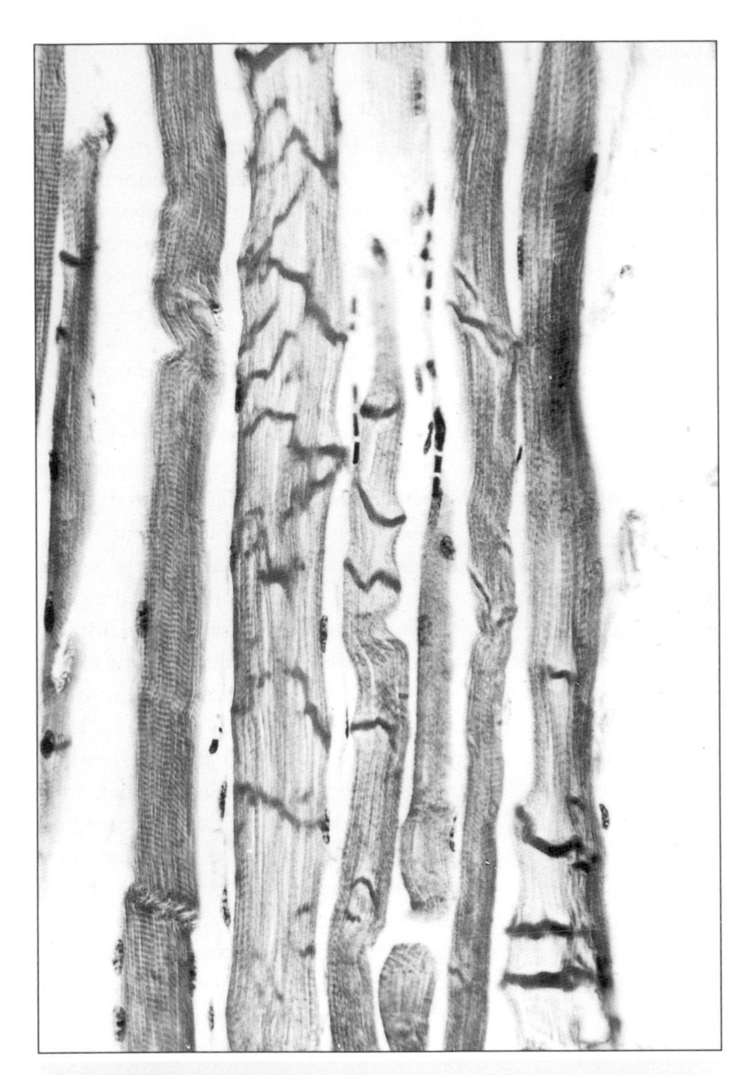

Figure 2.65 Acute myopathy in a pig with malignant hyperthermia (porcine stress syndrome) with characteristic **segmental hypercontraction**. (Courtesy of TJ Hulland.)

hyperthermia are similar to those seen in other MH-susceptible species.

Bibliography

Aleman M, et al. Association of a mutation in the ryanodine receptor 1 gene with equine malignant hyperthermia. Muscle Nerve 2004;30:356–365.

Claxton-Gill MS, et al. Suspected malignant hyperthermia syndrome in a miniature pot-bellied pig anesthetized with isoflurane. J Am Vet Med Assoc 1993;203:1434–1436.

Duncan KL, et al. Malignant hyperthermia-like reaction secondary to ingestion of hops in five dogs. J Am Vet Med Assoc 1997;210:51–54.

Fujii J, et al. Identification of a mutation in porcine ryanodine receptor associated with malignant hyperthermia. Science 1991;253:448–451.

Gaschen FP, et al. Lethal peracute rhabdomyolysis associated with stress and general anesthesia in three dystrophin-deficient cats. Vet Pathol 1998;35:117–123.

Hartmann S, et al. Influences of breed, sex, and susceptibility to malignant hyperthermia on lipid composition of skeletal muscle and adipose tissue in swine. Am J Vet Res 1997;58:738–743.

Heffron JJA, et al. Muscle fiber type, fiber diameter and pH values of m. longissimus dorsi of normal, malignant hyperthermia – and PSE-susceptible pigs. Br Vet J 1982;138:45–50.

Lewis PJ, et al. Effect of exercise and pre-slaughter stress on pork muscle characteristics. Meat Sci 1989;26:121–129.

Lopez JR, et al. Myoplasmic free [Ca2+} during a malignant hyperthermia episode in swine. Muscle Nerve 1988;11:82–88.

Lundström K, et al. Effect of halothane genotype on muscle metabolism at slaughter and its relationship with meat quality: a within-litter comparison. Meat Sci 1989;25:251–263.

MacLennan DH, Phillips MS. Malignant hyperthermia. Science 1992;256:789–794.

Manley SV, et al. Malignant hyperthermia-like reactions in three anesthetized horses. J Am Vet Med Assoc 1983;183:85–89.

O'Brien PJ. Etiopathogenetic defect of malignant hyperthermia: hypersensitive calcium-release channel of skeletal muscle sarcoplasmic reticulum. Vet Res Commun 1987;11:527–559.

O'Brien PJ, et al. Canine malignant hyperthermia susceptibility: erythrocyte defects-osmotic fragility, glucose-6-phosphate dehydrogenase deficiency and abnormal Ca2+ homeostasis. Can J Comp Med 1984;48:381–389.

O'Brien PJ, et al. Use of a DNA-based test for the mutation associated with porcine stress syndrome (malignant hyperthermia) in 10,000 breeding swine. J Am Vet Med Assoc 1993;203:842–851.

Rand JS, O'Brien PJ. Exercise-induced malignant hyperthermia in an English Springer spaniel. J Am Vet Med Assoc 1987;190:1013–1014.

Somers CJ, McLoughlan JV. Malignant hyperthermia in pigs: calcium ion uptake by mitochondria from skeletal muscle of susceptible animals given neuroleptic drugs and halothane. J Comp Pathol 1982;92:191–198.

Sosnicki A. Histopathological observation of stress myopathy in M. longissimus in the pig and relationships with meat quality, fattening and slaughter traits. J Anim Sci 1987;65:584–596.

Wingertzahn MA, Ochs RS. Control of calcium in skeletal muscle excitation-contraction coupling: implications for malignant hyperthermia. Molec Genet Metab 1998;65:113–120.

CIRCULATORY DISTURBANCES OF MUSCLE

Skeletal muscle is a highly vascular tissue with an abundant capillary bed that forms an extensive system of anastomoses. It is generally not possible to induce muscle fiber necrosis by ligation of, or damage to, intermuscular arteries, because most muscles receive small collateral arterioles from tendons, fascial sheaths, and major nerve trunks. Naturally occurring examples of ischemic muscle necrosis are most often due to vascular occlusion secondary to pressure. Occlusion of major arteries such as aortic-iliac thrombosis ("saddle thrombi") can also cause ischemic muscle necrosis.

Each muscle fiber is served, at any given level, by three to 12 capillaries that run mainly longitudinally in the endomysium. Type 1 fibers are served by slightly more capillaries than are type 2 fibers of comparable size. Muscles such as those of mastication are particularly well supplied; nearly twice as many capillaries serve each of these fibers than is the case for the major thigh or shoulder muscles.

Maximum myofiber diameter is limited to some extent by the distance from the capillary to the center of the fiber(s) supplied. When the distance becomes abnormally great, the fiber is likely to form a longitudinal cleft down one side (*fiber splitting*) into which a capillary slips, effectively serving the fiber interior (Figs 2.16, 2.17). Complete or incomplete longitudinal fiber division appears to be a mechanism primarily initiated to improve the capillary-to-fiber ratio.

Ischemic damage to muscle fibers, and the capacity to repair, will depend on the completeness and duration of oxygen and nutrient deprivation.

- Least damaging is *transient hypoxia* of a few hours duration, which causes coagulation of muscle contractile proteins but does little harm to the other cellular components or to the satellite cells. Muscles are ordinarily restored to normal function in about 16–20 days by myoblast activation, division and fusion to form myotubes (see Degeneration and repair of muscle, Fig. 2.22) that mature to myofibers.
- The next level of injury is induced by *episodes of ischemia lasting 6–24 hours*, which cause death of both myofiber and satellite cell nuclei and coagulative necrosis of long segments of myofibers. The capacity for regenerative muscle fiber repair is lost or greatly reduced and reaction is largely local proliferation of fibroblasts and endothelial cells within the endomysium. The repair process is quite rapid but leads to a randomly distributed mixture of regenerated or original fibers interspersed with fibrosis.
- The *third level of ischemic injury is that lasting for more than 18–24 hours*, which leads to death of all cells within an area of muscle. The tissue response in this case is confined to a slow peripheral sequestration followed by phagocytic removal of dead muscle and fibroblastic proliferation that can take months to complete. The end result is a mass of scar tissue that can include adipose tissue, with a peripheral narrow zone of distorted muscle fibers.

During the *acute phase of ischemic muscle destruction*, a relatively orderly sequence of functional and morphological changes can be expected. After as little as 1 h of ischemia, the ability of the muscle fiber to contract in response to any stimulus is lost. Ultrastructurally, changes in subcellular components begin after about 6–7 h of ischemia when the tubular systems become dilated and begin to disintegrate. Some mitochondria may show evidence of swelling and disarray at 8 h, but even after 24 h many mitochondria may be well preserved. Z bands begin to disintegrate at about 12 h. Other components of the sarcomere, including thick and thin myofilaments, remain intact for at least 48 h, and it is only after this time that an amorphous hyaline mass forms, free of cross or longitudinal striations. Degeneration of the fiber at the Z bands occurs after 48 h and may be an extension of the earlier Z band disintegration.

Regardless of the duration and extent of the ischemic change, *the muscle fiber plasma membrane becomes permeable to enzymes and myoglobin*. Serum creatine kinase activity is markedly increased but often returns to near normal in 4–5 days, even when destruction of muscle is extensive. Myoglobin is released from damaged muscle and the amount released will vary directly with the severity and extent of damage. When a large mass of muscle is physically injured or when ischemic degenerative changes are extensive, large amounts of myoglobin are released into the bloodstream. Much of this is excreted by the kidneys. Myoglobin has a direct toxic effect on convoluted tubules leading to nephrosis. Perhaps more importantly, renal ischemia due to shock will contribute to the potential for severe renal damage and renal shutdown. Hyperkalemia due to massive muscle fiber breakdown can result in acute heart failure.

Four syndromes of ischemic muscle necrosis are recognized in humans and animals, namely, compartment syndrome, downer syndrome, muscle crush syndrome, and vascular occlusive syndrome. The distinctions among these syndromes are not always clear. In veterinary medicine, *hypotensive myopathy in anesthetized horses constitutes a fifth syndrome.* In the compartment syndrome, the downer syndrome, and the muscle crush syndrome, ischemia is caused by increasing intramuscular pressure. The vascular occlusive syndrome results from physical obstruction of the blood supply to muscle, and hypotension leading to poor muscle perfusion is thought to be the cause of hypotensive myopathy in horses.

Compartment syndrome

Muscles that are surrounded by either a heavy aponeurotic sheath or by bone and sheath are vulnerable to ischemia when muscle fibers are subjected to moderately vigorous but not exhaustive contraction. This syndrome occurs in well-conditioned athletes, but nowhere is the syndrome more clearly primary and specific than in the infarction that occurs in the *supracoracoid muscles of some breeds of broiler chickens and in some breeds of turkeys*. In these birds, a brief, vigorous flapping of the wings increases intramuscular pressure of the supracoracoid muscle within the inelastic breastbone and the outer muscle sheath. Muscle in full contraction increases in volume up to 20% and this causes partial or transient collapse of the venous outflow. At the same time, muscle activity increases arterial blood flow to the muscle. Subsequent muscle contractions tend to build internal pressure until the intramuscular pressure exceeds first venous and then arterial blood pressure. Metabolites of the muscle fibers exerting an increased osmotic tension coupled with increased arteriolar blood pressure cause accumulation of interstitial water early in the process and this further increases intramuscular pressure. Once blood flow has stopped, ischemic changes of both muscle and vessels begin, and further water escapes from damaged endothelial cells. Pressure builds for 1–4 h after muscle exercise and the extent and severity of damage to muscle increases with time. In both humans and birds, early fasciotomy releases intramuscular pressure and restores the potential for complete regenerative repair.

The so-called *spontaneous rupture of the gastrocnemius muscle of Channel Island breeds of cattle* may represent an example of compartment syndrome leading to ischemia and subsequent rupture (Fig. 2.66). Similarly, the swelling of muscle that can occur in dogs and horses with *masticatory myopathy*, and in horses with *exertional rhabdomyolysis*, may occur at least partly due to compartment syndrome, with initial muscle damage leading to increased pressure against thick overlying fascia.

Downer syndrome

Humans and most of the domestic species share a muscle ischemia syndrome that is initiated by external pressure of objects or by pressure created by the weight of body, torso, or head on a limb tucked under the body for prolonged periods. This condition in humans is usually related to drug overdose, while in animals it is induced by prolonged anesthesia, muscle, joint, or bone damage causing prostration, or metabolic or neurologic disease causing paresis. Absolute size and body weight has some influence on the incidence of the disease. Animals in good condition are particularly susceptible, and thin animals seldom suffer from ischemic muscle necrosis. Rams and heavy ewes, boars and sows, and even large dogs are occasionally susceptible, but this disorder does not occur in cats. *Cows are the species most frequently affected*, partly because of their weight and their muscle bulk and

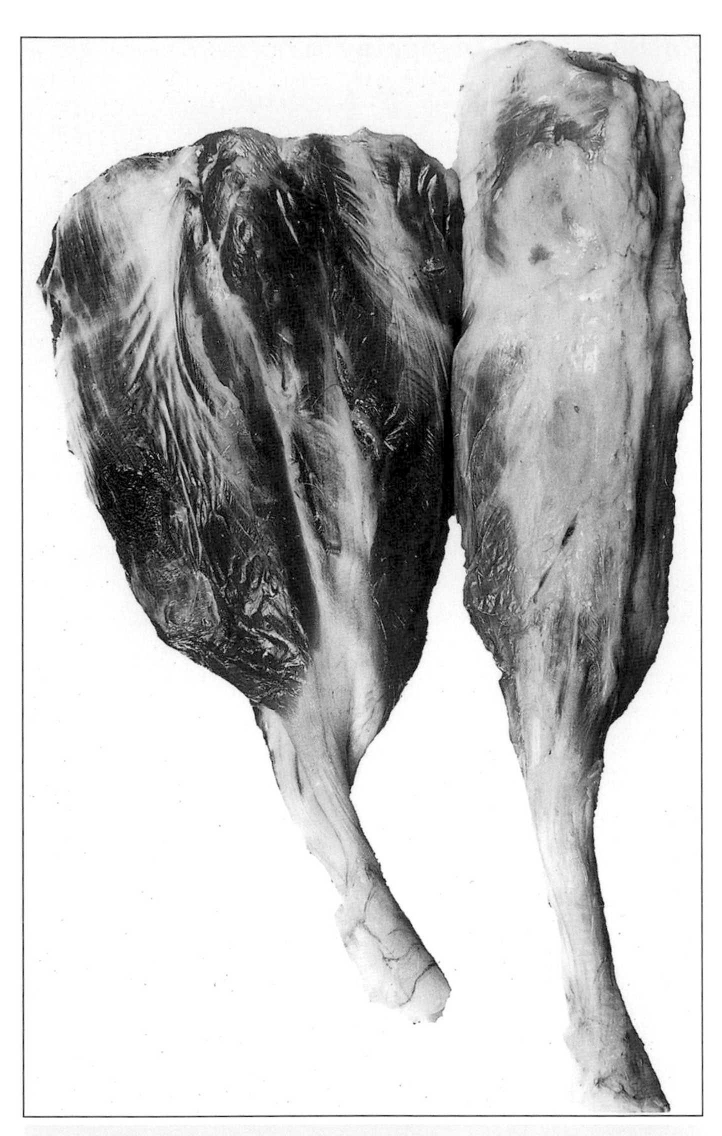

Figure 2.66 Rupture of the gastrocnemius muscle in a Channel Island cow, probably due to **compartment syndrome**. Affected muscle is on the right; normal muscle is on the left. (Courtesy of TJ Hulland.)

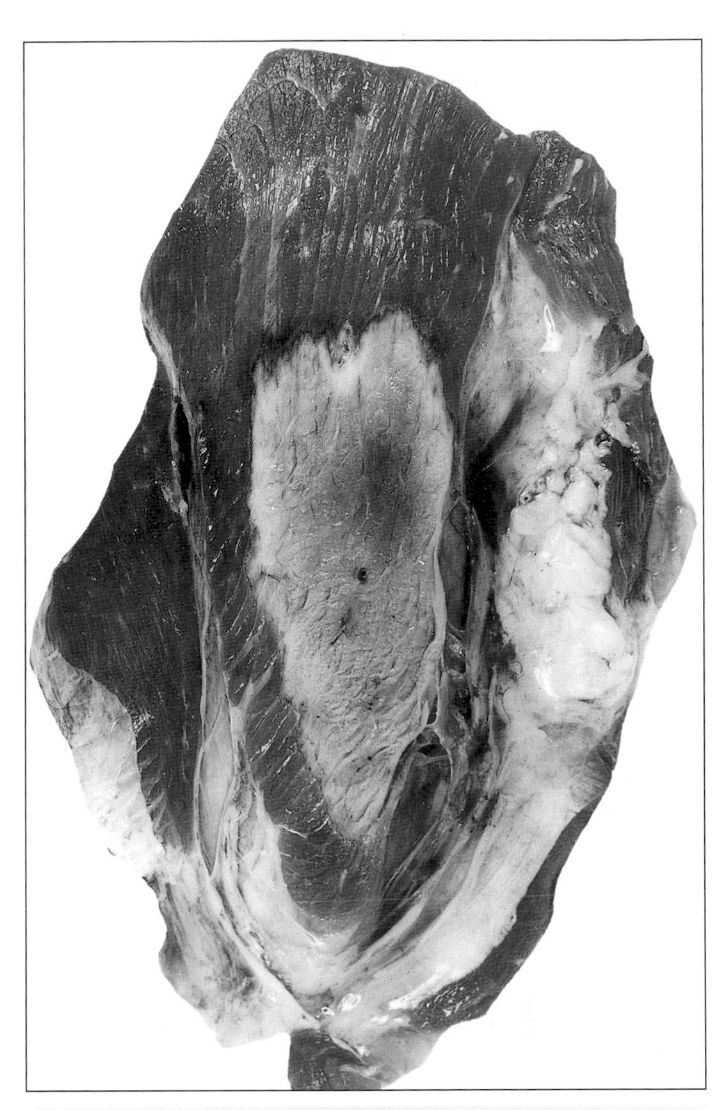

Figure 2.67 Locally extensive pale zone of infarcted thigh muscle due to ischemia in a **downer cow**. (Courtesy of TJ Hulland.)

partly because they are subject to diseases in which paresis is common (Fig. 2.67).

The pathogenesis of the downer syndrome depends upon the fact that the weight of the body can cause pressure within muscles to rise to levels considerably higher than both venous and arterial pressure. Muscles of limbs in a flexed or tucked position are particularly susceptible. The intramuscular pressure soon serves to collapse veins of the fascial sheaths and skin, causing congestion, and then collapses arteries. In cows and horses, extensive ischemic lesions are sometimes created by a period of inertia as short as 6 h, while some cows seem to be able to tolerate 12 or even more hours of immobility with minimal residual lesions. As time passes and as the pressure is removed, the affected limb continues to swell as edema fluid increases under returned arterial flow. *Reperfusion injury is likely to contribute to ischemic damage in the downer syndrome.* The extent of lesions within a muscle mass is quite variable but seldom involves more than half of the mass. The degree of damage will reflect the extent, duration, and severity of the ischemic episode as well as the extent and rapidity of reflow.

The clinical presentation of downer syndrome can be complicated by *pressure-induced peripheral nerve injury*. Even 6 h of anesthesia or comparable inactivity in horses and cows can cause sciatic or other nerve damage leading to *peroneal nerve paralysis* and a flexed rear fetlock, or a dropped shoulder and elbow due to *radial paralysis*. This neuropathy is, however, more often due to nerve conduction block than to structural nerve damage, allowing for the possibility of a relatively rapid recovery. If there is actual structural damage to nerves, effective recovery and mobilization may be delayed until nerves to muscles are regenerated, and complete recovery is not always possible.

Muscle crush syndrome

This form of muscle ischemia has characteristics in common with downer syndrome. *It is usually initiated by acute accidental trauma, often including bone fracture.* It occurs less frequently in animals than in humans, but has been seen in the dog and perhaps the cow. Initial events center on the *traumatic laceration of muscle*, which leads to a combination of high osmotic tension and hyperemia that result in accumulation of abundant edema fluid in the area. Edema causing increased pressure can exacerbate the muscle damage. If the damaged muscle and bone are still confined within a relatively firm sheath, conditions resembling those of compartment syndrome are set up. The limb swells and extends, and becomes turgid. Ischemia of variable extent ensues but, because of the great amount of myoglobin released, *renal dysfunction* may dominate the syndrome.

Vascular occlusive syndrome

When a *major vessel to a limb is occluded* the limb becomes cool, the arterial pulse is lost, skin over the limb loses its ability to sweat, and some limitation of movement may be apparent. When this occurs as a result of *aortic-iliac artery thrombosis in the horse* the effects are usually transient, apparently due to effective collateral circulation. Some muscle degeneration probably occurs but is repaired rapidly and completely. In the *cat with aortic-iliac thrombosis* associated with underlying cardiomyopathy, more of the aorta is likely to be occluded than is the case in the horse, and collateral circulation may be less effective at restoring circulation to hindlimb muscles. Muscle lesions vary from mild to severe (Fig. 2.68). The *anatomic pattern of degeneration* varies from one case to another and more distal muscles are not necessarily more vulnerable. Hindlimb muscle from cats with aortic-iliac thrombosis can also exhibit chronic myopathic changes indicative of previous bouts of subclinical ischemic myopathy.

An ischemic lesion of muscle seen in *sheep in advanced pregnancy* appears also to be caused by arterial occlusion. Ewes carrying twins or triplets sometimes suffer from ischemic necrosis of the internal abdominal oblique muscle without evidence of congestion or hemorrhage. This muscle does not have a confining sheath thus the necrosis is not part of a compartment syndrome. The arterial supply to the abdominal oblique is via a tortuous branch of the internal iliac artery which turns back on itself inside the iliac tuberosity, and it may be vulnerable to stretch and/or trauma. Ischemia of the muscle is followed by rupture, and subsequently the other abdominal muscles also rupture. In spite of all of this, the ewes sometimes lamb at term without difficulty.

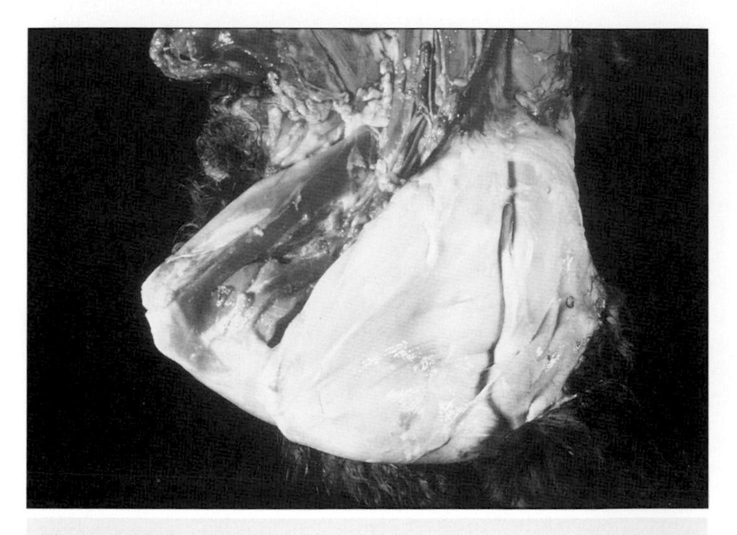

Figure 2.68 Pale thigh muscle due to infarction in a cat with **ischemic myopathy** due to aortic-iliac thrombosis.

Postanesthetic myopathy in horses

Postoperative weakness due to neuromuscular dysfunction occurs with some regularity in horses. A *variety of etiologies* are possible. Heavily muscled horses anesthetized and laid on poorly padded surfaces can develop *pressure-induced ischemic damage* to muscle similar to downer syndrome. *Compartment syndrome* affecting selected muscles can also occur. Cases of compartment syndrome in which a hemorrhagic infiltrate is prominent suggest predominantly venous occlusion. Pressure-induced neuropathy is a frequent complication. Horses with underlying myopathy, such as hyperkalemic periodic paralysis (HYPP) (see Myotonic and spastic syndromes) and polysaccharide storage myopathy (see Metabolic myopathies) are particularly prone to postanesthetic myopathy. A hyperthermia-like condition is also possible, especially in horses with HYPP.

A syndrome of ischemic myopathy due to hypotension and decreased muscle perfusion occurs in horses, most often associated with *halothane anesthesia*. This syndrome can be reproduced experimentally. Marked increases in serum CK and AST activities and lactate concentration occur. Swelling is most common in downside muscles, with increased intracompartmental pressure indicative of associated compartment syndrome.

Fibrotic myopathy

Fibrotic myopathies occur in a number of species including horses, dogs, cats, and humans, and most commonly involve the semitendinosus muscles. *Fibrotic myopathy is nonspecific and may be a consequence of intramuscular injections, primary myopathies, or peripheral neuropathies.* It may occur spontaneously in Quarter Horses and Greyhounds that rupture muscles upon explosive exercise, but is predisposed in conditions such as hemophilia where repeated hemorrhage into muscles leads to extensive fibrosis. *Affected muscles are replaced by contracted bands of dense scar tissue.*

Bibliography

Cox VS, et al. The role of pressure damage in pathogenesis of the downer cow syndrome. Am J Vet Res 1982;43:26–31.

Friend SCE. Postanesthetic myonecrosis in horses. Can Vet J 1981;22:367–371.

Gomez-Villamandos R, et al. Tenotomy of the tibial insertion of the semitendinosus muscle of two horses with fibrotic myopathy. Vet Record 1995; 136:67–68.

Grandy JL, et al. Arterial hypotension and the development of postanesthetic myopathy in halothane-anesthetized horses. Am J Vet Res 1987;48:192–197.

Hilton-Jones D. The clinical features of some miscellaneous neuromuscular disorders. In: Walton J, et al., eds. Disorders of Voluntary Muscle. 6th ed. New York: Churchill-Livingstone, 1994:976–977.

Lindsay WA, et al., Equine postanesthetic forelimb lameness: Intracompartmental muscle pressure changes and biochemical patterns. Am J Vet Res 1980;41:1919–1924.

Lindsay WA, et al. Induction of equine postanesthetic myositis after halothane-induced hypotension. Am J Vet Res 1989;50:404–410.

Martindale L, et al. Effects of subfascial pressure in experimental deep pectoral myopathy of the fowl: An angiographic study. Avian Pathol 1979;8:425–436.

Maxie MG, Physick-Sheard PW. Aortic-iliac thrombosis in horses. Vet Pathol 1985;22:238–249.

Moore RW, et al Fibrotic myopathy of the semitendinosus muscle of four dogs. Vet Surgery 1981;10:169–174.
Mubarak S, Owen CA. Compartmental syndrome and its relation to the crush syndrome: A spectrum of disease. Clin Orthop 1975;113:81–89.
Norman WM, et al. Postanesthetic compartmental syndrome in a horse. J Am Vet Med Assoc 1989;195:502–504.
Rorabeck CH, McGee HMJ. Acute compartment syndromes. Vet Comp Orthopaedics Traumatol 1990;3:117–122.
Steffey EP, et al. Effects of five hours of constant 1.2 MAC halothane in sternally recumbent, spontaneously breathing horses. Equine Vet J 1990;22:433–436.

PHYSICAL INJURIES OF MUSCLE

Traumatic injuries of muscle (*laceration, contusion, tearing, penetrating wounds*) are common and may be the result of external trauma, or they may be a result of a muscle rupture or tear of the fascia as occurs occasionally in violent contraction, rarely in overextension. The effects of external trauma are very variable and depend on the qualities of the applied force, the presence or absence of concomitant fracture of the adjacent bones, and especially on the degree of hemorrhage, injury to blood vessels, and injury to motor nerves. The principles governing the outcome of these types of lesions have been discussed above.

Violent contraction of muscle may result in either hernia or rupture with hemorrhage. A hernia occurs when the belly of the muscle protrudes through a rent in the overlying fascia and epimysium. The hernia can be reduced by pressure when the muscle is relaxed and it hardens and bulges further when the muscle contracts, providing thereby a point of useful distinction between hernia and tumor of soft tissue.

Actual rupture of muscle tissue may also occur during violent exercise and is probably more common than rupture of the tendon. The muscle bulges at the end opposite to that which is torn. Such ruptures are not necessarily complete from the outset, but may become so later from additional strain or degeneration caused by infiltrating hemorrhage with pressure and ischemia. Regeneration in large defects is ineffective and the gap is filled in by scar tissue. The muscle most frequently ruptured in animals is the *diaphragm*. Trauma, with acute abdominal compression, is the usual excitant in the dog. In cattle, it tends to follow diaphragmatic myositis secondary to traumatic reticulitis. In horses it is a consequence (in foals) of abdominal compression at parturition, and diaphragmatic rupture occurs occasionally with acute gastric dilation. *Acquired ruptures must be differentiated from congenital and postmortem ruptures by attention to the edges of the cleft and the disposition of abdominal viscera.* Muscles subjected to continuous pressure undergo degeneration, necrosis, and fibrous replacement. It is possible that pressure can have a direct effect on the fibers by disorganizing their internal structure, but the principal effect is to interfere with circulation.

The histologic appearance of traumatic injury depends on the age of the lesions. Initially it includes sarcolemmal rupture with adjacent intact fibers showing hyaline and granular degeneration, accompanied by edema and hemorrhage and neutrophilic infiltration. Reparative changes are conventional, but if the endomysial tubes are extensively disrupted, regeneration will be by "budding" with accompanying fibrosis. Bleeding into muscle, whether caused by trauma or spontaneous hemorrhage, as in some hemorrhagic diatheses, is often sufficient in volume to result in hematoma, the fate of which will depend largely on its volume. Metaplastic bone may form in the capsule of the hematoma. Severe trauma-induced swelling in muscle will result in secondary ischemic injury, which causes muscle necrosis. Primary healing is by regeneration by budding and extensive fibrosis because endomysial tubes are transected.

Ossifying fibrodysplasia

Also termed *myositis ossificans or fibrodysplasia ossificans*, this infrequent condition of the dog, cat, pig, and horse represents heterotopic mineralization within the connective tissues of skeletal muscle. It occurs as either a localized or a generalized form. The generalized form is described under Fibromatous disorders of tendons and aponeuroses.

The *localized form* of myositis ossificans occurs in the dog and horse. In the dog, the lesion often, but not always, occurs secondary to trauma and results in firm swollen areas in the affected muscles generally in the caudal hip, shoulder, quadriceps, or neck. Microscopically, the lesion typically has *three zones* – a central area of actively proliferating undifferentiated connective tissue, a middle zone with osteoid and immature bone, and an outer zone of mature trabecular bone.

Strains/tears/ruptures/fibrotic myopathies/contractures

Strains are the result of *overstretching of muscles* that have disrupted muscle fibers, most commonly at the muscle–tendon junction. The severity of damage varies from mild localized disruption to complete rupture of muscle fibers. Hemorrhage and edema accompany the muscle damage and healing is by fibrosis.

Fibrotic myopathy of the semitendinosus, semimembranosus, and gracilis muscles occurs most often in Quarter Horses performing sliding halts. Physical tearing and hemorrhage from these abrupt maneuvers initiates the damage with fibrous replacement as an outcome. Additionally, some cases are the result of denervation injury.

Several syndromes of limb muscle dysfunction, possibly associated with trauma, are described in dogs. A variety of names have been applied including *infraspinatus contracture, quadriceps contracture, gracilis contracture, fibrotic myopathy of semitendinosus, and gracilis-semitendinosus myopathy*. The contractures are the result of functional shortening of affected muscles following injury and healing by fibrosis. German Shepherds, especially males, are involved with the gracilis/semitendinosus fibrotic myopathy. The affected muscle may contain a thin fibrous band.

A myopathy of the tail muscles in hunting dogs ("limber tail" or "frozen tail") appears to be associated with overwork and environmental stresses.

Bibliography

Beech J. Myopathies in horses. Aust Eq Vet 1990;8:138–145.
Bone DL, McGavin MD. Myositis ossificans in the dog: A case report and review. J Am An Hosp Assoc 1985;21:135–138.
Braund KG. Idiopathic and exogenous causes of myopathies in dogs and cats. Vet Med 1997;92:629–634.

Capello V, et al. Myopathy of the "gracilis semitendinosus muscle complex" in the dog. Eur J Comp An Pract 1993;3:57–68.
Fitch RB, et al. Muscle injuries in dogs. Compend Contin Educ Pract Vet 1997;19:947–957.
Kramer M, et al. Diagnosis and therapy of contractures of the gracilis and infraspinatus muscles. Kleinteirpraxis 1996;41:889–896.
Lewis DD. Gracilis-semitendinosus myopathy. In: Bonagura JD, ed. Kirk's Current Veterinary Therapy XIII Small Animal Practice. Philadelphia, PA: W.B. Saunders, 2000:989–992.
Lewis DD, et al. Gracilis or semitendinosus myopathy in 18 dogs. J Am An Hosp Assoc 1997;33:177–188.
Luttgen PJ. Miscellaneous myopathies. Sem Vet Med Surg (Small Anim) 1989;4:168–176.
Seibold HR, Davis CL. Generalized myositis ossificans (familial) in pigs. Pathol Vet 1967;4:79–88.
Steiss JE, Braund KG. Frozen tail or limber tail in working dogs. Vet Rec 1997;141:179.
Tirgari M. Ventral hernia in the sheep. Vet Rec 1979;106:7–9.
Valberg SJ. Muscular causes of exercise intolerance in horses. Vet Clin N Am: Eq Pract 1996;12:495–513.
Valentine BA, et al. Fibrodysplasia ossificans progressiva in the cat. J Vet Int Med 1992;6:335–340.
Valentine BA, et al. Denervation atrophy in three horses with fibrotic myopathy. J Am Vet Med Assoc 1994;205:332–336.
Warren HB, Carpenter JL. Fibrodysplasia ossificans in three cats. Vet Pathol 1984;21:495–499.
Watt PR. Posttraumatic myositis ossificans and fibrotic myopathy in the rectus femoris muscle in a dog: A case report and literature review. J Am An Hosp Assoc 1992;28:560–564.

NUTRITIONAL MYOPATHY

Nutritional myopathies (also named nutritional myodegeneration, nutritional muscular dystrophy, white muscle disease, stiff-lamb disease) are *principally diseases of calves, lambs, swine, and foals*. They infrequently affect carnivores. *The nutritional deficiencies are principally selenium and vitamin E*. Various environmental factors may, at times, also contribute to the muscle lesions historically associated with selenium/vitamin E deficiency. The clinical syndrome was first produced experimentally in 1928 in the suckling young of female rats fed a diet deficient in vitamin E but the skeletal muscle lesions were not identified until further studies in 1938 when the disease was incorrectly called a "dystrophy," a term appropriately applied to some inherited diseases of muscle. Selenium was established as an essential nutrient and implicated in nutritional myopathy in the late 1950s. Muscle fiber degeneration, as seen in nutritional myopathy, was discussed earlier (see Degeneration and repair of muscle); *it is a selective, segmental polyfocal and polyphasic degeneration of contractile components of the muscle cell* which leaves the ensheathing basal lamina and satellite cells intact, and therefore enables a rapid and efficient regenerative repair to take place. Myoglobinuria is usually absent in the enzootic disease of young animals but may occur in the sporadic cases in young adult animals, as those have a higher concentration of myoglobin in skeletal muscle. Frequently, skeletal muscle damage is concurrent with myocardial lesions.

Etiology and pathogenesis

Nutritional myopathy is a problem around the world but it occurs most often in those countries with intensive livestock agriculture operations. *Selenium moves through a soil–plant–animal cycle*. Sedimentary rocks provide most of the Se that becomes incorporated into soils. Alkaline and well-aerated soils provide much higher amounts of Se available to growing plants than acid, poorly aerated soils. This difference in availability from soils is related to the chemical form of Se and not to the Se concentration in the soil. *Soluble selenates* predominate in alkaline soils, and sparingly soluble *selenites* complexed with iron salts are in acid soils. As Se moves from soils into growing plants, it is largely incorporated into organic compounds, mainly in those selenoproteins with abundant selenomethionine. The Se content in the lush forage of heavily fertilized and watered soils is low because of dilution by the abundant plant tissue. Surveys of plants grown in soils throughout the USA and other countries have provided data and have been used to map areas of Se deficiency and excess. Deficient areas include the southeastern, northeastern, midwestern, and far northwestern portions of the US. The prevalence of Se-E deficiency diseases in animals throughout the USA correlates closely with the areas having low ($<$0.05 ppm dry weight) plant Se concentrations. Animals are able to utilize Se from inorganic salts (selenites and selenates) as well as from the organic forms in plants. Further, the Se of compounds in feedstuffs of plant origin has a much higher biological availability than Se found in compounds of animal products (e.g., fish meals). Other inorganic Se sources, elemental Se, and selenides, have little or no biological value for animals. In most of the studies that compared the efficacy of various chemical forms of Se to prevent deficiency disease in animals, *organic Se was found to have greater protection than inorganic Se (selenite)*. However, because selenite is readily available and inexpensive, this form is commonly used as a dietary Se supplement.

Selenium is distributed widely in animal tissues, and the concentration is directly related to dietary intake. Highest concentrations are found in kidney and liver, intermediate amounts are found in heart and skeletal muscle, and low content is found in blood and fat. Animals fed rations in which small amounts (0.1–0.2 ppm) of Se are added to meet their nutritional requirements do not develop large increases in tissue Se content; therefore, human consumption of the tissues of animals so fed offers no risk of causing Se toxicosis.

Selenium deficiency in animals may be induced by the incorporation of high but nontoxic amounts of certain elements that antagonize Se. *Copper, silver, tellurium, and zinc in rations can induce typical lesions of Se-E deficiency in animals fed diets containing amounts of Se ordinarily considered adequate*. Also, a role for high amounts of dietary sulfur as a Se antagonist has been claimed. The importance of Se antagonists in field, rather than laboratory, conditions remains to be established. However, such a mechanism should be considered when animals fed a selenium supplement develop lesions of Se-E deficiency.

Vitamin E content of compounded animal feeds is generally low because many of the feedstuffs used are poor sources of that vitamin. Rich sources of vitamin E include wheat bran, many vegetable oils, and legumes such as alfalfa. The biological activity of vitamin E is concentrated in the α-tocopherol fraction, and thus determinations of total tocopherol content of feeds may be of limited value for determining their vitamin E potency, to prevent deficiency disease. Diets that contain large amounts of polyunsaturated fats (e.g., those in fish oils) will require greater amounts of vitamin E, which limits oxidation and the development of rancidity. Also, if diets with low Se content are fed, vitamin E supplements will need to be increased to prevent deficiency disease.

Of the domestic mammals, *cattle, sheep, and pigs are most susceptible to nutritional myopathy*. Horses and goats are moderately susceptible, and occasional cases have been reported in dogs and cats. Most zoo ungulates should be regarded as susceptible to the disease. Historically, nutritional myopathy has been thought of as a disease of young animals, particularly the very young. *Rapid postnatal growth seems to predispose*, a problem perhaps of outgrowing a scarce resource or of biochemical transition as fiber types develop into the adult patterns. Although nutritional muscle degeneration does occasionally occur in mature animals, it is rare.

In cattle, spontaneous nutritional myopathy may occur in utero in 7-month-old fetuses, and muscle lesions are seen in lambs and calves at birth. However, lesions may not occur in calves or lambs born of cows or ewes, which themselves have extensive lesions of nutritional myopathy prior to, or at the time of, parturition. It is equally true that dams of calves or lambs with extensive lesions seldom show clinical disease or even clinicopathological evidence of muscle fiber breakdown.

Nutritional myopathy occurs in all of the susceptible domestic species on widely variable planes of nutrition. Neonatal disease usually affects the thrifty, well-grown suckling animal and the sporadic disease in yearlings and adults usually occurs in animals in good physical condition. The adult disease affects animals fed marginal-quality rations, such as turnips or poor-quality hay, and can appear as clinical or subclinical disease in animals in very poor condition because of neglect or chronic disease. Animals with nutritional myopathy often lose condition rapidly and appear to be very unthrifty even when the muscle disease is not clinically severe.

One of the most perplexing aspects of these myopathies is the irregularity and unpredictability of their occurrence. Natural disease is seldom a serious problem in consecutive years, yet sometimes it will occur in most years in any given region. A good deal of correlative and circumstantial evidence indicates that climate-related conditions, such as the length and the amount of sunshine of the growing season, and the length of the housing season, may be very important. Since the disease often occurs while animals are consuming stored feeds, the condition and duration of storage of the fodder can be relevant. Detailed investigation sometimes reveals comparable concentrations of vitamin E and selenium in forage from one year to the next, yet the incidence of nutritional myopathy in animals consuming it may be quite different. Grazing of dry pastures may be associated with an increase in the incidence of disease and may also have an influence later through the stored hay or grain harvested from them. On the other hand, ingestion of lush pasture may also cause problems. The leaves of some pasture plants have moderately high levels of polyunsaturated fatty acids and these fatty acids are absorbed largely intact in herbivores. They are almost certainly antagonistic to selenium and vitamin E, thus the requirements for these nutrients may be raised considerably when animals first graze new pasture. *In most parts of the world, nutritional myopathy occurs in late winter or early spring*, but in sheep it may occur more often in the fall, in both pastured and feedlot animals that are immature.

The patterns of nutritional myopathy seem, in a general way, to obey the rules of straightforward deficiency of one or two essential nutrients. The metabolism of vitamin E and selenium is incompletely understood. Understanding of factors involved in membrane integrity and membrane alterations in disease has elucidated the role of the subcellular changes, which seem to be a basic result of deficiency of these substances.

In many cells, *vitamin E- and selenium-containing enzymes are required as physiologic antagonists to a group of chemically varied substances known as free radicals*. **Free radicals** are molecules with an odd number of electrons; they can be either organic or inorganic. Some free radicals are products of normal cell function, and several participate in, or are products of, oxidative metabolism. They may also be produced outside the cell as products of tissue radiation, drug reactions, and inflammation. One of the major sources of free radicals is the cell detoxification process, which renders materials less harmful by converting them to epoxides. Many intracellular and extracellular free radicals contain oxygen, and are involved in electron transfer reactions. They are highly reactive and this is responsible for their rapid alteration (instability), which occurs in oxidation-reduction reactions within a wide range of cellular structures and enzyme systems.

Free radicals may initiate cellular injury by causing peroxidation of membrane lipids and by causing physicochemical damage to protein molecules including those of mitochondria, endoplasmic reticulum, and cytosol. Protection against the effects of free radicals is provided partly by the constant presence of *small scavenger molecules* such as tocopherols, ascorbate, and beta-carotene. These "quench" free radicals, but both free radicals and scavengers are consumed in the process. Protection is also provided in part by selenium-containing enzymes of the *glutathione peroxidase/glutathione reductase system*. This system is capable, under normal circumstances, of more or less constant renewal by a complex sequence that makes use of several enzymes, although some consumption of the selenium-containing component does occur.

From the above, certain conclusions seem to emerge. *Although vitamin E- and the selenium-containing glutathione system perform many similar functions at the cellular level in quenching destructive metabolites and byproducts, they may function independently*. The circumstantial clinical evidence that one can relieve the need for the other in the prevention of muscle disease is also reasonably explained. The need for some of both at all times within the cell, and vitamin E outside the cell, perhaps is explained by the fact that the two mechanisms quench a different array of free radicals and that tocopherol operates both outside and inside the cell while the glutathione system operates only inside the cell. The practical interpretation of deficiency of vitamin E or selenium should relate to the consumption of these elements during a steady intracellular production of free radicals, rather than an interpretation of these nutrients as structural cellular components that may be deficient.

In the absence of sufficient protection by selenium and/or vitamin E, cellular membranes are modified by free radicals, and the ability of those membranes to maintain essential differential gradients for one or more ions is diminished or lost. The normal inward flow of calcium ions from the extracellular compartment to the cytosol, where calcium levels are one quarter to one half as high as extracellularly, causes a greatly increased demand for energy to move calcium away from the calcium-sensitive myofilaments and into mitochondria which act as sumps. As a result, mitochondria may accumulate up to 50 times their normal amount of calcium, and this results in reduction in their ability to produce energy. It also initiates the sequence of events identified earlier (see Degeneration and repair of muscle) as "mitochondrial calcium overload" which proceeds to calcium-induced hypercontraction of myofibrils and degeneration of myofibers.

The explanations of intracellular dynamics and myofiber degeneration outlined above indicate that *segmental muscle fiber degeneration with mineralization is not a specific lesion.* Any event which can trigger the cascade of degenerative events in the muscle fiber could produce a similar lesion. Starvation, or poor-quality rations, or rations in which vitamin E and/or selenium have been destroyed, could produce muscle lesions simply by not providing enough protective scavenger molecules. Metallic toxicants or other chemicals, including therapeutic agents, might produce disease by binding selenium and inducing a higher than normal demand for antioxidant molecules such as tocopherols or glutathione. The relationship between unaccustomed exercise or cold weather and nutritional myopathy, which is frequently observed in all ages and all susceptible species, may be explained by an energy depletion at the intracellular level rather than by membrane alteration, especially in those instances of nutritional myopathy in which levels of tissue vitamin E and selenium are near normal. Excepting those cases exacerbated by driving, transport, or other forced exercise, serum and tissue concentrations of vitamin E and selenium generally correlate well with levels in the feed of the animals concerned. *This by itself seems to indicate that the naturally occurring disease is a true deficiency.*

Once the myofiber cell membrane (plasmalemma) has been altered, the stage has been set for leakage of intracellular enzymes into the extracellular space. *The concentration of activity of muscle enzymes in blood is a rough indication of the extent of muscle fiber destruction.* It is clear that increase in concentrations of enzymes in plasma may accompany extensive athletic use of muscles and indicate physiologic disruption of muscle fibers. When monitored by muscle biopsies in animals and man, however, such increase in enzyme concentrations is associated with degeneration of fibers or at least of some fiber segments (segmental degeneration).

The concentration of creatine kinase in plasma is the enzyme that seems to be most specific in indicating muscle damage although, in animals, plasma concentrations of aspartate aminotransferase is quite specific for muscle as well. Its activity in serum tends to rise later and disappear much later than creatine kinase and therefore, its evaluation is most useful in establishing the time and duration of the muscle injury. Serum glutathione peroxidase activities are reliable indicators of selenium availability. Tissue concentrations of selenium may not reflect metabolic availability if selenium is stored in complex form. Mineral supplements often contain a variety of metals as contaminants. Those that have been shown experimentally to have a myopathy-inducing effect include iron, silver, tellurium, cobalt, copper, zinc, and cadmium. The complicity of such metals in the production of natural disease is undetermined but worthy of examination.

Nutritional myopathy of cattle

Clinicopathologic descriptions of the disease in calves appeared in the 1890s and the disease was well known at that time in Germany, France, Switzerland, and Scandinavia. *Nutritional myopathy occurs, sometimes in endemic proportions, in calves, mostly of beef type and 4–6 weeks old.* It is also common in animals up to 6 months of age and occurs sporadically in older cattle. In calves there is often a typical history indicating that the dam has been housed at least 3–4 months and had been fed poor-quality hay or not enough hay. Similar problems occur in calves in the USA, Australia, and New Zealand when legume hay alone or irrigated legume pasture is fed. Sulfur fertilizers applied to the pasture, and copper deficiency in the dam, may be contributing factors. *The precipitating event in many cases is unaccustomed physical activity that converts subclinical to clinical disease.* The feeding of cod liver oil that has become rancid destroys vitamin E in the ration and has been blamed for producing the disease. The presenting sign in calves is often stiffness or dyspnea, but a shuffling gait, a dropping of the chest between the shoulders, and outward rotation of the forelimbs have also been noted. Some calves become recumbent and die rapidly with signs of respiratory failure. Calves over 3–4 months of age may show myoglobinuria.

Postmortem lesions in calves are usually dominated by marked mineralization of necrotic skeletal and/or cardiac muscle. When the heart is extensively affected, intercostal muscles and the diaphragm are usually also affected, but other skeletal muscle lesions may not be widespread. *Heart lesions in calves usually involve the left ventricle more than the right.* Small lesions just under the epicardium or endocardium may appear as scattered white "brush" strokes. The mineralized lesions are creamy white and opaque. Small streaks of hemorrhage may also be seen. Lungs are often filled with pink frothy fluid and an excess of fluid may be present in the thorax indicating heart failure. Acute pneumonic changes sometimes develop as a complication of pulmonary edema. *In those cases where skeletal muscle lesions predominate, the most extensive lesions can be found in the large weight-bearing muscles of the thigh and shoulder,* but many others are affected and the lesions are bilaterally symmetrical.

Suckling animals often have extensive lesions in the *highly active tongue and neck muscles,* and occasionally in the voluntary muscles of rectum, urethra, and esophagus. Affected muscles are pale, irregularly opaque and yellow to creamy-white. The longitudinal divisions of muscle (primary bundles of 40–200 fibers) often have an indistinct appearance in most severely affected areas and sometimes streaks of hemorrhage and moderate local edema are present. Minimal myocardial lesions are sometimes present, but not accompanied by evidence of cardiac failure.

In older calves and young adult cattle, the patterns of disease vary considerably and are unrelated to age. Dairy and beef calves 6–12 months of age show stiffness and lethargy just after winter housing, or sometimes while they are housed. *The disease is often related to poor-quality feed.* In similar circumstances, extensive myopathy occurs in pregnant heifers and they may suffer a high incidence of abortion, stillbirth, placental retention, and parturient recumbency. Feedlot steers fed high-moisture corn, which has been treated with propionic acid to control fungal growth and stored for 6–8 months, show initial signs of diarrhea and unthriftiness and become recumbent for 2 or 3 weeks. Many have lesions in muscles at slaughter. Most mature animals with extensive skeletal muscle lesions have myoglobinuria.

Young adult cattle with bilateral dorsal scapular displacement ("*flying scapula*") have rupture of the serratus ventralis muscle and this may be of sufficient duration to have extensive fibrosis and multifocal osseous and cartilaginous metaplasia underlying the displaced scapulae. Presumably, nutritional myopathy of the subscapular muscles has preceded rupture and displacement.

Histologic lesions of nutritional myopathy are varied only slightly by age of the lesion. The earliest lesion visible by light microscopy is *hypercontraction*, recognizable in fiber segments with tightly contracted sarcomeres or no striations. In cross-section, hypercontracted fibers are large, round, and stain strongly with eosin. This is the change which is usually described as *hyaline*, implying an amorphous structure, but striations may be visible for 3–4 days when examined by electron microscopy. Eventually these hypercontracted fiber segments will be phagocytosed but not as quickly as other fibers that undergo fragmentation with or without mineralization. In both types of degeneration, the processes of degeneration and repair are essentially those described earlier and allowance needs to be made in histological examination for the incremental changes of chronic deficiency. Thus, the typical histologic findings will be a *polyphasic, polyfocal myopathy*.

By electron microscopy, the earliest detectable change is *degeneration of mitochondria* and this is followed by loss of some parts of the sarcomere and then disintegration of the tubular systems. By histochemical examination it can be determined that *type 1 fibers in the interior of primary bundles degenerate preferentially but not exclusively*. Apart from this preference, the pattern of degeneration appears to be random. This random pattern is helpful in distinguishing this from other muscle diseases such as ischemic degeneration.

Changes in *myocardium* are very similar to those seen in skeletal muscle. Mineralization of hyalinized fibers is often pronounced and the coagulated, mineralized myofibrils appear to be rapidly removed by macrophages. Necrotic myocardial fibers are not regenerated; they are replaced by condensed fibrous stroma.

Nutritional myopathy of sheep and goats

Nutritional myopathy in **sheep** *is probably more prevalent in more areas of the world than the disease in cattle.* The disease was first described in Germany in 1925. The names white muscle disease, rigid lamb disease, and stiff lamb disease were coined to describe the most frequently encountered clinical patterns in 2–4-week-old lambs, which very often are *spring lambs, recently turned out onto the first green pasture.* Congenital nutritional myopathy does occur in lambs, but not often. The typical disease may occur as an outbreak among lambs from 1 day to 2 months of age or beyond. Mortality at this stage may be very low or may reach 50%. The next peak of incidence occurs at 4–8 months of age as weaned lambs are put onto lush pastures following mowing or into feedlots. Mortality is not usually very high, but the incidence of minimal clinical disease may be moderately high and that of subclinical disease may be higher. Beyond these age groups, nutritional myopathy in more mature sheep is clinically apparent sporadically, but subclinical disease may involve from 5–30% of a group. Under special circumstances, the incidence of clinical disease and mortality may rise dramatically. Thus, in various parts of the world, the disease has been precipitated by stress from bad weather, prolonged winter feeding, subsistence on root crops, or forced activity, as well as feeding on stubble, legume pastures, dry pastures, and pastures with too much copper. Outbreaks in lambs and yearlings have also occurred on pastures on which copper had been made unavailable by top-dressing with molybdenum.

Deficiency in sheep is attributed to deficiency of vitamin E or selenium, but seldom of both. In certain regions of the world, one nutrient does not seem to be able to replace the other to any extent, while in others the addition of either vitamin E or selenium is rapidly curative.

Lesions and their corresponding clinical signs are as varied as the circumstances under which myopathy occurs. The lesions may be detectable in lamb fetuses at least 2 weeks prior to parturition. In the congenital disease, *tongue and neck muscles* used in suckling movements often contain the most severe lesions. When the lesions occur in lambs a few days older, they are likely to be much more extensive and involve primarily the *major muscles of the shoulder and thigh but also back, neck, and respiratory (diaphragm and intercostal) muscles*. The gross appearance of affected muscles is similar to that described for calves, although *the likelihood of muscle mineralization is probably greater.* Lambs normally have pale muscles, consequently the recognition of the mineralized flecking in primary bundles is almost essential if diagnosis is to be made grossly with any confidence. It is necessary to confirm the gross diagnosis by histological examination.

In older sheep, lesions are more varied in distribution, location, and extent, but some similarity to the distribution in young animals may exist. For example, bilaterally symmetrical lesions of the thigh muscles may occur but they may predominate in or be confined to the intermediate head of the triceps, or the tensor fascia latae. Lesions in pregnant ewes may be more or less confined to the abdominal muscles subjected to increased work load from supporting the pregnant uterus and may rupture allowing viscera to herniate.

Microscopically, the changes seen in affected muscle over a period of several days follow the expected sequence of *necrosis, mineralization, phagocytosis, and regeneration characterized by satellite cell proliferation and myoblast formation*. Because the basal laminae of myofibers are intact, all of this can be completed within about 16–18 days, leaving little in the way of residual lesions, but often repair lesions of several days evolution can be seen side by side with more recent ones (*polyphasic, polyfocal myopathy*). Repair can take place in the face of continuing deficiency, but even normal activity during the early repair phase is likely to lead to more myofiber necrosis.

Reports of nutritional myopathy in **goats** are relatively few but this may be due to the fact that the goat is less often reared under intensive animal agriculture practices. Caprine nutritional myopathy has been observed in Europe, the Middle East, New Zealand, Australia, and North America. In most instances it appears in goats on pasture, and clinical and pathological changes are similar to those seen in sheep.

Nutritional myopathy of pigs

Nutritional myopathy in swine has been reported as a spontaneous disease wherever intensive pig rearing is practiced, but particularly in northern, central and eastern continental Europe, the UK, the US, and Canada. Classical lesions involving only skeletal muscles are less common than some of the other expressions of porcine vitamin E/selenium deficiency such as hepatosis dietetica and mulberry heart disease, but *systematic microscopic study of muscles has revealed a much higher incidence of muscle lesions than was thought to exist.* Since the pig is an easily managed experimental animal, much more is known about experimental vitamin E/selenium deficiency in this species than in others.

Naturally occurring nutritional myopathy is not known to be congenital in pigs but piglets as young as 1 day may have extensive

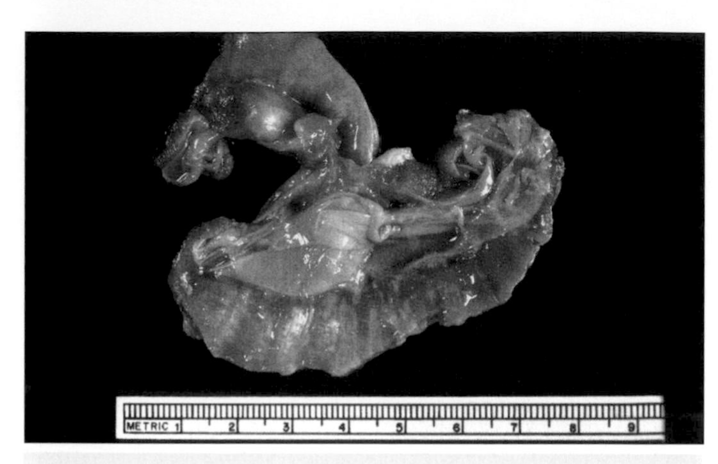

Figure 2.69 White streaks with necrosis radiate in diaphragm from a pig with **nutritional myopathy**.

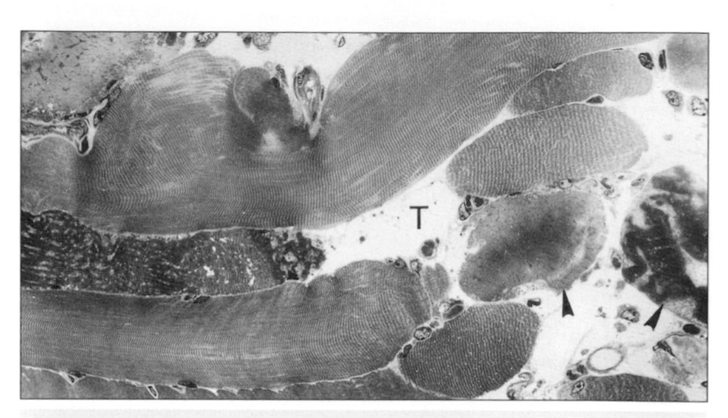

Figure 2.70 Segmental myodegeneration in a pig with nutritional myopathy. T = tube of external lamina; arrowheads = clumps of disrupted contractile material. (Reprinted from Van Vleet JF et al. Am J Vet Res 1976;37:911.)

lesions, which cause paresis or extreme weakness. Growing pigs of all sizes up to 65 kg may be affected in outbreaks, but *most commonly affected are weaned pigs of 6–20 weeks of age.* A special circumstance is that caused in pigs a few days old by the *injection of iron dextran products*, which precipitates acute widespread degenerative and usually fatal myopathy. It is believed that iron acts as a catalyst for lipid peroxidation of cell membranes. Older pigs, and particularly sows that have recently farrowed, are occasionally susceptible to widespread nutritional myopathy of sufficient severity to cause prostration, although more often clinical signs, if present at all, consist of lethargy and slowness of movement.

Apart from deficiencies in diet, the factors that trigger the disease in pigs seem to be relatively few. Unaccustomed exercise does not seem to play a part, but *feeding rancid or oxidized fish liver oils, which destroy vitamin E, may do so.* Newly harvested grain sometimes seems to contain a myopathy-inducing factor, and pigs fed quantities of peas (*Pisum sativum*) may be particularly prone to the disease. Metals occurring as contaminants in ground mineral mixes can induce an increased requirement for vitamin E and/or selenium. Silver, copper, cadmium, cobalt, vanadium, tellurium, and zinc, and possibly other metals, in some way bind selenium or prevent its participation in free radical protective activities. This leads to a twofold or greater demand for selenium to prevent lesions that can be only partly alleviated by vitamin E supplementation.

Mineralization of degenerate fibers is often not abundant and even when it is present and visible, it is difficult to detect grossly in the naturally pale muscles of the pig. This, and the fact that lesions in heart and liver are much more dramatic, may explain why there are relatively few reports of skeletal muscle lesions in natural outbreaks of vitamin E/selenium deficiency disease. In the experimental disease in pigs, gross lesions may be seen (Fig. 2.69) but many skeletal muscle lesions are microscopic, while the liver and heart lesions are grossly visible.

Microscopic muscle lesions are similar to the polyphasic, polyfocal myopathy seen in lambs and calves (Figs 2.70–2.75). Type 1 fibers are principally affected and in view of the orderly central arrangement of type 1 fibers within muscle fascicles in the pig, this leads to a *distinct central degeneration of primary muscle bundles.* Regeneration is often rapid and complete in surviving piglets, but the mortality rate may be as high as 80% of a litter, and usually 100% when secondary to iron injection. The survival rate for older pigs is higher

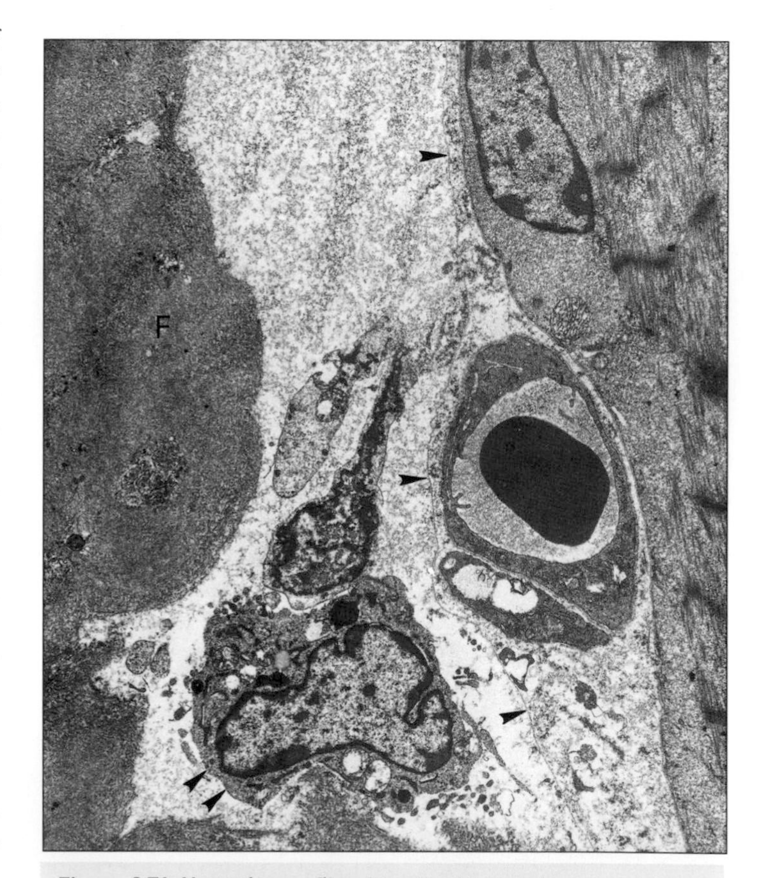

Figure 2.71 Necrotic myofiber is outlined by persistent basal lamina (arrowheads) in a pig with nutritional myopathy. Double arrowhead = invading macrophage. F = disrupted fibrils. (Reprinted from Van Vleet JF et al. Am J Vet Res 1976;37:911.)

except in those instances in which the cardiac lesions are prominent. Relatively few pigs survive mulberry heart disease.

Myocardial degeneration (mulberry heart disease) is the most common manifestation of vitamin E/selenium deficiency in growing weaned pigs 6–20 weeks of age. It is described in Vol. 3, Cardiovascular system.

The liver lesions associated with vitamin E/selenium deficiency are referred to as *nutritional hepatic necrosis or hepatosis dietetica* and are described in Vol. 2, Liver and biliary system.

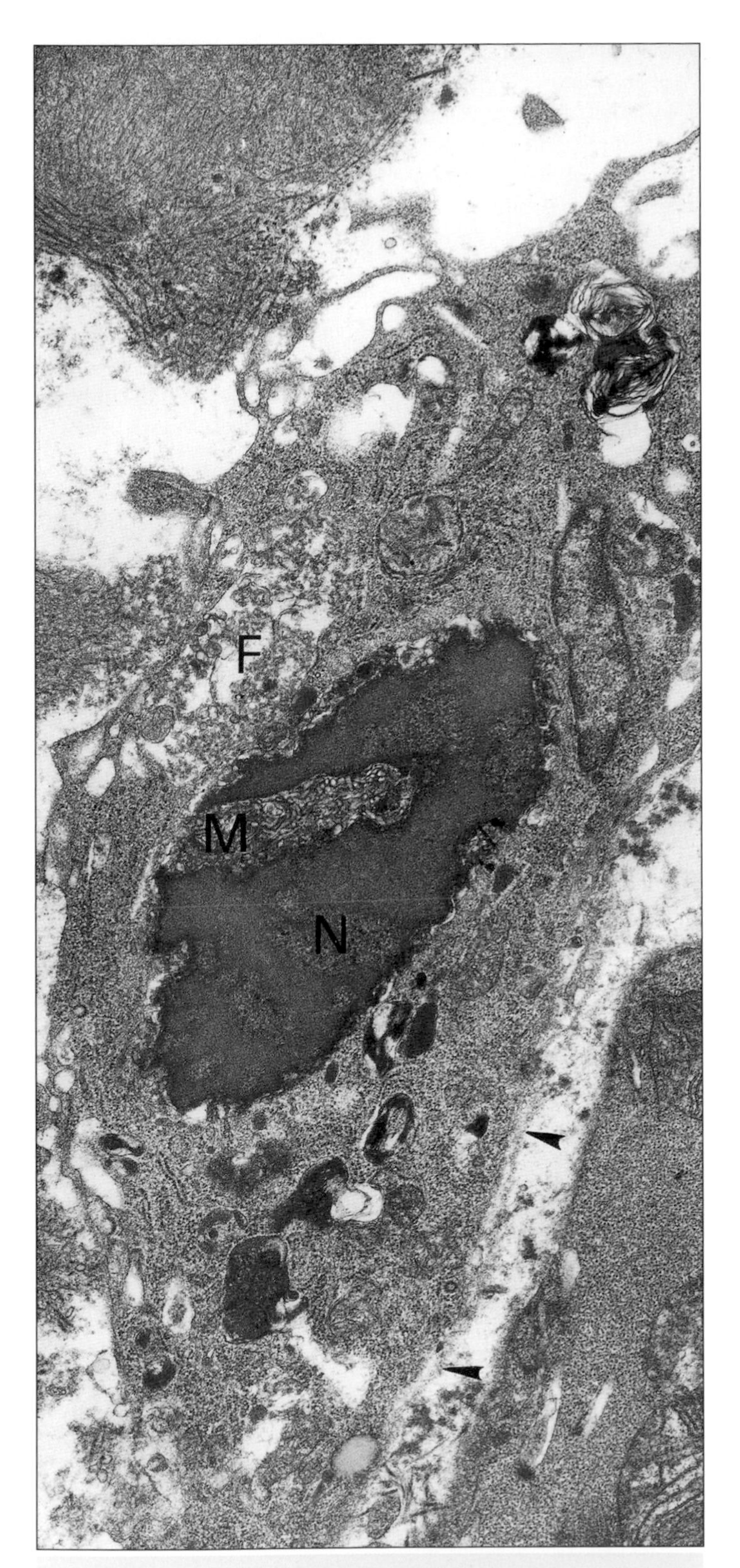

Figure 2.72 Macrophage within necrotic fiber contains engulfed cellular debris, from a pig with nutritional myopathy. Arrowheads = basal lamina, F = disrupted fibrils, M = mitochondria, N = pyknotic myofiber nucleus. (Reprinted from Van Vleet JF et al. Am J Vet Res 1976;37:911.)

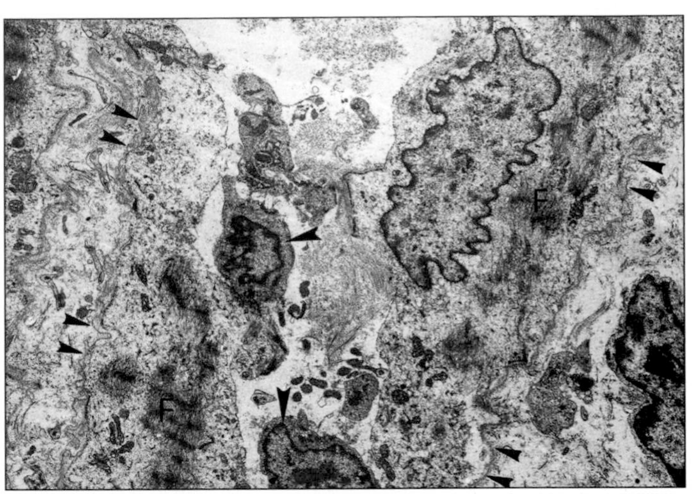

Figure 2.73 Regenerating myofiber, outlined by basal lamina (double arrowheads), has large nucleus and forming myofibrils (F), from a pig with nutritional myopathy. Arrowheads = macrophages. (Reprinted from Van Vleet JF et al. Am J Vet Res 1976;37:911.)

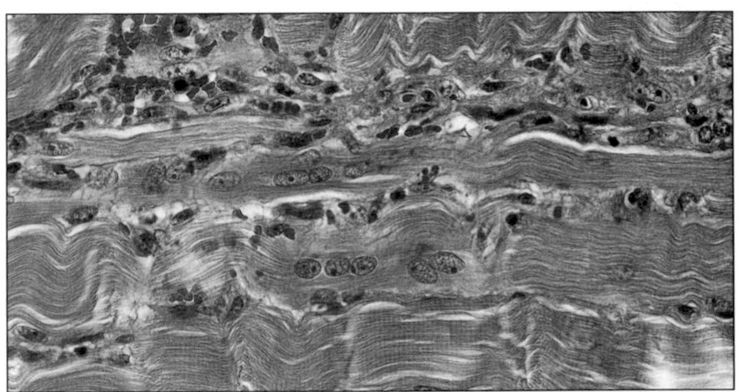

Figure 2.74 Late stage of regeneration has central rows of myonuclei and formed myofibrils in a pig with nutritional myopathy. (Reprinted from Van Vleet JF et al. Am J Vet Res 1976;37:911.)

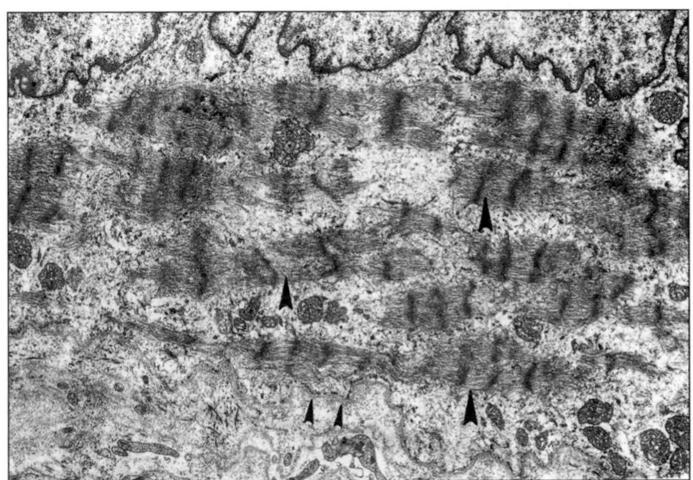

Figure 2.75 Ultrastructural appearance of **late stage of regeneration** in a pig with nutritional myopathy. Forming myofibrils (arrowheads). Basal lamina (double arrowheads). (Reprinted from Van Vleet JF et al. Am J Vet Res 1976;37:911.)

Nutritional myopathy of horses

A disease in *foals* that is, in many respects, comparable to vitamin E/selenium deficiency myopathies in other species, has been recognized for many years. *The usual age range is 1 day to 12 weeks and it may be present at birth.* Cases have been reported from North America, Europe, and Australia in most breeds of light horses and in pony, zebra, and donkey foals. The similarities of lesions and circumstances of the equine syndrome and nutritional myopathy of ruminants has led to the conclusion that the disease is due to a deficiency of vitamin E and/or selenium, but this has not been confirmed. Tissue concentrations of selenium and glutathione peroxidase in affected foals are often no lower than those in healthy foals, however, and selenium and vitamin E appear to have little or no curative value, and in a few instances, little or no preventive value. Serum creatine kinase concentrations may be very high; over 2 million IU/L in nonsurviving cases, and as high as 200 000 IU/L in surviving animals.

Postmortem lesions of nutritional myopathy in foals are similar in many respects to those in calves and lambs – a *polyphasic, polyfocal myopathy*. Foals dying acutely may have myocardial lesions. In the *subacute syndrome, shoulder, neck, and thigh muscles* may be bilaterally and extensively involved and this usually accounts for an inability to rise or to assume certain postures such as the one for suckling. Involvement of the lingual, pharyngeal, and masticatory muscles results in dysphagia. Involvement of digital flexors and extensors may be more frequent than in calves but typical lesions are the *chalky opaque flecking of muscle*. Myoglobinuria may be present and reflects the severity of muscle damage. Sometimes in poorly nourished stabled horses, there is involvement of the masticatory and tongue muscles. This lesion has been called *masticatory myositis* in foals and *polymyositis* in older animals, but based on clinical and pathological grounds *the syndromes seem to be part of nutritional myopathy.*

The distinction between true nutritional myopathy and other diseases is more difficult in older horses than it is for foals, because circumstances and lesions are not as distinctive and because the history is often fragmentary. Nutritional myopathy occurs in animals ranging from less than 1 year to middle age. *The clinical signs may be nonspecific* and may be mistaken for evidence of colic, cardiac failure, wry neck, or general depression, but *the most common features are stiffness and muscular weakness.* Lesions are seldom widespread enough to cause severe crippling although lethargy may be secondary to skeletal muscle degeneration. A willingness to eat is retained in downer animals. *The most convincing indications of nutritional myopathy are the myocardial lesions that are similar to those seen in other species. The presence of myocardial necrosis separates the syndrome from the exertional and ischemic myopathies.*

As is the case with foals, the vitamin E and/or selenium status of older horses with lesions is sometimes difficult to reconcile with information in other species. Low concentrations of blood selenium or glutathione peroxidase are not always present in horses with lesions. Blood tocopherol and glutathione peroxidase concentrations do not seem to be related in individual animals, and selenium and vitamin E may not be curative or, in some cases, not preventive. There is, however, indirect evidence of a need for one or both of the nutrients for optimal muscle function.

Histologic lesions in both foals and older horses are similar to those seen in calves or pigs – a *polyphasic, polyfocal myopathy*. The repair process in foals is rapid and usually complete in 2 weeks if the foal survives, but some lasting retardation of growth may result. Older animals may have the same capability for regeneration especially in subclinical disease, but it is expected that in older animals the repair process may be less effective, and healing will be by scarring in severely affected muscles and this may be responsible for limitations of gait or deviation of the neck.

Steatitis is apparently not seen in older horses with nutritional myopathy but it is common in foals and may, in the healing stage, lead to lumpiness in subcutaneous adipose tissue, especially along the nuchal crest and over the gluteal muscles and the abdominal wall. The affected fat is firm and yellow-brown. Microscopically, neutrophilic infiltration and necrosis and mineralization of fat cells are present.

Nutritional myopathy of other species

Nutritional myopathy is unusual in carnivores and primates. Clinical, morphological, and therapeutic evidence suggests that it does occur. There are several reports in dogs fed prolonged diets unusually low in vitamin E and selenium, and dogs with chronic biliary fistulas developing nutritional myopathy and myocardial damage. *Cats fed vitamin E-deficient diets develop steatitis (yellow fat disease).*

Nutritional myopathy in *ranch mink*, usually accompanied by steatitis, had been a periodic but costly problem. With the introduction of commercial feeds in which vitamin E is added to counteract the effects of oxidized fish oils or other lipid peroxides, it has largely disappeared. It is unlikely that the disease occurs in wild mink.

A number of *zoo animals* appear to be susceptible to nutritional myopathy, but details are scarce and evidence largely circumstantial. A small nocturnal wallaby, the Rottnest quokka (*Setonix brachyurus*), and the nyala (*Tragelaphus angasi*) seem to be exquisitely susceptible. Problems of diagnosis arise in such populations in which capture myopathy is a complication (see Exertional myopathies), but cases that circumstantially appear to be due to nutritional myopathy are reported in several species of gazelle and antelope in Africa, roe deer in Scotland, and white-tailed deer and Rocky Mountain bighorn sheep in North America.

Bibliography

Allen JG, et al. A study of nutritional myopathy in weaned sheep. Aust Vet J 1986;63:8–13.

Allen WM, et al. Degenerative myopathy with myoglobinuria in yearling cattle. Br Vet J 1975;131:292–308.

Anderson PH, et al. The sequence of myodegeneration in nutritional myopathy of the older calf. Br Vet J 1977;133:160–167.

Andrews ED, et al. Selenium-responsive diseases of animals in New Zealand. NZ Vet J 1968;16:3–17.

Beech J. Myopathies in horses. Aust Eq Vet 1990;8:138–145.

Bradley R, et al. Changing patterns of nutritional myodegeneration (white muscle disease) in cattle and sheep in the period 1975–1985 in Great Britain. Bov Pract 1987;22:38–45.

Bradley R, Fell BF. Myopathies in animals. In: Walton J, ed. Disorders of Voluntary Muscle. New York: Churchill -Livingstone, 1981:824–872.

Brigelius-Flohe R, Traber MG. Vitamin E: function and metabolism. FASEB 1999;13:1145–1155.

Buergelt CD, et al. Nutritional myodegeneration associated with dorsal scapular displacement in beef heifers. J Comp Pathol 1996;114:445–450.

Clark IA. Tissue damage caused by free oxygen radicals. Pathology 1986; 18:181–186.
Dodd DC, et al. Muscle degeneration and yellow fat disease in foals. NZ Vet J 1960;8:45–50.
Hadlow WJ. Disease of skeletal muscle. In: Innes JRM, Saunders LZ, eds. Comparative Neuropathology. San Diego, CA: Academic Press, 1962:147–243.
Hadlow WJ. Myopathies of animals. In: The Striated Muscle. International Academy of Pathology Monograph No. 12. Baltimore, MD: Williams & Wilkins Co., 1973:364–409.
Hamliri A, et al. Evaluation of biochemical evidence of congenital nutritional myopathy in two-week prepartum fetuses from selenium-deficient ewes. Am J Vet Res 1990;51(7):1112–1115.
Hosie BD, et al. Acute myopathy in horses at grass in east and southeast Scotland. Vet Rec 1986;119:444–449.
Hutchinson LJ, et al. Nutritional myodegeneration in a group of Chianina heifers. J Am Vet Med Assoc 1982;181:581–584.
Kennedy S, et al. Experimental myopathy in vitamin E- and selenium-depleted calves with and without added dietary polyunsaturated fatty acids as a model for nutritional degenerative myopathy in ruminant cattle. Res Vet Sci 1987; 43:384–394.
Kubota J, et al. Selenium in crops in the United States in relation to selenium-responsive diseases of animals. Agric Food Chem 1967;15:448–453.
Lofstedt J. White muscle disease of foals. Vet Clin N Am Eq Pract 1997;13:169–185.
Owen R, et al. Dystrophic myodegeneration in adult horses. J Am Vet Med Assoc 1977;171:343–349.
Patterson DSP, et al. The toxicity of parenteral iron preparations in the rabbit and pig with a comparison of the clinical and biochemical responses to iron-dextrose in 2 day-old and 8 day-old piglets. Zentralbl Veterinaermed [A] 19871;18:453.
Peet RL, Dickson J. Rhabdomyolysis in housed, fine-wooled merino sheep, associated with low plasma alpha-tocopherol concentrations. Aust Vet J 1988;65:398–399.
Radostits OM, et al. Selenium and/or vitamin E deficiencies. In: Radostits OM, et al., eds. Veterinary Medicine. A Textbook of the Diseases of Cattle, Sheep, Pigs, Goats, and Horses. 9th ed. New York: W.B. Saunders Co., 2000:1515–1533.
Rice DA, McMurray CH. Use of sodium hydroxide treated selenium deficient barley to induce vitamin E and selenium deficiency in yearling cattle. Vet Rec 1986;118:173–176.
Roneus B. Glutathione peroxidase and selenium in the blood of healthy horses and foals affected by muscular dystrophy. Nord Vet Med 1982;34:350–353.
Ross AD, et al. Nutritional myopathy in goats. Aust Vet J 1989;66(11):361–363.
Ruth GR, Van Vleet JF. Experimentally induced selenium-vitamin E deficiency in growing swine: selective destruction of type 1 skeletal muscle fibers. Am J Vet Res 1974;35:237–244.
Smith DL, et al. A nutritional myopathy enzootic in a group of yearling beef cattle. Can Vet J 1985;26:385–390.
Van Vleet JF. Experimentally induced vitamin E-selenium deficiency in the growing dog. J Am Vet Med Assoc 1975;166:769–774.
Van Vleet JF. Comparative efficacy of five supplementation procedures to control selenium-vitamin E deficiency in swine. Am J Vet Res 1982;43:1180–1189.
Van Vleet JF, Ferrans VJ. Etiologic factors and pathologic alterations in selenium-vitamin E deficiency and excess in animals and humans. Biol Trace Elem Res 1992;33:1–21.
Van Vleet JF, et al. Induction of lesions of selenium-vitamin E deficiency in weanling swine fed silver, cobalt, tellurium, zinc, cadmium and vanadium. Am J Vet Res 1981;42:789–799.
Wilson TM, et al. Myodegeneration and suspected selenium/vitamin E deficiency in horses. J Am Vet Med Assoc 1976;169:213–217.
Wrogemann K, Pena SDJ. Mitochondrial calcium overload: a general mechanism for cell-necrosis in muscle diseases. Lancet 1976;1:672–673.
Zhang J, et al. Selenium deficiency in horses (1981–1983). In: Combs GF, Jr., et al, eds. Selenium in Biology and Medicine. Part B. New York: AVI Publishing Co., 1987:843–848.

TOXIC MYOPATHIES

A large group of chemical and biological agents are recognized as producing skeletal muscle degeneration and necrosis, either experimentally in laboratory animals or as sporadic clinical occurrences in human patients treated with various therapeutic agents. However, in veterinary medicine, naturally occurring toxicities are largely limited to disease syndromes associated with ingestion of *ionophores, toxic plants, and plant-origin toxins*.

Skeletal muscle susceptibility to toxicants appears in part related to the specialized metabolism of muscle and the increased demands on the metabolic process from contraction. In addition, sensitivity to toxicants may be enhanced because many of the substances tend to bind to skeletal muscle fibers. Skeletal muscle dysfunction or damage has been induced by altered neurogenic function (increased motor nerve activity, neuromuscular blockade, acetylcholine accumulation, and denervation atrophy); immunologic modulations; alterations in various subcellular sites centered on cell membranes, myofilaments, lysosomes, microtubules, and sarcoplasmic reticulum; altered intracellular calcium concentration; altered protein synthesis; and altered muscle cell differentiation. Some agents, such as oxytetracycline, cause direct local injury at injection sites.

Clinical expression of myotoxicities is highly variable and ranges from lack of overt clinical signs but elevated serum concentrations of skeletal muscle origin enzymes, stiffness and muscle pain with or without myoglobinuria, and severe muscle weakness accompanied by recumbency usually with myoglobinuria. Mortality rates may be high in severely affected animals; death is often caused by concurrent myocardial damage by the same toxin.

Ionophore toxicosis

Ionophores *used in agriculture are monensin, lasalocid, salinomycin, narasin, and maduramicin.* Ionophores are compounds that alter membrane permeability to electrolytes by influencing transmembrane transport. In excess, all of these agents damage skeletal and cardiac muscle but *horses are uniquely susceptible*. Most reports of toxicosis involve monensin, an ionophore used widely for years.

Monensin, an antibiotic produced by the fermentation of *Streptomyces cinnamonensis*, has a growth-promoting effect in ruminants and is an efficient coccidiostat in birds and other animals. Monensin is produced commercially in very large quantities in North America and Europe where it is added, as a concentrated premix, to pelleted or bulk feeds fed to cattle, sheep, and other ruminants. Toxicity develops when monensin is fed to monogastric animals, which have a much reduced tolerance for the drug, or when human or mechanical error leads to concentrations of monensin in the ration that are abnormally high for the species being fed. Toxic effects have been recorded in horses, donkeys, mules, zebras, cattle, sheep, dogs, wallabies, camels, blesbok, Stone sheep, turkeys, and chickens. Many episodes of monensin poisoning have been caused by mixing errors in packaged, pelleted, commercial animal feeds, either concentrates or final mix which has put hundreds or thousands of animals at risk, sometimes over wide geographic areas. In North America alone, such mixing errors have been reported in horse, cattle, dog, and zoo feeds. Some indication of susceptibility of different species is provided by the *estimated LD_{50} for different animals*. Horses and other equids that are sensitive have an LD_{50} of 2–3 mg of monensin/kg body weight. LD_{50} values for other species are: dogs, 5–8 mg/kg; sheep and goats, 12–24 mg/kg; cattle, 50–80 mg/kg; and various types of poultry 90–200 mg/kg. Pigs, which may be given the drug for its coccidiostatic properties or are exposed by mistake, have an LD_{50} of 16–50 mg/kg body weight. The toxic effects of monensin or salinomycin are potentiated by the addition of tiamulin, triacetyloleandomycin, or sulfonamides to the ration, usually for therapeutic purposes.

Ingestion of **maduramicin**, an ionophore antibiotic utilized as a coccidiostat in poultry, has caused *cardiotoxicity in cattle and sheep*. Cases occurred in South Africa and Israel where dried poultry litter was used as a source of protein for ruminants. The clinical and pathological features of this toxicosis are similar to those of monensin cardiotoxicity.

When a single large toxic dose of an ionophore is fed to an animal, clinical signs of *lethargy, stiffness, muscular weakness, and recumbency* occur within 24 hours. Horses and other equids are likely, in the early stages, to show marked signs of colic, apprehension, shifting or fidgeting, sweating, myoglobinuria, and muscle tremors. Dogs show apprehension and progressive weakness. If sublethal doses are fed, the toxic effect will be cumulative, and the clinical onset may be delayed for 2–3 days to weeks depending on the total amount and the period over which it is fed, but the debility is likely to be more pronounced. Animals on low-level toxicity experiments often have delayed progression of the toxic signs because consumption of these feeds is reduced. These animals frequently scour and lose weight. At dose levels capable of inducing clinical signs of toxicity in a few days, many animals show evidence of *progressive cardiac failure due to a high incidence of myocardial lesions*. Animals recovering from the acute disease may subsequently develop within several months signs of progressive cardiac insufficiency from myocardial fibrosis, and sometimes renal failure, in addition to poor growth or poor weight gain, although the signs referable to skeletal muscle injury may disappear.

Postmortem lesions of ionophore toxicity may be difficult to detect in acute cases dying within 24 hours. *In horses, myocardial damage predominates, in sheep and swine the skeletal muscles are the main site of damage and myoglobinuria is generally present* (Figs 2.76, 2.77), *and in cattle skeletal and cardiac muscle are about equally affected*. Skeletal muscle may lack normal rigor, and ill-defined pale streaks may be visible in both myocardium and skeletal muscle. Later, the white streaking and local atrophy of affected skeletal muscles becomes more prominent. Hindlimb muscles may be the sites of major degenerative changes. Cases with terminal cardiac damage will have features of congestive heart failure including fluid accumulations in body cavities, pulmonary congestion and edema, and hepatic congestion.

Microscopic lesions of ionophore toxicity typically are *monophasic, multifocal degeneration* by 48 hours after exposure and thus differ from the polyphasic, multifocal lesions of nutritional myopathy. One of the earliest electron-microscopically visible lesions in muscle fibers is *marked swelling and disintegration of mitochondria*. Monensin is an ionophore that distorts membrane transport of sodium and potassium. This apparently leads to distortions of the electrolyte-modulated calcium gating mechanism and then mitochondrial failure, energy exhaustion, failure of calcium ion removal from the cytosol, and eventually myofibrillar hypercontraction and segmental degeneration. *Both type 1 and type 2 fibers are involved with hyaline necrosis and macrophagic infiltration* (Figs 2.78–2.83).

Myofiber nuclei and satellite cell nuclei as well as endomysial cells apparently survive acute toxicity, and the early stages of regeneration

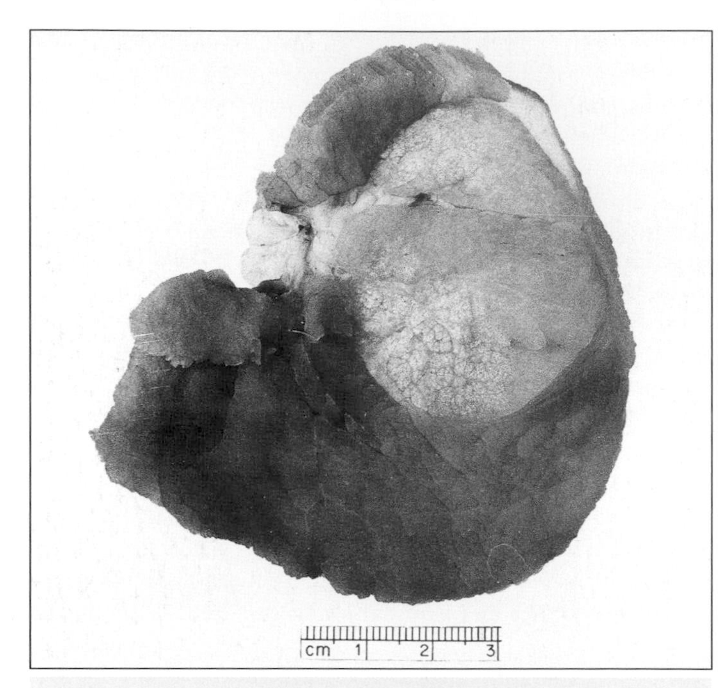

Figure 2.76 Pale area of necrosis in cross-section of caudal thigh muscles from a pig with **monensin toxicosis**. (Reprinted from Van Vleet JF et al. Am J Vet Res 1983;44:1460.)

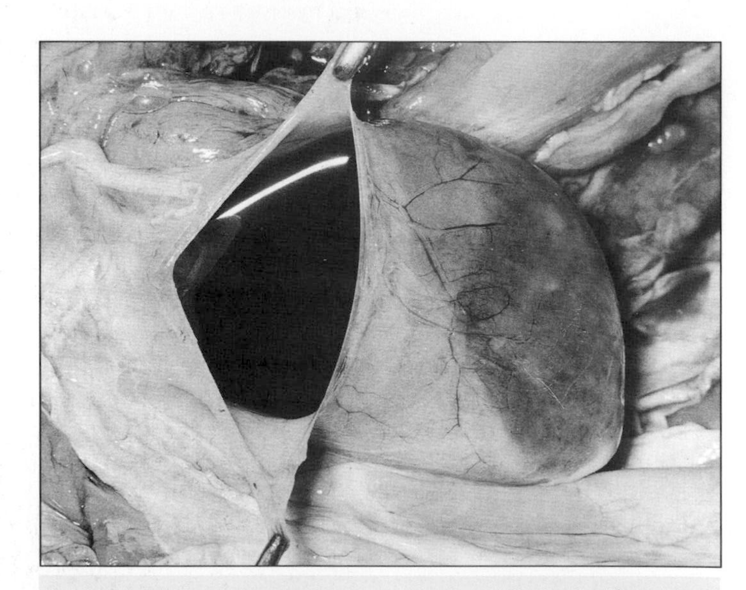

Figure 2.77 **Myoglobinuria** in a pig with monensin toxicosis. (Reprinted from Van Vleet JF et al. Am J Vet Res 1983;44:1460.)

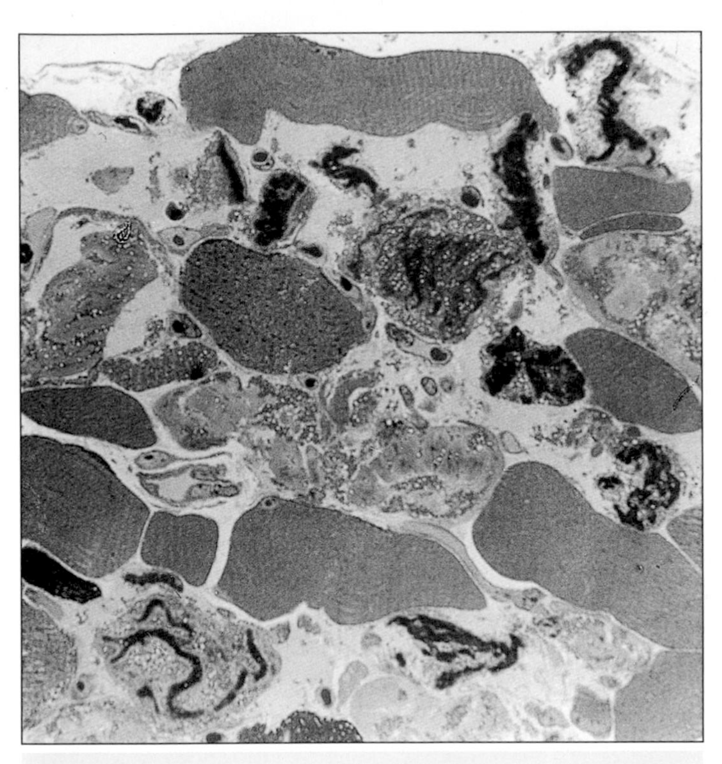

Figure 2.78 Acute myonecrosis of diaphragm of a pig one day after monensin toxicosis. (Reprinted from Van Vleet JF et al. Am J Pathol 1984;114:461.)

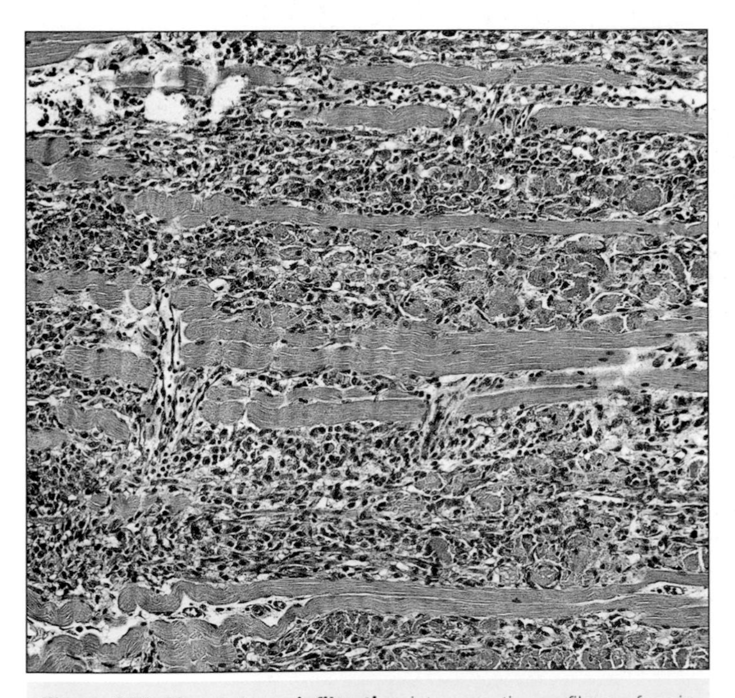

Figure 2.79 Macrophage infiltration into necrotic myofibers of a pig four days after monensin toxicosis. (Reprinted from Van Vleet JF et al. Am J Vet Res 1983;44:1460.)

are initiated during the first few days following exposure (Figs 2.82–2.85).

Myocardial lesions in monensin toxicity are not reparable and, particularly in a growing animal, the probability of lasting cardiac insufficiency is high.

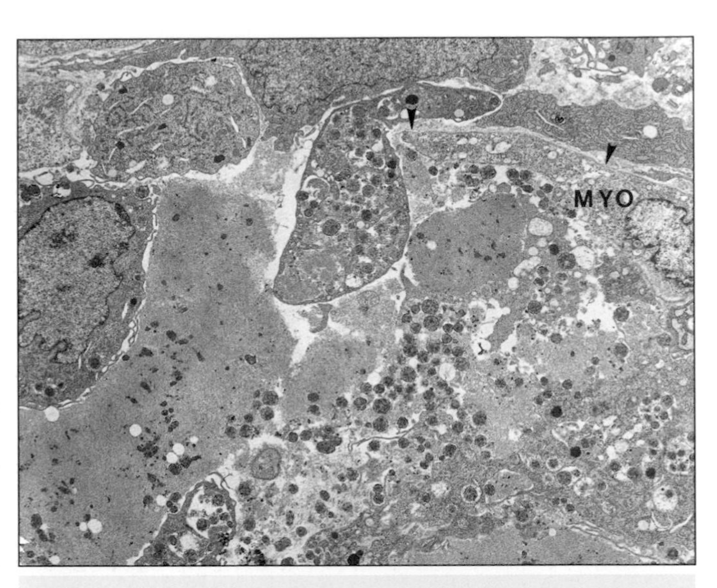

Figure 2.80 Necrotic myofiber with mineralized mitochondria and infiltrated macrophages in a pig with monensin toxicosis. Arrowheads = external lamina. MYO = presumptive myoblast. (Reprinted from Van Vleet JF et al. Am J Pathol 1984;114:461.)

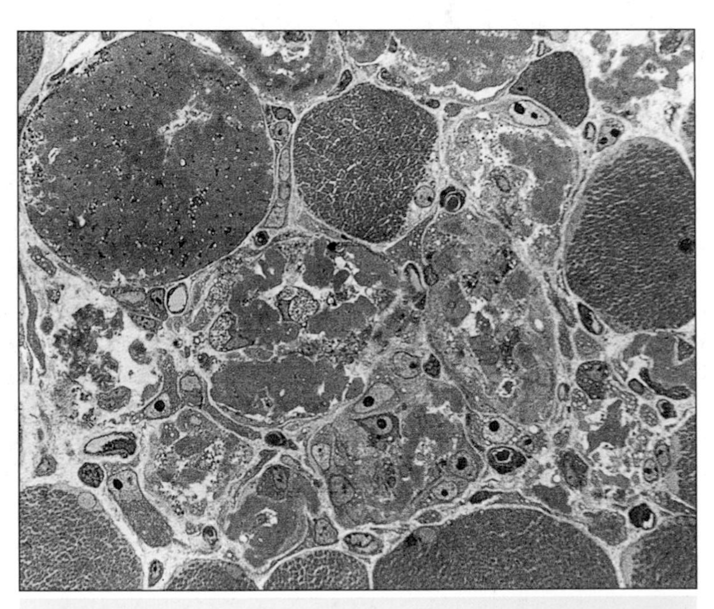

Figure 2.81 Cross-sectioned necrotic myofibers with **macrophage infiltration** in a pig with monensin toxicosis. (Reprinted from Van Vleet JF et al. Am J Vet Res 1983;44:1469.)

Toxic plants and plant-origin toxins

Cassia spp. toxicity – ruminants

In the southern USA, mature cattle and goats on pasture may ingest the beans of the **senna or coffee senna plant** (*Cassia occidentalis* or *C. obtusifolia*) or **coyotillo** (*Karwinskia humboldtiana*) late in the year, after a killing frost has made the plant more palatable than normal. Horses and pigs may also be affected. After eating the plant for a few days, animals develop diarrhea, show evidence of weakness, and display a swaying, stumbling gait that is related to the developing muscle lesions. The disease progresses rapidly and most of the animals affected become recumbent and develop myoglobinuria and

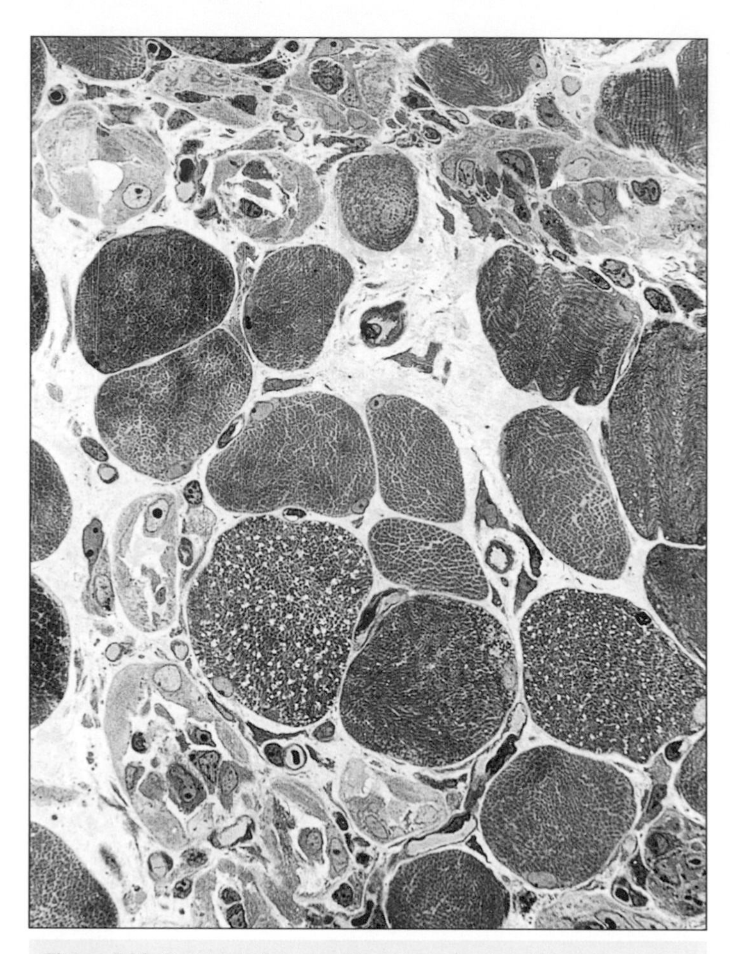

Figure 2.82 Regenerating myofibers have peripheral ring of myoblasts in the diaphragm of a pig with monensin toxicosis. (Reprinted from Van Vleet JF et al. Am J Pathol 1984;114:461.)

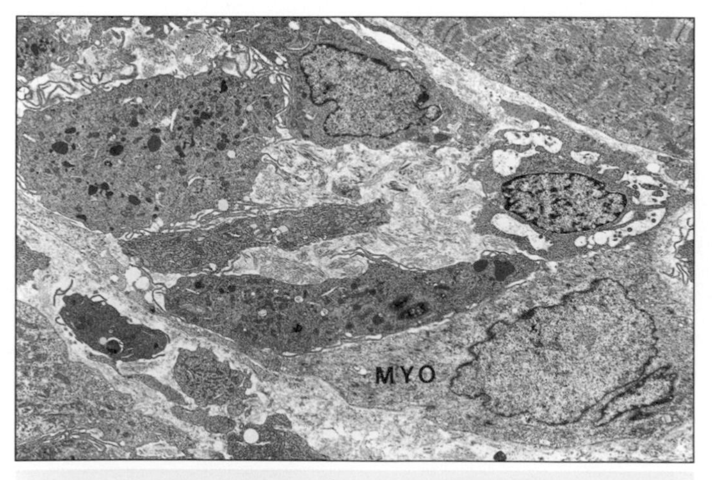

Figure 2.83 Regenerating myofiber has myoblast (MYO) and macrophages in the semitendinosus muscle of a pig with monensin toxicosis. (Reprinted from Van Vleet JF et al. Am J Pathol 1984;114:461.)

high concentrations of muscle-origin enzymes in serum. Recumbent animals usually do not recover but may live for several days. The morbidity rate may reach 60%.

Postmortem lesions in recumbent animals consist of *ill-defined pallor of much of the muscle mass*. Histologic changes are typically *monophasic multifocal myopathy*. The destruction of muscle fibers is

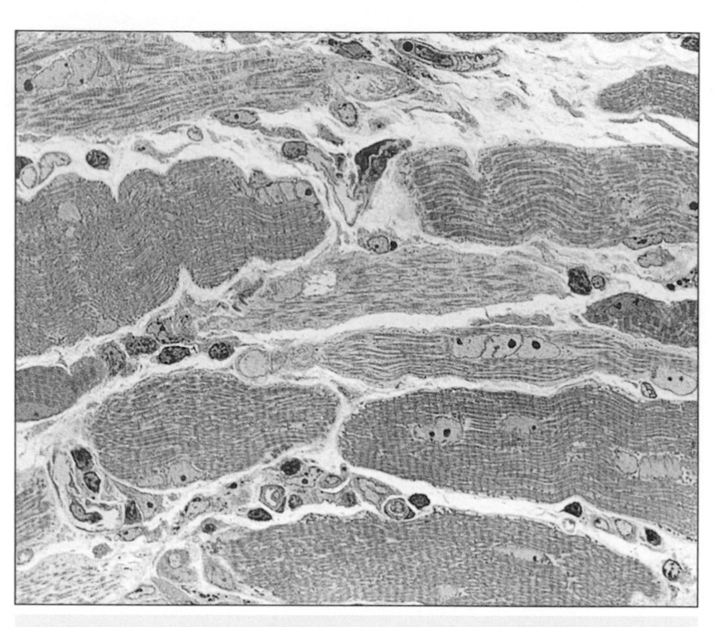

Figure 2.84 Late stage of myofiber regeneration with central rows of nuclei in the diaphragm of a pig with monensin toxicosis. (Reprinted from Van Vleet JF et al. Am J Pathol 1984;114:461.)

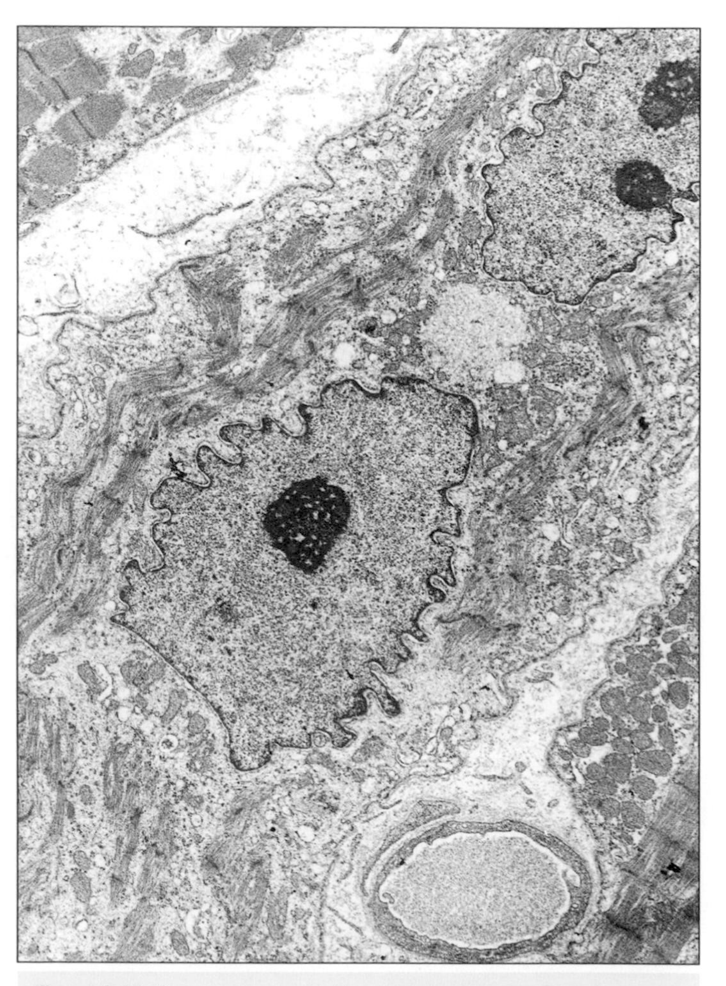

Figure 2.85 Central row of nuclei in **regenerating myofiber** from a pig with monensin toxicosis. (Reprinted from Van Vleet JF et al. Am J Pathol 1984;114:461.)

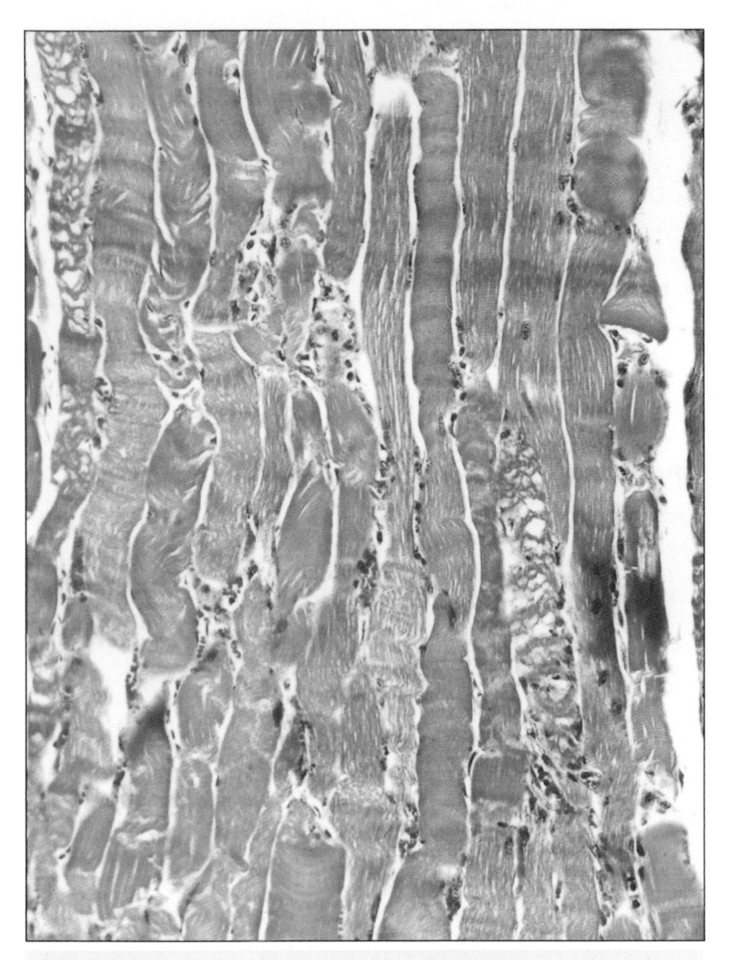

Figure 2.86 Myodegeneration caused by ***Cassia occidentalis*** **poisoning** of a heifer. (Courtesy of KR Pierce.)

segmental, but sarcolemmal sheaths and muscle nuclei remain, enclosing the floccular degenerate contractile elements (Fig. 2.86). Myocardium is not extensively involved but animals dying acutely show some myocardial lesions. Apparently recovered animals have not been examined, and the specific toxin has not been characterized.

Cassia spp. toxicity – swine

Natural outbreaks of toxicity on several pig farms occurred when animals were fed grain contaminated with *C. occidentalis* seeds. Several pigs died after a short period of reduced weight gain and a progressively wobbly, unsteady gait. Experimentally, the clinical disease was reproduced after 40 days with diets with as little as 1% of ground seeds. Postmortem examination revealed no gross lesions, but microscopic degeneration of the myocardium and diaphragm were characterized by *vacuolation and segmental hypercontraction of fibers*. The lesions were unexpectedly limited in the skeletal musculature, considering the marked locomotor clinical signs.

Gossypol toxicity

Gossypol *is a yellow, pigmented, polyphenolic substance present in cottonseeds* (*Gossypium* spp.). It is toxic to swine, and toxicosis occurs when swine are fed cottonseed cake or meal at a concentration of 10% or more of rations to which it is added as a protein supplement.

Lesions occur after feeding such rations for a month or more, which suggests that the toxic effects are cumulative. Gossypol is toxic to experimental lambs and calves at concentrations of less than 450 ppm in the feed (the level of free gossypol permitted in human and some animal foods). Dogs may also be affected. Lesions are present in several organs, including the heart, skeletal muscles, liver, and lungs, and *death is due to cardiac failure*, which causes fluid accumulation in body cavities. Histologically, *segmental necrosis of skeletal muscle and myocardium* is present, the liver has centrilobular necrosis and the lungs are congested and edematous. Affected animals are pot-bellied and poorly grown, and most die acutely. Natural outbreaks of disease in calves and lambs circumstantially linked to cottonseed meal ingestion have similar patterns of poor growth and sudden death. Serum enzyme concentrations are generally not significantly increased, which seems to confirm that the heart is the only striated muscle generally affected. Other circumstantial evidence suggests, however, that in calves, skeletal muscle lesions can be locally extensive but unpredictable in distribution. *Both type 1 and 2 muscle fibers appear to be affected in a selective, segmental myopathy* generally indistinguishable from the lesions of other toxic myopathies except that both myofiber types are equally involved.

Other toxic myopathies

Myopathies are reported in sheep with **lupinosis** (*Diaporthe toxica*), in sheep with **water hemlock** (*Cicuta douglasii*) toxicosis, in calves with **false lupine** (*Thermopsis montana*) toxicosis, in horses with **white snakeroot** (*Eupatorium* spp.) toxicosis, and in pigs, cattle, sheep, and other species with **selenium** toxicosis.

Bibliography

Anderson PH, et al. Suspected selenium poisoning in lambs. Veterinary Record 1985;116:647.

Anderson TD, et al. Acute monensin toxicosis in sheep: Light and electron microscopic changes. Am J Vet Res 1984;45:1142–1147.

Argov Z, et al. Toxic and iatrogenic myopathies and neuromuscular transmission disorders. In: Karpati G, et al., eds. Disorders of Voluntary Muscle. 7th ed. New York: Cambridge University Press, 2001:676–688.

Argov Z, Mastaglia FL. Drug-induced neuromuscular disorders in man. In: Walton J, et al., eds. Disorders of Voluntary Muscle. 6th ed. New York: Churchill-Livingstone, 1994:989–1029.

Barth AT, et al. Coffee senna (*Senna occidentalis*) poisoning in cattle in Brazil. Vet Hum Toxicol 1994;36:541–545.

Bastianello SS, et al. Cardiomyopathy of ruminants induced by the liter of poultry fed on rations containing the ionophore antibiotic, maduramicin. II. Macropathology and histopathology. Onderstepoort J Vet Res 1995;62:5–18.

Bastianello SS, et al. A chronic cardiomyopathy in feedlot cattle attributed to toxic levels of salinomycin in the feed. J South Afr Vet Assn 1996;67:38–41.

Bezerra PS, et al. Monensin poisoning in Brazilian horses. Vet Hum Toxicol 1999;41:383–385.

Blanchard PC, et al. Lasalocid toxicosis in dairy calves. J Vet Diag Invest 1993;5:300–302.

Boemo CM, et al. Monensin toxicity in horses. An outbreak resulting in the deaths of ten horses. Aust Eq Vet 1991;9:103–107.

Colvin JM, et al. *Cassia occidentalis* toxicosis in growing pigs. J Am Vet Med Assoc 1986;189:423–426.

Dewan ML, et al. Toxic myodegeneration in goats by feeding mature fruits from the coyotillo plant (*Karwinskia humboldtiana*). Am J Pathol 1965;46:215–226.

Dollahite JW, Henson JB. Toxic plants as the etiologic agent of myopathies in animals. Am J Vet Res 1965;26:749–752.

East NE, et al. Apparent gossypol-induced toxicosis in adult dairy goats. J Am Vet Med Assoc 1994;204:642–643.

Goedegebuure SA. Spontaneous primary myopathies in domestic mammals. A review. Vet Quarterly 1987;9:155–171.

Hazlett MJ, et al. Monensin/roxarsone contaminated dog food associated with myodegeneration and renal medullary necrosis in dogs. Can Vet J 1992; 33:749–751.

Holmberg CA, et al. Pathological and toxicological studies of calves fed a high concentration cottonseed meal diet. Vet Pathol 1988;25:147–153.

Jones LA. Gossypol toxicosis. J Am Vet Med Assoc 1988;193:292–293.

Karsai F, et al. Several cases of poisoning of dogs with the growth promoter narasin. Tieraztliche Umschau 1990;45:316, 319–324.

Keeler RF, Baker DC. Myopathy in cattle induced by alkaloid extracts from *Thermopsis montana, Laburnum anagyroides* and a *Lupinus* sp. J Comp Pathol 1990;103:169–182.

Lane RJM. Toxic and drug-induced myopathies. In: Lane RJM, ed. Handbook of Muscle Disease. New York: Marcel Dekker, 1996:379–389.

Lightfoot RM. The musculoskeletal system. In: Turton J, Hoosen J, eds. Target Organ Pathology. London: Taylor and Francis, 1998:239–272.

Mastaglia FL, Argov Z. Drug-induced myopathies and disorders of neuromuscular transmission. In: Manzo L, et al., eds. Advances in Neurotoxicology. Oxford: Pergamon Press, 1986:319–328.

Miller RE, et al. Acute monensin toxicosis in Stone sheep (*Ovis dalli stonei*), blesbok (*Damaliscus dorcus phillipsi*), and a Bactrian camel (*Camelus bactrianus*). J Am Vet Med Assoc 1990;196:131–134.

Morgan S, et al. Clinical, clinicopathologic, pathologic, and toxicologic alteration associated with gossypol toxicosis in feeder lambs. Am J Vet Res 1988; 49:493–499.

Panter KE, et al. Water hemlock (*Cicuta douglasii*) toxicosis in sheep: pathologic description and prevention of lesions and death. J Vet Diag Invest 1996;8:474–480.

Plumlee KH, et al. Acute salinomycin toxicosis of pigs. J Vet Diag Invest 1995;7:419–420.

Rowe LD, et al. Cassia-induced myopathy. In: Keeler RF, Tu AL, eds. Handbook of Natural Toxins. vol. 6. Toxicology of Plant and Fungal Compounds. New York: Marcel Dekker, 1991:335–351.

Salyi G, et al. Ionophore antibiotics caused poisoning in swine herds. Magyar Allatorvosok Lapja 1994;49:140–146.

Schweitzer D, et al. Accidental monensin sodium intoxication of feedlot cattle. J Am Vet Med Assoc 1984;184:1273–1276.

Scimeca JM, Oehme FW. Postmortem guide to common poisonous plants of livestock. Vet Hum Toxicol 1985;27:189–199.

Shlosberg A, et al. Cardiomyopathy in cattle induced by residues of the coccidiostat maduramicin in poultry litter given as a feedstuff. Vet Res Commun 1992;16:45–58.

Shortridge EH, et al. Acute selenium poisoning in cattle. N Z Vet J 1971;19:47–50.

Smith GM, Allen JG. Effectiveness of alpha-tocopherol and selenium supplements in preventing lupinosis-associated myopathy in sheep. Aust Vet J 1997;75:341–348.

Stowe HD, et al. Selenium toxicosis in feeder pigs. J Am Vet Med Assoc 1992;201:292–295.

Todd GC, et al. Comparative toxicology of monensin sodium in laboratory animals. J An Sci 1984;58:1512–1517.

Umemura T, et al. Enhanced myotoxicity and involvement of both type I and II fibers in monensin-tiamulin toxicosis in pigs. Vet Pathol 1985;22:409–414.

Van Vleet JF, et al. Clinical, clinicopathologic, and pathologic alterations in acute monensin toxicosis in cattle. Am J Vet Res 1983;44:2133–2144.

Van Vleet JF, et al. Monensin toxicosis in swine: potentiation by tiamulin administration and ameliorative effect of treatment with selenium and/or vitamin E. Am J Vet Res 1987;48:1520–1524.

Van Vleet JF, et al. Cardiovascular and skeletal muscle system. In: Haschek-Hock WM, Rousseaux CG, Wallig MA, eds. Handbook of Toxicologic Pathology. 2nd ed. Vol. 2. San Diego, CA: Academic Press, 2002:363–455.

Van Vleet JF, Ferrans VJ. Ultrastructural alterations in skeletal muscle of pigs with acute monensin myotoxicosis. Am J Pathol 1984;114:461–471.

Wouters ATB, et al. Experimental narasin poisoning in cattle. Pesquisa Vet Brasileira 1997;17:82–88.

Zelski RZ, et al. Gossypol toxicity in preruminant calves. Aust Vet J 1995; 72:394–398.

MYOPATHIES ASSOCIATED WITH ENDOCRINE DISORDERS

Hypothyroidism

Some dogs with hypothyroidism may develop clinical signs of weakness, stiffness, reluctance to move, decreased exercise tolerance, and *muscle wasting* in addition to the traditional signs of alopecia and obesity. The likelihood of development of myopathy is increased if concomitant endocrinopathies are present such as diabetes mellitus and hyperadrenocorticism. Peripheral neuropathy with axonal degeneration may also be produced in hypothyroidism (and hyperadrenocorticism) with subsequent atrophy of type 1 and type 2 fibers.

Muscle biopsies reveal *atrophy and loss of type 2 fibers*. The atrophic fibers appear oval or angular in outline and are present throughout all muscle fascicles. Nemaline rods may be found, especially in type 1 fibers. No evidence of muscle fiber degradation or inflammatory cell infiltration is present. Initiation of thyroid hormone replacement therapy leads to resolution of the lesions. Selective involvement of type 2 fibers has been attributed to alterations in carbohydrate metabolism with subsequent loss of energy from glycolysis and glycogenolysis.

Hyperthyroidism

Affected cats may exhibit muscular tremors, ventroflexion of the neck, disturbances in gait, generalized weakness, and collapse. Microscopic alterations usually are absent, but *nonspecific fiber damage may be present.*

Hyperadrenocorticism

Cushing's disease from pituitary-dependent hyperadrenocorticism, adrenal-dependent hyperadrenocorticism, and iatrogenic hyperadrenocorticism may result in muscular weakness, stiff stilted gait, *muscle atrophy,* and inability to walk in dogs. The pelvic limbs are mainly affected.

In muscle biopsies, there are *selective type 2 fiber atrophy, fiber splitting, and focal necrosis*. Medical or surgical treatment of Cushing's disease may lead to resolution of the muscle lesions unless severe atrophy or contracture was present in the pelvic limb musculature. The muscle fiber alterations are attributed to *increased catabolism and inhibited synthesis of muscle proteins from glucocorticoid excess.*

Hypoadrenocorticism

Addison's disease in dogs and cats often results in muscle weakness presumed to be related to accompanying *hyperkalemia*. Muscle alterations have not been characterized.

Increased growth hormone exposure

Beagle dogs given exogenous porcine growth hormone had hypertrophy of types 1 and 2 fibers. However, skeletal muscle alterations have not been described in dogs or cats with acromegaly.

Bibliography

Blot S, Fuhrer L. Myopathies in domestic carnivores. Part 2. Review of conditions. Eur J Compan An Pract 1996;6:56–69.

Braund KG. Endogenous causes of myopathies in dogs and cats. Vet Med 1997;92:618–628.

Braund KG, et al. Subclinical myopathy associated with hyperadrenocorticism in the dog. Vet Pathol 1980;17:134–148.

Cuddon PA. Feline neuromuscular disease. Feline Pract 1994;22:7–13.

Goedegebuure SA. Spontaneous primary myopathies in domestic mammals: A review. Vet Quart 1987;9:155–171.

LeCouteur RA, et al. Metabolic and endocrine myopathies of dogs and cats. Sem Vet Med Surg (Small Anim) 1989;4:146–155.

Molon-Noblet S, et al. Effect of chronic growth hormone administration in skeletal muscle in dogs. Tox Pathol 1998;26:207–212.

Orrell RW, et al. Muscle dysfunction in endocrine disease. In: Lane RJM, ed. Handbook of Muscle Disease. New York: Marcel Dekker, 1996:365–378.

Platt SR. Neuromuscular complications in endocrine and metabolic diseases. Vet Clin North Am Small Anim Pract 2002;32:125–146.

Shelton GD. Differential diagnosis of muscle diseases in companion animals. Prog Vet Neurol 1991;2:27–33.

MYOPATHIES ASSOCIATED WITH SERUM ELECTROLYTE ABNORMALITIES

Hypokalemia in cats

In 1984, a *polymyopathy* was identified in cats and in over half of the affected animals, there was a coexisting hypokalemia. Subsequently, a distinct syndrome of **hypokalemic myopathy** was characterized and the disorder was also termed *feline kaliopenic polymyopathy-nephropathy syndrome* and *sporadic feline hypokalemic polymyopathy*.

Clinically, the affected cats had generalized weakness, ventroflexion of the neck, a stiff stilted gait, exercise intolerance, reluctance to walk, and muscle pain. Serum activity of skeletal muscle origin enzymes (CK, AST) was elevated and serum potassium levels were low (<3 mEq/L). Hypokalemia was attributed to low dietary intake or excessive renal loss. Low intake occurred in cats fed potassium-depleted regular diets or high-protein vegetarian diets. Excessive renal loss of potassium was present in cats with chronic renal disease and in those fed acidic diets to prevent urolithiasis. Also, the syndrome reported in Burmese kittens 2–6 months of age with intermittent hypokalemia, is presumed to be heritable.

In general, *the skeletal muscle lesions have been either mild or absent.* Lesions have been described as a *polyphasic myopathy with concurrent necrosis and regeneration.* The skeletal muscle damage was attributed to influx of sodium with a decrease in resting membrane potential and hypopolarization, altered glycogen metabolism in skeletal muscle fibers, and ischemic injury from hypokalemia-induced vasoconstriction. Treatment with potassium supplementation is generally successful but the syndrome may recur unless supplementation is maintained.

Hypokalemia in cattle

In 1997, a hypokalemic syndrome with *muscle weakness and myopathy* was reported. Affected cattle were weak, recumbent, and were unable to elevate their heads off the ground and instead held them against their flanks. They were post-parturient and had moderate to severe ketosis with hypokalemia (1.4–2.3 mEq/L). The animals were treated with isoflupredone, a glucocorticoid with high mineralocorticoid activity. The skeletal muscle damage involved the hindlimbs and included vacuolar degeneration, necrosis with macrophagic infiltration, and variably present secondary ischemic injury.

Hypernatremia in cats

Muscle weakness evident as ventroflexion of the neck has been observed with hypernatremia and hypodipsia in the cat.

Hypophosphatemia in dogs

Muscle weakness occurs in dogs with hypophosphatemia. Necrosis of skeletal muscle with myoglobinuria was present in severe acute phosphorus depletion.

Bibliography

Braund KG. Endogenous causes of myopathies in dogs and cats. Vet Med 1997;92:618–628.

Edwards CM, Belford CJ. Hypokalemic polymyopathy in Burmese cats. Aust Vet Pract 1995;25:58–60.

Leon A, et al. Hypokalemic episodic polymyopathy in cats fed a vegetarian diet. Aust Vet J 1992;69:249–254.

Fettman MJ. Feline kaliopenic polymyopathy/nephropathy syndrome. Vet Clin North Am Small Anim Pract 1989;19:415–432.

Knochel JP. Skeletal muscle in hypophosphatemia and phosphorus deficiency. Adv Exp Med Biol 1978;103:357–366.

Le Couteur RA, et al. Metabolic and endocrine myopathies of dogs and cats. Sem Vet Med Surg (Small Anim) 1989;4:146–155.

Sielman ES, et al. Hypokalemia syndrome in dairy cows: 10 cases (1992–1996). J Am Vet Med Assoc 1997;210:240–243.

EXERTIONAL MYOPATHIES

The term **exertional myopathy** *is indicative of myofiber damage occurring due to exercise stress.* Acute myofiber injury is precipitated by exercise in a broad group of myopathies, including X-linked muscular dystrophy, nutritional myopathy, metabolic myopathies, malignant hyperthermia, and myopathy due to hypokalemia. In such cases, the initiation of abnormal excitation–contraction coupling, inadequate energy metabolism, ionic imbalance, or simply the mechanical stresses occurring during contraction are thought to lead to myofiber damage of predisposed muscle.

Historically, the syndrome of passage of *myoglobin-pigmented urine (myoglobinuria)* was recognized long before it was determined that massive *skeletal muscle necrosis (rhabdomyolysis)* was the cause. Small wonder that so many names exist for the varying manifestations of exertional myopathy. In a broad sense, *exertional myopathy has included the group of diseases in which acute muscle fiber necrosis is initiated by muscle activity of the major muscle groups but in which the underlying cause is unknown or poorly understood.* Such activity may be intensive or exhaustive, but in susceptible individuals exertional myopathy may occur with only minimal exercise. Continued research into causes of exertional rhabdomyolysis is clearly warranted and, as is true of equine exertional rhabdomyolysis (see below), may lead to better understanding of causes and preventive measures.

Exertional myopathy (rhabdomyolysis) in the horse

Various manifestations of exertional myopathy have been recognized in horses for many, many years. There are numerous names for the disorder, including *azoturia* (presumably named for nitrogen-containing compounds in the urine, and possibly related to the resemblance of myoglobin to the red-purple azo dyes), *black water, paralytic myoglobinuria, Monday-morning disease, set fast, and tying up.* Various classifications have distinguished the disorder in heavy horse breeds that are prone to severe and often life-threatening muscle injury, particularly when worked after a day of rest and full grain ration (hence the term Monday-morning disease), from the often less severe disorder in light horse breeds. Muscle injury severe enough to result in myoglobinuria, profound weakness, and recumbency is common in heavy horse breeds, hence the terms azoturia, black water, and paralytic myoglobinuria. Exertional myopathy in light horse breeds is typically less severe, resulting in episodic muscle pain, sometimes associated with swelling, and reluctance to move, hence the names set fast and tying up. Given the recent recognition of a metabolic myopathy leading to exertional rhabdomyolysis in both heavy and light breeds (see below), it becomes clear that *the same underlying disorder can result in a spectrum of clinical signs.*

It has long been suspected that the clinical disorder represents a syndrome with multiple possible etiologies. It has been proposed that exertional myopathy in the horse be classified as either sporadic exertional rhabdomyolysis or recurrent exertional rhabdomyolysis, with sporadic exertional rhabdomyolysis possible due to muscle exhaustion or electrolyte depletion in any horse, and recurrent exertional rhabdomyolysis occurring in horses somehow predisposed to this disorder. Studies of serum activities of CK and AST following exercise have shown, however, that subclinical exertional myopathy is common in horses. As exertional myopathy can occur without obvious clinical signs other than, perhaps, poor performance, it is possible that so-called sporadic cases really represent recurrent disease, and therefore this classification is difficult to justify based on current knowledge of equine muscle disease.

Previously, *etiologies* proposed for equine exertional rhabdomyolysis have included muscle lactic acidosis, hypothyroidism, electrolyte imbalance, and vitamin E and/or selenium deficiency. Of these, *only electrolyte imbalance, in particular hypokalemia, is still considered possible.* Extensive studies have shown that lactic acid levels in the muscle of exercising horses prone to exertional rhabdomyolysis are no different than those of control horses, removal of thyroid glands results in poor cardiac output and performance without evidence of muscle damage, and vitamin E and selenium status varies widely in affected horses. More recently, a *metabolic myopathy* thought to involve abnormal starch and sugar metabolism (equine polysaccharide storage myopathy, see the Metabolic myopathies section) has been shown to be the most common cause of exertional rhabdomyolysis in many breeds of horses, including Quarter Horse, Warmblood, draft, Arabian, Standardbred, Tennessee Walker, Morgan, and Welsh pony-related breeds. It is possible that a similar metabolic disorder is the cause of recurrent exertional rhabdomyolysis in Thoroughbreds, although this is controversial, with one group reporting evidence for abnormal calcium handling in muscle fibers of affected Thoroughbreds. Defective ryanodine receptor function similar to malignant hyperthermia has not, however, been found in affected Thoroughbreds. Whether the abnormal muscle contracture testing reported in in vitro studies of muscle from Thoroughbreds with recurrent exertional rhabdomyolysis is a primary or secondary abnormality is still unknown. *There is strong evidence that there is an inherited basis for the predisposition to exertional rhabdomyolysis in horses.* Both autosomal recessive and autosomal dominant inheritance have been proposed, depending on the breed studied. Although further studies are needed, *it is now accepted that exertional rhabdomyolysis in horses is most often due to underlying metabolic abnormalities of muscle rather than simply due to poor management of diet and exercise.*

Although diets high in starches and sugars (grains) are associated with increased severity of exertional rhabdomyolysis, clinical signs can still occur in horses fed only forage. Despite differing opinions regarding cause, *almost all horses with recurrent exertional rhabdomyolysis respond positively following a diet change to one that is high in fat, high in fiber, and low in starches and sugars.* Stall rest appears to exacerbate the signs of equine exertional rhabdomyolysis, however the mechanism by which daily exercise benefits such horses is still unknown.

Weakness and/or pain in the hindlimbs occur suddenly, and the animal soon becomes unable or very reluctant to move. This may be accompanied by sweating and generalized tremors. The affected muscles, which are typically those of the *gluteal, femoral, and lumbar groups*, may be swollen and board-like in their rigidity. *Myoglobinuria* can appear early in the disease, causing dark red-brown discoloration of the urine. Severely affected horses become recumbent, a sign that is often a prelude to death from myoglobinuric nephrosis or problems associated with being down and attempting to rise. Considerable variation occurs between cases as to the nature and duration of the initiating exercise and severity of clinical signs. Recovery from mild attacks in quiet animals may occur in a few hours. Recovery from severe episodes may take days. But, if an animal continues to struggle and is unable to rise, death or euthanasia is the most likely outcome. *Atrophy of the gluteal muscles* may be a feature of recovery in moderate to severe cases. Exertional rhabdomyolysis occurs in both males and females, although *females appear to be predisposed.* The activity of the ovarian hormones estrogen and progesterone does not, however, appear to be directly related to onset of exertional rhabdomyolysis in females, and ovariectomy is not an effective therapy.

The apparent pain and muscle swelling associated with many cases of equine exertional rhabdomyolysis is curious, as muscle necrosis per se is neither painful nor does it cause muscle swelling. It is suspected that *increased intramuscular pressure, perhaps exacerbated by oxidative membrane injury, may cause painful muscle injury in this disorder.*

This may explain the often-reported improvement obtained following vitamin E and selenium supplementation in affected horses.

Muscle fiber membrane injury leads to release of sarcoplasmic proteins, most notably myoglobin, creatine kinase (CK), and aspartate aminotransferase (AST). Serum activity of CK peaks at approximately 4–6 hours post-injury and declines rapidly, with a half-life of approximately 6–10 hours. Therefore, if serum CK activity is not reduced by at least 50% every 24 hours this is evidence of continued muscle injury. Serum activity of AST increases more slowly, with a peak at about 48 hours post-injury and a very long half-life that can lead to persistent AST increases for days to weeks. The degree of CK and AST increase does not, however, correlate with severity of clinical signs. It is possible that muscle cramping or stiffness in the absence of overt necrosis may occur in some horses.

Grossly visible changes in muscle may be inapparent. In severe cases they are most obvious in the gluteal, lumbar, and caudal thigh regions but lesions often are widespread. *Muscles may be moist, swollen, and dark, and streaks of pallor may be visible in the more extensively involved muscles.* If ischemic complications occur, the muscles also may show blotchy or linear hemorrhage. In animals that have survived for 2–3 days, muscles may become paler and, although edema may surround larger muscle divisions, the locally damaged areas appear dry compared to normal muscle.

Necrosis affects primarily the strongly glycolytic fibers (type 2B glycolytic and type 2A oxidative-glycolytic fibers; Fig. 2.87), in contrast to the primary involvement of type 1 oxidative fibers in the nutritional myopathies. The timing and sequence of events are not clear, but *damaged fiber segments generally undergo hypercontraction and hyaline degeneration* (Fig. 2.88) *followed by coagulative necrosis.* Mineralization is not typically seen. There is also potential for perpetuation of myofiber injury due to release of free radicals from damaged membranes and subsequent oxidative membrane injury. This sequence of events may reduce the capacity of muscle protein to hold water, consequently water is lost to the interstitial compartment where it raises local pressure and predisposes to ischemia (*compartment syndrome*), particularly if moderate muscle movement is continued (see Circulatory disturbances of muscle). Oxidative injury to muscle capillary endothelium may also contribute to intramuscular edema and increased pressure. Cardiac involvement is rare.

The early irreversible fiber change as monitored by electron microscopy consists of myofibrillar waving and architectural loss, irregular mitochondrial swelling, and interfibrillar edema. After 12 h, more marked sarcomere destruction occurs along with streaming of Z-bands. Histologically, the lesions are characterized by scattered single or small groups of necrotic fiber segments admixed with intact fibers. In the more severe, acute tying-up cases, 1–5% of muscle fibers in a biopsy sample may be affected. In the less severe cases, the amount of fiber damage involves less than 0.2% of fibers in irreversible change but many more fibers can undergo hypercontraction that is potentially reversible. If muscle is examined days after injury, fiber regeneration will be apparent. Lesions are often monophasic and multifocal, but can be polyphasic in horses with repeated bouts of necrosis or on-going injury (Fig. 2.89).

In horses with *polysaccharide storage myopathy*, abnormal inclusions of pale blue-gray complex polysaccharide may be seen within scattered myofibers on H&E stain (see Fig. 2.60). Inclusions may be numerous or very rare, and have been shown to occur only within type 2A and type 2B fibers. *Inclusions stain intensely with periodic acid-Schiff (PAS) for glycogen and resist amylase digestion.* In severe chronic cases, interstitial aggregates of complex polysaccharide-laden macrophages may be seen, indicative of previous necrosis of polysaccharide-laden segments, and marked fatty infiltration is possible (see Fig. 2.60). Subsarcolemmal aggregates of amylase-sensitive glycogen are also a feature of this disorder, and may occur in the absence of complex polysaccharide in some affected horses (see Fig. 2.62). Chronic myopathic changes, including excessive fiber size variation due to fiber hypertrophy and atrophy and increased numbers of internal nuclei are common. Given the high incidence of underlying equine polysaccharide storage myopathy in horses with histories of exertional rhabdomyolysis or postanesthetic myopathy (see below), *PAS staining and careful evaluation of muscle from all such cases for evidence of chronic myopathy and abnormal glycogen and complex polysaccharide storage is warranted.*

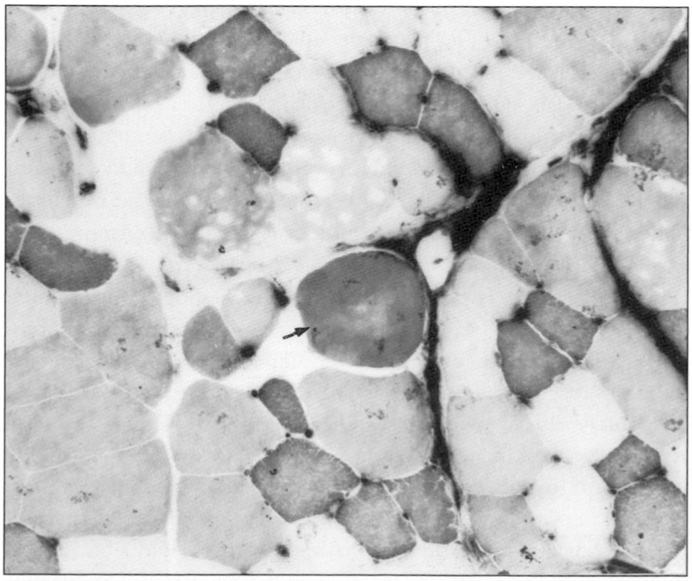

Figure 2.87 Equine exertional rhabdomyolysis with selective necrosis of type 2 (dark staining) fibers (arrow). Frozen section, ATPase, alkaline preincubation. (Courtesy of TJ Hulland.)

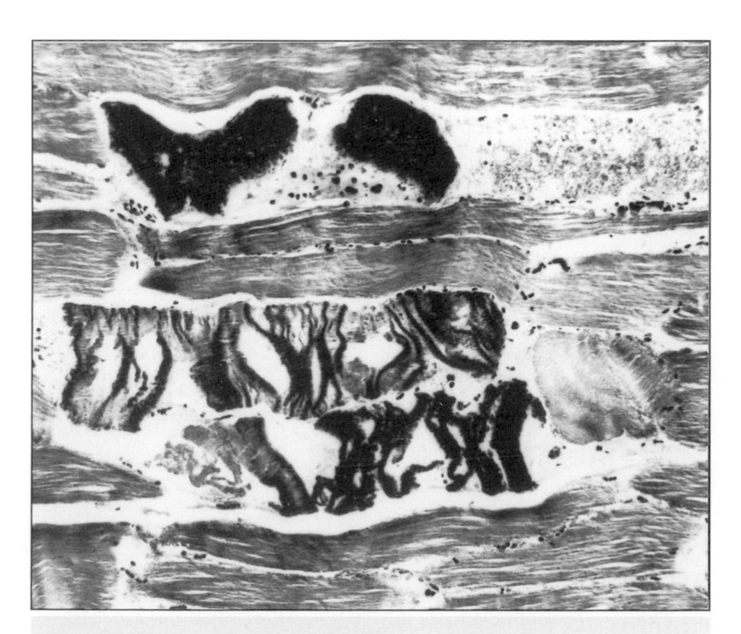

Figure 2.88 Segmental hypercontraction and acute necrosis in myofibers in a horse with **exertional rhabdomyolysis**. (Courtesy of TJ Hulland.)

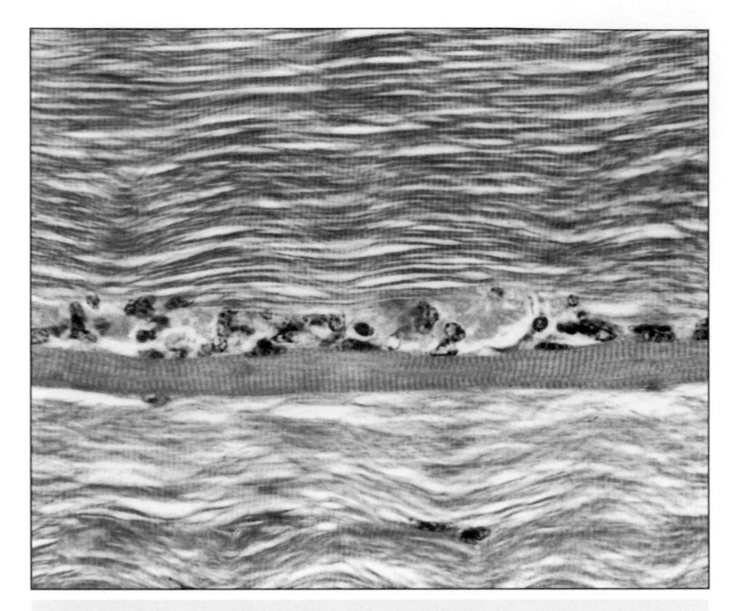

Figure 2.89 Concurrent myofiber necrosis and regeneration in a horse with **recurrent exertional rhabdomyolysis** with episodes 12 days apart. (Courtesy of TJ Hulland.)

Other equine degenerative myopathies

In addition to nutritional myopathy and exertional rhabdomyolysis, *degenerative myopathy can occur in horses recovering from general anesthesia*. This syndrome of **postanesthetic myopathy** has been recognized most often in heavy horse breeds. Although experimental induction of hypotension during general anesthesia will cause postanesthetic myopathy in any horse (see Circulatory disturbances of muscle), recent studies of clinical cases indicate that *many occur due to underlying polysaccharide storage myopathy*. Persistently high CK serum levels can occur in horses with postanesthetic myopathy due to polysaccharide storage myopathy, indicative of on-going muscle injury occurring even after the horse has stood up. A form of malignant hyperthermia has also been proposed as a cause of anesthetic-related myopathy in horses. This may be appropriate for those cases in which hyperthermia occurs during inhalant anesthesia, but most affected horses develop myopathy during recovery rather than during anesthesia. Although such horses may develop dangerously high body temperatures during recovery, this condition is best considered to be a hypermetabolic state rather than malignant hyperthermia. Underlying myopathy of any type may be a predisposing factor in horses that develop life-threatening hyperthermia either during or following general anesthesia.

Nutritional myopathy in horses causes a degenerative myopathy (see Nutritional myopathy), as do various *plant toxins and ionophores* (see Toxic myopathies). A myoglobinuric disease of pastured horses has also been described in Britain, in which extensive myolysis is triggered by an as yet unknown factor.

Exertional myopathy in dogs

Exertional rhabdomyolysis *is recognized as a syndrome affecting racing Greyhounds and racing sled dogs*. Given the vast difference in type of exercise (i.e., sprint vs endurance racing) in these two breeds of dog, there are likely to be differing underlying etiologies.

In *racing Greyhounds*, the disorder primarily affects longissimus, quadriceps, and biceps femoris muscles. Affected dogs may display distress and generalized muscle pain associated with a stiff gait. Myoglobinuria can lead to death due to renal failure. In less severe cases, myoglobinuria is not evident, and muscle pain may only be mild to moderate. Similar to exertional rhabdomyolysis in horses, affected muscles may be swollen as well as painful, indicative of mechanisms besides simple muscle necrosis as a cause of pain and swelling. Predisposing factors proposed include an *excitable nature, lack of physical fitness, hot and humid conditions, and overexertion of physically fit dogs*. Gross lesions are not often seen in affected muscles, although histopathologic evidence of acute degenerative changes is found in susceptible muscles.

Racing sled dogs may undergo massive rhabdomyolysis during racing that can lead to *sudden death*. There is often selective involvement of certain muscle groups; in one case studied there were moderate to severe polyfocal and monophasic necrotizing lesions involving quadriceps, psoas, deep digital flexor, and gastrocnemius muscles, with sparing of triceps brachii, epaxial, and cranial tibial muscles. Gross lesions are not typically seen, and sampling of multiple muscle groups may be necessary to determine the extent of injury. It has been suggested that prolonged endurance-type exercise leads to increased lipid peroxidation and reduced plasma antioxidant concentrations, however vitamin E supplementation does not appear to ameliorate exercise-induced muscle injury in racing sled dogs, and pre-race plasma vitamin E levels do not appear to correlate with risk of exertional rhabdomyolysis. As in horses, dietary management is likely to play a role in canine exertional rhabdomyolysis, as a high-fat and low-carbohydrate diet has been reported to reduce exercise-induced muscle injury in these dogs.

Exertional myopathy in other species ("capture myopathy")

Massive muscle injury associated with exertion reported in other domestic animals such as sheep and cattle can occur due to overexertion. Underlying nutritional myopathy (see the section on Nutritional myopathy) or metabolic myopathy (see the section on Metabolic myopathies) is also possible. *Of special interest is exertional myopathy occurring in wild animals following capture and/or immobilization, an entity known as* "**capture myopathy**." First described in wild ungulates, this disorder has been seen in multiple species, including wild ruminants, captured otters, cetaceans, mustelids, canids, marsupials, and wild birds. Clinically affected animals can exhibit *dyspnea, weakness, muscle tremors or muscle rigidity, hyperthermia, collapse, and, often, death*. Thigh muscle rupture may occur. Those that do not die acutely show myoglobinuria and increased levels of muscle enzymes in the blood and may subsequently die of renal failure. When the animal is down, ischemic complications may be secondary (see Circulatory disturbances of muscle). The muscle lesions are capable of more or less complete repair over a few weeks unless infarction has intervened.

Capture myopathy is associated with stress to the affected animal, and *increased circulating catecholamines may play a role*, particularly in the cardiac damage that can be seen. Hyperthermia and metabolic acidosis have also been associated with capture myopathy. Extreme overexertion likely also contributes. In some cases, marginal selenium status or electrolyte abnormality such as hypokalemia or hyperkalemia may be predisposing factors.

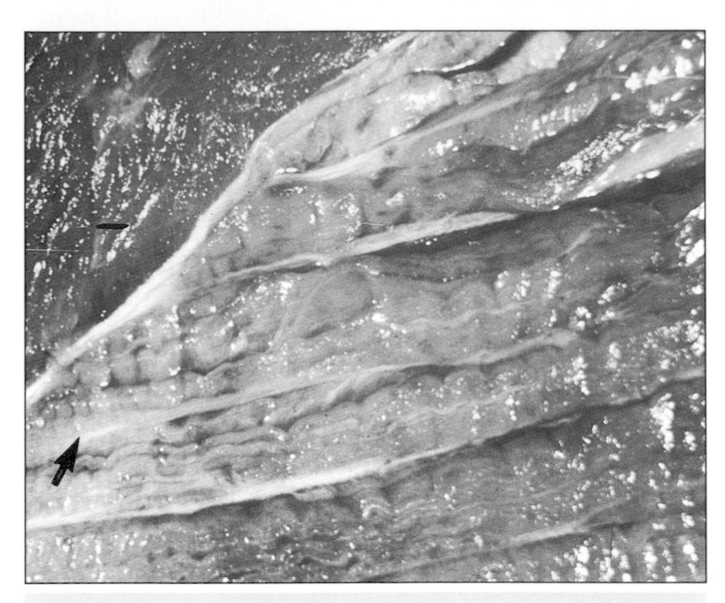

Figure 2.90 Marked pallor of affected muscle (arrow) in **bovine transport myopathy**. (Courtesy of TJ Hulland.)

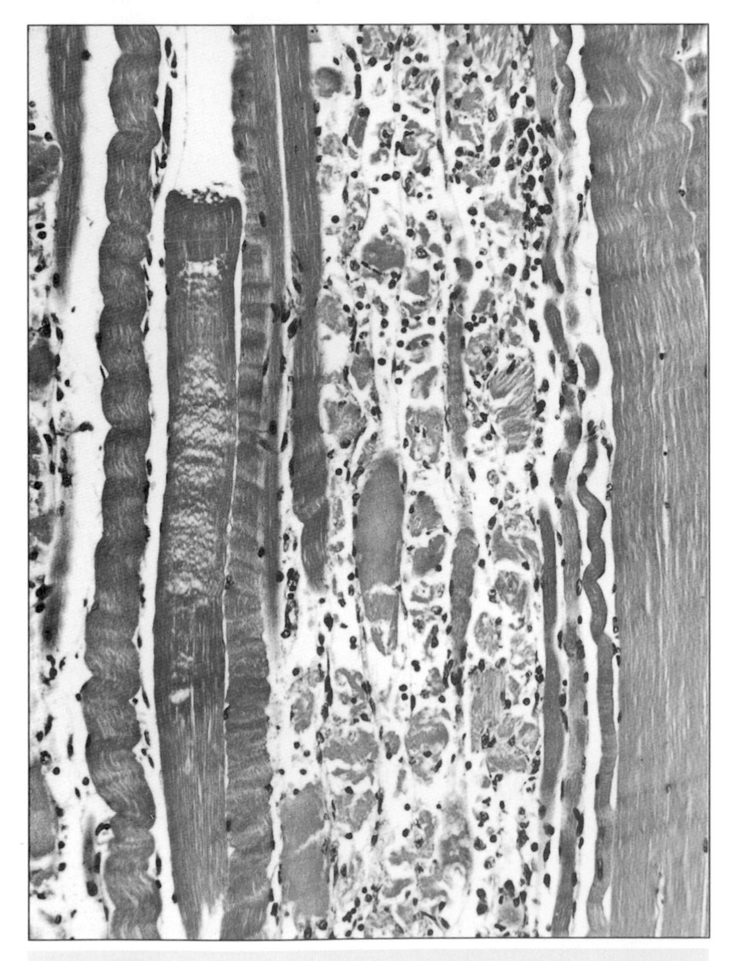

Figure 2.91 Extensive myofiber necrosis in a bighorn sheep with **capture myopathy**. (Courtesy of T Spraker.)

Gross and histologic lesions are often similar to those occurring due to other causes of severe exertional myopathy. They may also resemble those of hyperthermia in pigs, with *prominent muscle edema* in animals dying acutely. Muscles may contain *indistinct pale streaks* (Fig. 2.90), and *hemorrhagic streaking* is not uncommon. Degenerative lesions in skeletal muscle are typically *monophasic and polyfocal*. In most cases, death occurs during the degenerative phase and therefore acute myodegeneration, often with macrophage invasion of affected segments, is seen affecting various muscles (Fig. 2.91). Cardiac lesions, when present, are most often acute, although animals that survive capture myopathy may die acutely at a later date due to myocardial fibrosis. Myoglobinuric nephrosis may be seen.

Bibliography

Bartsch RC, et al. A review of exertional rhabdomyolysis in wild and domestic animals and man. Vet Pathol 1977;14:314–324.

Beech J. Equine muscle disorders 1: Chronic intermittent rhabdomyolysis. Equine Vet Educ 2000;12:163–167.

Bloom BA, et al. Postanaesthetic recumbency in a Belgian filly with polysaccharide storage myopathy. Vet Rec 1999;144:73–75.

Blythe LL, et al. Metabolic disorders of racing greyhounds. In: Abilene KS, ed. Care of the Racing Greyhound. Portland: American Greyhound Council, 1994:267–274.

Frauenfelder HC, et al. Changes in serum muscle enzyme levels associated with training schedules and stage of the oestrous cycle in Thoroughbred racehorses. Equine Vet J 1986;18:371–374.

Freestone JF, Carolson GP. Muscle disorders in the horse: a retrospective study. Equine Vet J 1991;23:86–90.

Gericke MD, Hofmeyr JM. Aetiology and treatment of capture stress and myopathy in springbok, *Antidorcas marsupialis*. S Afr J Sci 1976;72:28.

Harris P, Colles C. The use of creatinine clearance ratios in the prevention of equine rhabdomyolysis: a report of four cases. Equine Vet J 1988;20:459–463.

Harthoorn AM, Young E. A relationship between acid-base balance and capture myopathy in zebra, *Equus burchelli* and an apparent therapy. Vet Rec 1974;95:337–342.

Hartup BK, et al. Exertional myopathy in translocated river otters from New York. J Wildlife Dis 1999;35:542–547.

Hildebrand SV, et al. Contracture test and histologic and histochemical analyses of muscle biopsy specimens from horses with exertional rhabdomyolysis. J Am Vet Med Assoc 1990;196:1077–1083.

Hinchcliff KW, et al. Oxidant stress in sled dogs subjected to repetitive endurance exercise. Am J Vet Res 2000;61:512–517.

Kock MD, et al. Effects of capture on biological parameters in free-ranging bighorn sheep (Ovis canadensis): evaluation of normal, stressed and mortality outcomes and documentation of postcapture survival. J Wildl Dis 1987;23:652–662.

Lentz LR, et al. Abnormal regulation of muscle contraction in horses with recurrent exertional rhabdomyolysis. Am J Vet Res 1999;60:992–999.

Lewis RJ, et al. Capture myopathy in elk in Alberta, Canada: a report of three cases. J Am Vet Med Assoc 1977;171:927–932.

Lindholm A, et al. Acute rhabdomyolysis ("tying-up") in Standardbred horses. A morphological and biochemical study. Acta Vet Scand 1974;15:325–339.

Lindsay WA, et al. Induction of equine postanesthetic myositis after halothane-induced hypotension. Am J Vet Res 1989;50:404–410.

MacLeay JM, et al. Heritability of recurrent exertional rhabdomyolysis in Thoroughbred racehorses. Am J Vet Res 1999;60:250–256.

Martin BB, et al. Causes of poor performance of horses during training, racing, or showing: 348 cases (1992–1996). J Am Vet Med Assoc 2000;216:554–558.

McEwen SA, Hulland TJ. Histochemical and morphometric evaluation of skeletal muscle from horses with exertional rhabdomyolysis (tying-up). Vet Pathol 1986;23:400–410.

Munday BL. Myonecrosis in free-living and recently-captured macropods. J Wildl Dis 1972;8:191–192.

Peet RL, et al. Exertional rhabdomyolysis in sheep. Aust Vet J 1980;56:155–156.
Piercy RJ, et al. Vitamin E and exertional rhabdomyolysis during endurance sled dog racing. Neuromusc Dis 2001;11:278–286.
Spraker TR. Pathophysiology associated with capture of wild animals. In: Montali RJ, Migaki G, eds. The Comparative Pathology of Zoo Animals. Washington, DC: Smithsonian Institutional Press, 1980:403–414.
Valberg S, et al. Muscle histopathology and plasma aspartate aminotransferase, creatine kinase and myoglobin changes with exercise in horses with recurrent exertional rhabdomyolysis. Equine Vet J 1993;25:11–16.
Valberg SJ, et al. Familial basis of exertional rhabdomyolysis in Quarter Horse-related breeds. Am J Vet Res 1996;57:286–290.
Valberg SJ, et al. Skeletal muscle metabolic response to exercise in horses with "tying up" due to polysaccharide storage myopathy. Equine Vet J 1999; 31:43–47.
Valentine BA, et al. Severe polysaccharide storage myopathy in Belgian and Percheron draught horses. Equine Vet J 1997;29:220–225.
Valentine BA, et al. Muscle biopsy diagnosis of equine motor neuron disease and equine polysaccharide storage myopathy. Equine Vet Educ 1998;10:42–50.
Valentine BA, et al. Dietary control of exertional rhabdomyolysis in horses. J Am Vet Med Assoc 1998;212:1588–1593.
Valentine BA, et al. Polysaccharide storage myopathy in Morgan, Arabian, and Standardbred related horses and Welsh-cross ponies. Vet Pathol 2000;37:193–196.
Van den Hoven R, Breukink HJ. Normal resting values of plasma free carnitine and acylcarnitine in horses predisposed to exertional rhabdomyolysis. Equine Vet J 1989;21:307–308.
Ward TL, et al. Calcium regulation by skeletal muscle membranes of horses with recurrent exertional rhabdomyolysis. Am J Vet Res 2000;61:242–247.
Whitwell KE, Harris P, Farrington PG. Atypical myoglobinuria: an acute myopathy in grazing horses. Equine Vet J 1988;20:357–363.
Williams ES, Thorne ET. Exertional myopathy (Capture Myopathy). In: Faribrother A, Locke LN, Hoff GL, eds. Noninfectious Diseases of Wildlife. Ames, IA: The Iowa State Press, 1996:181–193.

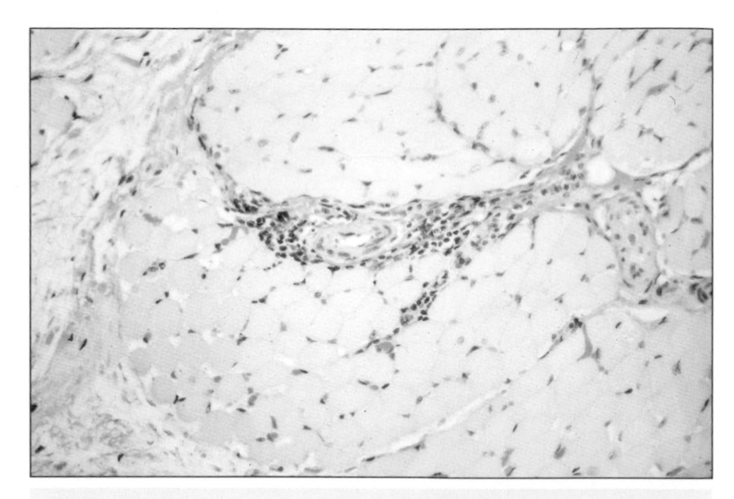

Figure 2.92 Interstitial and perivascular infiltration of mononuclear inflammatory cells characteristic of **immune-mediated myositis** in the temporal muscle of a dog.

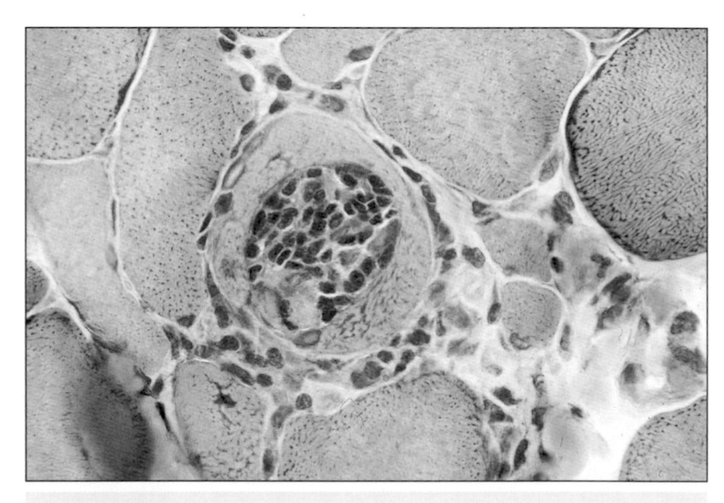

Figure 2.93 Mononuclear inflammatory cell infiltrate at the periphery and "coring out" the interior of an otherwise intact myofiber characteristic of **immune-mediated myositis** in a dog. Frozen section, modified Gomori's trichrome.

IMMUNE-MEDIATED CONDITIONS

Immune-mediated disorders are those in which abnormal activation of the immune system results in tissue damage. *Immune-mediated muscle damage can involve circulating antibodies directed against muscle cell components, cytotoxic T lymphocytes that infiltrate and attack muscle cells, or immune-complex deposition that subsequently exposes muscles to inflammatory mediators and ischemia.*

It is important to distinguish primary immune-mediated myositis from florid degenerative myopathy in which cellular infiltrates, primarily composed of macrophages, can mimic those of true inflammatory disease. It may be necessary to employ special procedures to identify the type of infiltrating cells or to detect specific antibody binding to muscle components. *Immune-mediated disease of muscle is characterized by interstitial and perivascular infiltration of lymphocytes and/or plasma cells* (Fig. 2.92). These cells may be mixed with macrophages and with eosinophils and neutrophils, particularly in cases accompanied by severe myofiber necrosis. *The diagnosis is dependent on determining that cellular infiltrates actually cause the myofiber necrosis and are not secondary to the muscle damage.* The finding of mononuclear leukocytic invasion of otherwise intact myofibers is the hallmark of primary myositis. Infiltrating cells may be seen surrounding intact myofibers, or may be seen centrally, causing a characteristic "coring out" of myofibers with otherwise intact peripheral myofibrils (Fig. 2.93). Lymphocytic myositis must be distinguished from infiltration of skeletal muscle by malignant lymphoma.

Masticatory myositis of dogs

An immune-mediated myositis localized to the masticatory muscles occurs in dogs. The masseter, temporal, and pterygoid muscles are selectively affected. Although previously designated as two separate disorders – *eosinophilic myositis and atrophic myositis – these are now recognized to be two ends of the spectrum of a single disease known as* **masticatory myositis**. Given the thick fascia of the masticatory muscles in dogs, the swelling that can occur in masticatory myositis may be due, at least in part, to ischemic damage due to compartment syndrome initiated by increased pressure within inflamed muscle. *Atrophic myositis is the result of prominent atrophy of temporal and masseter muscles.* The masticatory muscles of dogs have a unique myosin isoform, known as *type 2M myosin*. This unique myosin isoform results in an inability to achieve muscle fiber type reversal of canine masticatory muscle sections with an acid preincubation ATPase reaction. *Antibodies in dogs with masticatory muscle myositis are directed against this unique myosin isoform*, and diagnostic testing for type 2M antibodies in canine serum is available. It has been proposed that various bacterial infections may result in antibodies that cross-react between bacterial antigens and type 2M myosin.

Affected dogs are unable to fully open the mouth (*trismus*). Muscle swelling or atrophy is most obvious in the temporal and masseter muscles and is bilateral. Pain upon opening the jaw is common, and jaw immobility persists during general anesthesia. Swelling of muscle may result in a degree of exophthalmos. Attacks, if untreated, last up to 2–3 weeks and the periods between attacks may be a few weeks, months, or 2–3 years. If left unchecked, *this inflammatory myopathy leads to progressive destruction of the muscles of mastication and permanent inability to fully open the jaw*. Muscle atrophy gradually becomes very obvious and the head appears to have a fine fox-like contour with unusual prominence of the zygomatic arches (Fig. 2.94A, B).

This disorder occurs in many breeds, although the *German Shepherd breed* appears to be predisposed. Serum activities of CK and AST may be normal, or may be mildly to moderately increased. Masticatory myositis with a strong eosinophilic inflammatory component may be accompanied by peripheral blood eosinophilia, but this is not a consistent finding. Clinical response to immunosuppressive doses of corticosteroids may be rapid, but cases may relapse once corticosteroid therapy is discontinued. *Masticatory myositis is progressive*, but now that this disorder is often recognized and treated in early stages, fewer chronic cases are presented for postmortem examination. Affected dogs may, however, develop aspiration pneumonia or complications of corticosteroid therapy leading to death or euthanasia.

Grossly visible changes in the muscle vary with the stage of disease. The acutely affected muscles are swollen, dark red, doughy or hard, and the cut surface reveals hemorrhagic streaks and irregular yellow-white patches. In the late stages, there is advanced atrophy and fibrosis. Some areas consist only of pink-gray, semitranslucent, mature, connective tissue subdivided by the whiter residual tendons (Fig. 2.95).

Histologically, this disorder most often has a *multifocal and polyphasic pattern. Inflammatory infiltrates are interstitial and often perivascular.* Necrotic and regenerating myofibers are common in acute and active stages of the disease. Previous corticosteroid therapy can reduce and alter the inflammatory component present. Eosinophils may or may not be the predominant cell type seen in affected muscle, but *eosinophils will always be admixed with lymphocytes*. Eosinophils can be seen in muscle damaged by a variety of insults. The primary inflammatory cells causing destruction of myofibers in masticatory muscle myositis of dogs are lymphocytes, presumably recruited following binding of antibody. Lymphocytes may be admixed with plasma cells, and plasma cells may predominate in some cases. Macrophages will also be prominent in cases with marked myofiber necrosis. Fiber atrophy is common, and atrophic fibers can be seen associated with inflammation (Fig. 2.96) or with dense fibrosis.

Histologic examination of muscle from suspect masticatory myositis dogs can often be frustrating. The inflammatory lesions are patchy in some cases, and biopsy may reveal only generalized fiber atrophy. *Any evidence of fiber degeneration or regeneration, even in the absence of obvious inflammation, should be considered suspicious if the clinical history is consistent with myositis.* Examination for evidence of endomysial and perimysial fibrosis is important, as severe fibrosis will negatively impact on the prognosis for return of full jaw mobility

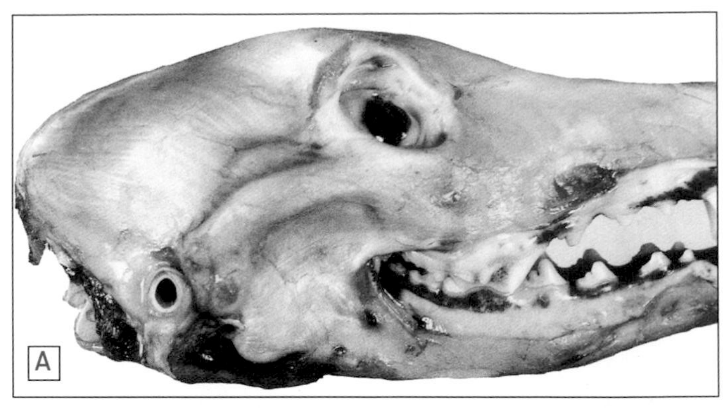

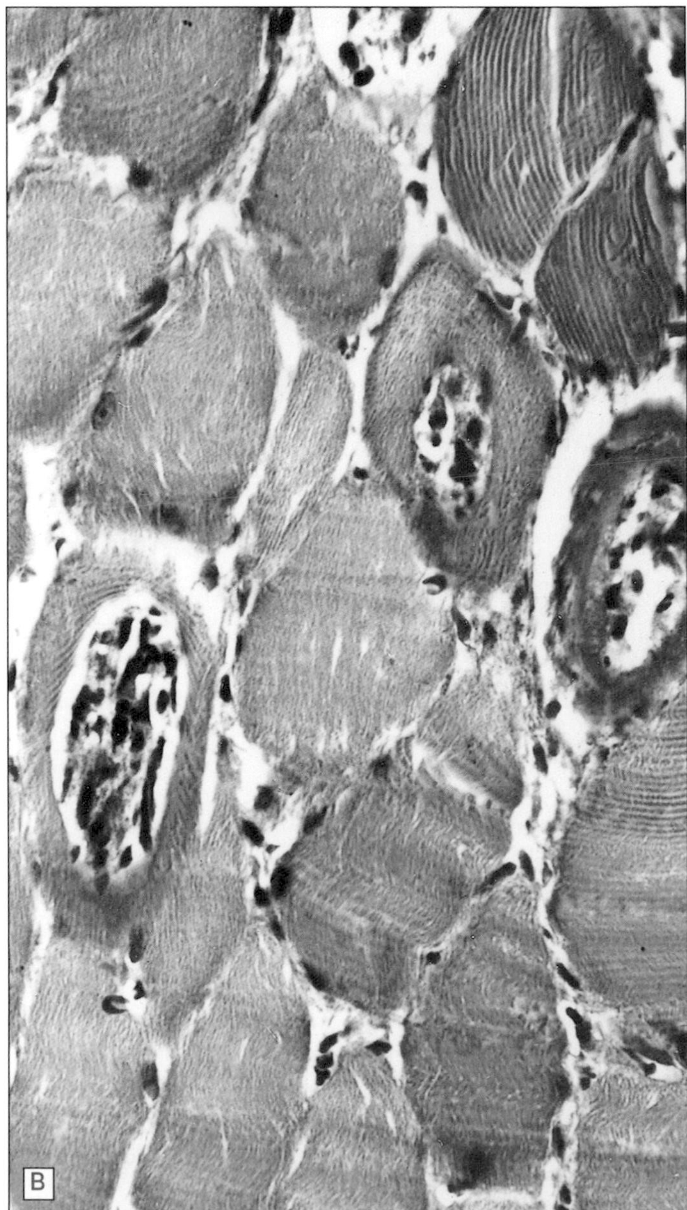

Figure 2.94 Chronic masticatory myositis in a dog. **A.** Severe atrophy of masticatory muscles. **B.** Multiple fibers being "cored out" by mononuclear inflammatory cells. (Courtesy of TJ Hulland.)

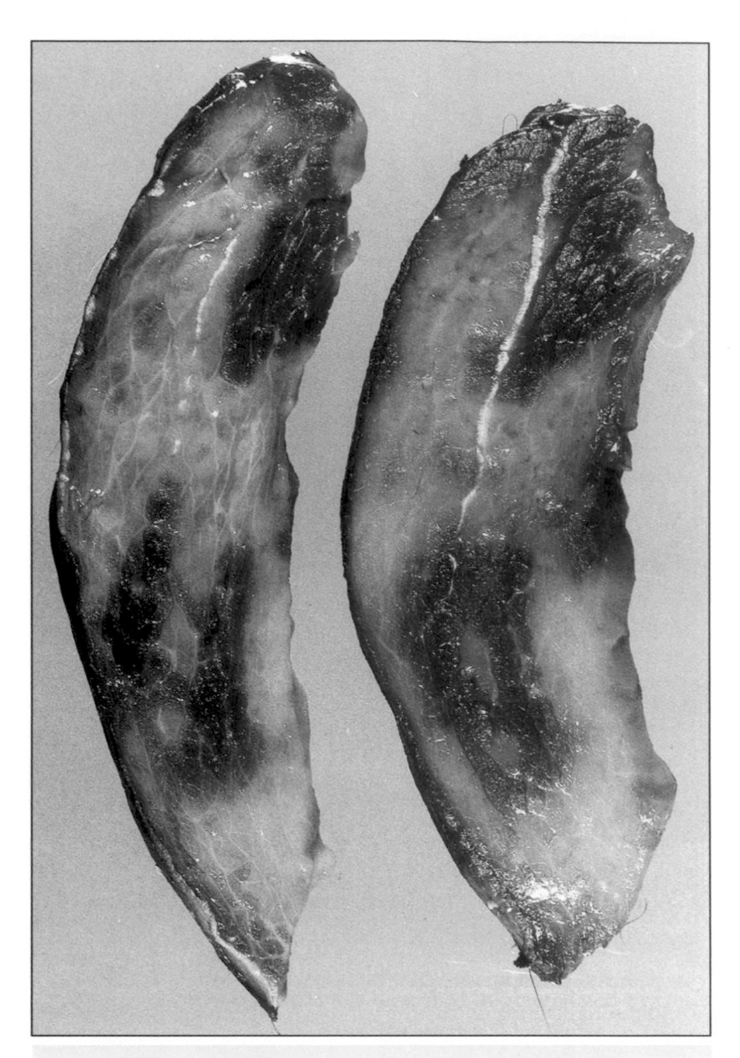

Figure 2.95 Large pale areas of fibrosis in temporal muscle from a dog with **chronic masticatory myositis**. (Courtesy of TJ Hulland.)

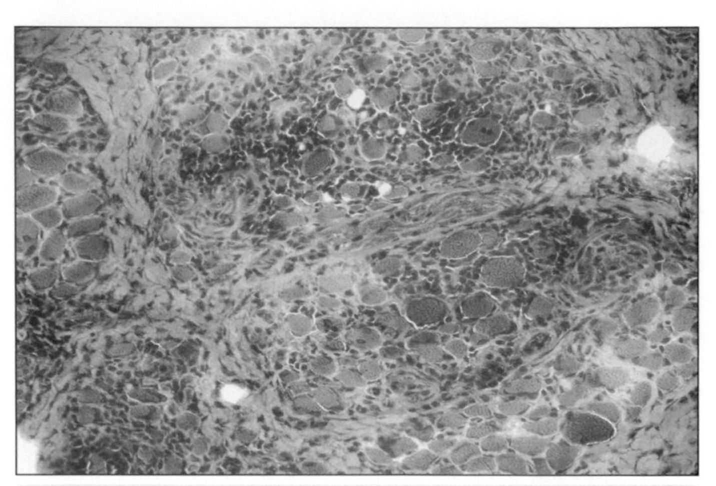

Figure 2.96 Masticatory myositis in the temporal muscle of a dog. Dense infiltrates of mononuclear inflammatory cells are admixed with atrophic and degenerating myofibers. Frozen section, modified Gomori's trichrome.

and muscle mass. Those cases with numerous inflammatory cells and minimal fibrosis are more likely to recover with corticosteroid therapy than cases in which inflammatory infiltrates are minimal and fibrosis is the predominant finding. An apparent increase in connective tissue may also occur due to loss of damaged myofibers and condensation of existing fibrous stroma.

The masticatory muscles of dogs, especially the temporal muscles, appear to be particularly prone to a variety of generalized myopathic and systemic disorders. Dogs with X-linked muscular dystrophy have prominent atrophy of the temporal muscle and are unable to fully open their mouths, although this condition is not painful. Labrador Retrievers with inherited myopathy also have prominent temporal muscle atrophy. Polymyositis (see below) may appear primarily as a problem with muscles of mastication, although careful evaluation will reveal abnormalities in other muscles. Dogs with any generalized illness often develop rapid atrophy of the temporal muscles that resolves with treatment for the primary problem. Persistent bilaterally symmetric atrophy of masticatory muscles not associated with pain, immobility of the jaw, or generalized disease also occurs in dogs. These latter cases of masticatory muscle atrophy appear to be idiopathic and are not associated with inflammation. If atrophy of temporal and/or masseter muscle occurs unilaterally, denervation atrophy is most likely.

Polymyositis of dogs

Immune-mediated polymyositis occurs most commonly in dogs. Dogs with polymyositis may be presented with primary signs of masticatory muscle involvement, and both masticatory myositis and polymyositis should be considered in the differential diagnosis of such dogs. Testing for serum antibodies to type 2M myosin may be useful, as *most dogs with polymyositis do not have serum antibodies to 2M myosin*. It is possible, however, for nonspecific myosin antibodies to be found in the serum of dogs with polymyositis or other myopathies associated with myofiber necrosis. *Muscle fiber damage in polymyositis is mediated by T lymphocytes*.

Polymyositis occurs mostly commonly in *adult dogs of various breeds*, although large breeds are over-represented and German Shepherds may be predisposed. *A breed-associated polymyositis has been recognized in Newfoundlands* in which signs of muscle weakness may be apparent in dogs as young as 6 months of age. *Clinical signs of polymyositis are variable*, and include exercise intolerance, overall muscle weakness, stiff gait, and muscle atrophy. Muscle pain, elicited by deep muscle palpation, may be evident. Esophageal muscle involvement leads to regurgitation. Fever may also occur. Increase in serum activities of CK and AST is quite variable, and values may be within normal limits. Polymyositis may occur as part of the spectrum of disease in dogs with *systemic lupus erythematosus*, which is often accompanied by a positive anti-nuclear antibody (ANA) titer. Treatment with immunosuppressive doses of corticosteroids often results in resolution of signs, although if esophageal muscle fibrosis has occurred there will be persistent esophageal dysfunction.

Gross pathologic findings include mild to severe generalized muscle atrophy. In cases with esophageal involvement, *dilation of the esophagus may be evident*. Examination of multiple samples from different sites on the head and limbs may be necessary to detect inflammatory lesions. The disorder is *multifocal and polyphasic. The most common finding is of interstitial and perivascular lymphocytic infiltration in affected muscle. Invasion of otherwise intact skeletal muscle fibers by lymphocytes is*

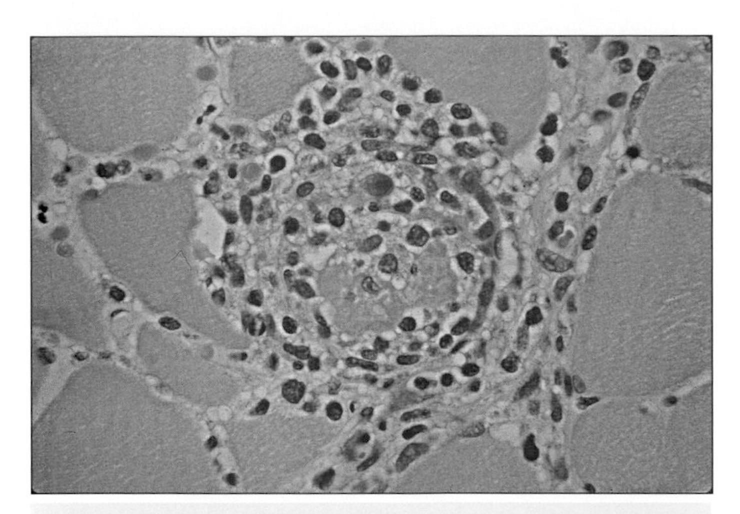

Figure 2.97 Polymyositis in a dog. Mononuclear inflammatory cells surround and invade myofibers causing necrosis. (Courtesy of BJ Cooper.)

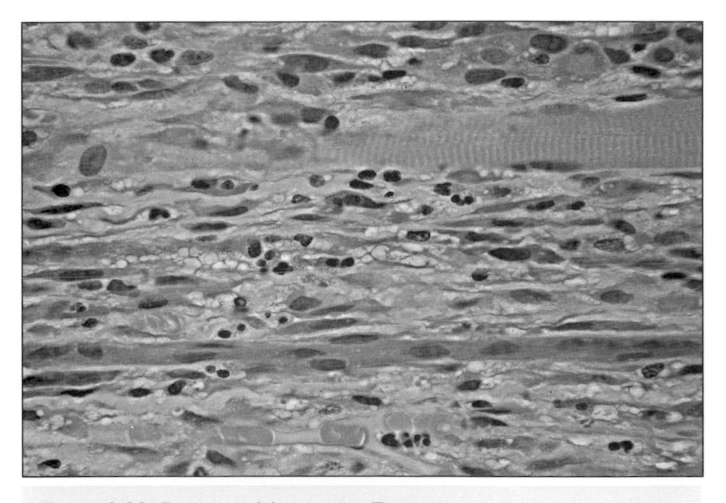

Figure 2.98 Polymyositis in a dog. There is a regenerating myotube as well as active inflammation consisting of eosinophils and mononuclear cells. (Courtesy of BJ Cooper.)

characteristic (Fig. 2.97). Regenerating fibers as well as degenerating fibers are common (Fig. 2.98), and severe chronic disease may result in some degree of endomysial/perimysial fibrosis. Fibrosis may be most apparent in masticatory muscles and in the esophageal wall. Immunophenotypic studies have confirmed that, similar to polymyositis in humans, *invading lymphocytes in canine polymyositis are primarily cytotoxic (CD8+) T cells.* An admixture of inflammatory cells, however, including eosinophils and neutrophils, can be seen in particularly florid lesions.

Extraocular muscle myositis of dogs

A bilateral polymyositis involving only the **extraocular rectus and oblique muscles** *has been described in dogs.* The retractor bulbi and all other skeletal muscles are normal. Golden Retriever dogs appear to be predisposed. This disorder affects young to young-adult dogs, with age range of onset from about 6–18 months. *Clinical signs are of sudden onset of bilateral nonpainful exophthalmos.* Gross lesions of swelling and pallor can be seen within extraocular muscles. *Interstitial lymphocytic inflammatory cell infiltrates are associated with myofiber necrosis and regeneration in a multifocal polyphasic pattern.* Given the localization within extraocular muscles, an immune-mediated disorder directed at a unique epitope within these muscles is suspected. Corticosteroid therapy is usually curative, which supports an immune-mediated basis for this disorder.

Polymyositis of cats

Most reported cases of polymyositis in cats have instead proved to be degenerative polymyopathy due to hypokalemia. A lymphocytic polymyositis associated with retroviral disease has been identified in adult cats experimentally infected with *Feline immunodeficiency virus* (FIV). Clinical signs of neuromuscular dysfunction are not apparent, but serum activity of CK is moderately increased. Inflammation has the typical interstitial and perivascular pattern of immune-mediated myositis. Infiltration of muscle and myofiber necrosis of multiple muscles is mediated by cytotoxic CD8+ T lymphocytes. Other lymphocyte subsets are not found. Pelvic limb musculature is more commonly affected than thoracic limb muscles. This disorder in cats is similar to HIV-associated polymyositis in people and SIV-associated polymyositis in monkeys. A severe chronic polymyositis associated with progressive weakness and muscle atrophy has been reported in a captive Bengal tiger. Histopathologic evidence of a multifocal and polyphasic myositis characterized by interstitial infiltrates of lymphocytes and invasion of intact myofibers by mononuclear cells typical of polymyositis were seen. As this case occurred prior to the recognition of FIV infection in cats, it is tempting to speculate that this may also have been viral-associated.

Immune-mediated myositis of horses

Although exertional and postanesthetic myopathies in horses are often called "myositis," this term is not appropriate for these conditions. These disorders are degenerative myopathies and are not primary inflammatory conditions.

Hemorrhagic necrosis of muscle due to vascular injury occurs in horses with immune-complex disease due to *Streptococcus equi*-associated *purpura hemorrhagica.* In some cases, the involvement of skeletal muscle is severe enough for neuromuscular dysfunction to be the primary presenting sign. Affected horses typically have markedly increased serum activities of CK and AST associated with muscle weakness and pain. Dependent edema can also be seen. *Hemorrhagic infarcts can be found within affected muscles, and fibrinoid necrosis of vascular walls and vasculitis are seen in tissue sections* (Fig. 2.99). Inflammatory infiltrates are not seen except at the periphery of necrotic zones. Infarcts in other organs, such as lung and intestine, are common. *Streptococcus equi* can often be isolated from lymph nodes or guttural pouches. Immune complexes in purpura hemorrhagica are composed of IgA and streptococcal M protein.

Another syndrome of degenerative myopathy and rapid muscle atrophy occurs in young to young-adult Quarter Horses following exposure to *Streptococcus equi.* Skeletal muscle appears to be the only tissue affected in these horses. The cause is not yet known, although cross-reacting antibodies to streptococci affecting skeletal muscle myosin have been proposed.

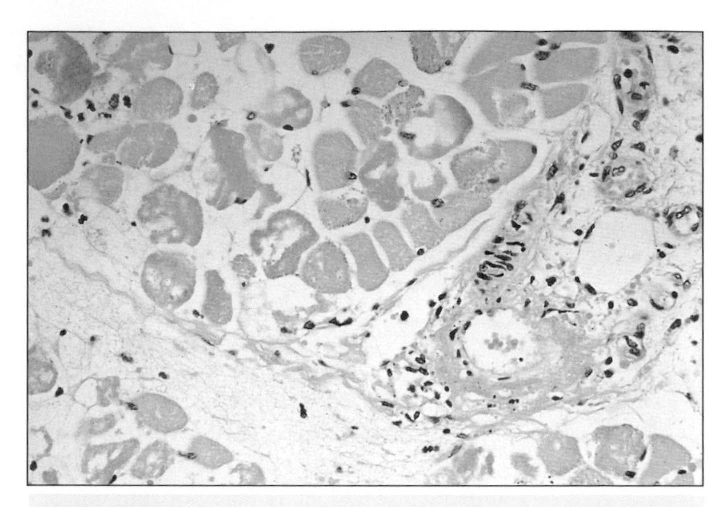

Figure 2.99 *Streptococcus equi*-associated **purpura hemorrhagica** involving skeletal muscle. Acute myofiber necrosis is associated with fibrinoid necrosis of the wall of an interstitial blood vessel. (From McGavin MD, Zachary JF. Pathologic Basis of Veterinary Disease, 2006, with permission of Elsevier Ltd.)

Acquired myasthenia gravis

Two clearly defined types of myasthenia gravis occur in dogs and cats. The *congenital disease* is due to abnormal neuromuscular junction formation and is discussed in the section on Congenital myasthenia gravis. The *acquired disease* occurs when circulating antibodies to motor end plate acetylcholine receptors bind and form immune complexes at the neuromuscular junction. The cross-linking of bound antibodies leads to increased endocytosis of acetylcholine receptors and therefore reduction in receptor density.

As in people, a link between thymic abnormalities and development of acquired myasthenia gravis occurs in dogs and cats. *Thymic follicular hyperplasia or thymoma is associated with development of myasthenia gravis in people, and thymoma is associated with myasthenia gravis in dogs and cats.* The normal thymus contains myoid cells that express muscle proteins and acetylcholine receptors. The presence of these cells is thought to be important for induction of self-recognition of these proteins. Myoid cells are readily seen by light microscopy in the thymus of neonatal or late-term aborted ruminants. Myoid cells occur in the thymic medulla and consist of large round cells with central euchromatic nuclei and abundant eosinophilic cytoplasm. These cells are scattered amongst the epithelial cells of Hassall's corpuscles, and will be found to express muscle actin and myoglobin with immunocytochemical procedures. It is thought that abnormal immune regulation occurs due to thymoma. Removal of the thymic mass often results in resolution of signs of thymoma-induced myasthenia gravis.

Acquired myasthenia gravis in dogs has also been *associated with concurrent hypothyroidism*, and sporadic cases have occurred apparently *associated with malignant neoplasia*. In most cases, myasthenia gravis occurs unassociated with an underlying neoplastic or systemic disease process.

Three clinical forms of acquired myasthenia gravis are recognized in dogs.

- The classic form is the *generalized form*, in which episodic weakness, primarily of appendicular muscles, leads to exercise-induced collapse. Signs of weakness are alleviated by rest. Generalized myasthenia may also appear as selective and persistent weakness primarily of pelvic limbs. Megaesophagus is common in generalized myasthenia gravis in dogs.
- A *localized form* with selective involvement of esophageal, facial, and pharyngeal muscle leads to megaesophagus and regurgitation without generalized weakness.
- The third form is a *fulminating form* in which rapid development of sustained generalized weakness occurs.

Only generalized myasthenia gravis has been described in the *cat*.

Breeds at risk for development of acquired myasthenia gravis include German Shepherds, Golden Retrievers, Akitas, terrier breeds, German Shorthaired Pointers and Chihuahuas. An inherited predisposition to myasthenia gravis has been described in Newfoundland dogs. A bimodal age distribution occurs in dogs, with peak incidences of acquired myasthenia gravis occurring at about 3 years of age and at about 10 years of age. There does not appear to be a sex predisposition in dogs. A generalized form of myasthenia gravis occurs in cats, and Abyssinian cats may be predisposed.

Diagnosis of myasthenia gravis can be made in many cases with *electrodiagnostic testing* of repetitive nerve stimulation response, in which a decremental response in the compound motor action potential is demonstrated. A positive response to anticholinesterase therapy (edrophonium) is also considered diagnostic. *Detection of circulating anti-acetylcholine receptor antibodies is considered the most definitive test.*

Abnormalities are not seen in muscle or peripheral nerves by light microscopy, but immune complexes can be detected at neuromuscular junctions using immunocytochemical procedures. Reduction in acetylcholine receptor density due to increased internalization of receptors can be demonstrated with specialized techniques such as bungarotoxin binding assay. Alteration in morphology of synaptic clefts is seen on ultrastructural examination. Dogs with associated megaesophagus often have concurrent aspiration pneumonia.

To date, thymic follicular hyperplasia has not been described as a cause of myasthenia gravis in animals. Thymoma can be associated with either the generalized form or the fulminant form of myasthenia gravis in dogs, and with generalized myasthenia gravis in cats.

Bibliography

Carpenter JL, et al. Canine bilateral extraocular polymyositis. Vet Pathol 1989;26:510–512.

Cuddon PA. Breed associated polymyositis of young Newfoundlands. J Vet Int Med 1999;13:239.

Dardenne M, et al. Thymomatous epithelial cells and skeletal muscle share a common epitope defined by a monoclonal antibody. Am J Pathol 1987;126:194–198.

Dewey CW, et al. Clinical forms of acquired myasthenia gravi in dogs: 25 cases (1988–1995). J Vet Int Med 1997;11:50–57.

Duncan ID, et al. Inflammatory myopathy in a captive Bengal tiger. J Am Vet Med Assoc 1982;181:1237–1241.

Engel AG, Arahata K. Mononuclear cells in myopathies: quantitation of functionally distinct subsets, recognition of antigen-specific cell-mediated cytotoxicity in some diseases, and implications for the pathogenesis of the different inflammatory myopathies. Human Pathol 1986;17:704–721.

Flagstad A, et al. Congenital myasthenic syndrome in the dog breed Gammel Dansk Hønsehund: clinical, electrophysiological, pharmacological and immunological comparison with acquired myasthenia gravis. Acta Vet Scand 1989;30:89–102.

Goebel HH, et al. Recent advances in the morphology of myositis. Path Res Pract 1985;180:1–9.

Joseph RJ, et al. Myasthenia gravis in the cat. J Vet Int Med 1988;2:75–79.

King LG, Vite CH. Acute fulminating myasthenia gravis in five dogs. J Am Vet Med Assoc 212:830–834, 1998.

Kornegay JN, et al. Polymyositis in dogs. J Am Vet Med Assoc 1980;176:431–438.

Krotje LJ, et al. Acquired myasthenia gravis and cholangiocellular carcinoma in a dog. J Am Vet Med Assoc 1990;197:488–490.

Krum SH, et al. Polymyositis and polyarthritis associated with systemic lupus erythematosus in a dog. J Am Vet Med Assoc 1977;170:61–64.

Lennon VA, et al. Acquired and congenital myasthenia gravis in dogs – a study of 20 cases. In: Satoyoshi E, ed. Myasthenia Gravis – Pathogenesis and Treatment. Tokyo: University of Tokyo Press, 1981:41–54.

Lipsitz D, et al. Inherited predisposition to myasthenia gravis in Newfoundlands. J Am Vet Med Assoc 1999;215:956–958.

Moore AS, et al. Osteogenic sarcoma and myasthenia gravis in a dog. J Am Vet Med Assoc 1990;197:226–227.

Orvis JS, Cardinet GH. Canine muscle fiber types and susceptibility of masticatory muscles to myositis. Muscle Nerve 1981;4:354–359.

Podell M, et al. Feline immunodeficiency virus associated myopathy in the adult cat. Muscle Nerve 1998;21:1680–1685.

Scott-Moncrieff JC, et al. Acquired myasthenia gravis in a cat with thymoma. J Am Vet Med Assoc 1990;196:1291–1293.

Shelton GD, Cardinet GH, III. Pathophysiologic basis of canine muscle disorders. J Vet Intern Med 1987;1:36–44.

Shelton GD, et al. Expression of fiber type specific proteins during ontogeny of canine temporalis muscle. Muscle Nerve 1988;11:124–132.

Shelton GD, et al. Canine and human myasthenia gravis autoantibodies recognize similar regions on the acetylcholine receptor. Neurology 1988;38:1417–1423.

Shelton GD, et al. Acquired myasthenia gravis, selective involvement of esophageal, pharyngeal, and facial muscles. J Vet Int Med 1990;4:281–284.

Shelton GD, et al. Risk factors for acquired myasthenia gravis in dogs: 1,154 cases (1991–1995). J Am Vet Med Assoc 1997;212:1428–1431.

Taylor SM. Selected disorders of muscle and the neuromuscular junction. Vet Clin North Am Small Anim Pract 2000;30:59–75, vi.

Valberg SJ, et al. Myopathies associated with *Streptococcus equi* infections in horses. Proc Am Assoc Eq Prac 1996;42:292–293.

MYOSITIS

Myositis means inflammation of muscle, but it is often difficult to determine whether the process is part of a classical inflammatory response that happens to be active in muscle or whether some components of inflammation are activated by a process that is primarily degenerative. The cause of myositis is often not evident except in the obvious cases in which the inflammatory nature of the reaction is signaled by a suppurative or granulomatous response or where it is a component of a systemic infectious disease, such as *Bluetongue virus* infection in sheep, foot and mouth disease, and toxoplasmosis (see Vol. 2, Alimentary system).

Infectious agents and parasites are frequently the cause of mild myopathy (as distinct from myositis) in animals, in which case, the degenerative muscle changes are an almost incidental and often unnoticed part of systemic infection or toxemia. There are, however, some systemic and local infections that cause myositis rather than myopathy, and they will be considered here. *Living muscle is an inhospitable site for almost all bacteria*, and consequently myositis is rarely a complication of bacterial infections even when they are overwhelmingly septicemic or repeatedly bacteremic. Pyogenic organisms sometimes give rise to solitary muscle abscesses, particularly in pigs and goats, but *bacterial polymyositis is a feature of only a few infections*, such as *Histophilus somni* in lambs and cattle, and *Actinobacillus equuli* in foals. *Clostridium* spp., on the other hand, are very well adapted to growing in muscle once damage to muscle fibers provides them with an opportunity.

Other diseases of muscle with an inflammatory response are presented under immune-mediated conditions and include several canine conditions (masticatory myositis, extraocular muscle myositis, polymyositis) and an equine disease (purpura hemorrhagica).

Suppurative myositis

Abscesses in muscle may sometimes be hematogenous in origin, but more often they result from *inoculation* (penetrating wound, contaminated injection, contamination of surgical site or laceration), or by *extension from a suppurative focus* in adjacent structures, such as joints, tendon sheaths, or lymph nodes. The most common causes of abscesses in muscle are *Arcanobacterium* (*Actinomyces, Corynebacterium*) *pyogenes* in cattle and swine, *Corynebacterium pseudotuberculosis* in sheep, goats, and horses, and *Streptococcus equi* in horses. A variety of streptococci and staphylococci are retrieved from such lesions in many species.

The natural development of suppurative myositis is comparable to abscessation elsewhere. The early stage consists of *local, ill-defined, cellulitis*. Healing may take place after this with a minimum of scarring, or it may proceed to the formation of a *typical abscess with a liquefied center, a pyogenic membrane, and an outer fibrous sheath* (Fig. 2.100). The lesion may slowly organize if it is effectively sterilized, expand if it is not or, alternatively, fistulate to the surface, collapse, and heal. In the healing process, damaged muscle fibers will participate in fiber regeneration to only a very limited extent.

In cats and horses particularly, the early stage of local cellulitis may give rise to a rapidly expanding cellulitis of muscle and adjacent fibrous and fat tissue. This phlegmonous inflammation leads to extensive destruction of muscle fibers that are subsequently mostly replaced by scar tissue. The organisms involved may vary, but *Pasteurella multocida* has been incriminated in cats, while staphylococci appear to be the most common in other domestic species. Acute cellulitis and myositis may occur in *Haemophilus parasuis* infection (Glasser's disease) in swine.

Malignant edema (gas gangrene)

The muscles, especially if devitalized in some manner, are highly susceptible to bacteria of the genus Clostridium, and these organisms, when they proliferate, are highly toxigenic and cause extensive necrosis of muscle, with blood-stained edema and the formation of gas. Once the bacteria become established, the toxins they elaborate provide a suitable and expanding environment for further bacterial growth. Death occurs as a result of *systemic intoxication*.

These bacteria are gram-positive bacilli, to a greater or lesser degree anaerobic, and they exist in the environment as resistant spores. Germination of the spores and vegetative growth requires

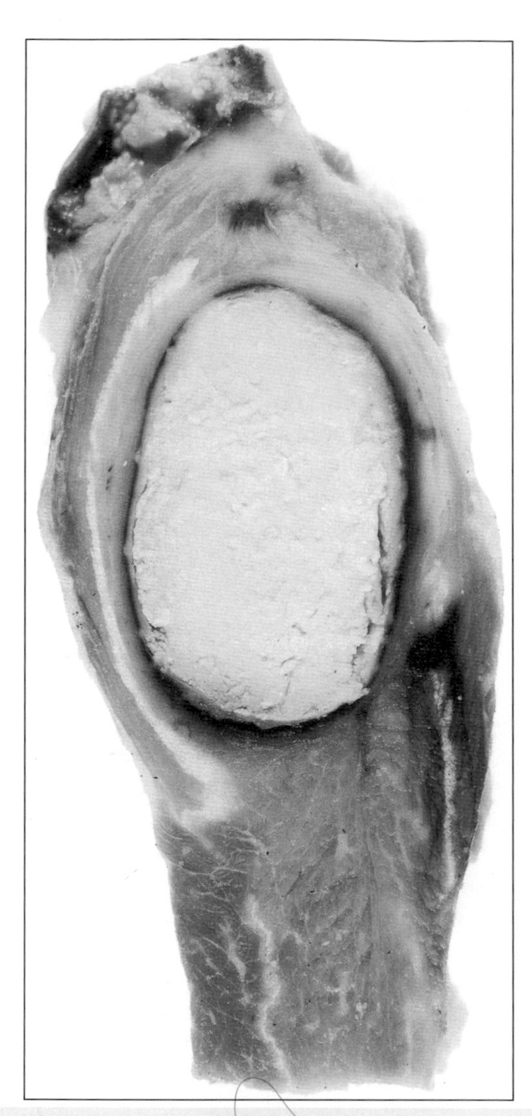

Figure 2.100 Abscess in the gluteal muscles of a goat. (Courtesy of W Hadlow.)

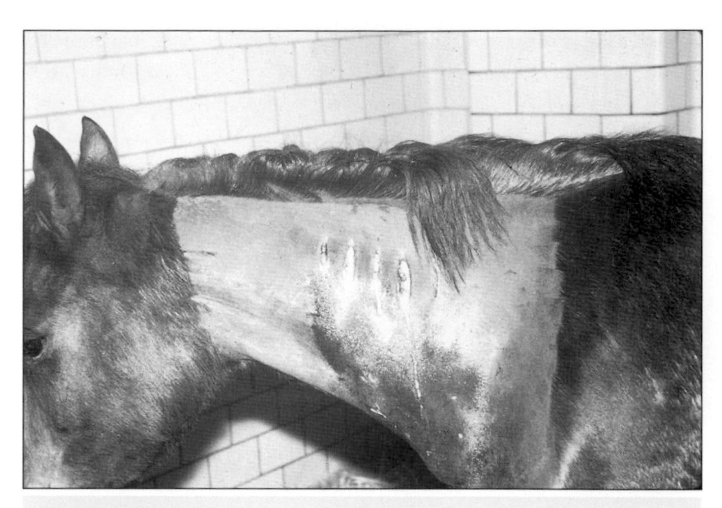

Figure 2.101 Subcutaneous swelling over neck due to **clostridial myositis** in a horse. (Courtesy of W Rebhun.)

fairly precise local conditions, chiefly a low oxidation-reduction potential and an alkaline pH. These conditions are best produced by deep penetrating wounds and the lesions that result from the activity of the anaerobes are called "*malignant edema*," "*gas gangrene*," and "*anaerobic cellulitis*." Since the pathogenic clostridia are frequently found in soil and feces, *any contamination of an open wound is likely to introduce those potential pathogens*. Although their presence in a wound always carries a threat of gas gangrene, the very great majority of wounds thus infected heal without ill effect; in these, the local conditions in the wound must be regarded as unsuitable for germination, vegetation, or the production of toxins.

The species of the genus *Clostridium* that are of most importance as the agents of gas gangrene are *C. septicum, C. perfringens, C. novyi,* and *C. chauvoei*. These organisms not only cause gas gangrene, which is usually a mixed infection, but in animals they are, as pure infections, responsible for a number of specific diseases that are not associated with surface wounding and, with one exception, not associated with primary lesions in muscle. The exception is *C. chauvoei, which* causes bacterial myositis – *blackleg* – in ruminants. The other specific diseases include *black disease* caused by *C. novyi* (see Vol. 2, Liver and biliary system), *braxy* caused by *C. septicum,* and the *clostridial enterotoxemias* caused by *C. perfringens* (see Vol. 2, Alimentary system).

Gas gangrene and malignant edema are essentially wound infections in which *C. septicum, C. perfringens, C. novyi, C. sordelli*, and *C. chauvoei* are the principal pathogens acting alone, or in combination with each other or with a variety of other aerobes and anaerobes, the latter being saprophytes with proteolytic and putrefactive properties. *Ruminants, horses, and swine are highly susceptible to these infections*, whereas carnivores are rarely affected with gas gangrene. Since deep wounds are the ones most suitable to the development of gas gangrene, the common causes of such susceptible wounds in animals are castration, shearing, penetrating stake wounds, injuries to the female genitalia during parturition and, especially in swine, inoculation sites. The distinctive characteristics of these local infections are *severe edema* (Fig. 2.101), the formation of *gas bubbles* that give crepitation, *discoloration* of the overlying skin, *coldness* of the affected part, and, in particular, the constitutional signs of *profound toxemia* with prostration, circulatory collapse, and sudden death.

Malignant edema is included in this title to distinguish certain cases of clostridial myositis of which gas gangrene is not a part; indeed, in animals, the non-gangrenous form of clostridial myositis is much more common than is the gangrenous form. *Malignant edema is more typically a cellulitis than a myositis*, and the muscles may escape significant injury even in fulminating, highly toxigenic infections of the sort that are fatal in 48 h. All of the factors that determine whether gangrene develops in these infections are not known. Even when the primary pathogens present are the same, the relative potencies and the amounts of the toxins produced may vary, and it is expected that accompanying nonprimary organisms will, to some extent, influence the local course of the infection. One factor that is probably of much importance in determining whether the inflammation will be confined to the connective tissues (malignant edema) or will directly involve muscle (myositis) is the adequacy of the blood supply to the muscle. If the muscle is devitalized by the initial trauma, or subsequently as a result of toxic injury to the blood vessels, the development of true gangrene is in order; in this manner, *malignant edema or anaerobic cellulitis may develop into gangrene*.

The pathogenesis of clostridial myositis and cellulitis is obviously not simple and is not initiated merely by the presence of spores or vegetative forms in the wound; it may begin only when the organisms have produced enough toxin to immobilize and destroy any adjacent leukocytes and enough toxin to cause death of tissue. Once the bacteria are established and producing toxins, they are capable of creating spreading conditions suitable for their advance. The progression is longitudinal, up and down fascial planes; transverse progression is very limited. The spread is facilitated by increased capillary permeability, the edema fluid separating the muscle fibers and fascia, assisted in this by gas bubbles (Fig. 2.102). This fluid also allows for further diffusion of the toxins and spread of the bacteria. Venous and capillary thrombosis result in local circulatory disturbances and these, in turn, result in further devitalization of tissue. *Once the process is started, it may progress with extraordinary rapidity*. If clostridial myositis is to develop in a wound, there is usually evidence of it within 24 hours.

In gas gangrene, there is extensive disintegration of muscle and saturation of the tissues with exudate that is in part serous and in part profusely sanguineous. When lysis of exuded red cells occurs, the tissues become stained darkly with hemoglobin. The tissues have a rancid odor in the beginning and an exceedingly foul odor in the end.

Histologically, *edema fluid*, poor in protein, separates the muscle fibers from each other and the endomysium. The *degenerating muscle fibers* stain intensely with eosin, the sarcolemma and its nuclei degenerate, but the striations are unduly persistent. Such a histologic picture is always seen at the advancing margin of the lesion. *Neutrophils are never numerous*; a few are loosely scattered at the advancing margin of the lesion and slightly greater numbers in the dermis, but they are rapidly and effectively immobilized and destroyed by the toxins. Deeper within the lesions, muscle fibers are fragmented, but this is probably an indication of physical forces having been applied to necrotic fiber segments at a stage in which the animal is still mobile. Fragmentation is by no means a constant feature of gas gangrene and the absence of it at the periphery of lesions indicates only that, in the later stages of the disease, muscle activity is drastically reduced in a recumbent animal. *Bacteria are seldom numerous in the lesions*, but collections of them may be seen either in muscle fibers or in connective tissue. Involvement of adjacent adipose tissue by the necrotizing process liberates fat droplets that may become embolic.

It is not uncommon for animals to die within 24 h of the onset of local signs of gas gangrene. Invasion, sometimes massive, of the bloodstream occurs shortly before death, or shortly after, and the offending organisms can then be obtained from most tissues. As well as the local lesion, there is at postmortem *severe pulmonary congestion* and evidence of *profound toxic degeneration of the parenchymatous organs*. By very few hours postmortem, there is extensive gas formation in all organs and they crepitate. The liver, especially, may be honey-combed with bubbles, and cut blood vessels continuously release gas bubbles.

There are some variations in the gross appearance of the lesion depending on the species of the principal pathogen. *Putrefaction is the property of contaminating saprophytes* since the primary pathogens are poorly endowed in this regard; the latter are, however, saccharolytic and that is the origin of the *gas bubbles* in the lesions. The exotoxin of *C. novyi* has a rather specific action on vascular endothelium and serous membranes, and relatively pure infections with this organism produce very extensive edematous infiltration of connective tissues. There is no putrefaction, only slight or no discoloration of muscle, and the gelatinous edema fluid is quite clear or at most pink. The toxic potency of this organism is shown by the fact that in fatal infections the organisms are so few as to be difficult to locate even in the primary focus, from which site they show little inclination to move.

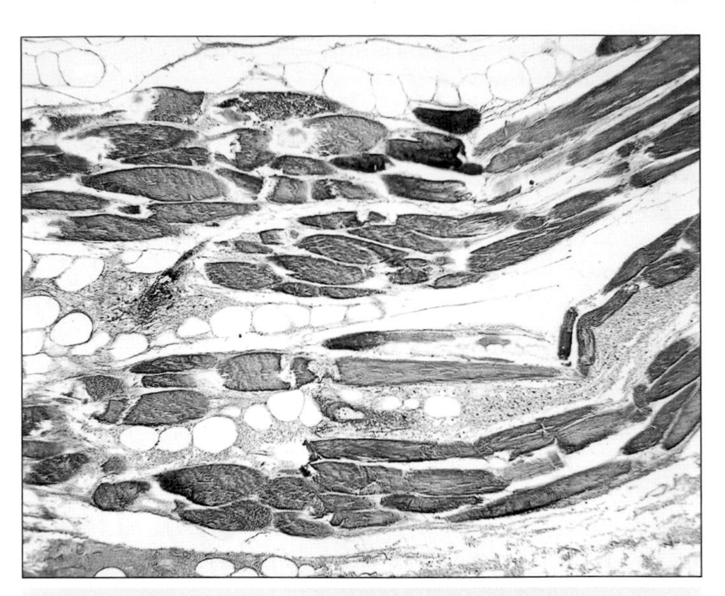

Figure 2.102 Lysed red blood cells and gas bubbles in sublingual muscle in **malignant edema** in a cow. (Courtesy of W Hadlow.)

A typical wound infection by *C. novyi* is that known as "**swelled head**" in rams, the wounds being acquired on the top of the head during fighting. This is a quickly fatal condition, death usually occurring within 48 h. There is extensive infiltration with clear, gelatinous fluid in the tissues of the head, throat, neck, and cranial thorax and sometimes also in the pleural and pericardial sacs. There is no discoloration of muscle and no, or scant, extravasation of erythrocytes. The bacilli are very few in number and cultivable only from the primary focus of infection. *Clostridium novyi* may also predominate in wound infections of horses and, when it does, these lesions too are a nonhemorrhagic variety of malignant edema. *Clostridium chauvoei* as a wound infection always produces heavily sanguineous edema fluid and much gas. *Clostridium septicum* produces large quantities of gelatinous exudate, which is, however, intensely stained with blood. The muscular tissue may be discolored dark red-to-black and, although gas is present, the bubbles are very small. Dark blood exudes freely from veins in the perimysium, and hemoglobin stains narrow collars of surrounding tissue at the margin of the lesions. *Clostridium perfringens* is the usual cause of gas gangrene in man and produces similar lesions in animals. It shows much less tendency than *C. chauvoei* and *C. septicum* to invade the bloodstream terminally or after death. The most frequent cause of malignant edema is *C. septicum*.

Blackleg

Blackleg, also known as black quarter and emphysematous gangrene, is a gangrenous myositis of ruminants caused by C. chauvoei and characterized by the activation of latent spores in muscle. This definition of blackleg separates it from gas gangrene in which, if *C. chauvoei* is involved, it is as a wound contaminant.

Blackleg can sometimes be mimicked closely by the syndrome known as "stable blackleg" or "pseudo-blackleg" caused similarly by germination of latent spores of *C. septicum* in cattle. For diagnostic, prognostic, and epidemiologic reasons, it is important to make a distinction between disease of the blackleg pattern of pathogenesis and disease of the much less complex pathogenesis of gas gangrene and malignant edema. The latter diseases occur sporadically wherever cattle and sheep are raised but appear as a confined outbreak only when groups of animals have been subjected to similar traumatic procedures such as shearing wounds or intramuscular injections. *Blackleg on the other hand is, in spite of a worldwide distribution, peculiarly localized to regions, and within regions to farms.* Within these locales, it is persistently but irregularly enzootic, but rather selective of its hosts, and controllable only by vaccination. *The muscle lesion produced is not distinctive for the blackleg pathogenesis*, nor is the presence of *C. chauvoei* in a typical gangrenous lesion, because *C. chauvoei* can also be a wound contaminant. Identification of the blackleg syndrome should be made on a freshly dead cadaver or preferably on more than one in an outbreak. In the confirmation of blackleg and of pseudo-blackleg particularly, attempts at distinguishing syndromes must be tempered by the knowledge that *C. septicum proliferates rapidly after death while C. chauvoei does not.* The probability of overgrowth is great when a few hours have elapsed between death and bacteriological examination.

Blackleg occurs most often in cattle and sheep and rarely in other domestic animals. Blackleg in **cattle** primarily affects animals 9 months to 2 years of age with a reduced incidence at 6–9 months and 2–3 years, and an even lower incidence in animals over 3 years of age. It affects animals in good condition, and often selectively causes death in the best-grown or best-fattened animals in a group. *Blackleg is chiefly a disease of pastured animals with a tendency to be seasonal in summer.* It is often associated with moist pastures and rapid growth of both forage and cattle, but it is also a problem on some arid ranges. Because the source of *C. chauvoei* organisms appears to be persistent on certain fields, *it has been assumed that the organism is soilborne*, but it is unlikely that it grows in soil. Growth does take place readily in the intestinal tract of cattle, and it is now thought that soil contamination persists by a process of constant replenishment by fecal contamination.

The detailed pathogenesis of blackleg is still somewhat uncertain, but many of the critical points in the following proposed sequence of events have been confirmed in the natural disease and in experimental infections in cattle. *The infection is acquired by the ingestion of spores*, and either these spores, or spores produced following one or more germinative cycles in the gut, are taken across the intestinal mucosa in some way. Macrophages may be responsible for this passage, but it may be possible for the spores to enter natural or transient apertures at tips of villi or in lymphoid crypts or be taken in by lymphoepithelial cells of the ileal domes by endocytosis. *Spores are distributed to tissues where they may be stored for long periods in phagocytic cells.* There may be a certain dynamic turnover, for example in and out of Kupffer cells in the liver, but spores can be found in many tissues of normal animals, including muscle. *The latent spores in muscle are stimulated to germinate when a local event creates muscle damage or low oxygen tension.* This last step is difficult to produce experimentally, but circumstantial evidence seems to confirm its inclusion in the sequence. Parallels exist in other clostridial diseases about which there is much less doubt. It may be that all that is required to establish a medium for the organisms to multiply is a small intramuscular hemorrhage or a degenerative focus initiated by traumatic damage to muscle as part of forced exercise.

The clinical manifestations of blackleg are often not observed and because of the rapid clinical course, *animals are often found dead.* When animals are seen ill, signs consist of lameness, swelling, and crepitation of the skin over a thigh or shoulder if the lesion is superficial, and fever. It is typical for swellings to increase rapidly in size and to be hot initially and cold later. Affected animals subsequently show depression and circulatory collapse. *Death rapidly ensues and seldom does an animal survive more than 24–36 h after the onset of any signs of lameness.* If the muscle lesions are deep within a muscle mass or in the diaphragm, no localizing signs may be evident and no palpable changes detectable. Similarly, lesions in the tongue, heart or sublumbar muscles may escape clinical detection.

An animal that has died of blackleg swells and bloats rapidly, but on incision it is often not as putrid as its external appearance would suggest. Blood-stained froth flows from the nose but not usually from other orifices. Blotchy hemorrhages may be present on the conjunctivae. A poorly circumscribed swelling may be visible on superficial inspection and crepitation detectable on palpation. The skin overlying crepitant swellings is taut and resonant, but normal or dark in color and of normal strength. The subcutaneous tissues and fascia around the lesion are thick with yellow gelatinous fluid that is copiously blood-stained close to the lesion. Gas bubbles may be apparent in the fluid. The affected muscles present slightly different appearances at different distances from the center of the lesion. *Towards the periphery of the lesion, the muscle is dark red, and moist with edema fluid* (Fig. 2.103). *Towards the center, it is red-black, occasionally with putty-colored islands, and the tissue is dry, friable, and porous where gas bubbles separate the primary bundles of fibers* (Fig. 2.104A, B). If this tissue is squeezed, it crepitates and a small amount of thin red fluid oozes out. When the tissue is exposed to air, it takes on a light red

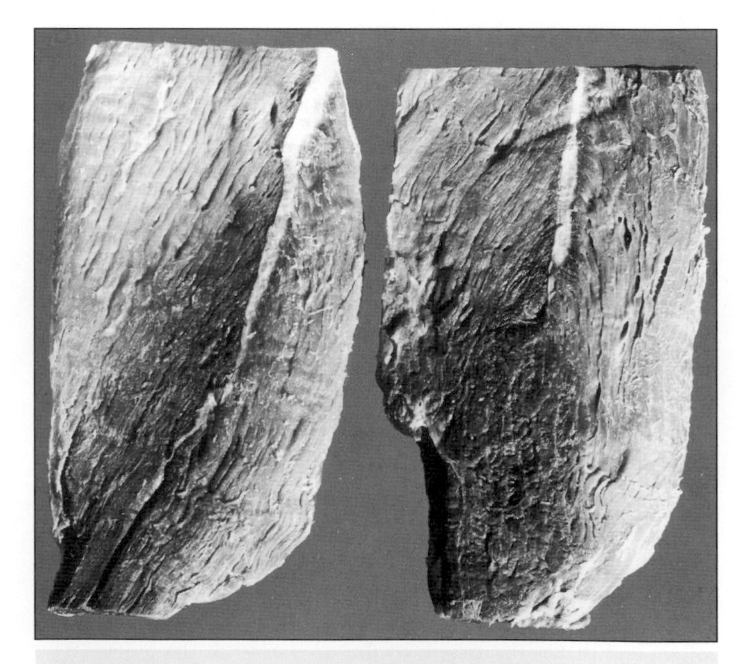

Figure 2.103 Dark areas of hemorrhage on cut surface of muscles in **blackleg** in a calf. (Courtesy of W Hadlow.)

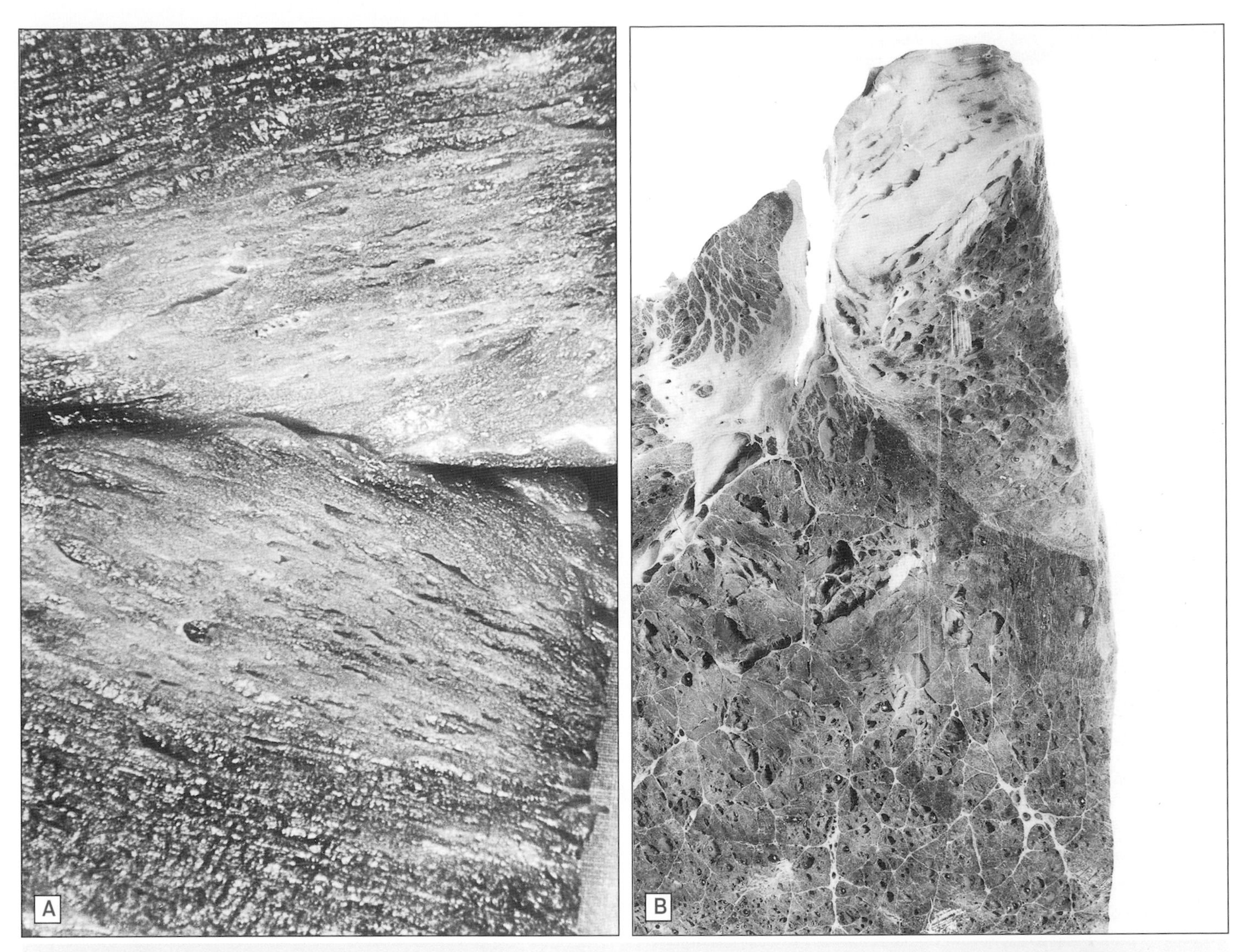

Figure 2.104 Blackleg in a cow. **A.** Dry appearance of affected muscle. **B.** Muscle bundles separated by gas bubbles. (Courtesy of TJ Hulland.)

color and watery exudate drips from cut surfaces. *The odor which emanates from the muscle is sweet and butyric, like rancid butter.*

The initial bacterial lesion in blackleg is cellulitis with copious edema and hemorrhage. Degeneration of the muscle fibers is caused by both diffusing toxin and injury to blood vessels; the extent of ischemic muscle fiber death probably determines how quickly and how extensively tissue gangrene extends through the muscle. Gangrenous lesions expand longitudinally with the long axis of muscles more readily than in a lateral direction, but "skip" areas may create necrotic zones that are highly irregular in contour. The expansion is enhanced by the edema fluid between fibers. At the time of death, animals with a single muscle lesion may have relatively small or very large areas of gangrene. Gas is not produced until muscle fibers die and are penetrated by bacteria and toxins. *The exudate and gas bubbles separate bundles of fibers and individual fibers and these undergo necrosis with preservation of striations in the center of the focus, and fatty and granular degeneration towards the periphery* (Figs 2.105, 2.106). Leukocytes are sparse, being destroyed by diffusing toxins, and only a scattering of debris is found at the periphery of the lesion.

The lesions of blackleg are usually found in the large muscles of the pectoral and pelvic girdles, but they may be found in any striated muscle including

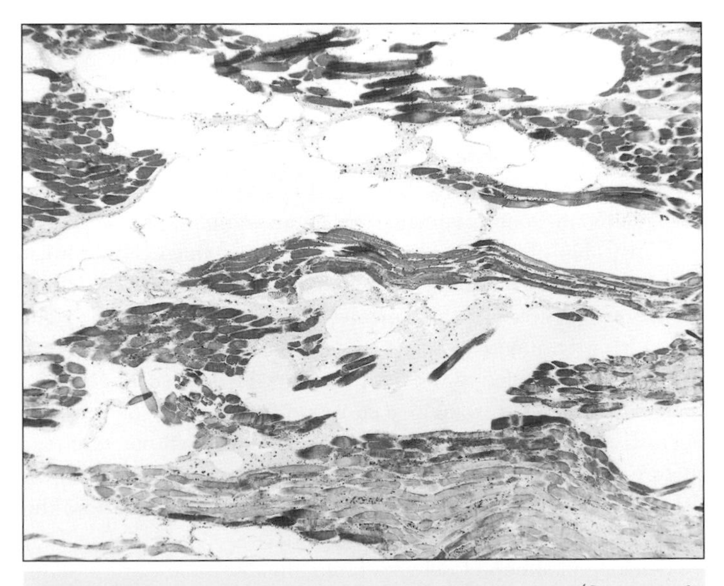

Figure 2.105 Gas bubbles in muscle in **blackleg** in a cow. (Courtesy of W Hadlow.)

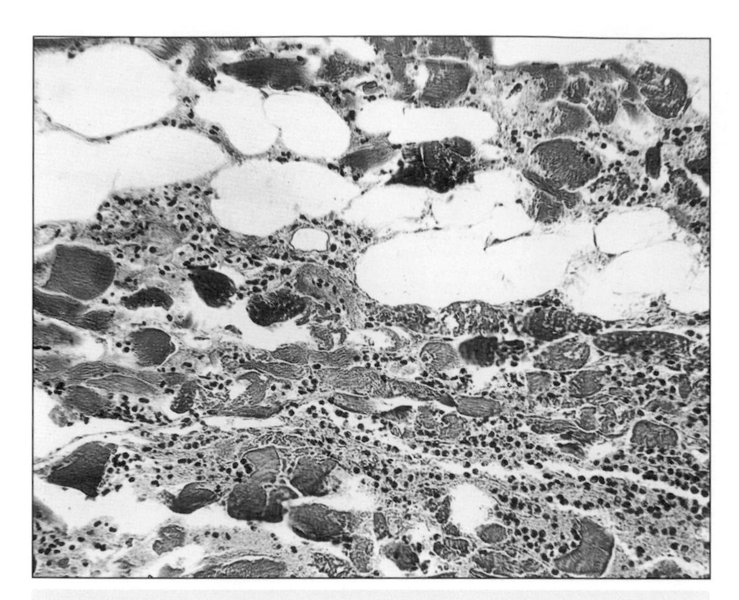

Figure 2.106 Necrosis of myofibers, neutrophilic infiltrate, and gas bubbles in **blackleg** in a cow. (Courtesy of W Hadlow.)

the myocardium. Lesions in the crura of the diaphragm and in the tongue are quite common, and if lesions are present in two or three sites simultaneously, they may be lethal before any of them is very large. This makes their clinical detection more difficult, and their detection at postmortem dependent on detailed examination of many muscles. Even with small widely separated lesions, however, the rancid butter odor may be pervasive.

In addition to the specific muscle lesions of blackleg, changes are present in the rest of the carcass. *There is severe parenchymatous degeneration of liver, kidney, and endocrine glands*, and while this is like conventional postmortem change, the rapidity of its development can suggest blackleg-related toxemia or bacteremia. There is often *fibrinohemorrhagic pleuritis* and, as a generality, when this lesion is present without severe pneumonia, blackleg should be suspected. The parietal pleura is hemorrhagic, and large or delicate blood-stained clots of fibrin overlie the ventral mediastinum and epicardium. Pneumonia is not part of the intrathoracic lesion, but the lungs are congested, and they may be quite edematous. The myocardium may be pale and friable, or dark red; some of the latter areas contain foci of *emphysematous myocarditis and necrosis*. It is these areas that give rise to fibrinohemorrhagic pericarditis; they may be primary or metastatic blackleg lesions. Endocardial lesions sometimes occur, particularly in young animals. The endocardium is hemorrhagic and may be ulcerated or contain built-up fixed, endocardial thrombi in the atrium or on the outer wall of the right ventricle. If there is atrioventricular valve involvement, it is usually on the right side. The peritoneum is intact and normal unless an underlying myositis has extended to it. The spleen may be normal, or enlarged with congested, mushy, pulp. Pale round foci of early putrefactive necrosis may be found in the liver and kidney without reaction; these enlarge with the postmortem interval and become porous. Organisms can often be recovered from many organs and from the blood shortly after death.

Blackleg in **sheep** closely resembles the disease in cattle and the causative organism is the same. *The disease in sheep, however, is much less common than in cattle*, and, although there is some overlap in enzootic distribution, *the disease in sheep usually occurs in locales quite apart from those where it occurs in cattle*. The clinical signs are similar to those in cattle except that crepitation may not be palpable during life, and there is usually dark discoloration of the overlying skin. The lesions resemble those in cattle, but there are usually fewer gas bubbles, and the muscle remains more moist.

Pseudo-blackleg

Pseudo-blackleg mimics blackleg very closely. This disease of cattle produces lesions, which are deep, like those of blackleg. A *diagnosis* of pseudo-blackleg can only be made when there is no detectable wound, the lesion is deeply located, and *C. septicum* is demonstrated in the lesions of a carcass examined immediately after death. This latter precaution is necessary to avoid, as far as possible, misdiagnosis based on the postmortem invasion of *C. septicum* and other organisms from the alimentary tract.

The lesions of pseudo-blackleg differ quantitatively and somewhat qualitatively, from those of blackleg. They tend to be multiple in widely separated muscles. There is very extensive blood-stained gelatinous exudate in the connective tissues, and this exudate contains only occasional small gas bubbles. The lesions may become confluent as very large patches throughout the connective tissues. By contrast, *the muscle lesions, although always present, are less extensive than in blackleg*. The muscles are dark red and moist, and only after examination by multiple incisions is the lack of a distinct primary focus evident. When bubbles of gas are present in necrotic muscle, they are smaller and not as numerous as they are in blackleg.

Pseudo-blackleg is reported in *pigs* in which the muscle lesions are part of a generalized body invasion by *C. septicum* organisms following entry via a primary gastric focus.

Specific infectious diseases with muscle alterations

Muscle lesions are specific findings in *foot-and-mouth disease* of calves (see Vol. 2, Alimentary system), *bluetongue* of sheep (see Vol. 2, Alimentary system), *Teschen disease* of swine, *Coxsackie virus infections* in suckling mice, and leptospirosis (*Leptospira icterohaemorrhagiae*) of dogs. In 5–10% of calves affected with foot-and-mouth disease, pale areas with or without white streaks of mineralization are present (Fig. 2.107) and represent areas of hyaline degeneration histologically. Myocarditis may also be found in calves. Sheep with bluetongue may have scattered small hemorrhagic lesions in skeletal muscle. Microscopic findings are hyaline degeneration, vasculitis, and hemorrhage.

Granulomatous lesions

Various diseases discussed elsewhere may also display granulomatous lesions in skeletal muscle. *Actinobacillosis* ("wooden tongue" in cattle) (see Vol. 2, Alimentary system), *actinomycosis* ("lumpy jaw in cattle") (see Vol. 1, Bones and joints), and *tuberculosis* (see Vol. 3, Hematopoietic system) are examples.

Beef cattle given injections of oil-adjuvant bacterins into paravertebral muscles may develop pyogranulomatous myositis with extension into the vertebral canal. Affected cattle showed lameness and paraparesis.

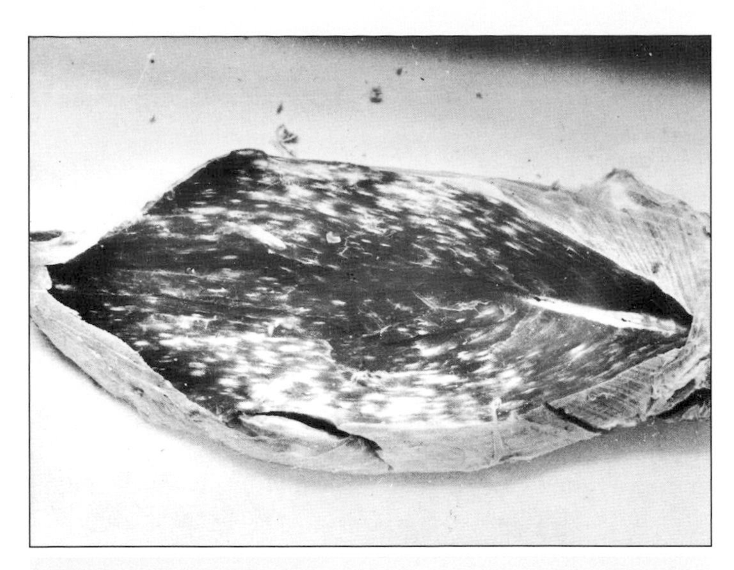

Figure 2.107 Disseminated pale areas of myonecrosis in **foot-and-mouth disease** in a calf. (Courtesy of W Hadlow.)

Other diseases with granulomatous lesions in skeletal muscle are *botryomycosis* and *Roeckl's granuloma* described in detail below.

Staphylococcal granuloma

Chronic granulomas of muscle or connective tissue caused by staphylococci, and referred to as **botryomycosis** in early literature, are much less common than they once were, but they still occur, particularly in the *horse and pig*. They represent a persistent, low-grade infection by *Staphylococcus aureus,* but it is not clear why the same organism at other times produces a conventional abscess or a gangrenous phlegmon. In horses, lesions are most frequent on the neck and pectoral region ("breast boils"), while in the pig, castration wounds and the mammary glands are the most common sites.

The lesion begins as a microabscess around a small colony of organisms and progresses rapidly, sometimes to a very large size. The *fully formed granuloma* is a hard, nodular, gray-white mass of dense, fibrous tissue, irregularly cavitated by small abscesses. The abscesses may be joined by tracts or they may fistulate to the surface. They contain a small quantity of thick, orange-yellow pus, which in turn contains minute granules. The granules consist of a central colony of the organisms while the bulk of the granule mass is made up of "clubs" of reactive protein material; hence the *typical club colony of botryomycosis*. Histologically, the organisms are readily visible in tissues since they stain with hematoxylin and are relatively large. Variable numbers of neutrophils, lymphocytes, and plasma cells are present in the loose fibrous tissue outside of the club colony. Muscle is involved at the periphery of the expanding granulomatous lesion where fibrous septa surround fibers causing atrophy and segmental degeneration.

Roeckl's granuloma of cattle

This nodular lesion of skeletal muscle is apparently specific for cattle, and it may be associated with similar lesions in liver, lungs, lymph nodes, and testes. The lesion is sometimes referred to as "*nodular necrosis*," and it is well known in Europe but rare elsewhere. Included in the list of suggested causes are tuberculosis, pseudotuberculosis, sarcocystosis, blastomycosis, and larvae of *Hypoderma bovis*, but none has been regularly found in typical lesions. Acid-fast organisms are usually not present, and although *Arcanobacterium pyogenes* is sometimes recovered, it is not considered to be the cause of the multiple granulomas.

The lesions occur in cattle of all ages. In any single animal, nodules are all of the same size but the size varies from one animal to the next, from 0.5–5.0 cm in diameter, in or under the skin. *Sites of predilection are the skin around the base of the tail, the limbs, the withers, and the abdominal wall* but lesions are seldom seen deep in muscle masses.

When nodules are cut, surfaces tend to bulge and consist of three zones. The *central zone* is dry, dull, necrotic-looking, and often distinctly yellow. The *reactive zone* is gray-pink, semitranslucent and elastic. The *outer layer* is thin, white fibrous tissue that radiates out along trabecular divisions in adjacent muscle. Larger nodules may be laminated, indicating periodic growth, and small nodules may be reduced to a hard scar with or without mineralization.

Histologically, the early stages of Roeckl's granuloma are small abscesses surrounded by granulation tissue that may contain abundant eosinophils. In other animals, the predominant inflammatory cell may be the lymphocyte. Epithelioid cells and a few giant cells may be present in the reactive zone. The capsule is made up of mature collagen. *These lesions seem to be the modified or exaggerated response of a sensitized animal to a persistent or repetitively introduced antigen.*

Changes in muscle secondary to systemic infections

Lesions in muscle caused by the specific presence of an infectious agent are described elsewhere. More common than these lesions of muscle are the degenerative changes of muscle fibers that occur in acute systemic infections such as pneumonic pasteurellosis of cattle ("shipping fever"); these may be the result of endotoxemia. The lesions, although widespread, cannot be appreciated grossly and consist of *segmental degeneration of a few or many fibers with retraction of fiber segments*. The extent of the degeneration of contractile substance may be very slight, and for this reason floccular or mineralizing changes may be sparse. Some fibers show the distinct hyaline change of Zenker's degeneration with retraction cups visible but not frequent. The fiber breaks lead to *minimal reactive cellularity* since there is little call for extensive clean-up by macrophages or for regenerative proliferation by satellite cells. The changes may be easily overlooked, but a clue to their presence is corrugation of only some fibers or groups of fibers in a longitudinal section of muscle. Although the corrugated fibers may appear otherwise normal, the recoil can be traced to proximal or distal transverse separations. Endomysium and blood vessels are intact, although occasionally there are petechial or larger hemorrhages, and infiltrating lymphocytes or neutrophils are few or absent. *Since the degeneration is almost exclusive to sarcoplasm, survival of the animal should allow complete restoration.*

Bibliography

Emslie-Smith AM, et al. Major histocompatibility complex class 1 antigen expression, immunolocalization of interferon subtypes, and T cell-mediated cytotoxicity in myopathies. Human Pathol 1989;20:224–231.

Engel AG, Arahata K. Mononuclear cells in myopathies: quantitation of functionally distinct subsets, recognition of antigen-specific cell-mediated cytotoxicity

in some diseases, and implications for the pathogenesis of the different inflammatory myopathies. Human Pathol 1986;17:704–721.
Goebel HH, et al. Recent advances in the morphology of myositis. Path Res Pract 1985;180:1–9.
Hadlow WJ. Diseases of skeletal muscle. In: Innes JRM, Saunders LZ, eds. Comparative Neuropathology. New York: Academic Press, 1962:147–243.
Hoefling DC. Acute myositis associated with *Haemophilus parasuis* in primary SPF sows. J Vet Diag Invest 1991;3:354–355.
Hole NH. Three cases of nodular necrosis (Roeckl's granuloma) in the muscles of cattle. J Comp Pathol 1938;51:9–22.
McAllister MM, et al. Myositis, lameness, and paraparesis associated with use of an oil-adjuvant bacterin in beef cows. J Am Vet Med Assoc 1995;207:936–938.
McLaughlin SA, et al. *Clostridium septicum* infection in the horse. Equine Pract 1979;1:17–20.
Oakley CL, Warrack GH. The soluble antigens of *Clostridium oedematiens* type D (*C. haemolyticum*). J Pathol Bact 1959;78:543–551.
Orfeur NB, Hebeler HF. Blackquarter in pigs. Vet Rec 1953;65:822.
Podell M. Inflammatory myopathies. Vet Clin North Am, Small Anim Pract 2002;32:147–167.
Rebhun WC, et al. Malignant edema in horses. J Am Vet Med Assoc 1985;187:732–736.
Ringel SP, et al. Quantitative histopathology of the inflammatory myopathies. Arch Neurol 1986;43:1004–1009.
Seddon HR, et al. Blackleg in sheep in N.S.W. Aust Vet J 1931;7:2–18.
Sojka JE, et al. *Clostridium chauvoei* myositis infection in a neonatal calf. J Vet Diagn Invest 1992;4:201–203.
Sterne M, Edwards JB. Blackleg in pigs caused by *Clostridium chauvoei*. Vet Rec 1955;67:314–315.
Walton J. The inflammatory myopathies. J Royal Soc Med 1983;76:998–1010.

PARASITIC DISEASES

Sarcocystosis

***Sarcocystis* spp.** *are protozoal parasites of animal muscle that in many respects resemble coccidia, the main difference being their obligatory development in two hosts.* The sexual stages develop in a predator host, while the asexual phases develop in the prey animal. Some animals, such as the opossum and man, are vehicles for both parts of the *Sarcocystis* spp. cycle but not for the same species, there being considerable specificity on the part of both the intermediate and definitive hosts. There is, however, some latitude. For example, several individual parasites develop in dogs, or coyotes, or foxes, or wolves as a definitive host, and a number of intermediate host species of the same general type may be "accidentally" infected at low level. Currently over 90 *Sarcocystis* species are recognized in mammals, birds, and reptiles, and 14 of these are regularly found in muscles of domestic animals as part of the intermediate host infection. The prevalence of infection in cattle, sheep, and horses approaches 100%. Where it was once thought that the muscle phase of infection was asymptomatic and safe for the intermediate host, it is now known that particularly *the schizogonous phase may cause severe clinical disease and death* under both natural and experimental conditions. The production of enteric disease by the sexual phase in the predator host is considered elsewhere (see Vol. 2, Alimentary system). Fetal infection with abortion and neonatal mortality is described in Vol. 3, Female genital system.

The very substantial differences between *Sarcocystis* species in respect of the intermediate host response appears to be a parasite characteristic, not a difference in host immunologic response, although clinical disease may be modified by immunity.

Consideration here is primarily given to those *Sarcocystis* spp. infections affecting the muscles of domestic animals as intermediate hosts. *Sporocysts* are ingested when herbage contaminated by carnivore or human fecal material is consumed. *Sporozoites* are released and these invade many tissues. One or two generations of *schizogony* take place within endothelial cells, the first in small arterioles, the second (if there is one) in capillaries. The second or third generation of *schizonts* develops within striated muscle fibers as thin-walled cysts initially containing round *metrocytes*, which repeatedly divide to produce numerous banana-shaped *bradyzoites*. The much-enlarged mature cyst persists in muscle for long periods and the cycle is completed when muscle is consumed by the predator host and the *sexual cycle* of the parasite is developed in the intestinal epithelial cells.

Clinical disease in an intermediate host may occur at either of two stages of the developmental cycle. It may take the form of fever, petechiation of mucous membranes, edema, icterus, and macrocytic hypochromic anemia 3–5 weeks after initial infection and lasting for 6–8 weeks during the *schizogonous (parasitemic) stage*. These signs seem to be related to many small episodes of intravascular coagulation, although endothelial schizonts are not the site of thrombus formation. The parasites are also present in perivascular macrophages. The second stage in which clinical signs and death may occur comes as the *schizonts enter muscle at about 40 days*, sometimes with extensive fiber degeneration and marked enzyme release which attracts macrophages and plasma cells. Another wave of muscle disease may be associated with enlargement of the cysts in a massive infestation and this can cause lameness. Maturation of cysts may take 60–100 days, by which time any tissue reaction has subsided; this may account for the earlier impression that the parasite was an innocuous passenger in muscle.

Two species of *Sarcocystis* have been recognized in the muscles of the **horse;** *S. bertrami* (*S. equicanis*) and *S. fayeri*. Both species complete their cycle in the dog. *S. bertrami* seems to cause the greatest tissue response but neither seems to cause clinical disease and both are therefore, judged "non-pathogenic." Cysts in horse muscle are microscopic in size and rarely numerous, but occasionally there is massive involvement of skeletal muscles.

Sarcocystis species in **cattle** are presently considered to be: *S. cruzi* with a cycle completed in domestic and wild Canidae; *S. hirsuta* with a cycle completed in the domestic cat; and *S. hominis* with a cycle completed in man. Two additional species are found in the water buffalo; *S. fusiformis* with a cat–buffalo cycle, and *S. levinei* with a dog–buffalo cycle. Only *S. cruzi* seems to be capable of causing significant clinical disease in cattle. Clinical signs exhibited during the schizogonous stage may include evidence of hemolysis as described above as well as progressive debility, abortion, drooling, lymphadenitis, sloughing of the tip of the tail and, in some outbreaks, death in a high proportion of affected animals. See also Eosinophilic myositis of cattle and sheep.

Four species of *Sarcocystis* regularly affect **sheep,** namely *S. tenella* (*S. ovicanis*) and *S. arieticanis,* which have a sheep–dog cycle, and *S. gigantea* and *S. medusiformis,* which have a sheep–cat cycle. *Sarcocystis tenella* is quite virulent in lambs if infective doses are large, and naturally occurring encephalomyelitis in mature sheep with neurological disease has been blamed on this organism. Chronically debilitated sheep often have an enormous number of cysts in their muscles. This ought to have some effect on muscle performance, but lameness is not apparent. *Sarcocystis gigantea* cysts are very large (1–3 mm) and distend segments of esophageal striated muscle fibers well above the adventitial surface of the esophagus (Fig. 2.108A, B). It is the only *Sarcocystis* of domestic animals that is visible with the naked eye.

Two species (*S. capricanis* and *S. hericanis*) have a goat–dog cycle, and another (*S. moulei*) has a goat–cat cycle. None appears to be pathogenic for **goats** as natural infections but, experimentally, even moderate levels of infectious sporocysts led to death of some animals.

Three species of *Sarcocystis* are found in **swine;** *S. miescheriana* with a pig–dog and pig–wild Canidae cycle, *S. porcifelis* with a pig–cat cycle, and *S. suihominis,* which completes its cycle in humans. Of the three, only *S. miescheriana* is known to produce clinical signs of diarrhea, myositis, and lameness.

Sarcocystis organisms have been observed in the muscles of **dogs** and **cats** from time to time. It was thought that these represented erratically traveling parasites in an abnormal site, but it now appears that such cysts are morphologically unlike the species that originate in the cat or dog and complete their cycle in the sheep, horse, or cow. A new identity has not yet been given to these sarcocysts.

Sarcocystosis occurs in many wild species; for example, deer have at least five distinct species all of which complete their cycle in the dog or in wild Canidae.

Histologically, *Sarcocystis* organisms are rarely accompanied by an acute inflammatory reaction, and *schizonts in endothelial cells cause little or no evidence of endothelial cell destruction*. As the organisms enter muscle, a wide range of change may be encountered. Usually there is no muscle fiber degeneration but there may be thin, linear collections of lymphocytes between fibers in the region. Sometimes the muscle fiber undergoes segmental hyaline change in the region of the invading parasite and rarely, extensive floccular degeneration of muscle fibers occurs. The extent of muscle change bears little relationship to the numbers of developing cysts, but generally, very low numbers of *Sarcocystis* produce no reaction.

As cysts mature, and the contained bradyzoites become more distinct, the cyst capsule within the enlarged muscle fiber becomes

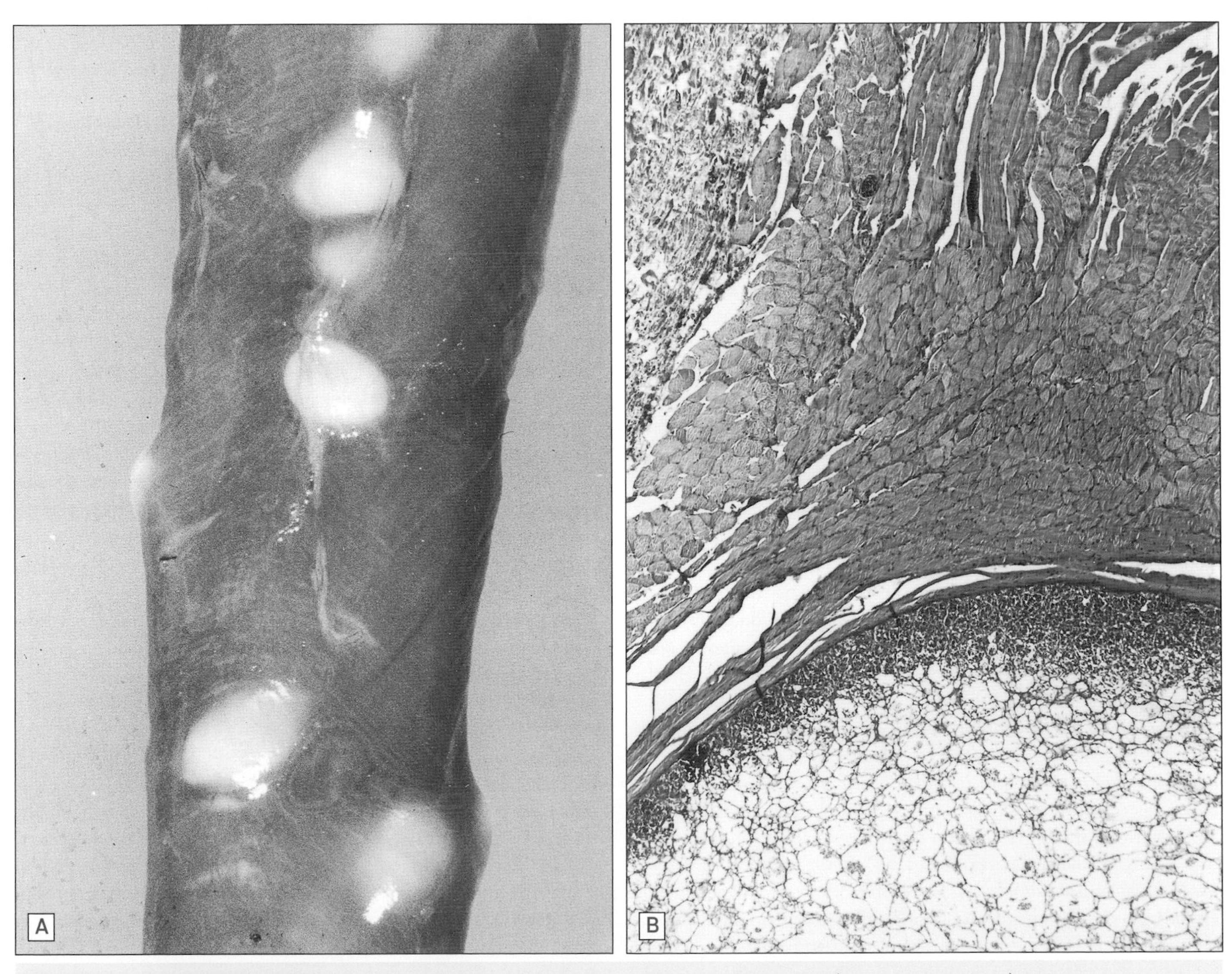

Figure 2.108 A. *Sarcocystis gigantea*. A. In the esophagus of a sheep. **B.** Cyst margin in muscle section. (Courtesy of TJ Hulland.)

thicker and more clearly differentiated from the muscle sarcoplasm. Muscle sarcoplasm and muscle nuclei gather around the parasite in the early stages. In some parasitic species, the outer capsular zone develops distinct radial striations, which, on electron microscopy, prove to be complex convolutions of the cyst wall. Small pores allow communication between cyst contents and muscle cell content, but apart from the obvious nutritional dependence of the parasite on muscle fiber, little is known of the biochemical interplay which must take place.

Microscopic inspection of *Sarcocystis*-infected muscle often reveals occasional degenerate parasitic cysts surrounded by variable numbers of inflammatory cells (very few of which are eosinophils), or, at a later state, macrophages and granulation tissue. It is not known whether these represent "over-age" cysts or simply random changes in an easily modified host–parasite relationship. Such reactions in muscle increase with host age.

Eosinophilic myositis of cattle and sheep

Eosinophilic myositis *is a relatively rare condition in cattle and sheep of all ages* that has some significance for meat inspection because the lesions are usually discovered in skeletal muscle and myocardium of animals slaughtered for human consumption. *Sudden deaths in cattle and sheep have been ascribed to the myocarditis.* The disease is included here because *there is good evidence that eosinophilic myositis in sheep and cattle may be caused by degeneration of* Sarcocystis *spp. The converse is not true and, in some cases of eosinophilic myositis, no degenerating parasites can be found.* *Sarcocystis* spp. remnants are often found in the center of the myositis lesions, and IgE specific for the parasite is associated with degranulated eosinophils. Animals with parasites but not myositis have serum levels of IgE comparable to those in animals with lesions, suggesting that the inflammatory reaction in eosinophilic myositis is stimulated by independent parasite tube rupture or by trauma to muscle fibers. There are reports of traumatic muscle rupture in cattle initiating an eosinophilic response. A heat-stable, eosinophil-chemotactic substance has been isolated from affected bovine muscle in which eosinophilic myositis lesions were present. The substance has a molecular size less than bovine albumin, and its activity seems to correlate with lesion size and severity.

The gross lesions of eosinophilic myositis in cattle are characteristic, being well-demarcated, green, focal stripes or patches that fade to off-white when exposed to air. Some lesions have a brown-green or gray-green color. Single muscles or groups of muscles may be involved or the lesions may be widespread through all muscles, including the heart. Individual lesions may be 2–3 mm to 5–6 cm in diameter in both heart and skeletal muscle, and no part of the muscle mass seems to be exempt.

Histologically, both acute and more chronic fibrous reactions may exist side by side. *The reaction is characterized by large numbers of eosinophils, and it is these that impart the green color to the lesion.* Dense masses of mature eosinophils separate adjacent endomysial sheaths and perimysial trabeculae. Muscle fiber degeneration is not an obvious feature of the disease, but *occasional segments of fibers do undergo hypercontraction and degeneration.* These may be later evident only as endomysial sheaths stuffed with eosinophils rather than muscle fibers because muscle fiber regeneration seems to be impaired or modified.

With time, fibroplasia is evident. In the chronic lesion, dense collagenous tissue is prominent and the inflammatory cell population changes from eosinophils to a smaller population of lymphocytes, plasma cells, and histiocytes.

In some cases, individual lesions may take on some of the characteristics of a *granuloma* in which central muscle fibers along with adjacent eosinophils undergo degeneration. This central necrotic mass acquires a fringe of epithelioid cells and giant cells, and fibrous tissue becomes circumferentially oriented. The central eosinophilic mass may gather calcium salts while the edge of the lesion consists of infiltrating eosinophils and fibroblasts that radiate into adjacent muscle. Granulomatous lesions will leave a small scar, but it is likely that the more diffuse lesions of eosinophilic myositis in cattle can disappear in time with very little residual lesion.

Eosinophilic myositis in *sheep* tends to occur in young animals under 2 years of age. Lesions are comparable in distribution and type to those in cattle although the frequency of the granulomatous type of change may be higher.

Toxoplasma and *Neospora* myositis

In addition to *Sarcocystis,* two apicomplexan parasites, *Toxoplasma* and *Neospora*, produce myopathy in several species. Both infections are dealt with more fully elsewhere (see Vol. 2, Alimentary system; and Vol. 1, Nervous system, respectively).

Toxoplasma gondii infections, particularly in puppies and kittens, or in any species of farm animal naturally immunosuppressed, or in animals on immunosuppressive therapy, may massively involve skeletal muscle fibers. *Myositis with mononuclear leukocytic infiltration, myofiber necrosis, and myofiber atrophy is accompanied by polyradiculoneuritis.* In the majority of toxoplasma infections, however, muscle lesions are rare. In muscle fibers, both tachyzoites and thin-walled cysts (bradyzoites) may be present but the former are generally transient, spherical, and nonreactive.

Neospora caninum infections occur worldwide mainly in dogs, but the organisms are also found in cats, and the disease may have originated in the latter species. *The disease is associated with abortion and perinatal mortality in cattle with nonsuppurative encephalitis, myocarditis, and periportal hepatitis in affected animals.* Neosporosis appears to have been present in the US for over 30 years and many of the organisms originally identified in tissue sections as *Toxoplasma* are now recognized as *Neospora*. The two organisms can be distinguished definitively by immunoperoxidase procedures, and presumptively by microscopic appearance. *Neospora* cysts are thick-walled; *Toxoplasma* cysts are thin-walled and found in several tissues, including muscle. Serologic tests can detect antibodies to *N. caninum* and to *T. gondii*.

Neospora caninum has a much greater tendency to produce *myositis* because the tachyzoites form large fusiform packets in muscle after the second division stage of meronts. When these escape from the muscle fiber in a partially immunized host, an inflammatory reaction, abundant and predominantly histiocytic and plasmacytic, separates individual fibers. There is also segmental muscle fiber degeneration, which may be a response to direct parasite invasion, but is likely the result of a local release of free radicals from dying inflammatory cells. At this stage, clinical signs of muscle weakness may be obvious and at necropsy, muscles over the entire body may be pale, streaky, and atrophic. Inflammatory lesions often also affect nerves and nerve roots and result in denervation atrophy.

The life cycle and source of infection for neosporosis are unknown. The only known mode of natural infection is transplacental in persistently infected bitches, with affected litters having distinctive clinical features of progressive pelvic limb weakness, muscle atrophy, and joint contracture. The disease has been produced experimentally in immunocompetent cats, but the lesions are more severe in cats given corticosteroids.

Trichinellosis

Muscle is the habitat for encysted larvae of the nematode *Trichinella* spp., which may survive there for many years (Fig. 2.109). The muscle belongs to the animal that earlier harbored the adult worm in its duodenum, and *since animal-to-animal transmission of infection is accomplished by the consumption of infected muscle, most of the species regularly involved are carnivores or scavenger species.* Man, dogs, and a variety of wild Canidae, cats and wild Felidae, pigs, rats, mustelids, bears, polar bears, raccoons, and mice become hosts to the adult and their persistent larvae. Other species including horse and birds may become infected when muscle tissue is included in their feed; horsemeat has been a natural source of trichinellosis in man. *Trichinellosis is a zoonotic disease sometimes occurring in spectacular outbreaks in man and animals.* Humans become infected when they consume uncooked or incompletely cooked meat of pigs, bears, or aquatic mammals. In those regions of the world where inspection of meat is routine, the incidence of infection is very low, but even in countries such as Canada and the USA, the incidence in wild carnivores is 1–10%.

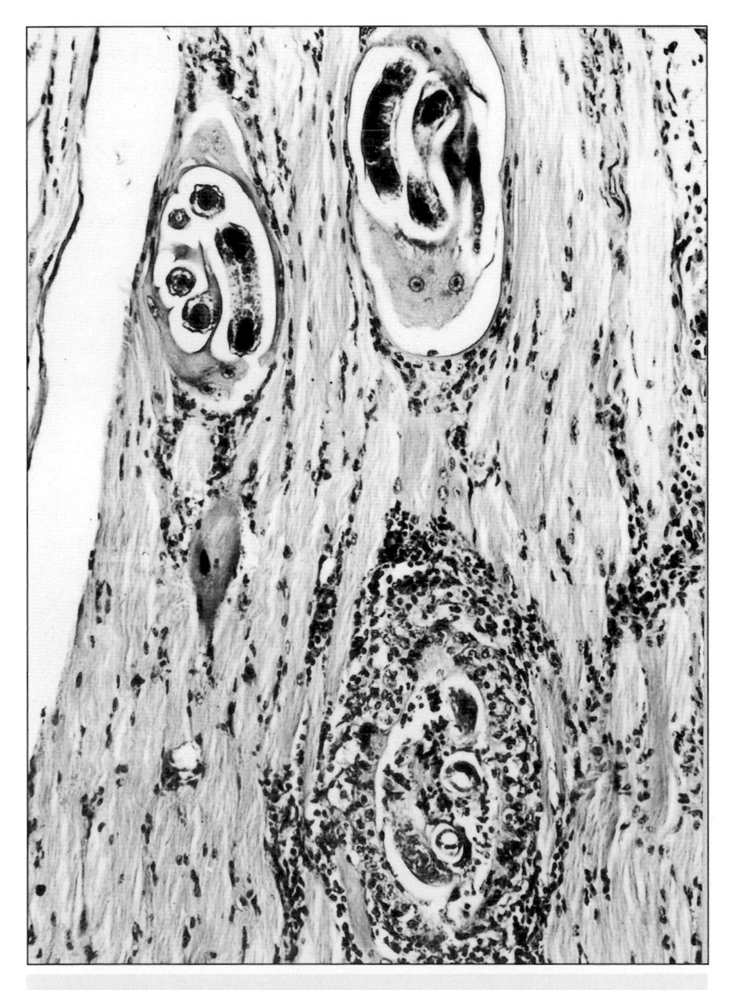

Figure 2.109 ***Trichinella spiralis*** larvae encysted in muscle of a pig.

The parasitic cycle for *T. spiralis* begins with ingestion of infected meat fibers. Gastric juices liberate the encysted larvae, which then molt twice, grow to a length of 1–4 mm as threadlike fourth-stage worms, and molt again. Maturity is reached in about 4 days following ingestion, the adults copulate and the male dies. The ovoviviparous females penetrate via the crypts of Lieberkuhn to the submucosal lymphatics where they deposit 0.1 mm long larvae into lymph vessels. The persistence of females in the duodenum is dependent on the state of surface immunity (probably IgA antibody produced locally in the gut wall) and varies from days to 5–6 weeks. Some larvae may be passed in feces as the female moves out of the duodenal crypts. The remaining larvae migrate with the lymph, then the blood, to reach the pulmonary and systemic circulations. Those that find their way to muscle may achieve a safe haven away from developing immunity by entering a muscle fiber; those that arrive elsewhere may survive for a brief period but are soon destroyed. In a previously sensitized host, few of the approximately 500 larvae produced by each female are able to enter a muscle fiber in time to ensure survival.

Within the muscle fiber, the larva grows, coils and enlarges a segment of the host muscle fiber, which is induced to develop some unusual changes as the "nurse cell." Nuclei enlarge, myofibrils are greatly reduced, the basal lamina is very greatly increased in its thickness and number of folds around the affected segment of muscle fiber, and the sarcoplasmic reticulum, which is in intimate contact with the worm, proliferates. Mitochondria in the immediate vicinity increase in number as they are reduced in size. After a month, the larvae are up to 100 μm long and coiled in a figure of eight. There is usually one per fiber. *Larvae are not normally visible by naked eye inspection of muscles unless they are old and mineralized.* On routine microscopic examination of muscle, larvae lie in bulging glassy segments of muscle fiber that may be loosely encircled by eosinophils, and in due course, by a scattering of lymphocytes, plasma cells, and macrophages. If the parasitized muscle segment degenerates, the larva is exposed and soon dies to become the center of a more acute inflammatory, but still predominantly eosinophilic, reaction. Segments of muscle fiber adjacent to the encysted larva may show evidence of degeneration or subsequent regenerative repair with basophilia and centrally located nuclei. In a heavy infestation, a large proportion of the muscle fibers in predilective muscle sites may be taken up with either the parasite or adjacent reactive zones. Purely physical replacement of functional muscle accounts for most of the clinical signs of infestation when they are present, though usually they are absent.

In 2–3 months, the cellular reaction subsides and the muscle fibers enclosing larvae become further modified to give the impression, on light microscopy, of a fibrous capsule. Since parasite survival can only be assured by intracellular seclusion, the "capsule" is, in reality, modified muscle cell components or, perhaps more correctly, modified satellite cells and basal lamina. Once the larvae are encysted in this way, further change, apart from muscle fiber degeneration, is usually confined to deposition of mineral in the encapsulating muscle structure, but this does not seem to affect parasite viability. *The larvae may survive more than 20 years* although the average life span is probably a good deal less depending on host longevity and the occurrence of fiber degeneration.

Several features of this parasitism are unexplained, including the distribution of larvae within the host. Certain muscles such as the respiratory and masticatory muscles are preferentially and heavily infected while other muscles contain a reduced burden. Activity alone is not responsible because a paralyzed diaphragm is still preferentially susceptible. Concentration of larvae in preferred sites may be influenced by blood distribution, increased larval survival, the presence of some needed nutrient, or preferential shielding from normal body defense mechanisms. Heart muscle is sometimes involved, but not heavily; *the muscles most involved are tongue, masseter and laryngeal muscles, diaphragm, intercostal muscles, and muscles of the eye*, but no striated muscle is exempt. Since some of the selectively involved muscles are small, heavy infestation may have a significant clinical effect in the form of muscle weakness, paralysis, or reduced responsiveness. Usually parasitic infestations of muscle are asymptomatic, and this feature enhances the transfer of infection from animals to man.

Five species of *Trichinella,* with eight genotypes identified by DNA analysis, are parasites of muscle:

- *Trichinella spiralis* is the parasite of pigs, rodents, and man in temperate and tropical climates, and is the most prevalent strain. It is moderately resistant to short-term freezing, and its infectivity is not reduced by freezing and thawing.
- *Trichinella nativa* is found in colder climates and is the species most often encountered in polar bears, bears, aquatic mammals, and the Inuit. Its cycle is similar in most respects to that of *T. spiralis* but the larval form is much more resistant to freezing for long periods.
- *Trichinella nelsoni* is found in carnivores in eastern and southern Africa and also in central and eastern Europe.
- *Trichinella britovi* has been reported in southern Europe.
- *Trichinella pseudospiralis* is found in northeastern Europe and differs from the other species in its failure to encyst in muscle. The species migrates through muscle more or less continuously under experimental conditions, but appears otherwise to have a cycle similar to that of *T. spiralis.*

Cysticercosis

Many of the larval forms of tapeworms of carnivores develop and are temporarily stored in the viscera or other tissues of prey species. A few have a special predilection for skeletal muscles and myocardium, and this much smaller group is dealt with here. The pathological effects of adult tapeworms in the intestinal tract of the carnivorous host are described in Vol. 2, Alimentary system.

Taenia solium is a large tapeworm (up to 8 m long) common in many parts of the world and resident in the intestinal tract of humans and sometimes other primates. The larvae (or metacestode form) usually develop in the pig or wild pig, but for this species of tapeworm humans can sometimes be host to both the tapeworm and the larval cysticercus. Gravid tapeworm segments are passed in feces, and because they are nonmotile, the 40 000 eggs in each segment tend to be concentrated over a small area. Susceptible pigs having access to infected human feces are easily infected. Eggs resist destruction for relatively long periods in soil, moist ground surfaces or sewage sludge, and survive in flowing water for a while. Following ingestion, the outer shell is digested in the stomach releasing and activating the tiny *oncosphere*, which penetrates the intestinal blood vessels and reaches the general circulation. *Most of the larvae in the pig find their way to heart, masseter, tongue, or shoulder muscles.* When they migrate in humans, they are distributed to connective tissues, brain, and viscera. The larvae become *cysticerci* (*Cysticercus cellulosae*), enlarge to a cyst with a single inverted scolex, which, when mature, measure 1–2 cm and are easily visible between muscle fibers. Cysticerci are rapidly ensheathed at first in a loose, and then a more dense, connective tissue capsule derived from endomysium. A few lymphocytes and a few or many eosinophils lie in the outer regions of the capsule. The cysticercus seems to avoid effective immune-mediated destruction for some time by converting elements of the complement system to inactive products, although in a strongly immunized animal the larvae are eventually destroyed, mineralized, and removed (Fig. 2.110A). In order to allow themselves growing room within developing inelastic collagenous capsules, the cysticerci create a crescentic zone of degenerative lysis (presumed to be induced enzymatically); this can often be seen in histologic sections of encysted metacestodes, as can parts of the scolices and hooks in those species which have them. *Cysticercus cellulosae* has rostellar hooks. The survival time in muscle for *C. cellulosae* is not known, but the question is usually not relevant since *pigs are normally slaughtered at a young age when virtually all cysticerci in muscle are viable.* Humans complete the cycle and become infected when they consume raw or incompletely cooked pork.

Taenia saginata is probably the *most common tapeworm in humans; its larvae are in cattle,* and are found in most regions of the world. Transfer of the very resistant eggs from the fecund proglottids to calves or cattle is often enhanced by contamination of open water by sewage, or by use of sewage as fertilizer on fields. It also occurs directly by contamination of animal feeds with human feces or from soiled human hands. The life cycle is similar to that described above for *T. solium* and *the larval form (Cysticercus bovis) similarly preferentially infests heart and masticatory muscles,* although cysts are often widespread throughout the muscles. Histologically the reaction to the parasite involves few eosinophils. *Cysticercus bovis* does not have rostellar hooks. Following a period of growth and development of about 10 weeks the larvae become infective. After about another 30 days the cysticerci begin to die, but some larvae may be viable 9 months after infection. Death of the larvae is probably the result of development of an immune reaction. Cattle that have acquired resistance to the invasion of oncospheres across the gut apparently do not have an enhanced capability to cause degeneration of preexisting muscle cysticerci. Humans acquire infection when they consume inadequately cooked beef or veal.

Taenia ovis is a tapeworm commonly found in dogs and wild carnivores throughout the world that, in its larval form, has a cysticercus (*Cysticercus ovis*) that develops in the heart and skeletal muscles of sheep and goats (Fig. 2.110B). The cycle is similar to that for *T. saginata* but the larvae do have rostellar hooks, which may sometimes be an aid to histologic identification in lesions even after the cysticercus has begun to disintegrate.

Taenia krabbei is a tapeworm in *wild carnivores* in temperate and arctic climates whose larval form (*Cysticercus tarandi*) is found in reindeer, gazelle, moose, and other wild ruminants. Lesions produced in the intermediate host are similar to those seen in cattle with *C. bovis,* and a similar cycle is assumed.

Hepatozoonosis

Myositis caused by *Hepatozoon americanum* (initially classified as *H. canis*) was a consistent feature of 15 natural cases of infection in

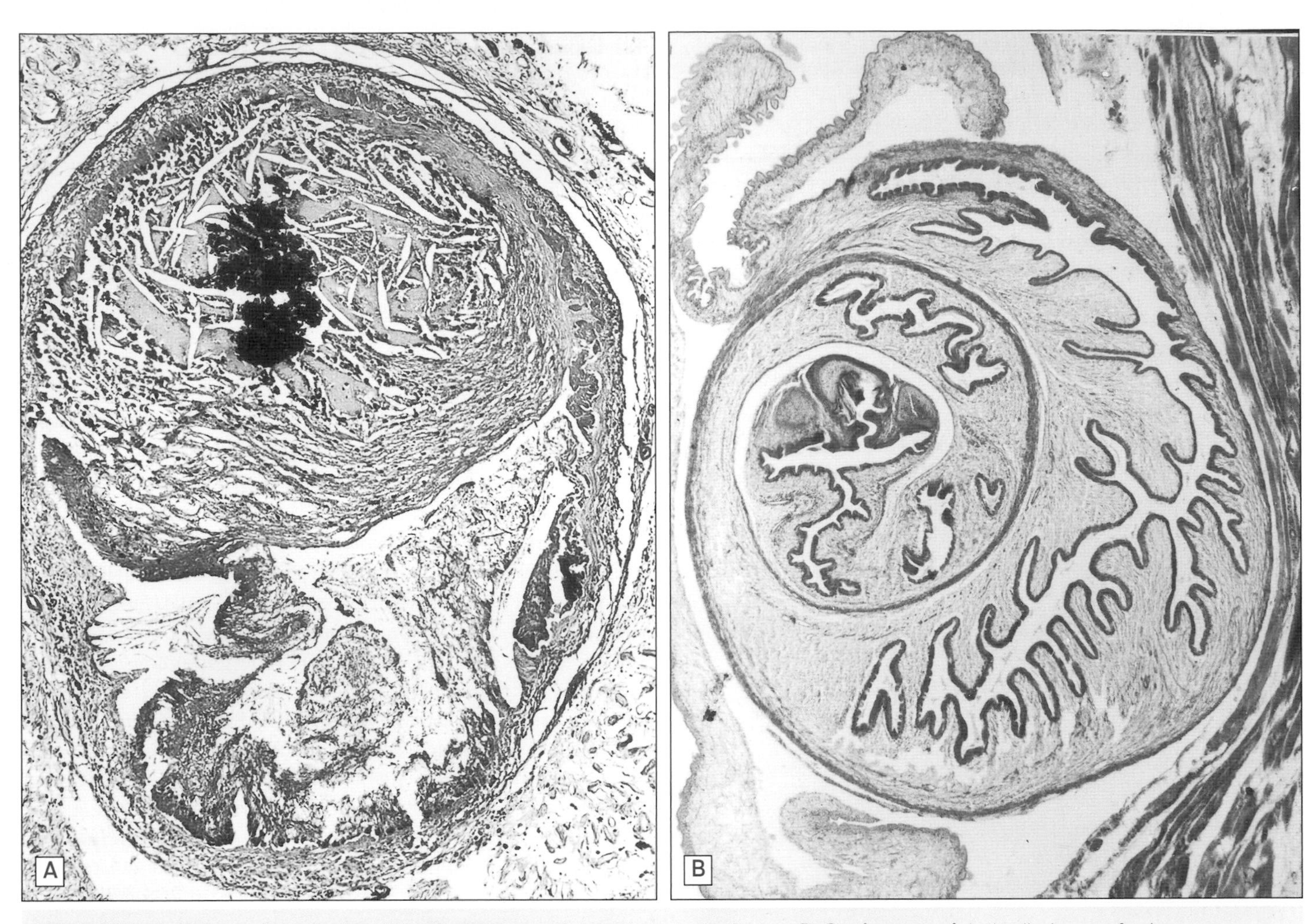

Figure 2.110 **A.** Degenerating and mineralizing ***Cysticercus cellulosae*** in the brain of a dog. **B.** ***Cysticercus ovis*** in the diaphragm of a sheep.

dogs in the southern USA. Cases have been limited mainly to the Gulf Coast area of Louisiana and Texas and from Oklahoma. The disease occurs in a variety of Canidae and Felidae in South Africa and the Middle East, and has become established in the dog and brown tick (*Rhipicephalus sanguineus*) populations in North America. Animals become infected by ingesting an infected tick or possibly another infected arthropod; sporozoites are released, invade the gut wall, and *undergo schizogony in many tissues of the host, including skeletal muscle*. Rupture of schizonts in time leads to an inflammatory reaction, but the subsequent stage, a large 250 μm, thick-walled, single-celled cyst does not stimulate a body response.

Affected dogs (generally less than 6 months old) show fever, anorexia, weight loss, general body pain, and gait abnormalities, and many show respiratory signs. Concurrent disease may be needed to facilitate infection. The clinical disease is often prolonged by spontaneous remissions. Radiographs may show irregular periosteal proliferations. Most dogs have marked leukocytosis and a slight increase in serum creatine kinase activity. The organism in gametocyte form may be present in neutrophils, and muscle biopsy may demonstrate the cysts, or the typical pyogranulomatous reaction in response to the release of merozoites, or the schizonts themselves.

At postmortem, muscle lesions consist of *multiple acute granulomas* interspersed with rows of neutrophils between muscle fibers. Developing stages of the parasite are usually abundant. Dogs may die with *secondary amyloidosis and glomerulonephritis*.

Chagas' disease (American trypanosomiasis)

The disease in dogs has prominent lesions of myocarditis but may also have skeletal muscle involvement. Affected muscle has *myofiber necrosis with infiltrates of lymphocytes and macrophages*. See Vol. 3, Hematopoietic system for further information.

Bibliography

Barrows PL, et al. Experimental *Sarcocystis suicanis* infections: disease in growing pigs. Am J Vet Res 1982;43:1409–1412.

Barton CL, et al. Canine hepatozoonosis: a retrospective study of 15 naturally occurring cases. J Am Anim Hosp Assoc 1985;21:125–134.

Boireau P, et al. *Trichinella* in horses: a low frequency infection with high human risk. Vet Parasitol 2000;93:309–320.

Braun U, et al. Regurgitation due to megaesophagus in a ram. Can Vet J 1990;31:391–392.

Braund KG. Idiopathic and exogenous causes of myopathies in dogs and cats. Vet Med 1997;92:629–634.

Braund KG, et al. Toxoplasma polymyositis/polyneuropathy: A new clinical variant in two mature dogs. J Am Anim Hosp Assoc 1988;24:93–97.

Bundza A, Feltmate TE. Eosinophilic myositis/lymphadenitis in slaughter cattle. Can Vet J 1989;30:514–516.

Craig TM. Parasitic myositis of dogs and cats. Sem Vet Med Surg (Small Anim) 1989;4:161–167.

Dick TA, et al. Sylvatic trichinosis in Ontario, Canada. J Wildl Dis 1986;22:42–47.

Dubey JP, Carpenter JL. Histologically confirmed clinical toxoplasmosis in cats: 100 cases (1952–1990). J Am Vet Med Assoc 1993;203:1556–1566.
Dubey JP, et al. Sarcocystosis in goats: clinical signs and pathologic and hematologic findings. J Am Vet Med Assoc 1981;178:683–699.
Dubey JP, et al. Repeated transplacental transmission of *Neospora caninum* in dogs. J Am Vet Med Assoc 1990;197:857–860.
Dubey JP, Lindsay DS. Neosporosis – a newly recognized protozoan disease. J Vet Parasitol 1996;10:99–145.
Dubey JP, et al. Neosporosis in cats. Vet Pathol 1990;27:335–339.
Edwards JF, et al. Disseminated sarcocystosis in a cat with lymphosarcoma. J Am Vet Med Assoc 1988;193:831–832.
Faull WB, et al. Toxoplasmosis in a flock of sheep: some investigations into its source and control. Vet Rec 1986;119:491–493.
Frelier PF, et al. Bovine sarcocystosis: pathologic features of naturally occurring infection with *Sarcocystis cruzi*. Am J Vet Res 1979;40:651–657.
Gajadhar AA, Marquardt WC. Ultrastructural and transmission evidence of *Sarcocystis cruzi* associated with eosinophilic myositis in cattle. Can J Vet Res 1992;56:41–46.
Hadlow WJ. Diseases of skeletal muscle. In: Innes JRM, Saunders LZ, eds. Comparative Neuropathology. San Diego, CA: Academic Press, 1962:147–243.
Jensen R, et al. Eosinophilic myositis and muscular sarcocystosis in the carcasses of slaughtered cattle and lambs. Am J Vet Res 1986;47:587–593.
Kirkpatrick CE, et al. *Sarcocystis* sp. in muscles of domestic cats. Vet Pathol 1986;23:88–90.
LeCount AL, Zimmermann WJ. Trichinosis in mountain lions in Arizona. J Wildl Dis 1986;22:432–434.
Leek RG, et al. Sheep experimentally infected with *Sarcocystis* from dogs. I. Disease in young lambs. J Parasitol 1977;63:642–650.
Levine ND, Tadros W. Named species and hosts of *Sarcocystis* (protozoa: Apicomplexa: Sarcocystidae). Syst Parasitol 1981;2:41–59.
Lindberg R, et al. Canine trichinosis with signs of neuromuscular disease. J Small Anim Pract 1991;32:194–197.
Lindsay DS, Dubey JP. Immunohistochemical diagnosis of *Neospora caninum* in tissue sections. Am J Vet Res 1989;50:1981–1983.
McIntosh A, Miller D. Bovine cysticercosis, with special reference to the early developmental stages of *Taenia saginata*. Am J Vet Res 1960;21:169–177.
McManus D. Prenatal infection of calves with *Cysticercus bovis*. Vet Rec 1960;72:847–848.
O'Toole D. Experimental ovine sarcocystosis: sequential ultrastructural pathology in skeletal muscle. J Comp Path 1987;97:57–60.
Panciera RJ, et al. Comparison of tissue stages of *Hepatozoon americanum* in the dog using immunohistochemical and routine histologic methods. Vet Pathol 2001;38:422–426.
Pozio E. New patterns of *Trichinella* infection. Vet Parasitol 2001;98:133–148.
Savini G, et al. Sensitivities and specificities of two ELISA tests for detecting infection with *Sarcocystis* in cattle of Western Australia. Prevent Vet Med 1997; 32:35–40.
Schad GA, et al. *Trichinella spiralis* in the black bear (*Ursus americanus*) of Pennsylvania: distribution, prevalence and intensity of infection. J Wildl Dis 1986;22:36–41.
Tenter AM. Current research on *Sarcocystis* species of domestic animals. Int J Parasitol 1995; 25:1311–1130.
Tinling SP, et al. A light and electron microscopic study of sarcocysts in a horse. J Parasitol 1980;66:458–465.
Traub-Dargatz JL, et al. Multifocal myositis associated with *Sarcocystis* sp. in a horse. J Am Vet Med Assoc 1994;205:1574–1576.

NEOPLASTIC DISEASES OF MUSCLE

Primary tumors of striated muscle are uncommon in domestic animals and include tumors of cardiac as well as of skeletal muscle. Myogenic tumors do not arise from fully differentiated muscle fibers and rarely arise from satellite cells. *In most cases, myogenic tumors are thought to originate from uncommitted pluripotential mesenchymal stem cells,* which can also give rise to mixed tumors containing myogenic elements as well as neurogenic, epithelial, or other mesenchymal elements. Such mixed tumors are quite rare in animals.

The cell types encountered in tumors of skeletal muscle reflect the developmental stages of embryonic and regenerating muscle. That is, *tumor cell morphology varies from a round cell resembling a satellite cell or myoblast, to spindle cell, to multinucleate cell.* Historically, the *diagnosis of skeletal muscle tumors has relied heavily on the identification of cross striations within tumor cells.* Cross striations may be identified in elongate multinucleate cells with central chains of nuclei, the so-called "strap cells," or in ovoid cells such as the so-called "racquet cells." Cross striations may be more readily identified following staining with phosphotungstic acid hematoxylin (*PTAH*). Cells with such cross striations are often rare or nonexistent within skeletal muscle tumors, and this approach is time consuming and often frustrating. Identification of primitive sarcomeric structures such as filaments arranged in parallel with associated electron dense Z bands by *electron microscopy* has been somewhat more rewarding. More recently, given the specificity of myogenic markers and relative ease of immunohistochemical identification of muscle tumors, *immunohistochemistry has largely replaced electron microscopy and PTAH staining. Desmin and muscle actin* are proteins expressed early in skeletal muscle differentiation and are expressed by many or most skeletal muscle tumor cells. Desmin will often highlight cross striations in skeletal muscle tumors far better than PTAH stain. These markers will not, however, differentiate tumors of skeletal and cardiac muscle origin from tumors of smooth muscle origin. *Myoglobin and sarcomeric actin* are specific markers of striated muscle differentiation that are expressed later in myocyte differentiation. Typically, fewer tumor cells will express these proteins, and often only the most differentiated skeletal muscle tumor cells will express myoglobin.

When evaluating tumors involving skeletal muscle, *be aware that nonmyogenic tumors infiltrating or metastatic to skeletal muscle can cause extensive damage and bizarre regenerative fibers that often mimic neoplastic cells.* This is especially true of tumors with extensive sclerosis. These bizarre cells should not be mistaken for tumor cells. Entrapped skeletal muscle fibers within a nonmyogenic tumor will also stain with immunohistochemical markers for skeletal muscle and can cause confusion.

Both benign (rhabdomyoma) and malignant (rhabdomyosarcoma) skeletal muscle tumors occur in domestic animals. As in people, rhabdomyoma and rhabdomyosarcoma often occur in young animals. Classification of these tumors, particularly rhabdomyosarcoma, has been difficult and often confusing. The classification presented here is based on the current scheme of classification of myogenic tumors in people.

Rhabdomyoma

Benign tumors of striated muscle origin are most common in the *heart of pigs* and involving the *larynx of dogs*. In pigs, the red wattle pig breed appears to be predisposed. Rare cases of cardiac rhabdomyoma have also occurred in sheep, cattle, and dogs. Females may be predisposed. **Cardiac rhabdomyomas** *are incidental findings* most often involving the left ventricular wall. Tumors can also occur in the septum, and least commonly involve the right ventricular wall. These lesions are present in young animals, and current opinion suggests that they are *most likely hamartomas or dysplastic lesions rather than true neoplasms*. These lesions occur as smooth-surfaced nodular masses up to about 3 cm diameter embedded in the myocardium. These lesions are circumscribed but nonencapsulated, and are formed by *large vacuolated myocytes with pale eosinophilic cytoplasm*. Mitoses are not seen.

Laryngeal rhabdomyomas have been reported in dogs from 2 to 10 years of age. Tumors most often occur as nodular masses protruding into the lumen of the larynx, resulting in clinical signs of dyspnea, stridor, or altered bark. One tumor occurred in the laryngeal pharynx. *Laryngeal rhabdomyoma cells are large, round, and moderately pleomorphic, and contain abundant vacuolated to granular eosinophilic cytoplasm* (Fig. 2.111). Scattered multinucleate and elongate strap cells may be seen. Intracytoplasmic glycogen may be revealed by PAS staining. Ultrastructural features include numerous mitochondria, and these tumors were initially misdiagnosed as laryngeal oncocytomas. Ultrastructural identification of *primitive myofilaments and Z band type material* (Fig. 2.112), and *positive immunostaining for skeletal muscle markers* (Fig. 2.113), has confirmed the striated muscle origin of these tumors. Although there are reports of invasive tumors classified as laryngeal rhabdomyosarcoma, *these tumors typically exhibit minimal invasion and mitotic figures, metastasis has not been seen*, and the vast majority of these tumors are thought to be benign and cured by wide surgical excision.

Rhabdomyoma is rare in other sites and other species. Rhabdomyoma of the *skin* has been reported to occur on the convex surface of the pinna in four white cats aged 6–7 years. Rarely, rhabdomyoma occurs in the skin of the trunk or legs. A cystic rhabdomyoma attached to the *diaphragm* by a stalk has been reported in the mediastinum of a 2-year-old filly.

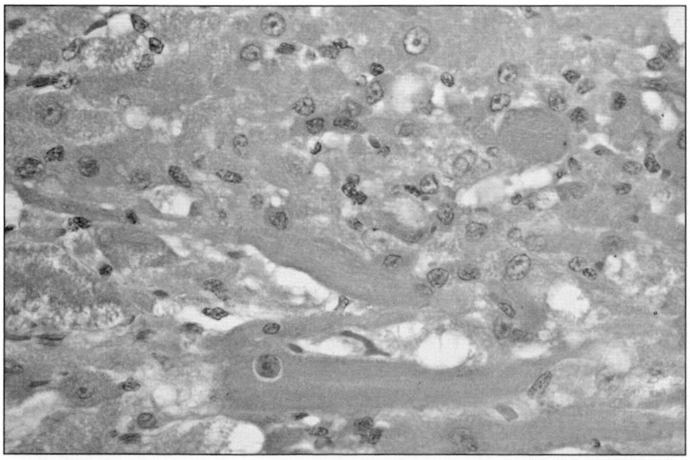

Figure 2.111 Canine **laryngeal rhabdomyoma** with characteristic moderately pleomorphic plump round-to-elongate cells with euchromatic nuclei. (Courtesy of BJ Cooper.)

Rhabdomyosarcoma

Rhabdomyosarcomas are most often fleshy growths that may form within skeletal muscle or grow into the lumen of tubular organs of the urogenital tract. Growth is often rapid, resulting in central areas of hemorrhage and necrosis.

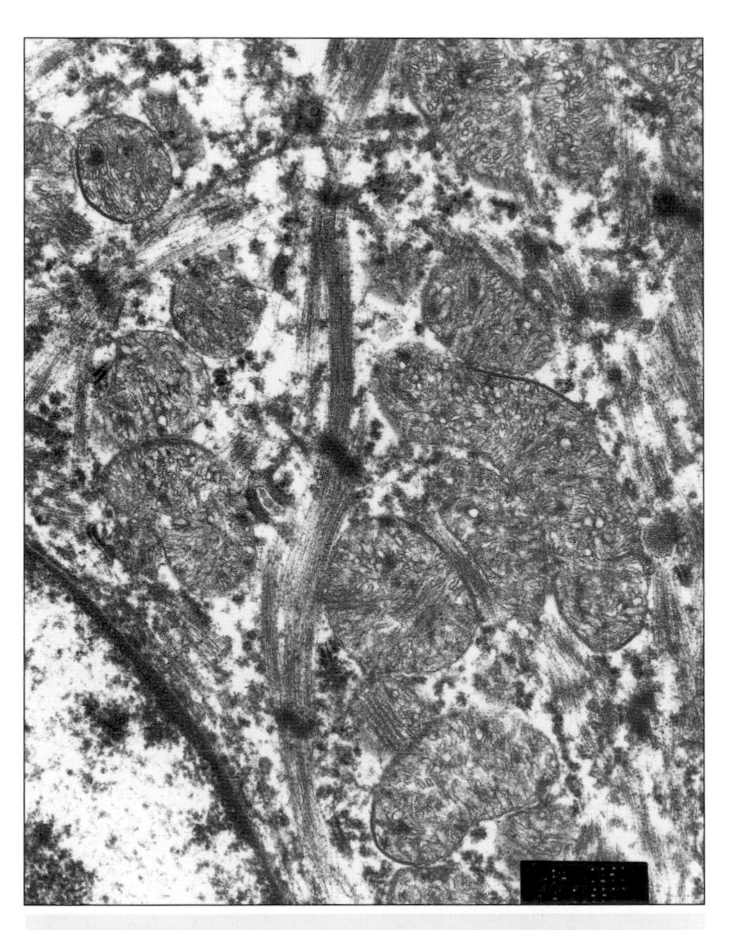

Figure 2.112 Ultrastructural features of canine **laryngeal rhabdomyoma** demonstrating characteristic Z-band type material and associated myofilaments. Mitochondria are also prominent. (Courtesy of DJ Meuten.)

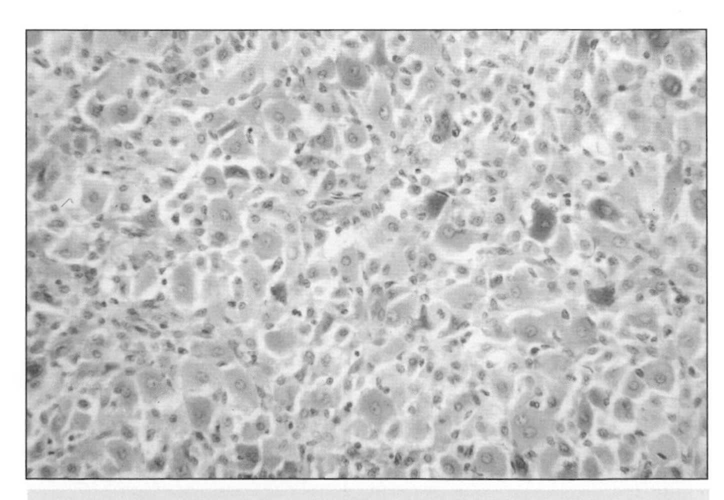

Figure 2.113 Positive myoglobin immunostaining of the cytoplasm of many cells of a canine **laryngeal rhabdomyoma**. (Courtesy of BJ Cooper.)

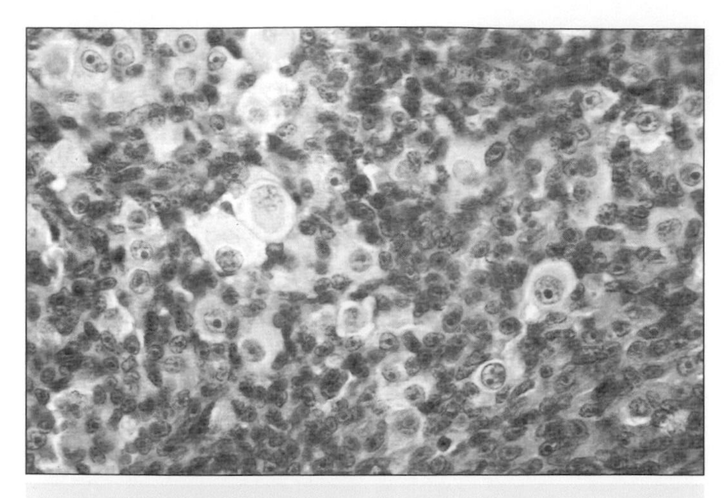

Figure 2.114 Admixed small basophilic cells and larger rhabdomyoblast cells in a feline **embryonal rhabdomyosarcoma**. (From McGavin MD, Zachary JF. Pathologic Basis of Veterinary Disease, 2006, with permission of Elsevier Ltd.)

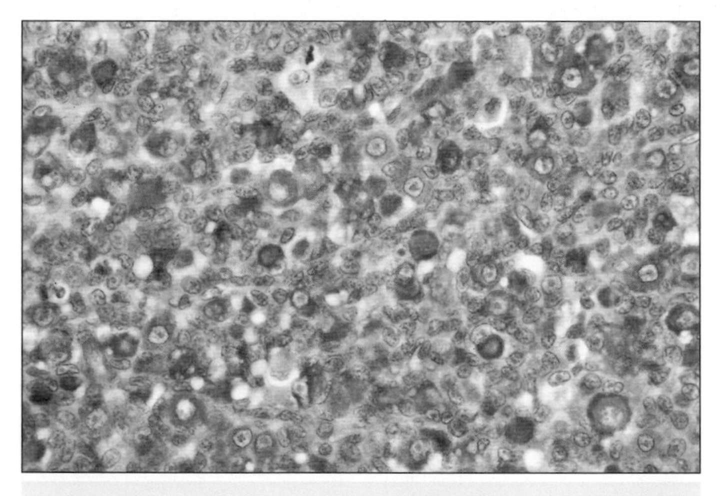

Figure 2.115 Positive immunostaining for desmin in rhabdomyoblast cells of a feline **embryoneal rhabdomyosarcoma**. (From McGavin MD, Zachary JF. Pathologic Basis of Veterinary Disease, 2006, with permission of Elsevier Ltd.)

Rhabdomyosarcoma in people has been classified histologically as *embryonal* rhabdomyosarcoma, *alveolar* rhabdomyosarcoma, and *pleomorphic* rhabdomyosarcoma. *Botryoid* rhabdomyosarcoma, a tumor most common in the urogenital tract, is considered a variant of embryonal rhabdomyosarcoma. *Embryonal rhabdomyosarcoma, and the botryoid variant, are the most common forms in people and, it would appear, in animals.* The alveolar variant is less common in both people and animals, and pleomorphic rhabdomyosarcoma, often thought to be the most classic and most common form, is actually the least common tumor. A review of the veterinary literature revealed that most tumors designated as pleomorphic variants actually had histologic features warranting designation as embryonal rhabdomyosarcoma.

Embryonal rhabdomyosarcoma is composed of primitive cells that may be either round and myoblast-like, or elongate and myotube-like ("strap cells"), and can be binucleate or multinucleate. Tumors may consist entirely of one cell type or may contain a mixture of these cell types. Embryonal rhabdomyosarcoma occurs most commonly in *young animals* and often *involves the head or neck, including the oral cavity*, although occurrence at other sites is possible. The round cell form is the most common, and embryonal rhabdomyosarcoma should be considered in the differential of any nonhistiocytic and nonlymphoid round-cell tumor of the head or neck of a young animal. The *round cell embryonal rhabdomyosarcomas* consist either of small cells with large central euchromatic nuclei, often with a single prominent nucleolus, and indistinct cytoplasm, or of larger round cells with similar nuclei and prominent eosinophilic cytoplasm (*rhabdomyoblast cells*); there is often an admixture of these two cell types (Fig. 2.114). Muscle markers are most often expressed by the larger rhabdomyoblast cells (Fig. 2.115). Scattered cells may have prominent cytoplasmic vacuolation resulting in a "spider-web" cell. The *botryoid variant* – a "grape-like" tumor – occurs most often in the trigone area of the urinary bladder in young large breed dogs. In these tumors the cells consist of elongate multinucleate myotube-like cells, often in a myxoid stroma (Fig. 2.116A, B). A similar embryonal rhabdomyosarcoma with prominent myxoid stroma can occur at subcutaneous sites and can be misdiagnosed as myxosarcoma. Although embryonal rhabdomyosarcoma is most common in dogs, this type of tumor also occurs in cats, sheep, cattle, pigs, and horses.

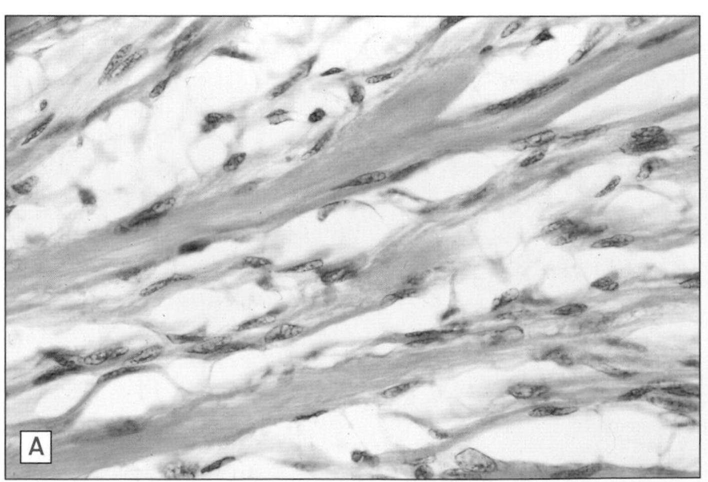

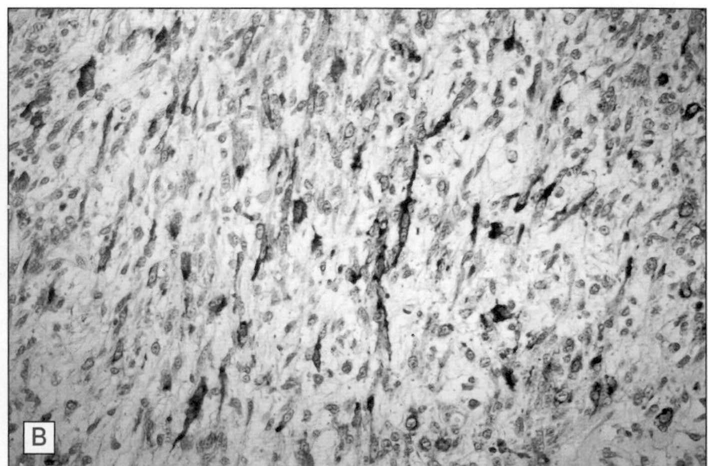

Figure 2.116 Urinary bladder embryonal rhabdomyosarcoma in the trigone of a 1-year-old large breed dog. **A.** Characteristic elongate myotubes. (From McGavin MD, Zachary JF. Pathologic Basis of Veterinary Disease, 2006, with permission of Elsevier Ltd.) **B.** Positive immunostaining for desmin. (Courtesy of BJ Cooper.)

Embryonal rhabdomyosarcoma in all species often occurs in young to young-adult individuals. There appears to be a female predominance, especially for the botryoid variant in the urogenital tract. Cytogenetic abnormalities are commonly associated with childhood rhabdomyosarcomas in people, and a similar situation has been seen in pigs in which a cluster of rhabdomyosarcomas in young pigs was found to have a *genetic basis*.

Alveolar rhabdomyosarcoma is also a tumor of adolescent and young adult people. This tumor consists of sheets of uniformly small, undifferentiated round cells in which tumor cells are supported on a fibrous framework and often *form alveolar-like structures due to loss of cohesiveness in the center of cell nests*. Multinucleate cells can be seen, but cross-striations are rare. A *solid alveolar pattern* is also possible, with sheets of small, undifferentiated round cells that resemble embryonal rhabdomyosarcoma but that lack any differentiation towards the larger eosinophilic rhabdomyoblast cells (Fig. 2.117). This form of rhabdomyosarcoma has been seen in dogs, horses, and a cow.

Virtually all rhabdomyosarcomas exhibit some degree of cellular pleomorphism. Pleomorphic rhabdomyosarcoma is often diagnosed, however *only tumors lacking any areas with features of embryonal or alveolar rhabdomyosarcoma should be designated as pleomorphic variants*. In people, pleomorphic rhabdomyosarcoma is a tumor of adults, most often occurring in major muscle groups such as the muscles of the thigh. Pleomorphic rhabdomyosarcoma has been seen arising in the neck muscle of a 3-year-old dog and in the tongue of a 5-year-old horse. Pleomorphic rhabdomyosarcoma consists of plump spindle cells in a haphazard arrangement that may be admixed with scattered multinucleate cells, strap cells, racket cells, and large, round rhabdomyoblasts (Fig. 2.118A, B).

Cardiac rhabdomyosarcomas occur, but are rare, with all cases to date reported in dogs. The age range of affected dogs was 14 months to 7 years. Clinical signs of cardiac failure can occur, although one tumor was found as an incidental finding. Histologic features of poor differentiation, cellular pleomorphism, mitotic activity, and local invasion warrant the diagnosis of rhabdomyosarcoma rather than rhabdomyoma.

The behavior of rhabdomyosarcoma in animals parallels that of humans, in which aggressive local invasion and frequent metastasis are seen. Although the data regarding pattern of metastasis is scanty in animals, metastasis to atypical sites such as to other skeletal muscle sites, to cardiac muscle, and to spinal cord have been seen.

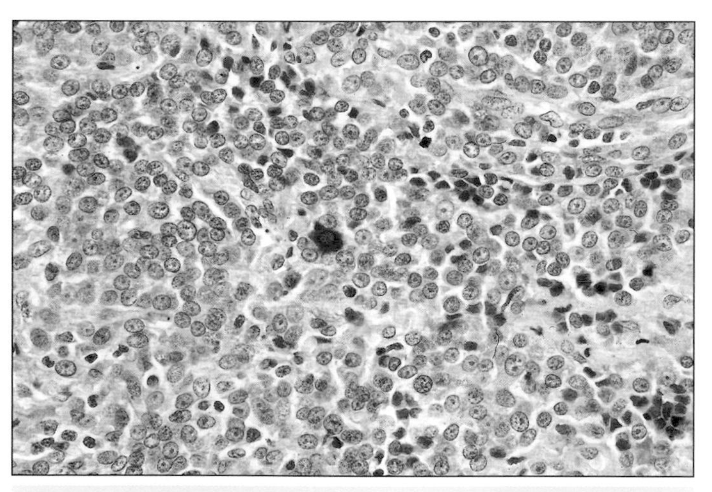

Figure 2.117 Solid sheets of undifferentiated small cells with focal intense cytoplasmic staining for myoglobin in a **solid alveolar rhabdomyosarcoma** in the hip muscle of a 7-year-old dog. (Courtesy of BJ Cooper.)

Nonmuscle primary tumors of muscle

These tumors arise from supporting mesenchymal tissues of muscle. Malignant tumors are far more common than benign tumors.

- *Poorly differentiated sarcomas* and *giant cell sarcomas* occur within muscle, especially at the site of intramuscular vaccinations in predisposed cats. These tumors may be mistaken for rhabdomyosarcoma but rarely express skeletal muscle cell markers, and are most often variants of fibrosarcoma.
- *Hemangiosarcoma* arising within skeletal muscle occurs most frequently in the dog and in the horse (Fig. 2.119). Due to the large amount of hemorrhage and scanty tumor cells, these tumors are often difficult to diagnose from biopsy specimens. Intramuscular hemangiosarcoma is often mistaken clinically for intramuscular hematoma. Intramuscular hemangiosarcoma is an aggressive tumor, exhibiting both local invasion and distant metastasis, such as to lung.

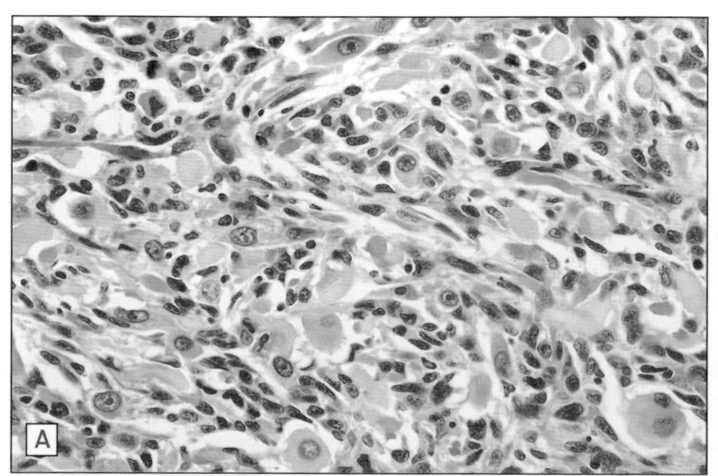

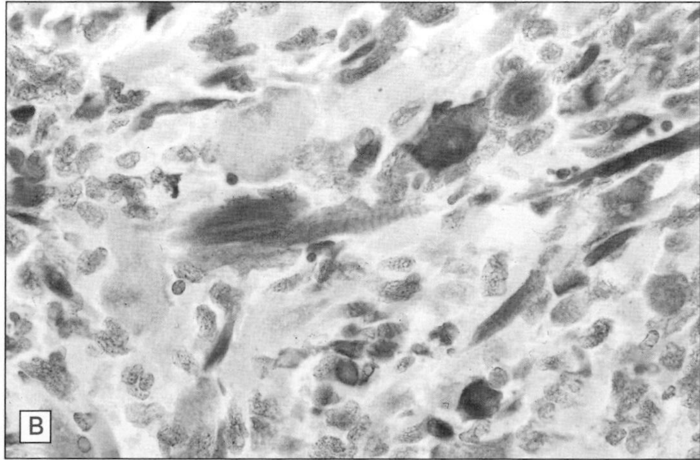

Figure 2.118 Pleomorphic rhabdomyosarcoma in the neck muscle of a 3-year-old dog. **A.** Characteristic mixed plump and pleomorphic spindle cells and round-to-ovoid cells. **B.** Positive immunostaining for desmin that highlights cross striations in spindle cells and in round-to-ovoid cells. (Courtesy of BJ Cooper.)

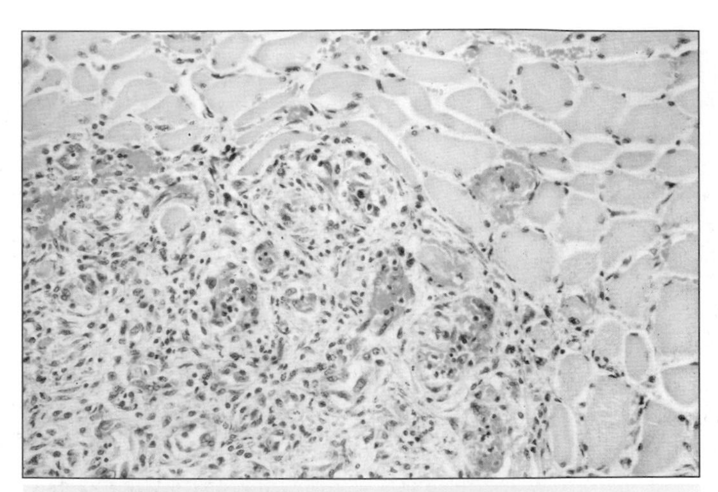

Figure 2.119 Proliferating invasive neoplastic endothelial cells forming irregular vascular channels typical of **hemangiosarcoma** within the skeletal muscle of an adult horse.

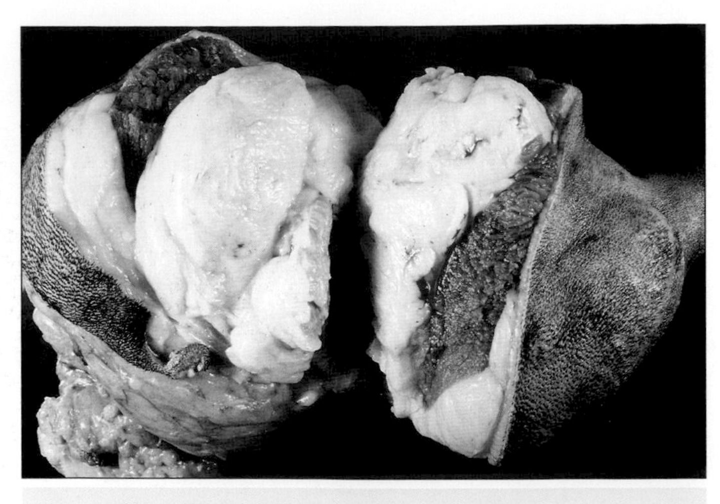

Figure 2.121 **Infiltrative lipoma** invasive into skeletal muscle of an adult dog. (Courtesy of BJ Cooper.)

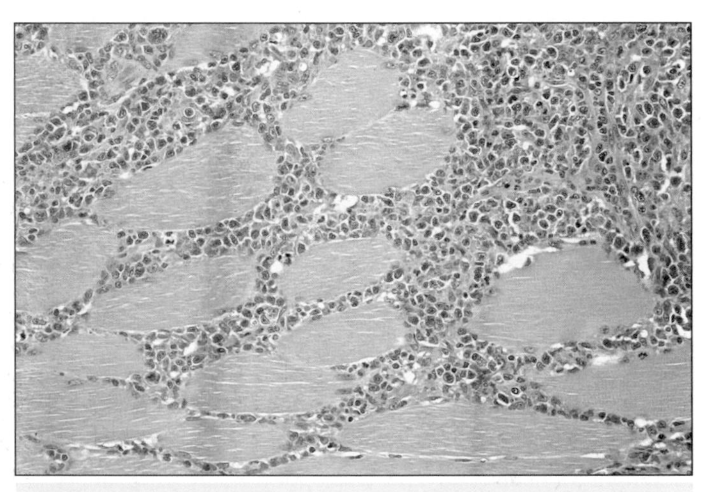

Figure 2.120 Intramuscular invasion of **lymphoma** in an adult cat.

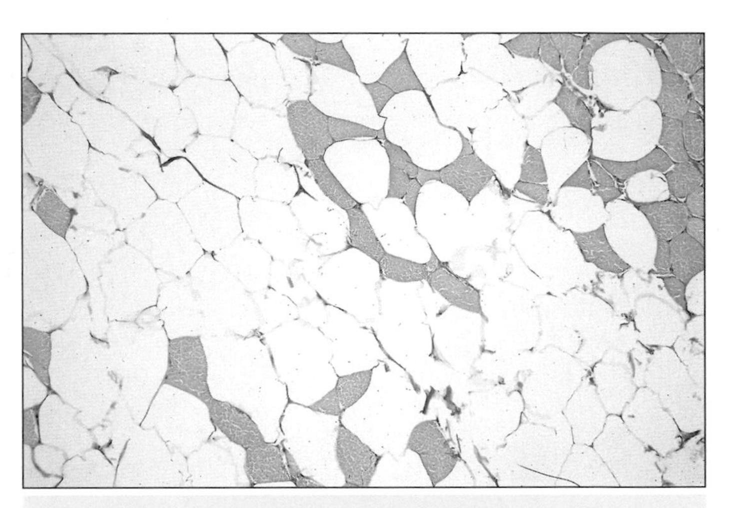

Figure 2.122 Invasion of skeletal muscle by mature adipose tissue typical of **infiltrative lipoma** in an adult dog. (Courtesy of BJ Cooper.)

- *Nerve sheath neoplasms* can arise from major nerve trunks within skeletal muscle but are typically localized to intramuscular nerves without infiltration of adjacent muscle.
- *Granular cell tumor* ("myoblastoma") is a tumor that can occur in the musculature of the tongue of dogs and cats and, rarely, within cardiac muscle. Granular cell tumor consists of closely packed round cells with prominent intracytoplasmic PAS-positive, amylase-resistant granules. Ultrastructurally, these granules consist of secondary lysosomes. Although previously thought to be of skeletal muscle origin, more recent studies have refuted this theory, and granular cell tumor appears to be most often a tumor of Schwann cell origin.
- *Malignant lymphoma* may occur within skeletal muscle, but whether this represents primary intramuscular tumor or local or metastatic spread is not always certain. Infiltration of skeletal muscle by neoplastic lymphocytes must be distinguished from lymphocytic infiltration due to immune-mediated myositis. Lymphoma cells are typically relatively homogeneous and often atypical, and surround myofibers and efface skeletal muscle architecture without obvious myofiber necrosis or "coring out" of myofibers (Fig. 2.120).

Secondary tumors of skeletal muscle

The *infiltrative variant of lipoma* arising within the subcutis is characterized by prominent intramuscular invasion (Figs 2.121, 2.122). This tumor, although locally invasive, does not metastasize, and wide surgical excision is generally curative. Infiltrative lipoma occurs most often in dogs and horses. Although uncommon, *subcutaneous mast cell tumors* can invade underlying skeletal muscle. *Other soft tissue sarcomas* arising in the subcutis, such as fibrosarcoma and hemangiopericytoma, can also extend into adjacent skeletal muscle. *Carcinomas,* such as squamous cell carcinoma, are often seen invading and destroying adjacent skeletal muscle.

In general, tumor metastasis to skeletal muscle is less common than metastasis to other organs. There is evidence to suggest that tumor cells in skeletal muscle microvasculature are destroyed at a higher rate than tumor cells within other organs, such as liver. Dermal melanoma of older gray horses often metastasizes to the muscle fascia, but less commonly involves the muscle itself. Skeletal muscle metastasis of canine prostatic carcinoma can result in foci of intramuscular fibroplasia, sometimes with associated chondroid differentiation, that can mimic focal or multifocal myositis ossificans (see Physical injuries

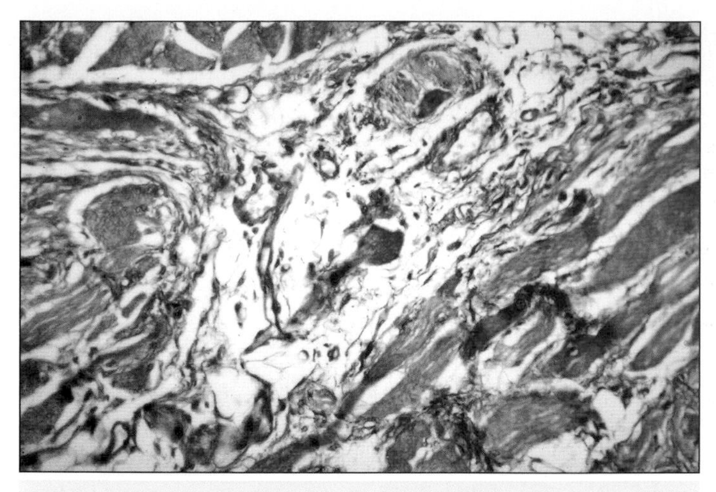

Figure 2.123 Irregular myofiber orientation with associated endomysial fibrosis in a **muscle pseudotumor** from a Great Dane dog. Masson trichrome stain.

of muscle). Diaphragmatic muscle is often a site of intraabdominal or intrathoracic tumor spread by "seeding."

Muscle pseudotumors

Muscle pseudotumors include a group of reactive lesions that can mimic neoplasia. *Localized myositis ossificans* and *musculoaponeurotic fibromatosis* qualify as muscle pseudotumors but are discussed in the sections Physical injuries of muscle and Tendons and aponeuroses, respectively. An *unusual muscle pseudotumor* has been seen in two dogs, both Great Danes, in which a localized swelling in the dorsal scapular area was found to be associated with skeletal muscle. These lesions were composed of irregularly arranged mature skeletal muscle fibers with marked cytoarchitectural alterations and associated endomysial fibrosis (Fig. 2.123). Muscle pseudotumors in man are most often thought to be *associated with muscle trauma*, and a similar etiology seems logical for animals.

Bibliography

Andreasen CB, et al. Desmin as a marker for canine botryoid rhabdomyosarcomas. J Comp Pathol 1988;98:23–29.

Bergman PJ, et al. Infiltrative lipoma in dogs: 16 cases (1981–1992). J Am Vet Med Assoc 1994; 205:322–324.

Blomqvist G, et al. Differences in lodgement of tumour cells in muscle and liver. Clin Expl Metastasis 1988;6:285–289.

Brown PJ. Immunohistochemical localization of myoglobin in connective tissue tumors in dogs. Vet Pathol 1987;24:573–574.

Bundza A, Greig AS. Cytological, cytochemical, light and ultrastructural studies of a bovine rhabdomyosarcoma. Bov Prac 1981;2:24–27.

Carter RL, et al. Comparative phenotypes in rhabdomyosarcomas and developing skeletal muscle. Histopathology 1990;17:301–309.

Clegg PD, Coumbe A. Alveolar rhabdomyosarcoma: an unusual cause of lameness in a pony. Eq Vet J 1993;25:547–549.

Cooper BJ, Valentine BA. Tumors of muscle. In: Meuten DJ, ed. Moulton's Tumors of Domestic Animals. Ames, IA: Iowa State University Press 2002:319–363.

Dallman MJ, et al. Feline lymphosarcoma with cutaneous and muscle lesions. J Am Vet Med Assoc 1982;181:166–168.

Enzinger FM, Weiss SW. Soft Tissue Tumors. 2nd ed. Washington, DC: CV Mosby Co. 1988.

Folpe AL, et al. Tenosynovial giant cell tumors: Evidence for a desmin-positive dendritic cell subpopulation. Mod Pathol 1998;11:939–944.

Gonin-Jmaa D, et al. Pericardial effusion in a dog with rhabdomyosarcoma in the right ventricular wall. J Small Anim Pract 1996;37:193–196.

Hanson PD, et al. Rhabdomyosarcoma of the tongue in a horse. J Am Vet Med Assoc 1993;202:1281–1284.

Hollowood K, Fletcher CDM. Rhabdomyosarcoma in adults. Sem Diagn Pathol 1994;11:47–57.

Kakulas BA. Muscle trauma. In: Mastaglia FL, Walton J, eds. Skeletal Muscle Pathology. New York: Churchill-Livingstone, 1982:599–602.

Kim DY, et al. Juvenile rhabdomyosarcomas in two dogs. Vet Pathol 1996;33:447–450.

Kramek BA, et al. Infiltrative lipoma in three dogs. J Am Vet Med Assoc 1985;186:81–82.

Ladds PW, Webster DR. Pharyngeal rhabdomyosarcoma in a dog. Vet Pathol 1971;8:256–259.

Lepage OM, et al. Infiltrative lipoma in a Quarter horse. Cornell Vet 1993; 83:57–60.

Madewell B, et al. Canine laryngeal rhabdomyosarcoma: an immunohistochemical and electron microscopic study. Jap J Vet Sci 1988;50:1079–1084.

Martín de las Mulas J, et al. Desmin and vimentin immunocharacterization of feline muscle tumors. Vet Pathol 1992;29:260–262.

Matsui T, et al. Bovine undifferentiated alveolar rhabdomyosarcoma and its differentiation in xenotransplanted tumors. Vet Pathol 1991;28:438–445.

McEwen BJE. Congenital cardiac rhabdomyomas in red wattle pigs. Can Vet J 1994;35:48–49.

Meuten DJ, et al. Canine laryngeal rhabdomyoma. Vet Pathol 1985;22:533–539.

Newton WA, Jr. Classification of rhabdomyosarcoma. In: Harms D, Schmidt D, eds. Current Topics in Pathology. Berlin, Springer-Verlag, 1995.

Patnaik AK. Histologic and immunohistochemical studies of granular cell tumors in seven dogs, three cats, one horse and one bird. Vet Pathol 1993;30:176–185.

Roth L. Rhabdomyoma of the ear pinna in four cats. J Comp Pathol 1990;103:237–240.

Sarnelli R, et al. Alveolar rhabdomyosarcoma of the greater omentum in a dog. Vet Pathol 1994;31:473–475.

Southwood LL, et al. Disseminated hemangiosarcoma in the horse: 35 cases. J Vet Intern Med 2000;14:105–109.

Tanaka K, Stromberg PC. Embryonal rhabdomyosarcoma in a sheep. Vet Pathol 1993;30:396–399.

Tanimoto T, Ohtsuki Y. The pathogenesis of so-called cardiac rhabdomyoma in swine: a histological, immunohistochemical and ultrastructural study. Virchows Arch 1995;427:213–221.

Turnquist SE, et al. Botryoid rhabdomyosarcoma of the urinary bladder in a filly. J Vet Diagn Invest 1993;5:451–453.

Tsokos M. The diagnosis and classification of childhood rhabdomyosarcoma. Sem Diagn Pathol 1994;11:26–38.

Vos JH, et al. Rhabdomyosarcomas in young pigs in a swine breeding farm: a morphologic and immunohistochemical study. Vet Pathol 1993; 30:271–279.

Yanoff SR, et al. Tracheal defect and embryonal rhabdomyosarcoma in a young dog. Can Vet J 1996;37:172–173.

Young HE, et al. Human reserve pluripotent mesenchymal stem cells are present in the connective tissues of skeletal muscle and dermis derived from fetal, adult and geriatric donors. Anat Record 2001;264:51–62.

Tendons and aponeuroses

GENERAL CONSIDERATIONS

Tendons are derived from the same pool of embryonic mesenchymal cells as muscle fibers and it is very likely that although commitment occurs early, the differentiation of myoblastic and tenoblastic cells occurs relatively late. In some tendons, notably the suspensory ligaments of the limbs of the foal, the first wave of differentiation is as a muscle and only subsequently does further development produce a tendon. As might be suspected, the two end products have many structural similarities. *The basic structural units of tendons are bundles of collagen that cluster around a central elongated collection of tendon fibroblasts or tenocytes and capillaries.* Multiples of these units combine to form *fascicles* somewhat like primary muscle bundles, and fascicles in turn combine in clusters to form the *complete tendon*, which is ensheathed by a looser fibrous tissue called the *peritenon*.

Tendons are quite completely, though sparsely, supplied with blood vessels but in keeping with low nutritional requirements once the tendon is formed, relatively wide distances may separate adjacent parallel vascular channels in mature animals. Segments of long tendons may appear to be almost avascular at times, if flow volume is used as an indicator of vascularity.

At birth, tendons are cellular and vascular, as tenoblasts or tenocytes elaborate the orderly, synchronously kinked, parallel collagen bundles. The kinking provides a mechanism for absorbing stretch impact and provides an interlocking adhesive strength for adjacent fibers, which is enhanced by the presence of an amorphous, noncollagen ground substance that acts as a "glue." The physical properties of tendons are largely dependent on cross-linking of collagen molecules.

TENDON AGING AND INJURY

As tendons age, they change color from pearly white to yellow-tan and may acquire an even darker brown or red-gray center. Some of these color changes are related to repeated minor episodes of capillary hemorrhage that occur even in normal, unworked horses or cattle. The distinction between normal and abnormal is often a difficult one to make, but *it is normal (in the sense of usual and harmless) for tendons to undergo focal cartilaginous metaplasia.* Osseous metaplasia in tendons, however, is distinctly pathologic.

An important issue in the process of tendon aging and injury relates to predisposing lesions. Cartilaginous metaplasia, ischemia, and local fibroblastic proliferations have been regarded as predisposing changes, but they are frequently found in normal animals. It now seems that preparatory events need not be postulated to explain most of the lesions seen. *The predilection sites for tendon damage are predictably those with anatomic weakness or that receive disproportionate stretch forces.* The subsequent changes relate to stretching of tendon collagen and vessels.

When a tendon is stretched beyond load capacity, fibrils are very likely to be pulled out of kink register and even if no fibrils break, the tendon will be subsequently weaker at that point. Such *stretch lesions* are usually accompanied by ruptured collagen as well, although it may be only microscopically detectable. The sequence of events that follows involves the rupture of capillaries, release of fibrin, stimulation of tenocytes and/or peritenon cells to form myofibroblasts, and the formation of scar collagen that in many ways resembles the original tendon. In the acute stages, this process makes the tendon swollen, warm, and painful; in the chronic stage, the tendon is larger and longer than normal. Original tendon is uniquely constructed entirely of type I collagen. *When tendon repairs, the mature scar will no longer consist only of type I collagen since 20–30% of the replacement tissue will be type III collagen, a form of fiber less able to withstand stretch forces than type I.* It is likely that alterations in the proportions of the component glycosaminoglycans (e.g., hyaluronic acid, dermatan sulfate, chondroitin sulfate) occur following injury and during repair. The differences between a minor sprain and incomplete or even complete tendon rupture are differences in quantity not form. In larger lesions, there is a greater chance for tendon necrosis and sequestration, and a greater chance for the formation of a fibrin clot that is not longitudinally oriented by tension. This may lead to misalignment of the scar fibrils, adhesions to adjacent sheaths, and irregular contours of the tendon. Since myofibroblastic scar tissue is capable of contracting as it matures, the result of tendon repair is not necessarily a longer tendon but, inevitably, a weaker tendon.

PARASITIC DISEASES OF TENDONS AND APONEUROSES

Nematodes of the family Onchocercidae make connective tissue, vessel walls, or tendons of cattle and horses their preferred habitat. Most of these, and especially those that live in tendons, belong to the genus *Onchocerca*, although not all *Onchocerca* parasites have an affinity for tendons. Three different parasites infect domesticated cattle, *Onchocerca gibsoni, O. gutturosa,* and *O. lienalis,* but full investigation may eventually increase the number. Three different parasites, *O. gutturosa, O. reticulata,* and *O. cervicalis* infect horses. *Onchocerca gibsoni* infects cattle in Africa, Asia, and Australia. *Onchocerca gutturosa* occurs in cattle and horses in North America, Africa, Australia, and Europe. *Onchocerca lienalis* is considered to be a separate species by some and synonymous with *O. gutturosa* by others; it is not as widespread as is *O. gutturosa,* but is seen in cattle in Australia and North America. *Onchocerca reticulata* infects horses in Europe and Asia, and *O. cervicalis* infects horses worldwide. The prevalence of onchocerciasis can be very high, ranging from 20–100% of the population in endemic areas, but *infection by these connective tissue parasites has been greatly reduced by widespread use of ivermectin as an anthelmintic.*

The adult worms, less than 1.0 mm thick and 50–80 cm long for the female, much shorter for the male, live in tendons, tendon sheaths, or connective tissues of the brisket or abdominal wall from which site they liberate *microfilariae* over long periods. The larvae make their way to skin where they are picked up by a blood-sucking parasite in which the next phase of development takes place.

Onchocerca gibsoni characteristically provokes and inhabits a "worm nodule" or "worm nest" on the *brisket or external surfaces of the hindlimbs* that may reach 3 cm in diameter. These fibrous lesions are important in the meat industry because the worms must be manually removed and this is time consuming if several dozen are present. The nodules may be palpable or moveable in the skin or they may be fixed to the dermis or ribs. Those in the flank are usually beneath the fascia lata and are not externally palpable. The adult worms inhabit fine tunnels in the discrete nodules of dense fibrous tissue where they form a tangled mass in a milky fluid. Female worms are just grossly visible but the smaller males are not. Sometimes old hemorrhages, or mineralized remnants of worms, are contained in the larger nodules, and microscopically many larvae may also be seen in the capsule as they exit, perhaps via lymphatic vessels. Microfilariae are rarely seen in lymph nodes or blood vessels, but these routes may be used to reach the skin where they collect in large numbers without stimulating a reaction. The intermediate blood-sucking host is probably a simulid or a culicoid insect.

Onchocerca gutturosa is most frequently located on the surface of the *ligamentum nuchae* of cattle adjacent to the thoracic vertebral spines and less frequently on the scapula, humerus, or femur. It is sometimes found in the horse. The adult worms, which are found in pairs, do not stimulate the formation of a nodule as is the case for *O. gibsoni*, but lie in loose connective tissue. They apparently cause no disease or reaction and in spite of their wide distribution around the world they are rarely dissected out or even detected. The intermediate hosts are not all known, but simulids can transfer the infestation.

Onchocerca lienalis lies in delicate tunnels in the gastrosplenic ligament and in the splenic capsule of cattle.

Adult worms of *Onchocerca cervicalis* live between the fibers of the ligamentum nuchae over the shoulder or neck of the horse or in loose connective tissues nearby. A second very similar parasite, *O. reticulata,* resides at a much lower level of frequency in the tissue around tendon sheaths adjacent to the carpus or suspensory ligaments or at the fetlock where a low-grade tissue reaction is initiated by the presence of adult worms. When the worms die, they mineralize and are engulfed by a poorly defined, dense, fibrous reaction. The infestation usually goes undetected and most horses are apparently asymptomatic. The long threadlike female worm is less than 1 mm thick but 50–70 cm long. Larvae are hatched from eggs prior to their release from the uterus, and they make their way through connective tissue to the skin where they presumably travel in the dermal lymph vessels. Larvae (microfilariae), which are about 4 μm wide and 200–250 μm long, tend to aggregate in certain skin regions, particularly the skin of the ventral abdominal midline, the inner thighs, and the eyelids. Living microfilariae seem to stimulate no reaction whatever, but dead larvae are capable of stimulating a response that involves lymphocytes and eosinophils. These local nodular responses may be seen in skin accompanied by pruritus, alopecia, and scaliness, and they may be seen histologically in areas where larvae are particularly numerous. Living larvae can be quite readily detected as loosely curled structures just under the epidermis and adjacent to adnexal skin structures in histological sections. Microfilariae of *O. cervicalis* and *O. reticularis* are transported to another horse by blood-sucking insects in which an obligatory stage of development occurs. Several different insects may be suitable hosts, but only *Culicoides* midges and mosquitoes of the *Anopheles* species have been confirmed in the role.

FIBROMATOUS DISORDERS OF TENDONS AND APONEUROSES

A number of degenerative disorders resulting in proliferation of fibrous, cartilaginous, and osseous tissue within tendons and aponeuroses are described in man and animals. Some such disorders are inherited, whereas others are acquired. For the most part, little is known regarding the pathogenesis of these processes.

Fibromatoses *are defined as progressive, infiltrative, nonmetastasizing fibroblastic lesions.* A variety of such disorders are recognized in humans, and a similar disorder occurs in the horse. These lesions, although considered nonneoplastic by most investigators, can exhibit marked local infiltration and distortion of affected muscle.

Musculoaponeurotic fibromatosis (desmoid tumor) of the horse

A peculiar progressive fibrosing disorder, **musculoaponeurotic fibromatosis (desmoid tumor)**, occurs in the horse. Although most cases involve the *pectoral region*, other sites are possible. Affected horses develop progressive distortion and induration of affected musculature due to proliferation of fibroblasts, myofibroblasts, and subsequent fibrosis dissecting between muscle fibers and fascicles that is often accompanied by foci of lymphocytic infiltration (Fig. 2.124). Although wide surgical excision may be curative, in most cases the extent of the lesion at diagnosis precludes effective surgical intervention. Studies of a small number of horses have revealed fluid-filled pockets of apparently sterile inflammation deep within the lesion, suggesting that this disorder in horses may be a peculiar response to trauma such as from an injection or ruptured bursa.

Fibrodysplasia ossificans progressiva (FOP)

Fibrodysplasia ossificans progressiva *(FOP) is a progressive fibrosing and ossifying lesion of tendons and muscle-associated aponeuroses that occurs in humans and cats.* This disorder was previously referred to as myositis ossificans progressiva, which is incorrect, as the disorder involves muscle-associated connective tissue and is not a primary myopathy (see Physical injuries of muscle). Fibrodysplasia ossificans progressiva in man is a devastating disease of children and young adults. Progressive fibrosis and ossification of muscle-associated connective tissue, including tendons and fascia, result in eventual incapacitation. This disorder is inherited as a dominant trait.

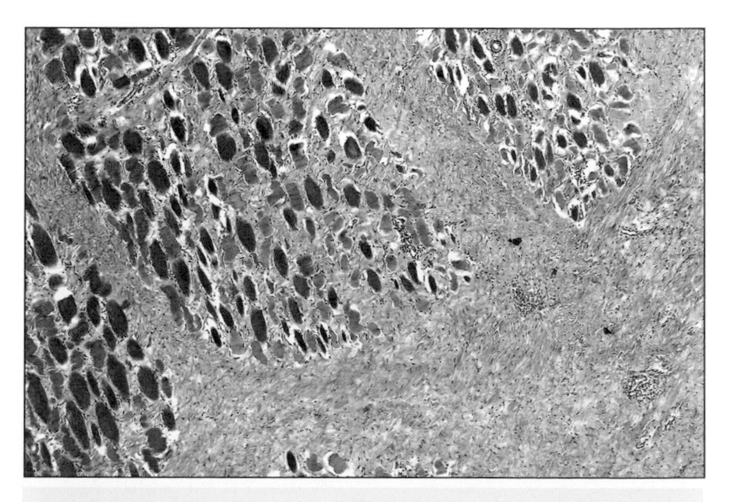

Figure 2.124 Perimysial and endomysial connective tissue dissecting between muscle bundles and myofibers in a horse with **musculoaponeurotic fibromatosis**. Foci of lymphocytes are also visible within the perimysial connective tissue. Masson trichrome stain. (Courtesy of BJ Cooper.)

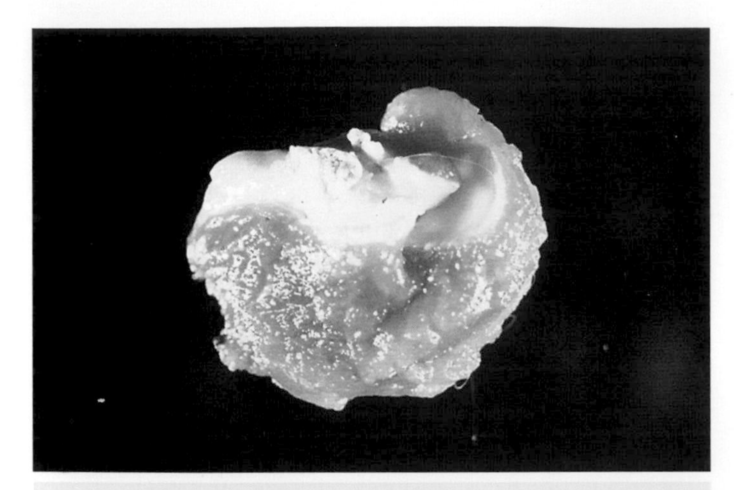

Figure 2.125 Marked thickening of the gastrocnemius muscle fascia of a young adult cat with fibrodysplasia ossificans progressiva. (Courtesy of L. Fuhrer.)

A similar disorder occurs sporadically in young to young-adult *cats*. Age at diagnosis in the cat has ranged from 10 months to 6 years. To date, inheritance of FOP has not been confirmed in the cat. Clinical signs include progressive stiffness of gait, decreased joint mobility, increased bulk and firmness of muscle, and pain upon handling. Radiography and gross pathology reveal *characteristic thickening with mineralization and ossification of muscle fascia* (Fig. 2.125). The histopathologic features are of fibroblastic proliferation within fascia with subsequent cartilage and bone formation. Early lesions may have an associated mild lymphoid infiltrate.

An inherited form of what was described as generalized myositis ossificans has been described in young *pigs*. The lesion in these pigs, however, was a proliferation of periosteal bone involving vertebrae, ribs, and tarsal bones, suggesting that this may be a primary bone disorder.

Bibliography

Baer E, et al. Hierarchical structure in polymeric materials. Science 1987;235:1015–1022.

Birch HL, et al. Age-related changes to the molecular and cellular components of equine flexor tendons. Equine Vet J 1999;31:391–396.

Goodship AE, et al. The pathobiology and repair of tendon and ligament injury. Vet Clin North Am Equine Pract 1994;10:323–349.

Kobayashi A, et al. Morphological and histochemical analysis of a case of superficial digital flexor tendon injury in the horse. J Comp Pathol 1999;120:403–414.

Lichtenfels JR. Helminths of domestic equids. Proc Helminth Soc Washington 1975;42:1–92.

McCullagh KG, et al. Tendon injuries and their treatment in the horse. Vet Rec 1979;105:54–57.

Michna H. Organisation of collagen fibrils in tendon: changes induced by an anabolic steroid. Virchows Arch [Cell Pathol] 1986;52:75–86.

Ottley ML, et al. Equine onchocerciasis in Queensland and Northern Territory of Australia. Aust Vet J 1983;60:200–203.

Scott DW. Parasitic diseases. In: Large Animal Dermatology. Philadelphia, PA: W.B. Saunders Co, 1988:255–259.

Seibold HR, Davis CL. Generalized myositis ossificans (familial) in pigs. Path Vet 1967;4:79–88.

Stannard AA, Cello RM. *Onchocerca cervicalis* infection in horses from the western United States. Am J Vet Res 1975;36:1029–1031.

Valentine BA, et al. Intramuscular desmoid tumor (musculoaponeurotic fibromatosis) in two horses. Vet Pathol 1999;36:468–470.

Valentine BA, et al. Fibrodysplasia ossificans progressiva in the cat. J Vet Intern Med 1992;6:335–340.

Webbon PM. A post mortem study of equine digital flexor tendons. Equine Vet J 1977;9:61–67.

3 Nervous system

M. Grant Maxie and Sameh Youssef

ACKNOWLEDGMENTS

We gratefully acknowledge the foundation laid for this chapter by previous authors, including Drs. Ken Jubb, Clive Huxtable, and Neil Sullivan. We also appreciate the useful suggestions made by Drs. Ron Slocombe and Murray Hazlett during the current revision.

CYTOPATHOLOGY OF NERVOUS TISSUE

Nervous tissue is highly specialized and structurally complex, and neuropathology has always tended to be set apart as an arcane specialist area, to be entered only by a select few. However, the veterinary pathologist cannot escape having to deal with it frequently, and we attempt in this section to provide a contemporary basis for understanding veterinary neuropathology.

The principal cells of the central nervous system (CNS) are *neurons* and *glia*, plus cells of the meninges and blood vessels. *Macroglia* (astrocytes, oligodendrocytes, ependymal cells) are of neuroectodermal origin; *microglia* are derived from bone marrow.

Neuron

The **neuron** *is the fundamental cell of the nervous system, and ultimately all neurologic disease must involve functional disturbances in neurons.* In conventional histopathology, the term "neuron" refers to the cell body of the nerve cell that often is only a small part of the total cell volume. For the purposes of comprehending pathogenetic mechanisms, it is important to remember always that the neuron comprises both the *cell body* ("soma" or "perikaryon") and the cell processes, in particular the *axon*. The whole cell constitutes a structure concerned with the generation, conduction, and transmission of impulses, and in some cases a single cell performs this task over a very long distance. For example, in a lumbar dorsal root ganglion of a horse, the cell body of a sensory neuron may project a process distally to the extremity of the hind foot and centrally to the caudal brain stem, making it without doubt the largest cell in the body. If the soma were enlarged to the size of an orange, the processes would have the dimensions of a garden hose and would be over 20 km in length. Pathologic reactions within one cell may therefore be separated by considerable distance. Also, neurons function in hierarchical chains organized into anatomic systems.

The soma is the metabolic factory for the whole cell and the great bulk of synthetic and degradative operations take place there. The axons are serviced throughout their length by a bidirectional transport system that moves components both away from and towards the soma (anterograde and retrograde transport respectively). The transport mechanisms are fuelled by the consumption of energy along the course of the axon. Many components are moved in the anterograde direction within 25 nm vesicles by a "fast" transport system at a rate of 20–30 mm/h. The motor for this system, intimately associated with the neurotubules, is an ATPase called *kinesin*. Larger vesicles of about 500 nm are transported retrograde by this fast pathway, and the translocator is an isoform of dynein, the ATPase which powers cilia and flagella in other types of cell. Mitochondria are also moved by fast transport, but at a somewhat slower rate. Neurofilaments, neurotubules, and some soluble proteins move by slow transport in the anterograde direction only, at a rate of about 1–3 mm/day, and are degraded when they reach the terminus. Should the operations of the soma or the transport systems be impaired, the health of the axon will suffer and, appropriately, in most instances the largest and longest axons are most vulnerable. Equally, *when a neuron is fatally damaged the whole cell dies*, and the consequent changes will spread over the whole extent of its domain. However, long lengths of the axon may degenerate without compromising the viability of the remainder of the cell and without inducing dramatic morphologic change in the soma, and there is often scope for adequate regeneration of the lost axonal extremity. These issues will be addressed more fully below, under *axonopathy*.

The vitality of individual neurons is sustained by their active relationship with other neurons, or other types of cells with which they interact. If a neuron dies, surviving neurons with which it has synaptic connections may regress due to lack of activation, undergo atrophy, and eventually die. This process is called *transynaptic degeneration* and it will progress along specific anatomic pathways. It is useful also to realize that neurons are extremely diverse pharmacologically and biochemically; this is well illustrated by the highly selective and regionalized effects of different toxins and metabolic disturbances. The selective effects of tetanus and botulinum toxins are good examples.

During organogenesis, vast numbers of neuroblasts proliferate and immature neurons migrate to their final destinations. As large numbers of developing neurons are superfluous, there is a need to select amongst them and eliminate the excess by apoptosis. Discrimination between those that will survive and those that are effete will depend on the transfer of trophic factors between cells including from glia to neurons. Around the time of birth, and for variable periods afterwards, the latter stages of the process may still be extant, particularly in the cerebellar cortex and paravertebral ganglia. It is probable that the signals between cells during growth and physiological activity are the same as those which if overloaded may lead to neuronal injury. The margin of safety between proper levels of transmitter and too little or too much is very narrow.

The mature neuron is a postmitotic cell and there is a net loss throughout adult life, especially during senescence. Thus in a thorough scan of a histologic section from a senile animal, it might be expected that a few degenerate neurons will be found, even when fixation artifacts are minimal. There is however continuous postnatal generation of neurons in some parts of the brain and in at least some species. In species so far examined, neuroblasts generated in the dentate gyrus of the hippocampus and from the progenitor cells of the subependymal zone between the lateral ventricle and the caudate continue to migrate postnatally to the olfactory bulb. These migrations do not depend on guidance from radial glia as in the embryonic brain. Rather the postnatal neuroblasts migrate in a chain designated as the "rostral migratory stream" strictly delineated by rows of astrocytes. There is evidence that new neurons are generated in the olfactory bulb. Axonotomy procedures that sever the pituitary stalk in the rat and some other mammalian species are known to be followed by re-establishment of functional hypothalamic–hypophyseal connections within a few weeks. Cells with neuron-like characters appear to migrate through the neuropil of the median eminence to congregate on its surface. The functional significance of these migrations and the dynamics of these populations are obscure. It is assumed that the olfactory migrants and their proliferation in situ in the bulb may have a bearing on the development of olfactory neuroblastomas.

Degenerative changes of the nerve cell body

Nuclear margination – the neuronal nucleus is usually single and centrally located (Fig. 3.1), and its *margination can be taken to indicate*

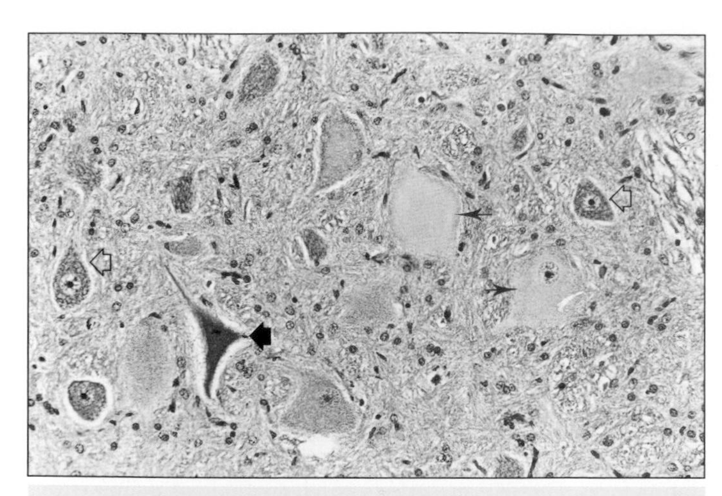

Figure 3.1 Red nucleus in swayback in a goat. Normal neurons (open arrows); **central chromatolysis** (arrows); shrunken, necrotic neuron (closed arrow).

nonspecific degeneration, especially when combined with loss of staining affinity. However, an eccentric nucleus can be normal in some groups of smaller neurons, and is often present in the large cells of the periventricular gray matter such as the mesencephalic nucleus of the trigeminal nerve and the olives. These cells also tend to have a "chromatolytic" appearance.

Chromatolysis is a change in appearance of the soma brought about by the *dispersal of the rough endoplasmic reticulum* (Nissl granules), and is subclassified as *central* or *peripheral* according to its locus within the cell body. Its assessment depends upon an appreciation of the prominence and distribution of Nissl granules seen normally at the particular location. There are no artifactual changes that mimic chromatolysis and, provided it is accurately identified, it can always be regarded as a lesion. A number of special stains, such as cresyl violet, will demonstrate it better than routine hematoxylin and eosin.

Central chromatolysis is best appreciated in large neurons of some of the brain stem nuclei, in the spinal motor neurons, and peripheral ganglia. The chromatolytic cells are swollen and rounded, rather than having the normal angulated appearance, and the nucleus becomes eccentric. Nissl granules clear from the central region of the cell body, leaving this zone with a smooth ground-glass appearance (Fig. 3.1). Central chromatolysis occurs in a number of pathologic situations. It is often seen in bulbo-spinal motor neurons and sensory neurons whose peripherally projecting axons are injured, and especially when the injury occurs close to the cell body. The reaction follows such injury quickly, beginning within 24 hours, and becoming maximal in 1–3 weeks. When the dynamics of axonal flow are remembered, it can be appreciated that such an event will have a major feedback on the soma. In effect, the cell must rearrange its metabolism to adapt to its changed circumstances, and organize for a regenerative effort, involving the reconstruction of an axonal segment greater in volume perhaps than its surviving volume. In this context, *central chromatolysis has been termed the* **axon reaction**, *and represents an anabolic adaptive response*. In this reaction, the nucleus becomes extremely eccentric, and develops a prominent nucleolus and a basophilic cap of RNA on its cytoplasmic aspect. The Nissl substance disperses, and the cytoplasm becomes rich in free ribosomes, lysosomes, and mitochondria. There may also be some increase in the number of neurofilaments. All these changes reflect a shift in metabolic activity, with a switch towards increased synthesis of structural cellular proteins, and a marked decline in synthesis of transmitters. With completion of successful axonal regeneration, the chromatolytic soma returns to normal, sometimes passing through a densely basophilic phase in which it is packed with Nissl granules.

In some circumstances following axonal injury, central chromatolysis may proceed to cell death or permanent atrophy, and this is usually the case in neurons whose axons project entirely within the central nervous system (CNS). *In general, the closer to the cell body the axonal lesion, the more likely is the cell to die*. Those cells destined to die have swollen achromatic cytoplasm depleted of organelles.

Central chromatolysis is also induced in more overtly neuronopathic conditions, most notably the numerous motor neuron degenerations described in various species, and it is a feature of the pathology of perinatal copper deficiency in the sheep and goat (Fig. 3.1). Similarly, it is a striking feature in autonomic ganglia in equine and feline dysautonomias. In all such cases, the affected cells often proceed to necrosis and dissolution (Gudden's atrophy). In many of these degenerative neuronopathies, the cytoplasmic alteration is due to massive accumulation of neurofilaments in the soma (see Progressive motor neuron diseases, p. 372). Nuclear margination is not as marked as in the axon reaction, and the prominent nucleolus and nuclear cap are not evident. These differences distinguish a regressive state from a regenerative one.

Peripheral chromatolysis indicates clearing of the periphery of the soma, with Nissl granules persisting around the nucleus. This change is generally associated with slight cellular shrinkage rather than swelling. It is a nonspecific lesion and can often be regarded as an early stage en route to necrosis.

In both forms of chromatolysis, microglia and astrocytes may proliferate and cover large expanses of the cell surface, thereby separating terminal boutons from the neuronal surface.

Neuronal atrophy – loss of cytoplasmic bulk and reduction in size (Fig. 3.2A) might be expected in situations of permanent loss of synaptic connections (see transynaptic degeneration above), as when central axons undergo Wallerian degeneration but fail to regenerate.

Ischemic necrosis – in this *characteristic acute degenerative change*, the cytoplasm of the neuronal soma becomes shrunken and distinctly acidophilic (Fig. 3.2B), and the nucleus progresses through pyknosis and rhexis to lysis, leaving the coagulated cytoplasmic remnants to undergo liquefaction without undergoing phagocytosis. The remnant "ghosts" may persist for several days. *The reaction is not confined to ischemia*, and may be seen in the cerebral cortex in hypoxia, hypoglycemia, the encephalopathy of thiamine deficiency, and in some chemical intoxications, such as organomercurialism and indirect salt poisoning. Following seizures, it may frequently be found in the dentate gyrus of the hippocampus and the cerebellar Purkinje cells. There are usually obvious proplastic changes in astrocytes and capillary endothelia in the vicinity of the affected neurons.

This raises the concept of **excitotoxicity**, in which neuronal degeneration and death are considered to result from excessive stimulus by an excitatory neurotransmitter. This phenomenon is thought to operate particularly in those neuronal systems utilizing glutamate as a transmitter, such as the cells in the hippocampal areas mentioned above. Paradoxically, glutamate is potentially highly toxic to neurons, and normally is rapidly cleared by the glia following its release. Excessive release or defective clearance of glutamate from the environment of postsynaptic neurons predisposes to excitotoxicity, and

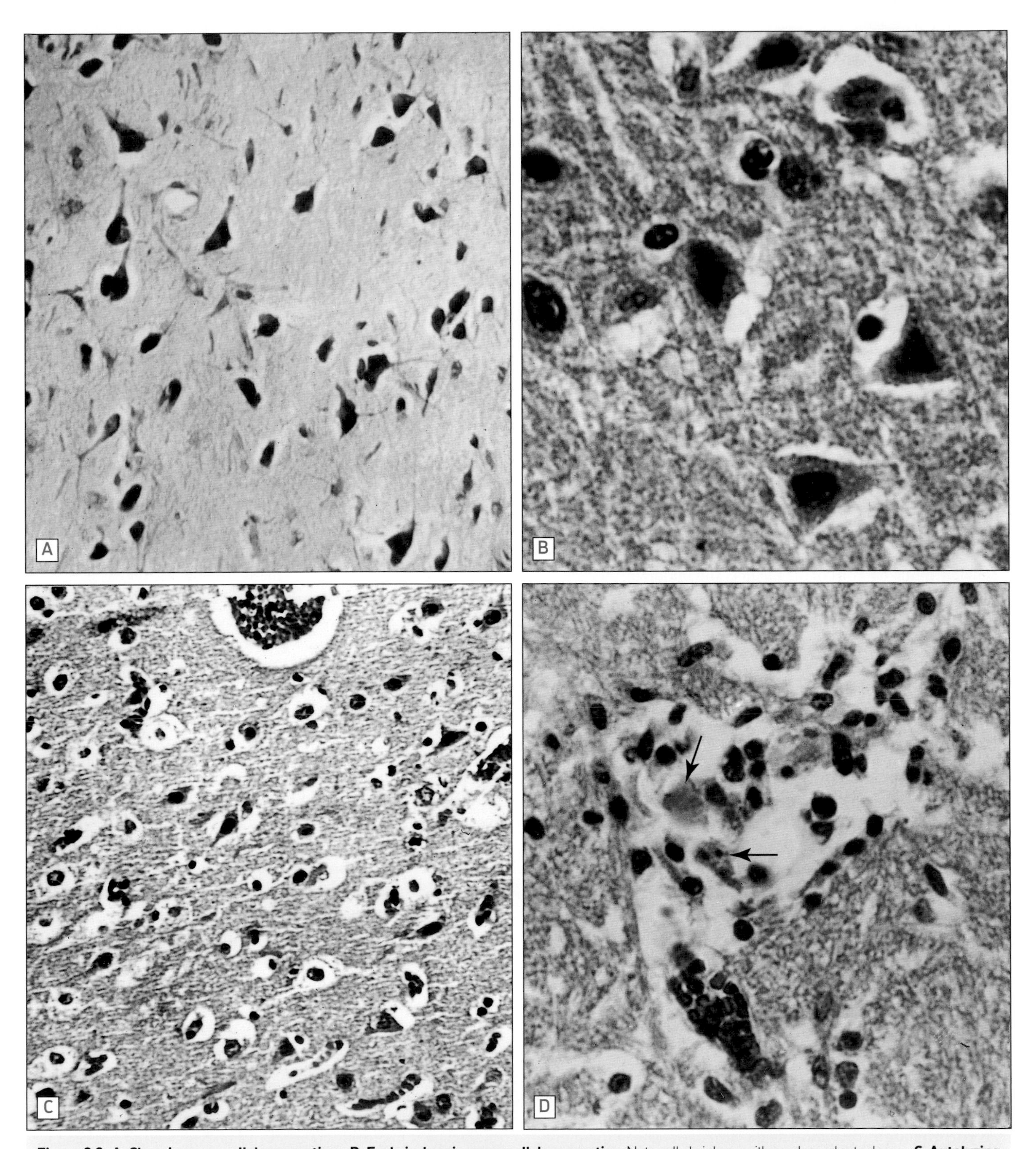

Figure 3.2 A. Chronic nerve cell degeneration. **B. Early ischemic nerve cell degeneration**. Note cell shrinkage with condensed cytoplasm. **C. Autolyzing cerebral cortex** easily misinterpreted as liquefactive necrosis. **D. Neuronophagic nodule** in equine encephalitis; fragmented neuron (arrows).

such circumstances are provided by hypoxia and hypoglycemia. The pathogenesis is thought to involve ionic overloading of the cell, acute swelling, and then cell death with cytoplasmic coagulation and eosinophilia.

Neuronal necrosis may occasionally be expressed as cytoplasmic shrinkage and basophilia with nuclear dissolution (Fig. 3.1). Shrunken basophilic neurons with normal nuclei ("*dark neurons*") are generally taken to be artifactual, and are often numerous.

Liquefactive necrosis is often at risk of being misinterpreted as autolytic change and fixation artifact, particularly shrinkage artifact (Fig. 3.2C). A lesion can sometimes be distinguished from an artifact by the presence or absence of significant alterations in other tissue cells, for instance the swelling of capillary endothelium or indications of glial proliferation.

Necrosis with neuronophagia – in many viral infections, the death of neurons provokes the gathering of phagocytes around the cell body (**satellitosis**), and removal by them of the debris, forming **neuronophagic nodules** (Fig. 3.2D). This is usually a response of the microglia, although satellite perineuronal oligodendrocytes may also proliferate in response to neuronal injury. Neuronophagia may also be seen in metabolic or toxigenic neuronal degenerations, but is generally not as extensive as in viral infection.

Vacuolar degeneration – neurons in the early stages of acute injury inflicted by viruses, toxins, or metabolic derangements, such as excitotoxicity, may develop numerous small cytoplasmic vacuoles, usually reflecting *mitochondrial swelling*. However, *artifactual peripheral vacuolation is very common*, giving the periphery of the cytoplasm a foamy web-like appearance. This is particularly so in the cerebellar Purkinje cells and large neurons of some of the brain stem nuclei.

Large neuronal vacuoles, few in number per cell, are occasionally observed in otherwise normal brains, and may be seen in the red and oculomotor nuclei of aged cattle and sheep. When they occur at high frequency in the neurons of the medulla and midbrain, they are virtually pathognomonic of *scrapie* in sheep and goats (Fig. 3.3). Widespread neuronal vacuolation with single or multiple large vacuoles, unexplained as to pathogenesis, is occasionally seen in dogs and cattle with progressive neurological dysfunction.

Vacuolar change is strikingly evident in those *lysosomal storage diseases* in which the stored material is extracted during processing, or is unstained by the routine methods. In these situations, the neuron can become dramatically bloated by the accumulation of myriad secondary lysosomes that displace the normal organelles and distend the soma with a foamy mass of apparently empty vacuoles. In most cases, the storage process involves other cell types inside and outside the nervous system, and is accompanied by additional neuropathological manifestations (see Storage diseases).

Storage of pigments and other materials – neurons may accumulate large quantities of **ceroid/lipofuscin** or other pigments, either as a consequence of aging, or in storage disorders involving such substances. The pathogenesis of the *ceroid/lipofuscinoses* remains unclear but, as is discussed elsewhere, there is a genetic basis in some instances, while in others unspecified environmental factors may be involved. The complex storage material accumulates as granules in a manner analogous to the other lysosomal storage diseases, although a clearly defined limiting membrane is not usually apparent ultrastructurally. When the process is intense, rusty-brown discoloration of the gray matter and ganglia may be evident grossly.

Neuromelanins may also accumulate excessively in those midbrain nuclei where they are usually present in modest amounts, and extensive neuromelanosis can occur in sheep chronically poisoned by *Phalaris* sp. In extreme cases, the gray matter and ganglia may have macroscopic green discoloration.

Siderotic pigmentation of neurons, in which the cells become encrusted with basophilic complexes of iron, calcium, and phosphorus, may be found near contusions and hemorrhages. It is not known, however, whether the iron is derived from the hemoglobin or from intracellular iron-containing respiratory enzymes. The neurons may be otherwise normal, or their degeneration may produce small lakes of basophilic deposit. The latter are common in the neonatal cerebellar cortex.

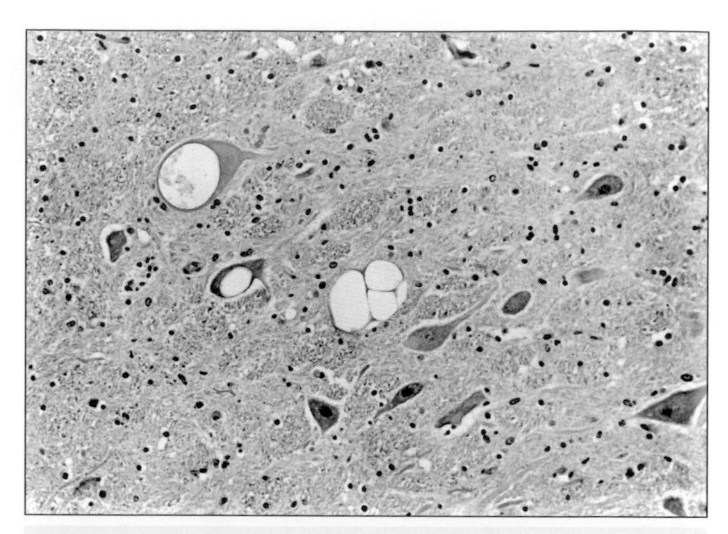

Figure 3.3 Neuronal vacuolation in scrapie in a sheep. (Courtesy of RF Slocombe.)

Viral inclusion bodies – the best known is the *Negri body* of rabies, which is eosinophilic and intracytoplasmic. Herpesvirus inclusions are characteristically intranuclear, while those of the paramyxoviruses such as *Canine distemper virus* may be intracytoplasmic or intranuclear. The use of specific immunostains has greatly facilitated the identification of viral inclusions.

Non-viral eosinophilic cytoplasmic inclusion bodies also occur. Sometimes they are an incidental finding in otherwise normal brains at sporadic locations; in cats, they can sometimes be found in the pyramidal cells of the hippocampus and lateral geniculate nuclei.

More specific inclusions have been described in people and animals in neuronal degenerative diseases. In humans, ultrastructural differences define several types of inclusion: **Hirano**, **Pick**, **Lewy**, **Lafora**, and **Bunina bodies**. *Hirano-like bodies*, appearing histologically as elongated eosinophilic inclusions and, ultrastructurally, as masses of beaded filaments, are reported in horses and dogs, together with other structures having some of the features of Bunina bodies. Further definition of these types of inclusions in animals is required, and their pathogenetic significance is not understood; they are a feature of equine motor neuron disease (Fig. 3.4). *Bunina bodies* are small eosinophilic inclusions of 2–5 μm, sometimes in small clusters or chains that characterize human *amyotrophic lateral sclerosis*; similar inclusions are occasionally observed in degenerative and inflammatory neurological disease in animals.

Lafora bodies are occasionally observed in neurological disease, but most frequently are incidental findings in aged animals. They are basophilic to amphophilic inclusions that are strongly PAS positive and metachromatic, 5–20 μm in size, intracytoplasmic or in processes or free in the neuropil (Fig. 3.5). They represent an abnormality of carbohydrate metabolism producing glucose polymers called *polyglucosans*. In the very rare *Lafora disease* (see Storage diseases), they occur in massive numbers throughout the brain within the neuronal soma, the dendrites, and less commonly the axons; they are associated with severe myoclonus epilepsy.

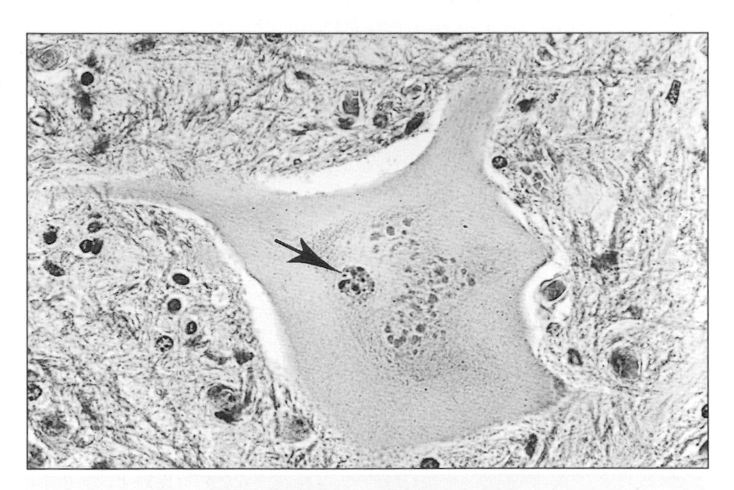

Figure 3.4 Spinal motor neuron in **motor neuron disease** in a horse. Chromatolysis, nuclear dissolution (arrow) and cytoplasmic inclusions.

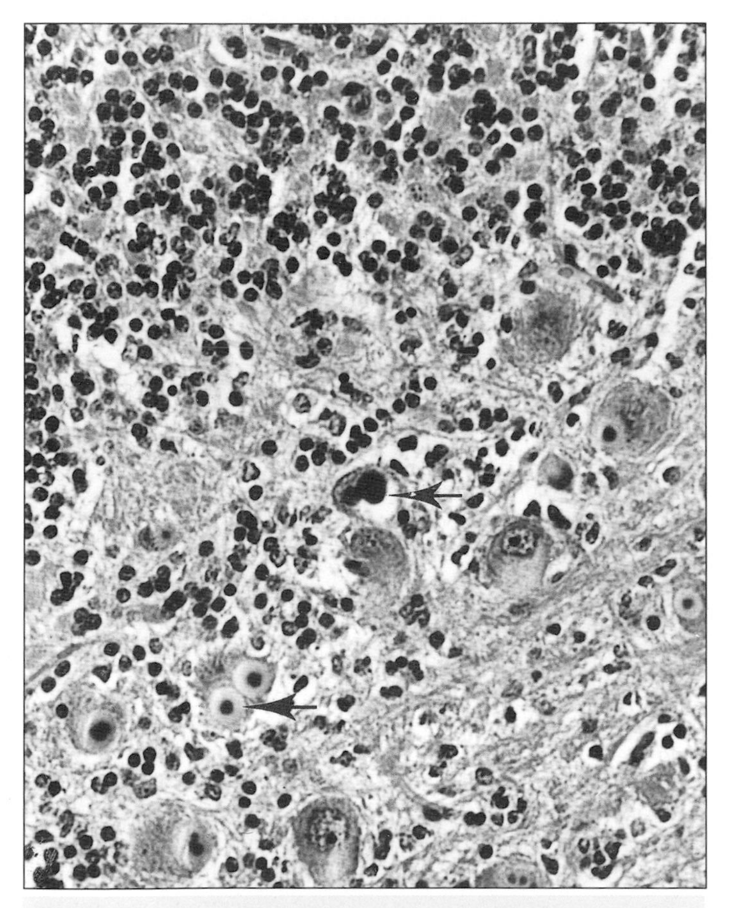

Figure 3.5 Lafora bodies in Purkinje cells (arrows) in a dog.

Mucocyte (Buscaino body) is the term applied to glassy, pale gray-blue bodies of variable size and shape, roughly the same size as neurons, seen on routinely processed and stained sections of brains. These are usually dispersed in the neuropil, typically in major white matter tracts and are considered by most to be an *artifact* of fixation and processing. They may be PAS positive, but are not always so, and there are rare reports of the accumulation of mucocytes associated with disease.

Axon

The axon acts as the solitary efferent extension of all neurons except those sensory neurons in the spinal ganglia whose peripherally directed myelinated axons function as dendrites, in that they conduct impulses towards the cell body. Axons may branch extensively towards their terminations.

The first part of the axon is called the *initial segment* and it has distinctive ultrastructure, related to its being the site of membrane ion channels critical for the initiation of a propagated action potential. The axoplasm contains mitochondria, endosomes, intermediate filaments (neurofilaments), microtubules (neurotubules), and secretory vesicles or granules containing neurotransmitters appropriate for the particular cell. The axoplasm will also contain soluble macromolecules such as enzymes.

Axons are sustained by their parent cell bodies and by the cells that invest them along their course. The axoplasm is devoid of ribosomes, and axoplasmic proteins are provided by the soma. Similarly, the lysosomal apparatus is limited in the axon, in terms of digestive capacity, and many obsolete materials and organelles are returned by retrograde transport to the cell body for complete degradation. The role of neurotubules in transport mechanisms has been mentioned above, and is critically important for the maintenance of the axon. Axonal diameter is distinctly reduced at the nodes of Ranvier, and these "strictures" are probably the reason that paranodal swellings filled with transported vesicles and organelles are a feature of many axonopathies in which transport has been disturbed.

Neurofilaments are responsible for the maintenance of axonal size and geometry, and are part of the generic cytoskeletal intermediate filament family. The proteolytic destruction of neurofilaments, triggered by the influx of calcium ions, is a common pathway for the collapse and disintegration of damaged axons. Larger axons are invested in a segmental manner by a *myelin sheath*, interrupted at the *nodes of Ranvier,* and penetrated at intervals by incisures.

All this sophistication is not resolved in routine light microscopic examination of paraffin-embedded tissues. The course of axons can be highlighted by the use of silver staining techniques, which emphasize the shrinkage artifact and distortion produced by routine tissue preparation. Nonetheless, with experience, many lesions in paraffin-embedded tissue can be interpreted but, particularly for peripheral nerves, plastic embedding of specimens is far preferable.

Types of **axonopathy** have been grouped according to whether they begin in the *proximal* or the *distal* portion of the axon, and whether they involve central or peripheral axons or both. Thus, for example, one may distinguish central and peripheral distal axonopathy, or central proximal axonopathy. The principal categories of axonopathy can now be discussed in broad terms.

Wallerian degeneration *denotes the changes that follow acute focal injury to a myelinated axon*, such that distal to the injury it becomes nonviable. When the soma is uninjured, there is potential for regeneration and, in peripheral nerves, this may be complete. Should the acute injury involve death of the cell body, then Wallerian degeneration of the axon will proceed as part of the dissolution of the entire neuron. The classical scenario for Wallerian degeneration is *acute focal mechanical injury in a peripheral nerve*, which effectively transects axoplasmic flow. Within 24 hours, the distal segment begins to degenerate fairly evenly along its length. Focal eosinophilic swellings occur, often containing accumulations of degenerate organelles, and

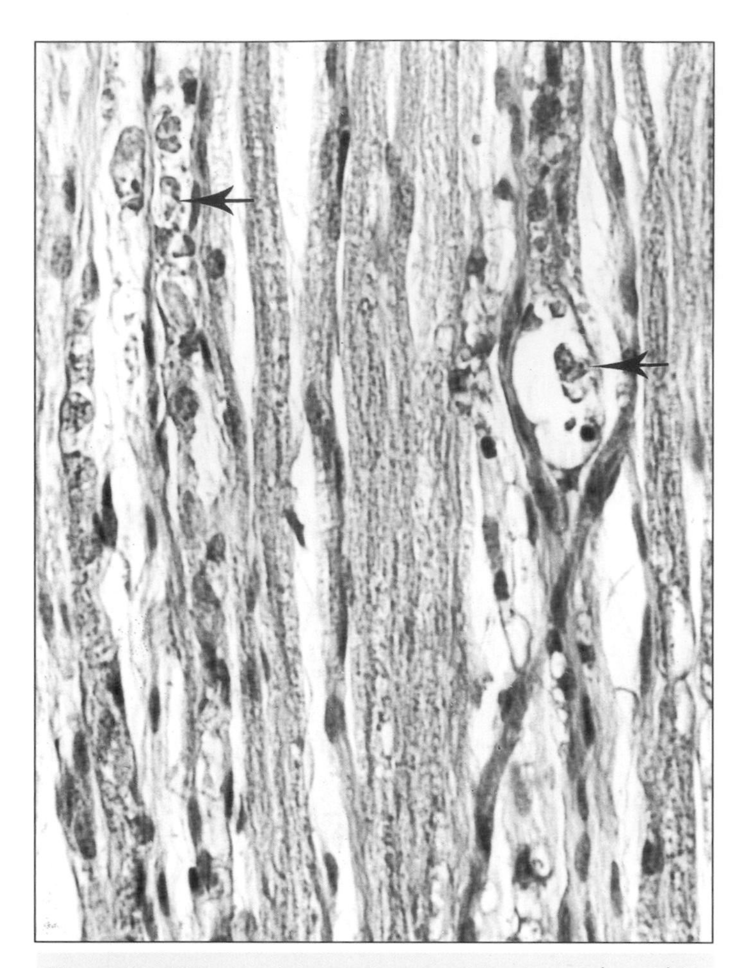

Figure 3.6 Wallerian degeneration in peripheral nerve (arrows) in copper deficiency in a goat.

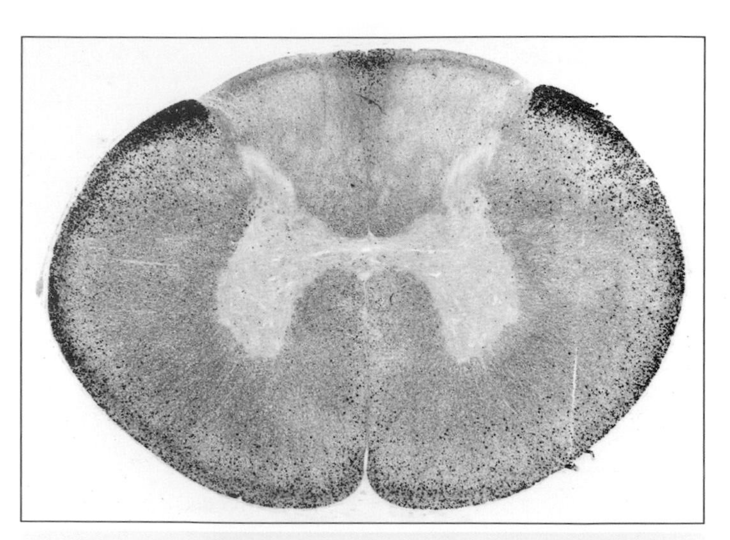

Figure 3.7 Degeneration of myelin in spinal cord in a pig with copper deficiency. Stained with Marchi. Note selective involvement of tracts, namely the fasciculus gracilis and dorsal and ventral spinocerebellar tracts. (Courtesy of MD McGavin.)

then fragmentation becomes evident by 48 hours or so. Schwann cells respond rapidly as myelin sheaths are made redundant by disintegration of the axon. Initially, myelin retracts from the nodes and then forms into *ellipsoids*, regarded originally as "*digestion chambers*" for the enzymic lysis of the axonal fragments (Fig. 3.6). The myelin itself condenses into aggregates and fragments and, together with remaining axonal debris, becomes the target of invading macrophages. Prior to this, the complex myelin lipids are progressively transformed into simpler neutral lipids over a period of 10–20 days, and this is reflected in the reaction to specific lipophilic stains. Macrophages enter the sheath and soon become filled with sudanophilic droplets. These lipid-laden cells may persist in the interstitium for many weeks. Some of the myelin debris is phagocytosed by Schwann cells themselves, and they begin to proliferate. As the debris is cleared away, proliferating Schwann cells form bands along the former course of the myelinated axons (*Bungner's bands*). Similar Wallerian changes occur proximal to the site of injury over several internodes. If conditions are favorable at the site of injury, sprouts from the axonal stump will find their way along the Schwann cell bands and be directed to their correct destinations. In most instances, the *growing axonal sprouts* advance at a rate of 2–4 mm/day, and the new axon will be invested by Schwann cell cytoplasm. Sprouting from individual axons is initially multiple and, by an unknown mechanism, one sprout is selected for the completion of regeneration. Thus a new axon may arise from a different soma than did the original. *The regenerated axon is remyelinated by Schwann cells*, although the new sheath is thinner than the original and nodal length variable and shorter. Should axonal regeneration be prevented, Schwann cell bands persist, and endoneurial fibrosis usually develops. *Abortive regeneration can lead to a tangled clump of neurites, Schwann cells, and fibrocytes at the injury site.* This will happen after transection if too great a distance separates the severed ends of the nerve fibers.

The effectiveness of regeneration in peripheral nerves is related to the comparatively simple axon/Schwann cell relationship, the presence of a basal lamina tube around each myelinated axon, and the replicative ability and metabolic resilience of the Schwann cells.

These conditions do not apply in the **CNS**, where the oligodendrocyte/axon relationship is far more complex – the oligodendrocyte is a relatively poorly regenerative cell type, there is no basal lamina scaffold, and the debris from central myelin is thought to inhibit axonal sprouting. The initial regressive changes of Wallerian degeneration are similar to those described for the peripheral nerves, although they proceed over a longer time-course. This is because the involvement of hematogenous macrophages is slower and less intense in the CNS, and activated microglial cells undertake most of the work. Axonal sprouting and some remyelination can occur. However, the poverty of the regenerative response results mostly in the *permanent disappearance of the axons, myelin, and oligodendrocyte cell bodies*. Some of the myelin debris may be phagocytosed by reactive astrocytes, and their processes extend to fill the vacancy, creating a ramifying network of astroglial scar tissue. Wallerian degeneration in the CNS is most commonly seen in the spinal cord, the optic tract, and the brain stem. Probably the best-known association is with the focal compressive myelopathies in the horse and dog (the wobbler syndromes).

During the active degenerative phase, recently phagocytosed and partially digested myelin debris may be distinguished in paraffin sections by the use of the Luxol fast blue/periodic acid Schiff stain. Degenerate myelin is well visualized by the Marchi technique (Fig. 3.7), or by immunostaining of myelin basic protein (MBP). End-stage plaques of astrogliosis may be demonstrated by traditional gliophilic stains or by the use of immunostaining for glial fibrillary acidic protein (GFAP – intermediate filament protein).

The destruction of myelin in Wallerian degeneration is known as **secondary demyelination** and is to be distinguished from **primary demyelination** in which the axon is initially undamaged (see below).

Distal axonopathy is seen in a number of chronic intoxications and genetically determined entities. It begins with degenerative changes in the distal reaches of the affected fibers and fairly characteristically involves the largest and longest, such as the proprioceptive and motor tracts of the spinal cord, the optic tract, and the recurrent laryngeal and other long peripheral nerves. Implicit in this pattern is a disturbance of anterograde axonal transport, upon which the maintenance of axonal wellbeing depends. In general, the process begins with the formation of focal axonal swellings containing degenerate organelles. These swellings are ovoid or circular eosinophilic structures commonly referred to as **spheroids**. This may progress to axonal fragmentation and attempted regeneration that may be abortive and is succeeded by further degeneration. These changes may develop focally in the distal regions of the axon and may extend more proximally with time. Diagnostically, the key is the recognition of the pattern of degenerative changes towards the terminations of long tracts (see Cycad poisoning, p. 364). The lesion is a feature of intoxication with certain of the organophosphates for example.

Proximal axonopathy is the contrasting situation in which focal swellings and degeneration begin in the proximal axonal regions. It is a pattern less likely to be encountered in natural animal disease than the distal variety. It is perhaps best exemplified by the large fusiform swellings, **torpedoes**, seen on the proximal axonal segments of cerebellar Purkinje cells in the mycotoxicosis of perennial rye grass poisoning and some storage diseases (Fig. 3.8). Such lesions may develop in central or peripheral axons and be associated with genetically determined or acquired disease. Proximal axonal swellings caused by the accumulation of neurofilaments are a feature of several neurodegenerative diseases described elsewhere in this chapter. A defect in the transport of phosphorylated neurofilaments results in the accumulation of masses of them, where they cause large, amphophilic axonal swellings. The fundamental pathogenesis remains undefined.

Axonal dystrophy is a term used to describe an axonopathic process characterized by the occurrence of *large focal swellings, often concentrated in the terminals and preterminals of long axons.* They are therefore frequently seen in and around relay nuclei in the brain, and in peripheral endings. The spheroids in axonal dystrophy can become extremely large, over 100 μm in diameter, and are filled with accumulations of normal organelles, degenerate organelles, and abnormal membranous and tubular structures. In hematoxylin and eosin sections, their appearance can be variable (Fig. 3.9A, B); some are densely eosinophilic, and either smooth or granular or vacuolated; others may be pale with central denser-staining cores; some may have a basophilic hue and evidence of focal mineralization. However, the swellings are not usually associated with any marked reaction on the part of surrounding elements and only rarely are seen to be undergoing fragmentation and dissolution. They are long-lasting, in contrast to the spheroids of acute axonal degeneration. Thinning of the myelin sheath around spheroids will occur as lamellae slip to accommodate the focal axonal enlargement (Fig. 3.10). The pathogenesis is unclear, but evidence points to a *disturbance of retrograde axonal transport.* The lesion is a common finding in the relay nuclei of the caudal brain stem in old age, and is a frequent accompaniment to neuronal storage diseases. It is the principal feature of diseases known as **neuroaxonal dystrophies**, of which several are recorded in the veterinary literature. In several such diseases, the topography of the axonal dystrophy seems to fit the clinical deficits but there is evidence that, in many situations, even intense development of the lesion has no functional significance. This seems generally so in regard to axonal dystrophy in the gracilis and cuneate nuclei.

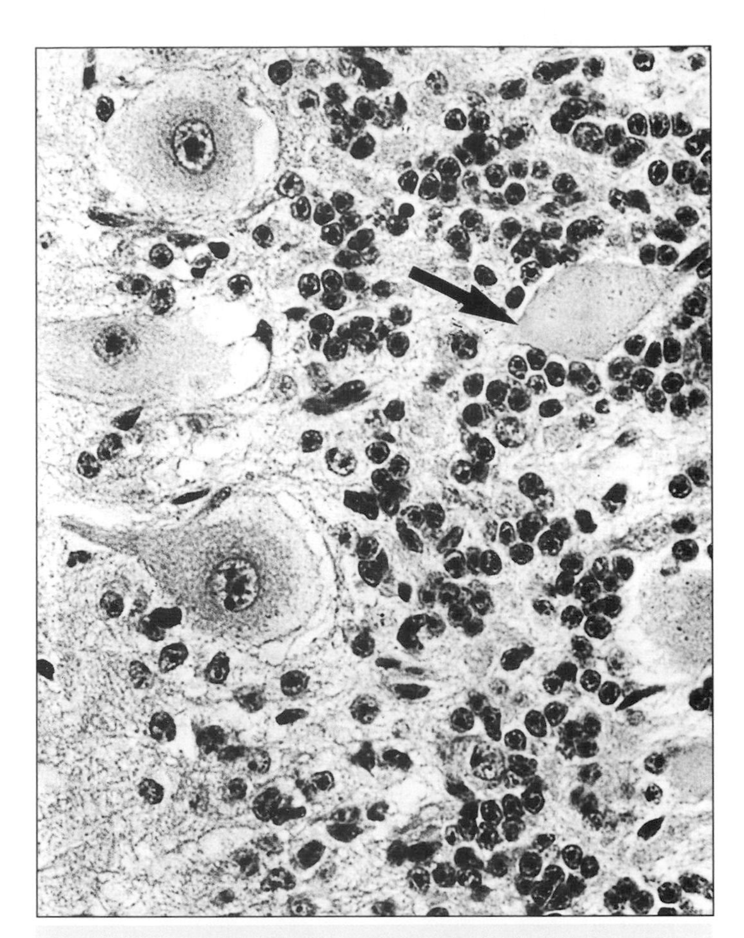

Figure 3.8 Proximal axonal enlargement - "**torpedo**" (arrow) - of a Purkinje cell, in mannosidosis in an Aberdeen Angus calf.

Oligodendrocytes, Schwann cells, and the myelin sheath

The **oligodendrocyte** is one of the close companion cells of the neuron in the CNS. One population of these cells occurs as satellites to nerve cell bodies and may proliferate in the event of injury to the neurons, but the role of the satellites is essentially unknown. *The role of oligodendrocytes is to provide and maintain the myelin sheaths around those axons with a diameter greater than about 1 μm.* They are accordingly located in the myelinated tracts amongst the fascicles of axons and are referred to as *interfascicular oligodendrocytes*. Particularly in neonates and in cases of hypo- or delayed myelinogenesis, distinction histologically between astrocytes and oligodendrocytes can be uncertain. Oligodendrocytes are smaller than astrocytes, nuclear density is greater, and the cells are arranged in rows between fascicles. In immature animals, nuclei of oligodendrocytes are morphologically

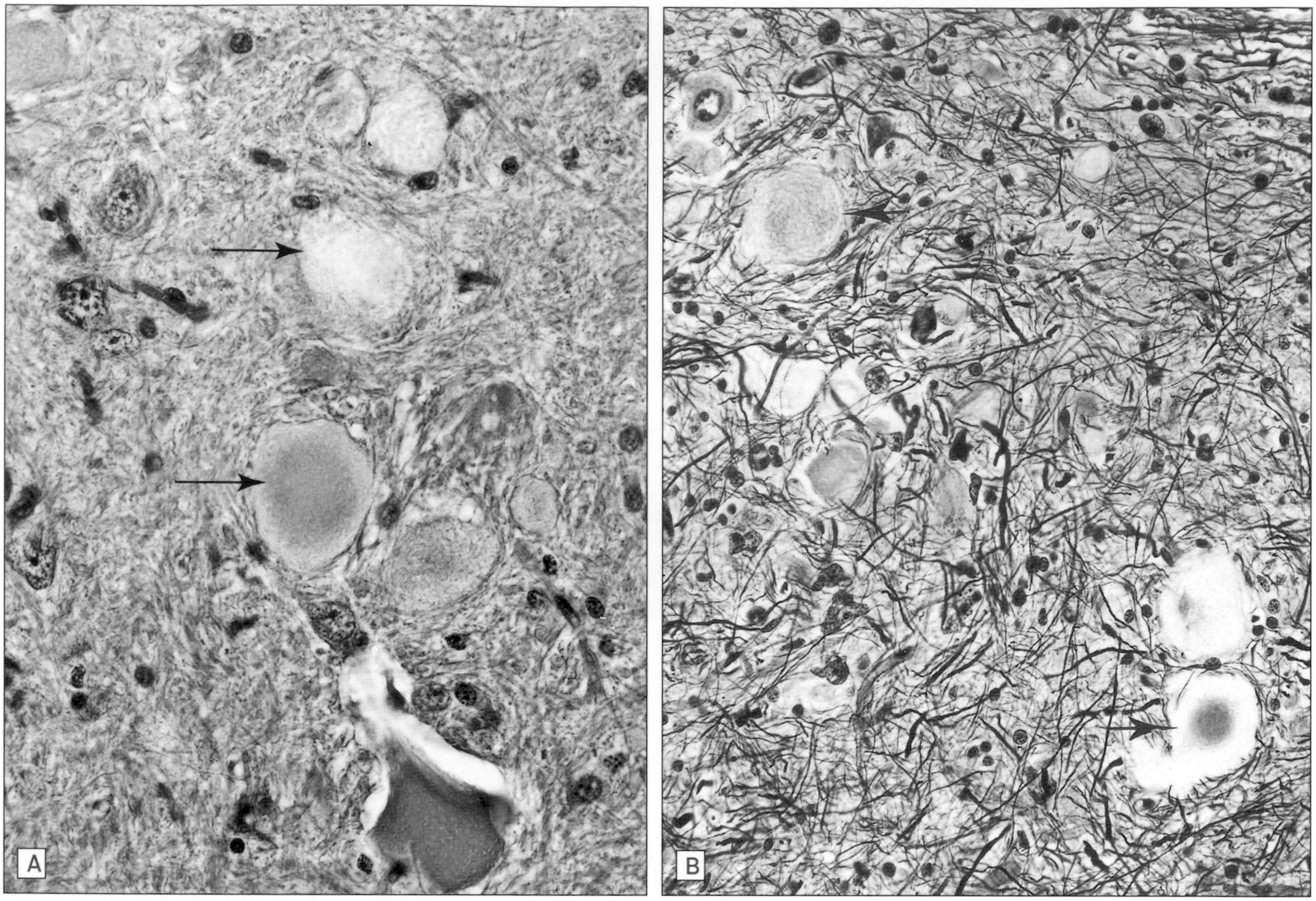

Figure 3.9 Axonal dystrophy in a Rottweiler. **A.** Focal axonal swellings (arrows); H&E stain. **B.** Silver stain reveals varying content of neurofilaments in swellings. (Courtesy of LC Cork.)

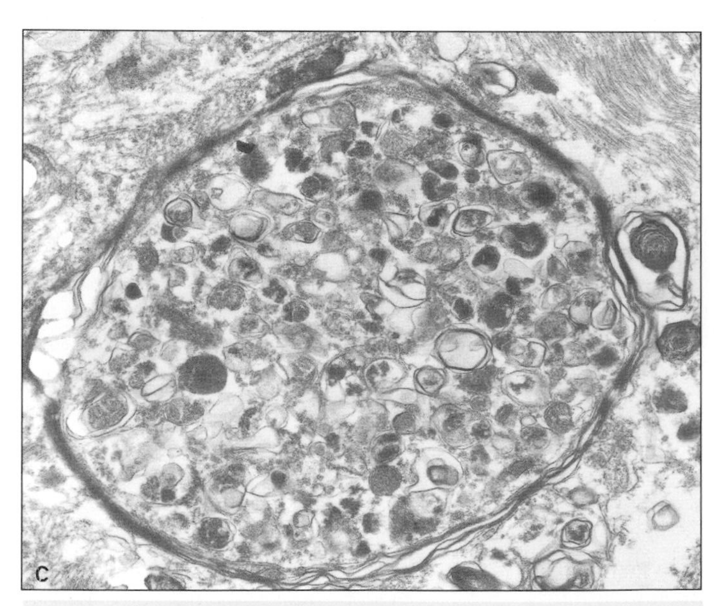

Figure 3.10 Axonal dystrophy in a cat with mannosidosis. Focal axonal swelling containing degenerate organelles; note thinning of myelin sheath. (Courtesy of SU Walkley.)

heterogeneous and those with large nuclei and clear nucleoplasm and not readily distinguished from astrocytes are probably immature and capable of division or synthesis of membrane myelin.

Oligodendrocytes arise from precursor cells in the subventricular zone of the developing forebrain and from the floor plate of the neural tube in brain stem and spinal cord. These progenitors migrate extensively to settle along fiber tracts of the developing white matter where they go through a series of maturation changes to produce myelin.

Each mature oligodendrocyte has a compact cell body of characteristic ultrastructural appearance, and a dozen or so thin processes each of which connects the perikaryon to a segment of myelin some distance away. Each segment of myelin covers one axonal internode, and is an extended and compacted sheet of specialized oligodendroglial plasma membrane bilayers, wound concentrically and spirally around the axon, like a rolled-up newspaper. In the formation of this compacted membrane, both the intracellular and extracellular spaces are obliterated, creating the major and minor dense lines of myelin lamellae as seen with the electron microscope. In some axons, a sheath of 100 or so bilayers may be formed. A portion of intact cytoplasm remains at the innermost and outermost lamellae, known as the "inner" and "outer" tongues respectively. Tracts of uncompacted cytoplasm course through the sheath to form the "incisures," and also occur where the myelin lamellae terminate at the paranodal region, as the "terminal loops." The lamellated myelin sheath is a relatively stable but plastic structure, whose lipid and protein components are supplied and turned over by the oligodendrocyte.

For light microscopy, myelin is well demonstrated by several special stains, with osmium tetroxide being particularly effective. Biochemically, central myelin is largely composed of cholesterol, galactocerebroside, and phospholipids, together with a number of distinctive protein constituents. The most abundant of these is the proteolipid protein (PLP), with lesser amounts of myelin basic protein (MBP), and myelin-associated glycoprotein (MAG). PLP is concentrated at the intraperiod line, MBP on the cytoplasmic face of the major dense line, and MAG at the axoplasmic/myelin interface. They probably play an important role in maintaining the stability of the sheath.

It is thus apparent that one oligodendrocyte myelinates several axonal internodes, that the myelin sheath is part of the oligodendrocyte, and that death of the oligodendrocyte will result in the demise of all the myelin sheath segments supplied by that cell. However, destruction of one or more myelin sheath segments does not necessarily result in death of the parent oligodendrocyte, but may stimulate it to withdraw its remaining myelin. The dynamics of the oligodendrocyte population are still not absolutely clear, but it is becoming accepted that there is a system of undifferentiated reserve cells able to take on to some extent regenerative and reparative tasks. These cells may originate from the perineuronal satellite oligodendroglia.

Myelination occurs relatively late in the development of the CNS, and maturing oligodendrocytes invest axons with myelin by replacing an initial ensheathment of astrocytic processes. Once this is completed, most of the cells assume the characteristics of maturity, while some do appear to remain in a less mature state. The ability of oligodendrocytes to synthesize myelin at specific times and in specific tracts that are specific for the animal species must require signaling mechanisms that wait to be clarified.

Oligodendrocytes do not exhibit a range of reactions for the light microscopist, generally undergoing rapid lysis when injured. Acute injury may be manifested by hydropic swelling of the perikaryon. On occasion, mitotic activity and an increase in numbers may be observed when a primary demyelinating process is operating, but this seems to be very rare in veterinary pathology. Their numbers may be increased by condensation in linear rows in interfascicular gliosis. Inclusion bodies may be present in the nuclei in some viral diseases such as canine distemper. Excepting oligodendroglial tumors, damage to the cells is expressed in disordered myelin.

The process of myelination is dependent on close interaction between the axon and the myelinating cell. The two act as a unit, and signals are exchanged between them for all aspects of the process. While the axon may survive for a long period without its myelin sheath, loss of the axon provokes immediate disintegration and removal of the myelin sheath. *This situation of axonal degeneration with secondary myelin loss is termed Wallerian degeneration*, and has been discussed above under axonopathy.

Myelination in peripheral nerves is the responsibility of **Schwann cells**, and they have a distinctly different relationship with axons to that of oligodendrocytes. Each peripheral internode is myelinated by a single cell, and the myelinated axon is invested by a basal lamina tube of Schwann cell origin, and by endoneurial collagen. Signals from Schwann cells influence the development of all components of the nerve and endo- and epineural connective tissue and the Schwann cells themselves. Schwann cells develop from the neural crest as two different cell types, *myelinating* and *nonmyelinating*. This differentiation is reversible, which is consistent with the absence of precursors in mature nerves regenerating after injury. If mature Schwann cells lose contact with axons, as occurs in nerve injury, the cells undergo regression and the myelin disintegrates. The dedifferentiated cells multiply and provide growth factors that support the regrowth of axons.

The cell body of the Schwann cell directly apposes the axon. Peripheral myelin is also chemically distinct from central myelin and this can be appreciated by the tinctorial difference between the two in appropriately stained sections of the spinal cord/spinal nerve interface. This chemical difference is reflected in antigenic differences; the major protein is termed Po and is distinct from PLP, as is the basic protein P1 from MBP. *Schwann cells are able to replicate prolifically, to phagocytose damaged myelin, and to remyelinate newly regenerated or previously demyelinated axons.* This replicative ability means that the loss of a proportion of the cells may be compensated. The peripheral myelinated axon is therefore a much more resilient structure than its central counterpart. The general principles of the axon/myelin relationship, as outlined for CNS, still apply however. *Destruction of Schwann cells will result in the disintegration of the dependent myelin.* Destruction of axons will cause myelin degradation, Schwann cell proliferation and, in time, endoneurial fibrosis.

In paraffin sections of normal nerve, Schwann cells appear as ovoid nuclei closely apposed to the axon. Proliferating Schwann cells in longitudinal section often appear as bands (*Bungner's bands*) of spindle-shaped cells resembling fibroblasts. In cross-section, they form concentric whorls called "*onion bulbs.*" Nodular proliferations of Schwann cells are referred to as *Reynaud bodies*. Large Reynaud bodies are a common incidental finding in nerves of horses.

A number of diseases primarily involve the myelin sheath, and may frequently leave the myelinating cell body intact. These diseases usually require ultrastructural evaluation for adequate investigation.

In **demyelinating diseases**, the sheath is removed from the axons, leaving them naked over variable lengths and providing potential for serious slowing of impulse conduction. In peripheral nerves, the removal of myelin from randomly scattered internodes gives rise to segmental demyelination, which is best appreciated in teased fiber preparations. Demyelination is frequently carried out by macrophages that insinuate cytoplasmic processes into the intraperiod lines and strip the sheath from the axonal internode, ingesting and digesting myelin debris. In other situations, myelin appears first to be disrupted by humoral factors and undergoes splitting and vesiculation prior to phagocytosis. Myelinophagy can be identified by the use of stains such as the Luxol fast blue/periodic acid Schiff technique. Degenerate myelin can be visualized by the Marchi technique (see Fig. 3.7).

In the CNS, there is some scope for remyelination, but the complex arrangement and limited replicative capacity of the oligodendrocytes limits the reparative potential. Regenerated myelin sheaths are thinner than the originals, appearing to the experienced eye as being too narrow for the diameter of the axon they ensheath. Remyelinated internodes are also shorter. In the peripheral nervous system, the potential for remyelination is much more favorable. Repeated bouts of demyelination may result in "onion bulb" and

Reynaud body formations, and in the production of thin and irregular myelin segments.

In **hypomyelinating diseases**, myelinating cells fail, for various reasons, to provide adequate myelination during the development phase, and the affected individual suffers transient or permanent myelin deficiency, varying in extent and severity according to the particular disease (Fig. 3.11A, B, C, D). The majority of these conditions involve the CNS only (see Myelinopathies). Myelin sheaths are thin or absent, but myelinophagy is generally minimal or nonexistent. Oligodendrocytes may be few, or present in normal numbers, and may exhibit features of immaturity.

In **dysmyelinating diseases**, there is a qualitative defect in the myelin produced, and the quantity may also be reduced. A large variety of these disorders has been produced for research purposes in inbred strains of laboratory mice.

Myelinic edema *is disruption of the lamellar structure by reopening of the extracellular space along the intraperiod line*. It may occur in both central and peripheral myelin. It is caused by a number of chemical agents, e.g., hexachlorophene, and leads to a spectacular state of spongy degeneration of white matter, one form of status spongiosus. With some causal agents, there are associated degenerative and reactive changes, but with other causes there is, remarkably, no apparent response on the part of other tissue elements including the oligodendrocytes themselves. The lesion does not necessarily cause functional disturbances even when well developed; it seems that this may depend on the number of intact lamellae left in place. It may resolve over a period of weeks with no evidence of breakdown of the affected myelin (see Spongiform myelinopathies).

Astrocytes

Astrocytes may be regarded as the interstitial cells of the CNS, as their processes occupy most of the space between and around the neuronal and oligodendroglial elements, and the perivascular and subpial zones. Astrocytes are of two types: the **protoplasmic** (type 1), located mainly within the cerebral gray matter, and the **fibrous** (type 2), located mainly within white matter tracts. Evidence suggests a common progenitor cell, the 011A cell, for the type 2 astrocyte and the oligodendrocyte. Indeed, there is evidence for several different functional types of astrocyte, the functional diversity reflecting diverse locational needs. Radial glial cells, which are the precursors of astrocytes, guide the migration of neurons from the subependymal generative zones to their final positions; astrocytes guide axons into their proper fiber tracts; astrocytes are important in the regulation of ionic exchanges between cells of the nervous system; astrocytes form functional connections by production of molecules that are tropic for other specialized cells of the nervous system.

The intercellular space of CNS tissue is a 20-nm cleft between astrocytes and the other elements, and is interrupted by loose junctions and zonulae adherentia between the former. The astrocytic perikaryon is sparse and barely evident in routine paraffin sections, and the numerous and ramifying processes are invisible. The nuclei appear, therefore, as naked and spherical, and about the size of those of small to medium-sized neurons; they usually lack a nucleolus, but sometimes have a chromatic dot, the centrosome. Immunochemical demonstration of *vimentin* is used to confirm the identity of immature astrocytes, and *glial fibrillary acidic protein* (GFAP) to confirm identity of mature astrocytes including neoplastic astrocytes. However, GFAP is not entirely specific for astrocytes. Ultrastructurally, the astrocytic cytoplasm throughout is relatively devoid of organelles and appears largely empty and watery. The chief features are bundles of intermediate filaments, clusters of glycogen granules, and a few mitochondria and lysosomes.

All capillary blood vessels in the CNS are closely invested by the expanded ends of astrocytic processes, the *end feet*. There is also a dense network of processes at the surface beneath the pia mater, the *glia limitans*. A specialized population of astrocytes occurs in the Purkinje cell layer of the cerebellum and is known as *Bergmann's glia*. These cells have long straight processes that extend out through the molecular layer to the surface.

Astrocytes and their processes are well visualized by the application of special stains, such as the Cajal method (Fig. 3.12A, B), or immunostaining for the intermediate filament glial fibrillary acidic protein (GFAP) (Fig. 3.13A, B). Astrocytes are considered to play an important role in the movement of cations and water, to be much involved in maintenance of conditions favorable for the electrical activity of neurons, and to be a source of cytokines and growth factors that support neurons and neuronal activity. Type 2 cells have a major role in this regard at the nodes of Ranvier where they form a close relationship with both the axon and the terminal myelin loops. They are also involved in the detoxification of ammonia, and perhaps other metabolites.

When lethal astrocytic injury occurs, the cytoplasm swells and becomes visible, albeit faintly, and the nucleus becomes eccentric and pyknotic. Disintegration of cytoplasm and nucleus follows rapidly. Astrocytes, however, are capable of a number of reactive responses when they, or cells around them, are damaged. *A frequent response is swelling and eosinophilia of the cytoplasm, with some cells acquiring two or more nuclei. These plump reactive astrocytes are called* **gemistocytes** (Fig. 3.14). In a mild response, cytoplasmic swelling may be minimal but some proliferation of both cells and processes generally occurs (*astrogliosis*). With cessation of injury, cytoplasmic swelling regresses but there may be a permanent residuum of extra cells and processes. Around the borders of severe lesions, such as malacic foci, the proliferation of processes may become extremely dense (Fig. 3.15). Astrocytic proplasia is limited to surviving tissue however, and post-malacic cavities cannot be filled by astrocytic processes.

Reactive astrogliosis is expected in Wallerian degeneration, following neuronal loss, and in sustained cerebral or spinal edema, and is a feature of many viral encephalitides in which viral infection of astrocytes is probably a prime stimulus. This is certainly the case in canine distemper, in which inclusion bodies are common in reactive astrocytes. Astrocytes are the cells primarily responsible for repair and scar formation in the brain.

In acute cerebral or spinal vasogenic edema, swollen astrocytes and their processes undergo a type of hydropic degeneration. This can only be resolved satisfactorily with the electron microscope, when the clear distension can be seen, particularly in the perivascular end-feet.

An acute astrocytic reaction known as the formation of **Alzheimer type II cells** is best exemplified by the metabolic disturbance in *hepatic encephalopathy* resulting from liver failure (Fig. 3.16). The nucleus becomes distinctly enlarged and vesicular but remains rounded; the cytoplasm swells and may become visible. This change does not involve the generation of large masses of cytoplasmic intermediate filaments, and there is a weak reaction to GFAP

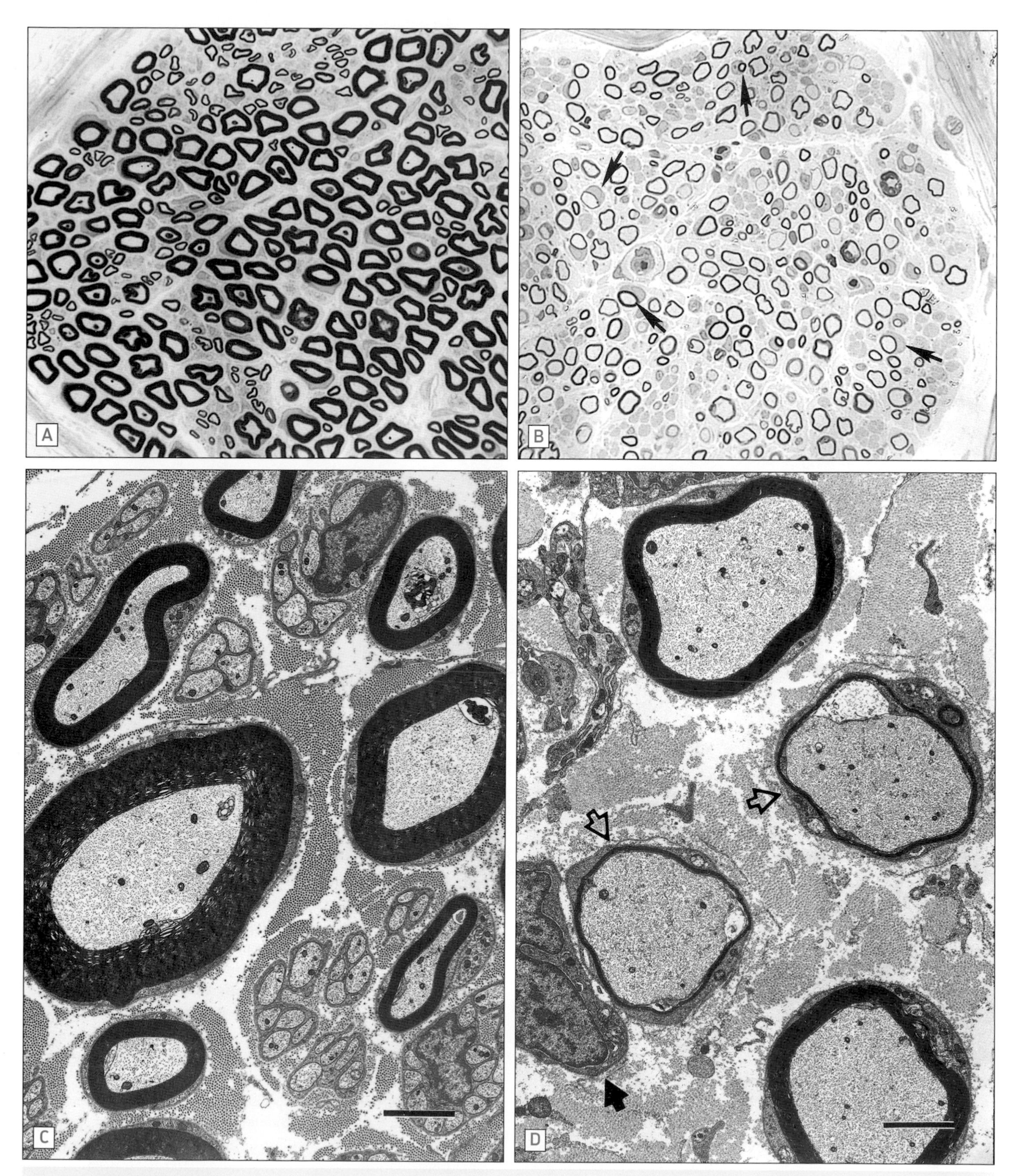

Figure 3.11 Polyneuropathy in a Golden Retriever. Comparison of normal (**A**) and hypomyelinated (**B**) peripheral nerve. Voluminous Schwann cell cytoplasm (arrows). (**C**) and (**D**) corresponding ultrastructure: normal (**C**), hypomyelinated (**D**). Thinly myelinated fibers (open arrow). Schwann cell nucleus (black arrow). Bar = 2 μm. (Reprinted with permission from Braund KG, et al. Vet Pathol 1989:26:202.)

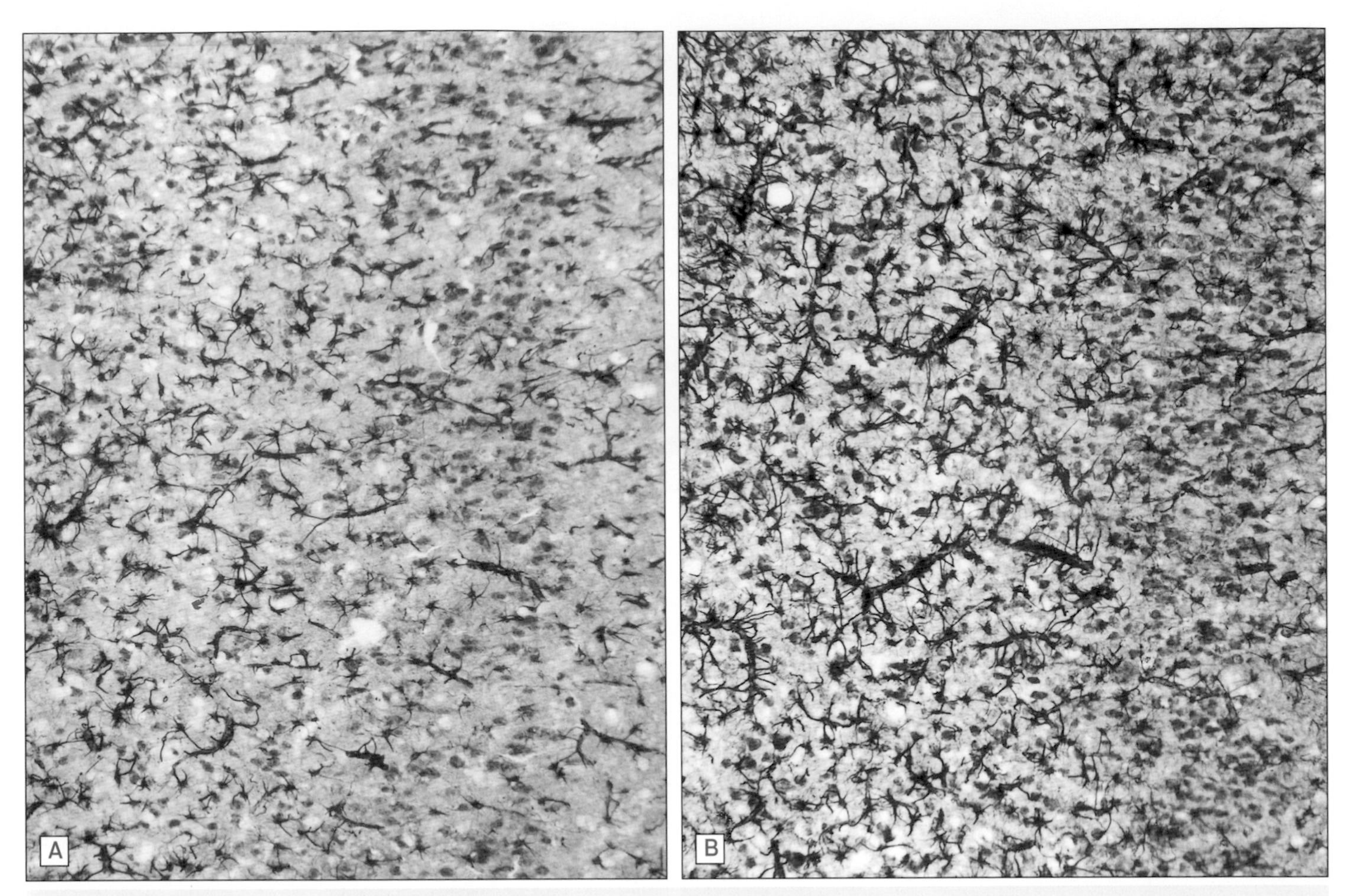

Figure 3.12 Astrocytes in the cerebral cortex of a goat with scrapie, stained by the Cajal method. **A.** Normal. **B.** Fibrous astrogliosis. (Reprinted with permission from Hadlow WJ, Race RE. Vet Pathol 1986;23:593.)

immunostains. It is caused by the accumulation of ammonia and other endogenous toxins, and would therefore also be expected in cases of exogenous ammonia intoxication. In some circumstances, cells suggested to be astrocytes are capable of *phagocytosis of tissue debris*, particularly myelin. This can be seen in Wallerian degeneration in the optic nerves when the bulk of myelinophagy may be performed by astrocytes. It has also been observed in other regions of the brain and cord.

A bizarre and rare astrocytic response is the formation of **Rosenthal fibers**; these are irregularly shaped, hyaline eosinophilic structures of undetermined composition, formed within the cell bodies and processes. The massive production of Rosenthal fibers is a feature of *Alexander disease*, an idiopathic entity described in humans and dogs, now regarded as the only primary genetic disease of astrocytes.

Microglia

Microglia are derived from the mononuclear phagocyte lineage, and function as the *fixed macrophage system* of the CNS. In the normal brain and cord, they appear by routine microscopy as *inconspicuous, small hyperchromatic nuclei, often wedge-shaped, and with no visible cytoplasm.* However, special staining techniques reveal extensive thin cytoplasmic processes and, with the electron microscope, dense perikaryal cytoplasm with elongated strands of rough endoplasmic reticulum and lipofuscin-like granules are characteristic. They are most frequent in the gray matter where they may group in the vicinity of neurons, and in both gray and white matter they are most numerous adjacent to blood vessels. During organogenesis, they are derived from blood monocytes that also give rise to the rich population of leptomeningeal and perivascular histiocytes that can migrate into the neuropil when significant vascular damage has occurred. Microglia are the primary immune effector cells of the central nervous system. Activated microglia at the site of injury express increased levels of major histocompatibility antigens and, like other macrophages, microglia release inflammatory cytokines that amplify the inflammatory response by recruiting other cells to the site of injury. They may also be important in the persistence of some viral infections.

The simplest microglial response to tissue injury is a *hypertrophic reaction* in which the nucleus becomes rounded and the cytoplasm visible as a narrow, often eccentric, eosinophilic rim. In routinely stained preparations, such cells may be difficult to distinguish from astrocytes. They may also proliferate, although their ability to do so seems limited, and many of the cells in proliferative foci are probably derived from immigrant histiocytes. Focal proliferation gives rise to nodules of 30–40 or more cells, while diffuse proliferation creates an overall impression of increased cellularity in the microscopic field (Fig. 3.17). *Microglial nodules are very commonly a feature of viral encephalitides*, occurring in both gray and white matter, but are

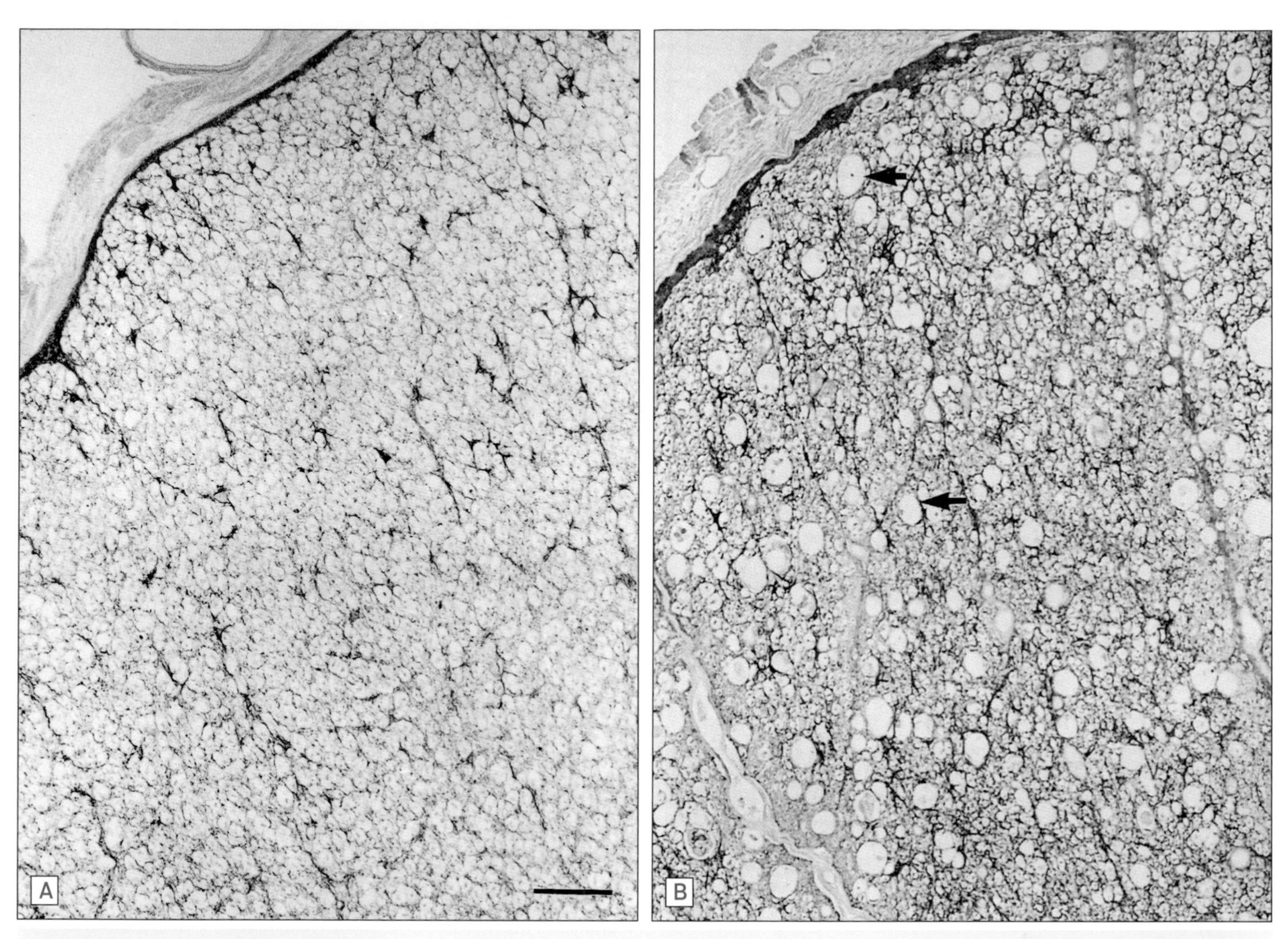

Figure 3.13 Glial fibrillary acidic protein (GFAP) staining of equine spinal cords. **A.** Normal. **B. Wobbler**. Astrogliosis at site of compressive injury; axonal degeneration (arrows). (Courtesy of JV Yovich.)

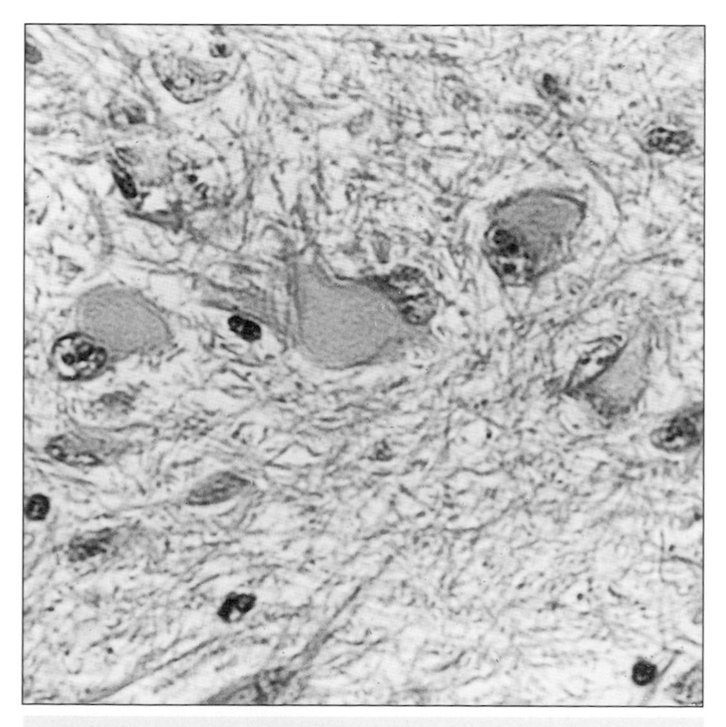

Figure 3.14 Reactive astrocytes (gemistocytes) near malacic focus.

not specific for viral infections. Reactive microglia may develop greatly elongated and sometimes tortuous nuclei, in which case they are called *rod cells*. These again are often seen in viral diseases. Activated microglia release cytokines and chemokines that aid in defense against CNS infections, as well as contributing to neurodegenerative conditions.

The most vigorous response of the microglia is their *transformation to macrophages*, when they assume the morphology typical of cells engaged in phagocytosis. When ingesting myelin debris, their cytoplasm becomes foamy as they load themselves with lipid vacuoles. Often the nucleus becomes pyknotic, and they are referred to as **gitter cells, compound granular corpuscles**, or **fat-granule cells** (Fig. 3.18A, B). In severe lesions, many of the gitter cells will have arisen from blood monocytes as well as from microglia. Lipid-laden cells may persist for months around focal lesions, but slow migration to the perivascular spaces and the meninges does take place. Some of the cells may be found at these locations after even longer periods, with the ingested lipid transformed to lipofuscin.

Microglial phagocytes are usually responsible for **neuronophagia**, in which phagocytic cells gather around fragmenting degenerate neuronal cell bodies (see Fig. 3.2D). This response is a feature of many viral infections in which neurons die, but is uncommon in ischemic or other forms of neuronal necrosis.

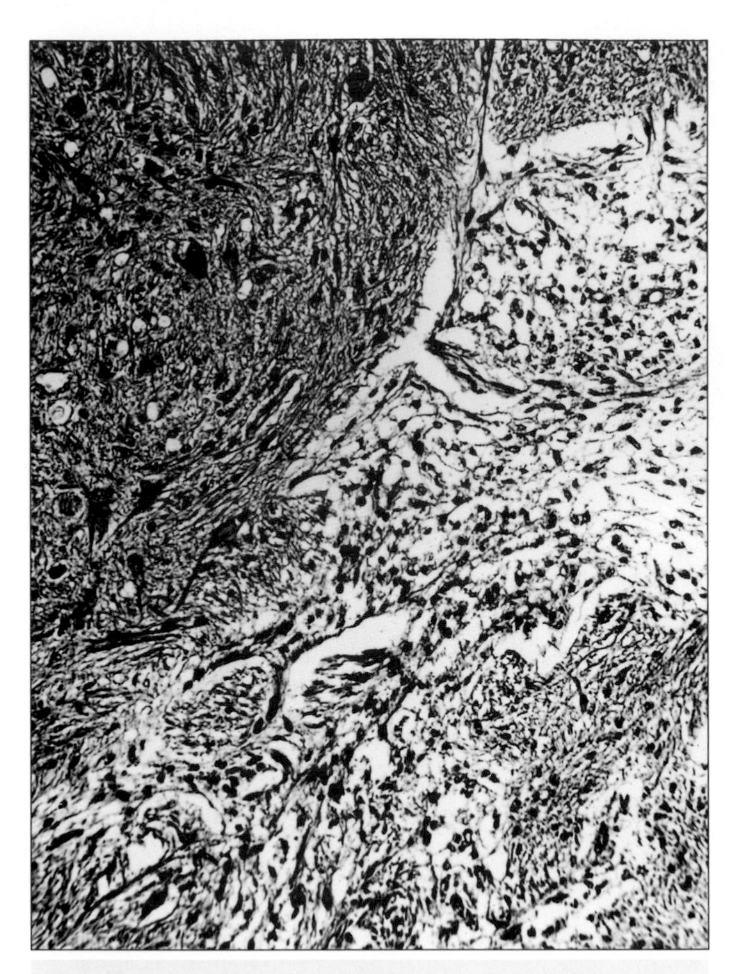

Figure 3.15 Astrogliosis forming wall to residual cyst.

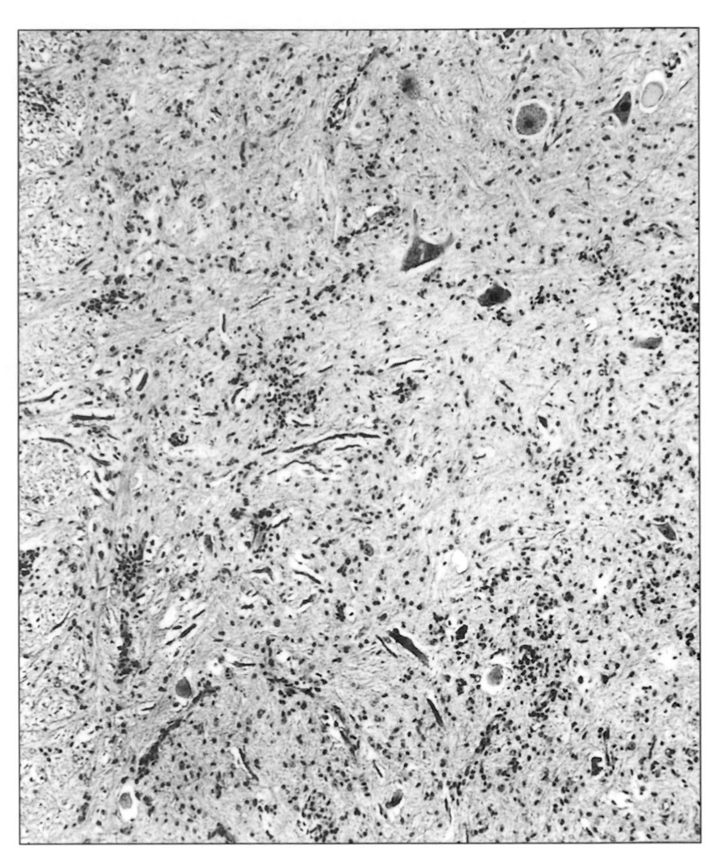

Figure 3.17 Focal and diffuse **gliosis** in the poliomyelitis of louping in a sheep.

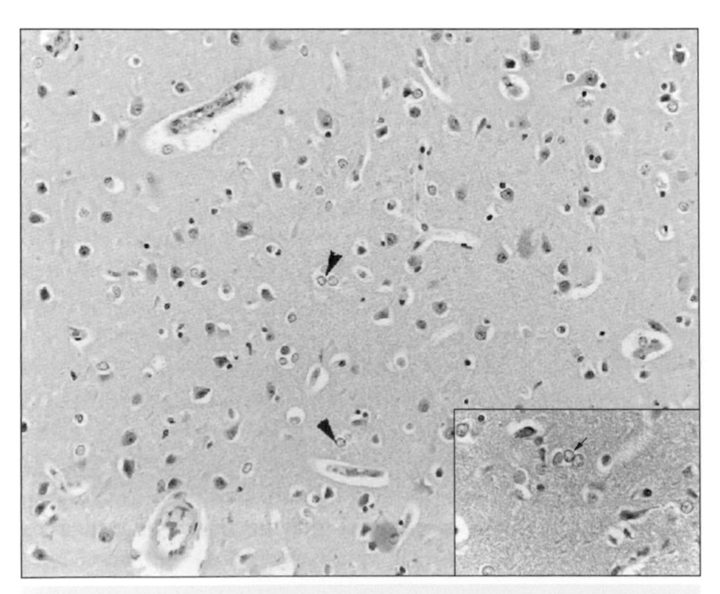

Figure 3.16 Marked **Alzheimer type II astrocytosis** in equine hepatic encephalopathy (arrowheads). Inset: Alzheimer type II cells are often arranged in pairs (cuddling cells) or clusters (arrow): pony.

Microcirculation

There are some structural peculiarities of blood vessels in the CNS that have a bearing on the development of pathologic processes. The capillaries differ from those in other tissues by being surrounded by an investment of astrocytic end-feet. Also, the endothelial cells are sealed together by tight junctions, and the basement membrane divides to incorporate pericytes into the capillary wall. This arrangement in its totality creates the **blood–brain barrier** that selectively limits the entry of many molecules into the neuropil in most of the brain. The barrier is lacking in a few locales, such as the area postrema and certain other periventricular nuclei.

The distribution of brain capillaries varies considerably, but they are more abundant in the gray matter than the white. Their concentration is higher in some parts of the gray matter, such as the supraoptic and paraventricular nuclei and the area postrema, especially where neuroendocrine activity is concentrated. It is in these areas that the blood–brain barrier is lacking.

Regional variations in the concentrations of capillaries do not appear to influence local pathologic processes. The capillary and venular endothelium is highly labile and responds to a variety of injuries by swelling and proliferating (Fig. 3.18B). However, in spite of fairly vigorous proplasia, *cerebral capillaries seem to be almost incapable of budding, so reactive neovascularization is minimal.* The formation of new capillaries is probably limited to situations where granulation tissue is derived from the mesenchyme of the meninges.

Both arterioles and venules of the CNS are thin walled, especially the latter whose walls are composed mainly of a thin layer of fibrous tissue with very little elastica and no muscle. They are thus susceptible to injury and prone to hemorrhage and, in the cerebral white matter, leukocytes tend to sequester in them in bacterial

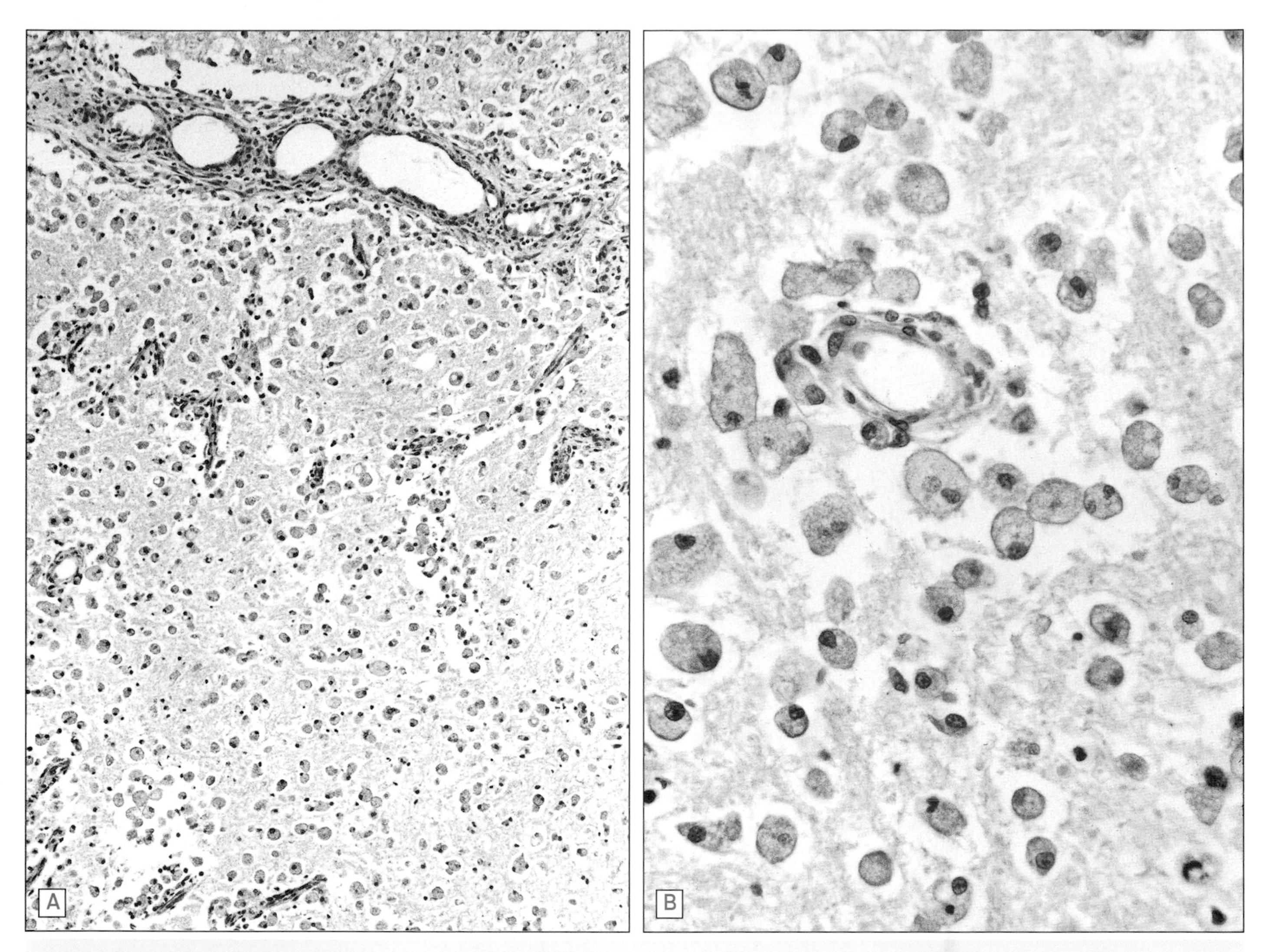

Figure 3.18 A. Gitter cells and reactive capillaries in recent cerebral infarct in a dog. **B.** High-power view of gitter cells.

infections. The veins are valveless and, as backflow of blood after death is usual, cerebral venous congestion can be difficult to assess.

Both arteries and veins have an outer adventitial layer of variable thickness, and a **perivascular Virchow–Robin space**. The space around veins is continuous with the subarachnoid space and is lined by an invagination of the pia-arachnoid. Around cortical arteries however, there is an investment of leptomeninges in a single layer, an arrangement by which the intracortical perivascular space communicates with the perivascular space about arteries in the leptomeninges. Arteries that enter through the rostral perforated substance may differ from those in the dorsal cortex in that the arteries are surrounded by two leptomeningeal layers with a space between them that communicates with the perivascular space around arteries in the subarachnoid space. The varied arrangements may reflect the need to allow passage of interstitial fluid to the local lymphatics.

In diffuse inflammatory or neoplastic diseases, this space, more potential than real under normal conditions, becomes patent and accumulates reactive and invading cells. The tendency for these cells to be confined to the space gives rise to the neuropathologic term **perivascular cuffing** (Fig. 3.19). The size of cuffs is usually related to the size of the space, and they may vary from one cell thick about the smallest venules to 10–12 or more cells thick around the larger vessels. *Perivascular cuffing is classically seen in inflammatory conditions*, and all classes of reactive leukocyte may be seen depending on the cause. While most of the cells are of hematogenous origin, there is no doubt that in some diseases, enteroviral infections for example, they may arise largely from the proliferation of adventitial cells or resident histiocytes. Lymphoid perivascular cuffing is a feature of many viral encephalitides. Some diseases too are characterized by the production of cerebral and/or spinal vasculitis, but these changes are discussed in a following section.

Mention must be made of the *nests of residual glia (islands of Calleja)* that are seen beneath the ependyma of the lateral ventricles and in the dentate fascia of the hippocampus. These cells are relics of the developmental period and possibly act as a supply of replacement cells in the adult. They occur in small aggregations and often as eccentric cuffs around vessels. Generally they are monomorphic and appear as small dark nuclei and may be mistaken for inflammatory cells.

Bibliography

Baumann N, Pham-Dinh D. Biology of oligodendrocyte and myelin in the mammalian central nervous system. Physiol Rev 2001;81:871–927.

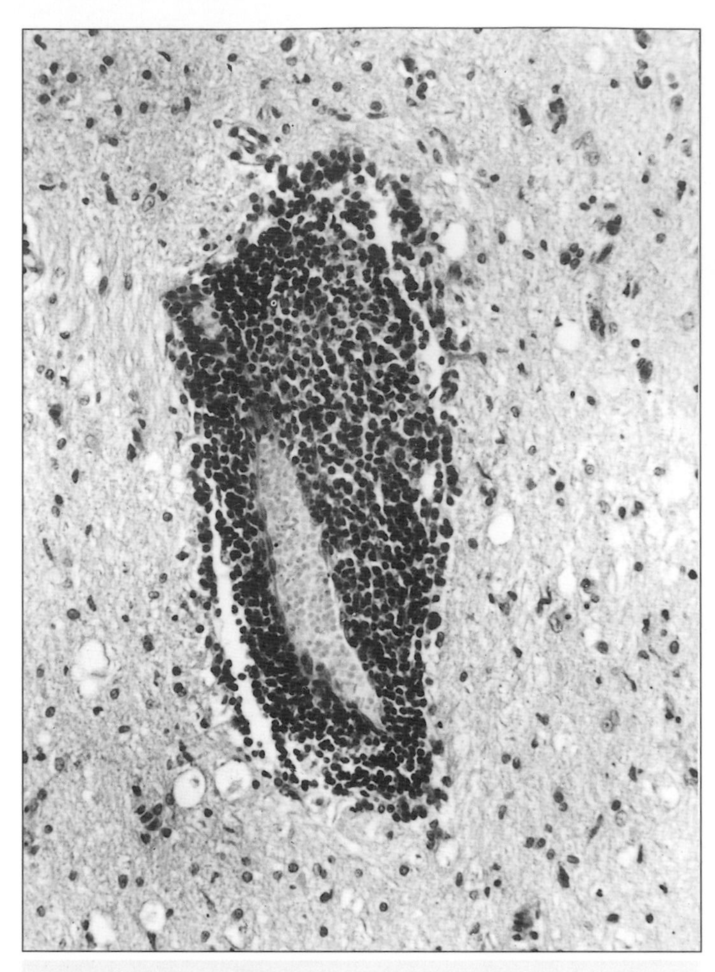

Figure 3.19 Perivascular cuff in a dog with encephalitis. Lymphocytes are confined to the Virchow–Robin space.

Gonzalez-Scarano F, Baltuch G. Microglia as mediators of inflammatory and degenerative diseases. Annu Rev Neurosci 1999;22:219–240.

Graham DJ, Lantos PL, eds. Greenfield's Neuropathology. 7th ed. London: Arnold Publishers, 2002.

Hess DC, et al. Hematopoietic origin of microglial and perivascular cells in brain. Exp Neurol 2004;186:134–144.

Hirano A. Hirano bodies and related neuronal inclusions. Neuropathol Appl Neurobiol 1994;20:3–11.

Jessen KR, Mirsky R. Schwann cells and their precursors emerge as major regulators of nerve development. Trends Neurosci 1999;22:402–410.

Rock RB, et al. Role of microglia in central nervous system infections. Clin Microbiol Rev 2004;17:942–964.

Simard AR, Rivest S. Bone marrow stem cells have the ability to populate the entire central nervous system into fully differentiated parenchymal microglia. FASEB J 2004;18:998–1000.

Simard AR, Rivest S. Role of inflammation in the neurobiology of stem cells. Neuroreport 2004;15:2305–2310.

Sosunov AA, et al. Inclusions similar to Hirano bodies in urinary bladder neurons of dogs. Zentralbl Pathol 1994;139:471–476.

Yokoyama A, et al. Microglia, a potential source of neurons, astrocytes, and oligodendrocytes. Glia 2004;45:96–104.

MALFORMATIONS OF THE CENTRAL NERVOUS SYSTEM

Malformations of the central nervous system (CNS) are common in domestic animals, and their variety is perhaps greater than the variety of malformations in other tissues. There is abundant field and experimental evidence that the effects of teratogens are manifested in the nervous system with disproportionately high frequency. One explanation is that the high degree of differentiation and complexity of the CNS give it an increased susceptibility to developmental disturbances. In addition to inherited diseases, a large number of infectious and toxic environmental agents are capable of causing anomalies. The cause of malformation in an individual domestic animal fetus is seldom determined, in part because of the long time lapse between the initiating event and the fetal presentation. The most frequent sporadic anatomic abnormalities are neural tube defects, and these are initiated in a narrow time range: embryonic days 8.5–10.5 in the mouse, days 15–18 in the pig, days 21–28 in humans.

Congenital abnormalities of the CNS consist of deviations in either the nature or velocity of the developmental process. Several main patterns of abnormal development can be recognized.

- The largest category includes those disorders with a morphological basis that are a consequence of *failure or disorder of structural development.* Many such abnormalities are recognizable by distinctive gross changes, but others require microscopic examination.
- Some conditions appear to represent *retardation of normal development* rather than structural aberrations.
- Disturbance of the normal development may also manifest as *premature senescence or degeneration of formed tissues* such as the various forms of neuronal abiotrophy.
- Some congenital abnormalities appear to represent *primary disturbances of function* rather than of tissue structure. The most frequently recognized functional disorders are those that arise as a consequence of inherited biochemical defects and that cause distinctive neurohistologic changes. This category is exemplified by the various lysosomal storage diseases and the leukodystrophies.
- Neither an anatomical nor a biochemical basis has yet been identified for a number of congenital neurological diseases that often *appear to be inherited*, e.g., idiopathic epileptiform conditions in various species.

The initial steps in the formation of the CNS take place early in embryogenesis. As soon as the germ layers are established, the **neural plate**, a thickened band of ectoderm, develops along the mid-dorsal line of the embryo, and is the primordium for the brain and spinal cord. Differential growth at the margins and in the midplane result in folding of the plate to form a *neural groove* bounded on each side by an elevated *neural fold*. The groove continues to deepen, and the neural folds meet dorsally and fuse, likely beginning at multiple sites, to form the **neural tube**, which simultaneously separates from the superficial ectoderm. Physical properties of cells and tissues both inside and outside the neural plate determine the formation of the neural tube (*neurulation*). Cellular proliferative activity within the neural tube is concentrated within an inner subependymal or germinal layer of actively dividing neuroectodermal cells that, with differentiation and outward migration, gives rise first to neurons and later to glia.

The neural tube extends the full length of the embryo and is the progenitor of the entire CNS. **Neural tube defects** (NTD), which result from failure of a portion of the neural tube to close or from reopening of a successfully closed segment, may be cranial or spinal or concurrent in both locations. Shortly after formation of the neural tube, the rudiments of the cranium and vertebrae appear in accord with the fundamental plan of segmental organization. *Segmentation and development of the axial skeletal investment of the nervous system depend on the developmental integrity of the neural tube.* Hence, NTDs also involve malformations of overlying bony or soft tissues. The spectrum of NTDs includes anencephaly, encephalocele, spinal dysraphism, and meningomyelocele. Incomplete closure of a raphe, especially the neural tube, is referred to as *dysraphism*.

The genes controlling neurogenesis are very strongly conserved in evolution and much effort is placed on analysis of responsible genes and gene actions in human embryos and in the many models of NTD in mutant and transgenic mice. Notwithstanding the shared gene arrays of the many mouse models and humans, only one mouse phenotype, the *curly tail* mouse, exhibits the anencephaly/meningomyelocele phenotype that is the most frequent NTD in human fetuses. The phenotype results from failure of closure of cranial and caudal neuropores, the ends of the neural tube. The *Sonic hedgehog gene* (Shh), secreted initially from the notochord and later from the floorplate, is implicated in inducing development of the floor of the neural plate and differentiation of neurons in the ventral sections of the developing cord. Development of the dorsal roof plate of the cord, differentiation of neural crest cells and formation of neurons within the dorsal cord are the responsibility of members of the *bone morphogenetic protein* (BMP) family derived from surface ectoderm.

The normal pattern of development of the CNS is not smoothly progressive but comprises a complicated interdependent series of growth spurts of organs and tissues. Birth does not mark a single stage in the structural development of the brain and there is considerable species variation in the stage of CNS development at birth. *Cattle, horses, sheep, and pigs are born with nervous systems having a remarkable degree of structural and functional maturity; kittens and puppies are born with their nervous systems relatively immature.* After the nervous system is fully formed, the capacity for further production of nerve cells is lost and subsequent development comprises mainly progressive lengthening and myelination of axons and extension of neuronal dendrites and glial processes.

For each species, neural development thus proceeds along a characteristic predetermined pathway. When mature, the nervous system possesses considerable inherent stability, but a time-linked process of decay is also part of the total system of development. Aging neurons tend to accumulate ceroid pigments that almost certainly reduce their functional efficiency. There is also a continual normal loss of neurons, and in normal animals neuraxonal degeneration is an insignificant but not infrequent finding.

Abiotrophy *designates the occurrence of intrinsic premature degeneration of cells and tissues.* In the hereditary abiotrophies affecting the nervous systems of animals, such premature loss of vitality is manifested by accelerated and exacerbated degeneration of neurons and their processes.

Investigation of the etiology of neural effects is complicated by the fact that *the same type of abnormality may be produced by both genetic and exogenous causes*, and in many instances, particularly those of sporadic occurrence, the cause remains unidentified. A variety of transplacental viral infections of the fetal nervous system at critical stages of gestation may result in neurological defects. Some viruses can produce changes such as symmetrical cavitating lesions that lack pathological features that suggest antecedent infection and resemble malformations thought to be of genetic or toxic cause.

The outcome of fetal interactions with agents potentially teratogenic for the nervous system depends on the species and age of the fetus and the nature of the agent. For the various patterns of malformations, there are corresponding critical periods during which developing neural tissue is vulnerable. The teratogenicity of the agent is dependent on its cellular tropism, which is commonly directed towards immature rapidly dividing cells but which often involves specific subpopulations of these cells. Thus, time sets the stage and presents the array of vulnerability, but the agent chooses from among the parts at risk those it has special affinities for damaging.

The most common mode of action for teratogens is selective destruction of cells. Such cytolytic effects have been demonstrated with neural defects induced by *viruses* and *chemicals* as well as by *physical agents* such as hyperthermia. In the case of viruses, cellular destruction can be a direct consequence of infection but may develop as part of the inflammatory reaction. The toxicities of many drugs are mediated not by the compounds themselves but by highly reactive metabolites. If they are not detoxified, these unstable metabolites interact covalently with cell macromolecules and may kill affected cells. Cytolysis seems to be the common operative mechanism in a number of important malformations that often have gross features such as the cavitating cerebral defects and cerebellar hypoplasia. Teratogens may sometimes act by inhibition or distortion of normal cellular development and function to produce more subtle developmental deviations such as hypomyelinogenesis. Infection of calves with *Bovine viral diarrhea virus*, of lambs with *Border disease virus*, and of piglets with *Classical swine fever virus* may provide instances of noncytolytic disturbance of fetal neural development of this type.

Some drug metabolites, rather than killing cells, result in mutations through binding to nucleoprotein. In view of the multiplicity of pathogenetic pathways that have been identified, it is not surprising that a spectrum of pathogenic effects can result from the action of one teratogen. All of the lesions may result from an exposure or any one effect may develop either alone or in combination. Such diversity of teratogenic expression is illustrated by the wide variety of neural and extraneural defects found in kittens born to cats exposed to griseofulvin in pregnancy. *A particular abnormality may arise as an expression of many different causes, sometimes disparate in character.* The cavitating cerebral defects provide examples of this.

Several attributes of fetal neural tissue are pertinent to the interpretation of malformations. Necrosis of groups of cells occurs in normal development and may be seen in association with remodeling processes. The immature nervous system does not react to damage in the same way as adult tissue. Parts may be absorbed without trace of connective tissue or neuroglial repair. Furthermore, severe malformations are unlikely to proceed directly from destructive processes since destruction of parts of the embryonal structure removes the inductor and inhibitor influences on neighboring cell groups. This may, in some instances, lead to arrest of normal processes and, in others, to exuberant reparative proliferation of neuroepithelium that is indicated histologically by the formation of distinctive neuroepithelial rosettes. *Thus, malformations may be compounded of degeneration, necrosis, inhibition, overgrowth, and repair.* There is at best only a general correlation between the nature of an anomaly and the time in development when it was initiated. In retrospective studies of malformations of unknown cause, it is only possible to identify the latest time at which the malformation may have been produced based on the normal development of the nervous system of the species in question.

In the event of infection of the developing nervous system by potentially teratogenic viruses, the outcome is determined primarily by age-related cellular susceptibility. However the immunological status of the fetus, particularly its capacity to produce neutralizing antibody, is likely to be important in determining the character of the neural lesions resulting from viral infection. *Lesions leading to major anomalies tend to occur prior to the fetal age at which the fetus can mount a serum neutralizing antibody response to infectious agents.* The fetal brain, especially in the early stages of development, has limited inflammatory potential, but viral-induced destruction of neural tissue in the early fetus may be accompanied by an intense macrophage reaction despite lack of immunological maturity. Such necrotizing processes typically produce gross anatomical defects with little or no evidence of inflammation because of subsidence of the inflammatory changes. In older fetuses, cytolytic processes are reduced mainly by absence of a susceptible cell population rather than by immune mechanisms, but nonsuppurative encephalitis frequently persists as a residual lesion.

Destruction of developing neural tissue may be effected by mechanisms other than those directly cytopathic for primitive neuroectodermal cells. *Vascular damage* with consequential edema and necrosis is one such mechanism. Although the fetus is resistant to hypoxia, except if prolonged or profound, there is evidence of the potential of circulatory disturbances in the genesis of cavitating CNS malformations such as hydranencephaly.

There are additional poorly understood pathogenetic influences that doubtless contribute to the outcome of fetal interactions with teratogens. Such factors include *maternal and fetal genotype*, and experimental evidence suggests that *pharmacogenetic differences* among fetuses of a particular species are important determinants of the results of in utero drug exposure. With viral infections, teratogenic potential may vary markedly depending on the *strain of the virus* and upon the *immune status* of the maternal host.

The detailed discussions of CNS malformations that follow are organized on an anatomical basis, from cranial to caudal.

Bibliography

Costa LG, et al. Developmental neuropathology of environmental agents. Annu Rev Pharmacol Toxicol 2004;44:87–110.

de Lahunta A. Abiotrophy in domestic animals: a review. Can J Vet Res 1990;54:65–76.

Dennis SM. Congenital defects of the nervous system of lambs. Aust Vet J 1975;51:385–388.

George TM, Fuh E. Review of animal models of surgically induced spinal neural tube defects: implications for fetal surgery. Pediatr Neurosurg 2003;39:81–90.

Grooms DL. Reproductive consequences of infection with bovine viral diarrhea virus. Vet Clin North Am Food Anim Pract 2004;20:5–19.

Harding BN, Copp AJ. Malformations. In: Graham DI, Lantos PL, eds. Greenfield's Neuropathology. 7th ed. London: Arnold Publishers, 2002:357–483.

Hewicker-Trautwein M, et al. Brain lesions in calves following transplacental infection with bovine-virus diarrhoea virus. Zentralbl Veterinarmed B 1995;42:65–77.

James LF, et al. Biomedical applications of poisonous plant research. J Agric Food Chem 2004;52:3211–3230.

King CT, et al. Antifungal therapy during pregnancy. Clin Infect Dis 1998;27:1151–1160.

Leipold HW, et al. Congenital defects of the bovine central nervous system. Vet Clin North Am Food Anim Pract 1993;9:77–91.

McIntosh GH, et al. The effect of maternal and fetal thyroidectomy on fetal brain development in sheep. Neuropathol Appl Neurobiol 1983;9:215–223.

Oberst RD. Viruses as teratogens. Vet Clin North Am Food Anim Pract 1993;9:23–31.

Panter KE, Stegelmeier BL. Reproductive toxicoses of food animals. Vet Clin North Am Food Anim Pract 2000;16:531–544.

Rousseaux CG. Congenital defects as a cause of perinatal mortality of beef calves. Vet Clin North Am Food Anim Pract 1994;10:35–51.

Santos-Guzman J, et al. Antagonism of hypervitaminosis A-induced anterior neural tube closure defects with a methyl-donor deficiency in murine whole-embryo culture. J Nutr 2003;133:3561–3570.

Sarnat HB, Flores-Sarnat L. Integrative classification of morphology and molecular genetics in central nervous system malformations. Am J Med Genet A 2004;126:386–392.

Smith MS, et al. The induction of neural tube defects by maternal hyperthermia: a comparison of the guinea-pig and human. Neuropathol Appl Neurobiol 1992;18:71–80.

Spielberg SP. Pharmacogenetics and the fetus. N Engl J Med 1982;307:115–116.

Summers BA, et al. Malformations of the central nervous system. In: Veterinary Neuropathology. St. Louis, MO: Mosby, 1995:68–94.

Wintour EM, et al. Experimental hydranencephaly in the ovine fetus. Acta Neuropathol (Berl) 1996;91:537–544.

Woollen NE. Congenital diseases and abnormalities of pigs. Vet Clin North Am Food Anim Pract 1993;9:163–181.

Cerebrum

Cerebral aplasia, anencephaly

True **anencephaly**, which means *absence of brain*, is a rare event, and the term has been misapplied to cases of **cerebral aplasia**, or *prosencephalic hypoplasia*, in which the cerebral hemispheres are absent, but components of the brain stem (midbrain, pons, medulla) have formed (Fig 3.20). Anomalies of the same general or specific pattern vary considerably from case to case in the details of their expression, various

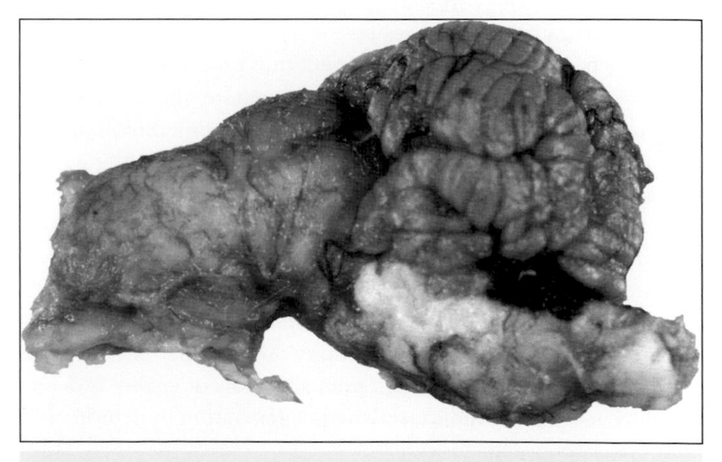

Figure 3.20 Cerebral aplasia ("anencephaly") in a calf. The cerebral hemispheres have failed to form, and only brain stem and cerebellum are present. (Courtesy of RF Slocombe.)

combinations of typical malformations occur, and there is considerable variability in the development of morphological sequelae.

The primary defect in cerebral aplasia is arrest of closure of the rostral portion of the neural tube. There is, in consequence, failure of development of the cranium and, with skin lacking over the lesion, the dysplastic rudiments of neural tissue are exposed to the exterior. Cerebral aplasia is seldom complete from the beginning because the eyes, either well developed or present as rudimentary vesicles, are present. When the eyes are rudimentary, ganglion cells and optic fibers may be missing. The cranial and neural defects are probably more or less proportionate. With severe degrees of cerebral aplasia, or true anencephaly, there may be complete failure of cranial development (**acrania**) or there may be rudimentary development of the occipital and adjacent bones. In those cases of cerebral aplasia in which the rostral portion of the brain stem is present, there may be a greater degree of cranial development but failure of fusion (**cranioschisis**). The base of the cranium is well developed, but there are a variety of anomalies of basal bones and no sella turcica. The neurohypophysis is absent and the adenohypophysis is either absent or unidentifiable. Failure of development of the neurohypophysis can be responsible for the failure of the adenohypophysis to develop normally, and this in turn may be responsible for prolonged gestation of some anencephalics. The caudal extent of the neural tube defect varies greatly. There may be involvement of the cervical vertebrae or of the entire neural tube (**craniorhachischisis totalis**); the defect is always continuous, not segmental. Even when the spinal cord is closed, it may be hypoplastic. When the cord is well developed, it is still small because of the absence of descending tracts.

In cerebral aplasia, the cerebral hemispheres are reduced to a tough formless mass of tissue on the exposed basal bones. The tissue is composed largely of blood vessels with some intermingled neural tissue and is termed the *area cerebrovasculosa*. Choroid plexuses may be recognizable, and the whole may be covered by a thin layer of squamous epithelium.

Bibliography

Colas JF, Schoenwolf GC. Differential expression of two cell adhesion molecules, Ephrin-A5 and Integrin alpha6, during cranial neurulation in the chick embryo. Dev Neurosci 2003;25:357–365.

Dias MS, Partington M. Embryology of myelomeningocele and anencephaly. Neurosurg Focus 2004;16:E1.

Dennis SM. Congenital defects of the nervous system of lambs. Aust Vet J 1975;51:385–388.

Finnell RH, et al. Pathobiology and genetics of neural tube defects. Epilepsia 2003;44(Suppl 3):14–23.

Harris MJ, Juriloff DM. Mini-review: toward understanding mechanisms of genetic neural tube defects in mice. Teratology 1999;60:292–305.

Zohn IE, et al. Cell polarity pathways converge and extend to regulate neural tube closure. Trends Cell Biol 2003;13:451–454.

Encephalocele, meningocele

Encephalocele *(meningoencephalocele, cephalocele) is protrusion of the brain through a defect in the cranium* (**crania bifida**). The defect is termed **meningocele** if only fluid-filled meninges protrude. In *exencephaly*, the brain may be either exposed or protruding. These anomalies can be inherited in pigs and in Burmese cats, and have been associated with treatment of the pregnant queen with griseofulvin.

The morphogenesis of these defects is not simply a problem of defective ossification of the skull with secondary herniation of preformed intracranial tissue but, instead, *depends on a primary neural tube defect by which there is focal failure of dehiscence of the neural tube from the embryonic ectoderm* and, in consequence, focal failure of development of the axial skeletal encasement. The herniations are related to suture lines and are almost always median. They vary from 2–10 cm in diameter, and the largest diameter is always much larger than the diameter of the cranial opening. The skin forms the hernial sac, and ectopic bits of disorganized neural tissue may be attached to it; the dura mater does not form in the areas of defect. Encephalocele and meningocele occur usually in the frontal regions (Fig. 3.21) but some are occipital (Fig. 3.22), and these latter tend to be located below the

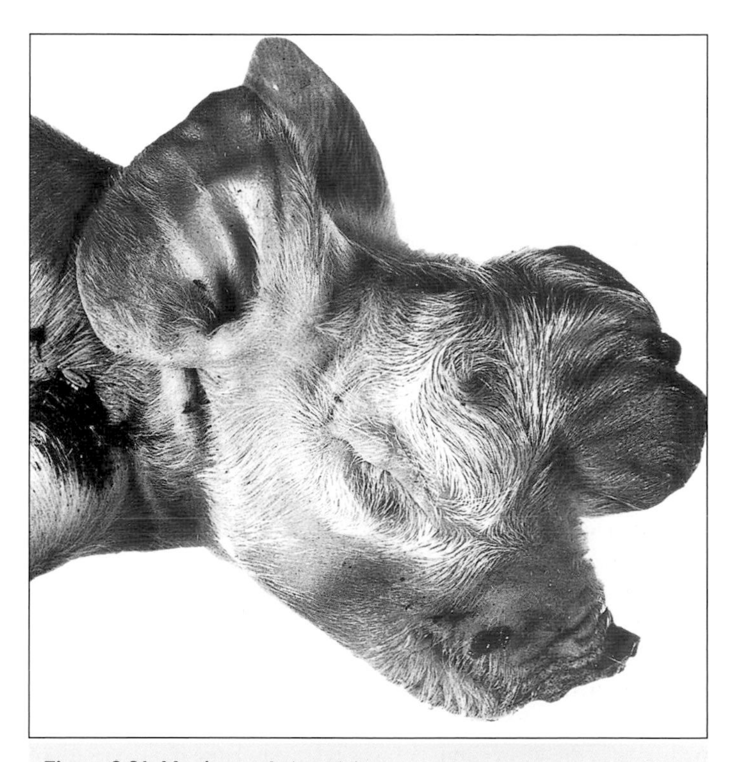

Figure 3.21 Meningocele in a piglet.

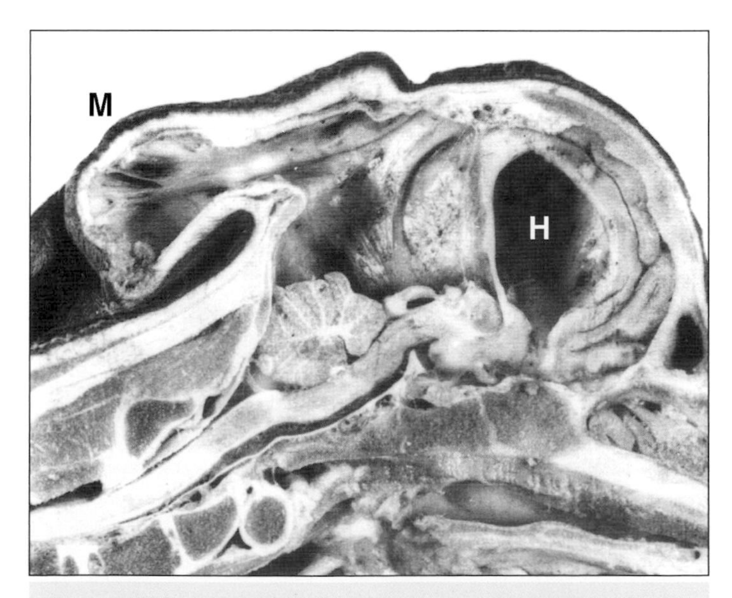

Figure 3.22 Hydrocephalus (H) and occipital **meningocele** (M) in a calf.

occipital crest. Occipital encephaloceles may also be associated with spina bifida of the upper cervical region, sometimes with enlargement of the foramen magnum and absence of the arch of the atlas.

Less well known in animals are *frontonasal or frontoethmoidal encephaloceles* that coexist with facial deformities.

Bibliography

Sponenberg DP, Graf-Webster E. Hereditary meningoencephalocele in Burmese cats. J Hered 1986;77:60.

Vogt DW, et al. Congenital meningocele-encephalocele in an experimental swine herd. Am J Vet Res 1986;47:188–191.

Defects in cerebral corticogenesis

These malformations have their teratogenetic period early in fetal life following closure of the neural tube, and usually occur in association with other neural anomalies. With the establishment of the telencephalic vesicles, cortical neurogenesis begins from the germinal epithelium lining the neural tube, especially in those parts destined to become the lateral ventricles. Initially, cell division gives rise to similar daughter cells that also act as progenitors so that cell numbers increase geometrically. Later, the cell divisions become increasingly asymmetric as an increasing proportion of progenitors produce postmitotic precursors of neurons. The first postmitotic neurons migrate to the subpial plate along guides produced by radial glia that extend from the periventricular zone to the cortical surface. Successive waves of migratory neurons will leapfrog the preceding waves such that the first waves will reside in the deeper layers of the cortical plate corresponding to layer 6 of the mature cortex and the later waves will migrate to form the more superficial layers. Errors of proliferation of germinal epithelial cells may result in microencephaly or macroencephaly; errors of migration result in various patterns of disorder affecting the cerebral gyri.

Microencephaly *refers to an abnormally small brain.* The diminution affects particularly the cerebrum. The hypoplastic brain is accommodated within the cranial cavity, which is often smaller than normal so that the cerebellum appears relatively large. The gyri are of normal size but simplified pattern, and the brain stem structures are normal. *The deficiency is of cerebral gray and white matter.* It may be an isolated defect or associated with any of a variety of other defects. Microencephaly is manifested externally by an abnormally flattened and narrowed frontal part of the cranium. The cranial bones, particularly the frontal bones, are thicker than normal. Microencephaly occurs in fetal infections by *Akabane virus* in lambs and calves, *Bovine viral diarrhea virus* in calves, *Border disease virus* in lambs, and *Classical swine fever virus* in piglets. The condition has been produced experimentally in lambs exposed to prenatal hyperthermia.

Megalencephaly *refers to an abnormally large brain or excessive volume of the intracranial contents.* Enlargements as a result of excessive germinal cell proliferation are rare and tend to be asymmetrical with exaggerated degrees of heterotopia.

Cortical dysplasia *encompasses defects in the architecture of the cerebral cortex.* In its mildest expression, there is only histological evidence of lack of the normal orderly layered appearance of the cerebral cortex. *Neuronal heterotopia* is the presence of clusters of nerve cells at a site where they are normally absent, such as subcortical white matter. This condition represents incomplete migration of neuroblasts during fetal life and is usually associated with dysplastic development of the cortex. Scattered, rather than clustered, neurons are commonly present in subcortical white matter and are not of clinical significance. *The presence of aggregations of small dark primitive neuroglial cells is a normal finding in periventricular locations and in the rhinencephalic cortex.* Heterotopia may also involve glial elements, here taking the form of aberrant nests of glial cells.

In **microgyria** *(polymicrogyria), convolutions are small and unusually numerous, and the normal gyral pattern is lost in affected areas.* The lesion may be asymmetrical or patchy, abruptly demarcated from normal cortex, but its real extent may only be revealed on cut surfaces. It may be present near the margins of cavitating lesions such as hydranencephaly. **Ulegyria** also imparts a wrinkled appearance to the cortex but arises as a consequence of scarring and atrophy in otherwise topographically normal gyri. It is a *result of laminar necrosis*, particularly affecting sulci, caused by prolonged ischemic/anoxic injury in the perinatal period.

In **lissencephaly** (agyria), the primitive pattern of the telencephalon persists due to arrested migration of neuroblasts from the ventricular zone along radial glial fibers to the appropriate cortical lamina. *Convolutions are almost entirely absent* and the brain surface may be smooth except for slight grooves in which the meningeal vessels are situated. The cerebral cortex is excessively thick. In humans with *LIS1* or *DCX* gene mutations, failure of dynein-mediated nucleus–centrosome coupling leads to abnormal neuronal migration. Lissencephaly occurs in Lhasa Apso dogs.

Pachygyria (macrogyria) is characterized by *excessively broad brain convolutions* resulting from fewer secondary gyri and increased depth of the gray matter underlying the smooth part of the cortex. Pachygyria is a transitional malformation of the cortex, less severe than agyria but akin to it.

Bibliography

Crino PB. Malformations of cortical development: molecular pathogenesis and experimental strategies. Adv Exp Med Biol 2004;548:175–191.

Franklin RJ, et al. An inherited neurological disorder of the St Bernard dog characterised by unusual cerebellar cortical dysplasia. Vet Rec 1997;140:656–657.

Pilz D, et al. Neuronal migration, cerebral cortical development, and cerebral cortical anomalies. J Neuropathol Exp Neurol 2002;61:1–11.

Saito M, et al. Magnetic resonance imaging features of lissencephaly in 2 Lhasa Apsos. Vet Radiol Ultrasound 2002;43:331–337.

Tanaka T, et al. Lis1 and doublecortin function with dynein to mediate coupling of the nucleus to the centrosome in neuronal migration. J Cell Biol 2004;165:709–721.

Disorders of axonal growth

As neurons migrate from the periventricular germinal zone along radial glia, they begin to form axonal and dendritic processes. The growth and direction of growth of these processes are guided by complex cues including molecules of the extracellular matrix and there is an extensive literature relating to the molecular genetics that regulate these processes.

Agenesis or hypoplasia of the corpus callosum is an *uncommon anomaly* but is recorded in most domestic species. It is the most studied of the disorders of axonal growth in human and animal models. It may occur alone or in association with other anomalies of the brain (Fig. 3.23). The septum pellucidum is absent as a collateral

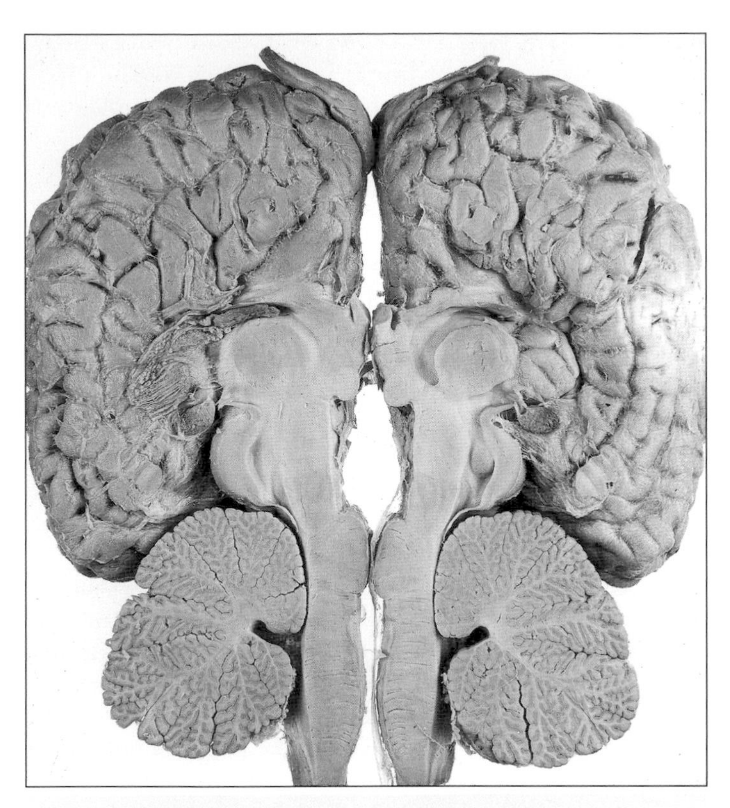

Figure 3.23 Agenesis of corpus callosum in a horse.

defect; the leaves are separated and displaced laterally to the roof of the lateral ventricles. There is no cingulate gyrus, the interhemispheric gyri appearing to radiate from the roof of the third ventricle.

The corpus callosum is formed by the crossing-over of fibers from one hemisphere to the other, a migration that begins at the lamina terminalis, which is the most rostral point of the neural tube. Dysgenesis of the prosencephalic vesicle in its midline may impair the lamina terminalis, or there may be disordered outgrowth of axons from the cerebral cortex. The migration of fibers is guided by a glial scaffold, which may be absent as the primary defect. The corpus may be entirely absent or the commissures may be present and the corpus defective in its central part.

The development of the septum lucidum is linked to that of the corpus callosum and its residue may form a **cystic septum pellucidum**. The cavum septi pellucidi is always present in the fetus as a midline cavity that originates within the commissural plate by tissue resorption. In the normal course, the cavity is obliterated, resulting in a glial midline raphe, but *failure of fusion of the leaflets results in a cystic fluid-filled cavity that varies from a thin slit to a rounder cavity*. The cyst is covered externally by ependyma and lined by a glial mesh. This condition occasionally accompanies defects caused by fetal infections with viruses such as those of Akabane disease, bluetongue, bovine viral diarrhea, and Border disease.

Holoencephaly

Immediately on closure of the rostral neuropore, the rostral end of the tube enlarges to form three vesicles, the rostral of which, or *prosencephalon*, will become the forebrain, the intermediate vesicle will form the *mesencephalon* or midbrain, and the caudal vesicle will form the hindbrain or *rhombencephalon*. The dorsal wall of the rostral vesicle becomes thickened dorsally in the midline to form the commissural plate, eventually the corpus callosum, and the vesicle expands laterally to form the paired cerebral vesicles, which will become the cerebral hemispheres.

Holoencephaly (holoprosencephaly) refers to a spectrum of deformities involving the hemispheres and typically including aplasia of the olfactory bulbs and tracts (arhinencephaly), as a result of failure of cleavage of the prosencephalon. The dysplasia is typically associated with facial deformities, and the extent of the nervous and facial deformities correspond closely. The most severe expression is cyclopia (synophthalmus), but the spectrum ranges through intermediate expressions such as cebocephaly to lesser deformities in which the orbits and nose may be normal or the nares are retruded with variably expressed clefts of lips and palate.

Cyclopia, referring to the presence of a *single large median eye*, emphasizes the most obvious and remarkable abnormality of a very complicated defect. The condition is not uncommon in domestic animals, especially pigs, and it can be reproduced experimentally simply and in many different ways.

The causes of sporadic cases are largely unknown, but many instances in humans are due to chromosomal anomalies. Various degrees of cyclopia are present in Guernsey and Jersey fetuses that are the subjects of *prolonged gestation*. *Veratrum californicum* is responsible for congenital cyclopian malformations that occur endemically in lambs in the western livestock grazing areas of the USA. The teratogenic agent in the plant is *cyclopamine*, a steroidal alkaloid. Induction of the cyclopian deformity in lamb fetuses is dependent on pregnant ewes ingesting *V. californicum* on day 14 of gestation. Cyclopia has also been produced experimentally in cattle and goats, with a similar narrow interval of susceptibility to maternal ingestion of *Veratrum* on or about day 14 of gestation. Cyclopamine-induced teratogenesis may result from antagonism of Sonic hedgehog gene signal transduction that is necessary for normal dorsoventral patterning of the neural tube and somites. The primary defect occurs at the neural plate stage of development and involves the rostral extremity of the notochord and the mesoderm immediately surrounding it. Failure of proper induction accounts for the changes in the skull, in soft tissues of the face, and in the brain. The optic defect, consisting of greater-or-lesser division of a single anlage, is probably secondary to the defects of the forebrain.

The orbits may be approximated (Fig. 3.24) but, typically, there is one large orbit and a single optic foramen. Several bones, including the ethmoids, nasal septum, lacrimal bones, and premaxillae, are usually absent. The globe may be absent, rudimentary, or may form a single structure of near-normal conformation, or be partially divided or completely duplicated. The nose is a proboscis or tube that does not communicate with the pharynx and that is typically situated above the median eye. The forebrain is always severely malformed; the hemispheres are not fully cleft but are present instead as a single thin-walled vesicle with a smooth surface and common ventricle and lacking olfactory nerves and tracts, corpus callosum, septum pellucidum, and fornix.

The hindbrain is usually normal. The pituitary may be displaced or absent and fetal gigantism associated with prolonged gestation (see Vol. 3, Female genital system) occurs in some deformed lambs and calves. The optic nerve is single, atrophic, or absent. The oculomotor and abducens nerves are hypoplastic or absent. There is internal hydrocephalus.

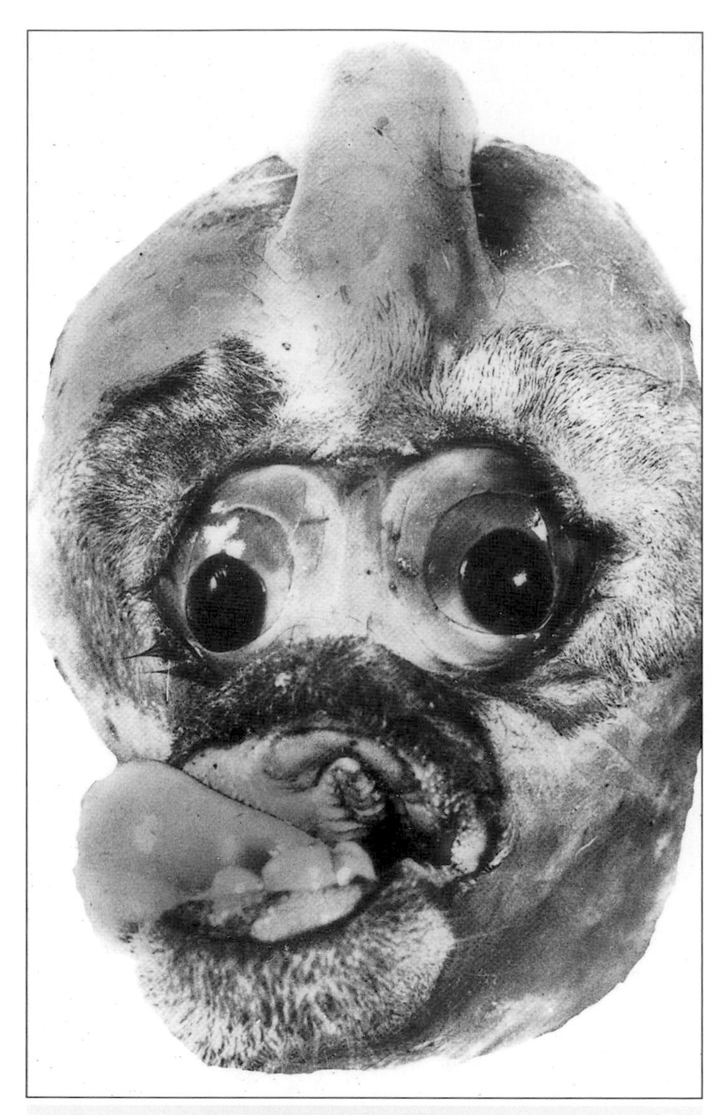

Figure 3.24 Cyclopia (synophthalmus) in a calf with inherited prolonged gestation.

Veratrum californicum also causes embryonic death. A wide range of other defects has been produced experimentally in lambs, with abbreviation of the metacarpal and metatarsal bones being the most distinctive.

Cebocephaly (monkey face) *is anatomically comparable to cyclopia, and probably represents a less severe expression of the same basic defects.* There are two eyes, severely hypoplastic, in separate but approximated orbits. The nose is in the normal position, but deformed and may not protrude. There is a single, small nasal cavity or a proboscis with no communication with the pharynx. The brain appears as in cyclopia but may have a slight median sulcus.

Bibliography

Cho DY, et al. Holoprosencephaly in a bovine calf. Acta Neuropathol (Berl) 1985;67:322–325.

Cho DY, Leipold HW. Agenesis of corpus callosum in calves. Cornell Vet 1978;68:99–107.

Hahn JS, Pinter JD. Holoprosencephaly: genetic, neuroradiological, and clinical advances. Semin Pediatr Neurol 2002;9:309–319.

Incardona JP, et al. The teratogenic *Veratrum* alkaloid cyclopamine inhibits sonic hedgehog signal transduction. Development 1998;125:3553–3562.

Sullivan SA, et al. Lobar holoprosencephaly in a Miniature Schnauzer with hypodipsic hypernatremia. J Am Vet Med Assoc 2003;223:1783–1787.

Hydrocephalus

Hydrocephalus is characterized by abnormal accumulation of fluid in the cranial cavity. In **internal hydrocephalus**, the fluid is within the ventricular system; in **external hydrocephalus**, the fluid is in the arachnoid space; and in **communicating hydrocephalus**, the excess fluid is present in both locations. The communicating and external types of hydrocephalus, the latter to be distinguished from cerebral atrophy, are quite rare in animals. Internal hydrocephalus, which is denoted by variably dilated ventricular cavities lined by ependyma, is quite common, may be congenital or acquired, but both forms may be considered here for convenience.

Cerebrospinal fluid (CSF) is produced by the ventricular choroid plexuses by means of filtration and secretion. There are significant contributions by ependyma and extraventricular structures. Because of the permeable nature of the ependymal lining of the ventricular system, the CSF is in effect an extension of the extracellular fluid of the CNS, and its composition is affected by metabolic and pathological changes within the brain.

The flow of CSF is from the lateral ventricle through the interventricular foramen to the third ventricle and then via the mesencephalic aqueduct to the fourth ventricle. From here, most of the fluid leaves the ventricular system and passes by way of the lateral cerebellomedullary apertures into the subarachnoid space. A small amount of CSF passes into the central canal of the spinal cord from the fourth ventricle. The greater part of the fluid flows forward into the cerebral subarachnoid spaces and basal cisterns; the balance circulates in a restricted fashion in the spinal subarachnoid space. The energy required to circulate CSF is imparted largely by the choroid plexuses through their production of fluid. The arterial pulse also contributes to CSF movement through associated variations in hemispheric volume. Venous resorption of CSF occurs where arachnoid villi form in the walls of the larger meningeal veins. Transfer of fluid is effected by hydrostatic pressure, with reflux being prevented by the valvular nature of the villi. The arachnoid villi are normally highly permeable, being able to permit the passage of red blood cells. Impedance of this resorption appears to contribute to the increased intracranial pressure of hypovitaminosis A in calves. Some outflow in dogs can occur via the cribriform plate and in cats along the subarachnoid space of olfactory, optic, and acoustic nerves, but significant outflow may possibly occur only in association with raised intracranial pressure. The spinal subarachnoid space appears to communicate freely with the lymphatic system opening in the intradural nerve roots.

Familiarity with the normal directional flow of CSF is basic to an understanding of the pathogenesis of hydrocephalus because in most cases it is probably of obstructive origin. Certainly, *an obstruction can be demonstrated in most instances of acquired hydrocephalus in animals.* In congenital hydrocephalus, obstruction is quite often not demonstrable, but stenotic aqueductal malformations may be found (Fig. 3.25). Obstructive hydrocephalus has been induced experimentally in many species of immature laboratory animals with a range of viruses ubiquitous in animals and man. The selective destructive action of these viruses on ependymal cells with subsequent reparative gliovascular

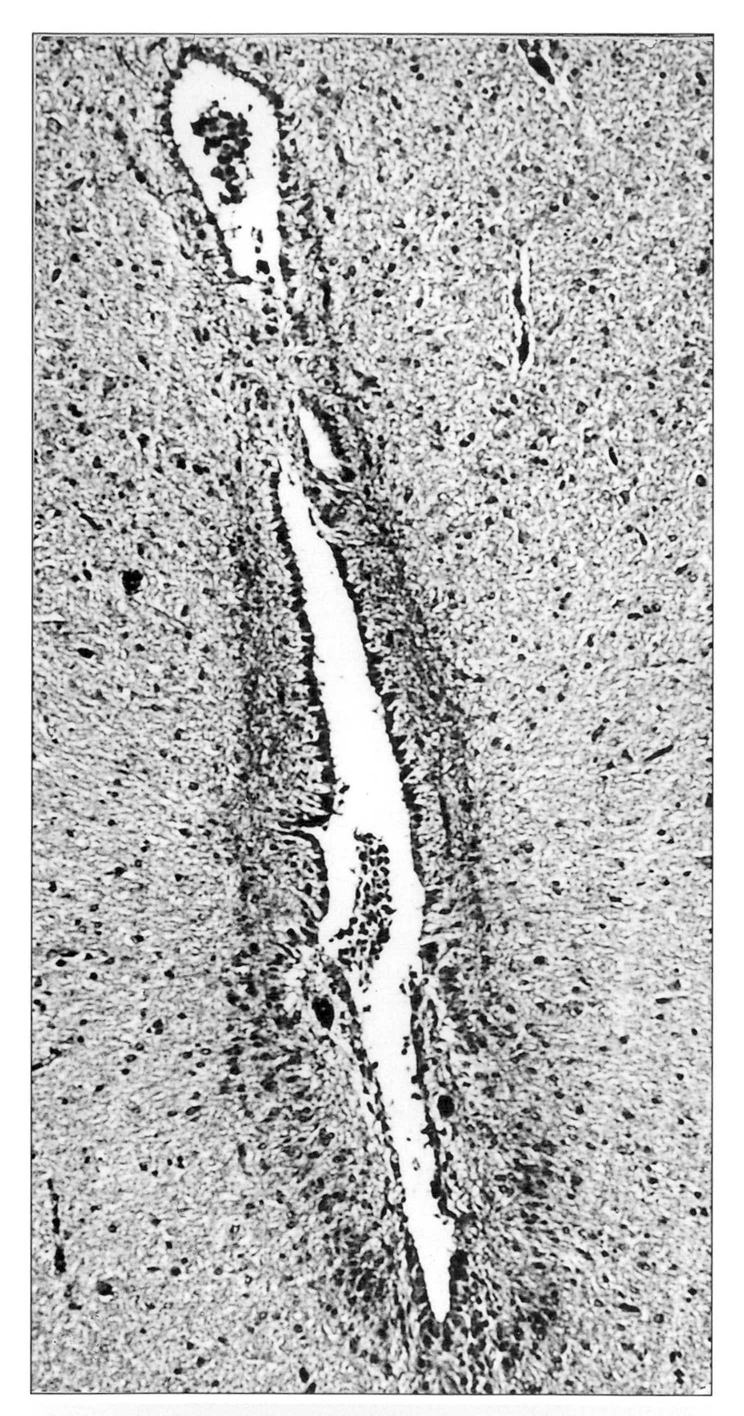

Figure 3.25 Malformation of aqueduct in a calf.

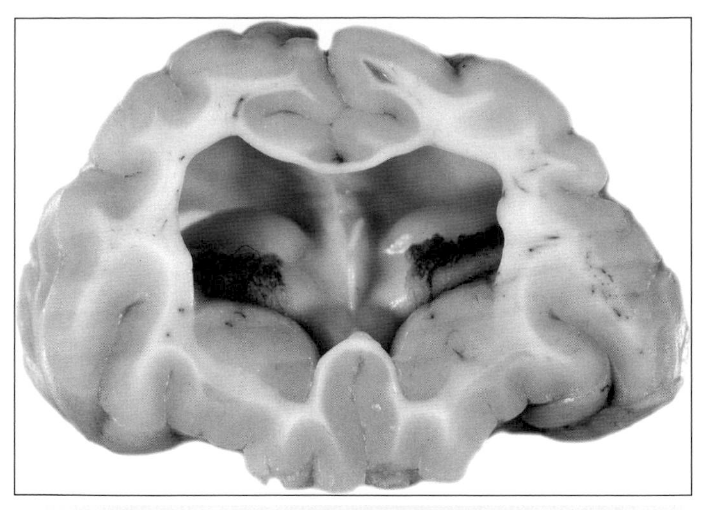

Figure 3.26 Hydrocephalus in a cat, due to vitamin A deficiency. (Courtesy of RF Slocombe.)

proliferation results in obstruction of CSF pathways, usually in the mesencephalic aqueduct. Thus far in domestic animals, viral-induced hydrocephalus of this genesis has been demonstrated only in experimental canine parainfluenza virus infection in dogs.

Hydrocephalus is "physiological" in the early fetus when the hemispheres are largely thin-walled vesicles. *Congenital hydrocephalus exaggerates this physiological degree of ventricular dilation*. Even in the absence of obstruction, physiological hydrocephalus may persist or be exaggerated in instances of neural dysplasia such as, for example, in cyclopia and cebocephaly. The cavitating cerebral defects, hydranencephaly and porencephaly, are associated with internal hydrocephalus. This is likely to be an *ex vacuo* or compensatory hydrocephalus occurring secondary to loss of cerebral tissue as in the inherited leukodystrophies and storage diseases, but a hydrostatic component arising from deranged circulation of CSF is also possible. Hydrocephalus may accompany other neural anomalies, but chiefly the rather rare Arnold–Chiari and Dandy–Walker malformations in which hydrocephalus is obstructive in origin and associated with abnormalities of the cerebellum and medulla.

With the exception of the few examples just given, *congenital hydrocephalus remains anatomically obvious but pathogenetically obscure*, and such cases are common. Pups, calves, foals, and piglets are chiefly affected, with a familial incidence, possibly genetic, in pigs. The defect is quite uncommon in cats.

Congenital hydrocephalus is well known in **pups**, especially those of the brachycephalic breeds. This should not imply that the hydrocephalus is correlative to, or a product of, brachycephaly because within breeds there is not much variation in the degree of the skeletal defect, and no obvious relation between it and the presence and severity of hydrocephalus. Malformation of the mesencephalic aqueduct may be a significant pathogenetic factor. The anatomic expression of the hydrocephalus also varies considerably; one lateral ventricle may be involved or both may be dilated symmetrically or asymmetrically, the third ventricle and rostral portion of the aqueduct are usually, but not always, involved, and the fourth ventricle is normal.

Sporadic cases of congenital hydrocephalus occur widely in **cattle**. Many appear to be secondary to aqueductal stenosis. An autosomal recessive gene is considered responsible for many apparently hereditary cases, but the possible roles of fetal infections and nutritional factors must be considered.

Outbreaks of congenital hydrocephalus are recorded in calves in which slit-like deformation of the aqueduct of Sylvius was associated with lateral narrowing of the midbrain, in the peripheral areas of which there was vascular proliferation and perivascular gliosis. Hydrocephalus also occurs in association with chondrodysplasias, especially of the "bulldog" type, but the primary neural defect in these is not known. Several hydrocephalic syndromes have been described in Hereford and Shorthorn cattle; features include cerebellar hypoplasia, microphthalmia, myopathy, and ocular anomalies.

Experimentally, *dietary deficiency of vitamin A* can cause congenital and neonatal hydrocephalus (Fig. 3.26), but spontaneous outbreaks occur only in cattle which have fed for prolonged periods on dry pasture or in feedlots. The hydrocephalus is ascribed to functional impairment of absorption of fluid from arachnoid villi but there is frequently severe compression of the brain and herniations in the caudal fossa, which is expected to provide mechanical obstruction to drainage.

Acquired hydrocephalus is fairly common in animals. It does not approach in severity the congenital defect. The causes are almost always obstructive, but minor degrees of ventricular dilation occur in association with cerebral atrophy in old dogs. Meningeal lesions that destroy the arachnoid villi can lead to external hydrocephalus. This is, however, quite rare, although it has been observed in diffuse meningeal carcinomatosis. Most diffuse meningeal lesions are inflammatory, but these are typically associated with internal rather than external hydrocephalus because meningitis tends to involve the basilar regions and the caudal fossa chiefly and there interferes with the patency of the lateral cerebellomedullary apertures. Most cases of bacterial meningitis are fatal before the changes of hydrocephalus develop unless, as frequently happens, concurrent inflammation of the choroid plexuses extends to the ependyma of the aqueduct and obstructs that channel. Even relatively chronic cases of meningitis, such as may be observed in cryptococcosis, are associated with internal rather than communicating or external hydrocephalus. Additional causes of acquired hydrocephalus are intracranial neoplasms, usually primary but sometimes metastatic, and including papillomas and carcinomas of the choroid plexus, parasitic cysts such as hydatids and coenurids, and the late effects of chronic or healed inflammation that involve the ependyma or cause inflammatory softening or atrophy of paraependymal tissue. The pyogranulomatous ependymitis and meningoencephalitis of feline infectious peritonitis occasionally results in hydrocephalus. In horses, the so-called cholesteatomas or cholesterol granulomas that develop in the choroid plexuses of the lateral ventricles may occlude the interventricular foramen and cause internal hydrocephalus.

Hydrocephalus does not regress. Whether it progresses or not is difficult to determine. Congenital hydrocephalus cannot be easily diagnosed in the newborn in the absence of secondary changes in the cranium, and diagnosable cases seldom live long enough for the course of the defect to be ascertained. Probably, however, congenital hydrocephalus of mild or moderate degree can remain static because, although a severe and fatal defect is common enough in puppies, *hydrocephalus in brachycephalic breeds of dogs is frequently an incidental finding at necropsy*, and the degree of ventricular dilation may be minor or moderate irrespective of the age of the animal. Acquired hydrocephalus in postnatal life tends to be progressive when of obstructive type, the course depending on the site and nature of the obstructing lesion. Compensatory hydrocephalus occurring as a response to cerebral atrophy is static or at the most slowly progressive; it is never severe, except perhaps in familial lipofuscinosis of dogs.

Congenital hydrocephalus is frequently associated with malformation of the cranium. The degree of cranial malformation varies from slight doming, which may be difficult to appreciate, to enormous enlargement, which may cause dystocia. Cranial malformation is not invariable however, and many cases of congenital hydrocephalus of considerable severity may occur with a skull of normal contour. Whether cranial malformation occurs or not probably depends on the time of onset of the hydrocephalus relative to the degree of ossification of the cranial bones and the development and strength of the sutures, and also on the rate at which the fluid is accumulated.

It is often difficult to be certain of the presence of minor degrees of hydrocephalus. The soft brains of the newborn collapse when removed from the skull so that dilation of ventricles may not be apparent. In older, firmer brains, asymmetry of the lateral ventricles and relative dilation of the rostral end of the aqueduct when compared with the caudal end are useful indices. *The septum pellucidum, however, is the structure most sensitive to the effects of fluid accumulation*; it may be fenestrated or may persist as an irregular lacework of connective tissue, but typically, it is absent. Even in mild hydrocephalus, there is usually atrophy in Ammon's horn readily detectable by the ease with which the piriform lobes dimple under slight pressure. With hydrocephalus of greater severity, there is ventricular dilation of corresponding degree. The lateral and third ventricles are most severely affected, and there may be no alteration in the fourth. With ventricular dilation, parenchymal atrophy affects chiefly the white matter and the cerebral cortices; ventrally, the increased pressure is buttressed by the basal ganglia. The corpus callosum is elevated and thinned, and the cerebral cortices over the vertex may be reduced to thin shells of gray matter. The floor of the third ventricle is extremely thinned, the hypophysis is atrophied, and the cerebellum is compressed and displaced caudally.

The extensive cranial malformation of congenital hydrocephalus can occur only if the sutures are ununited. The temporal, frontal, and parietal bones are enlarged and thin and are separated from each other by broad membranes of connective tissue in which accessory bones may form. In these severe cases, the base of the cranium is flattened, the fossae are enlarged and smoothed out, and the orbits are separated but individually reduced in size so that the eyes may protrude.

Gray matter is remarkably resistant to the effects of the pressure exerted by the fluid, but the subcortical white matter degenerates rapidly. It is edematous, the oligodendrocytes and astrocytes are reduced in number, and compound granular corpuscles can be found sometimes in short bands lying deep and parallel to the ependyma. The ependyma, tela choroidea, and meninges are usually not altered significantly.

Bibliography

Baumgartner WK, et al. Ultrastructural evaluation of acute encephalitis and hydrocephalus in dogs caused by canine parainfluenza virus. Vet Pathol 1982;19:305–314.

Brinker T, et al. Dynamic properties of lymphatic pathways for the absorption of cerebrospinal fluid. Acta Neuropathol (Berl) 1997;94:493–498.

Cantile C, et al. Hydrocephalus with periventricular encephalitis in the dog. Zentralbl Veterinarmed A 1997;44:595–601.

Dubey JP, et al. Hydrocephalus associated with *Neospora caninum* infection in an aborted bovine fetus. J Comp Pathol 1998;118:169–173.

Harrington ML, et al. Hydrocephalus. Vet Clin North Am Small Anim Pract 1996;26:843–856.

Hewicker-Trautwein M, et al. Brain lesions in calves following transplacental infection with bovine-virus diarrhoea virus. Zentralbl Veterinarmed B 1995;42:65–77.

Jackson CA, et al. Neurological manifestation of cholesterinic granulomas in three horses. Vet Rec 1994;135:228–230.

Johnson RP, et al. Familial cerebellar ataxia with hydrocephalus in bull mastiffs. Vet Radiol Ultrasound 2001;42:246–249.

Leipold HW, Dennis SM. Congenital defects of the bovine central nervous system. Vet Clin North Am Food Anim Pract 1987;3:159–177.

Luciano MG, et al. Cerebrovascular adaptation in chronic hydrocephalus. J Cereb Blood Flow Metab 2001;21:285–294.

Nykamp S, et al. Chronic subdural hematomas and hydrocephalus in a dog. Vet Radiol Ultrasound 2001;42:511–514.
Rivas LJ, et al. Cervical meningomyelocele associated with spina bifida in a hydrocephalic miniature colt. J Am Vet Med Assoc 1996;209:950–953.
Smith HJ, Stevenson RG. Congenital hydrocephalus in swine. Can Vet J 1973;14:311–312.
van der Lugt JJ, Prozesky L. The pathology of blindness in new-born calves caused by hypovitaminosis A. Onderstepoort J Vet Res 1989;56:99–109.
Wunschmann A, Oglesbee M. Periventricular changes associated with spontaneous canine hydrocephalus. Vet Pathol 2001;38:67–73.

Hydranencephaly, porencephaly

In **hydranencephaly**, *there can be complete or almost complete absence of the cerebral hemispheres, leaving only membranous sacs filled with CSF and enclosed by leptomeninges.* The cranial cavity is always complete, in contrast to hydrocephalus, and usually of normal conformation, although occasionally there is mild doming of the skull or thickening of the cranial bones. The dorsal, and often the caudal parts of the hemispheres, are the portions most severely defective (Fig. 3.27A, B, C). The leptomeninges may easily be damaged on removing the calvaria but are in their usual position and form sacs enclosing CSF, the fluid occupying the space normally occupied by parenchyma. Discrete remnants of parenchyma may be present in the meninges. When the leptomeninges are incised, it is apparent that the brain stem is of near-normal conformation with well-developed hippocampus and choroid plexuses. The rostral portion of the corpus callosum and septum pellucidum may be intact although attenuated. Cerebellar hypoplasia may be present as a concurrent defect as may the histologic deficits of hypomyelinogenesis.

Hydranencephaly is the residual lesion of full-thickness necrosis of the cerebral hemisphere. In animals, the lesion develops in early fetal stages and before the mature arrangements of the cortex are present. The marginal tissue is dysplastic, flat, and microgyric or the gyri have a radial arrangement from the defect. Although a diagnosis of hydranencephaly is readily made on macroscopic inspection, histological study

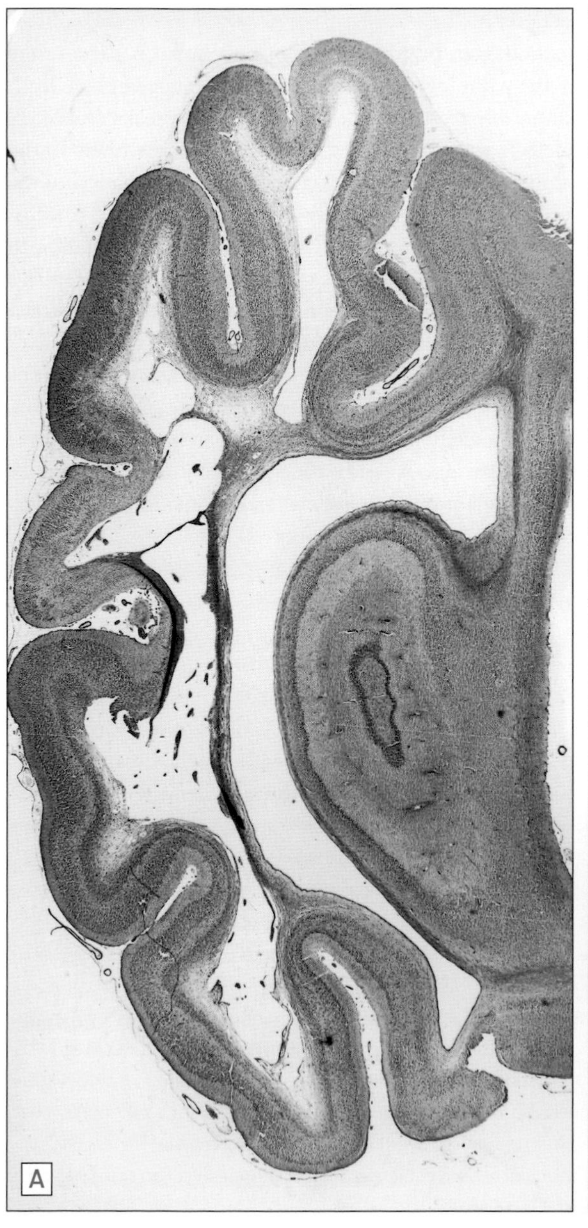

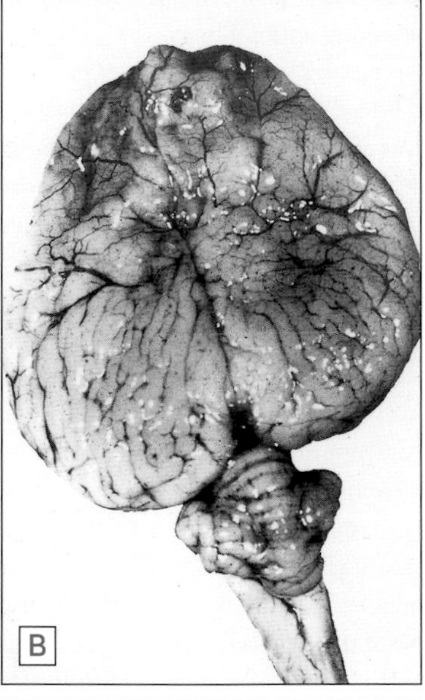

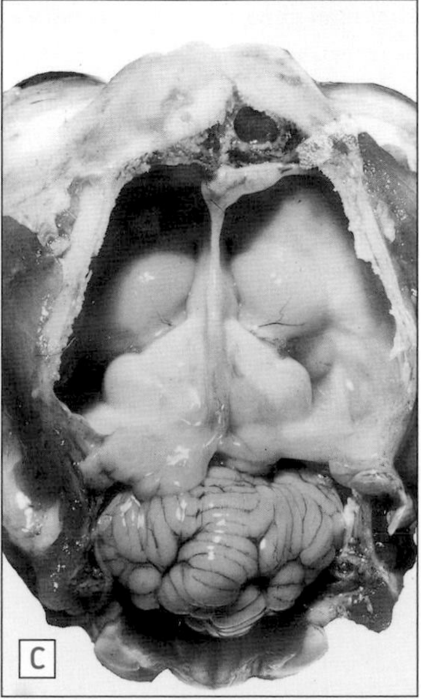

Figure 3.27 A. Hydranencephaly in a lamb with swayback. (Courtesy of J McC Howell.) **B. Hydranencephaly** and cerebellar hypoplasia in a lamb, subsequent to intrauterine *Bluetongue virus* infection. **C. Hydranencephaly** in a cat; meninges removed to expose the brain stem structures.

may provide some insight into the nature of the disease process. The membranous coverings of the remnants of the hemispheres comprise arachnoid, pia, and a thin mantle of residual cortex in normal juxtaposition. The residual cortical tissue may be lined by attenuated ependyma displaced outwards with expansion of the lateral ventricles, but this ependymal lining is frequently incomplete or absent, and the cavity abuts directly on cortical tissue which may be unremarkable except for mild astrocytosis.

Hydranencephaly occurs in all species but is most common in calves, in which it occurs either sporadically or as minor epizootics. The lesion occurs similarly although less frequently in *lambs*. The species occurrence of hydranencephaly reflects its etiological associations with certain viruses infecting the fetus at a critical stage of gestation. In these cases, *hydranencephaly is often part of a spectrum of neural lesions*, the expression of which depends mainly on the age of the fetus at infection. Viruses that are well established as causes of hydranencephaly tend to be either arboviruses, such as *Akabane virus, Bluetongue virus, Rift Valley fever virus* and *Wesselsbron virus*, or pestiviruses, such as *Bovine viral diarrhea virus* and *Border disease virus*.

The *pathogenesis* of hydranencephaly has been clarified through studies of the cavitating encephalopathies caused by fetal viral infections, particularly bluetongue and Border disease in lambs. These infections at critical periods of gestation produce *subventricular zones of necrosis* of the developing cerebral hemispheres. These zones, which may have a vascular basis, involve the neuroblasts in their outward migration and result in cavitation and deprive the cortex of its normal complement of neurons. These cavitations range in size from small cysts with only minor changes in the overlying cortex (porencephaly) to large confluent spaces with the hemispheres reduced to fluid-filled sacs (hydranencephaly). During the necrotizing process, there may be an intense macrophage response, but it is usual for this reaction to have subsided by the time the animal is born and examined.

Mechanical factors also contribute to the development of hydranencephaly. A dissecting effect associated with escape of CSF into the parenchyma may also be important since segmental loss of ventricular ependyma is an early feature of the cavitating process.

Compensatory expansion of the lateral ventricles secondary to loss of brain substance occurs and rapid expansion of the fetal calvaria during the gestation period allows stretching and rupture of residual cortical tissue. In less severely affected areas, the outer rim of cortex overlies a band of subependymal tissue, the intervening cavity being occupied by trabecular parenchymal remnants. Rosette formations of cells that resemble ependymal epithelium may be found in the subependymal area. Accumulations of mineralized debris may be present in the meninges.

Porencephaly *is cystic cavitation of the brain evolving from a destructive process in prenatal life.* The defect typically involves the white matter of the cerebral hemispheres. An affected brain may contain a single cyst or there may be multiple cystic lesions. The temporal portion of the cerebral hemispheres is an area of predilection, but porencephalic change may be found throughout the cerebral hemispheres, although typically sparing the basal nuclei. Occasionally, lesions are found in brain stem and cerebellum. The cysts are usually randomly located, but evidence of bilateral symmetry is sometimes apparent, particularly in well-developed lesions of the cerebral hemisphere. Rarely cysts may communicate with ventricular cavities or with the subarachnoid space. The cysts may be apparent from the meningeal aspect as focal fluctuant areas of attenuated cerebral cortex or as superficial, clear submeningeal cysts. The cysts range in size from microscopic to several centimeters in diameter. The cysts are variable in shape, but roughly spherical or cleft-like outlines are common. On section, they are filled with clear fluid and are smooth walled, but are traversed by variable numbers of trabeculae. Less well-developed lesions may appear as gelatinous softenings.

The porencephalic cavities, particularly the larger defects, are often unremarkable microscopically, being lined by a layer of flattened glia. Apart from some mild marginal astrocytosis, they show surprisingly little evidence of reactive or inflammatory change. In other cases, there is accumulation of hemosiderin-containing gitter cells about the margins of the cyst and within the cavity. The trabeculae comprise residual brain parenchyma, usually oriented about a blood vessel. Some small lesions, evident grossly as focal gelatinous areas, appear as focal leukomalacia comprising white matter in the process of dissolution associated with accumulation of macrophages and gitter cells. Sometimes the inflammatory nature of the lesions is indicated by the presence of mild nonsuppurative meningoencephalitis with gliosis, perivascular cuffing and focal mineralization about the margins of the cysts, and mononuclear infiltration in the meninges overlying the defects.

The etiopathogenesis of porencephaly parallels, but is a less severe expression of, the pathological process seen in hydranencephaly. Both lesions are commonly recorded in the course of outbreaks of cavitating cerebral defects and may occur together in the same brain. In the case of cavitating viral infections of the fetal brain, termination of the disease process in either porencephaly or hydranencephaly is influenced by gestational age at infection, with porencephaly tending to follow infection at a later stage than is the case with hydranencephaly.

Porencephaly is a common manifestation of prenatal infection of *lambs* with some strains of *Border disease virus* and is seen in calves infected in utero by *Bovine viral diarrhea virus*. The cystic or gelatinous transformations of the cerebral white matter that occur in some cases of copper deficiency in lambs (swayback) are porencephalic in nature. The lesion has also been induced experimentally in lambs by exposure of pregnant ewes to hyperthermia during the last two-thirds of pregnancy.

Bibliography

Chung SI, et al. Congenital malformations in sheep resulting from in utero inoculation of Cache Valley virus. Am J Vet Res 1990;51:1645–1648.

Hartley WJ, et al. Brain cavitation and micrencephaly in lambs exposed to prenatal hyperthermia. Teratology 1974;9:299–303.

Hewicker-Trautwein M, et al. Brain lesions in calves following transplacental infection with bovine-virus diarrhoea virus. Zentralbl Veterinarmed B 1995;42:65–77.

Hewicker-Trautwein M, Trautwein G. Porencephaly, hydranencephaly and leukoencephalopathy in ovine fetuses following transplacental infection with bovine virus diarrhoea virus: distribution of viral antigen and characterization of cellular response. Acta Neuropathol (Berl) 1994;87:385–397.

Hunter P, et al. Teratogenicity of a mutagenised Rift Valley fever virus (MVP 12) in sheep. Onderstepoort J Vet Res 2002;69:95–98.

Kitani H, et al. Preferential infection of neuronal and astroglia cells by Akabane virus in primary cultures of fetal bovine brain. Vet Microbiol 2000;73:269–279.

MacLachlan NJ, Osburn BI. Bluetongue virus-induced hydranencephaly in cattle. Vet Pathol 1983;20:563–573.

Tsuda T, et al. Arthrogryposis, hydranencephaly and cerebellar hypoplasia syndrome in neonatal calves resulting from intrauterine infection with Aino virus. Vet Res 2004;35:531–538.

Wintour EM, et al. Experimental hydranencephaly in the ovine fetus. Acta Neuropathol (Berl) 1996;91:537–544.

Periventricular leukomalacia of neonates

Interrelated lesions dominated by intraventricular hemorrhage, ventriculomegaly, and malacia of white matter are quite frequent in neonates. In domestic animals, the lesion has not been distinguished from hydrocephalus and hydranencephaly, which is the reason for considering it here with the malformations from which it needs to be distinguished, rather than with malacic diseases. The application of imaging technology has identified a surprising incidence of the complex in human neonates with later minimal to severe neurological deficits. The lesions in human neonates are most frequently associated with placentitis, prematurity, and growth retardation, suggesting that placental insufficiency may be critically important. In lambs, there is an association with placentitis of toxoplasmosis, tick-borne fever, and chlamydiosis.

Periventricular leukomalacia typically refers to necrosis of white matter adjacent to the lateral ventricles that results in the formation of cysts in the cerebrum or in more extensive lesions simulating hydranencephaly or hydrocephalus *ex vacuo*. In animals, the lesion is not limited to the cerebrum but may extend to affect also periventricular white matter of the cerebellum, cerebellar roof nuclei, and white matter of the cerebellar folia.

Intraventricular hemorrhage may extend caudally as far as the central canal of the spinal cord causing ventricular dilation. The hemorrhage of variable severity may remain intramural in the hemispheral white matter.

Periventricular leukomalacia may allow survival in pups for several weeks. The cavitating cerebral lesion, and the cerebellar lesion if present, is lined internally by ependyma and a thin layer of white matter. There may be local defects allowing communication with the dilated ventricle. Clustered cases are observed in kids and lambs. Affected neonates tend to be small for age, stillborn, or die immediately after delivery, although some with minor neurologic defect may survive and develop normally.

The pathogenesis of these defects is unknown. The mechanisms appear to involve the structural fragility of blood vessels in the periventricular subependymal zone and instability of blood flow in the vulnerable areas. Perivascular hemorrhages may be confined to this zone. The malacic lesion in white matter is coagulative necrosis with vacuolation of the tissue and acidophilic swollen retraction balls on axonal fragments. Microglia provide the only inflammatory cells. Cystic lesions have peripheral sprigs of capillaries and marginal and luminal macrophages expected to contain hemosiderin. In individual cases in lambs and kids, the lesions may be of different ages and, in clustered cases in these animals, some may show hemorrhage only and some may show established cavities.

Bibliography

Back SA, Rivkees SA. Emerging concepts in periventricular white matter injury. Semin Perinatol 2004;28:405–414.

Chianini F, et al. Neuropathological changes in ovine fetuses caused by tickborne fever. Vet Rec 2004;155:805–806.

Kuban K, et al. White matter disorders of prematurity: Association with intraventricular hemorrhage and ventriculomegaly. J Pediatr 1999;134:539–546.

Marumo G, et al. Generation of periventricular leukomalacia by repeated umbilical cord occlusion in near-term fetal sheep and its possible pathogenetical mechanisms. Biol Neonate 2001;79:39–45.

Cerebellum/caudal fossa

The cerebellum develops from the lips of the rhombencephalon in the region of incomplete closure of the neural tube. There are *two major germinative zones*. The rostral lips give rise to precursors of the cerebellar granule cells. In their first migration, granule cell precursors cover the whole of the cerebellar pial layer at about the time of closure of the rostral neuropore. This is a germinative layer that produces a second generation of germinal cells, some of which remain as daughter cells and others undergo lateral migration in the developing molecular layer. In a third migratory wave, postmitotic cells send axons vertically down through the molecular and Purkinje-cell layers under guidance of radial glia; the cell body then moves along the axon to the maturing granular layer.

Disorder of the granule cell layer is frequently part of the disruption caused by fetal viral infections. *Focal heterotopias* are frequent in neonates usually without clinical effect. These cells may be the origin of the medulloblastomas of young animals.

The caudal rhombic lips produce a highly proliferative neuroepithelium from which neuronal precursors migrate along several pathways to form the Purkinje cells of the cerebellar cortex, the cerebellar roof nuclei, and to the precerebellar nuclei including the olivary, cuneate, and reticular nuclei of the medulla, and to the pontine and tegmental nuclei of the pons; axons from these nuclei project back into the cerebellum.

The cerebellum has three functionally distinct regions. The *vestibulocerebellum* regulates balance and eye movements. It is the oldest part of the cerebellum (paleocerebellum) and occupies the flocculonodular lobules where it receives afferents from the vestibular nuclei. The *spinocerebellum* regulates limb and body movements, receiving somatosensory information via the spinocerebellar tracts and precerebellar nuclei, and occupies the vermis and medial aspects of the hemispheres. The lateral hemispheres, the *cerebrocerebellum*, receive input from the cerebrum via pontine nuclei and are involved in the composition of complex movements. Within these main cerebellar regions, there is further regional patterning corresponding to body parts.

Disorders of migration and survival of Purkinje cells underlie many of the cerebellar malformations, and premature loss is the most common component of the abiotrophies. Correlative changes may be present in the precerebellar nuclei and in the cerebellar roof nuclei.

Cerebellar defects are among the more important of the developmental anomalies of the CNS because of their frequent occurrence and almost invariable accompaniment by significant and distinctive clinical manifestations. They may be expressions of failure of intercellular communication and support whereby a defect in one cell lineage may adversely affect the organizational pattern and function and viability of other cell types. *Cerebellar defects are quite common in cats and calves, relatively so in pigs, dogs, and lambs, but uncommon in foals.* Most defects of morphogenesis can be divided into two broad categories and the entities are discussed below as being examples of either *cerebellar hypoplasia* or *cerebellar abiotrophy (atrophy)*. This distinction into hypoplastic and atrophic types is somewhat artificial, because it is apparent that many cases are compounded by both processes.

Minor dysplastic lesions of no consequence are quite common in young animals but are fewer or less conspicuous in adults. They are most common in the flocculonodular lobules and where the cortex terminates at the peduncles. The foci are microscopic and consist of tangled islands of germinal, molecular, and granular layers with Purkinje cells distributed haphazardly. The dysplasias of the Arnold–Chiari and Dandy–Walker syndromes, of copper deficiency, and the metabolic storage disorders are discussed separately.

The name of the teratological condition merely emphasizes the major component, in these cases the cerebellar defect. There may, however, be coincident malformations such as agenesis of the corpus callosum or hydranencephaly. *There are always correlative changes*, this term grouping together those structural changes that occur in nuclear masses that send fibers to, or receive fibers from, the cerebellum as well as in the particular tract of fibers themselves. The term implies that there is a causal connection, the cerebellar defects being primary and the subcerebellar defects being secondary, but such an implication is less likely to be valid for the cerebellar hypoplasias than for the cerebellar atrophies. Anatomic classifications of the cerebellar hypoplasias tend to take into account the distribution and severity of correlative changes, especially those in the deep cerebellar nuclei, the pontine nuclei, the inferior olives and in the cerebellar brachia, the restiform bodies, and the spinocerebellar tracts. The pattern of correlative changes varies from case to case, and there is not a quantitative correspondence between the cerebellar defects and the correlative defects. There are also very wide variations in the severity of the cerebellar hypoplasias, which is reasonable if the severity is properly to be related to the time of onset, duration, and severity of the arrest of development. From these viewpoints, *anatomical classification of cerebellar hypoplasias is artificial because the defects are quantitative.*

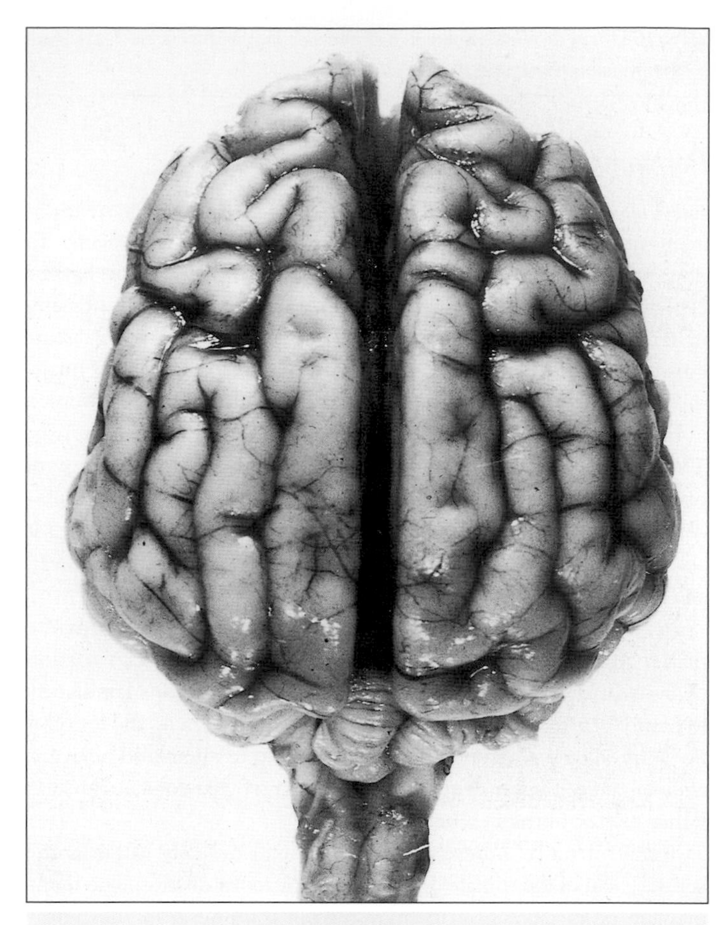

Figure 3.28 Cerebellar hypoplasia in a dog.

Cerebellar hypoplasia, abiotrophy

Cerebellar hypoplasia *is one of the most common congenital nervous system defects of domestic animals and is seen in all domestic species* (Fig. 3.28). There is persuasive evidence for genetically determined occurrence of the disease in calves of various breeds, particularly beef shorthorns, in Arabian and Arabian cross foals, and in Gotland ponies and Chow Chow dogs. A novel form of cerebellar hypoplasia with intraneuronal inclusions is reported from New Zealand in Cocker Spaniel dogs with progressive ataxia and seizures. Cerebellar hypoplasia has been reported in piglets born to sows treated with the organophosphate trichlorfon during pregnancy, and may be detected microscopically in goat kids and lambs affected by hypocuprosis. The most prevalent and best-defined cerebellar hypoplasias are those that follow infection of the developing cerebellum by *Feline panleukopenia virus, Bovine viral diarrhea virus, Border disease virus,* and *Classical swine fever virus.* Canine parvoviral DNA has been detected in cerebellar hypoplasia in dogs. The occurrence of cerebellar hypoplasia as a consequence of viral infections of the developing nervous system is further discussed in the section Viral causes of developmental defects of the central nervous system.

Cerebellar growth patterns determine the gestational or perinatal periods during which cerebellar hypoplasia may follow the action of a teratogen and influence the nature and scope of the structural aberrations marking the hypoplastic process. The cerebellum originates as a dorsal growth of the alar plate of the metencephalon over the fourth ventricle. Germinal cells adjacent to the fourth ventricle differentiate into neurons that migrate into the developing cerebellum to form the deep nuclei and Purkinje neurons. This differentiation occurs prior to mid-gestation. A population of germinal cells migrates to the surface of the developing cerebellum and forms a layer several cells thick. This is the external granular layer that covers the folia as they develop. In this layer, cells proliferate rapidly and differentiate into microneurons such as basket cells, stellate cells and granule cells, which migrate into the folium to their definitive locations. This proliferation, differentiation, and migration begins late in gestation and continues for a few weeks postnatally in most species. Normal cerebellar cytoarchitectural development, including the maturation and localization of Purkinje cells, is dependent upon these microneurons establishing orderly synaptic connections.

It is the actively mitotic germinative cells of the external granular layer that are especially vulnerable to the effects of teratogenic agents. *Feline panleukopenia virus, Bovine viral diarrhea virus, and Border disease virus cause selective necrosis of external granular layer cells.* That the destructive process may be augmented by vascular damage has been demonstrated for *Bovine viral diarrhea virus. Classical swine fever virus* possibly acts through inhibition of cell division and maturation. In puppies, segmental cerebellar dysplasia may result from postnatal infection with canine herpesvirus. Since the growth behavior of the subependymal cell plate has features in common with the external granular layer of the cerebellum, residual lesions attributable to this site of infection, such as cavitating defects, may be associated with cerebellar hypoplasia, particularly in cases of viral origin.

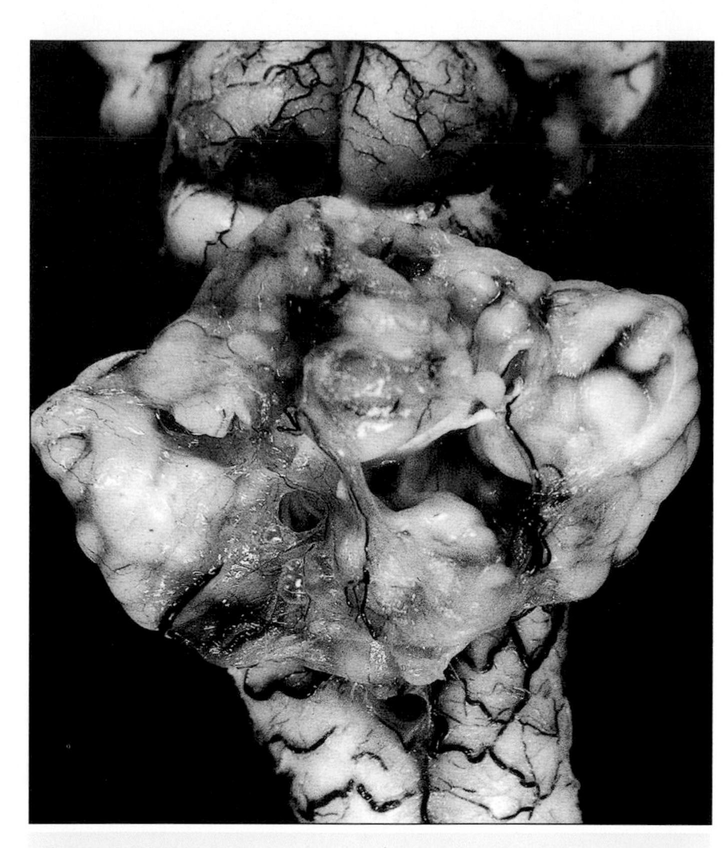

Figure 3.29 Cerebellar hypoplasia (cerebrum removed to expose cerebellar lesion) in a cow; asymptomatic over 5 years.

The anatomic expressions of hypoplasia, both in the cerebellum and subcerebellar structures, are very variable in degree. In some cases, the cerebellum may appear grossly normal, the hypoplastic defects being detectable only on microscopic examination. In such cases, the defects are irregular in distribution although there is a more or less severe loss of Purkinje cells. The granular layer is here and there narrowed and deficient in cells, but the molecular layer is normal. Correlative lesions may be present or absent and when present may be asymmetrical; they occur chiefly in the deep cerebellar nuclei, olives, and cerebellar peduncles. At the other extreme, the cerebellum may be represented only by a small nubbin of tissue or two unconnected nubbins each related to a hypoplastic peduncle (Fig. 3.29). In these severe defects, there is no folial pattern or division into lobes. Intermediate degrees of cerebellar hypoplasia are, however, the most common. It is usually possible to recognize with the naked eye that the cerebellar peduncles are diminished in size, especially the brachium pontis, that the medullary pyramids are flattened and that the small size of the restiform bodies gives the fourth ventricle a flattened appearance. Microscopically, the cerebellar cortex is disorganized. A brief description is not possible because the pattern varies greatly from case to case and place to place in the one animal. The Purkinje cells and the cells of the granular layer are the most obviously deficient and, in those that are present, regressive changes are common.

Cerebellar atrophy (or **abiotrophy**) *refers to premature or accelerated degeneration of formed elements, presumably caused by some intrinsic metabolic defect.* The Purkinje cells appear particularly susceptible to spontaneous degeneration; there may be secondary depletion of granule cells but other cortical layers are normal.

Cerebellar atrophy occurs in lambs, dogs, cats, various breeds of cattle, piglets, and foals. The disease in **lambs**, which are commonly known as "*daft lambs*," is reported from England and Canada. It is not restricted to any breed but is presumed to be inherited. The dams are normal. Affected lambs show signs of cerebellar dysfunction at birth, which include abnormalities of muscle tone, disorders of equilibrium, and tremors. The cerebellum is however normal in size and gross form. The histological changes affect primarily the Purkinje and Golgi cells, and these especially in the median lobe. Degeneration and loss of these cells leave some empty baskets and a replacement astrogliosis. In the early stages of degeneration, the Purkinje and Golgi cells are shrunken and hyperchromatic or swollen and pale with cytoplasmic vacuolation. They ultimately undergo lysis and disappear, leaving a spongy zone between the granular and molecular layers. There is, simultaneously, a diminution in the population of granule cells. Regressive changes with gliosis may be apparent in the deep cerebellar nuclei and olives.

Progressive cerebellar degenerations are common in **dogs,** and abiotrophic defects have been recorded in a variety of breeds including Airedales, Gordon Setters, rough-coated Collies, Border Collies, Finnish Terriers, Beagles, Australian Kelpies, and Bernese Mountain Dogs. Signs in the pups become evident at about 3 months of age. The cerebellum may be normal in size and shape or slightly diminished in size and somewhat flattened. Microscopically, there is degeneration and loss of Purkinje cells and granule cells (Fig. 3.30A, B). The Purkinje cells degenerate, being either shrunken and hyperchromatic or pale, swollen and vacuolated (Fig. 3.31A); most disappear, leaving empty baskets and a fenestrated ground layer (Fig. 3.31B). The atrophic process may show evidence of regional predilection. In Gordon Setters, the dorsal portions of the median lobe and vermis are most severely affected, while in Collie dogs selective involvement of the rostral folia of the vermis is reflected in macroscopic diminution of this area. Collateral changes in the subcerebellar nuclei are minor, but in this regard it may be pertinent that affected dogs are usually euthanized shortly after the defect becomes apparent. Nonprogressive cerebellar ataxia noted at 2 weeks of age is reported in Coton de Tulear dogs.

Hereditary striatonigral and cerebello-olivary degeneration occurs in the *Kerry Blue Terrier.* Pedigrees of affected dogs indicate autosomal recessive inheritance. Clinical signs begin between 9 and 16 weeks of age and are characterized by ataxia and dysmetria. *The inherent defect is neuronal degeneration,* and the brain changes follow a definite anatomical and temporal pattern of development. Degeneration and loss of Purkinje cells in the cerebellar cortex is evident at the onset of clinical signs. Subsequently there is sequential involvement of the olivary nuclei, caudate nuclei and putamen, and finally the substantia nigra. In the cerebellar cortex, chromatolytic degeneration and loss of Purkinje cells is attended by astrocytosis involving Bergmann's glia and depletion of granule cells. In the cerebellar white matter and contained nuclei, there is status spongiosus and axonal swelling. Changes in the olivary nuclei, basal nuclei, and substantia nigra tend to be symmetrical and initially (Fig. 3.32) feature neuronal degeneration, axonal swelling, spongiosus and fibrous astrocytosis, with progression to malacia and cavitation. Olivary neurons undergo chromatolysis, while in the remaining nuclear structures the nerve cells accumulate intracytoplasmic eosinophilic granules and undergo ischemic change.

Macroscopic evidence of the disease process in the cerebellum is limited to a modest degree of folial atrophy but, with progression

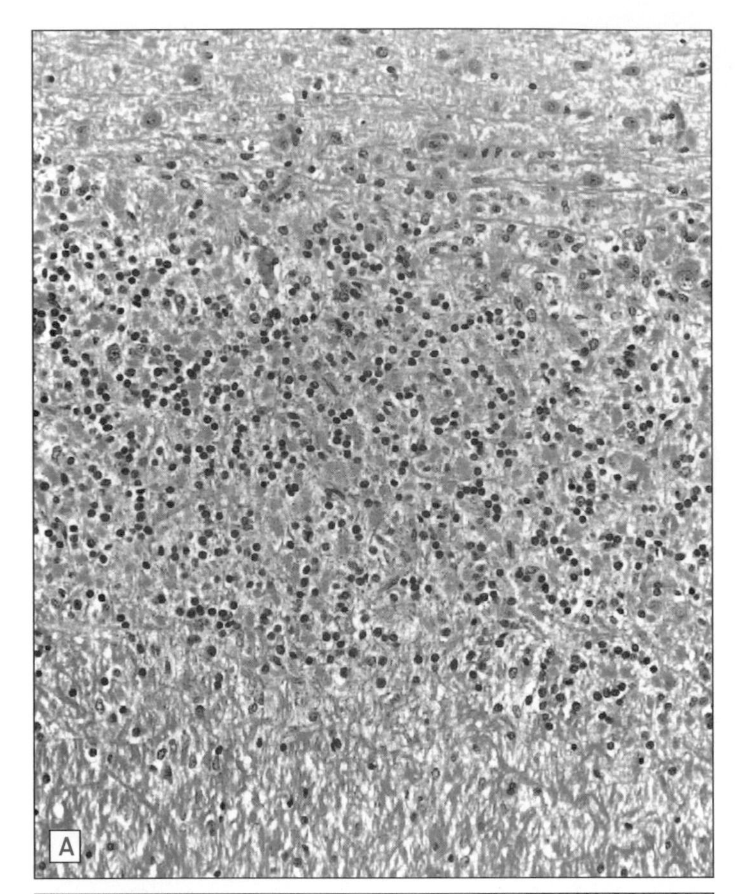

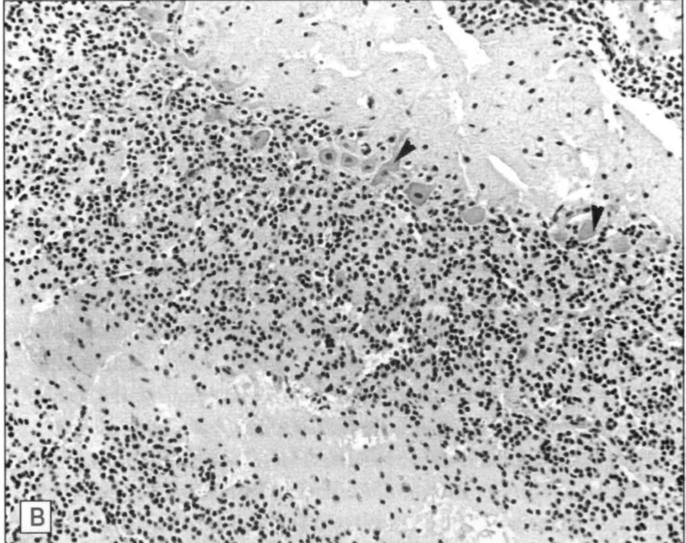

Figure 3.30 A. Cerebellar abiotrophy in a puppy; note severe hypoplasia of the molecular layer with almost complete absence of Purkinje cells. **B.** Cerebellar cortex of an age-matched puppy showing normal molecular layer and abundance of Purkinje cells (arrowheads).

of the condition, involvement of the basal and brain stem nuclei is manifest grossly by bilateral focal malacic lesions. Gross lesions are most severe in the caudate nucleus, which, after 7–8 months of clinical illness, may be reduced to numerous microcystic cavities. *It is proposed that the cerebellum and basal nuclei are the primary areas of involvement*, with the lesions in the olivary nucleus and substantia nigra being attributed to transynaptic neuronal degeneration along glutaminergic neurotransmission pathways.

The Kerry Blue Terrier condition is not the sole cerebellar abiotrophy in which accompanying extracerebellar lesions may be found. Olivary nuclei may be affected in the Bernese Mountain Dog, the cerebral cortex in the miniature Poodle, and spinal Wallerian degeneration may be found in rough-coated and Border Collies and in Merino sheep. In the Swedish Lapland Dog, there is a neuronal abiotrophy involving Purkinje cells; however, the effects of this are overshadowed by motor neuron degeneration and the disease is discussed below with others of that group.

Bovine familial convulsions and ataxia *is a heritable disorder of purebred and crossbred Aberdeen Angus cattle in the United Kingdom*. The clinical syndrome is characterized by intermittent episodic seizures in newborn and young calves and by the gradual development of ataxia with spasticity and hypermetria in calves surviving bouts of seizures extending over 2–3 months. The distinctive microscopic change is Purkinje cell axonal swelling in the cerebellar granular layer. There is also degeneration and loss of Purkinje cells. An apparently similar disorder has been described in Charolais cattle in the United Kingdom.

Sporadic cases of various forms of juvenile and adult-onset cerebellar degeneration, including **olivopontocerebellar atrophy**, have been reported in **cats**.

Cerebellar abiotrophy occurs in **horses**, particularly Arabian and part-Arabian horses, as well as in the Swedish Gotland pony and the American miniature horse, and is an inherited, likely autosomal recessive, condition. Head tremors and ataxia develop in affected Arabian foals between birth and 6 months of age, as a result of loss of Purkinje cells and granule cells from the cerebellar folia. An additional finding in an American miniature horse was degeneration of dorsal accessory olivary and lateral (accessory) cuneate nuclei and focal necrosis in the putamen.

Gomen disease *is a cerebellar degeneration and ataxia of horses in New Caledonia*. Some folial atrophy in the cerebellar vermis may be evident on gross examination. Microscopically, there is thinning of the cerebellar molecular layer and loss of Purkinje and granule cells. There is also considerable deposition of a pigment resembling lipofuscin in many of the surviving Purkinje cells as well as in the neurons of the brain and spinal cord. This material is also present in macrophages seen in areas where Purkinje cells are missing. The cause is unknown, but is thought to be an environmental toxin.

Bibliography

Barlow RM. Morphogenesis of cerebellar lesions in bovine familial convulsions and ataxia. Vet Pathol 1981;18:151–162.

Berry ML, Blas-Machado U. Cerebellar abiotrophy in a miniature schnauzer. Can Vet J 2003;44:657–659.

Bildfell RJ, et al. Cerebellar cortical degeneration in a Labrador retriever. Can Vet J 1995;36:570–572.

Carmichael KP, et al. Clinical, hematologic, and biochemical features of a syndrome in Bernese mountain dogs characterized by hepatocerebellar degeneration. J Am Vet Med Assoc 1996;208:1277–1279.

Carmichael S, et al. Familial cerebellar ataxia with hydrocephalus in bull mastiffs. Vet Rec 1983;112:354–358.

Clark RG, et al. Suspected inherited cerebellar neuroaxonal dystrophy in collie sheep dogs. N Z Vet J 1982;30:102–103.

Coates JR, et al. Neonatal cerebellar ataxia in Coton de Tulear dogs. J Vet Intern Med 2002;16:680–689.

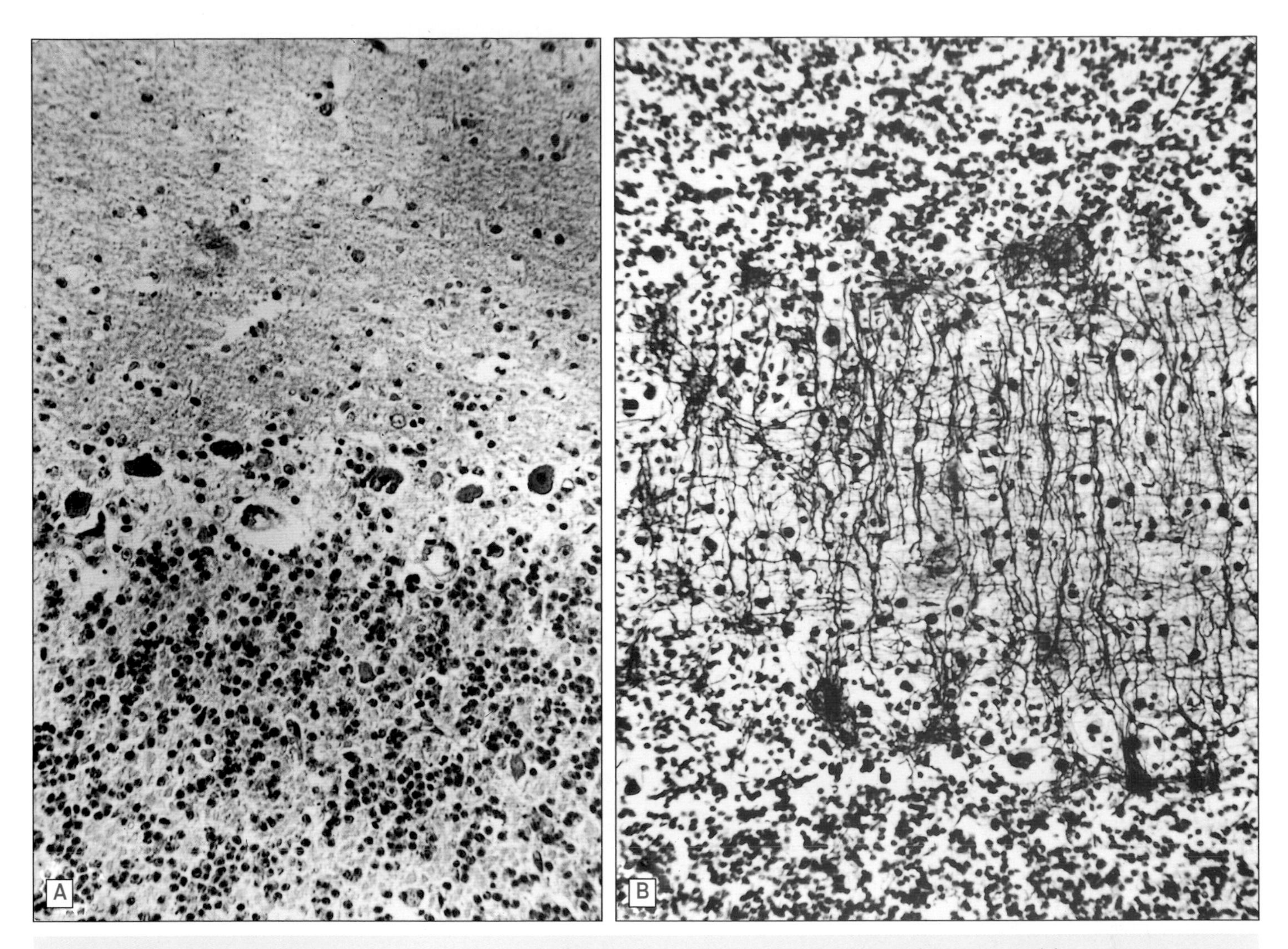

Figure 3.31 A. Degenerating Purkinje cells in **congenital cerebellar atrophy** in a dog. **B. Empty basket cells**; same case as (**A**).

Cummings JF, de Lahunta A. A study of cerebellar and cerebral cortical degeneration in miniature Poodle pups with emphasis on the ultrastructure of Purkinje cell changes. Acta Neuropathol (Berl) 1988;75:261–271.

DeBowes RM, et al. Cerebellar abiotrophy. Vet Clin North Am Equine Pract 1987;3:345–352.

Fox J, et al. Cerebello-olivary and lateral (accessory) cuneate degeneration in a juvenile American miniature horse. Vet Pathol 2000;37:271–274.

Franklin RJ, et al. An inherited neurological disorder of the St Bernard dog characterised by unusual cerebellar cortical dysplasia. Vet Rec 1997;140:656–657.

Hartley WJ, et al. The pathology of Gomen disease: a cerebellar disorder of horses in New Caledonia. Vet Pathol 1982;19:399–405.

Jolly RD, et al. Progressive ataxia and seizures in a Cocker Spaniel: a new type of neurodegenerative disease with novel intra-neuronal inclusions. N Z Vet J 2002;50:203–206.

Kemp J, et al. Cerebellar abiotrophy in Holstein Friesian calves. Vet Rec 1995;136:198.

Montgomery DL, Storts RW. Hereditary striatonigral and cerebello olivary degeneration of the Kerry blue terrier. Vet Pathol 1983;20:143–159.

Osburn BI, Castrucci G. Diaplacental infections with ruminant pestiviruses. Arch Virol Suppl 1991;3:71–78.

Pope AM, et al. Trichlorfon-induced congenital cerebellar hypoplasia in neonatal pigs. J Am Vet Med Assoc 1986;189:781–783.

Resibois A, Poncelet L. Olivopontocerebellar atrophy in two adult cats, sporadic cases or new genetic entity. Vet Pathol 2004;41:20–29.

Riond JL, et al. Bovine viral diarrhea virus-induced cerebellar disease in a calf. J Am Vet Med Assoc 1990;197:1631–1632.

Roeder PL, et al. Pestivirus fetopathogenicity in cattle: changing sequelae with fetal maturation. Vet Rec 1986;118:44–48.

Schatzberg SJ, et al. Polymerase chain reaction (PCR) amplification of parvoviral DNA from the brains of dogs and cats with cerebellar hypoplasia. J Vet Intern Med 2003;17:538–544.

Sharp NJ, et al. Hydranencephaly and cerebellar hypoplasia in two kittens attributed to intrauterine parvovirus infection. J Comp Pathol 1999;121:39–53.

Tago Y, et al. Granule cell type cerebellar hypoplasia in a beagle dog. Lab Anim 1993;27:151–155.

Thomas JB, Robertson D. Hereditary cerebellar abiotrophy in Australian kelpie dogs. Aust Vet J 1989;66:301–302.

Tsuda T, et al. Arthrogryposis, hydranencephaly and cerebellar hypoplasia syndrome in neonatal calves resulting from intrauterine infection with Aino virus. Vet Res 2004;35:531–538.

van der Merwe LL, Lane E. Diagnosis of cerebellar cortical degeneration in a Scottish terrier using magnetic resonance imaging. J Small Anim Pract 2001;42:409–412.

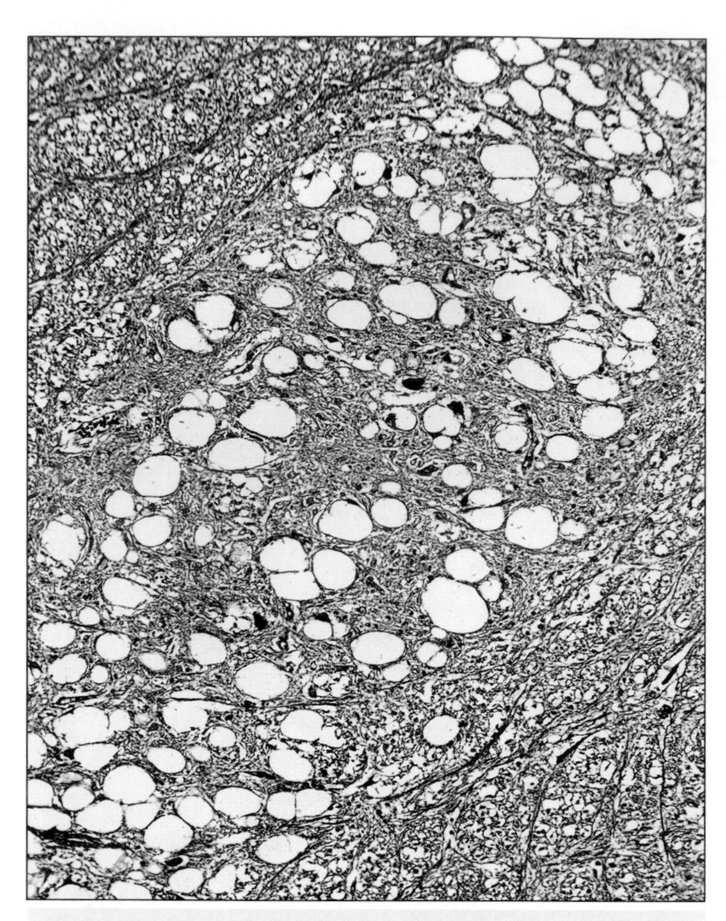

Figure 3.32 Neuronal degeneration and spongiosus, in inferior olive in a Kerry Blue Terrier with cerebellar abiotrophy.

Wessels ME, et al. Daft lamb disease. Vet Rec 2003;152:477–478.

Whittington RJ, et al. Cerebellar abiotrophy in crossbred cattle. Aust Vet J 1989;66:12–15.

Arnold–Chiari malformation

In the Arnold–Chiari malformation (Chiari type II malformation), the cerebellar vermis is herniated as a tongue-like process of tissue into the foramen magnum and cranial spinal canal where it overlies an elongated medulla that is also displaced caudally (Fig. 3.33). The cranial nerves from the medulla alter their trajectory. The tentorium is inserted caudally towards the foramen magnum, the tentorial hiatus is shallow and wide, and the pons and occipital poles are displaced through it. The displaced occipital poles show sagittal, parallel gyri. Internal hydrocephalus may be a secondary effect, and spina bifida or meningomyelocele may be concurrent.

The caudal fossa in particular, but perhaps also the rostral fossa, is too small for the normal volume of brain tissue, suggesting that there has been failure of neurogenic induction of osseous growth. The defect is observed occasionally in calves. In the Cavalier King Charles Spaniel dog, occipital bone hypoplasia with obstruction of the foramen magnum and secondary syringomyelia is common, and is similar to human *Chiari type I malformation*.

Bibliography

LeClerc S, et al. Central nervous system and vertebral malformation resembling the Arnold-Chiari syndrome in a Simmental calf. Can Vet J 1997;38:300–301.

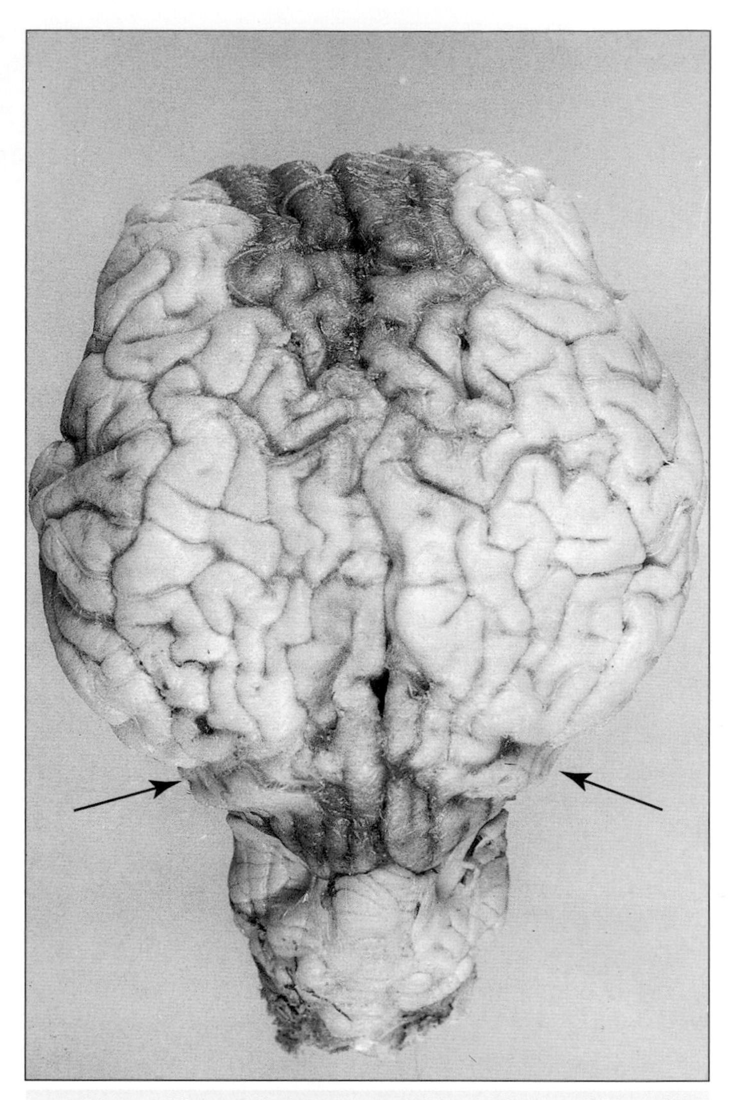

Figure 3.33 Arnold-Chiari malformation in a calf. Cerebellar deformity and coning accompanying spina bifida. Compression and hemorrhage of the occipital lobes (arrows). Pigmentation of rostral brain is normal.

Madarame H, et al. Cerebellar hypoplasia associated with Arnold-Chiari malformation in a Japanese shorthorn calf. J Comp Pathol 1991;104:1–5.

Rusbridge C, Knowler SP. Inheritance of occipital bone hypoplasia (Chiari type I malformation) in Cavalier King Charles Spaniels. J Vet Intern Med 2004; 18:673–678.

Dandy–Walker syndrome

In the Dandy–Walker syndrome, seen in various species, *there is a midline defect of the cerebellum with the vermis largely absent and the cerebellar hemispheres widely separated by a large fluid-filled cyst in an enlarged caudal fossa.* The roof of the cyst, which ruptures easily when the brain is removed, consists of ependyma, a disorganized layer of glial tissue, and an outer layer of leptomeningeal tissue. An expanded fourth ventricle forms the floor of the cyst. The vermal malformation is thought to be the result of a primary midline developmental defect.

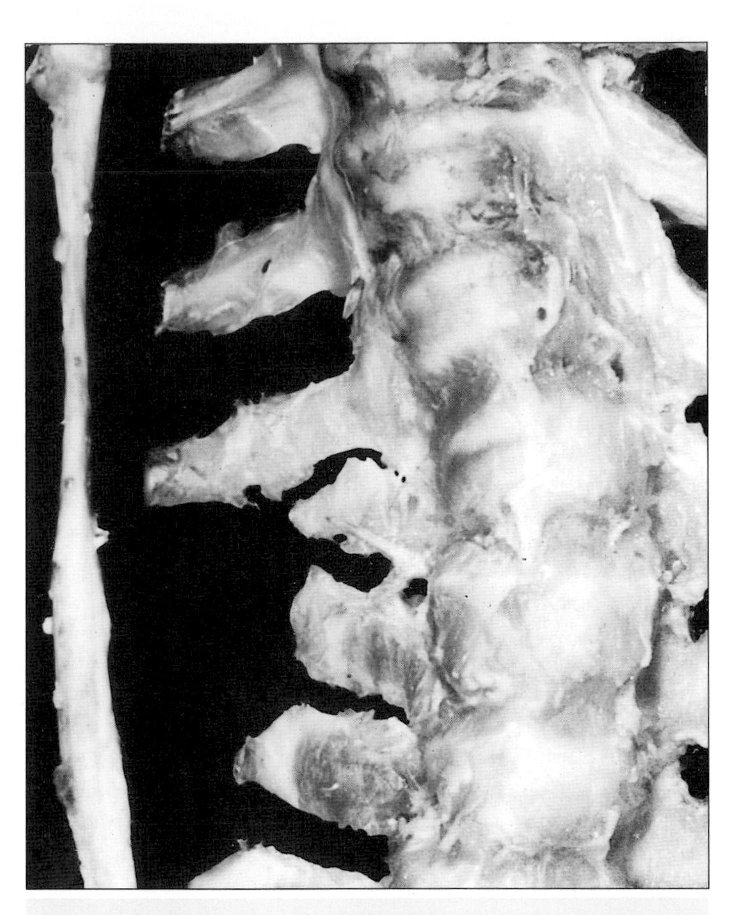

Figure 3.34 Constriction of spinal cord in congenital scoliosis in a calf.

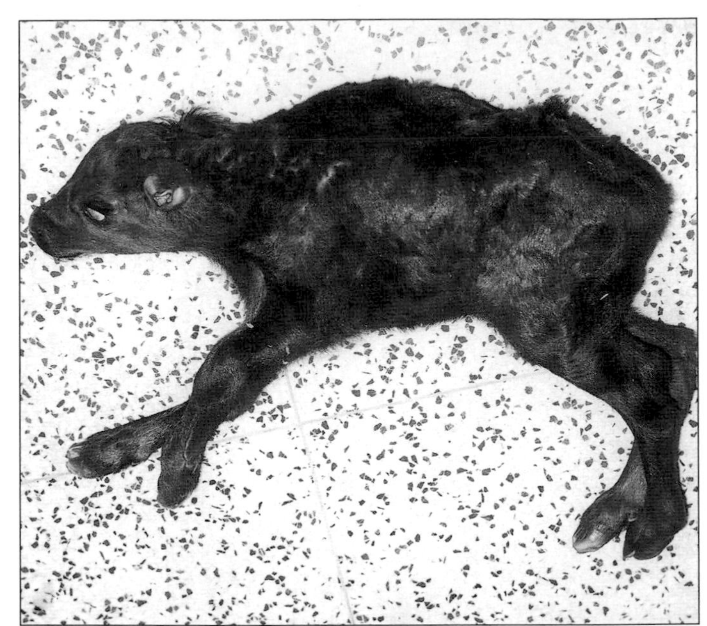

Figure 3.35 Perosomus elumbus in a calf.

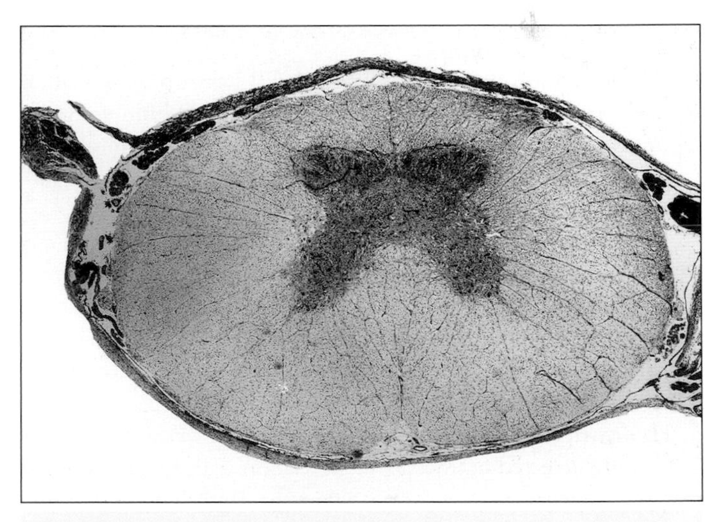

Figure 3.36 Absence of central canal of spinal cord in **dysraphism** in a dog.

Bibliography

Cudd TA. Agenesis of the corpus callosum with cerebellar vermian hypoplasia in a foal resembling the Dandy-Walker syndrome: pre-mortem diagnosis by clinical evaluation and CT scanning. Equine Vet J 1990;22:328.

Jeffrey M, et al. Dandy-Walker malformation in two calves. Vet Rec 1990;126: 499–501.

Kornegay JN. Cerebellar vermian hypoplasia in dogs. Vet Pathol 1986;23:374–379.

Noureddine C, et al. Ultrasonographic appearance of Dandy Walker-like syndrome in a Boston terrier. Vet Radiol Ultrasound 2004;45:336–339.

Spinal cord

Myelodysplasia

Myelodysplasia refers to abnormal development of the spinal cord. **Segmental aplasia** and **hypoplasia** may occur at any level of the spinal cord (Fig. 3.34), but *the lumbar region is most frequently affected*. Some cases are associated with fetal *Akabane virus* infection.

Perosomus elumbus, which occurs in calves and lambs, *is characterized by partial agenesis of the spinal cord*. The lumbar segment is involved, and there is failure of induction of the related vertebrae. The cranial part of the body is normal, but *the vertebral axis ends at the caudal thoracic region, and lumbar, sacral, and coccygeal vertebrae are absent* (Fig. 3.35). The spinal cord ends in the thoracic region in a blind vertebral canal. The caudal part of the body remains attached to the cranial part by soft tissue only; the limbs are arthrogrypotic and their muscles atrophic. Atypically, only some lumbar segments are absent, or severely hypoplastic with absence of arches and spinal muscle, and a remnant of cauda equina may be found in the sacral region.

The most severe forms of myelodysplasia, affecting especially the potential dorsal regions of the cord, occur *in association with the forms of spina bifida* described below. Myelodysplasia, not associated with the skeletal manifestations of spina bifida but probably best included in this classification, occurs quite commonly in animals particularly *in association with arthrogryposis in calves and lambs*. The dysplasia, which is readily detectable by the presence of *aberrant central canals* (sometimes as many as six), chiefly involves limited lengths of the lumbar segment of the cord but occasionally is localized to cervical or thoracic regions. *Denervation atrophy of appendicular muscle is constantly present and is the probable basis of the arthrogrypotic changes*. The degree of dysplasia is quite variable, but it is characterized by aberrations of the central canal (Fig. 3.36), by the absence of dorsal or ventral septa, the presence of ectopic septa and clefts, and by distortion, asymmetry, and

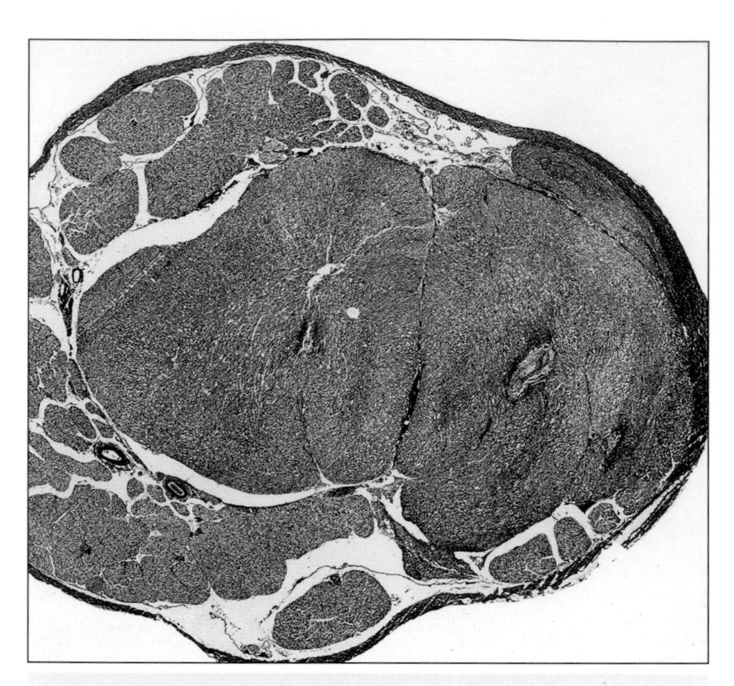

Figure 3.37 Diplomyelia in a dog.

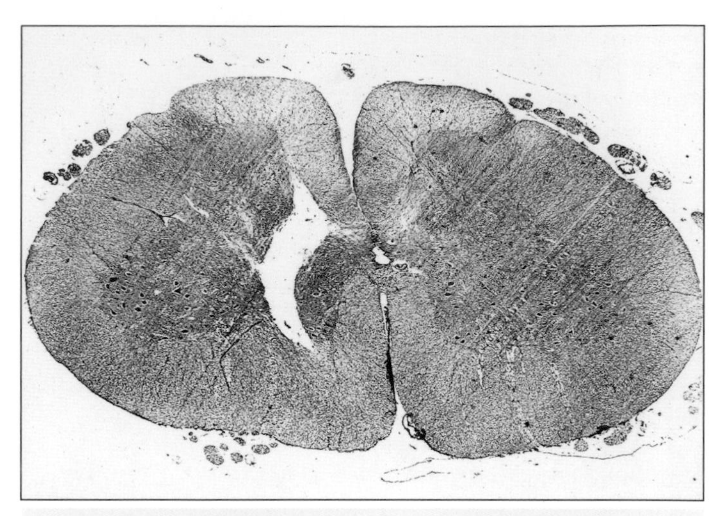

Figure 3.38 Syringomyelia in a dog.

partial duplication of the ventral and dorsal horns of gray matter. In some cases the cord is duplicated completely within common leptomeninges and dura (*diplomyelia*) (Fig. 3.37), or within separate meningeal coverings and vertebral canals separated by a bony partition (*diastematomyelia*).

Syringomyelia *is tubular cavitation of the spinal cord that extends over several segments*; it is an uncommon anomaly in animals. Syringomyelia is rarely acquired and is best known as one of the lesions associated with the familial disorder of young Weimaraner dogs described below. When the cavitation involves the medulla, the defect is termed *syringobulbia*. Syringomyelia and syringobulbia may occur together.

Hydromyelia *is dilation of the central canal of the spinal cord*. It is not commonly detected but occurs in association with spina bifida and may be a precursor lesion for syringomyelia. Both hydromyelia and syringomyelia are found in the dysraphic spinal cord of arthrogrypotic Charolais calves. Hydromyelia may be acquired as a consequence of obstruction of cerebrospinal fluid flow in the central canal.

A syndrome of pelvic limb gait disturbance in young **Weimaraner dogs** is a manifestation of a spectrum of myelodysplastic and dysraphic lesions, and is inherited in a co-dominant mode with variable penetrance. The trait is lethal in the homozygous state. Affected animals exhibit a gait deficit from the time they begin to walk, but clinical signs in some cases may be barely noticeable. Severely affected dogs typically are unable to completely extend the hindlimbs so that their normal attitude is crouched. When walking, the hindlimbs are moved together in a "bunny-hopping" or "kangaroo-gait" fashion. Additionally, affected animals may show thoraco-lumbar scoliosis, depression of the sternum, and abnormal hair streams in the dorsal cervical region. There is no significant progression or regression of clinical signs with age, and there is not a good correlation between clinical signs and the degree of structural malformation.

Pathologically, the exposed spinal cord is grossly normal in size and conformation, but *a range of dysraphic defects may be present* including: anomalies of the dorsal septum, which may be absent; hydromyelia and other anomalies of the central canal, which may be absent; duplication or displacement of the central canal; anomalies of extent and distribution of the central gray matter; anomalies of the ventral horns consisting of deficient delineation and development of medial cell groups, and aberrant collections of neurons and gray neuropil; deficiency of the ventral median fissure, which may be total. Histologic studies on affected embryos suggest that the primary lesion is related to aberrantly positioned mantle cells ventral to the central canal in the floor plate area.

Syringomyelia is not present until about 8 months of age and involves lumbar segments. Cavitation may be barely visible to the naked eye. Microscopically, the cavity is usually found in the central gray matter dorsal and lateral to the central canal (Fig.3.38). There is not much encroachment on the white matter except for that in the white commissures when the cavitation extends from one side to the other. Connection with the central canal is difficult to demonstrate but may be found in serial sections. Ependyma does not line the cavity, the walls of which are formed of frayed nervous tissue with an appearance suggesting that the cord has been squashed or torn at necropsy. The tissue around the cavity is edematous and stains poorly.

Spina bifida and related defects

Spina bifida *refers to absence of the dorsal portions of the vertebrae*. It is, however, a rather imperfect name as the various forms of the defect represent differences in degree of defective closure of the neural tube, its separation from the ectoderm, and its induction of a skeletal investment. It is convenient to divide the defect into several classes on the basis of severity: *myeloschisis, spina bifida occulta, spina bifida cystica with meningocele, and spina bifida with myelomeningocele apply to the vertebral defect; amyelia, diastematomyelia, hydromyelia, and dysraphism apply to the spinal cord*.

In **total myeloschisis**, *neurulation does not occur*, the neural plate remaining open. By total is meant a defect that involves the whole of the vertebral axis with anencephaly an expected accompaniment. There is virtual amyelia (absence of spinal cord), neural tissue being present only as soft red masses in the residual groove. *Local myeloschisis* is a localized defect due to failure of closure of the neural tube. One or more vertebral segments may be defective. The defect may occur in any portion of the vertebral axis but is expected to be lumbosacral.

The defect occurs most frequently in brachycephalic breeds of dogs and is inherited as an autosomal dominant condition in Manx cats. Affected cats are heterozygotes of variable expression, while the homozygous state is lethal. *Sacrococcygeal agenesis* occurs in association with spina bifida in Manx cats, calves, dogs, and sheep.

Spina bifida occulta is perhaps the least rare form of the defect in animals, and it is occult because *it is not apparent except for the presence of dimpling or deeper invagination of the skin*. It may accompany defects in other remote tissues but the defect is otherwise limited to the absence of one or more vertebral arches. The cord may be grossly normal but dysplastic microscopically, usually with diastematomyelia. The spinous processes may be bifid or absent.

In **spina bifida cystica**, a cystic swelling protrudes through the vertebral defect. Because of differential growth of the vertebral and neural axes, the cranial–caudal position of the skin and bone lesions may not correspond, especially in the caudal regions where the defects are expected to occur.

When meninges protrude (**meningocele**), the roof of the cyst is comprised of skin and condensed meninges, including dura mater. The spinal cord may be normal grossly but dysplastic segments are detected microscopically. Macroscopic lesions in the cord include partial duplication and cystic distension of the central canal that communicates with the endodural space via a cleft in the dorsal funiculi. A meningocele may contain a large accumulation of adipose tissue (**lipomeningocele**).

When meninges and spinal cord protrude (**meningomyelocele**), the cyst tends to be broad-based. *Failure of dehiscence of the neural crest from surface ectoderm provides for a central area without epithelial covering.* This *medullovasculosa* corresponds to the cerebrovasculosa of anencephaly and consists of vascularized meninges, heterotopic cord tissue, and connective tissue. The defects in the cord include those mentioned as occurring with meningocele and, in severe cases, duplication or absence of the cord in affected segments. The *tethered cord* syndrome refers to attachment of the meningomyelocele that prevents the normal ascent of the spinal cord as the vertebral column grows.

A **dermoid sinus** is a congenital abnormality, inherited in Rhodesian Ridgeback dogs, in which incomplete separation of the neural tube from the overlying dorsal midline ectoderm allows persistence of a sinus connecting the skin surface to the supraspinous ligament, or it may extend as deep as the dura mater of the spinal cord.

Bibliography

Bailey CS, Morgan JP. Congenital spinal malformations. Vet Clin North Am Small Anim Pract 1992;22:985–1015.

Boyd JS. Unusual case of spina bifida in a Friesian cross calf. Vet Rec 1985;116:203–205.

Deforest ME, Basrur PK. Malformations and the Manx syndrome in cats. Can Vet J 1979;20:304–314.

Engel HN, Draper DD. Comparative prenatal development of the spinal cord in normal and dysraphic dogs: Embryonic stage. Am J Vet Res 1982;43:1729–1743.

Gopal T, Leipold HW. Lipomeningocele in a calf. Vet Pathol 1979;16:610–612.

Gruys E, Bethlehem M. The dysraphic state in the calf, lamb and piglet. Zentralbl Veterinarmed A 1976;23:811–818.

Kirberger RM, et al. Hydromyelia in the dog. Vet Radiol Ultrasound 1997;38:30–38.

Klekamp J. The pathophysiology of syringomyelia - historical overview and current concept. Acta Neurochir (Wien) 2002;144:649–664.

Leipold HW, et al. Arthrogryposis and associated defects in newborn calves. Am J Vet Res 1970;31:1367–1374.

Ohfuji S. Spinal dysraphism in a newborn Holstein-Friesian calf. Vet Pathol 1999;36:607–609.

Plummer SB, et al. Tethered spinal cord and an intradural lipoma associated with a meningocele in a Manx-type cat. J Am Vet Med Assoc 1993;203:1159–1161.

Ruberte J, et al. Malformations of the vertebral bodies and the ribs associated to spinal dysraphism without spina bifida in a Pekingese dog. Zentralbl Veterinarmed A 1995;42:307–313.

Rusbridge C, et al. Syringohydromyelia in Cavalier King Charles spaniels. J Am Anim Hosp Assoc 2000;36:34–41.

Shamir M, et al. Surgical treatment of tethered spinal cord syndrome in a dog with myelomeningocele. Vet Rec 2001;148:755–756.

van Hoogmoed L, et al. Surgical repair of a thoracic meningocele in a foal. Vet Surg 1999;28:496–500.

Wilson JW, et al. Spina bifida in the dog. Vet Pathol 1979;16:165–179.

Viral causes of developmental defects of the central nervous system

Akabane virus

Akabane virus (AKAV), a species of the genus *Orthobunyavirus*, is among the most potent of the viral teratogens of domestic animals, but the infection is otherwise asymptomatic. **Iriki virus**, a strain of AKAV, has similar pathogenic potential. Following maternal infection at critical stages of gestation, AKAV produces a range of predominantly neural abnormalities in calves, lambs, and kids, but *AKAV is best known for producing outbreaks of arthrogryposis and hydranencephaly in calves*. Epizootics of Akabane virus disease in cattle have been reported in areas of Japan, Israel, and Australia. The vector in Australia is the biting midge *Culicoides brevitarsis*, and the virus has also been isolated from mosquitoes in Japan. Buffaloes, horses, and pigs are additional vertebrate hosts. Although arthrogryposis and hydranencephaly may be the most obvious manifestations in field epizootics of bovine AKAV disease, a range of overlapping syndromes is observed in calves in affected herds. The pattern of fetal disease corresponds to the gestational age of the fetus at the time of infection. Infection late in gestation may cause abortion. The initial manifestation of neural abnormality in a field outbreak is the birth of incoordinate calves and, in this group, nonsuppurative encephalomyelitis is evident on histological examination. *Microencephaly* and *cerebellar hypoplasia* occur occasionally as manifestations of late infection. *Arthrogryposis*, sometimes associated with spinal deformities, appears early in the outbreak following fetal infection at 5–6 months of pregnancy. In arthrogrypotic calves, there is loss of spinal ventral horn neurons, loss of myelin in the motor tracts of the spinal cord and in ventral spinal nerves, and denervation atrophy together with fibrous and adipose replacement of skeletal musculature.

At least some strains of AKAV have the capacity to cause *polymyositis*, particularly in the early myotubular phase of skeletal muscle development, suggesting the possible involvement of this process in the arthrogrypotic change. *Severe hydranencephaly*, manifest clinically as blindness and stupidity, is seen towards the end of the epizootic, being the result of fetal infection at 3–4 months of gestation. With increasing age of the fetus at the time of infection, the cavitating cerebral changes are less severe and grade towards *porencephaly*.

The teratogenic potential of AKAV in **sheep and goats** is qualitatively the same as for cattle. Cavitating cerebral defects, arthrogryposis, microencephaly, and agenesis or hypoplasia of the spinal cord have been produced in lambs born of ewes inoculated on days 29–48 of pregnancy. Field observations in Australian flocks suggest that, in sheep, *microencephaly* is relatively more common as a consequence of AKAV infection than it is in cattle.

Aino virus, a serotype of species *Shuni virus*, genus *Orthobunyavirus*, can cause arthrogryposis, hydranencephaly, and cerebellar hypoplasia in bovine fetuses infected experimentally, and is suspected to be the teratogen in field cases of congenital bovine malformations in Japan.

Cache Valley virus (CVV), a serotype of species *Bunyamwera virus*, genus *Orthobunyavirus*, is a mosquito-borne bunyavirus that is endemic in North America. CVV is capable of infecting a variety of mammals, generally as subclinical infections but it is occasionally teratogenic in fetal lambs. The nature and pathogenesis of the abnormalities produced are comparable to those of *Akabane virus* in sheep. Three other members of genus *Orthobunyavirus* – **LaCrosse virus** and **San Angelo virus** (serotypes of *California encephalitis virus*), and **Main Drain virus** – also express bunyaviral tropism for fetal tissue infection and can induce lesions including arthrogryposis, hydrocephalus, fetal death, axial skeletal deviations, anasarca, and oligohydramnios.

Chuzan virus (CHUV), a strain of species *Palyam virus*, genus *Orbivirus*, family Reoviridae, is transmitted by *Culicoides* sp. CHUV is infective for several ruminant species, and in Japan has been incriminated as a teratogen of fetal calves with features similar to those of *Akabane virus* infection.

Bibliography

Bishop AL, et al. Effects of altitude, distance and waves of movement on the dispersal in Australia of the arbovirus vector, *Culicoides brevitarsis* Kieffer (Diptera: *Ceratopogonidae*). Prev Vet Med 2004;65:135–145.

Charles JA. Akabane virus. Vet Clin North Am Food Anim Pract 1994;10:525–546.

Edwards JF. Cache Valley virus. Vet Clin North Am Food Anim Pract 1994;10:515–524.

Edwards JF, et al. Ovine fetal malformations induced by in utero inoculation with Main Drain, San Angelo, and LaCrosse viruses. Am J Trop Med Hyg 1997;56:171–176.

Haughey KE, et al. Akabane disease in sheep. Aust Vet J 1988;65:136–140.

Kitani H, et al. Preferential infection of neuronal and astroglia cells by Akabane virus in primary cultures of fetal bovine brain. Vet Microbiol 2000;73:269–279.

Kitano Y, et al. A congenital abnormality of calves, suggestive of a new type of arthropod-borne virus infection. J Comp Pathol 1994;111:427–437.

Liao YK, et al. The isolation of Akabane virus (Iriki strain) from calves in Taiwan. J Basic Microbiol 1996;36:33–39.

Miura Y, et al. Hydranencephaly-cerebellar hypoplasia in a newborn calf after infection of its dam with Chuzan virus. Nippon Juigaku Zasshi 1990;52:689–694.

Tateyama S, et al. An outbreak of congenital hydranencephaly and cerebellar hypoplasia among calves in South Kyushu, Japan: a pathological study. Res Vet Sci 1990;49:127–131.

Tsuda T, et al. Arthrogryposis, hydranencephaly and cerebellar hypoplasia syndrome in neonatal calves resulting from intrauterine infection with Aino virus. Vet Res 2004;35:531–538.

Bluetongue virus

Hydranencephaly and porencephaly have been reported in lambs and calves whose dams received a live attenuated bluetongue vaccine or contracted *Bluetongue virus* (BTV, species of the genus *Orbivirus*, family Reoviridae) infection during pregnancy (Fig. 3.27B). The type of congenital anomaly found depends on the fetal age at the time of infection with BTV. Lambs infected with bluetongue vaccine virus at 50–55 days gestation develop severe necrotizing encephalopathy and retinopathy, which at birth is manifest as *hydranencephaly and retinal dysplasia*. Infection of lambs at 75 days gestation causes multifocal encephalitis and selective vacuolation of white matter that is manifest as porencephalic cysts in the newborn; ocular lesions are not observed in these newborn lambs. Lesions in brains of lambs infected after 100 days gestation are confined to mild focal meningoencephalitis. BTV infection of fetal calves can cause hydranencephaly.

Bibliography

Flanagan M, Johnson SJ. The effects of vaccination of Merino ewes with an attenuated Australian bluetongue virus serotype 23 at different stages of gestation. Aust Vet J 1995;72:455–457.

Housawi FM, et al. Abortions, stillbirths and deformities in sheep at the Al-Ahsa oasis in eastern Saudi Arabia: isolation of a bluetongue serogroup virus from the affected lambs. Rev Sci Tech 2004;23:913–920.

MacLachlan NJ, et al. Bluetongue virus-induced encephalopathy in fetal cattle. Vet Pathol 1985;22:415–417.

Rift Valley fever virus and Wesselsbron virus

These infections are considered more fully in Vol. 2 Liver and biliary system. In addition to *Wesselsbron virus* (WESSV), there are several other mosquito-borne flaviviruses (genus *Flavivirus*, family Flaviviridae) in South Africa, including *West Nile virus* and *Banzi virus*, to which sheep are experimentally susceptible and which result in abortion, stillbirths, and neonatal deaths; anomalies include *hydranencephaly, porencephaly, and internal hydrocephalus*.

Rift Valley fever virus and WESSV are mosquito-borne and tend to circulate together. They are both primarily hepatotropic, but the wild strain of WESSV and attenuated strains of both are neurotropic, and vaccine strains may be responsible for most outbreaks of congenital neurologic disease. The presenting features are similar to those of Akabane disease, but the high incidence of hydrops amnii and prolonged gestation is especially a feature.

The destructive changes in the CNS produced by one or other of these viruses, or both together, can be more severe than with other teratogenic viruses and result in segmental aplasia of the cord, aplasia of the cerebellum, and anencephaly. It is more usual, however, that the defects include brachygnathia, hydranencephaly or porencephaly, hypoplasia of cerebellum and spinal cord, and varied musculoskeletal stigmata of arthrogryposis.

Bibliography

Barnard BJH, Voges SF. Flaviviruses in South Africa: pathogenicity for sheep. Onderstepoort J Vet Res 1986;53:235–238.

Coetzer JAW. Brain teratology as a result of transplacental virus infection in ruminants. J S Afr Vet Assoc 1980;51:153–157.

Hunter P, et al. Teratogenicity of a mutagenised Rift Valley fever virus (MVP 12) in sheep. Onderstepoort J Vet Res 2002;69:95–98.

Oberst RD. Viruses as teratogens. Vet Clin North Am Food Anim Pract 1993;9:23–31.

Bovine viral diarrhea virus

The diseases caused by *Bovine viral diarrhea virus* (BVDV), genus *Pestivirus*, family Flaviviridae, are considered in detail in Vol. 2, Alimentary system. The ecology of BVDV depends on transplacental transmission and the establishment of immune tolerance and persistent infections. Horizontal transfer of infection occurs readily, but is seldom clinically significant. Persistently infected fetuses that survive to become pregnant transmit BVDV to the conceptus. Although viral strains differ in their pathogenicity, infection of susceptible cows during early and middle stages of gestation is likely to result in either fetal death or a variety of developmental defects, predominantly neural and ocular. Some congenitally affected calves also have erosive lesions in the upper alimentary tract and abomasum resembling those seen in adult cattle; brachygnathism also occurs.

The outcome of infection of the fetal calf is related to gestational age, advancing fetal maturity being associated with increased resistance to the virus. Infections occurring within the first 100 days of fetal life tend to be lethal resulting in *abortion or mummification*. Although the gross pathologic changes seen in these lethal infections lack unique features, the patterns of tissue response are characteristic, but are rarely seen as such fetuses die in utero and undergo autolysis. Necrotizing inflammation can involve a variety of tissues. The reactive changes are dominated by mononuclear, predominantly macrophage, infiltration of hepatic portal areas, myocardium, spleen, and lymph nodes, which is reflected grossly in enlargement, nodularity and mottling of the liver and enlargement of spleen and lymph nodes (Fig. 3.39). The presence of *growth-arrest lines in long bones* suggests that the fetus undergoes one or more intrauterine crises before death. Affected fetuses may have partial alopecia that spares the tail, the lower portion of the limbs, and the head, these being points of initial hair growth during fetal development. The microscopic skin changes that evolve from the initial necrotizing dermatitis and correlate with the alopecia are hypoplasia of hair follicles and cystic distension of adnexal glands.

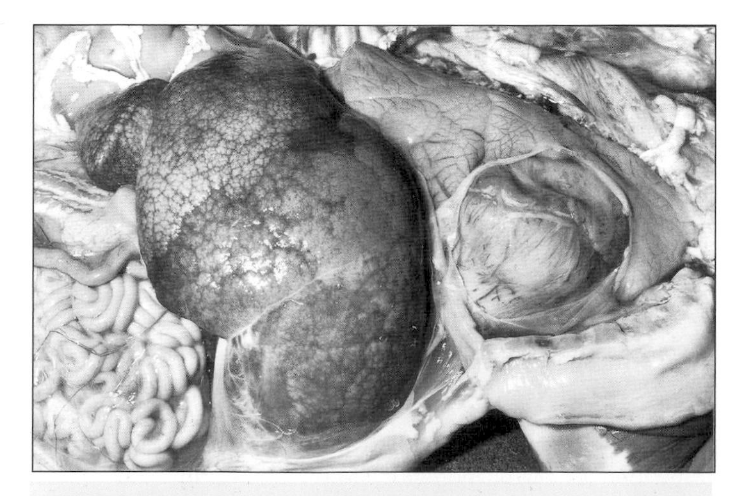

Figure 3.39 Myocardial pallor due to myocarditis and myocardial degeneration, and chronic hepatic congestion with ascites in a bovine fetus due to ***Bovine viral diarrhea virus* infection**, although *Neospora caninum* infection must also be ruled out in such cases.

The teratogenic effects of BVDV are manifest during the 100–170 day period. The period of susceptibility presumably varies with the strain of virus. *Cerebellar hypoplasia is the most characteristic defect* (Fig. 3.40). Gross cerebellar changes range from more or less uniform atrophy to irregular folial atrophy and agenesis accompanied by cavitation. The hypoplastic process is compounded by the effects of necrosis of external granular layer cells and parenchymal destruction as a consequence of folial edema resulting from vasculitis. The relative contribution of these processes is quite variable, but it appears that the vasculopathy may be more prominent in older fetuses. The nature and extent of involvement of individual folia also varies considerably. The evolution of the cerebellar changes has been studied experimentally. Acute lesions are evident 2 weeks after infection. Cellular necrosis in the external granular layer is accompanied by nonsuppurative meningitis. Vasculitis, marked by endothelial proliferation and perivascular leukocytic infiltration, is associated with folial edema, and there may be focal hemorrhages in the cerebellar white matter and cortex.

Folial edema, depending on its severity, may result in total folial destruction, cavitation or focal, often linear, areas of folial white matter deficient in myelin and axons. Where necrosis of the external granular layer predominates, the result is irregular atrophy of affected folia. Features of the atrophic process are marked depletion

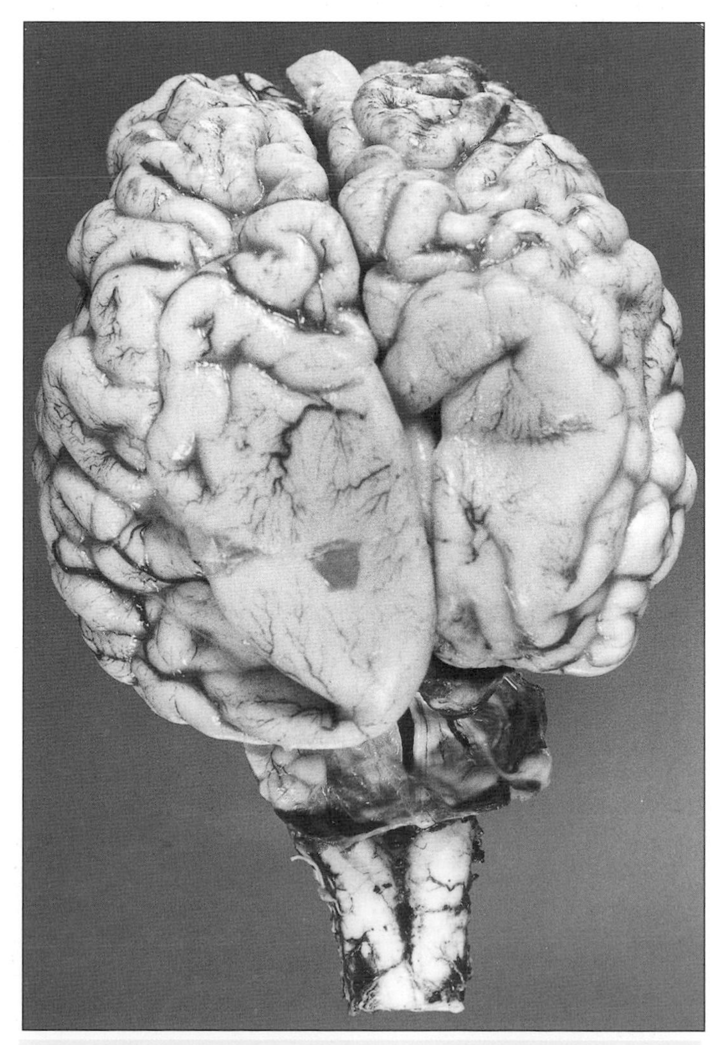

Figure 3.40 Cerebellar hypoplasia and **hydrocephalus** in a calf.

of granule cells, ectopia of Purkinje cells, and the presence of swollen Purkinje cell axons in the granular layer. The evolution of the cerebellar lesion in the fetal calf extends over 6 weeks and, by 10 weeks after maternal infection, inflammatory changes are not evident in the brain.

Other CNS defects that may be a consequence of fetal infection are porencephaly, hydranencephaly, microencephaly, hydrocephalus, cystic septum pellucidum, and dysmyelination. Ocular anomalies commonly accompany cerebellar defects, and include retinal dysplasia and atrophy, cataract, optic neuritis and atrophy, microphthalmia, and persistent pupillary membrane.

Infection of the fetus later than 170 days is unlikely to cause either intrauterine death or malformation. This increased resistance coincides with the fetus acquiring the capacity to produce neutralizing antibody to the virus. However, BVDV also has the capacity to induce more subtle developmental aberrations such as *intrauterine growth retardation* and *atrophy of the thymus and lymphoid tissues*. The regressive changes in thymus and lymphoid tissues offer a morphological basis for the immunological suppression and tolerance phenomena associated with congenital infections with BVDV.

Bibliography

Brownlie J. The pathogenesis of bovine virus diarrhoea virus infections. Rev Sci Tech Off Int Epiz 1990;9:43–59.

Grooms DL. Reproductive consequences of infection with bovine viral diarrhea virus. Vet Clin North Am Food Anim Pract 2004;20:5–19.

Hewicker-Trautwein M, et al. Brain lesions in calves following transplacental infection with bovine-virus diarrhoea virus. Zentralbl Veterinarmed B 1995;42:65–77.

Nettleton PF. Pestivirus infections in ruminants other than cattle. Rev Sci Tech Off Int Epiz 1990;9:131–150.

Border disease virus

Border disease (BD) of lambs was first described from the border counties of England and Wales, and is now recognized in many countries. Affected lambs show gross tremors and long hairy birth coats ("hairy-shaker," or "fuzzy" lambs).

BD is caused by *Border disease virus* (BDV), genus *Pestivirus*, family Flaviviridae, which is very closely related to *Bovine viral diarrhea virus* (BVDV) and less closely to *Classical swine fever virus*. These viruses possess a similar host spectrum experimentally, and interspecies transmission, especially between ruminants, does occur naturally but the clinical expression in recipients may be modified or absent. The ecology of BDV and the pathogenesis of BD depend on the ability of the virus to cross the placenta and then either to produce disease in the fetus or a state of immunotolerance and *persistent infection (PI) that allows excretion of the virus continuously in postnatal life*. Strain variations of BDV, differing host responses depending on breed and genotype, and gestational age at which infection occurs contribute to the varied manifestations of the disease. Congenital disease and persistent infection are typically caused by the *noncytopathic biotype* of BDV; mucosal disease-like syndrome is caused by a *cytopathic biotype* of BDV. Sheep can also be infected naturally with BVDV types 1 and 2, and BVDV is capable of producing the BD syndrome in sheep and goats. Pigs can be naturally infected by BDV, e.g., strain Frijters, which can confuse identification of classical swine fever.

Primary infection of postnatal sheep by BDV is usually subclinical, immunity develops and the virus is eliminated. In pregnant ewes, the virus infects the fetus within the first week of exposure and is not then influenced by the immune status of the ewe.

BDV is a potential cause of a variety of developmental disorders, including *hypomyelinogenesis, cavitating cerebral defects such as porencephaly, hydranencephaly, and cystic septum pellucidum; cerebellar dysplasia; arthrogryposis and skeletal defects; mandibular brachygnathism, and thymic hypoplasia*. The pathogenicity of the virus is most freely expressed in experimental infections, the cavitating cerebral lesions and cerebellar dysplasia being common sequelae of experimental infections but only occasionally encountered in the natural disease.

Bovine viral diarrhea virus is capable of producing the Border disease syndrome in sheep and goats, and the syndrome in piglets caused by congenital infection with *Classical swine fever virus*.

The ovine fetus is liable to significant damage if the dam is infected with BDV between days 16–80 of gestation. *The age-related immune capacity of the fetus is the important determinant of the nature of the disease produced.* In the case of infections occurring within the first half of gestation, the result may be *fetal death and abortion*. Alternatively, the fetus may survive, frequently carrying an immunologically tolerated infection. In this event, the virus persists in fetal tissues and postnatally the lamb fails to produce specific antibody. Such PI sheep harbor the virus for prolonged periods, are chronic excretors of the virus, and readily transmit infection. Lateral spread is important in the field and, although the virus can be transmitted experimentally by a number of routes, the mode of lateral transfer of infection under natural conditions has not been identified.

Infections in the second half of gestation elicit both humoral and cell-mediated immune responses and it is this acquisition of immunocompetence that endows the fetus with substantial resistance to infection after day 80 of gestation. In the case of infections initiated between day 90 of gestation and the early days of postnatal life, the cell-mediated immune response is expressed morphologically as *nodular periarteritis*. The periarteritis affects medium to small arterioles, particularly in the meninges and substance of the CNS, but also occurs mildly in a wide range of other tissues.

The developmental anomalies arising from fetal infection are also related to the gestational stage at which the fetus encounters the virus, but lesions produced also vary markedly according to virus strain, dose, route of infection, and host genetic factors. *Hypomyelinogenesis, the characteristic neural lesion*, is diffuse in fetuses infected early in gestation but becomes progressively milder and more restricted to higher, later myelinating regions of the CNS in infections initiated later in gestation. The occurrence of porencephaly and cerebellar dysplasia has been confined to infections initiated at days 45–72 of gestation. The development of the cutaneous lesion requires that infection be initiated before day 80 of gestation.

Hypomyelinogenesis and clinical tremors may substantially resolve during the first few months of life notwithstanding that the animals have persistent replicating infection, suggesting that the normal processes of myelin deposition have been delayed or that cellular injury has been slowly repaired. The virus does infect myelinating oligodendroglia, astroglia, and glial progenitor cells, and it is reasonable to assume a direct effect on the differentiation or maturation of oligodendroglia. However, the virus also infects many non-neural cells, including thyroid epithelium. There are no morphological changes in the thyroid epithelium, but reduction in circulating thyroid hormone levels may contribute to delayed maturation.

The cavitating cerebral defects and cerebellar dysplasia arise from inflammatory destruction of developing neural elements, possibly secondary to vasculitis. These lambs may have severe locomotor and behavioral abnormalities and defects of vision, the latter probably of central origin rather than due to focal retinal dysplasias that may be present. They are serologically positive but not persistently infected.

The *abnormality of birth coats* occurs in fetuses infected before ~90 days gestation. There are no cytological changes in the papillae that can be ascribed to direct viral action. The primary follicles revert to a more primitive type, are enlarged and produce heavily medullated fibers that are most prominent after about 3 weeks. There are fewer secondary follicles and their development is retarded.

BDV infection also interferes with pre- and postnatal development of skeleton, musculature, and viscera. Tissues most affected are those that have their main growth spurt in the fetal period. *Growth-arrest lines in long bones* suggest periods of interrupted intrauterine development.

Lambs that are persistently infected at birth remain so but not all show neurological signs. Growth and viability may be depressed. Some PI sheep develop oculonasal discharges and respiratory distress or severe diarrhea and die in 2–4 weeks with inflammatory lymphoproliferative lesions in many organs. In the brain, these reactions occur particularly in the choroid plexuses and periventricular substance. Proliferative metaplastic changes in the intestinal mucosa affect mainly the cecum and colon, the hyperplastic glands penetrating the muscular mucosa. *The delayed disease has features resembling those of mucosal disease of cattle,* which is considered to be due to superinfection by a different strain of BVDV or by minor mutation of homologous virus in animals that are persistently infected.

Infection by BDV is widespread in **goats** but disease attributable to this virus is not. The characteristics of the natural and experimental disease are similar to those in sheep, but spontaneous neurological disease is not a feature. The fetal goat may be much more susceptible to infection than the fetal lamb; a high incidence of fetal death, mummification, and abortion is reported.

Bibliography

Becher P, et al. Cytopathogenicity of border disease virus is correlated with integration of cellular sequences into the viral genome. Virol 1996;70:2992–2998.

Braun U, et al. Border disease in a flock of sheep. Schweiz Arch Tierheilkd 2002;144:419–426.

Caffrey JF, et al. Morphometric analysis of growth retardation in fetal lambs following experimental infection of pregnant ewes with border disease virus. Res Vet Sci 1997;62:245–248.

Monies RJ, et al. Mucosal disease-like lesions in sheep infected with Border disease virus. Vet Rec 2004;155:765–769.

Nettleton PF, et al. Border disease of sheep and goats. Vet Res 1998;29:327–340.

Pratelli A, et al. Pestivirus infection in small ruminants: virological and histopathological findings. New Microbiol 1999;22:351–356.

Thur B, et al. Immunohistochemical diagnosis of pestivirus infection associated with bovine and ovine abortion and perinatal death. Am J Vet Res 1997;58:1371–1375.

Vilcek S, Belak S. Genetic identification of pestivirus strain Frijters as a border disease virus from pigs. J Virol Methods 1996;60:103–108.

Vilcek S, et al. Molecular characterization of ovine pestiviruses. J Gen Virol 1997;78(Pt 4):725–735.

Classical swine fever virus

The disease is discussed in detail in Vol. 3, Cardiovascular system.

Both vaccine and certain low-virulence field strains of *Classical swine fever virus* (CSFV, hog cholera virus) are teratogenic for the fetal piglet. Fetuses are susceptible to infection regardless of the immune status of the sow. The apparent induction of immune tolerance results in the delivery of chronically infected piglets lacking antibody. The gestational interval during which fetal piglets are susceptible to the teratogenic effects of CSFV extends at least from day 10 to 97 of gestation, but the occurrence of malformation is favored by infection around day 30. The most characteristic anomalies involve the nervous system. The combination of *hypoplasia and dysplasia of the cerebellum and CNS hypomyelinogenesis*, most severe in the spinal cord, comprises one form of the *congenital tremor syndrome* of piglets. *Microencephaly* is also a rather characteristic sequel. The mechanism by which these lesions evolve is compatible with a persistent neural infection resulting in selective inhibition of cell division. Additional effects noted in affected litters include fetal mummification, stillbirth, pulmonary hypoplasia, nodularity of the liver, ascites, anasarca, cutaneous purpura, arthrogryposis, and micrognathia.

Bibliography

Bradley R, et al. Congenital tremor type A1: light and electron microscopical observations on the spinal cords of affected piglets. J Comp Pathol 1983;93:43–59.

Johnson KP, et al. Multiple fetal malformations due to persistent viral infection. 1. Abortion, intrauterine death, and gross abnormalities in fetal swine infected with hog cholera vaccine virus. Lab Invest 1974;30:608–617.

Paton DJ, Greiser-Wilke I. Classical swine fever – an update. Res Vet Sci 2003;75:169–178.

Feline panleukopenia virus

This disease is discussed in detail in Vol. 2, Alimentary system.

Feline panleukopenia virus (FPLV), a species of the genus *Parvovirus*, family Parvoviridae, is pathogenic to the cerebellum of kittens before and shortly after birth, at which time the cerebellum is growing and differentiating rapidly. FPLV has tropism for cells that have a high mitotic rate, and its site of action is the external germinal layer of the cerebellum. The formation of *intranuclear inclusion bodies* is an early feature of the infection; they disappear by day 14 of infection. The infected cells are destroyed and with them the growth potential of the cerebellum; hence *cerebellar hypoplasia* results. The Purkinje cells, which are postmitotic but immature, are also affected although inclusion bodies do not form in them. The nuclei of the Purkinje cells show vesicular ballooning, eosinophilia, and condensation of the membrane. One or more large vacuoles form in the cytoplasm. Some Purkinje cells undergo coagulative necrosis.

In view of the tropism of FPLV for rapidly replicating cells, a wide spectrum of abnormalities might be expected to result from infection of kittens in utero. The virus will cross the placenta and produce generalized infection of the fetus as indicated by the distribution of inclusion bodies. The subependymal cell plate shares growth behavior with the external granular layer of the cerebellum, and, although heavily infected, only one instance of hydranencephaly attributable to damage at this site of infection has been recorded. In visceral organs, only slight degrees of renal hypoplasia have been observed in infected kitten fetuses.

Bibliography

Parrish CR. Pathogenesis of feline panleukopenia virus and canine parvovirus. Baillieres Clin Haematol 1995;8:57–71.

van Vuuren M, et al. Feline panleukopenia virus revisited: molecular characteristics and pathological lesions associated with three recent isolates. J S Afr Vet Assoc 2000;71:140–143.

STORAGE DISEASES

As most storage diseases involve neurons and neurologic impairment, they are discussed here. Within all cells, except mature erythrocytes, normal catabolism directs a steady stream of endogenous macromolecules into vesicular compartments for degradation to simple molecules that may be re-used or excreted. These essentially autophagic pathways, through which each cell recycles its own constituents, may also receive endogenous and exogenous molecules from the extracellular milieu, taken up by endocytosis or phagocytosis.

Storage states, or disorders, are characterized by the accumulation of material(s) resistant to or exceeding the capacity of the machinery of intracellular digestion, disposal, or transport. Hemosiderosis and some types of hepatic lipidosis are common examples of the storage of physiologically normal substances due to the overloading of essentially normal, biochemically competent cells. A storage disease, by contrast, can be regarded as a storage process with a primary pathologic basis within the storing cells, and with potential for the perturbation of their function. The implication is that the catabolic machinery of the cells is fundamentally incompetent. This is generally demonstrable, but it is difficult to provide a neat definition that clearly distinguishes this situation in all circumstances.

Practically all cell types are potentially vulnerable to storage-induction, but those most vulnerable are long-lived postmitotic cells, such as neurons and cardiac myocytes. Cells in dynamic renewal systems, such as enterocytes, scarcely have the chance to become involved before their time is over.

The lysosomal apparatus provides the machinery for a great deal of intracellular degradation; most storage diseases involve intralysosomal accumulation and are hence termed **lysosomal storage diseases**. The 40 or so lysosomal acid hydrolases are capable of digesting completely the complex macromolecules synthesized for cell membranes, organelles, secretory products, etc. This enzymic destruction must be sequestered away from the rest of the cell, and is carried out in vesicles provided with an ion pump in their limiting membranes that maintains an acidic interior, or lysosol, for the optimal activity of the hydrolases.

Newly synthesized lysosomal enzymes are carried from the trans-Golgi region within primary lysosomal vesicles, and are delivered to substrate-containing vesicles (endosomes, heterophagosomes, autophagosomes, secretory vesicles) by fusion of vesicle membranes. The end products of digestion, which are simple lipids, amino acids, and sugars, are transported from the vesicular lysosol back into the cytosol. There may be small quantities of indigestible residues that, in cells such as hepatocytes, may be extruded by a process of exocytosis.

The lysosomal hydrolases tend to be "*exoenzymes*," sequentially breaking linkages at the ends of large molecules, but unable to act on linkages within them. This means that if the sequence is blocked at some point, further digestion cannot proceed. Should the digestive sequence be impaired, the cell will steadily accumulate a mass of vacuoles containing undegraded substrate. One type of molecule will be the major stored substance, but often the stored material will be somewhat heterogeneous, as the enzymes are linkage-specific rather than substrate-specific. Thus, *the morphologic hallmark of lysosomal storage disease is the presence of distended cells, crowded with vacuoles bounded by single membranes containing the stored material*; these vacuoles react enzyme-histochemically for acid phosphatase or other lysosomal hydrolases. They represent the adaptive hypertrophy of the lysosomal apparatus. In some cases, the morphology and histochemical reactivity of the stored substance may fairly clearly indicate its nature, for example glycogen. Lectin histochemistry may also be useful for characterizing stored material, exploiting the avid carbohydrate-binding properties of these agglutinating proteins in combination with a visualizing system.

Lysosomal digestion can be impaired in several ways. The most relevant here is *deficient activity of a specific lysosomal hydrolase because of a* **genetic defect**. This is the basis of the inherited lysosomal storage diseases in humans and animals, most of which are transmitted as autosomal recessive, and some as X-linked, traits. The deficiency in activity may come about via a total absence of enzyme protein, via the production of a defective or unstable enzyme, or via the absence of a specific activator protein required by some enzymes for the initiation of activity. These activators are small-molecular-weight, heat-stable proteins that function as detergents. They may interact with either the enzyme or its substrate. In the category of defective enzyme protein, one could also include the rare mechanism in which the enzyme lacks the specific molecular tag required to direct it, following its synthesis, to the lysosomal compartment; it is therefore immediately excreted from the cell, and the lysosomes remain deficient in that enzyme activity.

In most *autosomally inherited conditions*, the gene dose effect results in heterozygous individuals being generally phenotypically normal, but usually having demonstrably subnormal tissue activity of the particular enzyme in question. Tissues of homozygous affected individuals will contain swollen vacuolated cells, and chemical analysis reveals large amounts of the stored substance, and variable amounts of other metabolically related substances. *Multisystem involvement is likely to occur*, with storage being evident in many cell types in many organs. The cells and tissues most affected will be those most active in turning over the substrate in question, but usually the fixed and mobile macrophages are also prominently involved. This is because they avidly accumulate substrate from tissue fluids and plasma. The process begins in utero and in many cases is well developed at birth, although clinical impairment may be mild at that time. The age of onset and speed of progression of disease can vary, probably on the basis of the amount of residual enzyme activity, and often involving the ratio between various isoenzymes. In several human entities, subtypes are described on this basis.

As pointed out above, the *in vitro* tissue activity of the enzyme involved can usually be demonstrated to be negligible. However, if there was, for example, *deficiency of an activator protein*, the in vitro assay of tissues for the subject enzyme might reveal paradoxically high levels of activity, reflecting the hypertrophy of the lysosomal apparatus. The enzyme, however, would be inactive in vivo in the absence of the activator protein. In addition, and especially if the assay involves synthetic substrates, various isoenzymes may give the impression of adequate activity in vitro, which has no relation to the in vivo situation. In spite of this, assay of enzyme activity in skin fibroblasts or peripheral blood leukocytes has been diagnostically useful in many genetic storage diseases, identifying both homozygous and heterozygous individuals. Molecular genetic methods can be expected to play an increasingly important role in this area.

In an alternative mechanism of storage, *an* **exogenous toxin** *may specifically inhibit a lysosomal enzyme*, and temporarily induce a state analogous to a genetic enzyme deficiency. This is the established basis of at least one plant intoxication, "locoism," and is suspected in others. The morphologic and chemical characteristics are typical, but tissue activity of the subject enzyme may be quite high when it is separated from the inhibitor and assayed.

In a final general mechanism, *substrate that is resistant to a normal and intact enzymic battery may enter degradative pathways*. This may be an exogenous substrate, or a modified endogenous substrate. By this mechanism, several amphophilic drugs, such as chloroquine, have been found to induce storage diseases by complexing with endogenous molecules to produce indigestible products. Theoretically this mechanism could also have a genetic basis, by which an indigestible substrate is produced.

The lysosomal basis of some storage diseases is uncertain, and *non-lysosomal entities*, such as several of the glycogenoses, are clearly defined. Further, although many storage diseases have been defined in molecular terms, some have not and, in most cases, the basis of cellular dysfunction is far from clarified. There is more involved than simply the mechanical crowding out of other organelles. In most instances the storage process seems to have little primary cytotoxic effect. It seems rather that the induction of secondary and tertiary metabolic and structural effects is responsible for functional disturbances.

In many of the **neuronal storage diseases**, the process is multisystemic, and all neurons are involved, including those of the retina and peripheral ganglia, together with cells in most other organs. But neither of the two preceding conditions is invariable. When neurons are involved in storage disease, clinical signs of neurologic impairment eventually become evident, but, in general, this does not correlate with significant neuronal death, and the mechanisms of dysfunction are still largely unresolved. Regional neuronal death begins at an early stage in a few storage diseases and is progressive; it probably contributes significantly to functional disturbance at the end stage of many storage diseases.

In the face of a progressive storage process, neurons have no recourse but to accumulate storage vacuoles until they, or the animal, die. It seems probable that there is some limited capacity to discharge some of the stored load by exocytosis but, *in general, intractable constipation is inevitable as long as enzymic activity is deficient*. In spite of this, the cell limits the sites of storage to the soma and some of the larger dendritic stems. As a result, the soma becomes greatly distended and the cell outline rounded and swollen, rather than angular (Fig. 3.41). However, even within the soma, storage may be somewhat polarized, often adjacent to the axon hillock; differing planes of section may suggest that some neurons are not affected, particularly if examined early in the course of the disease. The multitude of storage vacuoles crowds and displaces other organelles, and the neuron takes on a chromatolytic and foamy appearance. Glial, endothelial, and perithelial cells are generally similarly affected.

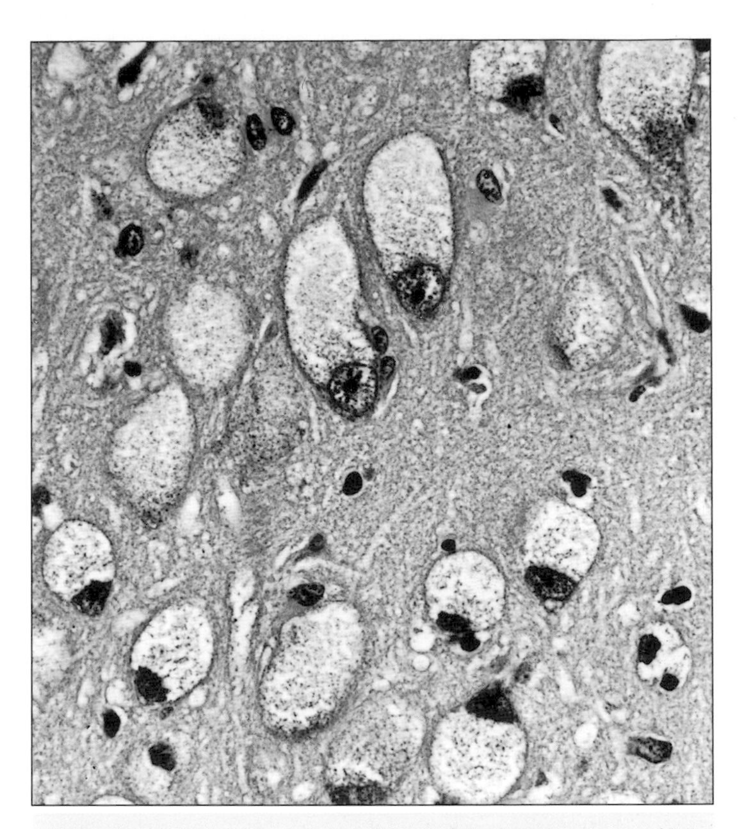

Figure 3.41 Swollen neurons in a **lysosomal storage disease** (GM_1 gangliosidosis) in a sheep. (Reprinted with permission from Murnane RD, et al. Vet Pathol 1991;28:332.)

In several ganglioside storage diseases, certain populations of neurons, particularly in the pyramidal system of the cerebral cortex and thalamic relay nuclei, undergo a form of *focal hypertrophy* in order to generate more "storage space." These cells develop large swollen compartments between the axon hillock and the initial axonal segment, dubbed "*meganeurites*." In addition, cells in these regions may sprout *aberrant dendritic spines*, whether or not they have meganeurites. The spines arise from the axon hillock and from meganeurites and form synaptic contacts. The origin of the presynaptic elements of these contacts has not been determined, but such abnormal neuronal connections could well contribute to malfunction. They may be permanent in the induced storage diseases in which otherwise the stored material may be catabolized and removed if the toxic inhibition of the enzymes is removed. These changes, dramatic as they are, cannot be appreciated without the use of special techniques, most notably the Golgi impregnation method. In addition, focal swellings may develop along the course of axons, appearing as eosinophilic spheroids, similar to those described for axonal dystrophy (see Fig. 3.9). They are often very prominent in some nuclear groups, exhibiting a tendency to form in the terminal presynaptic regions of axons, but they can be seen anywhere in the white matter and also in the peripheral nerves. They do not contain specific storage material, but are crowded with degenerate organelles and/or abnormal tubules and vesicles. They probably reflect a secondary effect of the storage process on retrograde axonal transport. The functional significance of this secondary axonal dystrophy is not resolved, but it is a prominent pathologic feature in many storage diseases.

Bibliography

Folkerth RD. Abnormalities of developing white matter in lysosomal storage diseases. J Neuropathol Exp Neurol 1999;58:887–902.

Futerman AH, van Meer G. The cell biology of lysosomal storage disorders. Nat Rev Mol Cell Biol 2004;5:554–565.

Jolly RD, Walkley SU. Lysosomal storage diseases of animals: an essay in comparative pathology. Vet Pathol 1997;34:527–548.

Meikle PJ, et al. Diagnosis of lysosomal storage disorders: current techniques and future directions. Expert Rev Mol Diagn 2004;4:677–691.

Nixon RA, Cataldo AM. The lysosomal system in neuronal cell death: a review. Ann N Y Acad Sci 1993;679:87–109.

Walkley SU. Cellular pathology of lysosomal storage disorders. Brain Pathol 1998;8:175–193.

Inherited storage diseases

Virtually all the inherited storage diseases of animals are proven or assumed to be lysosomal in nature. This applies to all those to be described below with the exceptions of the canine glycogenoses analogous to types 3 and 7 glycogenoses in humans. They are classified into broad groups, according to the class of macromolecule whose degradation is defective. As many of these diseases were first described in humans, the catalog is replete with eponyms, mostly derived from the names of the eminent people who provided those first descriptions. Within the broad groups, individual entities are defined by the nature of the dominant storage material, which reflects the specific enzymic deficit. Not all the storage diseases documented in humans have been found to have analogs in domestic animals, but the list is growing and the prevalence of inbreeding makes it likely that this will continue. *The general clinical characteristic is the onset of progressive neurologic impairment at a young age.*

In the descriptions of pathology that follow, variations in the patterns of lesions are likely to surface as more cases are described. A useful practical distinction can be made between those diseases in which the vacuoles appear empty in both paraffin and resin sections (Fig. 3.42A), and those in which they contain residual material (Fig. 3.42B). The former reflect water-soluble substrates leached out during processing, and point to certain diseases as described below.

Sphingolipidoses

Sphingolipidoses are lysosomal storage diseases caused by a genetic defect in catabolism of *glycosphingolipids*, which are important normal components of cell membranes.

In general, **gangliosidoses** are characterized clinically by the *onset at an early age of discrete head and limb tremors and dysmetria*. Worsening locomotor deficits and mentation terminate eventually

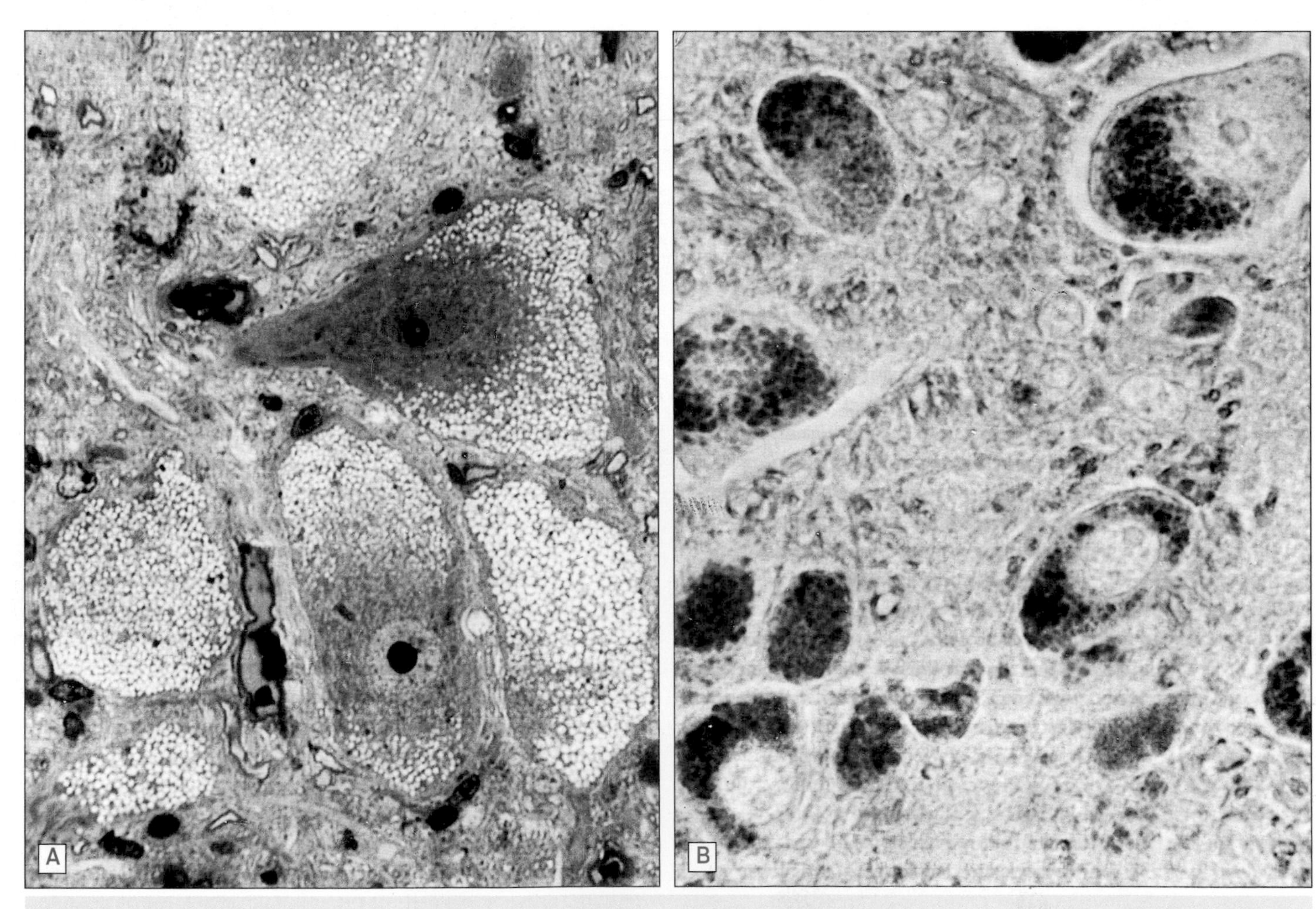

Figure 3.42 Neuronal **lysosomal storage disease**. **A.** Resin section showing "empty" vacuoles in bovine mannosidosis. (Courtesy of RD Jolly.) **B.** Dense granules, Sudan black positive, in gangliosidosis in a German Shorthaired Pointer dog. (Courtesy of E Karbe.)

in blindness, somnolence, seizures, and quadriplegia. Data indicate *autosomal recessive inheritance*.

In **GM_1 gangliosidosis** (generalized gangliosidosis), deficiency of *β-galactosidase* leads to accumulation of GM_1 ganglioside and some oligosaccharides. GM_1 gangliosidosis has been documented in cats (domestic shorthair, Korat, Siamese), dogs (Alaskan Husky, Beagle, English Springer Spaniel, Portuguese Water Dog, Shiba), Friesian cattle, and sheep (Coopworth-Romney, Romney, Suffolk).

In **GM_2 gangliosidosis**, GM_2 ganglioside accumulates due to deficient lysosomal degradative activity of *hexosaminidase*, which exists as a dimer in two forms, αβ (hexosaminidase A) or ββ (hexosaminidase B), or of an *activator protein*. Globoside may also accumulate. GM_2 gangliosidosis has been documented in domestic shorthair and Korat cats (β subunit deficiency), German Shorthaired Pointer dog, Golden Retriever (β subunit deficiency), Japanese Spaniel dog (GM_2 activator protein deficiency), and Yorkshire pigs. Variants of GM_2 gangliosidosis in humans are Tay–Sachs and Sandhoff diseases, and activator deficiency.

Neuronal storage in gangliosidoses is manifested in routine paraffin sections as marked distension of the soma, with *foamy, faintly eosinophilic cytoplasm* (Figs 3.41, 3.43A). The stored material is strongly PAS-positive in frozen sections, and is evident in plastic sections as 1–3 μm osmiophilic granules. Ultrastructurally, these are seen as *characteristic membranous cytoplasmic bodies*, consisting of concentric membranous whorls with a periodicity of about 5 nm (Fig. 3.43B). Vacuolated macrophages may also be found around blood vessels in the CNS, and storage also occurs in glial cells. Axonal spheroids may be reasonably numerous. Gliosis, demyelination and neuronal loss are not apparent until end stage. In those instances where hepatic storage occurs, hepatocytes and Kupffer cells contain large, empty vacuoles, the site of storage of a water-soluble glycopeptide.

GM_1 gangliosidosis in Suffolk sheep is associated with a dual enzyme deficiency, with βl-galactosidase deficiency being profound (5% residual activity), and α-neuraminidase deficiency less so (20% residual activity). Progressive ataxia in affected lambs first becomes evident at 4–6 months of age. Histologically, there is intense storage in most central and peripheral ganglionic neurons (Fig. 3.41), and in the kidney, liver, and lymph nodes, and cardiac Purkinje fibers. Stored material in neurons stains PAS and Luxol fast blue positive, but Sudan black negative. Axonal spheroids are frequent in cerebral and cerebellar white matter.

Glucocerebrosidosis (glucosylceramidosis) has been described in the Sydney Silky Terrier, and is the counterpart to *Gaucher disease* of humans. It results from deficient activity of *glucocerebrosidase*, which

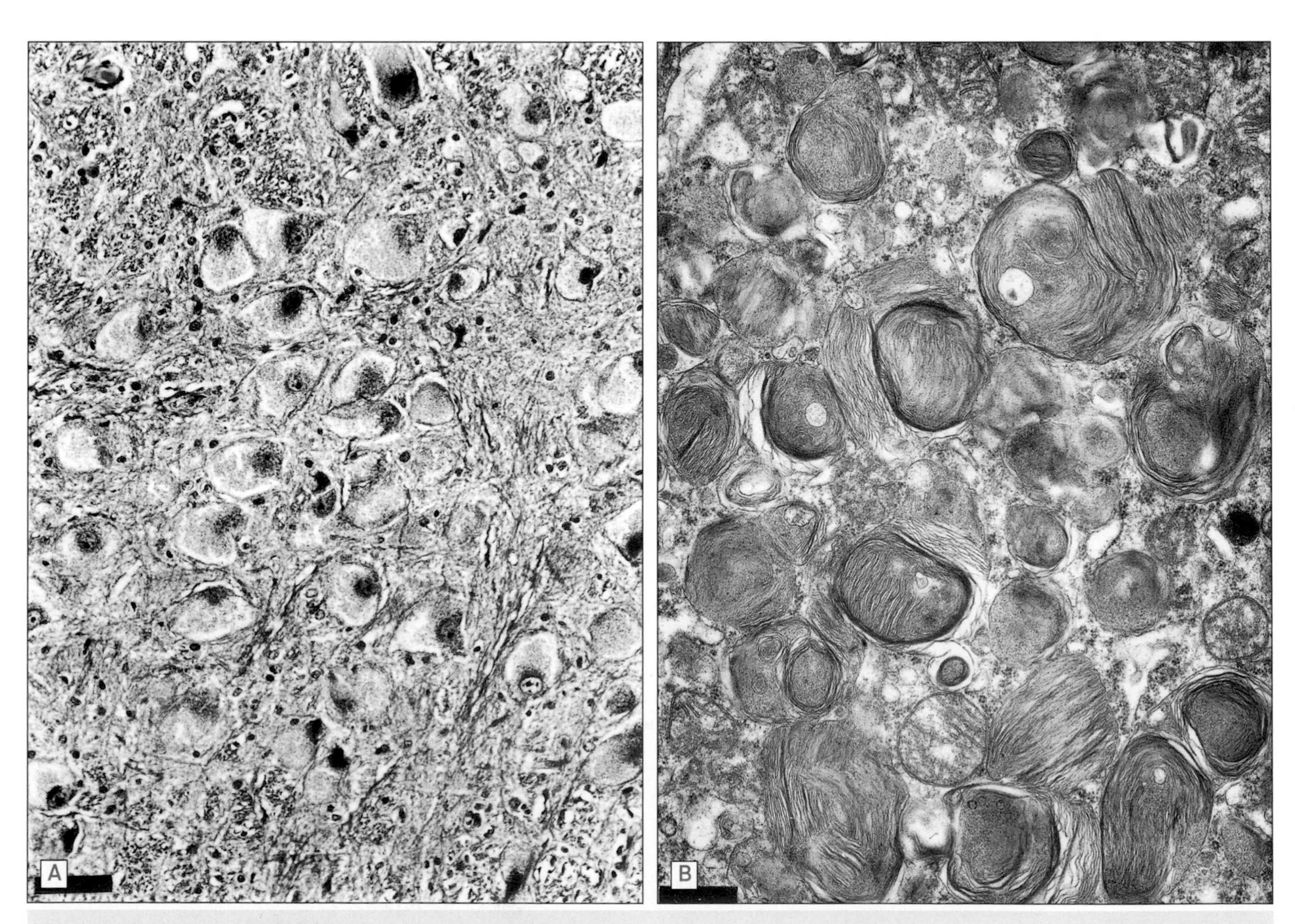

Figure 3.43 GM_1 gangliosidosis in a Portuguese Waterdog. **A.** Pale swollen neurons. Bar = 63 μm. **B.** Storage bodies showing concentric lamellae or parallel stacks of membranes. Bar = 0.6 μm. (Reprinted with permission from Saunders GK, et al. Vet Pathol 1988;25:265.)

catalyzes the conversion of glucocerebroside to ceramide. The former is derived from the catabolism of gangliosides.

Storage in the dog is expressed in macrophages in the hepatic sinusoids and lymph nodes, and in neurons in some parts of the brain but, interestingly, not in Purkinje cells and not in the spinal cord. Swollen cells have weakly eosinophilic cytoplasmic vacuoles, which are PAS-positive in the macrophages but PAS-negative in neurons. Degenerating neurons occur in the cerebral and cerebellar cortices, and Wallerian degeneration in related white matter.

Ultrastructurally, the macrophage storage material has a *characteristic twisted branching tubular structure*, and the cells in the human disease are known as *Gaucher cells*. In neurons, the storage granules are either lamellated membranous cytoplasmic bodies, resembling the Zebra bodies of mucopolysaccharidoses, or bilamellar wisps. In Gaucher variants in humans, storage may not occur in neurons.

Sphingomyelinosis has been recognized in Siamese, domestic shorthair and Balinese cats, and Poodle and Boxer dogs, and is regarded as the counterpart of *Niemann–Pick disease* in people, of which there are several variants. In types A and B, deficient activity of *sphingomyelinase* results in storage of sphingomyelin, cholesterol, and gangliosides in most neurons, and in macrophages in the liver, spleen, lymph nodes, adrenals, bone marrow, and lungs. The type C variant is caused by defective activity of a cholesterol transporter, NPC1 protein, or in the soluble lysosomal cholesterol-binding NPC2 protein. In animals, most cases are analogous to human type A; type C is described in cats and Boxer dogs.

At necropsy there is enlargement and pallor of the liver, splenomegaly, and gray nodules in the lungs. Microscopically, the visceral organs mentioned are packed with foamy macrophages, and the neurons are distended by masses of light gray, 1–2 μm autofluorescent granules. In frozen sections, the reactivity of vacuoles to oil-red-O and PAS stains is variable.

Type C Niemann–Pick disease is also characterized by numerous axonal spheroids in many areas of the neuraxis. Ultrastructurally, neuronal storage granules are concentric multilamellar structures or dense bodies.

Galactosialidosis, which results from combined deficiency of β-galactosidase and α-neuraminidase enzyme activity, is reported in a Schipperke dog. A similar combined enzyme deficiency in inbred Suffolk sheep resembled GM1 gangliosidosis phenotypically.

Galactocerebrosidosis (*galactosylceramide lipidosis, globoid cell leukodystrophy; Krabbe disease*), due to deficiency of *galactocerebrosidase*, is a member of this group, but involves storage in macrophages rather than neurons. It is discussed later under myelinopathies.

Bibliography

Alroy J, et al. Canine GM1-gangliosidosis. A clinical, morphologic, histochemical, and biochemical comparison of two different models. Am J Pathol 1992;140:675–689.

Brown DE, et al. Feline Niemann-Pick disease type C. Am J Pathol 1994;144:1412–1415.

De Maria R, et al. Beta-galactosidase deficiency in a Korat cat: a new form of feline GM1-gangliosidosis. Acta Neuropathol (Berl) 1998;96:307–314.

Donelly WJ, Sheahan BJ. GM1 gangliosidosis of Friesian calves: a review. Irish Vet J 1981;35:45–55.

Kamiya S, et al. Lectin histochemistry of feline sphingomyelinosis. Histol Histopathol 1991;6:21–24.

Knowles K, et al. Adult-onset lysosomal storage disease in a Schipperke dog: clinical, morphological and biochemical studies. Acta Neuropathol (Berl) 1993;86:306–312.

Kosanke SD, et al. Morphogenesis of light and electron microscopic lesions in porcine GM2 gangliosidosis. Vet Pathol 1979;16:6–17.

Kuwamura M, et al. Type C Niemann-Pick disease in a boxer dog. Acta Neuropathol (Berl) 1993;85:345–348.

Muller G, et al. GM1-gangliosidosis in Alaskan huskies: clinical and pathologic findings. Vet Pathol 2001;38:281–290.

Murnane RD, et al. Clinical and clinicopathologic characteristics of ovine GM-1 gangliosidosis. J Vet Intern Med 1994;8:221–223.

Neuwelt EA, et al. Characterisation of a new model of GM2 gangliosidosis (Sandhoff's disease) in Korat cats. J Clin Invest 1985;76:482–490.

Ozkara HA. Recent advances in the biochemistry and genetics of sphingolipidoses. Brain Dev 2004;26:497–505.

Prieur DJ, et al. Ovine GM-1 gangliosidosis. Am J Pathol 1991;139:1511–1513.

Ryder SJ, Simmons MM. A lysosomal storage disease of Romney sheep that resembles human type 3 GM1 gangliosidosis. Acta Neuropathol (Berl) 2001;101:225–228.

Satoh H, et al. Increased concentration of GM1-ganglioside in cerebrospinal fluid in dogs with GM1- and GM2-gangliosidoses and its clinical application for diagnosis. J Vet Diagn Invest 2004;16:223–226.

Saunders GK, et al. GM1 gangliosidosis in Portuguese water dogs: pathologic and biochemical findings. Vet Pathol 1988;25:265–269.

Singer HS, Cork LC. Canine GM2 gangliosidosis: morphological and biochemical analysis. Vet Pathol 1989;26:114–120.

Skelly BJ, et al. A new form of ovine GM1-gangliosidosis. Acta Neuropathol (Berl) 1995;89:374–379.

Wang ZH, et al. Isolation and characterization of the normal canine beta-galactosidase gene and its mutation in a dog model of GM1-gangliosidosis. J Inherit Metab Dis 2000;23:593–606.

Yamato O, et al. Sandhoff disease in a golden retriever dog. J Inherit Metab Dis 2002;25:319–320.

Yamato O, et al. GM2-gangliosidosis variant 0 (Sandhoff-like disease) in a family of Japanese domestic cats. Vet Rec 2004;155:739–744.

Glycoproteinoses

This group includes diseases in which there is *defective degradation of the carbohydrate component of N-linked glycoproteins*. These carbohydrate moieties are rich in mannose, N-acetyl glucosamine and fucose, and in particular diseases this is reflected in the storage residues that are detectable in the urine.

α-Mannosidosis has been the most economically important of the inherited storage diseases of animals, as it once occurred at high frequency in some populations of Angus cattle and the derivative Murray Grey breed. It is also recorded in the Galloway breed. The characterization and study of the disease in New Zealand led to effective carrier detection and certification schemes for its elimination and the incidence declined significantly. Inheritance is autosomal recessive, and affected calves have retarded growth, increasingly severe ataxia, and behavioral changes. The disease reaches end-stage by about 18 months of age.

Due to the synthesis of a defective enzyme protein, such individuals have *deficient lysosomal α-mannosidase* activity in virtually all cells except hepatocytes. All but the final mannose molecule of the glycans destined for digestion by this enzyme are alpha-linked. As a result, mannose/N-acetylglucosamine oligosaccharides accumulate in storage vacuoles that appear empty by light microscopy (Fig. 3.42A), as the material is extracted during tissue processing. Ultrastructurally, the vacuoles are seen to contain sparse membranous fragments and some floccular material (Fig. 3.44).

Neuronal storage is widespread and severe, but neuronal loss is not conspicuous until the terminal stages. Axonal spheroids are numerous in both gray and white matter, but especially in the cerebellar roof nuclei, the caudal brain stem proprioceptive nuclei, and on the proximal parts of Purkinje cell axons. The striking extent of storage in secretory epithelia, such as in pancreas and kidney, endothelia, fixed macrophages and fibrocytes is best appreciated in plastic-embedded sections.

α-mannosidosis has also been described in Persian and domestic shorthair and longhair cats. In the first two breeds, kittens are clinically affected very early in life, having retarded growth, facial dysmorphism, ataxia, tremor, and hepatomegaly. Intense and universal neuronal storage is accompanied by hypomyelination in the cerebrum, and widespread occurrence of axonal spheroids. Extensive storage in other tissues is as described for the bovine disease.

In the domestic longhair cat, nervous signs are reported to be milder and more slowly progressive, and there are no ocular abnormalities, hepatomegaly, myelin deficiency, or pancreatic acinar cell involvement. However, intense loss of Purkinje cells is evident and there is great diversity in the morphology of the storage cytosomes, with many membranous cytoplasmic bodies in caudal brain stem nuclei.

β-Mannosidosis has been described in the Anglo-Nubian goat, and in Salers cattle. The final mannose residue of the glycoprotein glycans is beta-linked to N-acetylglucosamine; its hydrolysis normally follows that of the alpha linkages described above. Deficiency of *β-mannosidase* leads therefore to the storage of di- or trisaccharides containing one molecule of mannose.

The disease has been most comprehensively documented in Nubian goats; inheritance is autosomal recessive. Clinical signs are severe at birth, affected kids having small palpebral fissures, facial dysmorphisms, domed skulls, joint contractures, intention tremors, and deafness. They are generally unable to stand and, even with intensive care, will survive for only a few months.

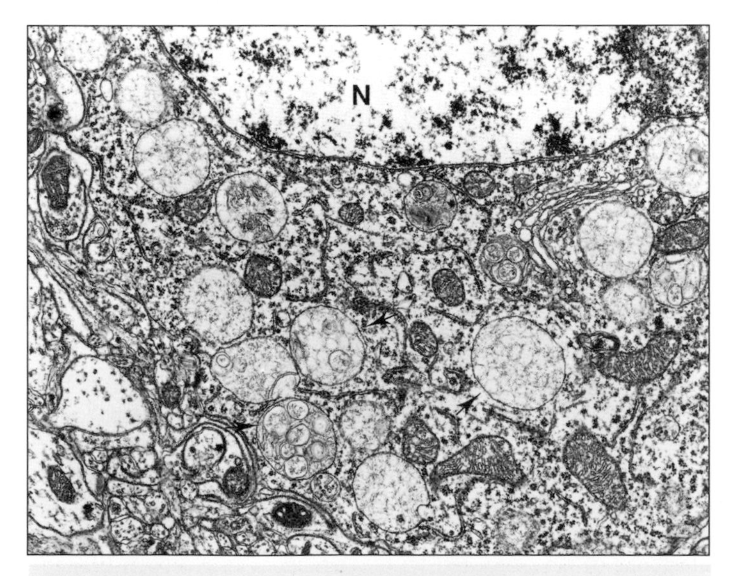

Figure 3.44 Cortical neuron in **feline mannosidosis**; storage vacuoles (arrows) contain either sparse floccular material or membranous arrays. Nucleus (N). (Courtesy of SU Walkley.)

Grossly, there is dilation of the ventricles and hypomyelination of the cerebrum and cerebellum. The latter may be the result of congenital hypothyroidism, due to storage-mediated interference with thyroid function, and it accounts for the congenital syndrome. Microscopically, neuronal vacuolation is ubiquitous and axonal spheroids numerous, especially in the internal capsule, cerebellar white matter, and basal ganglia. Vacuolated macrophages occur around some blood vessels in the brain, and there may be focal mineralization in the cerebellum and cerebrum. Large focal swellings filled with neurofilaments are sometimes present in the proximal axons of spinal motor neurons, and spheroids are numerous in sensory endings in mucous membranes and conjunctivae. Intense storage in most other tissues is similar to that described for α-mannosidosis, as is the ultrastructure of the storage vacuoles.

α-L-fucosidosis occurs in the English Springer Spaniel. As the result of deficient activity of *α-L-fucosidase*, water-soluble, fucose-containing compounds are stored as glycosylasparagines. Autosomal recessive inheritance is established, and the disease has a somewhat delayed clinical onset, with wasting, ataxia and proprioceptive deficits beginning at about 6 months of age, and becoming severe by about 2 years. A striking gross lesion is marked swelling, up to 10 mm diameter, of the cervical portion of the vagus nerves, the cervical nerves, and dorsal root ganglia.

As in mannosidosis, storage is intense in most tissues, cells becoming distended with apparently empty vacuoles. In the CNS, it is present in all neurons and in astrocytes and microglial cells; there are numerous perivascular accumulations of vacuolated macrophages. Axonal spheroids are present in the cerebellar white matter. In the thickened nerves, there is heavy infiltration of macrophages and the accumulation of myxoid perineurial ground substance.

Bibliography

Bryan L, et al. Bovine beta-mannosidosis: pathologic and genetic findings in Salers calves. Vet Pathol 1993;30:130–139.

Healy PJ, Malmo J. Roles for biochemical and polymerase chain reaction technologies in diagnosis and control of bovine alpha-mannosidosis. Aust Vet J 1998;76:699–700.

Jolly RD. The mannosidoses and ceroid-lipofuscinoses: experimental studies on two types of storage disease. Pathol 1997;29:51–56.

Lovell KL, et al. Biochemical and histochemical analysis of lysosomal enzyme activities in caprine beta-mannosidosis. Mol Chem Neuropathol 1994;21:61–74.

Skelly BJ, et al. Genomic screening for fucosidosis in English Springer Spaniels. Am J Vet Res 1999;60:726–729.

Vite CH, et al. Histopathology, electrodiagnostic testing, and magnetic resonance imaging show significant peripheral and central nervous system myelin abnormalities in the cat model of alpha-mannosidosis. J Neuropathol Exp Neurol 2001;60:817–828.

Mucopolysaccharidoses

This group of diseases is defined by *defective catabolism of glycosaminoglycans (GAG, mucopolysaccharides)* and has major expression in the skeleton and connective tissues. These diseases are therefore also discussed with Bones and joints. Glycosaminoglycans – dermatan sulfate, heparan sulfate, keratan sulfate, chondroitan sulfate – are extremely large and complex molecules, and many enzymes are involved in their degradation. As a result, 11 are entities defined in humans; four have been reported in domestic animals, and in three of these there is major involvement of neurons. General features include facial and skeletal dysmorphisms, degenerative joint disease, corneal clouding, thickening and distortion of heart valves, and thickening of the leptomeninges. Large quantities of heparan and dermatan sulfates are excreted, and are detectable, in the urine.

In animals, deficiency of **α-L-iduronidase** has been observed in the domestic shorthair cat and the Plott Hound, and is regarded as the counterpart of *mucopolysaccharidosis type I* (**MPS I**) *in man*, variants of which include the *Hurler and Scheie syndromes*. The macroscopic features described above are subtended by intense storage in fibroblasts, fixed macrophages, chondrocytes, myocytes, and pericytes in most organ systems. Glandular epithelial cells are consistently less affected than mesoderm-derived cells. The involvement of chondrocytes is associated with dysplasias of endochondral ossification, and with degeneration of articular cartilage.

Neuronal storage is universal, but neuronal loss is not conspicuous. Storage vacuoles are ultrastructurally pleomorphic; they may appear largely empty, or to contain sparse floccular to granular amorphous material, or lamellar membranous structures termed *Zebra bodies*. The latter appear to be lipid in nature, and probably represent induced secondary storage of sphingolipids. There is thus a somewhat variable reaction to tissue staining for GAG and lipid. There is some suggestion that affected cats may have a high incidence of cranial meningiomas.

In the Nubian goat, **N-acetylglucosamine-6-sulfatase deficiency** gives rise to a counterpart of human **MPS III**, *Sanfilippo disease*. Clinical features encompass delayed ability of the neonate to stand and walk, persistently ataxic gait, marked bowing of the forelimbs, and corneal clouding. Gross changes include dwarfism, kyphoscoliosis, scapular hypermobility, and cartilaginous and bony abnormalities. Two main types of lysosomal storage bodies occur microscopically. The primary storage material is *heparan sulfate*, which appears as lucent floccular material in lysosomes in arterial smooth muscle and cardiac myocytes, fibroblasts, macrophages, hepatocytes, Kupffer cells, and chondrocytes. Neurons, in contrast, are packed with PAS-positive multilamellar bodies representing secondary storage of *gangliosides* induced by interference with neuraminidase activity. Mucopolysaccharidoses IIIA and IIIB are reported in several dog breeds.

In Siamese and domestic shorthair cats, **arylsulfatase-B deficiency** produces a counterpart to human **MPS VI** (*Maroteaux–Lamy syndrome*). The disease has the same general features as described above, but neuronal storage does not occur. Storage in peripheral blood neutrophils is detected as metachromatic cytoplasmic granules.

A **β-glucuronidase-deficient MPS** has been described in dogs and cats, and is considered analogous to human **MPS VII** (*Sly disease*). The general features of the clinical disease are as described above, and there is excessive urinary excretion of chondroitin-4-sulfate and chondroitin-6-sulfate. There is *widespread neurovisceral storage*, with cytoplasmic inclusions appearing largely empty or containing sparse granular or lamellar material.

Bibliography

Crawley AC, et al. Prevalence of mucopolysaccharidosis type VI mutations in Siamese cats. J Vet Intern Med 2003;17:495–498.

Ellinwood NM, et al. A model of mucopolysaccharidosis IIIB (Sanfilippo syndrome type IIIB): N-acetyl-alpha-D-glucosaminidase deficiency in Schipperke dogs. J Inherit Metab Dis 2003;26:489–504.

Haskins M, et al. Animal models for mucopolysaccharidoses and their clinical relevance. Acta Paediatr Suppl 2002;91:88–97.

He X, et al. Identification and characterization of the molecular lesion causing mucopolysaccharidosis type I in cats. Mol Genet Metab 1999;67:106–112.

Jolly RD, et al. Screening for the mucopolysaccharidosis-IIIA gene in Huntaway dogs. N Z Vet J 2002;50:122.

Jones MZ, et al. Caprine mucopolysaccharidosis IIID: fetal and neonatal brain and liver glycosaminoglycan and morphological perturbations. J Mol Neurosci 2004;24:277–291.

Macri B, et al. Mucopolysaccharidosis VI in a Siamese/short-haired European cat. J Vet Med A Physiol Pathol Clin Med 2002;49:438–442.

Schultheiss PC, et al. Mucopolysaccharidosis VII in a cat. Vet Pathol 2000; 37:502–505.

Silverstein Dombrowski DC, et al. Mucopolysaccharidosis type VII in a German shepherd dog. J Am Vet Med Assoc 2004;224:553–557.

Glycogenoses

A number of enzymes are involved in the catabolism of glycogen, but only one of these, *α-1,4-glucosidase*, is a lysosomal enzyme. The lysosomal pathway degrades any glycogen that finds its way into autophagic vacuoles, while the other pathways are more related to metabolic mobilization of glycogen. In humans, eight different glycogen storage diseases have been identified, with the lysosomal type being classified as **type II**, *Pompe disease*. As the storage process is very widespread in this disease, it is also referred to as *generalized glycogenosis*. In most other types, storage is concentrated in liver and muscle.

α-1,4-glucosidase deficiency has been well documented in Shorthorn and Brahman beef cattle. The disease has autosomal recessive inheritance, and affected calves have severe clinical signs by about a year of age. The most damaging effects are produced in the skeletal and cardiac muscle; weakness and congestive cardiac failure are clinically dominant, and cardiomegaly and hepatomegaly evident at necropsy. There is *widespread glycogen storage*, much of which occurs in typical lysosomal storage vacuoles, but some of which is intracytoplasmic. Swollen, vacuolated cells contain diastase-sensitive, PAS-positive material, which is ultrastructurally typical of glycogen. Vacuolar myopathy and cardiomyopathy are prominent (Fig. 3.45); *neuronal storage is universal and severe* and is accompanied by glial storage, with numerous axonal spheroids in the vestibular and cuneate nuclei, terminal fasciculus gracilis, and throughout the spinal cord gray matter (see Fig. 3.8). Mild Wallerian degeneration may be present in the lateral and ventral columns of the spinal cord and in some peripheral nerves.

Type II glycogenosis has also been documented in the Lapland dog, and suspected on morphologic grounds in the domestic cat and Corriedale sheep.

Amylo-1,6-glucosidase deficiency is recorded in the German Shepherd Dog, as a counterpart of glycogenosis **type III** (Cori disease). Cytoplasmic glycogen storage occurs in liver, muscle, and myocardium, and in neurons and glia in the brain and spinal cord.

Polyglucosan body disease (glycogen storage disease **type IV**) is reported in a mixed-breed dog as the result of an inherited metabolic defect associated with a deficiency of glycogen-branching enzyme. Periodic acid Schiff (PAS)-positive polyglucosan bodies (abnormal glycogen) were present in neurons, liver, and myocardium.

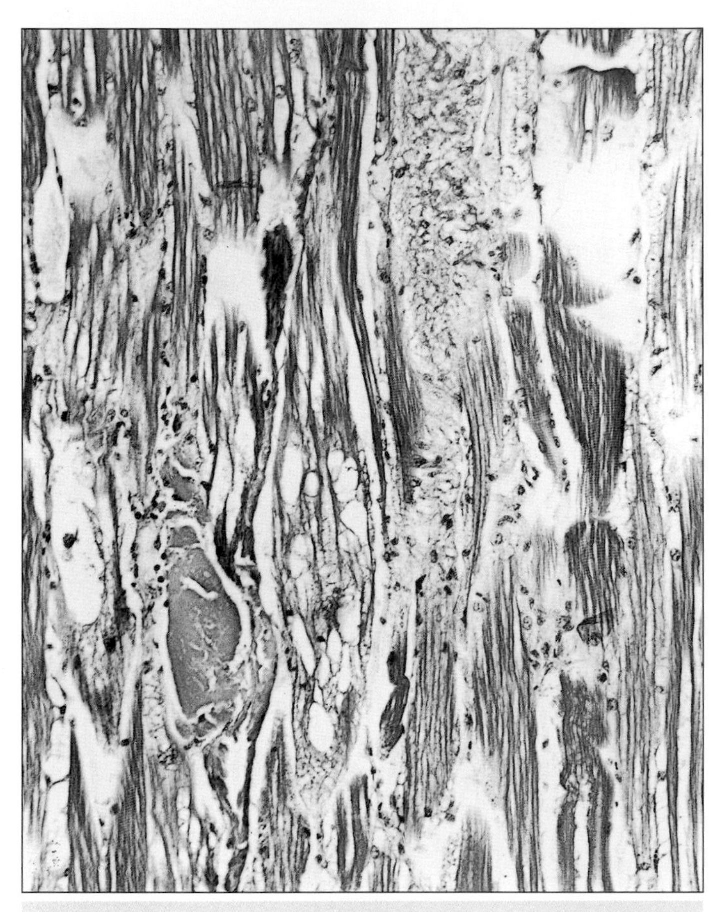

Figure 3.45 Vacuolated and degenerate skeletal muscle fibers in **generalized glycogenosis** in a Shorthorn calf.

Bibliography

Ceh L, et al. Glycogenosis type III in the dog. Acta Vet Scand 1976;17:210–222.

Cook RD, et al. Changes in nervous tissue in bovine generalised glycogenosis type 11. Neuropath Appl Neurobiol 1982;8:95–107.

Dennis JA, et al. The bovine alpha-glucosidase gene: coding region, genomic structure, and mutations that cause bovine generalized glycogenosis. Mamm Genome 2000;11:206–212.

Jolly RD, et al. Polyglucosan body disease in a mixed-breed dog. N Z Vet J 2002;50:32–35.

Palmer DG, et al. Bovine glycogenosis type II: the molecular defect in Shorthorn cattle. Neuromuscul Disord 1994;4:39–48.

Reichmann KG, et al. Clinical, diagnostic and biochemical features of generalised glycogenosis type II in Brahman cattle. Aust Vet J 1993;70:405–408.

Mucolipidoses

Mucolipidosis describes a disease with the features of both sphingolipidoses and mucopolysaccharidoses. **Mucolipidosis II** (ML II), also called *I-cell (inclusion-cell) disease*, is a lysosomal storage disease caused by deficient activity of *N-acetylglucosamine-1-phosphotransferase*. The condition is inherited as an autosomal recessive in domestic shorthair cats. Affected kittens fail to thrive and have behavioral dullness, facial dysmorphia, and ataxia. Diffuse retinal degeneration leads to blindness. Storage lysosomes containing oligosaccharides, mucopolysaccharides, and lipids are most common in bone, cartilage, skin, and other connective tissues; a few cerebral cortical neurons have lipid inclusions, and some sciatic nerve axons are affected.

Bibliography

Bosshard NU, et al. Spontaneous mucolipidosis in a cat: an animal model of human I-cell disease. Vet Pathol 1996;33:1–13.

Mazrier H, et al. Inheritance, biochemical abnormalities, and clinical features of feline mucolipidosis II: the first animal model of human I-cell disease. J Hered 2003;94:363–373.

Ceroid-lipofuscinoses

With advancing age and senility, intracytoplasmic granules of the autofluorescent lipopigment, **lipofuscin**, accumulate in neurons, fixed phagocytes, macrophages and muscle cells. This *"wear and tear" pigment* is familiar to all pathologists, and has a characteristic histochemical profile and ultrastructure; the irregularly shaped granules have a high-density component punctuated with vacuoles of low density. For many years, in the group of diseases known as the "ceroid-lipofuscinoses," it has been assumed that a similar pigment is stored in lysosomes. However, other compounds, such as the hydrophobic lipid-binding protein subunit c of mitochondrial ATP synthase are also complexed with lipid and may predominate; hence at least some of these conditions might better be termed **proteinoses**.

In animals, neuronal ceroid-lipofuscinoses (NCL, Batten disease) of proven or presumptive **inherited** nature have been described in Siamese cats, South Hampshire sheep, Devon cattle, Nubian goats, and many breeds of dog including English Setter, Chihuahua, Dachshund, Saluki, Dalmatian, Blue Heeler, Border Collie, Tibetan Terrier, and crossbred. In general, *although storage may be widespread in several organs, it is most damaging in neurons of the cerebral cortex, retina, and cerebellar Purkinje system*. Thus there is frequently extensive cellular loss and atrophy in these regions, and correlating dementia, blindness, and ataxia. Macroscopically, atrophied areas may have a distinctly brown tinge. Microscopically, the storage granules are brightly autofluorescent under ultraviolet light, pale brown-red or colorless with hematoxylin and eosin, weakly acid-fast, magenta with PAS, and intensely positive with Luxol fast blue. Ultrastructurally, they appear as *membrane-bound cytosomes* up to 15 nm in diameter, irregular in outline, and with a variety of forms (Fig. 3.46). Some have membranous material arranged as *"curvilinear bodies" and "fingerprint bodies,"* which are considered characteristic. Others may have *laminated stacks of membranes* akin to zebra bodies, membranous stacks, or dense granular deposits.

The variation in features of NCL is illustrated by comparing the disease in various species and breeds. In Devon cattle, the major clinical deficit is profound blindness at about 14 months of age, with death usually due to misadventure by about 2 years. There is severe retinal atrophy but only mild loss of neurons from the cerebral and cerebellar cortices. In Tibetan Terriers, blindness is again the dominant sign, but the onset is delayed to middle life and is accompanied terminally by stupor. In the Border Collie and some other dog breeds, there are gait and visual deficits by 18–24 months of age, accompanied by increasing aggression and dementia. Retinal lesions are mild and blindness is central in origin. Neuronal loss and gliosis are particularly severe in the cerebellar Purkinje cell layer, and significant in the limbic system.

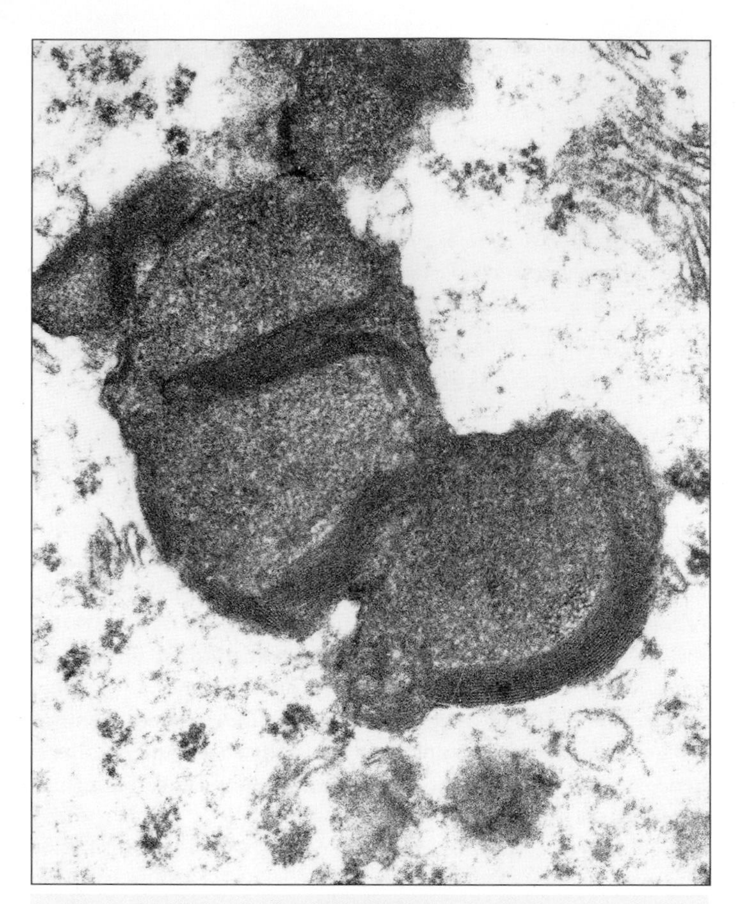

Figure 3.46 Ceroid lipofuscinosis in a Tibetan Terrier. Granular and membranous storage body in a Purkinje cell. (Courtesy of JF Cummings.)

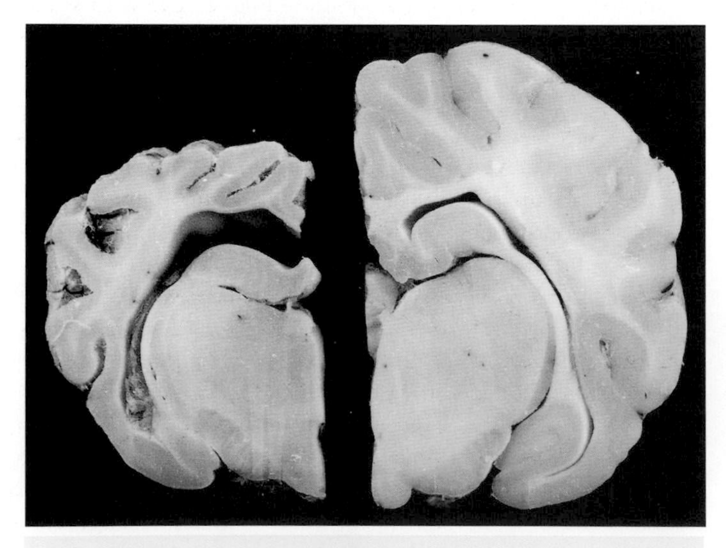

Figure 3.47 Ceroid lipofuscinosis in a South Hampshire lamb. Marked cerebral atrophy at 4 months; control right. (Courtesy of RD Jolly.)

The pathogenesis of at least some forms of NCL may involve a defect in mitochondria rather than a defect in lysosomal catabolism, and may involve accumulation of hydrophobic protein. The NCL in South Hampshire sheep has been thoroughly studied. The brains of affected lambs grow normally until 4 months of age, and then undergo atrophy (Fig. 3.47). Half of the material stored in lysosomes is the lipid-binding protein subunit c of mitochondrial ATP synthase. NCL in Merino sheep is also a subunit c-storing disease, clinically and pathologically similar to NCL in South Hampshire sheep. The NCL in both breeds (OCL6 form) apparently results from a mutation at the same gene locus in chromosomal region OAR7q13-15, and both breeds are potential animal models for the human late infantile variant CLN6. CLN proteins are coded by *NCL* genes.

Bibliography

Cook RW, et al. Neuronal ceroid lipofuscinosis in Merino sheep. Aust Vet J 2002;80:292–297.

Gardiner RM. The molecular genetic basis of the neuronal ceroid lipofuscinoses. Neurol Sci 2000;21(3 Suppl):S15–19.

Jolly RD, Walkley SU. Ovine ceroid lipofuscinosis (OCL6): postulated mechanism of neurodegeneration. Mol Genet Metab 1999;66:376–380.

Jolly RD, et al. Neuronal ceroid-lipofuscinosis in Borderdale sheep. N Z Vet J 2002;50:199–202.

Koie H, et al. Magnetic resonance imaging of neuronal ceroid lipofuscinosis in a border collie. J Vet Med Sci 2004;66:1453–1456.

Minatel L, et al. Ceroid-lipofuscinosis in a Cocker Spaniel dog. Vet Pathol 2000; 37:488–490.

Rossmeisl JH Jr, et al. Neuronal ceroid-lipofuscinosis in a Labrador Retriever. J Vet Diagn Invest 2003;15:457–460.

Sisk DB, et al. Clinical and pathologic features of ceroid-lipofuscinosis in two Australian cattle dogs. J Am Vet Med Assoc 1990;197:361–364.

Siso S, et al. Adult onset thalamocerebellar degeneration in dogs associated to neuronal storage of ceroid lipopigment. Acta Neuropathol (Berl) 2004; 108:386–392.

Url A, et al. Equine neuronal ceroid lipofuscinosis. Acta Neuropathol (Berl) 2001; 101:410–414.

Miscellaneous genetic storage diseases

The apparent lysosomal storage of lipid material in spinal motor neurons is described in English Pointer dogs, and is discussed under motor neuron diseases.

A counterpart to the autosomal recessive human **Lafora disease** has been recorded in Basset Hound, Poodle and Beagle dogs. Progressive myoclonus epilepsy is associated with *widespread intraneuronal storage of a complex polyglucosan*, which appears as characteristic *Lafora bodies* (see Fig. 3.5). They are most numerous in Purkinje cells, and neurons of the caudate, thalamic, and periventricular nuclei. They are non-membrane-bound spherical structures with a central basophilic core and a peripheral halo of radiating filaments. They are strongly PAS-positive and are found in both perikaryon and dendrites; they vary greatly in size, ranging up to 15–20 μm. Human LD is caused by mutation in the *EPM2A* gene that encodes for laforin and the *EPM2B* gene that encodes for malin. Lafora bodies are occasionally found incidentally in otherwise normal brains and spinal cords, especially in older dogs.

Bibliography

Chan EM, et al. Laforin preferentially binds the neurotoxic starch-like polyglucosans, which form in its absence in progressive myoclonus epilepsy. Hum Mol Genet 2004;13:1117–1129.

Gredal H, et al. Progressive myoclonus epilepsy in a beagle. J Small Anim Pract 2003;44:511–514.

Schoeman T, et al. Polyglucosan storage disease in a dog resembling Lafora's disease. J Vet Intern Med 2002;16:201–207.

Induced storage diseases

Numerous types of storage process have been successfully produced experimentally, and there is a group of naturally occurring disorders related to the ingestion of plants, in which induced storage disease is proven or suspected.

Swainsonine toxicosis

Swainsonine, *an indolizidine alkaloid*, is the active principle of several species of toxic plants that have caused considerable problems for all classes of grazing livestock. These include poison pea (*Swainsona* sp.) of Australia, locoweeds (*Astragalus, Oxytropis* sp.) of North America, broomweed (*Sida carpinifolia*) of Brazil, and shrubby morning glory (*Ipomoea carnea*) of Mozambique. Endophytic fungi, such as *Embellisia,* that grow on locoweed can induce the same toxicity. As a *potent inhibitor of lysosomal α-mannosidase*, swainsonine induces a form of **α-mannosidosis** that is a close copy of the genetic disease of cattle and cats. Continued ingestion of toxic material over a period of 4–6 weeks and more results in failure to thrive and, ultimately, ataxia, proprioceptive deficits and behavioral abnormalities ("locoism" in North America, "pea-struck" in Australia). Necropsy examination during, or within a short time after, exposure to the plant reveals microscopic and ultrastructural lesions identical to those of genetic α-mannosidosis. Within 2 weeks of last exposure, much of the storage disease resolves, but axonal spheroids may persist in large numbers in areas such as the cerebellar roof nuclei and caudal brain stem. Swainsonine-induced mannosidosis has been experimentally compared in the cat with genetic mannosidosis in order to determine the reversibility of changes such as meganeurite and aberrant synapse formation in higher neurons (see introductory section). Clinical recovery may or may not occur following cessation of exposure, and the persistence of secondary neuronal changes suggests that they, rather than the storage process, may underlie neuronal malfunction. Exposure of young growing animals is more likely to produce irreversible disease than exposure of adults.

The induced disease is, however, biochemically distinct from the genetic, as *the alkaloid also inhibits Golgi mannosidase II*, an enzyme involved in the post-translational trimming modifications of the glycan moiety of glycoproteins. As a result, abnormal proportions of different types of glycoproteins are produced, and the storage oligosaccharides are larger than those in the genetic disease. No modification of the storage disease appears to result from this difference.

In swainsonine intoxication of pregnant animals, both dam and fetus are affected, and *abortion and terata are well recognized in ovine locoweed toxicosis.* Suppressive effects on fertility are also recognized.

Trachyandra poisoning

Ingestion of *Trachyandra divaricata* or *T. laxa* for several weeks has been associated with severe neurologic disease and **lipofuscinosis** in sheep, horses, goats, and pigs in South Africa and Australia. The clinical syndrome is one of weakness, suggesting a neuromuscular disorder, and is often accompanied by *intense lipofuscin storage in all central and peripheral neurons* and, to a lesser extent, in macrophages of the intestinal lamina propria, hepatocytes, Kupffer cells, and renal tubular epithelium. Pigment storage may be sufficiently intense to cause macroscopic rusty-brown discoloration of central gray nuclei and peripheral ganglia. The pigment granules have all the histochemical and ultrastructural features of lipofuscin. The clinical signs appear to be irreversible and their relationship to the storage process is obscure; the basis of the storage process is unknown.

Phalaris poisoning

Extensive losses in sheep and cattle in Australia, New Zealand, South Africa, California, and Argentina have been due to grazing *Phalaris* sp., principally *P. aquatica* and *P. arundinacea*, but also *P. minor, P. caroliniana*, and *P. angusta*. Several syndromes of *Phalaris* toxicosis affect principally ruminants but occasionally horses – dramatic large-scale sudden mortalities occur in sheep, sudden deaths have been associated in horses, staggers syndromes of acute onset and recoverable or of chronic onset and not recoverable occur in sheep and occasionally in cattle. Onset of staggers syndromes may be rapid on exposure to immature plants or delayed for up to several months. It is probable that resistance to the toxicosis may be produced by catabolism of toxins by adapted ruminal microflora.

There are two acute neurological syndromes. *Sudden death* in sheep and horses without observable tissue changes is probably caused by cardiotoxic compounds, a mix of *methyl tryptamine* and *β-carboline indoleamines* chemically related to 5-hydroxytryptamine (serotonin). The second acute syndrome is in sheep and is referred to as a polioencephalomalacia-like syndrome, the result of edema of deep cortical gray matter laminae. Severe astrocytic edema in the cortex is similar to that seen in citrullinemia, and suggests peracute ammonia toxicity due to toxic impairment of urea-cycle enzymes.

The clinical onset of the staggers syndrome may be delayed for several months after exposure to toxic pasture has ceased. It is characterized by generalized muscle tremors progressing to stiffness, collapse on forced exercise, and tetanic seizures. In most cases, recovery does not occur and apparent recovery is followed by relapses.

In cases examined early in the course of the disease, there may be no gross or microscopic lesions but, in general, pathologic changes are present. Most characteristically, there is *storage of granular pigment within neurons* of the brain stem nuclei, spinal gray matter and dorsal root ganglia, and in macrophages of the cerebrospinal fluid. A similar pigment is also present within renal tubular epithelial cells. When storage is intense, the affected gray matter and kidneys may have distinct green discoloration on gross inspection (Fig. 3.48A). Histologically, the pigment granules are green-brown and present in a perinuclear distribution in neurons (Fig. 3.48B), although some granules may accumulate in dendrites. Ultrastructurally, the storage granules are composed of concentric membranous lamellae, sometimes interspersed with fine granular material. They are membrane bound and are considered to be lysosomal in nature. In most cases, there is also Wallerian degeneration concentrated in ventral, ventromedial, and lateral funiculi throughout the spinal cord, and in the medial longitudinal fasciculus. This distribution suggests selective damage to long descending motor tracts. Severely affected areas may also have intense diffuse astrogliosis. Intense reactive astrogliosis may also be seen in ventral spinal cord gray matter, along with mild neuronal loss.

Solanum poisoning

Ingestion of *Solanum kwebense* or *S. fastigiatum* is associated with neuronal degeneration and loss in the cerebellum, as discussed elsewhere.

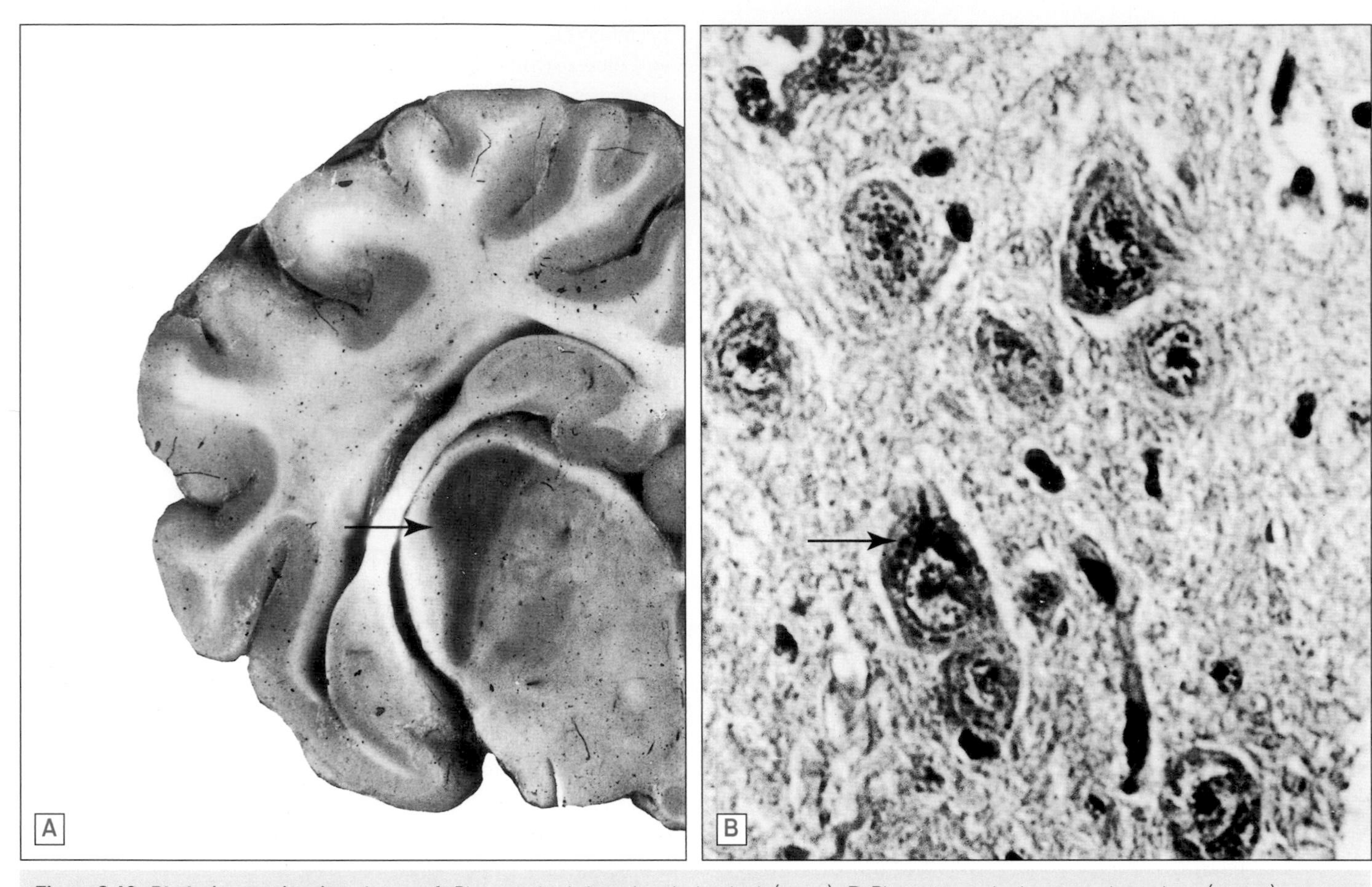

Figure 3.48 ***Phalaris* sp. poisoning** of a cow. **A.** Pigmentation in lateral geniculate body (arrow). **B.** Pigment granules in neuronal cytoplasm (arrows).

Purkinje cells and some other neurons are vacuolated, and lamellated lipid material is stored in endoplasmic reticulum or lysosomes. The lectin-binding pattern is consistent with a glycolipid storage disease.

Gomen disease

As discussed elsewhere, this is a suspected toxicosis of horses in New Caledonia, in which there is cerebellar neuronal degeneration, and associated lipofuscin storage in neurons and phagocytic cells.

Bibliography

Bourke CA, et al. Clinical observations and differentiation of the peracute *Phalaris aquatica* poisoning syndrome in sheep known as 'polioencephalomalacia-like sudden death'. Aust Vet J 2003;81:698–700.

Colegate SM, et al. Suspected blue canary grass (*Phalaris coerulescens*) poisoning of horses. Aust Vet J 1999;77:537–538.

Huxtable CR, et al. Neurological disease and lipofuscinosis in horses and sheep grazing *Trachyandra divaricata* (branched onion weed) in south Western Australia. Aust Vet J 1987;64:105–108.

Loretti AP, et al. Lysosomal storage disease in *Sida carpinifolia* toxicosis: an induced mannosidosis in horses. Equine Vet J 2003;35:434–438.

McLain-Romero J, et al. The toxicosis of *Embellisia* fungi from locoweed (*Oxytropis lambertii*) is similar to locoweed toxicosis in rats. J Anim Sci 2004;82:2169–2174.

Michael JP. Indolizidine and quinolizidine alkaloids. Nat Prod Rep 2004;21:625–649.

Odriozola E, et al. Neuropathological effects and deaths of cattle and sheep in Argentina from *Phalaris angusta*. Vet Hum Toxicol 1991;33:465–467.

Paulovich FB, et al. Lectin histochemical study of lipopigments present in the cerebellum of *Solanum fastigiatum var. fastigiatum* intoxicated cattle. J Vet Med A Physiol Pathol Clin Med 2002;49:473–477.

Schumaher-Henrique B, et al. The clinical, biochemical, haematological and pathological effects of long-term administration of *Ipomoea carnea* to growing goats. Vet Res Commun 2003;27:311–319.

Stegelmeier BL, et al. Dose response of sheep poisoned with locoweed (*Oxytropis sericea*). J Vet Diagn Invest 1999;11:448–456.

INCREASED INTRACRANIAL PRESSURE, CEREBRAL SWELLING, AND EDEMA

Normally only a narrow space separates the brain from the dura mater. Both the dura and skull are unyielding so that only a relatively small increase in the volume of the intracranial contents is permissible without increasing intracranial pressure. When the pressure is increased, something has to yield. The following refers particularly to the brain, but the principles apply equally to the spinal cord, especially in cases of trauma.

The causes of increased intracranial pressure are many and varied. One component of almost all of them is edema. **Brain edema** is an increase in water content of brain tissue. Brain tissue is about 75% water, a little more for gray matter and a little less for white matter. The edema may be more or less localized and geographically related to local lesions, or it may be diffuse. In addition to the pathogenetic mechanisms to be discussed here, acquired hydrocephalus and vitamin A deficiency in young animals can be responsible for increased intracranial pressure. In vitamin A deficiency, there is increased secretion of cerebrospinal fluid by the choroid plexus and decreased absorption by arachnoid villi, effects that may be quickly repaired by administered vitamin. Also important in domestic animals is impaired growth and remodeling of cranium and vertebrae that leads to disproportion between the volume of the growing nervous system and volume of the cranial cavity and spinal canal.

The local lesions that may result in **local edema** of the brain or spinal cord include: neoplasms, inflammations, parasitic cysts, focal necrosis of various causes, trauma, hemorrhages of parenchyma and meninges, and space-occupying lesions of the meninges that cause pressure on the brain. In each example, the edema may be mild or extensive and may contribute more than the primary or inciting lesion to the clinical signs, and to the swelling of the brain or spinal cord and increase of intracranial pressure.

Generalized cerebral edema and swelling of the brain also occurs in relation to a variety of *systemic conditions*. Some degree of swelling can be anticipated as a *postmortem change*, especially in the brain of young animals, and is probably to be related to the imbibition of fluid in autolysis. Cerebral edema with swelling occurs with diffuse *meningitis*, moderately so in the diffuse *viral encephalitides*, *acute bacterial toxemias* such as clostridial enterotoxemia, and *chemical intoxications* such as lead and organomercurial poisoning, and quite severely in the pathologic syndrome of sheep and cattle known as *polioencephalomalacia*. Generalized edema of moderate degree is expected in the many metabolic and toxic conditions which are characterized by disturbances of cellular osmoregulation, in particular disturbances which interfere with intracellular and extracellular concentrations of sodium and potassium; the acute-onset neurologic disease which occurs in *salt poisoning* of pigs and in *water intoxication* in young ruminants given water *ad libitum* after a period of deprivation would be in this category.

There are differences between gray and white matter in their susceptibility to edema, and different areas of gray substance or of white differ in their vulnerability. The considerations of edema here recognize several types of edema but are limited for descriptive purposes to the cytotoxic and vasogenic varieties. **Congestive brain swelling** is an increase in volume, especially in capillaries and post-capillary venules, as a result of loss of autoregulation of arterial input. In vivo imaging techniques can identify this edematous pattern but it is not easily evaluated at postmortem because of the valveless character of intracerebral veins. **Interstitial edema** that affects the central white matter in hydrocephalus and the spinal cord in hydromyelia and syringomyelia is considered with those diseases, the edema is a result of acutely raised intraventricular pressure. Hypo-osmotic edema follows a reduction of serum osmolality, usually as a result of fluid administration or ingestion.

A distinction is maintained here between **cytotoxic edema** and **vasogenic edema**, notwithstanding that the endothelial barrier between blood and brain may be functionally deranged in each type. *Intracellular* or **cytotoxic edema** depends on direct or indirect noxious injury to cells and interference with the mechanisms that control cell volume. For cells in non-nervous tissues, the swelling would represent hydropic change, the movement of water from interstitial tissues into cell cytoplasm. There is, however, in nervous tissue no significant interstitial tissue or intercellular space. The intercellular space in the brain is not more than 10–20 nm. There is a layer of material that stains as glycoprotein or glycosaminoglycan on cell membranes, but there is doubt as to whether it is the counterpart of other interstitial gels. The net increase in water in the brain in cytotoxic edema must represent a movement from plasma, and the regulatory mechanisms must therefore reside in the capillary endothelium and the brain cells. The basic disturbance is in osmoregulation, which depends mainly on the efficiency of the sodium/potassium pump and adenosine triphosphate as an energy source.

In cytotoxic edema, the swelling is in neurons but mainly in the astrocytes. Simple swelling of astrocytes is the most obvious structural change in gray matter. Swelling of the astrocytes involves the nucleus and processes. Glycogen granules accumulate in the watery protoplasm. If mild edema persists, the astrocytes react as described in an earlier section. If the edema is severe, the astrocyte nucleus is much enlarged, the chromatin is dispersed against the nuclear membrane, and the processes are voluminous. Death of acutely swollen astrocytes may not be accompanied by changes in the adjacent neuropil. Neurons may swell as a brief prelude to lysis. Satellite oligodendroglia are generally spared.

However, in cytotoxic edema, oligodendrocytes in white matter degenerate. The nucleus is swollen and less dense than normal; the nucleolus is hypertrophied, and the cytoplasm is enlarged and often visible in routine material. Changes in oligodendroglial processes that are wrapped as myelin are difficult to evaluate histologically except in those instances of specific cytotoxic edema in which there is splitting of the intraperiod line and the accumulation of water in intermyelinic clefts.

Vasogenic edema *is the term used to distinguish the extracellular accumulation of fluid from cytotoxic edema.* The basis of vasogenic edema is injury to vascular endothelium of sufficient severity to allow leakage or permeation of plasma constituents including, if the injury is sufficient, plasma proteins. The fluid spreads between cells in response to hydrostatic pressures in the cerebral circulation and those in the tissue. Vasogenic edema is a common complication of traumatic, inflammatory, and hemorrhagic lesions of the nervous system. It is not a conspicuous change in gray matter, because the dense tangle of neuropil resists the passage of fluid. There are exceptions such as in the periventricular nuclei where vasogenic edema occurs rather selectively in thiamine deficiency. The structure of white matter offers less resistance to the passage of edema fluid of this origin, and the comparison between the susceptibility of gray and white matter can be seen readily with local lesions near their junction in the cortex. The long fiber tracts such as the spinal cord, internal capsules, and optic tracts tend to be spared. The density and disposition of these tracts probably exert a considerable influence on the spread of edema about local lesions as, for example, the corpus callosum seems effectively to prevent spread from one hemisphere to the other.

The histological appearances are similar to those in cytotoxic edema with the addition of dissecting changes along fiber tracts. The white matter is loosely textured, the myelinated fibers being spread apart. The spaces created may be clear or they may, depending on the degree of permeability, contain homogeneous proteinaceous fluid (Fig. 3.49). Plasma droplets that stain brightly with periodic acid-Schiff are frequently present in perivascular clefts (Fig. 3.50).

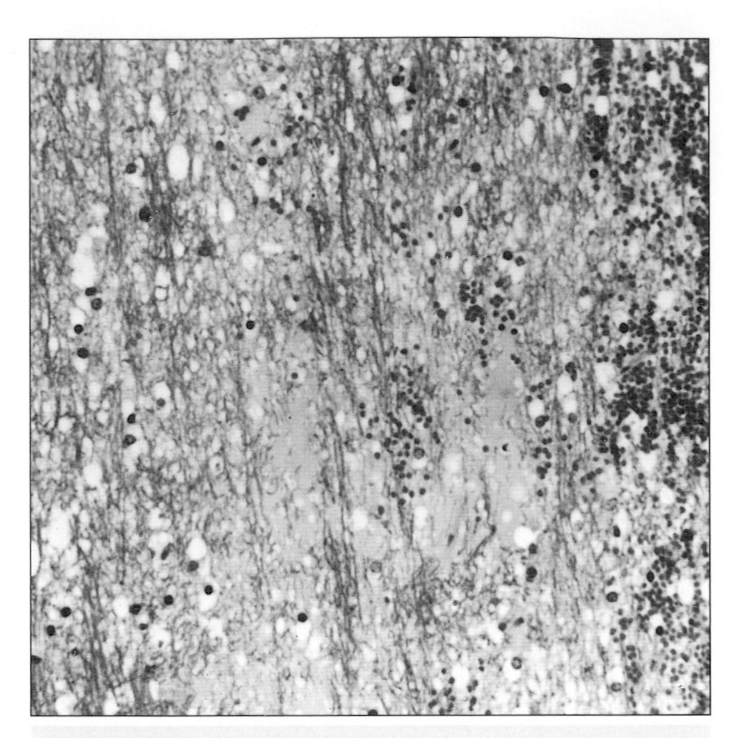

Figure 3.49 Vasogenic edema and hemorrhage with degeneration of white matter.

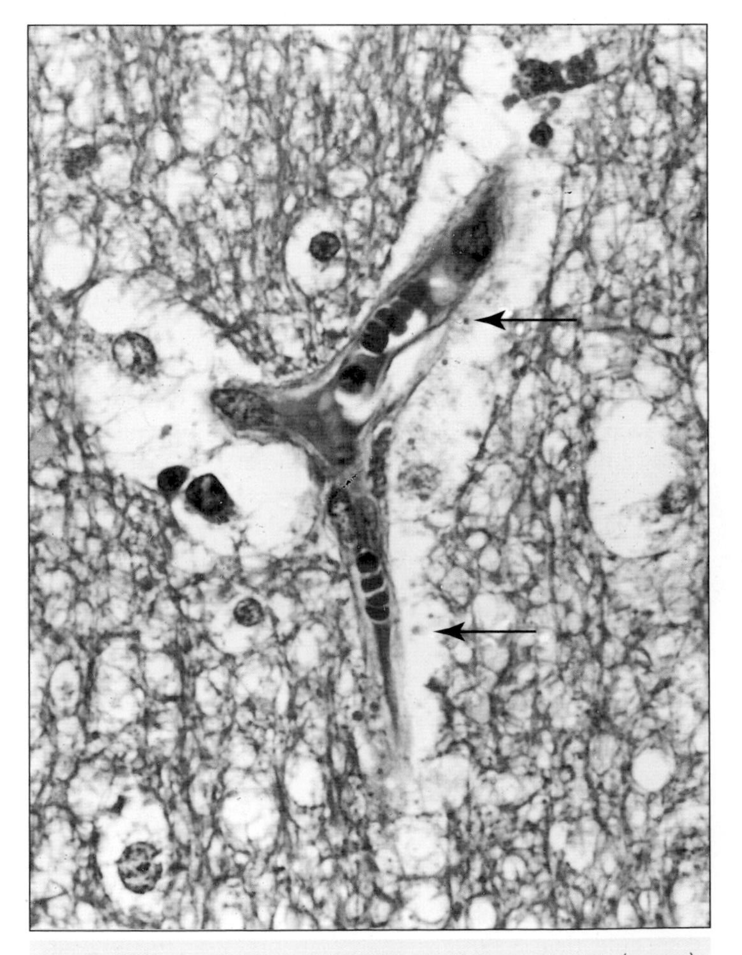

Figure 3.50 Accumulation of clear **edema** with protein droplets (arrows) around a vessel in a pig with mulberry heart disease.

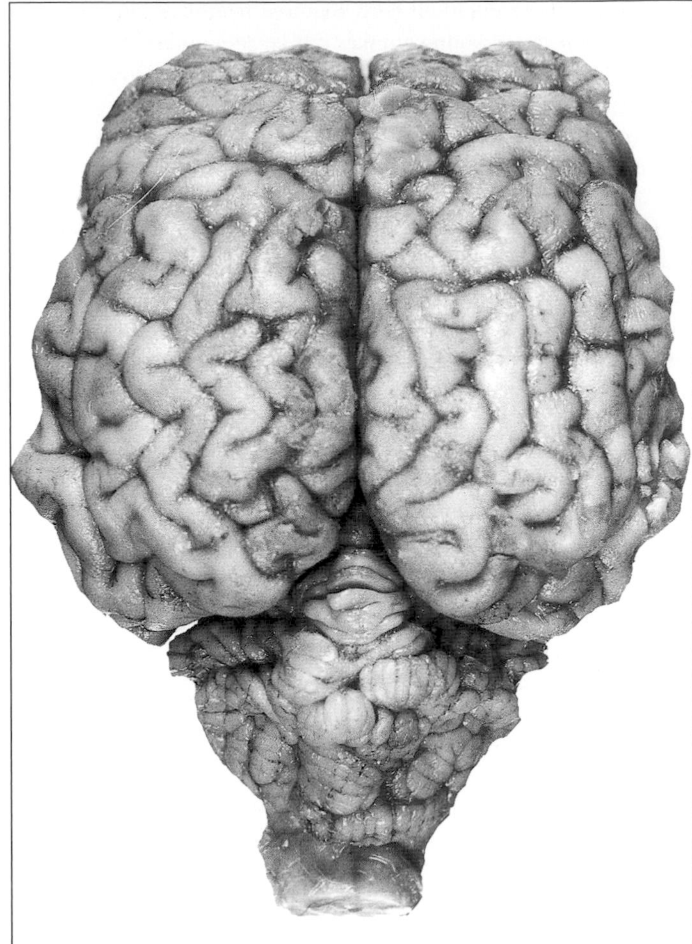

Figure 3.51 Cerebral edema with displacement and coning of cerebellum in a calf.

Diffuse cerebral edema that is mild or moderate may be difficult to recognize grossly. More severe degrees are readily recognized although easily overlooked. *The brain is swollen, pale, soft, and wet* and, because of its softness, the cerebral hemispheres tend to droop over the edges of the parietal bones when the calvaria is removed. With these severe and rapid swellings, the course is short, and there may not be signs of displacement or flattening of the gyri. When the swelling is less severe, and of longer duration, the brain may be relatively firm and dry, the gyri are pale or a faint-yellow color, and the brain is displaced caudally so that it appears unusually elongate. The displacement is most obvious where it involves the cerebellum and medulla (Fig. 3.51). With moderate displacement, the caudal surfaces of the cerebellar hemispheres are depressed by contact with the occipital bones. When the displacement is of greater degree, the *medulla and caudal portion of the vermis are herniated through the foramen magnum*. The displaced vermis is flattened and lies like a tongue over the medulla (so-called lipping of the cerebellum). The rhomboid fossa is flattened. The rostral portion of the vermis is pressed against the rostral medullary velum and may occlude the opening of the cerebral aqueduct to cause internal hydrocephalus. The brain stem is displaced caudally, and this is especially evident in the displacement of the corpora quadrigemina well into the caudal fossa. Perhaps because the tentorium rather closely embraces the brain stem in animals, herniation of the occipital lobes through the tentorial space into the caudal fossa is seldom observed. It may, however, be observed in cerebral edema of long standing in horses and cattle, especially if the brain is fixed in situ so that the pressure grooves produced by the free edge of the tentorium are retained. Impaction of tissue in the tentorial space interferes with the flow of cerebrospinal fluid from the caudal to the rostral fossa and contributes to hydrocephalus.

Displacements in the rostral fossa in diffuse cerebral swelling are of lesser degree and significance. The nerves may be stretched and flattened, but pareses are seldom observed. The vasculature must be compromised in all cases. Occasionally there is thrombosis of the superior sagittal sinus with venous infarction in the dorsal cortex, ischemic necrosis in the caudomedial surface of the occipital lobe referable to compression of the caudal cerebral arteries, and pontine hemorrhage referable probably to occlusion of small veins in this area.

Localized edematous changes reach their most extensive development in the centrum semiovale of the cerebrum and in the deep white matter of the cerebellum surrounding local lesions in these areas. The edematous area may be recognized by the swelling, which may be greater in volume than that produced by the primary lesion and have a soft, depressed and damp or watery appearance on the cut surface. The extent of the edema cannot be appreciated on gross inspection because the margins are indefinite, and the same difficulty in delineating the edematous area is experienced at microscopy. When the lesion is of prolonged duration, the extent of the edematous areas can be appreciated a little better by yellow discoloration that develops.

The combination of edema with a local lesion may displace the brain in one or more directions. Caudal displacement through the caudal fossa may occur as it does in diffuse swelling. The displacements may be more local, involving lateral shifts of the base of the brain or medial displacement of one hemisphere so that the falx cerebri is displaced laterally or the cingulate gyrus is herniated beneath the free margin of the falx and the lateral and third ventricles are depressed.

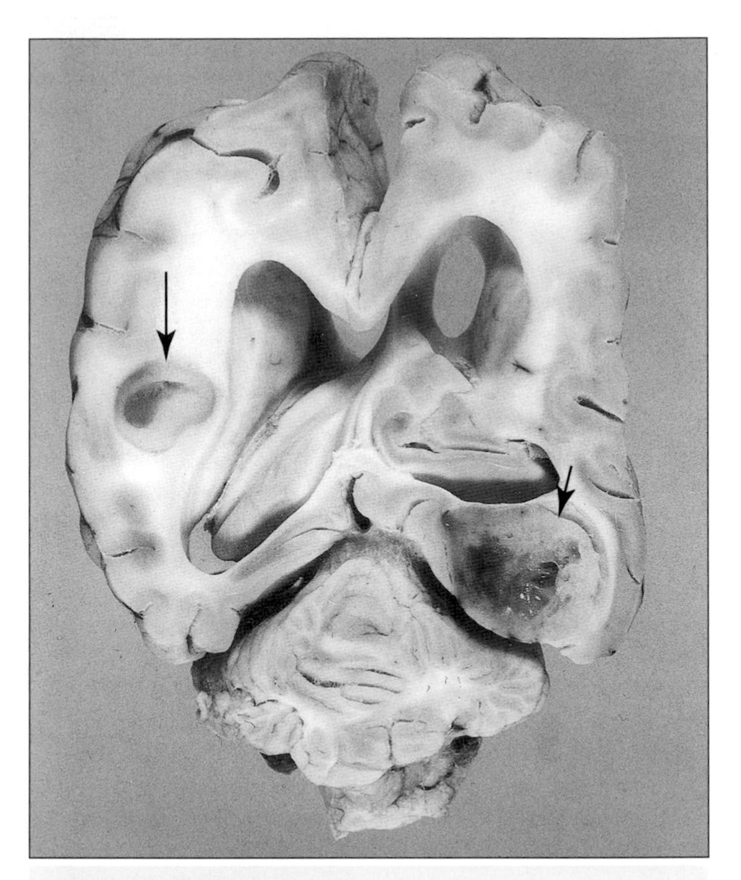

Figure 3.52 Tumor metastases (arrows) at the junction of gray and white matter in a dog.

LESIONS OF BLOOD VESSELS AND CIRCULATORY DISTURBANCES

Diseases of blood vessels are considered in detail with the Cardiovascular system. This section deals with some special features of cerebrospinal circulation and the lesions, usually ischemic or hemorrhagic, which result from vascular injury.

The blood supply to the brain is derived from the *internal carotid and vertebral arteries*, these sources anastomosing under the brain stem and at the *circle of Willis*. The major cerebral vessels, derived from the carotid and vertebral arteries, anastomose quite freely in the pia-arachnoid, but once an artery or arteriole penetrates the substance of the brain, it becomes an *end artery* although there are some anastomoses at the capillary level. Although these anastomoses can be demonstrated readily, even those of arteriolar size in the meninges are probably of little value. Under normal circumstances, the cerebral arteries have rather set fields of supply. If one vessel is occluded, some collateral circulation develops, but it does not take over more than the periphery of the area of supply of the occluded vessel. In the brain, there may be influences governing collateral circulation in addition to those operating in other tissues, but the basic considerations still apply. The development of collateral circulation will be influenced by the anatomic arrangements of vessels, the volume of ischemic tissue, the rate at which the vascular occlusion develops, the size of the occluded vessel, and, importantly, the quantity of blood flow, which is referable to the state of the systemic circulation, and the quality of blood flow, which is referable to such matters as the oxygen tension and viscosity of plasma. For complete cessation of blood flow in an area of brain, it is probably not necessary that there be complete occlusion of the corresponding artery because flow is expected to cease, especially in peripheral twigs, while the intravascular pressure is still above zero. For this reason, ischemic injury in the brain localized to the field of distribution of one or other major cerebral artery may result from occlusion of a carotid vessel. Extracranial anastomoses between the major arterial vessels are, however, effective in the event of vascular occlusion occurring proximal to the circle of Willis.

Arteries entering the substance of the brain are relatively small and arise at right angles from the parent vessels in the pia-arachnoid. There are abrupt changes in caliber when the meningeal vessels divide and this provides an entrapment mechanism for large emboli. The vessels that enter the brain are progressively attenuated to capillaries in both gray and white matter, but many capillaries loop back into the cortex from near the gray–white junction. Many small emboli lodge at the gray–white junction, although expansion of the embolic or metastatic lesions is predominantly in the white matter (Fig. 3.52).

The *arterial supply to the spinal cord* is derived from the vertebral artery in the cervical region and from radicular arteries in the lumbar region anastomosing as the ventral spinal artery. There is some doubt as to the direction of flow in cervical, thoracic, and lumbar portions of the spinal artery and it is possible that there is a border zone in the caudal cervical and cranial thoracic region that is particularly vulnerable to ischemia if flow is impaired in the vertebral artery or the caudal portions of the ventral spinal artery.

In the spinal cord, the central gray matter is supplied by branches of the ventral spinal artery that enter the ventral sulcus, and lesions of these branches affect the gray matter of the cord rather selectively. The white matter is supplied by an anastomotic complex in the meninges that produces many small vessels that penetrate directly as end-vessels and are susceptible to compression or hypotension.

Cerebral veins have abundant and useful anastomoses. Untoward effects are not expected to follow occlusion of single veins because absence of valves permits reflex flow. The venous sinuses of the dura mater empty into the jugular veins, but they also communicate freely through the bones with extracranial veins. Because of these communications, the effects of obstruction of a dural sinus may be relatively slight, unless there is venous stagnation of the head or venous stagnation within the cranium produced by cerebral swelling or occlusion of more than one major sinus. The venous system of the spinal cord is freely anastomotic and drains via the radicular vessels to the paravertebral plexuses. These vessels are also valveless and allow very free communication up and down the spinal canal such that an embolus arising in caudal veins may bypass the caudal vena cava in passing to the lungs. These arrangements of veins may assist in temperature and pressure control in spinal and cerebral vessels. The arrangements have disadvantages. Infiltrating neoplasms may extend from extradural positions to the cord along the venules. In the cranial cavity, infections may extend from the face to the basal meninges. In cattle, sheep, and dogs, pyogranulomatous processes that are occasionally found in the hypothalamic–hypophyseal region are introduced in migrating intravenous foreign bodies that enter the cranial cavity in veins passing through the ophthalmic foramen.

Disturbances in the cerebrospinal vasculature with impaired blood flow may be composed of obstructive and hemorrhagic lesions, or they may be part of global cerebral ischemia with failure of adequate total perfusion. Diseases associated with abnormality of the circulating blood, such as the anoxias, hypoglycemia, and hyperviscosity, are discussed later with neurodegenerative diseases.

Ischemic lesions

The outcome of vascular obstructions depends on the type and size of the vessel obstructed, the degree and duration of ischemia, and the relative vulnerability of the tissues to anoxia. The injury may vary in severity from a temporary functional disturbance to the other extreme of infarction and necrosis. *Neurons and oligodendroglia are the most sensitive of the neural structures to ischemia, astrocytes are moderately resistant, and microglia and the blood vessels are quite resistant and may survive in small areas in which all else dies.* Gray matter, with its high metabolic rate and dependence on oxygen, is more sensitive than is white matter, but there are regional differences in the sensitivity of gray matter.

Obstructive lesions of cerebrospinal vessels are not commonly observed in animals, and ischemic changes may be absent even when the vessels are profoundly altered. On the other hand, lesions which are regarded as being of ischemic type are quite commonly observed in the absence of demonstrable vascular occlusion. These cases tend to be individual in their occurrence and without particular pattern.

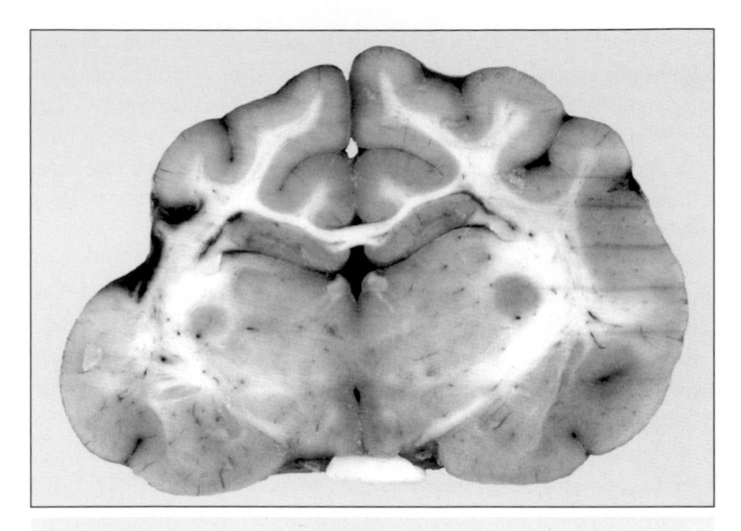

Figure 3.53 Focal loss of gray matter from left parietal cerebral cortex, in **feline ischemic encephalopathy.** (Courtesy of RF Slocombe.)

Global ischemia is occasionally observed in animals suffering cardiac arrest under anesthesia, and in neonatal "barking foals and piglets." Purkinje cells, the hippocampal cortex, and neurons of the cerebral cortex are the most sensitive of all, and, within the cerebral cortex, the deeper laminae are more sensitive than the superficial laminae. Necrosis is accentuated over boundary zones at the margins of distribution of the rostral, middle, and caudal cerebral arteries. Similar regional susceptibility can be demonstrated in the cerebellar cortex. The deeper laminae of the cortex may be selectively destroyed in ischemia, producing a distribution of necrosis that is known as **laminar cortical necrosis**. Lesions are expected to be symmetrical but may not be. In severe and prolonged global ischemia, necrosis may involve all of the cortex and other nuclei such as globus pallidus and lateral thalamus. The sensitivity to necrosis parallels that in severe hypoglycemia except that hypoglycemic injury spares the cerebellar Purkinje cells. The assumption that the injury is a result of anoxia and energy deficit does not recognize the complex biochemical perturbations set in train by cellular anoxia.

Feline ischemic encephalopathy is recognized in mature cats, and results from aberrant migration of *Cuterebra* larvae in the brain. While larval migration tracks may be present, the ischemic lesions may be the result of toxin-induced vasospasm. The extent and distribution of degeneration vary from case to case. Milder lesions occur in superficial cortical laminae as multiple foci. More severe or extensive lesions tend to be in the distribution area of the middle cerebral artery and may be bilateral but asymmetrical (Fig 3.53). In some cases, there may be ischemic lesions in the brain stem.

Ischemic and hemorrhagic cerebral lesions occur in the **neonatal maladjustment syndrome of foals**, also known as the "barker" or "convulsive foal" syndrome, which is discussed with congenital atelectasis in Vol. 2, Respiratory system. The nature of the circulatory derangement is not understood but the lesions are presumed to reflect cerebral ischemia and variably delayed reflow. There is ischemic laminar necrosis of the cerebral cortex (Fig. 3.54), sometimes accompanied by necrosis in the paired gray nuclei of the midbrain and brain stem, and by multiple small hemorrhages. In some foals affected by

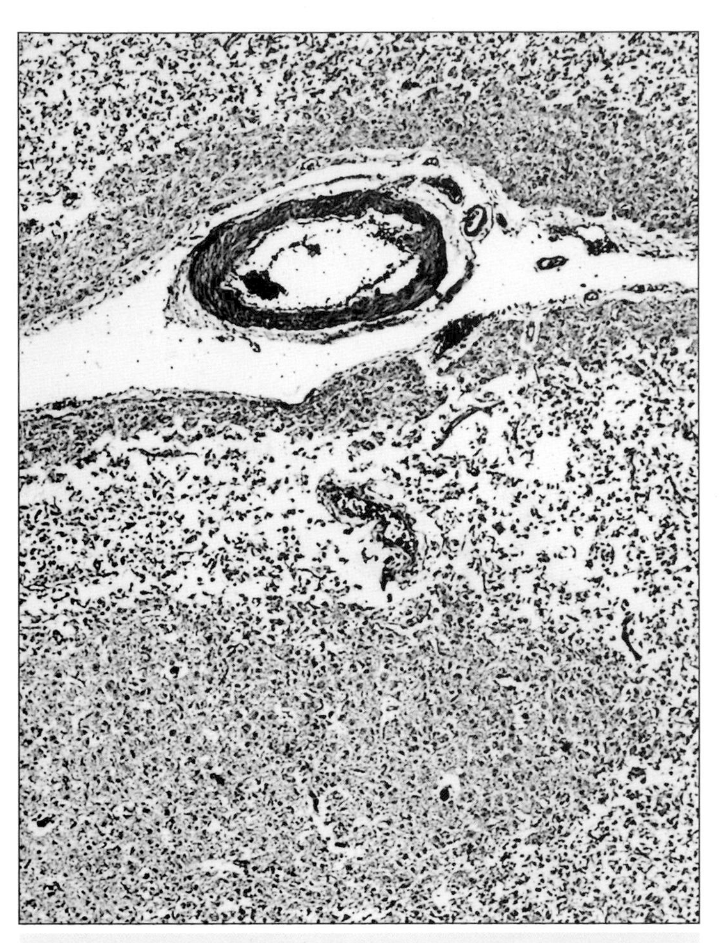

Figure 3.54 Polioencephalomalacia of cerebral cortex in a foal with neonatal maladjustment syndrome.

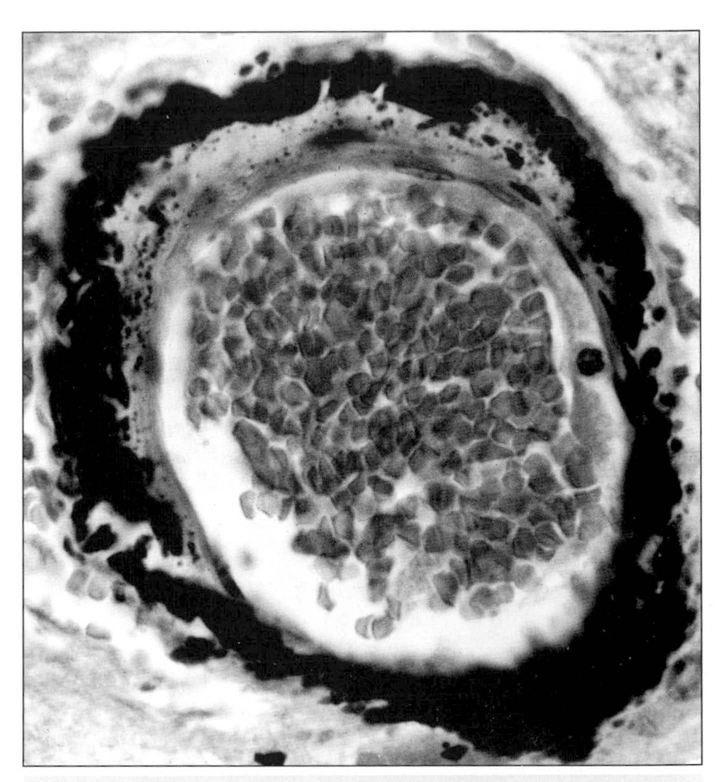

Figure 3.55 Siderosis of cerebral vessel in a horse.

this neonatal syndrome, there is minimal ischemic necrosis but instead a profuse distribution of small perivascular and petechial hemorrhages in the cerebrum, cerebellum, and brain stem.

Degenerative vascular disease of arteriosclerotic type is not important in animal disease. *Atheroma* occurs in some hypothyroid dogs. *Siderosis* of the walls of the arterioles occurs commonly as a change associated with advancing age in horses. The calcium and iron salts may be deposited in amounts capable of converting the vessels to rigid pipes (Fig. 3.55). The patency of the vessels is well maintained. There is no thrombosis, and vascular stenosis probably proceeds slowly enough for adaptive circulatory changes to occur because small areas of softening, presumably ischemic, are unusual.

Hyaline necrosis in meningeal vessels, which is observed in swine with hepatosis dietetica, is not usually associated with secondary lesions. The hyaline necrosis in meningeal vessels in pigs with organomercurial poisoning is associated with severe cerebral injury that may be, in part, due to reduced perfusion (Fig. 3.56). *Amyloid degeneration* of meningeal and intracerebral vessels occurs in aged dogs and the thickenings of the meningeal arteries may be visible grossly. Senile argyrophilic plaques that contain amyloid deposits may be associated with the vascular lesions. The systemic distribution of amyloid is minimal. Petechial hemorrhages occur in relation to the diseased vessels in about 50% of cases and, exceptionally, there is massive hemorrhage.

Cerebrospinal angiopathy is an important cause of neurological disease in pigs. It occurs in the alimentary enterotoxemia known

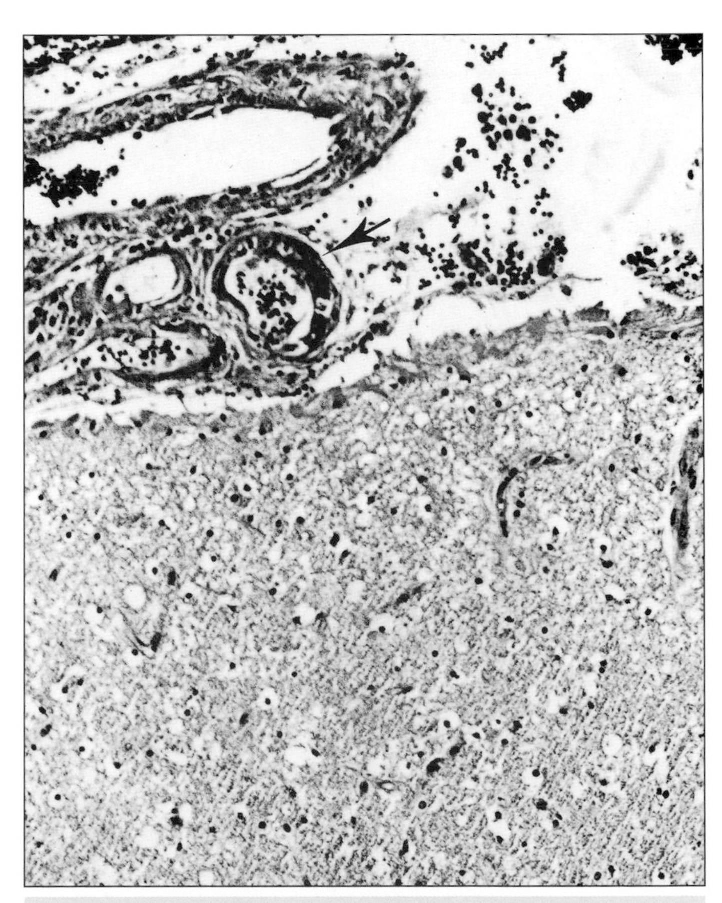

Figure 3.56 Necrosis of meningeal arterioles (arrow) due to organomercurial poisoning in a pig.

as **edema disease** of pigs with similar lesions in vessels of brain and other tissues (Fig. 3.57). The lesions are described in detail in Vol. 2, Alimentary system. In groups of older pigs, arteritis or periarteritis can develop and may represent a chronic or persistent expression of the acute angiopathy.

Vascular permeability changes provide a basis for **annual ryegrass toxicosis** of sheep and cattle in Australia, South Africa, and formerly in the USA. The distribution of the disease is governed in part by the distribution of annual ryegrasses, *Lolium rigidum* and hybrids, in winter rainfall areas, although the disease can occur in other areas by the use of transported fodder. The distribution is also governed by the distribution of toxin-producing *Clavibacter toxicus* (*Corynebacterium rathayi*) and infection by the bacterium of galls produced in the seed head by the nematode *Anguina agrostis*. In addition to *Lolium* spp., known host plants include *Polypogon monspeliensis* (annual beardgrass), *Festuca nigrescens* (chewings fescue), and *Agrostis avenacea* (blowngrass).

The nematode *Anguina agrostis* emerges from fallen galls following first autumn rains, migrates into the growing points of the ryegrass seedlings, and later penetrates the florets to produce galls. The nematodes are harmless to animals but may carry on the cuticle the bacterium that will proliferate in the gall, forming a yellow slime. The active principle, *corynetoxin*, is closely related to the tunicamycin antibiotics produced by some strains of *Streptomyces*. Indeed, tunicamycin-like metabolites have been detected in mycotoxicosis in pigs. Corynetoxins and tunicamycins inhibit lipid-linked N-glycosylation of glycoproteins, which compromises cell membrane integrity.

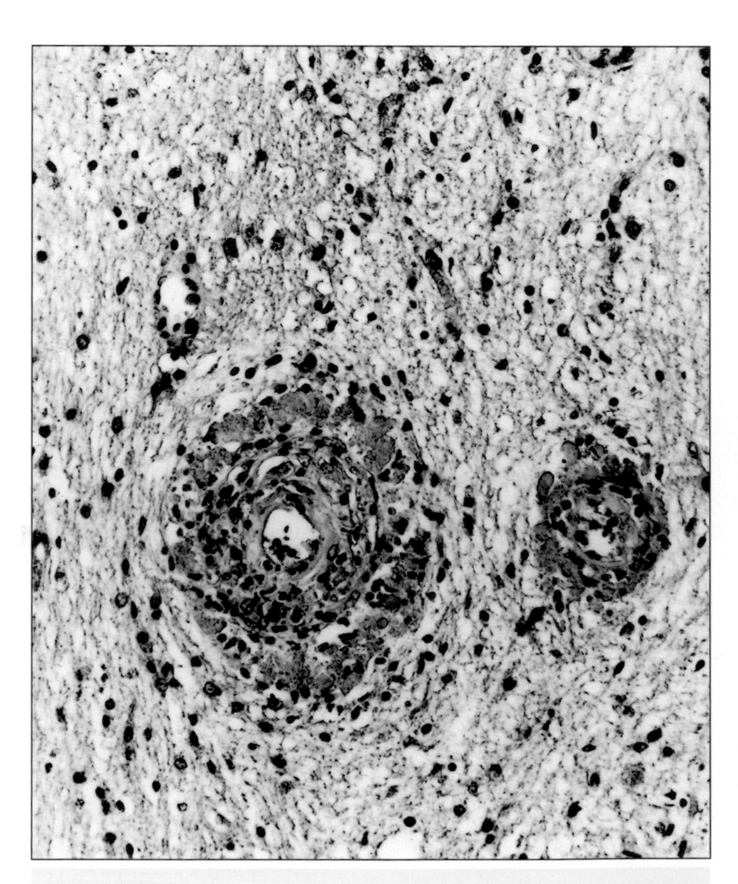

Figure 3.57 Necrosis and inflammation of vessels in brain stem in a pig with **edema disease**.

The toxicosis is characterized clinically by neurologic signs and high mortality. Pregnant ewes may abort. The pathogenesis of abortion has not been examined but the occurrence of hemorrhages in various organs, pulmonary edema and swelling of endoplasmic reticulum of hepatocytes indicates systemic intoxication, notwithstanding the prominence of neurologic signs.

The clinical signs, which are severe, include excitability, aggression in cattle, disturbances of gait and convulsions. The clinical course may be less than 12 hours. Gross changes include pulmonary edema and a pale swollen liver, and occasionally there are hemorrhages in various organs.

Microscopic changes in nervous tissue are subtle, especially following routine fixation by immersion, which may not preserve transudates. Tracer injections show widespread alterations to cerebrovascular permeability in the brain and meninges, indicating endothelial damage and disruption of the blood–brain barrier. The perivascular transudate resembles plasma (Fig. 3.58) in staining properties, and may be present as perivascular lakes or droplets that stain strongly with PAS stain. Only occasionally can fibrin be demonstrated, but extravasation of red cells from capillaries may be present in neuropil. Astrocytes are

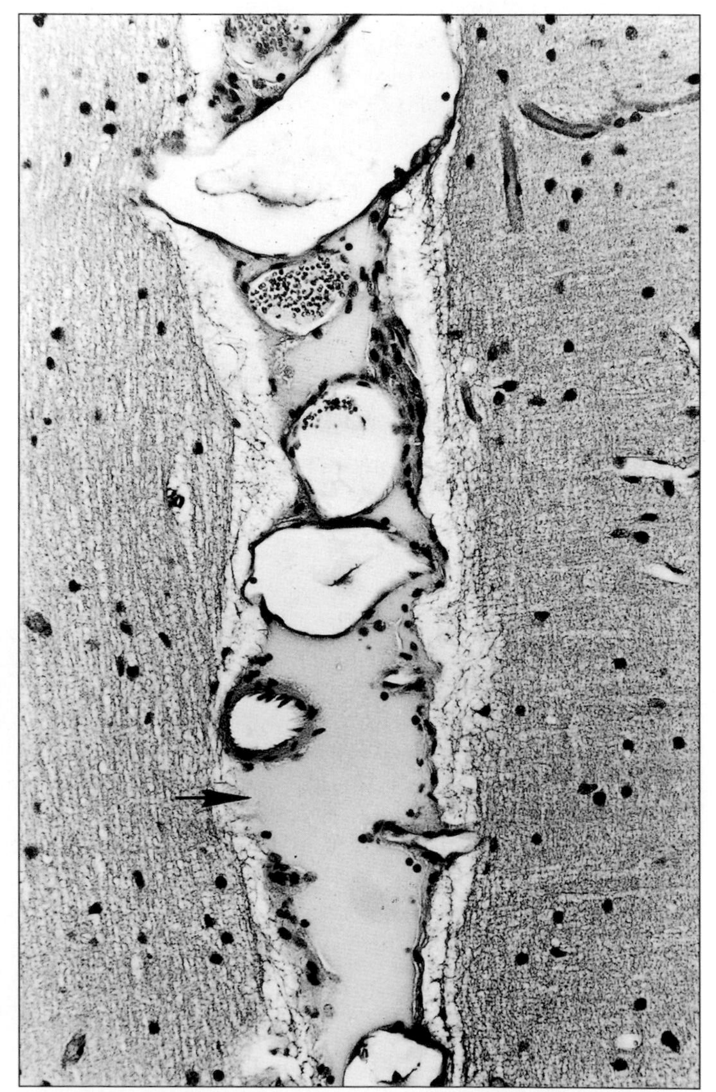

Figure 3.58 Vascular leakage (arrow) in the leptomeninges of the cerebellum of a sheep with annual ryegrass toxicity. (Courtesy of J McC Howell.)

swollen with acidophilic cytoplasm, and there may be widespread necrobiosis of oligodendroglia in the cerebral gray matter.

The capillary endothelium shows ultrastructural evidence of injury. Endothelial cells are swollen and electron-lucent, the cisternae of rough endoplasmic reticulum are distended, mitochondria are swollen with disorganization of cristae, and capillary lumina sometimes contain platelet aggregations. The changes are best seen in cerebellar cortex and meninges. Neuronal change is minimal but there may be patchy loss of Purkinje cells and scattered small foci of malacia.

Cerebrospinal vasculitis, affecting both arterioles and veins, occurs in a number of specific diseases. *Polyarteritis* (periarteritis nodosa) appears to have some predilection for the cerebral arteries, especially in the pig, and for the spinal arteries in the dog in which it is cited as **steroid-responsive meningo-arteritis**. Vasculitis is a rather specific feature of classical swine fever (Fig. 3.59), sporadic bovine encephalomyelitis (Fig. 3.60), and malignant catarrhal fever; the agents of these diseases have no predilection for neural tissue, and parenchymal degeneration, which is sometimes observed, is secondary to occlusion of vessels; this occlusion, in turn, is secondary to inflammatory lesions of the vascular adventitia. Adventitial proliferations and perivascular infiltrates are common to many of the encephalitides, both bacterial and viral, and focal softenings of the brain and cord in these inflammatory diseases can frequently be related to occlusive vasculitis. The occlusive lesions are not solely related to the acute phase of inflammation, but adventitial fibrosis and vascular stenosis may be prominent in the healed phase of encephalitis and may lead eventually to ischemic damage and softenings.

Thrombosis and embolism in the cerebrospinal arterioles is very seldom observed in animals. Thrombosis of an internal carotid vessel or ventral spinal artery may accompany atrial and aortic thrombosis, especially in cats (Fig. 3.61). Bone marrow emboli form after trauma and fractures, most commonly in dogs (Fig. 3.62). *Emboli composed of fibrocartilage or nucleus pulposus* occur in spinal arteries and veins in most species, and cause hemorrhagic and ischemic infarcts of sudden onset (Fig. 3.63). The cervical or lumbar segments may be affected. The pathogenesis is discussed with Diseases of bones and joints. *Bacterial thrombi* may develop in a variety of bacteremic diseases such as erysipelas, shigellosis, pasteurellosis, and the septicemias caused by *Histophilus, Streptococcus*, and the coliforms. Abscessation develops rapidly about these bacterial colonies, but in the early stages perivascular zones of softening may be observed.

Perhaps the least morphological expression of arteriolar obstruction is death of neurons in a narrow zone of cortex representing the central portion of a field of distribution of a single arteriole. In the early stage, there is acute ischemic necrosis of neurons and oligodendroglia. There is no softening in these minimal lesions, but they are readily visible at low power as narrow zones of pallor. At higher magnification, the affected zone is seen to be unusually cellular, this being due in the early stages to microgliosis and later to astrogliosis.

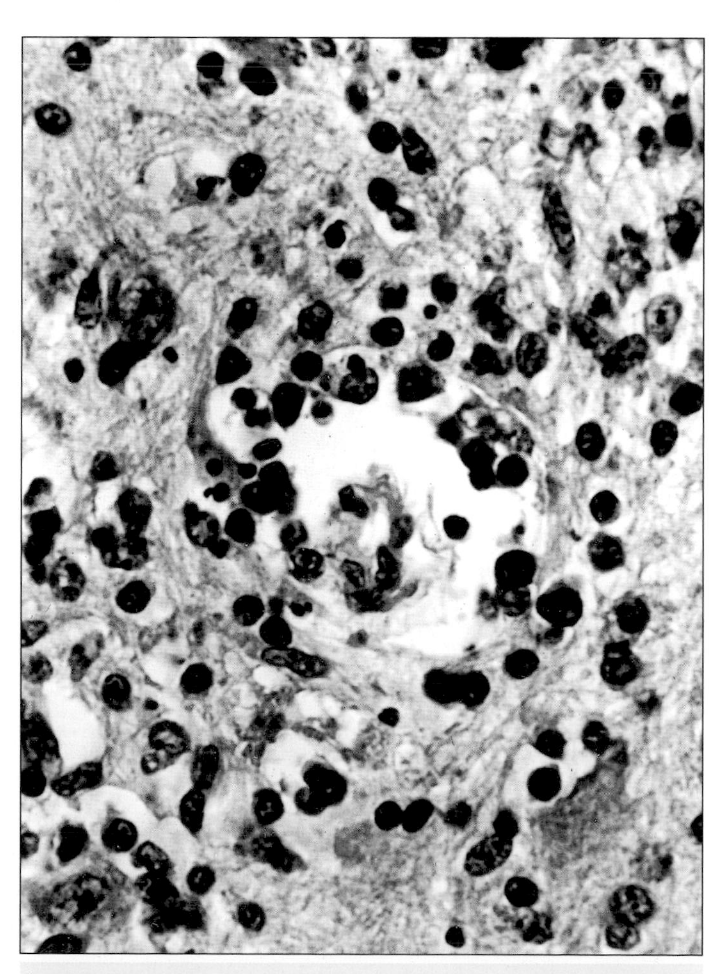

Figure 3.59 Gliosis around a degenerate vessel in classical swine fever.

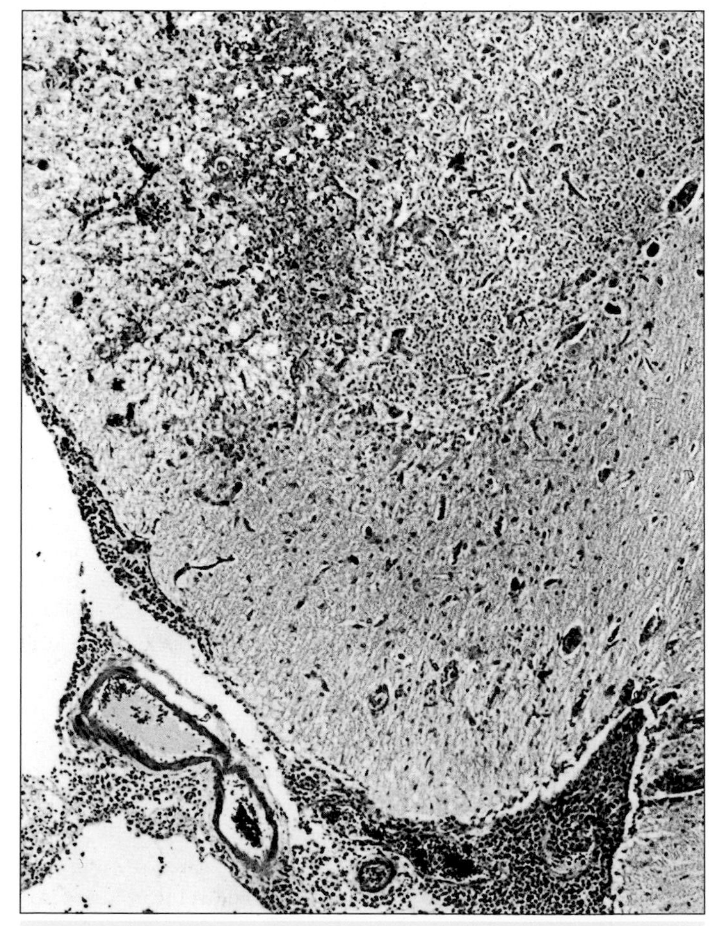

Figure 3.60 Necrosis of cerebellar cortex and meningitis in **sporadic bovine encephalomyelitis**.

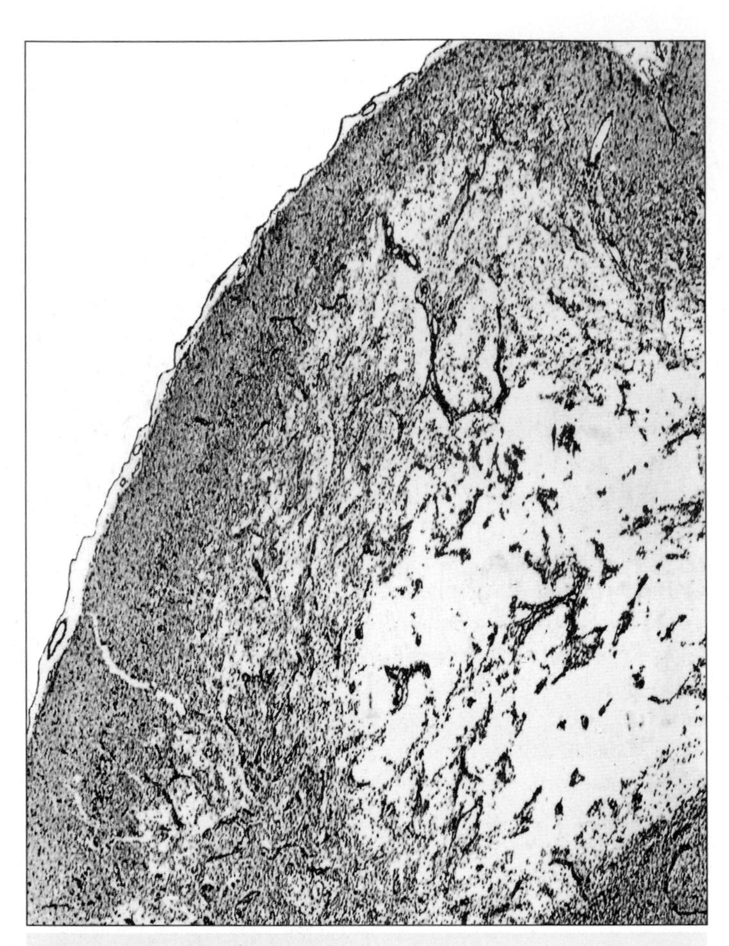

Figure 3.61 Residual cyst in cerebral cortex, the result of carotid thrombosis and ischemic infarction in a cat.

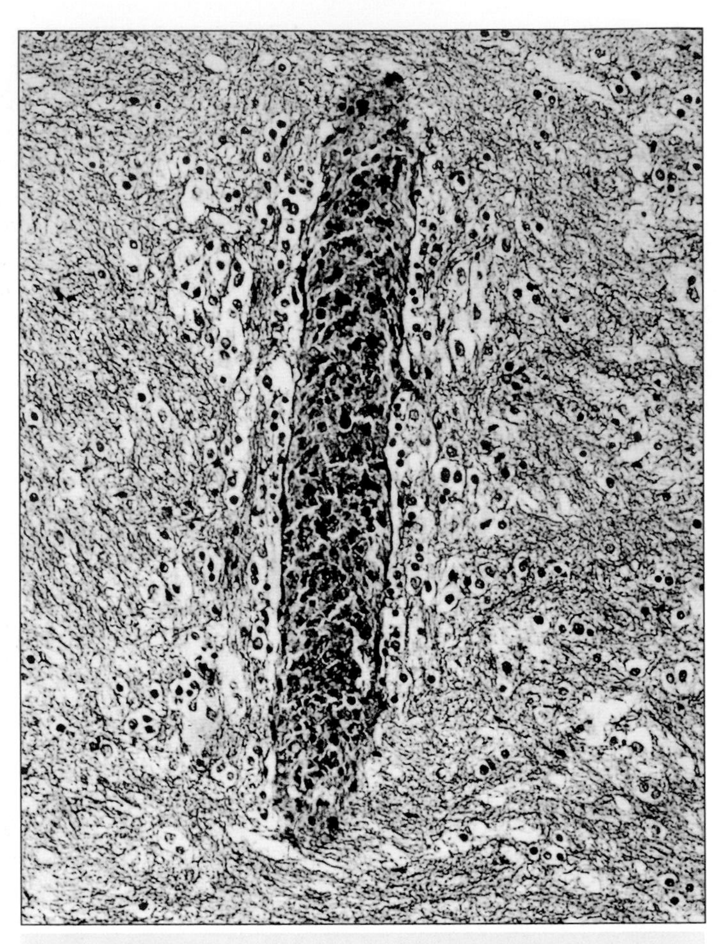

Figure 3.62 Marrow embolus and surrounding intracellular edema following trauma and femoral fracture in a dog.

Obstruction of an artery or arteriole results typically in *infarction*, and infarcts involve both gray and white matter. In the early stages, affected areas swell, and the involved gray matter may be hemorrhagic (Fig. 3.64). At the center of an infarct, there is coagulative and liquefactive necrosis and around the periphery there is a zone of minimal ischemic injury with the characters mentioned above. Many capillary vessels survive, partly because of their relative insensitivity to anoxia and partly because they benefit first from the collateral circulation that develops. Surviving vessels show endothelial and adventitial proliferation, and the astrocytes around the margin of the lesion react. The necrotic tissues are removed from the periphery by liquefaction and microglial phagocytosis, and a cyst remains (Fig. 3.61). The cyst contains fluid, and distended microglia, so-called *compound granular corpuscles*, may be found in it for very long periods. The wall of the cyst is ragged and irregular and is formed by reactive astrocytes. When the defect extends to the meninges, it may be partially filled in by proliferated leptomeningeal tissue.

Obstruction of cerebrospinal veins is the result either of pressure or inflammation with thrombosis, although rarely it may be due to neoplastic invasion and permeation of the dural sinuses. *Thrombophlebitis* is usually bacterial and the associated meningitis is more conspicuous and important than the venous thromboses; isolated venous obstructions are not of much significance.

Intracranial thrombophlebitis can be due chiefly to retrograde spread of inflammation from an extracranial primary focus, but thrombophlebitis of this type is uncommon. Such primary foci may occur in the orbital or nasal cavities, the paranasal sinuses, or the middle ear. Intracranial inflammations have little tendency to cause thrombosis of the dural sinuses. In verminous infestations of the brain, especially those caused by *Strongylus* larvae in horses, there is some tendency for the larvae to migrate to the superior sagittal and transverse sinuses and to cause thrombosis of these. Spinal thrombophlebitis results from ascending infections from docking wounds in lambs and from bite wounds of the tails of pigs.

Noninflammatory thrombosis of the cranial dural sinuses occurs chiefly in the superior sagittal sinus. It occurs in polioencephalomalacia of cattle, in which it is probably secondary to severe and prolonged swelling of the brain. Sinus thrombosis may also be observed following head injuries, even those not accompanied by lacerations (Fig. 3.65).

Venous infarcts differ from arterial infarcts by the more extensive hemorrhage in the affected areas and by the diffusion of blood into the adjacent subarachnoid space. The superficial veins are engorged and the congested area is edematous and swollen. The hemorrhages are perivenular and petechial or larger, and are present in the gray matter and to a lesser extent in the white matter. The subsequent course and reaction are similar to those following arterial obstruction, and the residual lesion is a depressed and shrunken or cystic area that is dark brown-yellow.

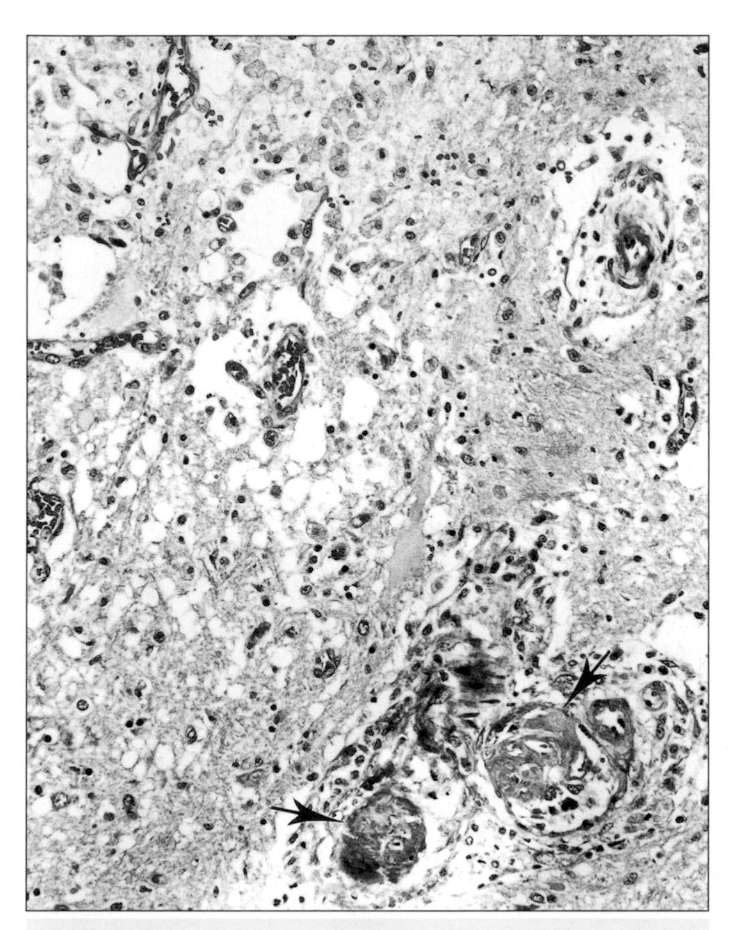

Figure 3.63 Cartilaginous emboli (arrows) causing spinal myelomalacia in a dog.

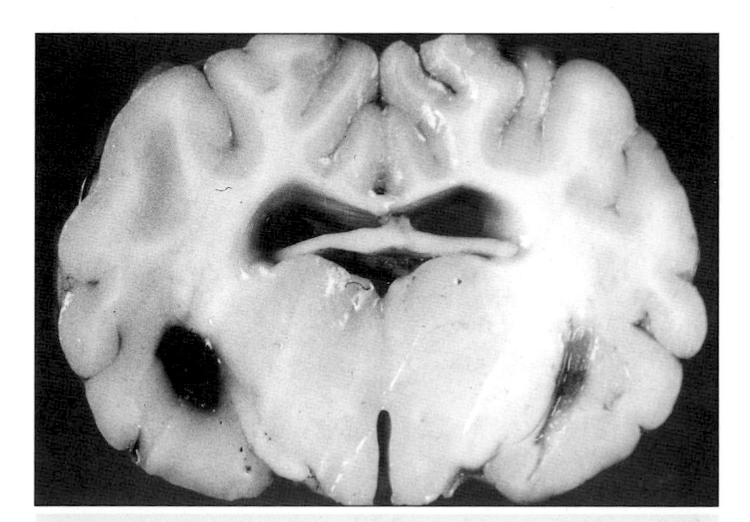

Figure 3.64 Hemorrhage (left) and malacia (right) in cerebrum of a pig with **mulberry heart disease**.

Hemorrhagic lesions

Hemorrhages in the CNS may be *traumatic or spontaneous* and may be restricted to the meninges or the parenchyma or involve both. Hemorrhages accompanying periventricular leukomalacia in neonates are discussed earlier. The causes are, in general, the same and are of much variety. They can be broadly grouped into those affecting the integrity of the vessel wall and those that reduce the coagulability of the

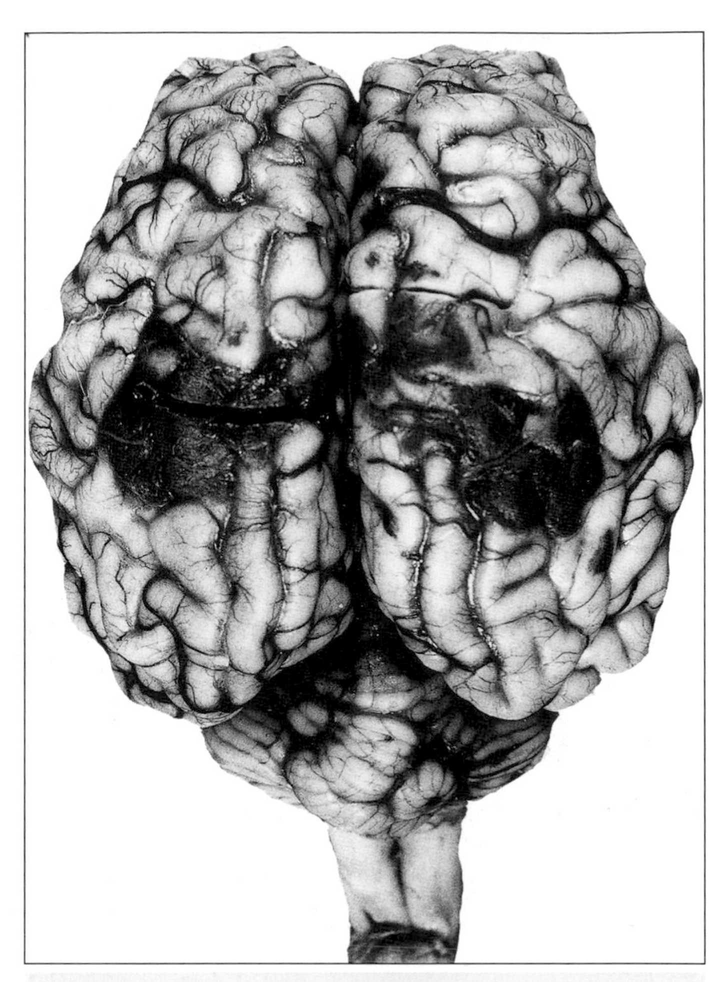

Figure 3.65 Venous infarcts in cortex secondary to thrombosis of sagittal sinus in a calf.

blood. Care is necessary in deciding whether observed extravasations are significant because they can be produced readily as *artifacts at postmortem*. Quite extensive spread of blood into the basal meninges commonly occurs from the venous sinuses when the head is removed at the atlanto-occipital junction, and into the spinal meninges when the spinal column is transected. Hemorrhages of petechial size in the parenchyma can be largely avoided as artifacts if the brain or cord is fixed before slicing. The microscopic distinction of antemortem from postmortem hemorrhages can also be difficult because, apart from minor degenerative changes of the parenchyma, terminal hemorrhages provoke very little reaction, even on the part of the microglia.

Spontaneous hemorrhages in the brains of animals are almost invariably of petechial or slightly larger size occurring in the hemorrhagic diatheses, especially the symptomatic purpura of septicemic infections (see Vol. 3, Hematopoietic system). Such hemorrhages occur typically from capillaries as well as small venules and are found in meninges and brain. There is no specificity in the geographic distribution of purpuric hemorrhages except in infectious canine hepatitis in which intracranial hemorrhage, although not consistently present, has a predilection for the midbrain and medulla. In "focal symmetrical encephalomalacia" (see Vol. 2, Alimentary system) the lesions are grossly visible only when hemorrhagic; they are regularly bilateral and symmetrical and have a rather specific pattern in which the internal capsules, dorsolateral thalamus, cerebral aqueduct, and pons may all be involved. Hemorrhages also characterize thiamine deficiency in dogs and cats and have a specific distribution and symmetry, being regularly present in the inferior colliculi and less consistently present in the mammillary bodies and other periventricular nuclei.

Isolated hemorrhages or hematomas are quite rare in animals. The hemorrhages may extend to the ventricles and induce hydrocephalus, or involve the central canal of the cord to produce hematomyelia.

Meningeal hemorrhages, both epidural and subdural, are common in lambs and calves that have required obstetric assistance and probably reflect hemodynamic disturbances in dystocia. Hemorrhages of similar distribution occur in calves born unassisted from cows exposed to the coumarins of moldy sweet clover.

Microcirculatory lesions

A range of changes affecting the microcirculation in the nervous system may not produce ischemia or hemorrhage. They are associated with extravasation of formed or fluid elements, are not disease-specific in their character although their distribution may be specific, and result from degenerative changes especially in capillaries and venules. Sludging of leukocytes is frequently observed in venules of cerebral and cerebellar hemispheres in diseases causing leukocytosis, including a range of infectious diseases with neutrophil leukocytosis and the rather rare endotheliotropic lymphoma. Sludging of white cells is frequent in East Coast fever caused by *Theileria parva*, and sludging of red cells infected by *Babesia bovis* and possibly other protozoa; the pathogenesis of sludging may not be the same as for falciform malaria in which adhesion seems to be important in pathogenesis. Viral infections, such as classical swine fever and canine adenovirus, are frequent causes of capillary hemorrhage.

Diapedesis of red cells is a common event in sudden death of many causes and is frequently mimicked in postmortem trauma. The interval between diapedesis and death may be too short for reactive changes, visible by light microscopy, to develop in the vessels. With some delay, swelling of endothelial cells and their nuclei develops. The hemorrhages may be from arterioles, with the red cells remaining in the perivascular space. Diapedesis from capillaries and small venules depends on disruption of endothelium and astrocytic processes and, depending on relative pressures, the red cells may spread in the intercellular spaces.

Diapedesis of red cells occurs in periventricular nuclei in thiamine-deficiency encephalopathy, and in the brain stem in concussion, contrecoup injury, and in hypomagnesemia in sheep and cattle (Fig. 3.66). The white matter of the cerebral and cerebellar hemispheres is susceptible to diapedesis. The hemorrhages are sometimes large enough to be visible as petechiae in diverse conditions including infectious purpuras, anoxia, fat and other microembolism, in diseases associated with erythrocyte sludging, and in disseminated intravascular coagulation.

Leakage of plasma, usually from small venules, may occur in any part of the CNS. It is seen most frequently surrounding areas of traumatic injury or in the conditions noted above that lead to erythrocyte diapedesis. The plasma will contain some fibrinogen, and polymerized fibrin in its usual form may be demonstrated around the vessels. It is more usual, however, for the fibrin to be in its unpolymerized or molecular form, and the plasma both within and outside the vessels to be transformed into a homogeneous gel that

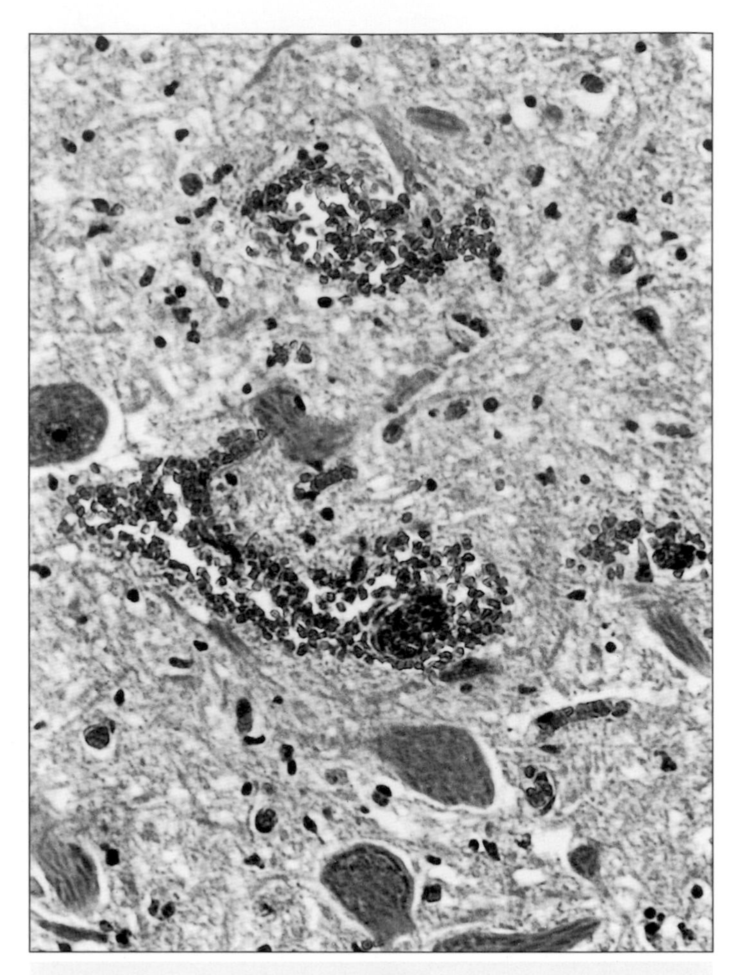

Figure 3.66 Perivascular hemorrhage in a cow with hypomagnesemia.

stains brightly by the PAS technique. The plasma gel may appear as capillary plugs or as perivascular droplets that appear to incite very little reaction.

Vascular injury that allows diapedesis of plasma will also allow passage of serum or protein filtrate (Fig. 3.67). In fields of injury, the differences in levels of permeability change may be evident from the protein content of transudate. While plasma will routinely stain because of its fibrinogen content, the amount of protein in serum may be too low for preservation and staining (see Fig. 3.50). The perivascular changes occur especially about capillaries and venules in the white matter and have the characteristics described earlier for vasogenic edema. Prolonged survival or recovery may leave *focal glial scars* as residue (see Fig. 3.15).

Bibliography

Benson JE, Schwartz KJ. Ischemic myelomalacia associated with fibrocartilaginous embolism in multiple finishing swine. J Vet Diagn Invest 1998;10:274–277.

Berry PH, et al. Morphological changes in the central nervous system of sheep affected with experimental annual ryegrass (*Lolium rigidum*) toxicity. J Comp Pathol 1980;90:603–616.

Cheeke PR. Endogenous toxins and mycotoxins in forage grasses and their effects on livestock. J Anim Sci 1995;73:909–918.

Finnie JW, O'Shea JD. Effect of tunicamycin on the blood-brain barrier and on endothelial cells *in vitro*. J Comp Pathol 1990;102:363–374.

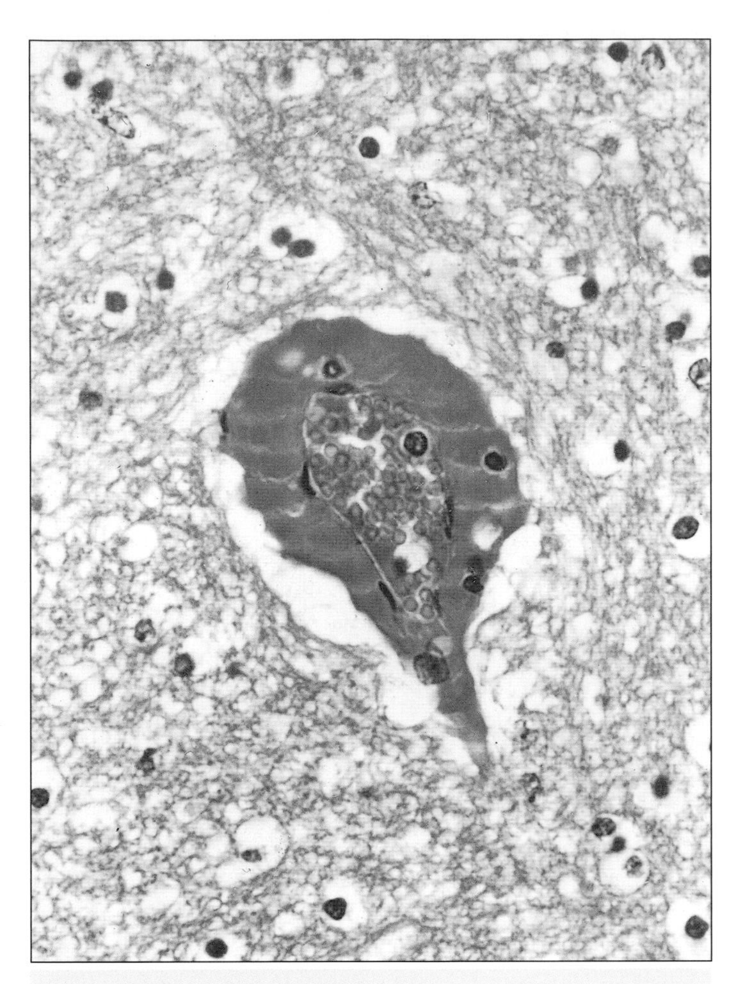

Figure 3.67 Accumulation of proteinaceous fluid around vessel in a sheep with **focal symmetrical encephalomalacia**.

Font A, et al. Acute paraplegia associated with vasculitis in a dog with leishmaniasis. J Small Anim Pract 2004;45:199–201.

Gandini G, et al. Fibrocartilaginous embolism in 75 dogs: clinical findings and factors influencing the recovery rate. J Small Anim Pract 2003;44:76–80.

Jago MV, Culvenor CC. Tunicamycin and corynetoxin poisoning in sheep. Aust Vet J 1987;64:232–235.

Landolfi JA, et al. Fibrocartilaginous embolic myelopathy in a calf. J Vet Diagn Invest 2004;16:360–362.

Nakamura K, et al. Swine cerebrospinal angiopathy and demyelination and malacia. Vet Pathol 1982;19:140–149.

Nakamura S, et al. Deposition of amyloid beta protein (A beta) subtypes [A beta 40 and A beta 42(43)] in canine senile plaques and cerebral amyloid angiopathy. Acta Neuropathol (Berl) 1997;94:323–328.

Palmer AC, Rossdale PD. Neuropathological changes associated with the neonatal maladjustment syndrome in the thoroughbred foal. Res Vet Sci 1976;20:267–275.

Riley IT, et al. Poisoning of livestock in Oregon in the 1940s to 1960s attributed to corynetoxins produced by *Rathayibacter* in nematode galls in chewings fescue (*Festuca nigrescens*). Vet Hum Toxicol 2003;45:160–162.

Sebastian MM, Giles RC. Fibrocartilaginous embolic myelopathy in a horse. J Vet Med A Physiol Pathol Clin Med 2004;51:341–343.

Williams KJ, et al. Cerebrospinal cuterebriasis in cats and its association with feline ischemic encephalopathy. Vet Pathol 1998;35:330–343.

TRAUMATIC INJURIES

Trauma to the head and vertebral column are of importance because of the effects that such injuries have on the contained brain and spinal cord. Both the brain and spinal cord are well protected from external injurious forces by the bony encasements. The more or less rounded shape of the skull favors glancing blows and the lateral diffusion of lines of force; the diploe and sutures are capable of absorbing considerable amounts of shock; and the internal system of bony ridges directs lines of force to the base of the skull. The spinal column is well protected by the surrounding soft tissues, by its own highly cancellous structure, system of ligaments, and intervertebral disks. The nature of acquired injuries is quite varied and is determined by many factors including: the relative vulnerability of the soft tissues, the direction in which the injurious force is applied, the physical rigidity of the bones, the ability of the part to move in response to the applied force, and the mass and velocity of the force.

Concussion

Concussion is a transient loss of consciousness and reflex activity following a sudden injury to the head. Full recovery is expected, and it is assumed that in mild cases there is no morphological injury. In experimental animals, however, degenerative changes are found in the nuclear masses of the brain stem, and these are probably responsible for the clinical features. Following single injuries, chromatolysis develops in many of the larger neurons of the brain stem, and in a proportion of affected cells the degeneration is progressive. With repeated episodes of concussion, affected neurons have a wider distribution that includes the cerebral cortex, and the proportion of cells irreversibly injured is increased. These changes in the brain stem and reticular formation occur if the impact forces are substantial and the brain is subject to rapid acceleration/deceleration; in these cases direct injury in the hemispheres is to be expected. The mildest degrees of concussion produce no visible structural damage when examined with the light microscope, but there is some experimental evidence that plasma substances including proteins may be transported in vesicles through the endothelial cells, and the brain and cord may lose their capacity for autoregulation of blood flow in local areas of static injury.

While the dynamics of the disturbances in neurons that are responsible for the concussion are unclear, some of the physical qualities of the reaction between the head and the applied force have been elucidated. The vibrations that travel back and forth in the brain from the point of impact appear not to be important. If the head is firmly immobilized, quite a considerable force may be suddenly applied to it with relatively minor effect, the force of the blow (**coup**) being absorbed by the skull. Force of much lesser magnitude will cause concussion if the head is capable of moving in response to the blow. The principle to be obtained from these observations is that *a degree of acceleration or deceleration is necessary to produce concussion*, neural injury being due to displacement of the cranium relative to its contents. The brain of an adult animal is normally a little smaller than the cranial cavity and being suspended in the cavity, is capable of slight independent movement. If the head is freely movable and struck a heavy blow, it moves away from the point of impact and collides at the area of impact (coup) with the brain that is momentarily static. As the brain moves suddenly within the skull toward the point of impact, leptomeningeal blood vessels may be torn as the brain pulls away from the skull (**contrecoup**), and *the contrecoup injury may be greater than the coup injury*. In young animals, the brain closely fits the cranial cavity, so relative displacement of the whole brain is expected to be minimal. However, the brain is plastic, so sudden acceleration or deceleration leads to internal deformation. Displacements and transient deformations of the brain result in neuronal changes and unconsciousness probably through the effect of shearing strains on neurons, axons, dendrites, synapses, and blood vessels, as well as direct pressure effects when the brain is displaced across bony ridges.

Contusion

In contusion, the architecture of the nervous tissue is retained but there is hemorrhage into the meninges and about the blood vessels in the parenchyma. Contusions may be diffuse or focal injuries, although often those coexist.

The pathogenetic factors in diffuse contusions are generally the same as those operating in causing concussion, but the applied force, the displacements, and the induced shearing and direct forces are all of greater magnitude. Typically in diffuse injuries, *some of the most severe hemorrhages occur on the surface of the brain opposite the point of impact*. Hemorrhages of this distribution are known as *contrecoup*, and their development depends on the sudden movement of the brain to the point of impact (*coup*) with tension and tearing of pial and cortical vessels opposite the point of impact, and with direct or rotational displacement of brain over bony prominences, where the vessels become exposed to tensile and shear forces.

Focal contused injuries develop typically at the point of impact, and the mechanism of development is somewhat different from that of the diffuse injuries. In focal injuries, movement of the head is not sufficient to cause significant displacement of the brain. Instead, the applied force, usually with relatively high velocity and relatively low mass, causes fracture or deformation of the skull at the point of impact. The deformation of the skull may only be transient but sufficient to cause bruising of the tissue immediately beneath.

Laceration

Laceration is a traumatic injury in which there is disruption of the architecture of the tissue. The mechanics of lacerations are in general the same as those of contusion. Penetrating injuries are analogous to, but more severe than, those that result in focal contusions. Lacerations may also occur with blunt injuries of the type that cause displacement of the brain. In such cases, contrecoup lacerations occur typically on the surfaces of gyri where these are displaced over bony prominences. Shear forces developed during deformation or molding of the brain may be adequate to cause deep hemorrhages and even the cleavage of the gray from the white matter over small areas of the cortex.

Lacerations caused by penetrating injuries are always liable to *secondary infections*, especially when fragments of skin and soft tissue and spicules of bone from the internal plates are displaced into the brain. In the absence of infection, repair takes place in the manner that is usual for defects of nervous tissue. The detritus of blood and nervous tissue is removed by microglia and meningothelial macrophages. If the defect is small, an astrocytic scar forms, but usually a cyst remains, lined by proliferated astrocytes. Adhesions between the glial tissue and pia mater produce meningocerebral scars that are notably epileptogenic.

Fracture of the skull

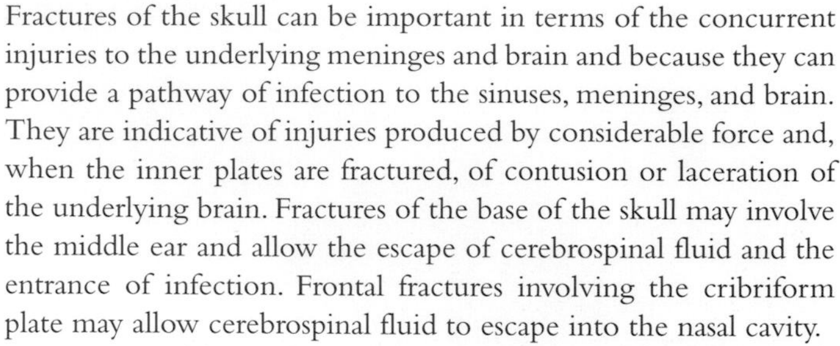

Fractures of the skull can be important in terms of the concurrent injuries to the underlying meninges and brain and because they can provide a pathway of infection to the sinuses, meninges, and brain. They are indicative of injuries produced by considerable force and, when the inner plates are fractured, of contusion or laceration of the underlying brain. Fractures of the base of the skull may involve the middle ear and allow the escape of cerebrospinal fluid and the entrance of infection. Frontal fractures involving the cribriform plate may allow cerebrospinal fluid to escape into the nasal cavity.

Fractures of the skull are usually quite easy to detect by virtue of the displacement of bone and meningeal hemorrhage. Some, however, may be difficult to detect. This applies especially to fissures that develop during transient deformation of the skull and to impacted basilar fractures, such as occur in horses that rear backward and strike the nape of the neck and occiput. With these fractures, hemorrhages may be scant and basilar fractures are revealed only when the dura is carefully dissected away.

Injuries to the spinal cord

It is possible for direct injuries to the spinal cord to occur without obvious injury to the vertebrae. Such spinal injuries are necessarily lacerations caused by penetrating foreign bodies. Wandering parasites as causes of traumatic injury are discussed later. Much more common are indirect injuries to the cord acquired in the course of vertebral luxations or fractures with dislocation. *The most common of indirect injuries to the cord are produced by extruded nucleus pulposus in dogs, and by compression of the cervical cord in the syndrome known as "wobbler"* (see Vol. 1, Bones and joints).

Vertebral subluxations are the result of trauma, but *fracture dislocation* may be pathological as well as traumatic, and frequently is in swine and ruminants when the fracture occurs through an area of vertebral osteomyelitis or osteochondrosis. The injuries to the cord occur chiefly at the time of accident and are due mainly to the stresses to which the cord is subjected and partly to impediment to the blood supply. Cumulative injury may occur, especially in dislocations when continued pressure on the cord or stretching of the cord over bony prominences causes intermittent ischemia.

Subluxations are largely restricted to the cervical column, where there is relative mobility of the ligaments. In the thoracic and lumbar spine, comparable forces are more likely to cause fracture because of the brevity of the ligaments. The fractures may involve only a lamina, the odontoid process, or an articular process, and therefore be difficult to detect. *Fracture dislocations of the vertebral column occur chiefly in the caudal cervical region and about the thoracolumbar junction.* Most injurious are those fractures that involve the vertebral body because there is usually displacement of a fragment caudodorsally into the spinal canal. Both in luxation and fracture displacement, pressure may be exerted over several segments of cord by epidural and endodural blood clots (Fig 3.68).

Traumatic injuries to the spinal cord may be slight enough to be satisfactorily recoverable, or they may, at the other extreme, cause transection and an extensive length of necrosis. Early contused

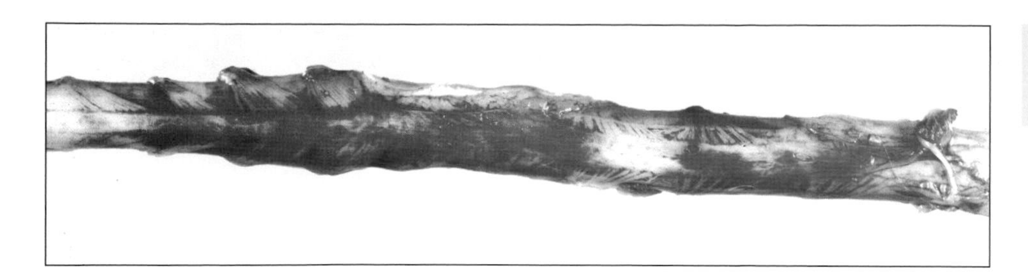

Figure 3.68 Extensive **subdural hemorrhage** of the spinal cord in a dog, caused by physical trauma. (Courtesy of RF Slocombe.)

lesions cause swelling of the cord over one or two vertebral segments. The swelling may be easier to palpate by gently stroking the cord than to appreciate by inspection. Later, the cord is shrunken at the level of injury, and this also may be best detected by palpation. In the swollen zone, dark points of hemorrhage may be detected on section, and these occur usually in the central gray matter and at its junction with the white. If the demarcation of gray from white matter is obscured, it can be expected that softening of some degree is present. Cores of softening may be recognizable grossly, and the fact that they are extending up and down the cord from the point of injury is explained as tracking of exudate, especially serum or edema fluid, along the fiber tracts and the path of least resistance since, because the meninges are usually intact, the amount of local swelling is limited.

With severe compression, the cord may be entirely necrotic at the point of injury and over several segments. *Necrosis is probably due to vascular injury*, and, for the same reason, isolated segments of necrosis may occur apart from the main injury. When the cord is necrotic, it is initially swollen, but after a lapse of some weeks the dura forms a narrowed, collapsible tube containing debris.

Microscopically, in the mildest injuries there is swelling of axons and myelin sheaths. The injured axons become beaded, but they are possibly not irreversibly injured unless fragmentation follows the beading, because functional recovery can follow minor and transient paralytic injuries. Where the axons are severed, there is bulbous swelling of the retracted ends. Degenerative neuronal changes consisting of the clumping of Nissl substance and central chromatolysis are constantly present. Ultimately, there is some loss of neurons. When softening occurs, the sequence of changes is the same as occurs in any neural lesion with loss of substance. The hemorrhage is usually slight and perivascular, but it may enter the central canal and pass along it for a considerable distance.

In long-standing spinal injuries, adhesions may be found between the meninges and between the dura mater and periosteum. In the injured zone of cord, there may be loss of fibers and myelin sheaths with astrogliosis or, in the more severe injuries with loss of substance, there may be cysts, pial-glial or collagenous scars, or the cord may be converted to a thin sclerotic band.

DEGENERATION IN THE NERVOUS SYSTEM

Foregoing sections dealing with cytopathology and the effects of circulatory disturbances and trauma are discussions of changes that are largely degenerative. The same will be true of many sections in later parts of this chapter because neural injury, regardless of cause or severity, is characterized chiefly by degeneration. Discussed in this section are those lesions and diseases of the CNS that are expressed as degenerations of nervous tissue.

Meninges

Age changes in the meninges may advance to such a degree as to be pathological. *Collagenous and osseous metaplasia* occurs commonly in the cranial dura mater of dogs and cats. The process begins in the frontal region and extends to the temporal and occipital areas. The plaque-like thickenings of the surface meninges tend not to extend to the basal or cerebellar meninges. Ossification, which is detectable as small intradural plaques, follows hyalinization of the connective tissues and may or may not be preceded by mineralization. The dura adheres firmly to the periosteum. Perhaps by an independent process, *spherical mineralized nodules* form in the basal dura beneath the medulla in some aging dogs. Histologically, these nodules show a whorled pattern of fibroblastic cells often enclosing small concretions known as **psammoma bodies**.

Hyalinization of dural collagen occurs also in the spinal dura mater with aging and may be preliminary to the osseous metaplasia of the dura observed frequently in large breeds of dogs. The latter condition is referred to as **ossifying pachymeningitis** but, in spite of the frequency of the dural change, little is known of its pathogenesis or effects. *Dural ossification* is found in older age groups of some large breeds and varies in its expression from multiple separate plaques to rigid ossification over several segments of the cord. The changes are best developed in the lumbar region but may involve much of the spinal dura. The basic change appears to be degenerative and metaplastic rather than inflammatory. Locomotor dysfunction in affected animals is more likely to be attributable to concurrent spondylosis and degenerative/reactive changes in joints. The plaques consist of lamellar bone that is mature in appearance and that from the earliest stages contains cancellous spaces and active bone marrow.

Degenerative changes in leptomeninges are less well identified than those in the dura and are limited to collagenization and hyalinization. They are not functionally significant, but the opacities produced, especially the focal thickening in arachnoid granulations in old animals, can be misinterpreted as inflammatory change.

Choroid plexuses

With advancing age, there is *hyaline degeneration of the connective tissues of the choroid plexuses*, especially those of the lateral ventricles (Fig. 3.69). The basement membranes of the capillaries are also involved. The hyaline tissues may become mineralized.

Cholesteatosis of the choroid plexuses in the form of tumor-like nodules, usually termed *cholesteatomas* or *cholesterol granulomas*, occurs in 15–20% of old horses. They are more frequent in the plexuses of the fourth ventricle than in the lateral ventricles, but those in the lateral ventricles are the more important because they may attain large size and, by obstructing the interventricular foramen,

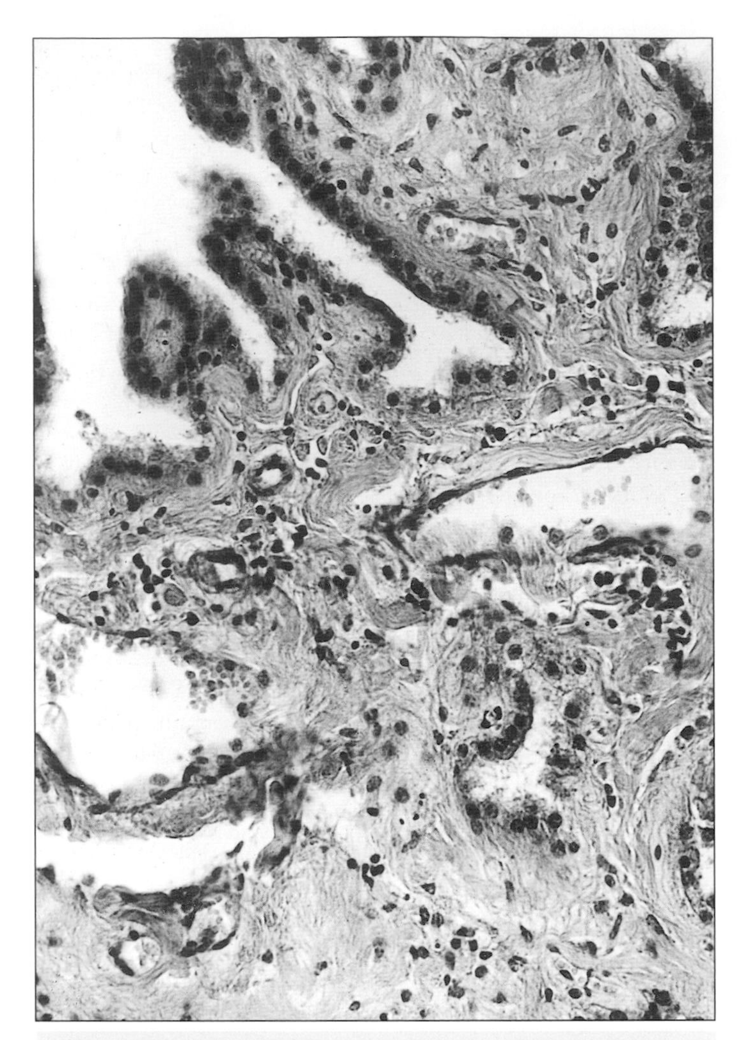

Figure 3.69 Senile hyalinization in the choroid plexus of a horse.

cause hydrocephalus leading to dilation and pressure atrophy of the walls of the ventricles (Fig. 3.70A).

The development of cholesteatosis appears to be related in some manner to chronic or intermittent congestion and edema with congestive hemorrhages in the choroid plexuses. During an edematous episode, the plexuses are slightly swollen, yellow, and soft. The interstitial tissues are edematous and infiltrated lightly by macrophages containing lipid and hemosiderin. The crystals of cholesterol are deposited in the tissue spaces and apparently act as foreign bodies to stimulate low-grade productive inflammation (Fig. 3.70B).

The affected plexus is swollen, and small areas or the whole of it may be occupied by the cholesterol granulomas. These are firm but crumbly, gray nodules with a gleaming, pearly appearance on cut surface. The crystals can be expressed from the cut surface by slight pressure.

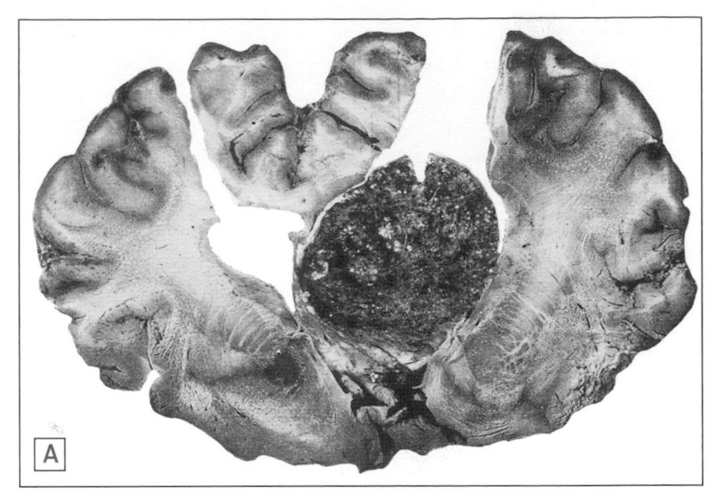

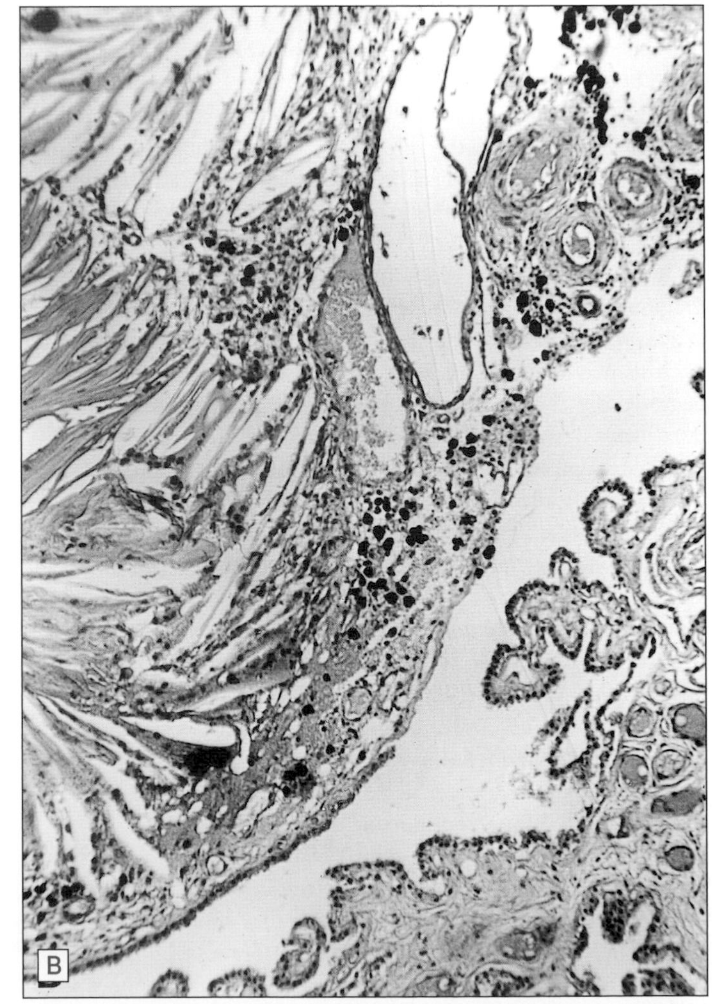

Figure 3.70 A. Cholesterol granuloma in the choroid plexus of the right lateral ventricle of a horse. (Courtesy of P Olafson.) **B. Cholesterol granuloma** in the choroid plexus of a horse.

Atrophy in the brain and spinal cord

The most spectacular atrophy of the cerebrum occurs in cases of congenital lipofuscinosis and of progressive internal hydrocephalus. **Senile atrophy** of the brain and cord is frequently obvious but seldom severe in animals. The atrophy is most marked when it is associated with the combined influences of senility and marasmus, and it occurs more frequently in sheep than in other species. The pachymeninges are thickened and those of the cranium are partially adherent to the periosteum. The leptomeninges are thickened, tough, and granular. The brain is reduced in volume and weight and may be discolored a darker gray-yellow. The convolutions are narrowed and wrinkled and the sulci are shallow and widened. Both brain and cord are much firmer than is normal. The ventricles are moderately dilated. Histologically, the neurons, especially of the cortex, are shrunken, distorted, and dark staining and their numbers are depleted. The amount of Nissl substance is reduced and the neuronal nuclei stain diffusely. Lipochromes are increased in amount and satellitosis is prominent; macrophages laden with lipochrome are present in the perivascular spaces. There is a diffuse increase in glial fibers, which is responsible for the increased firmness of the tissue. The gliosis is most prominent about Virchow–Robin spaces, and there is a general tendency for protoplasmic astrocytes to transform into fibrous ones. The Virchow–Robin spaces are dilated, and some may be visible to the naked eye. The media of the vessels contain increased amounts of collagen.

Focal atrophy of the brain and cord is the result of slight but long-continued pressure. The loss of function is often disproportionately large as the result of acute pressure lesions compared with the extent of pathologic change. The reverse is often true in chronic pressure, and function may be retained to a surprising degree. Hydrocephalus is common as a cause of chronic pressure, and other sources of pressure are space-occupying lesions of the meninges or bony vault.

The pathogenesis of the changes produced by chronic pressure is unclarified. Because the immediate effects of pressure are more likely to be felt by veins than by arteries or solid tissue, the atrophic changes are usually attributed to venous stasis and edema. More acute pressure effects grade into circumstances and consequences discussed under trauma. Whatever the mechanism, myelin is the most vulnerable component of the tissue and undergoes slow progressive degeneration. There is also slow progressive atrophy and loss of neurons, especially of the Purkinje cells when pressure is exerted on the cerebellum, the neurons of the deeper laminae when pressure is exerted on the cerebrum, and of the ventral horn cells in the spinal cord. The degenerating myelin is replaced by glial fibers.

Segmental cerebellar atrophy is common in pigs following a variety of nervous diseases. The rostral vermis and adjacent portions of the lateral lobes are affected, these being within the distribution of the rostral cerebellar artery. There is no acute change but, instead, a gradual loss of granule and Purkinje cells with secondary changes in the white matter and reactive gliosis. The lesion is asymptomatic.

Anoxia and anoxic poisons

The neuropathological effects of anoxia are seldom observed in animals or perhaps seldom looked for. Since most cases die acutely, there may be very little to see. The pathological effects of anoxia, not only in the CNS, but in general, are expressions of "vulnerability," a property which differs from organ to organ and between parts and cells of one organ. *The components of the nervous system are vulnerable in a rather fixed order*, which is neuron, oligodendroglia, astroglia, microglia, and blood vessels in that diminishing order of sensitivity. The neurons are not a uniform population, and there are regional differences in their susceptibility to anoxia, those of the cerebral cortex and the Purkinje cells being the most sensitive. Within the cerebral cortex, the neurons of the deeper laminae are more sensitive than those in the superficial laminae. Beneath these levels, there is a gradient of susceptibility through the geniculate bodies, hypothalamus, thalamus, paleocortex, and caudate nucleus. The various patterns of vulnerability are relative; they are established largely by experiments in animals and are subject to some variation depending in part on the experimental species and on the type of anoxia induced. They do nevertheless emphasize the problem of selective vulnerability at the cellular level. There are, in addition, broader regional differences in vulnerability to anoxia such as those that allow parts of the cerebral cortex to be necrotic while adjacent parts survive intact and that allow the same agent or anoxic insult to cause, leukomalacia on some occasions, and poliomalacia on other occasions. The basis of these regional differences in vulnerability, and the apparent differences in the patterns of degeneration following different types of anoxia, is still to be established.

The pathological effects of anoxia on nervous tissue are of two types, which are to some extent differences in degree. The least clear morphological expression is *selective neuronal necrosis*. The neuronal necrosis is typically of the ischemic type, and it is followed by glial repair. Greater degrees of anoxia, sufficient to kill astroglia as well as neurons, result in *softening*. These are the expected changes in anoxic anoxias such as might occur with cardiac arrest or periods of apnea in grand mal epilepsy.

As a response in some episodes of anoxia, such as may be induced, for example, in the histotoxic variety of cyanide poisoning, the degeneration and necrosis may affect the white matter with only minimal changes in the gray. The reason for this is not known. The malacic changes in the white matter of the cerebral hemispheres are preceded by edema, which suggests that local circulatory disturbances contribute to its development. Clearly the attribution of selective vulnerability on the basis of local metabolic demand for oxygen is inadequate, and a fuller explanation will probably require, in addition, consideration of vascular architecture, the autoregulation of blood pressure and flow, and local metabolic factors in the maintenance of myelin and axons.

Cyanide poisoning

The anoxia produced by cyanide is classified as *histotoxic* because the action of the poison is to *inhibit intracellular respiratory enzymes*. The cyanides are particularly rapid in their action, and death usually occurs from a few minutes to an hour after the onset of clinical signs. In the most acute cases, the clinical course occupies only a few minutes and is characterized by dyspnea, drooling, trembling, and recumbency; it terminates in convulsions. The *blood is bright red* owing to its high degree of oxygen saturation. In cases that survive for an hour, the clinical signs are the same with, in addition, vomiting, especially in pigs, nystagmus and cyanosis. In these cases, the blood is often dark owing to anoxemia.

The morbid changes are those associated with anoxia. Because most cases survive for half an hour to one hour, the blood is dark and does not clot and the tissues are dark. There is congestion in the lungs and hemorrhages of dyspneic type in the tracheal mucosa. Ecchymoses of the epicardium are usual. In pigs, there is pulmonary edema and hydropericardium, and there may be capillary hemorrhages deep in the myocardium by the coronary grooves. Severe pulmonary edema is present in some dogs.

Descriptions of lesions in the nervous system of animals in cyanide poisoning are largely limited to experimental observations in dogs and cats. In many natural cases of the poisoning, there is no significant alteration in the brain. The degenerative lesions in the brain in experimental poisoning may involve predominantly the gray matter or the white. When in gray matter, there is patchy necrosis and laminar loss of cells in the cerebral cortex, and necrosis in the head of the caudate nucleus, paleocortex, substantia nigra, and thalamus. There is edema in the cerebral white matter, sometimes in the absence of cortical change. On the other hand, single graded exposures of rats may produce the principal lesions in white matter, especially in the corpus callosum. In this species, there are gradients of injury in the callosum reflecting gradients of susceptibility, the most severe degeneration occurring in the caudal core of the callosum. The gradients are attributed to regional differences of blood supply, which are expected to reinforce the histotoxic anoxia of cytochrome oxidase inhibition by cyanide. The earliest change described in the callosal lesion is axonal swelling producing a spongy appearance by light microscopy; alterations of myelin, and oligodendrocytes are second in time.

Plants containing toxic levels of hydrocyanic acid bound as glucosides are common and widespread and are the usual source of cyanide poisoning. The compounds are in general the β-glycosides of α-hydroxynitriles and are activated by endogenous glucosidases in the plant, or in other plants, or by ruminal microorganisms. For these reasons, cyanide poisoning occurs chiefly in ruminants. Toxin generation of this type does not occur at the low pH of the monogastric stomach, but a lethal amount may be absorbed from the large bowel if there has been a large intake of toxigenic material.

Both sheep and cattle are capable of detoxifying cyanide in the liver to form *thiocyanate*. Thiocyanate itself is toxic but in a manner different from that of cyanide; if thiocyanate is present in low concentrations over prolonged periods, it is goitrogenic. The cyanide concentration in a stated species of plant varies considerably with stage and rate of growth and with the fertility of the soil. Plants that are growing rapidly contain the highest concentrations of the glucosides, especially if the growth phase follows one of retardation caused, for example, by wilting, frostbite, or close grazing. The glucosides are regarded as being metabolic by-products.

Plants of many species contain cyanogenetic glucosides but only a few are important in this regard. The majority of cyanogenetic plants are usually harmless either because of low palatability or low concentration of the glucosides. The important cultivated toxic plants are the sorghums (*Sorghum* spp.), and the star grasses (*Cynodon* spp.). Those of the cherry family are also potently cyanogenetic. Linseed concentrates can be dangerous, especially if eaten in large quantities.

Chronic cyanide intoxication is not recorded, but extended periods of grazing the cyanogenetic sorghum and sudan grass may lead to ataxia in cattle and horses, cystitis and urinary incontinence, and abortion in mares. Attempts to link the clinical syndrome to cyanogenetic compounds in the plants are inconclusive, and a causal association with cyanides seems unlikely. There is axonal degeneration and demyelination at all levels of the cord but most prominent caudally in ventral and lateral funiculi. Ataxic syndromes occur in sheep grazing *Sorghum* sp. may involve large numbers of animals in syndromes that differ from those in horses and cattle. Urinary incontinence does not occur. There is limb paresis with knuckling, incoordination and disturbance of equilibrium, and head and body tremors. Pregnant ewes may produce stillborn, weak, or arthrogrypotic lambs. While the lesions in horses and cattle are of Wallerian type in the spinal cord, those in sheep are of an axonopathy with proximal spheroids in the major nuclei of the brain stem and ventral horns of the cord.

Nitrate/nitrite poisoning

Ruminants are also vulnerable to *phytogenous nitrates*, when intraruminal microbial conversion of nitrates to nitrites exceeds the rate of conversion of the latter to ammonia. The nitrate sources again include many crop plants as well as weeds; plant nitrate concentrations are influenced by soil nitrogen level, and physiologic stresses on the plants, such as water stress and herbicide damage. Occasionally, high nitrate concentration in drinking water is the problem. *Absorbed nitrites convert hemoglobin to methemoglobin*, which imparts a *dark "chocolate" color* to the blood, and causes dyspnea, cyanosis, weakness, tremors, collapse, and coma. There are no gross or histological brain lesions. The condition is discussed more fully in Vol. 3, Hematopoietic system.

Fluoroacetate poisoning

Fluoroacetate is toxic by virtue of its ability to form fluoracetyl-CoA, which potently inhibits the Kreb's cycle enzymes *cis*-aconitase and succinate dehydrogenase, thereby paralyzing cellular respiration. Herbivores are usually poisoned by ingesting *fluoroacetate-containing plants*, while other animals may be affected by accident or design by being exposed to sodium fluoroacetate formulated as a *pesticide*. The clinical signs are of the same general character as those described above but, in the dog, frenzied hyperactivity is reported. As with cyanide, the myocardium is highly vulnerable, and multifocal necrosis may be seen. Fluoroacetate poisoning is discussed in Vol. 3, Cardiovascular system.

Carbon monoxide poisoning

This is rarely observed and is discussed in the interests of completeness. Carbon monoxide has an affinity for hemoglobin which is several hundred times the affinity of oxygen for hemoglobin. The carboxyhemoglobin produced prevents oxygen exchange and causes anoxic anoxia. The anoxia is reinforced by a histotoxic component due to the affinity of carbon monoxide for iron-containing respiratory enzymes.

Carboxyhemoglobin and, therefore, the blood and tissues of poisoned animals are *bright pink*. All organs are congested, but especially the brain, in which the veins and capillaries are much dilated. The dilated vessels are observed especially in the white matter and hemorrhages occur from them. Acute fatalities are not expected to be associated with neural lesions. Survival is expected to be followed by complete recovery, but there may be residual lesions of anoxic type, especially neuronal loss.

Carbon monoxide poisoning is reported occasionally in animals in confined quarters that are heated by petroleum fuels. Most of the reported instances are in pigs, and poisoning is associated with a high level of stillbirth and neonatal mortality. Following experimental exposure, patchy or extensive leukomalacia may be present in the hemispheres in the newborn.

Hypoglycemia

It is useful to extend the classification of anoxia to include hypoglycemia, which causes a *disturbance of intracellular respiration*. Oxygen is available to the nervous tissue, but, in the absence or reduction of the amount of substrate, the oxygen is not utilized.

Hypoglycemia may occur as a result of a functioning *tumor of the pancreatic islets* or as a response to insulin overdosage in the treatment of diabetes. It is also part of the metabolic disturbance of *ketosis in cows* and *pregnancy toxemia in ewes*, and arguments have been advanced for regarding the irreversibility of pregnancy toxemia as being due to hypoglycemic encephalopathy. Piglets in the first week of life readily develop hypoglycemia if there is dietary restriction from any cause. Effective gluconeogenesis does not develop in piglets until about the seventh day of life, and during this first week their glycemic levels are rather precise reflections of dietary intake. In spite of the severe convulsions and deep coma that occur in hypoglycemia, conspicuous changes do not occur in the brain. It is probable that biochemical disturbances in the neurons precede histological signs of degeneration by a considerable period. For this reason, acute hypoglycemic death is not expected to produce cerebral lesions. When the period of coma is prolonged, it is probable that all neurons are to some extent altered, but the differentiation of hypoglycemic from autolytic and nonspecific changes can seldom be made with confidence. Although classified with the anoxias, hypoglycemia does not produce the ischemic type of neuronal degeneration characteristic of the usual sorts of anoxia. There is, instead, a tendency for the severe type of neuronal degeneration to occur, characterized by rapid and complete chromatolysis, disappearance of the cytoplasmic margins, and then fading of the cytoplasm, with pyknosis, eccentricity and fading of the nucleus. The regional susceptibility of neurons to hypoglycemia, exclusive of the Purkinje cells, parallels that of susceptibility to anoxia.

Bibliography

Anderson RW, et al. Impact mechanics and axonal injury in a sheep model. J Neurotrauma 2003;20:961–974.

Bourke C. *Sorghum* spp neurotoxicity in sheep. Aust Vet J 1995;72:467.

Bradley GA, et al. Neuroaxonal degeneration in sheep grazing *Sorghum* sp pastures. J Vet Diagn Invest 1995;7:229–236.

Calabresi P, et al. Cellular factors controlling neuronal vulnerability in the brain: A lesson from the striatum. Neurology 2000;55:1249–1255.

Dimakopoulos AC, Mayer RJ. Aspects of neurodegeneration in the canine brain. J Nutr 2002;132(6 Suppl 2):1579S–1582S.

Finnie JW, Blumbergs PC. Traumatic brain injury. Vet Pathol 2002;39:679–689.

Funata N, et al. A study of experimental cyanide encephalopathy in the acute phase–physiological and neuropathological correlation. Acta Neuropathol (Berl) 1984;64:99–107.

MacKay RJ. Brain injury after head trauma: pathophysiology, diagnosis, and treatment. Vet Clin North Am Equine Pract 2004;20:199–216.

McKenzie RA, McMiking LI. Ataxia and urinary incompetence in cattle grazing sorghum. Aust Vet J 1977;53:496–497.

Okeda R. Concept and pathogenesis of "hypoxic-ischemic encephalopathy". Acta Neurochir Suppl 2003;86:3–6.

Penney DG. Acute carbon monoxide poisoning: animal models: a review. Toxicology 1990;62:123–160.

Soto-Blanco B, et al. Physiopathological effects of the administration of chronic cyanide to growing goats–a model for ingestion of cyanogenic plants. Vet Res Commun 2001;25:379–389.

Vink-Nooteboom M, et al. Computed tomography of cholesterinic granulomas in the choroid plexus of horses. Vet Radiol Ultrasound 1998;39:512–516.

Malacia and malacic diseases

Necrosis of individual elements of nervous tissue is described earlier under Cytopathology. **Encephalomalacia** and **myelomalacia** refer to necrosis in the brain and cord respectively. *Malacia means softening*, and is used interchangeably with that term to signify necrosis of tissue in the CNS. It is sometimes, as imprecise practice, used interchangeably with demyelination. There is no sharp line to be drawn between demyelination and malacia, especially in the early stages of development of the degenerative process, but the term demyelination should probably be restricted to those lesions in which the myelin sheath is primarily or selectively injured to leave the axons naked but intact. When neurons and neuroglia degenerate and die as part of the primary response, the term malacia is applicable.

The *sequence of events* in softening or malacia is specific only for the tissue. The morphological changes in necrosis, in the removal of dead tissue, and in healing are the same regardless of the insult. The insults can be varied, and *malacia, alone or as part of another change, is one of the most common lesions in the brain and cord*. It is discussed in the sections dealing with vascular accidents and trauma, it occurs in many instances of encephalomyelitis, is discussed elsewhere in these volumes as a lesion of mulberry heart disease, of antenatal *bluetongue virus* infections in lambs, and of clostridial enterotoxemia in lambs that escape apoplectic death and live for some days. Malacic lesions are probably the basis of most cases of hydranencephaly.

Although the nature of the malacic process is not specific for cause, there is some specificity in the localization of lesions and in their particular pattern of distribution. These features may allow the recognition of known associations or causes, such as the nigropallidal distribution of lesions in horses poisoned by yellow star thistle, and the focal symmetrical lesions of the internal capsule in lambs with clostridial enterotoxemia. Although these and some other associations have been determined, the pathogenesis of the lesions and the problems of selective injury to certain parts of the brain remain to be resolved.

The sequence of changes in malacic foci is approximately the same in all cases and is outlined below. The rapidity of change is quite variable and depends on the species and age of the animal, the location of the necrosis, the volume of tissue affected, and the inciting cause. The speed of resolution is also affected by the quality of vascular perfusion in adjacent nervous tissue, whether the necrosis is ischemic or hemorrhagic and on the time over which the cause acts.

The malacic process, once initiated, appears to proceed very rapidly in the fetal and immature nervous system, and to leave cystic structures and hydranencephaly without much evidence of continuing reaction at the time these animals are available for necropsy examination (see Fig. 3.27). The reasons for the rapidity of change in immature nervous tissue are not clear, but contributing factors may involve the paucity of myelin that is difficult to remove, the paucity of mature mesenchyme in meninges and about vessels, and the plasticity of vascular arrangements in the developing brain. The rapidity of change in gray matter is generally greater than in the white. Autolytic liquefactive changes depend on continued enzymatic activity that, in turn, depends on availability of oxygen either by diffusion from surrounding tissue or by reflow in the local vessels. Small foci of necrosis are expected to resolve more quickly than large. Malacic lesions in the neocortex where diffusion from collateral vessels is available are expected to resolve more rapidly than those in the paleocortex where the vascular supply is more strictly of the end-artery type. Some causes of malacia, such as vascular occlusion, act promptly and the pathological changes are directly consequential. The cause may act continuously over a period, as in leukoencephalomalacia of horses, and the changes may be incremental. The process, once established, may itself initiate progressive change as in traumatic injury to the cord in which swelling within the confines of the meninges assists the spread of edema and vascular response beyond the site of the original injury.

A malacic lesion that develops acutely may not, in the absence of hemorrhage, be demonstrable before about the twelfth hour of onset. The early change is in texture, with the affected part being soft, and in color, with the affected part being gray. Within 2–3 days, the malacic foci begin to disintegrate, the softness is more evident, and the surrounding tissue is swollen by edema, and pale in gray matter or yellow in white matter. Subject to the above qualifications, *the necrotic area eventually liquefies and a cyst remains*. The cyst may be loculated or traversed by vascular strands that have survived the episode.

Histologically there is, in acute episodes, reduced staining affinity by about 12 hours. The cellular elements show the changes described earlier. The early active response involves circulating neutrophils, which may enter in large numbers, but this response is replaced in 3–4 days by macrophages. The first appearance of macrophages is about blood vessels, their peak activity occurs in about 2 weeks, but a few will survive for a very long time. Astrocytic gliosis replaces or surrounds the resolved necrotic area (see Fig. 3.61).

In the specific syndromes to be discussed below, the degenerative changes tend to be restricted to, or to affect principally, either the gray matter or the white matter. Softening of gray matter is known as **poliomalacia** and softening of white matter is known as **leukomalacia**; each may be qualified as to whether cerebral (encephalo-) or spinal (myelo-). The diseases to be described below are specific, but malacia is not exclusive to them. Necrosis of cerebral cortex, is rare in horses except in the neonatal "barker syndrome" (see Fig. 3.54). In ruminants, poliomalacia is, in the early stages, expected to respond to thiamine, but it also occurs in lead poisoning, in water intoxication, and in other, ill-defined, circumstances. Lead also causes poliomalacia in dogs. Convulsive episodes in dogs, some associated with distemper, may leave malacic changes especially in parietal and temporal cortex. Idiopathic necrosis and malacia of the hippocampus and piriform lobe in cats is reported from Europe as a cause of seizures. Metronidazole intoxication of dogs and cats can result in brain stem leukomalacia. In pigs, polioencephalomalacia is usually due to salt poisoning, but individual cases occur in meningitis or without other association. The isolated case of malacia can be difficult to explain.

Focal symmetrical poliomyelomalacia syndromes

This disease, as described from Kenyan **sheep**, is characterized by focal softening of the gray matter of the spinal cord, most consistent and severe in the cervical enlargement. A similar syndrome occurs in parts of West Africa. There is no information on the cause or pathogenesis, although the distribution of necrosis in relation to the cross-section of the cord and the irregular segmental involvement of the gray matter, especially in the cervical region, are consistent with a *vascular component* in the pathogenesis. Lesions of similar distribution and character are occasionally met with in dogs and cats with inflammatory or thrombotic occlusion of the ventral spinal artery. Affected sheep suddenly develop flaccid or spastic paresis that always involves the forelimbs and sometimes the hindlimbs as well. There are no cerebral signs. Affected animals are lambs or up to 18 months old. There are no gross lesions to be observed except in cases of long standing, in which some brown discoloration may be noted in the malacic areas. Microscopically, there are bilateral lesions of remarkable symmetry in the ventral horns of the spinal cord. The dorsal horns are spared, as is a narrow rim of gray substance around the periphery of the ventral horns, and the commissural gray matter. The affected areas undergo dissolution with the usual reaction on the part of the microglia. At a later stage, proliferating capillaries in small numbers criss-cross the microcavitations, and the astrocytes at the margins proliferate. The malacic foci are found in the cervical and lumbar enlargements as "skip" lesions involving a few segments and, when the necrosis is extensive, similar foci may be found in the medulla.

A similar syndrome has been responsible for heavy losses in native sheep in Ghana and Ivory Coast. All ages are affected but mainly adult ewes. Clinical progression is rapid, from initial stumbling to ataxia and recumbency, opisthotonos and nystagmus and ultimately flaccid paralysis. There are microscopic changes of cytotoxic edema, especially affecting oligodendrocytes widely in the nervous system and also perivascular astrocytes and capsule cells of spinal ganglia. Foci of spongy degeneration and malacia, bilateral but not always symmetrical, are of patchy distribution and most frequent in the spinal intumescence, cerebellar roof nuclei, and large nuclei of the brain stem.

Encephalomyelomalacia of similar character is reported in young individual **goats** in California. The lesions are bilaterally symmetrical and affect particularly the lumbar and cervical enlargements and the inferior colliculi. Other brain stem nuclei are inconsistently involved. The similarity of these malacic lesions to those which can be produced experimentally by nicotinamide antagonists has been noted.

Focal symmetrical poliomyelomalacia of pigs is clinically and pathologically similar to the spontaneous poliomalacias of sheep and goats. The presenting signs are spinal with ataxia progressing to forelimb or hindlimb paresis or quadriplegia in a few days. In field cases, malacic foci are found, symmetrically in the ventral horns of the cervical and lumbar enlargements. The malacic foci are visible grossly as yellow-brown areas of softening or gray depressed areas of liquefaction. The histologic changes are typical of malacia (Fig. 3.71). There is heavy loss of neurons, and endothelial and glial proliferation in older lesions. Similar changes may be present in medullary nuclei.

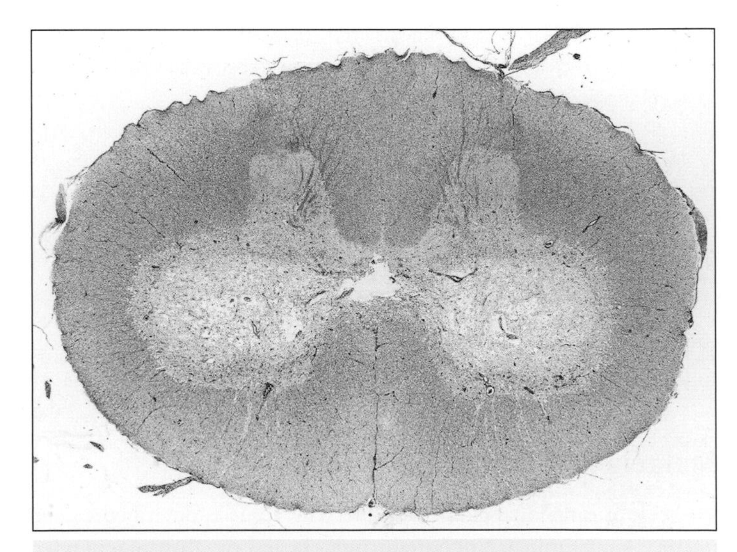

Figure 3.71 Focal symmetrical poliomyelomalacia involving ventral horns of cervical cord in a pig with selenium toxicity. (Courtesy of TM Wilson.)

Affected animals may show changes associated with *selenium toxicoses*, including scurfiness of skin, hair loss and separation of horn at the coronet. Dietary selenium, whether as sodium selenite added to rations or the feeding of selenium-accumulator plants, reproduces the syndrome, although there is some inconsistency in the lesions produced, with degeneration being more frequent in the nuclear masses of the medulla and brain stem. *Astragalus bisulcatus*, a selenium-accumulator plant, will cause concurrent polioencephalomalacia. The mechanism of neurotoxicity of selenium is obscure, but may occur through the generation of reactive oxygen species during reaction of thiols, and is expected to be influenced by other nutritional and metabolic interactions.

Focal symmetrical poliomyelomalacia, the lesion limited to the sacral and lumbar enlargements, is described in **Ayrshire calves**. The malacia affects the ventral horns, sparing the dorsal horns and the central gray matter. The cause is not known.

Bibliography

Bonniwell MA, Barlow RM. Ataxia/paresis syndrome of sheep in West Africa associated with bilateral multifocal cerebrospinal poliomalacia. Vet Rec 1985;116:94–97.

Brini E, et al. Necrosis of hippocampus and piriform lobe: clinical and neuropathological findings in two Italian cats. J Feline Med Surg 2004;6:377–381.

Cordy DR, et al. Caprine encephalomyelomalacia. Vet Pathol 1984;21:269–273.

Dow SW, et al. Central nervous system toxicosis associated with metronidazole treatment of dogs: five cases (1984–1987). J Am Vet Med Assoc 1989;195:365–368.

Nogueira CW, et al. Investigations into the potential neurotoxicity induced by diselenides in mice and rats. Toxicology 2003;183:29–37.

Palmer AC, et al. Focal symmetrical poliomalacia of the spinal cord in Ayrshire calves. Vet Pathol 1986;23:506–509.

Panter KE, et al. Comparative toxicity of selenium from seleno-DL-methionine, sodium selenate, and *Astragalus bisulcatus* in pigs. Fundam Appl Toxicol 1996;32:217–223.

Penrith ML, Robinson JT. Selenium toxicosis with focal symmetrical poliomyelomalacia in postweaning pigs in South Africa. Onderstepoort J Vet Res 1996;63:171–179.

Focal symmetrical encephalomalacia in swine

Aeschynomene indica is a common weed in irrigated rice fields and may be fed with rice and screenings of broken rice. Signs of neurologic disorder develop in a few days. Lesions are restricted to the brain, are symmetrical, involve especially the vestibular and cerebellar roof nuclei, nuclei of the midbrain, and the paleocortex. The toxic factor is unknown, but pathogenesis may depend on primary damage to microvasculature.

Bibliography

Oliveira FN, et al. Focal symmetrical encephalomalacia in swine from ingestion of *Aeschynomene indica* seeds. Vet Hum Toxicol 2004;46:309–311.

Polioencephalomalacia of ruminants

Polioencephalomalacia (PEM) as used in practice applies especially to softenings restricted to the cerebrocortical gray matter of laminar distribution. The lesion may alternatively be designated as "cerebrocortical necrosis" or "laminar cortical necrosis." Necrosis of this distribution is the basis of the well-recognized syndrome of cattle, sheep, and goats known as PEM. It is also the lesion of salt poisoning in swine, is occasionally observed in lead poisoning of cattle, and is described among the residual neurologic lesions of cyanide poisoning. Apart from these known associations or causes, laminar cortical necrosis is observed sporadically in swine, dogs, and cats.

The disease, PEM of sheep, goats, and cattle and other managed ruminants, is similar in its clinical and pathologic aspects in the several species, but the course in sheep and goats is, as a rule, shorter, with fewer survivors from the stage of overt brain swelling. Merino sheep appear to be much more resistant than other breeds.

The incidence is highest in sheep in the age group from weaning to 18 months, but sporadic cases occur in older animals. This general statement of incidence applies to pastured animals as well as to those in feedlots or barns. It is a disease of young cattle, the age incidence depending on the population exposure. As originally described in Colorado, affected animals are mainly 1–2 years of age but, elsewhere, the incidence is highest in younger stock of 3–8 months of age. The severity of the disease is rather less in pastured than in feedlot or housed cattle and sheep. Its least clinical expression, occasionally observed in outbreaks in sheep, is blindness and dullness, a tendency to head press against obstacles, and cessation of feeding. There are no ocular abnormalities in this, or in any other, grade of the disease, and the blindness is cortical. Animals showing these mild signs usually recover completely in the course of several days. If they are killed for examination, malacic changes may be found to be minimal or absent but there is widespread neuronal necrosis of ischemic type in the deeper laminae of the cerebral cortex. Animals affected more severely may remain on their feet and show, in addition to the above signs, muscular tremors especially of the head, and intermittent opisthotonos; if they survive, they become partially decorticate and remain blind and stupid.

In severe cases of PEM, the animals are recumbent. There is twitching of the face, ears, and eyelids, intermittent grinding of teeth, drooling, and bulbar paralysis in some. Opisthotonos is present and some animals are convulsive. In the early stages, the neurologic signs are intermittent, but later they become more constant with persistent opisthotonos and nystagmus. Flaccidity is usual, although there may be transient periods of spasticity, and clonic convulsions are intermittent. Death occurs in coma after a course of one to several days. These signs are entirely referable to the nervous system; other systems are undisturbed except for the very occasional case in which massive hemoglobinuria after excess water intake precedes the onset of neurologic signs.

The **lesions** are qualitatively the same in all cases, but they differ in their degree and in the ease with which they may be detected, this depending on severity and duration. Young animals usually die more rapidly than old ones and may show cerebral edema and swelling only. The swelling affects the cerebral hemispheres, which are pale, slightly soft, and droop over the cut edges of the cranium. In these cases of short course, there may be no obvious displacement of the brain. When the fresh cortex is sectioned, it usually shows a laminar paleness about 0.5–1 mm wide following the contour of the gray matter at the junction between gray and white. This change may be most easily visible in the gyri rather than in the depths of the sulci. Its extensiveness varies considerably from case to case but remains within the boundaries of the supply area of the middle cerebral and caudal cerebral arteries. In the rostral distribution of these vessels, the lesions are patchy but are more extensive caudally towards and

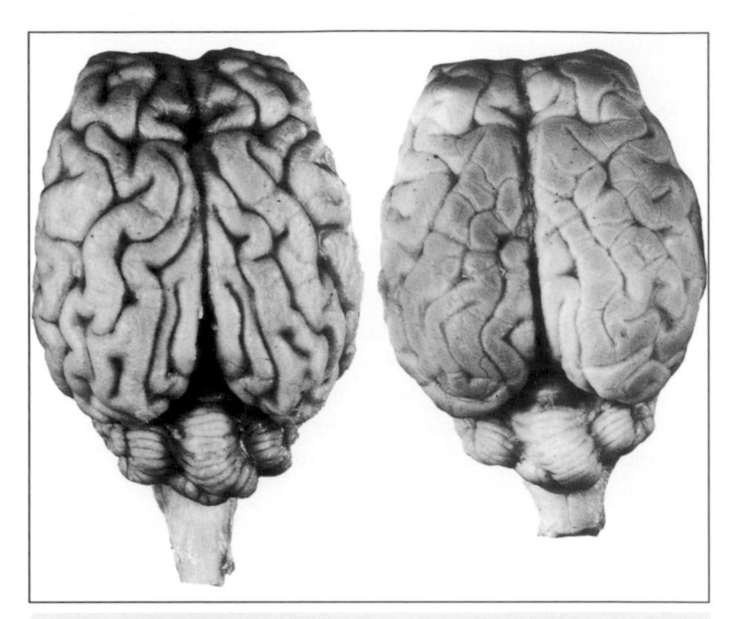

Figure 3.72 Polioencephalomalacia in a sheep. Normal brain (left), and affected brain with flattened gyri (right).

over the caudal poles of the hemispheres. The dorsal surfaces of the hemispheres are involved, and the distribution is approximately symmetrical. In either fresh or formalinized material, the gross lesions of cortical necrosis autofluoresce under ultraviolet light, due to the presence of lipid metabolites in macrophages, or of high-molecular-weight, collagen-like material.

In cases that survive for several days, the necrosis becomes more and more obvious. The brain is grossly swollen (Fig. 3.72), and, almost without exception, it is displaced caudally with herniation of the medulla and cerebellum into the foramen magnum. The dorsum of the hemispheres is palpably quite soft and the normal turgidity of the brain is gone. The surfaces of the gyri are a characteristic yellow-brown and the normal adhesion of leptomeninges to the gyral surfaces may not be present. On the cut surface of the cerebrum, there will be areas of minimal change resembling those described above. The necrotic zones can usually be appreciated to be narrow and pale or yellow instead of gray, and they are friable and shrink away from the cut surface (Fig. 3.73). Lines of cleavage between the gray and the white matter can be discerned. These are present especially over and extending down the sides of the gyri but seldom extend around the depths of the sulci. In some cases, yellow foci of softening can be found in the herniated portion of the cerebellar vermis. Hemorrhage is insignificant and usually not apparent in the cerebrum and cerebellum, but hemorrhagic foci of softening may be found in the collicular region, thalamus, and caudate nuclei. In some cases, there is thrombosis of the dorsal longitudinal sinus.

Animals that survive for 2 weeks or longer are decorticate over more or less extensive areas. The white cores of the gyri are largely intact and project nakedly or with an irregular covering of softened friable gray matter. Over some gyri, the gray matter is intact. The subarachnoid space is widened and the meninges droop over the enlarged sulci. Subpial cysts may be evident where the devastation is not complete and the meninges are adherent. The brain is smaller than normal and not displaced, the lateral and third ventricles are dilated, and there is an excess of cerebrospinal fluid.

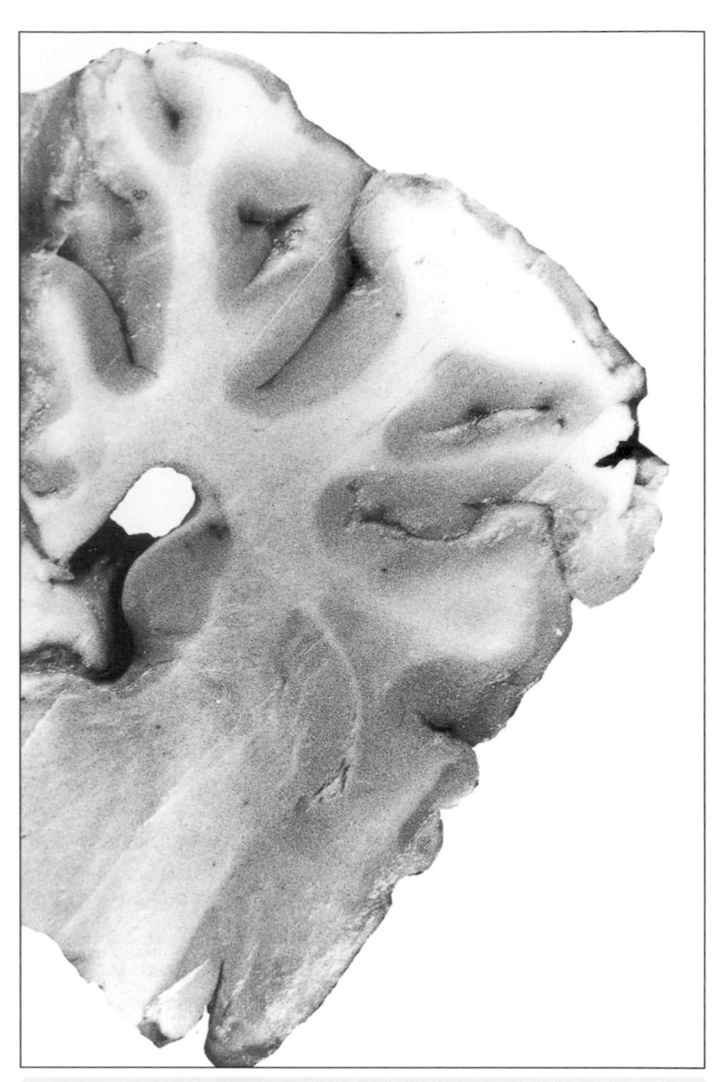

Figure 3.73 Chronic lesion in **polioencephalomalacia** in an ox; note the marked irregular narrowing of cerebral cortex.

The **microscopic changes** are of the same type in all affected parts but vary in distribution and severity. The least change is one of laminar necrosis of neurons affecting especially the deeper laminae. The neurons are shrunken, acidophilic, and surrounded by a clear space; in 2–3 days, many are converted to eosinophilic globules without nuclear remnants. Healing, if it occurs, is with intense astrogliosis.

The malacic areas are laminar (Fig. 3.74). The deepest laminae are consistently involved. Frequently, the superficial lamina is involved. The softened laminae do not necessarily overlie one another although there is usually considerable overlapping. When two distinct laminae of necrosis overlie one another, they frequently merge in the depths of the sulci to produce necrosis of the total width of the gray stratum (Fig. 3.74). Necrosis of the superficial lamina is first recognizable as a rather uniform sponginess. The layer then disintegrates and the middle laminae, if intact, are separated from the pia by a moat of gitter cells in which vessels are very sparse (Fig. 3.75). The leptomeninges are thickened and contain many activated histiocytes.

The middle laminae may remain structurally intact for considerable periods. The neurons therein die acutely, but the glia are rather persistent. The vessels are prominent, with swollen proliferating endothelial and adventitial cells and a perivascular clear space.

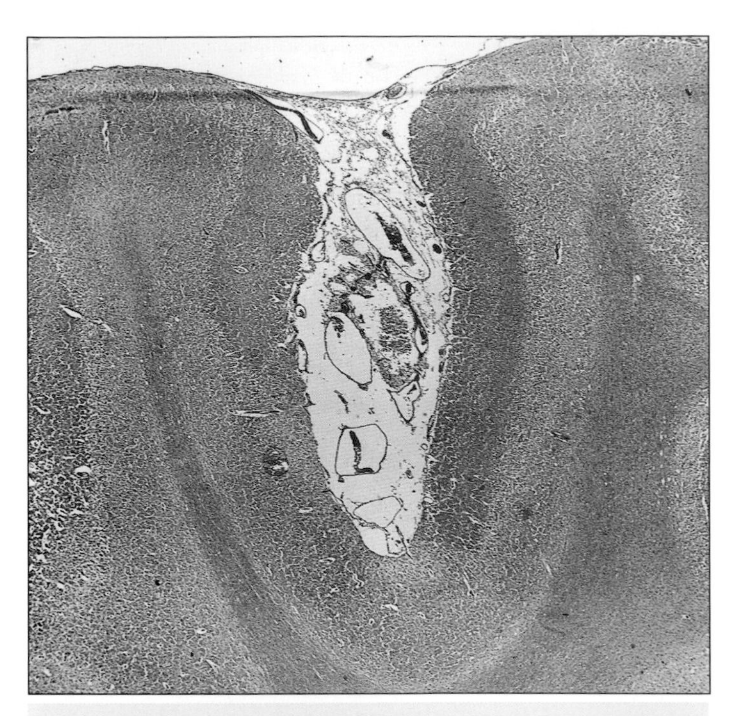

Figure 3.74 Polioencephalomalacia in an ox. Pallid areas of degeneration involving full width of cortex in depth of sulcus.

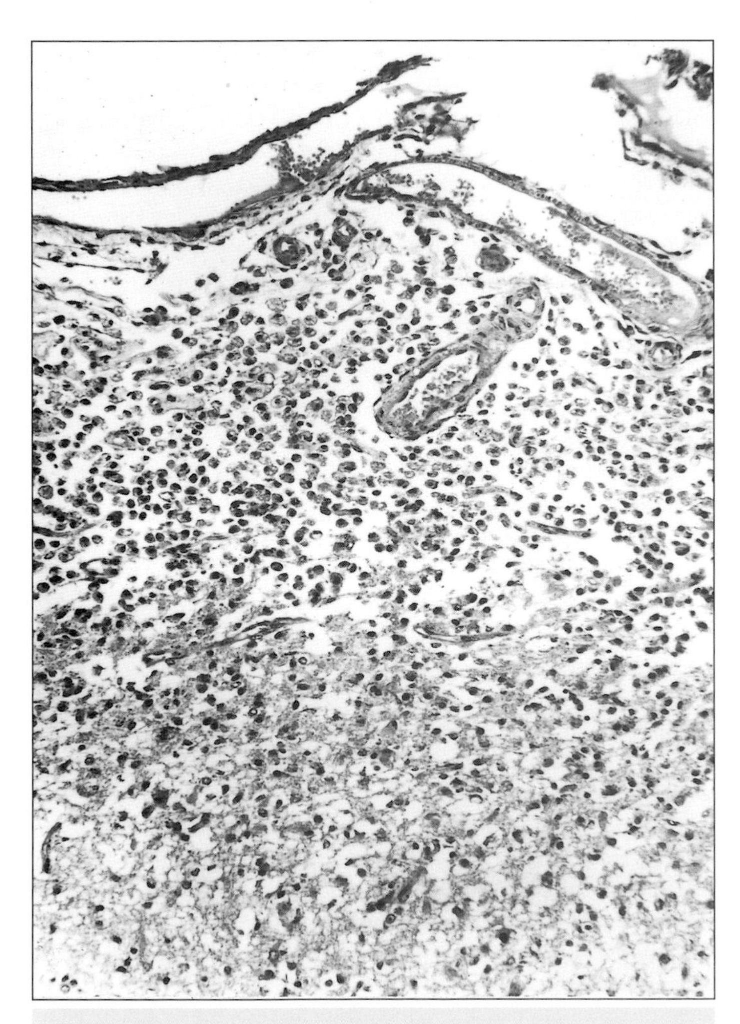

Figure 3.75 Collapse of meninges, with gitter cells replacing necrotic cortex in **polioencephalomalacia** in an ox.

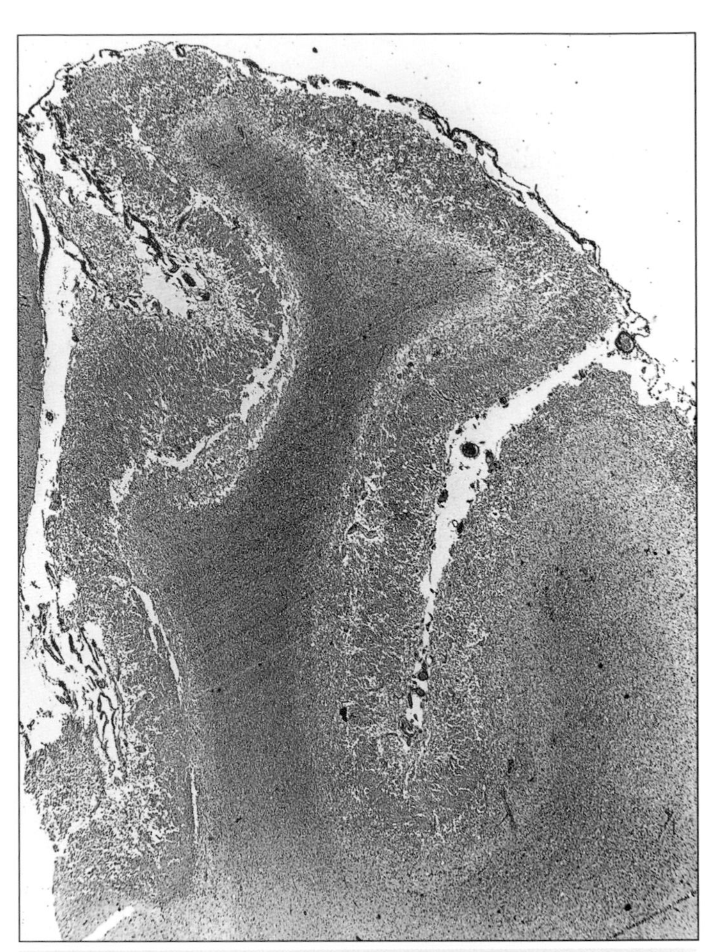

Figure 3.76 Subtotal cortical necrosis with separation in **polioencephalomalacia** in an ox.

There is *early edema and neuronal necrosis in the deepest laminae* and the edema extends to the adjacent white matter, giving the zone a pale washed-out, fibrillary appearance in sections (Fig. 3.74). There is demyelination in the edematous white matter, but the glia survive fairly well, and the astrocytes react and swell. The microglia become active and concentrate in the deep laminae, which disintegrate to cleave overlying cortical remnants from the subjacent white matter (Fig. 3.76).

The macroscopic lesions observed in the cerebellum and subcortical areas are typical foci of softening. Microscopic changes of less severity are more common. They occur in the herniated portion of the vermis and consist of acute degeneration of Purkinje cells with more or less extensive cytolysis in the granular layer.

The chronic lesions of surviving animals resemble those described earlier in ischemic infarcts. The dead tissue is removed by microglia. In zones where the gray matter has been entirely necrotic, the pia may be separated from the white matter by a clear space or be in contact with the white and partially adherent as a glial–pial scar formed by connection with the proliferated astrocytes that line the defect. Where the superficial laminae have remained intact, elongate cystic spaces lined by astrocytes remain where the necrotic parenchyma has been removed.

The areas of softening quite clearly have a distribution related to the field of supply of the middle cerebral artery. When the lesion is of restricted distribution, it is related to the periphery of the field of distribution

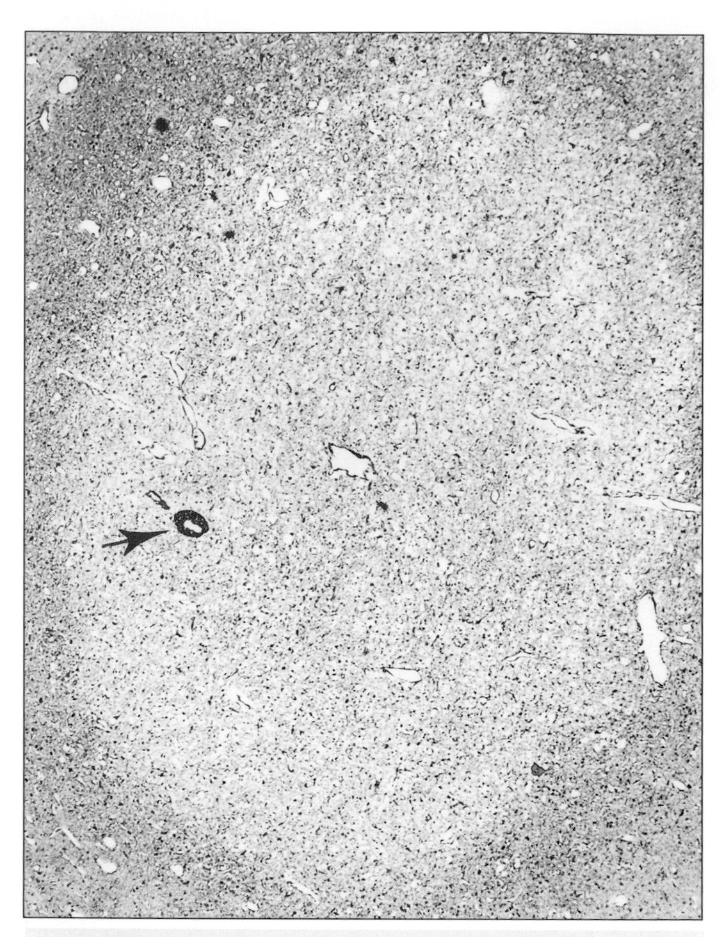

Figure 3.77 Edema in inferior colliculus with ring hemorrhage (arrow) in **polioencephalomalacia** in a sheep.

of this vessel over the dorsal cerebral cortex and, when the lesion is more extensive, it covers more of the field of supply of this vessel, but necrosis is seldom found ventral to the caudal ectosylvian fissure. The cortex rostral to the transverse sulcus and in the field of supply of the rostral cerebral artery escapes significant injury. Necrosis may be observed in the distribution area of the caudal cerebral artery, but only when the swelling and displacement is severe, a fact suggesting that necrosis in this distribution is secondary to tentorial herniation with compression of the caudal vessels against the free edge of the tentorium.

Degenerative changes in periventricular nuclei of type and distribution typical of thiamine deficiency in other species are present in some cases of PEM (Fig. 3.77) and their histologic appearances suggest that their development precedes the cortical necrosis. This observation applies also to the experimental disease produced by amprolium.

The **cause** of PEM in ruminants is often unknown, as the lesion of PEM lacks etiologic specificity. Sporadic cases and outbreaks are observed in animals given access to water after a period of deprivation suggesting that these cases may be expressions of *water deprivation–sodium ion toxicosis* developing in the manner discussed later for salt poisoning in swine. It has been observed in sheep eating the nardoo, *Marsilea drummondi*, and associated with the *thiaminase* present in that fern. The disease has been produced experimentally with analogues of thiamine with impaired activity, and by the feeding of rhizomes of bracken fern, which are known to contain thiaminase.

Deficiency of thiamine or a disturbance in its metabolism is implicated in PEM. Thiamine, if administered early, may lead to prompt clinical recovery. Calves examined early in the course of the disease may have elevated blood pyruvate, reduced blood transketolase, and reduced levels of thiamine in liver and brain. Cerebral edema and laminar necrosis have also developed in lambs and calves given the thiamine antagonist, amprolium. Thiaminolytic enzymes can be found in rumen contents in some cases of PEM, and it is accepted that they are produced as exoenzymes of some rumen microbes. Degradation of thiamine may reduce the amount available and simultaneously produce analogues of the vitamin. The thiamine-responsive disease is sporadic.

Sulfur compounds have emerged as important causes of morbidity. Sulfite, an intermediate in the reduction of sulfate, can cleave thiamine into pyrimidine and thiazole constituents thereby rendering it inactive. Diets and drinking water containing high levels of sulfates can increase the incidence of PEM in cattle, and in sheep fed diets high in sulfur. Sulfur compounds, mainly sulfur dioxide, used to color meat can precipitate a thiamine deficiency syndrome in dogs and cats. The sources of sulfur to ruminants are varied. There is a high incidence of PEM in cattle in feedlots especially when they are fed diets based on molasses, which can be high in sulfur. Inappropriate use of ammonium sulfate for urine acidification in feedlot cattle and sheep is recorded. The high incidence of the disease in animals fed sugarbeet pulp and the occasional outbreak in cattle fed thiocyanate-containing *Brassica* plants may be ascribed to high sulfur content. Groundwater in many areas has a high content of calcium sulfate. The NRC recommended dietary sulfur level for ruminants is less than 0.3%; the maximum tolerated intake is 0.4%; water sulfate concentrations >2000 ppm are associated with the occurrence of PEM. The molecular pathogenesis of sulfur-related PEM is unclear, as is its relationship to thiamine activity and to the malacic lesions in the corpus striatum not seen in thiamine-responsive disease.

Bibliography

Cebra CK, Cebra ML. Altered mentation caused by polioencephalomalacia, hypernatremia, and lead poisoning. Vet Clin North Am Food Anim Pract 2004;20:287–302.

Gould DH. Polioencephalomalacia. J Anim Sci 1998;76:309–314.

Gould DH. Update on sulfur-related polioencephalomalacia. Vet Clin North Am Food Anim Pract 2000;16:481–496.

Haydock D. Sulfur-induced polioencephalomalacia in a herd of rotationally grazed beef cattle. Can Vet J 2003;44:828–829.

Hill FI, Ebbett PC. Polioencephalomalacia in cattle in New Zealand fed chou moellier (*Brassica oleracea*). N Z Vet J 1997;45:37–39.

McAllister MM, et al. Sulphide-induced polioencephalomalacia in lambs. J Comp Pathol 1992;106:267–278.

Niles GA, et al. The relationship between sulphur, thiamine and polioencephalomalacia – A review. Bov Pract 2002;36:93–98.

Thiamine deficiency

Thiamine (vitamin B1) is a *dietary requirement of carnivores*. Herbivores are capable of synthesizing their own requirements, the synthesis being microbial and taking place in the rumen, and probably in the large intestine of horses. Experimental deficiency can be produced in calves and lambs, but only when they are very young and before they have established a useful ruminal flora; neurologic signs, including ataxia, cerebellar tremors, and convulsions, occur in these experimental deficiencies (see also Polioencephalomalacia of ruminants). Horses are poisoned by eating bracken fern and horsetail (*Equisetum arvense*), both of which plants contain a *thiaminase*. The plants are unpalatable, but poisoning may occur when they are included in pasture hays. The disease in horses is characterized by incoordination, which may be severe and lead to recumbency and bradycardia. Affected animals respond rapidly to thiamine. The nervous system has never been suitably examined for lesions.

Thiamine deficiency has been produced in most domestic species and in others. It has been an important natural disease in foxes and cats and continues to be of some importance in mink. In these carnivorous species, the deficiency is induced by a *thiamine-splitting enzyme naturally present in many species of fish*. Metabolic analogues of thiamine are known and have been used experimentally to produce the deficiency, but there are no known naturally occurring competitive analogues. Processed foods for dogs and cats can easily be made deficient in thiamine as the vitamin is susceptible to heating at 100°C or above in a medium of neutral or alkaline pH. The feeding to cats and dogs of meat that has been exposed to sulfur dioxide to preserve the fresh appearance can lead to thiamine deficiency; *thiamine is destroyed by sulfates.*

The syndrome, originally described as *Chastek paralysis*, produced by thiamine deficiency in foxes and mink is comparable to that in cats and may develop in 2–4 weeks of being fed the deficient diet. The onset of neurological signs is indicative of severe depletion of thiamine; the clinical and pathological consequences of marginal deficiency are not known. Initially, there is reluctance to eat, and drooling and anorexia may be present for up to one week before distinct clinical signs occur. Neurologic signs first consist of ataxia, incoordination, pupillary dilation, and sluggish pupillary reflexes. Convulsions are easily induced and are characterized by strong ventroflexion of the head. At this stage, animals usually respond rapidly and fully to thiamine, but there may be residual mild ataxia. After 2–3 days of neurological signs, animals pass into an irreversible phase of semicoma, opisthotonos, continual crying, and spasticity.

The *lesions of thiamine deficiency in carnivores* pass through the sequence of vacuolation of neuropil, vascular dilation, hemorrhage, and necrosis. These changes are occasionally observed in the middle laminae of the occipital and temporal cortex as poliomalacia, but *the areas of remarkable vulnerability are in the periventricular gray matter*. The periventricular lesions are always bilaterally symmetrical. The only consistency in the pattern of the lesions in the periventricular system is the involvement of the inferior colliculi (Fig. 3.78A). Next to the inferior colliculi, lesions are most commonly found in the medial vestibular, red and lateral geniculate nuclei, but they may be found in any of the periventricular nuclei. In contrast with Wernicke encephalopathy in man, with which the disease in carnivores can be compared, cats and foxes only irregularly develop hemorrhages in the mammillary bodies.

The initial morphological change is *vacuolation in nuclei of special susceptibility*. This is easiest to detect in the lateral geniculate bodies, inferior colliculi, and red nuclei (Fig. 3.78B, C, D). The vacuolation develops in cats at about the time they become susceptible to the induction of convulsions and at about the time that alterations in the permeability of the blood–brain barrier become demonstrable. This altered permeability, which may result from free-radical injury, is limited to those nuclear masses that are known to be vulnerable to injury in this deficiency. The case may not progress beyond this stage but, instead, pass to recovery. In the event of recovery, *intense astrogliosis* develops and remains to indicate the past presence of thiamine deficiency. With the development of vacuolation it is also possible to recognize vascular dilation especially affecting venules and especially in the susceptible nuclei. *Hemorrhage* occurs from both capillaries and venules, consistently in fatal cases. The hemorrhages may be large enough in the colliculi and vestibular nuclei to be visible to the naked eye (Fig. 3.78A, B).

Thiamine deficiency appears to affect most severely the relay systems from the eye and ear, but the histogenesis of the changes is vague. Phosphorylated thiamine is the coenzyme, *cocarboxylase*, and it participates probably in all oxidative decarboxylations as well as in some other metabolic transformations. It is a cofactor for transketolase, α-ketoglutarate dehydrogenase, pyruvate dehydrogenase, and branched-chain α-keto acid dehydrogenase. It may also have a function in axonal conduction and synaptic transmission. In all animals in which thiamine deficiency has been produced, the deficiency is attended by an *elevation of the pyruvate levels of blood*. This is to be anticipated from what is known of the function of the vitamin, but cannot be connected in any way to the nature of the nervous signs or the nature or distribution of the neural lesions. There is decreased glucose utilization by the brain and shortly before the development of lesions the vulnerable areas suffer a burst of metabolic activity with local production of lactate, and it is possible that the focal lesions, initially, are the result of focal lactic acidosis. The bradycardia is explainable on the basis of impaired carbohydrate metabolism because cardiac muscle depends for its energy supplies on carbohydrate, chiefly pyruvate, and in this differs from skeletal muscle. *Myocardial degeneration* is described in the experimental disease in several species and in the spontaneous disease in cats, dogs, and foxes; focal myocardial necroses are more prominent in the right than in the left ventricle.

Although it is not possible to correlate thiamine deficiency and its lesions with the distribution and activity of pyruvate decarboxylase, there is some correlation between thiamine deficiency and the distribution of transketolase activity in the nervous system. Transketolase is a thiamine pyrophosphate-dependent enzyme active in the hexose monophosphate shunt. The enzyme is active in white matter and apparently important in the metabolism of oligodendrocytes. During progressive thiamine depletion, brain transketolase activity declines before signs of the deficiency develop, and the decline is greater than for pyruvate decarboxylase. Moreover, the decline of brain transketolase is greatest in those areas in which lesions develop in rats.

The relation of transketolase deficiency to the evolution of lesions is unclear, as is the sequence of morphological changes. The spongy change appears to be a primary event, and vascular changes secondary. The hemorrhages are a terminal event. Fine-structural studies suggest that changes in vessels in selective areas of injury are secondary to degenerative changes in regional glia. The glia are edematous – swollen with clear cytoplasm – and their rupture leads to increase of extracellular spaces. Additional studies have shown early damage in the neuropil with degenerative and hypertrophic changes and axonal degeneration with preservation of neurons. Increased release of glutamate in vulnerable brain structures may result in N-methyl-D-aspartate receptor-mediated excitotoxicity; apoptotic cell death may result from increased expression of immediate early genes such as *c-fos* and *c-jun*.

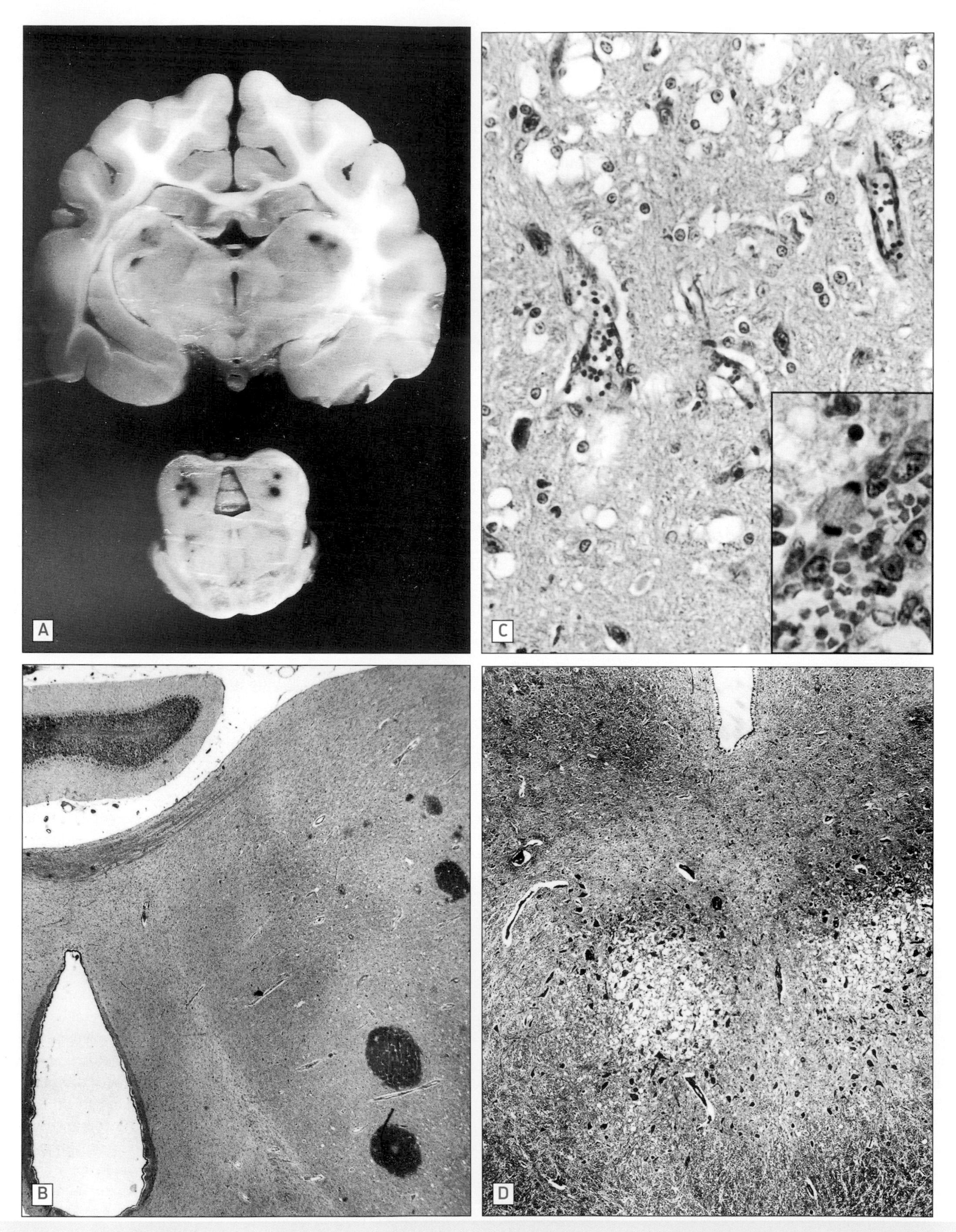

Figure 3.78 Thiamine deficiency in a cat. **A.** Hemorrhage in lateral geniculate bodies and inferior colliculi. **B.** Focal hemorrhages with edema in inferior colliculus. **C.** Edema, gliosis, and vascular reaction in inferior colliculus. Inset: mitosis in endothelial cell. **D.** Edema in oculomotor nuclei.

Bibliography

Anderson WI, Morrow LA. Thiamine deficiency encephalopathy with concurrent myocardial degeneration and polyradiculoneuropathy in a cat. Cornell Vet 1987;77:251–257.

Hazell AS, et al. Mechanisms of neuronal cell death in Wernicke's encephalopathy. Metab Brain Dis 1998;13:97–122.

Meng JS, Okeda R. Neuropathological study of the role of mast cells and histamine-positive neurons in selective vulnerability of the thalamus and inferior colliculus in thiamine-deficient encephalopathy. Neuropathol 2003;23:25–35.

Okada HM, et al. Thiamine deficiency encephalopathy in foxes and mink. Vet Pathol 1987;24:180–182.

Studdert VP, Labuc RH. Thiamine deficiency in cats and dogs associated with feeding meat preserved with sulphur dioxide. Aust Vet J 1991;68:54–57.

Nigropallidal encephalomalacia of horses

Prolonged ingestion of yellow star thistle, *Centaurea solstitialis*, or Russian knapweed, *Centaurea repens*, produces encephalomalacia in horses. It is a disease of dry summer pastures in which the thistle, which remains green, provides most of the forage. The putative neurotoxin is *repin*, a principal sesquiterpene lactone present in aerial parts. Repin appears to cause glutathione depletion, which leads to oxidative damage, mitochondrial dysfunction, and neuronal cell death.

The onset of the disease is sudden and may occur as early as 1 month after initial exposure to star thistle. The syndrome is characterized by idle drowsiness, persistent chewing movements, and difficulty in prehension, the latter apparently related to incoordination of the lips and tongue. Sensation and reflexes are normal. Death is due to starvation, dehydration, or intercurrent disease. *Malacic lesions are consistently present in the brain and affect specifically the pallidus and substantia nigra.* There is some variation of the pattern depending on whether the lesions are symmetrical or not and involve both pallidus and substantia nigra or only one of the structures. Usually both structures are symmetrically involved. The pallidal foci involve the rostral portion of the globus pallidus, are lenticular in form, and 1–1.5 cm in size. The core of necrotic tissue in the substantia nigra is ~0.5 cm in diameter and extends from about the level of the mammillary bodies to the point of emergence of the oculomotor nerve (Fig. 3.79). The affected areas are evident as slightly bulging, yellow, gelatinous foci. The softening progresses rapidly, and in about 3 weeks the lesion is sharply demarcated as a *pseudocystic cavity*. The microscopic changes are those ordinary in malacia and do not give a clue to the immediate pathogenesis.

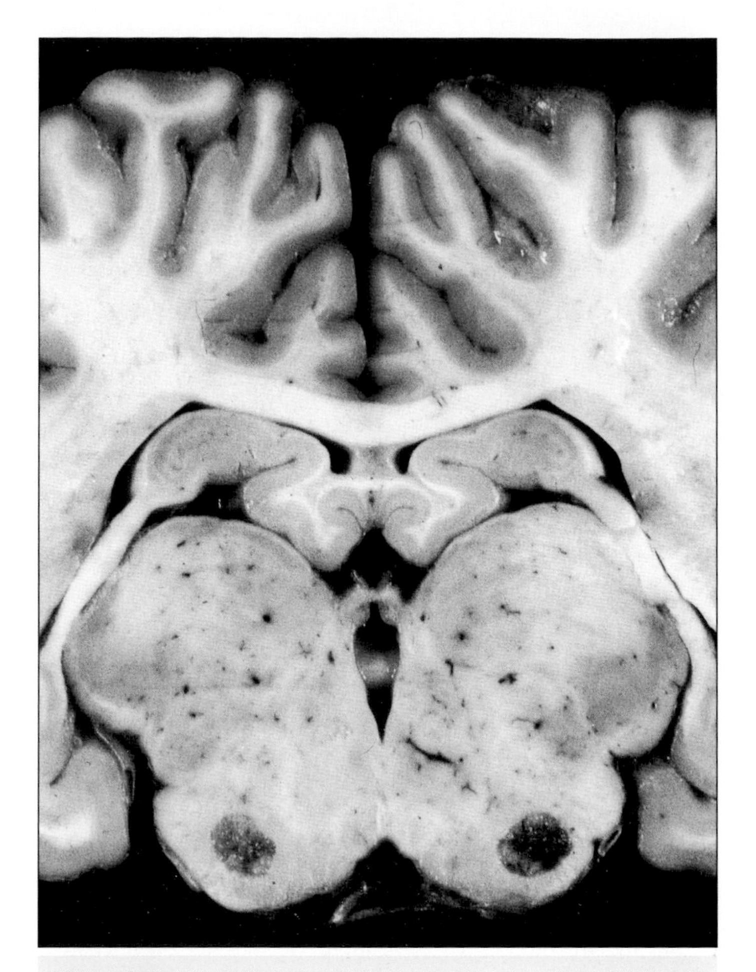

Figure 3.79 Bilaterally symmetric foci of malacia in substantia nigra in **nigropallidal encephalomalacia** in a horse.

Bibliography

Robles M, et al. Cytotoxic effects of repin, a principal sesquiterpene lactone of Russian knapweed. J Neurosci Res 1997;47:90–97.

Sanders SG, et al. Magnetic resonance imaging features of equine nigropallidal encephalomalacia. Vet Radiol Ultrasound 2001;42:291–296.

Tukov FF, et al. Characterization of the role of glutathione in repin-induced mitochondrial dysfunction, oxidative stress and dopaminergic neurotoxicity in rat pheochromocytoma (PC12) cells. Neurotoxicol 2004;25:989–999.

Salt (NaCl) poisoning

Salt poisoning may be a *direct and immediate* result of excessive ingestion of salt, or it may be *indirect and delayed*, developing only after several days of excessive salt intake and restricted water intake. These two types of salt poisoning are pathogenetically dissimilar, and neither will occur if animals are always provided with free access to water of low saline content.

Direct salt poisoning is largely a problem of salinity of drinking water. Excessive saline content of fodder is not a concern, except in terms of palatability, if an abundance of fresh water is available; for example, sheep may take rations containing up to 13% sodium chloride for prolonged periods without ill effects. This high tolerance for salt in fodder is utilized to restrict food intake during periods of scarcity and also to encourage water intake in the control of urolithiasis.

The salinity of drinking water is important, not only in terms of the concentration of sodium chloride or total salts, but also in terms of what salt and what acid radicals are present. It is difficult to provide figures for acceptable salinity of drinking water for livestock because of the variations in the proportions and concentrations of the various salts present, but the usual recommendation is that the concentration of sodium chloride or total salt should be <1.7% for sheep, <1.0% for cattle, and <0.9% for horses, and preferably not more than one half of these concentrations.

Acute, direct salt poisoning occurs chiefly in cattle, especially if they are very thirsty when first given access to saline water. Poisoning may also occur in cattle if they are given free access to salt supplements after a prolonged period of salt restriction such as occurs in cattle grazing on mountain pastures. *Clinical signs in cattle are referable to the alimentary tract and nervous system*, and include vomiting, polyuria, diarrhea, and abdominal pain with paresis, knuckling of the fetlocks, and blindness. Death may occur in 24 hours.

At autopsy, there is severe congestion of the mucosa of the abomasum and excessive, dark, fluid intestinal content. The alimentary changes are probably in large measure due to osmotic disturbances in the gut, but the neurological signs are unaccounted for. Also unexplained is the development of moderate anasarca in animals that survive for some days.

Indirect salt poisoning is a neurologic disease. There are circumstantial reasons for believing that it occurs in cattle and sheep and that it is occasionally responsible for PEM in these species, but *the disease is proven to occur only in swine*. Toxicity is related to the sodium ion; the clinical and pathological features of this disease are not duplicated in any other.

Apparent blindness and deafness initiate the clinical syndrome in indirect salt poisoning in swine. The animal is oblivious to its environment and cannot be provoked to squeal. There is head pressing suggestive of increased intracranial pressure, arching or pivoting, and these signs usually lead to the convulsive syndrome. The convulsions are very characteristic in their pattern and in the regularity of the time intervals in which they recur. They begin as tremors of the snout and rapidly extend as clonic spasms of the neck muscles with jerky opisthotonos that causes the pig to walk backwards and sit down. The animal passes into lateral recumbency and generalized clonic convulsions.

The lesions of this intoxication are restricted to the brain. There is moderate cerebral edema but no displacement. The basic changes in the brain are laminar loss of cortical neurons and laminar (middle laminae) malacia. These are the changes described earlier for PEM of cattle and sheep. The specificity of the lesion is given by the *abundance of eosinophils that are infiltrated into the meninges and Virchow–Robin spaces*. This particular lesion and its frequent relation to excessive intake of salt have been recognized for many decades, but until the cause was established, the syndrome was designated as "eosinophilic meningoencephalitis" on account of the relatively pure infiltrations of eosinophils that were found. Eosinophils tend to infiltrate in the meninges and perivascular spaces in the brains of pigs with other cerebral lesions, such as the leukomalacia of mulberry-heart disease and various encephalitides, but *the combination of laminar change and cerebral eosinophilia is pathognomonic of salt poisoning*.

The amount of salt in the diets of pigs varies considerably, but toxicity does not occur if plenty of water is available. The critical level of salt in the fodder is approximately 2% when water intake is restricted. Signs of poisoning may occur when the water supply is replenished after a period of restriction.

Although excessive intake of salt over a period of several days sets the stage, which is reflected in elevated plasma levels of sodium and chloride, the disease is precipitated by water so that it may equally well be regarded as a *form of water intoxication*. Beyond this, the pathogenesis of the lesions remains obscure. It is noteworthy that they are anoxic in character and distribution.

Bibliography

Baars AJ, et al. A case of common salt poisoning in slaughtering pigs. Tijdschr Diergeneeskd 1988;113:933–935.

Scarratt WK, et al. Water deprivation-sodium chloride intoxication in a group of feeder lambs. J Am Vet Med Assoc 1985;186:977–978.

Senturk S, Huseyin C. Salt poisoning in beef cattle. Vet Hum Toxicol 2004;46:26–27.

Mycotoxic leukoencephalomalacia of horses

A neurological syndrome occurs in horses fed moldy corn for ~1 month or longer. The neurological signs are of fairly sudden onset and consist of drowsiness, impaired vision, partial or complete pharyngeal paralysis, weakness, staggering, and a tendency to circle. The course is from a very few hours to about a month, but death usually occurs on day 2 or 3. Recovery from clinical signs apparently does not occur; chronic cases with static signs are dummies.

The mycotoxin responsible is *fumonisin B1*, a product of *Fusarium verticillioides* (*Fusarium moniliforme*) and *F. proliferatum*, which grow on corn (maize) in warm moist conditions, circumstances in which outbreaks of the disease occur. Sporadic cases occur in circumstances involving moldy fodder. The neurological disease occurs in donkeys and mules as well as in horses.

The neurological signs described in the spontaneous disease are related to the encephalomalacia, which may be due to fumonisin-induced microcirculatory damage as well as impairment of cardiovascular function. In the experimental disease and a small proportion of spontaneous cases, nervous signs may include mania rather than neurological deficit; these dramatic cases may be icteric and the nervous signs are those usual in the horse in acute hepatic failure. In natural and experimental cases, there may be *hepatic lesions* varying greatly in severity. The hepatic lesions when present are similar to those produced in other species by aflatoxin (see Vol. 2, Liver and biliary system).

The lesion usually described is *necrosis of the white matter of the cerebral hemispheres* (Fig. 3.80). The surface of the brain may be unaltered on inspection, but palpable softness may be detected in the cortex overlying large areas of leukomalacia. Grossly, there is no cerebral edema or brain swelling, although the overlying gyri might be slightly flattened and discolored. The foci of softening may be of microscopic dimensions, but usually they are readily visible on the cut surface. The softenings occur at random in the white matter of the cerebral hemispheres. They may be bilateral but are not necessarily symmetrical. The malacic foci are soft, pulpy, gray depressions distinct by virtue of

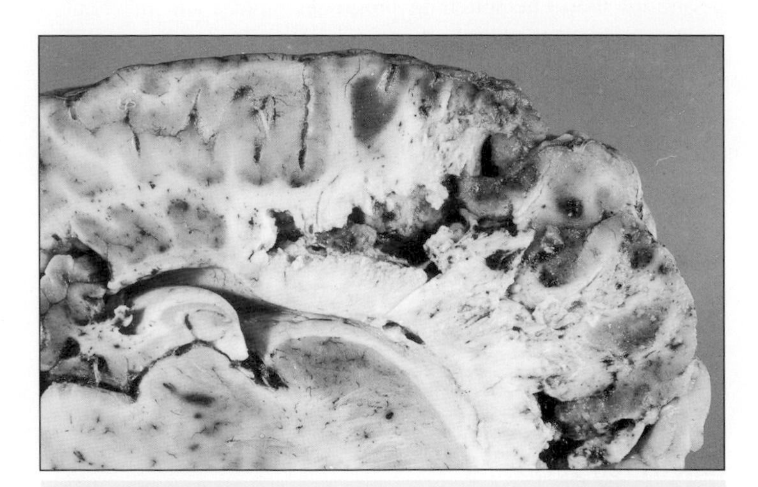

Figure 3.80 Irregular malacia and hemorrhage in cerebral hemisphere in a horse with **mycotoxic leukoencephalomalacia.** (Courtesy of TM Wilson.)

numerous small hemorrhages in a peripheral zone of a few millimeters' breadth. Depending on the duration, there may be diffuse, yellow, edematous swelling of the adjacent white matter.

In small foci, and probably initiating them all, there is severe edema of the white matter. The white matter is spread apart by fluid, and the myelin sheaths, axons, and glia disintegrate to form a structureless, acidophilic, semifluid mass to which the microglia react. The edematous change is not confined to the cerebrum but is reported to occur in all parts of the spinal cord. Foci of softening also occur in the brain stem and spinal cord, but here, in contrast with the brain, the necrosis affects the gray matter chiefly (Fig. 3.81).

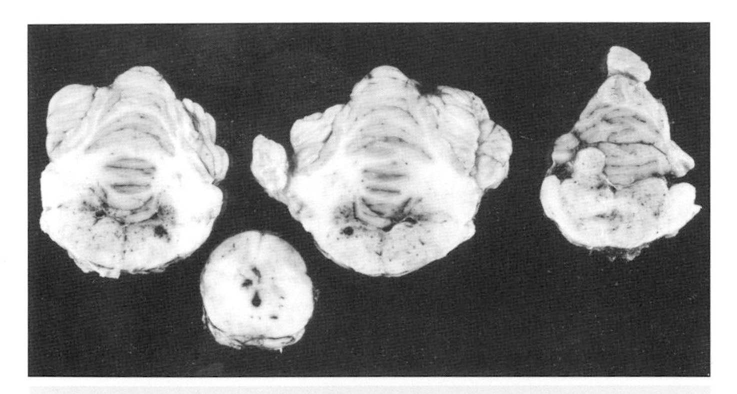

Figure 3.81 Focal hemorrhage and malacia in brain stem of a horse with **mycotoxic leukoencephalomalacia.** (Courtesy of TM Wilson.)

Microscopically, *the areas of malacia are widely distributed and irregular in their form*, mainly in the white matter but a few small foci may be seen in the cortex. The irregular cavitations tend to surround and follow the course of the blood vessels, and there is edematous separation of tissue extending from the periphery of the cavitations (Fig. 3.82A). Cellular infiltrations, mainly of eosinophils but with some plasma cells, are present in the walls of vessels, in the perivascular spaces, and lightly in the edematous parenchyma (Fig. 3.82B). The adventitia of the vessels, especially in the brain stem, may be remarkably thickened. There is abundant lipofuscin pigment in macrophages.

Bibliography

Plumlee KH, Galey FD. Neurotoxic mycotoxins: a review of fungal toxins that cause neurological disease in large animals. J Vet Intern Med 1994;8:49–54.

Ross PF, et al. Experimental equine leukoencephalomalacia, toxic hepatosis, and encephalopathy caused by corn naturally contaminated with fumonisins. J Vet Diagn Invest 1993;5:69–74.

Smith GW, et al. Cardiovascular changes associated with intravenous administration of fumonisin B1 in horses. Am J Vet Res 2002;63:538–545.

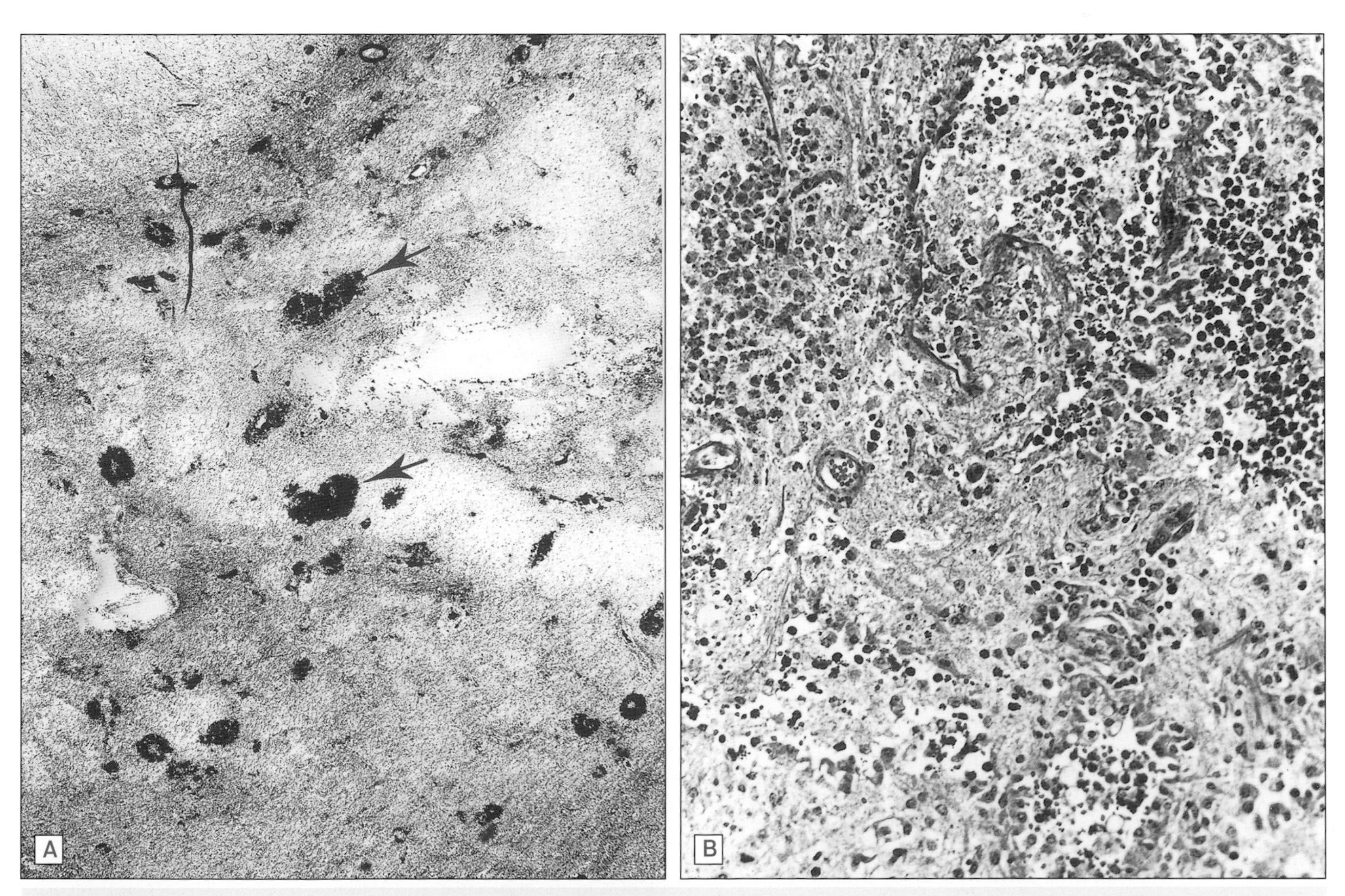

Figure 3.82 A. Malacia and hemorrhage (arrows) in a horse with **mycotoxic leukoencephalomalacia**; myelin sheath stain. (Courtesy of EW Hurst.) **B.** Vascular degeneration in malacic foci in a horse with **mycotoxic leukoencephalomalacia**. Infiltrating cells are eosinophils and hypertrophied microglia (compound granular corpuscles).

Lead poisoning

Lead is perhaps the most consistently important poison in farm animals. Poisoning is common and fatal in cattle, is less common but fatal in sheep, is occasionally observed in horses, dogs, and cats, and is rare in swine. The disease in cattle is probably always acute whereas that in horses is virtually always chronic. The signs are almost exclusively neurologic even though the amount of lead deposited in nervous tissue is relatively small.

The usual sources of lead for cattle are *paint* and *metallic lead in storage batteries*. Adult cattle are most frequently poisoned at pasture by licking paint or putty cans from rubbish dumps. Calves are usually poisoned when from boredom or allotriophagia they lick painted pens, troughs, etc. Metallic lead does not reliably produce poisoning in ruminants under experimental conditions but frequently does so naturally, perhaps because the metal, when well weathered, contains soluble salts on its surface. Lead, chronically ingested, does accumulate in the tissues of ruminants, but it is not a cumulative poison in these species. Under conditions of chronic assimilation in ruminants, large amounts of lead may be stored in tissues, including the brain, without causing lesions or clinical disease. Cows have been shown to tolerate 2 g of lead daily for as long as 2 years without apparent harm. Sheep may accumulate large amounts of lead in the course of grazing over abandoned lead-mining areas that have been converted to pasture; the severe osteoporosis that may develop cannot be attributed to the accumulated lead, but may be related to copper deficiency.

The situation in horses is largely the reverse of that in ruminants because in horses lead poisoning is usually chronic. This probably represents in part species susceptibility, but is in part due to the manner of exposure in that horses are usually poisoned by prolonged inhalation of fumes from lead smelters or by prolonged ingestion of pastures contaminated by such effluent; such pasture exposure of course also occurs in cattle. Contaminated pastures may contain as much as 100–200 mg Pb/kg foliage.

Lead poisoning may occur in circumstances additional to those cited above. Boiled linseed oil contains lead and it is occasionally mistakenly used as a laxative for animals. Dogs are occasionally poisoned by drinking gasoline that contains tetra-ethyl lead. Lead pipes may yield significant amounts of lead to soft water. Lead arsenate, widely used as an orchard spray, is commonly responsible for poisoning of cattle and sheep, but the signs and lesions refer largely to activity of the arsenate.

Lead is usually obtained by ingestion but only a small proportion of the ingested dose is absorbed, something of the order of 1–2% even of a soluble salt such as lead acetate. The limitation of absorption is due largely to formation of insoluble complexes in the alimentary tract. Absorbed lead is slowly excreted in bile, milk, and urine, and is deposited in tissues, especially in liver and kidneys in acute poisoning and in bones in chronic poisoning. The turnover of deposited lead is slow but continuous with gradual elimination in bile and urine; the half-life of lead in blood can range from months to years.

The *relative neurotropism of lead* is not well explained. Most metals exert their most deleterious effects at the sites of absorption and elimination, but lead largely spares these and affects nervous tissue with a high degree of specificity. Lead exerts toxicity by a number of mechanisms, including binding to calcium- and zinc-binding proteins, by random hydrolysis of nucleic acids, and by inducing RNA catalysis through activation of ribosomal 5S RNA, a natural leadzyme.

The various species differ in their sensitivity to lead, and the **clinical syndromes** produced also differ somewhat, although they are always chiefly neurologic. There seems to be remarkably little correlation between the doses of lead that will produce experimental poisoning and the very small amounts that induce toxicity naturally. Young animals are relatively more susceptible than adults.

The acute poisoning in *cattle* usually leads to death in 12–24 hours. Calves stagger, develop muscle tremors, and rapidly become recumbent. Convulsions are intermittent until death, and between convulsions there is opisthotonos, muscular tremors, champing of the jaws, and hyperesthesia to touch and sound. Adults show less tendency to early recumbency. In these there is frenzy, head pressing, and apparent blindness, with death in convulsions. When the poisoning is less acute, cattle may survive for 4–5 days. They are dull and apathetic, apparently blind, and without appetite. There may be drooling, intermittent grinding of teeth, and hyperesthesia, but dullness and immobility predominate. Ruminal agony is fairly constant and dark fetid feces may be passed terminally. Death occurs quietly or in convulsions or from misadventure. The manifestations of lead poisoning in sheep are similar to those of the subacute syndrome in cattle.

The disease in *horses* is paralytic. When horses ingest large amounts of lead, they develop severe depression and general paralysis, sometimes with clonic convulsions and abdominal pain. In chronic poisoning, usually known as *chronic plumbs*, the characteristic signs are those of specific nerve pareses affecting chiefly the cranial nerves and expressed particularly as laryngeal and pharyngeal paralysis. The clinical manifestations in dogs are also neurologic, but their pattern is not characteristic. There is anorexia, emaciation, mental irritability, muscular tremors, ataxia, and intermittent convulsions.

Specific **lesions** are not observed in lead poisoning in cattle. In cases that survive for 4–5 days, the ruminal contents may be foul because of immotility and the lower gut may contain a small volume of dark fetid feces, the color attributed to lead sulfide. There is no gastroenteritis and any clinical signs of colic are probably related to nervous dysfunction. There may be mild degenerative changes in the parenchymatous organs, but these cannot be attributed to lead.

There is moderate brain swelling, but probably never severe enough to cause displacement and not often severe enough to be appreciated grossly. Even microscopically, the cerebral edema is not easy to appreciate or to distinguish from early autolytic change. The capillaries and venules are congested and there may be petechial hemorrhages. The prominence of capillaries in the gray matter is due largely to congestion, but there may be some endothelial swelling and proliferation to make them more conspicuous. Neuronal changes are equivocal. In some subacute cases in which the course is prolonged for several days, there may be *laminar cortical necrosis*. The best explanations of laminar necrosis are still based on ischemia-anoxia, implying that lead is not directly neurotoxic in terms of neuronal injury. Indeed, lead tends not to accumulate in nervous tissue. The capillary alterations may therefore be of considerable functional importance and probably precede the swelling of glia. The capillary changes are best seen in thick sections stained by a Nissl stain and in the cerebellum better than in the cerebrum. In the cerebellum, the vascular lesion in the molecular and Purkinje layer is often accompanied by astro- and microgliosis.

The histological basis of the paralytic changes in lead poisoning in horses probably has the same basis as the peripheral neuropathy of chronic plumbs in man, in which the paralysis affects those muscles that are used most constantly and is due to segmental degeneration of axons and myelin in the distal parts of motor fibers. In humans, the peripheral neuropathy of lead poisoning is purely motor.

In dogs, there is edema of the white matter of the brain and cord. Degenerative changes in myelin sheaths occur almost universally but are somewhat less severe in heavily myelinated tracts such as the optic tract, corpus callosum, and peduncles than in lightly myelinated areas, such as the deep white matter of the cerebellum and cerebrum. There is spongy degeneration in the subthalamus, head of the caudate nucleus, and deep cortical laminae with extensive loss of neurons in such areas. Reaction on the part of astrocytes and microglia is slight.

Mild degenerative changes occur in the liver and kidneys of dogs chronically poisoned with lead, and can be overlooked in routine examinations. Most conspicuous is enlargement and vesiculation of the nuclei in the convoluted tubules. *Irregular, acid-fast, intranuclear inclusion bodies can be found in the renal tubules in some cases.* These inclusions are irregularly present in cases of lead poisoning, but when present, they have diagnostic value. They may develop in any species poisoned, but in dogs, they must be distinguished from the brick-like, acidophilic inclusions that can be present in the nuclei of renal tubules and hepatic cells. These inclusions are also acid-fast, but have no specificity for lead poisoning and are present in the nuclei of apparently healthy dogs. In cattle, the degree of tubular epithelial degeneration is slight in most cases, but there is often a surprising degree of mitotic activity and there may be severe nephrosis with extensive fibrosis in young calves.

The **diagnosis** of lead poisoning is necessarily chemical because lesions are either absent or nonspecific. Because of the variability of pathogenetic factors and species susceptibility discussed above, precise figures cannot be given for the concentration of lead in tissues that can be regarded as indicating lead poisoning. As little as 4–7 μg lead/g liver has been found in horses dying of chronic intoxication. In cattle, levels of lead (on a wet weight basis) of 40 μg/g or more in the kidney and 10 μg/g or more in the liver are accepted as confirmatory of lead poisoning.

Bibliography

Barciszewska MZ, et al. 5S rRNA is a leadzyme. A molecular basis for lead toxicity. J Biochem (Tokyo) 2003;133:309–315.

Knight TE, Kumar MS. Lead toxicosis in cats - a review. J Feline Med Surg 2003;5:249–255.

Lemos RA, et al. Lead poisoning in cattle grazing pasture contaminated by industrial waste. Vet Hum Toxicol 2004;46:326–328.

Marchetti C. Molecular targets of lead in brain neurotoxicity. Neurotox Res 2003;5:221–236.

Morgan RV. Lead poisoning in small companion animals: an update (1987–1992). Vet Hum Toxicol 1994;36:18–22.

Palacios H, et al. Lead poisoning of horses in the vicinity of a battery recycling plant. Sci Total Environ 2002;290:81–89.

Rumbeiha WK, et al. A retrospective study on the disappearance of blood lead in cattle with accidental lead toxicosis. J Vet Diagn Invest 2001;13:373–378.

Neurodegenerative diseases

There are some significant neurologic diseases in which dramatic clinical disturbances are not matched by equivalent morphologic alteration in nervous tissue. For instance, *toxins that interfere with synaptic function can have fatal consequences,* yet leave neurons normal in appearance to routine examination. **Botulism, tetanus**, and **strychnine toxicosis** are well-known examples. In the latter two conditions, the release of spinal motor neurons from the inhibitory influence of "Renshaw cells" (inhibitory neurons) leads to the extensor spasms and hyperesthesia that characterize them. The activity of the inhibitory neurotransmitter glycine is blocked – in the case of tetanus by pre-synaptic blockade of its release, in the case of strychnine by post-synaptic blockade of its receptors. An inborn metabolic equivalent of these poisonings is *hereditary myoclonus* of Poll Hereford calves and of Peruvian Paso horses, in which there is an absence of glycine receptors on spinal motor neurons. In the Hereford disease, the calves are born normally, but suffer severe tetanic spasms on stimulation, are unable to stand, and are nonviable.

A distinctive locomotor disturbance in Australian sheep (Coonabarabran staggers, "cathead" staggers) has been associated with grazing of the zygophyllaceous plant *Tribulus terrestris*. The clinical disease is characterized by asymmetric atrophy of pelvic limb extensor muscles, and irreversible asymmetric para- or tetraparesis without ataxia. There are no significant structural lesions in the nervous system. Evidence has been presented to suggest that the syndrome is caused by β-carboline alkaloids acting on dopaminergic upper motor neurons in the nigrostriatum. The long-term nature of the deficits may be the result of the ability of such compounds to form adducts with DNA sequences of genes associated with the synthesis of dopamine. Locomotor disturbances have also been documented in sheep and cattle grazing other zygophyllaceous plants in North America and Africa.

A large number of plant intoxications cause acute neurologic disease without morphologic alterations; **tremorgenic mycotoxicoses** are discussed below.

Inherited **spasticity syndromes** are described in cattle as "spastic paresis" and "spastic syndrome" and in Scottish Terriers as "Scotty cramp." Various inherited **myotonic syndromes** are referred to in Vol. 1, Muscle and tendon. The common **tetanic/paretic syndromes** that accompany hypocalcemia and hypomagnesemia are not associated with significant neural lesions.

This section will deal with noninflammatory diseases in which there is selective neuronal degeneration, involving either neurons in their entirety (**neuronopathies**) or restricted to axons (**axonopathies**). In reality, this division is somewhat arbitrary, as the axon is a wholly dependent part of any neuron, but the concept is useful for the classification of various diseases.

In general, when entire neurons or just their axons are lost in these circumstances, there are reactions by adjacent tissue elements but, as there is often minimal tissue loss overall, the predominant pathologic change is microscopic. At the end-stage of severe chronic diseases, macroscopic atrophy may become evident (see Cytopathology of nervous tissue).

The diseases have been grouped into *three categories of neuronopathies and axonopathies: "central," "peripheral," and "central and peripheral,"* according to the distribution of the lesions in the central and peripheral nervous systems. The choice of category for a particular disease is based on the predominant pattern of morphological change seen in a typical case, and the criteria are not absolute. There will inevitably be some overlap and the naming and lesion topography of each may not necessarily be fully justified or complete. Some of the diseases are rare, and, because they are inherited, are highlighted by research workers aiming to use them as experimental model systems. New entities are progressively being identified. Sampling of the nervous system in diseases such as these should be as comprehensive as possible. The pattern and extent of lesions are important criteria in the diagnosis of known diseases, and in the documentation of new ones.

Bibliography

Bourke CA, et al. Locomotor effects in sheep of alkaloids identified in Australian *Tribulus terrestris*. Aust Vet J 1992;69:163–165.

Gundlach AL, et al. Deficit of inhibitory glycine receptors in spinal cord from Peruvian Pasos: evidence for an equine form of inherited myoclonus. Brain Res 1993;628:263–270.

Harper PA, et al. Inherited congenital myoclonus of Poll Hereford calves: a clinical, pathological and biochemical study. Vet Rec 1986;119:59–62.

Osweiler GD. Mycotoxins. Vet Clin North Am Equine Pract 2001;17:547–566.

Pierce KD, et al. A nonsense mutation in the alpha1 subunit of the inhibitory glycine receptor associated with bovine myoclonus. Mol Cell Neurosci 2001;17:354–363.

Central neuronopathies and axonopathies

Compressive optic neuropathy

Compression of optic nerves in the optic foraminae is a well-known manifestation of vitamin A deficiency in the calf and pig due to stenosis of the foraminae. In poisoning by plants of the genera *Stypandra* and *Helichrysum* and by halogenated salicylanilides, the foraminae are of normal size.

These conditions are discussed fully under myelinopathies, but one usual feature of their pathology is *intense Wallerian degeneration of the optic nerves and tracts*, which may be due to swelling and compression of the nerves within the optic canals. The acute phase of the lesion would be expected to show severe ischemic necro-degenerative changes involving all the nervous tissue elements localized within the optic canals, with acute axonal degeneration extending along the optic nerves, through the chiasm and into the optic tracts of the midbrain. Retrobulbar segments of the optic nerves should be minimally affected. With the passage of time, the site of compression should exhibit malacic alterations, gitter-cell infiltration and astrogliosis, while the progression of Wallerian changes in the optic nerves and tracts should lead to extensive loss of myelinated axons and oligodendrocytes, with reactive astrogliosis. In the long term, retrograde degenerative changes lead to the loss of retinal ganglion cells and their axons, retinal atrophy, and gliosis.

Bibliography

van der Lugt JJ, Prozesky L. The pathology of blindness in new-born calves caused by hypovitaminosis A. Onderstepoort J Vet Res 1989;56:99–109.

Organomercurial poisoning

Mercurial compounds are cumulative poisons. The syndromes produced by the organic and inorganic salts are quite different, but the differences are probably not qualitative.

The toxicity of the organic salts depends on their solubility and the syndrome produced depends on the size and chronicity of dosage. Poisoning by inorganic salts is expected to be by ingestion, but percutaneous absorption is possible. *Poisoning by inorganic mercury is quite rare in animals.* Acute toxicity following ingestion is characterized by severe abdominal pain, vomiting, and diarrhea caused by the coagulative effect of mercury in the lining of the gut. Death may occur in a few hours. If the animal survives the initial episode, death may occur several days later from nephrosis with uremia. There may at this stage be ulcerative colitis due to the concentration of mercury in the colonic mucosa by which route it is in part eliminated. Chronic cumulative poisoning probably does not occur in animals.

Mercurialism in animals is usually caused by the organic salts, such as ethyl mercury phosphate and mercury p-toluene sulfonanilide, which are applied to seed grains for the purpose of controlling fungal diseases of the germinating plants. Toxicity may not be manifested if the treated grain is consumed for a short period only. Chronic mercurialism occurs chiefly in swine and is occasionally observed in cattle, but is most unusual in other domestic species. The manifestations are almost solely neurological. Mechanisms of organomercurial toxicity include inhibition of protein synthesis, disruption of microtubules, disturbance of neurotransmitter function, oxidative stress, and triggering of excitotoxicity mechanisms.

"*Minamata disease*" is a mercurialism of cats, birds, and man in the Minamata Bay area of Japan, associated with the eating of fish and shellfish from the bay. The fish contain large amounts of organomercurials, which probably spilled into the bay with industrial effluent. Similar environmental disease occurs in other countries.

The **clinical syndrome** of mercurialism in cattle closely resembles that of lead poisoning, but the signs, which are of sudden onset, may not occur for several weeks after the first of continuous exposures. Because degeneration of the conducting system of the heart is common, cardiac irregularities are to be expected. Signs may occur in swine as early as 15 days after being fed treated grain. There is loss of appetite, wasting, dullness, blindness, severe weakness, and incoordination, progressing rapidly until the animal can no longer stand. The dullness passes to coma, which may last for several days with intermittent episodes of clonic-tonic convulsions. Both swine and cattle may be moderately uremic.

Gross **lesions** are minimal. In both swine and cattle, the kidneys may be moderately swollen, pale, and wet, and in pigs there is often hydropericardium. Poisoned cattle have mild to moderate cerebral swelling and displacement. The cerebral cortices are soft and pale, and occasionally there is juxtasagittal venous infarction. The pallor of the cortex is visible on the cut surface so that there may be no clear distinction between gray and white matter; this change is irregular in distribution. Where the gray matter is distinct from the white, a narrow pallid band separating them may be visible. In swine, the dead white color of the cortex is often striking, especially when it is emphasized by the ischemia that may be present. The appearance of the two hemispheres may be different, that uppermost being pallid and ischemic and that of the side on which the animal is lying having congested meningeal veins. The brain is swollen and the gyri are flattened, although this is difficult to appreciate in pigs in which swelling is never severe.

Microscopically, there is *nephrosis* of mild to moderate degree usually without clear evidence of significant tubular epithelial necrosis although this is dependent on dosage. The tubular epithelium is swollen to such an extent that it may obliterate the tubular lumen. There is microscopic proteinuria. *Degeneration of the Purkinje network in the heart* is observed fairly consistently in cattle, but it may

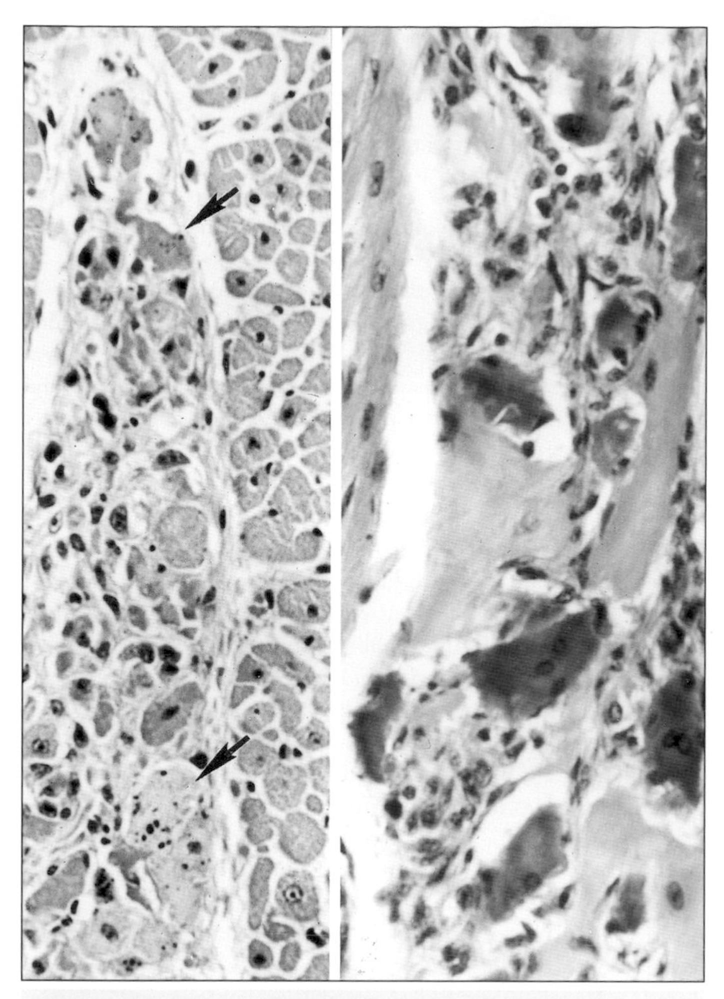

Figure 3.83 Organomercurial poisoning in an ox. Degeneration of Purkinje network in myocardium (left, arrows). Fibrosis and mineralization of Purkinje network (right).

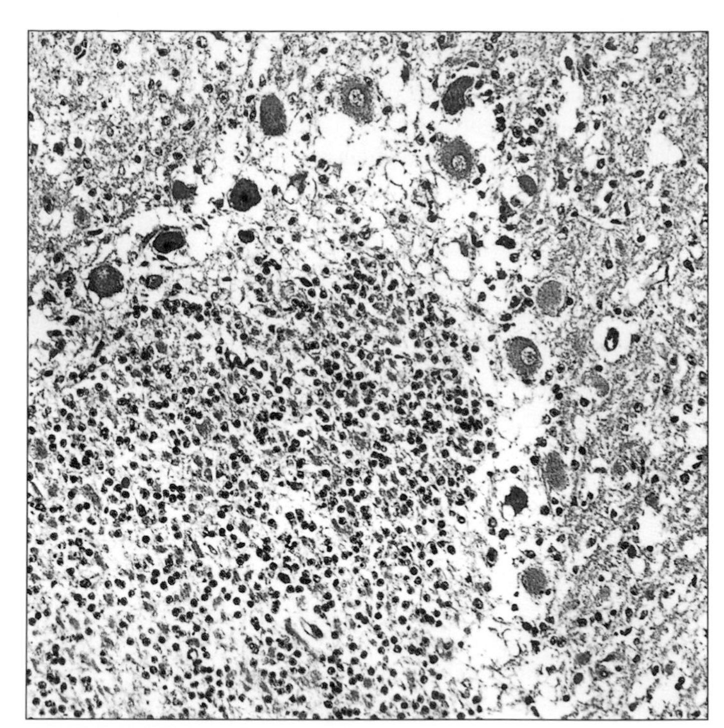

Figure 3.84 Organomercurial poisoning in an ox. Purkinje cell necrosis and degeneration in granular layer of cerebellar cortex.

not be present when the course of the toxicity is short and seems not to occur in swine. There is acidophilic, coagulative necrosis, irregularly but extensively distributed in the Purkinje network (Fig. 3.83A). The degenerate substance fragments and is removed by histiocytes and replaced by connective tissue. Mineralization is common (Fig. 3.83B). There are no clearly demonstrable degenerative changes in the myocardium.

Degenerative changes are consistently present throughout the nervous system in both cattle and swine. They differ quantitatively from case to case but are qualitatively the same. The lesions are rather more rapidly catastrophic in cattle than in swine. There is *acute neuronal degeneration*. This is of ischemic type and largely of ischemic distribution, the neurons of the middle laminae of the cerebral cortex being extensively injured. However, shrunken, acidophilic neurons can be found at all levels of the brain and cord and, with time, there is extensive cell loss from all cortical laminae. Moderate gliosis accompanies the neuronal degeneration and is expected to be most prominent in those areas of the cortical gray matter that, on gross inspection of the cut surface, are pallid. The *gliosis* is in part astrocytic and in part microglial. Compound granular corpuscles are not formed, the reactive microglia being prominently rod-shaped. There is edema in the subjacent white matter. In swine, the edema leads in time to demyelination, but in this species there is no softening. In cattle, the edema of white matter is more severe and, in the multiform layer and middle laminae, frequently produces a spongy degeneration, which may be visible grossly. This occasionally leads to laminar necrosis in cattle.

In both cattle and swine, *fibrinoid necrosis of the media of leptomeningeal arteries* is quite characteristic (see Fig. 3.56). The change probably occurs in all cases, affecting both cerebral and spinal vessels, but it is well marked in a few cases only. Swine are more prone to the vascular lesions than are cattle. Accompanying the vascular lesions, there is an outpouring of much fibrin into the meningeal spaces.

Organomercurials appear rather selectively to damage the *granule cells of the cerebellum* in all species (Fig. 3.84). Cattle are more sensitive to this degeneration than are swine. In swine, the Purkinje cells remain fairly intact, but in cattle they are often lost from about the tips of the folia. The degeneration of Purkinje cells is accompanied by microgliosis in the molecular layer and may be a response to swelling and pressure rather than a direct response to mercury.

Perhaps because the course is usually short in cattle, the spinal neurons are only mildly injured. In swine, there is often extensive ischemic necrosis of individual relay neurons. This, together with peripheral neuropathy, accounts for paralytic phenomena in swine. There is axonal degeneration and demyelination in peripheral nerves, the degenerative changes being more severe when the course is prolonged.

Bibliography

Davies TS, et al. The pathology of subacute methylmercurialism in swine. Cornell Vet 1976;66:32–55.

Herigstad RR, et al. Chronic methylmercury toxicosis in calves. J Am Vet Med Assoc 1972;160:173–182.

Sanfeliu C, et al. Neurotoxicity of organomercurial compounds. Neurotox Res 2003;5:283–305.

Solanum poisoning

Several of the many hundreds of species of the plant genus *Solanum* (family Solanaceae; nightshade family) are toxic to livestock by a variety of means. The disease of cattle in southern Africa known colloquially as *maldronksiekte* is associated with grazing *Solanum kwebense*. Affected animals show little abnormality at rest, but when moved exhibit head tilt, muscle tremors, incoordination, and convulsions.

The brain at necropsy may show gross evidence of cerebellar atrophy, uniformly affecting all lobes. Histologically there is diffuse loss of Purkinje cells, gliosis in the molecular layer, and atrophy of both molecular and granular layers. Surviving Purkinje cells are swollen, with strongly acidophilic cytoplasm, which contains numerous small "empty" vacuoles. Neurons elsewhere in the brain may show similar but far less intense vacuolation. Morphologically the vacuolation is suggestive of a lysosomal storage process and, ultrastructurally, there are membranous cytoplasmic inclusions similar to those seen in the sphingolipidoses. The nature of any stored material has not been reported to date.

Similar signs and lesions in cattle have been associated with the grazing of *S. bonariensis* in Uruguay, *S. dimidiatum* in the USA, and *S. fastigiatum* in Brazil, and in goats grazing *Solanum cinereum* in Australia.

Bibliography

Bourke CA. Cerebellar degeneration in goats grazing *Solanum cinereum* (Narrawa burr). Aust Vet J 1997;75:363.

Pienaar JG, et al. Maldronksiekte in cattle: a neuronopathy caused by *Solanum kwebense*. Onderst J Vet Res 1976;43:67–74.

Cycad poisoning

The primitive palm-like plants of this family (genera *Cycas, Zamia, Bowenia, Macrozamia*) occur in tropical and subtropical environments, and have been associated with the intoxication of both people and animals. Cycad toxicity is proposed as a cause of the amyotrophic lateral sclerosis–parkinsonism–dementia complex in humans. The seeds and young fronds of cycads contain the toxic glycosides, *cycasin* and *macrozamin*, and, following ingestion, the hepatic metabolism of the aglycone, *methylazoxymethane*, may cause neuronal apoptosis and acute zonal hepatic necrosis.

In tropical Australasia, chronic exposure of cattle is associated with a neurological syndrome known as "*Zamia staggers*." The syndrome is characterized by pelvic limb ataxia that may become severe. Pathologically there is distal axonopathy in the spinal cord. The ascending fasciculus gracilis and dorsal spinocerebellar tracts have axonal degeneration most intense in the cervical segments, while the same is true of descending ventrolateral tracts (Fig. 3.85A, B, C). Typical Wallerian changes lead eventually to loss of myelinated axons and reactive fibrous astrogliosis.

Bibliography

Albretsen JC, et al. Cycad palm toxicosis in dogs: 60 cases (1987–1997). J Am Vet Med Assoc 1998;213:99–101.

Hall WT. Cycad (zamia) poisoning in Australia. Aust Vet J 1987;64:149–151.

Shaw CA, Wilson JM. Analysis of neurological disease in four dimensions: insight from ALS-PDC epidemiology and animal models. Neurosci Biobehav Rev 2003;27:493–505.

Yasuda N, Shimizu T. Cycad poisoning in cattle in Japan–studies on spontaneous and experimental cases. J Toxicol Sci 1998;23(Suppl 2):126–128.

Tremorgenic neuromycotoxicoses

Perennial rye-grass staggers is a common mycotoxicosis in parts of Australia, New Zealand, and Europe, and is occasionally reported in the USA and southern Africa. Sheep, cattle, and horses may be affected. It occurs in the summer and autumn on dry, short pastures of *Lolium perenne*, and clinical signs appear 5–10 days following exposure. Animals develop fine head tremors and head nodding and weaving at rest and, if forced to move, have a stiff-legged, incoordinate gait, and are inclined to collapse in tetanic spasms, from which they recover quickly. There is low mortality, and total recovery will take place within 3 weeks of removal from toxic pasture. The disease is a due to indolic *lolitrems* produced by the endophytic fungus *Neotyphodium (Acremonium) lolii*. The toxins are known collectively as *tremorgens*.

There are no gross lesions in lolitrem toxicosis and microscopic change is limited to the occurrence of fusiform enlargement of the proximal axons of some cerebellar Purkinje cells. These axonal swellings are known as *torpedoes* and represent a proximal axonopathy, but their relationship to the clinical signs is unclear, and they have not been reported in any other tremorgenic diseases. The axonal lesions are best demonstrated by the use of silver staining techniques, such as the Holmes method.

Other tremorgenic neuromycotoxicoses are described in which lesions may be absent. *Claviceps paspali*, the ergot of *Paspalum*, produces tremorgenic paspalitrems that cause intoxication in cattle, occasionally in sheep and rarely in horses. Tremorgenic mycotoxin intoxication occurs in dogs from penitrem A or roquefortine produced by *Penicillium* spp. and ingested in moldy food, and in horses consuming mycotoxins in dallis grass.

Bibliography

Botha CJ, et al. A tremorgenic mycotoxicosis in cattle caused by *Paspalum distichum* (L.) infected by *Claviceps paspali*. J S Afr Vet Assoc 1996;67:36–37.

Bourke CA. The clinical differentiation of nervous and muscular locomotor disorders of sheep in Australia. Aust Vet J 1995;72:228–234.

Odriozola E, et al. Ryegrass staggers in heifers: a new mycotoxicosis in Argentina. Vet Hum Toxicol 1993;35:144–146.

Osweiler GD. Mycotoxins. Vet Clin North Am Equine Pract 2001;17:547–566.

Plumlee KH, Galey FD. Neurotoxic mycotoxins: a review of fungal toxins that cause neurological disease in large animals. J Vet Intern Med 1994;8:49–54.

Young KL, et al. Tremorgenic mycotoxin intoxication with penitrem A and roquefortine in two dogs. J Am Vet Med Assoc 2003;222:52–53.

Equine degenerative myeloencephalopathy

Equine degenerative myeloencephalopathy (EDM) is a *chronically progressive syndrome of symmetrical ataxia of unknown cause in equids* of several breeds and strains, including zebras. Predisposing factors include *vitamin E deficiency, hereditary predisposition*, inadequate exposure to green pasture, and possible exposure to wood preservatives or insecticides. A role for copper deficiency has not been substantiated. A familial hereditary pattern is recognized for Appaloosa, Standardbred, and Paso Fino horses with EDM.

The average age of horses at initial presentation is about 6 months, but may be as much as 24 months. The clinical presentation is

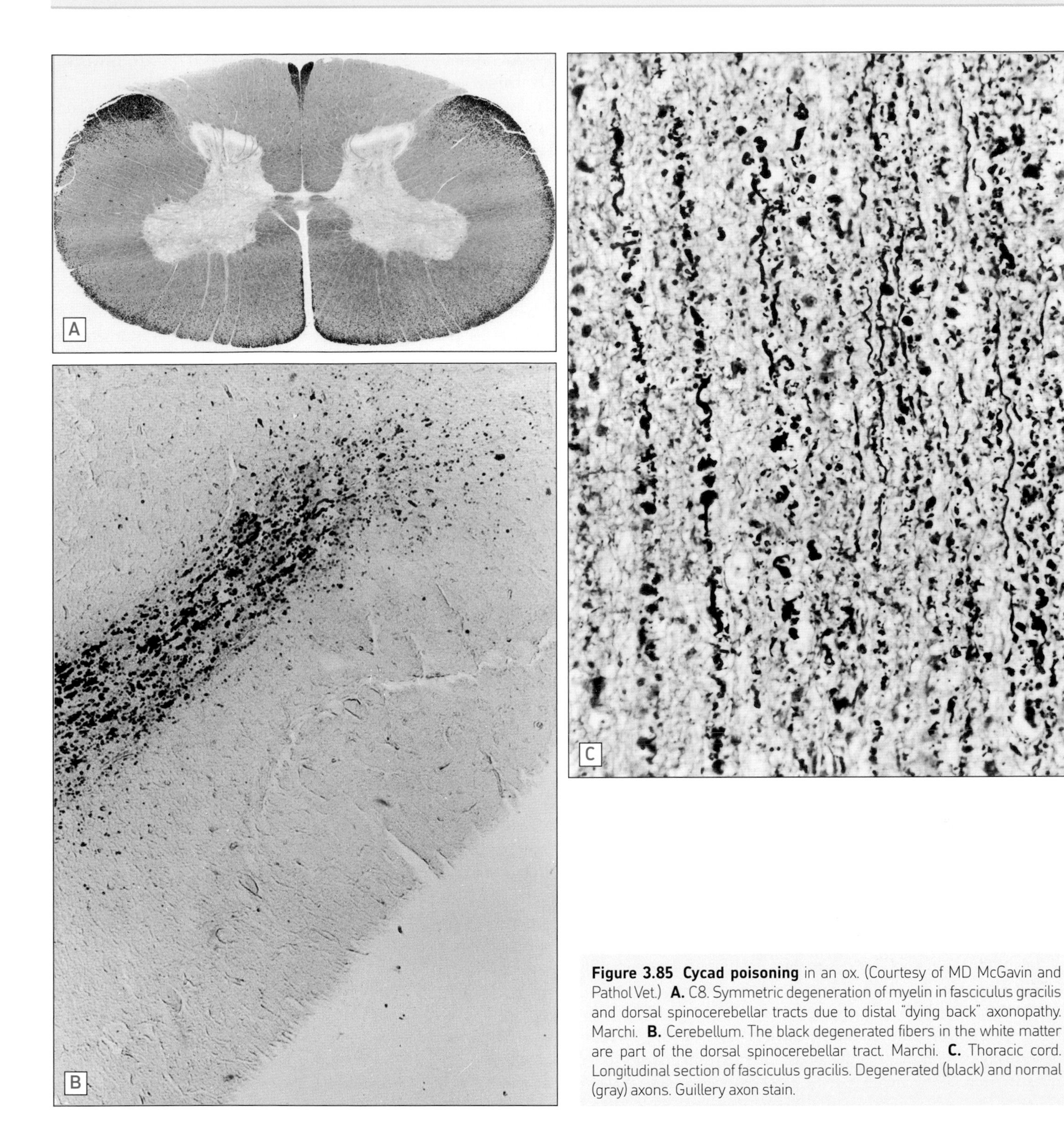

Figure 3.85 Cycad poisoning in an ox. (Courtesy of MD McGavin and Pathol Vet.) **A.** C8. Symmetric degeneration of myelin in fasciculus gracilis and dorsal spinocerebellar tracts due to distal "dying back" axonopathy. Marchi. **B.** Cerebellum. The black degenerated fibers in the white matter are part of the dorsal spinocerebellar tract. Marchi. **C.** Thoracic cord. Longitudinal section of fasciculus gracilis. Degenerated (black) and normal (gray) axons. Guillery axon stain.

dominated by disturbances of general proprioception and upper motor neuron function referable to the spinal cord, and thus closely resembles focal compressive myelopathy of the mid-cervical region. However, no skeletal or other gross lesions can be demonstrated.

Pathologically, there is evidence of *ongoing Wallerian degeneration and post-Wallerian astrogliosis in all funiculi throughout the spinal cord*, but concentrated in the ascending dorsolateral (spinocerebellar) and descending ventromedial (motor) funiculi of the cranial cervical and mid-thoracic segments. The changes are often most severe in the thoracic segments. Similar but mild changes are present in myelinated tracts of the caudal medulla and caudal cerebellar peduncles.

When well established in the thoracic cord segments, the process leads to considerable loss of myelinated axons and dense reactive astrogliosis that also involves the adjacent glia limitans. In some cases, the destructive process seems to reach an endpoint, with dense gliosis but little or no active Wallerian change. Chromatolytic and necrotic neurons, and axonal spheroids, can be found in Clarke's column (the nucleus of the dorsal spinocerebellar tract), which is located just dorsolateral and immediately adjacent to the central canal of the cord between the first thoracic and mid-lumbar segments. The disease involves total destruction of many neurons in this system, and macrophages containing a lipoidal pigment can also be found in this location. Disruption of axonal transport likely plays a crucial role in the pathogenesis of dystrophic axons in EDM.

The origin of the degenerating descending axons in the ventromedial tracts is uncertain, and there have been no reports of neuronal degeneration in the midbrain nuclei likely to be the source of these fibers. It is possible that the descending tract lesion is purely an axonopathy. Axonal spheroids and vacuoles have also been described in the lateral cuneate and gracilis nuclei of the caudal brain stem. These are the relay nuclei receiving the long ascending proprioceptive tracts of the spinal cord. However, even though this disease occurs in young horses, the changes in these nuclei may be nonspecific as they are commonly seen in a variety of situations, including animals with no overt clinical neurologic disease. In contrast to compressive cervical myelopathy (the wobbler syndrome), *there is simultaneous involvement in multiple cord segments of ascending* **and** *descending tracts*. This excludes focal compression of the cord as an etiologic factor. There is no obvious pathogenetic link between the various neuronal systems involved.

Bibliography

Cummings JF, et al. Endothelial lipopigment as an indicator of alpha-tocopherol deficiency in two equine neurodegenerative diseases. Acta Neuropathol (Berl) 1995;90:266–272.

Gandini G, et al. Equine degenerative myeloencephalopathy in five Quarter Horses: clinical and neuropathological findings. Equine Vet J 2004;36:83–85.

Miller MM, Collatos C. Equine degenerative myeloencephalopathy. Vet Clin North Am Equine Pract 1997;13:43–52.

Siso S, et al. Abnormal synaptic protein expression in two Arabian horses with equine degenerative myeloencephalopathy. Vet J 2003;166:238–243.

Axonal dystrophies

Diseases in which the pathology is characterized by axonal dystrophy, as described under cytopathology (see Figs 3.9, 3.10), have been described in sheep, horses, dogs, and cats.

One of the earliest axonal dystrophies documented occurred in **Suffolk sheep**. In this disease, described in California, lambs normal at birth develop progressive ataxia at 1–6 months of age. The lambs eventually become recumbent after a course of 10–12 weeks. It is virtually certain that the disease is inherited and appears to be a recessive trait. There are no specific gross changes, and *the diagnostic histologic lesion is the presence of numerous axonal spheroids*, in and adjacent to several gray matter areas. The consistently affected areas are as follows: the entire spinal gray matter, with spheroids in greatest numbers at the base of the dorsal horns, in Clarke's column and in the intermediolateral nuclei; the caudal brain-stem nuclei, gracilis, cuneate, accessory cuneate, inferior olivary, lateral reticular and lateral vestibular; the cerebellar roof nuclei with the exception of the dentate; and the rostral colliculi and lateral geniculate nuclei. The spheroids are the focally swollen terminations of sensory axons, and represent a genuine axonal dystrophy. The pattern of lesions indicates the involvement of two sensory systems, one visual and the other proprioceptive and possibly exteroceptive, and the clinical signs could be accounted for by perturbation of the latter.

An identical condition has been described in **Coopworth, Romney, and Perendale sheep** in New Zealand, while in Australia a disease in **Merino sheep** has been reported as an axonopathy, although the lesions described are consistent with axonal dystrophy. In this disease, as reported from localized areas of eastern Australia, sheep aged 1–4 years develop severe caudal gait abnormalities that are progressive and irreversible. Axonal spheroids are present in large numbers, predominantly in myelinated tracts in the mid- and hindbrain and throughout the spinal cord, being more abundant in the dorsal funiculi than the ventral. Wallerian changes are mild. In the brain, areas of predilection are the cerebellar peduncles, transverse pontocerebellar fibers, dorsolateral thalamic tracts, cuneate fasciculus, median longitudinal fasciculus and corticospinal tracts. Rather than being concentrated at terminal regions, the spheroids appear to be multiple along the course of individual axons. The cause remains undefined but seems likely to be a heritable defect.

In horses, neuroaxonal dystrophy is thought by some investigators to be a localized form of equine degenerative myeloencephalopathy. Affected breeds include Morgans, Haflingers, and Quarter Horses. In the **Morgan horse**, a clinical syndrome of pelvic limb dysmetria and incoordination is accompanied by intense axonal dystrophy in the accessory cuneate nuclei. Breeding experiments suggest a familial component, but no definitive inheritance pattern has been demonstrated.

In **Haflinger horses**, a report describes an ataxia syndrome first evident at about 4 months of age, with ataxia in the pelvic limbs more severe by about 2 years of age. A familial hereditary basis is proposed. Neuroaxonal dystrophy was evident as numerous spheroids in the nuclei gracilis, cuneate, solitary tract and intermediomedialis, and in Clarke's column. These changes were accompanied by astrogliosis and lipofuscin pigmentation of neurons and macrophages, and significantly reduced serum tocopherol values.

Canine diseases classified as axonal dystrophies have been described in a growing list of breeds, including Rottweilers, Collie sheepdogs, Chihuahuas, English Cocker Spaniels, Jack Russell Terriers, and Papillons.

In the **Rottweiler**, neuroaxonal dystrophy is a *familial progressive sensory ataxia*, with a pattern of occurrence suggestive of autosomal recessive inheritance. Abnormal expression of various proteins leads to severe disruption of axonal transport in dystrophic axons. Neurologic signs may be expressed before 12 months of age, often being first noticed as abnormal clumsiness. With time, there is steadily progressing ataxia and distinct hypermetria, particularly in the forelimbs, in which there is also toe-dragging and knuckling. Mild head tremor and incoordination may also become evident. By 4–6 years of age, nystagmus, crossed-extensor reflexes, and a positive Babinski sign may be present, but dogs remain alert and responsive. Strength and conscious proprioception are maintained throughout, and the signs are related mainly to a disturbance of unconscious proprioceptive input to the cerebellum.

At necropsy there may be mild patchy cerebellar atrophy, and the optic nerves appear small. The characteristic histologic feature is the presence of *massive numbers of axonal spheroids* (see Fig. 3.9A, B) in the nerve root entry zone of the dorsal horn throughout the spinal cord, in the vestibular, lateral, and medial geniculate, and sensory trigeminal nuclei, and in Rexed's laminae of the spinal cord. Fewer spheroids are present in the inferior olivary, trochlear, and oculomotor nuclei, and in the spinal cord ventral horn. Occasional spheroids are found in the globus pallidus, hippocampus, thalamus, hypothalamus, caudate nucleus, and reticular substance. In the cerebellum, lesions are concentrated in the vermis. Spheroids are present in the granular layer, white matter, and roof nuclei. There is some loss of Purkinje and granule cells.

Affected **Collie sheepdogs** have progressive ataxia and gait abnormalities first apparent at 2–4 months of age. The disease is strongly suspected to be inherited as an autosomal recessive trait. The lesions are purely microscopic and confined to the deep cerebellar and vestibular areas. Many axonal spheroids are present in the central cerebellar white matter and adjacent roof nuclei, and in the lateral vestibular nuclei. Wallerian degeneration is minimal and the cerebellar cortex unaffected.

In the **Chihuahua**, affected animals are normal until about 7 weeks of age, when there is sudden onset of tremor and gait disturbances. The pathogenesis remains undefined. Large numbers of axonal spheroids are present in the white matter of the internal capsule, cerebellum, lateral geniculate nucleus, rostrodorsal thalamus, acoustic tubercle, olivary nuclei, and the corticospinal and spinothalamic tracts.

In the **cat**, several axonal dystrophies have been reported. A GABAergic neuroaxonal dystrophy occurs in *feline Niemann–Pick disease type C*, an autosomal recessive lysosomal storage disease. An *autosomal recessive hereditary condition* has been as described in domestic shorthaired cats in association with an unusual lilac coat color. Clinical signs first become evident at 5–6 weeks of age as head bobbing. In the ensuing 8–10 weeks, there is progressively worsening ataxia, and possibly visual impairment and vestibular deficits. The process may then stabilize, and animals may survive to adulthood, but are poorly grown. Gross neuropathological change is confined to slight cerebellar atrophy, most obvious in the caudal vermis. Histologically there are numerous spheroids in the inferior olivary and lateral cuneate nuclei. Lesser numbers of spheroids are in the lateral mid-brain tegmentum, lateral and rostral ventral thalamic nuclei, and the cerebellar vermis. An additional feature is diffuse swelling of axons in the above locations and in the medial lemniscus, medial longitudinal fasciculus, central tegmental tract, and spinal nerve dorsal roots. Neuronal loss and gliosis can be found in the inferior olivary and lateral thalamic nuclei, and in the Purkinje and granule cell layers in the cerebellar vermis. Spheroids and neuronal loss are also evident in the spiral ganglion and organ of Corti in the inner ear.

Bibliography

Adams AP, et al. Neuroaxonal dystrophy in a two-year-old quarter horse filly. Can Vet J 1996;37:43–44.

Baumgartner W, et al. Neuroaxonal dystrophy associated with vitamin E deficiency in two Haflinger horses. J Comp Pathol 1990;103:113–119.

Franklin RJ, et al. Neuroaxonal dystrophy in a litter of papillon pups. J Small Anim Pract 1995;36:441–444.

Harper PAW, Morton AG. Neuroaxonal dystrophy in Merino sheep. Aust Vet J 1991;68:152–153.

Harper PAW, Healy PJ. Neurological disease associated with degenerative axonopathy of neonatal Holstein-Friesian calves. Aust Vet J 1989;66:143–149.

March PA, et al. GABAergic neuroaxonal dystrophy and other cytopathological alterations in feline Niemann-Pick disease type C. Acta Neuropathol (Berl) 1997;94:164–172.

McLellan GJ, et al. Clinical and pathological observations in English cocker spaniels with primary metabolic vitamin E deficiency and retinal pigment epithelial dystrophy. Vet Rec 2003;153:287–292.

Nuttall WD. Ovine neuroaxonal dystrophy in New Zealand. N Z Vet J 1988;36:5–7.

Resibois A, Poncelet L. Purkinje cell neuroaxonal dystrophy similar to nervous mutant mice phenotype in two sibling kittens. Acta Neuropathol (Berl) 2004;107:553–558.

Sacre BJ, et al. Neuroaxonal dystrophy in a Jack Russell terrier pup resembling human infantile neuroaxonal dystrophy. Cornell Vet 1993;83:133–142.

Siso S, et al. Juvenile neuroaxonal dystrophy in a Rottweiler: accumulation of synaptic proteins in dystrophic axons. Acta Neuropathol (Berl) 2001;102: 501–504.

Congenital axonopathy in Friesian/Holstein calves

A series of cases is described from Australia in which calves were recumbent from birth, and exhibited spastic paresis and a variety of other neurologic signs. The characteristic microscopic lesion is *active Wallerian degeneration in all funiculi throughout the spinal cord*, especially at the periphery. Similar changes are evident in the cerebellar peduncles, the median longitudinal fasciculus, spinocerebellar and rubrospinal tracts, and in the roots of cranial nerves III, V, VII, and VIII. In a few cases, mild degeneration occurs in the midbrain and some peripheral nerves. The Wallerian changes are accompanied by a very mild glial response and it is likely that the disease begins in utero shortly before birth. The pathogenesis is unknown, and an autosomal recessive trait is suspected.

Bibliography

Harper PAW, Healy PJ. Neurological disease associated with degenerative axonopathy of neonatal Holstein-Friesian calves. Aust Vet J 1989;66:143–149.

Myeloencephalopathy in Brown Swiss cattle

The first clinical sign of *bovine progressive degenerative myeloencephalopathy*, known colloquially as *weaver syndrome*, is slight ataxia, appearing at 5–8 months of age and worsening progressively over the ensuing 12–18 months. At the advanced stage, there is severe truncal ataxia and pelvic limb dysmetria, with distinct proprioceptive deficits. This terminates in recumbency with its secondary complications. The condition is inherited as a simple autosomal recessive trait; the weaver gene is closely associated with a microsatellite locus for milk production on bovine synteny group 13.

The major and primary lesion is in the spinal cord white matter. At all stages of the disease, there is *active axonal degeneration, with both axonal lysis and spheroid formation*. Axonolysis imparts an appearance of status spongiosus to affected white matter, and advanced lesions have myelin loss and moderate gliosis. The axonopathy is present in both ascending and descending tracts at all levels of the cord, but is most severe in the thoracic segment. The process may begin in the thoracic segment and extends anterograde and retrograde from this site. Ultrastructural changes indicate disturbed axoplasmic transport and subsequent axonal degeneration. Mild axonal lesions of a similar character occur in the brain stem, but are inconsistent in their location. However, a consistent additional lesion is degeneration and loss of Purkinje cells from the cerebellar cortex.

Bibliography

el Hamidi M, et al. Ultrastructural changes in Brown Swiss cattle affected with bovine progressive degenerative myeloencephalopathy (Weaver syndrome). Zentralbl Veterinarmed A 1990;37:729–736.

Georges M, et al. Microsatellite mapping of the gene causing weaver disease in cattle will allow the study of an associated quantitative trait locus. Proc Natl Acad Sci USA 1993;90:1058–1062.

Multisystem neuronal degeneration of Cocker Spaniel dogs

In this condition, reported from Switzerland, red-haired Cocker Spaniel dogs of both sexes develop slowly progressive neurologic signs from about 6 months of age. The clinical picture is dominated by behavioral changes, disorders of gait and balance, tremors, and sometimes seizures. Ultimately, the severity of signs necessitates euthanasia. The cause remains undefined, but a genetic basis seems likely.

Neuropathologic changes are bilaterally symmetrical and involve loss of neurons, predominantly in the septal nuclei, globus pallidus, subthalamic nuclei, substantia nigra, tectum, medial geniculate nuclei, and cerebellar and vestibular nuclei. The neuronal loss is accompanied by gliosis and axonal spheroids. In addition, the white matter of the fimbriae of the fornix, central cerebellum, corpus callosum, thalamic striae, and subcallosal gyri have intense gliosis, axonal spheroids, loss of myelin, and perivascular macrophages.

Bibliography

Jaggy A, Vandevelde M. Multisystem neuronal degeneration in cocker spaniels. J Vet Int Med 1988;2:117–120.

Neuronal inclusion-body disease of Japanese Brown cattle

An acute neurologic disease of Japanese Brown cattle is described from the island of Kyushu, in which there is hyperexcitability, fever, profuse sweating, and usually sudden death. The cause is unknown, but cases recorded have all been in females. Neuronal cytoplasmic inclusions have been demonstrated in the CNS of humans dying with multiple system atrophy.

There are no gross lesions of significance, but a large percentage of affected cattle have single, or sometimes multiple, *eosinophilic cytoplasmic inclusion bodies in large neurons of the midbrain, pons and medulla*. The inclusions are mostly in the axon hillock region, are oval in shape and about 18 μm in greatest diameter. Ultrastructurally, they appear as sequestrations of degenerate mitochondria, with associated aggregations of rough endoplasmic reticulum and lipofuscin bodies.

Bibliography

Fukuda T, Kishikawa M. Intraneuronal eosinophilic bodies of beef cattle (Japanese Brown). Neuropath Appl Neurobiol 1989;15:357–369.

Sugiura K, et al. Distribution of neuronal cytoplasmic inclusions in multiple system atrophy. Nagoya J Med Sci 1995;58:117–126.

Central and peripheral neuronopathies and axonopathies

Organophosphate poisoning

The toxicity of organophosphates (OPs) is based on their ability to phosphorylate and inactivate a number of esterases for which they can act as substrates. The acute inactivation of acetylcholinesterase is a well-known effect, exploited for pesticidal and anthelmintic purposes. Our concern here is with *delayed neurotoxicity* that follows 2–25 days after exposure and that involves the inactivation of esterases within neurons. Inactivation of esterases tends to be irreversible and recovery depends upon synthesis of new enzyme, and this will vary with the compound and the particular enzyme(s) inactivated. There is also wide individual and species variability in sensitivity to neurointoxication. OPs are derivatives of phosphoric, thiophosphoric, and dithiophosphoric acids, and are used not only as poisons but also in industrial applications in hydraulic systems, as high-temperature lubricants, and as plasticizers. Delayed neurotoxicity, which may be induced by OPs that have no acute effect on acetylcholinesterase, is particularly a property of the *arylphosphates*, the best known being *triorthocresyl phosphate* (TOCP).

The clinical presentation is characterized by the onset of ataxia, weakness and proprioceptive deficits, and ultimately paralysis. Severe dyspnea and loss of vocalization are often present in cattle and pigs, and hypomyelinogenesis is described in piglets and laryngeal nerve degeneration in horses given organophosphate anthelmintics.

The pathology and pathogenesis of delayed OP intoxication have been studied quite thoroughly. OPs are not cumulatively toxic, but a single threshold dose will induce central and peripheral distal axonopathy. *Multifocal degenerative changes develop in distal regions of axons*, with accumulations of organelles in the regions of proximal paranodes producing marked swellings. Axonolysis then follows and there may be cycles of attempted regeneration and further degeneration. In peripheral nerves, these changes are most intense in the intramuscular segments, and involvement of the recurrent laryngeal nerves makes *aphonia* a prominent sign in many cases. In the CNS, axonal degeneration is focused at the distal extremities of the long descending and ascending spinal tracts. The picture is dominated by axonal swellings, microcavitation, and secondary myelin loss.

Bibliography

Coppock RW, et al. A review of nonpesticide phosphate ester-induced neurotoxicity in cattle. Vet Hum Toxicol 1995;37:576–579.

Coyotillo poisoning

The coyotillo or buckthorn shrub, *Karwinskia humboldtiana*, is indigenous to the southwest USA, Mexico, and Central America, and its fruits are toxic to many species, including humans. The neurotoxin present in the fruit is *tullidinol*. Goats are most commonly affected, and intoxication is first manifested as hyperesthesia, which is followed by ataxia, gait abnormalities, and weakness, with signs developing over a couple of weeks. If the polyneuropathy is mild, recovery may occur.

Pathologically there is a *severe, predominantly motor, distal peripheral axonopathy* that appears to be the major pathological event, although there is significant segmental demyelination as well. Denervation atrophy becomes apparent in skeletal muscle. In the CNS, numerous swellings may develop in the proximal axons of cerebellar Purkinje cells, appearing in the granule cell layer and the folial white matter. Swollen axons may also be found in the lateral and ventral funiculi of the spinal cord.

Bibliography

Munoz-Martinez EJ, et al. Depression of fast axonal transport in axons demyelinated by intraneural injection of a neurotoxin from *K. humboldtiana*. Neurochem Res 1994;19:1341–1348.

Mesquite toxicosis in small ruminants

Various species of mesquite (*Prosopis*) are widespread on rangeland in the southwestern USA, Mexico, and Central and South America. Goats are more likely to be exposed given their browsing habits. Ingestion of the leaves, pods, and seeds of *Prosopis glandulosa* (honey mesquite) and *P. juliflora* (velvet mesquite) can cause mandibular tremors, tongue protrusion, drooling, dysphagia, and weight loss due to selective toxicity to cranial nerve nuclei. Histologic lesions consist of fine vacuolation of the perikaryon of neurons in the trigeminal nuclei and occasionally the oculomotor nuclei. Wallerian degeneration occurs in the mandibular and trigeminal nerves, with resultant denervation atrophy of muscles that they innervate.

Bibliography

Tabosa IM, et al. Neuronal vacuolation of the trigeminal nuclei in goats caused by ingestion of *Prosopis juliflora* pods (mesquite beans). Vet Hum Toxicol 2000;42:155–158.

Washburn KE, et al. Honey mesquite toxicosis in a goat. J Am Vet Med Assoc 2002;220:1837–1839.

Aspergillus clavatus toxicosis

An acute clinical syndrome of cattle and sheep has been reported from several countries associated with a mycotoxicosis caused by *Aspergillus clavatus.* Most outbreaks are caused by fungal growth on industrial organic waste or stored products or by plants grown in hydroponics. The fungus is known to produce a variety of toxic metabolites including patulin, kojic acid, cytochalasins, and tremorgenic mycotoxins. The toxic syndromes observed in animals are suggested to result from synergistic action of these toxins. The clinical syndrome is dominated by acute onset of drooling and ataxia that progresses to recumbency and death. The neuropathology is characterized by *acute central chromatolysis of neurons* in the red and vestibular nuclei, and in spinal ventral horn gray matter and ganglia. Wallerian degeneration and myelin edema are evident in all tracts of the spinal white matter.

Bibliography

McKenzie RA, et al. *Aspergillus clavatus* tremorgenic neurotoxicosis in cattle fed sprouted grains. Aust Vet J 2004;82:635–638.

Sabater-Vilar M, et al. Patulin produced by an *Aspergillus clavatus* isolated from feed containing malting residues associated with a lethal neurotoxicosis in cattle. Mycopathologia 2004;158:419–426.

Arsenic poisoning

Animals may be poisoned by arsenic by ingestion or percutaneous absorption, the toxic dose by the latter route being considerably less than the toxic oral dose. The commonest sources of arsenic are fluids used as insecticides and herbicides. Most arsenical dips and sprays for animals contain sodium arsenite and, after these operations, a considerable but nontoxic amount of arsenic is absorbed through the skin. Percutaneous absorption is increased if the animals are hot at dipping and kept hot afterwards, and if they are not allowed to dry quickly. Absorption is rapid through shear wounds and through hyperemic skin such as of the thighs and scrotum of rams in the breeding season. Local high concentrations of arsenic on the skin also cause local acute dermatitis.

Herbicides of most importance are those containing *sodium arsenite, lead arsenate, and arsenic pentoxide,* and poisoning occurs usually when animals get access to recently contaminated pasture. A variety of mistakes and accidents commonly expose animals to these compounds. Paris green (cupric acetoarsenite), used as poison for grasshoppers and other parasites of plants, is occasionally responsible for poisoning. Ore deposits frequently contain large amounts of arsenic, and chronic arsenical poisoning can occur when pasture and drinking water are contaminated by the exhaust from smelters.

The toxicity of arsenicals varies considerably depending on the solubility of the salt and, in the case of organic arsenicals, on the rate at which the arsenic is released from organic bondage. The syndromes of arsenic poisoning differ according to acuteness or chronicity and also according to whether the arsenic is organic or inorganic, but these latter differences are probably not qualitative. One, and perhaps the main, *mechanism of action of arsenicals is combination with, and inactivation of, sulfhydryl groups* resulting in general depression of metabolic activity. The organs most susceptible to metabolic decline are the brain, lungs, liver, kidney, and alimentary mucosa. In poisoning by inorganic arsenic, the pattern of signs and lesions is the same regardless of the route of absorption, thus indicating that, although alimentary tract signs may dominate the clinical disturbance, they are part of the systemic intoxications. In poisoning by organic arsenic, which is observed in pigs, the signs are referable entirely to the nervous system.

The ingestion of very large amounts of a soluble **inorganic arsenical** may result in death in less than 24 hours. There is profound depression and peripheral circulatory collapse; at postmortem in such cases, there are usually no lesions, or at most, slight edema of the abomasum.

With poisoning of lesser severity, 1–2 days lapse between the ingestion of arsenic and the onset of clinical signs. The onset is sudden with acute abdominal distress, nervous depression, circulatory weakness, and, after some hours, terminal diarrhea and convulsions. Some cases may survive for several days and show additional neuromuscular signs of tremor and incoordination. In chronic poisoning, the signs are nonspecific, being those of unthriftiness, capricious appetite and loss of vigor. Pregnant cows may abort. Visible mucous membranes and the muzzle may be hyperemic and inflamed.

Lesions produced by *acute poisoning by inorganic arsenicals* can be largely explained on the basis of *vascular injury*. There is splanchnic congestion with petechial hemorrhages of serous membranes. The mucosa or submucosa of the stomach or abomasum is intensely congested, and the abomasal plicae are usually thickened by edema fluid. There are intramucosal and submucosal hemorrhages of patchy distribution, and these lead quickly to more or less extensive ulceration of the stomach and intestine. The intestinal content is very fluid and may contain shreds of mucus and detritus. There is mild, usually fatty, degeneration of the parenchymatous organs, sometimes with hepatocellular necrosis and edema of the kidney. Lesions in the brain develop in the course of 3–4 days and consist of moderate diffuse cerebral edema and petechiation. The hemorrhages, which are of capillary type and apparently due to necrosis of the walls of these vessels, are distributed throughout the white matter.

The anatomical changes in *chronic arsenical poisoning* have the same distribution as in the acute poisoning. The stomach and gut remain mildly congested, edematous, and ulcerated, and there are prominent fatty changes in the heart, liver and kidneys. Neural lesions may not be found in the CNS except for those changes that are secondary to peripheral neuropathy. In both sensory and motor components of peripheral nerves, there is degeneration of myelin and axons.

The application of arsenic to the skin may cause acute and chronic dermatitis if cutaneous circulation is poor, but if the circulation is good the arsenic tends to be absorbed and to cause systemic rather than local toxicity. Dermatitis, when it develops, is characterized by intense erythema, necrosis, and sloughing; the residual ulcerative lesions are indolent.

Organoarsenical phenylarsonic acid derivatives are commonly used as feed additives for swine, for growth promotion and the control of enteric disease. Poisoning is thus largely confined to this species, and is caused by accident or careless management; however, the margin of safety can be quite low when arsanilic acid is used to control swine dysentery. Two syndromes are recognized, caused by p-aminophenylarsonic acid (**arsanilic acid**), and 3-nitro-4-hydroxyphenylarsonic acid (**3-nitro**).

In *arsanilic acid poisoning*, there is usually acute onset of cutaneous erythema, hyperesthesia, ataxia, blindness, vestibular disturbances and, terminally, muscular weakness. There are no gross neural lesions but, microscopically, mild edema of the white matter may be present in the brain and cord, and a few shrunken and degenerate neurons in the medulla. Extensive Wallerian degeneration frequently develops in the optic and peripheral nerves, but may not be present in spite of severe clinical signs.

In *3-nitro poisoning*, there is a syndrome of repeated clonic convulsive seizures following exercise, with progression to paraplegia, but no blindness. Pathologically there is Wallerian degeneration consistent with distal axonopathy in the spinal cord. The lesion is intense in the dorsal proprioceptive and spinocerebellar tracts of the cervical cord, and lateral and ventral funiculi of the caudal cord. Optic and peripheral neuropathy are mild.

Bibliography

Kennedy S, et al. Neuropathology of experimental 3-nitro-4-hydroxyphenylarsonic acid toxicosis in pigs. Vet Pathol 1986;23:454–461.

Neiger R, et al. Bovine arsenic toxicosis. J Vet Diagn Invest 2004;16:436–438.

Neonatal copper deficiency (swayback, enzootic ataxia)

It is generally accepted that maternal/fetal copper deficiency is a major factor in a characteristic neurologic disease of lambs, goat kids, and piglets. The syndrome has been most studied in the lamb, and the terms "*swayback*" and "*enzootic ataxia*," used to describe the signs shown by affected animals, are entrenched as names for the disease. The provision of adequate copper supplementation of pregnant animals at risk can effectively eliminate the disease in their offspring, and treatment of affected animals with copper may produce some remission of signs. Supplementation of unaffected lambs at risk has also been claimed to be effective in prevention. Other manifestations of copper deficiency, such as "steely wool," osteoporosis, and hypopigmentation of black wool, could be expected in affected sheep flocks.

The bioavailability of and physiologic requirement for copper are influenced by many factors, and a functional deficiency state is often determined by overall availability rather than actual copper intake. Thus there may be *absolute primary deficiency*, or *conditioned secondary deficiency*, brought about by reduced absorption from the gut, reduced availability in tissues, or enhanced excretion. The interactive roles in copper metabolism of soil and dietary molybdenum, sulfate, iron, and zinc are important. *Molybdenum* is a prime antagonist for copper and, in the presence of adequate sulfate, limits the capacity to absorb copper from the gut and the capacity to store absorbed copper in the liver. This antagonism is unique to ruminants and is provided by the formation in the rumen of *thiomolybdates*, a series of anions in which sulfur progressively substitutes for oxygen in the molybdate ion. Copper complexed to thiomolybdate forms insoluble complexes that are poorly absorbed; this is primarily an effect of maximally substituted tetrathiomolybdate; lesser substituted thiomolybdates may be absorbed and be responsible for reducing copper availability at the local tissue level.

Iron is an antagonist to copper, although the mechanism is not known. Experimental exposure of ruminants to high intakes of iron induces severe hypocupremia, but a role for iron in naturally occurring copper deficiency syndromes is not of known importance.

Copper is required for the catalytic activity of enzymes that are essential for neural function and include tyrosinase for melanin synthesis, cytochrome oxidase for electron transport in mitochondrial respiration, copper/zinc superoxide dismutase for antioxidant activity, dopamine hydroxylase for catecholamine synthesis, and ceruloplasmin for iron homeostasis. Other copper-containing enzymes, such as lysl oxidase, are important in animal disease but anomalous relationships between copper analyses and actions and the occurrence of prenatal and neonatal disease suggest that there are as yet unidentified enzymes or functions required for developing lambs and kids.

Species and breed differences, pregnancy, plant/soil relationships, fiber content of the diet, and seasonal conditions will govern nutritional requirements. Aspects of copper metabolism differ significantly between sheep and goats. It is also possible that undefined factors may bear significantly on metabolic availability. In spite of this, the copper content of CNS tissue in affected neonates tends to be consistently below normal values, and represents the most reliable tissue assay. It is also true that some individuals with similarly low copper values can be clinically normal, although this holds more for goat kids and piglets than lambs. As the ability to metabolize copper is not impaired, tissue concentrations in affected animals may return to normal fairly rapidly after dietary correction, with concentration in the liver recovering more rapidly than in the CNS.

The effects of copper deficiency on the CNS occur in utero and during early neonatal life. Despite intensive investigation, the biological role of copper in the developing nervous system remains unclarified and contentious. Copper is a component of the enzymes cytochrome oxidase and superoxide dismutase, and of the protein ceruloplasmin. Interference with the functions of these has variously been proposed as the molecular basis of the disease via suppression of mitochondrial respiration and phospholipid synthesis or via damage inflicted by superoxide radicals. It should be added that lambs with no clinical signs have been found to have neuronal degenerative lesions, and lambs with clinical signs have minimal lesions.

Clinical swayback in lambs occurs in a congenital form and a delayed form, also called "enzootic ataxia" in which, after being normal at birth, lambs suddenly develop signs at any time between 1 week and several months of age. The clinical signs are dominated by motor

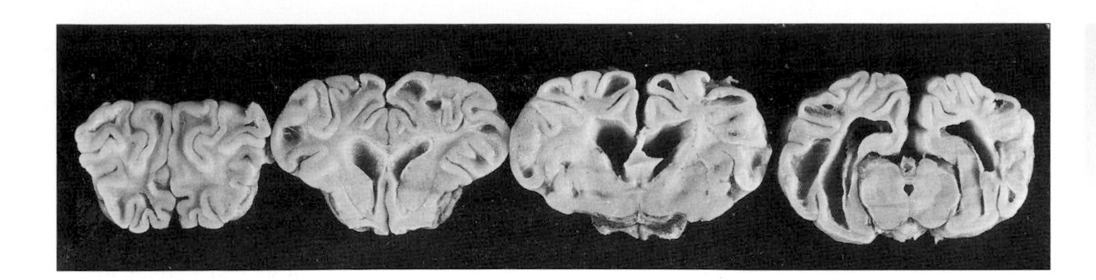

Figure 3.86 Bilaterally symmetrical cavitation of cerebral white matter in **swayback** in a lamb. (Reprinted with permission from Innes JRM, Saunders LZ. *Comparative Neuropathology*. Academic Press, New York, 1962.)

disturbances, with staggering and ataxia. Congenital cases may be blind and unable to stand.

Some lambs with *congenital swayback* have an extensive structural lesion grossly evident in the *cerebral white matter*, but all have some degree of the neuronal degenerative changes described below for the delayed disease. The former lesion is bilateral and symmetrical gelatinous softening or cavitation (Figs 3.27A, 3.86), which may be restricted to the occipital pole or may involve the entire corpus medullare, sparing only a thin rim of white matter adjacent to gray. Histologic and ultrastructural descriptions of the gelatinous lesion are meager, but marked edema with mild fibrillary astrogliosis and a paucity of myelin can be expected. Some myelin degradation products are usually present, but never in great quantity, and gitter cells are sparse. It seems likely that many axons are initially spared, but that rapid dissolution of all elements leads to cavitation. The pathogenesis of this lesion remains obscure; it seems that both hypomyelination and demyelination may be involved but the basis of the tissue lysis is unexplained.

Although lambs with *delayed swayback* do not have lytic lesions in the cerebral white matter, they consistently have changes in both gray and white matter in other parts of the neuraxis. Most investigators consider that these changes largely develop and progress after birth, but this is not absolute, as pointed out above. Extensive Wallerian degeneration is concentrated in dorsolateral and ventromedial tracts throughout the spinal cord. *The pattern of tract degeneration is suggestive of a distal axonopathy*. In addition, conspicuous degenerative changes are present in neurons in the red, lateral vestibular, medullary reticular, and dorsal spinocerebellar nuclei in Clarke's column, and in the spinal motor neurons, particularly in the intumescences (see Fig. 3.1). Many such neurons are undergoing central chromatolysis, and some have nuclear rhexis and lysis. A few may be undergoing neuronophagia. Swollen neurons have been shown by immunocytochemistry to contain masses of phosphorylated neurofilament epitopes. Sites of neuronal loss are marked by fibrous astrogliosis.

Wallerian degeneration may be apparent in ventral spinal nerve exit zones and rootlets, and in peripheral nerves (see Fig. 3.6), although this finding has not been highlighted as much as in goat kids. The pattern of axonal changes is consistent with the degenerating axons being those arising from the nuclei where neurons are also degenerate. Opinion favors the hypothesis that the lesions represent primary neuroaxonal degeneration with secondary myelin loss, although the myelin has been shown to be qualitatively abnormal and therefore theoretically unstable.

A very small number of lambs may have a *cerebellar lesion*, or *cerebrocortical necrosis*, as described below for goat kids. A further variant reported in lambs with delayed swayback is the occurrence of *acute cerebral edema* that is sometimes unilateral and involves both gray and white matter. Small gelatinous or cystic foci may be present at the corticomedullary junction. The pathogenesis is unexplained.

There is no unifying explanation for the spectrum of changes found in swayback, nor for the molecular mechanisms relating to the role of copper. It has been proposed that the spectrum reflects a critical level of copper deficiency, cytotoxic at particular times when different regions of the developing brain/spinal cord are undergoing growth spurts. It has also been suggested that the lesions reflect oxidative damage concentrated in particular vascular fields.

In **goat kids**, the clinicopathologic spectrum is similar, but has different emphasis. The great majority of reports describes delayed swayback, with a high incidence of cerebellar degeneration/dysplasia, and of peripheral motor axon degeneration. The cerebellar changes include necrosis and dystopia of Purkinje cells, depletion of internal granule cells, and Wallerian degeneration in folial white matter. The lesions tend to be multifocal and may involve vermis and hemispheres or be restricted to the vermis. In a very few cases, congenital swayback is reported in kids, and in only two individuals were cerebral gelatinous and cavitating changes found. An additional variant reported in both lambs and kids is the occurrence of diffuse cerebrocortical necrosis.

Lesions in **piglets** have the same general character in regard to Wallerian changes as described above for delayed swayback, but chromatolytic neurons are not evident. A swayback-like disease has also been documented in adult captive *red deer*, but the role of copper is uncertain.

Bibliography

Alleyne T, et al. Cytochrome-c oxidase isolated from the brain of swayback-diseased sheep displays unusual structure and uncharacteristic kinetics. Mol Chem Neuropathol. 1998;34:233–247.

Handeland K, Flaoyen A. Enzootic ataxia in a Norwegian red deer herd. Acta Vet Scand 2000;41:329–331.

Howell JM, et al. Observations on the lesions in the white matter of the spinal cord of swayback sheep. Acta Neuropath (Berl) 1969;21:33–41.

Pletcher JM, Banting LF. Copper deficiency in piglets characterized by spongy myelopathy and degenerative lesions in the great blood vessels. J S Afr Vet Assoc 1983;54:45–46.

Suttle NF. The role of comparative pathology in the study of copper and cobalt deficiencies in ruminants. J Comp Pathol 1988;99:241–258.

Waggoner DJ, et al. The role of copper in neurodegenerative disease. Neurobiol Dis 1999;6:221–230.

Wouda W, et al. Delayed swayback in goat kids, a study of 23 cases. Vet Q 1986;8:45–56.

Progressive axonopathy of Boxer dogs

This progressive disorder is inherited as an autosomal recessive trait, and begins in early life. Defects in slow axonal transport are involved in the pathogenesis of this condition; myelin lesions may then occur in response to primary axonal changes, and represent adaptive remodeling to alterations in axonal caliber and metabolism.

Clinical signs first become apparent at about 2 months of age and progress fairly rapidly until 12 or 18 months, when they may either become static or advance very slowly. The dominant clinical sign is *hindlimb ataxia*, with proprioceptive deficits, hypotonia, and areflexia often being evident.

Degenerative lesions have been described in the spinal cord, caudal brain stem, optic nerves, spinal and cranial nerves, and major autonomic nerve trunks. *Morphologic changes are most obvious in the spinal cord and caudal brain stem*, and their intensity seems to parallel the clinical progression. Axonal spheroids develop in the spinal cord and are concentrated in the ventral and ventrolateral funiculi in the cervical and thoracic segments. A few axons undergoing Wallerian degeneration are also evident, but are always in a minority. Myelin sheaths are thinned around the spheroids, as would be expected, but attenuated sheaths may also occur around axonal segments not obviously swollen. Vacuolation of myelin segments is also a feature. These white matter changes have no obvious tract distribution. In the gray matter, spheroids are found in many nuclei of the caudal brain stem, and to a small extent in the spinal cord. However, from the diencephalon forward, there are virtually no gray matter lesions. Axonal swellings and myelin vacuolation are prominent in the optic nerves in the area of the chiasm.

In spinal nerve roots, there are, early in the disease, focal axonal swellings and a range of myelin abnormalities, including vacuolation, thinning, and segmental loss. With time, the involvement of ventral roots is appreciably more severe than dorsal roots. As the disease advances, such changes progress distally down the nerves, but axonal degeneration is accompanied by regeneration, and denervation of muscle is not significant. Changes of a similar character have been described in cranial nerves and large autonomic trunks.

Bibliography

Griffiths IR, et al. Progressive axonopathy: an inherited neuropathy of boxer dogs. An immunocytochemical study of the axonal cytoskeleton. Neuropathol Appl Neurobiol 1989;15:63–74.

Degenerative radiculomyelopathy of German Shepherds and other dogs

This idiopathic condition is a slowly progressive, irreversible, adult-onset disease, characterized by paraparesis and truncal ataxia. The condition is not completely defined, but may be hereditary, and the neurodegeneration appears to have an immune-mediated component. Vitamin E deficiency seems unlikely to be involved.

Some studies describe lesions in spinal nerve roots and cord, whereas others restrict changes to the cord; secondary degenerative changes have been noted in brain nuclei. In about 10–15% of cases, there is loss of patellar reflexes and degeneration in femoral nerves. Arguments have been advanced for and against a distal dying-back type of pathogenesis, and the affliction of dogs of large breeds other than the German Shepherd.

Axonal degeneration and evidence of demyelination are present in the spinal cord and probably, on occasion, in the spinal nerves. While there have been descriptions of symmetrical degenerative changes at the distal extremities of long tracts in the cord, a separate study documented myelin vacuolation, myelin deficiency, a few spheroids and some Wallerian degeneration, distributed randomly and asymmetrically, and most intense in the thoracic segments.

Bibliography

Barclay KB, Haines DM. Immunohistochemical evidence for immunoglobulin and complement deposition in spinal cord lesions in degenerative myelopathy in German shepherd dogs. Can J Vet Res 1994;58:20–24.

Fechner H, et al. Molecular genetic and expression analysis of alpha-tocopherol transfer protein mRNA in German shepherd dogs with degenerative myelopathy. Berl Munch Tierarztl Wochenschr 2003;116:31–36.

Johnston PE, et al. Central nervous system pathology in 25 dogs with chronic degenerative radiculomyelopathy. Vet Rec 2000;146:629–633.

Giant axonal neuropathy of the German Shepherd Dog

This uncommon disease is a *distal axonopathy* in which disorderly clumps of neurofilaments accumulate towards the extremities of long axons, and their most distal regions eventually degenerate completely. The *neurofilamentous accumulations create the very large argentophilic axonal swellings* that give the disease its name.

The clinical onset is at about 15 months of age and there is progression to paraparesis, ataxia, and megaesophagus within a few months. The disease is apparently inherited in an autosomal recessive manner.

In the CNS, the giant swellings are found in the rostral regions of the ascending fasciculus gracilis and the dorsal spinocerebellar tracts, and in the caudal regions of the descending lateral corticospinal tracts. In the peripheral nervous system, they are found in both myelinated and unmyelinated large fibers in the more distal regions of the major nerves of the limbs and the recurrent laryngeal nerves. Small focal axonal swellings are also scattered through various regions of the brain from the cerebral cortex back to the caudal brain stem, and on to the dorsal and intermediate gray columns of the cord. Some Wallerian changes accompany the small swellings in these areas.

Bibliography

Duncan ID, Griffiths IR. Canine giant axonal neuropathy: some aspects of its clinical, pathological and comparative features. J Small Anim Pract 1981;22:491–501.

King RH, et al. Axonal neurofilamentous accumulations: a comparison between human and canine giant axonal neuropathy and 2,5-HD neuropathy. Neuropathol Appl Neurobiol 1993;19:224–232.

Progressive motor neuron diseases

There is a group of neurodegenerative diseases, described in several species, which have a common clinical and pathological theme, and which can therefore be dealt with together. They appear to have as a counterpart *amyotrophic lateral sclerosis in humans*. Diseases with this basic theme have been described in Brittany Spaniels, Swedish Lapland Dogs, Rottweiler dogs, domestic shorthaired cats, various breeds of horses, Yorkshire and Hampshire pigs, and in Brown Swiss, Danish Red, Piedmont, and Holstein-Friesian calves.

The clinical presentation in **horses** is dominated by progressive lower motor neuron paralysis which usually ends in tetraplegia and muscle atrophy. There is preferential damage to type 1, high-oxidative fibers, reflected in wastage especially of postural muscles. The pathological findings are dominated by denervation atrophy of pelvic and pectoral muscle groups, and by regressive changes in spinal motor neurons. Other neurons in the motor hierarchy may be afflicted, including the pyramidal cells of the motor cortex. In some instances, neurons in the brain stem and peripheral ganglia are also involved. In the earlier stages of neuronal degeneration, there may be chromatolytic swelling of the soma, with reduced basophilia, and fading of the nucleus, which tends to remain centrally located. In many of the diseases, the swollen cell bodies are often crowded with neurofilaments. Eosinophilic inclusions may be present in the cytoplasm, usually representing clustered remnants of normal organelles trapped amongst arrays of neurofilaments (see Fig. 3.4). In some cases, these inclusions may be found to have the characteristics of Hirano, Lewy, or Bunina bodies described in human neuropathology. The neuronopathy progresses eventually to neuronal death on a cell-by-cell basis, with individual neurons in different stages of the process at any one time. Ultimately there may be considerable neuronal loss, with residual gliosis, and Wallerian change in motor nerves and spinal white matter.

These diseases are considered to be primary metabolic dysfunctions of the nerve cell body; most have an apparently *genetic basis* and an early-age onset. Hereditary spinal muscular atrophy in calves may result from a defect in the survival motor neuron gene. A series of horses is reported from the northeast United States in which the epidemiology strongly suggests an environmental cause. Horses particularly at risk are those that for long periods do not have access to green pasture. Vitamin E status is deficient, which suggests that the lesion is a result of *free radical injury*. The presence of lipofuscin pigments in vascular endothelium and in the retinal pigment epithelium in some affected horses supports the concept of *vitamin E deficiency*. It should be noted also that the neuronal lesions in congenital copper deficiency have many of these features (see Fig. 3.1). Variations on the basic theme are provided in terms of the age of onset and speed of progression of signs, the extent and pattern of frank neuronal degeneration, involvement of nuclei in the mid- and hindbrain, and the presence of Wallerian degeneration in the spinal white matter and peripheral nerves.

Probably the most comprehensively described condition is **hereditary spinal muscular atrophy of Brittany Spaniels**, and it will serve as a generic example. In the Spaniels, there is *autosomal dominant* inheritance and three phenotypic variants: chronic, intermediate, and accelerated. The latter leads to quadriplegia at about 3 months of age, the others over several years, if at all. At the end-stage, there is pronounced denervation atrophy of pectoral and pelvic muscle groups, as well as of the tongue and masseter muscles.

The neuropathology is marked by degenerative change in spinal motor neurons, focused in the intumescences, with similar involvement of the hypoglossal and trigeminal motor nuclei. Particularly in the accelerated, homozygous variant, there are numerous pale, swollen, and chromatolytic motor neurons, with occasional cells undergoing fragmentation and necrosis. Swollen neurons are depleted of ribosomes and a few are packed with neurofilaments (Fig. 3.87). Most characteristically, large argentophilic swellings are present in the proximal segments of many axons close to the affected cell bodies. These have been shown by electron microscopy to be *tangles of disorganized neurofilaments* (Fig. 3.88A). All these changes are much less evident in the more chronic, heterozygous, forms of the disease and clinical weakness is only mild in many cases. Although it is established that there is a defect in the metabolism of neurofilaments as they move from the cell body into the proximal axon of individual neurons, it is not yet clear that this is the primary molecular lesion. Recent studies have shown that there is growth arrest of spinal motor neurons and, initially, affected pups have a greater than normal number of these cells, with a shift to a smaller cell size. Ventral root axons undergo atrophy, which may be followed by loss of entire neurons.

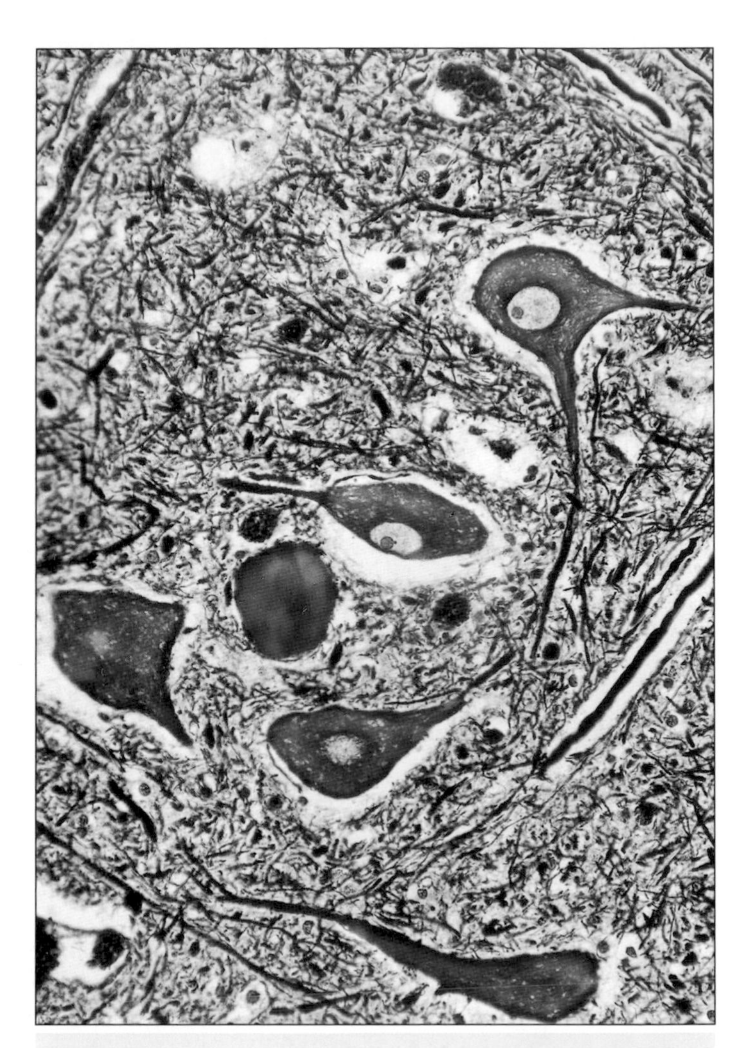

Figure 3.87 Proximal axonal swelling packed with neurofilaments in a spinal motor neuron of a Brittany Spaniel with **motor neuron disease**; silver impregnation. (Courtesy of LC Cork.)

In the **Swedish Lapland Dog**, the pattern of lesions is different, there being degeneration of spinal motor neurons only in the lateral aspects of the intumescences; neuronal degeneration also occurs in spinal ganglia and cerebellar Purkinje cells, but not in brain stem nuclei. The disease has been termed *neuronal abiotrophy*, and is included here because of the dominance of denervation atrophy of muscle in the clinical presentation. The atrophy is concentrated in the more distal muscle groups of the limbs, in keeping with the topography of degenerate spinal motor neurons. Any cerebellar deficits are probably over-ridden by the lower motor neuron impairment.

In the **English Pointer** dog, a strikingly different motor neuron disease has been described in which weakness and muscle atrophy become obvious at about 5 months of age and severe by about 9 months. There is correspondingly severe distal degeneration of peripheral motor nerves and denervation of muscle. However, rather than the changes described above, spinal motor neurons are

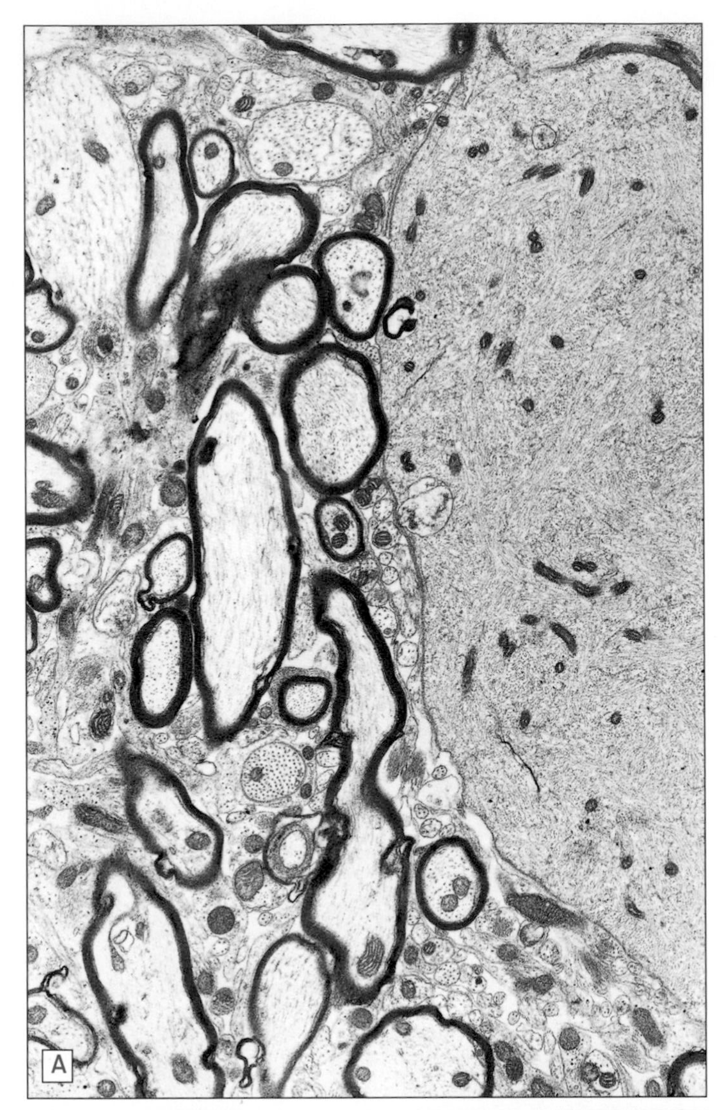

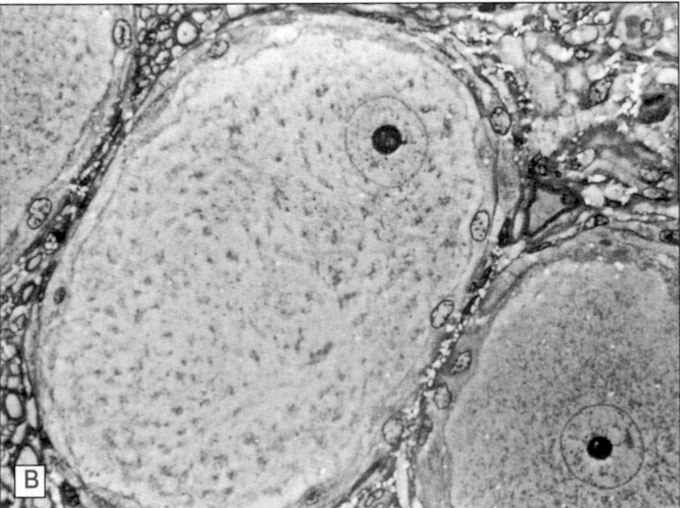

Figure 3.88 A. Proximal axonal swelling packed with neurofilaments in a spinal motor neuron of a Brittany Spaniel with **motor neuron disease**. (Courtesy of LC Cork.) **B.** Swollen neuron in a spinal ganglion of a "**shaker calf**"; Nissl substance is dispersed by neurofilamentous masses. (Courtesy of CG Rousseaux.)

filled with *cytoplasmic lipid inclusions* reminiscent of those seen in the gangliosidoses and mucopolysaccharidoses, and in some drug-induced conditions. No significant loss of motor neurons is apparent, and similar inclusions are present in the hypoglossal and spinal accessory nuclei, but not elsewhere.

Focal, asymmetrical spinal motor neuron degeneration with acute onset and a rapid course is described in **German Shepherd** pups. The affected neurons are within the cervical spinal cord intumescence, and exhibit peripheral chromatolysis or vacuolation. There is secondary denervation and wasting of forearm muscles. Progressive lower motor neuron disease has also been reported in **Saluki** and **Griffon Briquet Vendeen** pups.

Bibliography

Braund KG. Degenerative causes of neuropathies in dogs and cats. Vet Med 1996;91:722–739.

Carrasco DI, et al. Activity-driven synaptic and axonal degeneration in canine motor neuron disease. J Neurophysiol 2004;92:1175–1181.

Green SL, et al. Canine motor neuron disease: clinicopathologic features and selected indicators of oxidative stress. J Vet Intern Med 2001;15:112–119.

Inada S, et al. Canine storage disease characterized by hereditary progressive neurogenic muscular atrophy: breeding experiments and clinical manifestation. Am J Vet Res 1986;47:2294–2299.

Izumo S, et al. Morphological study on the hereditary neurogenic amyotrophic dogs: accumulation of lipid compound-like structures in the lower motor neuron. Acta Neuropathol (Berl) 1983;61:270–274.

Kent M, et al. Motor neuron abiotrophy in a saluki. J Am Anim Hosp Assoc 1999;35:436–439.

Longeri M, et al. Survival motor neuron (SMN) polymorphism in relation to congenital arthrogryposis in two Piedmont calves (piemontese). Genet Sel Evol 2003;35(Suppl 1):S167–175.

Mandara MT, Di Meo A. Lower motor neuron disease in the Griffon Briquet Vendeen dog. Vet Pathol 1998;35:412–414.

Polack EW, et al. Concentrations of trace minerals in the spinal cord of horses with equine motor neuron disease. Am J Vet Res 2000;61:609–611.

Verhulst D, et al. Equine motor neuron disease and retinal degeneration. Equine Vet Educ 2001;13:59–61.

Neurodegeneration of horned Hereford calves

The term "**shaker calf**" refers to a disease in which newborn horned Hereford calves are unable to stand without assistance and develop generalized fine tremors and profound muscular weakness. While they often die in the neonatal period because of secondary complications, some, after a short period of apparent remission, show relentlessly progressive spastic paraparesis, but remain alert and may survive for some months. The disease is presumed to be inherited on the basis of pedigree analysis. The fundamental metabolic defect remains to be characterized.

The pathology is characterized by dramatic swelling of the cell bodies and processes of neurons throughout the spinal cord. Swelling is due to the *accumulation of masses of neurofilaments* that impart a faintly fibrillar, amphophilic appearance in routine sections. This lesion involves ventral horn motor neurons, sensory neurons of the substantia gelatinosa, Clarke's column, and the intermediolateral (sympathetic) nuclei. Neuronal necrosis is minimal, although the site of occasional cell loss can be found as nodules of reactive glia. Some

Wallerian degeneration is evident in ventral spinal nerve roots and the ventromedial spinal white matter.

The neuronal lesion is also present in the major motor nuclei of the brain stem, the reticular formation and the cerebellar Purkinje cells, and to a slight degree in the lateral geniculate nucleus and layer 5 of the frontal cortex. Some affected cells are evident in peripheral ganglia (Fig. 3.88B), including the myenteric plexus, and in the retinal ganglion cells.

Bibliography

Rousseaux CG, et al. "Shaker" calf syndrome: a newly recognised inherited neurodegenerative disorder of horned Hereford calves. Vet Pathol 1985;22:104–111.

Sillevis Smitt PA, de Jong JM. Animal models of amyotrophic lateral sclerosis and the spinal muscular atrophies. J Neurol Sci 1989;91:231–258.

Neuropathy in Gelbvieh calves

A familial, and likely hereditary, condition has been reported in Gelbvieh calves that had developed hindlimb ataxia and paresis, and were found histologically to have peripheral neuropathy and proliferative glomerulopathy; skeletal muscle degeneration was prominent in some cases. Degeneration was severe in peripheral nerves, dorsal and ventral spinal nerve roots, and less marked in dorsal fasciculi of the spinal cord.

Bibliography

Moisan PG, et al. A familial degenerative neuromuscular disease of Gelbvieh cattle. J Vet Diagn Invest 2002;14:140–149.

Panciera RJ, et al. A familial peripheral neuropathy and glomerulopathy in Gelbvieh calves. Vet Pathol 2003;40:63–70.

Progressive neuronopathy of the Cairn Terrier

Progressive neuronopathy occurs only in Cairn Terriers and is suspected to be inherited. This multisystem chromatolytic degeneration clinically resembles globoid cell leukodystrophy, from which it can be differentiated clinically by the exercise-induced deterioration of neurological signs in progressive neuronopathy. Animals of both sexes develop hindlimb weakness, tetraparesis, ataxia, head tremor, and loss of reflexes between 5 and 7 months of age.

Both central and peripheral chromatolysis of neurons are evident, and occur in Clarke's column and dorsal and ventral horn cells in the spinal cord, in sensory ganglia, and in the cuneate, lateral cuneate, glossopharyngeal, vagus, reticular, lateral vestibular, mesencephalic trigeminal, red and cerebellar roof nuclei. Wallerian degeneration is present in lateral and ventral funiculi of the cord, to various degrees, and also in dorsal and ventral spinal nerve roots.

Ultrastructural studies on one case suggested that the chromatolytic change was associated with depletion of ribosomes and increased numbers of mitochondria in perikarya, and that Wallerian degeneration was probably secondary to the metabolic disturbance in the cell body. This case was also marked by onset of signs at 11 weeks of age, bouts of cataplectic collapse, and thoracolumbar myelomalacia.

Bibliography

Cummings J, et al. Multisystemic chromatolytic neuronal degeneration in Cairn terriers. J Vet Int Med 1991;5:91–94.

Zaal MD, et al. Progressive neuronopathy in two Cairn terrier litter mates. Vet Q 1997;19:34–36.

Primary hyperoxaluria in the cat

In this inherited metabolic disorder in cats, profound deficiency in the activity of D-glycerate dehydrogenase is associated with L-glyceric aciduria, hyperoxaluria and the heavy deposition of oxalate crystals in the renal tubules. This leads to *oxalate nephrosis* and renal failure before a year of age.

An accompanying neuronal lesion occurs in the form of large swellings in the proximal axons of spinal motor neurons, ventral roots, intramuscular nerves, and the dorsal root ganglia. These swellings are caused by *neurofilamentous accumulations*, and are accompanied by some Wallerian degeneration in peripheral nerves. There is no obvious metabolic link between the neuronal lesions and the other biochemical disturbances, and the syndrome may represent a dual genetic defect.

Bibliography

McKerrel RE. Primary hyperoxaluria (L-glyceric aciduria) in the cat: a newly recognized inherited disease. Vet Rec 1989;125:31–34.

The dysautonomias

The term dysautonomia denotes a profound failure of both sympathetic and parasympathetic functions across several organ systems. Domestic animals affected include horses (**equine grass sickness**), cats (**Key–Gaskell syndrome**), and dogs. *Clostridium botulinum* is thought to play a role in equine dysautonomia and perhaps in the feline syndrome, which may hence be toxico-infectious forms of botulism.

Particularly in the cat, it is considered that there is a single episode of injury to neurons, with acute degeneration and subsequent reparative reactions if the animal survives for a number of weeks. There is a good correlation between the clinical signs and the extensive destruction in autonomic ganglia, and *autonomic denervation would account for the major functional disturbances*. The occasional expression of mild proprioceptive and lower motor neuron deficits may be explained by the lesions in dorsal root ganglia and spinal motor neurons respectively.

In the equine disease, the clinical picture is primarily the result of neurogenic obstruction of the alimentary tract with various parts of the tract involved to differing degrees, with distinct acute, subacute, and chronic forms. Clinical differential diagnosis can be exceedingly difficult. The outcome is usually fatal; some chronic cases may recover with intensive care.

In the cat, there is acute onset of clinical disease that in a few cases may resolve after many months, but many animals die or require euthanasia early in the course. Onset is marked by dilated pupils, prolapsed nictitating membrane, dry mucous membranes, megaesophagus, constipation, vomiting, and dehydration. In the dog, the most severe and consistent loss of autonomic neurons occurs in the pelvic, mesenteric, and ciliary ganglia. Minimal changes are reported in the CNS. Differential diagnoses in dogs include ganglioradiculitis (sensory neuronopathy).

In the acute phase, *extensive chromatolysis and death of ganglion cells* is present throughout the peripheral autonomic ganglia (Fig. 3.89), with axonal degeneration in autonomic nerve fibers. There is also neuronal

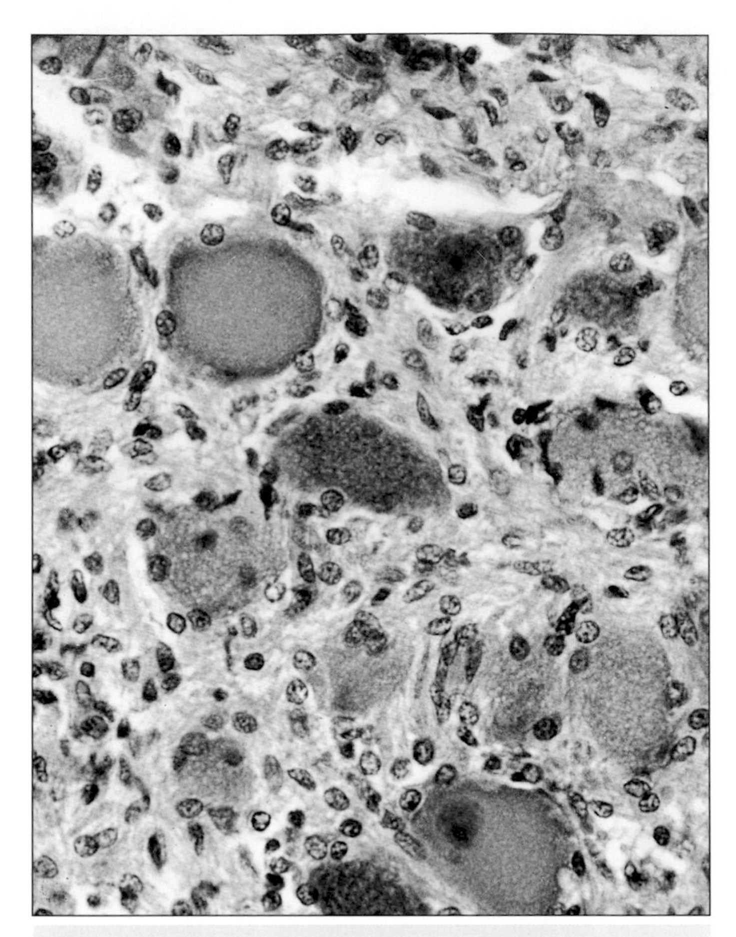

Figure 3.89 Central chromatolysis in ganglionic neurons of a horse with grass sickness.

degeneration in the nuclei of cranial nerves III, V, VII and XII, the dorsal motor nucleus of the vagus, and the nucleus ambiguus. Some neuronal degeneration may be found in dorsal root ganglia, and in the ventral horn and intermediolateral areas of the spinal gray matter. In later phases of the disease, depletion of neurons at the above sites is evident, with reactive and proliferative changes on the part of non-neuronal elements.

Bibliography

Hahn CN, et al. Central neuropathology of equine grass sickness. Acta Neuropathol (Berl) 2001;102:153–159.

Harkin KR, et al. Dysautonomia in dogs: 65 cases (1993–2000). J Am Vet Med Assoc 2002;220:633–639.

McCarthy HE, et al. Equine grass sickness is associated with low antibody levels to *Clostridium botulinum*: a matched case-control study. Equine Vet J 2004;36:123–129.

Nunn F, et al. Association between Key-Gaskell syndrome and infection by *Clostridium botulinum* type C/D. Vet Rec 2004;155:111–115.

O'Brien DP, Johnson GC. Dysautonomia and autonomic neuropathies. Vet Clin North Am Small Anim Pract 2002;32:251–265.

Sensory neuropathies in the dog

Sensory neuropathies are reported in an increasingly long list of various dog breeds. A small number of **English Pointer** pups from a particular mating developed a syndrome of acral mutilation and analgesia. The size of spinal ganglia was reduced, with reduced numbers of neurons, and reduced fiber density in the dorsolateral fasciculus of the spinal cord (Lissauer`s tract). These clinical and morphologic findings are consistent with a *specific deficit in nociceptive pathways*. It is suggested that the presumably genetically based disorder involves both hypoplasia of the system and continued degeneration postnatally.

In **longhaired Dachshunds**, proprioceptive, nociceptive, and urinary deficits are associated with a *distal degenerative axonopathy*. Distal cutaneous nerves have marked loss of large myelinated fibers, and degenerative changes in both myelinated and unmyelinated fibers. In the spinal cord there is axonal degeneration in the fasciculus gracilis, of greatest intensity at its distal extremity in the cervical region.

Progressive myelopathy and neuropathy causing progressive ataxia in littermate **New Zealand Huntaway** dogs is described as a *central–peripheral distal axonopathy*, in which there is degeneration of axon and myelin in sensory, proprioceptive, and motor tracts of the spinal cord and to a mild degree in some peripheral nerves.

In dogs of **various breeds**, there are reports of diffuse ganglioneuritis, with destruction of primary sensory neurons and subsequent Wallerian degeneration and axonal loss in peripheral nerves in the spinal dorsal funiculi, spinal tract of the trigeminal nerve, and solitary tract. These cases are mentioned here as the *extensive axonal degeneration* is the more likely lesion to be routinely noted, and its pattern should immediately draw attention to the primary involvement of dorsal root ganglia. The pathogenesis of this ganglioneuritis is not known but may be similar to that of Guillain–Barré syndrome, a post-infectious syndrome in people.

Bibliography

Braund KG, et al. Distal sensorimotor polyneuropathy in mature Rottweiler dogs. Vet Pathol 1994;31:316–326.

Cummings JF, et al. Hereditary sensory neuropathy. Nociceptive loss and acral mutilation in pointer dogs: canine hereditary sensory neuropathy. Am J Pathol 1983;112:136–138.

Duncan ID, et al. The pathology of a sensory neuropathy affecting long haired Dachshund dogs. Acta Neuropath (Berl) 1982;58:141–151.

Jolly RD, et al. Progressive myelopathy and neuropathy in New Zealand Huntaway dogs. N Z Vet J 2000;48:188–191.

Peripheral axonopathies

Lesions involving single peripheral nerves are termed **mononeuropathies**. They are usually the result of focal compression or contusion by trauma, tumor masses, or similar lesions, and involve centrifugal Wallerian degeneration about the lesion. If several nerves are randomly involved in such a way, the term **mononeuropathy multiplex** may be applied. **Polyneuropathy** describes bilaterally symmetrical involvement of several nerves, and carries the implication of a systemic disturbance.

From the clinical point of view, most peripheral polyneuropathies occur in association with polyneuritis or demyelination, but in this section our focus is on **noninflammatory axonopathies**, and the other types of disease are discussed elsewhere. Intense Wallerian degeneration of peripheral motor axons will of course accompany degeneration of the ventral spinal motor nerve cell bodies, as occurs in the motor neuron diseases previously discussed. Similarly, in the very rare primary sensory polyneuropathies, peripheral sensory fibers will degenerate, but the degeneration will also extend, with the central projections of these cells, into the dorsal funiculi of the spinal cord. In some intoxications, delayed organophosphate for example, peripheral neuropathy will be accompanied by central axonopathy, as has been illustrated above. All the foregoing emphasizes the unity of the nervous system and the inconsistencies involved in deciding where neurons begin and end, but nonetheless certain diseases have a clear central or peripheral focus.

With the exception of equine recurrent laryngeal neuropathy, *noninflammatory peripheral polyneuropathies are uncommon and are generally to be regarded as distal axonopathies of the spinal neurons*. Motor axon involvement means that *denervation muscle atrophy* is a frequent concurrent lesion. It should be remembered too that with advancing age, subclinical degenerative changes are to be expected in peripheral nerves and spinal roots.

Equine laryngeal hemiplegia

The clinical manifestations of this common and well-recognized disease are the consequence of *denervation atrophy of the intrinsic muscles of the left side of the larynx*. The resultant inability to adduct the arytenoid cartilage and the vocal fold leads to partial obstruction of the airway on inspiration, and inspiratory stridor on exertion, referred to as "*roaring*."

The underlying lesion is *idiopathic degeneration of the left recurrent laryngeal nerve*, suggested to result from progressive degeneration of large myelinated axons, which increases in intensity towards the distal extremities of the nerve. During active degeneration, localized axonal swellings result from paranodal and internodal accumulations of granular dense bodies and degenerate mitochondria, although numerous atrophied axonal segments have also been described. Loss of axons is indicated by the presence of Bungner's bands, which may contain fragments of axonal and myelin debris, and permanent axonal loss is reflected in considerable endoneurial fibrosis. Some axonal regenerative activity may be apparent. There is also evidence of recurrent demyelination and remyelination, considered to be secondary to axonal degeneration.

The cause of this axonopathy remains unknown. Young, tall male horses with long necks seem predisposed and there is a high incidence in Thoroughbred and draft breeds. *Mechanical factors* operating on the left recurrent laryngeal nerve have been proposed, such as stretching of the anchored nerve, or pressure exerted where it reflects around the aorta. However, subclinical involvement of the right recurrent nerve seems to be the rule. Studies of clinically normal horses have revealed bilateral neuropathy with more severe denervation of the laryngeal adductor muscles as compared to the abductors, and this pattern also holds true for horses with laryngeal hemiplegia. The factors determining progression of the subclinical disease, the mechanism for the preferential adductor involvement, and the reason for the greater severity on the left side are unexplained.

One study suggested that similar distal degenerative changes also occur in the long axons of the hindlimbs, but only a few horses were sampled. Such a finding implies a *systemic metabolic or toxic disorder*, producing a polyneuropathy with maximal expression in the left recurrent laryngeal nerve. In New Zealand, laryngeal hemiplegia in association with stringhalt has occurred in seasonal outbreak form in horses grazing the plant *Hypochaeris radicata*. Laryngeal paralysis has occasionally been reported in cases of intoxication with *lead*, or *organophosphates*, as part of widespread axonopathy.

No convincing evidence of lesions in the CNS is available at present, although they have been sought in the nucleus ambiguus from which the recurrent laryngeal axons arise. It has been claimed that axonal spheroids in the lateral cuneate nucleus are more numerous in horses with laryngeal paralysis, but the significance of this is unclear. Such lesions are common and generally nonspecific, and it is difficult to see how they could be related pathogenetically to the rather different lesions in the motor axons supplying the larynx.

Equine stringhalt

Stringhalt is the name given to a clinical condition of horses characterized by *extreme exaggerated flexion of the hindlimbs*. It has been recognized for many years to occur in *sporadic* and *epizootic* forms, the latter associated with the grazing of certain plants, notably *Hypochaeris radicata* (false dandelion, flatweed). Stringhalt may develop subsequent to trauma to the dorsum of the metatarsus. Various degenerative changes have been reported in the spinal cord and peripheral nerves in stringhalt. Selective loss of large-diameter myelinated fibers in peripheral nerves in horses with Australian stringhalt is consistent with distal axonopathy leading to neurogenic muscle atrophy.

Equine suprascapular neuropathy

Mononeuropathy of the suprascapular nerve in the horse has been designated for many years by the old clinical term "*sweeney*." The nerve is prone to injury at its site of reflection around the wing of the scapula, and in many cases *trauma* at this site is probably the initiating cause. Evidence has been advanced to suggest, however, that *entrapment of the nerve* by a tendinous band may lead to degeneration in the absence of additional trauma. In cases of sufficient severity, axonal degeneration, demyelination, and endoneurial fibrosis will be associated with denervation of the spinatus muscle and chronic lameness.

Canine laryngeal neuropathies

Cases are described of neurogenic laryngeal muscle atrophy in old dogs of several breeds but, in the **Bouvier** breed, autosomal dominant inheritance has been proposed for a unilateral or bilateral condition with onset at an early age. Clinical laryngeal paresis/paralysis is evident and is accompanied by denervation atrophy of laryngeal muscles, and Wallerian degeneration of the distal recurrent laryngeal nerves. In this breed, laryngeal paralysis is attributed to an abiotrophic process in nucleus ambiguus in the medulla. Gliosis and neuronal atrophy have been recorded in vagal nuclei in **Siberian Huskies**. In **Dalmatian** dogs, the laryngeal paralysis–polyneuropathy complex is a generalized axonopathy with dying back of laryngeal and peripheral nerves. Neurogenic atrophy of muscles, including those of the larynx, is reported in related **Leonberger** dogs with a spontaneous distal, symmetrical polyneuropathy.

Endocrine neuropathies

Clinical polyneuropathy has been associated with *diabetes mellitus in the dog and cat* and is well recognized in people. In the cat, hindlimb weakness, poor postural reactions, depressed patellar reflexes and plantigrade stance are described. Axonal conduction velocity is reduced in the sciatic and ulnar nerves. Clinical remission often follows therapeutic management of the diabetic state.

The pathogenesis of diabetic neuropathy remains uncertain, but it is generally accepted that there is *distal axonopathy* with cycles of degeneration/regeneration and accompanying demyelination/remyelination. The distal degeneration may be due to impairment of axonal transport mechanisms secondary to reduced availability of glucose for the neuron. Lesions include axonal atrophy of myelinated and unmyelinated fibers, demyelination and, in some animals, intra-axonal accumulation of glycogen.

A peripheral neuropathy has also been associated with *canine hypothyroidism*.

Feline hyperlipoproteinemia

A series of cats has been described with a *genetically based deficiency of lipoprotein lipase activity* and a resulting severe hyperchylomicronemia. Amongst other manifestations, there is a high incidence of *mononeuropathy multiplex*, with clinical palsies related to various peripheral and cranial nerves, including instances of Horner's syndrome. Neurological deficits are related to multiple focal red/brown nodules in the perineurium of nerve trunks, which are organizing hematomas associated with a xanthomatous/granulomatous component. Xanthomatous masses extend between nerve fascicles and appear to compress and distort them, inducing Wallerian degeneration to various degrees of severity. The xanthomas arise from phagocytosis of cholesterol esters by macrophages. These lesions are generally located in loci where trauma is likely and also occur commonly at the emergence of spinal nerve roots.

"Kangaroo gait" of lactating ewes

This condition was first reported from New Zealand, and subsequently from the United Kingdom. There is a low flock incidence and only ewes in lactation or up to 1 month post-weaning are affected. The clinical syndrome is consistent with *bilateral radial nerve palsy*, and there is a characteristic bounding gait during attempted rapid movement. In most cases, there is gradual clinical improvement and eventual recovery. The cause is not known. There have been limited studies of pathology. Extensive Wallerian degeneration with regeneration has been described in the radial nerve trunks of chronically affected ewes, but in some acutely affected animals no radial nerve lesions could be demonstrated. In one study, there were additionally reported spongy change in the neuropil, dorsal root ganglionopathy, and neuronal degeneration in the hippocampus and cervical spinal cord, although these findings were variable.

Bibliography

Braund KG, et al. Idiopathic polyneuropathy in Alaskan Malamutes. J Vet Int Med 1997;11:243–249.

Cahill JI, Goulden BE. Further evidence for a central nervous system component in equine laryngeal hemiplegia. N Z Vet J 1989;37:89–90.

Clements AC, et al. Clinical and pathological investigations of 'kangaroo gait' in sheep. Vet Rec 2002;150:485–486.

Crabill MR, et al. Stringhalt secondary to trauma to the dorsoproximal region of the metatarsus in horses: 10 cases (1986–1991). J Am Vet Med Assoc 1994;205:867–869.

Dixon PM, et al. Laryngeal paralysis: a study of 375 cases in a mixed-breed population of horses. Equine Vet J 2001;33:452–458.

Duncan ID, et al. Subclinical entrapment neuropathy of the equine suprascapular nerve. Acta Neuropath (Berl) 1987;74:53–61.

Duncan ID, et al. Preferential denervation of the adductor muscles of the equine larynx II: nerve pathology. Eq Vet J 1991;23:99–103.

Jones BR, et al. Peripheral neuropathy in cats in inherited primary hyperchylomicronaemia. Vet Rec 1986;119:268–272.

Munana KR. Long-term complications of diabetes mellitus, Part I: Retinopathy, nephropathy, neuropathy. Vet Clin North Am Small Anim Pract 1995;25:715–730.

Shelton GD, et al. Inherited polyneuropathy in Leonberger dogs: a mixed or intermediate form of Charcot-Marie-Tooth disease? Muscle Nerve 2003;27:471–477.

Slocombe RF, et al. Pathological aspects of Australian stringhalt. Equine Vet J 1992;24:174–183.

Myelinopathies

Myelin sheaths in the central or peripheral nervous system may be the focus of various disease processes, but simultaneous central and peripheral involvement is rare. This is not surprising when one considers the fundamental differences between the two. As previously noted, myelin breakdown and removal in Wallerian degeneration will follow as a **secondary** consequence of axonal degeneration. On the other hand, in some inflammatory diseases, macrophages acting within the orchestration of the immune system will strip myelin from axons, leaving the latter intact for a time at least. In this context, antibodies or inflammatory mediators may bind to and destabilize the structure of the myelin lamellae, causing disruption of the sheath and provoking its phagocytosis. Such **primary demyelination** occurs for example in the CNS in canine distemper, and in the peripheral nerves in "coonhound paralysis." The demyelinating aspects of these entities are discussed elsewhere.

Attention in this section is on *noninflammatory diseases in which some disorder of myelin formation, maintenance, or stability is the primary event*. It should be remembered that the myelin sheath is a specialized extended process of oligodendrocyte or Schwann cell plasma membrane, and myelinopathies are therefore part of the cytopathology of these cells. Within the complex category of myelinopathies, we will discuss *leukodystrophies*, or disorders of myelin synthesis or maintenance; *hypomyelinogenesis,* which may be at one end of the spectrum of leukodystrophy; and *spongy degeneration* or spongiform myelinopathies.

Hypomyelinogenesis

The great majority of the hypomyelinogeneses are restricted to the CNS, and they have been described in most domestic species with the notable exception of the horse. Although in many cases a genetic basis has been demonstrated or strongly implied in hypomyelinogenesis, several viruses have been implicated, and the possibility of toxic or nutritional factors should be kept in mind. A common theme is sex-linked inheritance and affected males.

Myelinogenesis begins sometime after the middle of gestation and continues in the postnatal period for various times depending on the species. It is more advanced at birth in those species in which the young are able to stand and walk soon after, for it correlates with the overall maturity of the nervous system.

The process requires a complex unfolding of events in order to be successful. In the first place, there must be differentiation of competent myelinating cells in sufficient number, and they must migrate to, recognize, and contact the target axons appropriately. Second, the axon itself must send a specific signal to the myelinating cell to initiate its investment. The diameter of the axon dictates whether or not it is myelinated and how thick the sheath will be. The threshold size is about 1 μm in the CNS and 2 μm in the peripheral nerves. Finally, the molecular components of the myelin must be produced and delivered to their correct sites in the membrane. One or several of these processes may be perturbed to give rise to diseases characterized by hypomyelinogenesis.

Myelination does not occur synchronously throughout the nervous system, but in a distinctly regional sequence. Thus lesions of this type may involve some tracts more than others, or completely spare some tracts. There may be complete absence of myelin, or an inadequate amount of myelin that may be either chemically normal or abnormal. For the latter case, the term *dysmyelination* has been coined but, as these conditions are characterized by a reduced quantity of myelin, **hypomyelination** is a suitable generic term. As would be expected, such diseases are manifested early in life, and a very common and dominant clinical feature is the onset of a severe generalized tremor syndrome. This has led to the use of names such as *congenital "tremor," "shaker," or "trembler"* to describe the clinical state. The severity of the clinical signs can vary from life threatening to mild.

The deficiency of myelin may in some instances be permanent, while in others it seems that myelination may be delayed, but eventually proceeds to the extent that clinical deficits resolve. In general, the pathologic picture is dominated by a paucity of myelin with little or no evidence of the breakdown and removal of previously formed sheaths. There may be other accompanying structural defects, notably cerebellar hypoplasia, particularly when a teratogenic virus is the cause.

When routine morphologic evaluations are being made on very young animals, reference should be made to age-matched controls. In the dog for instance, very little myelin is normally present prior to 2 weeks of postnatal age, whereas in the sheep myelination begins at about day 50 of gestation. The investigation of such conditions makes use of traditional stains for myelin and axons, plastic-embedded sections for light and electron microscopy, and immunostaining techniques for marker antigens, such as myelin basic protein. There needs to be some familiarity with the normal morphologic features of early myelination. Some of these are mentioned in the disease descriptions that follow.

Canine hypomyelinogenesis

A number of canine hypomyelinogeneses have been documented and several provisional conclusions can be made. All but one of the diseases involve the central myelin only, and it appears that they are not pathogenetically identical and can be divided into two broad groups according to severity. The most severe are those described in the Samoyed, Springer Spaniel, and Dalmatian breeds.

In the **Samoyed**, severe generalized tremors become apparent at about 3 weeks of age, with a predominance of males being affected. Inability to stand leads to severe incapacitation and a high mortality rate. A genetic basis is suspected. It has been suggested that a central pathogenetic event is *retardation of gliogenesis*, with oligodendrocytes failing to differentiate fully. Profound hypomyelination is suggested on gross inspection of the brain by a lack of contrast between gray and white matter throughout the CNS. The sparing of the peripheral nervous system is well appreciated macroscopically by comparing the myelin-deficient optic nerves to the other cranial nerves, in particular the adjacent oculomotor nerve.

By routine light microscopy, there is normal peripheral myelin but *almost total absence of central myelin, and diffuse microgliosis*. Silver stains suggest axons to be present in normal number. Electron microscopy reveals a few axons to have thin and poorly compacted myelin sheaths, the presence of numerous astroglial processes, and a large number of microglia. Oligodendrocytes are greatly reduced in number and appear immature. Axons, by contrast, are normal in number and morphology but the great majority are devoid of a myelin sheath.

In the **Springer Spaniel**, severe generalized tremor in male pups is evident at 10–12 days of age ("*shaking pups*"). The condition is inherited as an *X-linked recessive*, and severe myelin deficiency is caused by the shaker pup (*shp*) mutation of the myelin proteolipid protein (*Plp*) gene. Central hypomyelination is profound but less severe in the spinal cord than in the brain and optic nerves. In contrast to the Samoyed, microgliosis is not prominent, but in other respects the gross and histologic features are similar. The electron microscope, however, resolves some further differences. For example, some thin myelin sheaths are present that have lamellae of normal configuration. Some axons have a few internodes sheathed, many of which are shorter than would be expected for the axonal caliber, and many of which are single units terminating as "heminodes." Although some immature oligodendrocytes are evident, so too are normally mature ones. In animals 2 months old or more, there are also hallmarks of the early stages of normal myelination that persist well beyond their usual period of the first month of life. These include such features as large amounts of oligodendrocyte cytoplasm in lateral loops, and outwardly terminating lateral loops. In addition, many oligodendrocytes have lysosomal digestive vacuoles thought to relate to the degradation of abnormal myelin components.

The disease in the **Dalmatian** is reported in a male pup that developed severe tremors in the neonatal period and was destroyed at 8 weeks of age. Profound deficiency of central myelin was accompanied by reduced numbers of oligodendroglia, with a few axons having extremely thin and poorly compacted sheaths.

Disorders of lesser severity are described in the Chow Chow, Weimaraner, Bernese Mountain Dog, and in two crossbred ("Lurcher") dogs.

Affected **Chow Chow** dogs have marked impairment from 2 weeks of age, but progressive improvement leads to a virtual absence of clinical deficits by the end of the first year of life. At all stages, the animals remain ambulatory, bright, and responsive, in spite of a pronounced hypermetric gait with a distinctive "rocking horse" motion when trying to initiate movement. Tremors and head bobbing are exacerbated by excitement and disappear at rest. It has not been possible to establish a definite heritable basis for this disease, but it is suggested to be the result of a genetically determined delay in oligodendrocyte maturation.

In pups examined at about 3 months of age, no gross lesions are reported, but profound hypomyelination is evident histologically in the CNS. This is particularly so in the cerebral subcortical white matter, cerebellar folia, ventral half of the cerebral peduncles, optic tracts, and the peripheral zones of the ventral and lateral funiculi of the spinal cord. By contrast, the cerebellar peduncles and fasciculus proprius of the spinal cord are relatively well myelinated. Electron microscopy reveals mostly thin myelin sheaths in the least-affected areas, and mostly naked axons in the worst-affected areas. Oligodendrocytes are present in normal numbers and generally appear morphologically normal, although stellate cells containing intermediate filaments may be found.

In older dogs in clinical remission, the brain is well myelinated apart from some mildly deficient foci in subcortical white matter and corpus callosum. However, myelin deficiency is still marked in the lateral and ventral funiculi of the cord, which also has a few degenerate axons. Ultrastructurally, these areas contain a few well-myelinated or thinly myelinated axons separated by masses of astrocytic processes. Indications of immaturity are provided by poorly compacted sheaths and some massively oversized sheaths that fold away from the axon in redundant loops.

The **Weimaraner** syndrome is closely similar to the above but has only been studied pathologically in the early phase. The tremor syndrome, in evidence at 3 weeks of age, seems to resolve by a year. A heritable basis has been proposed but not confirmed, and delayed oligodendrocyte differentiation suggested as the underlying defect. Pups necropsied at 4–5 weeks of age have no gross abnormalities, but histologic staining reactions suggest myelin deficiency, and this is particularly obvious at the periphery of the lateral and ventral funiculi of the spinal cord. This contrasts with the relatively well-myelinated dorsal columns. Oligodendrocytes are reduced in number. Ultrastructurally, there is considerable evidence of myelin immaturity as described above. Astrocytic fibers are prominent and oligodendrocyte morphology seems normal.

The **Bernese Mountain Dog** "trembler pup" has a fine head and limb tremor that subsides with sleep and improves substantially by 9–12 weeks of age. An autosomal recessive mode of inheritance has been proposed. There are no gross lesions and hypomyelination is concentrated in the spinal cord, where axons are thinly sheathed by morphologically normal myelin. Oligodendrocytes in this case appear to be increased in numbers and morphologically normal. **Lurcher** pups were reported to have unmyelinated and thinly myelinated axons in the peripheral sections of the lateral funiculi of the spinal cord. The changes are subtle and not readily apparent unless plastic-embedded sections are employed. These animals are of interest as they are crossbred, making a genetic cause a more remote possibility.

Hypomyelination has been reported only rarely in **cats**.

The sole reported occurrence of **peripheral hypomyelination** in domestic animals involves the **Golden Retriever** breed. Two littermates, one male and one female, had ataxia, weakness, a crouched stance, and pelvic-limb muscle atrophy at about 2 months of age. Peripheral nerve samples revealed axons of all calibers to be thinly myelinated and Schwann cells to be increased in number and hypertrophied (see Fig. 3.11). There were no indications of demyelination.

Porcine hypomyelinogenesis

Syndromes of **congenital tremor** (CT, myoclonia congenita, dancing pig) are well recognized in pigs. CT has been classified on the basis of the presence (type A) or absence (type B) of myelin deficiency in the central or peripheral nervous system; CT type A has been subdivided into five subtypes, AI–AV. The various forms of CT are similar clinically; affected piglets may bounce on their digits, and have rhythmic whole-body tremors that worsen with excitement and cease with sleep.

CT type AI is caused by transplacental infection in the middle trimester with *Classical swine fever virus*, which causes significant hypomyelinogenesis in addition to other neural lesions in the fetus, most notably cerebellar hypoplasia. The cerebellar changes may be focal and are most likely to be detected in sagittal sections of the vermis and hemispheres. The myelin lesion is generally similar to that seen in lambs with Border disease.

CT type AII may be the result of *Porcine circovirus* type 2 infection, but the role, if any, of this virus remains controversial.

CT type AIII occurs in Landrace or Landrace-crossbreds, and is inherited as an X-*linked recessive* trait, afflicting male neonates, and due to a mutation in the proteolipid protein gene *Plp*. There is myelin deficiency throughout the CNS, but most obvious in the spinal cord, cerebellum, and cerebral gyri. Oligodendrocyte numbers are reduced; many small and medium-sized axons are unmyelinated or only thinly so. Large-diameter axons appear normally myelinated.

CT type AIV occurs in the British Saddleback breed; there is an *autosomal recessive* inheritance mode. Hypomyelination is present throughout the neuraxis with axons of all sizes affected. Many sheaths are poorly compacted and vacuolated. Oligodendrocytes are numerous, and many appear immature ultrastructurally, and sometimes contain cytoplasmic intermediate filaments. Still others contain autophagosomes and dense bodies. The neuropil also contains excessive astrocytic fibers and lipid-laden macrophages. These findings, together with biochemical evidence of myelin degradation, suggest that newly formed myelin is unstable and is rapidly broken down.

CT type AV occurs in piglets of sows exposed to the organophosphate *trichlorfon* between days 45 and 63 of pregnancy.

CT type B is idiopathic, and lacks structural or neurochemical defects.

Ovine and caprine hypomyelinogenesis

Border disease in lambs has become the model for the several pestivirus-induced myelin disorders of animals. *Border disease virus* can cause transplacental infection, which, if on or after day 50, has the potential to produce a range of terata. In the classical syndrome, newborn lambs are often referred to as "*hairy shakers*," due to the combination of generalized tremor and hairy birth coat. There is *diffuse hypomyelination in the CNS,* which is especially prominent in the spinal cord, particularly the more caudal regions. Some myelination is present, but has ultrastructural features of immaturity, in that lamellae remain uncompacted and axons retain the angulated profiles they normally acquire just before myelination and lose soon after. There are also compact sheaths abnormally thin for axonal diameter, and intramyelinic and periaxonal vacuoles.

While glial cell numbers may appear normal by light microscopy, there are in fact reduced numbers of mature oligodendrocytes and increased numbers of microglia. Many microglia are packed with lipid droplets, the origin of which does not appear to be degraded myelin. It is suggested that maturation of oligodendrocytes is delayed, and that although the time of onset of myelination is close to normal, its rate is greatly reduced. The blockade of glial maturation may be the result of virus-induced fetal hypothyroidism; abundant viral antigen can be found in the thyroid, and circulating thyroxin is significantly depressed, but this alternative hypothesis remains unproven.

Severe hypomyelinogenesis is a feature of neonatal goat kids with **β-mannosidosis**. Hypothyroidism has been proposed as the underlying mechanism, as a consequence of the lysosomal storage disease.

Bovine hypomyelinogenesis

Myelination in calves proceeds between gestational week 20 and postnatal week 8. A spectrum of terata and spinal hypomyelinogenesis similar to that in piglets and lambs may develop in calves infected with *Bovine viral diarrhea virus* in utero after day 100 of gestation.

Bibliography

Anderson CA, et al. Border disease virus-induced decrease in thyroid hormone levels with associated hypomyelination. Lab Invest 1987;57:168–175.

Baumann N, Pham-Dinh D. Biology of oligodendrocyte and myelin in the mammalian central nervous system. Physiol Rev 2001;81:871–927.

Baumgartner BG, Brenig B. The role of proteolipid proteins in the development of congenital tremors type AIII: a review. Dtsch Tierarztl Wochenschr 1996;103:404–407.

Binkhorst GJ, et al. Neurological disorders, virus persistence and hypomyelination in calves due to intra-uterine infections with bovine virus diarrhoea virus. Vet Quart 1983;5:145–155.

Braund KG, et al. Congenital hypomyelinating polyneuropathy in two golden retriever littermates. Vet Pathol 1989;26:202–208.

Choi J, et al. Sequence analysis of old and new strains of porcine circovirus associated with congenital tremors in pigs and their comparison with strains involved with postweaning multisystemic wasting syndrome. Can J Vet Res 2002;66:217–224.

Cummings JF, et al. Tremors in Samoyed pups with oligodendrocyte deficiencies and hypomyelination. Acta Neuropathol (Berl) 1986;71:267–277.

Jeffrey M, et al. Immunocytochemical localization of border disease virus in the spinal cord of fetal and newborn lambs. Neuropathol Appl Neurobiol 1990;16:501–510.

Kornegay JN. Hypomyelination in Weimaraner dogs. Acta Neuropathol (Berl) 1987;72:394–401.

Mayhew IG, et al. Tremor syndrome and hypomyelination in Lurcher pups. J Small Anim Pract 1984;25:551–559.

Nadon NL, Duncan ID. Molecular analysis of glial cell development in the canine 'shaking pup' mutant. Dev Neurosci 1996;18:174–184.

Palmer AC, et al. Recognition of 'trembler', a hypomyelinating condition in the Bernese mountain dog. Vet Rec 1987;120:609–612.

Segales J, et al. Pathological findings associated with naturally acquired porcine circovirus type 2 associated disease. Vet Microbiol 2004;98:137–149.

Stoffregen DA, et al. Hypomyelination of the central nervous system of two Siamese kitten littermates. Vet Pathol 1993;30:388–391.

Vandevelde M, et al. Dysmyelination in chow chow dogs: further studies in older dogs. Acta Neuropathol (Berl) 1981;55:81–87.

Leukodystrophic and myelinolytic diseases

This section will address those diseases characterized by degeneration and loss of myelin, not as a result of, or in association with, inflammation but due to some failure of myelinating cells to sustain and maintain their sheaths in an intact and ordered condition. The implication is that sheaths are initially formed, but then deteriorate, leaving their axons intact for a time at least. The use of terminology in this area is of course somewhat arbitrary. For our purposes, **primary demyelination** is taken to imply the removal from around intact axons of structurally and chemically normal myelin, usually by macrophages and often in an inflammatory setting. The term **leukodystrophy** is applied to diseases with a heritable basis, early onset in life, lack of inflammation, symmetry of lesions, and in which some inherent qualitative defect in myelin (*dysmyelinogenesis*) leads to its dissolution and removal. **Myelinolysis** refers to the initial disruption of myelin structure by extensive decompaction of lamellae as a prelude to its breakdown and removal, and as such could be involved in many processes. There is scope for considerable overlap and liberal interpretation of definitions. The diseases discussed in this section will not include any which could easily be classified as demyelinating, in the sense indicated above, or as malacic in the sense indicated elsewhere in this chapter, in spite of the propensity for focal softening and even cavitation in some of the leukodystrophies.

Globoid cell leukodystrophy

This disease, also known as *galactocerebrosidosis*, *galactosylceramide lipidosis*, and *Krabbe disease*, has been documented in the Cairn and West Highland White Terrier, miniature Poodle, Bluetick Hound, Bassett Hound, Beagle, domestic cat, and polled Dorset sheep. It is due to a genetically determined deficiency, usually autosomal recessive, in the activity of lysosomal *galactocerebrosidase*, and as such falls within the *sphingolipidosis group of lysosomal storage diseases*. However, it has special characteristics that make it more appropriate to be discussed as a leukodystrophy, and it was so named before the lysosomal defect was recognized. Neurologic impairment begins at an early age and progresses rapidly to a fatal conclusion. The enzymic deficit blocks the catabolism of the galactocerebrosides (galactosylceramides). These compounds are major components of myelin, and the disorder thus principally affects the metabolic well-being of oligodendrocytes and Schwann cells.

Early in the disease, during active myelination, the myelinating cells store galactocerebroside within lysosomes. However, the enzyme is also involved in the breakdown of other metabolites, most notably galactosylsphingosine (psychosine), which is also normally synthesized by oligodendrocytes. This substance is highly cytotoxic to oligodendrocytes when it accumulates, and causes their extensive degeneration and death. Myelination ceases and formed myelin degenerates. During this process, macrophages accumulate to ingest the degenerate myelin but are also unable to degrade galactocerebroside. They give rise to the distinctive, swollen, PAS-positive "*globoid cells*," which form large cuffs around blood vessels in the central white matter, and are also found in the leptomeninges and in the endoneurium of peripheral nerves (Fig. 3.90). Their presence at the latter site is useful for premortem diagnosis by nerve biopsy. At end-stage, the pathology of the disease is marked by the presence of these cells, together with diffuse demyelination, axonal loss, and dense astrogliosis in the brain and spinal cord.

Dalmatian leukodystrophy

Reported only from Norway, this cavitating leukodystrophy has a probable autosomal recessive inheritance and a clinical onset at around 3–6 months of age. The signs are progressive and variable, and

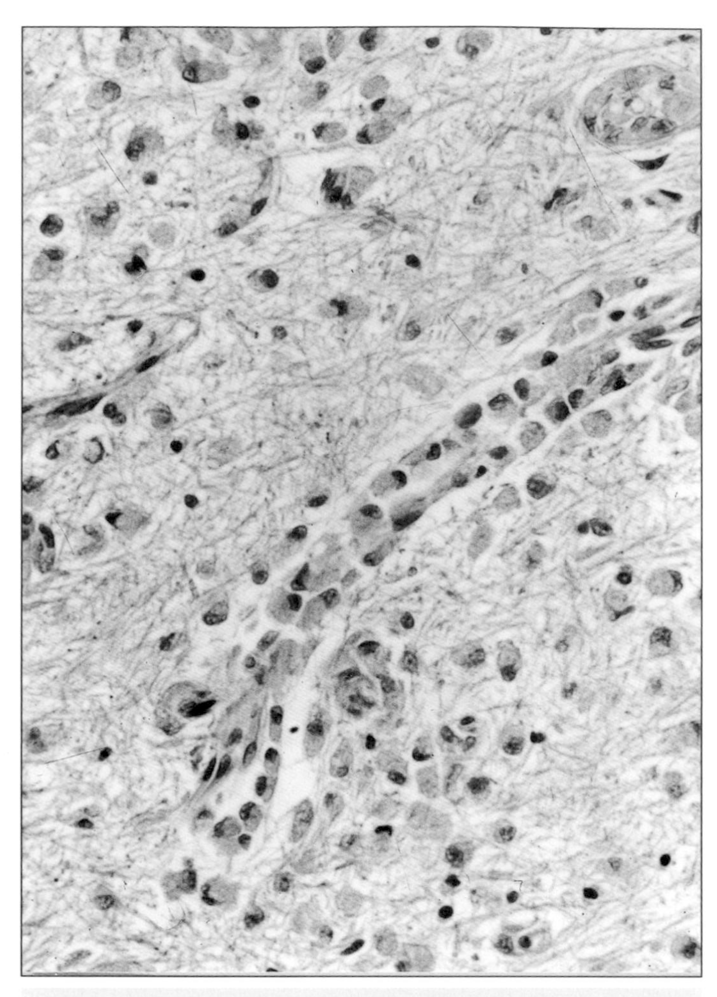

Figure 3.90 Macrophages, filled with degenerate myelin products, aggregating around vessels in **globoid cell leukodystrophy** in a Cairn Terrier.

include either gait deficit or visual impairment or both. The former begins as pelvic and then thoracic limb ataxia and dysmetria, with eventual paraparesis. Mental status remains unimpaired throughout.

The neuropathology is characterized by *bilateral, symmetrical, focal areas of intense loss of myelin* in the centrum semiovale, corpus callosum, internal capsule, caudate nucleus, optic nerves, and thoracic cord white matter adjacent to the ventral horns. Initially axons remain intact. The myelin destruction appears to begin with lamellar vesiculation followed by phagocytosis, and gitter cells are abundant. Fibrous astrogliosis becomes prominent around advanced plaques. The intensity of the process is variable, but lesions are usually visible macroscopically in the central cerebral white matter, appearing as gray depressed areas or, in advanced cases, as cavitations. In some animals, the brain is small and the lateral ventricles enlarged.

Afghan Hound hereditary myelopathy

The initial reports of this disease described acute necrotizing myelomalacia, but subsequent studies indicated a mechanism involving *florid myelinolysis and cavitation*, but essentially sparing axons. It has an apparent recessive inheritance, pre-adult onset, symmetry of lesions, and is noninflammatory, all of which allow for classification as a leukodystrophy. The fundamental pathomechanisms remain undefined. The age of clinical onset is between 3 and 12 months, and caudal ataxia and weakness progress rapidly to paraplegia in a few days. Within 2 weeks there is thoracic limb weakness and phrenic paralysis. A similar syndrome is reported in Kooiker dogs.

The lesions (Fig. 3.91A, B) are focused in the *thoracic spinal cord* where cribriform and spongiotic changes are present in all funiculi (Fig. 3.91B) and are grossly discernible as discoloration and softening or cavitation. Caudally the lesions extend into the lumbar segments, but only in the ventral funiculi; they extend cranially to the midcervical level in the dorsal and/or ventral funiculi (Fig. 3.91A). In some cases there may be lesions in the superior olivary nuclei.

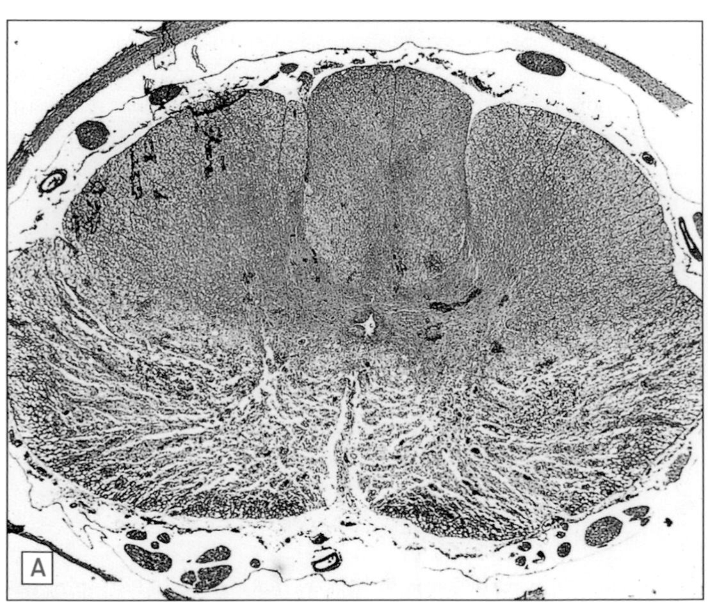

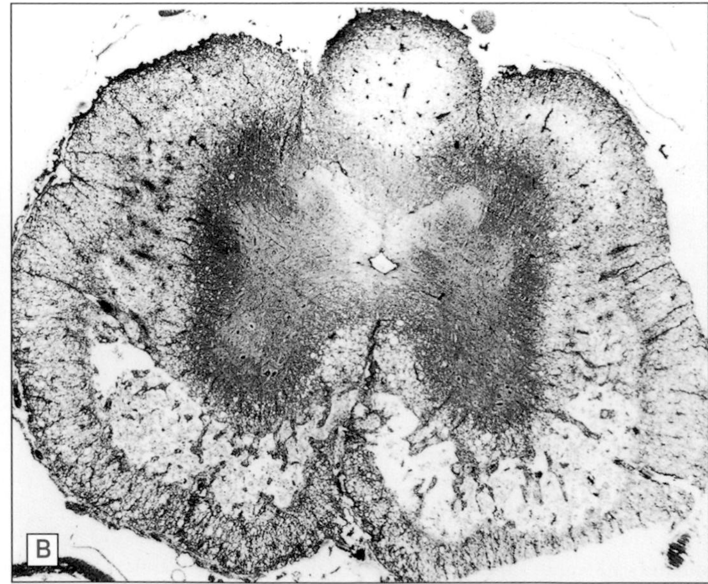

Figure 3.91 Afghan myelopathy. A. Caudal cervical spinal cord. **B.** Thoracic spinal cord.

The sparing of axons is reflected in the paucity of distal Wallerian degeneration in tracts ascending or descending through the lesions.

Light and electron microscopic examination has revealed initial vacuolation of myelin by splitting of lamellae at the intraperiod line and expansion of the extracellular space. Fragmented and degenerate myelin is phagocytosed by gitter cells, leaving surviving axons and reactive astrocytes within microcavities. The cavities are traversed by blood vessels associated with delicate glial strands. Some focal axonal swelling and disintegration are evident, but myelinolysis following vacuolation is the dominant change.

Rottweiler leukoencephalomyelopathy

Some difficulties arise in classifying this disease as a true leukodystrophy, as the onset is delayed until after 12 months of age. However, there is the probability of autosomal recessive inheritance, and the lesions involve progressive noninflammatory symmetrical myelin degeneration and removal. Clinically there are slow, but relentlessly progressive, ataxia, hypermetria, and paresis of all limbs, especially the forelimbs, and ultimately severe proprioceptive loss.

The principal locus of the disorder is the *cervical spinal cord*, which on gross inspection may have extensive dull white discoloration of the dorsal and lateral funiculi. Histologic examination reveals lesions to be present in these funiculi, and also in the deep cerebellar white matter and in other regions of the cord. Lesions are marked by significant loss of myelin (Fig. 3.92), with preservation of most axons, either naked or thinly myelinated, and fibrous astrogliosis. There is some evidence that vesicular degeneration of myelin is an early change. In the cervical cord, there may additionally be focal microcavitation deep within the affected areas, edema, numerous gitter cells, and vascular prominence. A narrow rim of intact white matter usually survives immediately deep to the glia limitans. These severe changes may on occasion extend into the thoracic cord and pyramidal tracts.

Fibrinoid leukodystrophy (Alexander disease)

This rare and unusual *myeloencephalopathy*, analogous to Alexander disease in humans, has been reported in the Scottish Terrier, Labrador Retriever, Miniature Poodle, and sheep. The clinical signs of progressive tetraparesis and ataxia are associated with spongy white matter lesions, astrocytic gliosis, and accumulation of eosinophilic refractile bodies (*Rosenthal fibers*) within the processes of astrocytes disposed around blood vessels in the CNS.

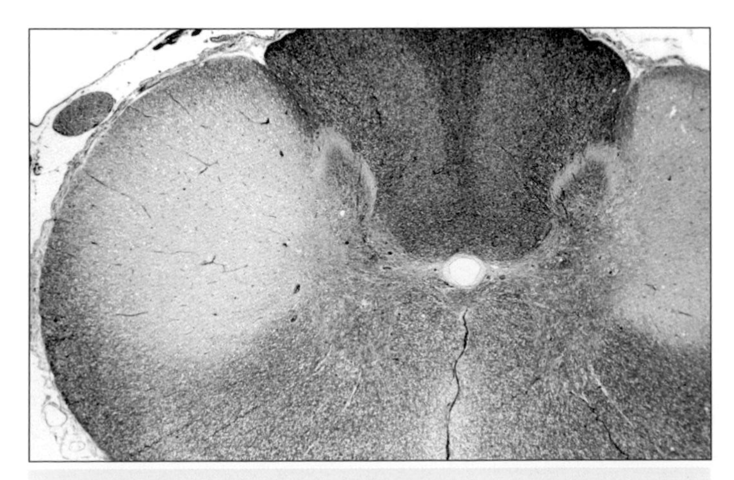

Figure 3.92 Bilateral demyelination of lateral funiculi in the cervical spinal cord in **Rottweiler leukoencephalomyelopathy**. (Courtesy of RF Slocombe.)

Progressive spinal myelinopathy of Murray Grey cattle

Reported in calves of the Murray Grey breed in Australia, this disease may afflict animals at birth, or not become expressed until about 12 months of age. The clinical syndrome is one of spinal ataxia, manifested as incoordination of the pelvic limbs and lateral swaying of the hindquarters at rest. A consistent sign is collapse of one hindlimb, with a tendency to fall to one side. These pelvic limb deficits are progressive and lead to increasing impairment. A similar condition is reported in Simmental calves.

The characteristic lesions are microscopic only, symmetrical, and consistently occur in the *lateral and ventral funiculi throughout the spinal cord*. There is a *distinct deficit of myelin* in the lateral funiculi beneath the dorsal root entry zone, and in ventral funiculi adjacent to the ventral median fissure. In some cases, the fasciculi gracilis and cuneatus are also involved. The process appears to involve ballooning degeneration of myelin sheaths, which may impart a distinctly spongy appearance to the lesion. The progressive loss of myelin is not accompanied by large numbers of myelinophages, and Wallerian degeneration is minimal. There is substantial astrogliosis and thickening of the glia limitans.

In the brain, similar white matter lesions may be found in the spinocerebellar tracts, tectospinal tracts, and medial longitudinal fasciculus. Some neurons undergoing central chromatolysis are present in ventral spinal gray matter, Clarke's column, the red nuclei, lateral vestibular nuclei, reticular formation, and cerebellar roof nuclei.

Progressive ataxia of Charolais cattle

This disease is pathologically unique amongst the domestic species, and appears to represent a progressive inability on the part of some oligodendrocytes to maintain the paranodal extremities of their myelin domains; it may represent oligodendroglial dysplasia. The disease is presumably genetically determined, but has been reported in three-quarter crossbred animals. Both sexes may be affected and clinical signs become evident between 8–24 months of age.

The clinical spectrum involves increasing ataxia and dysmetria, head tremor and some tendency to aggressive behavior. The mental status remains bright and alert. Affected females often urinate in a series of short spurts. The clinical signs progress slowly but steadily, and the animals can be expected to become recumbent by 3 years of age at the latest.

There are no specific gross lesions, but the microscopic findings are distinctive and unprecedented, and are located mainly in the cerebellar white matter and peduncles, the internal capsule, corpus callosum, optic tract, lateral lemniscus, median longitudinal fasciculus, pontine decussation, and ventral and lateral funiculi of the spinal cord. In these white matter tracts, there are *multifocal, granular eosinophilic plaques* about 30 μm in diameter (Fig. 3.93). The plaques are traversed by axons and stain with many, but not all, of the features of normal myelin. There is no sign of myelin degradation or

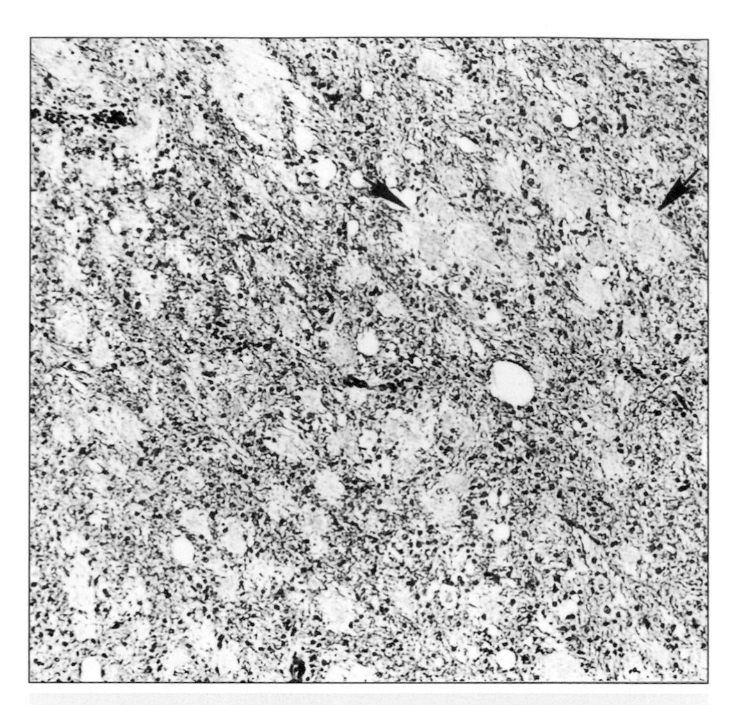

Figure 3.93 Plaques in white matter (arrows) in **progressive ataxia** of Charolais cattle.

phagocytosis. Immediately around the plaques there appears to be an increased number of astrocytes and oligodendrocytes. Some very minor axonal degeneration may be found in some plaques and in normal white matter. It has been concluded that early plaques can be distinguished from old ones. Electron microscopy reveals them to be complex. The ultrastructure suggests great disorder at the myelin paranodes, with relatively normal internodal regions. New plaques reveal axons encompassed, near abnormally long nodes of Ranvier, by hypertrophied oligodendrocyte tongues and processes within a thin myelin sheath. Old plaques contain demyelinated axons (some of which are swollen), surrounded by disorganized myelin lamellae and masses of oligodendrocyte processes. It is suggested that each plaque represents the territory of one oligodendrocyte, and reflects its failure to maintain normal paranodal myelin loops, in the course of which a massive hypertrophy of its processes occurs.

Multifocal symmetrical myelinolytic encephalopathy of Simmental, Limousin, and Aberdeen Angus calves

Reports from Australia, New Zealand, the USA, and Britain describe similar diseases in calves of these breeds, in which *spongy vacuolation of white matter progresses focally to lysis and cavitation*, but with the initial sparing of many axons and nerve cell bodies. In Limousin calves, such foci are present in the cerebellar peduncles and optic chiasm; in Simmental calves, in the internal capsule, caudate nucleus, putamen, periaqueductal white matter, lateral cuneate nucleus, and inferior olive. The distribution extends more widely in Aberdeen Angus and in some cases will include the spinal gray matter. In Limousins and Aberdeen Angus, blindness and dysmetria appear at about 1 month of age, and some animals develop seizures and opisthotonos, while others remain stable. In Simmentals, the clinical onset is between 5 and 8 months of age. There is progressive ataxia, weight loss and eventual dullness and emaciation, with death usual by 12 months of age. The pathogenesis of these diseases is uncertain; similarities exist with Leigh disease of humans, and familial syndromes in Australian Cattle Dogs and Alaskan Huskies.

Feline spinal myelinopathy

An adult-onset condition involving progressive noninflammatory myelin loss in the spinal cord has been reported in cats in California. The pathomechanism is undefined. Myelin deficiency develops in the absence of significant axonal degeneration, and is accompanied by astrogliosis. The lesions occur in all funiculi, and are most intense in the thoracic and lumbar segments.

Tibetan Mastiff hypertrophic neuropathy

This recessively inherited condition affects *peripheral nerves* and is considered to reflect a primary metabolic defect of Schwann cells, with failure to maintain myelin during axonal elongation in postnatal growth. The CNS is not involved. The clinical onset is consistently between 7 and 10 weeks of age. There is rapid progression of generalized weakness with hyporeflexia, slowed nerve conduction velocity, and ultimately tetraplegia in many cases.

In peripheral nerves and their spinal roots, there are changes consistent with *demyelination, remyelination, and endoneurial fibrosis*. Thus many axons are denuded, while some have a thin sheath; proliferating Schwann cells form onion bulbs, and endoneurial collagen is prominent. Axonal degeneration is not a feature. The most characteristic features are revealed ultrastructurally. Schwann cell cytoplasm contains *dense accumulations of 6–7-nm filaments*, occurring at sites where the myelin sheath has separated along the major dense lines, and in the adaxonal cytoplasm. There are also anomalous incisure patterns within the sheaths, with many incisural openings staggered through the entire thickness of the sheath.

Bibliography

Bjerkas I. Hereditary "cavitating" leucodystrophy in Dalmatian dogs. Acta Neuropathol (Berl) 1977;40:163–169.

Cooper BJ, et al. Defective Schwann cell function in canine inherited hypertrophic neuropathy. Acta Neuropathol (Berl) 1984;63:51–56.

Cordy DR. Progressive ataxia of Charolais cattle - an oligodendroglial dysplasia. Vet Pathol 1986;23:78–80.

Edwards JR, et al. Inherited progressive spinal myelinopathy in Murray Grey cattle. Aust Vet J 1988;65:108–109.

Harper PA, et al. Multifocal encephalopathy in Limousin calves. Aust Vet J 1990; 67:111–112.

Hindmarsh M, Harper PAW. Congenital spongiform myelinopathy of Simmental calves. Aust Vet J 1995;72:193–194.

Mandigers PJ, et al. Hereditary necrotising myelopathy in Kooiker dogs. Res Vet Sci 1993;54:118–123.

Philbey AW, Martel KS. A multifocal symmetrical necrotising encephalomyelopathy in Angus calves. Aust Vet J 2003;81:226–229.

Pritchard DH, et al. Globoid cell leukodystrophy in polled Dorset sheep. Vet Pathol 1980;17:399–405.

Sigurdson CJ, et al. Globoid cell-like leukodystrophy in a domestic longhaired cat. Vet Pathol 2002;39:494–496.

Slocombe RF, et al. Leucoencephalomyelopathy in Australian Rottweiler dogs. Aust Vet J 1989;66:147–150.

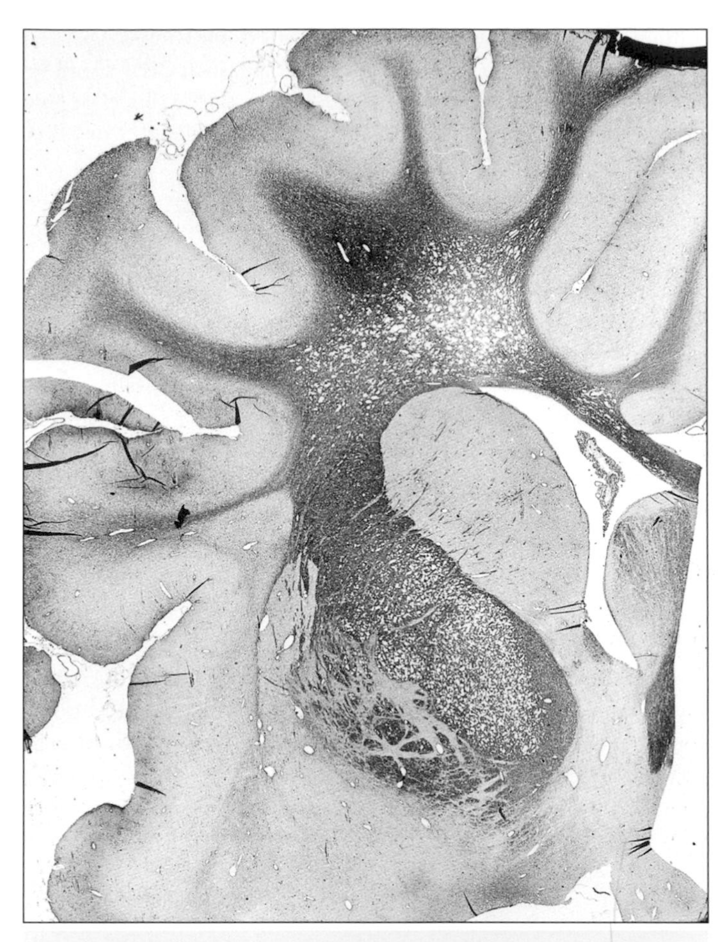

Figure 3.94 Status spongiosus of central cerebral white matter in spongiform myelinopathy in a silver fox. (Reprinted with permission from Hargen G, Bjerkas I. Vet Pathol 1990;27:187.)

Sorjonen DC, et al. Myeloencephalopathy with eosinophilic refractile bodies (Rosenthal fibers) in a Scottish terrier. J Am Vet Med Assoc 1987;190:1004–1006.

Steffen DJ, et al. Multifocal subacute necrotizing encephalomyelopathy in Simmental calves. J Vet Diagn Invest 1994;6:466–472.

Targett M, McInnes E. Afghan hound myelopathy. Vet Rec 1998;142:704.

Wenger DA, et al. Globoid cell leukodystrophy in cairn and West Highland white terriers. J Hered 1999;90:138–142.

Spongiform myelinopathies

There is a group of diseases in which the dominant pathological feature is *dramatic vacuolation of myelin* that often occurs without any overt indication of large-scale myelin breakdown or phagocytosis. There is still the familiar problem, however, of deciding how to categorize some diseases that have overlapping features of myelin vacuolation and myelin degeneration and it is acknowledged that some of the conditions described below could be placed elsewhere.

Myelin vacuolation is one of several different morphological changes encompassed by the term "**status spongiosus**" of nervous tissue (Fig. 3.94). Although producing a striking light microscopic picture when well developed, electron microscopy is required for its fine definition (Fig. 3.95A, B, C). Histologic changes suggestive of this lesion are a fairly common postmortem artifact.

Vacuolation of myelin may come about in several ways, the most frequent of which involves *separation of lamellae along the intraperiod*

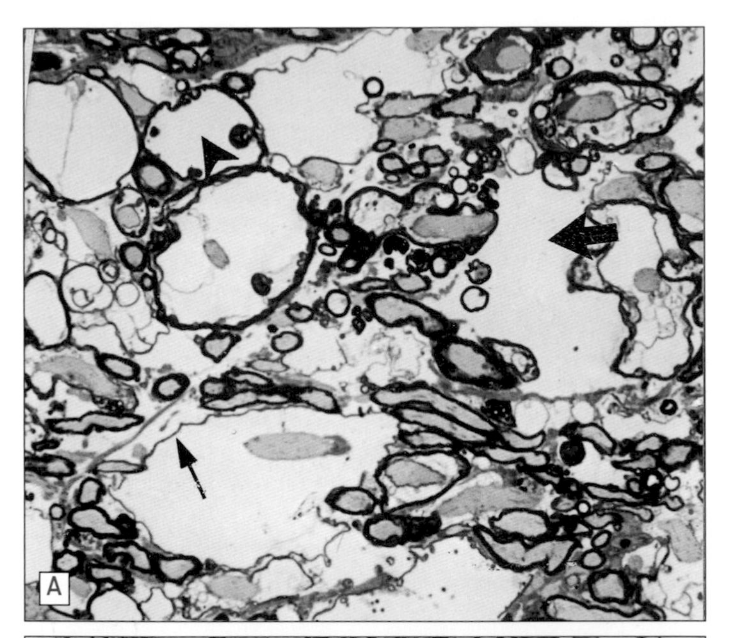

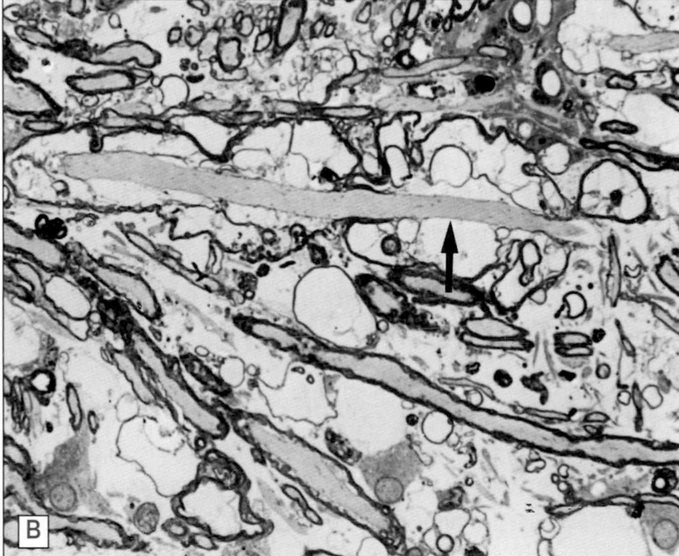

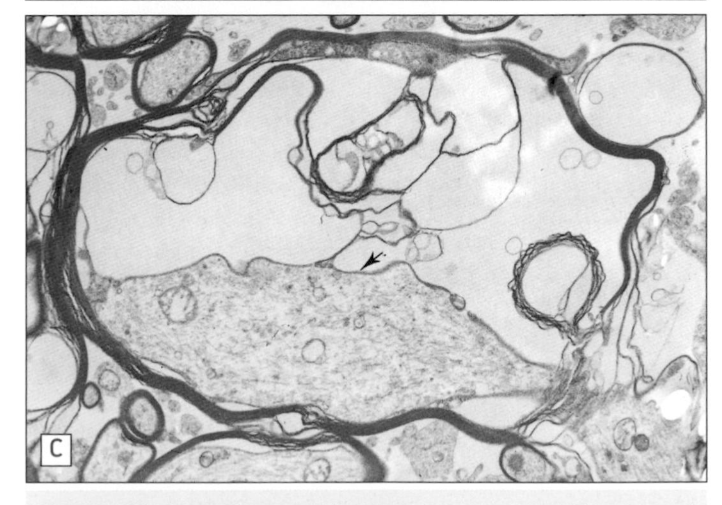

Figure 3.95 Spongiform myelinopathy in a silver fox. **A.** Note thin and dilated myelin sheath around normal axon (small arrow), empty myelin-bound vacuole (arrowhead), and expanded extracellular space (large arrow). **B.** Disrupted myelin around normal axon (arrow). **C.** Electron micrograph demonstrating periaxonal vacuolation and split myelin lamellae around normal axon (arrow). (Reprinted with permission from Hagen G, Bjerkas I. Vet Pathol 1990;27:187.)

line, thereby reopening the extracellular space originally obliterated within the spiraling processes of the myelinating cell. This mechanism can produce vacuoles within the sheath at multiple levels and multiple loci along an internode. In experimental situations, this type of vacuolation has been associated with an increase in tissue water and electrolytes, consistent with simple edema, and accounts for the brain swelling which may occur in severe cases. The vacuoles therefore contain no stainable material. A variety of associated functional disturbances has been described but, remarkably, the lesion may have little functional impact, even when quite intense and prolonged. It seems likely that the myelin lesion is one facet of a complex metabolic disturbance, whose ramifications vary according to basic causes. In humans, the classical disease of this type is *Canavan's disease*, with congenital and infantile forms due to an autosomal recessive trait, and a rare juvenile form with no demonstrable familial association.

Vacuolation may also arise by separation of lamellae at the major dense line, reopening the intracellular compartment of the myelinating cell, or by ballooning of the periaxonal space. Depending on the particular disease, the vacuolation of the myelin may or may not be accompanied by structural changes in other elements of the tissue, including the myelinating cell bodies, and, in general, these are more likely to occur if vacuolation has been prolonged. In some instances too, prolongation of the process is associated with a reduced quantity of myelin. In those cases where there is no indication of myelin degradation, its steady withdrawal by the normal catabolic pathways with concurrent suppression of synthesis is implied.

The spongiform myelinopathies of animals fall into two broad groups: those that are **idiopathic**, and those that have a defined **metabolic** or **toxic** basis.

Idiopathic spongiform myelinopathies

This group is documented in a small number of case reports involving calves, pups, and kittens, and most are suspected to have a heredofamilial basis. Several conditions involving newborn **Hereford** calves have been described over the years, with some conflicting and confusing aspects. Earlier reports proposed a condition, dubbed "hereditary neuraxial edema," to be a single entity with a variable clinical and pathological expression – the pathogenesis of several of these conditions has been unraveled, including *inherited congenital myoclonus* and *branched chain ketoacid dehydrogenase deficiency* (BCKD). The former is recognized in several countries in newborn polled Herefords that have violent myoclonic muscle spasms that prevent them from standing. There are no structural lesions, but biochemical studies have revealed an absence of glycinergic receptors on spinal inhibitory neurons. The functional disturbance is thus analogous to strychnine poisoning and is equally fatal. BCKD is discussed below.

From New Zealand, a disease of **horned Hereford** calves has been named *congenital brain edema*. Newborn calves are unable to stand after birth and have coarse tonic muscle contractions. Vacuolation of myelin is diffuse, extends into the gray matter, and is accompanied by elevated brain water content. Hydropic degeneration of astrocytes and expansion of the extracellular space are detectable ultrastructurally. There is also considered to be a deficiency of myelin.

In Britain, a very similar picture is recorded in **polled Hereford** calves. There may remain an entity in Hereford calves, severely neurologically impaired at birth, in which myelin vacuolation is extensive in the CNS, is confined to the white matter, and is not associated with hypomyelinogenesis. For the time being, such cases could be classified as hereditary neuraxial edema in the absence of any demonstrable metabolic disturbance suggestive of BCKD or other aminoacidopathy.

In **Samoyed** pups, a generalized tremor syndrome occurs in the first few weeks of life, with a severe and ultimately fatal outcome. Myelin vacuolation is diffuse throughout the CNS and there is no change in any other tissue element.

Labrador pups are described to have initial episodes of extensor rigidity, tremor, and dorsal flexion of the neck at 4–6 weeks of age, and then progressive dysmetria. Intense vacuolation of myelin is confined to the white matter in the CNS, but occurs to a mild degree in peripheral nerves as well. Throughout the CNS, the myelin lesion is accompanied by fibrous astrogliosis and prominence of capillary blood vessels. A similar condition with a familial pattern (familial spongiform leukodystrophy) is recognized in **Shetland Sheepdogs**. Clinical signs usually start at 3 weeks of age and include progressive seizures and dysphagia. Spongiform degeneration is most prominent in the cerebellum and corona radiata.

In a **Silky Terrier** pup, a myoclonic syndrome is described, with vacuolation of myelin occurring in the brain but not the spinal cord, together with the presence of Alzheimer type II astrocytes. In **Egyptian Mau** kittens, there is progressive ataxia and hypermetria; vacuolar change extends from white into gray matter throughout the CNS. Spongiform CNS myelinopathy has been reported in a group of related **African dwarf goats**.

Spongiform myelinopathy of silver foxes

A hereditary nervous disease occurs in farmed silver foxes in Norway. The presenting sign is hindlimb ataxia appearing between 2–4 months of age, and progressing over the next 4–8 weeks, after which time clinical improvement seems to occur.

No gross lesions are present, and histologically there is *symmetrical myelin vacuolation* affecting white matter of the cerebrum, cerebellum, brain stem, and spinal cord (Fig. 3.94). The extent and severity of vacuolation vary from case to case. In long-standing cases, vacuolation seems to resolve to a large extent, with residual intense astrogliosis.

Ultrastructurally, early features of the disease include intramyelinic vacuolation due to lamellar separation at the intraperiod line, large cytoplasmic vacuoles in oligodendrocyte cytoplasm, demyelination, expansion of extracellular space, and astrocytic hypertrophy (Fig. 3.95A, B, C). Late in the disease, there is evidence of remyelination in gliotic areas.

Toxic/metabolic spongiform myelinopathies

Hepatic and renal encephalopathy

Endogenous intoxications associated with hepatic and, to a lesser extent, renal failure, are recognized to induce brain lesions of this type, the former quite frequently, the latter less so.

The familiar clinicopathologic term, *hepatic encephalopathy*, designates a complex autointoxication, in which accumulations of ammonia and other metabolites reflect the inability of the liver to carry out its normal detoxifying role. This may in turn reflect reduced liver mass, portosystemic shunting, or both. *The neural lesions of hepatic encephalopathy are several and variable.*

Clinical evidence of nervous dysfunction may be accompanied by extensive and well-developed *spongy vacuolation of myelin* (Fig. 3.96), which tends to be most intense at the junction of the cerebral cortex and adjacent white matter, and often around the deep cerebellar nuclei. The lesion is to be expected in ruminants with subacute or chronic phyto- or mycotoxic liver injury, and in small animals with developmental portosystemic shunts or acquired liver disease. In sheep, copper toxicosis may lead to massive myelin vacuolation. There may also be *Alzheimer type II astroglial cells* (see Fig. 3.16) although, with the notable exception of the horse, this is generally less a feature in animals than in humans. In the horse, hepatic encephalopathy is characterized by the presence of Alzheimer type II cells, with no significant myelin vacuolation.

Although myelin vacuolation may be induced experimentally with ammonia alone, the syndrome is *not simple ammonia intoxication*, but may also involve perturbed monoamine neurotransmission, imbalance between excitatory and inhibitory amino acid neurotransmission, and accumulation of an endogenous benzodiazepine-like substance.

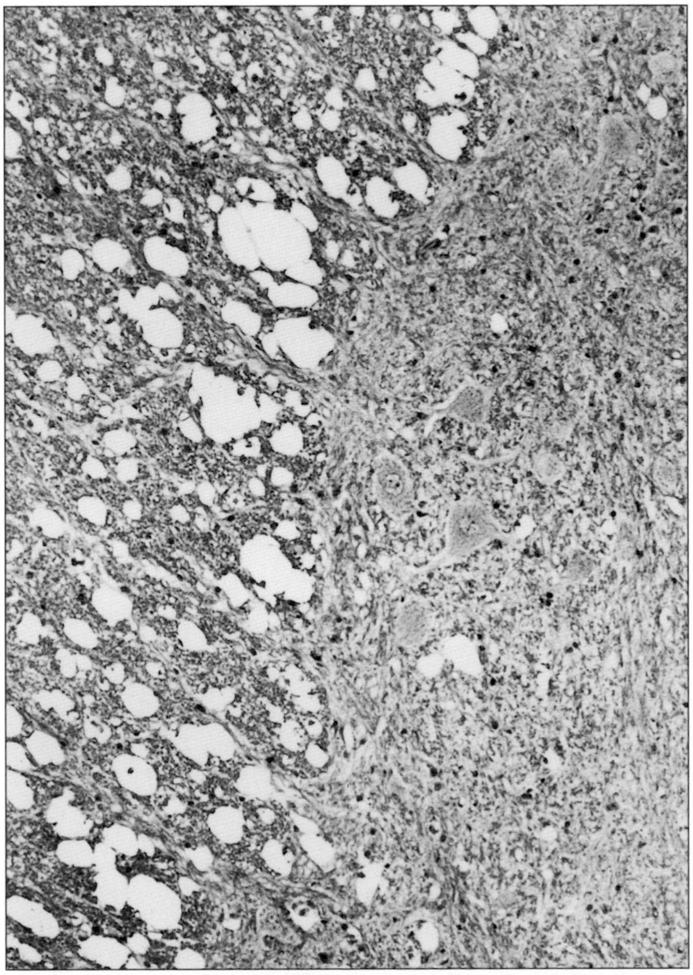

Figure 3.96 Intramyelinic edema and spongiform change surrounding spinal gray matter in **hepatic encephalopathy** in a sheep.

Branched chain α-ketoacid decarboxylase deficiency

This disease, also known as **maple syrup urine disease**, has been described in Hereford, polled Hereford, and polled Shorthorn calves, and is inherited as an *autosomal recessive* character. This mutation causes deficiency of the mitochondrial branched-chain α-ketoacid dehydrogenase (BCKD) complex. Deficiency of BCKD leads to the accumulation of the branched-chain amino acids leucine, isoleucine, and valine and their respective ketoacids, ketoisocaproic, keto-β-methylvaleric, and ketoisovaleric acids. The molecular mechanism of the intoxication remains to be precisely defined, but probably involves toxic metabolites.

The disease may be expressed in utero, and calves become dull and recumbent by 2–4 days of age, and finally develop opisthotonos. The urine in many cases has the smell of maple syrup, the characteristic which gave the disease its common name in affected children. Branched chain amino acids are found to be in abnormally high concentrations in plasma, cerebrospinal fluid, and tissues.

Pathologically, there may be gross evidence of brain swelling expressed as flattened cerebral gyri and, histologically, *severe spongy vacuolation of myelin in the CNS*. The spongiotic change is pronounced in the large myelinated tracts of the cerebral hemispheres and cerebellum (Fig. 3.97), and in myelinated tracts abutting brain-stem nuclei and spinal gray matter. Most of the spinal white matter is not affected. In cases that survive for a week or more, a modest number of axonal spheroids may be found in affected white matter. The

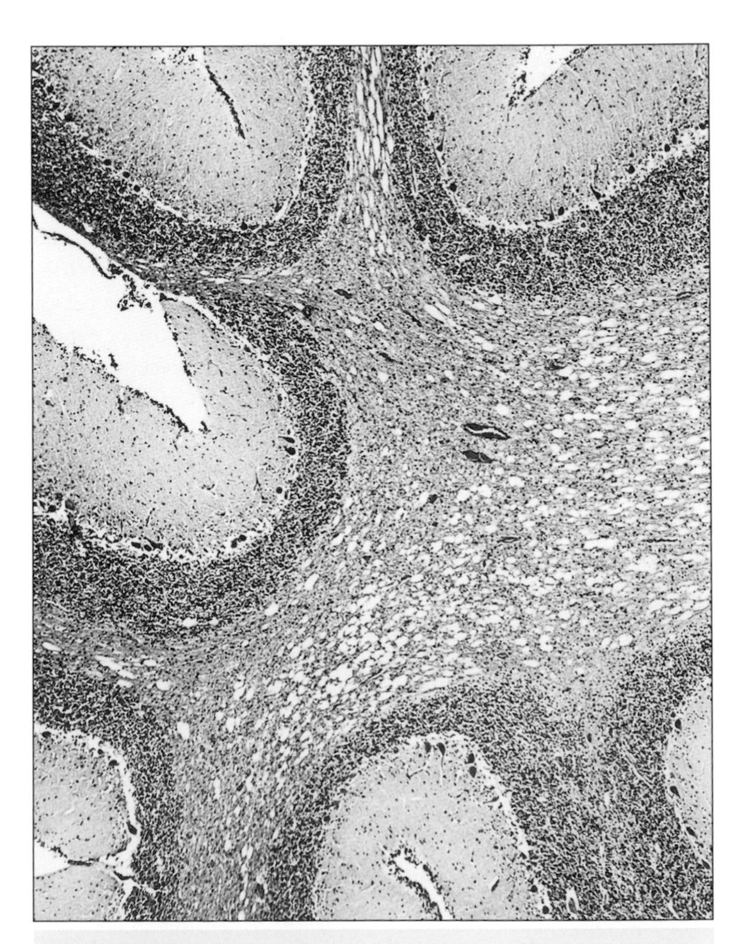

Figure 3.97 Status spongiosus in the central cerebellar white matter of a calf with **maple syrup urine disease**.

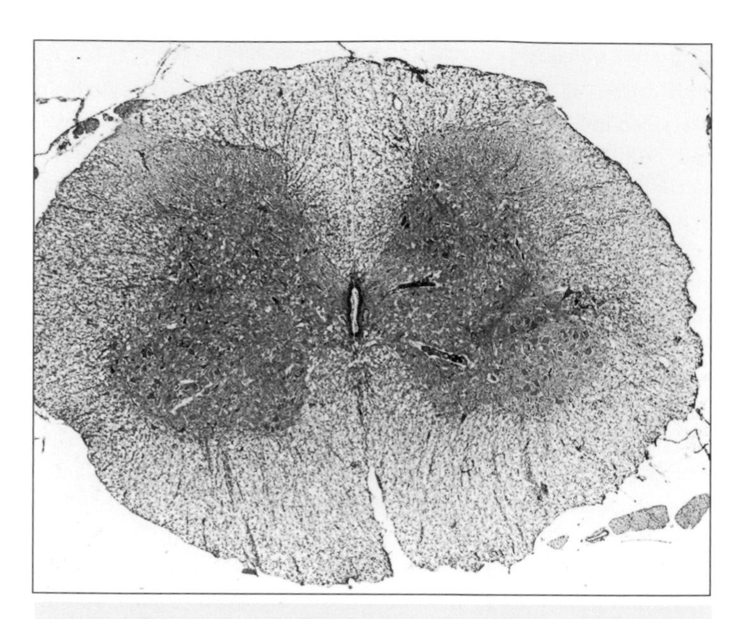

Figure 3.98 Intramyelin edema and diffuse spongiform change in the spinal cord white matter of a dog with **hexachlorophene poisoning**.

brain water content is elevated, and the electron microscope reveals splitting of myelin lamellae at the intraperiod line.

Hexachlorophene toxicosis

Hexachlorophene is a polychlorinated phenolic compound with useful topical antiseptic properties, and is sometimes given orally against *Fasciola hepatica*. Intoxication has usually been associated with repeated application to the skin of very young animals, whence absorption is rapid, and systemic accumulation may cause effects within several days. The clinical features of severe intoxication are shaking, shivering, excitement, tonic-clonic convulsions, and terminal coma.

The major lesion is *spongy vacuolation of central and peripheral myelin* (Fig. 3.98), with lamellar splitting at the intraperiod line, and no associated degenerative or reactive changes. This lesion may persist for many weeks, even after clinical signs have abated. Under experimental conditions, vacuolation of the retinal photoreceptor outer segments is also evident, but this has not been a reported feature of accidental intoxication.

Halogenated salicylanilide toxicosis

The halogenated salicylanilides are long-acting anthelmintics used in sheep and goats, and include closantel and rafoxanide. Accidental overdosing has led to intoxication expressed as ataxia, depression, and blindness, which may be permanent. The response appears to be inconsistent, and unknown predisposing factors are possibly involved.

Microscopically, there is *spongy vacuolation of myelin in both the CNS and peripheral nerves*, without any accompanying reaction or degeneration. The lesion in the brain is most intense in the brain stem. This change may persist for several weeks. Acute degenerative changes may be found in the optic nerves and in the retinal ganglion cell layer, where hemorrhage has also been described. The syndrome has some similarities to stypandrol poisoning, described below.

Stypandra toxicosis

The binaphthalene tetrol, **stypandrol**, is the toxic principle of the Australian liliaceous *Stypandra* sp. ("blindgrass") and also of the Asiatic *Hemerocallis* sp., hence the alternative name **hemerocallin**. Ingestion of toxic strains of such plants by grazing mammals or birds has an acute effect, usually manifested as moderate depression and blindness, although a high dose may produce prostration and death.

In acutely affected animals, *myelin vacuolation* caused by lamellar splitting at the intraperiod line is extensive throughout the CNS, and may persist for many weeks or even months, without apparent functional effect. Blindness, however, tends to be permanent and is associated with Wallerian degeneration of the optic nerves and tracts, and degeneration of retinal photoreceptors. Degeneration of the optic nerves may be the result of compression within the optic canals secondary to swelling caused by the myelin edema, and there may be a separate direct toxic effect on the photoreceptors.

Tylecodon toxicosis

Tylecodon wallichii is the cause of **krimpsiekte, a** neurotoxicosis of small ruminants in South Africa. The toxic principle is **cotyledoside**, a neurotoxic bufadienolide that can produce either acute or chronic poisoning, the latter probably as a cumulative effect of the toxicosis. Affected animals assume a posture with back arched, display torticollis, and then prolonged paralysis. Edema and formation of large vacuoles are particularly prominent in the optic radiations and thalamic white matter. A similar syndrome has been reported in small ruminants poisoned by *Ornithogalum toxicarium* in Namibia.

Helichrysum toxicosis

The many plant species of this genus are widely distributed, and distinct syndromes of toxicity in ruminants occur in Australia and South Africa: *Helichrysum blandoskianum* in Australia produces acute hepatic necrosis, presumptive hepatic encephalopathy, and spongiform change in the white matter of the brain stem, with a high mortality rate; *H. argyrosphaerum* in South Africa is associated with paresis, paralysis, and permanent blindness.

Intense spongy vacuolation of myelin in the brain is sufficient to cause grossly visible swelling of the optic nerves and chiasm, and gelatinous swelling of the periventricular white matter and corpus callosum. Focal hemorrhages may occur in the optic nerves and chiasm. Microscopically, the spongiform myelin lesion in the optic nerves is accompanied by Wallerian degeneration, suggesting compression within the optic canals. Myelin vacuolation is less severe in the spinal cord and peripheral nerves. The syndrome has similarities to stypandrol toxicosis.

Diplodia toxicity (diplodiosis)

Diplodiosis is a mycotoxicosis of cattle and sheep grazing on maize lands towards the end of the growing season in various countries in southern Africa and in Argentina. The causative fungus is *Diplodia maydis*. The fungus is extremely fetotoxic and causes neonatal mortality in lambs of ewes ingesting the toxin during late pregnancy. The spongy change is due to separation of myelin along the intraperiod line and may progress to lysis of myelin.

Bromethalin toxicity

Diffuse white matter spongiosus is described in dogs and cats given a single oral dose of this highly neurotoxic rodenticide.

Bibliography

Botha CJ, et al. A krimpsiekte-like syndrome in small stock poisoned by *Ornithogalum toxicarium* Archer & Archer. J S Afr Vet Assoc 2000;71:6–9.

Botha CJ, et al. Seasonal variation in cotyledoside concentration of *Tylecodon wallichii* (Harv.) Tolken subsp. *wallichii* sampled in a krimpsiekte-prevalent region. Onderstepoort J Vet Res 2001;68:1–9.
Dennis JA, Healy PJ. Definition of the mutation responsible for maple syrup urine disease in Poll Shorthorns and genotyping Poll Shorthorns and Poll Herefords for maple syrup urine disease alleles. Res Vet Sci 1999;67:1–6.
Dorman DC, et al. Neuropathologic findings of bromethalin toxicosis in the cat. Vet Pathol 1992;29:139–144.
Hagen G, et al. Ultrastructural findings in spongy degeneration of white matter in silver foxes (*Vulpes vulpes*). Acta Neuropathol (Berl) 1990;80:590–596.
Jolly RD. Congenital brain oedema of Hereford calves. J Pathol 1974;113:199–204.
Kelly DF, Gaskell CJ. Spongy degeneration of the central nervous system in kittens. Acta Neuropathol (Berl) 1976;35:151–158.
Maddison JE. Hepatic encephalopathy. Current concepts of the pathogenesis. J Vet Intern Med 1992;6:341–353.
Main DC, et al. *Stypandra imbricata* ("blindgrass") toxicosis in goats and sheep – clinical and pathologic findings in 4 field cases. Aust Vet J 1981;57:132–135.
McAuliffe OR, White WE. "Woolly everlasting daisy" (*Helichrysum blandoskianum*) toxicity in cattle and sheep. Aust Vet J 1976;52:366–368.
Morita T, et al. Severe involvement of cerebral neopallidum in a dog with hepatic encephalopathy. Vet Pathol 2004;41:442–445.
Obermaier G, et al. Spongiform central nervous system myelinopathy in African dwarf goats. J Comp Pathol 1995;113:357–372.
Poppenga RH, et al. Hexachlorophene toxicosis in a litter of Doberman pinschers. J Vet Diagn Invest 1990;2:129–131.
Prozesky L, et al. Perinatal mortality in lambs of ewes exposed to cultures of *Diplodia maydis (=Stenocarparella maydis)* during gestation. A study of the central-nervous-system lesions. Ond J Vet Res 1994;61:247–253.
Sheahan BJ, et al. Structural and biochemical changes in a spinal myelinopathy in twelve English foxhounds and two harriers. Vet Pathol 1991;28:117–124.
Swan GE. The pharmacology of halogenated salicylanilides and their anthelmintic use in animals. J S Afr Vet Assoc 1999;70:61–70.
Taboada J, Dimski DS. Hepatic encephalopathy: clinical signs, pathogenesis, and treatment. Vet Clin North Am Small Anim Pract 1995;25:337–355.
van der Lugt JJ, et al. Status spongiosis, optic neuropathy, and retinal degeneration in *Helichrysum argyrosphaerum* poisoning in sheep and a goat. Vet Pathol 1996;33:495–502.
Wood SL, Patterson JS. Shetland sheepdog leukodystrophy. J Vet Int Med 2001;15:486–493.
Zachary JF, O'Brien DP. Spongy degeneration of the central nervous system in two canine littermates. Vet Pathol 1985;22:561–571.

Spongiform encephalomyelopathies

The term "**status spongiosus**" applies to a variety of lesions in which the microscopic appearance of the neural tissue is transformed by numerous vacuoles or microcavities. As discussed above, one form of this state results from the vacuolation of myelin, and is the most common. In this section will be discussed diseases in which the change results from either the *swelling of astrocytes* or the *vacuolation of neurons and neurites*. Astrocytic swelling may occur nonspecifically in, or adjacent to, any area of neural tissue acutely injured by trauma, or ischemia, or in which vascular permeability is disturbed. In the absence of such circumstances, its occurrence suggests some direct toxic or metabolic influence upon the astrocytes themselves. It can thus be a feature in hepatic encephalopathy. Spongiform vacuolation of neurons and their processes may occur to a limited degree as an incidental change in the red nucleus and nuclei of the caudal brain stem, and also as an artifact of fixation. It needs to be interpreted against this background, and is usually considered in the context of the diagnosis of scrapie and related conditions. It is distinctly different from the foamy vacuolation seen in the lysosomal storage diseases.

Prion diseases

Prions (the word "prion" is a combined form of "proteinaceous" and "infectious") are believed to be the cause of fatal neurologic diseases in humans and several other mammalian species. Prion diseases (*prionoses*) are characterized by chronic progressive fatal neurologic manifestations, with both sensory and motor deficits and spongiform encephalopathy, and result from accumulation of an abnormal isoform (PrP^{Sc}, Sc refers to scrapie) of the host prion protein (PrP). The gene (*PRNP*) encoding the prion protein is highly conserved in animals and humans. Transmissible prion diseases result from infection with an external PrP^{Sc} and accumulation of host-produced PrP^{Sc}, and are called **transmissible spongiform encephalopathies** (TSEs) to differentiate them from prion diseases originating from genetic mutation, e.g., familial Creutzfeldt–Jacob disease in humans. The prion protein is widely distributed in tissues but concentrated in nervous tissue where normal prion protein (PrP^{c}, c is for cellular) is a glycolipid-anchored glycoprotein located on the surface of neuronal plasma membranes; its exact function in mammals is unknown. PrP^{Sc} is not only membrane anchored, but it can also be demonstrated in lysosomes using immunohistochemistry and electron microscopy. PrP^{Sc} almost never triggers an immune response.

Prion diseases in animals include *scrapie* of sheep and goats, *bovine spongiform encephalopathy* (BSE), *chronic wasting disease* (CWD) of deer and elk, *transmissible mink encephalopathy* (TME), *feline spongiform encephalopathy* (FSE), and *exotic ungulate encephalopathy* of captive wild ruminants. Human prion diseases include *kuru; Creutzfeldt–Jacob disease* (CJD), which has four types, sporadic CJD, familial CJD, iatrogenic CJD, and variant CJD (vCJD); *Gerstmann–Straussler–Scheinker disease* (GSS); and *fatal familial insomnia* (FFI). The inherited prion diseases of humans are all of dominant inheritance and all are associated with coding mutations of the *PRNP* gene. Interest in the TSEs has increased greatly for several reasons. First, the discovery that these diseases may result from an infectious protein agent that is lacking nucleic acids contradicted the central dogma of modern biology that all living organisms use nucleic acids to reproduce. Second, the appearance of BSE in Great Britain and other parts of the world, and its presumed relationship to vCJD, triggered both scientific and public interest in these diseases. Despite extensive work on prions, our understanding of their pathogenesis and etiology is incomplete.

The *protein-only hypothesis* is currently the most accepted hypothesis for the pathogenesis of prion diseases. This hypothesis states that: (1) PrP^{Sc} is the etiologic agent of TSEs and other prion diseases; (2) the transformation of α-helical PrP to its misfolded β-pleated sheet isoform, the PrP^{Sc}, requires either a genetic predisposition or requires the help of unknown protein cofactors (protein X) that act as a molecular chaperone for this conversion; (3) PrP^{Sc} triggers the PrP gene (*PRNP*) to produce more PrP^{Sc} (self-replicating protein); and (4) PrP^{Sc} can be infectious itself and can be transmitted to other hosts and cause disease (transmissible protein). There is a species barrier to transmission of the TSE agent, but it is not complete. Less-accepted theories for the etiology of prion diseases include the virion or virus hypothesis, and the autoimmunity/allergic hypothesis, which states that TSEs could be autoimmune diseases resulting from ingestion of feedstuffs contaminated with certain bacteria, e.g., *Acinetobacter* spp., that show molecular mimicry between bacterial components and CNS tissue. *Spiroplasma mirum*, a cell-wall-deficient bacterium, has also been proposed as a trigger for TSEs.

The mechanism by which PrP^{Sc} causes nerve cell degeneration is complicated and several mechanisms have been proposed including: (1) mechanical destruction of nerve cell membranes from the excessive accumulations; (2) lysosomal accumulation of PrP^{Sc} may trigger apoptosis by release of cathepsin D into cytosol; and (3) PrP^{Sc} may be a direct neurotoxin. There are multiple strains of prions in scrapie of sheep, the strains distinguished by biological properties in defined strains of mice determined especially by incubation periods and lesion profiles, and the nature and patterns of neuropathological changes. In sporadic disease in humans, different strains or types of the agent are beginning to be related to clinical phenotypes, and in some of the diseases in animals, additional to scrapie, there is evidence for strain variation. The agent of BSE is exceptional in being, so far, monotypic. Prions have unusual resistance to physical and chemical agents and this unusual resistance makes inactivation of prion infectivity very difficult.

The pathogenesis of these diseases is further complicated by genetic variation among hosts whereby homozygosity at particular codons is known to confer susceptibility to the natural or experimental disease and heterozygosity confers survival advantage, although this is expressed mainly as prolonged incubation time. In heterozygotes, the outcome of exposure may be further modified by other polymorphisms. For example, sheep carry two alleles of the PrP gene and five different allelic variants. Sheep breeds that are homozygous for the variant VRQ/VRQ (valine (V) at codon 136, arginine (R) at codon 154, glutamine (Q) at codon 171) are the most susceptible to scrapie, whereas sheep with the ARR (alanine (A)) variant are most resistant and do not develop overt disease.

The transmission of prions between individuals or species in spontaneous disease remains a mystery, except for kuru for which there is strong evidence for ritualistic cannibalism, and vCJD for which there is compelling evidence of oral transmission from BSE. It is noteworthy that all cases of vCJD and kuru are homozygous for methionine at *PRNP* codon 129. The oral route is probably important for BSE, vCJD, and TME. The mode of transmission of scrapie and CWD remains unclear.

There are *no gross abnormalities* in the brain other than those expected in older animals with a wasting disease. Some elements of the histological picture are consistently present but variable in their neuroanatomical distribution and degree of expression. The most consistent pattern involves the medulla oblongata. Inflammatory change is absent. *Spongiform change is an important identifying feature.* It consists of small rounded vacuoles in the neuropil sometimes extending into neurites. The vacuoles in the neuropil may become confluent. The extracellular space is normal. The vacuoles are of variable distribution in cerebral gray matter and may be diffuse or clustered. The pathogenesis of the spongiform change is not known.

Neuronal vacuolation has long been the identifier for scrapie. It is a feature of the natural and experimental prion diseases of animals noted above. The vacuolation may occur in the soma, perikaryon, or neurites, but may not be accompanied by the spongy change described above. The empty vacuoles may be single, multiple, or in chains. Loss of neurons is difficult to assess and neuronophagia is absent. Descriptions of abnormal numbers of dark neurons may not be significant.

Astrocytic hypertrophy and hyperplasia varies in severity. Astrocytic nuclei may be paired or densely packed and may be without increase of fibers. Astrocytosis usually involves gray matter affected by spongiform change and may spread to adjacent white matter.

Although frequent and readily detected in kuru and in vCJD of humans, *amyloid plaques are sparse or absent in the animal diseases*. They may be difficult to demonstrate in hematoxylin-eosin-stained sections but are well demonstrated with Congo red and especially the periodic acid-Schiff method. The pathogenic prion isoform is subject to limited proteolysis to produce a smaller molecule, PRP27-30, which is protease resistant and deposited as intraneural amyloid in neurons and neuropil and around neurons and blood vessels.

Electron-microscopic examination of detergent extracts of infected brain reveals characteristic fibrils, termed "*scrapie-associated fibrils*" (SAF), which have PrP^{sc} as their major component. In many cases, plaques of this material may be present in the neuropil, as histochemically detectable amyloid deposits, and it can be detected more sensitively by specific immuno-staining as "scrapie immunoreactive amyloid." Cerebrovascular amyloidosis is also usually demonstrable in ovine scrapie.

Scrapie was the first prion disease to be recognized and described, around 1732 in the UK, and is endemic worldwide, except in Australia and New Zealand where it has been eradicated. The precise route of transmission is unclear but the disease spreads in an infectious-like pattern with rapid lateral communicability in a contaminated field. Infection mostly occurs around the time of birth, and probably via ingestion, but the question of vertical modes of transmission remains unclarified. The likelihood of ewe-to-lamb transmission is highly significant, in that a ewe could give birth to and infect several lambs before showing clinical signs. The scrapie agent can infect goats sharing the pasture with affected sheep; natural spread to species other than goats grazing the same pasture is not reported.

As discussed above, sheep breeds differ in their susceptibility to scrapie. The morbidity of the natural disease is low, except in some closed stud flocks, and clinically affected animals are usually in the 2–5-year age group. There is a long incubation period, and the disease, once clinically manifest, is progressive and ultimately fatal in from 10 days to several months. The agent proliferates initially in the lymphoid tissues and lower intestine, but may take up to 2 years to reach the nervous system. A further 2 years may lapse before clinical signs appear. The methods of spread of the agent between both cells and organ systems are still enigmatic, although there is good evidence that the nervous system is first infected via the splanchnic nerves, which carry the agent to the thoracic spinal cord. Once within the central nervous system, the presence of the agent seems to be of no consequence until it reaches "clinical target areas," where the expression of PrP^{Sc} in select neurons could presumably lead to progressive dysfunction.

Both clinical signs and pathologic changes are somewhat variable but, in general, affected sheep are initially alert but excitable, tremble when excited, and may have seizures. Later, paresthesias may appear, manifested as agitated rubbing against posts and trees, and nibbling at the feet and legs when lying down, behavior that gave rise to the colloquial name "scrapie." Self-trauma can cause extensive loss of wool

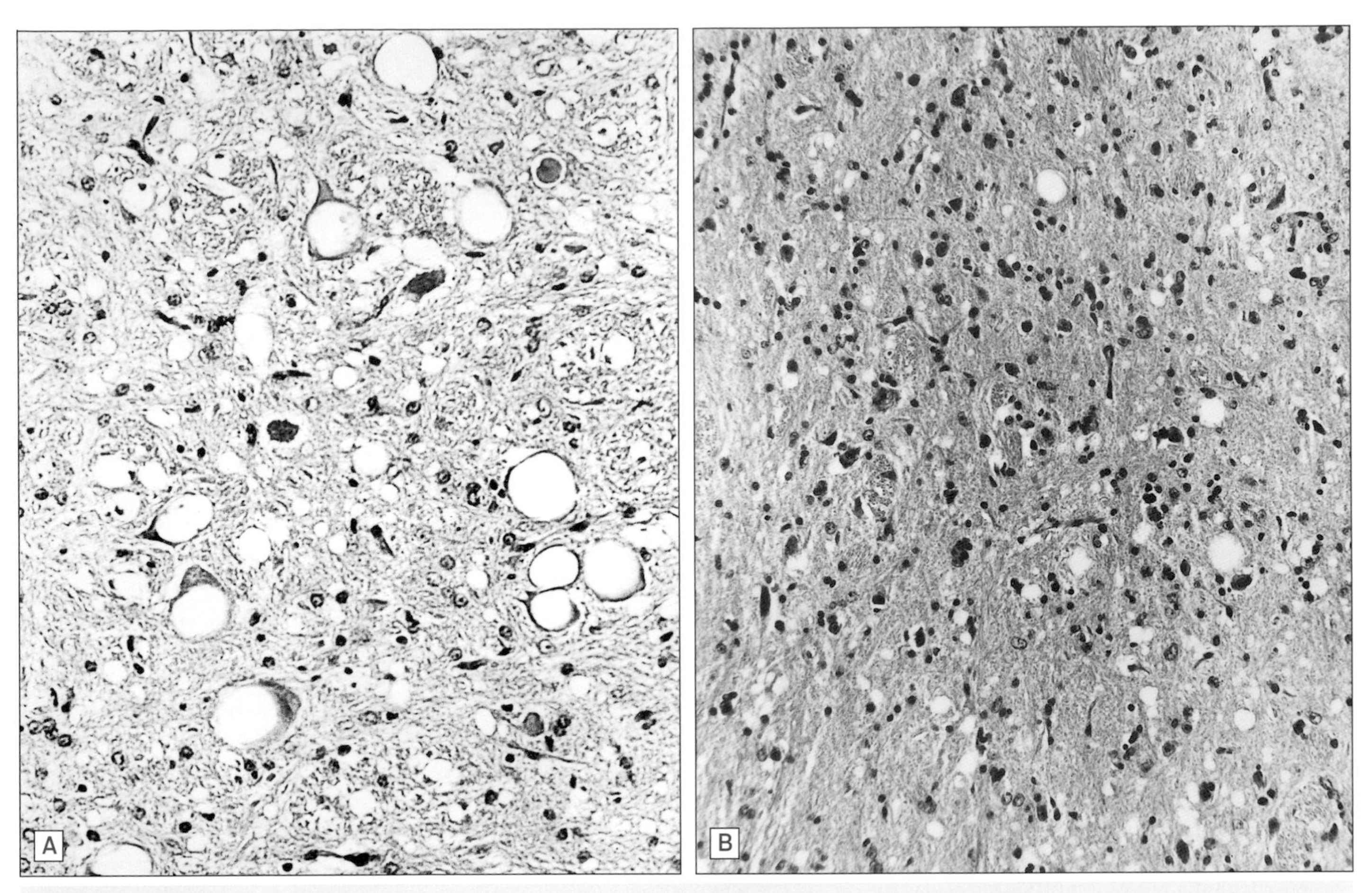

Figure 3.99 Scrapie in a sheep. **A.** Vacuolated neurons in the brain stem. **B.** Vacuolated neurons, loss of neurons, and gliosis in the medulla.

and abrasions of the skin. There is also progressive dysmetria and emaciation, and finally paralysis and death.

Apart from emaciation and self-trauma, there are no significant gross lesions, and no inflammatory changes. The most characteristic finding is the presence of *large intraneuronal vacuoles* in the medullary reticular, medial vestibular, lateral cuneate, and papilliform nuclei. The neuronal vacuolation may however be present throughout the brain stem and spinal cord (Fig. 3.99A). The vacuoles contain no stainable material and may considerably distort and displace the normal organelles. Although the vacuolated neurons do not generally appear degenerate in any other way, shrunken and apparently degenerate neurons may be found in mesencephalic, medullary, and deep cerebellar nuclei, and in the intermediolateral nucleus of the spinal cord. In late stages, neuronal loss may be evident, as well as diffuse fibrillary astrogliosis present mainly in the mesencephalon (Fig. 3.99B) and the molecular layer of the cerebellum. These lesions are bilaterally symmetrical, and the cerebral cortex is rarely involved (see Fig. 3.12A, B). *Spongy vacuolation of the neuropil* in gray matter is due to vacuolation of neuronal processes, but it is seldom a feature of the natural disease in sheep.

Bovine spongiform encephalopathy (BSE) causes cattle 3–6 years of age to become apprehensive, hyperesthetic, and dysmetric. The animals display fear and aggressive behavior, with progressive gait disturbances leading to frequent falling. Eventually, frenzied episodes or recumbency necessitate euthanasia. The origin of the rogue prion is still undetermined; however, ingestion of feed contaminated with infectious prion is the most likely origin for BSE. This contamination may have come from bone and meat meal from scrapie-infected sheep carcasses; however the BSE agent is different biologically than any of the known scrapie strains. Another source suggested is feed contamination with the remains of humans infected with CJD. Sporadic and genetically determined TSEs have not been detected in cattle. BSE is basically a food-borne epidemic; lateral or vertical transmission is highly unlikely. *The pathologic features of BSE resemble those of scrapie.* Scrapie-associated fibrils and immunoreactive amyloid are demonstrable. *Vacuolation of neuronal cell bodies and processes* is particularly prominent in the dorsal vagal, medullary reticular, vestibular, solitary, spinal trigeminal, and red nuclei, and is accompanied by moderate degrees of *spongiform change in neuropil.* The severity of neuropil and neuronal somatic vacuolation varies independently among anatomic locations, and the latter is sometimes accompanied by ceroid-lipofuscin granules. Occasional necrotic neurons and axonal spheroids may be present, as may mild astrogliosis.

Transmissible mink encephalopathy (TME) has caused high levels of morbidity and mortality in ranch mink in North America and northern Europe including Finland and Russia. The source of TME infection was not determined, but contamination of feed materials by the scrapie agent was suggested. The agent was experimentally pathogenic to a variety of wild carnivores, sheep, cattle, and primates. Neuronal vacuolation is sparse in this disease, which exhibits *spongy* *degeneration and astrocytosis* of parallel intensity. Neuronal vacuolation is mainly in brain stem. The lesions are especially well developed in the neocortex and amygdala, corpus striatum, caudodorsal thalamus, and medial geniculate bodies. The pathologic profile may differ between countries, perhaps due to strain differences of the agent or genotype of the captive mink.

Chronic wasting disease (CWD) of cervids affects mule deer (*Odocoileus hemionus*), white-tailed deer (*Odocoileus virginianus*), Rocky Mountain elk (*Cervus elaphus nelsoni*), and perhaps other cervids in several states in the USA and in western Canada. Although CWD was first diagnosed in the 1960s in captive cervids, it is now prevalent and possibly increasing among free-ranging and wild susceptible species and is considered to be the only TSE that occurs in free-ranging animals. The source of infection is unknown, but the disease is likely spread horizontally by ingestion of material contaminated with the CWD agent. CWD PrP^{Sc} is widespread not only in the CNS but also in various lymphoid tissues, including gut-associated lymphoid tissue (GALT). The presence of PrP^{SC} in GALT led to the presumption that PrP^{Sc} could be shed in feces causing pasture contamination and a health hazard to other animals or humans. Affected animals show slow progressive weight loss, dullness and depression, polydipsia and polyuria. Deer may show swallowing difficulty and esophageal dilation. Spongiform change, neuronal vacuolation, gliosis, and amyloid deposition are especially well developed in the olfactory tubercle, cortex hypothalamus, and vagal nuclei. Amyloid plaques are more frequently demonstrated in deer than in elk.

Feline spongiform encephalopathy (FSE) has been observed in domestic cats and captive felids in zoos. FSE was likely transmitted to captive felids by ingestion of BSE-infected cattle carcasses, and to domestic cats by ingestion of pet food contaminated with the BSE agent. The lesion pattern emphasizes the spongy change in deep laminae of cerebrum, the corpus striatum, thalamus, medial geniculate body, and cerebellar cortex. Neuronal vacuolation occurs mainly in medullary neurons but is not pronounced.

Transmissible spongiform encephalopathy of captive wild ruminants Several zoo members of the family Bovidae, e.g. nyala, Arabian oryx, and a bison, developed TSE at the time of the BSE epidemic in UK in association with ingestion of BSE-contaminated meat and bone meal.

Spongiform encephalopathy in nonhuman primates Lemurs and a rhesus macaque in France developed TSE naturally. The disease was likely a food-borne infection from ingestion of primate food containing BSE-contaminated beef.

Laboratory **diagnosis** of TSEs can be achieved by immunohistochemistry or by rapid tests such as ELISA or Western blot.

Bibliography

Bastian FO, et al. Linking chronic wasting disease to scrapie by comparison of *Spiroplasma mirum* ribosomal DNA sequences. Exp Mol Pathol 2004;77:49–56.

Baylis M, Goldmann W. The genetics of scrapie in sheep and goats. Curr Mol Med 2004;4:385–396.

Chesebro B. Introduction to the transmissible spongiform encephalopathies or prion diseases. Br Med Bull 2003;66:1–20.

Collinge J. Prion diseases of humans and animals: Their causes and molecular basis. Ann Rev Neurosci 2001;24:519–550.

DeArmond SJ. Discovering the mechanisms of neurodegeneration in prion diseases. Neurochem Res 2004;29:1979–1998.

Foster J, et al. Partial dissociation of PrP^{Sc} deposition and vacuolation in the brains of scrapie and BSE experimentally affected goats. J Gen Virol 2001;82: 267–273.

Foster JD, et al. Clinical signs, histopathology and genetics of experimental transmission of BSE and natural scrapie to sheeps and goats. Vet Rec 2001;148:165–171.

Hunter N, et al. Natural scrapie in a closed flock of Cheviot sheep occurs only in specific PrP genotypes. Arch Virol 1996;141:809–824.

Jeffrey M, et al. Oral inoculation of sheep with the agent of bovine spongiform encephalopathy (BSE). 1. Onset and distribution of disease-specific PrP accumulation in brain and viscera. J Comp Pathol 2001;124:280–289.

Lee HS, et al. Increased susceptibility to kuru of carriers of the PRNP129 methionine/methionine genotype. J Inf Dis 2001;183:192–196.

Prusiner SB. Shattuck lecture – neurodegenerative diseases and prions. N Engl J Med 2001;344:1516–1526.

Ryder SJ, et al. Immunohistochemical detection of PrP in the medulla oblongata of sheep: the spectrum of staining in normal and scrapie-affected sheep. Vet Rec 2001;148:7–13.

Soto C, Castilla J. The controversial protein-only hypothesis of prion propagation. Nat Med 2004;10 Suppl:S63–67.

Takemura K. An overview of transmissible spongiform encephalopathies. Anim Health Res Rev 2004;5:103–124.

Tiwana H, et al. Autoantibodies to brain components and antibodies to *Acinetobacter calcoaceticus* are present in bovine spongiform encephalopathy. Infect Immun 1999;67:6591–6595.

Wells GAH, et al. Preliminary observations on the pathogenesis of experimental bovine spongiform encephalopathy (BSE): an update. Vet Rec 1998; 142:103–106.

Wood JLN, et al. Neuropathology of scrapie: a study of the distribution patterns of brain lesions in 222 cases of natural scrapie in sheep, 1982–1991. Vet Rec 1997;140:167–174.

Bovine citrullinemia

This fulminating neurologic affliction of newborn Holstein-Friesian calves results from a blockade of urea cycle metabolism caused by *deficiency of arginosuccinate synthetase*. The enzyme deficiency leads to hyperammonemia and citrullinemia, and is due to an *autosomal recessive* genetic defect. Increased cross-breeding and screening of sires for the defect have reduced its prevalence to insignificant levels. Citrullinemia has also been reported in dogs.

Calves are affected within the first week of life, the clinical features being depression, head pressing, stupor, convulsions, terminal coma, and death. There are no gross neural lesions, but microscopically there is mild to moderate spongy vacuolation of the deep laminae of the cerebral cortex. *The spongy change is due to astrocytic swelling.* Hydropic astrocytes have enlarged vesicular nuclei, but their cell bodies and processes are vacuolated and give rise to the spongiform appearance of the neuropil, the creation of perineuronal spaces, and the enlargement of pericapillary spaces. The astrocytic reaction is believed to represent a stress on these cells in their attempts to detoxify ammonia. Astrocytes play a major role in ammonia detoxification via utilization of glutamine synthetase and glutamate dehydrogenase activities. In spite of the marked degenerative changes in astrocytes, other elements of the tissue remain morphologically normal, but neuronal function is obviously grossly disturbed.

Affected calves also have pale yellow-ochre discoloration of the liver, which is correlated microscopically and ultrastructurally with hydropic degeneration of hepatocytes.

Neuronal vacuolar degeneration of Angora goats

A scrapie-like neuronopathy is described in young Angora goats in Australia (where scrapie is not present), and is presumed to be genetically determined. Animals become ataxic at about 3 months of age, and progress to severe paresis. No significant gross lesions are present, but there is spectacular vacuolation of large neurons in the red nucleus and other brainstem nuclei, and in the spinal motor neurons. Some Wallerian changes are present in the brain stem, spinal cord and peripheral nerves.

Focal spongiform encephalopathy of dogs

A disease was originally described in **Bull Mastiffs** as familial cerebellar ataxia with hydrocephalus, but the main pathologic feature is spongy vacuolation of several gray matter nuclei. Clinical signs emerge between 6 and 9 weeks of age, and include ataxia and visual impairment, and a number of other variable deficits. An autosomal recessive genetic defect has been proposed.

Macroscopically, there is moderate to severe dilation of the ventricular system. Microscopically, bilaterally symmetrical spongy vacuolation and gliosis are evident in all three deep cerebellar nuclei, the posterior colliculi and, to a lesser extent, the lateral vestibular nuclei. The vacuolation is accompanied by axonal spheroids, but nerve cell bodies appear normal. Some of the vacuoles appear to involve myelin sheaths, but the lesions are essentially confined to the gray matter, and the cytologic basis of the vacuolation is not precisely defined.

Similar vacuolating lesions of these gray matter areas have been described in **Saluki** dogs.

Spongiform encephalopathy of unknown etiology and characterized histologically by neuronal vacuolation is recognized in **Rottweiler** dogs. The condition usually starts at 8 weeks of age and is characterized clinically by progressive laryngeal paralysis, tetraparesis, and cerebellar ataxia. Vacuolated neurons are prevalent in the cerebellar roof nuclei, nuclei of the extrapyramidal system, dorsal nerve root ganglia, myenteric plexus, and other ganglia of the autonomic nervous system.

A hereditary polioencephalomyelopathy of **Australian Cattle Dogs** is characterized histologically by neuronal, neuropilar, and astrocytic vacuolation, particularly in the ventral horn of the spinal cord, cerebellar, and brain stem nuclei. An autosomal recessive trait affecting the astrocytic mitochondria is suspected.

Alaskan Husky dogs can develop a hereditary familial encephalopathy (*Alaskan Husky encephalopathy*) similar to Leigh syndrome in humans and to the multifocal symmetrical myelinolytic encephalopathy of Simmental calves described above. Clinical signs usually start before 1 year of age and include seizures, ataxia, blindness, and behavioral abnormalities. Lesions are more prevalent in the basal nuclei, thalamus, midbrain, pons, and medulla oblongata, and include bilateral symmetrical malacia, status spongiosus, gemistocytic astrocytosis with marked intracytoplasmic vacuolation, gliosis, vascular hyperplasia, and mild infiltration of mixed inflammatory cells, with relative neuronal sparing. Similar but milder lesions occur in the cerebellar ventral vermis and the base of cerebral sulci. Neuronal sparing and marked astrocytic vacuolation suggests a role for astrocytes in the pathogenesis of this condition.

Bibliography

Brenner O, et al. Hereditary polioencephalomyelopathy of the Australian cattle dog. Acta Neuropathol (Berl) 1997;94:54–66.

Brenner O, et al. Alaskan Husky encephalopathy – a canine neurodegenerative disorder resembling subacute necrotizing encephalomyelopathy (Leigh syndrome). Acta Neuropathol (Berl) 2000;100:50–62.

Healy PG, et al. Bovine citrullinemia: a clinical, pathological, biochemical and genetic study. Aust Vet J 1990;67:255–258.

Johnson RP, et al. Familial cerebellar ataxia with hydrocephalus in bull mastiffs. Vet Radiol Ultrasound 2001;42:246–249.

Kortz GD, et al. Neuronal vacuolation and spinocerebellar degeneration in young rottweiler dogs. Vet Pathol 1997;34:296–302.

Lancaster MJ, et al. Progressive paresis in Angora goats. Aust Vet J 1987;64:123–124.

INFLAMMATION IN THE CENTRAL NERVOUS SYSTEM

Brain and infection

Organs defend against invading infectious organisms either by innate or adaptive immunity. Innate immunity is composed of resident components, e.g., pulmonary alveolar macrophages, or recruited components, e.g., neutrophils. Unlike parenchymatous organs, the brain depends solely on resident innate immunity to recognize and clear pathogens. In other words, under normal nondisease conditions, the brain does not rely either on adaptive immunity or the recruited components of innate immunity for defense. Innate immunity in the brain is diverse and composed of structural units, e.g., blood–brain barrier (BBB), plus cellular and chemical components.

The structural units that separate vulnerable brain cells from the blood stream are the **blood–brain barrier (BBB)** and the **blood–cerebrospinal fluid barrier (BCSFB)**, which is present at the choroid plexuses. The BBB is made up of endothelial cells lining the blood capillaries, pericytes embedded in the capillary basement membranes, and the foot processes of astrocytes. The endothelial cells of the BBB differ from other body endothelial cells, first by having significantly fewer endocytotic vesicles, thereby limiting the amount of transcellular flux, and second, they are connected by both *adherens junction* (e.g., cadherin) and *tight junction proteins*; the latter significantly reduce paracellular flux. Also, BBB endothelial cells are rich in several transport systems that selectively transport essential nutrients to the brain or harmful material back into the blood (efflux transport proteins). One of the most important efflux proteins is *P-glycoprotein*. Inhibition of P-glycoprotein increases the tissue invasiveness of *Listeria monocytogenes*. In addition to these protective properties of the BBB, the CSF side of the BCSFB is also rich in tight junctions, which restricts movement to the CSF. *The ability of organisms to breach these barriers determines their neurotropism.* Neurotropic viruses and bacteria have developed several strategies to breach or to cross these barriers. For example, several neurotropic viruses bypass the BBB and invade the brain via axons (e.g., *Rabies virus*); intracellular bacteria (e.g., *Mycobacterium bovis*) invade the brain as Trojan horses, hidden in infected leukocytes; and finally some bacteria have a direct cytotoxic effect on the endothelial cells of the BBB (e.g., *Histophilus somni*).

The cellular part of the brain's innate immunity is composed of perivascular **dendritic cells, microglia**, and **astrocytes**. These cells are rich in *pattern recognition receptors*, which bind directly and nonspecifically to *pathogen-associated molecular patterns*. For example, all three cell types are rich in *macrophage mannose receptor*, which is a lectin receptor that recognizes "nonself" sugars on the cell wall of gram-negative and gram-positive bacteria, parasites, and yeasts. Microglia cells also express several *tool-like receptors*, e.g., TLR 2 and 6, which have a major role as bridges between innate and adaptive immunity. Activated microglia express several receptors important for phagocytosis, e.g., CR3 and CR4; recognition of pathogens is followed by phagocytosis, largely by microglial cells and to a lesser extent by astrocytes. Finally, glial cells release several *cytokines* and *antimicrobial peptides*, for example, interleukin-1β, tumor necrosis factor-α, and the antimicrobial peptide *cathelicidin*. Inflammation of the brain starts once an infectious agent overcomes the resident innate immunity and recruiting begins of different components of adaptive immunity (leukocytes and humoral immunity), which are more specific and more effective but also more destructive.

Bibliography

Neudeck BL, et al. Intestinal P glycoprotein acts as a natural defense mechanism against *Listeria monocytogenes*. Infect Immun 2004;72:3849–3854.

Rubin LL, Staddon JM. The cell biology of the blood-brain barrier. Annu Rev Neurosci 1999;22:11–28.

Inflammation in the central nervous system

Inflammation of the brain is **encephalitis**, of the spinal cord **myelitis**, of the ependyma **ependymitis**, of the choroid plexus **choroiditis**, and of the meninges **meningitis**, qualified as **leptomeningitis** when it involves the pia-arachnoid and as **pachymeningitis** when it involves the dura. This is the area of neuropathology that is of most veterinary importance because it embraces many of the transmissible highly fatal infections of animals, because even the sporadic infections are common, and because there is always a pressing need for the pathologist to separate the inflammations into general or specific etiological categories. Most of the specific infectious diseases to be described in this chapter are caused by agents that demonstrate a remarkable or specific neurotropism. These are, however, only a segment of the list of agents that commonly, occasionally, or rarely involve the CNS (Table 3.1); neurologic lesions are also discussed with systemic infections elsewhere in these volumes.

Inflammatory processes in the CNS are basically the same as those in other tissues, but they derive some specific features from the special responsiveness and anatomic arrangements of the CNS. It is important to recognize the criteria of inflammation in the CNS and then to presume from that, as far as is possible, the nature of the infecting organisms because opportunities to intervene clinically are brief and the time frame for clinical intervention is less than required for definitive microbiological diagnosis.

The problem is not only one of why and how the CNS, of known high vulnerability to infection, is so frequently spared in systemic diseases; it is also one of why and how it is infected hematogenously. There is presently no better knowledge of why four out of five cases of Glasser's disease will have meningitis than why one of five will not, even though in the one case the pathologic syndrome is otherwise fully developed.

Infections that, in other organs or tissues, may be inconsequential and even asymptomatic frequently cause death or permanent disability when they involve the nervous system. There are several contributing factors, the most important of which is the *indispensability of most portions of the CNS*. The nervous tissue cannot reconstitute itself, but it may, if the lesion develops slowly, manage a considerable degree of functional compensation. Vascular responses may be more of an impediment than a help in the reaction to inflammation, because they lead consistently to edema and brain swelling that spreads the consequences of the inflammation far from the active focus. Vascular proliferation and fibrous tissue encapsulation may develop only when the inflammatory reaction involves the meninges and the larger blood vessels because these are the only source of reticulin and collagenous tissue. Investigation continues into how viruses spread in nervous tissue; bacteria and fungi can spread rapidly and extensively in the fluid of the ventricular system and meninges. Spread of infection from the ventricular fluid to the periventricular veins occurs readily across the ependyma, and spread from the meninges to the brain, or vice versa, can occur via the Virchow–Robin spaces. The special drainage of CSF is such that exudate rich in fibrin and cells is drained very poorly.

The structure of nervous tissue and meninges limits the anatomical types of inflammation that may occur. **Fibrinous inflammation** is confined to the meninges and larger perivascular spaces. Fibrin is usually indicative of a bacterial infection, but there are exceptions. Fibrinopurulent, largely fibrinous, exudate is caused by the mycoplasmas; fibrinous exudation is typical of the meningeal reaction in malignant catarrhal fever of cattle, and it is occasionally observed in organomercurial poisoning of swine and cattle. **Hemorrhagic inflammation** is not common except as examples of symptomatic purpura in infections such as porcine erysipelas and infectious canine hepatitis and in the infarcts of embolic infections. Hemorrhage is characteristic of helminthic infections, but these lesions are perhaps better regarded as traumatic malacias. **Suppurative or granulomatous inflammation** is the usual response to bacterial or mycotic infections. Viral infections are characterized by **nonsuppurative inflammation**, which is described in more detail later; it is typically composed of neuronal degeneration, perivascular cuffing by mononuclear cells, and focal or diffuse glial proliferations.

Applying these broad criteria, there is seldom much difficulty in deciding on the class of the infecting agent. *There is occasionally some difficulty in distinguishing between the reactions to degeneration and to viral infections*. While suppuration does not occur in either of these processes, early infiltration of neutrophils occurs in acute degenerations, such as the malacias, and a few neutrophils can be found migrating in affected gray matter in the first stages of many cases of viral encephalomyelitis. Acute demyelinating processes are associated with, and probably stimulate, perivascular cuffing. The cuffs tend to be quite distinct from those in viral infections by being relatively very thick (up to ten or more cells thick) and to be composed of pure populations of lymphocytes. *If there are proliferated adventitial cells with plasma cells or other leukocytes mixed in the cuffs of lymphocytes, then the cuffs are likely to be a response to infection*. Only three diseases in animals are caused by viruses and characterized by demyelination and these, namely canine distemper, leukoencephalomyelitis of goats, and visna of sheep, have their own distinguishing characteristics. A possible fourth is so-called "old dog encephalitis." Glial responsiveness occurs in a variety of degenerative and viral lesions, but *glial nodules are characteristic only of an infectious process*, usually viral but occasionally rickettsial or bacterial.

Bacterial and pyogenic infections of the nervous system

Epidural/subdural abscess and empyema

The brain and spinal cord are protected against direct penetration of infection by the skeletal encasement and by the dura mater; the dura is almost impermeable to inflammatory processes. However, infection of the epidural space or the bony encasement with pyogenic bacteria and occasionally fungi can occur and may lead to localized *abscessation* or to the collection of suppurative material in the epidural or subdural space without forming a discrete abscess (*epidural or subdural empyema*). Infection may be hematogenous from *distant sites of infection* (e.g., septic valvular endocarditis, lung abscess), *direct extension* (e.g., osteomyelitis, middle ear and tympanic bullae, eye, paranasal sinuses, ethmoid cells), *trauma* (e.g., bite wounds especially in cats), or by *direct incidental injection* (e.g., contaminated spinal needle). Most cranial epidural abscesses arise by direct extension from one of the paranasal sinuses. Spread from the middle ear and through the cribriform plate is usually directly to the leptomeninges and brain. Occasionally, epidural suppuration is observed to have tracked from a retropharyngeal or nodal abscess through cranial foramina. Epidural suppuration about the base of the brain usually does not become encapsulated.

Tail biting in pigs, docking of lambs, and tail fracture in cats are common etiologies for spinal epidural abscesses that develop either secondary to local venous bacterial invasion or by direct extension from septic osteomyelitis. In cattle, spinal epidural abscesses are usually secondary to osteomyelitis of the vertebral bodies, are more prevalent at the lumbosacral area, and are usually caused by *Arcanobacterium pyogenes* or *Fusobacterium necrophorum*. Migrating grass awns can cause osteomyelitis and epidural abscess in the thoracolumbar regions in dogs. Common bacterial etiologies for epidural abscess or empyema in dogs and cats include *Streptococcus*, *Staphylococcus*, *Brucella*, *Pasteurella*, *Bacteroides*, and *Fusobacterium*, and in horses include *Actinobacillus* and *Streptococcus*.

Clinical signs vary according to the area affected, and can range from mild pain and restlessness to blindness and ataxia. Epidural abscessation at the lumbosacral area in ruminants may lead to circling, which can be confused with encephalitic listeriosis. Spinal epidural abscesses usually cause compression malacia of the cord, if the osteomyelitis from which they originate does not first lead to pathologic fracture with displacement.

Subdural abscessation is seldom observed, but can result from local penetration, perhaps most frequently from the paranasal sinuses. Extension can occur from epidural abscesses or, because subdural suppuration is prone to cause local phlebitis, it may give rise to epidural suppuration. Subdural infection is liable to spread widely via the veins or after penetrating the outer layer of the arachnoid. Spread is also permitted by the slowness with which leptomeningeal fibrous tissue develops to encapsulate the reaction.

Leptomeningitis

Leptomeningitis can be classified according to *etiology* (e.g., bacterial, mycotic), according to *duration* (e.g., acute, chronic), and according to the *type of exudates* (e.g., fibrinous, purulent). Classification by type of exudate is very useful, not only because it indicates the expected histologic lesions, but also clinically because it indicates the possible etiology. *Purulent meningitis* is by far the most common meningitis in domestic animals, especially neonates. *Serocellular meningitis* is described later with viral inflammation. *Hemorrhagic meningitis* occurs in septicemic anthrax and very seldom in other septicemias. Purely *fibrinous meningitis* occurs in malignant catarrhal fever, chlamydiosis, and seldom in anything else. *Mycoplasma bovis* is a rare cause of fibrinous meningitis in calves. *Granulomatous meningitis* occurs in systemic infections of this type, such as tuberculosis and cryptococcosis. The nonsuppurative inflammations of the leptomeninges are described with the diseases of which they may be part. They are mentioned here to draw attention to the wide variety of infectious agents that may localize in and produce inflammation of the leptomeninges. We have also mentioned or discussed purulent leptomeningitis with the many specific diseases of which it can be part, but dwell on the purulent process here because it is common, lacks specificity, and is suitable for a "type" description.

Purulent leptomeningitis may arise by direct extension from an adjacent structure. Extension from an epidural abscess or inflammation may result in diffuse leptomeningitis but, in most of the few cases of this origin, the leptomeningitis is local and overshadowed by the brain abscess that usually forms. Leptomeningitis may arise by local extension from a brain abscess, either by direct permeation or by spread in the Virchow–Robin spaces. Such an origin is observed frequently in listeriosis and in association with very large cerebral abscesses, but most cerebral abscesses, which are usually small, track inwards to the white matter rather than out to the meninges. The reverse sequence in which meningitis spreads to the brain and cord is not unusual in granulomatous infections but is distinctly unusual in suppurative infections, and when it occurs it consists of invasion of the surface of the brain by neutrophils (Fig. 3.100A) rather than of abscessation.

Both purulent meningitis and cerebral abscesses are usually of hematogenous origin, but they are seldom concurrent, and one usually finds meningitis alone or abscessation alone. There are occasional exceptions including thromboembolic lesions and leptomeningitis complicated by choroiditis. Septic emboli are prone to localize in the brain but may localize in meningeal vessels (Fig. 3.100B). Although those in meningeal vessels may lead to diffuse suppurative meningitis, they are usually quickly walled off and prevented from spreading (Fig. 3.100C,D). In the other exception, that of choroiditis concurrent with leptomeningitis, encephalitis or cerebral abscesses may develop because choroiditis leads to exudation into the cerebrospinal fluid and the ependyma is virtually no barrier to infection. Even this combination of pathologic processes is unusual and, when choroiditis is complicated by ependymitis and suppurative encephalitis (Fig. 3.100E), there is usually little or no meningitis. Whether encephalitis develops by spread of meningitis may be largely a question of time, but it is not unusual for animals with purulent meningitis to survive for a week, and sometimes much longer. There is ample time for the inflammation to spread throughout the cranial and spinal meninges – and to the brain if it were going to do so – but it seldom does, and *there is seldom anatomic justification for the common diagnosis of suppurative meningoencephalitis.*

In the section on inflammatory diseases of joints and synovial structures, attention is drawn to the frequent concurrence of polyarthritis with choroiditis and leptomeningitis in fibrinopurulent infections. Erysipelas, in which arthritis is a typical lesion, is an

Table 3.1 Infectious agents/diseases inducing inflammatory changes in the nervous system

Species	Canine	Feline	Porcine	Bovine	Equine	Ovine/Caprine	Camelid	Remarks on brain lesions
a. Viral disease/agent								
Akabane virus	N	N	N	Y	N	S	SC	
Bovine herpesvirus 1	N	N	N	Y	N	N	N	
Bovine herpesvirus 5	N	N	N	Y	N	N	N	
Borna disease virus	Y	Y	N	Y	Y	Y	S	
Bovine paramyxovirus (unclassified)	N	N	N	S	N	N	N	
Canine adenovirus 2	S	N	N	N	N	N	N	Multiple hemorrhages particularly in brain stem/caudate nuclei.
Canine distemper virus	Y	N	N	N	N	N	N	
Canid herpesvirus 1	Y	N	N	N	N	N	N	Necrotizing meningoencephalitis which is most severe in cerebrum and brain stem.
Canine parvovirus 2	S	N	N	N	N	N	N	Vasculitis-induced lesions.
Classical swine fever virus	N	N	Y	N	N	N	N	Vasculitis-induced lesions.
Equine encephalitis viruses (EEEV, WEEV, VEEV)	SC/S	N	S	SC	Y	SC	?	
Equid herpesvirus 1 and EHV-4	N	N	N	N	Y	N	N	EHV 4 rarely causes encephalitis.
Equid herpesvirus 9	?	?	?	?	?	?	?	Natural disease only reported in deer.
Encephalomyocarditis virus	?	?	Y	S	S	?	S	Infection in some species (e.g., bovine) may be limited to myocarditis.
Equine infectious anemia virus	N	N	N	N	S	N	N	Multifocal to diffuse encephalomyelitis is a rare manifestation of EIAV infection; may also cause lymphohistiocytic periventricular leukoencephalitis.
Feline immunodeficiency virus	N	S	N	N	N	N	N	Nonsuppurative encephalomyelitis in some naturally infected cats; secondary *Toxoplasma* or *Feline infectious peritonitis virus* infections.
Feline leukemia virus	N	S	N	N	N	N	N	Non-inflammatory degenerative myelopathy.
Feline infectious peritonitis virus	N	Y	N	N	N	N	N	Fibrinopyogranulomatous periventriculitis, meningitis, and perivasculitis; chronic leukoencephalitis; segmental myelitis; choroiditis.
Hemagglutinating encephalomyelitis virus (HEV)	N	N	Y	N	N	N	N	
Highlands J virus	N	N	N	N	S	N	N	
Japanese encephalitis virus	SC	N	Y	SC	SC	SC	?	
La Crosse virus	S	N	N	N	N	N	?	

Species	Canine	Feline	Porcine	Bovine	Equine	Ovine/Caprine	Camelid	Remarks on brain lesions
Lentivirus encephalomyelitis	N	N	N	N	N	Y	N	
Louping ill virus	Y	?	Y	Y	Y	Y	Y	
Malignant catarrhal fever	N	N	S	Y	N	SC	?	
Nipah virus	Y	Y	Y	S	Y	Y	?	
Porcine arterivirus	N	N	Y	N	N	N	?	
Porcine circovirus-2	N	N	Y	N	N	N	?	
Porcine paramyxovirus (unclassified)	N	N	S	N	N	N	N	
Porcine rubulavirus	N	N	S	N	N	N	N	
Pseudorabies virus	Y	Y	Y	Y	S	Y	?	
Rabies virus	Y	Y	S	Y	Y	S	Y	
Porcine teschovirus (Teschen disease)	N	N	Y	N	N	N	N	
Tick-borne encephalitis virus	Y	?	?	?	?	?	?	
West Nile virus	Y	Y	SC	SC	Y	S	Y	
b. Protozoal diseases								
Acanthamoeba encephalitis	S	?	?	?	?	S	?	
Babesiosis	S	S	S	Y	S	Y	Y	Sludging of parasitized RBCs in blood capillaries.
Neospora caninum	Y	N	N	Y*	S	S	Y	* in bovine encephalitis, is only observed in aborted fetuses or very young calves infected in utero.
Neospora hughesi	N	N	N	N	Y	N	N	
Sarcocystis canis	S	N	N	N	N	N	N	
Sarcocystis neurona	N	S	N	N	Y	N	N	
Theileriosis	S	N	N	Y	S	Y	Y	
Toxoplasmosis	Y	Y	Y	SC/S	SC	Y	Y	
c. Bacterial diseases								
Listeria monocytogenes	S	S	S	Y	Y	Y	Y	
Histophilus somni	N	N	N	Y	N	Y	?	
d. Chlamydial and rickettsial diseases								
Chlamydophila pecorum	?	?	?	S	?	?	?	

Y The species is susceptible to natural infection and overt disease is reported regularly.
S The species is susceptible to natural infection but overt disease is reported only sporadically.
SC The species is susceptible to natural infection but the disease occurs subclinically without neurologic signs.
N The species is not susceptible to natural infection.
? No refereed papers about species susceptibility to natural infection.

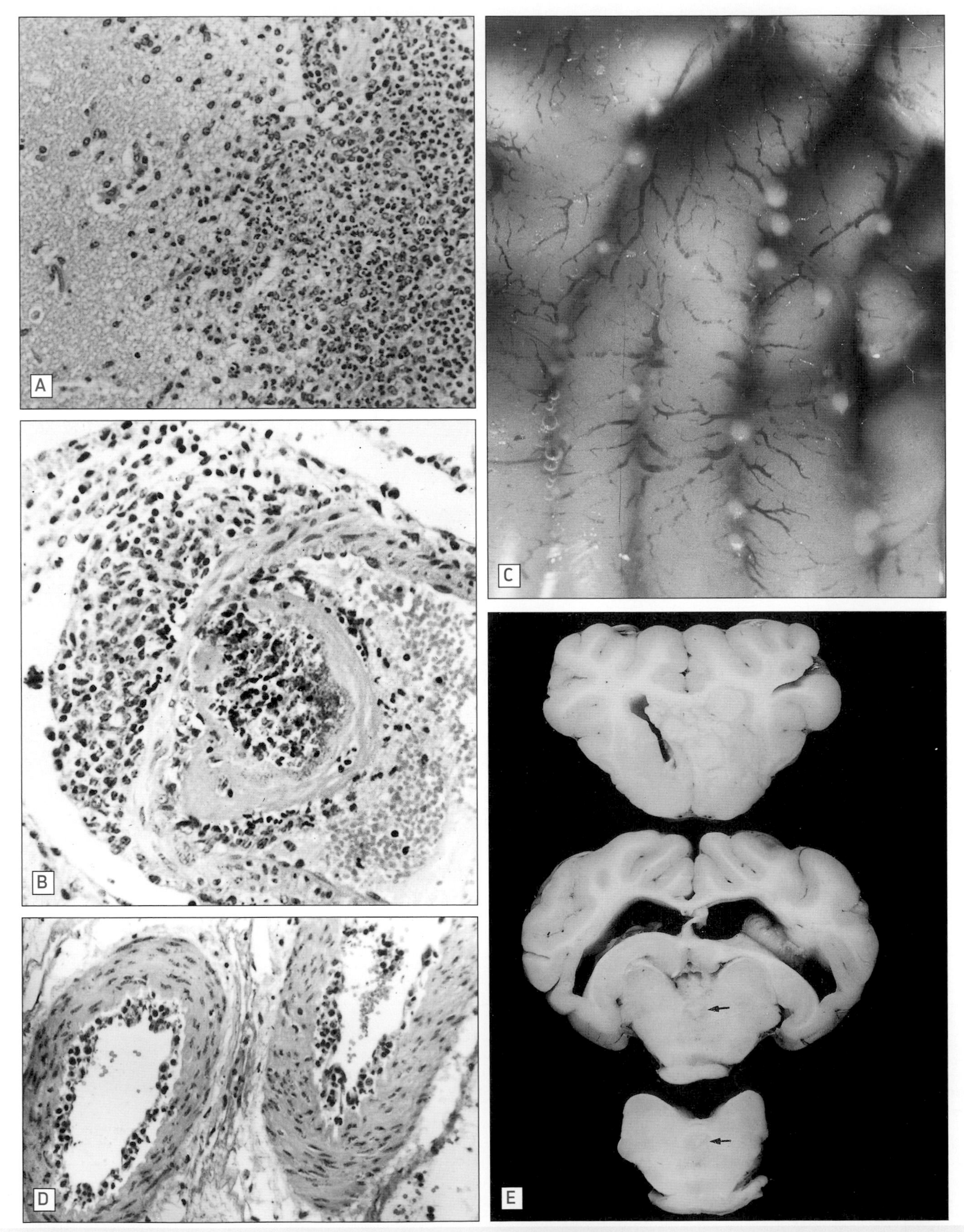

Figure 3.100 A. Suppurative meningitis with extension into cerebellar cortex. **B. Embolic meningeal arteritis** from streptococcal endocarditis in a pig. **C.** Miliary **meningeal abscesses** in a calf due to *Arcanobacterium pyogenes*. **D. Meningeal arteritis** with leukocytes beneath endothelium in coliform meningitis in a calf. **E.** Frontal sections to show periventricular abscess, early hydrocephalus, and occlusive ependymitis of aqueduct (arrows) secondary to **streptococcal choroiditis** in a pig.

exception in that it may produce septicemic and embolic lesions in the brain but it does not cause suppurative meningitis. Several bacteria, such as streptococci and *E. coli*, cause bacteremia and suppurative meningitis in neonates resulting in an important clinical entity, especially in ruminants and pigs, called **neonatal bacterial suppurative meningitis** (NBSM). Streptococcal NBSM in calves, lambs, and piglets (but not in foals), frequently has a combination of polyarthritis, purulent leptomeningitis, choroiditis and, in calves only, endophthalmitis (Fig. 3.101A, B). In pigs, *Streptococcus suis* types 1 and 2 (see Vol. 1, Bones and joints) cause NBSM that is usually accompanied by polyserositis; *S. suis* meningitis is suppurative in the acute stage, and lymphoplasmacytic in pigs that survive. *Streptococcus pneumoniae* usually produces fulminating septicemia in calves characterized only by very acute splenitis but, if the course of this infection is less fulminating than usual, polyarthritis and meningitis can be found. *E. coli*, another cause of NBSM of protracted course, commonly causes well-developed meningitis and polyarthritis in neonatal calves and lambs, but even in fulminating infections the mild changes of early inflammation can be found in these structures. On the other hand, both coliform and streptococcal infections in calves and piglets may avoid the joints and meninges and localize instead in the choroid plexuses and spread from there to the ventricles and brain, or localize in the brain alone. The coliforms and streptococci behave differently in calves with respect to the eyes; a combination of synovial, meningeal, and intraocular localizations is almost invariably of streptococcal origin (and the lesions can be well developed within 12 hours of birth, or even at birth according to farmers); the coliforms can, but only seldom do, cause endophthalmitis.

Mannheimia haemolytica and *P. multocida* are usually regarded only as causes of fibrinous pneumonia and hemorrhagic septicemia, but they are responsible for localized infections in other locations, including the meninges, in ruminants. When polyarthritis is present in septicemic or pulmonary pasteurellosis, *fibrinosuppurative leptomeningitis* can also be anticipated. Isolated cases and limited outbreaks of pasteurellosis that is entirely meningeal are observed in cattle and sheep, usually young ones. The course is asymptomatic until meningitis develops.

Once infectious agents gain access to the leptomeninges there is little resistance to spread in the meningeal spaces, and the inflammatory process becomes more or less diffuse in most cases. When the inflammatory process, excepting some that are granulomatous, remains localized, it is probable that only the inflammatory reaction, and not the infection, reaches the meningeal spaces. Cerebrospinal fluid is an excellent culture medium for many sorts of bacteria and these spread rapidly in the fluid, assisted to some slight extent by normal flow so that, although meningitis may appear grossly to have a limited distribution, its true distribution can be determined only microscopically.

The apparent gross distribution of meningitis varies somewhat with the cause. Thus in listeriosis, the process is confined largely or entirely to the meninges covering the medulla oblongata and upper cord, and in Glasser's disease and in malignant catarrhal fever the exudate is concentrated over the cerebellum and occipital poles of the cerebrum. In pyogenic meningitis, the basal meninges show the most obvious changes.

In the first day or so of suppurative meningitis before exudation is clearly recognizable, the meninges may be faintly opaque and hyperemic (Fig. 3.101C). After a few days, the appearance of the brain and cord is typical. The basal cisterns that accumulate the most exudate are filled with creamy pus or with gray-yellow fibrinopurulent exudate. The extreme exudation in these cisterns is due in part to their large size but in part also to sedimentation of particulate exudate. The exudate is in the arachnoid spaces and there is little if any on the outer surface of this membrane (Fig. 3.101D). The arachnoid appears stretched. *It is easy to overlook even copious exudates because their color is not very different from that of the brain.* A useful clue is that even the largest basilar vessels and the trunk of the oculomotor nerve are partially or completely buried and obscured by exudate and the filling-in of basal sinuses and grooves obliterates the normal topography. Over the hemispheres the exudate is usually confined to the fissures, where the arachnoid space is wide, and spares the surfaces of the gyri, where the arachnoid space is narrow. There is seldom frank pus over the hemispheres except in cases of unusually long survival.

The severe degree of exudation described above is what is usually seen in animals. In very acute or early cases, the exudation may be considerably less, and detectable only as congestion and cloudiness of the basal meninges extending towards the convexity of the hemispheres as fine gray sleeves about the arteries and veins. On careful inspection by naked eye, almost every case of purulent meningitis can be detected but the microscope may be necessary to confirm some cases.

The brain is swollen in every acute case of pyogenic meningitis, and the swelling is frequently severe enough to cause displacement with coning of the cerebellum. The pathogenesis of the edema and swelling is not known. The edema affects the white matter. It is possible that obstruction of the meningeal orifices of Virchow–Robin spaces by exudate and stasis of flow of meningeal fluid may contribute to the edema. The brain itself is normal except for softness and swelling and the rare cortical infarcts in the cerebrum or cerebellum.

Choroiditis commonly complicates leptomeningitis. It is usually quite obvious when it affects the plexuses of the fourth ventricles, but that affecting the plexuses of the lateral ventricle is not apparent until the ventricles are opened, although it may be expected if cloudy fluid escapes from the third ventricle when the infundibular process is opened. The CSF is cloudy, flakes of exudate overlie the plexuses and float in the fluid, and smeary sediments of pus lie on the walls of the ventricles (Fig. 3.101B). The exudate may be impacted in the aqueduct, occluding it and leading to ependymitis. Internal hydrocephalus then develops rapidly.

Microscopically, purulent meningitis does not differ in its character from pyogenic inflammation in other loose tissues, such as the lung. A few mononuclear cells are mixed with a very large number of neutrophils in the arachnoid spaces (Fig. 3.101E). The amount of fibrin in the exudate varies. There may be some infiltration for a short distance along the Virchow–Robin spaces about veins (Fig. 3.102). The pia mater as a rule remains intact, and it is only in exceptional cases that some microbial activity is observed in the adjacent parenchyma, or the pia is eroded to allow neutrophils to invade the surface of the brain. When the choroid plexuses are involved, they are swollen and infiltrated with leukocytes, many of them mononuclear. The plexus epithelium is eroded and covered by fibrin and cells. The ependyma is also eroded, there is edema of subependymal tissues, and the surrounding veins are infiltrated.

Internal hydrocephalus is a sequel to ependymitis and occlusion of the aqueduct, as a result of which the lateral and third ventricles are

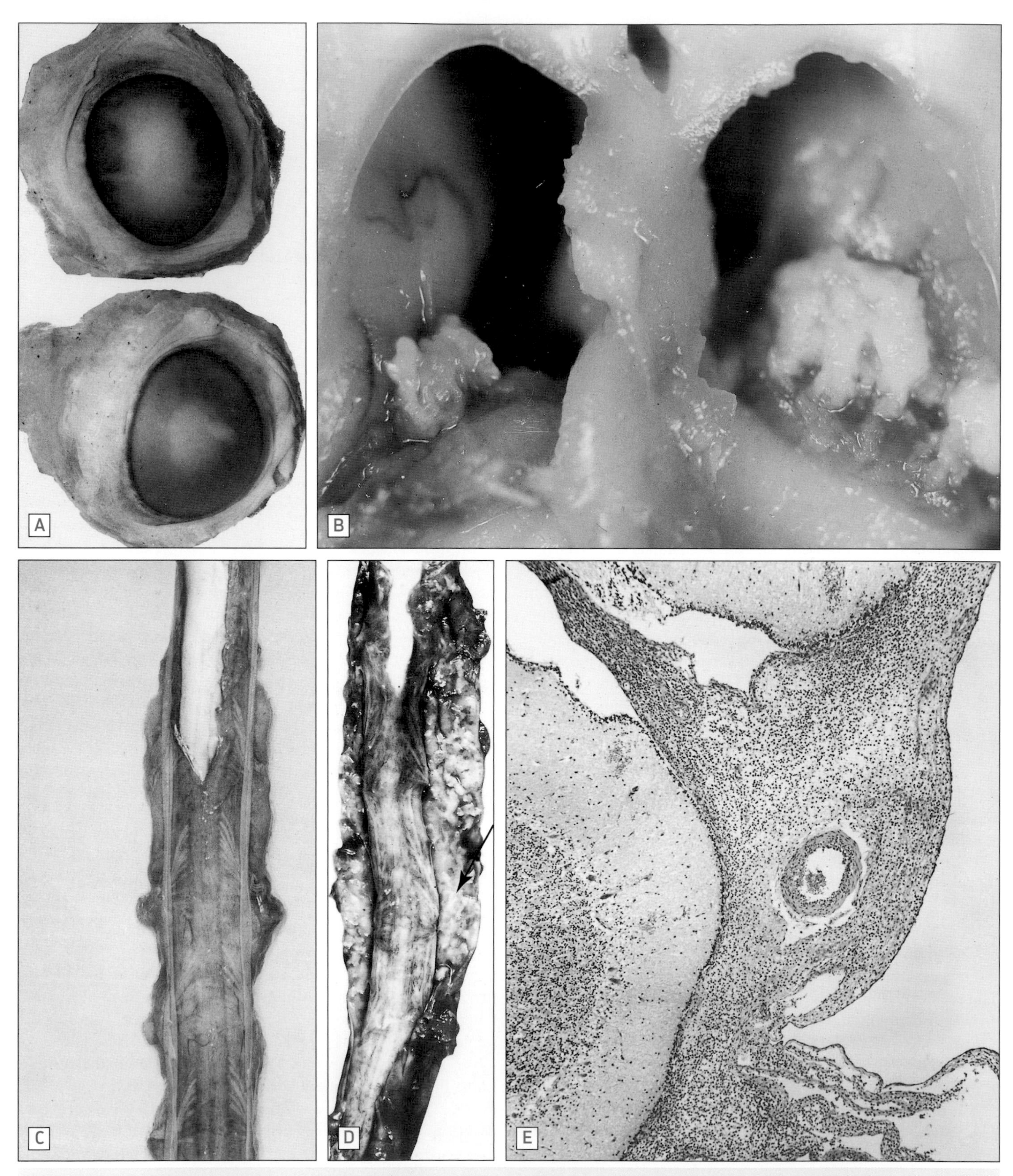

Figure 3.101 A. Hypopyon in streptococcal endophthalmitis in a calf. **B.** Horizontal slice through lateral ventricles to show **streptococcal choroiditis** and acquired hydrocephalus. **C. Spinal leptomeningitis** in a calf, due to *Escherichia coli*. (The dura is incised and reflected full length, the congested leptomeninges are incised at top.) **D. Spinal meningitis** in a dog: dura reflected to expose exudate (arrow). **E. Fibrinopurulent exudate** in leptomeninges in a pig, due to *Haemophilus parasuis*.

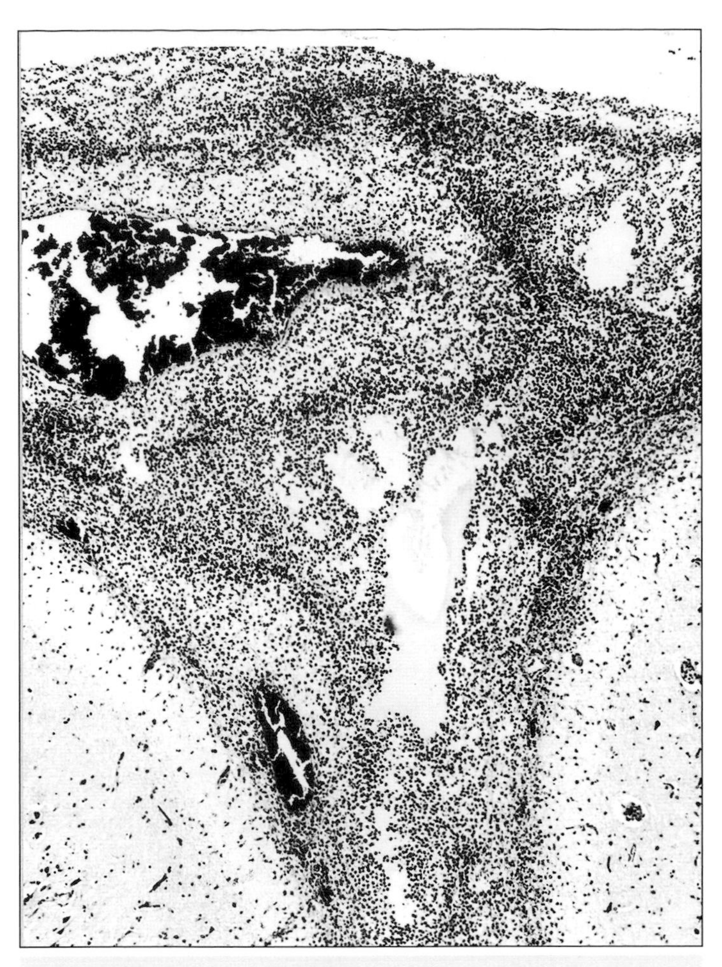

Figure 3.102 Purulent meningitis caused by *Haemophilus* spp. in a pig.

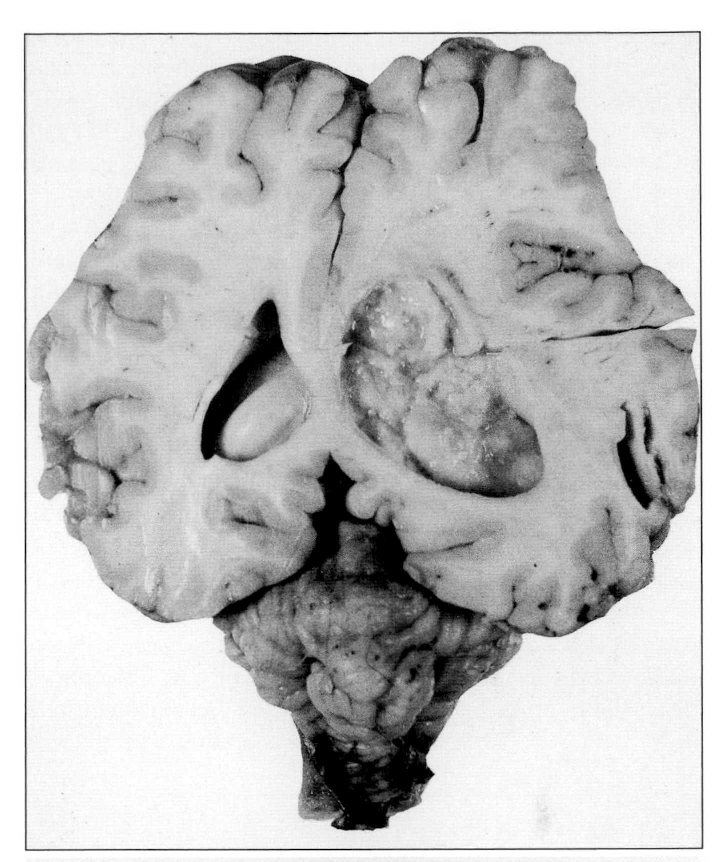

Figure 3.103 Necrobacillary abscess arising in **choroiditis** in an ox: swelling of hemisphere and caudal displacement with coning of cerebellum.

dilated (Fig. 3.103). This condition is a complication of choroiditis, but hydrocephalus may also be a sequel without choroiditis being present. The medullary foramina are frequently occluded as a result of inflammation in the tela choroidea so that CSF cannot escape from the ventricular system to the arachnoid spaces; the hydrocephalus is noncommunicating. Obstruction to the flow of fluid in the arachnoid spaces may occur as a result of brain swelling with impaction in the tentorial incisure, heavy deposits of exudate in the arachnoid space, or as a result of meningeal adhesions and thickenings in chronic inflammations. The hydrocephalus of this pathogenesis is communicating.

Chronic pyogenic leptomeningitis is rarely observed in animals. The process may sterilize itself or be sterilized by antimicrobials, but much of the injury is established in the early stages of the process and, once the diagnosis is evident clinically, *death is the expected outcome*. The early injury is exaggerated by the persistence of exudate even after the infection is controlled because there is no free drainage from the meningeal spaces. Healing occurs only after there has been considerable destruction of the meningeal framework with repair by fibrous tissue. Meningeal adhesions may produce cystic loculations in the arachnoid space, and obliterate the medullary foramen or basal arachnoid space and cause lingering death from hydrocephalus.

In a purulent process, *leptomeningeal vasculitis commonly occurs*. The expected sequelae of venous or ischemic infarcts are seldom observed even in those few cases with vasculitis in which thrombi can be found. This apparent discrepancy is probably due to the rate at which the vascular obstructions develop and on the type and size of vessel. Cases in which suppurative thrombophlebitis of the sagittal or transverse sinuses, or both, can be readily observed may not have venous infarcts in the brain. Thrombosis in the afferent circulation usually involves the smallest of meningeal vessels and usually develops at a rate that allows collateral circulation to develop. Inflammation of larger arteries (Fig. 3.100D) in which the endothelium is dissected from the intima by leukocytes has not been observed to lead to thrombosis.

Septicemic lesions, septic embolism, and cerebral abscess

The brain responds in septic or endotoxemic shock by releasing or controlling the release of several proinflammatory and anti-inflammatory cytokines; this major biochemical role is not always associated with a morphologic change in the CNS. *The CNS is injured to some extent in every episode of septicemia or sustained bacteremia.* The simplest and most common type of injury is inflicted on the venules, especially those of the cerebral white matter and to a lesser extent those of the cerebellar white matter. Injury of this type is not of much significance. There is sludging of leukocytes and probably of erythrocytes in these vessels, associated usually with degenerative and reactive changes in the endothelium. In the symptomatic purpuras, it is frequently possible to find the site of diapedesis in the brain, but not in other organs. Associated with endothelial injury there is often leakage of plasma into the perivascular space and, given time, adventitial proliferation and infiltration of a few lymphocytes or other leukocytes into the Virchow–Robin spaces. Commonly, the injury is more severe, the vessel wall is totally necrotic in its cross-section, and in these lesions a few bacteria may be demonstrable (Fig. 3.104).

Septic embolism in the CNS may be a complication of active endocarditis; the bacteria are usually gram-positive. The bacteria implicated most commonly are *Erysipelothrix rhusiopathiae* in pigs, streptococci in all species, and *Arcanobacterium pyogenes* in cattle.

The toxigenicity and pathogenicity of many infections by gram-negative bacteria in septicemic phase seem to depend largely on the number of organisms present, as has been demonstrated in sheep for septicemic pasteurellosis caused by *Mannheimia haemolytica*. In septicemic pasteurellosis of sheep, in infection of foals by *Actinobacillus equuli*, in infections of sheep and cattle by *Histophilus somni*, and in some coliform infections of calves, the blood literally swarms with bacteria because common to these infections is massive and widespread bacterial embolism. These are the principal infections in which bacterial embolism occurs in the CNS without there being a demonstrable primary focus such as endocarditis, pneumonia, or an abscess. The problem of cerebral embolism in these infections is not solely one of quantitative factors determined by the height of the bacteremia; qualitative factors of unknown nature are also involved.

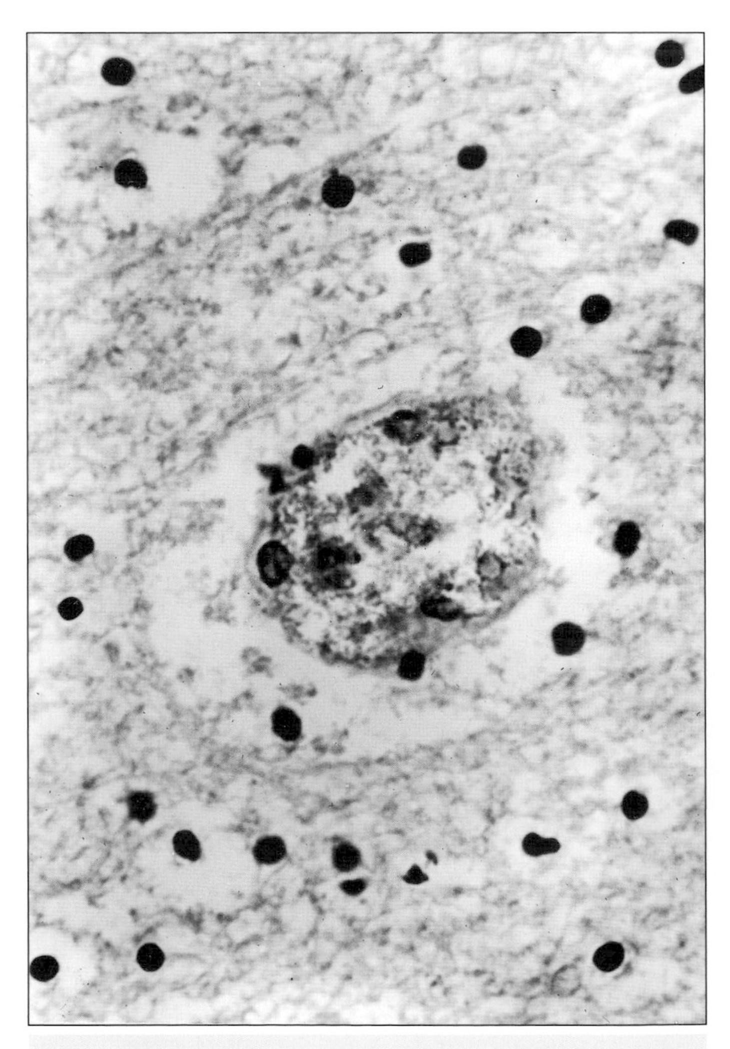

Figure 3.104 Necrosis of cerebral venule in *Escherichia coli* septicemia in a calf.

Septic thromboemboli and **bacterial emboli** lodge in the small cerebral vessels but, whereas thromboemboli tend to lodge particularly in small arterioles, bacterial emboli lodge in capillaries and venules. Consequences depend on the vessels involved, although the consequences are not particularly significant because abscessation occurs in either location. *Arterial emboli frequently cause ischemic infarcts, and venous and capillary emboli cause hemorrhagic infarcts.* The venular lesions also extend rapidly to involve large veins, whereas local spread in arteries does not occur.

Cerebral abscesses may arise in embolism, by direct implantation in wounds, or by direct invasion of the brain from an adjacent structure. Leptomeningitis rarely leads to abscessation, whereas choroiditis commonly leads to periventricular abscess. Abscesses in the spinal cord are seldom sought or observed; they may be hematogenous via arteries or veins (Fig. 3.105), and rarely do they enter through the dura.

Abscesses of hematogenous origin may occur anywhere in the brain, but there are two areas of remarkable predilection – the hypothalamus, and the cerebral cortex at the junction of gray and white matter (Fig. 3.106A, B). *Listeria monocytogenes* is an exception because it always demonstrates an affinity for the reticular formation in the brain stem. There may be only one abscess in the brain, or they may be multiple, especially when due to bacterial embolism. Multiple abscesses of septic thromboembolic origin tend often to be localized in one area of the brain. Some care is necessary in specifying the origin of multiple adjacent foci of suppuration because the *production of satellites*, each of which may be larger than the primary, is a natural attribute of brain abscesses.

Abscesses arising by direct invasion of the brain may develop in any location. There are two common sites of invasion, namely the *cribriform plate and inner ear*, and two somewhat less common, namely the *hypophyseal fossa and the paranasal sinuses*. Hypothalamic abscesses

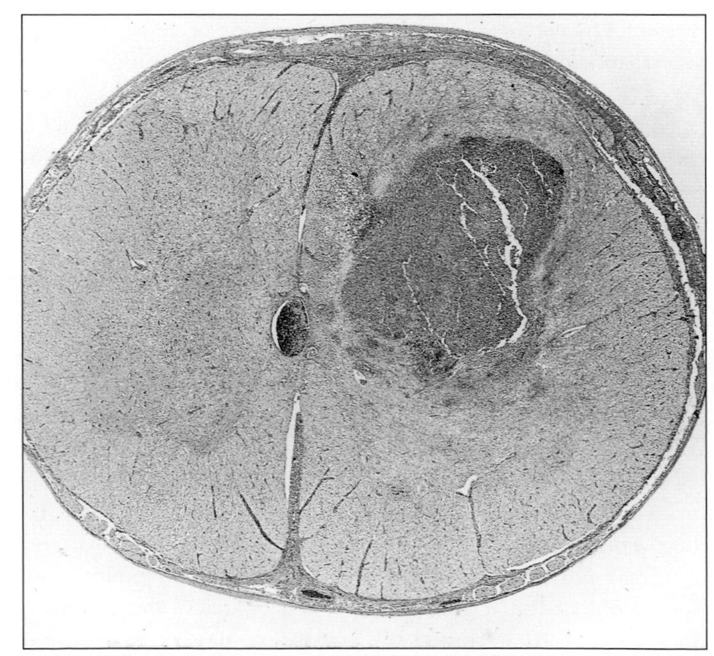

Figure 3.105 Meningitis, tracking abscess in dorsal horn, and ependymitis, complicating docking wound in a lamb.

are observed occasionally in cattle and dogs. At least some of those in dogs are caused by minute foreign bodies migrating with phlebitis through the orbital fissure or foramen rotundum and carrying actinomycetes. The importance of the cribriform plate and internal ear in the development of cerebral abscess is due to the frequency with which infections occur in those locations, that in neither site is there an actual or potential epidural space to protect the brain, and because nerves and vessels enter and leave through both.

Frontal abscesses of sinus origin occur occasionally in cattle as a complication of dehorning wounds, but abscesses in this site occur most commonly in sheep in which sinusitis, especially in the ethmoid cells, develops as a suppurative complication of myiasis (*Oestrus ovis*). *Arcanobacterium pyogenes* is the organism usually present. The olfactory bulb is destroyed and the first ventricle is opened, infection then spreading to the substance of the hemisphere (Fig. 3.107). There is little tendency to spread into the meninges from the point of entry or to invade the cortical gray matter, although both layers are usually secondarily involved by expansion of the abscess later.

Abscesses commonly develop at about the *cerebellopontine angle* as complications of suppurative otitis media. These are usually problems of pharyngitis, infection spreading via the Eustachian tube to the middle ear and from there to the brain, either by erosion of the bulla or extension along natural foramina.

Cerebellopontine abscesses are rarely, if ever, observed in horses in spite of the frequency of pharyngitis in this species. This exemption of horses may be due to the diversion of exudates from the Eustachian tube to the guttural pouches. Otogenic cerebral infections are very

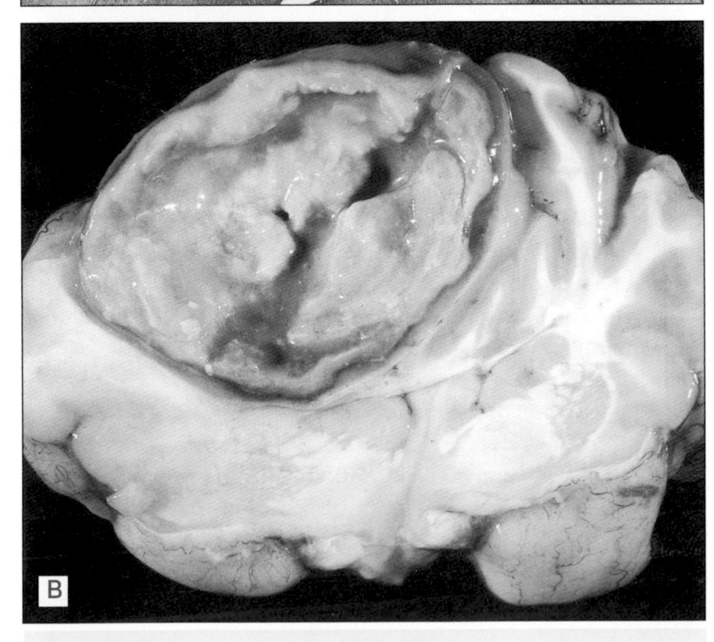

Figure 3.106 A. Hematogenous **abscesses** in cerebrum in a pig. **B. Abscess** distorting left cerebral hemisphere in a goat. *Pasteurella multocida* and *Fusobacterium necrophorum*.

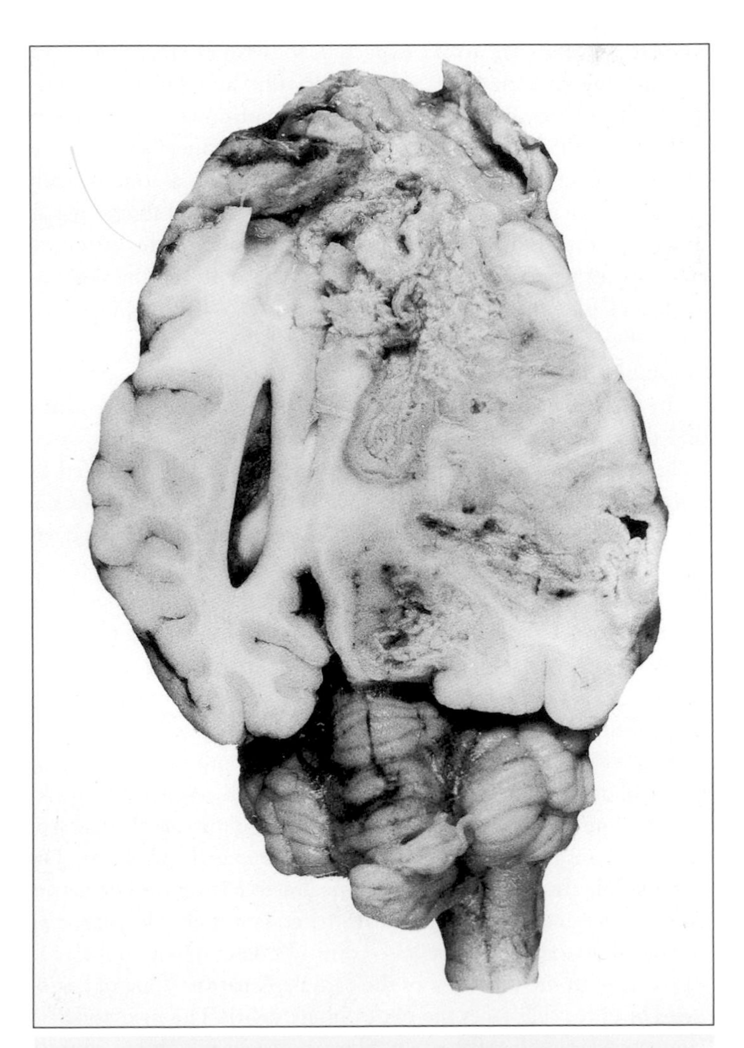

Figure 3.107 Arcanobacterial **abscess** arising from right ethmoid in a sheep.

seldom observed in dogs. Those observed have come via the auditory meatus rather than the Eustachian tube, and the cerebral reaction is nonspecifically granulomatous, usually without pus. Otitis media caused by *Pasteurella multocida* is fairly common as a complication of chronic cases of upper respiratory infection in cats and, when the infection extends to the cranial cavity, it produces diffuse purulent leptomeningitis and not, as expected, a cerebellopontine abscess. Most otogenic infections occur in sheep and swine; a few are observed in cattle, and in each species the outcome is an abscess of the brain.

Otic infections are commonly bilateral so that otogenic abscesses may be also. The usual organism in these abscesses is *Arcanobacterium pyogenes* alone or mixed with *Pseudomonas aeruginosa*, *Pasteurella multocida*, and mixed cocci. Affected pigs usually have several other chronic debilitating infections at the same time so that several animals in the herd may have otogenic abscesses. This pattern of infection in calves is uncommon and sporadic. In sheep on the other hand, the disease may be observed in limited outbreaks and there is an association with grazing on rough, dry, mature summer pastures. The reasons for this association are unknown.

Established abscesses are found much more commonly in the white matter than in the gray, in spite of the fact that they usually begin in the gray. There is no suitable explanation for this tendency to track into white matter, but once within white matter they do permeate along fiber tracts (Fig. 3.108). As a result of this activity, satellite abscesses are to be expected, sometimes chains of them. Connecting purulent tracts may be very thin and difficult to find.

An abscess may begin as an intense accumulation of neutrophils in and around a thrombosed vessel (Fig. 3.109A), or in a focus of septic encephalitis in which neutrophils lightly infiltrate a zone of early softening. The principal differences between a cerebral abscess and an abscess in some other location are the vulnerability of the surrounding nervous tissue to edema, which can destroy it, and the slowness with which encapsulation occurs (Fig. 3.109B). The meninges and larger blood vessels are the only sources of fibroblastic tissue for encapsulation.

In the *early stages*, the abscess cavity contains a liquefying center and the margins are irregular and poorly defined even microscopically. The surrounding brain tissue is edematous and infiltrated by neutrophils. The microglia and vessels are fairly resistant and reactive in a narrow peripheral zone, but the neurons and neuroglia degenerate. Most abscesses develop rather slowly and later become encapsulated. The capsule seems often to be formed more by condensation of vessels around an expanding focus than by proliferating fibroblastic tissue, but both contribute; the result is an irregular capsule thicker on the meningeal than on the ventricular aspect. Most capsules are very distinct and 1–3 mm wide. Their distinctness is due to the paucity of reticulin or collagen spreading out into the surrounding parenchyma or into the abscess cavity. In old abscesses with shrinkage, the core may separate from the capsule, and the capsule may separate extensively from the surrounding cerebral substance. The surrounding tissue is discolored yellow due to edema, the edematous zone often being much larger than the abscess itself. The *microscopic structure of the wall of a chronic abscess* does not differ much from case to case except in the thickness of the capsule. A narrow zone of histiocytes or gitter cells faces the neutrophilic debris. The next zone is a laminated layer of collagenous fibers between which are rows of gitter cells laden with debris. The outer zone is vascular, the vessels being large and usually nonreactive. The surrounding nervous tissue is severely edematous, with degeneration of myelin and fibers. Astrocytes are swollen and reactive about encapsulated abscesses, but it takes a long time for their fibrils to begin to intertwine with capsular reticulin. The veins are heavily cuffed by lymphocytes.

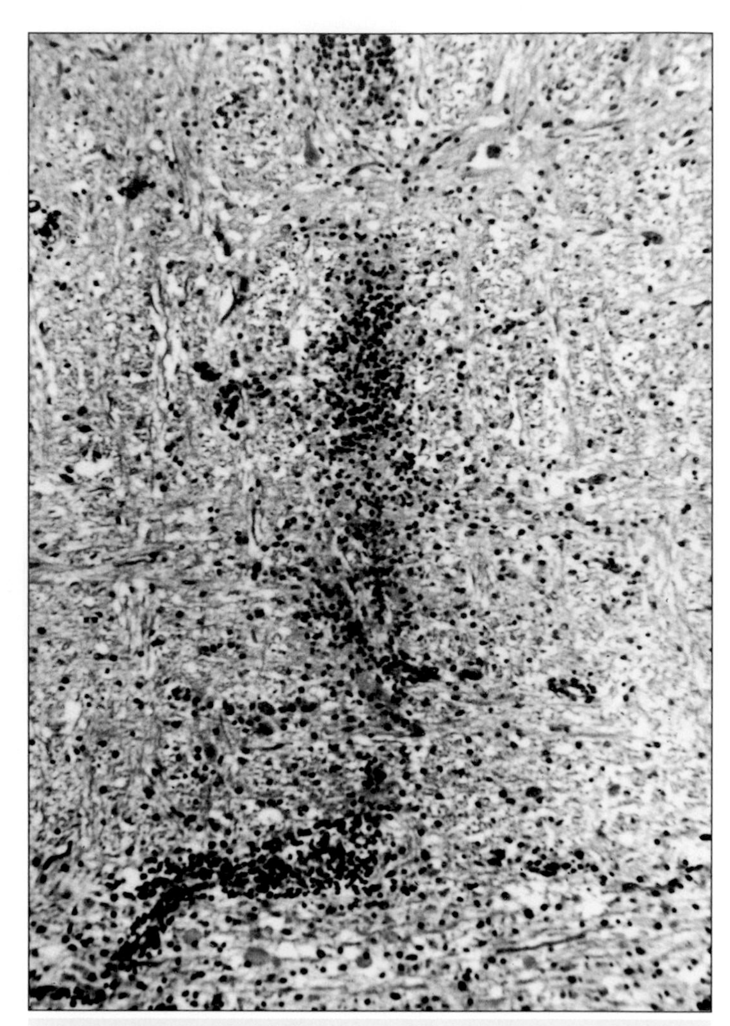

Figure 3.108 Spreading tract in suppurative (streptococcal) encephalitis in a pig.

When abscesses are multiple, death is the outcome after a short course. When they are isolated, they may permit prolonged survival. The course is usually short with medullary abscess, even when small, because it, or more usually the edema it provokes, interferes with vital centers. Abscesses in the hypothalamus or cerebrum may track through the white matter to the ventricles to produce pyencephaly that is quickly fatal (Fig. 3.110A, B, C, D). Large abscesses ultimately expand to the meninges to produce adhesive meningitis. Many abscesses act as space-occupying lesions by virtue of their size or the edema they provoke or both. The consequences of space occupation depend on the site and size of the lesion.

Bibliography

Fecteau G, George LW. Bacterial meningitis and encephalitis in ruminants. Vet Clin North Am Food Anim Pract 2004;20:363–377.

Gottschalk M, Segura M. The pathogenesis of the meningitis caused by *Streptococcus suis*: the unresolved questions. Vet Microbiol 2000;76:259–272.

Schroder-Petersen DL, Simonsen HB. Tail biting in pigs. Vet J 2001;162:196–210.

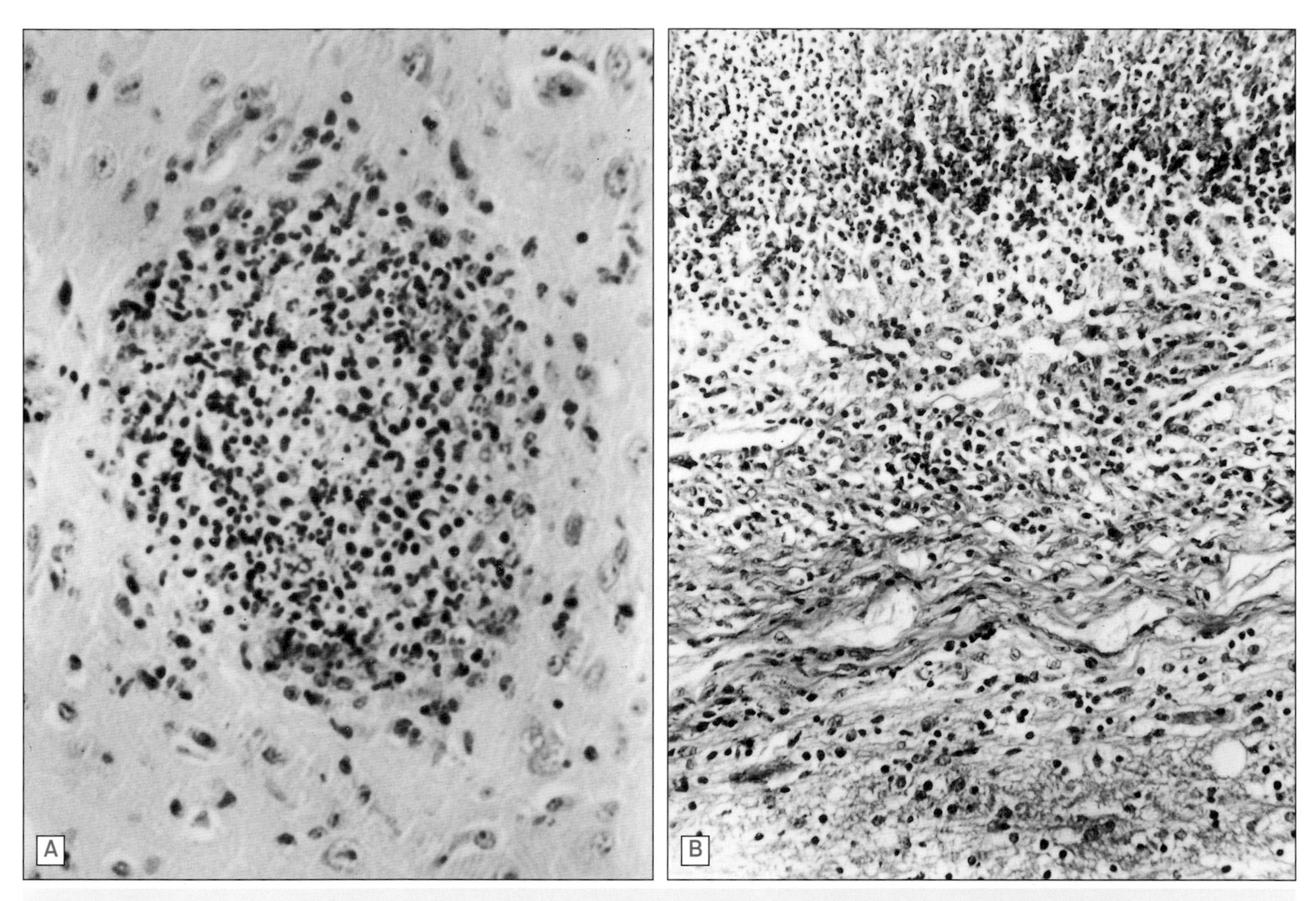

Figure 3.109 A. Early **cerebral abscess** from septic embolus in a pig. **B.** Structure of wall of **cerebral abscess**. Abscess (above) is separated from normal brain by a thin capsule.

Smith JJ et al. Bacterial meningitis and brain abscesses secondary to infectious disease processes involving the head in horses: seven cases (1980–2001). J Am Vet Med Assoc 2004;224:739–742.

Spoormakers TJ, et al. Brain abscesses as a metastatic manifestation of strangles: symptomatology and the use of magnetic resonance imaging as a diagnostic aid. Equine Vet J 2003;35:146–151.

Granulomatous and pyogranulomatous meningoencephalomyelitis

Granulomatous to pyogranulomatous meningoencephalomyelitis is observed in many systemic mycotic (e.g., blastomycosis, cryptococcosis) or algal (e.g., protothecosis) diseases, which are described elsewhere in this book. Granulomatous inflammation can also be caused by bacteria (e.g., *Mycobacterium bovis, Nocardia* sp.) (Fig. 3.111), and migrating helminths or arthropod larvae (see below). The diagnosis and differentiation among these etiologies requires culture or demonstration of the causative pathogen using histochemical or immunohistochemical stains.

Listeriosis

Listeriosis is caused by *Listeria monocytogenes*, a Gram-positive, facultative anaerobic bacillus that is ubiquitous in the environment and can multiply in diverse environmental conditions – it can grow in a temperature range from 4 to 45°C and at a pH range of 5 to 9. It is remarkably viable in the external environment, being able to survive in dried media for several months and in suitably moist soil for ~1 year. The organism is commonly isolated from tissues of normal animals, including tonsils and other gut-associated lymphoid tissue, and in large numbers from the feces of ruminants. *L. monocytogenes* has more than 11 serotypes; almost all animal infections are caused by serotypes 1/2a, 1/2b, and 4b.

Listeriosis is of worldwide distribution, possibly excepting the tropics. The organism has been isolated from diseased mammals and birds of many species and produces septicemia, meningitis, and abortion in humans. In domestic animals, the disease is most important in ruminants. *L. monocytogenes* is an intracellular pathogen of macrophages, neutrophils, and epithelial cells. Important virulence factor include the surface protein *internalin,* which internalizes with *E-cadherin*, an adherans junction protein, to overcome the intestinal, placental, and blood–brain barriers. Also, it relies on another virulence factor, *cholesterol-binding hemolysin*, to lyse phagocytic cell phagosomes and escape to the cytoplasm. The organism proliferates in the host cell cytoplasm and many migrate against the cell membrane to form protrusions that can then be taken up by other cells. It is one of the few organisms known to co-opt the host cell contractile actin to facilitate cell-to-cell transfer.

Listeriosis behaves as three separate diseases or syndromes. They seldom overlap so that each syndrome probably has a separate

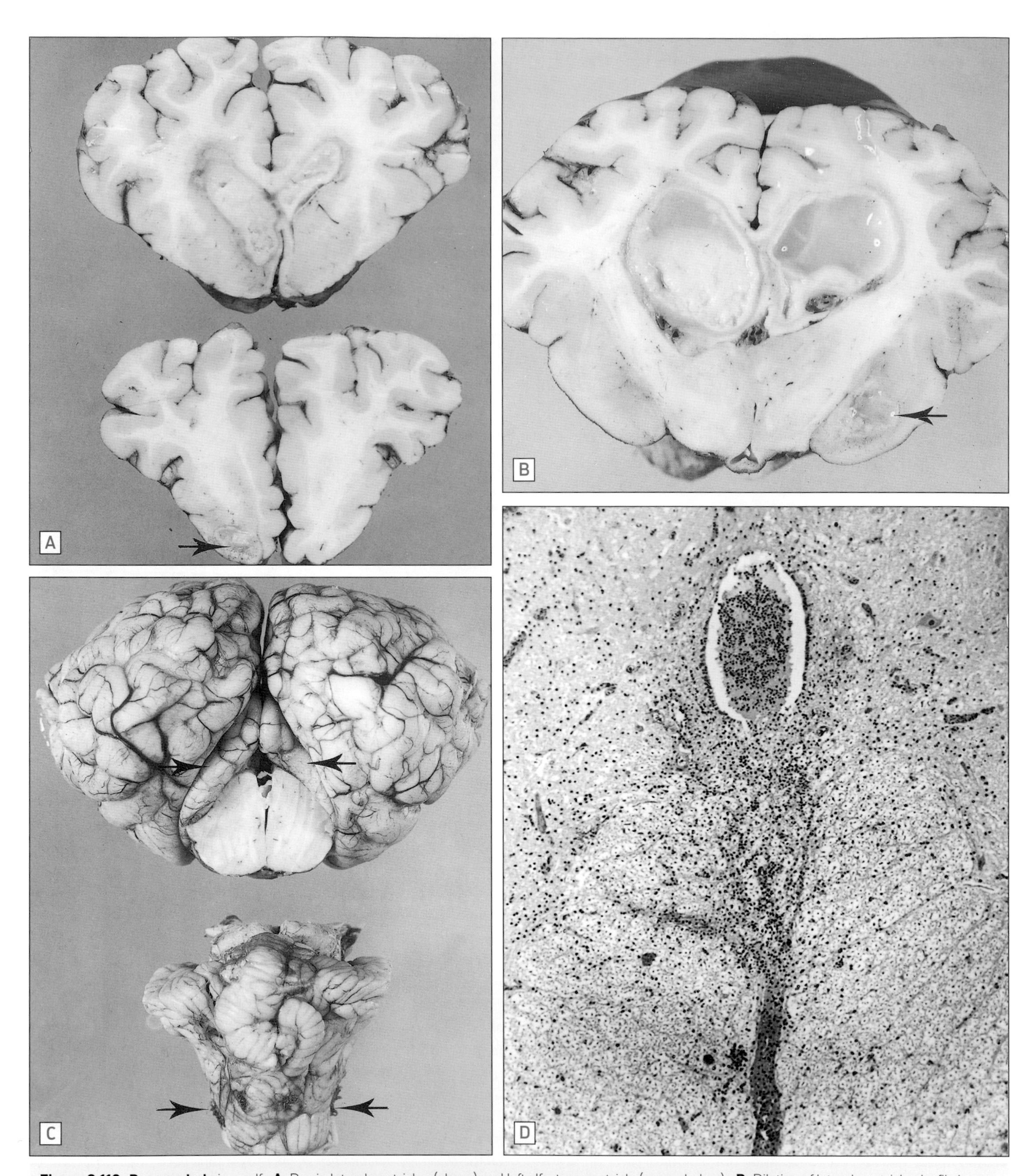

Figure 3.110 Pyencephaly in a calf. **A.** Pus in lateral ventricles (above) and left olfactory ventricle (arrow, below). **B.** Dilation of lateral ventricles by fibrinopurulent exudate (arrow). **C.** Brain swelling with cerebellar coning and hemorrhage (arrows, below) and subtentorial herniation of hemispheres (arrows, above). **D.** Inflammatory exudate in aqueduct.

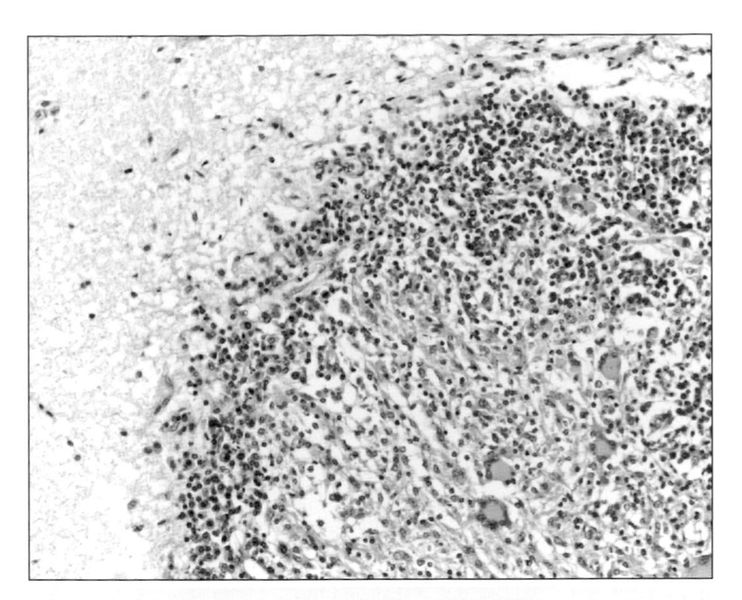

Figure 3.111 Granulomatous meningoencephalitis in bovine tuberculosis. (Courtesy of D Driemeier.)

pathogenesis. *The three recognized syndromes are: infection of the pregnant uterus with abortion, septicemia with miliary visceral abscesses, and encephalitis.* Additional syndromes of clinical significance in ruminants include conjunctivitis, possibly from contaminated silage dust, endocarditis, and mastitis. The uterine infection is discussed with Diseases of the pregnant uterus (see Vol. 3, Female genital system). Aborting ruminants are not usually ill, and abortion is usually late in gestation. The uterine infection is probably hematogenous and the bacteremic phase is asymptomatic, and localization occurs only in the uterus. Infection of the uterine contents can be established quite readily by oral exposure of pregnant animals and by intravenous inoculation.

Septicemic (systemic) listeriosis occurs in aborted fetuses and neonatal lambs, calves, and foals up to 1 week of age and in others that are several months of age, and is characterized by multisystemic bacterial colonization and multifocal multisystemic areas of coagulative necrosis or microabscess formation. The necrotic areas or microabscesses are miliary in distribution, very numerous in the liver, but much less numerous in the heart and other viscera, and characterized by tissue lytic necrosis with infiltration of neutrophils and fewer macrophages. Neonates generally become infected in utero.

Listerial encephalitis occurs almost solely in adult ruminants; its pathogenesis is partially understood. Listerial encephalitis may be sporadic or occur in outbreaks in which the morbidity may be 10% or higher. Outbreaks are usually associated with *heavy feeding of silage*, with disease most likely occurring in winter and early spring when the animals are indoors. This association of outbreaks of cerebral listeriosis with silage feeding is a circumstantial observation, but the association is so common that silage is fed as a calculated risk and removed from the ration when the first case occurs. The association with silage may indicate an acquired susceptibility of the animals or the provision of a growth medium that leads to heavy infection pressure. The organism will multiply in spoiled silage that is incompletely fermented and with a pH of 5.5 or above. Ingested *Listeria* is likely to breach the oral mucosal barrier through pathological or physiological wounds, e.g., erupted teeth wounds. *After invading the oral mucosa, the bacteria invade the trigeminal nerves and travel centripetally via axons to the brain. Listeria* can also breach the blood–brain barrier under experimental conditions; however the specific distribution of listerial encephalitis in the natural disease is inconsistent with a hematogenous infection. In animals, *Listeria has a remarkable affinity for the brain stem*, the lesions being most severe in the medulla and pons and less severe rostrally in the thalamus and caudally in the cervical parts of the spinal cord. Intravenous or oral dosing of pregnant ruminants will regularly produce intrauterine infection but seldom produce intracranial infection and probably never produce encephalitis of the specific distribution. Bacteremias with localization in the CNS regularly cause meningitis, choroiditis, and cerebral abscesses, which is what *L. monocytogenes* does, but only as an experimental hematogenous infection. When a pregnant animal dies of encephalitic listeriosis, the uterine contents are usually sterile.

Conjunctivitis and keratitis follow experimental conjunctival exposure, but this should not imply that the endophthalmitis of the natural disease is produced by local invasion. Rhinitis is clinically apparent in many cases of encephalitic listeriosis, but histological evidence does not support the idea that the olfactory nerves are a route of invasion of the brain. The position with respect to other cranial nerves and the internal ear has not been examined.

The *neurological signs* and lesions of listeriosis in the various ruminants are qualitatively the same, differing only in severity. The signs are combinations of mental confusion and depression, head pressing, and paralysis of one or more medullary centers. Characteristically, there is deviation of the head to one or other side without rotation of the head; when such an animal moves it does so in circles, hence the name "*circling disease*." There is frequently *unilateral paralysis of the seventh nerve* causing drooping of an ear, eyelid, and lips. There may also be paralysis of the masticatory muscles and of the pharynx. *Purulent endophthalmitis*, which is usually unilateral, is often present and has caused listeriosis to be confused with malignant catarrhal fever. The course of the disease in sheep and goats is a few hours to 2 days; survival occurs but usually with neurologic handicaps.

Listeriosis in *swine* is comparable to the disease in ruminants, but is relatively rare. Outbreaks of encephalitis may be observed with lesions of usual distribution in the brainstem. Alternatively, there may be abortion and neonatal death. The usual expression of the disease is visceral with miliary abscesses in the liver and heart.

The patterns of listeriosis in *other domestic species* appear to follow the general scheme but are rarely observed. The encephalitic form in adult horses, the septicemic form in foals, and abortions in mares are reported. Several cases of encephalitis caused by *L. monocytogenes* are reported in dogs.

Gross lesions are usually not observed in the brain in listerial encephalitis. Occasionally, the medullary meninges are thickened by green gelatinous edema, and gray foci of softening may be found in the cross-section of the medulla. The initial lesions are parenchymal; involvement of the meninges, which is almost constant, is secondary to the parenchymal lesions. Mild meningitis commonly affects the cerebellum and cranial cervical cord, and less commonly is found in patches over the cerebrum and down the spinal cord. *The characteristic parenchymal lesion is a microabscess.* It may begin in a tiny collection of neutrophils (Fig. 3.112A), but more usually begins in a minute focus of microglial reaction. The glial nodules may persist as such, the cells taking on the characters of histiocytes, but the tendency is always for the nodules to be infiltrated by neutrophils and for their centers to liquefy (Fig. 3.112B). The focal lesions do not

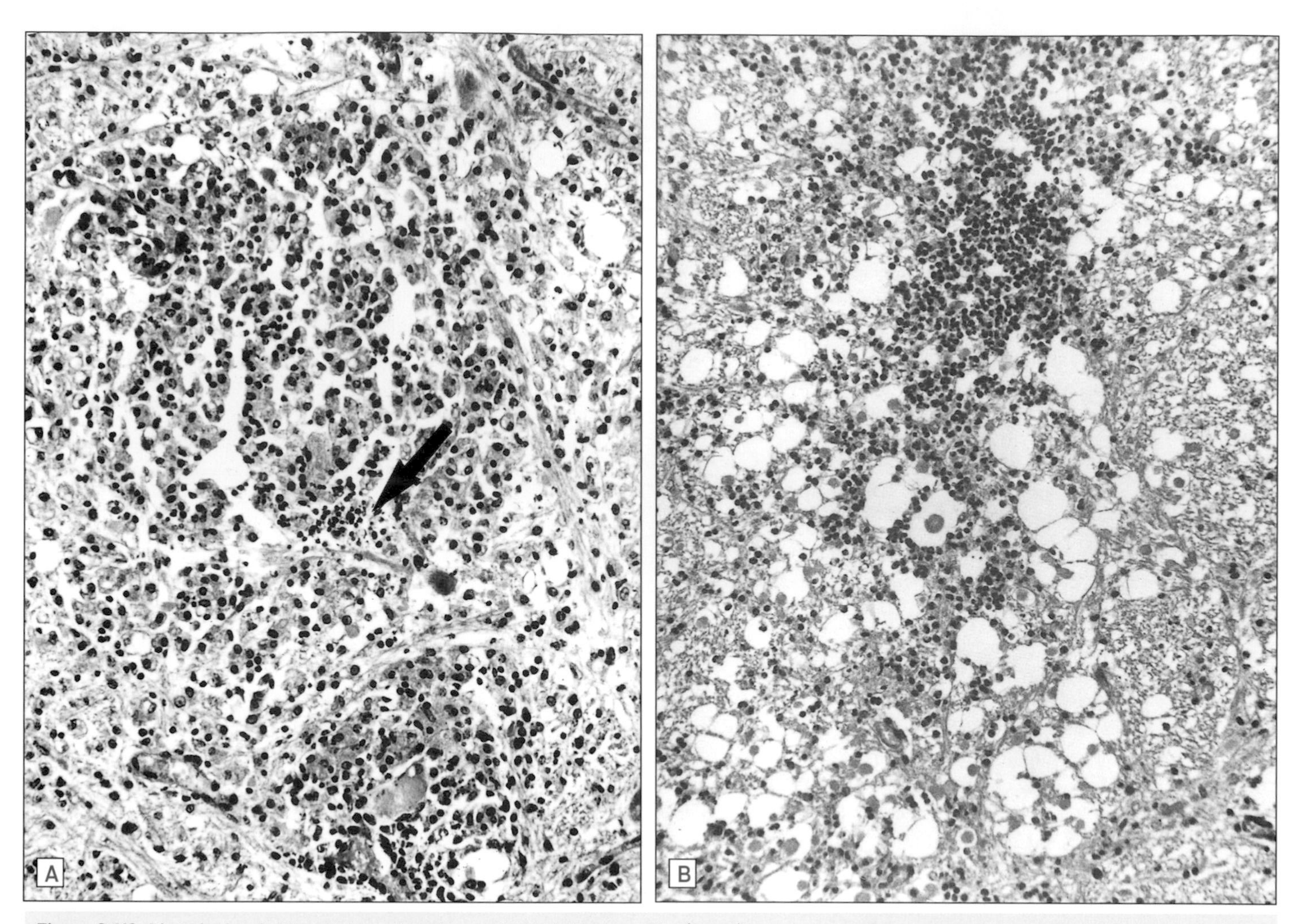

Figure 3.112 Listeriosis. A. Microglial reaction with small focus of **suppuration** (arrow) in a sheep. **B. Suppurative encephalitis** in an ox.

expand much, but suppurative foci may streak through the white matter. Apparently, the organism is not highly toxigenic because the parenchyma surrounding the glial nodules and focal abscesses may be little changed. Commonly however, the white matter is edematous and rarefied. Such areas may be large and lightly, but diffusely, infiltrated by neutrophils and hypertrophied microglia. Focal softening occurs and may coalesce. They are related to vessels that are occluded by inflammatory and thrombotic changes.

Acute vasculitis with exudation of fibrin occurs in the white matter in relation to suppurative foci. The vasculitis is secondary to drainage in the Virchow–Robin spaces from the primary parenchymal foci. It is in this manner that the meningeal infiltrates develop. Perivascular cuffing is heavy. The cuffs are composed mainly of lymphocytes and histiocytes with a few admixed neutrophils and eosinophils; granulocytes predominate in some cases.

Confirmation of the *diagnosis* is by culture, which is usually difficult and needs special procedures. Demonstrating gram-positive intramonocytic or intraneutrophilic bacilli in tissues in association with the aforementioned lesions is pathognomonic for listerial encephalitis.

Bibliography

Gyles CL, et al. Pathogenesis of Bacterial Infections in Animals. 3rd ed. Oxford, UK: Blackwell Publishing Ltd, 2004:99–107.

Otter A, Blakemore WF. Observations on the neural transport of *Listeria monocytogenes* in a mouse model. Neuropathol App Neurobiol 1989;15:590.

Popowska M, Markiewicz Z. Classes and functions of *Listeria monocytogenes* surface proteins. Pol J Microbiol 2004;53:75–88.

Histophilus somni infections (histophilosis, or *H. somni* disease complex)

Histophilus somni (formerly *Haemophilus somnus*) is the only species of the genus *Histophilus*, family Pasteurellaceae, and encompasses bacteria isolated from cattle and previously described as *Haemophilus somnus*, as well as ovine isolates formerly referred to as *Histophilus ovis* and *Haemophilus agni*. *H. somni* is a fastidious gram-negative coccobacillus, and a facultative anaerobic organism that is considered normal flora of the male and female bovine genital tract and to lesser extent the bovine nasal cavity. Calves are infected by carrier cows in the first months of life, and they in turn disseminate the infection in feedlots. The mechanism, site, and circumstance by which the bacteria invade the bloodstream are not known, but it is possible that organisms in genital discharges or aerosolized urine invade via the respiratory tract. Infection, especially the respiratory form, is usually preceded by stress factors such as transportation.

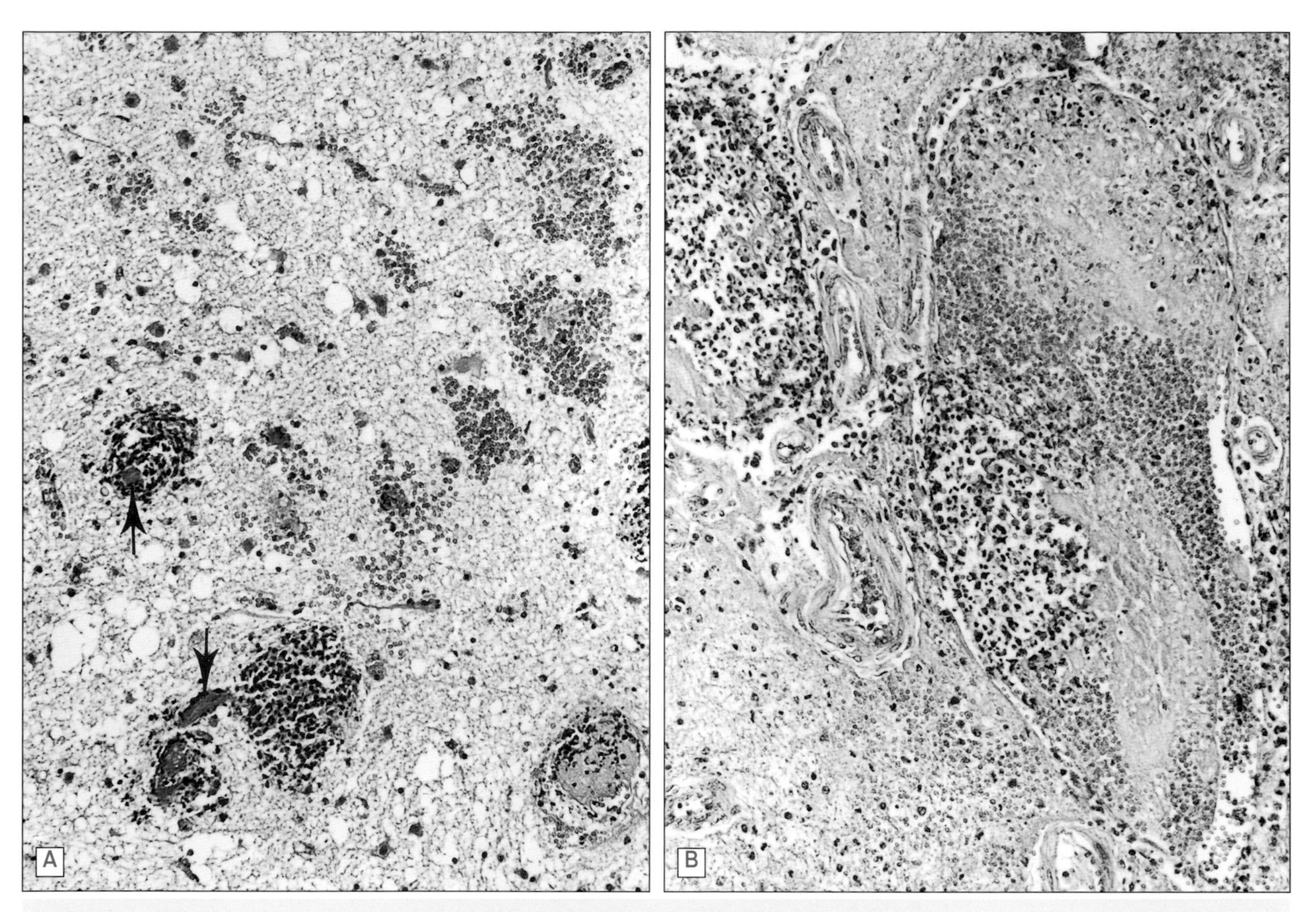

Figure 3.113 ***Histophilus somni*** infection in an ox. **A.** Thrombosis, hemorrhage, and bacterial colonies (arrows) in cerebral white matter. **B.** Thrombosis of meningeal vessels.

These bacteria have virulent and avirulent strains. Important *virulence factors* include lipo-oligosaccharide (LOS), immunoglobulin Fc binding proteins, inhibition of oxygen radicals, and intracellular survival. The mechanism of vasculitis in *H. somni* infection is complex but it can be partially explained by the effect of LSO on endothelial cells. LSO triggers apoptosis of bovine endothelial cells in vitro by caspase-3 activation. This effect is associated with the production of reactive oxygen and nitrogen intermediates. Cerebral blood vessels are particularly vulnerable to damage by the organism, but vasculitis can develop in most organs.

Histophilus somni causes a *septicemia* that may result in acute death or it may localize in one or several organs causing subacute or chronic, fatal or nonfatal disease. The septicemic phase of the disease is brief, and accompanied by fever and stiffness with few other signs. In some cases, the infection is controlled at this stage without localization, but often it leads to cerebral vasculitis with acute thrombosis, hemorrhage, and necrosis (Fig. 3.113A, B).

Histophilus somni can infect several bovine organ systems and cause infectious thrombotic meningoencephalitis (ITME), otitis externa, pneumonia, laryngitis/tracheitis, myocarditis, abortion, metritis/infertility, arthritis, mastitis, orchitis, and conjunctivitis. *Vasculitis with secondary thrombosis is the hallmark of the infection.* Bacterial embolism does not occur but may be simulated microscopically by intravascular proliferation of bacteria at sites of thrombosis. Thus, the former name "thromboembolic meningoencephalitis" is inaccurate. Histophilosis is an important disease of young cattle, but acute and chronic infections involving other organs are also economically significant.

Septicemia caused by *H. somni* develops in cattle of various ages maintained under various management systems, but in North America the disease is more prevalent in feedlots. It is most common in early winter, shortly after susceptible animals are moved there from pastures. Infection occurs in a large proportion of animals, but disease occurs in a minority. *H. somni* induces conditions in sheep identical to the bovine disease, i.e., septicemia, ITME, abortion, etc.

Cerebral localization produces a variety of neurologic signs, and without treatment affected animals become comatose and die within 1–2 days. The cerebral lesions are distinctive, and are visible in a large majority of untreated cases. The cerebrospinal fluid is cloudy and may contain pus and fibrin. *Scattered throughout the brain and spinal cord are multiple foci of hemorrhage and necrosis* (Fig. 3.114A, B). These foci may be 1–30 mm in diameter, and range from the bright red of recent hemorrhage to dark red-brown in older lesions. They have near-random distribution throughout the brain, but there may be some predilection for the thalamus and junction of the gray and white matter of the cerebral cortex. Meningitis is usually visible grossly and is most easily identified over the hemorrhagic foci. In animals that

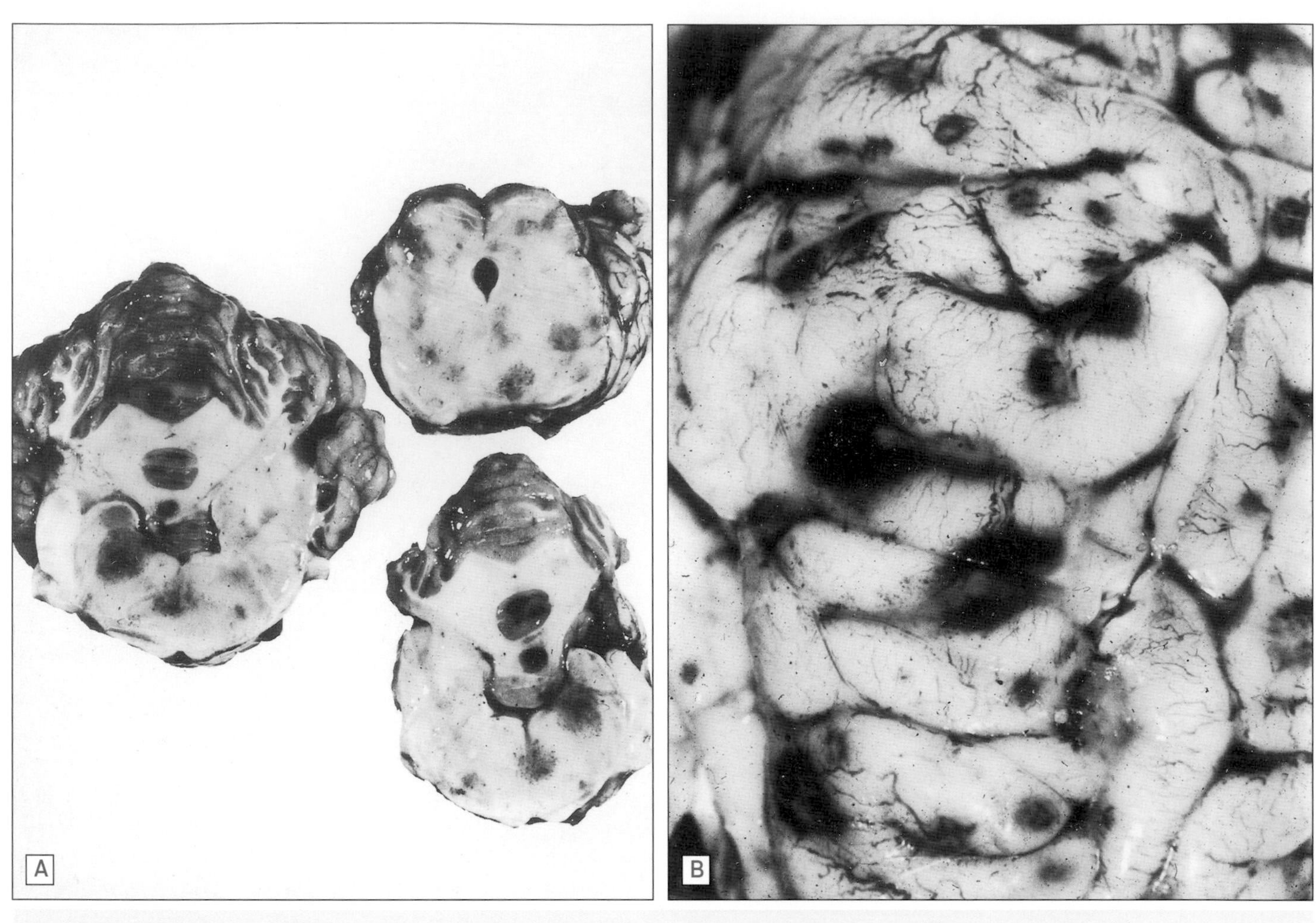

Figure 3.114 ***Histophilus somni*** infection in an ox. Multiple areas of hemorrhage and necrosis in brain stem (**A**) and cerebral cortex (**B**).

survive for a day or more, diffuse purulent leptomeningitis involves the basilar portions of the brain, and in these animals the older parenchymal lesions may have begun to soften.

The *histologic lesions* are similar in all organs but are usually most severe in the brain and consist of *intense vasculitis with thrombosis* and extension of the inflammation into the surrounding parenchyma, with or without infarction (Fig. 3.113A, B). Small venules (thrombophlebitis) are primarily affected, with thrombi often containing colonies of bacteria. The inflammatory response is neutrophilic, and cerebral lesions are quickly converted to abscesses.

Although cerebral vascular localization is a common and most dramatic result of the septicemia, *petechiation and evidence of inflammation are often visible throughout the body*, even in animals that die from fulminating disease. Foci of inflammation are easiest to identify in the renal medulla, skeletal muscle, lung, and laryngeal mucosa, but may also be visible in myocardium, intestine, and urinary bladder. Subacute to chronic disease develops commonly in some organs, especially joints, lungs, and heart, and is an important manifestation of *H. somni* infections.

In the acute disease, there is excess fluid in many *joints*, particularly the atlanto-occipital, where the capsule is distended by fluid that contains fibrin and sometimes blood. The synovial membranes and connective tissues around the affected joints are edematous and petechiated. The organism is sensitive to antimicrobials, and the course of the disease is often modified by therapy. The joints of animals that have survived several days contain thick mats of fibrin and pus, and the periarticular tissues are browned by old hemorrhage. Erosion of articular cartilages is rare.

Histophilus somni has been isolated from cattle with a variety of types of *pneumonia*, and its role in the bovine respiratory complex is discussed in the chapter on respiratory diseases. Pneumonia is an uncommon feature of the acute encephalitic form of the disease, but the lung can be involved as part of widespread vasculitis. *Ulcers of the larynx* occur in other diseases of feedlot animals, but, like atlanto-occipital arthritis, they are a regular enough feature of *H. somni* infection to serve as a valuable clue to the diagnosis and prompt a search for lesions in the brain. Similarly, *retinal hemorrhages* are grossly visible in a percentage of animals, and are of diagnostic assistance clinically and when gross brain lesions are absent.

A major manifestation of *H. somni* infection in some parts of North America, especially in western Canada, is *myocardial localization* following asymptomatic septicemia. Infarction, myocarditis, or abscess formation may result, and can lead to cardiac failure with or without mural and valvular endocarditis. In many animals, myocardial abscesses are found only when the myocardium of animals with chronic pneumonia or pleuritis is incised. Abscesses are most common in the left ventricular free wall, particularly in the papillary muscles.

Histophilus somni causes sporadic disease involving many other organs, including the ear, mammary gland, and those of the male and female genital tracts. It can also colonize the pregnant uterus and produce fetal disease and abortion (see The female genital system). The reported cases have not involved animals with cerebral localization, and may result from asymptomatic septicemia or transcervical invasion.

Bibliography

Angen O, et al. Proposal of *Histophilus somni* gen. nov., sp. nov. for the three species incertae sedis "*Haemophilus somnus*", "*Haemophilus agni*" and "*Histophilus ovis*". Int J Syst Evol Microbiol 2003;53:1449–1456.

Cassidy JP, et al. Thrombotic meningoencephalitis associated with *Histophilus ovis* infection in lambs in Europe. Vet Rec 1997;140:193–195.

Haines DM, et al. Immunohistochemical study of *Hemophilus somnus, Mycoplasma bovis, Mannheimia hemolytica*, and bovine viral diarrhea virus in death losses due to myocarditis in feedlot cattle. Can Vet J 2004;45:231–234.

Harris FW, Janzen ED. The *Haemophilus somnus* disease complex (haemophilosis): A review. Can Vet J 1989;30:816–822.

Lederer JA, et al. "*Haemophilus somnus*", a facultative intracellular pathogen of bovine mononuclear phagocytes. Infect Immun 1987;55:381–387.

Philbey AW, et al. Meningoencephalitis and other conditions associated with *Histophilus ovis* infection in sheep. Aust Vet J 1991;68:387–390.

Siddaramppa S, Inzana TJ. *Haemophilus somnus* virulence factors and resistance to host immunity. Anim Health Res Rev 2004;5:79–93.

Sylte MJ, et al. Caspase activation during *Haemophilus somnus* lipooligosaccharide-mediated apoptosis of bovine endothelial cells. Microb Pathog 2003;35:285–291.

Viral infections of the nervous system

Viral infections of the central nervous system are common, usually as part of systemic infections rather than examples of a specialized affinity for nervous tissue. Several viruses are neurotropic, however only a few are neurovirulent. A neurovirulent virus is a virus that multiplies in neural tissue and is able to induce lesions.

The **routes of invasion** of the nervous system available to viruses are *via nerves*, including the olfactory tracts, and *hematogenous*. Centripetal spread in axons does not depend on viral replication in axons, but passage is provided by the mechanisms of fast axoplasmic transport. Invasion by the olfactory route is theoretically simpler since olfactory receptors extend into and beyond the olfactory epithelium, and a cuff of arachnoid extends through the cribriform plate to the olfactory submucosa. This arrangement would allow viruses to spread along nerves without first penetrating to the submucosa or, having penetrated to the submucosa, to reach the CSF directly. This may be the route taken by *Bovine herpesvirus 1, Porcine teschovirus*, and Pseudorabies virus in young pigs. The olfactory route could be used following intranasal exposure or following hematogenous seeding of the olfactory epithelium or mucosa.

For most viruses, spread to the CNS is *hematogenous* after multiplication in some other tissue and the development of viremia of sufficient magnitude and duration. Viruses are susceptible to removal from blood by histiocytes, but viremia can be sustained if the viruses are small, associated with cells of blood, or replicated in endothelium or lymphatic tissues. Some viruses, such as *Canine distemper virus*, infect vascular endothelial cells whereas others infect surrounding glia suggesting transport across endothelium in pinocytotic vesicles. Invasion across the choroid plexus is not impeded by the fenestrated endothelial cells there but would require active infection of the epithelium and ependyma. There are areas of selective permeability to indicator dyes in the brain, such as the tuber cinereum and area postrema, but there is no evidence that these are selectively used by viruses.

The means by which viruses *spread in nervous tissue* are not known. Rapid dissemination can occur in the CSF, but some viruses, such as *Rabies virus*, extend rapidly through the parenchyma. The rate of spread of *Rabies virus*, assuming cell-to-cell growth and transmission, is probably more rapid than its generation time would permit, and permeation of the limited extracellular spaces of the brain by large viruses seems unlikely.

Separation of the specialized cells of the CNS into neurons, oligodendrocytes, astrocytes, and ependymocytes understates the diversity of cell populations in the brain and cord. Different cell populations may show different susceptibilities to infection by different viruses. Thus, Pseudorabies virus is nonselective in the destruction of cells in the rostral cortex of piglets, *Feline panleukopenia virus* selects rapidly proliferating cells of ependyma and cerebellar cortex, and *Porcine teschovirus 1* appears to affect particularly the spinal motor neurons.

Degeneration of neurons, reactivity of the glia, and perivascular reactions are the general hallmarks of viral infection of the CNS, and imply a sequence of viral cytopathogenicity and reaction to cellular degeneration. However, viruses that produce manifestations deviating from this rather simple system are many. *Classical swine fever virus* and *Bluetongue virus* at a suitably early fetal stage of development may produce **malformations** characterized by degeneration of tissue without reaction; later when the animal is immunologically competent, these viruses may produce ordinary encephalomyelitis. *Feline panleukopenia virus* causes cerebellar hypoplasia in the neonate but is without effect at a later stage of development.

Some viruses may produce *persistent tolerated infection* without clinical signs or lesions. At the other end of the spectrum is *Rabies virus*, which can cause death with minimal cytopathic effect and reaction, or no morphological change at all. Some virus infections are characterized by long latency and slow attrition, visna/maedi of sheep being the standard example expressed as either degeneration or chronic inflammation. *Transformation of nervous system cells by viruses* can be demonstrated in vitro, and a variety of tumors of the nervous system can be produced by viruses in experimental animals, but they have, as yet, no natural counterpart. The contribution of an immunological response to both the progress and morphology of encephalomyelitis is very difficult to determine.

General pathology of viral inflammation of the nervous system

Viral infections of the CNS typically induce **nonsuppurative inflammation**, a term that includes quite a variety of quantitative and qualitative changes. The changes are not specific for viral infections, being produced in some bacterial infections such as salmonellosis in swine, in the rickettsial infection, "salmon poisoning," of dogs, and probably in other rickettsioses. Nor are the lesions qualitatively the same in all viral infections, a fact that is of considerable usefulness in differential diagnosis. The differences are due in part to inherent characters of the agents, routes of invasion, patterns of localization, success of viral replication and release, duration and degree of cellular injury, and host defense reactions. As well as the differences, there are also the very considerable similarities that allow them all to be included with the "nonsuppurative encephalomyelitides."

The distribution of lesions in different viral infections is a reflection of the varied affinities of the viruses, and is useful in differential diagnosis but only generally applicable. The distributions of lesions or of inclusion bodies are only very rough guides to the distribution and activity of the virus.

Perivascular cuffing, or accumulation of cells in the adventitia of vessels and in the perivascular Virchow–Robin space, is almost constant in encephalitis, and, when present, is usually the most striking microscopic change. The accumulated cells are usually leukocytes, but in some diseases there may be very few hematogenous elements recognizable, the cuffs being composed instead of histiocytic cells that appear to have proliferated in situ from adventitial elements. These latter frequently fragment to resemble degenerate neutrophils if the postmortem interval is prolonged. Injury to the vessel wall proper is not constant, but when it occurs it may affect the arteries as a hyalinizing or fibrinoid change. This is characteristic of malignant catarrhal fever, for example, and occurs also in equine encephalitis. The endothelium may be selectively injured in classical swine fever and infectious canine hepatitis. The lesions associated with *Equid herpesvirus* infection may be limited to quite subtle endothelial swelling and proliferation in small blood vessels. When, in inflammation, the perivascular cuffs are large enough to disorganize the wall of the vessel and compress it, the endothelium frequently shows signs of swelling and proliferation, and there may also be altered adhesiveness so that leukocytes and red cells tend to stick to it. Thrombosis is incidental and very seldom observed, but compression of the vessels probably accounts for the ischemic parenchymal softenings that occur.

Infiltrating cells are predominantly lymphocytes, and they accumulate in the perivascular spaces (see Fig. 3.19). The earliest cells in the perivascular spaces may be neutrophils; in acute lesions, some of these can be found wandering in parenchyma or grouped in dense clusters. They soon disappear but may be found later for a short time in areas that soften. Lymphocytes remain in the cuffs and are admixed after a week or so with an increasing number of plasma cells and macrophages. A few eosinophils may also be found in pigs. Perivascular cuffing is not specific for viral infections. It is also a reaction to degeneration of neural tissue.

Glial reactions occur if the parenchyma is injured, even though the injury may not be appreciable, but the reaction may be absent in those infections that selectively involve the vessel walls. In inflamed areas, the oligodendroglia degenerate. Astrocytes degenerate or react depending on how strictly and severely they are injured – the stimuli for astrocytic reaction were discussed earlier in this chapter. *The gliosis that is so frequently a feature of nonsuppurative encephalomyelitis is almost solely microglial. The gliosis may be diffuse or focal but is commonly both* (see Fig. 3.17). Diffuse gliosis may be more apparent than real if due more to hypertrophy than to proliferation of these glia. Focal gliosis may occur anywhere in the parenchyma and may be related to small vessels and injury to microvasculature. When there are more than a dozen or so cells in such foci, some of the cells are likely to be lymphocytes, and occasionally there are a few plasma cells. The microglia in the center of a focus are frequently degenerate. There are two specifically named forms of microgliosis: "*neuronophagic nodules*" are foci of microglia about degenerating neurons (see Fig. 3.2D); "*glial shrubbery*" is an accumulation of these cells in the molecular layer of the cerebellum in relation to degenerating Purkinje cells (Fig. 3.115).

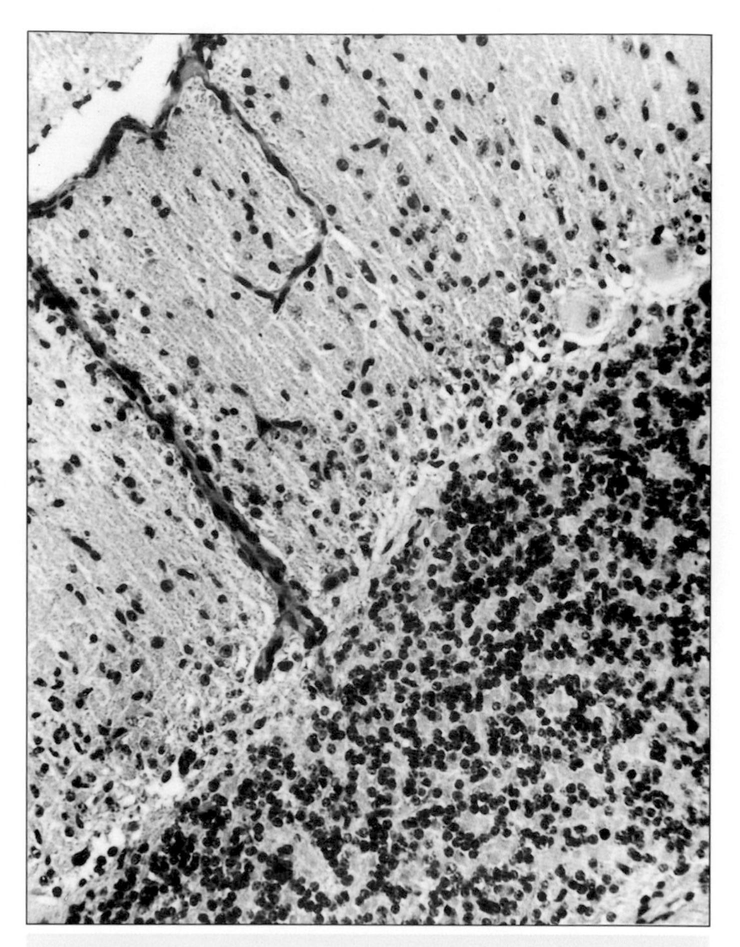

Figure 3.115 Encephalitis in **louping-ill** in a sheep. Destruction of Purkinje cells and gliosis in molecular layer of cerebellum ("glial shrubbery").

Neuronal changes must be the principal determinants of the outcome of the infection. The distribution of neuronal degeneration is to some slight extent specific, but the extensiveness is nonspecific and varies considerably. The morphological features of the degenerate cells are nonspecific. As a rule, the more severe degrees of neuronal degeneration are caused by viruses that are highly neurotropic, such as *Rabies virus*, but the severity of neuronal degeneration is not a dependable "lead" in differential diagnosis. The fact that *Rabies virus* can be lethal without morphological change in the CNS raises the possibility that other viruses may cause severe encephalopathy without inflammatory change. *The usual form of neuronal degeneration is central chromatolysis*, which may extend to completion with the cell then swollen, pale, and devoid of a nucleus. This is typical of the axonal reaction to injury, but the axons are intact. Many neurons appear as if coagulated, being shrunken, rounded, and isolated, and staining darkly with eosin. The nucleus is pyknotic or has disappeared. The coagulated neuron stimulates the formation of the neuronophagic nodule, but not all necrotic neurons elicit the reaction. Usually, intact neurons can be found adjacent to degenerate ones.

Lesions in white matter occur consistently even though many viruses are supposed to be specifically tropic for gray matter. Cuffing reactions are to be expected even if degeneration is limited to adjacent gray matter. *Microgliosis* is focal rather than diffuse and the nodules are small. Some degree of *disintegration of myelin* is inevitable, but conspicuous demyelination is a feature only of canine distemper, lentivirus leukoencephalitis of goats, and visna. Demyelination associated with viral diseases may be due to direct infection of melanin-forming cells, i.e., oligodendroglia, as in infection with *Canine distemper virus*, or may be a bystander lesion due to injury from inflammatory cytokines associated with viral infection.

Meningitis is seldom severe except in local distributions, and these tend to overlie parenchymal lesions. Some agents, of which typical examples are those of sporadic bovine encephalomyelitis (see Fig. 3.60) and malignant catarrhal fever, have a selective affinity for meningeal structures in the CNS. Others, such as *Canine distemper virus*, share the affinities so that leptomeningitis is part of the primary response. In the more purely neurotropic infections, such as rabies, the meningitis, or more precisely the meningeal infiltration, is due probably to drainage of products of reaction via the Virchow–Robin spaces from the brain or cord. The reacting cells in the meninges are of the same type as those in the brain, and they float freely in the arachnoid spaces.

No virus is known to be tropic for peripheral nerves in the sense of selectively producing direct lesions in them. Degenerative changes occur fairly early in the end plates and terminal parts of axons when the central cell body is destroyed. Foci of microglia and lymphocytes occur in the nerve roots quite commonly. Inflammation of the paravertebral ganglia, and especially the trigeminal (Gasserian) ganglia, is characteristic of rabies and of Teschen disease and related infections in pigs, but the frequency and distribution of this lesion in other viral encephalomyelitides and in other ganglia is unknown.

Inclusion bodies may form in neurons, neuroglia, or microglia and other mesenchymal cells. Inclusion bodies in the nervous system are usually acidophilic. They may be found only in neurons as in rabies, in glia, or in both. They may be cytoplasmic, nuclear, or both. Intranuclear inclusions, which must be distinguished from altered nucleoli, have considerable specificity; somewhat less reliance can be placed on intracytoplasmic inclusions. Cytoplasmic viral inclusions must be distinguished from normal inclusions.

Lyssavirus infections

Rabies is caused by *Rabies virus* (RABV), which belongs to the genus *Lyssavirus* of the family Rhabdoviridae. The RABV glycoprotein (RVG), which is a trimeric and surface-exposed viral coat protein, is responsible for RABV neurotropism by binding to several neural tissue receptors including the neuronal cell adhesion molecule (NCAM), and the p75 neurotrophin receptor (p75NTR). Evolutionary studies based on genes encoding the surface glycoprotein *suggest that RABV evolved first in bats*, possibly in vampire bats much more widely distributed than at present, and only later became adapted to terrestrial carnivores. There is a single major antigenic type with minor variations that allow epidemiological surveillance. *Seven genotypes* are defined by phylogenetic analysis. Type 1 is the classical *Rabies virus* of animals and vampire bats, and of all other bat lyssaviruses in North America. Type 2 (*Lagos bat virus*), type 3 (*Mokola virus*), type 4 (*Duvenhage virus*) are African genotypes. Types 5 (EBLV-1) and 6 (EBLV-2) are *European bat lyssavirus* 1 and 2, and type 7 (Ballina virus) is the *Australian bat lyssavirus*. The seven genotypes may further be allocated into *two major phylogroups* based on pathogenicity for mice and cross-neutralization. Phylogroup 1 includes genotypes 1, 4–7, and phylogroup 2 includes genotypes 2 and 3. Excepting *Mokola virus*, bats may be the preferential vector species for genotypes 2–7.

Rabies virus has two biotypes: "fixed" virus and "street" virus. *Fixed RABV*, which is the basis of vaccine strains, is a laboratory biotype stabilized in its properties by serial intracerebral passage. It is highly neurotropic, is not secreted in saliva, and does not produce Negri bodies. *Street RABV* is the feral biotype that circulates in enzootics and epizootics. In addition to neurotropism, it is tropic for salivary glands, in which it reaches high concentration, and possibly in other mucus-secreting epithelia, and produces Negri bodies.

The establishment of infection ordinarily depends on inoculation of the virus into a wound, such usually being inflicted by the bite of a rabid animal. Contamination of a fresh wound by infected saliva or tissues is much less dangerous. The virus replicates in myocytes around a bite wound for a short period of time, and then buds from the plasma membrane. Viral particles invade the local neuromuscular junction through conjugation of the RVG with the nicotinic acetylcholine receptor, and then invade neurotendinous spindles and ascend to the CNS and paravertebral ganglia via axoplasmic flow. Viral replication in the CNS is followed by centrifugal spread to major exit portals, such as the adrenal gland, nasal mucosa, and salivary glands; the virus is secreted with the saliva for a few days prior to the appearance of clinical signs. The incubation period is variable from weeks to months.

Although there are species differences in susceptibility, rabies is one disease to which *all mammals are susceptible*. The disease can be regarded as one of carnivores because it is almost always transmitted naturally only by bites, and man, herbivores, etc. are dead-end hosts. There are exceptions to the rule that RABV is bite-transmitted: *oral infection* can occur in diverse species and the application of modified RABV in "baits" utilizes this potential; *aerosol infection* can occur, as in dense congregations of colonial bats in bat caves, probably as droplet infection from salivary secretions; and a variety of aberrant circumstances may provide transfer opportunities for infectious virus, as has been reported for *corneal transplants*.

Reservoir hosts vary from time to time and from region to region. The principal reservoir vectors are: foxes and skunks in the USA and Canada, with the raccoon of importance on the Atlantic seaboard; foxes and dogs in northern Canada; foxes moving from east to west in Europe; wolves in eastern Europe and Iran; jackals in India and Northern Africa; the mongoose and genet cat in South Africa; and the mongoose in the Caribbean. *Sylvatic vectors* are responsible for most transmissions to man and domestic animals in countries where dog populations are controlled. Oral vaccination of wild carnivores, by using vaccine-laden baits, and routine vaccination of dogs have led to almost complete elimination of canine-transmitted rabies in developed countries. Rarely, vaccination of severely stressed animals with vaccines containing modified-live virus may induce post-vaccinal rabies. In tropical areas where domestic and feral dogs are not controlled, these animals are the principal hazards for man and livestock.

Bats present a special epidemiologic problem. Fructivorous and insectivorous bats as well as vampires are capable of transmitting RABV. Vampire bats inhabit South and Central America extending into northern Mexico and are, historically, responsible for a high incidence of rabies in mammals, especially cattle but including humans. When clinically affected, vampire bats manifest the disease as the furious form and show unnatural daylight activity.

The **clinical course** of rabies is usually acute, from 1–2 days, but can be as long as 10 days. It is seldom that a clinical diagnosis of rabies can be made with confidence. The terms "*furious rabies*" and "*dumb rabies*" place emphasis on particular features within a spectrum of behavioral changes and are inappropriate for noncarnivorous animals. *Aberrant behavioral patterns* can be recognized in affected animals during epizootics. The period of salivary excretion of virus before the onset of neurological signs is expected to be not more than a few days, vampire bats possibly excepted, and the duration of clinical disease to be a few days only. Once expressed clinically as neurologic disease, *rabies is almost invariably fatal*; recovery with or without neurologic deficit is quite rare but has been observed in several species following experimental exposure. Progressive infection and clinical disease do not inevitably follow exposure; up to 25% of feral populations may have specific antibodies as evidence that the infection provoked an immune response without progression to neurologic disease.

Specific gross lesions are not present at necropsy, but self-inflicted wounds and foreign bodies in the stomach of a carnivore should raise suspicion. The **histologic lesions** of rabies, when present, are *typical of nonsuppurative encephalomyelitis, with ganglioneuritis and parotid adenitis*. Inflammatory changes are usually present, but they may be very mild or absent. To some extent at least, the severity of lesions reflects the duration of the clinical disease. In the CNS, inflammatory and degenerative changes are most severe from the pons to the hypothalamus and in the cervical spinal cord, with relative sparing of the medulla. This relative sparing of the medulla appears to apply to all domestic species. The most severe lesions of the disease are generally found in dogs whereas other species, especially ruminants, which are highly susceptible, may show little more than an occasional vessel with a few cuffing lymphocytes and a few very small glial nodules (*Babès' nodules* in this disease), and this in spite of having numerous Negri bodies. These reactive phenomena probably reflect largely the degree of neuronal degeneration, and this may be remarkably slight in herbivores and remarkably severe in dogs.

The reaction is typically one of *perivascular cuffing and focal gliosis*. The cuffs are 1 to several cells thick and composed solely of lymphocytes (Fig. 3.116A); ring hemorrhages confined largely to the perivascular space are common about cuffed vessels. Hemorrhages are occasionally severe enough to be visible grossly in the spinal cord of horses and cattle (Fig. 3.116B). The Babès' nodules are composed of microglia, and they occur in both white and gray matter. The nodules vary greatly in size, some containing only six or seven cells and

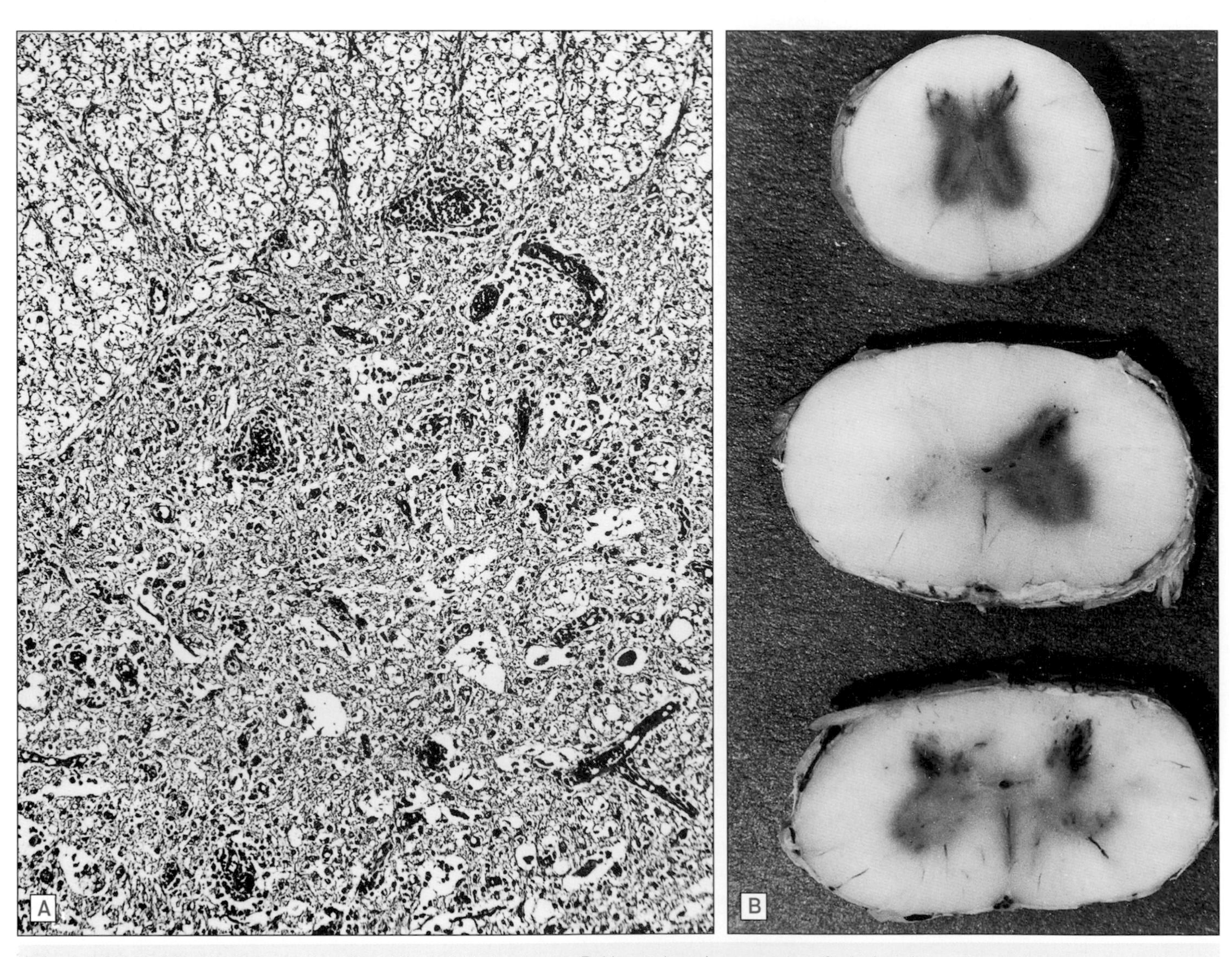

Figure 3.116 Rabies. A. Perivascular cuffs and focal gliosis in a horse. **B.** Hemorrhage in gray matter of spinal cord.

some containing 100 or more. Diffuse as well as focal gliosis occurs in areas of gray matter such as the pons and in the spinal cord, both horns of the latter being involved.

Neuronal degeneration in carnivores may be very extensive and quite out of proportion to the observed reactive changes, but may be very slight in pigs and herbivores. Neuronal and/or gray matter neuropilar vacuolation (*rabies-induced spongiform encephalopathy*) is reported to occur in experimental and natural rabies. The specificity of the neuronal changes and of the whole pathologic picture depends on the *inclusion bodies of Negri*. These are always *intracytoplasmic* and are present most commonly in the hippocampus of carnivores and in the Purkinje cells of herbivores. Fixed RABV does not produce Negri bodies, and street RABV fails to do so in up to 30% of cases. Neurons of any distribution may contain inclusion bodies, but they tend to be scarce where the inflammatory reaction is severe. Indeed Negri bodies may be found only in neurons that are otherwise histologically normal; they are not present in degenerate neurons. They have also been found, but rarely, in ganglion cells of the adrenal medulla, salivary glands, and retina. While the number of Negri bodies has little relation to the length of the incubation period, there is a relation to the duration of the clinical disease. They may not be found if the animal is killed instead of being allowed to die. They are produced consistently in white mice, the usual test animal.

Negri bodies are round or oval structures usually ~2–8 μm in diameter (Fig. 3.117A). They are plastic, their shape being molded to their environment. Those in the dendrites, seldom observed except in Purkinje cells, are oval and those in the cell body are usually rounded. There may be one or more per cell, and affected cells are otherwise only little changed. The inclusions are surrounded by a clear thin halo. Nonspecific homogeneous inclusions may be found in the pyramidal cells of the hippocampus in cats, skunks, and dogs. There may be several such inclusions per cell but each is minute, not measuring more than 1.5 μm. In old sheep and cattle, larger neurons, especially of the medulla and cord, may contain nonspecific inclusions. These have a dust-like distribution, are usually numerous, and are brightly acidophilic, angulated, and ~1.0 μm in size. Nonspecific inclusions that are indistinguishable from Negri bodies by light microscopy occur in the lateral geniculate neurons in cats. *Fluorescent antibody techniques are required for positive identification* and are essential in the rare chronic cases which may not yield virus on mouse inoculation.

If there is no *ganglioneuritis* in the paravertebral ganglia, then the possibility of the animal having rabies is very remote. If there is ganglioneuritis, it may be part of rabies or something else. Pigs, for example, get ganglioneuritis in the Teschen group of infections. Inflammatory changes in the trigeminal (Gasserian) ganglion in rabies may be present without inflammatory or neuronal changes being clearly evident in the brain. The ganglionic changes are of the same character as those in the brain, namely acute degeneration of ganglion cells, proliferation of capsule cells, and microglial nodules (Fig. 3.117B).

The natural transmission of RABV depends on virus being present in the saliva and, therefore, in the salivary glands. Fixed virus

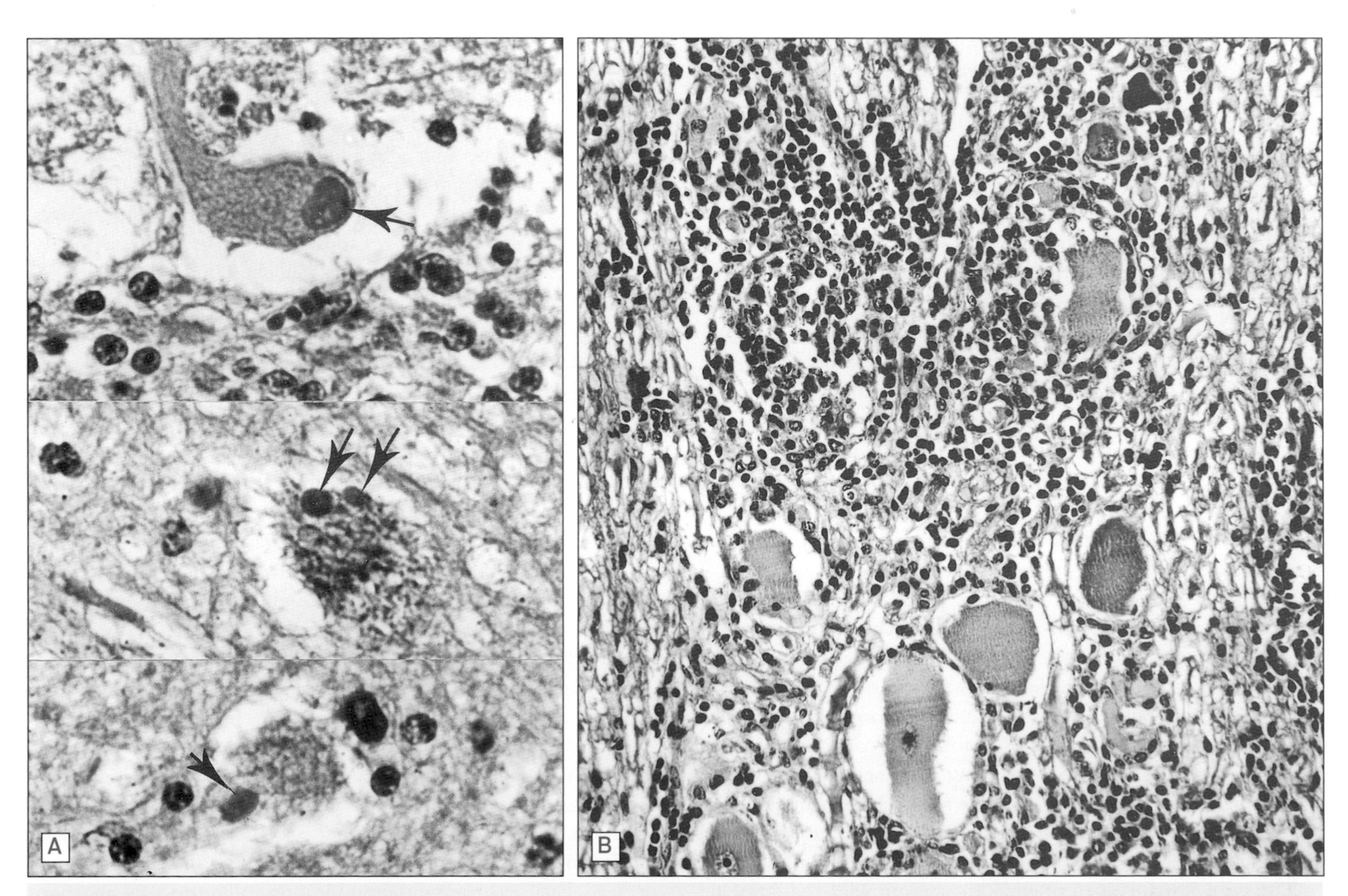

Figure 3.117 Rabies. A. Composite picture showing Negri bodies (arrows) in neuronal cytoplasm. **B.** Severe nonsuppurative inflammation of trigeminal ganglion.

has no affinity for the salivary glands, and none is present in some cases of infection with the street virus. Degenerative changes are reported in the epithelium of the mandibular salivary gland, but not in the parotid, in dogs.

The **diagnosis** of rabies is made by utilizing fluorescent antibody labeling on fresh or fixed tissue, or by virus isolation in cell culture.

Bibliography

Badrane H, et al. Evidence of two Lyssavirus phylogroups with distinct pathogenicity and immunogenicity. J Virol 2001;75:3268–3276.

Badrane H, Tordo N. Host switching in lyssavirus history from the chiroptera to the carnivora orders. J Virol 2001;75:8096–8104.

Charlton KM, et al. Experimental rabies in skunks and foxes. Pathogenesis of the spongiform lesions. Lab Invest 1987;57:634–645.

Esh JB, et al. Vaccine-induced rabies in four cats. J Am Vet Med Assoc 1982;180:1336–1339.

Langevin C, et al. Rabies virus glycoprotein (RVG) is a trimeric ligand for the N-terminal cysteine-rich domain of the mammalian p75 neurotrophin receptor. J Biol Chem 2002;277:37655–37662.

McColl KA, et al. Bat lyssavirus infections. Rev Sci Tech Off Int Epiz 2000;19:177–196.

McCormack JG, Allworth AM. Emerging viral infections in Australia. Med J Aust 2002;177:45–49.

Rosatte RC. Bat rabies in Canada: history, epidemiology and prevention. Can Vet J 1987;28:754–756.

Rupprecht CE, et al. Oral vaccination of wildlife against rabies: opportunities and challenges in prevention and control. Dev Biol (Basel) 2004;119:173–184.

Swanepoel R. Rabies. In: Coetzer JAW, et al, eds. Infectious Disease of Livestock with Special Reference to Southern Africa. 2nd ed. Vol 2. Oxford: Oxford University Press, 1994: 1123–1182.

Pseudorabies

Pseudorabies is also known as Aujeszky's disease, mad itch, infectious bulbar paralysis, and porcine herpesvirus infection. The causative agent, ***Suid herpesvirus 1*** (SuHV-1; Pseudorabies virus, PRV), belongs to the genus *Varicellovirus*, subfamily Alphaherpesvirinae, family Herpesviridae, but is unusual for a member of that group in its relative lack of host specificity and by being spread laterally as well as vertically in swine. A number of strains have been identified which exhibit a wide range of virulence. Pseudorabies virus is capable, as are other members of the family Herpesviridae, of establishing latent infection. Trigeminal ganglion, olfactory bulb, and tonsil are the most consistent sites of latency of PRV. In these organs, viral DNA can be detected in the absence of infectious virus. The pig is the only natural host, but the common domestic species are naturally susceptible; there are very few reports in horses and goats. Progressive infections do not occur in humans. The disease is reported worldwide, except for Canada and Australia. Natural infections occur in rats and mice and various species of wildlife and on fur farms. Of the laboratory animals, the rabbit is the most susceptible and is preferred for identification of the virus because of the fairly consistent development of intense local pruritus following subcutaneous inoculation. Guinea pigs are less susceptible and may resist subcutaneous inoculation but succumb to intracerebral and, occasionally, to intraperitoneal inoculation.

The virus is maintained in enzootic areas in wild and domestic swine, for which it is highly contagious but usually asymptomatic, and probably in brown rats. *Transmission* can occur by ingestion, but the usual method of spread between pigs is thought to be by contact of infective secretions with nasal mucosa or abraded skin. Animals are susceptible to intranasal inoculation and, regardless of the route of infection, the *virus can be found in nasal secretions*. The virus may also be present in saliva and urine. It is also present in blood, but this is of no significance for epidemiology or transmission. The infection will occur in pigs by contact very readily and probably by direct nose-to-nose transmission, but it does not appear to be contagious between individuals of other species and they probably acquire their infection by contact with swine or, possibly, rats. Pigs may harbor virus for many months in tonsils and nasopharyngeal secretions after exposure, but in other domestic species the virus is fairly strictly neurotropic, and therefore is not excreted unless given experimentally in large doses. Ingestion of *infected pig meat* is the usual source of infection for dogs and cats. Cattle and sheep may become infected by direct contact with carrier swine or by aerosol exposure, but there is strong circumstantial evidence implicating contaminated feed.

The *pathogenesis* of the infection following local inoculation is well established for the rabbit and is probably comparable in other species. The virus causes a local reaction at the site of inoculation if percutaneous and then spreads centripetally along the related nerve to the spinal cord; it then spreads outwards again along other peripheral nerves as other segments of cord are progressively invaded by spread within the CNS. Because of the progressive advance of infection along the cord, death may occur before demonstrable amounts of virus reach the brain and before lesions have time to develop there. Intracerebral inoculation produces encephalitis, and virus spreads to the cord and centrifugally along peripheral nerves to an extent that depends on survival time. Because the virus also circulates in the blood, there is some possibility but no evidence that it invades the brain directly, the evidence instead suggesting that it localizes in viscera and invades the nervous system along autonomic nerves. Following nasal or intraocular exposure, the virus spreads along the related nerves. The route of invasion following ingestion is by retrograde transneuronal infection. Transplacental infections occur in pigs causing abortion in about 50% of sows pregnant in the first month, and the delivery of macerated, mummified, and normal fetuses when infection occurs at later stages of gestation. The virus is reported to be present in the semen of carrier boars.

The *signs and course* of pseudorabies in pigs are very variable. Most cases are of mild febrile illness without pruritus or nervous signs, and with recovery expected in a week or so. Sows may subsequently produce mummified litters. Age is a very important factor governing the severity of the disease in swine; the mortality rate in nursing pigs and young weaners may be very high. Very young sucklings do not show specific nervous signs but rapidly become prostrate and die in 12–24 hours. In slightly older piglets, incoordination progresses rapidly to paralysis with muscular twitchings, tremors, and convulsions. Some pigs showing severe signs of encephalitis recover. Experimental peripheral inoculation will produce asymptomatic meningitis and encephalitis in swine, the inflammatory lesions being severe. The disease in older pigs is often characterized by fever, rhinitis, and coughing. There may be generalized pruritus in natural cases but it is not severe, being expressed usually by rubbing of the nose or head. Fetal resorption, mummification, stillbirths, and abortions are frequently reported.

The characteristic clinical sign of pseudorabies in animals other than pigs is *intense cutaneous irritation* developing at the point of inoculation or at the terminal distribution of a nerve trunk which passes the point of inoculation. This does not occur until the virus reaches the related segment of cord. Dogs may become frenzied, and besides the intense pruritus (mad itch) there may be jaw paralysis and drooling reminiscent of rabies. The clinical course in these species, which always ends in death, is frequently acute (a few hours) and never longer than 1 week. Pseudorabies may occur in sporadic, although significant, outbreaks in sheep and cattle. The mortality rate is very high. Death may occur without signs of illness or within 1–2 days of the onset of clinical signs. There is fever, and the itching may be on any part of the body but is most frequently about the head or hindlimbs. Other neurological signs are variable but constantly present.

There are *no specific gross lesions* of pseudorabies. At the site of cutaneous infection, there is acute serofibrinous inflammation, ballooning degeneration, and epithelial necrosis with rare intranuclear inclusions. Self-trauma due to intense itching may exacerbate these lesions. The intense pruritus at the site of inoculation is likely due to stimulation of regional sensory nerves by viral spread and multiplication. Gross changes are seen mostly in young pigs. There may be necrosis of tonsils and sometimes of the trachea and esophagus. Rhinitis with patchy epithelial necrosis is common. The lungs may be edematous. Tiny foci (1–2 mm) of hemorrhagic necrosis typical of alpha-herpesviral infection may be seen in liver, spleen, lung, intestines, adrenals, and placenta.

The **histologic lesions** reflect the neurotropic and epitheliotropic nature of the virus. Lesions are similar in all susceptible species, however, epitheliotropic lesions are more commonly seen in young, aborted, or stillbirth piglets and rarely seen in ruminants or carnivores, where the brain lesions are more common. In brain, the gray matter especially is affected, but death may occur before there are clear indications of neuronal degeneration or inflammatory reaction in the brain. With naturally acquired infections, the inflammatory changes are *nonsuppurative*. In addition, focal gliosis and lesions typical of neuronal degeneration (neuronophagia and satellitosis) are usually present (Fig. 3.118A, B). There is severe ganglioneuritis in paravertebral ganglia. The specificity of the reaction in the brain depends on the development of *acidophilic intranuclear inclusion bodies in neurons and astroglia* (Fig. 3.118C). These inclusion bodies occur in all species, including pigs; fixation in a mercurial fixative is helpful for their demonstration. Inclusions in swine are *solid and amphophilic*, but in other species the inclusions are granular and often small and multiple in an affected nucleus. By any route of infection, piglets tend to develop panencephalitis with most severe lesions in the cerebral cortex, brain stem, spinal ganglia, and basal ganglia of the brain (Fig. 3.118B); in other domestic species, the distribution of lesions in the CNS is local to, and determined by, the route of exposure. Lymphoplasmacytic inflammation with neuronal degeneration of the gastric myenteric plexi is also described.

Epitheliotropic lesions include the presence of tiny areas of coagulative or lytic necrosis in the liver, tonsils, lung, spleen, placenta, and adrenals with the presence of the characteristic intranuclear inclusions. Pulmonary lesions may be mild or severe. Edema and mild cellular infiltration may be diffuse and there may be focal or confluent necrotizing, hemorrhagic pneumonia (Fig. 3.118D). Hemorrhage and necrosis is present in lymph nodes, and foci of necrosis may be found in tonsils, liver, spleen, and adrenal. Necrotizing vasculitis is described in natural infections in sheep and experimentally in piglets. In aborted or stillborn piglets, which are suitable for examination, there is usually no evidence of encephalitis, but foci of necrosis may be found in liver and other parenchymatous tissues together with focal bronchiolar necrosis and interstitial pneumonia.

Rapid **diagnosis** can be achieved by fluorescent antibody tests on frozen sections of tissue, e.g., tonsils, liver, or brain. Isolation in eggs or tissue culture is also available.

Bibliography

Enquist LW, et al. Infection and spread of alphaherpesviruses in the nervous system. Adv Virus Res 1999;51:237–347.

Gortazar C, et al. Natural Aujeszky's disease in a Spanish wild boar population. Ann N Y Acad Sci 2002;969:210–212.

Mettenleiter TC. Aujeszky's disease (pseudorabies) virus: the virus and molecular pathogenesis – State of the art, June 1999. Vet Res 2000;31:99.

Narita M, et al. Enteric lesions induced by different pseudorabies (Aujeszky's disease) virus strains inoculated into closed intestinal loops of pigs. J Vet Diagn Invest 1998;10:36–42.

Schmidt SP, et al. A necrotizing pneumonia in lambs caused by pseudorabies virus (Aujeszky's disease virus). Can J Vet Res 1987;51:145–149.

Porcine hemagglutinating encephalomyelitis virus

Porcine hemagglutinating encephalomyelitis virus (HEV), a member of genus *Coronavirus*, family Coronaviridae, can be isolated from the respiratory tract of normal pigs, and is present worldwide. Other porcine coronaviruses include *Transmissible gastroenteritis virus*, *Porcine epidemic diarrhea virus*, and *Porcine respiratory coronavirus*. HEV is a group 2 species coronavirus antigenically related to *Bovine coronavirus, Human coronavirus OC43*, and *Murine hepatitis virus*. The pig is the only natural host for HEV. Although there is serological evidence of wide distribution in many swine-raising areas, clinical disease is rare because most piglets receive protective levels of colostral antibodies to HEV. Disease occurs in piglets 1–3 weeks of age and follows a clinical course of about 3 days to 3 weeks. The mortality rate is very high and survivors are usually unthrifty.

Following exposure, replication of virus occurs in the epithelium of nose, tonsil, lung, and small intestine, with spread to the CNS along peripheral nerves rather than hematogenously; viremia is not important in the pathogenesis. Viral antigen is detectable in alimentary ganglia during the incubation period of the disease. It is first demonstrable in the brain in trigeminal and vagal sensory nuclei, with later rostral spread in brain stem. Viral replication occurs in the myenteric plexus of the stomach, and involvement of the autonomic system probably can explain the predominant clinical signs of vomition and constipation.

Two *clinical syndromes* are recognized. Neurologic signs occur in 4–7-day-old piglets in some outbreaks and consist of stilted gait, hyperesthesia, progressive paresis, and convulsions in some cases. Clinical signs in 4–14-day-old piglets are dominated by anorexia and vomiting, and this syndrome is called "*vomiting and wasting disease*."

Lesions in the CNS may be found in some affected piglets that do not show clinical signs of nervous disease. The frequency with which inflammatory change is found is quite variable. Lesions when present are those of *nonsuppurative encephalomyelitis* affecting particularly the gray matter of medulla and brain stem. In such cases

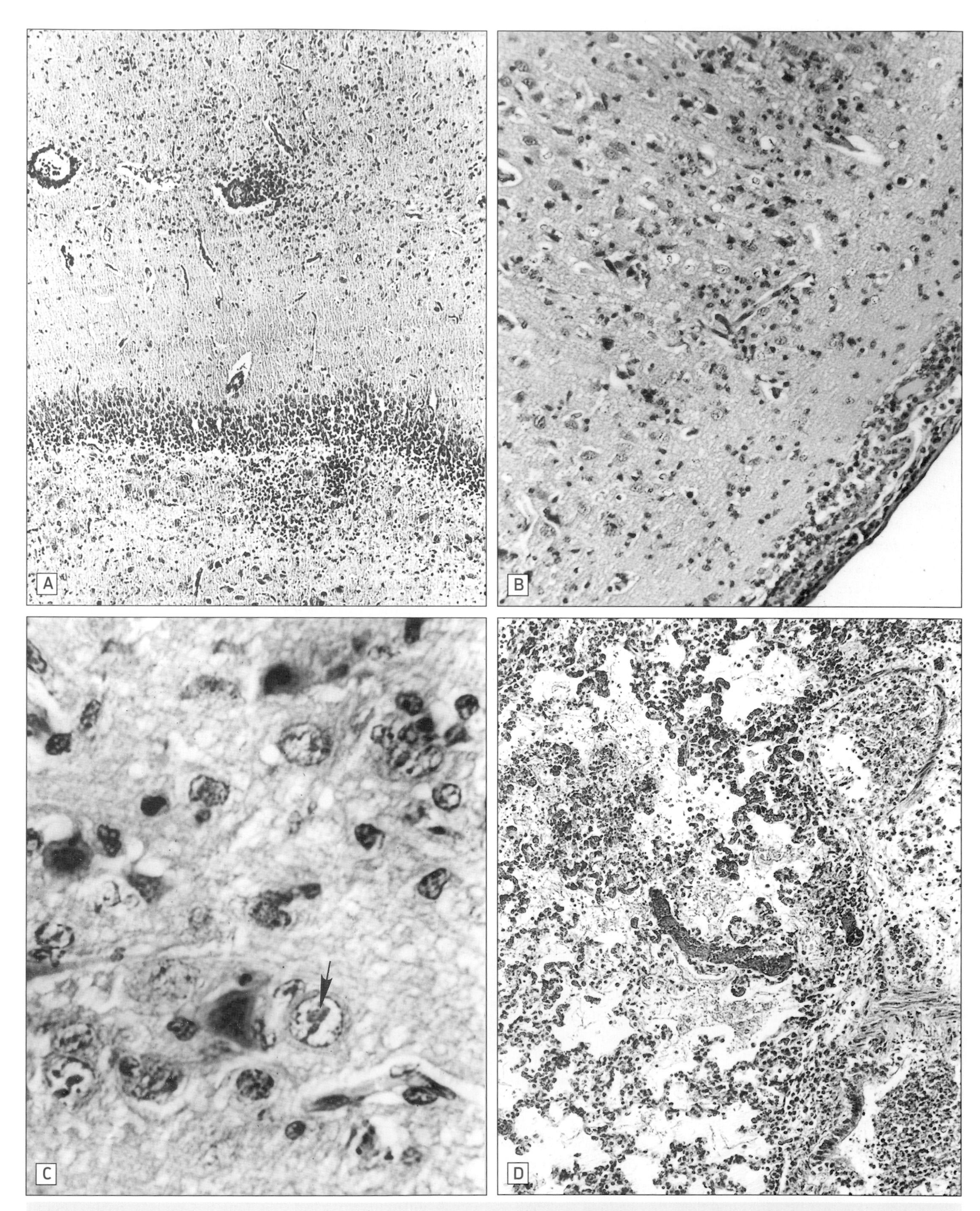

Figure 3.118 Pseudorabies in a pig. **A.** Perivascular cuffing, focal and diffuse gliosis in dentate gyrus. **B.** Meningitis and necrosis of cells in cerebrum. **C.** Neuronal necrosis and irregular inclusion bodies in nuclei (arrow). **D.** Necrotizing bronchopneumonia.

there is inflammation of the trigeminal, paravertebral, and autonomic ganglia. The gastric myenteric plexi are occasionally infiltrated with a few lymphocytes and plasma cells.

Diagnosis of HEV is problematic. Serology on acute and convalescent sera may help in detecting acute infection. Isolation of HEV can be attempted from brain stem of acutely ill piglets. Differential diagnoses of nervous conditions with high mortality in piglets include pseudorabies, classical swine fever, polioencephalomyelitis (Teschen disease), bacterial meningitis, streptococcal septicemia, and hypoglycemia.

Bibliography

Meyvisch C, Hoorens J. An electron microscopic study of experimentally-induced HEV encephalitis. Vet Pathol 1978;15:102–113.

Murphy AF, et al. Coronaviridae. In: Murphy FA, et al., eds. Veterinary Virology. London: Academic Press, 3rd ed. 1999:495–515.

Narita M, et al. Demonstration of viral antigen and immunoglobulin (IgG and IgM) in brain tissue of pigs experimentally infected with haemagglutinating encephalomyelitis virus. J Comp Pathol 1989;100:119–128.

Pensaert MB. Hemagglutinating encephalomyelitis virus. In: Straw BE, et al., eds. Diseases of Swine. 8th ed. Ames, IA: Iowa State University Press. 1999:151–157.

Enterovirus/teschovirus polioencephalomyelitis of pigs

Encephalomyelitis of pigs caused by porcine enteroviruses occurs in many countries and is distinguishable only by a study of the agents. Porcine enteroviruses are ubiquitous but are limited in their pathogenicity to swine. ***Porcine enterovirus** A* (PEV-A, formerly PEV serotype 8) and *Porcine enterovirus B* (formerly serotypes 9, 10) are in the genus *Enterovirus*, family Picornaviridae. Porcine enteroviruses serotypes 1–7 and 11–13 have been reclassified as ***Porcine teschovirus*** *1–7, 11–13*, genus *Teschovirus*, family Picornaviridae. Further reclassifications of picornaviruses can be expected. Infection by one enterovirus/teschovirus serotype does not confer protection against infection by another.

Infection is most commonly acquired by pigs after weaning due to waning maternal immunity and mixing of pigs from different sources. Infection follows the fecal–oral route and indirectly through contaminated fomites. Initial replication occurs in the tonsils and the intestinal epithelium, especially of ileum and colon; the enteric phase is not clinically significant or accompanied by tissue change. The enteric phase is followed by viremia and then invasion of the CNS. Viremia by some serotypes may lead to localization in the pregnant uterus and death of fetuses.

Infection with virulent virus may produce nervous signs as soon as 6 days after exposure. The virus is present in large amounts in tonsils and cervical lymph nodes by 24 hours, and in the mesenteric nodes and feces by 48 hours. The disease has two clinical forms: the highly fatal and severe form (**Teschen disease**) and a less virulent milder form (**Talfan disease**, poliomyelitis suum, benign enzootic paresis, Ontario encephalomyelitis, and polioencephalomyelitis.). Teschen disease, first recognized in 1929 in Teschen, Czech Republic, is caused by highly virulent ***Porcine teschovirus 1*** and is limited mostly to Europe, but sporadic epizootics occur in Africa. Talfan disease, caused by infection with less virulent strains of the virus, is more common than Teschen disease and occurs worldwide. Teschen disease is of high morbidity and high mortality affecting all age groups and expressed clinically as convulsions, opisthotonos, nystagmus and coma. Death commonly occurs in 3–4 days. Survivors may have residual paralysis. Talfan disease is characterized by lower morbidity and mortality, and the clinical signs are expressed as paresis and ataxia that seldom progresses to complete paralysis. The infection is asymptomatic in the absence of neurological signs, and up to 95% of exposed pigs develop latent or inapparent infections.

The *pathological changes* in these syndromes are the same although minor differences in severity and distribution of the lesions are reported. There are no gross changes. The histological changes are those of *nonsuppurative polioencephalomyelitis* extending throughout the cerebrospinal axis from the olfactory bulbs to the lumbar cord. Any series of cases of each of the syndromes provides a continuous spectrum of severity and distribution of the lesions. Lymphocytic meningitis is mild in the cerebral meninges and usually overlies areas of parenchymal injury in the cerebrum. In weaners and older animals in which the course is more prolonged than in very young pigs, intense lymphocytic meningitis develops over the cerebellum, usually in conjunction with inflammatory lesions in the underlying molecular layer (Fig. 3.119). Cerebellar meningitis is very slight if the course of the disease is 4–5 days or less, so that, although emphasized in reports of Teschen disease, it is not a feature in very young animals in which the course is short. The most severe lesions occur in the brain stem from the hypothalamus through the medulla and

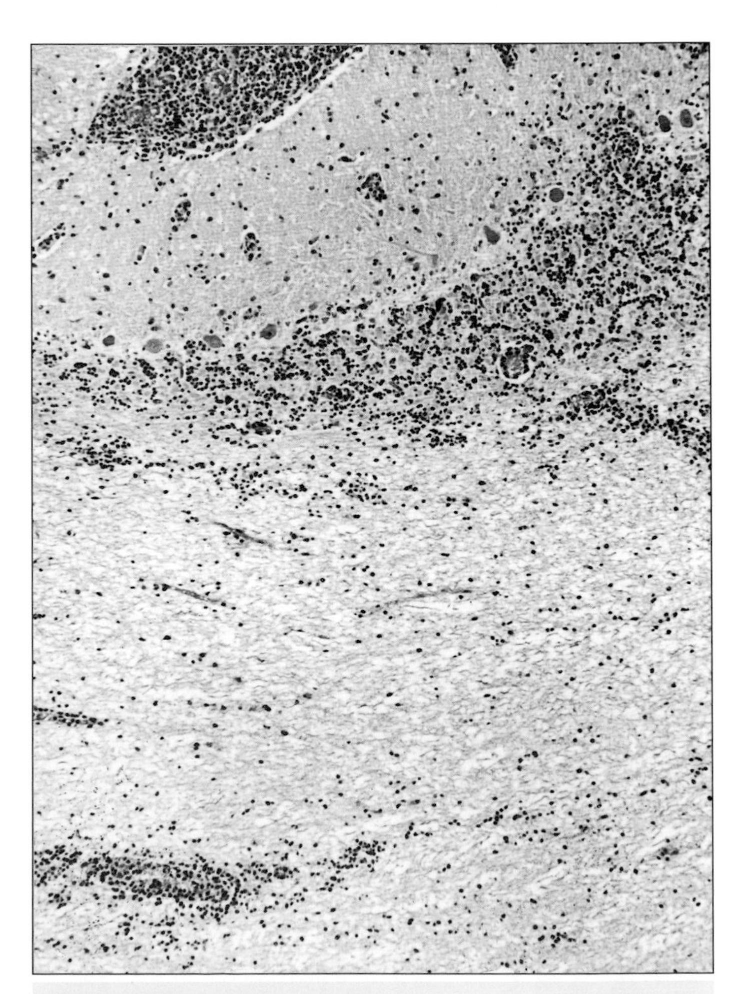

Figure 3.119 Nonsuppurative meningitis and encephalitis (cerebellum) in **enteroviral encephalomyelitis** in a pig.

decrease in intensity and diffuseness down the spinal cord. There is relative sparing of the cerebral and cerebellar cortices, but the deep substance of the cerebellum is consistently and often severely involved. Lesions in the spinal cord in each syndrome are largely confined to the gray matter, particularly the ventral horns, but may selectively involve the dorsal horns in very young pigs. Cord lesions are those of nonsuppurative myelitis and the motor neurons, particularly in gray matter of the ventral horns, experience different stages of neuronal degenerative and necrotic changes (neuronal swelling, chromatolysis, satellitosis, and finally neuronophagia). Lesions are consistently present in the dorsal root ganglia, and especially the trigeminal ganglia (Fig. 3.120).

Diagnosis can be achieved by virus isolation or immunohistochemistry.

Bibliography

Forman AJ, et al. The characterization and pathogenicity of porcine enteroviruses isolated in Victoria. Aust Vet J 1982;58:136–142.

Kaku Y, et al. Genetic reclassification of porcine enteroviruses. J Gen Virol 2001;82(Pt 2):417–424.

Krumbholz A, et al. Detection of porcine teschoviruses and enteroviruses by LightCycler real-time PCR. J Virol Methods 2003;113:51–63.

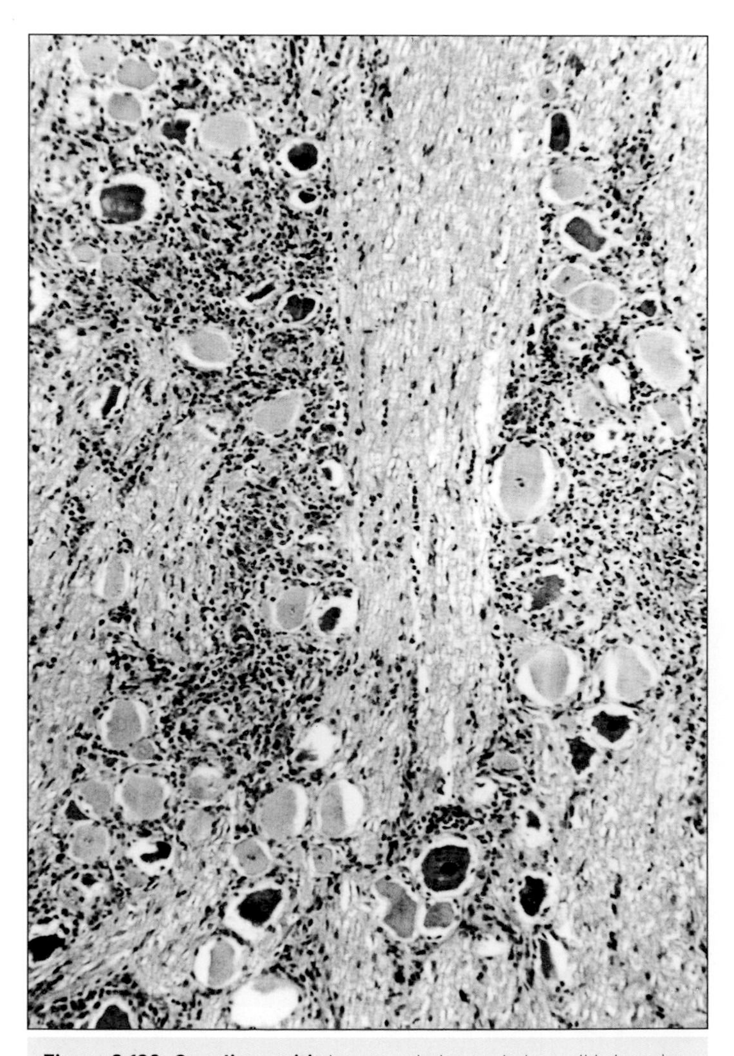

Figure 3.120 Ganglioneuritis in enteroviral encephalomyelitis in a pig.

Long JF. Pathogenesis of porcine polioencephalomyelitis. In: Olsen RG, et al, eds. Comparative Pathobiology of Viral Diseases. Vol 1. Boca Raton, FL: CRC Press Inc. 1985:179–197.

Narita M, et al. Demonstration of viral antigen and immunoglobulin (IgG and IgM) in brain tissue of pigs experimentally infected with haemagglutinating encephalomyelitis virus. J Comp Pathol 1989;100:119–128.

Oberste MS, et al. Genomic evidence that simian virus 2 and six other simian picornaviruses represent a new genus in Picornaviridae. Virology 2003; 314:283–293.

Pogranichniy RM, et al. A prolonged outbreak of polioencephalomyelitis due to infection with a group I porcine enterovirus. J Vet Diagn Invest 2003;15: 191–194.

Flaviviral encephalitides

The genus *Flavivirus* of the family Flaviviridae contains several important viruses that cause encephalitis in domestic and wild animals. Some of these viruses are emerging as very important not only for animal health but also for public health as they are highly zoonotic. The viruses of veterinary importance in this genus belong either to the *tick-borne virus group* or the *mosquito-borne virus group*. Viruses of both groups are maintained in a cycle involving ticks or mosquitoes respectively as invertebrate vectors, and wild vertebrate hosts as reservoirs. In most cases, infections of humans and/or domestic animals are incidental, and are not important for viral transmission or maintenance in the environment.

Diseases caused by tick-borne flaviviruses

Important veterinary viruses in this group include *Louping ill virus* and *Tick-borne encephalitis virus*; these two viruses are very closely related, and may have originated from a common ancestor. The group also includes several other viruses – *Langat virus, Kyasanur Forest disease virus*, *Omsk hemorrhagic fever virus*, and *Powassan virus* (POWV) – that are primarily of importance in humans. POWV causes severe encephalitis in humans in the USA, Canada, and Siberia, but induces encephalitis in animals only under experimental conditions.

Louping ill (ovine encephalomyelitis)

Louping ill is a tick-borne viral encephalomyelitis of sheep caused by *Louping ill virus* (LIV), which has been enzootic in England, Scotland, and Northern Ireland for more than a century and has been reported in Norway. The disease is named after the leaping (or louping) demonstrated by the diseased sheep. A similar disease has been reported in Spain, Greece, and Turkey affecting sheep or goats but because the etiologic viruses are different by nucleotide sequencing from LIV, each was considered a subtype of LIV but assigned different names: *Spanish sheep encephalomyelitis virus*, *Greek goat encephalomyelitis virus*, and *Turkish sheep encephalomyelitis virus*. Cattle, horses, goats, and deer pastured with affected sheep sometimes contract the disease, and nonfatal human infections are known. The virus causes fatal encephalomyelitis in red grouse (*Lagopus scoticus*). Outbreaks in piglets have followed the feeding of raw meat from lambs, and a case has been described in a dog.

The tick responsible for transmission in Great Britain is *Ixodes ricinus*, the castor-bean tick. Other species of *Ixodes*, and perhaps other arthropods, are potential vectors. *Ixodes ricinus* is parasitic on a variety of mammals in addition to sheep and on birds, however, the most significant wildlife host is the red grouse. Larval and nymphal ticks acquire the virus when feeding on infected sheep, and transmit the infection to new hosts in the succeeding nymphal and adult phases. Because of its natural mode of transmission, louping ill is most prevalent in early summer and early autumn when the ticks are active. After infection, the virus propagates in regional lymph nodes, proceeds to viremia, and then enters the CNS via the hematogenous route. Alternatively, the virus may localize indirectly from the blood in nasal structures and enter the brain via the olfactory nerves. Under experimental conditions, a number of factors may facilitate entry of virus into the brain, and facilitation is apparently given in natural cases by concurrent tick-borne fever, a rickettsiosis also transmitted by *I. ricinus*, and known to impair humoral and cellular defense mechanisms.

Although tick transmission is the usual mode of infection, the disease can be contracted in humans, monkeys, and mice by inhalation of infective droplets, but this route is not thought to be important naturally. Rabbits and guinea pigs are not susceptible even by intracerebral inoculation.

Louping ill is a systemic infection and, while it remains so, the disease is mildly febrile but otherwise of no consequence. When it invades the CNS and produces signs of encephalitis, the mortality rate is very high. The morbidity in endemic areas is quite low, and the disease is largely confined to either naïve lambs or to older lambs and yearlings whose colostral immunity is not reinforced by natural exposure. The viremic phase of louping ill is clinically silent or a febrile phase with dullness. Recovery may occur in a couple of days and leave solid immunity. If neurologic signs are to develop, they do so at about day 5 and are characterized by incoordination, tremors, cerebellar ataxia, and terminal paralysis.

There are no gross lesions. The disease is an *acute polioencephalomyelitis*. There is mild leptomeningitis corresponding to areas of inflammation of the parenchyma. Inflammation of the cerebellar leptomeninges may be quite severe when the cerebellar cortex is acutely affected (Fig. 3.115). The inflammatory lesions are more obvious than in most viral encephalitides, but are of the usual type, although unusually large numbers of neutrophils may be present in very severe cases, and largely restricted to gray matter, although cuffing and focal gliosis occur in the white matter. Neuronal degeneration may be severe and neuronophagia prominent. Some degree of selective vulnerability of the Purkinje and Golgi cells of the cerebellum is generally accepted and, although it can be demonstrated in many cases, its detection probably depends to a large extent on the duration of active infection. The spinal lesion is poliomyelitis affecting particularly the ventral horns (see Fig. 3.17). Inclusion bodies have not been observed in sheep but acidophilic, intracytoplasmic inclusions in neurons of the brain stem and cord are reported in experimentally affected monkeys and mice. Immunohistochemistry is available, and viral antigen can be identified easily, especially in the Purkinje cells of the cerebellum and their dendritic processes.

Encephalitis caused by *Tick-borne encephalitis virus*

Tick-borne encephalitis virus (TBEV) is a serious human threat that causes thousands of cases of encephalitis every year in endemic areas in Europe and Asia. Several wild and domestic animals are susceptible to infection but the infection is frequently subclinical, however TBEV is pathogenic for dogs and is able to cause fatal meningoencephalitis. The virus is transmitted to humans and animals mainly by *Ixodes ricinus* or *Ixodes persulcatus*. Humans can also become infected through consumption of milk from infected ruminants. Most infected dogs seroconvert without developing TBE, but the peracute disease in dogs has a high fatality rate. Affected dogs are usually euthanized due to associated severe convulsions, tremors, and ataxia. The histologic lesions are those of severe necrotizing lymphoplasmacytic and histiocytic meningoencephalomyelitis with severe glial nodule formation affecting mostly the basal ganglia, thalamus, mesencephalon, neuroparenchyma surrounding the fourth ventricle, and the medulla oblongata.

Bibliography

Callan RJ, Van Metre DC. Viral diseases of the ruminant nervous system. Vet Clin North Am Food Anim Pract 2004;20:327–362.

Charrel RN, et al. Tick-borne virus diseases of human interest in Europe. Clin Microbiol Infect 2004;10:1040–1055.

Gritsun TS, et al. Tick-borne encephalitis. Antiviral Res 2003;57:129–146.

Sheahan BJ, et al. The pathogenicity of louping ill virus for mice and lambs. J Comp Pathol 2002;126:137–146.

Stadtbaumer K, et al. Tick-borne encephalitis virus as a possible cause of optic neuritis in a dog. Vet Ophthalmol 2004;7:271–277.

Weissenbock H, et al. Tick-borne encephalitis in dogs: neuropathological findings and distribution of antigen. Acta Neuropathol (Berl) 1998;95:361–366.

Diseases caused by mosquito-borne viruses

The important veterinary viruses in this group include *West Nile virus* and *Japanese encephalitis virus*. Also included in the mosquito-borne, Japanese encephalitis virus group, are *Murray Valley encephalitis virus* and *St. Louis encephalitis virus*.

West Nile virus encephalomyelitis

West Nile virus (WNV) was first discovered in 1937 in the West Nile district of Uganda. In 1999 it was introduced into New York City where it caused a massive outbreak in animals and humans. During the period of 1999 to 2004, the virus spread rapidly to most of the USA and southern parts of Canada. It has been suggested that the virus was imported from the Middle East, due to genetic similarity between strains isolated in the Middle East and New York. The virus is now distributed throughout Africa, central and southern Asia, Australia (where it is called *Kunjin virus*), the USA, Canada, Mexico, and the Caribbean. The virus is divided genetically into two lineages – lineage 1 WNV is present in North America and some other parts of the world, lineage 2 is restricted to enzootic areas in Africa. Lineage 2 WNV strains are either nonpathogenic or occasionally cause mild human and equine disease. Some clades in lineage 1 (e.g., clade 1a) are highly virulent and are believed to be responsible for the recent outbreaks in North America. The virus has a wide host range, but is maintained in the environment mainly by a bird–mosquito–bird cycle. Wild birds, especially corvids, i.e., crows, are the main amplifying hosts. Wild birds usually develop prolonged viremia and the virus is distributed in almost every organ. In contrast, the viral antigen in infected horses, which is by far the most susceptible species of domestic animal, is sparse and limited to the CNS. Infection between birds or between birds and mammals or reptiles is mainly via mosquitoes. Mosquitoes of the *Culex* spp. are the main maintenance vectors. The virus is also found in other vectors such as ticks, but the biological importance of these vectors is yet to be determined. Rare methods of virus transmission include direct contact with infected materials and ingestion. Transplacental WNV transmission is only reported in human.

The *pathogenesis* of the encephalitis induced by WNV is not completely understood, however after the virus is injected by an infected mosquito, it probably propagates in regional endothelial cells and fibroblasts, viremia develops, and the virus reaches the brain hematogenously.

Equids, especially horses, are very susceptible to the infection. In naive areas, the first signs of WNV are the marked increase in cases of equine encephalitis and increased numbers of wild bird, especially corvid, mortalities. WN fever is a seasonal disease, related to the time of the year of mosquito activity, i.e., summer and fall. When naive horses are infected by the virus, mortality can reach up to 50% of affected horses, and clinical signs range from weakness and anorexia to severe acute ataxia or recumbency. However, the mortality rate decreases dramatically in the following seasons. Gross lesions are usually absent, but a few cases may have acute areas of hemorrhage or malacia affecting the thoracic and/or lumbar spinal cord. *Histologic lesions* are present mainly in the brain stem and thoracolumbar spinal cord, and to a lesser extent in cerebral cortex and cervical cord. The cerebellum is usually spared. *Lesions are those of nonsuppurative encephalomyelitis, gliosis, and glial nodule formation with occasional neuronal degeneration and necrosis* (Fig. 3.121A, B). Lesions are more pronounced in the gray matter. The glial nodules usually contain a few neutrophils amid the glial cells. Areas of hemorrhage and malacia are present in severe cases, especially in brain stem and the ventral horn of the thoracic and lumbar spinal cord. Axonal swelling and spheroid formation is frequent. The severity of lesions is greatly variable between outbreaks, and frequently the severity of clinical signs is not correlated with the severity of lesions. In most cases, the lesions are mild and confined to thin cuffs of a few blood vessels in the brain stem. Extraneural lesions, e.g., hepatitis, myocarditis, etc., which occur in avian WNV infection, do not occur in equine WNV infection.

The information about clinical signs and lesions in non-equine domestic species other than birds is very limited. Ruminants, canids, felids, and swine are far less susceptible to the disease than are horses or birds. These species are susceptible to the infection and develop very short viremia with subclinical disease; histologic lesions are very similar to those described in horses.

Diagnosis of WNV infection can be achieved by detection of WNV antigen in the brain using PCR or immunohistochemistry. WNV antigen in many cases can be very sparse, which makes the interpretation of IHC difficult. Positive IHC staining in most cases is limited to sparse axonal immunostaining.

Bibliography

Austgen LE, et al. Experimental infection of cats and dogs with West Nile virus. Emerg Infect Dis 2004;10:82–86.

Cantile C, et al. Pathologic and immunohistochemical findings in naturally occurring West Nile virus infection in horses. Vet Pathol 2001;38:414–421.

Mackenzie JS, et al. Emerging flaviviruses: the spread and resurgence of Japanese encephalitis, West Nile and dengue viruses. Nat Med 2004;12 Suppl:S98–109.

Yaeger M, et al. West Nile virus meningoencephalitis in a Suri alpaca and Suffolk ewe. J Vet Diagn Invest 2004;16:64–66.

Japanese encephalitis

Japanese encephalitis virus (JEV) is found through much of eastern, southern, and southeastern Asia, Papua New Guinea, and the Torres Strait of Northern Australia, where the disease is endemic with dramatic annual epidemics. In humans, there is a high ratio of subclinical to overt infections, with a case fatality rate of 10–15% and a high incidence of residual neurologic deficits in survivors. Transplacental infection followed by abortion occurs in humans and this is also the most serious expression of the disease in *pigs, the domestic species most importantly infected*.

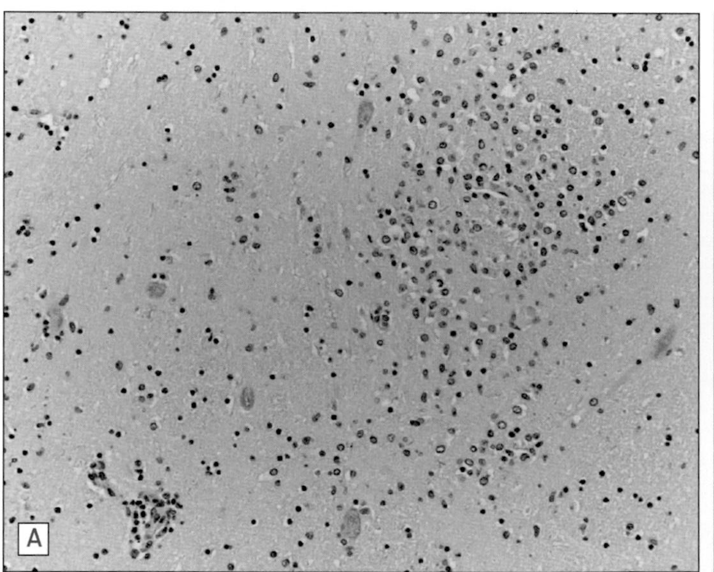

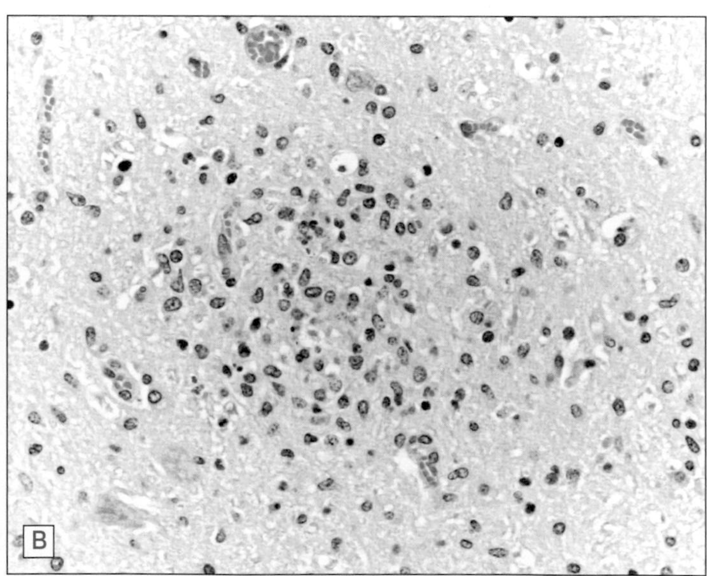

Figure 3.121 Brain stem of a horse with **West Nile viral encephalomyelitis. A.** Perivascular cuffs composed of lymphocytes and plasma cells are usually thin. **B.** Multifocal glial nodules are common and usually contain only a few neutrophils. (Courtesy of MJ Hazlett.)

The virus is maintained through mosquito–bird or mosquito–pig cycles. The virus is transmitted mainly by the mosquito, *Culex tritaeniorhynchus*, but other species of this genus and of the genera *Aedes* and *Armigeres* may be important as the virus is known to be vertically transmitted through some of them. *Ardeid water birds (e.g., herons and egrets) are the main maintenance reservoirs*. Many species of animals and birds are susceptible to mosquito-borne infection and develop antibody responses in timing with suitable climatic and habitat cycles. The pig is a very important domestic animal in many of the endemic areas and it is the most important amplifier host for the virus, developing sustained viremia of sufficient titer to infect feeding mosquitoes and indeed is probably the preferred host for *C. tritaeniohynchus*. Infection of humans and horses is incidental and both species are considered to be dead-end hosts.

Most horses, pigs, and cattle in endemic areas possess neutralizing antibodies against the virus. Intranasal and intracerebral inoculation can produce fatal encephalitis in calves, but natural cases of encephalitis in this species are quite rare. Among animals infected naturally with the virus, *only horses and donkeys develop clinical encephalitis*. There are no clinical signs of encephalitis in pigs, but pregnant susceptible sows may produce *stillborn piglets*. Infected stillborn and neonatal pigs may show hydrocephalus, cerebellar hypoplasia, and hypomyelinogenesis and anasarca; histological changes are restricted to the nervous system and may include *nonsuppurative encephalitis*. The lesions in these neonatal and stillborn piglets probably reflect the timing of infection in relation to the development of immune competence. Diffuse nonsuppurative encephalitis occurs in the brain and cord of piglets up to 6 months of age, but in the cerebellum it affects rather selectively the molecular and Purkinje layers. The histological pattern of Japanese encephalitis in pigs appears similar to that of Teschen and related diseases. In boars, the virus induces orchitis.

Severe epidemics of encephalitis have occurred in horses in Japan. The incubation period in horses ranges from 4–14 days, and case fatality is 5–15%. Lesions are confined to the CNS, are more prevalent in the cerebral hemispheres, and include extensive perivascular lymphoplasmacytic cuffing, gliosis, and areas of malacia with hemorrhage. The lesions in quality and distribution are the same as those produced by the *Eastern and Western equine encephalitis viruses*. Inclusion bodies are not reported in the Japanese disease. *Diagnosis* is best achieved by detection of viral RNA using PCR.

Bibliography

Ellis PM, et al. Japanese encephalitis. Vet Clin North Am Equine Pract 2000;16:565–578.

Mackenzie JS, et al. Emerging flaviviruses: the spread and resurgence of Japanese encephalitis, West Nile and dengue viruses. Nat Med 2004;10(12 Suppl):S98–109.

Rosen L, et al. Experimental vertical transmission of Japanese encephalitis virus by *Culex tritaeniorhynchus* and other mosquitoes. Am J Trop Med Hyg 1989; 40:548–556.

Williams DT, et al. Experimental infections of pigs with Japanese encephalitis virus and closely related Australian flaviviruses. Am J Trop Med Hyg 2001;65:379–387.

Yamada M, et al. Nonsuppurative encephalitis in piglets after experimental inoculation of Japanese encephalitis flavivirus isolated from pigs. Vet Pathol 2004;41:62–67.

Alphaviruses – equine encephalitides

Several members of the genus *Alphavirus*, family Togaviridae, cause either overt or subclinical encephalitis in horses or other animals. They all require an arthropod vector (frequently mosquitoes) for transmission.

Eastern, Western, and Venezuelan encephalitis in horses

Western equine encephalitis virus (WEEV), Eastern equine encephalitis virus (EEEV), and Venezuelan equine encephalitis virus (VEEV) are all members of the genus Alphavirus, family Togaviridae. Horses were originally regarded as the primary hosts of the EEVs, but horses are actually accidental and unfortunate hosts; birds for the American viruses (eastern and western type) or rodents for the Venezuelan virus are the most common vertebrate reservoir hosts, and mosquitoes are the principal vectors. Horses and humans, in both of which species the disease is of very considerable importance, are now known to be, in terms of transmission and often literally as well, dead-end hosts in which the titer of virus in blood is ordinarily too low to be a source of infection for mosquitoes.

Not all birds are capable of acting as reservoir hosts. Red-winged blackbirds, cardinals, sparrows, cedar waxwings, and the captive Chinese pheasant are highly susceptible to infection and nearly always die. Many other species, including adult domestic fowl and turkeys, are not sickened by the infection although fatalities can be produced in the young of these species.

EEEV is endemic along the North American Atlantic course, in the Caribbean, Central America, and along the northeastern coast of South America. The virus cycles between water birds and the mosquito, *Culiseta melanura*, which feeds on birds and does not feed on large mammals. Horses are likely to get infected by other mosquitoes, *Aedes sollicitans* and *A. vexans*, which feed on both horses and birds.

WEEV is present mostly in the valleys of western North American states, where the cycle is between wild birds, especially passerines, and the mosquito, *Culex tarsalis*. This mosquito feeds readily on animals, and human and animal cases occur regularly.

VEEV has two major different strain groups, the enzootic strains that are avirulent and cycle between *Culex* spp. mosquito and small rodents in the Caribbean areas, and the epizootic strains that are virulent to human and horse, found mainly in Venezuela, Colombia, and Peru, and circulate between several mosquito species and horses, which produce high titered viremia sufficient to infect the vector mosquitoes. Outbreaks of EEE and WEE occur in seasonal patterns related to the time of the year when mosquitoes are active. VEE outbreaks usually occur in a cyclical pattern approximately every 10 years.

Once infected, mosquitoes are known to remain so for life, and there is evidence that the virus is capable of multiplying in the insects. Arthropods other than mosquitoes may also be of some, but lesser, importance. The virus has been found in chicken mites (*Dermanyssus gallinae*), chicken lice (*Menopon pallidum, Eomenocanthus stramineus*), and assassin bugs (*Triatoma sanguisuga*). The spotted-fever tick, *Dermacentor andersoni*, is capable of transmitting the infection stage to stage and hereditarily. Transmission by aerosolization is reported only in humans; laboratory workers are at high risk of infection by aerosols.

Although humans and horses are the principal mammalian victims, other species are susceptible. Pigs readily develop asymptomatic infections but a few outbreaks have been reported in this species with histology typical of EEE. Pigs are not of significance for natural propagation of the virus because they do not develop significant viremia. Calves are susceptible to intracerebral inoculation but recover in 2 weeks. Guinea pigs and white mice are highly susceptible, rabbits are less so, and sheep, dogs, and cats are refractory.

The three viruses are similar in their pathogenesis. After the mosquito bite, the virus replicates in the regional blood vessels and lymph nodes, viremia develops, followed by secondary replication in lymph nodes and muscles. A second viremia then develops and is followed by brain invasion via the blood. In the CNS, the virus replicates in neurons, glial cells, and blood vessels. The virus causes neuronal necrosis, likely via stimulation of apoptosis.

Young horses are more susceptible than the old. Initially, there is viremia with fever and depression, usually unnoticed. The animal may then recover or the virus may invade the CNS, by which time the fever has subsided. The neurologic signs are characterized by derangements of consciousness and terminal paralysis. There may be early restlessness with compulsive walking, often in circles. There is central blindness. The animal becomes somnolent and assumes unnatural postures. At this stage, the course may remain static and the animal lives as a "dummy," or paralysis may develop, often first affecting cranial nerves but later general and flaccid. *The signs are largely cortical and the cortex is the principal site of the lesions.* The course, if fatal, is usually 2–4 days.

There are no gross changes. The microscopic changes are limited almost exclusively to *gray matter* (see Fig. 3.2D). When the course is short, 1 day or less, the reaction is largely on the part of neutrophils. These infiltrate the gray matter diffusely and may be found in foci suggestive of malacia (Fig. 3.122). There is early microglial reaction to produce rod cells. Endothelial cells, especially of veins are swollen, and hyaline or granular thrombi are common in these vessels. There are narrow cuffs of lymphocytes and neutrophils with perivenous hemorrhage and edema. After a couple of days, the neutrophils disappear, the cuffs are composed of lymphocytes, and there are both focal and diffuse microglial proliferations as in the standard nonsuppurative reactions. Neuronal degeneration and neuronophagia are common findings. Intranuclear inclusions similar to those in Borna disease may be present, but may be very difficult to identify.

The most severe lesions are in the cerebral cortex, especially the frontal, rhinencephalic, and occipital areas, with lesions of lesser intensity in the pyriform lobes. Severe lesions are also present in thalamus and hypothalamus. From the thalamus caudally, the intensity of inflammation diminishes but reveals no selectivity for particular nuclear masses. The cerebellum is less severely injured than other portions, although inflammatory changes may be found in the deep nuclei and spottily in the cortex. Mild changes occur in both dorsal and ventral horns of the cord, but their distribution is irregular. The trigeminal ganglia are not affected. The encephalomyelitis in the Venezuelan type may be purely nonsuppurative. Extraneural lesions are common in humans and birds but are rare in susceptible domestic mammals. Small intestinal lesions in a horse with EEE include multifocal myonecrosis and lymphomonocytic infiltration in the muscular layer and focal mild perivascular lymphocytic infiltration in the submucosa. Myocarditis is not uncommon in pigs suffering from EEE. Horses infected with VEEV can occasionally have some nonspecific extraneural lesions such as myeloid depletion in bone marrow and lympholysis in spleen and lymph nodes.

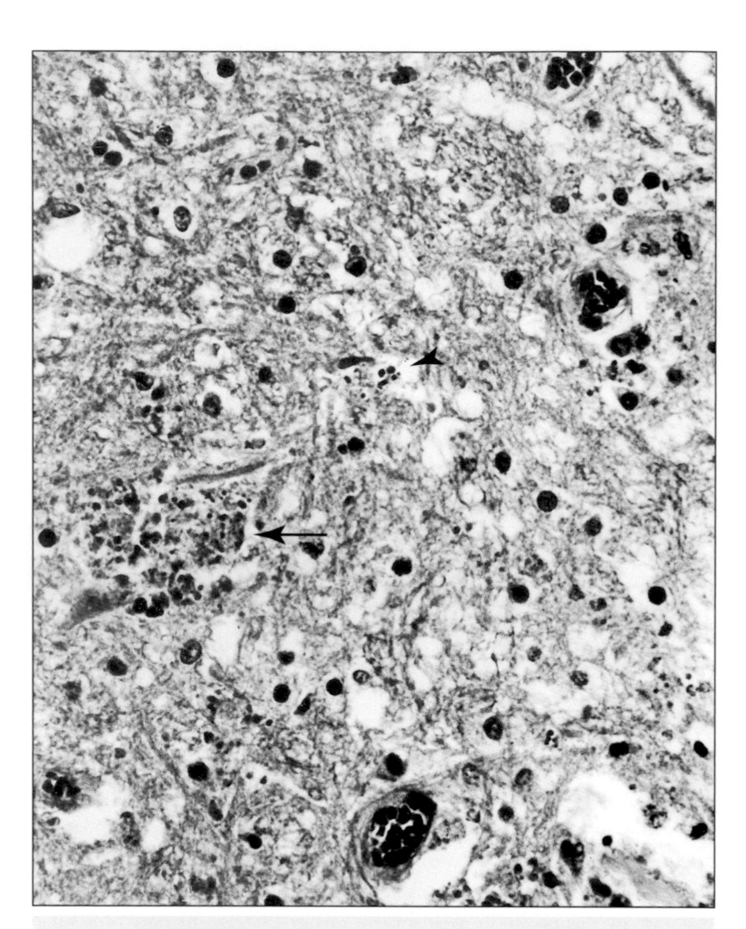

Figure 3.122 Neuronal necrosis (arrow), glial necrosis (arrowhead) in cerebrum in **equine encephalitis** in a horse.

Other *Alphavirus* encephalitides

Highlands J virus of America's east coast, ***Getah virus*** of southeast Asia, and ***Semliki forest virus*** of the Americas are all equine pathogens that are able to induce at least a febrile disease. All of these viruses are maintained in the environment by a mosquito–bird–mosquito cycle. Several mammals and birds seroconvert to these viruses, however overt disease is rare. *Highlands J virus* was reported as the cause of encephalitis in two horses. *Getah virus* does not induce encephalitis but clinical signs and lesions with some similarities to equine viral arteritis.

Bibliography

Elvinger F, et al. Prevalence of exposure to eastern equine encephalomyelitis virus in domestic and feral swine in Georgia. J Vet Diagn Invest 1996;8:481–484.

Gonzalez-Salazar D, et al. Equine amplification and virulence of subtype IE Venezuelan equine encephalitis viruses isolated during the 1993 and 1996 Mexican epizootics. Emerg Infect Dis 2003;9:161–168.

Jackson AC, Rossiter JP. Apoptotic cell death is an important cause of neuronal injury in experimental Venezuelan equine encephalitis virus infection of mice. Acta Neuropathol (Berl) 1997;93:349–353.

Karabatsos N, et al. Identification of Highlands J virus from a Florida horse. Am J Trop Med Hyg 1988;39:603–606.

Kramer LD, et al. Detection of encephalitis viruses in mosquitoes (*Diptera: Culicidae*) and avian tissues. J Med Entomol 2002;39:312–323.
Mackenzie JS, et al. Emerging flaviviruses: the spread and resurgence of Japanese encephalitis, West Nile and dengue viruses. Nat Med 2004;10(12 Suppl):S98–109.
McGee ED, et al. Eastern equine encephalomyelitis in an adult cow. Vet Pathol 1992;29:361–363.
Patterson JS, et al. Immunohistochemical diagnosis of eastern equine encephalomyelitis. J Vet Diagn Invest 1996;8:156–160.
Poonacha KB, et al. Intestinal lesions in a horse associated with eastern equine encephalomyelitis virus infection. Vet Pathol 1998;35:535–538.
Steele KE, et al. Comparative neurovirulence and tissue tropism of wild-type and attenuated strains of Venezuelan equine encephalitis virus administered by aerosol in C3H/HeN and BALB/c mice. Vet Pathol 1998;35:386–397.
Sudhir P, et al. Pathogenicity of a Venezuelan equine encephalomyelitis serotype IE virus isolate for ponies. Am J Trop Med Hyg 2003;68:485–494.
Weaver SC, Barrett AD. Transmission cycles, host range, evolution and emergence of arboviral disease. Nat Rev Microbiol 2004;2:789–801.

Borna disease

Borna disease, named after the village of Borna in Germany, is caused by *Borna disease virus* (BDV), which is the only member of the genus *Bornavirus*, family Bornaviridae. The virus exists worldwide in many vertebrates but most commonly infects horses, sheep, cattle, cats, dogs, and ostriches. The traditional endemic area is central Europe, but antibodies to the virus are found in horses outside Europe, including the USA and Japan. The mortality rate may be high (>80% in horses, 5–40% in sheep); surviving horses may be asymptomatic carriers, or may suffer relapses of disease. The virus has a controversial link to several human neuropsychiatric illnesses. In experimental hosts (tree shrews, rats), infection with BDV not only produces pathoanatomic changes, i.e., nonsuppurative encephalitis, but also behavioral changes and learning deficits.

The virus replicates in the nucleolus of the host cell without cytopathic effect, persistently infects cells, and induces brain lesions by *immune-mediated mechanisms*. In Lewis rats, acute (4–8 weeks post-infection) BDV infection is followed by massive infiltrates in the brain of CD4+ Th1, CD8+ T, and NK cells with a predominance of Th1 cytokines that favors cell-mediated immunity. In the chronic stage (beyond 15 weeks of infection), the aforementioned cellular infiltrates significantly decrease and the predominant cytokines are of Th2 type, favoring the shift to a humoral immune response; the resultant antibodies are not protective and have no significant effect on the disease. Due to this unique feature, infection of neonatal or immunocompromised animals does not lead to disease or to encephalitis.

The epidemiology of Borna disease, including reservoir, methods of transmission, and infection, remains obscure. Inflammation of the olfactory bulbs at the early stages of natural infection in humans suggests an intranasal route of infection followed by transaxonal migration to the olfactory bulb. Vertical transmission in horses and rats with life-long persistent infection is also suggested.

Clinically, the disease occurs sporadically or in clusters, however severe outbreaks are described in different species. *Equids and sheep are the most susceptible animals*, but natural disease is reported in many domestic species including but not limited to cattle, alpacas, cats, dogs, and ostriches. Most infections in horses remain subclinical and BDV-specific antibodies are frequently found in clinically healthy horses. The incubation period is not less than 4 weeks and introduces a clinical syndrome that is purely neurologic but of varied course, death occurring in 1–3 weeks. The mortality rate in diseased horses is 90–100%. Recurrent episodes at time of stress occur in surviving animals. Clinical signs include pharyngeal paralysis, hyperesthesia, standing in awkward positions, circling, muscular tremors, and spasms; blindness is common. Drowsiness and flaccid paresis develop terminally.

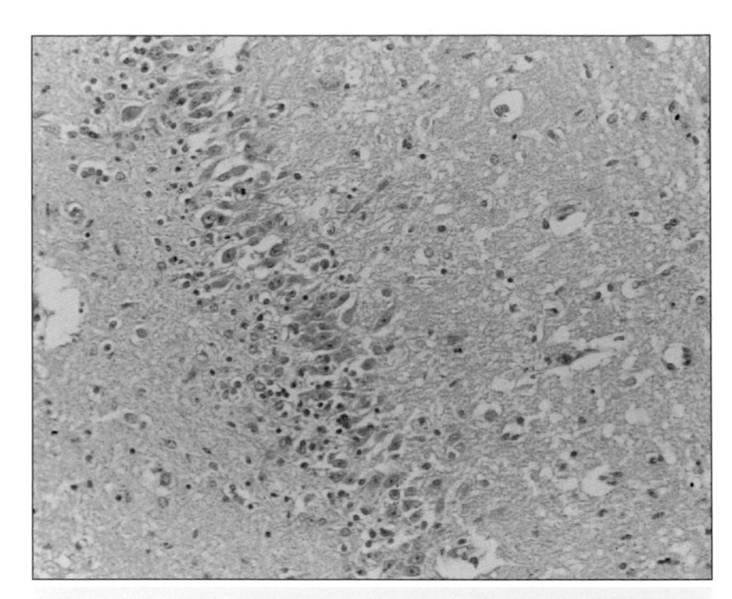

Figure 3.123 Nonsuppurative encephalitis and gliosis in the hippocampus of a horse with **Borna disease.**

There are no gross lesions. The distribution of lesions in Borna disease differs from that in other equine encephalomyelitides and parallels closely the distribution of viral antigen, as displayed by immunohistochemistry, and the distribution of infectivity, as determined by titration in cell cultures. Virus and lesions are present mostly in the gray matter of olfactory bulbs (early stage), hippocampus (Fig 3.123), limbic system, basal ganglia, and brain stem. The dorsal cerebrum and the cerebellum are relatively spared. Lesions may be present in optic nerves and retina. Histologic lesions are those of *nonsuppurative encephalomyelitis* with predilection for the aforementioned areas. Perivascular cuffs can be dramatically thick (>7 cell layer) and usually there are neuropilar clusters of lymphocytes and plasma cells. Other lesions include neuronophagia and focal gliosis. The presence of inclusion bodies (Joest–Degen bodies) is fairly pathognomonic; these are mainly in nuclei, especially in the hippocampus, and are very occasionally cytoplasmic. They stain well and red with Giemsa, and have a clear halo. Commercial PCR and immunohistochemistry kits are available for diagnosis.

Borna disease virus has been proposed as the cause of a chronic, slowly progressive neurologic disease affecting *cats* of all ages, sexes, and breeds. The disease is known clinically as *staggering disease,* and clinical signs include ataxia, paraparesis, and tetraparesis. Behavioral change is not a constant finding. Lesions are more prevalent in the gray matter of brain stem and in dorsal and ventral horns of the thoracic and/or cervical spinal cord segments. Lesions include mild to moderate lymphoplasmacytic cuffing with neuronophagia and neuronal degeneration and astrogliosis. Severe Wallerian degeneration is usually present in ventral and lateral columns of the cervical and thoracic spinal cord.

Bibliography

Bilzer T, et al. Immunopathology of Borna disease in the horse: clinical, virological and neuropathologic findings. Tierarztl Prax 1996;24:567–576.

Degiorgis MP, et al. Borna disease in a free-ranging lynx (*Lynx lynx*). J Clin Microbiol 2000;38:3087–3091.

Hornig M, et al. Borna disease virus. J Neurovirol 2003;9:259–273.

Lundgren AL, et al. Staggering disease in cats: isolation and characterization of the feline Borna disease virus. J Gen Virol 1995;76(Pt 9):2215–2222.

Lundgren AL, et al. Natural Borna disease in domestic animals others than horses and sheep. Zentralbl Veterinarmed B 1993;40:298–303.

Okamoto M, et al. Borna disease in a dog in Japan. J Comp Pathol 2002; 126:312–317.

Richt JA, et al. Borna disease in horses. Vet Clin North Am Equine Pract 2000; 16:579–595.

Lentiviral encephalomyelitis of sheep and goats

Caprine arthritis encephalitis virus (CAEV) of goats and *Visna/maedi virus* (VISNA) of sheep, in the genus *Lentivirus* of the family Retroviridae, are small-ruminant lentiviruses (SRLV). CAEV is the causative agent of caprine arthritis-encephalitis of goats and VISNA is the causative agent of the visna/maedi disease complex of sheep; at least some strains of the SRLV are transmissible between sheep and goats. In both natural hosts, *four clinical and pathological syndromes are recognized*, namely **mastitis, arthritis, interstitial pneumonia** (maedi and ovine progressive pneumonia) and **encephalomyelitis** (visna of sheep). Within endemic situations, any one or combination of the four syndromes may be present and when in combination one syndrome usually predominates.

Once infected, the virus is never eliminated and, while present, it is active even though there may be no clinical sign of neurologic deficit. Typically for this type of virus infection, the virus is highly cell-associated and replicates only slowly, infection persists for the life of the animal, the incubation period before seroconversion may be several months and before clinical disease may be months or years, the clinical disease is progressive, and the lesions are dominated by active mononuclear inflammatory cells. The pathogenesis and epidemiology of the various conditions are described in detail in Vol. 2, Respiratory system. Described below are the gross and histologic lesions and clinical signs found in the encephalomyelitis form of these diseases.

The encephalomyelitis form in sheep is called **visna** (Icelandic for wasting). As a natural disease, visna occurs in sheep of both sexes but clinical signs are seldom, if ever, observed in animals less than 2 years of age. Disease onset is insidious. The earliest sign may be barely perceptible caudal ataxia and fine trembling of the lips. The first sign to be noticed may be extensor paralysis of the hindlimbs. Once paralytic signs are evident, a fatal outcome appears certain. There is no fever and no sign of cerebral dysfunction, and death is due to starvation or secondary infection. The incidence of visna is relatively low. The course of the infection can be followed fairly well by routine examination of the CSF for lymphocytosis.

Normal sheep are expected to have $\leq 0.005 \times 10^9$ cells/L ($\leq 5/mm^3$) of CSF; in visna, cell numbers, chiefly lymphocytes, can be markedly elevated. After intracerebral inoculation, there is a latent period of up to 8 weeks, after which the CSF cell count begins to increase. The cell count may remain high for several months without other signs of disease. Thereafter, the animal may recover, as indicated by a drop in the CSF cell count, or the cell count may remain high, paralysis develops, and death follows.

The disease in the brain is chronic and demyelinating. There are no gross neural changes in this disease, and the histologic change is one of *patchy demyelinating encephalomyelitis*. The distribution of lesions, involving principally the white matter, is unlike the distribution produced by other neurotropic viruses. There is a mild to severe mononuclear type of cerebrospinal meningitis. The parenchymal lesion may be well-established by 1–2 months, and these early lesions are intensely inflammatory with perivascular cuffing and gliosis. They reveal clearly that the process begins in, and immediately beneath, the ependyma diffusely throughout the cerebrospinal axis. In this early stage, the myelinated fibers in the inflammatory foci remain remarkably intact; the gray matter of the cord is irregularly but often intensely affected by a nonsuppurative reaction even 2–3 months after inoculation. In the paralytic and terminal stages of the disease, the periventricular destruction of white matter in the cerebrum and cerebellum is extensive, and in some sections of the brain, especially in the cerebellum, almost every bit of white matter is destroyed leaving the gray matter free.

Destruction of myelinated fibers in the spinal cord is patchy and not due to progressive spread of the pericentral inflammation. The demyelinated plaques are characteristically peripheral and triangular in shape with a base on the pia mater. Although dorsal and lateral tracts are most frequently involved, there is no selectivity for particular fiber tracts and no symmetry. The degenerating foci are almost malacic in their severity, and the plaques contain numerous reactive microglia and astroglia. Spinal nerve roots share in the degenerative process. Germinal centers may form in the choroid plexus. In areas of intense inflammation, liquefactive foci of necrosis occur in the white matter and the loss of myelin is expected to be of Wallerian type. In the spinal cord, evidence of remyelination can be found indicating that oligodendrocytes are not target cells and that demyelination may be primary.

Caprine arthritis-encephalitis (CAE) appears to be widely distributed, but the expression of the infection is highly variable, and many infected goats show little or no clinical disease. Clinical disease of the nervous system affects kids 2–4 months of age and is frequently fatal. Animals that develop the early nervous disease or have early inapparent infections tend to develop synovitis and periarthritis in adulthood (see Bones and joints).

The clinical signs of CAE are referable to motor spinal dysfunction without signs of cerebral disease. Onset is indicated by hindlimb lameness and ataxia with paresis that progresses over several weeks to paralysis. The inflammatory lesions in the CNS may remain active for several years in goats that survive (see Fig. 3.124A, B). In the early clinical phase of the disease, changes are widely distributed in the white matter of the brain and cord, particularly in the subependyma and beneath the pia in the cord. The distribution and character of the lesions in the nervous tissue in the goat are, in general, similar to those in visna of sheep. There is, however, less tendency for the periventricular lesions to progress to gross cavitation of cerebral white matter. Instead, there is a tendency for the inflammatory and myelinoclastic areas to increase in number and severity caudally from the mesencephalon. As in visna, the spinal cord changes are discontinuous and, where present, involve the myelin in subpial plaques or in one or

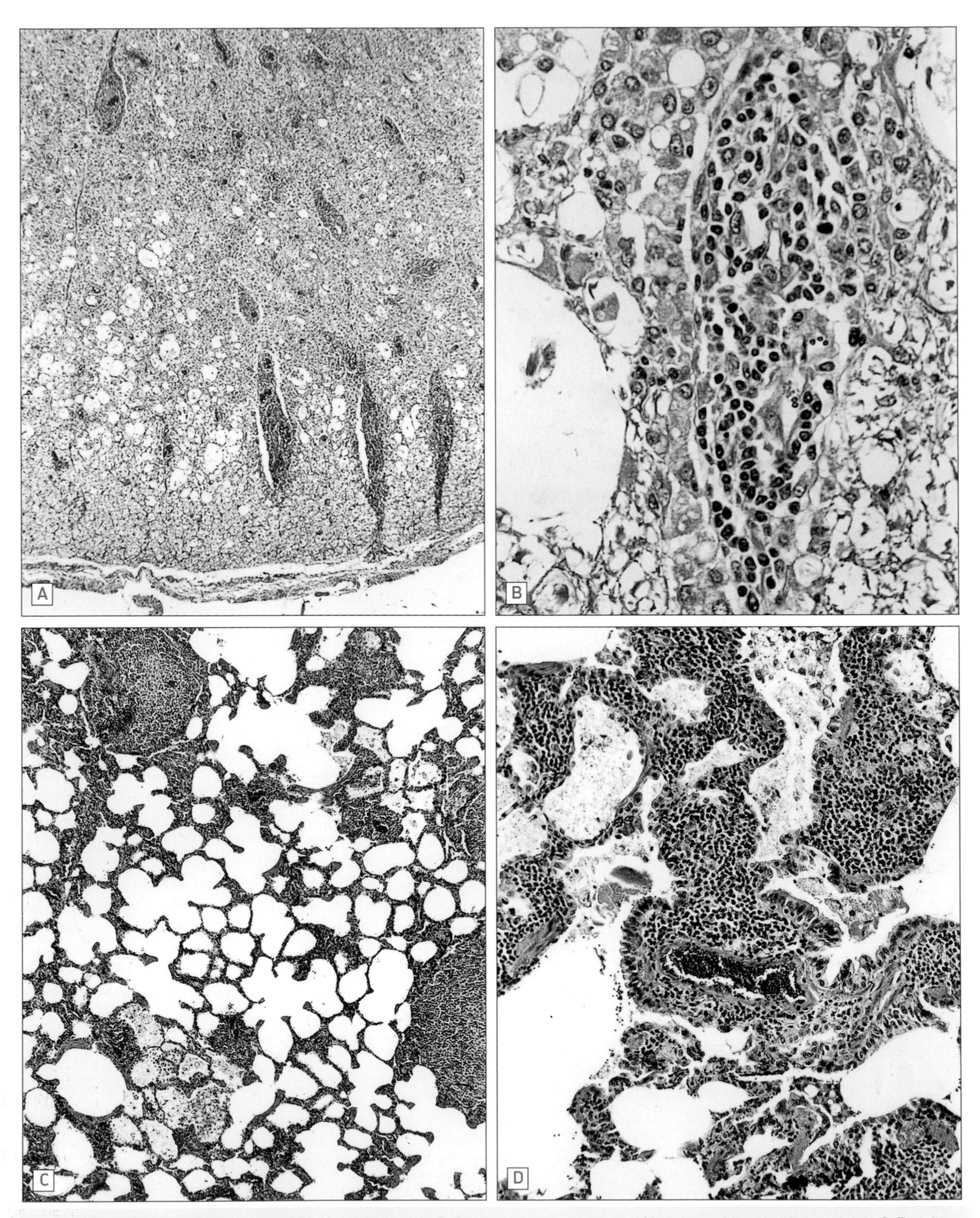

Figure 3.124 Caprine arthritis-encephalitis. A. Leukomyelitis. **B.** Detail of perivascular reaction. Note macrophages bordering vessel. **C.** Prominent perivascular and peribronchiolar lymphoid cuffs and focal interstitial pneumonia. **D.** Detail of (**C**) showing lymphocytes around vessels and bronchioles, and in alveolar walls.

more quadrants of the cord. The extent of perivascular infiltration by mononuclear cells (see Fig. 3.124B) is also greater in kids than in sheep. In addition to the encephalomyelitis, mastitis, and arthritis seen in CAE, interstitial pneumonia occurs in some natural and experimental cases (Fig. 3.124C, D).

Bibliography

Campbell RS, Robinson WF. The comparative pathology of the lentiviruses. J Comp Pathol 1998;119:333–395.

Craig LE, et al. Pathogenesis of ovine lentiviral encephalitis: derivation of a neurovirulent strain by *in vivo* passage. J Neurovirol 1997;3:417–427.

Georgsson G. Neuropathologic aspects of lentiviral infections. Ann N Y Acad Sci 1994;724:50–67.

Lavimore MD, et al. Lentivirus-induced lymphoproliferative disease. Comparative pathogenicity of phenotypically distinct ovine lentivirus strains. Am J Pathol 1988;130:80–90.

Perk K. Characteristics of ovine and caprine lentivirus infections. Leukemia 1995;9 (Suppl 1):S98–100.

Shah C, et al. Direct evidence for natural transmission of small-ruminant lentiviruses of subtype A4 from goats to sheep and vice versa. J Virol 2004;78:7518–7522.

Straub OC. Maedi-Visna virus infection in sheep. History and present knowledge. Comp Immunol Microbiol Infect Dis 2004;27:1–5.

Paramyxoviral encephalomyelitis of pigs

Porcine rubulavirus encephalomyelitis (blue eye disease)

Blue eye disease is caused by *Porcine rubulavirus* (La-Piedad-Michoacan-Mexico virus) of the genus *Rubulavirus*, family Paramyxoviridae. The disease is characterized by encephalomyelitis, reproductive failure, and corneal opacity. Outbreaks have been recorded in Mexico since 1980, but appear to be self-limiting in commercial pigs. In pregnant sows, the infection may be subclinical or responsible for *fetal death, mummification, and stillbirths,* and for the occasional appearance of corneal opacity in the sow. Piglets up to 2 weeks of age are most susceptible with up to 50% morbidity and very high mortality. The clinical signs are of encephalomyelitis leading to death within 2–4 days, although subclinical infections are also frequent and may be manifested only by corneal opacity.

The lesion is a typical *nonsuppurative encephalomyelitis* affecting mainly gray matter of the thalamus, midbrain, and cortex. Inclusion bodies have not been demonstrated. Anterior uveitis is mild, the inflammatory cells congregating in the iridocorneal angle and the corneoscleral junction. The corneal opacity is due to edema, which will resolve if the animal survives.

In mature male pigs, experimental exposure will result in epididymitis in almost all exposed and in a lesser number with orchitis and testicular atrophy. Interstitial pneumonia is part of the description.

Bibliography

Allan GM, et al. A sequential study of experimental porcine paramyxovirus (LPMV) infection of pigs: immunostaining of cryostat sections and virus isolation. J Vet Diag Invest 1996;8:405–413.

Mendoza-Magana ML, et al. Pig paramyxovirus of the blue eye disease binding to a 116 kDa glycoprotein expressed in pig neuronal membranes. J Vet Med B Infect Dis Vet Public Health 2001;48:489–499.

Nipah virus encephalitis

Nipah encephalitis, an emerging disease characterized by severe and rapidly progressive encephalitis, is caused by *Nipah virus* (NiV) of the genus *Henipavirus*, a novel genus in the family Paramyxoviridae. This genus also contains *Hendra virus*. Both are newly emerging viruses that can cause fatal encephalitis and pneumonia in humans and several animal species. The first severe outbreak of NiV encephalitis in humans occurred in 1998 near Ipoh, Malaysia, primarily among pig farmers and their families; the outbreak was preceded by an outbreak of encephalitis and pneumonia affecting pigs on many local farms. *Fruit bats* of the *Pteropid* species were later confirmed to be the natural reservoir host of NiV. Bats shed virus in their urine and saliva, which contaminates fruit that falls into pig pens and is eaten by pigs; bats in these trees also urinate directly on pigs. Initial human infection occurred in pig farmers by direct contact or aerosolization from infected pens. Pig-to-pig or pig-to-domestic-animal infections occur by direct contact with infected pig or mechanically by contact with contaminated utensils or feed. Direct transmission from bats-to-human or from human-to-human is controversial.

Pigs are the animals most susceptible to infection, but natural infection is reported in horses, cats, goats, and dogs; these species were infected by direct contact with infected pigs. Morbidity rates in pigs are ~10%, with case mortality rates of <15%. The incubation period is estimated to be 1–2 weeks. The virus targets two systems, the CNS and the respiratory system. Clinical signs are those of acute dyspnea (labored and harsh respiration, open-mouth breathing, severe cough) and acute nervous signs (trembling, seizures, or tetanus-like spasms). Abortion may occur to pregnant sows.

The lung is diffusely edematous with patchy acute hemorrhage. Meningeal blood vessels are severely congested. The histologic hallmark is *necrotizing vasculitis affecting arterioles, venules, and capillaries* with the presence of binucleated or multinucleated syncytial cells attached to the endothelium of affected blood vessels. Blood vessels undergo fibrinoid degeneration and leukocytoclastic vasculitis. Affected blood vessels are present most commonly in lung, brain, renal glomeruli, and lymphoid organs. Other pulmonary lesions include moderate lymphoplasmacytic bronchointerstitial pneumonia with mild necrotizing bronchiolitis and mild-to-moderate filling of alveoli with neutrophils, even in the absence of significant secondary bacterial infection. Severe lymphocytic and neutrophilic meningitis with mild lymphoplasmacytic encephalitis and occasional gliosis are consistent findings. Due to vasculitis, large areas of hemorrhage and infarction are common in affected organs. Occasionally, *eosinophilic intracytoplasmic and intranuclear inclusions* are present in neurons and syncytial endothelial cells. Syncytial cells can also be found attached within lymphatic vessels and to pulmonary alveolar septa.

Bibliography

Chua KB. Nipah virus outbreak in Malaysia. J Clin Virol 2003;26:265–275.

Hooper P, et al. Comparative pathology of the diseases caused by Hendra and Nipah viruses. Microbes Infect 2001;3:315–322.

Johnson RT. Emerging viral infections of the nervous system. J Neurovirol 2003;9:140–147.

Mackenzie JS, Field HE. Emerging encephalitogenic viruses: lyssaviruses and henipaviruses transmitted by frugivorous bats. Arch Virol Suppl 2004;18:97–111.

Other porcine paramyxoviral encephalitides

An outbreak of respiratory disease (necrotizing bronchointerstitial pneumonia) and encephalitis was recorded in a large pig farm affecting all ages. The etiologic agent was a previously unknown, as yet unclassified, paramyxovirus different than the other known porcine paramyxoviruses. CNS signs were characterized by recurring episodes of distress, head pressing, tremors, and hindlimb ataxia. No gross lesions were observed in brain. CNS lesions were lymphocytic perivasculitis and diffuse gliosis.

Bibliography

Janke BH, et al. Paramyxovirus infection in pigs with interstitial pneumonia and encephalitis in the United States. J Vet Diagn Invest 2001;13:428–433.

Akabane viral encephalitis

Akabane disease is caused by *Akabane virus* (AKAV) of the *Simbu virus group*, in the genus *Bunyavirus,* family Bunyaviridae. Iriki virus, a strain of AKAV, causes similar disease. The group also contains *Aino virus,* which causes congenital disease identical to that caused by AKAV. As mentioned earlier in this chapter, AKAV is a common cause of congenital CNS defects in infected bovine fetuses, however the virus has also been associated with nonsuppurative meningoencephalomyelitis in adult cows and young calves. Histologic lesions are more prominent in brain stem, pons, medulla oblongata, and the spinal cord ventral horn. Lesions are those of lymphohistiocytic cuffing with multifocal gliosis, neuronal necrosis, and occasional neuronophagia with microglial cells.

Bibliography

Lee JK, et al. Encephalomyelitis associated with akabane virus infection in adult cows. Vet Pathol 2002;39:269–273.
Liao YK, et al. The isolation of Akabane virus (Iriki strain) from calves in Taiwan. J Basic Microbiol 1996;36:33–39.

Bovine herpesviral encephalitis

Bovine necrotizing meningoencephalitis caused by *Bovine herpesvirus 5*

Bovine herpesvirus 5 (BoHV-5), the cause of bovine necrotizing meningoencephalitis, is antigenically related to *Bovine herpesvirus 1* (BoHV-1), the cause of infectious bovine rhinotracheitis. Both viruses are neurotropic, undergo latency in the trigeminal ganglia, and can be reactivated by natural or experimental stress; however, BoHV-1 rarely causes encephalitis. Both of these herpesviruses are in family Herpesviridae, subfamily Alphaherpesvirinae, genus *Varicellovirus*. Outbreaks of severe BoHV-5 necrotizing meningoencephalitis have occurred most frequently in South America, but the disease has been observed in other countries including the USA. Infection is by direct contact or aerosolization. Following intranasal inoculation, BoHV-5 reaches and invades the brain through the olfactory pathway. BoHV-5 envelope glycoproteins E (gE), gI, and Us9 convey viral neurovirulence and neuroinvasiveness by affecting anterograde viral spread via the olfactory pathway.

BoHV-5 encephalitis occurs as a sporadic disease or sometimes as outbreaks in calves and yearlings. The morbidity in herds may be as high as 50%, but is usually much lower; few recognizably sick animals survive. The incubation period is 1–2 weeks, followed by anorexia, apathy, circling, jaw chomping, and finally paddling and recumbency. These clinical signs may be associated with mild to severe rhinitis.

Gross lesions are usually absent, however in the severe form of the disease, bilaterally symmetrical areas of malacia, hemorrhage, and necrosis are described in the gray matter of the rostral cerebrum (Fig. 3.125). The hallmark histologic lesion is *severe cytonecrotizing nonsuppurative meningoencephalitis with marked gliosis* (Fig. 3.126A, B). Lesions are more commonly present in the gray matter of the rostral cerebrum, including olfactory bulb, and to a lesser extent in the cerebellum and diencephalon. Perivascular cuffs can be markedly thick (more than six layers of lymphocytes, plasma cells, and fewer histiocytes). Necrotic neurons are usually swollen, have lost their angularity, are basophilic, and have pyknotic nuclei. Typical *intranuclear alpha-herpesviral inclusions* are occasionally present in degenerate neurons and astrocytes (Fig. 3.126B). Trigeminal ganglioneuritis, neuronophagia, and satellitosis are commonly present. Necrotic or malacic areas can take the laminar cortical necrosis pattern of bovine polioencephalomalacia, however, the latter syndrome is not associated with the severe perivascular cuffing present in BoHV-5 encephalitis. Vasculitis affecting the cerebral microvasculature is only described in rabbits experimentally infected with the virus. The histologic lesions are fairly pathognomonic, however, confirmation of the diagnosis by PCR is recommended.

Bibliography

Al-Mubarak A, Chowdhury SI. In the absence of glycoprotein I (gI), gE determines bovine herpesvirus type 5 neuroinvasiveness and neurovirulence. J Neurovirol 2004;10:233–243.
Callan RJ, Van Metre DC. Viral diseases of the ruminant nervous system. Vet Clin North Am Food Anim Pract 2004;20:327–362.
Elias F, et al. Herpesvirus type-5 meningoencephalitis and malacia: histological lesions distribution in the central nervous system of naturally infected cattle. Pesq Vet Bras 2004;24:123–131.
Perez SE, et al. Primary infection, latency, and reactivation of bovine herpesvirus type 5 in the bovine nervous system. Vet Pathol 2002;39:437–444.

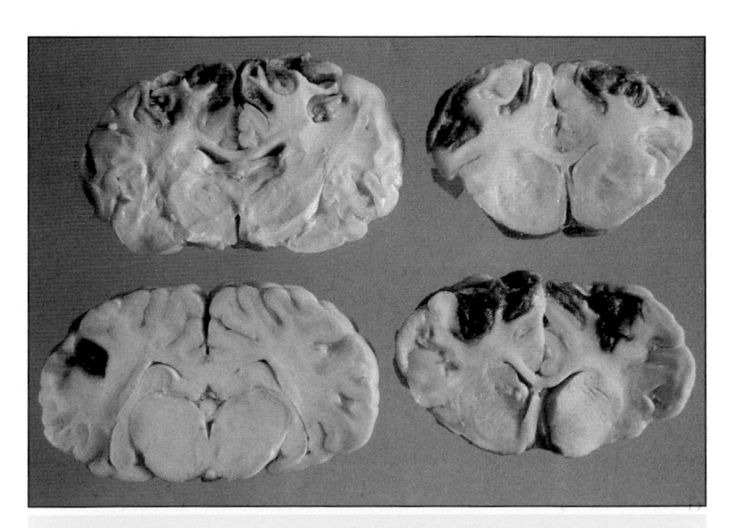

Figure 3.125 Areas of malacia, hemorrhage, and necrosis affecting the gray matter of the rostral cerebrum mostly in a bilaterally symmetrical pattern in **bovine necrotizing meningoencephalitis** caused by BoHV-5. (Courtesy of D. Driemeier.)

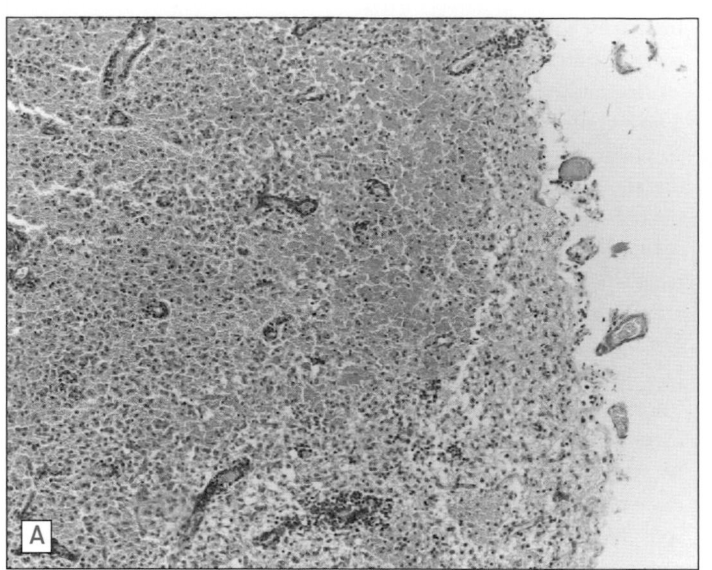

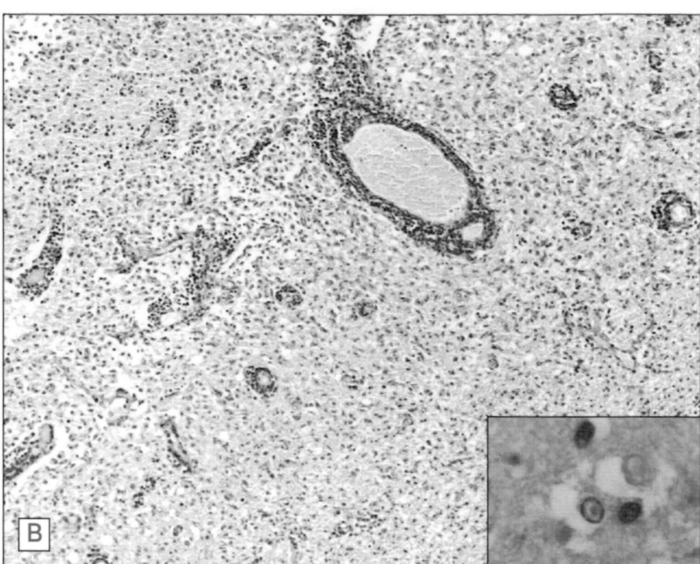

Figure 3.126 Severe hemorrhagic necrosis and malacia (**A**) with perivascular lymphocytic and plasmacytic cuffing (**B**) affecting the external cortical layers of the rostral cerebrum in **bovine necrotizing meningoencephalitis** caused by BoHV-5. Intra-astrocytic intranuclear herpesviral inclusion (inset in **B**). (Courtesy of D Driemeier.)

Spilki FR, et al. Neurovirulence and neuroinvasiveness of bovine herpesvirus type 1 and 5 in rabbits. Pesq Vet Bras 2002;22:58–63.

Bovine meningoencephalomyelitis caused by *Bovine herpesvirus 1*

Nonsuppurative encephalomyelitis due to *Bovine herpesvirus 1* (BoHV-1) is reported worldwide. BoHV-1 causes multiple and diverse conditions in cattle such as abortion, infectious bovine rhinotracheitis, infectious bovine vulvovaginitis, and balanoposthitis. Some BoHV-1 serotypes are neurovirulent and are able to induce encephalitis. Marked upper respiratory disease typically precedes or occurs concurrently with the encephalitis. The pathogenesis and clinical signs are similar to those described for BoHV-5. Histological lesions are those of *nonsuppurative encephalomyelitis with occasional intranuclear herpetic inclusions.* The massive neuronal necrosis and gliosis described in BoHV-5 are not usually seen in association with BoHV-1. BoHV-1 encephalitis is more prevalent in calves; however sporadic cases can affect adult cattle particularly in the Near and Middle East.

Bibliography

Meyer G, et al. Comparative pathogenesis of acute and latent infections of calves with bovine herpesvirus types 1 and 5. Arch Virol 2001;146:633–652.

Penny CD, et al. Upper respiratory disease and encephalitis in neonatal beef calves caused by bovine herpesvirus type 1. Vet Rec 2002;151:89–91.

Roels S, et al. Natural case of bovine herpesvirus 1 meningoencephalitis in an adult cow. Vet Rec 2000;146:586–588.

Malignant catarrhal fever

Malignant catarrhal fever (MCF) is a fatal multisystemic lymphoproliferative and inflammatory disease affecting many ruminant species. The details of MCF, including the lesions associated with its encephalomyelitic form, are described in Vol. 2, Alimentary system.

Nonsuppurative meningoencephalitis is reported in "malignant catarrhal fever" in *swine* in Europe resulting from infection with *Ovine herpesvirus 2*. *Caprine herpesvirus 2*, a gamma-herpesvirus, does not cause overt disease in goats, but causes fatal goat-associated MCF in certain species of deer.

Bibliography

Albini S, et al. Porcine malignant catarrhal fever: diagnostic findings and first detection of the pathogenic agent in diseased swine in Switzerland. Schweiz Arch Tierheilkd 2003;145:61–68.

Li H, et al. Caprine herpesvirus-2-associated malignant catarrhal fever in white-tailed deer (*Odocoileus virginianus*). J Vet Diagn Invest 2003;15:46–49.

Bovine paramyxoviral meningoencephalomyelitis

Sporadic cases of nonsuppurative meningoencephalomyelitis due to paramyxovirus are rarely reported. The causative virus is restricted to the European continent and is still not classified within the Paramyxoviridae but is distinct from the other bovine paramyxoviruses such as *Bovine parainfluenza virus 3*. The disease should be differentiated from the sporadic bovine encephalitis caused by *Chlamydophila* spp.

Bibliography

Bachmann PA, et al. Sporadic bovine meningoencephalitis – isolation of a paramyxovirus. Arch Virol 1975;48:107–120.

Theil D, et al. Neuropathological and aetiological studies of sporadic nonsuppurative meningoencephalomyelitis of cattle. Vet Rec 1998;143:244–249.

Porcine circovirus type 2 encephalopathies

Porcine circovirus type 2 (PCV2), the cause of porcine postweaning multisystemic wasting syndrome, produces nonsuppurative or granulomatous encephalitis with gliosis under experimental conditions, either alone or in association with porcine parvovirus. The PCV2 antigen has been identified in brain in these cases demonstrating neurotropism of the virus under experimental conditions. The role of PCV2 in encephalitis associated with natural infection is controversial. PCV2 antigen has been detected in brains of pigs with naturally occurring encephalitis but always in association with other pathogens that can cause encephalitis alone and under natural conditions (e.g., PRRSV or *Streptococcus suis*). Also, the PCV2 antigen was demonstrated in neonatal pigs in association with naturally occurring congenital tremor type A2 (see Porcine hypomyelinogenesis); however, the exact role of PCV2 in this condition is yet to be determined.

Bibliography

Kennedy S, et al. Reproduction of lesions of postweaning multisystemic wasting syndrome by infection of conventional pigs with porcine circovirus type 2 alone or in combination with porcine parvovirus. J Comp Pathol 2000;122:9–24.

Krakowka S, et al. Viral wasting syndrome of swine: experimental reproduction of postweaning multisystemic wasting syndrome in gnotobiotic swine by coinfection with porcine circovirus 2 and porcine parvovirus. Vet Pathol 2000;37:254–263.

Stevenson GW, et al. Tissue distribution and genetic typing of porcine circoviruses in pigs with naturally occurring congenital tremors. J Vet Diagn Invest 2001;13:57–62.

Porcine encephalitis associated with PRRSV infection

Porcine reproductive and respiratory syndrome virus (PRRSV) is neurovirulent especially in young pigs and can cause encephalitis under natural conditions, often in association with other PRRSV syndromes (e.g., interstitial pneumonia) (see Vol. 2, Respiratory system).

California encephalitis virus meningoencephalomyelitis

Several serotypes of species *California encephalitis virus* of genus *Orthobunyavirus*, family Bunyaviridae, usually cause only asymptomatic infections, but are capable of causing encephalitis. These include La Crosse virus (LACV), Snowshoe hare virus, and Jamestown Canyon virus.

La Crosse virus is maintained in the environment and transmitted between susceptible hosts by *Aedes triseriatus* mosquitoes. Chipmunks (*Tamias striatus*) and squirrels (*Sciurus carolinensis*) are the principal amplifying vertebrate hosts. Other wild mammals such as foxes (*Vulpes fulva* and *Urocyon cinereoargenteus*) and woodchucks (*Marmota monax*) may also contribute to virus maintenance. The virus causes encephalitis and secondary neurologic deficits in humans, particularly school-aged children. A few cases have been reported in dogs in Florida and Georgia, USA. The most predominant clinical signs in these dogs were seizures and head tilt. Gross lesions were usually unremarkable, but areas of malacia may be present in cortex. Histologic lesions are predominantly in the cerebral cortex and characterized by *histiocytic and lymphoplasmacytic meningoencephalitis* with fairly thick cuffs and multifocal necrotizing panencephalitis. The necrotic areas in the acute stage are histiocyte and neutrophil rich. The lesions of this disease are similar to those seen in idiopathic granulomatous meningoencephalomyelitis (GME) described below.

Antibodies to **Snowshoe hare virus** have been found in a wide range of wild and domestic mammals, but overt disease is very rare. Encephalitis in association with SSHV was reported in two horses from Canada, but the diagnosis was made based on detection of seroconversion; one horse recovered and the pathologic changes found in the second case were not described.

Bibliography

Black SS, et al. Necrotizing panencephalitis in puppies infected with La Crosse virus. J Vet Diagn Invest 1994;6:250–254.

Campbell GL, et al. Distribution of neutralizing antibodies to California and Bunyamwera serogroup viruses in horses and rodents in California. Am J Trop Med Hyg 1990;42:282–290.

Godsey MS Jr, et al. California serogroup virus infections in Wisconsin domestic animals. Am J Trop Med Hyg 1988;39:409–416.

Lynch JA, et al. California serogroup virus infection in a horse with encephalitis. J Am Vet Med Assoc 1985;186:389.

Tatum LM, et al. Canine LaCrosse viral meningoencephalomyelitis with possible public health implications. J Vet Diagn Invest 1999;11:184–188.

Canine herpesviral encephalitis

Canid herpesvirus 1 can cause an acute, highly fatal disease of neonates. Puppies after the age of 3 weeks are resistant to infection. The incidence is low, and the disease is only diagnosed at autopsy. Hypothermia predisposes to disease in neonates, in which the infection would otherwise be asymptomatic. Infection at birth is followed by cell-associated viremia and viral replication in vascular endothelium. This tropism is reflected in large hemorrhages at postmortem most apparent in renal surface, adrenal and serosa of gastrointestinal tract. Focal necroses occur in parenchymatous organs and inclusion bodies may be demonstrated in these foci. *Nonsuppurative meningoencephalitis* is most severe in cerebellum and brain stem. It may be accompanied by necrosis especially in the cerebellar cortex. Vascular endothelial hypertrophy and hyperplasia is accompanied by mononuclear infiltrates. There may be inflammatory changes in the retina, peripheral nerves, and ganglia.

Bibliography

Percy DH, et al. Pathogenesis of canine herpesvirus encephalitis. Am J Vet Res 1970;31:145–156.

Equine herpesviral myeloencephalopathy

Equid herpesvirus 1 (EHV-1) and *Equid herpesvirus 4* (EHV-4) are two antigenically related but distinct viruses in the genus *Varicellovirus*, subfamily Alphaherpesvirinae, family Herpesviridae. Both viruses are widespread in horses, have significant economic impact on the equine industry, and are responsible for several clinical conditions including respiratory disease, pulmonary vasculotropic disease, enteric disease, and abortion. *Equine myeloencephalopathy is an important neurological disease* characterized clinically by ataxia, paresis, and paralysis, and caused mainly by EHV-1 and incidentally by EHV-4. Almost all recent outbreaks have been associated with EHV-1 infection. Other members of equine alpha-herpesviruses that are pathogenic but do not cause neurologic disease include *Equid herpesvirus 3* (Equine coital exanthema virus) and *Equid herpesvirus 8*

(Asinine herpesvirus 8), which induces interstitial pneumonia in donkeys. *Equid herpesvirus 9* (Gazelle herpesvirus) causes severe encephalitis experimentally in several species of domestic animals; the natural outbreak of fulminant encephalitis has been reported in a herd of Thomson's gazelles that were in close association with zebra. The natural reservoir for EHV-9 is unknown, but zebras or other equidae have been suspected.

Most horses show serologic evidence of exposure to EHV-1 and EHV-4 but are asymptomatic, and vaccination does not necessarily confer protection from neurologic manifestations. Both viruses contain at least 13 glycoproteins, which are important virulence factors for attachment, entry to the host cell, and cell-to-cell dissemination. The natural spread of EHV-1 is through direct horse-to-horse contact, by inhalation of nasal aerosols from infected horses, or through direct contact with an infected aborted fetus or placenta. EHV-1 replicates first in upper respiratory tract epithelium and local lymph nodes, and then induces T-cell and monocyte-associated viremia that ends with invasion of endothelial cells of the CNS and pregnant uterus. This leukocyte-associated viremia protects the virus from humoral immunity. *The virus is endotheliotropic, epitheliotropic, and neurotropic, but not neurovirulent.* The replication of virus in endothelial cells of the CNS leads to initiation of the inflammatory cascade that ends in *thrombo-occlusive necrotizing vasculitis.* The resultant myeloencephalopathy is due to destruction of CNS tissue secondary to vasculitis. The vasculitis is either due to direct viral cytotoxic effect or due to an immune-mediated (Arthus-type reaction) mechanism. A similar mechanism is responsible for EHV-1-induced abortion and pulmonary vasculotropic disease. There are no genetic or antigenic differences between the EHV strains isolated from neurogenic cases versus abortigenic or respiratory cases.

EHV-1 and EHV-4 have life-long latency in T cells and in neural tissue such as trigeminal ganglia. Latent virus can be reactivated experimentally after very high doses of corticosteroids and naturally after stress (such as castration). In contrast to the extensive studies on EHV-1, the pathogenesis of EHV-4 infection is poorly documented.

The disease occurs sporadically, but in several recent outbreaks, most affected horses either died or were euthanized. The disease is common in late winter and spring, which is also the time of greatest prevalence of EHV-1 abortion outbreaks. The incubation period is 6–10 days and usually occurs in association with abortion and/or respiratory disease but can occur without preceding signs. All ages are susceptible, but *pregnant mares and mares nursing foals are over-represented.*

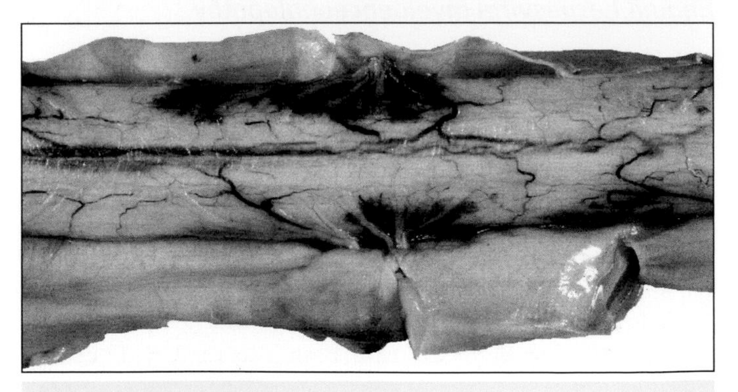

Figure 3.127 Acute spinal cord hemorrhage in a horse with **equine herpesviral myeloencephalopathy**. (Courtesy of RF Slocombe.)

Clinical signs start with fever and mild rhinitis. Neurologic signs are variable and depend on the part of the CNS affected by vasculitis, however common clinical signs include variable degrees of symmetrical ataxia and paresis that are more severe in pelvic limbs. Fecal and urinary incontinence are common, and clinical signs may end in hemi- or paraplegia. Gross and histologic lesions are sequelae to vasculitis. Gross lesions are not always present, but small (0.2–0.5 cm) random multifocal areas of hemorrhage may be present throughout the meninges, brain, and spinal cord (Fig. 3.127). In severe cases, multifocal necrohemorrhagic or malacic areas (up to 1.5 cm in diameter) can be present, especially in the white matter of spinal cord or the white or gray matter of the brain. *The characteristic histologic lesions are nonsuppurative necrotizing vasculitis and thrombosis*, with greater prevalence in the meningeal and parenchymal blood vessels of the brain stem and spinal cord. Perivascular edema, hemorrhage, focal areas of malacia, and infarction are present adjacent to the affected blood vessels. Occasionally, axonal swelling and mild nonsuppurative trigeminal ganglionitis are present. Extraneural lesions include uveal vasculitis and optic neuritis, especially in foals, and testicular and epididymal vasculitis in stallions.

Bibliography

Donaldson MT, Sweeney CR. Herpesvirus myeloencephalopathy in horses: 11 cases (1982–1996). J Am Vet Med Assoc 1998;213:671–675.

Reed SM, Toribio RE. Equine herpesvirus 1 and 4. Vet Clin North Am Equine Pract 2004;20:631–642.

Stierstorfer B, et al. Equine herpesvirus type 1 (EHV-1) myeloencephalopathy: a case report. J Vet Med B Infect Dis Vet Public Health 2002;49:37–41.

van Maanen C. Equine herpesvirus 1 and 4 infections: an update. Vet Q 2002; 24:58–78.

Wilson WD. Equine herpesvirus 1 myeloencephalopathy. Vet Clin North Am Equine Pract 1997;13:53–72.

Yanai T, et al. Experimental infection of equine herpesvirus 9 in dogs. Vet Pathol 2003;40:263–267.

Canine distemper and related conditions

Canine distemper is discussed in detail in Vol. 2, Respiratory system. Three neurologic conditions are discussed here: multifocal distemper encephalomyelitis in mature dogs, postvaccinal distemper, and old-dog encephalitis.

Multifocal distemper encephalomyelitis in mature dogs

This rare chronic progressive disease occurs when *Canine distemper virus* infects dogs at 4–8 years of age. This disease is not preceded by the classic form of canine distemper, and signs of systemic illness are often absent or transient. Clinical signs have a slow progressive course and include weakness of the pelvic limbs, generalized incoordination, but no seizures or personality changes, and occasionally head tremors. Lesions are restricted to the CNS and are most prevalent in the cerebellum and white matter of the spinal cord. The cerebral cortex is frequently spared. This distribution differentiates this condition from an extremely rare condition, old dog encephalitis, wherein the cerebral cortex is constantly affected. The lesions are those of *multifocal necrotizing nonsuppurative encephalitis* with rare canine distemper intranuclear intra-astrocytic inclusion bodies, and demyelination in the internal capsule and corona radiata.

Post-vaccinal canine distemper encephalitis

This condition occurs in young dogs 1–3 weeks after vaccination with attenuated *Canine distemper virus* vaccines and is characterized by an acute to subacute clinical course (1–5 days). The acute course is characterized by clinical signs reminiscent of the furious form of rabies including aggressive behavior and attempts to attack. It is not completely clear why some dogs develop this condition post-vaccination. Immune stimulation by other canine viruses (e.g., *Canine parvovirus*) at the time of vaccination was suggested. The lesions are not well documented, however, lesions are always restricted to the CNS and are reminiscent of the natural disease, but distinguished by the relative sparing of the white matter.

"Old dog" encephalitis

"Old dog" encephalitis (ODE) is rather rare. Most cases occur in dogs past middle age but it has been observed in dogs as young as 1 year of age. The disease is of insidious onset and is characterized by circling, swaying, and weaving. Compulsive walking with pushing against fixed objects is typical, but there is neither paralysis nor convulsions. The disease progresses over 3–4 months to coma or termination.

ODE is caused by *Canine distemper virus* (CDV), apparently as a consequence of long-term subclinical, persistent infection: CDV appears to persist in a replication-defective state. ODE does not appear to be simply a progression of the encephalomyelitis of canine distemper. Virus can be isolated from affected animals only by explantation of affected brain and then only with difficulty, and the disease is not transmissible by direct inoculation. Inclusion bodies are readily found in some cases, and their structure is identical with paramyxovirus nucleocapsids of CDV in nervous tissue. Antigen that responds to fluorescent antibody prepared against CDV is abundant in cells of the gray matter, and serum antibody titers can be very high.

Lesions are confined to the brain, which appears slightly reduced in size. The ventricles are moderately dilated. Lesions are diffusely distributed throughout the cerebral cortex, thalamus, and midbrain. The reaction is nonsuppurative, qualitatively always the same but varying in degree. The most obvious change is cuffing, and the cuffs are remarkable for their large size and the purity of the lymphocytic populations in them. Plasma cells are present in small numbers. The infiltrating cells are confined to the Virchow–Robin space and seldom spread into the parenchyma. The large cuffs occur in both gray and white matter but are most common at the junction of these two zones. Focal gliosis does not occur in this disease, but there is some proliferation of astrocytes about vessels and neurons. There is uniform and rather diffuse atrophic sclerosis of the cerebral white matter, which gives an impression of gliosis, but astrogliosis is not prominent. There is some demyelination, producing typical punched-out areas in the white matter, and distorted myelin sheaths in the heavily myelinated tracts are quite extensive when specially stained. Lymphocytes may be found in the choroid plexuses where they are inserted into the brain, and about vessels where they enter the parenchyma.

Nerve cells, especially in Ammon's horn and the pons, reveal chromatolysis with only a few remnants of Nissl substance in the periphery of the cytoplasm. The chromatolytic cytoplasm is slightly acidophilic. The neuronal nuclei in the forebrain are remarkably swollen in most of the altered nerve cells. In occasional nuclei, there is pink inclusion-like material. Neuronophagia does not occur. The astrocytic nuclei are remarkably swollen, have an irregular outline, and may contain traces of pink deposit in the nucleoplasm. In a proportion of cases, possibly those of longest duration, prominent *intranuclear and cytoplasmic eosinophilic inclusion bodies* may be found easily.

Bibliography

Axthelm MK, Krakowka S. Experimental old dog encephalitis (ODE) in a gnotobiotic dog. Vet Pathol 1998;35:527–534.

Cherpillod P, et al. DNA vaccine encoding nucleocapsid and surface proteins of wild type canine distemper virus protects its natural host against distemper. Vaccine 2000;18:2927–2936.

Guilford WG, et al. Fecal incontinence, urinary incontinence, and priapism associated with multifocal distemper encephalomyelitis in a dog. J Am Vet Med Assoc 1990;197:90–92.

Parasitic infections

Protozoal infections

The cerebral complications of infections by protozoa such as *Babesia, Theileria, Trypanosoma*, and *Toxoplasma* are discussed elsewhere in these volumes. *Acanthamoeba*, a free-living ameba, can produce granulomatous meningoencephalitis in dogs as part of an opportunistic generalized infection (Fig. 3.128).

From time to time and in individual cases, pathologists observe *sporozoan parasites* in neural tissues of fetuses, neonates, and adults and lesions presumed to be the consequence of their presence. There are, however, difficulties in specific identification of the parasites and in attribution of pathogenicity. The syndromes considered here are reasonably defined but are subject to revision as the parasites are identified and their lifecycles clarified.

Encephalitozoonosis

Encephalitozoon (Nosema) cuniculi is a microsporidian parasite capable of establishing infection in a wide variety of mammalian species and birds. It is rarely a zoonotic infection. Endemic infection is

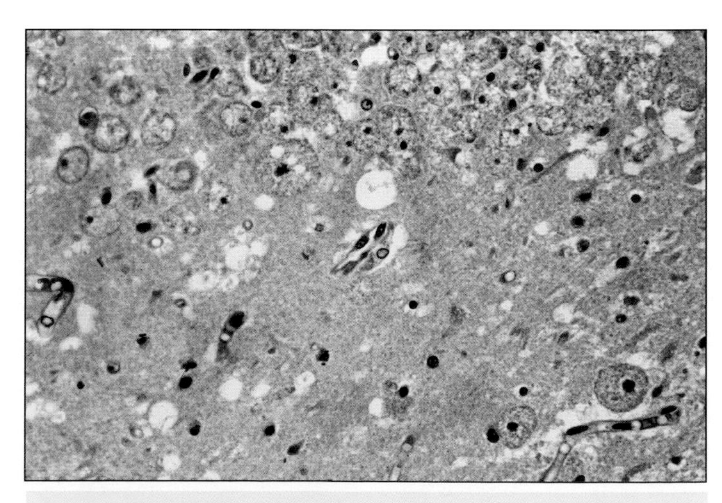

Figure 3.128 Amebic encephalitis in a dog: large numbers of amebae are present in this field, with only minimal reaction. (Courtesy of RF Slocombe.)

common in colonies of laboratory rodents in which the clinical consequences are mild but the pathologic changes may confuse other studies. Amongst domestic species, the disease is of interest in carnivores, especially farmed foxes in which serious mortalities occur, and occasionally in dogs and mink. The incidence of subclinical infection is not known, but a serological survey of an unselected population of asymptomatic stray dogs identified 10–15% to be seropositive.

The organism is an *obligate intracellular parasite* with a direct life cycle. It develops in parasitophorous vacuoles in cells of many tissues, especially endothelial cells, but is most easily found in brain and kidney in acute active infections. In chronic infections, the organisms can be sparse or impossible to find in microscopic sections, although it seems that animals once infected remain permanently so and excrete the organism mainly in urine.

Clinical disease occurs in dog and fox pups; the organism is shed in urine and feces of affected animals. In both hosts, transplacental infections appear to be important, but oral transmission, as by ingestion of infected rabbit carcasses, may occur. Experimental infection of mature dogs does not lead to clinical disease.

Tissue changes in encephalitozoonosis are most prominent in brain and kidney, but the organism selectively parasitizes vascular endothelium, and the *segmental vasculitis* that results is responsible for lesions in many tissues. Gross lesions may be limited to the kidneys as severe, nonsuppurative interstitial nephritis (Fig. 3.129A). Organisms are abundant in sections of kidney early in the disease but they are difficult to find at later stages. They are especially numerous in the epithelium and lumen of tubules, in glomerular capillaries and in the interstitium, and are present in small vessels and in the media and adventitia of intrarenal arteries. Fibrinoid necrosis affects some glomeruli and the arterial lesions resemble those of periarteritis nodosa. Focal hepatic necrosis and nonsuppurative portal infiltrations are associated with organisms in hepatocytes and Kupffer cells and with nodular vasculitis in the triads. Focal myocardial necrosis and inflammation are frequently associated with vasculitis.

The lesions in the nervous system are those of *widespread nonsuppurative meningoencephalomyelitis*. The severity of lesions varies unpredictably in different parts of the nervous system reflecting the random localization of the organism and the irregular distribution of inflammatory vascular change. Focal gliosis and microscopic granulomas surround small vessels (Fig. 3.129B). About larger vessels showing segmental fibrinoid change, mononuclear cells form cuffs involving the adventitia and perivascular space and eventually assume an epithelioid cell appearance. There is astrocytosis in the surrounding parenchyma. The vascular lesions in the meninges in the acute disease resemble those of polyarteritis nodosa and become dominated by sclerotic changes in the chronic disease in which perivascular cuffing and granulomatous reactions persist.

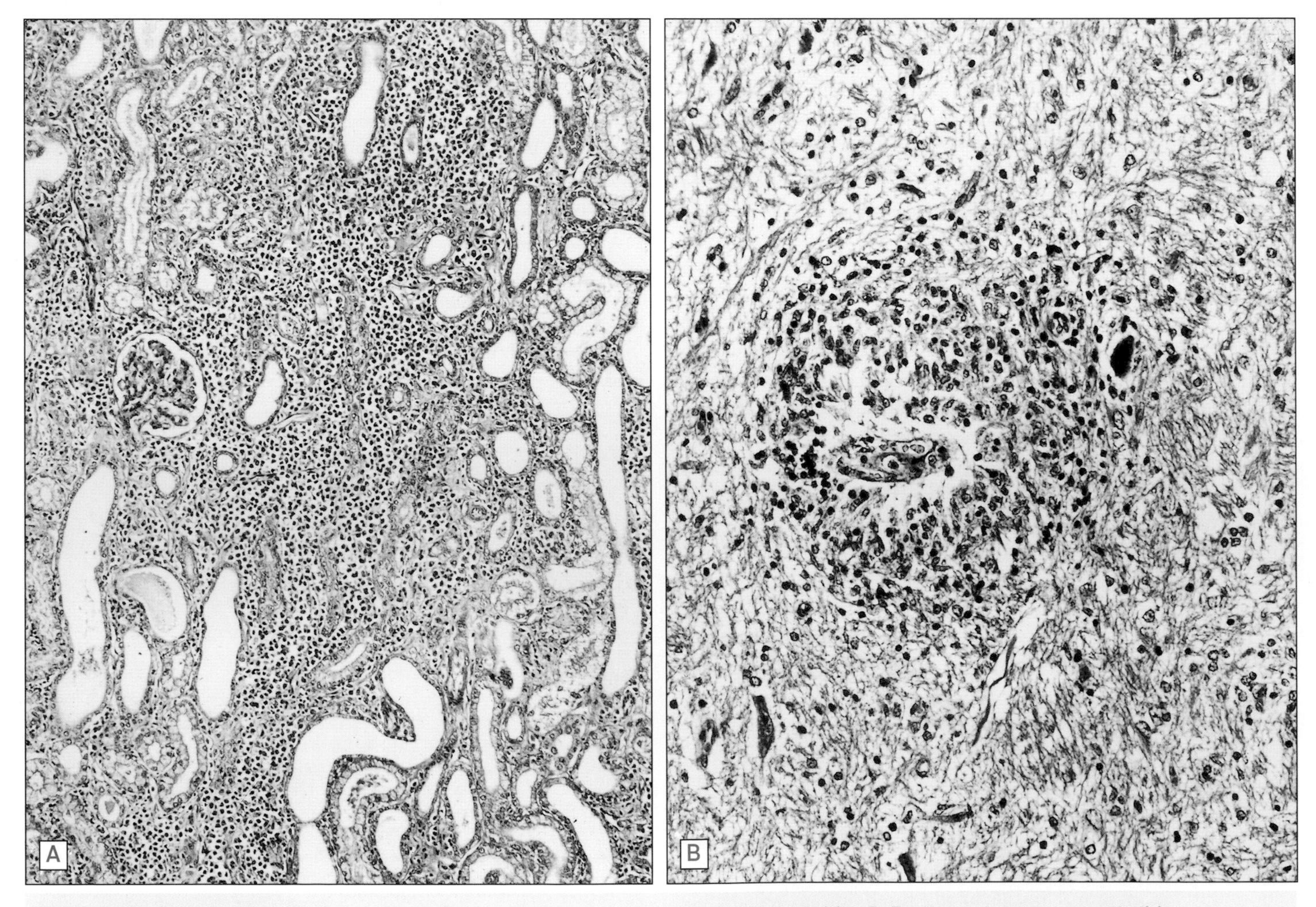

Figure 3.129 Encephalitozoonosis in a dog. **A.** Severe diffuse nonsuppurative interstitial **nephritis. B.** Focal granulomatous **encephalitis.**

Puppies which survive the early clinical disease may remain stunted and develop progressive renal disease. It is possible that encephalitozoonosis, as for any sporadic disease, is underdiagnosed especially in chronic infections in which the organism is difficult to demonstrate. Immunohistochemical methods help to identify sparse organisms and to distinguish them from similar parasites, particularly *Toxoplasma* and *Neospora*.

Bibliography

Bauer RW, et al. Isolation of *Acanthamoeba* sp. from a greyhound with pneumonia and granulomatous amebic encephalitis. J Vet Diagn Invest 1993;5:386–391.

Bjerkas I. Brain and spinal cord lesions in encephalitozoonosis in blue foxes. Acta Path Microbiol Immunol Scand 1987;95:269–279.

Snowden K, et al. *Encephalitozoon cuniculi* strain III is a cause of encephalitozoonosis in both humans and dogs. J Infect Dis 1999;180:2086–2088.

Wasson K, Peper RL. Mammalian microsporidiosis. Vet Pathol 2000;37:113–128.

Equine protozoal myeloencephalitis

Equine protozoal myeloencephalitis (EPM) is caused mainly by ***Sarcocystis neurona***, an apicomplexan protozoan parasite, however identical disease is reported in association with ***N. caninum*** and ***N. hughesi***. Opossums (*Didelphis* spp.) are the definitive host for *S. neurona,* and they are infected by eating intermediate host tissues that contain infective tissue cysts. *S. neurona*-induced EPM is restricted to the Americas in the geographical range of the opossum. Natural intermediate hosts (e.g., armadillos, sea otters, raccoons, skunks, cats) are infected by ingestion of food or water contaminated by sporocysts shed in opossum feces. Horses are assumed to be dead-end hosts, but may also act as intermediate hosts.

Exposure to *S. neurona* is widespread among horses, but the prevalence of the classic progressive disease is much lower. A seropositive horse is positive for exposure but not necessarily for the presence of the disease. However, the presence of seropositivity and the clinical signs of weakness and acute ataxia usually indicate active disease. Infection with *S. neurona* has no age predilection. Most EPM cases due to *S. neurona* infection appear in the summer and fall. Affected horses are presented with ataxia, limb weakness, lameness, and rarely seizures.

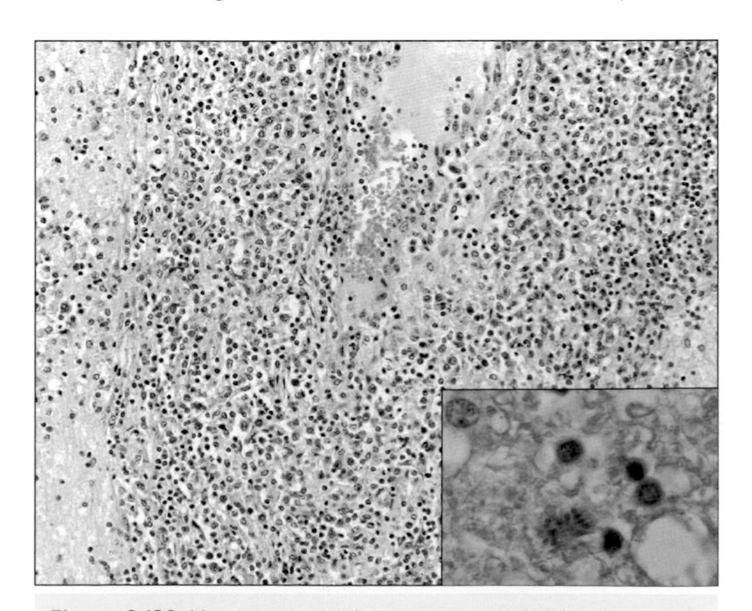

Figure 3.130 Massive mixed inflammatory encephalitis with variable numbers of eosinophils with rare intralesional ***Sarcocystis neurona*** schizonts (inset) in a horse with equine protozoal myeloencephalitis.

Gross lesions are present only in severe cases, and range from multifocal acute hemorrhage to the presence of discrete multifocal gray to dark yellow areas primarily in cross-sections of fixed brain stem, obex, pons, and cervical and thoracic cord. The histologic lesions are usually moderate to severe and characterized by multifocal areas of necrosis, malacia with aggregation of gitter cells, gliosis, and infiltration of large numbers of lymphocytes, histiocytes, plasma cells, and fewer eosinophils and neutrophils with severe involvement of the meninges (Fig. 3.130). The blood vessels in these areas have swollen activated endothelium with thick perivascular cuffs of mononuclear cells and occasional eosinophils. Also and particularly in cord sections, there is axonal swelling or loss besides the appearance of spheroids and some digestion chambers. In chronic cases, the inflammation can be predominantly histiocytic with occasional eosinophils and multinucleated giant cells.

Finding *S. neurona* merozoites or schizonts can be a challenge and serial sections must be examined in most cases. *S. neurona* schizonts are almost always present near areas of inflammation and necrosis, schizonts are oval or irregularly round, have very thin walls ($<0.5\,\mu m$), are up to $20\,\mu m$ in diameter, and contain a few basophilic ovoid merozoites $5\,\mu m \times 1.5\,\mu m$. The stage infective to the definitive host, i.e., sporocysts, can be found in tongue and other skeletal muscles. The *S. neurona* sporocyst is round (50–$100\,\mu m$) or elongate ($500\,\mu m$ long and $40\,\mu m$ wide), and contains a number of bradyzoites.

EPM-like disease can occur in other *S. neurona* intermediate hosts, including the cat, and this disease should be considered in the differential diagnosis of inflammatory encephalomyelitis in this species. Both *N. hughesi* and *N. caninum* can cause identical EPM lesions in horses. The complete life cycle and methods of transmission for *N. hughesi* have not been determined. *Neospora hughesi* tachyzoites are crescent-shaped, approximately $5 \times 2\,\mu m$. Definitive diagnosis of EPM in a live horse is challenging. Detection of *S. neurona* or *N. hughesi* antibodies in serum and cerebrospinal fluid by an immunoblot test is available. Positive results indicate exposure, but do not necessarily indicate that the horse has EPM. The postmortem diagnosis depends on finding characteristic lesions, especially in the presence of the characteristic protozoal stages. Immunohistochemistry kits for *S. neurona* and *N. caninum* are available commercially.

Bibliography

Dubey JP, et al. Clinical *Sarcocystis neurona* encephalomyelitis in a domestic cat following routine surgery. Vet Parasitol 2003;112:261–267.

Gillis KD, et al. Naturally occurring *Sarcocystis* infection in domestic cats (*Felis catus*). Int J Parasitol 2003;33:877–883.

Marsh AE, et al. Description of a new *Neospora* species (*Protozoa: Apicomplexa: Sarcocystidae*). J Parasitol 1998;84:983–991.

Packham AE, et al. Qualitative evaluation of selective tests for detection of *Neospora hughesi* antibodies in serum and cerebrospinal fluid of experimentally infected horses. J Parasitol 2002;88:1239–1246.

Sofaly CD, et al. Experimental induction of equine protozoan myeloencephalitis (EPM) in the horse: effect of *Sarcocystis neurona* sporocyst inoculation dose on the development of clinical neurologic disease. J Parasitol 2002;88:1164–1170.

Neosporosis

Neospora caninum is an apicomplexan coccidian parasite that is a major pathogen of cattle, in which it causes abortion, and for dogs. Other species, such as goats, sheep, deer, and horses, can be infected occasionally. Dogs are the primary definitive host, and they are also considered as an intermediate host. Other canids, e.g., coyotes (*Canis latrans*), may also be important definitive hosts. *N. caninum* has three infectious stages: tachyzoites, tissue cysts, and oocysts. Tachyzoites and tissue cysts are found both in intermediate hosts and the definitive host. However, oocysts are only present in the definitive host. Tachyzoites have been found in neurons, reticuloendothelial cells, hepatocytes, muscle cells including myocardium, and bovine placenta. Tissue cysts have been found in the CNS, muscles, and retina. The exact modes of transmission are not well understood. Dogs become infected by ingesting tissues contaminated with tissue cysts, and then shed oocysts in their feces. Cattle and other intermediate hosts become infected by ingesting sporulated oocyst-contaminated food, water, or soil. However, the principal route for infection in cattle is transplacental (vertical) transmission.

N. caninum does not cause significant clinical disease in adult **cattle**, however it causes abortion in both dairy and beef cows particularly at mid-term, although cows can abort at any time from 3 months to term. Infected fetuses may die in utero, be mummified, stillborn, or born alive with or without clinical signs. Extraneural lesions in bovine fetuses include *lymphocytic, plasmacytic and, to a lesser extent, histiocytic, hepatitis, pancarditis or myocarditis, myositis, and placentitis*. Cotyledonary necrosis may be associated with the placentitis. Intralesional *Neospora caninum* tachyzoites are occasionally present in the aforementioned organs. Tachyzoites appear in groups, either intracellular in neurons, endothelium or epithelial cells, or extracellular. Tachyzoites are spindle-shaped, 4–7 × 2 μm. Tissue cysts are primarily present in the CNS and rarely in skeletal muscles. Cyst diameter is up to 107 μm, with wall thickness of 1–4 μm, and containing numerous bradyzoites 8 × 2 μm.

The most frequent and almost pathognomonic CNS lesion in *bovine fetuses* is the presence of *multifocal discrete foci of necrosis* (~100–300 μm diameter), particularly in the brain and to a lesser extent in the cord (Fig. 3.131A, B). The necrotic areas are fairly well circumscribed, have necrotic centers and are surrounded by a rim of glial cells and macrophages. In advanced lesions, the necrotic area may be completely replaced by macrophages and a few glial cells, which make the lesions appear as discrete granulomas. The recognition of *N. caninum* tachyzoites and tissue cysts in aborted fetal brain or other fetal tissue is usually difficult on H&E stain, and immunohistochemistry must be performed to confirm the diagnosis of neosporosis. Other CNS lesions include mild nonsuppurative meningoencephalomyelitis. Fetal anomalies are not common in association with *Neospora* abortion.

Infection in **dogs** is transmitted either horizontally or vertically (transplacental). Dogs of any age can be affected and the infection can be generalized affecting any organs, including the skin, or can be localized. Infection in adult dogs is usually subclinical. Infection in young congenitally infected dogs is severe and characterized pathologically by encephalomyelitis and myositis/polyradiculoneuritis and clinically by hindlimb paresis that is followed by paralysis. CNS lesions are those of *necrotizing granulomatous, lymphoplasmacytic, and occasionally eosinophilic meningoencephalomyelitis* with diffuse gliosis, occasional axonal swelling, digestion chamber formation, and intralesional *N. caninum* tachyzoites and cysts (Fig. 3.132). These lesions are widely distributed in the brain and cord, however in the cortex the gray matter is affected predominantly. Lesions associated with the neuritis/polyradiculoneuritis is frequently severe, mostly affecting pelvic limbs, and characterized by severe lymphohistiocytic and occasional eosinophilic inflammation with associated secondary degenerative and necrotizing changes either in muscles or nerves with intralesional tachyzoites and rare cysts.

Experimental infection of pregnant **ewes** and **does** produces a disease that is identical pathologically to that observed in cattle, however natural disease is rare.

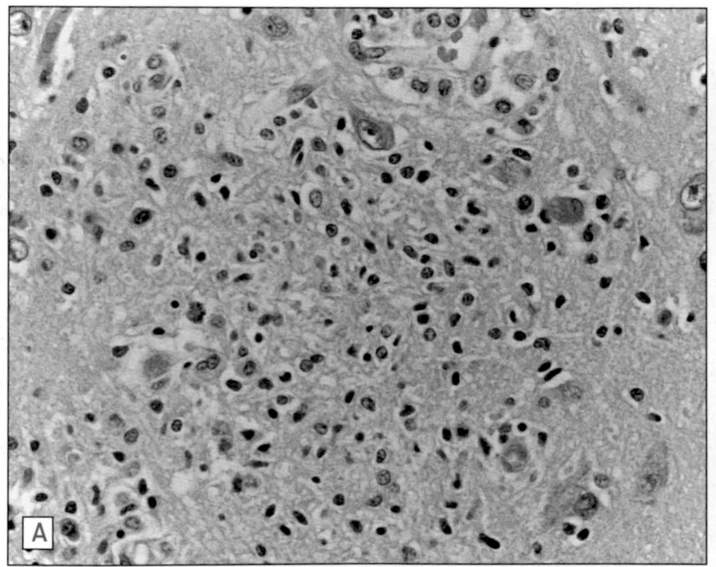

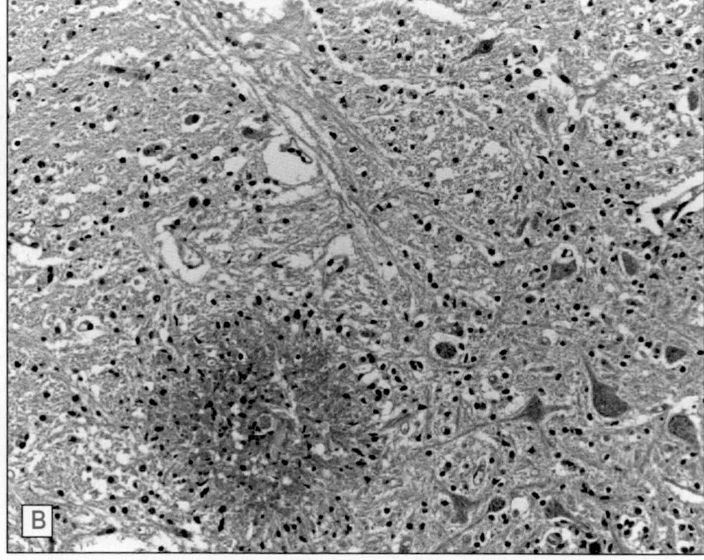

Figure 3.131 Lesions of neosporosis in fetal bovine brains may consist only of focal gliosis (**A**) or may occur as multifocal areas of neuropilar necrosis (**B**) encircled by glial cells and rarely giant cells. *Neospora caninum* cysts are rarely seen.

The epidemiology and methods of transmission of *N. caninum* and other *Neospora* in **horses**, e.g., *N. hughesi*, are not completely understood. Transplacental infection is suggested but not completely confirmed. *N. caninum* has been isolated from a few aborted fetuses. *N. caninum* and *N. hughesi* are rare causes of equine protozoal myeloencephalitis (see above).

Bibliography

Buxton D, et al. The comparative pathogenesis of neosporosis. Trends in Parasitol 2002;18:546–552.

De Marez T, et al. Oral infection of calves with *Neospora caninum* oocysts from dogs: humoral and cellular immune responses. Int J Parasitol 1999;29:1647–1657.

Dubey JP. Review of *Neospora caninum* and neosporosis in animals. Korean J Parasitol 2003;41:1–16.

Dubey JP, et al. Hydrocephalus associated with *Neospora caninum* infection in an aborted bovine fetus. J Comp Pathol 1998;118:169–173.

Hamir AN, et al. *Neospora caninum*-associated equine protozoal myeloencephalitis. Vet Parasitol 1998;79:269–274.

Illanes O, et al. *Neospora*-induced congenital myelitis and polyradiculoneuritis in a one-month-old Holstein calf. Can Vet J 1994;35:653–654.

MacKay RJ, et al. Equine protozoal myeloencephalitis. Vet Clin North Am Equine Pract 2000;16:405–425.

McAllister MM, et al. Dogs are definitive hosts of *Neospora caninum*. Int J Parasitol 1998;28:1473–1478.

Morales E, et al. Neosporosis in Mexican dairy herds: lesions and immunohistochemical detection of *Neospora caninum* in fetuses. J Comp Pathol 2001;125:58–63.

Toxoplasmosis

Toxoplasmosis is one of the most common protozoal diseases affecting humans and animals and is caused by ***Toxoplasma gondii***. Diseases caused by *T. gondii* are very similar in clinical presentation and pathology to those caused by *N. caninum*. Felids are the only definitive host and they also can act as an intermediate host. Other intermediate hosts include humans and other mammals. *T. gondii* has three infectious stages: tachyzoites, tissue cysts, and oocysts. Tachyzoites and tissue cysts are found in both intermediate and definitive hosts, however, oocysts are only present in the definitive host. Tachyzoites and tissue cysts are present more commonly in neural tissue and muscles, but can be present in virtually any tissue. Felids become infected by ingestion of tissues contaminated with tissue cysts, and shed oocysts in their feces. Human and other intermediate hosts including felids can become infected by ingesting sporulated oocyst-contaminated food, water, or soil. Transplacental transmission is important in cats, goats, and sheep. The extraneural pathology of toxoplasmosis is discussed elsewhere in these volumes. The nervous system lesions, including polyradiculoneuritis, are identical to those described above for neosporosis, however *the tissue cyst has a thinner wall (<0.5 μm), is 5–70 μm in size, and contains several bradyzoites 0.7–1.5 μm. Tachyzoites are 2–6 μm in size.* The encephalitic form of toxoplasmosis is most likely to occur in immunosuppressed dog and cats or kittens. Toxoplasmosis in pigs is generalized and can cause devastating disease with lesions including nonsuppurative encephalomyelitis with intralesional *T. gondii* stages.

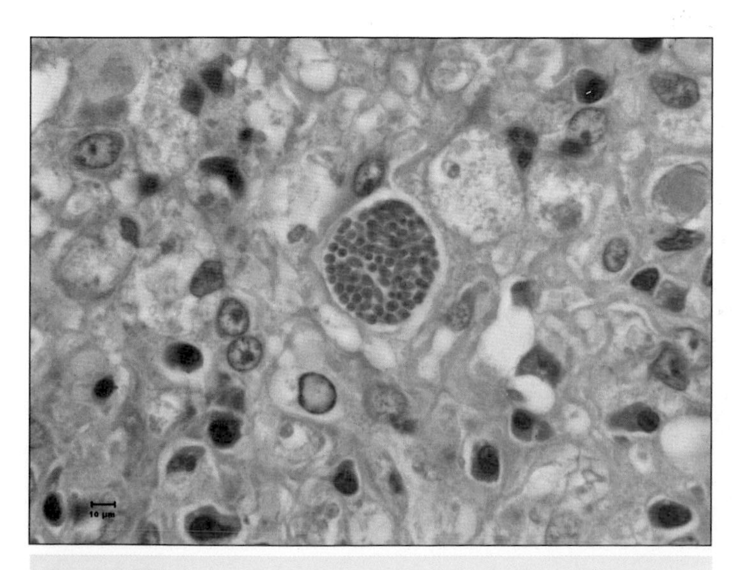

Figure 3.132 *Neospora caninum* cyst in the brain of a dog. (Courtesy of MJ Hazlett.)

Bibliography

Dubey JP. Toxoplasmosis – a waterborne zoonosis. Vet Parasitol 2004;126:57–72.

Gelmetti D, et al. Diagnostic investigations of toxoplasmosis in four swine herds. J Vet Diagn Invest 1999;11:87–90.

Sarcocystis canis encephalitis

A rare and generalized disease affecting dogs mostly in North America is caused by *S. canis* and characterized histologically by multisystemic vasculitis, hepatitis, and necrotizing lymphohistiocytic encephalitis in association with the presence of intralesional *S. canis* schizonts and merozoites (schizonts are 5–25 × 4–20 μm and contain 6–40 merozoites of 5–7 μm × 1 μm).

Bibliography

Dubey JP, Speer CA. *Sarcocystis canis* n. sp. (*Apicomplexa: Sarcocystidae*), the etiologic agent of generalized coccidiosis in dogs. J Parasitol 1991;77:522–527.

Trasti SL, et al. Fatal visceral and neural sarcocystosis in dogs. J Comp Pathol 1999;121:179–184.

Helminth and arthropod infestations

Nothing is known of what motivates and directs the migration of larval parasites. Those that migrate somatically are apt to go astray, and this appears especially likely when they wander in an alien host. Aberrant pathways include the nervous system with such frequency as to suggest that nematodes have a special propensity for wandering in the CNS. Whether this is indeed the case remains to be proven, but parasitic migrations in nervous tissue are more likely to be symptomatic than aberrant migrations in other tissues, and there is an impressive list of parasites that have been found in brain or cord. Many of these infestations and the parasites in question are discussed elsewhere in these volumes.

Cestodes

Adult cestodes live almost exclusively in the small intestines of the final host, however certain larval stages can infest the brain of the intermediate host. ***Coenurus cerebralis***, the larval stage of ***Taenia***

multiceps, which infests the small intestines of dogs and wild carnivores, is fairly common in the brains of sheep in Europe, less common in other herbivores, and rather rare in horses and humans. About 40% of pigs harboring ***Cysticercus cellulosae*** (the larval stage of the human tapeworm ***Taenia solium***) have cysts in the meninges and brain as well as in the muscle, and the same species has been identified in the brains of dogs. Possibly ***Cysticercus bovis*** (the larval stage of human tapeworm ***Taenia saginata***) and other cysticerci will invade nervous tissue with comparable frequency. Apparently, hydatids are seldom found in brain.

Nematodes

The term **cerebrospinal nematodiasis** is applied to nervous diseases resulting from aberrant nematode larval migrations. The few nematodes that produce the syndrome with any frequency are discussed below.

Parastrongylus *(Angiostrongylus)* ***cantonensis*** is a metastrongylid lungworm whose only known definitive host is the rat. It is widely distributed in the warm Pacific regions, but its distribution is much more limited than that of the gastropod intermediate hosts and the rat. The parasite resides in the pulmonary arteries of rats, eggs lodge as emboli in alveolar capillaries and the larvae, which hatch in about 6 days, and follow the tracheal–intestinal route to the exterior. First-stage larvae actively penetrate terrestrial and aquatic slugs and snails, which act as intermediate hosts. Transport hosts for third-stage larvae include frogs, crabs, and prawns. In addition to the rat, dogs, humans, and occasionally other species are infected by eating intermediate or transport hosts and, possibly, directly by ingestion of infective larvae that have emerged from intermediate hosts. Ingested larvae enter and are dispersed by the circulation to many tissues, but predominantly to brain, kidney, and muscle. Molting larvae in the brain produce a mild to severe inflammatory reaction before re-entering the venous circulation for return to the pulmonary arteries. Aberrant infections are important in humans and dogs, and are reported in horses and macropods. The human disease, eosinophilic meningoencephalitis, is usually mild and without sequelae, but infection in dogs can be accompanied by ascending paralysis. Larvae that enter the brain in dogs are probably inhibited in their development and destroyed there (Fig. 3.133). The lesions are granulomatous, randomly distributed in the cord and brain and are most frequent and severe in the cord (Fig. 3.134). Rarely, degenerate parasites are present in the granulomas, but apparently viable worms in the tissue are not accompanied by an inflammatory reaction. Eosinophils infiltrate the granulomas but are more numerous in affected meninges.

Parelaphostrongylus *(Pneumostrongylus)* ***tenuis*** is a metastrongylid parasite of white-tailed deer, *Odocoileus virginianus*, in North America. The intermediate hosts are terrestrial slugs and snails. Ingested larvae reach the spinal cord of the deer in ~10 days. They develop for up to 1 month in the dorsal horns of the cord at all levels and then migrate into the meningeal spaces. Some penetrate the dural veins and sinuses and mature. Eggs or larvae are carried in venous blood to the lungs. The larvae do very little to the cord in white-tailed deer, but the reaction is more severe in other species, including red deer, elk, moose, and sheep (Fig. 3.135). ***Elaphostrongylus panticola*** and ***E. rangifera*** of deer in northern Europe and Russia have a life cycle similar to that of *P. tenuis*, but infections are usually subclinical.

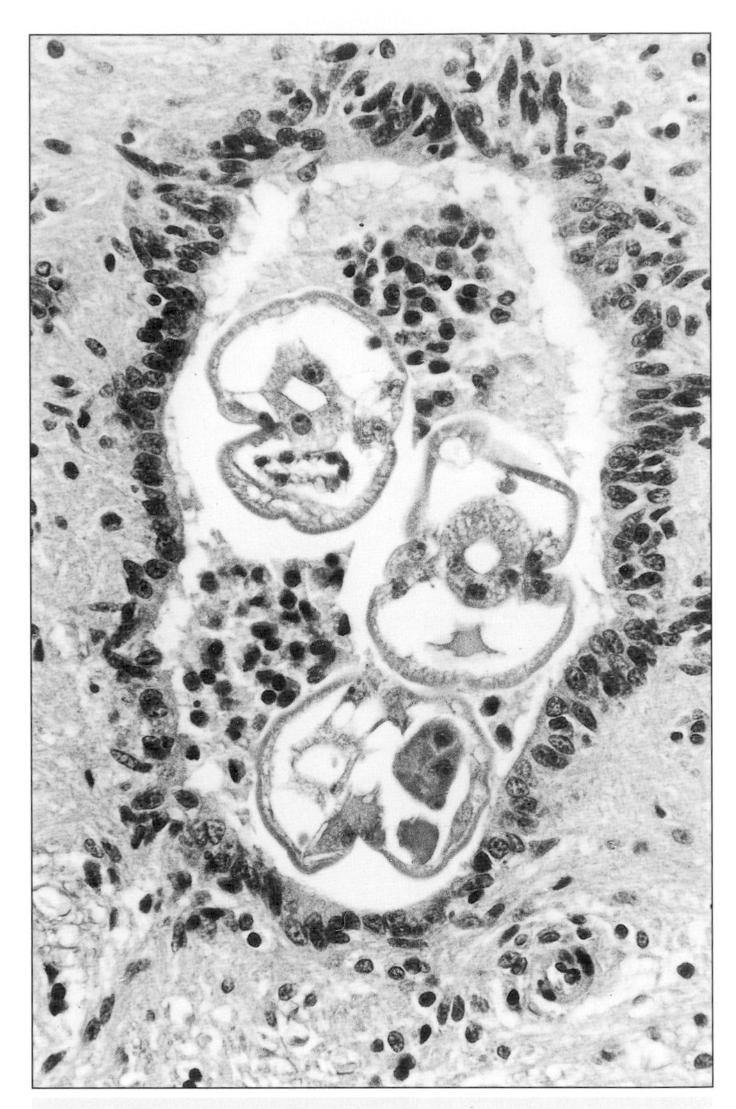

Figure 3.133 Larvae of ***Parastrongylus*** sp. in central canal of spinal cord in a dog.

When larvae of ***Elaeophora schneideri*** – a filarial parasite discussed in the Cardiovascular system – develop in the leptomeningeal arteries of various cervids, sheep and goats, they can cause ischemic necrosis of brain tissue.

Setaria digitata is normally found as an adult in the peritoneal cavity of cattle and buffalo in Asia (see also Peritoneum). Microfilariae can be carried to aberrant hosts such as horses, camels, sheep, and goats by mosquitoes, and larvae wandering in the brain and spinal cord are responsible for the neurological disease known as *kumri* (lumbar paralysis) in Asia. The migrating larvae apparently cause little or no damage in the natural host. The location of the lesions is variable, as are the clinical signs produced. Characteristically, the neurological signs are ataxia, weakness, or paralysis. The severity of the signs varies from slight weakness to quadriplegia, depending on the number and location of the wandering parasites; however, affected animals may remain bright and alert. The CNS lesions produced are fundamentally traumatic, and lead to microcavitation, as described below.

Halicephalobus gingivalis *(Micronema deletrix)* is a free-living nematode that is accidentally, but rarely, a parasite; this nematode is characterized by a rhabditiform esophagus. Massive intracranial invasion is reported in horses. The syndrome is acute and of short

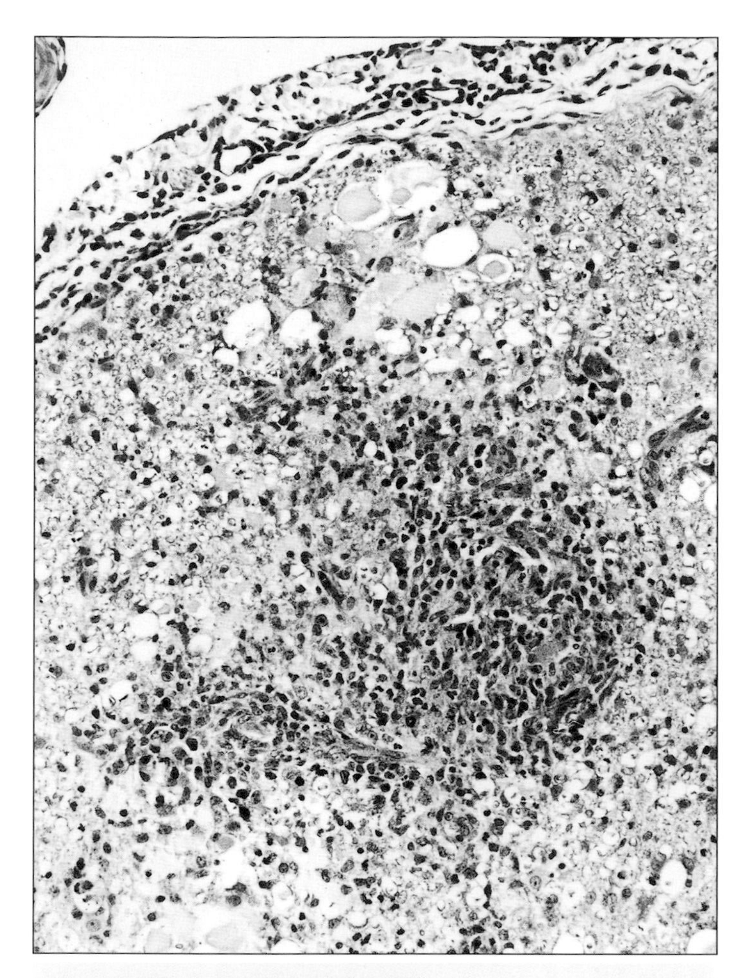

Figure 3.134 Granuloma formation, Wallerian degeneration, and spinal meningitis due to ***Parastrongylus*** infestation in a dog.

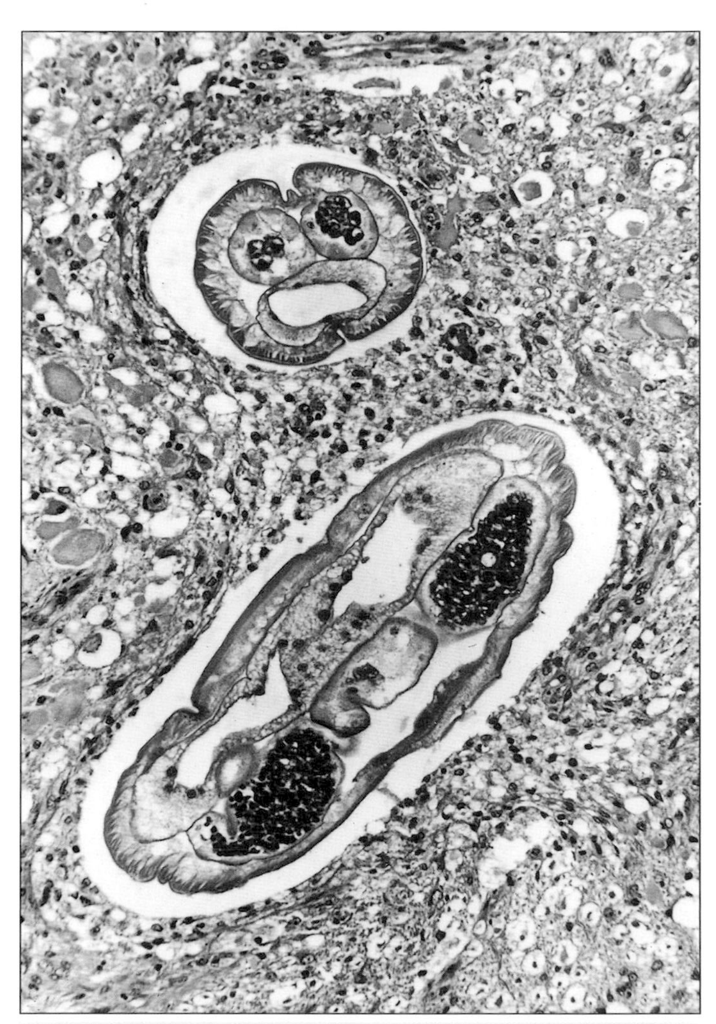

Figure 3.135 ***Parelaphostrongylus*** in spinal cord of a sheep.

duration. There are focal arachnoid hemorrhages and patchy meningeal thickenings. Only parthenogenetic female worms and larvae are found among the specimens in the brain, most easily in perivascular spaces (Fig. 3.136). Depending on the area of the CNS affected, lesions are granulomatous and eosinophilic meningoencephalitis, myelitis, polyradiculitis, or even cauda equine neuritis-like lesions. Parasitic granulomas in the kidney and gingiva may accompany the cerebral invasion. Little is known about the life cycle and method of transmission of this nematode. Oral ingestion or wound contamination then hematogenous distribution is suggested. Also, transmission from infected dam to her foal through milk is described in one case.

Gurltia paralysans, found in the spinal veins of cats, is reported to be responsible for a high incidence of paralysis in this host, and ***Angiostrongylus vasorum*** has caused hemorrhagic malacia in the brains of dogs. Aberrant hosts can develop severe cerebrospinal nematodiasis when they incidentally ingest the eggs of ***Baylisascaris procyonis*** (raccoon ascarid) or *Baylisascaris columnaris* (skunk ascarid).

Larval worms may also migrate aberrantly in the CNS of their natural hosts. ***Stephanurus dentatus*** quite frequently invades the spinal canal and may even encyst in the meninges in pigs. ***Strongylus* spp**. occasionally invade the brains of horses; Figure 3.137 shows the type of lesions that occur, and, although not identified in this case, the larvae were probably of *S. vulgaris* because these were identified in thrombi in the aortic bulb and carotid artery. **Ascarids** have a propensity for wandering in the brain of alien hosts and occasionally do so in their natural hosts.

Trematodes

Trematodes apparently have little tendency to invade nervous tissue. ***Troglotrema acutum*** may invade the brain from its normal habitat in the paranasal sinuses. The eggs of the lung flukes, ***Paragonimus* spp**., have been observed in the brains of dogs, possibly arriving there as emboli.

Arthropods

The only larval arthropods of interest are ***Hypoderma bovis***, which normally migrates through the spinal canal, and ***Oestrus ovis***, which may invade the brain from the nasal sinuses.

Cuterebra spp. (larva of a rodent or rabbit bot) in an abnormal host, i.e., cat and to a lesser extent dog, can undergo aberrant migration and has been reported in many organs including the eyes and CNS. Adult *Cuterebra* are nonparasitic and are seldom observed. Lesions in the brain are characteristic and indicative of vascular compromise and direct toxicity by toxin released from the larvae. These lesions include superficial laminar cerebrocortical necrosis, cerebral

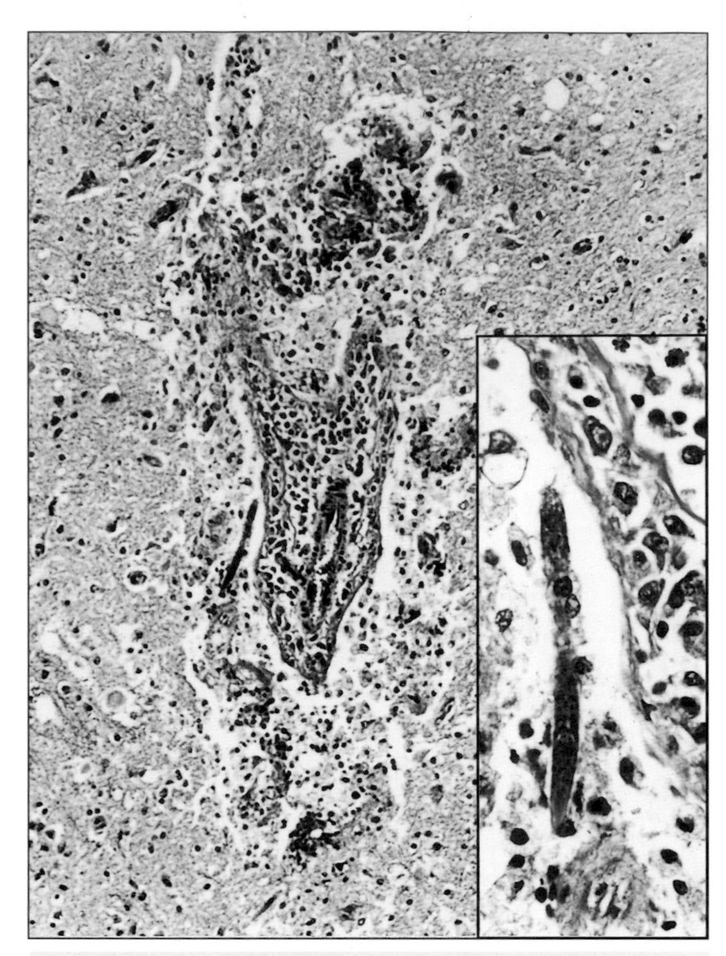

Figure 3.136 Perivascular inflammation in the brain of a horse caused by ***Halicephalobus gingivalis*** (*Micronema deletrix*). Inset: parasite with cellular reaction.

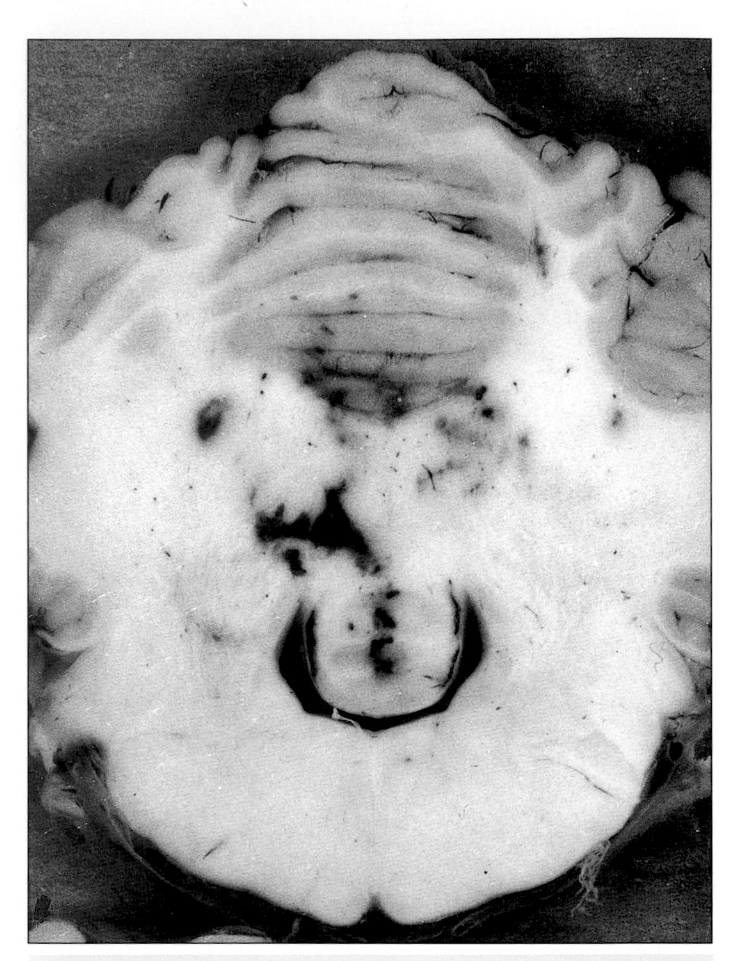

Figure 3.137 Hemorrhagic tracks in cerebellar white matter probably produced by ***Strongylus vulgaris*** in a horse.

(particularly at the olfactory bulbs and peduncles) and subependymal malacia and infarction, and finally larval migratory track lesions that are characterized by focal necrosis, hemorrhage, and infiltration of eosinophils, lymphocytes, plasma cells, and fewer neutrophils. Most of the track lesions are present in caudate nucleus or thalamus. Cuterebral larval migrans in the feline brain is thought to be the cause of *feline ischemic encephalopathy*.

The few parasites specifically mentioned are the most important in terms of neuropathology. Occasionally helminth larvae are discovered accidentally but rarely identified in sections of brain or cord, and it is somewhat more common to find lesions typical of those produced by migratory parasites without being able to locate the parasite. Some parasites, such as *Elaphostrongylus*, usually remain in the CNS whereas others, such as ascarids and strongyles, can be expected to keep moving. Finding the parasite is, therefore, largely a matter of luck, even when it is sought very early after the onset of clinical signs.

The lesions produced in nervous tissue by migratory larvae are mainly *malacic* and, although random, are fairly distinctive in their pattern. *Coenurus cerebralis* produces, in the invasion phase, purulent meningoencephalitis and later acts as a space-occupying lesion, but other invading parasites produce mainly traumatic lesions with very little inflammatory reaction except for a few eosinophils. The lesions produced by nematodes are sometimes grossly visible as *hemorrhagic foci or narrow, slightly tortuous tracks*. Brown, hemorrhagic discoloration depends on the parasite hitting a vein or arteriole, and it appears that some worms have a tendency to migrate along veins. There may be only one or several such tracks in the CNS, and they occur quite at random. Microscopically, the lesion is an irregular focus or pathway of traumatic malacia into which some hemorrhage may have occurred. There may be slight cellular infiltration in the adjacent meninges or nerve roots. The track is liquefied, and its margins not sharp, and apart from lymphocytes, gitter cells, and a few eosinophils, there is no significant reaction in the damaged tissue or in the adjacent vessels. The disruption, which is not selective in the tissues destroyed, leads to *microcavitation*. The disrupted axons, swollen, tortuous and as globose fragments, persist for some time in the microcavitations (Fig. 3.134). Gemistocytic astrocytes may be present in older lesions.

Bibliography

Boyce W, et al. Elaeophorosis in bighorn sheep in New Mexico. J Wildl Dis 1999;35:786–789.

Cooley AJ, et al. Heartworm disease manifested by encephalomyelitis and myositis in a dog. J Am Vet Med Assoc 1987;190:431–432.

Duncan RB Jr, Patton S. Naturally occurring cerebrospinal parelaphostrongylosis in a heifer. J Vet Diagn Invest 1998;10:287–291.

Furuoka H, et al. Neuropathological observation of rabbits (*Oryctolagus cuniculus*) affected with raccoon roundworm (*Baylisascaris procyonis*) larva migrans in Japan. J Vet Med Sci 2003;65:695–699.

Handeland K, et al. Experimental *Elaphostrongylus cervi* infection in sheep and goats. J Comp Pathol 2000;123:248–257.

Innes JRM, Pillai CP. Kumri, so-called lumbar paralysis of horses in Ceylon (India and Burma) and its identification with cerebrospinal nematodiases. Br Vet J 1955;111:223–235.

Johnson JS, et al. Radiculomeningomyelitis due to *Halicephalobus gingivalis* in a horse. Vet Pathol 2001;38:559–561.

Little PB. Cerebrospinal nematodiasis in Equidae. J Am Vet Med Assoc 1972;160:1407–1413.

Lunn J, et al. Antemortem diagnosis of canine neural angiostrongylosis using ELISA. Aust Vet J 2003;81:128–131.

Mahmoud OM, et al. An outbreak of neurofilariosis in young goats. Vet Parasitol 2004;120:151–156.

Mason KV. Canine neural angiostrongylosis: the clinical and therapeutic features of 55 natural cases. Aust Vet J 1987;64:201–203.

Nagy DW. *Parelaphostrongylus tenuis* and other parasitic diseases of the ruminant nervous system. Vet Clin North Am Food Anim Pract 2004;20:393–412.

Okolo MI. Cerebral cysticercosis in rural dogs. Microbios 1986;47:189–191.

Sartin EA, et al. Cerebral cuterebrosis in a dog. J Am Vet Med Assoc 1986;189:1338–1339.

Rudmann DG, et al. *Baylisascaris procyonis* larva migrans in a puppy: a case report and update for the veterinarian. J Am Anim Hosp Assoc 1996;32:73–76.

Tung KC, et al. Cerebrospinal setariosis with *Setaria marshalli* and *Setaria digitata* infection in cattle. J Vet Med Sci 2003;65:977–983.

Wilkins PA, et al. Evidence for transmission of *Halicephalobus deletrix (H gingivalis)* from dam to foal. J Vet Intern Med 2001;15:412–417.

Williams KJ, et al. Cerebrospinal cuterebriasis in cats and its association with feline ischemic encephalopathy. Vet Pathol 1998;35:330–343.

Wright JD, et al. Equine neural angiostrongylosis. Aust Vet J 1991;68:58–60.

Chlamydial disease

Sporadic bovine encephalomyelitis (SBE) occurs in calves less than 6 months of age, and is caused by ***Chlamydophila pecorum***. Identical disease is also reported due to infection with *Chlamydophila psittaci*. *Chlamydophila pecorum* also causes a wide range of other conditions in calves, including polyarthritis, metritis, conjunctivitis, and pneumonia. The disease occurs in the USA, Japan, Europe, and Australia; the agent probably has a worldwide distribution and most infections are asymptomatic. Encephalomyelitis is reported to occur naturally only in cattle and buffalo. As a rule, SBE is indeed sporadic, affecting only a few animals in a herd, however outbreaks of the disease with morbidity of 25% are described. Transmission appears to be by direct contact. The clinical syndrome is not particularly characteristic. It is composed of moderate fever and signs of catarrhal inflammation of the respiratory tract. There is some stiffness, weakness of the hindlimbs with staggering and knuckling of the fetlocks, and muscle tremors. There is some dullness; signs of excitement are not present. Death occurs in a few days to a few weeks.

The organism has a tropism for blood vessels, mesenchymal tissue and serous membranes, which make *vasculitis and polyserositis the hallmark of lesions*. Encephalitis is secondary to vascular damage. The gross morbid change that suggests a diagnosis of SBE is serofibrinous inflammation of serous membranes and synoviae. This is most consistently *peritonitis*, and in ~50% of fatal cases there is also *pleuritis and pericarditis*. The meninges appear congested and edematous and occasionally are covered with a few fibrin tags. Microscopically, there is a rather *severe and diffuse meningoencephalomyelitis* (see Fig. 3.60). The leptomeningitis is most severe about the base of the brain. The reactive cells are almost solely histiocytes and plasma cells, with only a few neutrophils. These cells infiltrate the meninges and perivascular spaces and mix with reactive adventitial cells of the vessel walls. The vascular endothelium proliferates secondary to lesions in the vascular walls, and ischemic changes may occur in the parenchyma. Reactive microglial nodules are widespread in the brain.

Cell culture of *Chlamydophila*, the gold standard diagnostic tool, is being displaced by detection by PCR. Elementary bodies produced by this organism occur in the cytoplasm of mononuclear cells in the exudates in the meninges and from serosal membranes and in microglia of nodules, but they are not numerous and their demonstration by special stains or immunohistochemistry is not usually rewarding.

Bibliography

Jee J, et al. High prevalence of natural *Chlamydophila* species infection in calves. J Clin Microbiol 2004;42:5664–5672.

Longbottom D. Chlamydial infections of domestic ruminants and swine: new nomenclature and new knowledge. Vet J 2004;168:9–11.

Piercy DW, et al. Encephalitis related to *Chlamydia psittaci* infection in a 14-week-old calf. Vet Rec 1999;144:126–128.

Idiopathic inflammatory diseases

Necrotizing meningoencephalitis of Pug and other small breed dogs

Canine necrotizing meningoencephalitis (NME), formerly "Pug dog encephalitis," is an idiopathic disease affecting mainly Pug dogs, but also reported rarely in Maltese, Pekingese, Shih Tzu, and Chihuahua. A similar condition, but with lesions more prevalent in the white matter, is reported in Yorkshire Terriers (distinct from *Yorkshire Terrier necrotizing encephalopathy*, which affects brain stem), named necrotizing leukoencephalitis. The cause of NME is unknown; several etiologic agents have been suggested as causes, including alpha-herpesvirus, but none has been confirmed. An autoimmune reaction against canine brain tissue has been suggested as a possible mechanism. A wide age range is affected. Generalized convulsions and their aftermath dominate the clinical picture, which may include lethargy, ataxia, and progression to coma. The clinical signs refer essentially to cortical disease that progresses rapidly over a few weeks, but which may extend to several months.

The lesions are particularly in the cerebral cortex, and are bilateral but asymmetric, often confluent over large areas, and extend to the adjacent white matter with relative sparing of the deeper periventricular tissue. The geography of the lesions therefore helps to distinguish this disease from other encephalitides of the dog. Grossly, localized swellings in the cerebrum contribute to asymmetry, and malacic foci may be seen as typical yellow areas of softening (Fig. 3.138) or, in cases of longer duration, as tiny cystic cavities.

The histological changes are necrotizing and with an affinity for the hemispheres. Numerous foci of meningitis, characterized by infiltrations of lymphocytes, plasma cells, and monocytes (Fig. 3.139), diminish caudally and may be absent in the caudal fossa and spinal cord. These infiltrates breach the pial barrier and destroy the superficial cortex to an extent and severity that is unusual. The evidence of

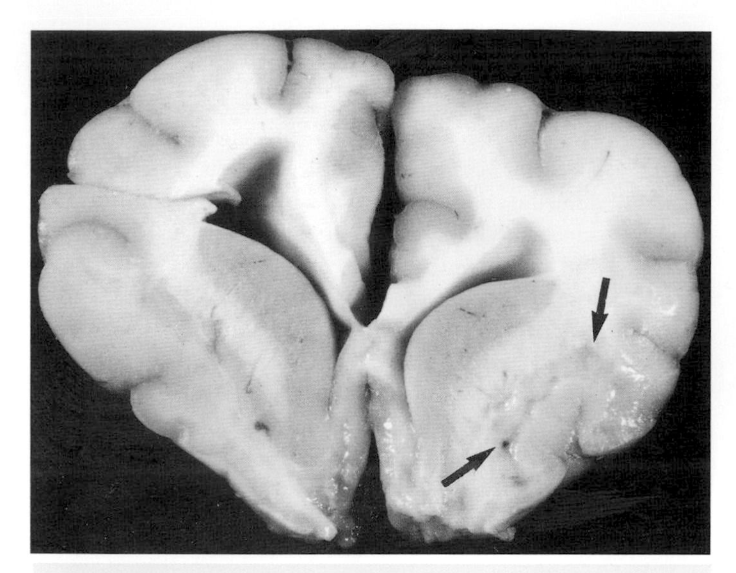

Figure 3.138 Malacic focus in ventrolateral cerebral hemisphere (arrows) in **Canine necrotizing meningoencephalitis**. (Reprinted with permission from Bradley GA. Vet Pathol 1991;28:91.)

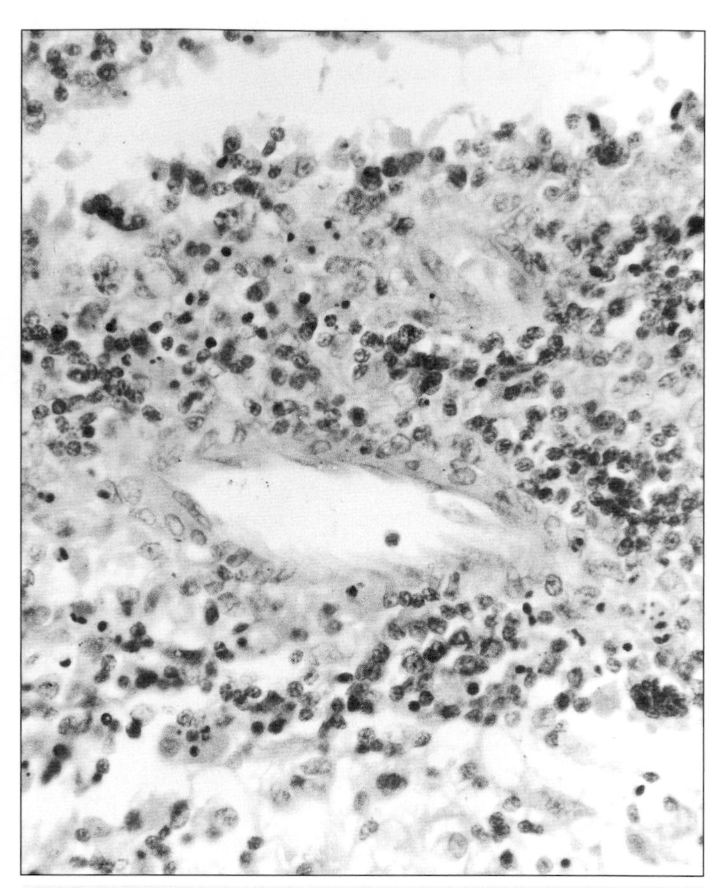

Figure 3.139 Meningeal arteriole surrounded by mixed mononuclear infiltrate in **Canine necrotizing meningoencephalitis**.

cerebral necrosis extends from selective neuronal necrosis to areas of malacia, the latter especially in chronic cases. Vascular endothelium in the cortex is reactive and associated with edema, occasional petechiae, and diffuse accumulation of mononuclear cells in parenchyma and vascular cuffs.

The differential features of this meningoencephalitis, in addition to its nonsuppurative nature, are the malacic degenerations and predilection for the cerebral cortex. This condition must be differentiated also from granulomatous meningoencephalomyelitis (GME). The inflammatory infiltrate in GME contains more histiocytes, which in the chronic stage transform to epithelioid cells that can form discrete cohesive sheets or granuloma-like lesions. Also, in GME, the reaction is predominantly in the white matter and is distributed in almost all parts of the CNS. In contrast, the reaction in NME is mostly in the cortical gray matter.

Bibliography

Cantile C, et al. Necrotizing meningoencephalitis associated with cortical hippocampal hamartia in a Pekingese dog. Vet Pathol 2001;38:119–122.

Hinrichs U, et al. A case of necrotizing meningoencephalitis in a pug dog (pug dog encephalitis–PDE). Tierarztl Prax 1996;24:489–492.

Granulomatous meningoencephalomyelitis

Granulomatous meningoencephalomyelitis (GME) is a sporadic disease of the CNS of dogs. GME appears to have a worldwide distribution and to occur mostly in *young to middle-aged dogs of small breeds*, e.g., terriers and toy breeds, however the disease can occur in any breed and in an age range of 6 months to 12 years. The cause of GME is unknown; several infectious causes have been suggested but not confirmed to be the cause of this condition. Based on the predominance of CD3+ T cells and MHC class II antigen-positive macrophages, an immune-mediated mechanism has been proposed.

Variations in the distribution and extent of the lesions result in a variety of clinical signs. Spinal lesions may be associated with ataxia, paresis, or paralysis (Fig. 3.140). Lesions in the brain stem frequently produce signs of vestibular dysfunction. Changes of behavior, forced movement and circling, depression and convulsions occur with supratentorial lesions. Macroscopic lesions, if evident, consist of gray-white discoloration of the white matter of the brain or spinal cord, and in those cases in which the cellular aggregations become confluent, there may be irregular areas of malacia (Fig. 3.141).

The histologic changes are patchy in distribution. There may be very few foci, or they may be disseminated, or they may be localized to one area and confluent, or there may, in the same animal, be both confluent and disseminated distributions. *The essential histologic feature is perivascular aggregation of cells rather selectively in the white matter.* The minimal lesion is cuffing of vessels by lymphocytes and plasma cells with small eccentric clumps of macrophages. The macrophages increase in number and may come to comprise the cuff, appearing as discrete granulomas, which, depending on the plane of section, may appear to be in the parenchyma. Occasional mitoses are present in these cells. Transformation to epithelioid cells occurs later. The perivascular aggregates expand in concentric arrangements and displace surrounding parenchyma (Fig. 3.142). Where the cuffing response is severe, edema and necrosis may occur in the adjacent white matter leading to a spillover of mononuclear cells into the parenchyma and to the usual reactive changes. Large malacic foci are unusual. In cases of prolonged duration, confluence of lesions occurs and reparative responses include the deposition of abundant reticulin and collagen in perivascular arrangements. Involvement of meninges is patchy and often related to lesions of white matter directly underlying.

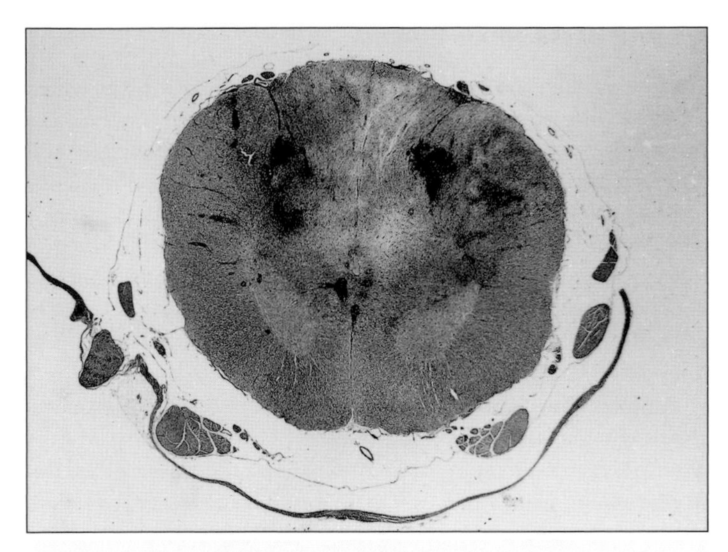

Figure 3.140 Focal lesions in the spinal cord of a dog with **granulomatous encephalitis**. (Courtesy of JB Thomas.)

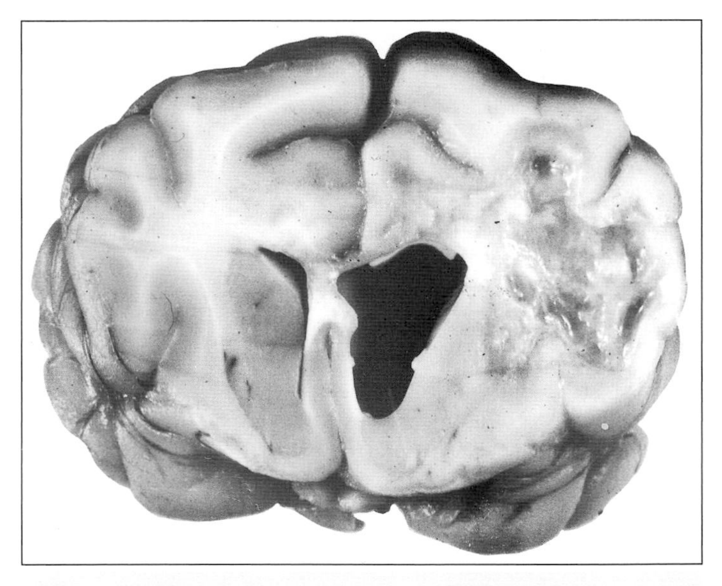

Figure 3.141 Malacia of cerebrum and hydrocephalus secondary to infarction in a dog with **granulomatous encephalitis**.

Cytological characterization of the cell aggregates can be difficult. In many, and perhaps most, cases, the cells are easy to classify, being well differentiated as lymphocytes, monocytes, plasma cells, and histiocytes (Fig. 3.143). Granulocytes may be present but are not numerous, and histiocytes often show epithelioid transformation and may form small syncytial masses. There may also be in some cases large immature cells of reticulohistiocytic type in which mitoses may be few or many. Differentiation between GME and brain malignant histiocytosis (BMH) can be problematic occasionally; BMH is frequently part of a multisystemic tumor and rarely occurs in isolation. Also, the absence of cellular atypia and the predominance of perivascular orientation should favor the diagnosis of GME.

Bibliography

Kipar A, et al. Immunohistochemical characterization of inflammatory cells in brains of dogs with granulomatous meningoencephalitis. Vet Pathol 1998;35:43–52.

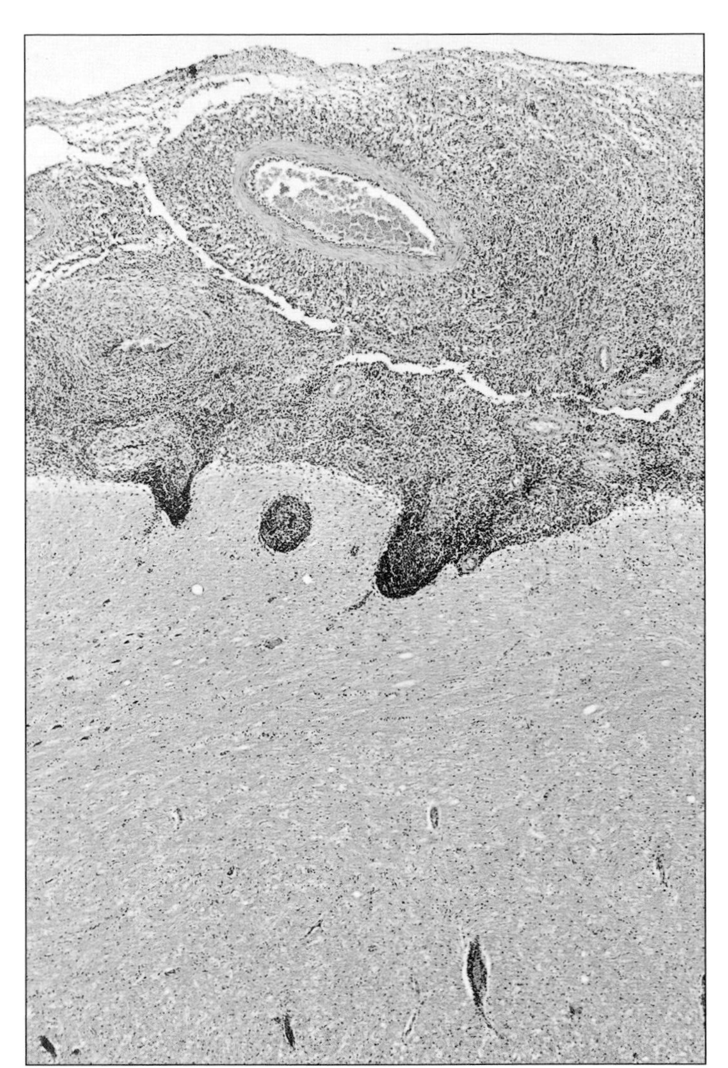

Figure 3.142 Dense perivascular meningeal infiltrate in **granulomatous encephalitis** in a dog.

Munana KR, Luttgen PJ. Prognostic factors for dogs with granulomatous meningoencephalomyelitis: 42 cases (1982–1996). J Am Vet Med Assoc 1998;212:1902–1906.

Suzuki M, et al. A comparative pathological study on granulomatous meningoencephalomyelitis and central malignant histiocytosis in dogs. J Vet Med Sci 2003;65:1319–1324.

Thomas JB, Eger C. Granulomatous meningoencephalomyelitis in 21 dogs. J Small Anim Pract 1989;30:287–293.

Acute polyradiculoneuritis (coonhound paralysis)

Acute polyradiculoneuritis, or polyradiculoneuropathy, affects primarily dogs, occasionally cats, and rarely horses, and has many similarities to Guillain-Barré syndrome in humans. The condition was named coonhound paralysis to reflect the fact that some affected dogs had been bitten or scratched by raccoons, although cases may have no known exposure to raccoons. Within 7–10 days, ascending flaccid paralysis, starting in the hindlimbs and progressing cranially to involve the forelimbs, leads to quadriplegia and rapid atrophy of muscle. There are no cerebral signs. Some dogs die of respiratory paralysis, but most will recover slowly if nursing is adequate. Dogs that have

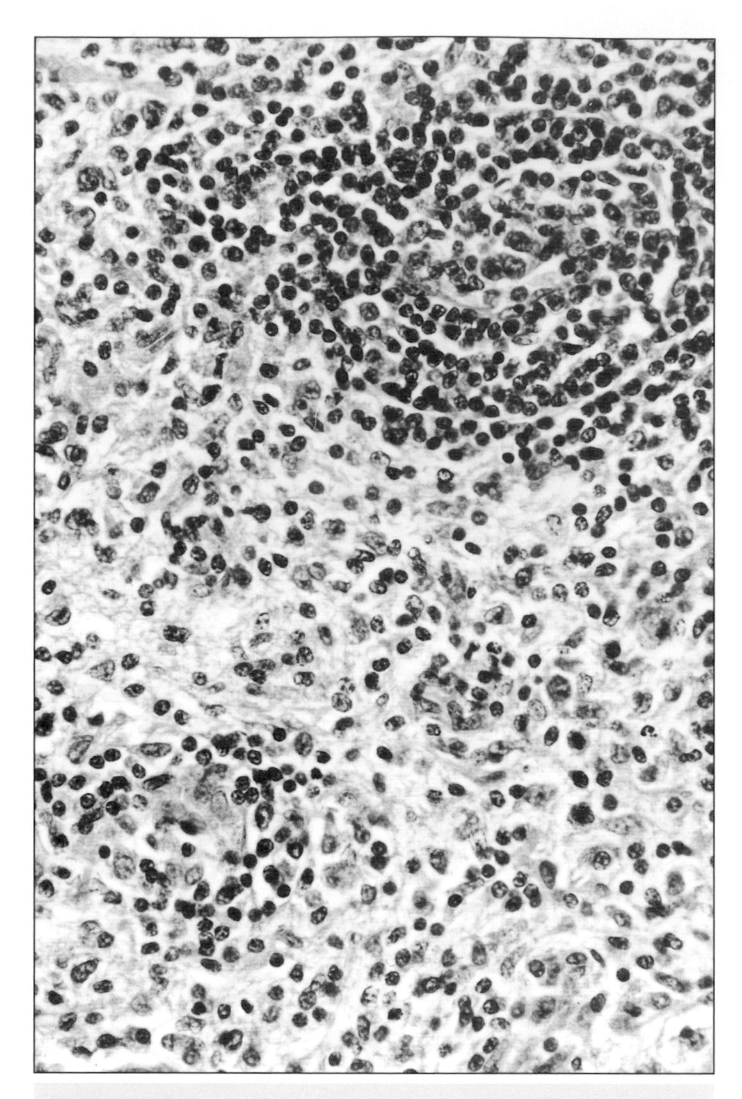

Figure 3.143 Detail of cellular infiltrate in brain in **granulomatous encephalitis** in a dog.

recovered appear to have increased sensitivity to subsequent exposure but may survive several bouts of paralysis. The disease has been transmitted using pooled saliva of raccoons, but the cause has not been identified; an autoimmune mechanism is suspected. Lesions are found in the *ventral roots of spinal nerves and in peripheral nerves*. Mononuclear and plasma cells infiltrate around venules, but the extent of the infiltrate is variable and not correlated with the course of the illness or the severity of nerve degeneration. There is primary and Wallerian degeneration afflicting ventral roots in particular, with axonal reaction in motor neurons and atrophy of denervation in muscle. This idiopathic polyradiculoneuritis is the most common inflammatory condition of peripheral nerves in dogs.

Bibliography

Cuddon PA. Electrophysiologic assessment of acute polyradiculoneuropathy in dogs: comparison with Guillain-Barré syndrome in people. J Vet Intern Med 1998;12:294–303.

Cummings JF, et al. Coonhound paralysis. Further clinical studies and electron microscopic observations. Acta Neuropathol (Berl) 1982;56:167–178.

Neuritis of the cauda equina

Neuritis of the cauda equina of horses is a polyneuritis in which the presenting signs are referable to the sacrococcygeal nerves and include perineal anesthesia, tail paralysis, urinary incontinence, fecal retention, weakness, atrophy of coccygeal muscles and, in longstanding cases, atrophy of the muscles of the hindlimbs. The neuritis is progressive. The cause is unknown, but the nature of the reaction suggests immune mediation, which may follow viral infection. The condition has been compared to experimental allergic neuritis in laboratory animals. *Halicephalobus gingivalis* is reported as a novel cause of cauda equina neuritis in one horse.

Although the pathologic changes emphasize the *sacral and caudal spinal nerve roots*, there may simultaneously be asymmetric pareses of other nerves producing isolated limb pareses, and paresis or paralysis referable to cranial nerves. The lesions in these other nerves are similar in character to, but much milder than, those in caudal nerve roots. Inflammatory changes are present in sensory and some autonomic ganglia, but changes in the spinal cord are limited to those that reflect peripheral nerve injury.

The gross changes affect in particular the extradural parts of the sacral and coccygeal nerves and may extend through the intervertebral foraminae into the adjacent muscle. The roots are thickened and fusiform and usually discolored by recent or old hemorrhage. The intradural segments of affected nerves are discolored but not usually enlarged.

Microscopically there is *granulomatous inflammation with extensive fibrosis*. The thickening and discoloration are attributable to hemorrhage, proliferation of epineural tissue, and inflammatory cell infiltrates. The infiltrating lymphocytes, plasma cells and macrophages are frequently disposed as to form granulomas, often with central epithelioid and giant cells; granulocytes do not feature in the infiltrates. Degenerative and regenerative changes are present in the myelin and axons of affected roots and appear to be more closely associated with endoneurial and perineurial fibroplasia than with leukocytic infiltrates.

Bibliography

Cummings JF, et al. Neuritis of the cauda equina, a chronic idiopathic polyradiculoneuritis in the horse. Acta Neuropathol (Berl) 1979;46:17–24.

Johnson JS, et al. Radiculomeningomyelitis due to *Halicephalobus gingivalis* in a horse. Vet Pathol 2001;38:559–561.

Wright JA, et al. Neuritis of the cauda equina in the horse. J Comp Pathol 1987;97:667–675.

Steroid-responsive meningitis-arteritis (Beagle pain syndrome)

Steroid-responsive meningitis-arteritis (SRMA) is a *polyarteritis of possible immune-mediated origin affecting mainly small to medium-sized leptomeningeal and myocardial arteries*, but arteries in many organs can be affected. Beagles, especially those in laboratory-bred colonies, are at high risk, but the disease is reported in Boxers, German Shorthaired Pointers, Nova Scotia Duck-tolling Retrievers, and rarely in other breeds. Affected dogs have fever, hyperesthesia, severe pain on manipulation, cervical rigidity, and anorexia. The clinical course of SRMA is usually acute, but a chronic form exists. Gross lesions are minimal, but areas of subarachnoid hemorrhage may be present along the brain stem and the spinal cord, especially the cervical part. Histologically, small to medium-sized leptomeningeal arteries, especially of the brain stem and spinal cord, and to a lesser extent heart and cranial mediastinum, have moderate to severe perivascular and transmural infiltrates of lymphocytes, plasma cells, histiocytes, and fewer neutrophils. Occasionally, neutrophils predominate. Also, there is severe fibrinoid necrosis, thrombosis, and occasionally periarterial fibrosis. Mild lymphocytic and histiocytic leptomeningitis is also a constant finding.

Distinct from SRMA, an unusual case of idiopathic vasculitis resembling "*isolated angiitis of the CNS*" in humans has been reported in a mixed-breed dog. The necrotizing vasculitis, with cuffs of mixed cell types including multinucleated giant cells, resulted in localized cerebral necrosis.

Bibliography

Sasaki M, et al. Vasculitis in a dog resembling isolated angiitis of the central nervous system in humans. Vet Pathol 2003;40:95–97.

Snyder PW, et al. Pathologic features of naturally occurring juvenile polyarteritis in beagle dogs. Vet Pathol 1995;32:337–345.

Shaker dog disease

Shaker dog disease is an idiopathic condition characterized clinically by *tremors* that worsen after stress or excitement. The condition was described first affecting solely young adult white-haired small dogs (little white shakers), but now is recognized in dogs of any size or coat color. Histologically, *mild diffuse, nonsuppurative encephalomyelitis* is present. No myelin disease is present.

Bibliography

Vanvooren N. A suspected case of idiopathic generalised tremor (shaker disease) in a shih tzu. Vet Rec 1995;136:568.

Yamaya Y, et al. A case of shaker dog disease in a miniature Dachshund. J Vet Med Sci 2004;66:1159–1160.

Sensory ganglioneuritis (sensory ganglioradiculitis)

Sensory ganglioneuritis (sensory neuronopathy) is a rare idiopathic disease of adult dogs characterized by *nonsuppurative inflammation of dorsal root (sensory) spinal ganglia and cranial sensory ganglia* with degeneration and necrosis of sensory neuronal cell bodies and proliferation of ganglionic satellite cells. The cause may be a cell-mediated immune mechanism. Secondary to sensory ganglion neuronal injury, Wallerian degeneration develops in the dorsal funiculi (fasciculus cuneatus and fasciculus gracilis) and the affected areas appear grossly as white V-shaped or triangular areas throughout the entire length of the spinal cord. Similar but milder lesions can be present in sympathetic ganglia, peripheral nerves, myenteric plexi, motor roots, and the spinal tract of the trigeminal nerve. Breed or sex predilection have not been observed. Clinical signs are variable and include generalized sensory ataxia, depression or absence of spinal reflexes, facial hypalgesia/paresthesia, megaesophagus, and dysphagia. Masticatory muscle atrophy is observed in a few dogs in association with this condition and is attributed to loss of motor fibers as they course through the trigeminal ganglion.

Bibliography

Cummings JF, et al. Ganglioradiculitis in the dog. A clinical, light- and electron-microscopic study. Acta Neuropathol (Berl) 1983;60(1–2):29–39.

Porter B, et al. Ganglioradiculitis (sensory neuronopathy) in a dog: clinical, morphologic, and immunohistochemical findings. Vet Pathol 2002;39:598–602.

Post-infectious encephalomyelitis

Neurological disease that follows, after a variable period, common viral infections or vaccination exposure is well known in children as post-infectious or post-vaccinal encephalitis, or acute disseminated encephalomyelitis. The common pathologic basis is a *demyelinating inflammatory process dominated by mononuclear inflammatory cells with a distinctive perivenous distribution*. Examples that meet the criteria have occurred in relation to rabies vaccination in dogs when such vaccines were prepared in neural tissue, and the pathologic process is the same as that in experimental allergic encephalomyelitis. The histologic changes are widely distributed in the brain and cord and affect mainly the white matter. Perivascular infiltrates of lymphocytes, plasma cells, and monocytes/macrophages widely distend the space and spread into the surrounding parenchyma. Proliferation of adventitial cells may be prominent. Although much descriptive emphasis has been given to demyelination, this is restricted to the perivascular areas of infiltration and to surrounding areas showing the usual degenerative and reactive changes.

Bibliography

Bennetto L, Scolding N. Inflammatory/post-infectious encephalomyelitis. J Neurol Neurosurg Psychiatry 2004;75(Suppl 1):22–28.

Shoenfeld Y, Aron-Maor A. Vaccination and autoimmunity-"vaccinosis": a dangerous liaison? J Autoimmun 2000;14:1–10.

Eosinophilic meningoencephalitis

Recognized causes of eosinophilic meningoencephalitis include nematode and protozoan parasites. **Idiopathic eosinophilic meningoencephalitis** has been reported in dogs, with Rottweilers and Golden Retrievers over-represented, and one cat. The condition is characterized clinically by behavioral changes such as inappropriate urination and lack of response to commands. In severe cases, episodes of sternal or lateral recumbency without loss of consciousness are described. Clinical pathology findings are mild to moderate peripheral blood eosinophilia and CSF pleocytosis with predominance of eosinophils. Grossly, there is thickening and green discoloration of the meninges. Histologic changes are those of eosinophilic and granulomatous meningitis of the cortex and cerebellum, and the underlying neural parenchyma appears pallid, occasionally spongiotic, and has mild eosinophilic and histiocytic cuffing with rare areas of axonal swelling and neuronal degeneration. Spinal cord lesions are poorly documented. The condition is usually responsive to steroid treatment, suggesting an immune-mediated mechanism.

Bibliography

Bennett PF, et al. Idiopathic eosinophilic meningoencephalitis in rottweiler dogs: three cases (1992–1997). Aust Vet J 1997;75:786–789.

Smith-Maxie LL, et al. Cerebrospinal fluid analysis and clinical outcome of eight dogs with eosinophilic meningoencephalomyelitis. J Vet Intern Med 1989;3:167–174.

Granulomatous radiculitis of the seventh and eighth cranial nerves of calves

This is a rare condition affecting young calves and characterized clinically by facial paralysis and pathologically by the presence of multifocal granulomas affecting mainly the roots of cranial nerves VII and VIII. The etiology is unknown; however, *Mycoplasma bovis* was suggested as a cause because some affected calves had concurrent mycoplasmal otitis media.

Bibliography

Maenhout D, et al. Space occupying lesions of cranial nerves in calves with facial paralysis. Vet Rec 1984;115:407–410.

Van der Lugt JJ, Jordaan P. Facial paralysis associated with space occupying lesions of cranial nerves in calves. Vet Rec 1994;134:579–580.

NEOPLASTIC DISEASES OF THE NERVOUS SYSTEM

Primary neoplastic disease of the CNS of animals is rare in species other than the dog and cat. Neoplasms derived from virtually every cell type in the nervous system are recorded.

The tumors may be *congenital*, and these do not differ in their characteristics from similar tumors in adult animals with the possible exceptions of: medulloblastoma, which is thought to be derived from the residual cells of the external granular layer of the cerebellum; craniopharyngiomas, which are thought to arise from remnants of Rathke's pouch, which forms the adenohypophysis; chordoma, which is thought to arise from remnants of notochord; intracranial teratoma, which is probably derived from germ cells; and cystic epidermoid tumors, which are thought to result from the inclusion of surface ectodermal cells at the time of closure of the neural groove. The relatively high incidence of tumors in Boxers and Boston Terriers may indicate a hereditary predisposition, which these breeds also have for endocrine neoplasia. The introduction of computerized tomography (CT) and magnetic resonance imaging (MRI), in addition to the use of immunohistochemistry, have improved our understanding of CNS tumors in various domestic animals and have helped in reaching more accurate diagnoses. Neoplasms of the CNS rarely metastasize to extraneural tissue, and their clinical importance depends on their destructive effect on host neural tissue and the resulting neurologic deficits.

The conventional tumors of the CNS are discussed here and classified according to the current histological classification published by the Armed Forces Institute of Pathology (AFIP) in cooperation with the World Health Organization (WHO). Tumors of the pituitary and nonchromaffin paraganglia are discussed with the Endocrine system.

Tumors of neuroepithelial tissue

Astrocytoma

Astrocytoma is the most common primary intracranial tumor (Fig. 3.144A–E). Astrocytomas are found most commonly in dogs, but are reported also in cats and cattle, and may occur in the brain or cord but are more prevalent in cerebrum, thalamus, hypothalamus, and midbrain. In dogs, astrocytomas are common in brachycephalic breeds but can occur in any breed. Astrocytomas have no age predilection, but are more prevalent in middle-aged or older dogs. The gross appearance varies, depending largely on the degree of malignancy. These tumors can be very difficult to detect grossly, especially when they involve white matter or grow slowly. They are then white and, because of their firmness, may be more readily palpable than visible. Their presence may be suspected only by deviation of some architectural feature (Fig. 3.144B, D). Larger and more malignant tumors are prone to vascular accidents and necrosis, and they are then easy to see (Fig. 3.144E), but the margins are never discrete, especially not when they are surrounded by edematous tissue. The extent of the tumor is always much greater than can be appreciated grossly.

Histologically, these tumors are very diverse and are classified as *low-grade astrocytoma* (well differentiated), *medium-grade astrocytoma* (anaplastic), and *high-grade astrocytoma* (glioblastoma).

Low-grade astrocytoma appears as an unencapsulated expansile and subtly invasive mass that replaces pre-existing tissues and has low to moderate numbers of bland round to oval cells. In most cases, the neoplasm appears as an increased population of fibrous astrocytes that individually are not clearly malignant (Fig. 3.144A). Variants of this neoplasm include **fibrillary astrocytoma** (neoplastic cells have scant cytoplasm but abundant fibrillary processes and filaments), **protoplasmic astrocytoma** (neoplastic cells have scant cytoplasm and few short processes and filaments), **gemistocytic astrocytoma** (neoplastic cells have abundant acidophilic cytoplasm and eccentric oval to round nuclei; Fig. 3.144C). Another variant, the **pilocytic astrocytoma** (neoplastic cells are bipolar, elongated (piloid or hair-like) astrocytes and have few Rosenthal fibers), has been reported in both dogs and cats.

In **medium-grade astrocytoma**, the population is denser; the nuclei are a little larger and darker and show slight but definite variations in size and shape but no mitoses. The cells are recognizable as astrocytes. The walls of the vessels may be slightly thickened.

In **high-grade astrocytoma**, or *glioblastoma multiforme*, hemorrhage and necrosis are expected and the adventitial and endothelial cells of the vessels proliferate forming glomeruloid blood vessels. Generally, only a few cells are recognizable as astrocytes. Neoplastic cells have a tendency for pseudopalisading around necrotic areas. Pleomorphism, giant nuclei, and multinucleated giant cells are common. Mitotic figures are common and atypical.

Astrocytomas exhibit positive immunostaining for glial fibrillary acidic protein (GFAP), S-100 protein, and vimentin. The staining pattern for GFAP varies from sparse to abundant.

Oligodendroglioma

This is the easiest of the glial tumors to recognize even when growing rapidly. This tumor is reported in dogs especially in brachycephalic breeds and rarely in cats. Grossly, it usually appears well demarcated, being gray, soft, and almost fluctuating (Fig. 3.145A). Hemorrhage and necrosis occur but are unusual. The tumor is densely cellular with almost no stroma. The nuclei are remarkably uniform and like those of normal oligodendroglia in size and shape. The cytoplasm does not stain, but its membrane does, so that the nucleus seems to lie in a clear

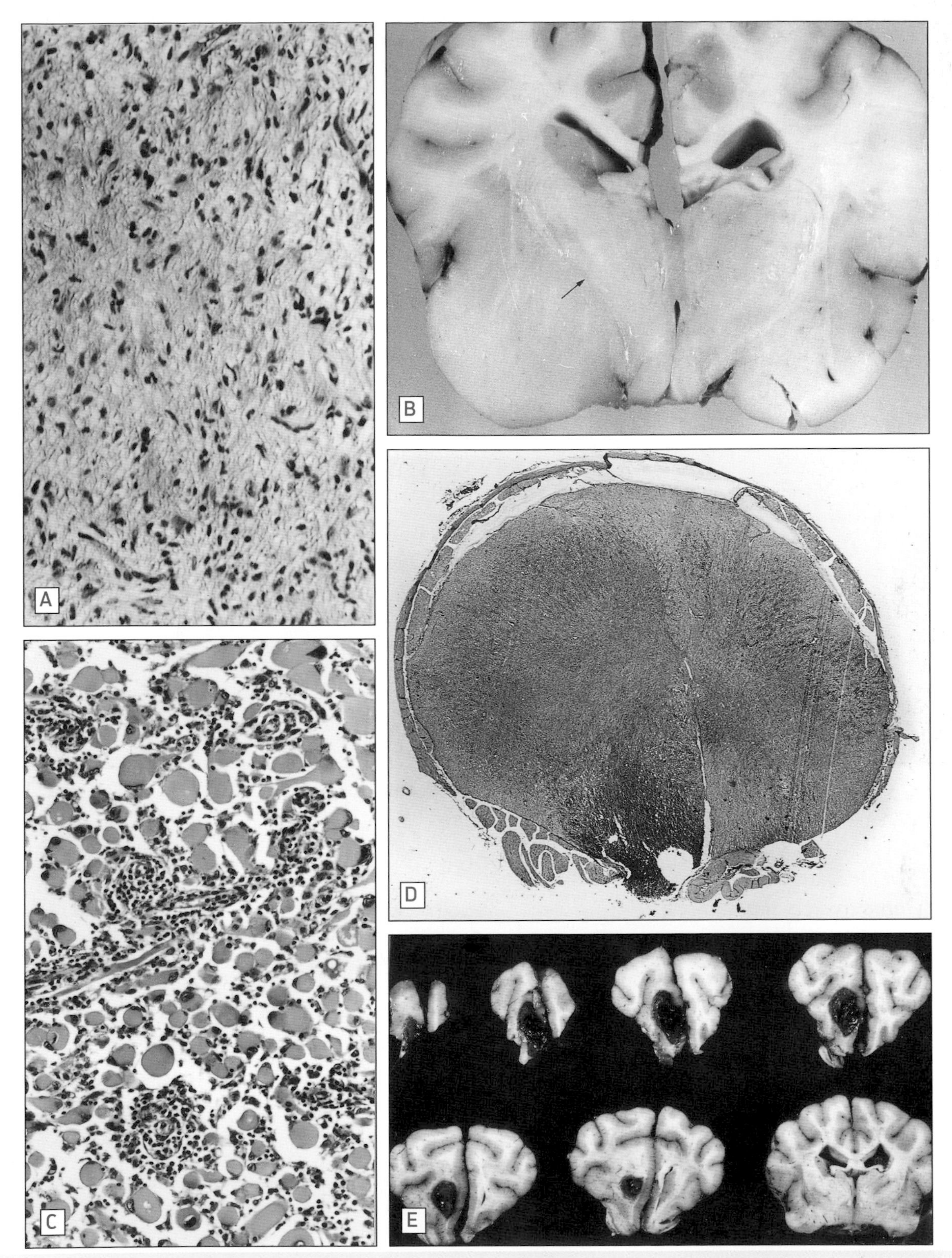

Figure 3.144 **A. Fibrous astrocytoma** in a dog. **B. Astrocytoma** in piriform lobe in a dog. Note lack of definition but displacement of internal capsule (arrow) by the homogeneous tumor. **C. Gemistocytic astrocytoma** in a dog. **D. Astrocytoma** of spinal cord in a dog. **E. Hemorrhagic astrocytoma** of left frontal lobe in a dog.

polyhedral or rounded halo (honeycomb cell pattern) (Fig. 3.145B). These tumors occur in white matter, and those near the third ventricle may contain areas distinguishable as astrocytoma or ependymoma. Blood vessels may proliferate especially at neoplasm margins to form glomeruli-like vessels. Mucinous degeneration and cyst formation may occur in these tumors and mineralization may occur in some of them. There are no clear indices of malignancy, although all must be regarded as malignant. Oligodendrogliomas do not stain with GFAP; however, the neoplastic cells are usually intermingled with some astrocytes that readily stain with GFAP.

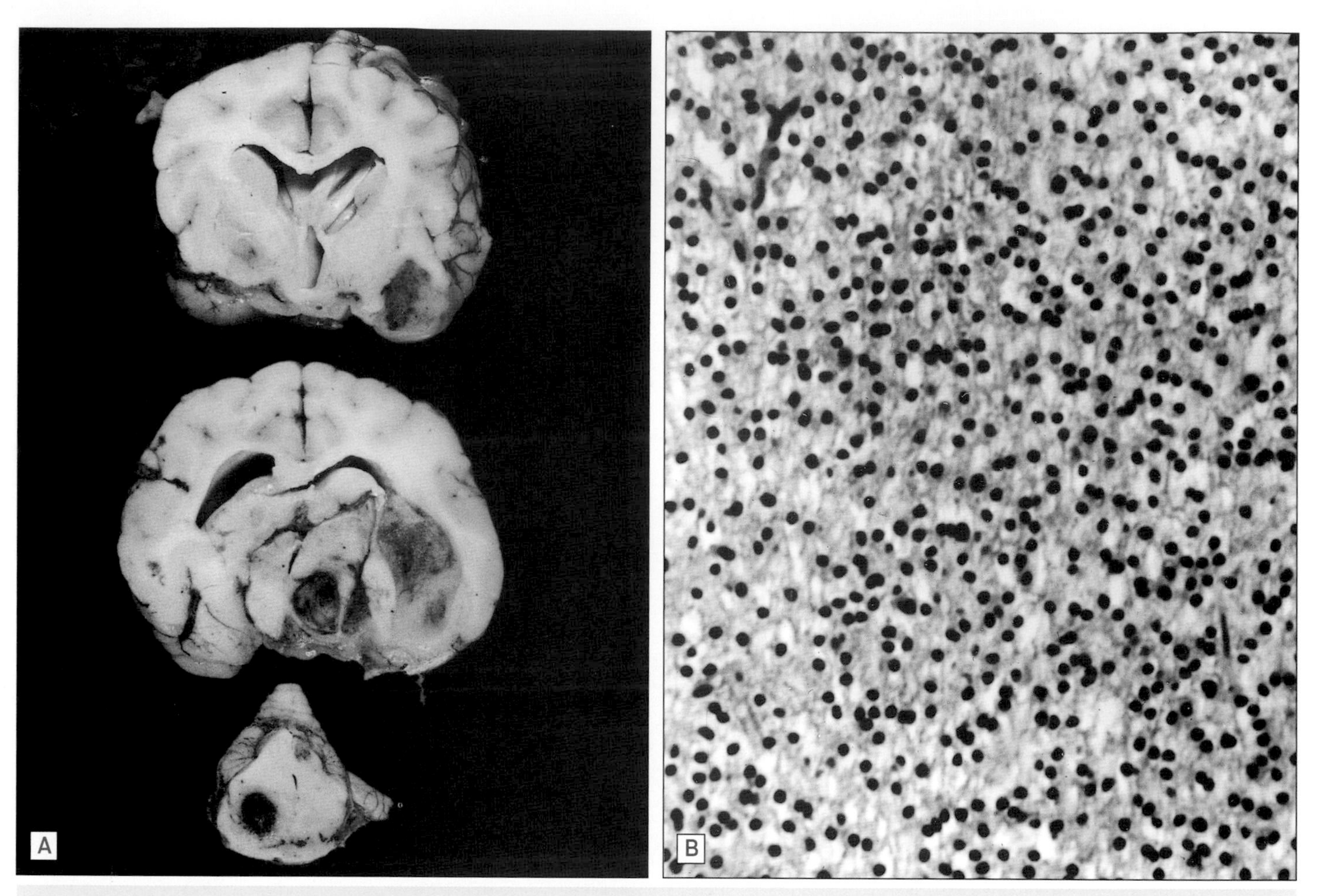

Figure 3.145 A. Oligodendroglioma involving right side of brain stem and piriform lobe in a dog. (Bottom section reversed to show caudal extension in brain stem.). **B.** Histologic pattern of oligodendroglioma.

Oligoastrocytoma (mixed glial tumor)

This glial neoplasm is composed of both neoplastic astrocytes and oligodendroglia.

Gliosarcoma

This rare glial tumor is composed of highly anaplastic glial cells with abundant sarcomatous components. Positive GFAP staining should differentiate this tumor from other spindle cell tumors, e.g., fibrosarcoma.

Gliomatosis cerebri

This is a diffuse infiltrating disease of dogs, predominantly of brachycephalic breeds, and humans characterized by an *infiltrative cell type reminiscent of astrocytes* rather than by the formation of a distinct tumor mass. The infiltrates involve the brain, often bilaterally but asymmetrically, with discontinuous areas also in the spinal cord. There is no tumor "mass," rather diffuse enlargement of affected regions, the cells insinuate among normal structures that remain intact with only slight damage to axons and neurons. Where the infiltrates involve the molecular layer of the cerebrum or the deep white matter, they spread in veils on leptomeninges and ependyma.

Gliomatosis cerebri is composed mainly of cells reminiscent of fibrillary astrocytic cells but there are also oligodendrocytes, cells of transitional character, and small unclassified cells (Fig. 3.146). The origin of the neoplastic cells in the canine cases is still controversial, as they do not stain with glial markers such as GFAP. The pattern of infiltration is unexplained, but involves participation of cell adhesion molecules.

Ependymoma

Ependymomas are neuroglial tumors derived from the lining epithelium of the ventricles and central canal of the spinal cord. Most arise about the third ventricle. They are gray and fleshy but may be dark from hemorrhage if they project into a ventricle. They are more prevalent in dogs and cats, but are reported in horses and cattle.

The tumors are usually densely cellular and those arising about the third ventricle may be difficult to distinguish from undifferentiated pituitary tumors. The nuclei are small, dark, and regular and the cytoplasm has no distinct boundaries. Pseudorosettes form around blood vessels, and are characterized by a perivascular nuclear-free zone. True rosettes are also present and appear as tubular cavities lined by cells of epithelial appearance. The cells forming true rosettes are bound together by desmosomes, have basally located nuclei, and

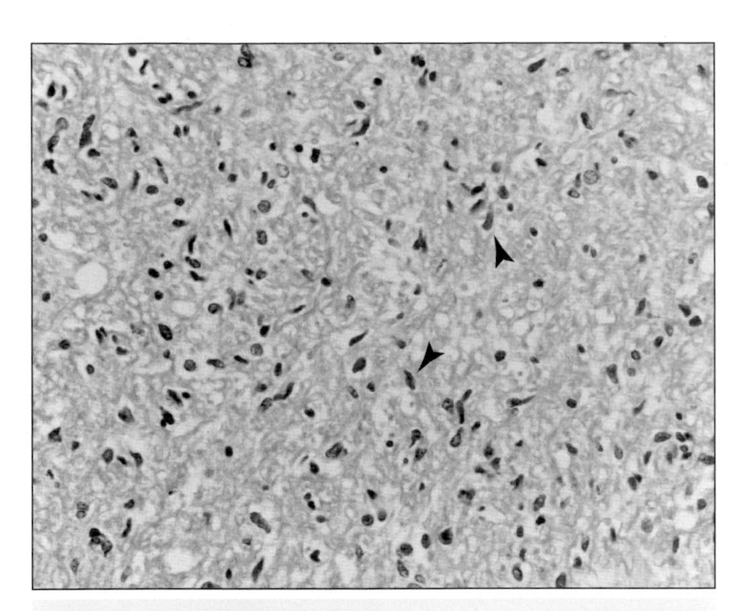

Figure 3.146 Gliomatosis cerebri appears as an increase in the cellularity of cerebrocortical white matter due to diffuse infiltration of neoplastic cells (arrowheads) that do not form a discrete mass or efface the preexisting tissue (Boxer dog).

have surface cilia anchoring phosphotungstic acid hematoxylin (PTAH)-positive blepharoplasts. A **papillary variant** does exist and is characterized by branching papillary stroma covered by recognizable, usually ciliated, ependymal cells (Fig. 3.147). Ependymomas of the spinal cord may be more papilliferous than those in the brain, with tumor cells attached to fronds that are supported by a delicate stroma and embedded in mucinous intercellular stroma. A **clear cell variant** resembling oligodendroglioma is only reported in humans. **Malignant ependymoma** is characterized by increased cellular atypia and mitoses.

Most canine ependymomas stain negatively for GFAP; however, feline and equine cases are reported to stain positively for this marker. Most ependymomas show slight positive staining for vimentin and cytokeratin. Human ependymomas stain strongly with anti-epithelial membrane antigen antibody (EMA); however, information about immunoreactivity of domestic animal ependymomas to EMA is not available.

Choroid plexus tumors

These are rare, reported in cats, horses, and cattle, and occur with higher frequency in dogs. They may be papillomas or carcinomas. They are vascular papillary growths that implant widely on the meninges. The cells retain recognizable choroidal character (Figs 3.148, 3.149). According to cellular atypia and invasiveness, these tumors can be classified as papilloma or carcinoma. Internal or communicating hydrocephalus is a complication. They express epithelial markers, e.g., pancytokeratin, but not glial markers, e.g., GFAP.

Neuronal and mixed neuronal glial tumors

These tumors of adult animals are composed of neurons and/or neurons admixed with glial cells.

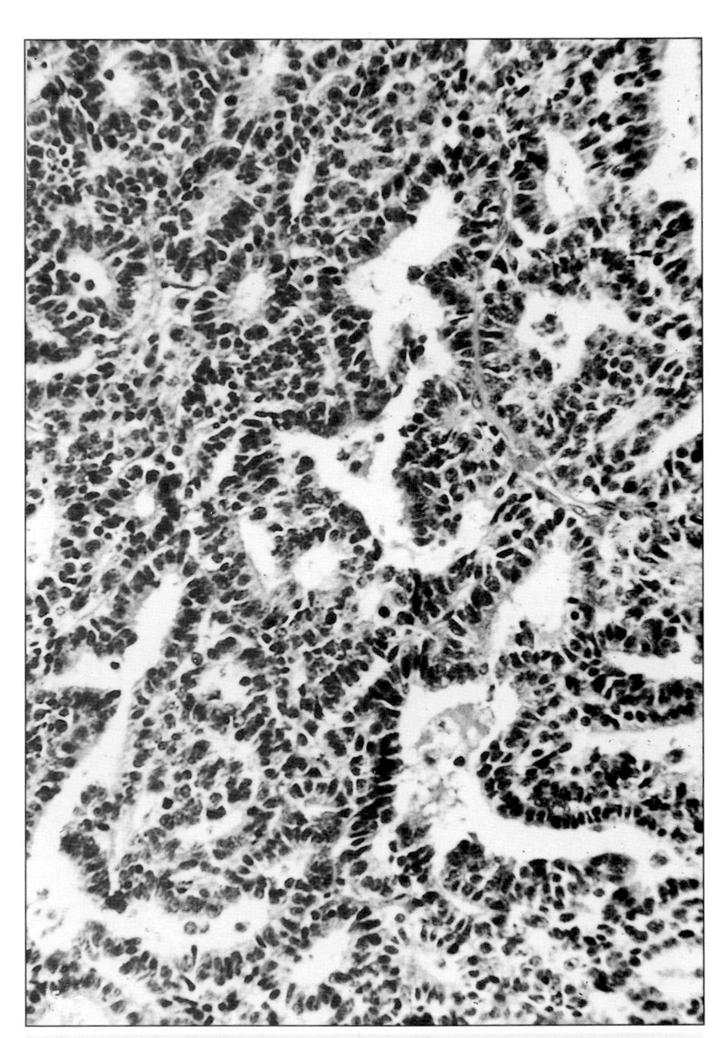

Figure 3.147 Typical branching papillary structure in an **ependymoma** in a dog.

Gangliocytomas

These are extremely rare tumors that are reported in dogs, a cow, and a horse. They appear to have a predilection for the cerebellum. The tumor is composed of cells reminiscent of large ganglion cells or mature pyramidal cells. Neoplastic cells do not stain with glial markers but show different reactivity with neuronal markers such as neuron-specific enolase (NSE) and synaptophysin.

Ganglioglioma

This is another rare bicellular tumor composed of neoplastic neuronal cells and neoplastic astrocytic cells. They have the same immunohistochemical staining pattern as gangliocytomas, but the astrocytic cells stain with GFAP.

Olfactory neuroblastomas (esthesioneuroblastoma)

This rare malignant tumor arises from primitive neurosensory cells present in the olfactory mucosa. They are uncommon but have been identified in various animal species, mainly dogs and cats. The olfactory epithelium is unique amongst neuronal structures in that the basal cells retain the ability to divide and differentiate to become

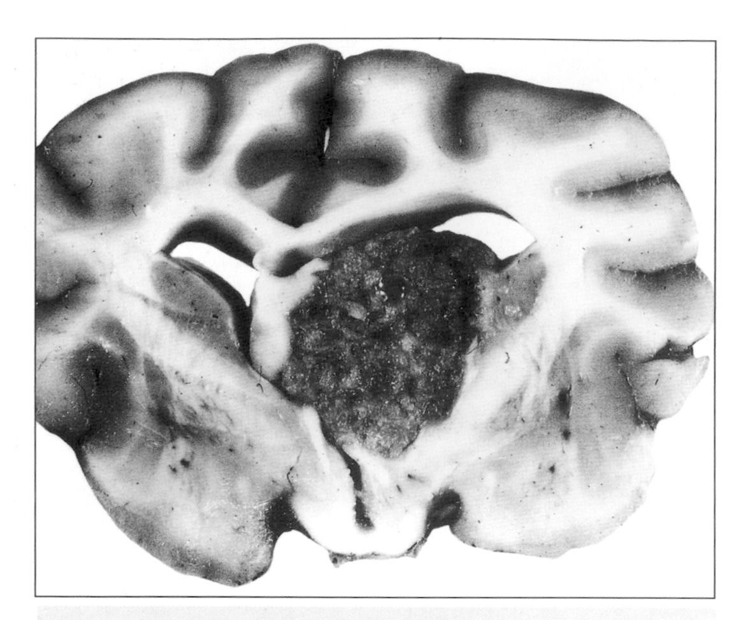

Figure 3.148 Choroid plexus papilloma in a dog.

sustentacular cells or bipolar neurosensory cells. The tumors are locally aggressive and may penetrate the cribriform plate. The dense cellular population is homogeneous, arranged in sheets or clusters but also forming true and pseudorosettes (Flexner-type rosettes and Homer Wright-type pseudorosettes). They may be palisaded on trabeculae, oval in shape with scant cytoplasm. Cytoplasmic processes may form an abundant, delicate fibrillary matrix. The detection of type C retroviral particles identified with feline leukemia in spontaneous olfactory neuroblastomas of cats is of interest. Neoplastic cells stain with different degrees of reactivity for both neuronal and epithelial immunohistochemical markers, e.g., NSE and cytokeratin respectively.

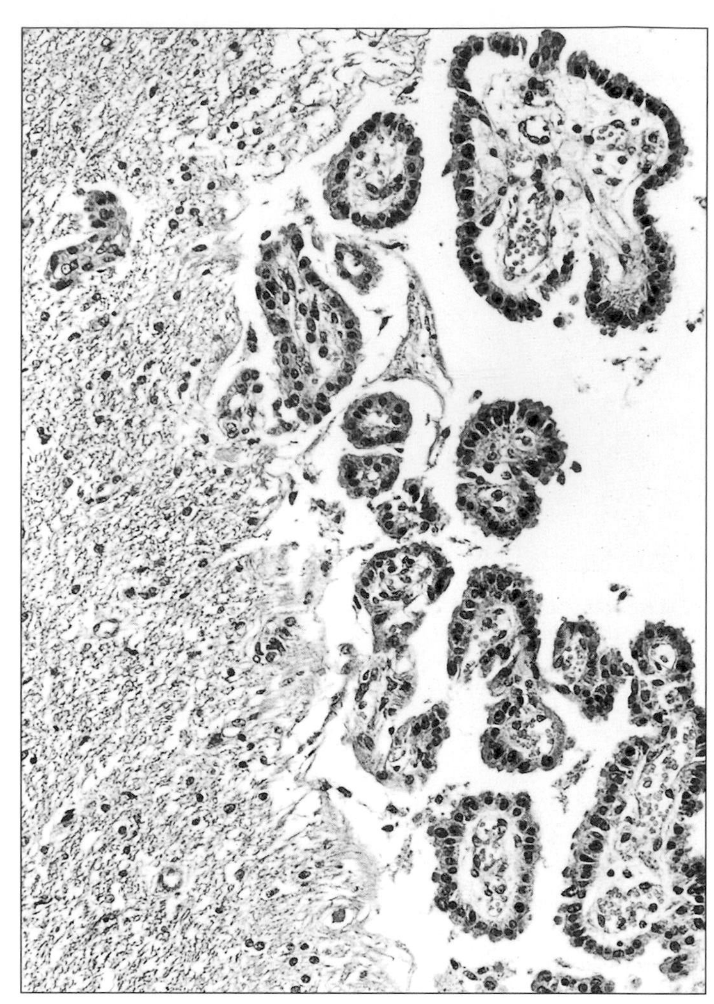

Figure 3.149 Invasion into the periventricular white matter of a dog by a **choroid plexus carcinoma**.

Embryonal tumors

These tumors arise from primitive or progenitor cells present in the nervous system and are capable of differentiating into different lineages including glial or neuronal cell lines.

Medulloblastoma (cerebellar primitive neuroectodermal tumor)

Medulloblastoma, well-known in children, is rare in animals, but occurs in the young of several species (Fig. 3.150), mainly calves and dogs. There is no such cell as a "medulloblast," the name invented for this tumor of unknown parentage. It is currently thought to arise from undifferentiated cells found in neonatal life beneath the cerebellar pia mater and thought to be the precursors of the cerebellar cortex. These tumors grow rapidly. Histologically, they are densely cellular with scant stroma and few vessels (Fig. 3.151A). The cells are small and classically "carrot-shaped" with oval or elongate nuclei and the cytoplasm tapering at one pole. They are also supposed to produce small perivascular palisades and pseudorosettes (Fig. 3.151B). These classical features are not always present, and then there is nothing by which this tumor can be identified except its location in the cerebellum. The term medulloblastoma should be limited to those embryonal tumors originated in the cerebellum. Tumors of this histological appearance in other sites in the brain of calves or other species are called *primitive neuroectodermal tumor* not medulloblastoma. Medulloblastomas stain positively for different neuronal markers including NSE and synaptophysin and some show positive staining for GFAP.

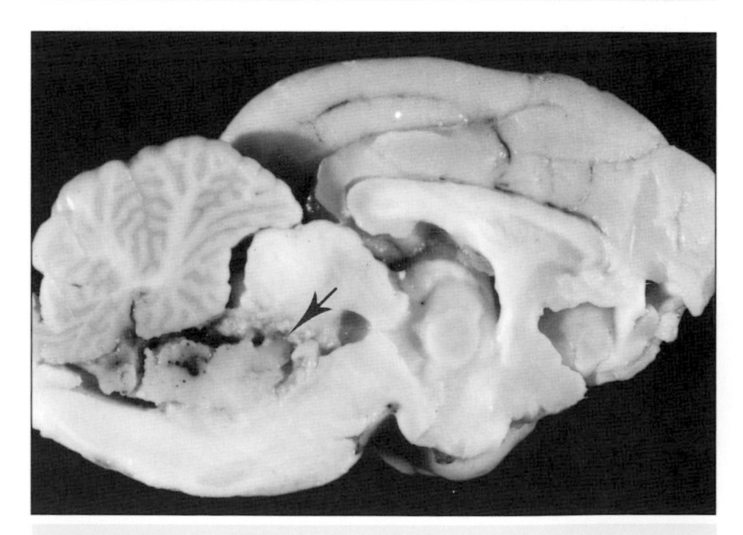

Figure 3.150 Medulloblastoma between cerebellum and fourth ventricle with extension into colliculus (arrow) in a cat.

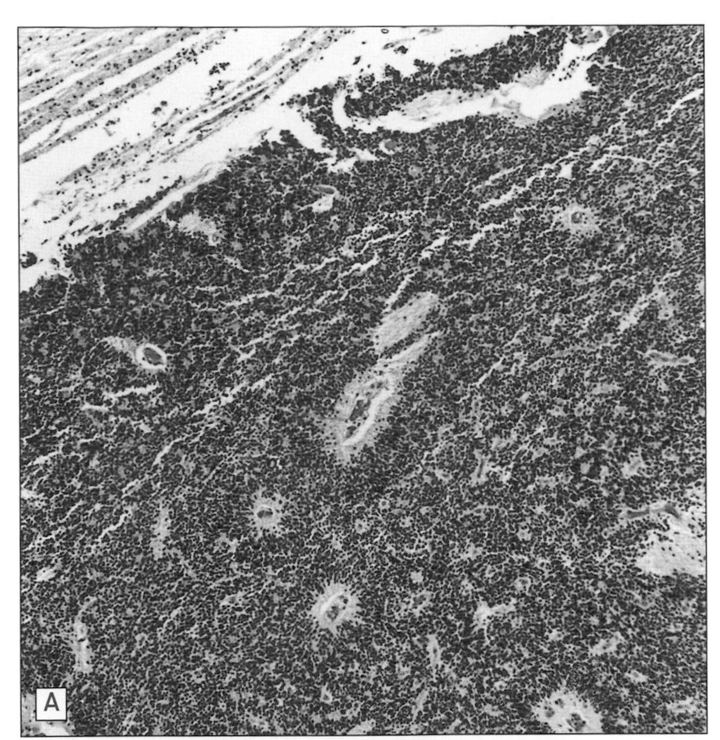

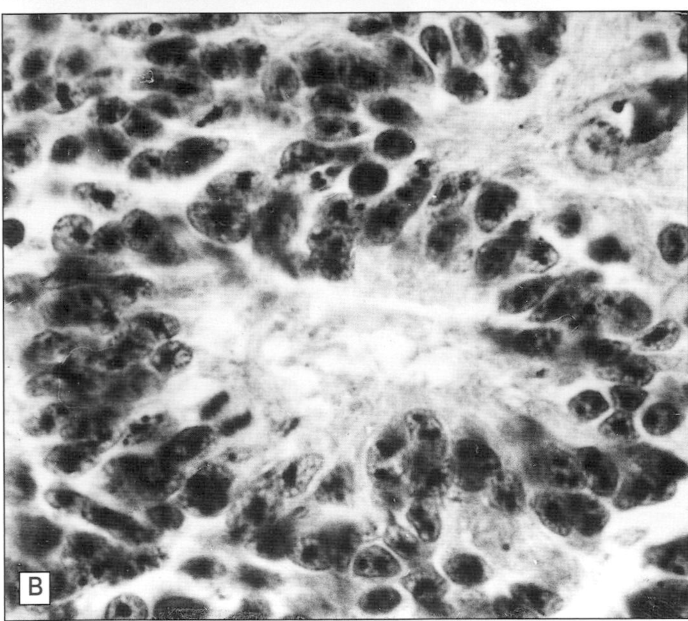

Figure 3.151 Histologic patterns of **medulloblastoma** in a calf. Pseudorosettes are visible in (**A**) and are detailed in (**B**), as circular groupings of dark tumor cells around a central pale area containing neurofibrils. (Courtesy of MD McGavin.)

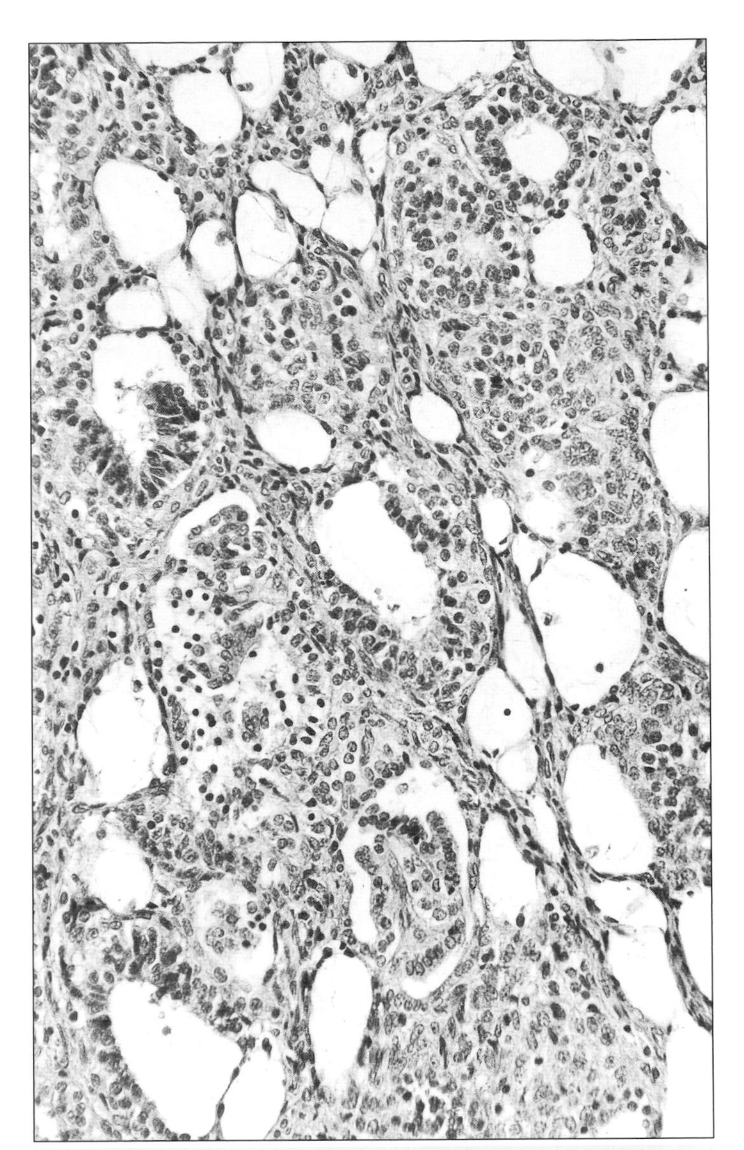

Figure 3.152 Neoplastic cells showing tubular structures with infoldings in **spinal nephroblastoma** in a dog.

Neuroblastomas

These tumors are rare and occur in any part of the CNS. Histologic criteria to distinguish them from other cellular neurogenic tumors are not satisfactory and identification must depend on other means. They are thought to arise from primitive neuroepithelial cells with differentiation towards postmitotic neuroblasts. The histologic appearances are similar to those of medulloblastoma, consisting of masses of small rounded cells that resemble lymphocytes, with hyperchromatic nuclei and scant cytoplasm. The presence of rosettes and pseudorosettes is helpful. Neoplastic cells stain positively with neuronal markers and negatively with glial markers such as GFAP.

Thoracolumbar spinal tumor of young dogs (spinal nephroblastoma)

These are single intradural masses occurring in young, large-breed dogs in the region between the tenth thoracic and second lumbar segments, and affected animals are presented with signs of cord compression. The tumor likely originates from the renal primordium, a renal ectopic embryonic remnant from which diverse nephron cell types are derived, present at this area. The histologic appearance is of glandular areas intermingling with cellular areas. The glandular areas consist of rosettes and tubules, the latter tortuous, branching and sometimes papilliferous, with infoldings reminiscent of embryonic glomerular capsules (Fig. 3.152). The cellular areas contain densely packed cells of blastema appearance with ovoid clear nuclei and indistinct cytoplasm. Some streaming is evident but muscle fibers are not present. In some of these tumors, glomerular structures can be recognized with confidence as can tubular cross-sections strongly

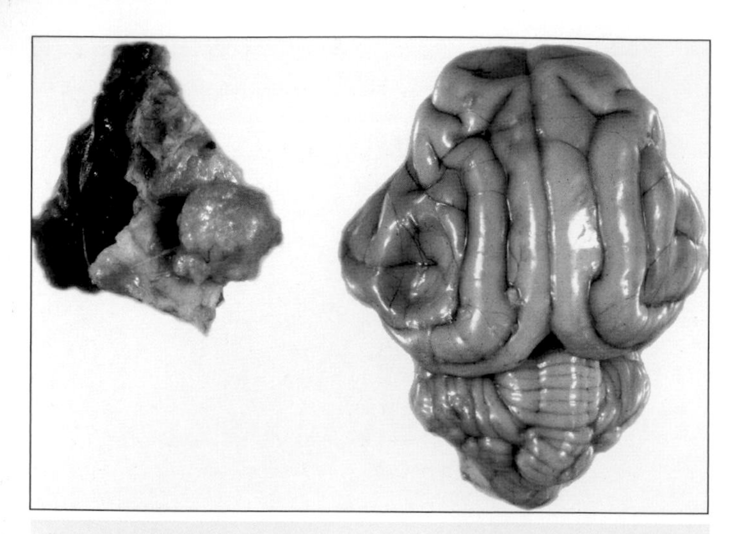

Figure 3.153 Meningioma attached to dura and calvaria (left), and leaving an indentation in the left parietal cerebral cortex of a cat. (Courtesy of RF Slocombe.)

suggestive of distal renal tubules. Presumably these tumors arise from ectopic embryonic remnants but notably the kidneys do not contain neoplasm although nephroblastomas are well recognized in dogs. From time to time, undifferentiated tumors of embryonic type and possibly derived from remnants of pronephros are seen in the cervical region of dogs and sheep. These tumors stain positive for cytokeratin and negative for glial and neuronal markers.

Pineal tumors

These tumors are rare. The benign variant is called *pineocytoma* and the malignant variant is called *pineoblastoma*. They are described in horses, cattle, and dogs. The diagnosis is based on the site of the tumor and its replacement of the pineal body. Other positive identifying characteristics are absent. Microscopically, there is a resemblance to medulloblastoma. The tumor may extend into midbrain and thalamus. Teratomatous tumors with characteristics of the gonadal teratomas are not described in the pineal gland of animals. Specific markers for tumors in animals are not reported.

Tumors of the meninges

These include the only tumor arising from meningothelial cells, **meningioma**, and those arising from nonmeningothelial cells, such as fibrosarcoma and sarcomatosis.

Meningiomas

Meningioma is the most common type of intracranial tumor in the cat and it is one of the commonest of the intracranial and intraspinal tumors in man, and is relatively common in dogs, rare in cattle, and not recorded in horses. It rises within the meninges, usually in close association with the dura, and grows expansively, compressing but seldom invading the brain (Fig. 3.153). Those in humans are presumed, by virtue of their site and structure, to arise mainly from the arachnoid granulations and also from islands of arachnoid cells that lie in the inner surface of the dura mater. A rare variant of meningioma is the **paranasal meningioma**, which arises from meningeal arachnoid cells that are trapped within or outside bone during development of the skull, and is reported in horses and dogs. The meningiomas observed in animals conform in histologic type to those observed in humans.

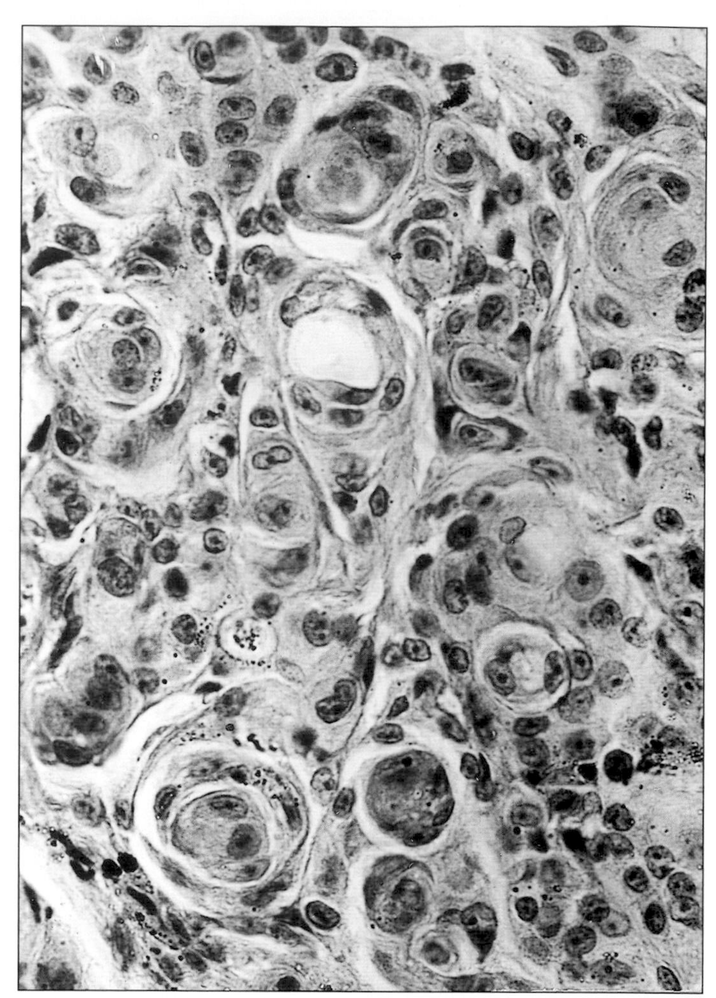

Figure 3.154 Histologic appearance of a **psammomatous meningioma.**

Meningiomas are globular, ovoid or tuberous, sometimes plaque-like, well circumscribed, and have a smooth surface. They are gray, sometimes yellow, on cut surface, firm, and may be gritty. Feline meningiomas are more easily separated from the brain parenchyma than are the canine ones, which are usually more interdigitated into the brain parenchyma. In cats, common locations include the tela choroidea of the third ventricle and the supratentorial meninges. They may be multiple in cats. There are several histologic varieties.

The **meningotheliomatous or epithelioid meningioma** is diffusely cellular with the cells in sheets or pseudo-alveoli. The stroma varies in amount, is richly vascular, and may contain much collagen. The cells are large with abundant finely granular pale cytoplasm without a distinct margin, and the nuclei are spherical or ovoid and rather vesicular. The **psammomatous meningioma** has the same general features as the foregoing, but the cells arrange themselves in whorls (Fig. 3.154). In the center of a whorl, lamellar hyaline tissue forms, derived possibly from cells, stroma, or a blood vessel. As the hyaline focus expands, it tends to be impregnated with salts of calcium and iron to form *psammoma bodies*. The **fibroblastic meningioma** is similar to fibroblastic tumors elsewhere. The **transitional or mixed type** has features of both epithelioid and fibroblastic meningioma.

Angioblastic meningiomas are highly vascular with prominent endothelial cells in formed vessels and lining vascular clefts. The vessels are surrounded by spindle cells giving a distinct resemblance to hemangiopericytoma. **Papillary meningiomas** are extremely rare in animals and composed of meningothelial cells arranged in papillary structures supported by fibrovascular cores. **Myxoid meningioma** is similar to myxoma elsewhere. There may be some difficulty in separating **hemangioma** from highly vascular meningiomas; both contain endothelial cells, pericytes, and stromal cells, the latter of uncertain parentage.

Granular cell meningiomas resemble granular cell tumors that occur elsewhere. They are included here because they do occur in the meninges and spinal nerve roots of dogs and the notion is attractive that some, at least, of the tumors are derived in common with cells of nerve sheaths and other neural crest mesenchyme. The tumors are usually small and well circumscribed but not well encapsulated. The cells are large and rounded, the cytoplasm clear apart from fine granules that may be few or numerous, and the nuclei small and rounded. The cytoplasmic granules are acidophilic and PAS-positive. Delicate stroma, in which amyloid may be deposited, separates the cells individually or in small groups. Stigmata of anaplasia are absent.

Most intracranial meningiomas are benign as indicated by low frequency of metastases and failure to invade the brain. By these criteria, ~2.5% are malignant and may metastasize. In contrast, extracranial meningiomas, which occur mainly in the paranasal region and orbit, are anaplastic and locally aggressive. Meningiomas stain positively for vimentin and negative for synaptophysin and GFAP. Staining for cytokeratin, NSE, and S-100 usually yield positive results but with sparse to moderate expression.

Fibrosarcoma

Fibrosarcomas may provide circumscribed or diffuse involvement of the meninges, or they may form local lesions of the brain or cord. They are not rare. Those of the brain and cord retain a perivascular orientation even though they are infiltrative. Histologically, some are acceptably fibrosarcoma but some are more pleomorphic and anaplastic spindle cell tumors. The histogenesis of these tumors is uncertain. They may arise from fibroblasts, pericytes, or resident reticuloendothelial cells of the monocyte-macrophage series. Some of the more anaplastic astroglial tumors provoke a remarkable degree of capillary endothelial hyperplasia and fibrosis of the vascular adventitia in brain and meninges. The proliferating fibroblastic cells are atypical, their appearance consistent with fibrosarcoma.

Meningeal sarcomatosis

Meningeal sarcomatosis is a rare condition reported only in dogs and characterized by diffuse infiltration of the leptomeninges, especially of the lumbar spinal cord, by pleomorphic neoplastic mesenchymal cells. Tumor may extend along the entire cerebrospinal axis from medulla to sacral cord. Neoplastic cells are present usually circumferentially in the subarachnoid space and may invade the subpial parenchyma of the spinal cord and to lesser extent the brain. Individual cells are pleomorphic, where the main neoplastic cells are large irregularly round cells (35–80 μm) with abundant cytoplasm and large round-to-ovoid hyperchromatic nuclei (20–65 μm). Neoplastic cells usually have a high mitotic rate and up to threefold anisokaryosis. In addition, several lymphoid, plasmacytoid, and histiocytic cells are present amid the neoplastic cells. A few multinucleated giant cells and intact neutrophils may also be present. The neoplastic large cells stain positively for vimentin. They usually stain positive, but with sparse to moderate expression, for CD18 and actin. They stain negatively for lymphocyte markers, S100, cytokeratin, and GFAP.

Hematopoietic tumors

Hematopoietic tumors such as lymphosarcoma, multiple myeloma, and malignant histiocytic tumors that originate in extraneural locations can metastasize to the CNS as part of their multisystemic metastasis, however in the following section we will describe those hematopoietic tumors that originate primarily in the CNS.

Lymphoma/lymphosarcoma

Primary CNS lymphomas are reported mainly in dogs and cats and sporadically in ruminants. They are mostly intraparenchymal and have an angiocentric (perivascular) pattern in contrast to lymphosarcomas metastatic from extraneural areas that are usually arranged diffusely in the meninges. Most primary CNS lymphomas are of T-cell type. Histologically, they follow the same morphology as extraneural lymphomas/lymphosarcomas.

Plasma cell tumor

A primary intracerebral intraparenchymal plasma cell tumor has been reported in a dog. An identical tumor was reported in a cat, but the diagnosis of primary neural plasma cell tumor was not confirmed due to incomplete postmortem examination.

Malignant histiocytosis

Primary neural malignant histiocytosis was reported in the right parieto-occipital lobe of a miniature Schnauzer as a poorly demarcated mass composed microscopically of histiocytic cells with many binucleate and multinucleate giant cells. Neoplastic cells stained positively for lysozyme.

Non-B, non-T leukocytic neoplasm (neoplastic reticulosis)

This controversial malignant neoplasm has a histologic resemblance to necrotizing meningoencephalitis (NME) of Pug dogs and granulomatous encephalitis (GME). The term "reticulosis" came into use because of aggregation of reticular fibers around neoplastic cells. Many cases diagnosed previously as reticulosis have been reclassified as lymphoma and a few as histiocytic tumors. The tumor may be single or multiple and can occur in any part of the CNS but is more prevalent in the cerebral white matter. The exact histogenesis of the neoplastic cells is yet to be determined, however, the neoplasm is composed histologically of angiocentric large (25–50 μm) round cells reminiscent of histiocytes and numerous non-neoplastic lymphocytes and macrophages. Multinucleate giant cells may predominate. Neoplastic cells usually show atypia and a moderate mitotic rate. The neoplastic cells stain positively with CD18 and negatively for lymphocyte markers, proving a leukocytic but non-lymphoid origin. The neoplasm has been reported in dogs and rarely in cats, cattle, and horses. The differentiation between neoplastic reticulosis and GME (formerly called inflammatory reticulosis) is difficult. The predominance of neoplastic histiocytic-like cells, cellular atypia, and high mitotic rate should favor the diagnosis of neoplastic reticulosis.

Microgliomatosis

The histogenic origin of the neoplastic cell in this rare neoplasm is controversial. The neoplasm diffusely infiltrates the cerebral white matter and brain stem with cells reminiscent of microglial cells. The infiltration in some cases can be limited to meninges or can be perivascular. In any case, this is a non-mass-forming neoplasm and the brain is almost unremarkable grossly. The neoplastic cells do not cause significant destruction of the pre-existing tissue. Neoplastic cells stain negatively for GFAP. There is strong overlap between microgliomatosis and gliomatosis cerebri. In human microgliomatosis, most neoplastic cells stain for CD18 and other monocyte/macrophage lineage markers. Similar studies on the immunohistochemical markers expressed by canine microgliomatosis are not available.

Tumors of the sellar region

Suprasellar germ cell tumors

Germ cell tumors are presumed to arise from ectopic embryonic germ cells which, intended for the developing gonad, may become widely distributed. They are responsible for a spectrum of tumors in humans, usually in the midline and according to histological features designated as *seminoma, choriocarcinoma, entodermal sinus tumor, and teratoma*. They are revealed early in life and the preferred locations in the cranial cavity are in the pineal region or in the hypothalamus above the sella. These are rare tumors in dogs. Their location and growth pattern is similar to that of pituitary adenomas and some may be misdiagnosed as craniopharyngioma.

The reported canine cases were suprasellar and classified on the basis of location, admixture of distinct cell types and patterns, and positive immunochemical staining for alpha fetoprotein. Sheets and nests of cells resembling seminoma were admixed with areas of vacuolated hepatoid cells, glandular formations similar to those in gonadal teratomas, and occasional foci of squamous epithelium.

Craniopharyngioma

Craniopharyngiomas are thought to arise from remnants of Rathke's pouch, which forms the adenohypophysis. Aberrant differentiation of Rathke's epithelium is common in dogs, expressed in cystic structures lined by respiratory-type epithelium. The craniopharyngioma, in contrast, consists of clumps of epithelial cells palisaded on collagenous stroma. Keratinization may be present to form pearls, as in well-differentiated squamous carcinoma. Degenerative foci contain cholesterol crystals and blood pigments. Neoplastic cells are positive for cytokeratin.

Other primary tumors and cysts

Epidermoid cysts

Epidermoid cysts in the brain are confined to the fourth ventricle and environs. They are rare, probably represent surface ectoderm misplaced at the period of closure of the neural groove, and are described only in humans, dogs, and a horse. The cystic structure is lined by squamous epithelium, and the cavities contain keratinaceous debris. They occur in young dogs and may develop to several centimeters in diameter. The clinical signs are determined by the location of the tumor.

Hamartoma or meningio-angiomatosis

Hamartoma or meningio-angiomatosis is a rare benign lesion, best regarded as a malformation or hamartoma producing circumscribed plaques on the surface of the brain. Blood vessels are in excess in the lesions and are cuffed by proliferating cells that are considered to be meningothelial. The lesion does extend into the underlying neural substance, which shows mixed degenerative and reactive changes.

Metastatic tumors

Secondary tumors can metastasize from extraneural tissue to the CNS. The most common examples include canine hemangiosarcoma, malignant histiocytosis, lymphosarcoma, and malignant melanoma of dogs and rarely other species.

Tumors affecting the CNS by extension or impingement

There are several tumors that do not arise directly from the CNS, but arise from structures adjacent to the CNS and sometimes impinge on the CNS, for example, vertebral osteosarcomas, nasal carcinomas, and chordomas.

Chordoma

Chordomas are rare tumors in animals with the exception of mink and European ferrets. In ferrets they are usually present at the tip of the tail. In humans, dogs, and cats, they are slow-growing persistent tumors mainly of the sacrococcygeal region with some occurring in paraspinal and cranial regions. On the basis of histological characters, *the tumor is presumed to arise from notochordal remnants*. Grossly, they are gelatinous, gray, friable, and lobulated. Histologically, the lobules are not encapsulated but are well defined by bands of connective tissue. The principal cell (physaliferous cells) types are large, clear, and vacuolated with a botanical appearance and some resemblance to cartilage (Fig. 3.155). The cytoplasm contains large clear vacuoles with distinct boundaries. At the periphery of the lobules there are smaller, stellate cells with eosinophilic cytoplasm; mitotic figures are rare in these but they may be the germinative cells. There may be islands of bone or cartilage. Mucinous substance can be demonstrated in the cytoplasmic vacuoles of the larger cells and between the cells; the smaller peripheral cells may contain PAS-positive granules. Differentiation from mucinous chondrosarcoma can be difficult without assistance of immunochemical methods. Chordomas will stain

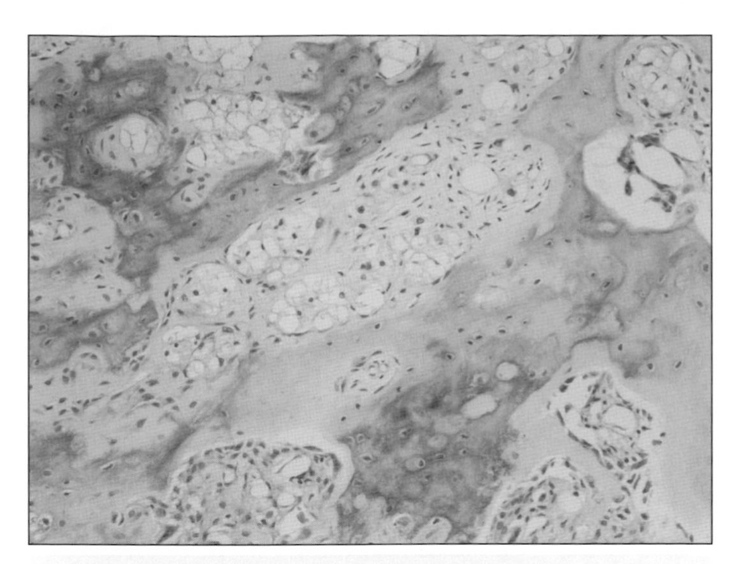

Figure 3.155 A **chordoma** in the tail of a ferret is composed of large, clear, vacuolated principal cells (physaliferous cells) in association with chondro-osteoid metaplasia.

immunohistochemically for cytokeratin, but chondrosarcomas will not. Chordomas also stain positively for vimentin and S-100.

Tumors of the peripheral nervous system

Ganglioneuroma and peripheral ganglioneuroblastoma

These rare tumors originate from the cranial and spinal ganglia and from sympathetic ganglia of the autonomic nervous system. They have been reported in cats, pigs, cattle, dogs, and horses. They can be solitary or multicentric. The few ganglioneuromas observed in cattle have developed in relation to the abdominal sympathetic plexuses. **Ganglioneuroma** is composed of ganglion cells and glial cells.

Ganglioneuroblastoma is composed of poorly to fairly well differentiated ganglion cells with more atypia and high nuclear-to-cytoplasmic ratio. The degree of differentiation of these tumors varies considerably, and they are a mixture of ganglion cells, Schwann cells, and nerve fibers. The ganglion cells show different degrees of differentiation from primitive neuroblasts to some that are remarkably mature. In the more primitive form, **neuroblastoma**, the neoplastic cells may form true or pseudorosettes. The adrenal medullary ganglioneuromas and ganglioblastomas are probably better regarded as hamartomatous malformations rather than as neoplasms.

Paraganglioma

This rare neuroendocrine tumor originates from extra-adrenal paraganglion chief cells associated with autonomic nervous system ganglia. The histologic picture resembles chemodectoma described in Vol. 3, Cardiovascular system. The neoplastic cells stain positive for neuroendocrine markers such as synaptophysin and chromogranin.

Peripheral nerve sheath tumors

These include the benign form (schwannoma, neurofibroma) or the malignant form (malignant schwannoma, neurofibrosarcoma) (Fig. 3.156A–E). The Schwann cell of the peripheral nervous system is accepted as the origin of these tumors. Most of these tumors are seen in the skin. The dermal tumors do pose problems of differentiation from fibrous and perivascular lesions (see the Skin and appendages). In skin, they do show some significant differences from the tumors of nerve trunks and roots.

Schwannomas may be largely solitary infiltrating lesions at any site on a nerve trunk. Those distant from the CNS are not encapsulated or well defined, are difficult to dissect cleanly, and have an ordinary fibrous appearance and texture. Schwannomas of nerve roots tend to be well-defined fusiform tumors. They probably arise from a single nerve and extend proximally and distally in conjunction with the nerve but external to it. In this way they may extend through the intervertebral foraminae and extend also to involve other nerves that have a plexus arrangement such as the brachial plexus. They may arise within and remain within the dura mater, and such tumors may be globose rather than fusiform and soft and discolored from hemorrhage. Expansive intradural growth may be slow and compress the brain or cord, but some of these tumors are malignant and invasive (Fig. 3.156D) and metastasize particularly to the lung.

Any cranial or spinal nerve root may be the site of growth, but in the dog, in which they are not rare, the brachial plexus is most frequently involved. In the thoracic region and on the acoustic nerve (Fig. 3.156A), the tumors tend to originate within the dura. The histologic appearance varies within and between tumors depending on the presence or absence of anaplastic change and the extent of hemorrhage, degeneration, fibrosis, and mineralization. Blood vessels are often prominent but ill formed. The anaplastic tumors consist of closely packed cells with oval or elongate nuclei that give an impression of interlacing streams not supported or guided by reticulin or collagen (Fig. 3.156B). In areas of tumors that are not anaplastic, two patterns are dominant and referred to as Antoni A and Antoni B. *Antoni A arrangements* are repetitive and give the tumor its character. Uniform, fusiform cells are arranged as bands, herring bones, whorls, or palisades (Verocay bodies) (Fig. 3.156C). *Antoni B tissue* is degenerative and may predominate in some sections. It is loose and myxoid, sometimes hyalinized and may be sparsely cellular (Fig. 3.156E). Microcysts may be present in areas of myxoid change. Cartilaginous and osseous metaplasia occur infrequently. A malignant variant is more invasive grossly and occasionally metastasizes to the lung and other organs. The neoplastic cells stain strongly for vimentin and usually stain positively but with varying intensity with S-100, GFAP, nerve growth factor receptor, and myoglobin. They stain negatively with α-smooth muscle actin, which stains hemangiopericytoma and rhabdomyosarcoma positively.

Neurofibromatosis of cattle is a well-recognized Schwannoma. It is common in abattoir material from old animals but has been observed in very young calves. The skin may be affected, but the lesions are usually restricted to deeper nerves of the thoracic wall and viscera. The brachial plexus, intercostal nerves, hepatic autonomic plexus, epicardial plexus, and autonomic nerves of the mediastinum are those most frequently affected in various collective patterns. Sympathetic ganglia, especially the stellate and others of the thorax, are also frequently involved. Affected nerves are thickened, firm, and gray, and may bear yellow-gray nodules. Affected ganglia may be enlarged to several centimeters and appear lobulated on section. The histologic appearances are as described above for Schwannomas, but anaplastic change is rare (Fig. 3.156C).

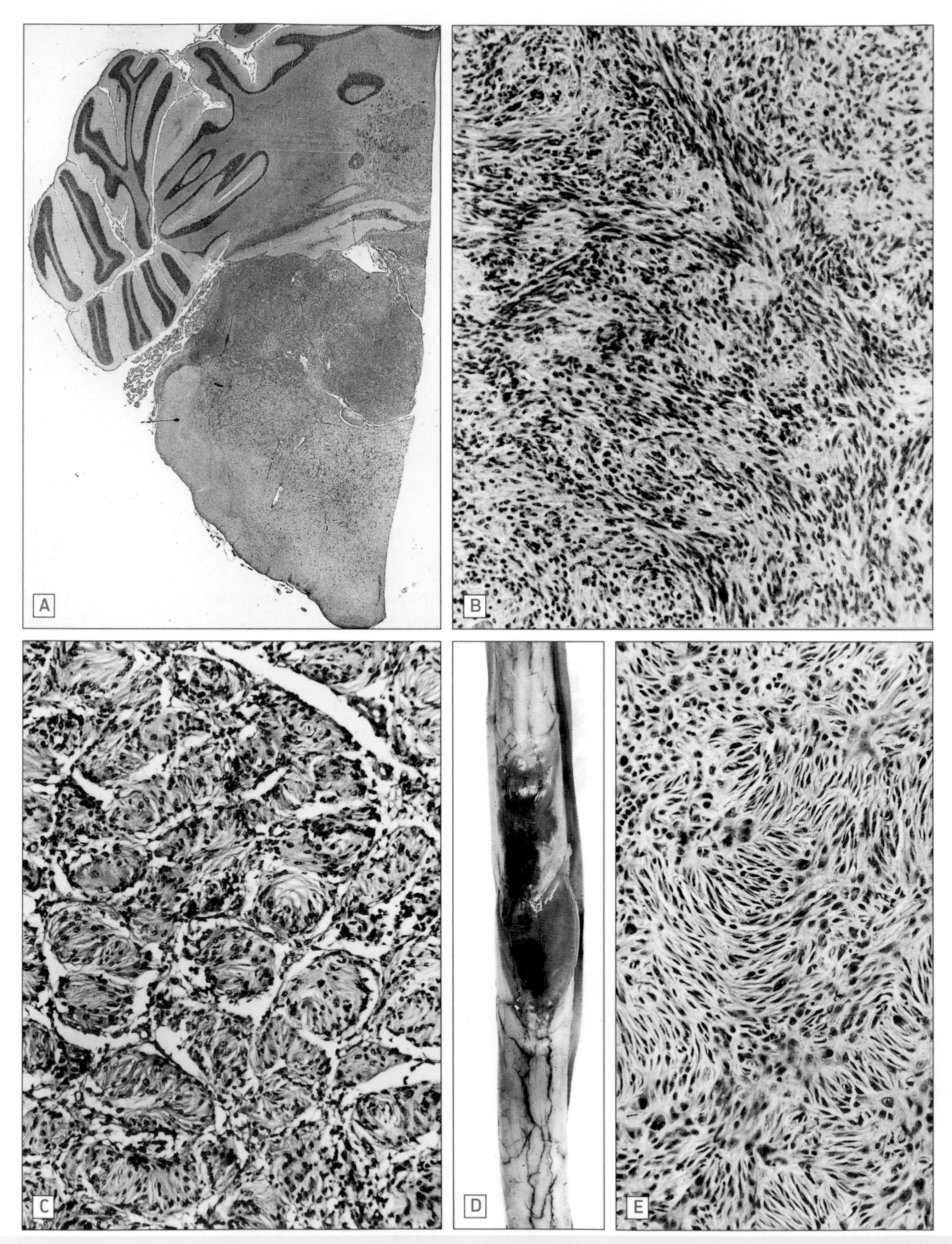

Figure 3.156 A. Acoustic schwannoma at cerebellopontine angle and filling the fourth ventricle of a dog. **B.** Section of (**A**). **C.** Patterns resembling Verocay bodies in neurofibromatosis in an ox. **D. Malignant schwannoma** in the spinal cord of a dog. **E. Schwannoma** in a cat.

Bibliography

Barnhart KF, et al. Immunohistochemical staining patterns of canine meningiomas and correlation with published immunophenotypes. Vet Pathol 2002;39:311–321.

Cantile C, et al. Pathological and immunohistochemical studies of choroid plexus carcinoma of the dog. J Comp Pathol 2002;126:183–193.

Capucchio MT, et al. Histological and immunohistochemical study of a neuroblastoma in a dog. Clin Neuropathol 2003;22:176–179.

Chandra AM, Ginn PE. Primary malignant histiocytosis of the brain in a dog. J Comp Pathol 1999;121:77–82.

Chijiwa K, et al. Immunohistochemical evaluation of canine peripheral nerve sheath tumors and other soft tissue sarcomas. Vet Pathol 2004;41:307–318.

Dickinson PJ, et al. Clinical and pathologic features of oligodendrogliomas in two cats. Vet Pathol 2000;37:160–167.

Fankhauser R, et al. Medulloblastomas in bovine twins of different sexes. Schweiz Arch Tierheilkd 1982;124:363–367.

Fondevila D, et al. Primary central nervous system T-cell lymphoma in a cat. Vet Pathol 1998;35:550–553.

Greenberg MJ, et al. Intracerebral plasma cell tumor in a cat: a case report and literature review. J Vet Intern Med 2004;18:581–585.

Hare WR. Primary suprasellar germ cell tumor in a dog. J Am Vet Med Assoc 1993;203:1432–1433.

Josephson GKA, Little PB. Four bovine meningeal tumours. Can Vet J 1990; 31:700–703.

Kimura K, et al. Anaplastic gangliocytoma with eosinophilic cytoplasmic granules in a cow. J Vet Med Sci 1999;61:983–985.

Koestner A, et al. eds. Histological Classification of the Tumors of the Nervous System of Domestic Animals. 2nd series, Vol 5. Washington, DC: AFIP and WHO, 1999.

Koperek O, et al. Value and limits of immunohistochemistry in differential diagnosis of clear cell primary brain tumors. Acta Neuropathol (Berl) 2004;108:24–30.

Kornegay JN, Gorgacz EJ. Intracranial epidermoid cysts in three dogs. Vet Pathol 1982;19:646–650.

Kreeger JM, et al. Paranasal meningioma in a horse. J Vet Diagn Invest 2002;14:322–325.

Kube SA, et al. Astrocytomas in young dogs. J Am Anim Hosp Assoc 2003;39:288–293.

LeCouteur RA. Current concepts in the diagnosis and treatment of brain tumours in dogs and cats. J Small Anim Pract 1999;40:411–416.

Lipsitz D, et al. Glioblastoma multiforme: clinical findings, magnetic resonance imaging, and pathology in five dogs. Vet Pathol 2003;40:659–669.

Liu CH, et al. Intracranial granular cell tumor in a dog. J Vet Med Sci 2004;66:77–79.

Lorenzo V, et al. Meningioangiomatosis in a dog: magnetic resonance imaging and neuropathological studies. J Small Anim Pract 1998;39:486–489.

Lu D. Concurrent benign and malignant multiple meningiomas in a cat: clinical, MRI and pathological findings. Vet Rec 2003;152:780–782.

Mamom T, et al. Oligodendroglioma in the cervical spinal cord of a dog. Vet Pathol 2004;41:524–526.

McKay JS, et al. Histological characterization of an ependymoma in the fourth ventricle of a cat. J Comp Pathol 1999;120:105–113.

Michimae Y, et al. Anaplastic ependymoma in the cervical spinal cord of a maltese dog. J Vet Med Sci 2004;66:1155–1158.

Nyska A, et al. Intracranial gangliocytoma in a dog. Vet Pathol 1995;32:190–192.

Park CH. Oligodendroglioma in a French bulldog. J Vet Sci 2003;4:195–197.

Patnaik AK, et al. Paranasal meningioma in the dog: a clinicopathologic study of ten cases. Vet Pathol 1986;23:362–368.

Peters M, et al. Intracranial epidermoid cyst in a horse. J Comp Pathol 2003; 129:89–92.

Porter B, et al. Gliomatosis cerebri in six dogs. Vet Pathol 2003;40:97–102.

Pye GW, et al. Thoracic vertebral chordoma in a domestic ferret (*Mustela putorius furo*). J Zoo Wildl Med 2000;31:107–111.

Reimer ME, et al. Rectal ganglioneuroma in a dog. J Am Anim Hosp Assoc 1999;35:107–110.

Ribas JL, et al. Comparison of meningio-angiomatosis in a man and a dog. Vet Pathol 1990;27:369–371.

Sale CS, et al. Spinal nephroblastoma in a crossbreed dog. J Small Anim Pract 2004;45:267–271.

Sant'Ana FJ, et al. Pilocytic astrocytoma in a cat. Vet Pathol 2002;39:759–761.

Schrenzel MD, et al. Type C retroviral expression in spontaneous feline olfactory neuroblastomas. Acta Neuropathol 1990;80:547–553.

Stober M, et al. Nerve sheath tumors in cattle: literature review and case report. Dtsch Tierarztl Wochenschr 2001;108:269–272.

Stoica G, et al. Morphology, immunohistochemistry, and genetic alterations in dog astrocytomas. Vet Pathol 2004;41:10–19.

Troxel MT, et al. Feline intracranial neoplasia: retrospective review of 160 cases (1985–2001). J Vet Intern Med 2003;17:850–859.

Valentine BA, et al. Suprasellar germ cell tumors in the dog: a report of five cases and review of the literature. Acta Neuropath 1988;76:94–100.

Willard MD, de Lahunta A. Microgliomatosis in a schnauzer dog. Cornell Vet 1982;72:211–219.

Yamada M, et al. Histopathological and immunohistochemical studies of intracranial nervous-system tumours in four cattle. J Comp Pathol 1998; 119:75–82.

Zimmerman KL, et al. A comparison of the cytologic and histologic features of meningiomas in four dogs. Vet Clin Pathol 2000;29:29–34.

4 Eye and ear

Brian P. Wilcock

Eye

Eye

GENERAL CONSIDERATIONS

The role of the veterinary pathologist in the diagnosis of ocular disease is usually restricted to histologic examination. Gross pathology of the eye is the realm of the clinical ophthalmologist. The sophistication of ocular clinical examination, including imaging techniques like ultrasound and magnetic image resonance, represents a substantial challenge for the ocular histopathologist. Especially when dealing with globes submitted from ophthalmic specialists, we are being asked to provide very precise histologic counterparts for some very specific macroscopic lesions detected by these increasingly sophisticated clinical examination techniques.

The reluctance of many pathologists to embrace ophthalmic pathology stems from the disappointing quality of sections made from formalin-fixed globes processed by routine methods, from unfamiliarity with ocular anatomy and histology, and from fear of the complex terminology shared by clinical ophthalmologists and ophthalmic pathologists. At least equally daunting is the need to be familiar with the ever-growing list of specific ocular syndromes, the correct identification of which has huge significance in terms of therapy and prognosis. There are many examples in which a perfectly adequate description and general morphologic diagnosis will nonetheless fail to communicate the appropriate prognostic or therapeutic information, simply because the clinician reading the report cannot make the connection between the histologic description and the specific clinical-pathologic syndrome. This is also true when dealing with the histologic manifestations of the innumerable inherited ocular disorders that occur in purebred dogs, the species that indisputably dominates veterinary ophthalmology. In many instances, the correct diagnosis requires the correlation of the lesion with the age, breed, and specific clinical features of the disease.

Ocular fixation

The eye undergoes very rapid postmortem/postenucleation change that not only obscures subtle degenerative lesions but also mimics genuine developmental or degenerative diseases. Even with a globe obtained within minutes of death or surgical removal, improper handling of the specimen frequently results in a section of poor quality. The globe can be speedily and gently removed by grasping the third eyelid with forceps and applying traction to the globe whilst making a circumferential incision at the fornix. Blunt curved scissors inserted through this incision may be used to sever the extraocular muscles and optic nerve, and allow the globe to be removed from the orbit. All orbital fat and extraocular muscles should be gently removed from the sclera to permit rapid penetration of fixative to the retina.

The choice of fixative depends upon the disease suspected and upon the type of examination to which the eye will be subjected. *Formalin* has the advantage of ready availability, ease of shipment, little danger of overfixation, and adequate preservation of color and macroscopic detail for photography. Also, it permits localization in the bisected globe of lesions identified ophthalmoscopically, and the use of electron microscopy should such examination be warranted by the findings of light microscopy. However, formalin penetrates the sclera slowly and there are postmortem changes, including retinal detachment, even in globes fixed immediately after death or surgery. Injection of formalin into the vitreous (0.25 ml for a dog or cat, 2.0 ml for a horse) greatly improves retinal fixation and helps prevent the almost inevitable retinal detachment that follows routine formalin fixation. Rapid-penetrating fixatives such as *Zenker's, Davidson's or Bouin's* are preferred for globes in which preservation of histologic detail (especially retinal detail) is paramount. All render the globe and its refractive media opaque and less suitable for macroscopic assessment and photography than does formalin. All require strict attention to the duration of fixation. *Regardless of the method of fixation, all eyes benefit from hardening in 70% ethanol over about 24 hours to prevent retinal detachment when trimming the globe for embedding.* A mixture of equal parts cold 4% buffered glutaraldehyde and 10% neutral formalin has been recommended as an ocular fixative for both light and electron microscopy.

In all domestic animals, *the preferred section for histology is made from a midsagittal slab which includes optic nerve*, thereby allowing examination of both tapetal and nontapetal fundus in the same section. **Attempting to slice the fixed globe with a scalpel blade is**

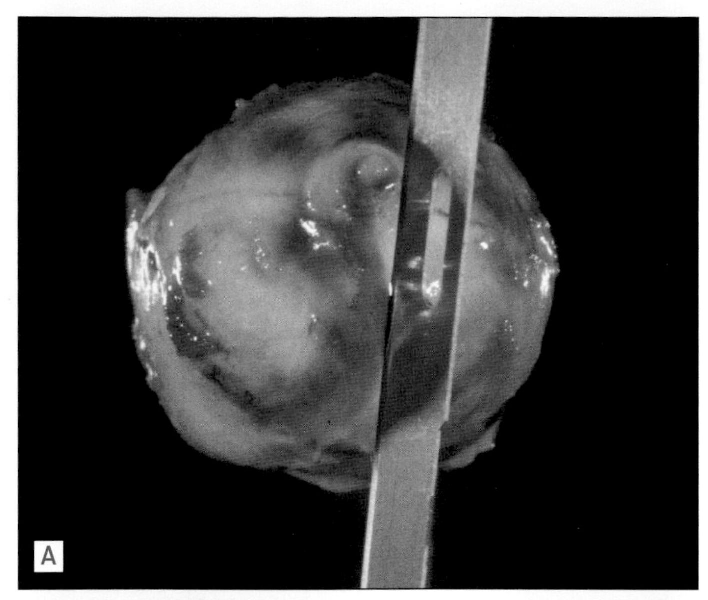

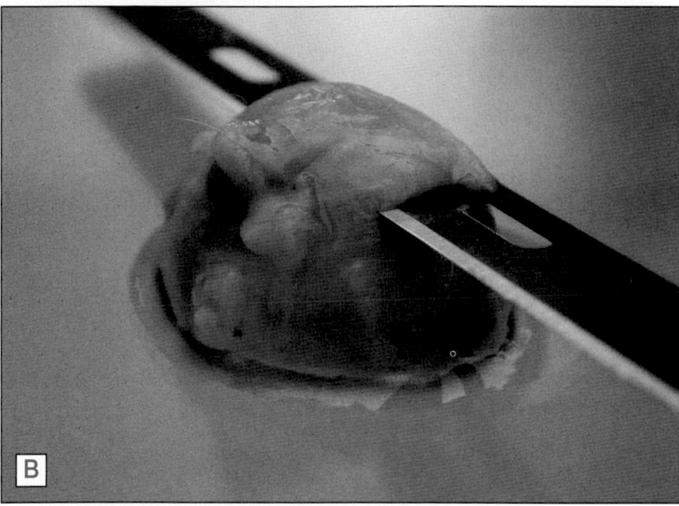

Figure 4.1 A. Trimming a fixed eye. The first incision is made from back to front, perpendicular to the posterior ciliary artery and just adjacent to the optic nerve. **B.** The second cut, made from front to back to avoid detaching the retina, is parallel to the first and far enough to the periphery to miss the lens.

perhaps the single biggest contributor to sections of poor quality. *The optimal cutting instrument is a new disposable microtome blade.* For small globes less than about 1 cm in diameter, an ordinary consumer razor blade is perfectly adequate.

Because there is no easily accessible instruction manual on how to obtain a good histologic section, those details are included here.

- The fixed globe, free of extraocular muscles and eyelids, is opened by a smooth sagittal incision beginning adjacent to the optic nerve and ending with the cornea.
- The correct 6:00–12:00 orientation, needed to capture tapetal and nontapetal fundus, is insured by making the incision at right angles to the orientation of the posterior ciliary artery (Fig. 4.1A).
- The open globe is then inspected for macroscopic lesions.
- A second cut, parallel to the first, is made from the cornea backward through the retina (Fig. 4.1B).
- That second cut should be far enough to the periphery to leave the already-bisected lens undisturbed (for a second cut through the lens will surely dislocate it).
- The resulting slab should be lifted carefully into a thick processing cassette or a tissue bag.
- Even though the piece of tissue is as much as 1 cm thick, it is hollow and thus presents no difficulty in terms of automated tissue embedding procedures.

Bibliography

Gelatt KN. Feline ophthalmology. Compend Cont Ed 1979;1:576–583.

Gelatt KN, ed. Veterinary Ophthalmology. Philadelphia, PA: Lea and Febiger, 1981.

Jensen HE. Histological changes in the canine eye related to aging. Proc Am Coll Vet Ophthalmol 1974:3–15.

Peiffer RL, ed. Comparative Ophthalmic Pathology. Springfield, IL: Charles C. Thomas, 1983.

Prince JH, et al. Anatomy and Histology of the Eye and Orbit in Domestic Animals. Springfield, IL: Charles C. Thomas, 1960.

Rubin LF. Inherited Eye Disease in Purebred Dogs. Philadelphia, PA: Williams & Wilkins, 1989.

Samuelson DG. Ophthalmic anatomy. In: Gelatt KN, ed. Veterinary Ophthalmology. 3rd ed. Baltimore, MD: Lippencott Williams & Wilkins, 1999:31–150.

Saunders LZ, Rubin LF. Ophthalmic Pathology of Animal. Basel, Switzerland: Karger, 1975.

Spencer WH, ed. Ophthalmic Pathology. Philadelphia, PA: W.B. Saunders, 1985.

Stryer L. The molecules of visual excitation. Scientific American 1987:42–50.

Yanoff M, Fine BS. Ocular Pathology. 3rd ed. Philadelphia, PA: J.B. Lippencott, 1989.

DEVELOPMENTAL ANOMALIES

Ocular developmental defects are common in domestic animals, particularly in purebred dog breeds in which extensive linebreeding has been used to increase the predictability of the phenotype. Many of the defects involve the eyelids and result from accentuation of anatomic peculiarities of the breed, such as entropion from deliberate enophthalmos or misdirected hairs from overly prominent facial folds. Such anomalies are clinically obvious and amenable to surgery, and rarely require the attention of a pathologist.

Anomalies of the globe are usually multiple, which reflects the stepwise induction and interdependence of the various parts of the developing eye. Without proper consideration of ocular embryology, any discussion of the lesions found in anomalous eyes threatens to be just a catologue of observations rather than a roadmap to understanding that such lesions are all predictable results of a relatively small number of possible errors in organogenesis. It is also important to recognize the differences in normal ocular structure among the various species, and the different rates at which mature form is attained. For example, the retina of carnivore eyes continues to develop for about 6 weeks postnatally, whereas that of ruminants and horses is mature at birth. Thus, something like retinal dysplasia is necessarily an in utero event in ungulates, but may be in response to early postnatal injury in carnivores.

Review of ocular organogenesis

The primary optic vesicle is an evagination of the forebrain that, with differential growth of brain and surface ectoderm, becomes separated from the presumptive diencephalon by the *optic stalk*. The

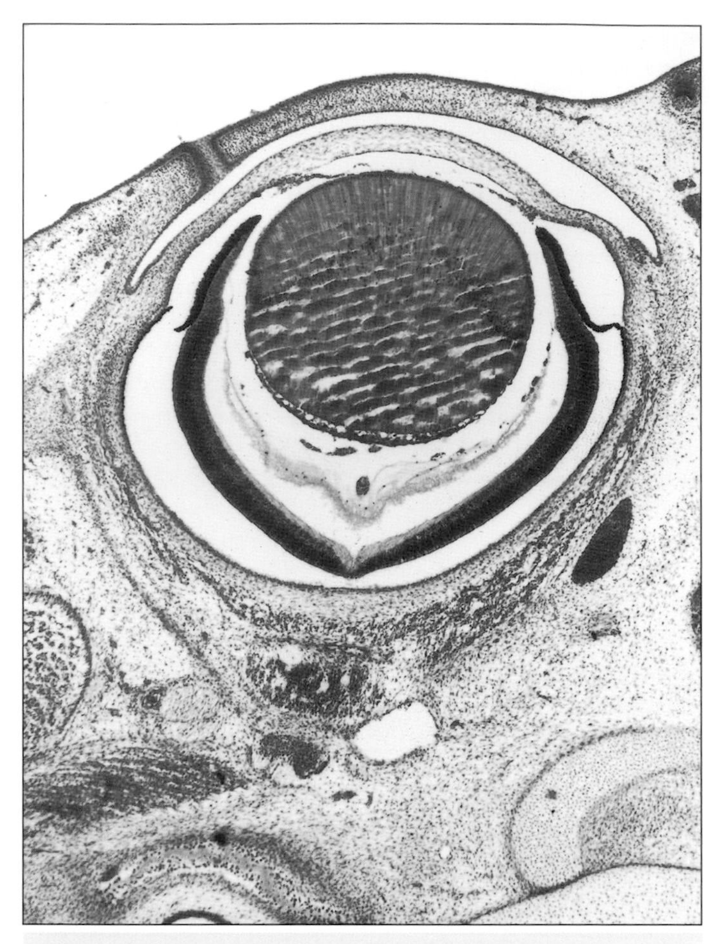

Figure 4.2 Canine embryo at 34 days gestation. Lids fused, cornea fully formed. Large lens surrounded by complete vascular tunic derived posteriorly from hyaloid artery and anteriorly from the future pupillary membrane. Iris not yet formed.

apposition of primary optic vesicle to overlying surface ectoderm induces a focal ectodermal thickening, the *lens placode*. The placode grows to form a primitive *lens vesicle*. It is the developing lens that orchestrates the invagination of the optic vesicle to form the bilayered *optic cup* and bring the lining neuroectoderm into the apposition that provides the future photoreceptor and pigment epithelial layers. Surrounding the optic cup is a mass of *mesenchyme*, derived from neural crest, which will form the vascular and fibrous tunics of the eye (iris and ciliary body stroma, corneal stroma and endothelium, choroid and sclera) under the induction of the differentiating neuroectoderm (Fig. 4.2). *Ocular adnexa and muscles* form independently and seem not to require normal development of the globe, as evidenced by the presence of normal lacrimal gland, lids, and extraocular muscles in most cases of severe microphthalmos.

Bibliography

Bellhorn RW. A survey of ocular findings in 8-to-10-month-old beagles. J Am Vet Med Assoc 1974;164:1114–1116.

Bistner SI. Embryology of the canine and bovine eyes. In: Gelatt KN, ed. Veterinary Ophthalmology. Philadelphia, PA: Lea and Febiger, 1981:3–11.

Cook CS. Ocular embryology and congenital malformations. In: Gelatt KN, ed. A Veterinary Ophthalmology. 3rd ed. Baltimore, MD: Lippincott Williams & Wilkins, 1999:3–30.

Dodds WJ, et al. The frequencies of inherited blood and eye diseases as determined by genetic screening programs. J Am Anim Hosp Assoc 1981;17:697–704.

Garner A, Griffiths P. Bilateral congenital ocular defects in a foal. Br J Ophthalmol 1969;53:513–517.

Gelatt KN, et al. Congenital ophthalmic anomalies in cattle. Mod Vet Pract 1976;57:105–109.

Huston R, et al. Congenital defects in foals. Equine Med Surg 1977;1:146–161.

Martin CL, Anderson BG. Ocular anatomy. In: Gelatt KN, ed. Veterinary Ophthalmology. Philadelphia, PA: Lea and Febiger, 1981:58–64.

Priester WA. Congenital ocular defects in cattle, horses, cats and dogs. J Am Vet Med Assoc 1972;160:1504–1511.

Saunders LZ, Rubin LF. Ophthalmic Pathology of Animals. An Atlas and Reference Book. Basel, Switzerland: Karger, 1975.

Selby LA, et al. Comparative aspects of congenital malformations in man and swine. J Am Vet Med Assoc 1971;159:1485–1490.

Defective organogenesis

Failure of the eye to attain even the stage of optic cup is a rare occurrence and is usually of unknown cause. The defect is usually bilateral but asymmetrical, and the severity of the defect relates to the stage of organogenesis at which the insult occurred. Failure of formation of the primary vesicle, or its early and complete regression, is *true anophthalmos* and is very rare. Failure of optic vesicle invagination gives rise to the very rare *congenital cystic eye*. Incomplete invagination results in *congenital retinal nonattachment*. Failure of division (or subsequent fusion) of the optic primordium as it grows from the telencephalon results in *cyclopia*, or *synophthalmos*, a single dysplastic midline globe.

Anophthalmos and microphthalmos

Anophthalmos, total absence of ocular tissue, is a very rare lesion, and almost all cases described are more correctly termed *severe microphthalmos,* in that some vestige of eye is found in serially sectioned orbital content. The usefulness of distinguishing between the two is questionable, and *many authors have adopted the term "clinical anophthalmos" for all such cases*. Concurrent anomalies of skeletal and central nervous systems are common.

Macroscopic examination of orbital content usually reveals a normal lacrimal gland and vestigial extraocular muscles. The globe is usually recognized as an irregular mass of black pigment, with structures such as cornea or optic nerve variably recognizable. Histologically, there is almost always a mass of pigmented neurectoderm, reminiscent of ciliary processes, and some effort at retinal differentiation (Fig. 4.3). There is frequently some remnant of lens, a finding that suggests regression of an embryonic globe that had reached at least the stage of optic cup. One or more plates of cartilage, presumably derived from third eyelid analog, are common.

Cyclopia and synophthalmos

Damage to the prosencephalon prior to the outgrowth of the optic vesicles may result in improper separation of paired cranial midline structures, including eyes. *Cyclopia is a fetal malformation characterized by a single median orbit containing a single globe.* Most specimens have some duplication of intraocular structures, such as lens, iris, or hyaloid

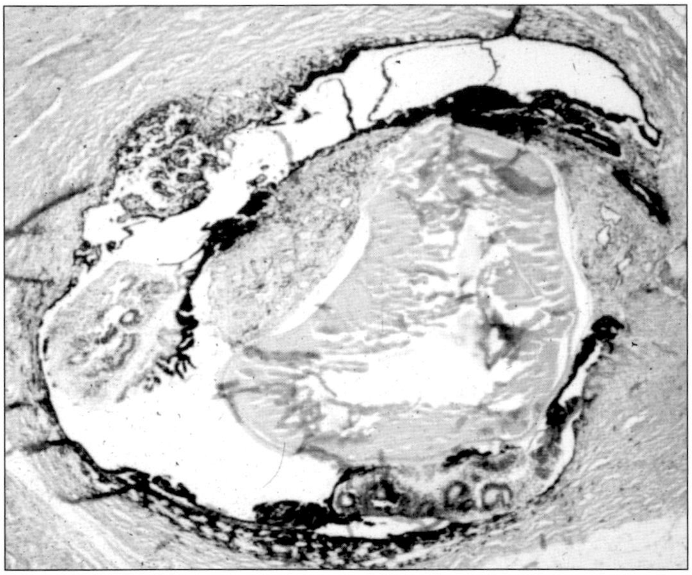

Figure 4.3 Secondary microphthalmia. The ciliary processes tend to be highly conserved even in the most disorganized globes.

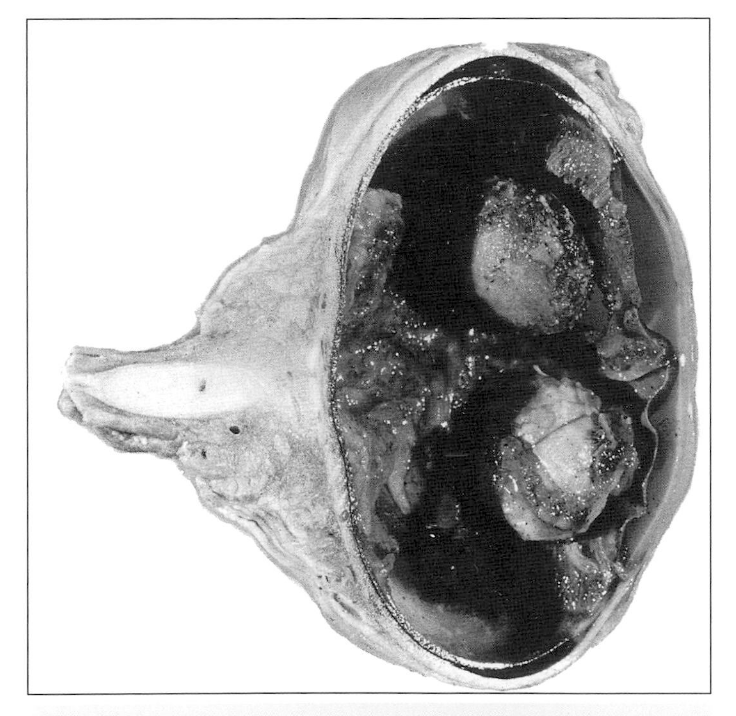

Figure 4.4 Globe from typical "cyclopian" calf. Duplication of lens and pupil indicates **synophthalmos** rather than true cyclopia.

vessels, and are thus more properly considered *incomplete separation or early fusion (synophthalmos)* (Fig. 4.4). Some specimens have two dysplastic globes within a single orbit. Severe cranial anomalies accompany cyclopia and synophthalmos, including absent or deformed ears, a median proboscis, cranioschisis, cleft palate, and brain anomalies ranging from microcephaly to hydranencephaly and hydrocephalus.

Cyclopian-like malformations have been reported in sheep, chickens, and dogs, and as inherited defects in cattle with the most thoroughly documented cases being in sheep grazing alpine pastures rich in the legume *Veratrum californicum*. Fresh and dried plants contain three steroidal alkaloids – jervine, cyclopamine, and cycloposine – capable of damaging the developing neural groove of the fetal lamb. Ewes eating the plant on gestational day 15 have lambs with the cyclopian malformation, for it is at that time that the neural groove has formed and the first cranial somites are forming. A similar syndrome has been produced in kids and calves by maternal feeding of the plant on day 14 of gestation. Ingestion of the alkaloids prior to day 15 in sheep may cause fetal death but no anomalies, and exposure soon after day 15 may cause various skeletal abnormalities but not cyclopia.

In naturally occurring outbreaks, affected lambs have deformities ranging from cyclopia with microcephaly to relatively normal lambs with harelip and cleft palate. Prolonged gestation is common in the case of severely malformed fetuses.

Cystic eye and retinal nonattachment

Failure of apposition of the optic vesicle to the cranial ectoderm results in failure of lens induction, which in turn removes the major stimulus for invagination of the optic vesicle to form the optic cup. *Persistence of the primary optic vesicle is seen as a cystic eye* (Fig. 4.5), consisting of a scleral sheet lined by neurectoderm of variable neurosensory and pigmentary differentiation. The absence of lens and of bilayered iridociliary epithelium distinguishes this rare lesion from the more common dysplastic eye of secondary microphthalmos.

Incomplete invagination of the optic vesicle allows persistence of the cavity of the primary optic vesicle and prevents attachment of the presumptive neurosensory retina to the developing retinal pigment epithelium. *In the postnatal globe, retinal nonattachment cannot easily be distinguished from acquired retinal separation.* In each instance, the retina is extensively folded and may have improper differentiation of neuronal layers. The diagnosis of retinal nonattachment is assisted if there is also lack of apposition between the two layers of neurectoderm covering the anterior uvea (destined to be iridal and ciliary epithelium) and if retinal rosettes are evident. In addition, since nonattachment is an early and fundamental error in organogenesis, such eyes usually lack a lens and probably will be microphthalmic with multiple anomalies.

Coloboma

The mildest and latest defect in organogenesis results from failure of complete fusion of the lips of the optic (embryonic) fissure, a slit-like but normal channel in the floor of the optic cup and stalk through which the vasoformative mesoderm and stromal mesenchyme enter the globe. Failure of closure of the fissure may occur anywhere along its length, but the channel persists most frequently as a notch-like defect of the caudal pole at, or just ventral to, the optic disk. Its exact location can vary substantially. It is lined by an outpouching of dysplastic neurectoderm. If the defect is sufficiently large, the outpouching of neurectoderm induces a similar bulge in the sclera, termed **scleral ectasia** (Fig. 4.6). Occasionally such ectasias are so large as to form a retrobulbar cyst as large as the globe itself (Fig. 4.7). Regardless of size, the lining of the scleral coloboma is formed by neurectoderm that bulged through the defect in the optic cup. Abortive neurosensory differentiation within the cyst wall is common and permits definitive

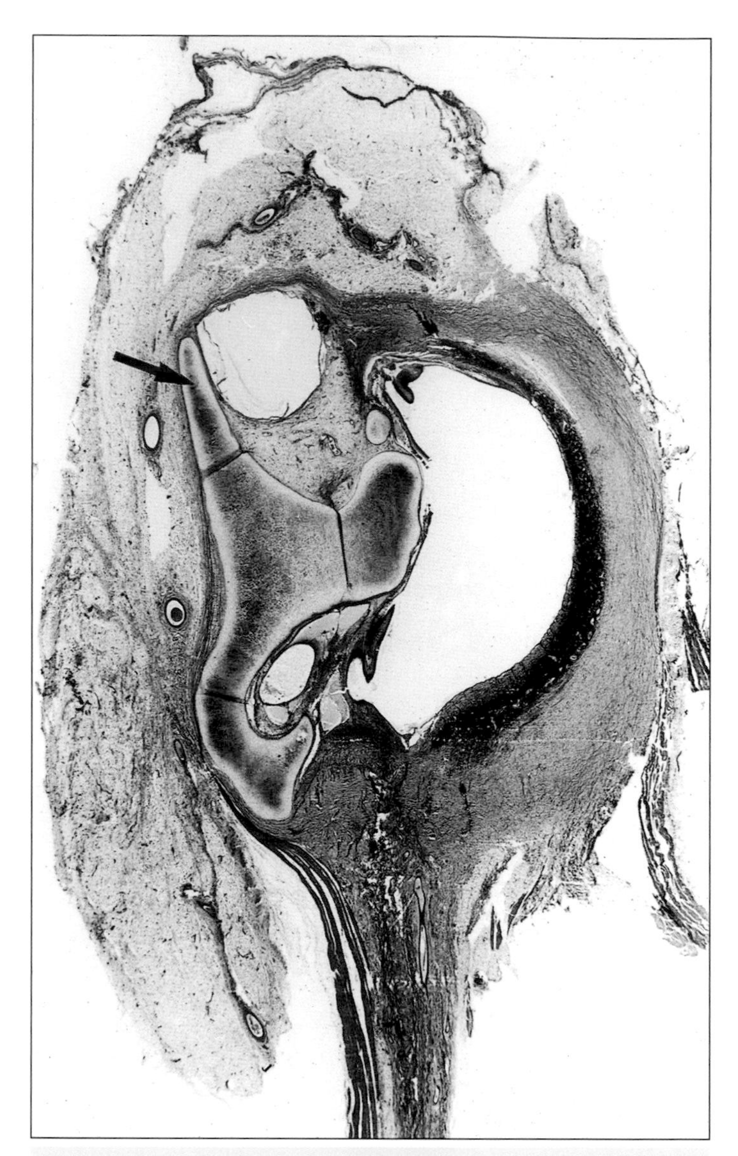

Figure 4.5 Severe **microphthalmos** in a foal. There is no lens, no apparent attempt at invagination, and no neurosensory retinal differentiation. Persistence of the cavity of the optic vesicle qualifies this as a cystic eye. Cartilage plate (arrow) is probably an analog of the third eyelid.

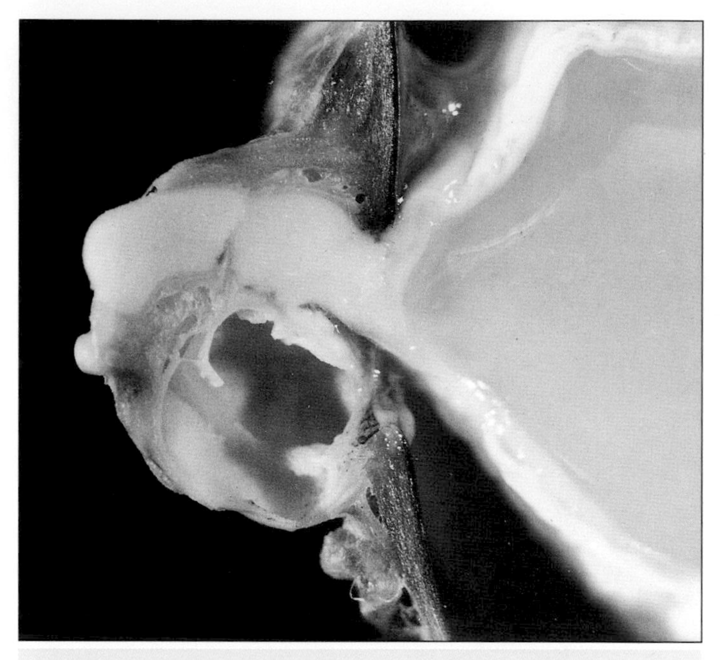

Figure 4.6 Coloboma adjacent to the optic disk, accompanied by retinal separation. Collie eye anomaly.

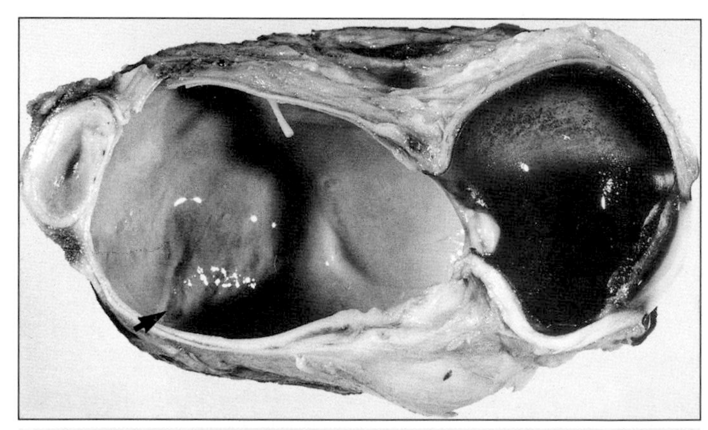

Figure 4.7 Retrobulbar cyst (arrow) formed by coloboma and massive scleral ectasia in a calf. The globe is small and the retina is completely separated.

identification of the retrobulbar cyst as being a **coloboma** (absence or defect of some ocular tissue) in terms of pathogenesis (Fig. 4.8).

Colobomas occur in all domestic species, but are especially frequent in Collie dogs as one manifestation of the Collie eye anomaly. In Collies, they usually arise within or just adjacent to the optic disk. They appear to arise as focal defects in maturation and/or induction of sclera and choroid by the retinal pigment epithelium (RPE) that is forming from the outer layer of the optic cup. Because the exact location of the embryonic fissure is somewhat variable, it is difficult to determine how many examples of coloboma are the result of delayed closure of that normal embryologic structure, and how many represent some more fundamental defect in the proper interaction of RPE and the developing periocular mesenchyme destined to form choroid and sclera. Proper maturation of the RPE, and in particular the normal acquisition of pigmentation, appears to be critical to the induction of normal mesenchymal migration and maturation. Its failure results in such varied anomalies as choroidal hypoplasia, segmental or diffuse iris and ciliary hypoplasia (known clinically as **iris coloboma**), and even microphthalmia. Because of its frequent association with the merle dilution defect in the coat color of dogs, the general syndrome is known as *merle ocular dysgenesis*. It is similar, but not identical, to Collie eye anomaly. The same defect occurs, with much less frequency, in color-dilute (incompletely albinotic) horses, cattle, non-merle dogs, and cats. A similar pathogenesis and spectrum of lesions, not proven to be associated with color dilution, occurs in Collie eye anomaly (see later). In Charolais cattle, colobomas of (or near) the optic disk are inherited as an autosomal dominant trait with incomplete penetrance. The lesion is bilateral but not necessarily equal in severity.

Defective differentiation

Subsequent to formation of the optic cup, ocular differentiation involves continued differentiation of neurectoderm into retinal and

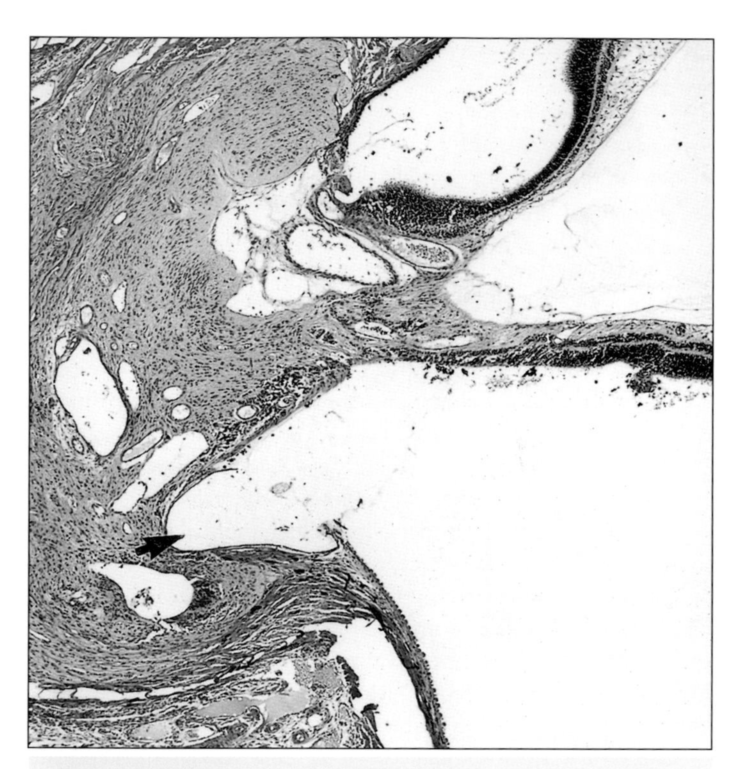

Figure 4.8 Coloboma (arrow) at the optic disk in a Collie pup with Collie eye anomaly. Dysplastic neurectoderm lines the defect and attempts to form sensory retina.

uveal neuroepithelium, and induction of primitive periocular neural crest mesenchyme to form the sclera and uvea. The normal development of retinal pigment epithelium from the neurectoderm of the posterior half of the optic vesicle seems prerequisite for these differentiations to occur.

It is traditional to present specific ocular anomalies as they relate to structures of the adult eye, and thus as anomalies of cornea, iris, lens, retina, and so on. This approach correlates well with the clinical examination of the eye but provides no understanding of the fundamental pathogenesis of the anomaly. *Here we will organize these "later" anomalies (occurring after the stage of optic cup formation) on the basis of the presumed pathogenesis: defective migration, proliferation, or remodeling of ocular mesenchyme, defective maturation of neurectoderm, and defective development of ectoderm.*

Bibliography

Bildfell R, et al. Bilateral optic disc colobomas in a Quarter Horse filly. Equine Vet J 2003;35:325–327.

Binns W, et al. Chronologic evaluation of teratogenesis in sheep fed *Veratrum californicum*. J Am Vet Med Assoc 1963;147:839–842.

Cook C, et al. Embryogenesis of posterior segment colobomas in the Australian Shepherd dog. Prog Vet Comp Ophthalmol 1991;1:163–170.

Dietz HH. Retinal dysplasia in dogs–a review. Nord Vet Med 1985;37:1–9.

Lee ST, et al. Development of an enzyme-linked immunosorbent assay for the veratrum plant teratogens: cyclopamine and jervine. J Agric Food Chem 2003;51:582–586.

Leipold HW, et al. Multiple ocular anomalies and hydrocephalus in grade beef shorthorn cattle. Am J Vet Res 1971;32:1019–1026.

Lowe JK, et al. Linkage mapping of the primary disease locus for collie eye anomaly. Genomics 2003;82:86–95.

McCormack J. Typical colobomas in Charolais bulls. Vet Med Small Anim Clin 1977;72:1626–1628.

Palludan B. The influence of vitamin A deficiency on foetal development in pigs with special reference to eye organogenesis. Int J Vitam Nutr Res 1976;46:223–235.

Wallin-Hakanson B, et al. Collie eye anomaly in the rough collie in Sweden: genetic transmission and influence on offspring vitality. J Small Anim Pract 2000;41:254–258.

Wheeler CA, Collier LL. Bilateral colobomas involving the optic discs in a Quarterhorse. Eq Vet J 1990;(Suppl 10):39–41.

Anomalies of mesenchyme

After formation of the optic cup and separation of the lens vesicle, the periocular mesenchyme undergoes a complex series of migrations, differentiations, and atrophies that determines the final structure of the vascular and fibrous tunics of the globe. At the anterior edge of the optic cup, one or more waves of mesenchymal invasion form corneal endothelium, corneal stroma, and the anterior half of the transient perilenticular vascular network, including the pupillary membrane. The posterior half of this perilenticular vascular tunic is formed by invasion of mesodermal endothelial cell precursors and supporting perivascular mesenchyme through the optic fissure to form the extensive but transient *hyaloid artery system* (see Fig. 4.2). Another mesenchymal wave accompanies the ingrowth of the neurectoderm at the anterior lip of the optic cup to form the iris stroma, although it is unclear which layer acts as the primary inducer. Its peripheral portion later atrophies to form the porous *filtration angle* of the anterior chamber, a process that may not be completed in carnivores until 6–8 weeks after birth. The choroid and sclera are induced by the developing retinal pigment epithelium to form from the mesenchyme surrounding the caudal half of the optic cup.

Anomalies of mesenchyme may result from defective ingrowth or differentiation, as with choroidal and iris hypoplasia, incomplete atrophy of the tunica vasculosa lentis or hyaloid artery system, or incomplete remodeling of the filtration angle to cause primary glaucoma.

Choroidal hypoplasia

This is a relatively common lesion in the eye of dogs by virtue of its prevalence in the Collie breed as the hallmark of Collie eye anomaly, and a very similar syndrome occurs in Australian Shepherd dogs and Shetland Sheepdogs. It is also seen in a variety of dog breeds in association with genes for color dilution (merle, dapple, and harlequin). *The hypoplasia is thought to result from induction failure by a defective retinal pigment epithelium.* The basic defect is not clearly established but may be related to defective pigmentation, a suggestion supported by the prevalence of iris and choroidal hypoplasia in white animals of all species, especially those with blue irises. Other anomalies linked to the choroidal hypoplasia/hypopigmentation include optic nerve coloboma, microphthalmia, and (with the merle ocular dysgenesis) cataract and segmental iris hypoplasia. Some degree of retinal dysplasia is also common. At least in theory, all of these defects are predictable outcomes of improper mesenchymal induction by a defective, inadequately pigmented retinal pigment epithelium. Even in otherwise normal (nonwhite) animals with a blue iris, there is usually hypoplasia of the tapetum and choroid.

Collie eye anomaly

This is a common disease of smooth and rough Collies, first reported in 1953 and at one time estimated to have affected 90% of North American Collies. During the period 1975–1979, the defect was still present in over 70% of 20 000 Collies examined in a voluntary screening program. Prevalence in Europe and the United Kingdom is lower (30–60%). *The basic defect, patchy to diffuse choroidal hypoplasia, is inherited as an autosomal recessive trait*, but the numerous associated defects are more unpredictable in their familial pattern. Similar syndromes are reported in Border Collies, Shetland Sheepdogs, and Australian Shepherd dogs, and are probably of similar pathogenesis. The prevalence in these breeds, as in rough Collies, has marked geographic variation.

The *ophthalmoscopic findings* include one or more of retinal vessel tortuosity, focal to diffuse choroidal and tapetal hypoplasia, optic nerve coloboma, and retinal separation with intraocular hemorrhage. Other observations that are occasionally made in eyes of affected dogs are enophthalmos, microphthalmos, and corneal stromal mineralization. The disease is always bilateral but not necessarily equal. Even the mild, visually insignificant lesion of focal choroidal hypoplasia is genetically significant.

Macroscopic examination of the bisected globe reveals abnormal pallor of the posterior segment of the globe. If the globe is transilluminated, the sclera and choroid are focally or diffusely more translucent than normal. The pallor and translucency imply choroidal hypoplasia. Within or adjacent to the optic disk there may be a colobomatous pit of variable size, the lining of which is continuous with the retina. Accompanying the larger type of pit is a bulge in the overlying sclera, called **scleral ectasia** or **posterior staphyloma.** If there is retinal separation, it is usually complete, with the only sites of attachment being at the abnormal optic disk and at the ora ciliaris (Fig. 4.9). In such cases, there may be extensive intravitreal hemorrhage and retinal tears. Almost all Collie eyes with retinal separation have large optic disk colobomas. Detachment from the ora ciliaris (so-called *retinal disinsertion*) may also occur, leaving the folded retina on the floor of the globe (Fig. 4.10).

The fundamental histologic lesion found in all affected eyes is choroidal hypoplasia. It is always diffuse, despite ophthalmoscopic observation of a lesion that may appear only to be focal within the dorsal temporal quadrant of the fundus. The choroid is thin and poorly pigmented, and the tapetum is thinner than normal or even absent (Fig. 4.11A, B). Retinal pigment epithelium is poorly pigmented, even in nontapetal fundus, and may be vacuolated. Because the choroid and tapetum in the normal dog do not reach adult thickness until about 4 months postpartum, age-matched control eyes are essential if overinterpretation of normal choroidal immaturity is to be avoided.

Histologic examination of eyes with optic disk colobomas reveals the bulging of dysplastic neurectoderm, continuous with retina, into the pit in the nerve head. The neurectoderm may show jumbled differentiation into ganglion cells, photoreceptor rosettes, glial cells, or pigment epithelium. Rosettes are common in the neurosensory retina adjacent to affected disks or embedded in the optic disk itself. In some specimens, there are degenerative retinal lesions overlying severely hypoplastic choroid. Edematous clefts are seen in the nerve fiber layer, and ganglion cells may be severely vacuolated.

Other retinal lesions include retinal folds and detachment. The folds are seen on histologic section as tubes of fully differentiated retina cut in cross-section or tangentially, and are thought to represent folds in a neurosensory retina that at least temporarily has grown in excess of the space available for it within the optic cup. These folds correspond to the clinically detectable vermiform streaks in the fundus, and gradually disappear as the dog (and eye) matures, allowing the growth of scleral shell to catch up with that of retina. Presumably it is a similar growth imbalance, but in the opposite direction, that causes retinal separation in about 10% of eyes with this syndrome. In this situation, a retina that is too small attempts to stretch from optic disk to ora ciliaris by the shortest route, rather than following the curvature of the scleral shell.

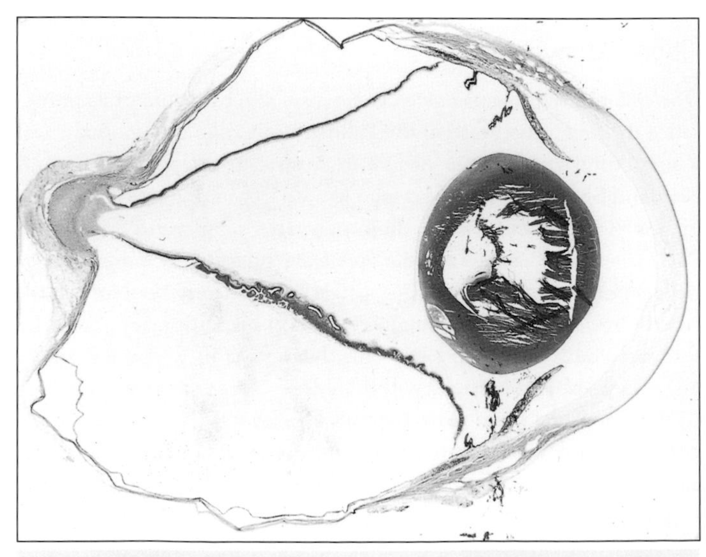

Figure 4.9 Retinal separation in Collie eye anomaly. There is coloboma at the optic disk. Choroid and sclera are thin. Retinal folding does not constitute dysplasia.

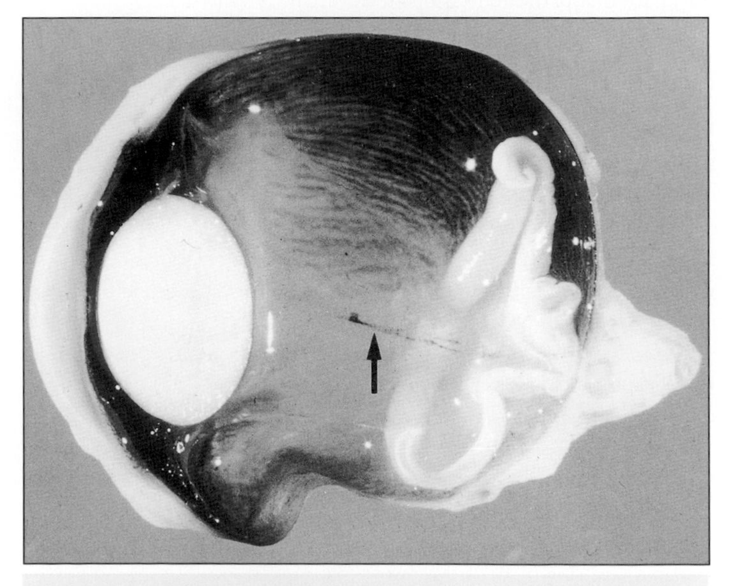

Figure 4.10 Retinal separation from ora ciliaris in Collie eye anomaly. Note hypopigmented choroid and prominent hyaloid artery (arrow).

Focal fibroblastic metaplasia and mineralization are occasionally seen in the subepithelial corneal stroma of dogs with Collie eye anomaly, but a similar defect is seen in anomalous eyes of other breeds; a genetic link to the Collie eye defect is not established. Tortuosity of retinal veins, a controversial clinical lesion sometimes considered part of Collie eye anomaly, has no described histologic counterpart.

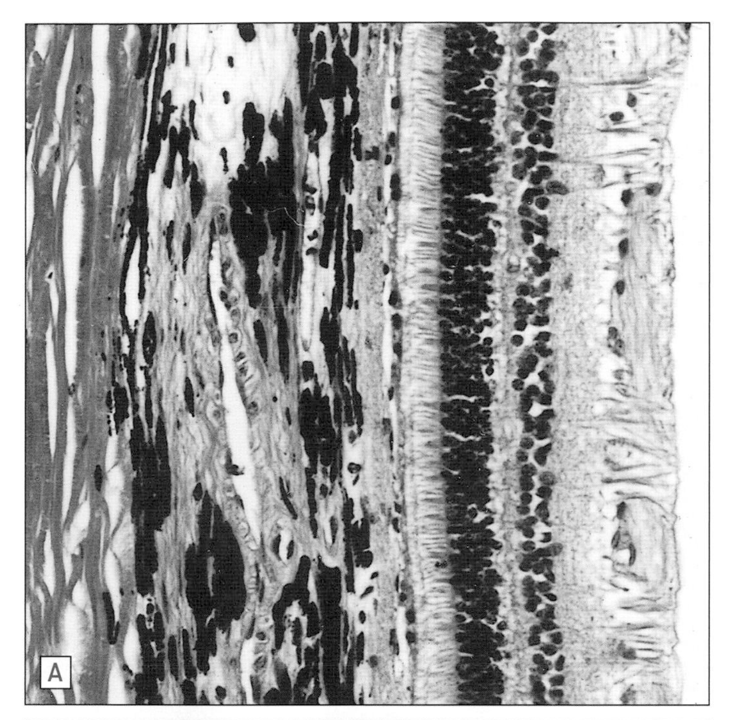

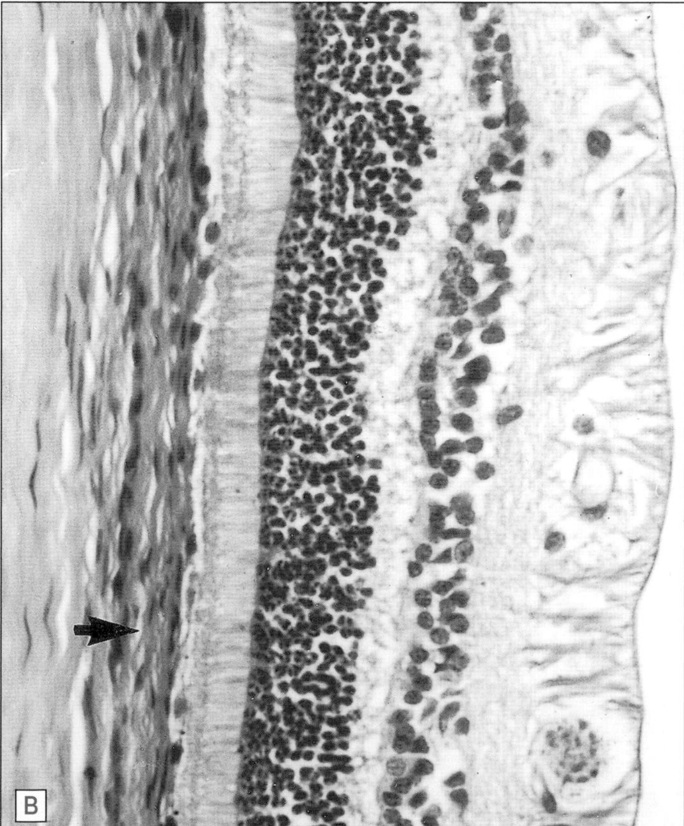

Figure 4.11 A. Normal posterior pole of the globe of a 13-week-old puppy. Tapetum present but thin (normal for puppy). Choroidal thickness approximates that of retina. **B.** Posterior pole just dorsal to the optic disk of a 13-week-old Collie with **Collie eye anomaly**. Tapetum is absent. Choroid (arrow) is severely hypoplastic.

The earliest lesion of this anomaly is defective differentiation of primitive retinal pigment epithelium to form rosette-like structures near the optic disk. Proper differentiation of both pigment epithelium and neurosensory retina requires obliteration of the lumen of the primary optic vesicle, which allows the two neurectodermal layers to come into apposition. Whether the earliest lesion of Collie eye anomaly results from inherently defective differentiation of pigment epithelium or from imperfect apposition of the two neurectodermal layers has not been resolved, but the central role of the pigment epithelium in determining ocular morphology suggests that the primary defect is in maturation of the presumptive retinal pigment epithelium. Anomalous development of choroid and sclera, including coloboma, is not seen in fetuses up to 45 gestational days, but is seen in neonates. This suggests that the defect is in choroidal maturation rather than in initial induction.

Another manifestation of mesenchymal maldevelopment in Collie eye anomaly, rarely noted clinically, is delayed atrophy and remodeling in the anterior chamber. The filtration angle may be closed, iris stroma may be attached to the corneal endothelium by a mesenchymal bridge, and remnants of anterior perilenticular mesenchyme are unusually prominent. Pigmentation of iridal neurectoderm is sparse. As these neonatal anterior segment lesions are not seen later in life (8–20 weeks) when puppies are examined ophthalmoscopically, it is presumed that they reflect only a minor delay in mesenchymal remodelling.

Defects primarily in anterior chamber mesenchyme

Hypoplasia of the iris *is a rare defect that may occur alone or in conjunction with multiple ocular defects.* It is relatively most frequent in horses, where it may be inherited and associated with cataract and conjunctival dermoids. The defect presumably results from incomplete inward migration of the anterior lip of the optic cup, with resultant lack of a neurectodermal scaffold to guide the subsequent migration of mesenchyme destined to form the iris stroma. The hypoplasia is usually severe and most cases are clinically described as *aniridia*. Histologic examination of such eyes usually reveals the vestigial iris as a triangular mesenchymal stump covered posteriorly by normal-appearing pigmented epithelium (Fig. 4.12A). The trabecular meshwork within the filtration angles may be malformed, but the ciliary apparatus is usually normal. The lens often is cataractous (Fig. 4.12B) and sometimes ectopic or hypoplastic. Glaucoma has been described as a sequel in horses (but not in other species), but it should be an expected sequel in severely affected eyes in any species because of the inevitable concurrent trabecular hypoplasia (Fig 4.12A).

Hypopigmentation of the iris may be unilateral or bilateral. When the loss of pigment is patchy in one or both irises, it is known as *heterochromia iridis*. The pigmentation may be diffusely absent in the iris stroma but present in the posterior iris epithelium (*subalbinotic*), or absent in both stroma and epithelium (*true albinism*). The iris is normal except for absence of visible pigment granules in the cytoplasm of otherwise normal stromal melanocytes and epithelial cells. Tapetum and, less reliably, choroid of affected eyes usually are hypoplastic as well as poorly pigmented.

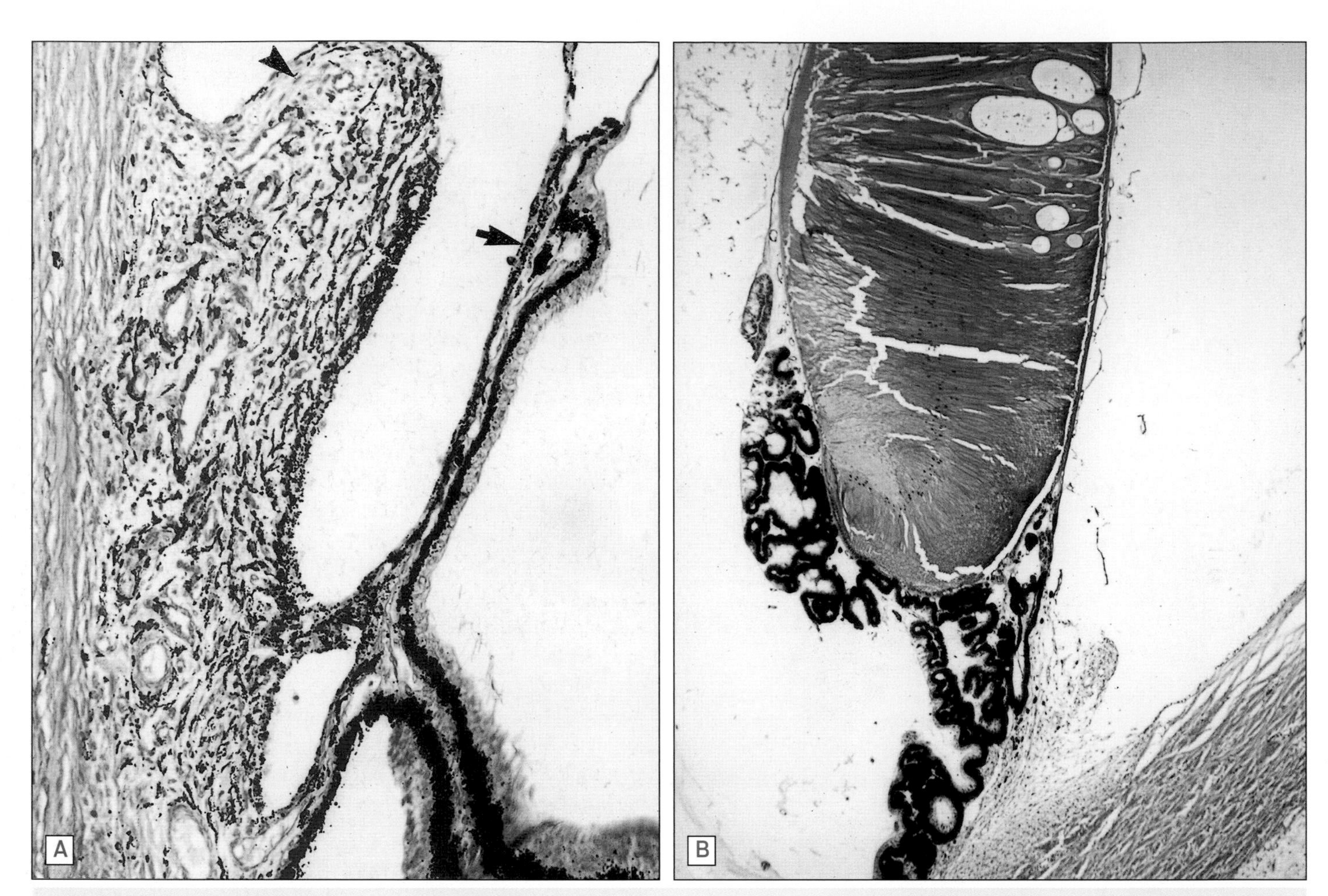

Figure 4.12 A. Iris hypoplasia (arrowhead) with hypoplasia of the trabecular meshwork in a dog. The ciliary processes (arrow) have developed normally. **B. Iris hypoplasia**, congenital cataract and dysplasia of ciliary processes in a piglet; one of three affected. The adherence of ciliary processes to the lens represents an arrest in remodeling rather than improper development.

Incomplete atrophy of the anterior chamber mesenchyme is relatively common in dogs and occurs occasionally in other domestic species. During organogenesis, waves of mesenchyme migrate between the surface ectoderm and the anterior rim of the optic cup. Some of the ingrowing mesenchyme forms corneal endothelium and stroma, while other portions of mesenchyme form the iris stroma and trabecular meshwork. Some of that mesenchyme occupies the anterior chamber and, as it matures, it forms a fibrovascular sheet stretching across the face of the lens and developing iris, known as the *pupillary membrane*. Its vascular component creates the anterior portion of an embryonic perilenticular vascular plexus, known as the *tunica vasculosa lentis*. Both the pupillary membrane and the tunica vasculosa lentis normally disappear late in gestation or in the early postnatal period. Failure of this anterior chamber fibrovascular mesenchyme to atrophy results in the very common anomaly of **persistent pupillary membrane** (persistence of the tunica vasculosa lentis alone is discussed later).

Atrophy of the pupillary membrane is frequently incomplete at birth and, in dogs, persistent remnants are common up to about 6 months of age. These insignificant and usually bloodless strands are seen as short, thread-like protrusions from the area of the minor arterial circle (iris collarette) and they may insert elsewhere on the iris, cross the pupil, or extend blindly into the anterior chamber (Fig. 4.13A). Persistent pupillary membranes achieve clinical significance in two ways. First, the size and number of strands crossing the pupil may be such that vision is obstructed. Second, strands that contact lens or cornea are associated with focal dysplasia of lens or corneal endothelium, clinically seen as opacity (Fig. 4.13B). Because the normal pupillary membrane never contacts the cornea, strands of pupillary membrane that extend from iris to cornea are considered to be minor versions of anterior segment dysgenesis (see below).

Histologic descriptions are mainly from studies in *Basenji dogs*, in which persistent pupillary membrane occurs as an autosomal recessive trait of variable penetrance. In this breed, atrophy of the pupillary membrane is abnormally slow even in dogs free of the defect in adult life, and remnants in puppies up to 8 months old are common. The membranes are seen as thin endothelial tubes, invested with a thin adventitial stroma, extending from vessels in the iris stroma near the collarette. The tubes are usually empty, but in severely affected eyes may contain erythrocytes, and the adventitia may contain melanin. The tubes weave in and out of the plane of section en route to corneal, iridic, or lenticular insertions. At sites of corneal insertion, corneal endothelium is either absent or dysplastic, with the latter manifested as fibrous metaplasia. Descemet's membrane is malformed or absent in the areas of attachment and there is associated deep stromal corneal edema to account for the clinically observed, minute

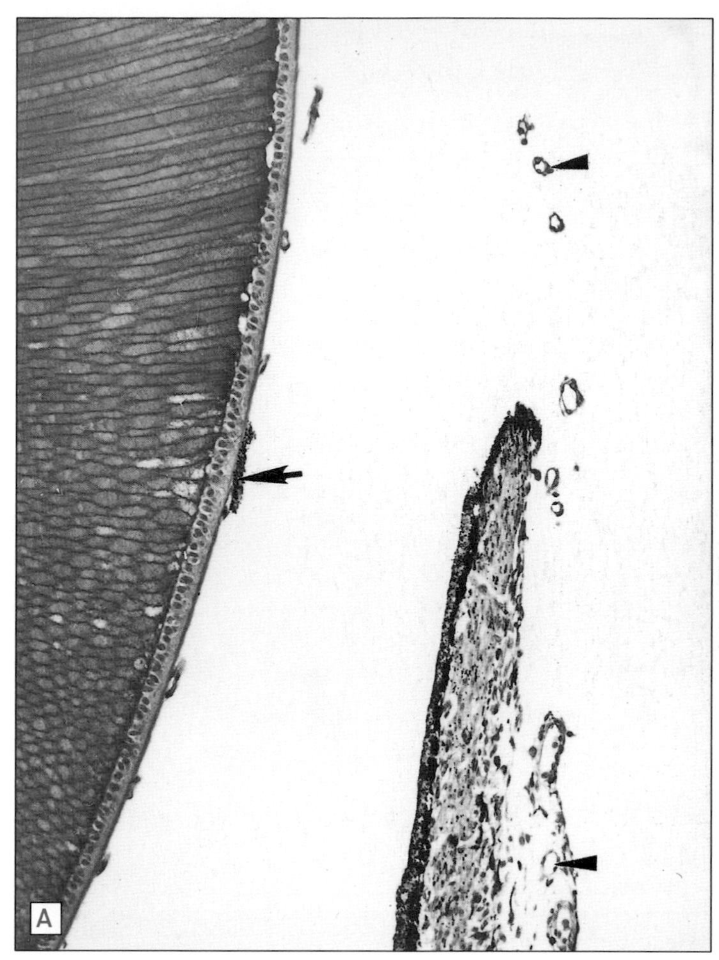

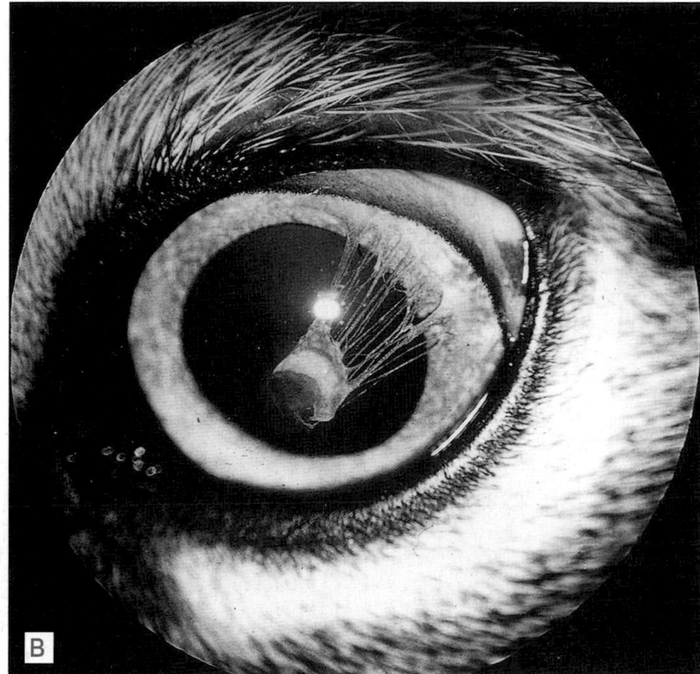

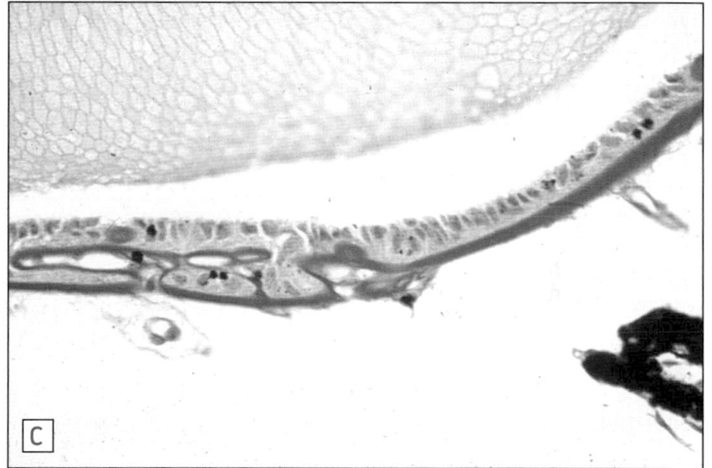

Figure 4.13 Persistent pupillary membrane. A. Persistence of the **anterior tunica vasculosa lentis** (arrow) and **pupillary membrane** (arrowheads), the latter continuous with the iris stromal vessels. **B. Central crescent insertion** of the persistent pupillary membrane in a dog is on the anterior pole of the lens, where it has induced a focal cataract. **C. Dysplastic development** of the anterior lens capsule as a consequence of adherence of persistent pupillary membrane.

gray stromal opacities. *Contact with the lens is accompanied by similar epithelial and basement membrane dysplasia, resulting in one or more epithelial, subcapsular, or polar cortical cataracts* (Fig. 4.13C). Some would classify this latter, more severe form of persistent pupillary membrane as a mild version of anterior segment dysgenesis (see below).

Much less common than persistent pupillary membrane are those defects grouped under the general category of **anterior segment dysgenesis** (or **anterior segment cleavage syndrome**). This group includes multiple anomalies of cornea, lens, and anterior uvea that stem from disordered development of anterior segment mesenchyme and/or improper separation of the developing lens from the overlying corneal mesenchyme. Such eyes are commonly microphthalmic and usually have microphakia, cataract, and congenital corneal opacities at sites of congenital anterior synechiae. The most severe cases have fusion of iris with corneal stroma without observed corneal endothelium or Descemet's membrane (forming a so-called "internal corneal ulcer"), and thus have no detectable anterior chamber (Fig. 4.14). *Most examples in dogs and cats probably result from perinatal corneal perforation from trauma or from progression of suppurative bacterial keratoconjunctivitis (ophthalmia neonatorum).* The

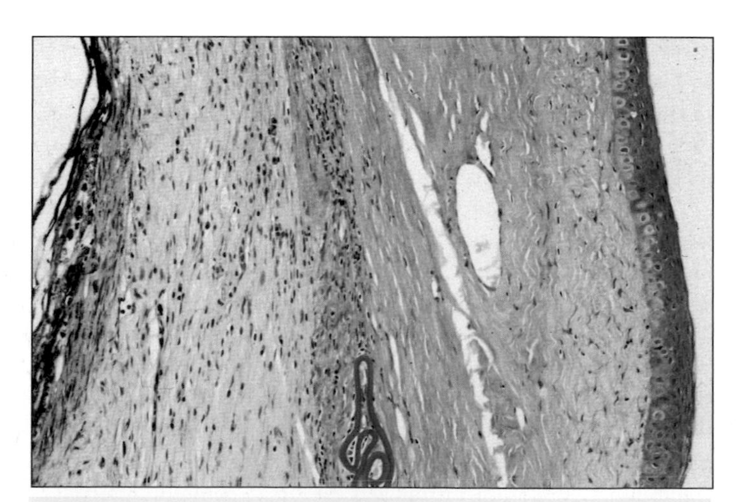

Figure 4.14 Anterior segment dysgenesis. Improper remodeling of anterior segment mesenchyme results in failure of formation of the anterior chamber. The iris is then fused to the cornea.

result is iris prolapse and incorporation of the iris into the developing cornea resulting in obliteration of the anterior chamber. Since the globe of dogs and cats continues to develop for many weeks after birth, this is yet another example of how difficult it can be to precisely distinguish idiopathic developmental disorders from those resulting from postnatal traumatic or inflammatory diseases.

Maldevelopment of the filtration angle (goniodysgenesis) occurs as a prevalent, inherited condition in dogs and in severely anomalous eyes of animals of any species. The defect may result from incomplete atrophy of mesenchyme that normally fills the fetal iridocorneal angle, or from inadequate posterior migration of the iris root. The defect is much more common in dogs than any other species. In the most severe cases, the trabecular meshwork may appear as a solid mesenchymal mass indistinguishable from the adjacent iris stroma (Fig. 4.15A). This rare lesion, known us *trabecular hypoplasia*, is a cause for truly congenital glaucoma. It is often accompanied by iris hypoplasia. Much more commonly, the error in remodeling is less profound and the lesion is seen as an imperforate or inadequately perforated mesenchymal sheet separating anterior chamber from a relatively normal trabecular meshwork (Fig. 4.15B). The only lesion may thus be a pectinate ligament that is thicker, more heavily pigmented and less fenestrated than normal. This has sometimes been referred to as *"pectinate ligament dysplasia."* (For a more complete discussion, see Glaucoma.)

Clinically noted ocular features of **bovine Marfan syndrome**, which are similar to human Marfan syndrome, are ectopia lentis, microspherophakia, and myopia. The human disease is caused by mutations in the fibrillin-1 gene; affected cattle have abnormal fibrillin metabolism. Eyes of affected cattle are characterized by megaloglobus, increased circumlental distance, asymmetrical ciliary processes, intact but fragile zonular fibers, and ectopia lentis. Affected animals have moderately hypoplastic ciliary bodies, compact filtration angles, and long thin irises with decreased fibrous stroma.

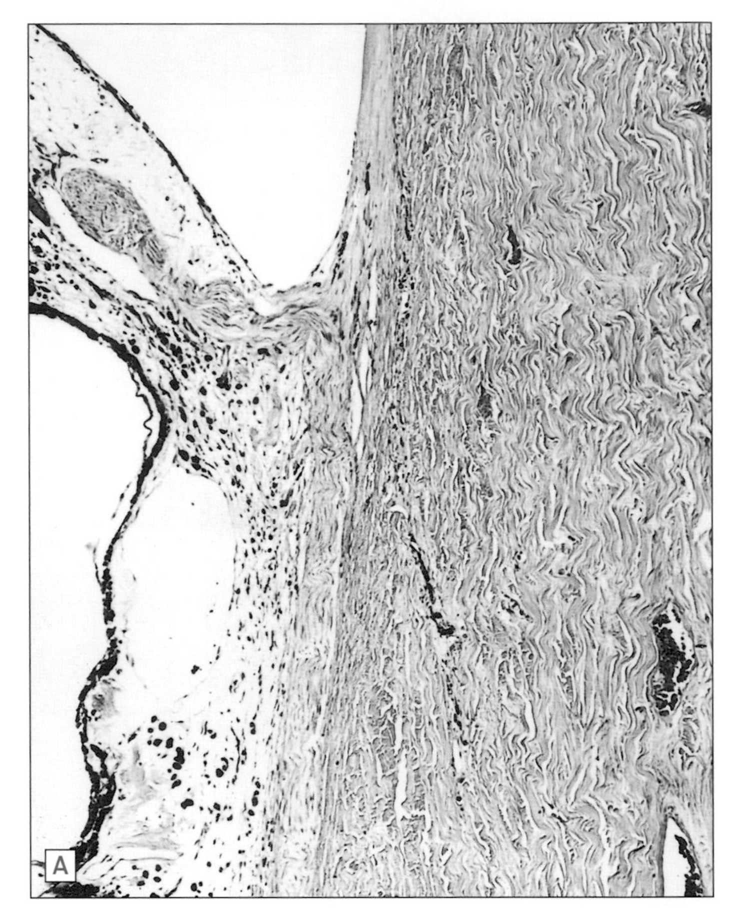

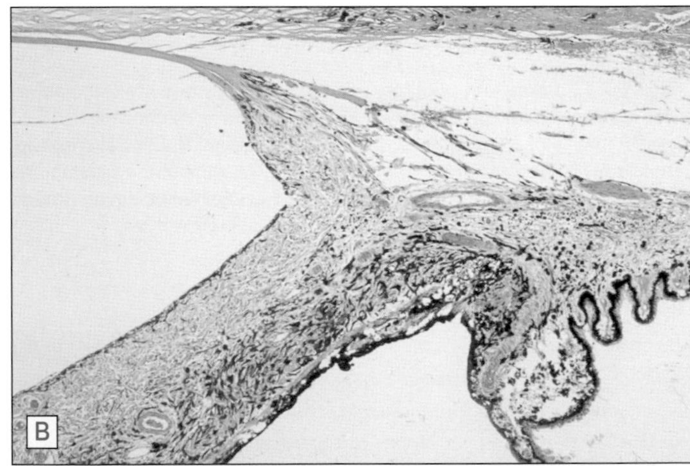

Figure 4.15 A. Goniodysgenesis. A primitive example (**trabecular hypoplasia**) with little maturation of the embryonic mesenchyme destined to form pectinate ligament and trabecular meshwork. **B.** A solid sheet of mesenchyme extends from the termination of Descemet's membrane into the iris stroma, with no obvious pectinate ligament. Other portions of the trabecular meshwork are relatively normal.

Incomplete atrophy of posterior segment mesenchyme

Incomplete atrophy of posterior segment mesenchyme may result in the mild and common lesion of **persistent hyaloid artery,** or in the much rarer but clinically more significant lesions of **persistent posterior perilenticular vascular tunic** with or without concurrent persistence of the primary vitreous. There is a tendency in clinical literature to group all of these defects under the umbrella of **persistent hyperplastic primary vitreous**, but histologically there is quite a wide range in the nature of the defect. Only the most severe qualify as true persistent hyperplastic primary vitreous.

The hyaloid artery and its branches are formed from mesenchyme and pre-endothelial mesoderm that enter the optic cup through the optic fissure prior to its closure. The vessel traverses the optic cup from optic disk to lens, where it ramifies over the posterior lens surface (posterior tunica vasculosa lentis). It joins with the vascular portion of the pupillary membrane (anterior tunica vasculosa lentis) to form a complete perilenticular vascular tunic. *As with its anterior chamber counterpart, the hyaloid system undergoes almost complete atrophy before birth.* Persistence of some vestige into adult life is common and clinically insignificant. In ruminants, the most common remnant is *Bergmeister's papilla*, a cone of glial tissue with a vascular core that extends from optic disk for a few millimeters into the vitreous (Fig.4.16). In calves up to about 2 months of age, the vestigial hyaloid system may still contain blood. In carnivores, it is the pupillary membrane that normally persists for several weeks postnatally. Bloodless remnants of the anterior termination of the hyaloid artery on the posterior lens capsule are known as *Mittendorf's dot*; it is a harmless anomaly, common in dogs and ruminants up to several years of age.

Much less common is undue persistence and even hyperplasia of the anterior end of the hyaloid system (**posterior tunica vasculosa lentis**). The normal tissue is a combination of blood vessels and

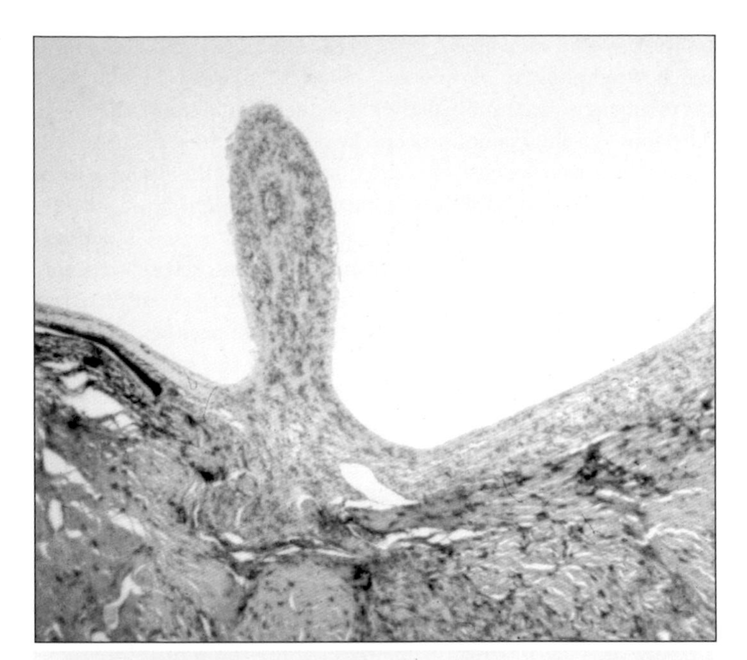

Figure 4.16 Bergmeister's papilla, the minimal histologic presentation of persistent hyaloid artery.

perivascular mesenchyme. Surrounding the hyaloid system is some primitive collagen, poorly characterized extracellular matrix, and a few macrophages. The combination of blood vessels and surrounding stroma is known as the *primary vitreous*. At least theoretically, *anomalous retention of the hyaloid artery and/or primary vitreous could therefore be separated into distinct entities of persistent hyaloid, persistent posterior tunica vasculosa lentis, persistent primary vitreous, and persistent hyperplastic primary vitreous*. Of these, the one most frequently reported (perhaps just because it is the most spectacular and significant) is **persistent hyperplastic primary vitreous**. In people, this rare anomaly is typically unilateral and is accompanied by microphthalmos, microphakia, retinal detachment, shallow anterior chamber, and embryonic filtration angles. The many reports of this anomaly in dogs have described a unilateral or bilateral retrolental vascular or fibrovascular network, usually without any other reported anomalies other than the expected posterior polar cataract. Such lesions are better described as *persistent posterior tunica vasculosa lentis*. In Doberman Pinschers, Bouviers and Staffordshire Bull Terriers, the classification as hyperplastic primary vitreous is more credible. In these breeds, the defect is inherited and forms a spectrum that includes persistent pupillary membrane, cataract, lenticonus, and microphthalmia as well as persistence of variable amounts of primary vitreous and posterior tunica vasculosa lentis (Fig. 4.17 A, B). The defects are detected as early as gestational day 30, at which time hyperplasia of posterior tunica vasculosa lentis is already obvious. Posterior polar cataracts and preretinal membranes are observed by day 37. The one report of two cases in cats was not supported by histopathology and its correct classification remains unknown.

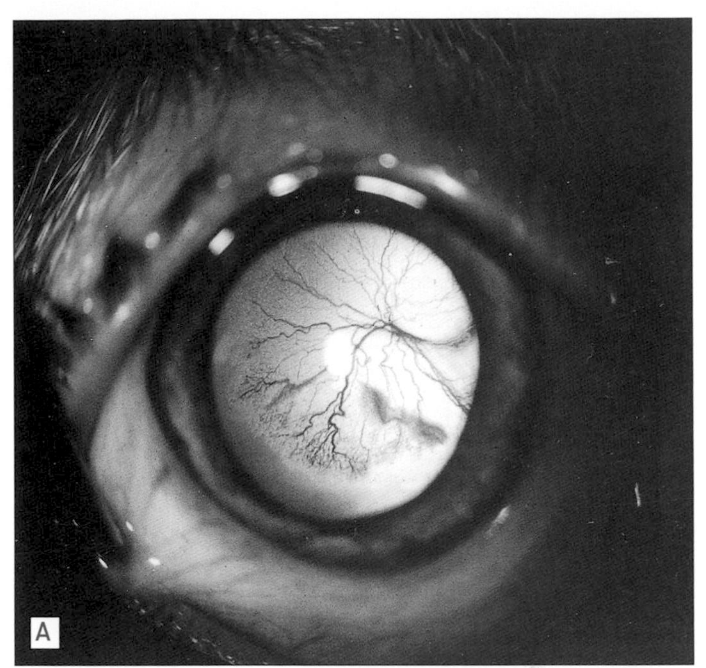

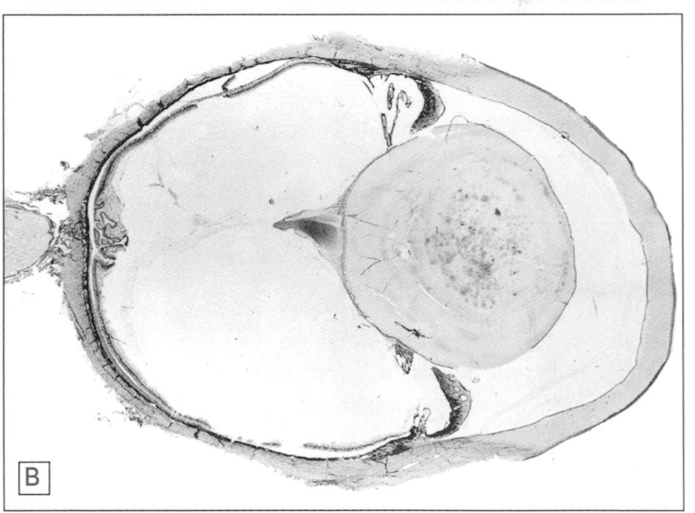

Figure 4.17 A. Persistence of hyaloid artery and posterior tunica vasculosa lentis in a dog. Posterior polar cataract is the almost inevitable consequence, as seen here. **B. Persistent hyperplastic primary vitreous**. A fibrocartilaginous plaque adheres to an elongated lens (lenticonus) and extends to the posterior pole. Retina is dysplastic near the optic disk, and the ciliary processes have not retracted from the lens capsule.

Bibliography

Allgoewer I, Pfefferkorn B. Persistent hyperplastic tunica vasculosa lentis and persistent hyperplastic primary vitreous (PHTVL/PHPV) in two cats. Vet Ophthalmol 2001;4:161–164.

Arnbjerg J, Jensen OA. Spontaneous microphthalmia in two Doberman puppies with anterior chamber cleavage syndrome. J Am Anim Hosp Assoc 1982;18:481–484.

Barnett KC, Knight GC. Persistent pupillary membrane and associated defects in the basenji. Vet Rec 1969;85:242–249.

Bayon A, et al. Ocular complications of persistent hyperplastic primary vitreous in three dogs. Vet Ophthalmol 2001;4:35–41.

Bertram T, et al. Ocular dysgenesis in Australian shepherd dogs. J Am Anim Hosp Assoc 1984;20:177–182.

Bistner S, et al. Diseases of the uveal tract (Part I). Compend Cont Ed 1979;1:868–876.

Boevé MH, et al. Persistent hyperplastic tunica vasculosa lentis and persistent hyperplastic primary vitreous in the dog: a comparative report. Prog Vet Comp Ophthalmol 1992;2:163–172.

Cook C, et al. Embryogenesis of posterior segment colobomas in the Australian Shepherd dog. Prog Vet Comp Ophthalmol 1991;1:163–170.

Crispin SM. Developmental anomalies and abnormalities of the equine iris. Vet Ophthalmol 2000;3:93–98.

Gelatt KN, et al. Ocular anomalies in incomplete albino cattle. Am J Vet Res 1969;30:1313–1316.

Joyce JR, et al. Iridal hypoplasia (aniridia) accompanied by limbic dermoids and cataracts in a group of related Quarterhorses. Eq Vet J 1990;(Suppl 10):26–28.

Lowe JK, et al. Linkage mapping of the primary disease locus for collie eye anomaly. Genomics 2003;82:86–95.

Martin CL. Development of pectinate ligament structure of the dog: Study by scanning electron microscopy. Am J Vet Res 1974;35:1433–1439.

Peiffer RL, et al. Persistent primary vitreous and pigmented cataract in a dog. J Am Anim Hosp Assoc 1977;13:478–480.

Pessier AP, Potter KA. Ocular pathology in bovine Marfan's syndrome with demonstration of altered fibrillin immunoreactivity in explanted ciliary body cells. Lab Invest 1996;75:87–95.

Roberts SR. Color dilution and hereditary defects in collie dogs. Am J Ophthalmol 1967;63:1762–1775.

Rubin LF, et al. Collie eye anomaly in Australian shepherd dogs. Prog Vet Comp Ophthalmol 1991;1:105–108.

Van der Linde-Sipman JS, et al. Persistent hyperplastic tunica vasculosa lentes and persistent hyperplastic primary vitreous in the Doberman pinscher. Pathological aspects. J Am Anim Hosp Assoc 1983;19:791–802.

Wood JL, et al. Pectinate ligament dysplasia and glaucoma in Flat Coated Retrievers. II. Assessment of prevalence and heritability. Vet Ophthalmol 1998;1:91–99.

Anomalies of neurectoderm

Included under this heading are anomalies of retina, optic nerve, and of neuroepithelium of iris and ciliary body. Of these, *retinal anomalies are by far the most frequent and most significant.*

Retinal dysplasia

Retinal dysplasia *is a general term denoting abnormal retinal differentiation characterized by jumbling of retinal layers and by glial proliferation.* In clinical practice, the term has been used incautiously to include genuine retinal dysplasia, postnecrotic retinal scarring of the developing retina, and retinal folding. Genuine retinal dysplasia results from failure of proper apposition of the two layers of the optic cup or from failure of proper induction by an inherently defective retinal pigment epithelium. Those examples clinically classified as retinal dysplasia that reflect disordered wound healing of developing retina, or just folding of retina that is otherwise perfectly formed, should not be considered examples of true retinal dysplasia. While there is no formal agreement on the issue, it seems most logical to divide so-called retinal dysplasia into three different categories: *retinal folds* within an otherwise normal retina, *postnecrotic dysplastic retinal wound healing*, and rare *"true" retinal dysplasia* that is a sequel to some fundamental developmental error in retinal induction or maturation.

Those examples of retinal dysplasia in which the only abnormality is **retinal folding** are by far the most common, and are seen primarily in dogs. The anatomic location, ophthalmoscopic appearance, and effect on vision vary from breed to breed but tend to be uniform within each breed, a fact used by clinical ophthalmologists when attempting to distinguish inherited dysplasias from those occurring as isolated anomalies or as sequelae to in utero infections. The most severe examples occur in dogs with retinal nonattachment. These have extensively folded retinas since the distance to be traversed from optic disk to ora ciliaris in a straight line is shorter than the convex route taken by attached retina, and redundant retina is therefore obliged to fold upon itself. Less severe examples, which are seen much more frequently and in the greatest variety of breeds, probably reflect inequity in growth rate between the retina and the outer layer of the optic cup (choroid and sclera). *The most common example is probably seen in Collie eye anomaly and in American Cocker Spaniels*, in which the defect may be transient. Presumably, the folds become flattened and disappear as continued choroidal and scleral growth eventually create a globe that can accommodate the retina. At least in Collies (and other related breeds with syndromes similar to Collie eye anomaly), *the retinal lesion is probably secondary to defective RPE.* Since the other defects of choroidal/scleral formation and maturation are attributed to faulty induction by a defective RPE, it is reasonable to attribute the retinal folding to the same mechanism (Fig 4.18).

A histologically similar retinal folding that may not depend on retinal:scleral growth imbalance is seen in English Springer Spaniels. Changes are seen as early as gestational day 45 and always by day 55. Focal infolding of the neuroblastic layer away from the retinal pigment epithelium and focal loss of the junctions between the neuroblasts (the outer limiting membrane) are the early changes, followed by overt focal retinal separation and extensive retinal folding. In all breeds in which this type of dysplasia has been adequately studied, it is inherited as a simple autosomal trait.

Retinal dysplasia as a sequel to **retinal necrosis** can occur as a sequel to a wide variety of viral and physical-chemical insults to the embryonic eye; naturally occurring examples are almost exclusively viral. Since the carnivore retina continues to develop for about 6 weeks after birth, the opportunity is great for postnatal injury in

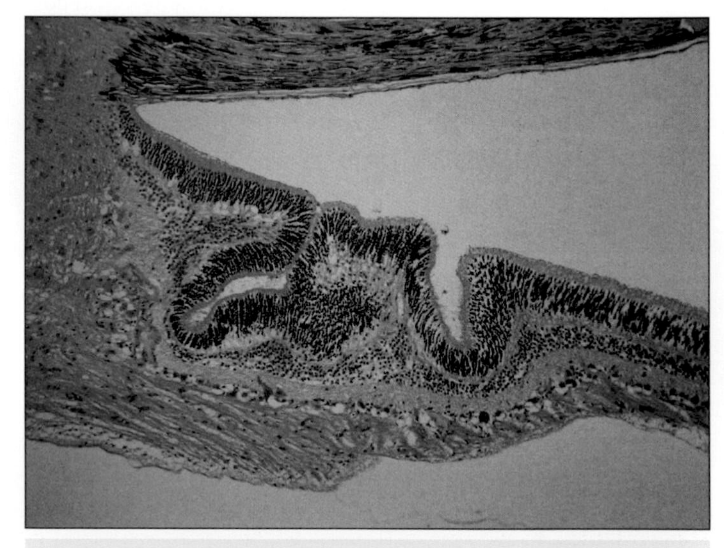

Figure 4.18 Retinal folding, presumably as a result of retinal redundancy that may eventually self-correct as the scleral shell grows to accommodate the retina. Retinal histologic organization is normal, distinguishing this from true retinal dysplasia.

puppies and kittens to produce retinal maldevelopment. Retinal maturation is most rapid in central (peripapillary) retina and progressively less towards the periphery, so that occasionally dysplastic lesions may be encountered only in peripheral retina – suggesting a viral (or other) injury quite close to the 6-week-old limit for dysplasia of this pathogenesis. Mature retina will scar but will not develop lesions of dysplasia.

The specific viruses implicated in domestic animals are *Bovine viral diarrhea virus* in cattle, *Bluetongue virus* in sheep, herpesvirus in dogs, and both parvovirus and leukemia virus in cats. The histologic lesion is similar for all diseases, with variation in lesions caused by the same virus in one species as great as the variation caused by different viruses in different species. *The most significant clue suggesting viral rather than genetic cause is the presence of residual inflammation and postnecrotic scarring in retina, optic nerve and, perhaps subtly, in choroid.* Injured retinal pigment epithelium undergoes one or more of reactive hyperplasia, migration into injured retina as discrete pigmented cells in areas of scarred retina, or metaplastic formation of multilayered fibroglial plaques in place of normal simple cuboidal epithelium (Fig. 4.19A, B). Disorganization of nuclear layers and rosette formation are seen as in other types of dysplasia.

Infection of calves with *Bovine viral diarrhea virus* between 79 and 150 days gestation is the most frequently encountered and thoroughly studied retinal dysplasia of known viral etiology. Work with other viruses has been too limited to allow definition of the susceptible period in fetal development or of the full range of resultant lesions. The limited descriptions of the other viral-induced retinal lesions suggest that the sequence of events is probably quite similar for all such agents.

The initial ocular lesion is nonsuppurative panuveitis and retinitis with multifocal retinal and choroidal necrosis. The acute inflammatory disease gradually subsides over several weeks, and most cases of spontaneous abortion or neonatal death retain scant vestige of previous inflammation. Those ocular structures already well differentiated at the time of the endophthalmitis (cornea, uvea, optic nerve) may undergo atrophy and scarring or be left virtually untouched. Other tissues, such as retina, are actively differentiating and exhibit a combination of the above atrophy and scarring as well as abortive regeneration and arrested differentiation. Retinal pigment epithelium in most examples (*Bluetongue virus* being an apparent exception) is infected and subsequently injured. *The result is a patchy alternation of abortive retinal regeneration, hyperplastic pigment epithelium, and postnecrotic glial scarring* (Fig. 4.19C). The lesions are usually more severe in nontapetal retina and are bilateral but not necessarily symmetrical. It seems reasonable to speculate that those naturally occurring cases in which the dysplasia is confined to peripheral retina represent late viral infection when only peripheral retina is still differentiating.

Because the virus has affinity for other neural tissues, *all calves with retinal dysplasia induced by Bovine viral diarrhea virus also have cerebellar atrophy, and some have hydrocephalus or hydranencephaly.* A similar association with hydrocephalus and other brain anomalies has been described for *Feline panleukopenia virus* infection in cats, *Bluetongue virus* infection in sheep, and in a possibly hereditary syndrome in white Shorthorn and Hereford cattle. In the latter two instances, the involvement of virus could not be excluded based upon published information.

Experimental irradiation of neonatal puppies (and, presumably, kittens) results in retinal necrosis and scarring virtually indistinguishable from postviral retinal dysplasia.

True retinal dysplasia, not associated with exogenous infection or teratogen, is rare. *It is characterized by retinal folds, retinal rosettes, patchy to diffuse blending of nuclear layers, loss of retinal cells and glial scars.* The folds and rosettes are the histologic counterparts of the vermiform streaks seen on the fundus with the ophthalmoscope. *The hallmark of retinal dysplasia is the rosette*, composed of a central lumen surrounded by 1–3 layers of neuroblasts. The three-layered rosette is the most common in naturally occurring cases in animals, and shows more or less complete retinal differentiation. Most such rosettes are probably retinal folds cut transversely (and, as mentioned above, should not be considered true dysplasia if no additional lesions are present). The lumen contains pink fibrils resembling photoreceptors and is bounded by a thin membrane resembling the normal outer limiting membrane. One- and two-layered rosettes are encountered infrequently and consist of a lumen surrounded by undifferentiated neuroblasts.

True retinal dysplasia occurs in combination with chondrodysplasia in several dog breeds, but particularly in Labrador Retrievers and Samoyeds. Cataract and persistent hyaloid remnants may accompany the retinal lesion. In Labradors, all the defects are the result of a single gene, with recessive effects on the skeleton and incompletely dominant effects on the eye.

Optic nerve hypoplasia

Hypoplasia is the most common anomaly of the optic nerve. The defect may be unilateral or bilateral, and usually occurs in eyes with other anomalies and particularly in eyes with retinal dysplasia. *In most instances, the so-called 'hypoplasia' is more likely to be atrophy* as the inevitable result of the destruction of ganglion cells in glaucomatous, viral, toxic, genetic, or idiopathic retinal disease (Fig. 4.20). The only clear example of an alternative pathogenesis is that associated with *maternal deficiency of vitamin A in cattle,* in which atrophy of the developing optic nerve results from failure of remodeling of the optic nerve foramen and subsequent stenosis. A similar lesion occurs in *pigs*, but in that species hypovitaminosis A seems more indiscriminately teratogenic, and optic nerve hypoplasia is accompanied by diffuse ocular dysplasia and multiple systemic anomalies. Hypoplasia is a relatively frequent clinical diagnosis in *toy breeds of dogs*, without apparent visual defects (and thus rarely receives histologic examination). Most examples are probably hypomyelination of the optic disk, which results from premature halt of myelinated nerve fibers at, or posterior to, the lamina cribrosa. The opposite, with myelin extending too far into the nerve fiber layer of the peripapillary retina, is also seen in dogs and is a frequent but insignificant occurrence in horses.

Inherited optic nerve hypoplasia is documented in one strain of laboratory mice, although it may accompany inherited retinal dysplasia or multiple inherited anomalies in any species. Histologic examination of affected eyes reveals few if any ganglion cells and a thin and moth-eaten nerve fiber layer.

Bibliography

Albert DM. Retinal neoplasia and dysplasia. I. Induction by feline leukemia virus. Invest Ophthalmol 1977;16:325–337.

Albert DM, et al. Canine herpes-induced retinal dysplasia and associated ocular anomalies. Invest Ophthalmol 1976;15:267–278.

Ashton N, et al. Retinal dysplasia in Sealyham terriers. J Path Bact 1968;96: 269–272.

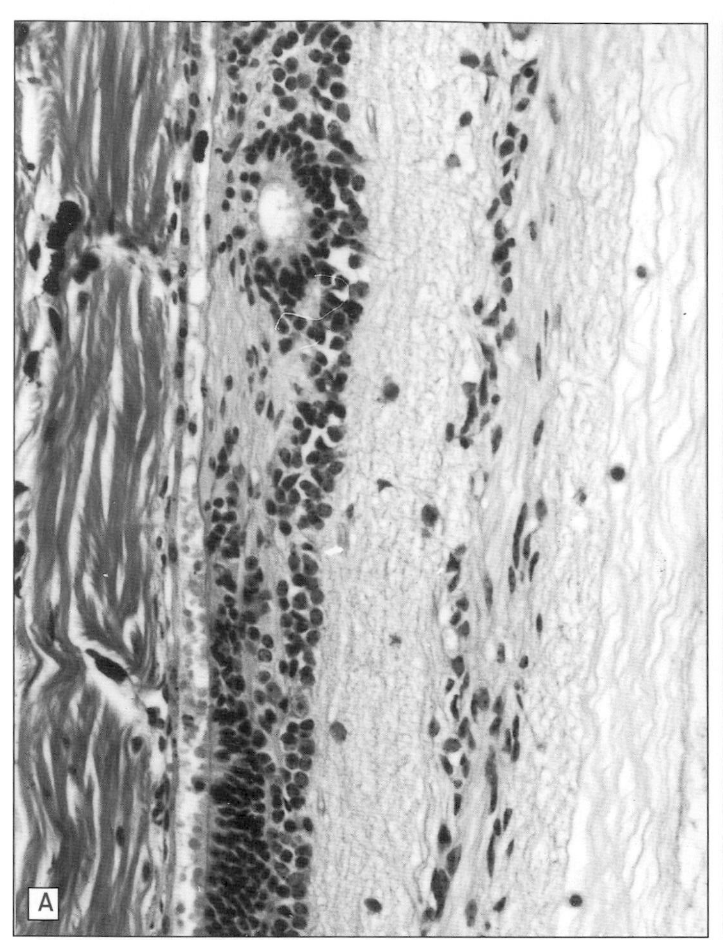

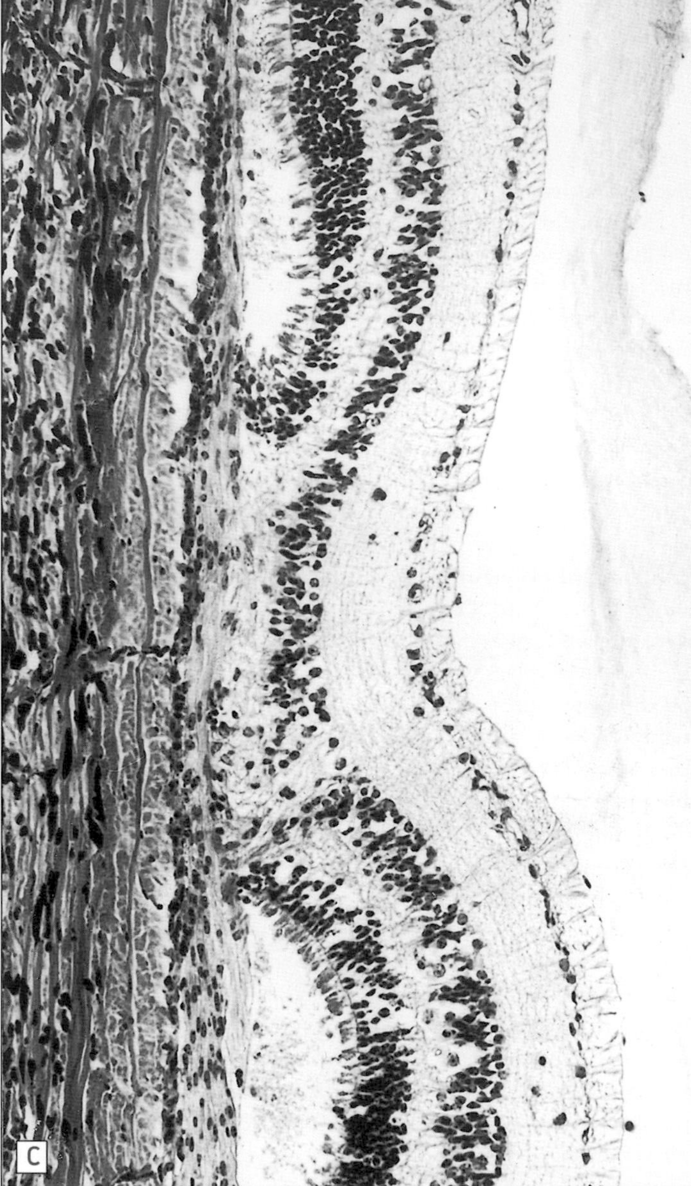

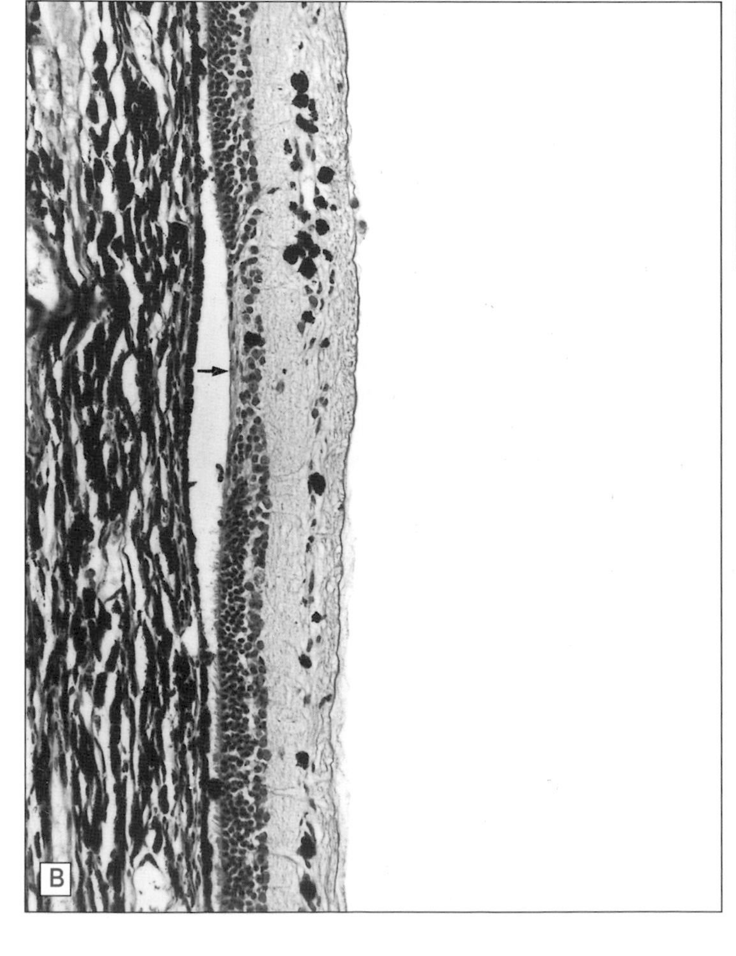

Figure 4.19 A. Postnecrotic retinal "dysplasia" due to *Bovine viral diarrhea virus* infection of a calf. Focal retinal scar with loss of outer nuclear layer and photoreceptors. Abortive regeneration with small rosette. Blending of inner and outer nuclear layers. Note lack of ganglion cells. **B.** Pigment-laden cells from retinal pigment epithelium have migrated into ganglion cell layer, in a calf with BVDV infection. **Post-necrotic scar** (arrow) with loss of photoreceptors and outer nuclear layer. **C. Focal chorioretinal scar** with loss of outer nuclear layer and fibrous metaplasia of adjacent retinal pigment epithelium, in a calf with prenatal BVDV infection.

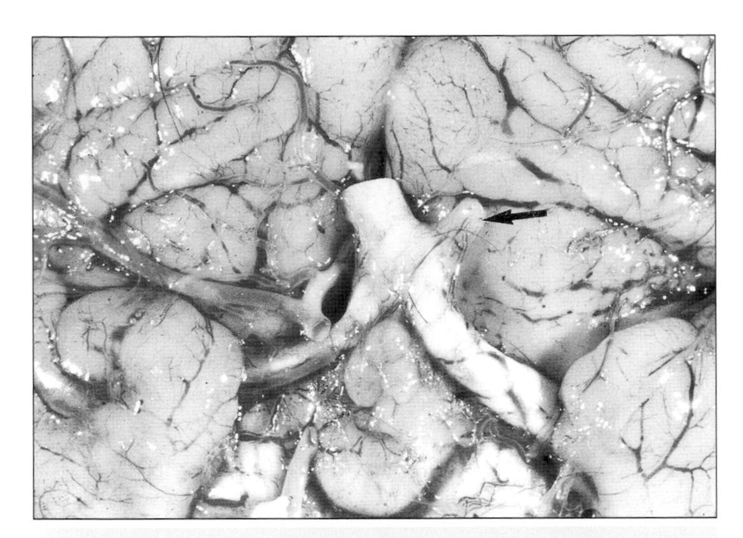

Figure 4.20 Optic chiasm in a foal with unilateral secondary (degenerative) microphthalmos. **Small left optic nerve** (arrow) due to prenatal atrophy following ganglion cell destruction.

Barnett KC. Comparative aspects of canine hereditary eye disease. Adv Vet Sci 1976;20:39–67.

Barnett KC, Grimes TD. Bilateral aplasia of the optic nerve in a cat. Br J Ophthalmol 1974;58:663–667.

Carrig CB, et al. Inheritance of associated ocular and skeletal dysplasia in Labrador retrievers. J Am Vet Med Assoc 1988;193:1269–1272.

Gelatt KN. Inherited retinopathies in the dog. Compend Cont Ed 1979;1: 307–313.

Gelatt KN, et al. Bilateral optic nerve hypoplasia in a colt. J Am Vet Med Assoc 1969;155:627–631.

Greene HJ, Leipold HW. Hereditary internal hydrocephalus and retinal dysplasia in shorthorn calves. Cornell Vet 1974;64:367–375.

Heywood R, Wells GAH. A retinal dysplasia in the beagle dog. Vet Rec 1970;87:178–180.

Kennedy PC, et al. Adenohypophyseal aplasia, an inherited defect associated with abnormal gestation in Guernsey cattle. Cornell Vet 1957;47:160–178.

Kern TJ, Riis RC. Optic nerve hypoplasia in three miniature poodles. J Am Vet Med Assoc 1981;178:49–54.

Lahav M, Albert DM. Clinical and histopathologic classification of retinal dysplasia. Am J Ophthalmol 1974;75:648–667.

Long SE, Crispin SM. Inheritance of multifocal retinal dysplasia in the golden retriever in the UK. Vet Rec 1999;145:702–704.

Narfstrom K. Hereditary and congenital ocular disease in the cat. J Feline Med Surg 1999;1:135–141.

Osburn BI, Castrucci G. Diaplacental infections with ruminant pestiviruses. Arch Virol Suppl 1991;3:71–78.

O'Toole D, et al. Retinal dysplasia of English springer spaniel dogs: Light microscopy of the postnatal lesions. Vet Pathol 1983;20:298–311.

Percy DH, et al. Retinal dysplasia due to feline panleukopenia virus infection. J Am Vet Med Assoc 1975;167:935–937.

Schweitzer DJ, et al. Retinal dysplasia and progressive atrophy in dogs irradiated during ocular development. Radiat Res 1987;111:340–353.

Turnquist SE, et al. Unilateral optic nerve hypoplasia and hydrocephalus in a Pekingese. Cornell Vet 1991;81:305–311.

van der Lugt JJ, Prozesky L. The pathology of blindness in new-born calves caused by hypovitaminosis A. Onderstepoort J Vet Res 1989;56:99–109.

Wallin-Hakanson B, et al. Collie eye anomaly in the rough collie in Sweden: genetic transmission and influence on offspring vitality. J Small Anim Pract 2000;41:254–258.

Whitely HE. Dysplastic canine retinal morphogenesis. Invest Ophthalmol Vis Sci 1991;32:1492–1498.

Anomalies of surface ectoderm

From fetal surface ectoderm are derived corneal epithelium, lens, lacrimal apparatus, and the epithelial portions of the eyelids and associated adnexa. Seldom are anomalies of the extraocular structures the subject of histopathologic study inasmuch as they are clinically obvious and of significance only if they result in corneal irritation, impaired vision, or unacceptable appearance.

Excessively large or small palpebral fissures are part of current fashion in some dog breeds. *Micropalpebral fissure frequently leads to entropion* as the lid margin curls inward, and resultant corneal abrasion necessitates surgical correction. Congenital entropion also occurs as sporadic flock epizootics in lambs, but whether this is a structural deformity or the result of eyelid spasm is unclear. Entropion associated with microphthalmos occurs in all species. Other eyelid defects include colobomas, which are focal to diffuse examples of eyelid agenesis, and delayed separation of the eyelid fusion, which is the normal state during organogenesis.

Disorders of cilia are very common in dogs, but uncommon in other species. Congenital defects include one or more of ectopic cilia, misdirected but otherwise normal cilia (**trichiasis**), the occurrence of a second row of cilia from the orifice of normal or atrophic Meibomian glands (**distichiasis**), and excessively large cilia (**trichomegaly**). In each instance, the significance of the anomaly depends on the presence or absence of corneal irritation.

The lacrimal gland and its ducts develop from an isolated bud of surface ectoderm and, while anomalies must surely exist, they have not been investigated. *Failure of patency of the lacrimal puncta* occurs in dogs and horses and manifests as excessive tearing. Ectopic or supernumerary openings have been reported in dogs and in cattle.

Corneal anomalies

Primary corneal maldevelopment is rare in all species. The category may be expanded to include *corneal dystrophies*, defined as bilateral, inherited, and usually central corneal opacities that, despite their typically adult onset, presumably have a congenital basis. These rare lesions will be discussed with degenerative diseases of the adult cornea.

Corneal anomalies may be ectodermal or mesenchymal, and may affect one or more of corneal size, shape, or transparency. **Microcornea** refers to a small but histologically normal cornea in an otherwise normal globe. A small cornea occurring in a microphthalmic globe is expected and does not merit a separate description. Mild microcornea of no clinical significance is reportedly common in certain dog breeds. **Megalocornea** has not been reported in domestic animals, except in predictable association with congenital buphthalmos.

Dermoid is a congenital lesion of cornea or conjunctiva characterized by *focal skin-like differentiation*, and as such is properly termed a **choristoma.** They occur in all species. There is one report of a geographically high prevalence of multiple, and sometimes bilateral, dermoids as an inherited phenomenon in polled Hereford cattle in the American midwest, but ordinarily they seem to occur as single, random anomalies of unknown pathogenesis. Defective induction (skin instead of corneal epithelium) by the invading corneal stromal mesenchyme is the most popular speculation.

The *degree of differentiation varies,* but most consist of stratified squamous keratinized and variably pigmented epithelium overlying an irregular dermis containing hair, sweat glands, and sebaceous glands. Very rarely, cartilage or bone is seen. The degree of adnexal differentiation varies widely but may approach that of normal skin (Fig. 4.21A, B, C). At the edge of the dermoid, the dermal collagen reorients to blend with the regular stroma of cornea, and the epidermis transforms itself to corneal epithelium. Surgical removal may be for cosmetic reasons, or may be required if dermoid hairs irritate cornea, or if the position of the dermoid interferes with vision. In most instances of corneal dermoid, the choristoma is attached to the surface of a corneal stroma of normal thickness, so excision of the dermoid should not risk perforation of the globe.

Congenital corneal opacities are *usually caused by anomalous formation of the anterior chamber, particularly congenital anterior synechiae and persistent pupillary membranes.* Adherence of anterior chamber structures to the corneal endothelium, or perhaps their interposition during ingrowth of the corneal endothelium, results in focal absence of the corneal endothelium and disorganization of adjacent corneal stroma. Grossly, the affected cornea has deep stromal opacity caused by stromal edema or fibrosis in the area of the defective endothelium. Pigment, originating from adherent uveal strands, may be found in the corneal stroma. The opacity may be diffuse or focal, depending on the extent of uveal–corneal adhesion. Many examples are part of a more widespread anterior segment dysgenesis (see under Defects primarily in anterior chamber mesenchyme).

Diffuse, congenital corneal opacity occurs in Holstein-Friesian cattle in England and Germany. The histologic lesion is diffuse corneal edema but its pathogenesis is unknown. The cornea remains permanently opaque.

Corneal opacity caused by noncellular depositions occurs in dogs and is usually of adult onset despite an apparently genetic basis. The exception is multifocal, subepithelial deposition of basophilic, PAS-positive material in the corneas of puppies with Collie eye anomaly or other mesodermal dysgeneses. The material is of unknown origin and may be the histologic counterpart of the transient, multifocal, subepithelial opacities seen quite commonly in 2–3-week-old puppies whose eyes are otherwise normal and thus unavailable for histologic examination.

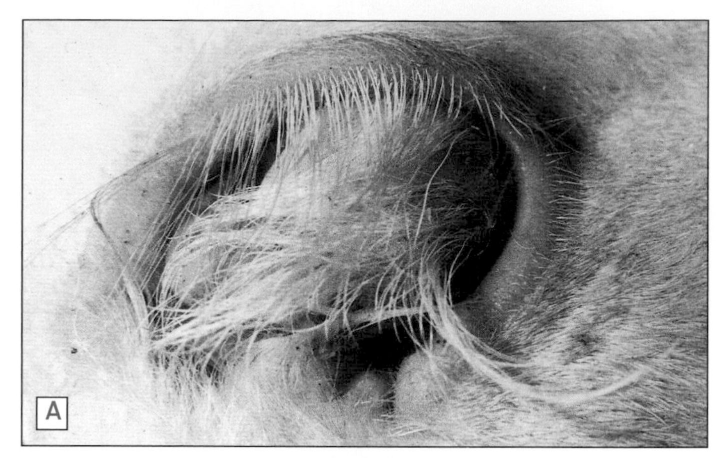

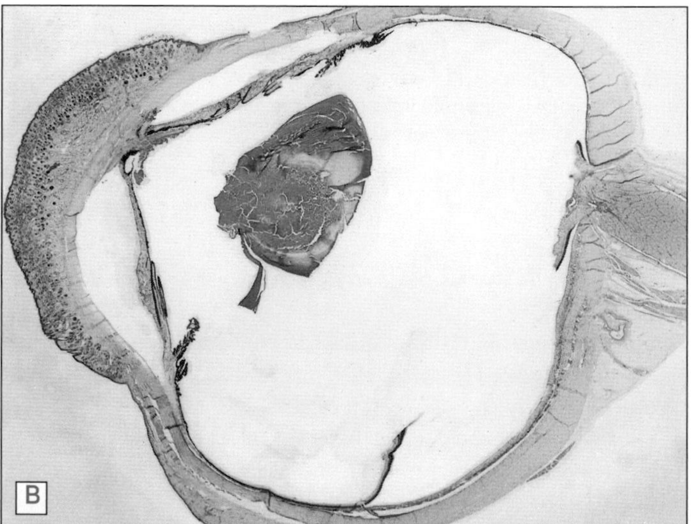

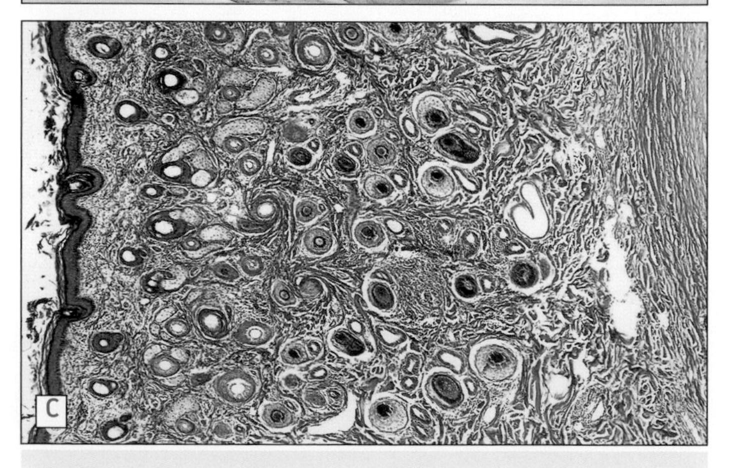

Figure 4.21 Corneal dermoid in a calf. **A.** Notch-like defect in lower lid is a coloboma. **B.** Anterior rupture of lens capsule with well-organized anterior synechia, probably from foreign-body perforation. **C. Corneal dermoid** in a calf; same eye as in (**A**) and (**B**). Development approaches that of normal skin. Note abrupt transition to dense regular corneal stroma at deep margin of the dermoid.

Anomalies of lens

The lens may be abnormally small, abnormally shaped, ectopic, or cataractous. Of these, *only ectopia and cataract are common.*

Aphakia *is the congenital absence of lens, and it may be primary or secondary.* It is claimed that primary aphakia is possible only in a rudimentary globe because of the central role of lens in the induction of invagination of the primary optic vesicle. Any globe with the structure of optic cup, regardless of how dysplastic, must have had a lens early in organogenesis and its absence later must be the result of degeneration. This assumption is an extrapolation from work done many years ago in chicken embryos; while no work has been published to refute this contention, there is no work in mammals to confirm it. In the one report of aphakia in modern literature that includes histologic examination, several other puppies had small lenses and all had invaginated optic cups with iris and retina. There was no conclusion about the nature of the injury to the developing eyes or the timing of such injury.

Microphakia, *or congenitally small lens*, is reported in dogs, calves, and cats, but is nonetheless rare. Most such reports describe the defect in association with ectopia lentis, microphthalmos, and anterior chamber mesenchymal anomalies. Such lenses are spherical and almost always are cataractous.

Lenticonus and **lentiglobus** *are rare defects of lens shape* characterized by an abrupt change in capsular configuration so that the lens acquires a globular or conical protrusion. The defect is usually polar and, in animals, usually posterior. From scattered and very old descriptions, it is difficult to define the "typical" histology of such lesions or their pathogenesis. The defect usually appears as a focal overgrowth of cortical lens fibers covered by thin posterior lens capsule and retained posterior epithelium. Of four relatively recent descriptions, all of canine eyes, all had congenital cataract but only in one did the cataract involve the protruding lens fibers themselves. Other ocular lesions reported include hyperplasia of tunica vasculosa lentis, rupture of the lens protrusion, and dysplasia of ciliary epithelium. At least in Doberman Pinscher dogs, the posterior lentiglobus or lenticonus accompanying hyperplastic tunica vasculosa lentis appears to be an acquired defect caused by the abnormal fibrovascular elements adherent to lens.

Congenitally ectopic lenses occur in all species, but are relatively common only in dogs and horses. *Much more common than congenital luxations are spontaneous luxations in adult dogs*, which may be associated with acquired lesions of the zonule. The reason for the particular susceptibility of small terriers and Poodles to spontaneous lens luxation is unknown.

Congenital cataract occurs in most severely anomalous eyes, but may occur as an isolated ocular lesion. When cataract is present in eyes with multiple anomalies, it usually results from persistence of some part of perilenticular vasoformative mesoderm, but may also result from intraocular inflammation or toxic degeneration. Persistence of pupillary membrane or hyaloid system frequently results in multiple epithelial defects and subcapsular opacities at the sites of mesodermal contact with the lens.

In dogs, congenital primary cataracts are frequently hereditary but, as with corneal and retinal diseases, most hereditary cataracts are not congenital. Subtle, nonprogressive nuclear or cortical opacities are common but clinically insignificant in dogs and are of unknown pathogenesis. Primary, and usually diffuse, cataract is the most common ocular anomaly of horses. The pathogenesis is unknown, but there is usually no other ocular lesion. Congenital nuclear cataracts have been described as an inherited lesion in Morgan horses in the United States.

Congenital cataract is rare in cattle, swine, sheep, and goats. In cattle, hereditary congenital cataract occurs in Holstein-Friesians and in Jerseys and is thought to be an autosomal recessive trait. It is also seen as an infrequent result of fetal infection with *Bovine viral diarrhea virus*.

There is a single report of bilateral, complete cataracts in a litter of Persian kittens, but there are no examples in swine or small ruminants except in association with multiple ocular defects.

The pathology of congenital cataract is the same as acquired cataract, and is discussed later. It may be nuclear, cortical or capsular, focal or diffuse, stationary or progressive depending upon the timing and pathogenesis of the original injury.

Bibliography

Aguirre GD, Bistner SI. Microphakia with lenticular luxation and subluxation in cats. Vet Med Small Anim Clin 1973;66:498–500.

Barkyoumb SD, Leipold HW. Nature and cause of bilateral ocular dermoids in Hereford cattle. Vet Pathol 1984;21:316–324.

Barrie KP, et al. Posterior lenticonus, microphthalmia, congenital cataracts and retinal folds in an old English sheepdog. J Am Anim Hosp Assoc 1979;15:715–717.

Beech J, et al. Congenital nuclear cataracts in the Morgan horse. J Am Vet Med Assoc 1984;184:1363–1365.

Bergsjo T, et al. Congenital blindness with ocular developmental anomalies, including retinal dysplasia, in Doberman Pinscher dogs. J Am Vet Med Assoc 1984;184:1383–1386.

Brightman AH, et al. Epibulbar solid dermoid choristoma in a pig. Vet Pathol 1985;22:292–294.

Gelatt KN. Cataracts in cattle. J Am Vet Med Assoc 1971;159:195–200.

Gwin RM, Gelatt KN. The canine lens. In: Gelatt KN, ed. Veterinary Ophthalmology. Philadelphia, PA: Lea and Febiger, 1981:435–473.

Lavach JD, Severin GA. Posterior lenticonus and lenticonus internum in a dog. J Am Anim Hosp Assoc 1977;13:685–687.

Martin CL. Zonular defects in the dog: A clinical and scanning electron microscopic study. J Am Anim Hosp Assoc 1978;14:571–579.

Martin CL, Leipold HW. Aphakia and multiple ocular defects in Saint Bernard puppies. Vet Med Small Anim Clin 1974;69:448–453.

Olesen HP, et al. Congenital hereditary cataract in cocker spaniels. J Small Anim Pract 1974;15:741–749.

Peiffer RL. Bilateral congenital aphakia and retinal detachment in a cat. J Am Anim Hosp Assoc 1982;18:128–130.

Peiffer RL, Gelatt KN. Congenital cataracts in a Persian kitten. Vet Med Small Anim Clin 1975;70:1334–1335.

Roberts SM. Congenital ocular anomalies. Vet Clin North Am Equine Pract 1992;8:459–478.

Rubin LF. Cataracts in golden retrievers. J Am Vet Med Assoc 1974;165:457–458.

Rubin LF, et al. Hereditary cataracts in miniature schnauzers. J Am Vet Med Assoc 1969;154:1456–1458.

Takei Y, Mizuno K. Electron microscopic studies on zonules. Graefes Arch Klin Exp Ophthalmol 1977;202:237–244.

Ocular adnexa

The adnexa include eyelids, nictitating membrane, lacrimal and accessory lacrimal glands. Developmental, degenerative, inflammatory, and neoplastic diseases of these structures are commonly encountered in clinical practice, but only the neoplasms and proliferative inflammatory lesions are regularly submitted for histologic examination.

Eyelids

Disorders of size and configuration of the palpebral fissure are common in purebred dogs, as are anomalies of number or placement of cilia. None requires histologic evaluation.

Blepharitis is *inflammation of the eyelid. Ordinarily, it refers to inflammation of the haired skin that covers the outer surface of the eyelid.* Diseases primarily affecting the palpebral conjunctiva that lines the bulbar surface of the eyelid would ordinarily be classified as conjunctivitis and are considered later. The diseases of the eyelid skin are, in general, exactly the same as diseases of skin elsewhere, and

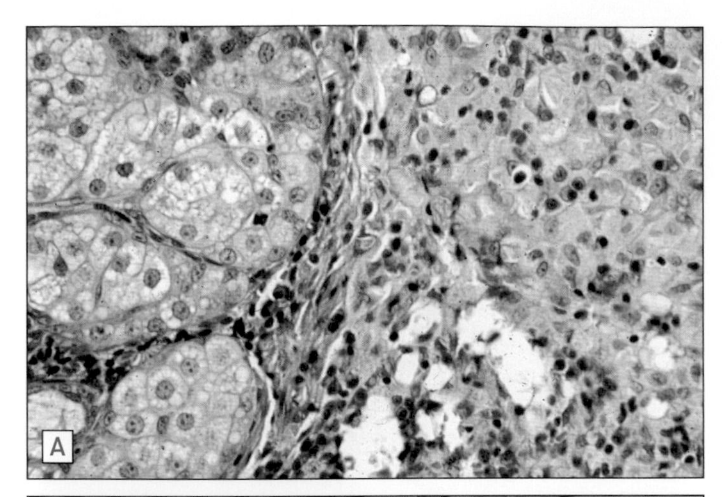

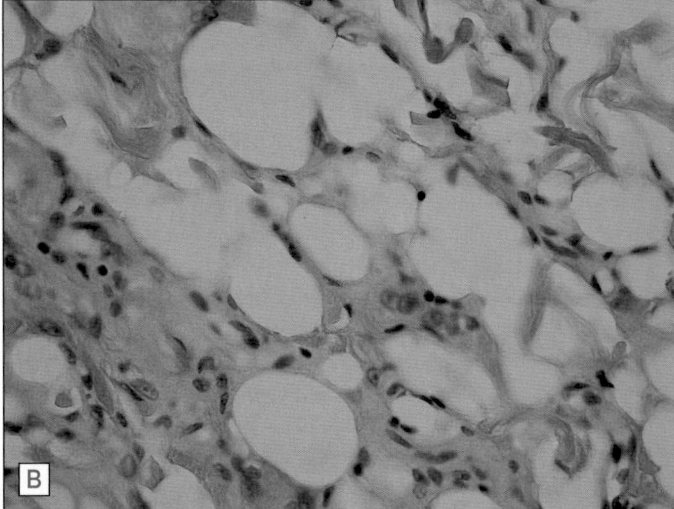

Figure 4.22 Chalazion. **A.** Leaking Meibomian gland or, more often, Meibomian adenoma surrounded by foamy macrophages. **B.** In this variant (particularly common in cats), the leaking secretion forms **lipid lakes** with a relatively inconspicuous granulomatous reaction.

are thus not considered here in any detail. Inflammatory lesions more or less unique to eyelid include hordeolum, chalazion, and idiopathic granulomatous marginal blepharitis.

External hordeolum or **stye** is *suppurative adenitis of the adnexal glands of Zeis or Moll.* **Internal hordeolum** is *suppurative inflammation of the Meibomian gland.*

Chalazion is *sterile granulomatous inflammation in response to the leakage of Meibomian secretion into the surrounding dermis.* While it can theoretically occur in response to any type of injury to the Meibomian gland, almost all cases are found adjacent to Meibomian adenomas. The histologic lesion is distinctive and comes in two forms that may occur independently or in conjunction with one another. The more common is an accumulation of large foamy macrophages and multinucleated cells around the abnormal Meibomian gland. The macrophages contain distinctive refractile intracellular slender elongated crystals that have a bright silvery-white appearance when examined with polarized light. Alternatively, the reaction may consist of a mixture of these macrophages and lakes of free lipid. In routine sections, these appear as clear empty spaces that could be confused with dilated lymphatics (Fig. 4.22A, B). This latter variant was originally described in cats as idiopathic lipogranulomatous conjunctivitis

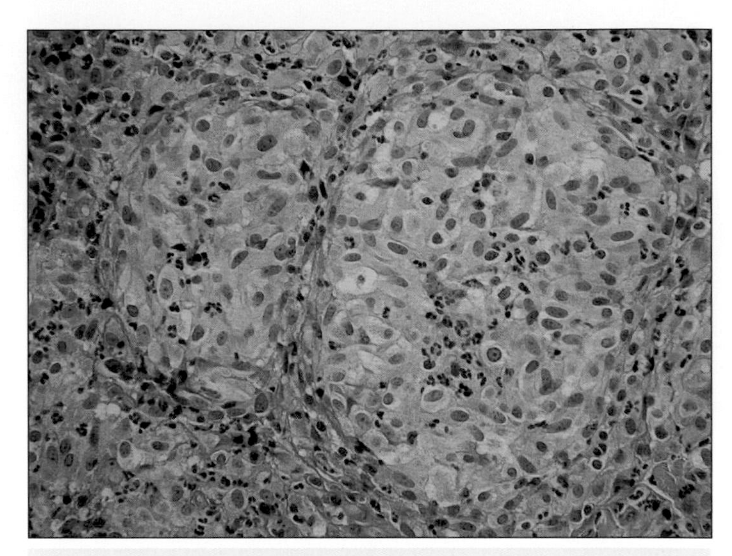

Figure 4.23 Granulomatous marginal blepharitis. Granulomas form around clear lipid vacuoles, sometimes with neutrophils. The location along the palpebral surface of the eyelid margin is critical to the diagnosis.

(see below), but current opinion is that it is just a feline version of chalazion.

Idiopathic granulomatous marginal blepharitis is a uniquely canine lesion. The macroscopic lesion varies from a single nodule to a series of coalescing nodules that create virtually diffuse thickening of one or both eyelid margins. *The histologic lesion is a coalescence of suppurating granulomas in the subconjunctival tissue of the eyelid margin, without any proven association with adnexal structures and without any identifiable etiologic agent.* The granulomas often form around a clear central lipid vacuole, with or without neutrophils at the interface between the vacuole and the surrounding macrophages (Fig. 4.23). The lesion bears considerable similarity to cutaneous sterile pyogranuloma syndrome and other idiopathic granulomatous panniculitis syndromes, all of which are equally mysterious in terms of pathogenesis. *The lesions differ from those of chalazion in that the latter does not form discrete granulomas, does not involve neutrophils, and is always found adjacent to Meibomian glands.*

Lacrimal system

Acquired disease of the lacrimal system is probably quite common in dogs if one includes keratoconjunctivitis sicca (see Keratitis) and eversion of the gland of the third eyelid.

Dacryoadenitis *is inflammation of the lacrimal gland,* and may result from involvement in orbital cellulitis or orbital trauma, spread from severe intraocular inflammation, incidental involvement in systemic diseases such as malignant catarrhal fever, feline infectious peritonitis, and canine distemper; or apparently specific immunologic assault. Specific dacryoadenitis caused by a coronavirus is extremely common in laboratory rats in which acute necrotizing inflammation of lacrimal, Harderian and salivary glands results in eventual fibrosis and squamous metaplasia of affected glands. Residual lesions in mildly affected rats are multiple lymphoid aggregates in the glandular interstitium. Similar changes are often seen in dogs with keratoconjunctivitis sicca, and in the absence of demonstrated viral cause, are assumed to represent autoimmune lacrimal adenitis. The analogous lesion in people with Sjögren's syndrome is associated with influx of numerous T-helper cells into the gland, but no studies have yet been published to prove this immune pathogenesis for canine lacrimal adenitis and atrophy. However, the efficacy of cyclosporine, which acts primarily by suppression of T-helper cells, in reversing canine lacrimal adenitis provides evidence for such a pathogenesis.

Protrusion of the nictitans gland is quite common in dogs, and is thought to reflect a congenital laxity in the connective tissue anchoring the gland to the cartilage of the third eyelid. Because the resultant eversion is unsightly and resembles a neoplasm, these lesions frequently are excised even though the membrana nictitans may be normal except for overlying conjunctival inflammation from exposure and abrasion. Since this gland sometimes supplies a significant proportion of total lacrimal secretion, its surgical removal may be followed by keratoconjunctivitis sicca in dogs that have less than optimal function of the primary lacrimal gland. In dogs with keratoconjunctivitis sicca, the gland may suffer the same lymphocytic interstitial adenitis, fibrosis, and atrophy as affects the lacrimal gland itself.

Conjunctiva

At the orifice of the Meibomian glands, the epidermis of the lid undergoes abrupt transition to the pseudostratified columnar mucous membrane typical of the palpebral conjunctiva. Goblet cells increase in number from the lid margin to the fornix, but ordinarily are absent in that portion of conjunctiva that extends from the fornix to the corneoscleral junction (bulbar conjunctiva). Lymphoid aggregates are common in the subepithelial connective tissue, particularly below the bulbar conjunctiva and the inner aspect of the nictitating membrane. These aggregates are more prominent in the conjunctiva of horses than other domestic species. Whether this is normal or a reflection of increased antigenic stimulation of the conjunctiva in the dusty environment of many horse stables is unknown. The transition from conjunctival to corneal epithelium occurs at, or slightly central to, the corneoscleral junction, and is marked by gradual loss of pigment, rete ridges, subepithelial blood vessels, and lymphoid tissue.

The general pathology of the conjunctiva is similar to that of other mucous membranes. Acute conjunctival injury, whether physical, chemical, or microbial, results in hyperemia and severe edema. Evacuation of goblet cells and cellular exudation from the very labile conjunctival vessels add to the excessive lacrimation caused by any ocular irritation. The ocular discharge progresses from serous to mucoid and perhaps purulent with increasing severity of insult. *Chronic irritation* results in epithelial hyperplasia, hyperplasia of goblet cells and lymphoid aggregates, or even squamous metaplasia progressing to keratinization. The goblet cell hyperplasia is a very uncommon lesion when compared to squamous metaplasia and lymphoid hyperplasia. Lymphoid hyperplasia may be so marked as to result in grossly visible white nodules that may require surgical or chemical removal to reduce irritation of the adjacent cornea. Although characteristic of a number of etiologically specific conjunctival diseases, *lymphoid hyperplasia is best considered a nonspecific response to any chronic antigenic stimulation*. Conjunctivitis frequently accompanies other ocular disease, notably keratitis, uveitis, and glaucoma. Conversely, conjunctival inflammation may spread to cornea, uvea, and orbit, although only secondary corneal involvement is common.

The causes of **conjunctivitis** *include every class of noxious stimulus, including allergy and desiccation*. Because conjunctival biopsy is rarely performed until all therapeutic measures have failed, it is rare to identify an etiologic agent associated with conjunctivitis. The etiologic significance of bacterial, fungal, and even viral agents should be considered very carefully in light of the normal bacterial flora, and the high prevalence of conjunctival carriage of several viral agents in clinically normal animals. At least in dogs, the isolation of gram-negative organisms, especially coliforms, *Pseudomonas* and *Proteus*, should be considered significant in light of the almost exclusively gram-positive flora of normal conjuctiva. Conjunctivitis occurs in a wide variety of multisystem diseases, such as canine distemper and ehrlichiosis, equine viral arteritis and babesiosis, bovine viral diarrhea, malignant catarrhal fever, classical swine fever, rinderpest, African swine fever, and others. Conjunctivitis accompanies most viral and allergic diseases of the upper respiratory tract. Only those diseases in which conjunctivitis is particularly prominent are discussed here.

Infectious bovine rhinotracheitis (IBR) is usually accompanied by serous to purulent conjunctivitis, which can be confused clinically with *infectious bovine keratoconjunctivitis* ('pinkeye') caused by *Moraxella bovis* (discussed below). However, corneal involvement with IBR is uncommon and is never the central suppurating ulcer typical of infectious keratoconjunctivitis. In an unpredictable number of animals, multifocal white glistening nodules, 1–2 mm in diameter, may be seen on the palpebral or bulbar conjunctiva. They appear as early as 3 days after instillation of *Bovine herpesvirus 1* into the conjunctival sac, and represent hyperplastic lymphoid aggregates. Overlying conjunctiva may be ulcerated and the defect filled with fibrin. IBR is discussed in Vol. 2, Respiratory system; Vol. 2, Alimentary system; Vol. 3, Female genital system.

In contrast to the situation in dogs, most cases of conjunctivitis in *cats* are probably caused by infectious agents. The agents incriminated include mycoplasma, chlamydia, or herpesvirus. The diagnosis is usually made based upon clinical characteristics, the presence of other clinical signs, and demonstration of the infectious agent via PCR or culture. Histologic lesions are not etiologically specific, and demonstration of the specific infectious agent in histology or cytology samples (even with the aid of immunofluorescence) becomes progressively more difficult as the lesions age.

Felid herpesvirus 1 causes a combination of conjunctivitis, keratitis, and upper respiratory disease when it first infects young cats, but it may cause conjunctivitis alone as a recurring infection in older cats that had recovered from the initial disease.

Mycoplasma felis and *M. gatae* have been reported to cause conjunctivitis unassociated with other signs in immunosuppressed cats, but instillation of organisms into the conjunctival sac of healthy cats without prior corticosteroid administration does not cause disease. In addition, many of the cats with putative mycoplasma conjunctivitis have had concurrent infection with herpesvirus or with chlamydia. It is likely that the mycoplasma, which is a member of the normal feline conjunctival flora, acts as a medically significant opportunist rather than as a primary pathogen. The conjunctivitis is pseudodiphtheritic and initially is unilateral. Histologically there is nonspecific erosive and suppurative conjunctivitis. Diagnosis requires the demonstration of coccoid bodies in the periphery of conjunctival epithelial cells.

Chlamydophila psittaci usually causes unilateral conjunctivitis in cats of any age, without any other associated disease. The conjunctivitis is initially neutrophilic, but rapidly becomes a nonspecific mixed infection with subepithelial neutrophils, macrophages, lymphocytes, and plasma cells. Early in the disease (between days 7 and 14), typical intracytoplasmic inclusion bodies can be seen, and their detection is enhanced by immunofluorescent staining. Because the clinical signs are characteristic and disease is easily treated with tetracycline, histologic assessment is rarely required. In cases that are resistant to therapy, the disease is usually chronic and histologically nonspecific by the time biopsy is eventually done.

Parasitic conjunctivitis

Parasitic conjunctivitis is relatively common worldwide and may be caused by members of the genera *Thelazia, Habronema, Draschia, Onchocerca,* and several members of the family Oestridae. Of these, only *Thelazia* is truly an ocular parasite; the others cause eyelid, conjunctival, or orbital disease incidentally in the course of larval migration.

Members of the genus ***Thelazia*** are thin, rapidly motile nematodes 7–20 mm in length that inhabit the conjunctival sac and lacrimal duct of a variety of wild and domestic mammals worldwide. Their prevalence is much greater than the prevalence of conjunctivitis, suggesting that their number must be greater than usual before signs of conjunctival irritation are observed. The species most commonly associated with conjunctivitis in domestic animals are *T. lacrymalis* in horses; *T. rhodesi, T. gulosa, T. skrjabini* in ruminants; *T. callipaeda* in carnivores and humans; and *T. californiensis* in many species including dog, cat, bear, coyote, deer, and man. Female worms are viviparous, and larvae free in lacrimal secretions are consumed by flies of the genus *Musca* in which they develop for 15–30 days. The third-stage infective larvae migrate to the fly's proboscis and are returned to the conjunctival sac as the fly feeds.

Ocular habronemiasis results from deposition of larvae by the fly intermediate host, usually *Musca domestica* or *Stomoxys calcitrans*, in the moisture of the medial canthus of horses. Larvae of *Habronema muscae, H. microstoma,* or *Draschia (Habronema) megastomum* are the culprits. The burrowing larvae cause an ulcerative, oozing lesion about 0.5–1.0 cm in diameter at the medial canthus, which becomes progressively more nodular as a granulomatous reaction to the larvae mounts. Mineralized granules may be found within the lesion along with caseous debris, liquefaction, and viable larvae. The histologic lesion is similar to that of cutaneous habronemiasis, namely chronic eosinophilic and granulomatous inflammation surrounding live or dead larvae and eosinophils (Fig. 4.24).

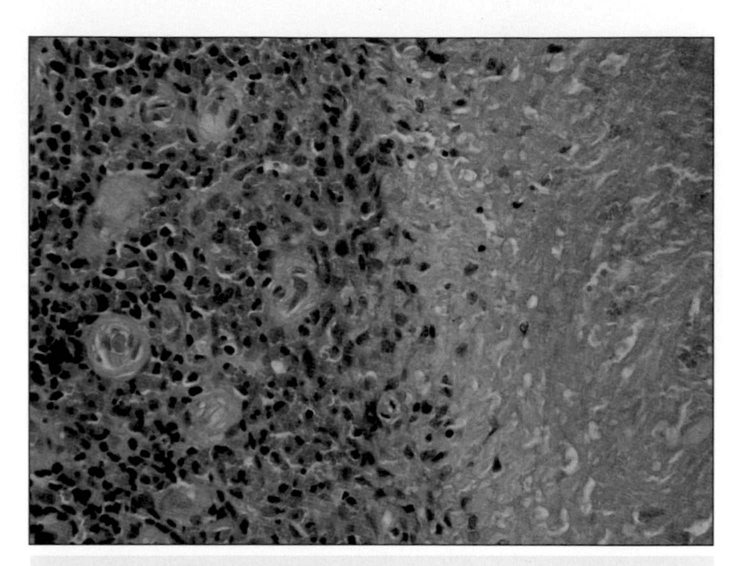

Figure 4.24 Conjunctival habronemiasis. Only rarely would fragments of larvae be detected within the center of these eosinophil-rich granulomas.

Ocular onchocerciasis results in the formation of granulomas and suppurating granulomas around fragmented or viable adult filarids within the sclera and subconjunctival lamina propria of dogs. Dogs are considered abnormal hosts for this parasite, which is much more commonly found in horses, cattle, and other ungulates. In horses, the infection causes a more diffuse eosinophilic and granulomatous conjunctivitis and peripheral stromal keratitis with a character similar to that in skin. Adults and microfilariae can be identified within the reaction.

Ophthalmomyiasis

A syndrome of periocular and even intraocular invasion by *fly larvae* occurs in various species including man. Its various manifestations are known collectively as ophthalmomyiasis. Specific *oculovascular myiasis*, "*uitpeuloog*," or "*gedoelstial myiasis*" is a disease of domestic ruminants and horses caused by invasion and migration of larvae of ***Gedoelstia*** spp. of Oestridae. The *Gedoelstia* are parasites of the blue wildebeest and hartebeest, the larvae being deposited in the eye, rather than in the nares as is the habit of *Oestrus ovis*. The most important member of the genus in terms of frequent aberrant parasitism in domestic species is *G. hassleri,* which in its natural antelope host migrates to the nasal cavity via the vascular system and cerebral meninges and subdural space. The parasitism is not clinically significant in the antelope, but in domestic species that are aberrant hosts, severe ocular and neural disease occurs, sometimes on a large scale. The disease is seasonal and occurs particularly in domestic ruminants in contact with wildebeest.

The ocular lesions vary from *transient mild conjunctivitis to destructive ophthalmitis* with orbital or periorbital edema or abscessation affecting one or both eyes. Neurological signs of varied pattern are common in sheep, partly due to the larvae directly and partly to thrombophlebitis marking their route of invasion. Thrombosis may be very extensive, may involve the jugular vessels and endocardium, and may cause sudden death when coronary vessels are affected.

Larval migration may be into the conjunctival sac, orbital tissues or into the eye itself. In the last instance, *ophthalmomyiasis interna*, the globe is often destroyed by the larval penetration. However, a syndrome of relatively harmless larval migration in the subretinal space or within vitreous has been reported in people. The characteristic subretinal linear tracks may be accompanied by focal retinal separation, preretinal and subretinal hemorrhage, and focal proliferations of retinal pigment epithelium. Two reported cases in cats had similar subretinal tracks, hyperplasia of pigment epithelium, and retinal hemorrhages. In one, the live motile larva was detected either on the face of, or just within, the retina. Subsequent examination failed to detect the larva, and the eye lesions resolved except for the subretinal tracks and pigment clumps.

The penetration is usually by a single larva despite numerous eggs or larvae within the conjunctiva. The larva may die within the globe or continue its migration by uneventful exit from the globe via sclera, optic nerve, or vessel adventitia.

Ophthalmomyiasis interna anterior has also been reported in a cat in association with infection with a first instar larva of ***Cuterebra*** spp. Severe anterior uveitis resolved after prompt surgical removal of the larva, but retinal degeneration and blindness ensued.

Immune-mediated conjunctivitis

Presumed allergic conjunctivitis occurs in all species but is most likely to be investigated in dogs (most examples of conjunctivitis in cats are assumed to have an infectious pathogenesis). Rarely is a specific allergen identified and, like its counterparts in allergic skin diseases, the diagnosis is based upon the failure to demonstrate infectious or mechanical causes, response to corticosteroid therapy, and sometimes a convincing association with environmental changes. Biopsy is rarely warranted, but when taken during the acute disease may show epithelial changes ranging from erosion to hyperplasia to squamous metaplasia, with eosinophils around dilated subepithelial blood vessels and percolating throughout the epithelium. Eosinophils are much more likely to be identified in cats than in dogs, a species difference that is also true of allergic skin disease in general. More chronic lesions, which are the more usual to be biopsied, have squamous metaplasia and lymphocytic-plasmacytic subepithelial infiltrates and the formation of lymphoid nodules.

There are a few histologically distinctive examples of conjunctivitis that are assumed to represent immune-mediated disease, mostly because they respond only to aggressive immunosuppressive therapy. In some dogs with chronic conjunctivitis (perhaps particularly German Shepherd Dogs), the infiltrate sometimes becomes particularly plasmacytic, diffuse, and thick in a fashion resembling an interface dermatitis. The bulbar surface of the third eyelid is the favorite location, and many believe this lesion (sometimes referred to as "*plasmoma*") to be the conjunctival variant of pannus keratitis.

Cats and horses may develop a severe **eosinophilic conjunctivitis** that is thought, by some, to be a conjunctival counterpart of the eosinophilic keratitis syndrome. Lesions may be unilateral or bilateral, and at least in cats there is almost always a concurrent ulcerative marginal blepharitis. Histologic changes include ulceration, epithelial hyperplasia, squamous metaplasia, and a heavy lymphocytic infiltration with a large proportion of eosinophils. Lesions in cats contain no detectable infectious agent, and no herpesviral DNA can be detected (the role of herpesviral infection in the pathogenesis of histologically similar eosinophilic keratitis in cats remains controversial). The clinical syndrome is rapidly responsive to topical corticosteroid administration.

Ligneous conjunctivitis is a distinctive clinical and histologic entity, thus far described only in Doberman Pinscher dogs. The clinical disease is bilateral and characterized by marked thickening and opacity of the palpebral conjunctiva and conjunctiva of the third eyelid. Histologically, the conjunctival lamina propria is thickened by massive deposition of hyaline material and a diffuse scattering of mononuclear leukocytes. Most of the leukocytes are T-lymphocytes, and the hyaline material stains weakly for IgG and IgA.

Feline lipogranulomatous conjunctivitis is probably the feline counterpart of canine chalazion. The lesion occurs almost exclusively in the lamina propria of the palpebral conjunctiva adjacent to the margin of either the upper or lower eyelid. The histology is very repeatable, consisting of a nodular accumulation of clear lipid lakes intermingled with large foamy macrophages and a few small or mononuclear leukocytes. Although the original report contained no mention of adjacent Meibomian lobules, the similarity between this entity and some cases of canine chalazion (or granulomatous dermatitis adjacent to injured cutaneous sebaceous glands) is striking and impossible to ignore (see Fig. 4.22B).

Bibliography

Allgoewer I, et al. Feline eosinophilic conjunctivitis. Vet Ophthalmol 2001;4:69–74.

Barrie KP, Gelatt KN. Diseases of the eyelids (part I). Compend Contin Educ Pract Vet 1979;1:405–410.

Barrie KP, Parshall CJ. Eyelid pyogranulomas in four dogs. J Am Anim Hosp Assoc 1979;14:433–438.

Basson PA. Studies on specific oculo-vascular myiasis (uitpeuloog) in sheep. V. Histopathology. Onderstepoort J Vet Res 1969;36:217–231.

Gardiner CH, et al. Onchocerciasis in two dogs. J Am Vet Med Assoc 1993;203:828–830.

Giangaspero A, et al. Occurrence of *Thelazia lacrymalis* (Nematoda, Spirurida, Thelaziidae) in native horses in Abruzzo region (central eastern Italy). Parasite 2000;7:51–53.

Harris BP, et al. Ophthalmomyiasis interna anterior associated with *Cuterebra* spp in a cat. J Am Vet Med Assoc 2000;216: 345, 352–355.

Hughes JP, et al. Keratoconjunctivitis associated with infectious bovine rhinotracheitis. J Am Vet Med Assoc 1964;145:32–39.

Kaswan RL, et al. Keratoconjunctivitis sicca: histopathologic study of nictitating membrane and lacrimal glands from 28 dogs. Am J Vet Res 1984;45:112–118.

Kerlin RL, Dubielzig RR. Lipogranulomatous conjunctivitis in cats. Vet Comp Ophthalmol 1997;7:177–180.

Lavach JD, Gelatt KN. Diseases of the eyelids (part II). Compend Cont Educ Pract Vet 1979;1:485–492.

Otranto D, Traversa D. Molecular characterization of the first internal transcribed spacer of ribosomal DNA of the most common species of eyeworms (Thelazioidea: *Thelazia*). J Parasitol 2004;90:185–188.

Pusterla N, et al. Cutaneous and ocular habronemiasis in horses: 63 cases (1988–2002). J Am Vet Med Assoc 2003;222:978–982.

Ramsey DT, et al. Ligneous conjunctivitis in four Doberman pinschers. J Am Anim Hosp Assoc 1996;32:439–447.

Raphel CF. Diseases of the equine eyelid. Compend Contin Educ Pract Vet 1982;4:S14–S21.

Read RA, Lucas, J. Lipogranulomatous conjunctivitis: Clinical findings from 21 eyes of 13 cats. Vet Ophthalmol 2001;4:93–98.

Van Halderen A, et al. The identification of *Mycoplasma conjunctivae* as an aetiological agent of infectious keratoconjunctivitis of sheep in South Africa. Onderstepoort J Vet Res 1994;61:231–237.

Whitley RD. Canine and feline primary ocular bacterial infections. Vet Clin North Am Small Anim Pract 2000;30:1151–1167.

CORNEA

The cornea of domestic mammals is a horizontal ellipse varying from 0.6–2.0 mm in thickness among the various species. In general, the larger and older the animal, the thicker is the cornea. It appears as a structural and physiologic modification of sclera, and when chronically injured may lose the specialized features of cornea and resemble sclera both ophthalmoscopically and histologically. Embryologically, the epithelium is derived from surface ectoderm; the stroma and corneal endothelium are from neural crest mesenchyme.

The major attribute of cornea is its clarity, and it is the loss of clarity that is the most obvious indicator of corneal disease. The clarity results from several highly specialized anatomic and physiologic features: an unusually regular, nonkeratinized and nonpigmented surface epithelium; an avascular, cell-poor stroma composed of very thin collagen (mostly type I) fibrils arranged in orderly lamellae separated by a critical distance to allow the uninterrupted passage of light (620–640 Angstroms); and a high degree of stromal dehydration maintained by the presence of epithelial tight junctions, endothelial tight junctions, and a Na-K-dependent ATP-ase pump in the cell membrane of the corneal endothelium (Fig. 4.25A).

The cornea exists in a privileged environmental niche, bathed in the nurturing and antimicrobial saline of the tear film and protected from other irritation by the movable eyelids. Within this protected niche, the cornea does therefore not require the protective attributes of skin (keratinization, leukocytes, blood vessels) to protect itself from the harsh external environment. If there is rapid deterioration in any component of this protective environment, the cornea is most likely to respond with ulceration and subsequent wound healing. If, on the other hand, the shift is of gradual onset, then the more likely response is adaptive metaplasia in which the cornea reaches into its embryologic cutaneous heritage and becomes skin-like.

Corneal injury may result from physical or chemical trauma, microbial agents, increased intraocular pressure and, rarely, from inborn errors of metabolism. Specific features of some of these injuries will be discussed later, but the general reactions to most corneal injuries are presented here.

Corneal edema

Corneal edema occurs rapidly following injury and results from imbibition of lacrimal water through damaged corneal epithelium, absorption of anterior chamber water at a site of corneal endothelial damage, or failure of electrolyte (and thus water) extrusion by the corneal endothelium. If the epithelial or endothelial defect is focal, the resultant edema is limited to the stroma adjacent to the defect. The edematous cornea is clinically opaque, and may be up to five times its normal thickness (Fig. 4.25B). At least experimentally, edema subsequent to endothelial damage tends to be more severe than edema secondary to epithelial injury. Edematous stroma stains less intensely than normal, and collagen lamellae are separated into a fine feltwork of pale-staining fibrils by excessive hydration of the glycosaminoglycan ground substance (principally keratan sulfate and chondroitin sulfate). Percolation of stromal fluid into the epithelium results in the intercellular and intracellular edema known as *bullous keratopathy* (Fig. 4.25C).

Edema may also be part of more chronic corneal disease. Corneal vascularization in response to severe injury is accompanied by edema, as the porous new capillaries leak fluid into the interstitial spaces. A small amount of perivascular corneal edema frequently accompanies the deep stromal vascularization seen in chronic anterior uveitis of any cause. Sometimes the edema is unexpectedly diffuse, severe, and may persist even after the uveitis itself has subsided. Such eyes have a neutrophilic or lymphocytic destructive endothelialitis, with leukocytes interspersed among the vacuolated, pyknotic endothelial cells (see later section Uveitis). Other examples of corneal edema are seen in glaucoma and anterior segment anomalies. In the former, it is assumed that the high aqueous pressure drives fluid into the hydrophilic corneal stroma to a degree that overcomes the endothelial ion pump that dehydrates the stroma under normal conditions. In anterior segment anomalies, persistent pupillary membranes or congenital anterior synechiae cause focal defects in endothelial continuity.

Persistent corneal edema seems to predispose to stromal vascularization and fibrosis, but numerous experimental models show that

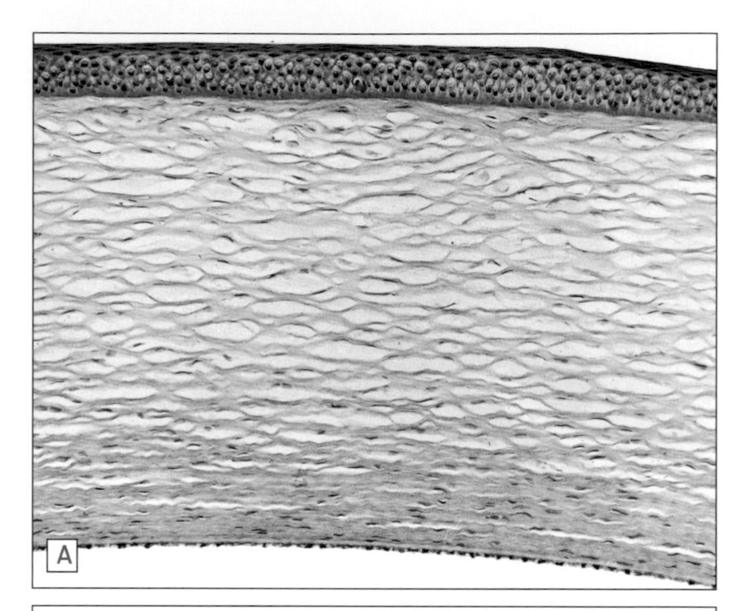

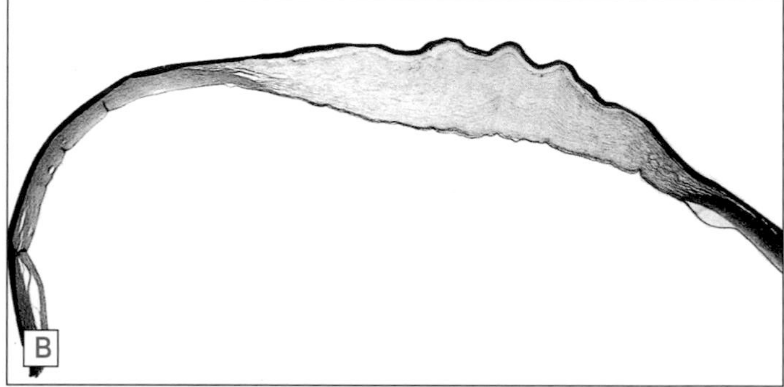

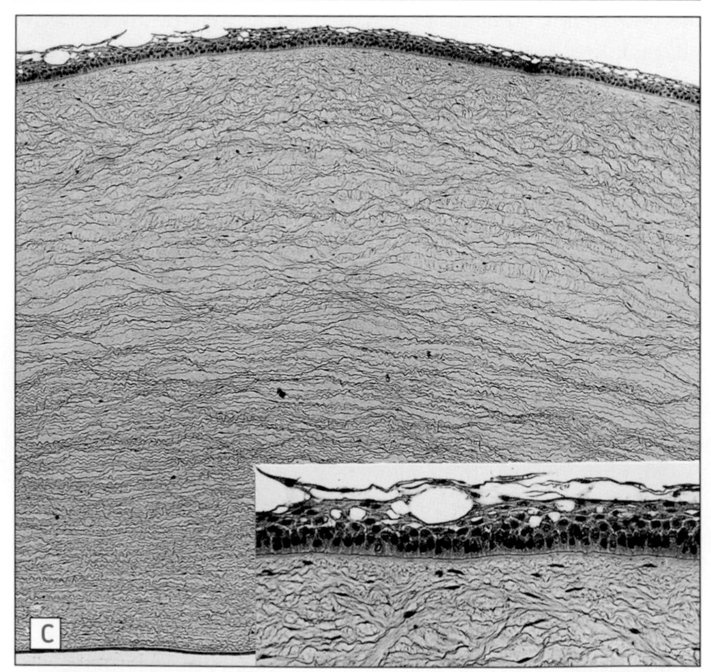

Figure 4.25 A. Normal canine cornea. Uniform, nonkeratinized epithelium without pigmentation or rete ridges. Stroma is poorly cellular. The clefts among the stromal fibers are unavoidable formalin fixation artifacts. **B. Central corneal edema** from abrasion of the corneal endothelium by lens. Foal, with congenital anterior lens luxation. **C. Severe corneal stromal edema**. Percolation of the fluid into the epithelium (insert) creates fluid vesicles known as **bullous keratopathy**.

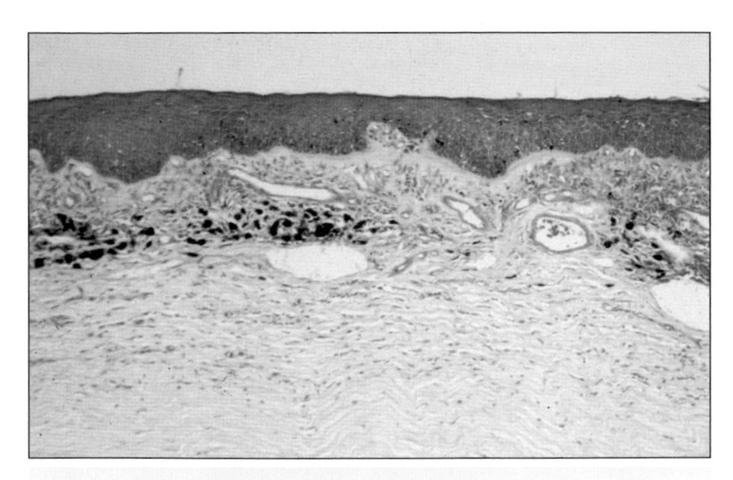

Figure 4.26 Corneal cutaneous metaplasia as a result of chronic keratoconjunctivitis sicca.

edema itself is not the stimulus. Instead, it is probably the infiltrating neutrophils that provide most of the angiogenic and fibroblastic cytokines. Damaged epithelium and stromal fibroblasts are alternative sources. A natural example of virtually permanent corneal edema, without accompanying vascularization, occurs in Boston Terrier and Chihuahua dogs with endothelial dystrophy.

Corneal cutaneous metaplasia

Injury to the corneal surface that exceeds the homeostatic ability of that epithelium resulting in corneal ulceration is described below. Less drastic change to the local environment that results in sublethal injury to the surface epithelium (qualitative or quantitative inadequacy of tears, irritation from misdirected eyelashes or from entropion) will result in adaptive cutaneous metaplasia. *The chronically irritated epithelium undergoes reactive hyperplasia with the appearance of rete ridges, melanin pigmentation, and surface keratinization.* The adjacent stroma undergoes dermis-like irregular fibroplasia and acquires vascularization via capillary migration from the limbus. These changes, while they enable the cornea to survive in a hostile environment and to combat the inflammatory stimulus, also deprive it of its transparency (Fig. 4.26).

Corneal wound healing

Corneal ulceration represents a loss of the surface epithelial barrier. It causes rapid osmotic imbibition of the tear film water, resulting in corneal edema. Neutrophils may be absorbed as well, and if present in large numbers they may initiate stromal lysis as they release their cytoplasmic enzymes. Persistent recruitment of neutrophils is usually a manifestation of sepsis, and is discussed further in the sections dealing with keratitis. In any corneal wound, however, there will be at least a few neutrophils.

The mechanisms of healing of corneal wounds vary with the severity of the injury, and involve an extremely complex interaction of epithelium, stroma, and innumerable cytokine growth factors derived from tear film, infiltrating leukocytes, and resident epithelium and stroma. Only the major elements will be described here, with an emphasis on histologically detectable events rather than on chemical mediators.

It is probably true that virtually any corneal injury results in at least some degree of both epithelial and stromal injury, but *from a purely histologic perspective one can sort corneal injuries into those involving primarily the epithelium and those involving a combination of the epithelium and underlying stroma. Those nonseptic defects involving epithelium alone, or epithelium and superficial stroma, heal by epithelial sliding followed after about 24 hours by mitosis.* One cannot claim that depth alone is the deciding factor, since even very deep wounds will sometimes heal just with epithelial sliding and eventual mitotic rebuilding, as long as the epithelium is satisfied with the quality of the underlying stroma. The sliding begins within a few hours, initially from wing cells from the immediately adjacent, viable cornea. Migration by basal cells rapidly follows. The sliding is preceded by lysis of the hemidesmosomes. Adhesion of the sliding epithelium is initially to adhesion molecules like fibronectin and laminin deposited along the exposed stromal surface. Reformation of the hemidesmosomes and their anchoring filaments may take weeks or even months, during which time epithelial adhesion remains precarious. Healing of shallow, uninfected corneal ulcers is rapid; experimentally induced 7-mm ulcers in horses heal within a mean of 11 days.

Persisting or reoccurring ulcers that cannot be healed just by sliding and replication of adjacent corneal epithelium may require the recruitment of cells from the epithelium at the corneoscleral junction, which is the site of the permanent replicative population. Such cells, when recruited for corneal wound healing, seem prone to retaining a conjunctival phenotype that includes pigmentation and a tendency to form rete ridges. One of the characteristics by which we recognize *chronic, stubborn corneal ulceration* is to observe this *conjunctival "metaplasia" of the surface epithelium.* Another is to recognize a *thickened basement membrane*, as the regenerating epithelium always seems to produce its own new basement membrane even if preexisting basement membrane still seems available. If the injurious stimulus disappears, the conjunctival character of the epithelium slowly fades, being replaced within a few weeks by a normal corneal epithelial configuration. Epithelial adhesion to the underlying stroma remains fragile for 6–8 weeks until the hemidesmosomal attachments of epithelium to basal lamina reform, and until the new epithelium secretes type VII collagen fibrils that anchor the basal lamina to the stroma. In the interim, the cells adhere to a mixture of fibrin and fibronectin derived from the inflamed conjunctival vessels via the tear film or from the injured cornea itself. In many cases, the only evidence of previous shallow ulceration is a thickened basal lamina resulting from secretion by the regenerating epithelium, and gentle undulation of the normally flat epithelial–stromal interface.

Stromal damage may be a direct result of the severity of the initial injury, but more often it is the result of neutrophil-mediated stromal lysis in those corneal injuries that were initially, or later became, septic. Shallow nonprogressive defects in the superficial stroma may be ignored, or may become filled by a thickened plaque of epithelial cells that create an epithelial facet. *Deeper defects that include more than the outer third of stroma will usually require rebuilding of the damaged stroma before epithelial sliding and regeneration can occur.* Within a few hours of the insult, neutrophils enter the wound via the tear film. They migrate into the stroma and control bacterial contamination, degrade damaged collagen, and stimulate both fibroplasia and vascularization via production of various cytokines, especially basic fibroblast growth factor derived from injured epithelium, stromal neutrophils, and injured stromal fibroblasts themselves. Viable stromal cells (keratocytes) adjacent to the wound undergo fibroblastic metaplasia and secrete large amounts of sulfated ground substance, particularly chondroitin sulfate. Most of the new stroma is usually produced by fibroblasts recruited from the limbus. Their ingrowth is always accompanied by a similar ingrowth of new blood vessels. This ingrowth begins about 4 days after substantial corneal injury, and migrates from the limbus centrally at a maximal rate of about 1 mm per day. This 4-day lag time is, presumably, a period of grace in which small or shallow defects can heal with epithelial regeneration alone, without the visual impairment that inevitably follows stromal fibroplasia. Once the epithelium seals the defect, there is immediate cessation of neutrophilic influx and, presumably, a similarly abrupt drop in the production of fibroblastic/angioplastic stimulatory cytokines. *The scarring and vascularization that are the manifestations of stromal rebuilding are permanent*, even though the fibrous tissue gradually becomes less cellular, the collagen fibrils reorient to resemble more closely the parallel arrays of normal stroma, and the ground substance gradually reverts from an embryonic configuration dominated by chondroitin sulfate to the normal predominance of keratan sulfate. Complete restitution of normal stroma, however, never occurs, although the residual scar may be subtle and better detected by clinical examination than by histology. Undesirable though such scarring may be, it is certainly better than the alternative of ineffective corneal healing and inevitable corneal rupture.

Healing of a corneal perforation involves the same events as does healing of a deep corneal ulcer, but there are some added challenges and complications. The cut edges of Descemet's elastic membrane retract from the wound and the transcorneal gap is initially plugged with fibrin and, sometimes, by prolapsed iris. If the gap is not closed by suturing or by a provisional matrix supplied by fibrin and/or iris stroma, there is the risk that the surface epithelium will grow downward along the cut surface of the stroma and into the anterior chamber (Fig. 4.27A). Its migration will be inhibited only by contact with viable corneal endothelium. If it does not encounter that endothelium, there is nothing to stop the epithelium from growing as a layer of stratified squamous epithelium all over the inside of the globe (Fig. 4.27B, C). Obstruction of the filtration angle inevitably causes glaucoma.

As with the surface epithelium, the corneal endothelium at the deep edge of the perforation attempts to bridge the defect by sliding over the fibrin scaffold to restore endothelial continuity. Replacement by mitosis begins within about 24 hours in some experimental models, but *the regenerative capability of the corneal endothelium in adult animals of most domestic species is very limited, and repair occurs by endothelial sliding and hypertrophy.* So potent is this capability that normal stromal dehydration can be maintained even in the face of a 50% reduction in endothelial cell density. The cut ends of Descemet's membrane make no apparent effort at regrowth, but rather the endothelium gradually secretes a new membrane that may eventually fuse with the old or remain separated from it by a layer of fibrous tissue.

The sequence of epithelial sliding and regeneration, remodeling stromal fibrosis and endothelial repair is not uniformly successful. Large gaping wounds fill with proliferating epithelium and stromal fibrous tissue that may protrude into the anterior chamber. The fibroblasts, most of which are probably derived from keratocytes but which may also evolve via endothelial metaplasia, tend to grow along the posterior surface of Descemet's membrane. Regenerating or sliding endothelium is then separated from the coiled remnants of the

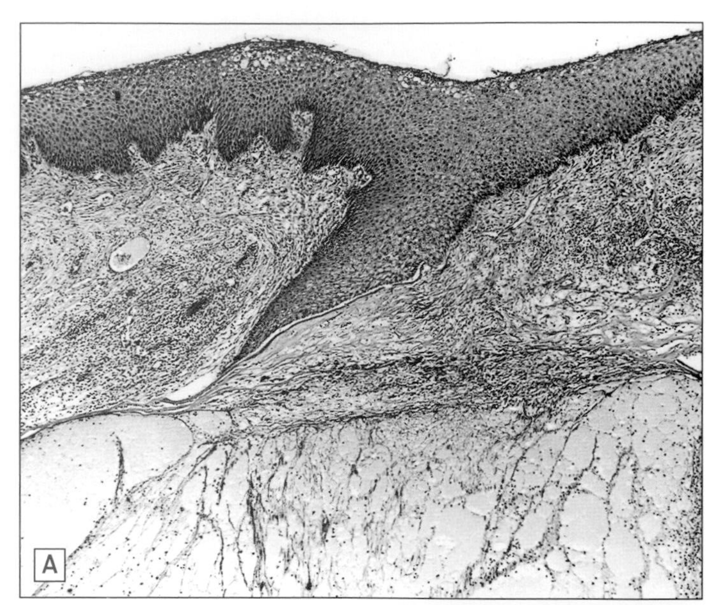

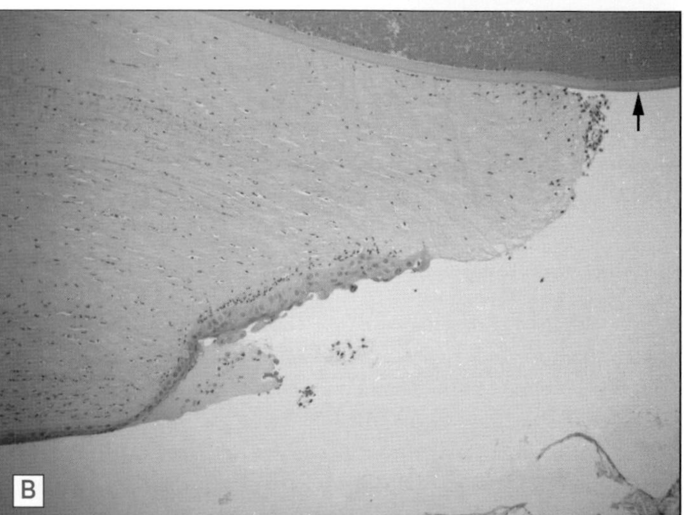

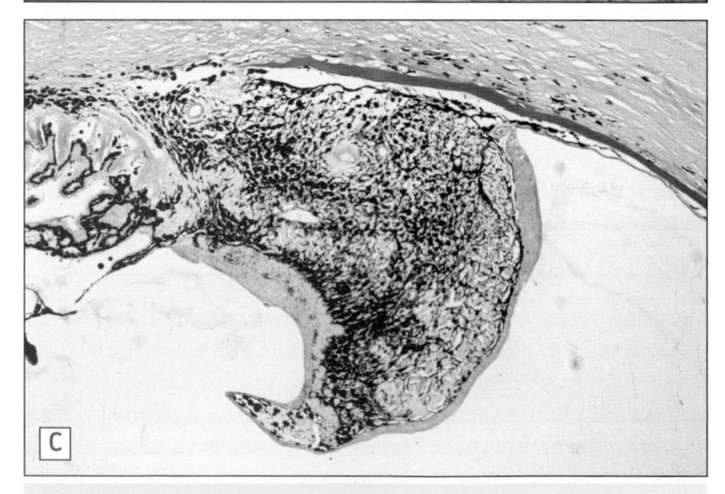

Figure 4.27 A. Corneal perforation in a steer. Defect filled by downgrowth of hyperplastic corneal epithelium. Adjacent stroma is vascularized and chronically inflamed. Edematous iris adheres to the innermost aspect of the lesion, creating focal anterior synechia. **B. Corneal epithelial downgrowth** along the gaping edge of an unsutured corneal laceration. Arrow points to Descemet's membrane that remains intact. **C. Corneal epithelial downgrowth** into the anterior chamber extends over the anterior and posterior surfaces of the iris.

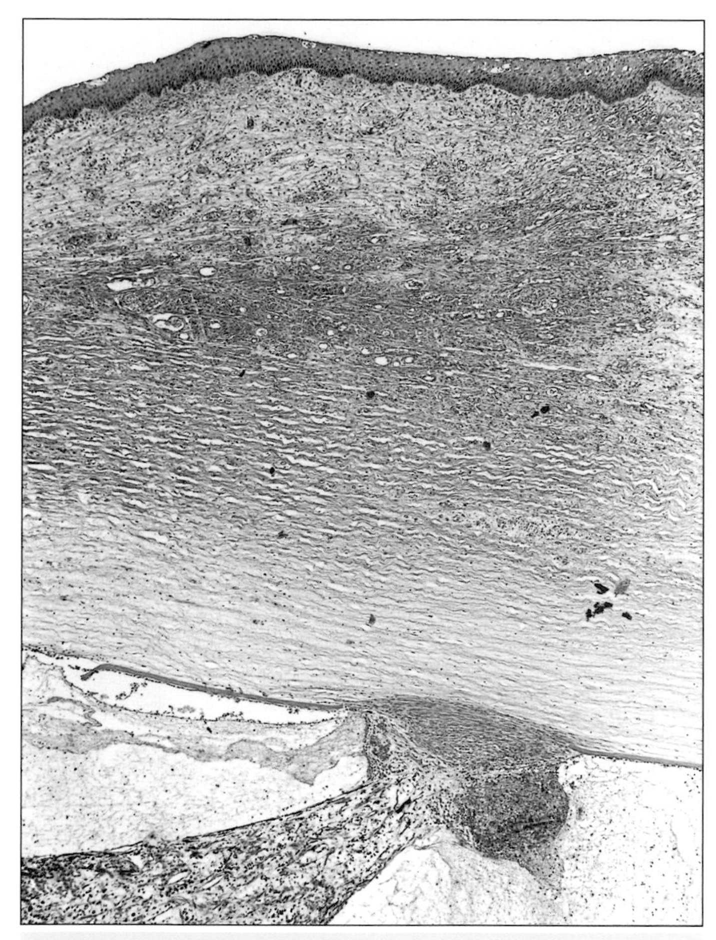

Figure 4.28 Corneal cutaneous metaplasia and chronic superficial stromal inflammation with vascularization. **Anterior synechia** adherent by fibrous plaque that is partly formed by metaplastic corneal endothelium.

original Descemet's membrane by a dense fibrous layer, called a *retrocorneal fibrous membrane*. Eventually, the corneal endothelium may regain continuity on the posterior surface of this membrane, secrete a new Descemet's membrane, and result in a cornea with two separate Descemet's membranes. Those perforations leading to iris prolapse will usually heal with permanent incorporation of the iris into the huge corneal scar, creating a permanent anterior synechia (Fig. 4.28).

Bibliography

Bahn CF, et al. Postnatal development of corneal endothelium. Invest Ophthalmol Vis Sci 1986;27:44–51.

Brogdon JD, et al. Effect of epidermal growth factor on healing of corneal endothelial cells in cats. Am J Vet Res 1989;50:1237–1243.

Cameron JD, et al. In vitro studies of corneal wound healing: epithelial–endothelial interactions. Invest Ophthalmol 1974;13:575–579.

Capella JA. Regenerating of endothelium in diseased and injured corneas. Am J Ophthalmol 1972;74:810–817.

HaveCintron C, et al. Morphologic analyses of proteoglycans in rabbit corneal scars. Invest Ophthalmol Vis Sci 1990;31:1789–1798.

Gipson IK, et al. Anchoring fibrils form a complex network in human and rabbit cornea. Invest Ophthalmol Vis Sci 1987;28:212–220.

Kay EP, et al. Modulation of endothelial cell morphology and collagen synthesis by polymorphonuclear leukocytes. Invest Ophthalmol Vis Sci 1984;25:502–512.

Kitazawa T, et al. The mechanism of accelerated corneal epithelial healing by human epidermal growth factor. Invest Ophthalmol Vis Sci 1990;31:1773–1778.

Landshman N, et al. Relationship between morphology and functional ability of regenerated corneal endothelium. Invest Ophthalmol Vis Sci 1988;29:1100–1109.

Lu L, et al. Corneal epithelial wound healing. Exp Biol Med 2001;226:653–664.

Mathers WD, et al. Dose-dependent effects of epidermal growth factor on corneal wound healing. Invest Ophthalmol Vis Sci 1989;30:2403–2406.

Neaderland MH, et al. Healing of experimentally induced corneal ulcers in horses. Am J Vet Res 1987;48:427–430.

Soubrane G, et al. Binding of basic fibroblast growth factor to normal and neovascularized rabbit cornea. Invest Ophthalmol Vis Sci 1990;31:323–333.

Van Horn DL, et al. Regenerative capacity of the corneal endothelium in rabbit and cat. Invest Ophthalmol 1977;16:597–613.

Watanabe K, et al. Stimulatory effects of fibronectin and EGF on migration of corneal epithelial cells. Invest Ophthalmol Vis Sci 1987;28:205–211.

Corneal dystrophy

Corneal dystrophies are bilateral, inherited (but not necessarily congenital) defects in structure or function of one or more corneal components. They are subclassified as epithelial, stromal, or endothelial. They are all uncommon, and almost all examples have been described in dogs. The list grows daily, with more than 30 different breeds affected. The least infrequent are the stromal dystrophies characterized by the deposition of lipids and/or minerals within an otherwise normal-appearing stroma. The deposition of mineral or lipid secondary to inflammatory disease or systemic metabolic abnormality should not be interpreted as corneal dystrophy.

Corneal endothelial dystrophy occurs in Boston Terriers, Chihuahuas, Dachshunds, and several other dog breeds, and causes slowly progressive bilateral corneal edema in mature dogs. The edema usually begins adjacent to the lateral limbus and may initially be unilateral and unaccompanied by other clinical signs. Later, epithelial fluid bullae may rupture to cause painful corneal ulcers and associated inflammation. Despite the persistent stromal edema, fibrosis and vascularization do not occur unless rupture of epithelial bullae initiates keratitis. *The primary lesion is spontaneous necrosis of corneal endothelium followed by hypertrophy, fibroblastic metaplasia, and sliding of viable endothelium.* A marked progressive decrease in overall endothelial cell density results, eventually, in what usually is severe bilateral corneal edema. The reason for the endothelial cell death is unknown. Focal irregularities in Descemet's membrane occur in areas of endothelial loss, presumably a result of new basement membrane production by adjacent reactive endothelium.

Posterior polymorphous dystrophy is characterized by multifocal random degeneration of corneal endothelial cells, accompanied by compensatory endothelial hypertrophy. Cellular loss causes exposure of Descemet's membrane, and adjacent deep stromal patchy edema.

A rare, juvenile-onset, genetically transmitted *endothelial dystrophy in Manx and domestic shorthair cats* is manifest as bilateral, progressive central epithelial and stromal edema. Fluid accumulates within superficial stroma and within the epithelium. Primary morphologic abnormalities are not described in the Manx, but in shorthairs there is irregularity and vacuolation of corneal endothelium.

Corneal stromal dystrophies include a wide range of breed-specific lipid and/or mineral deposits within the corneal stroma, with the exact age of onset, location, and clinical appearance being relatively specific in each breed. Specimens are rarely available for histologic assessment since the disease does not cause blindness and is not associated with any systemic abnormality. In most, the chemical nature of the deposit and character of the metabolic abnormality have not been determined.

Other corneal deposits

Deposition of mineral, lipid, or pigment within the cornea may occur secondary to chronic corneal injury or to systemic metabolic disease in any species.

Corneal hypermelanosis often accompanies *chronic corneal irritation in dogs* and less frequently in other species, particularly horses. The pigment is found in the basal layer of the corneal epithelium and in the superficial stroma. *It is the result of progressive ingrowth of new germinal cells that have retained pigment from the bulbar conjunctiva.* The clinical name, "*pigmentary keratitis*," is purely descriptive. The corneal epithelium is invariably hyperplastic and often has the other features of corneal cutaneous metaplasia, such as rete ridge formation, keratinization, and abnormally thick basement membrane. There is usually evidence of chronic stromal inflammation, including vascularization. Corneal stromal pigmentation without evidence of epithelial cutaneous metaplasia occurs infrequently, associated with previous iris prolapse that has contributed uveal melanin to the corneal stromal scar.

Other types of corneal pigmentation are rare. *Hemosiderin* will be found within corneal endothelial cells subsequent to anterior chamber hemorrhage or within stromal macrophages if there has been hemorrhage into the corneal stroma itself. Similar pigment may occur following implantation of corneal foreign bodies containing iron or other metals.

Diets high in cholesterol produce *diffuse corneal stromal lipidosis*, as well as focal lipid deposits in uveal epithelium and stroma. While hyperlipemia is not a documented prerequisite for most cases of corneal lipidosis in dogs (most of which are spontaneous dystrophies), *circumferential peripheral stromal lipidosis* is reported in dogs with hyperlipoproteinemia resulting from hypothyroidism and other causes.

Regardless of pathogenesis, the histologic lesion is similar. Cholesterol crystals and lipid vacuoles are found principally in anterior stroma, and are sometimes surrounded by lipid-laden macrophages and variable numbers of other leukocytes (Fig. 4.29). Vascularization is often present, but its pathogenesis is unknown. It appears that corneal vascularization can predispose to stromal lipidosis in animals with hyperlipemia, but it is also true that some animals with primary corneal lipidosis will develop secondary inflammation and vascularization.

Mineral deposition occurs primarily in the anterior stroma and the epithelial basement membrane. Predisposing corneal changes include desiccation, anesthesia, edema, or inflammation. *There are many methods for inducing deposition of calcium salts, but stromal edema seems to be the common denominator in almost all cases.* The edema may result from corneal epithelial desiccation (exposure keratitis), uveitis, corneal trauma, or chemical injury. Hypercalcemia from vitamin D toxicity or hyperparathyroidism exacerbates the mineralization and is essential to lesion development in some experimental models.

An unidentified corneal deposition is often seen in canine eyes suffering from multiple anomalies, particularly those involving uvea.

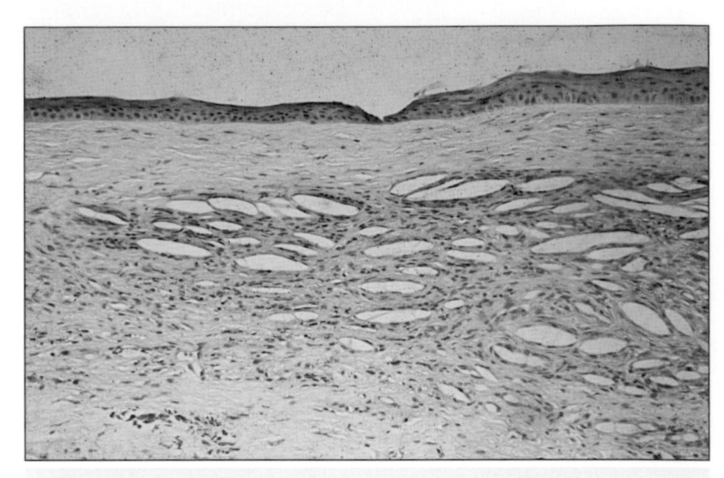

Figure 4.29 Lipid keratopathy. Clefts of cholesterol within the corneal stroma trigger mild nonseptic granulomatous inflammation.

Similar deposits are seen, with less regularity, in the horizontal midportion of the cornea of many normal puppies. Fine basophilic periodic acid-Schiff positive linear deposits are associated with the epithelial basement membrane or superficial stroma. There is some disarray of superficial stromal fibers but no inflammation. The nature and pathogenesis of the deposit are unknown, but most disappear after a few months.

Corneal degeneration

"Corneal degeneration" is a vague term sometimes used to describe those corneal lesions characterized by noninflammatory loss of epithelial or stromal viability. Diseases such as keratoconjunctivitis sicca and pannus keratopathy are sometimes considered primary degenerative lesions but their principal manifestation is inflammatory and they are discussed under keratitis.

The only degenerative, noninflammatory, acquired corneal lesions presented here are corneal sequestrum in cats and horses, and canine persistent erosion syndrome. It is quite possible that all three diseases have a similar pathogenesis, but for the moment they will be listed as three different diseases because of differences in clinical presentation.

Feline corneal sequestrum *is recognized clinically as a discrete orange-brown discoloration of the central cornea, affecting one or both eyes* (Fig. 4.30). Persian and Himalayan cats are more frequently affected than other breeds. Histologically, *the lesion is noninflammatory necrosis of stromal keratocytes, accompanied by pallor, hyalinization, and slight orange discoloration of the affected stroma.* The discoloration may be absent in very early cases. The overlying epithelium may be ulcerated or intact, but in those cases with an intact epithelium there is virtually always histologic evidence of previous ulceration. In older lesions, the periphery of the sequestrum may be marked by a zone of reactive mononuclear leukocytes and, perhaps, a few giant cells. The pigment is derived from porphyrins within the tear film, absorbed into the cornea as part of corneal edema that follows ulceration. *The sequestrum will eventually slough, and the defect heals by granulation* (although most lesions are treated by excision before that stage is reached).

The pathogenesis remains controversial. In flat-faced Persian and Himalayan cats, the pathogenesis probably involves corneal ulceration secondary to desiccation because of abnormal facial configuration. In

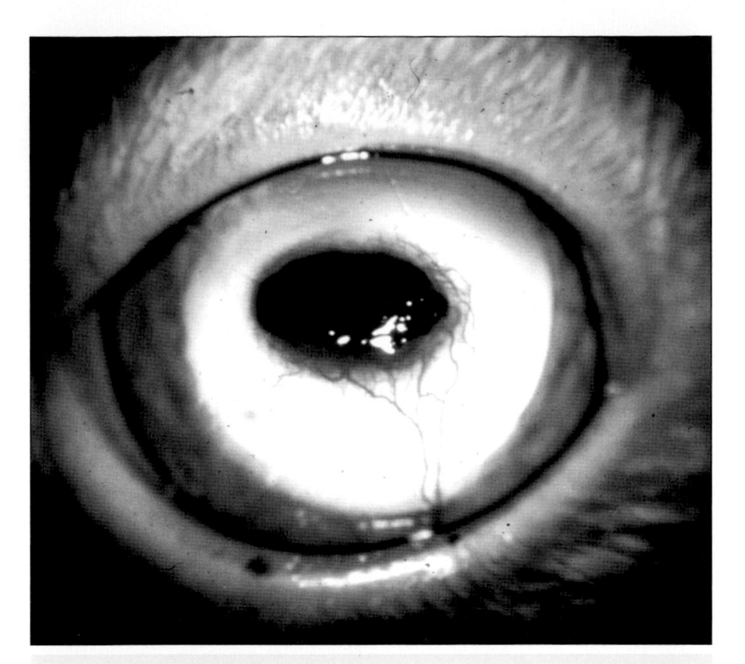

Figure 4.30 Feline corneal sequestrum.

non-Persian cats, there is a loose statistical association with herpesviral infection, and *it is reasonable to propose that corneal sequestrum is an uncommon sequel to any corneal ulceration in cats*. As will become clearer below, the brown discoloration is unique to cats and, for a long time, caused us to overlook the histologic similarity between the feline disease and similar histologic entities in horses and dogs. Not all feline cases acquire the characteristic brown pigmentation, and indeed some examples are virtually indistinguishable from canine and equine persistent ulcers described below.

Canine persistent (recurrent) ulcer syndrome was first described in Boxer dogs (hence the name "*Boxer ulcer*"). Although Boxers and related breeds may be predisposed, similar recurrent erosions are encountered in a wide variety of breeds. *The clinical syndrome is distinctive, characterized by a shallow central corneal erosion with scant edema and (at least initially) no vascularization*. The lesion refuses to heal, or repeatedly re-ulcerates, because of poor adhesion of the epithelium to the underlying stroma. The defect appears not to be in epithelial healing per se, since sliding and mitotic activity are normal in affected dogs. Keratectomy specimens reveal poorly adherent hyperplastic epithelium at the ulcer margins, usually with multiple clefts separating epithelium from stroma even in areas distant from the obvious ulcer (Fig. 4.31). The basal lamina is usually not visible with light microscopy, and the epithelium appears to be attempting to adhere to a thin zone of hypocellular, pale-staining stroma that could correctly be interpreted as a very shallow sequestrum qualitatively similar to what was described above in cats. *The observation of pyknotic and lytic keratocyte nuclei within this superficial zone suggests that the basic defect is degeneration of the superficial stroma*, so that epithelial hemidesmosomes and anchoring collagen fibrils attempting to reform after ulceration have no substrate in which to anchor. Very chronic cases usually acquire superficial stromal granulation tissue appropriate to any chronic ulceration, but its onset is much delayed in comparison to infectious or traumatic ulcers.

The lesion in **horses** is less frequent and less well characterized than in dogs or cats. It is histologically identical to what occurs in

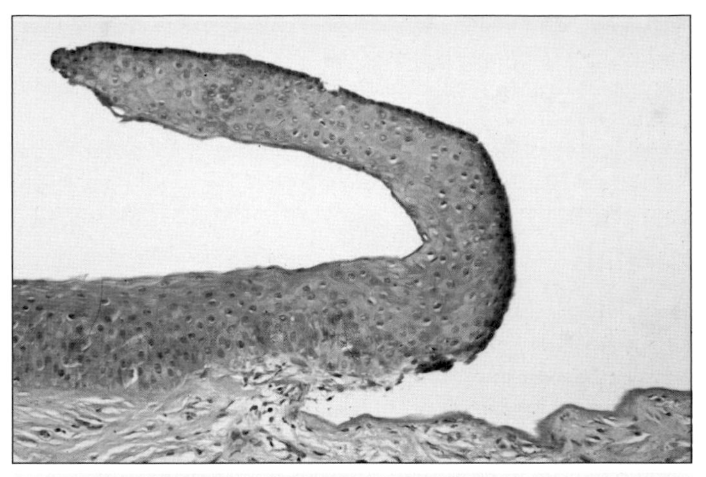

Figure 4.31 Canine persistent ulcer. Dysplastic, strongly regenerative epithelium is unable to adhere to the underlying superficial stroma.

dogs, although it seems to be more often complicated and thus disguised by superimposed fungal infection (see Fig. 4.35B).

Bibliography

Aguirre GD, et al. Keratoconjunctivitis sicca in dogs. J Am Vet Med Assoc 1971;158:1566–1579.

Cooley PL, Dice PF. Corneal dystrophy in the dog and cat. Vet Clin North Am: Small Anim Pract 1990;20:681–692.

Cooley PL, Wyman M. Indolent-like corneal ulcers in three horses. J Am Vet Med Assoc 1986;188:295–297.

Crispin SM. Crystalline corneal dystrophy in the dog. Histochemical and ultrastructural study. Cornea 1988;7:149–161.

Ekins MB, et al. Oval lipid corneal opacities in beagles: VI. Quantitation of excess stromal cholesterol and phospholipid. Exp Eye Res 1983;36:279–286.

Formston C, et al. Corneal necrosis in the cat. J Small Anim Pract 1974;15:19–25.

Gelatt KN, Samuelson DA. Recurrent corneal erosions and epithelial dystrophy in the boxer dog. J Am Anim Hosp Assoc 1982;18:453–460.

Gemensky AJ, Wilkie DA. Mineralized corneal sequestrum in a cat. J Am Vet Med Assoc 2001;219:1550, 1568–1572.

Gwin RM, Gelatt KN. Bilateral ocular lipidosis in a cottontail rabbit fed an all-milk diet. J Am Vet Med Assoc 1977;171:887–889.

Gwin RM. Primary canine corneal endothelial cell dystrophy: specular microscopic evaluation, diagnosis and therapy. J Am Anim Hosp Assoc 1982;18:471–479.

Hakanson NE, Dubielzig RR. Chronic superficial erosions with anterior stromal sequestration in three horses. Vet Comp Ophthalmol 1994;4:179–183.

Harrington GA, Kelly DF. Corneal lipidosis in a dog with bilateral thyroid carcinoma. Vet Pathol 1980;17:490–493.

Kirschner SE, et al. Idiopathic persistent corneal erosions: clinical and pathological findings in 18 dogs. J Am Anim Hosp Assoc 1989;25:84–90.

La Croix NC, et al. Nonhealing corneal ulcers in cats: 29 cases (1991–1999). J Am Vet Med Assoc 2001;218:733–735.

McLellan GJ, Archer FJ. Corneal stromal sequestration and keratoconjunctivitis sicca in a horse. Vet Ophthalmol 2000;3:207–212.

McMillan AD. Crystalline corneal opacities in the Siberian husky. J Am Vet Med Assoc 1979;175:829–832.

Martin CL, Dice PF. Corneal endothelial dystrophy in the dog. J Am Anim Hosp Assoc 1982;18:327–336.

Morgan RV. Feline corneal sequestration: a retrospective study of 42 cases (1987–1991). J Am Anim Hosp Assoc 1994;30:24–28.

Narfstrom K. Hereditary and congenital ocular disease in the cat. J Feline Med Surg 1999;1:135–141.

Startup FG. Corneal necrosis and sequestration in the cat: a review and record of 100 cases. J Small Anim Pract 1988;29:476–486.

Keratitis

Corneal inflammation is called **keratitis** *and has traditionally been divided into epithelial, stromal (interstitial), and ulcerative keratitis.* It is probably time to abandon this arbitrary classification, at least when dealing with ocular histopathology. In realistic terms, almost all corneal inflammatory lesions reaching a pathologist are chronic and severe, and it is difficult to determine how they started. By the time we see them, almost all are ulcerated or show extensive stromal scarring below a healed ulcer. Regardless of cause, corneal inflammation initially follows the stereotyped sequence of edema and leukocyte immigration from tears and distant limbic venules. With severe lesions, corneal stromal vascularization, fibrosis and epithelial metaplasia with pigmentation may occur.

Keratitis usually results from physical, chemical, or microbial injury to the cornea, but the cornea may also be affected by extension of disease from elsewhere in the eye, adnexa, or conjunctiva. The stroma and endothelium may become involved in diseases of the uvea by extension via the aqueous or by direct extension from iris root or ciliary apparatus across the limbus.

Purely **epithelial keratitis** is rarely encountered in histologic preparations, either because the clinical lesion is transient and so mild that eyes are unavailable for histologic examination, or because the lesion progresses to ulceration (as in acute keratoconjunctivitis sicca).

Ulcerative keratitis includes a large group of lesions caused by physical and chemical trauma, desiccation, bacterial, fungal or viral infection, and rarely from primary degeneration of the corneal epithelium itself. *Regardless of cause, the loss of epithelium initiates a predictable series of corneal reactions caused by tear imbibition, local production of cytokines, and opportunistic microbial contamination of the wound.* Imbibition causes superficial stromal edema below the ulcer and is followed by immigration of neutrophils from the tear film and, later, from the limbus. The leukocytes, while somewhat protective against opportunistic pathogens, also add their collagenases, proteases, and stimulatory cytokines to the wound and thereby may contribute to its progression. Epithelial and stromal repair proceeds as already described for corneal wound healing, but the repair fails in those cases in which microbial contamination is well established or in which the cause of the initial ulceration has not been corrected. Common examples of the latter are found in dogs in which corneal trauma by misdirected cilia or facial hair, or desiccation due to lacrimal gland dysfunction, persists.

The usual role of bacteria and fungi in the pathogenesis of corneal ulceration is opportunistic. However, these opportunists contribute significantly to the perpetuation and worsening of the lesion. Proteases and collagenases of microbial, leukocytic, or corneal origin progressively liquefy corneal stroma, a process termed **keratomalacia** (Fig. 4.32). Ulcers contaminated by *Pseudomonas* and *Streptococcus* spp. are particularly prone to rapid liquefaction because of the potent collagenases and proteases produced by these organisms. *Pseudomonas* ulcers have been extensively investigated because of the devastating liquefaction of cornea that commonly accompanies this infection. The bacteria themselves produce numerous proteases and other toxins that may be important in the establishment of the early infection, but most of the characteristic stromal malacia results from the action of proteases originating from leukocytes, reactive corneal epithelium, or injured stroma. The stroma contains a variety of proenzymes (for collagenases, elastases, gelatinases, and other stromal lysins) that are cleaved by the *Pseudomonas* toxins to produce the active enzymes. Which toxins are produced, and in what quantities, is very strain dependent. The stepwise degradation of stroma is seen histologically as a featureless eosinophilic coagulum, which occurs with progressive septic ulcers regardless of the species of bacterium. Neutrophils may encircle the liquefying focus as a thick wall of live and fragmented cells. The resulting localized suppurative keratomalacia is called a ring *abscess* (Fig. 4.33), although that terminology is rarely used today. It is seen more commonly in cattle than any other species, perhaps because of the prevalence of untreated, contaminated corneal ulcers in that species and the prevalence of septic corneal perforation.

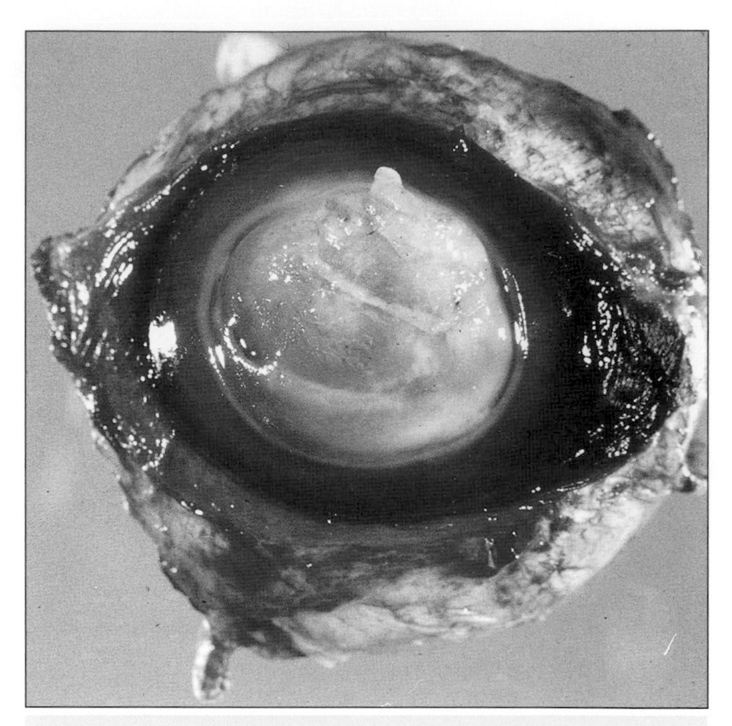

Figure 4.32 Keratomalacia in a horse with *Pseudomonas* keratitis.

The sequelae of ulcerative keratitis involve cornea, conjunctiva, and uvea. *The ulcer itself may heal with vascularization and scarring proportional to the severity of the initial lesion. It may persist as a stubborn but nonprogressive lesion, or it may progress to involve more of the stroma and epithelium.* Stromal liquefaction that reaches Descemet's membrane results in its forward bulging as a descemetocele. This membrane, while resistant to penetration of the microbial agents themselves, is apparently permeable to inflammatory mediators and microbial toxins that diffuse into the anterior chamber. These chemicals, combined with a vasoactive sensory neural reflex from irritated cornea, are responsible for the vasodilation and exudation in anterior uvea that are seen histologically in virtually all globes with deep ulcerative keratitis. Even in nonperforating keratitis, the anterior uveal inflammation may result in sufficient fibrin exudation so as to predispose to focal adhesions of iris to lens or (rarely) to cornea.

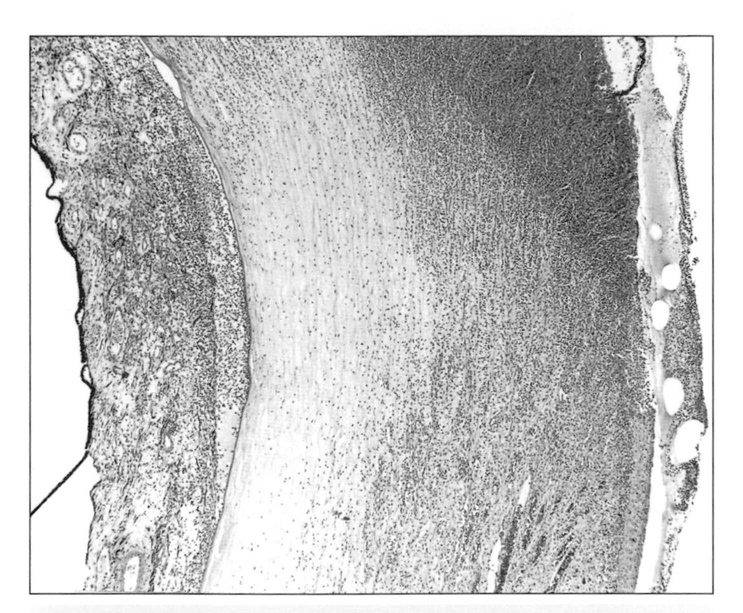

Figure 4.33 Severe suppurative keratomalacia accompanied by massive stromal edema, in a calf. The iris bows forward and almost obliterates the anterior chamber, a manifestation either of iris bombé or of nearby iris prolapse.

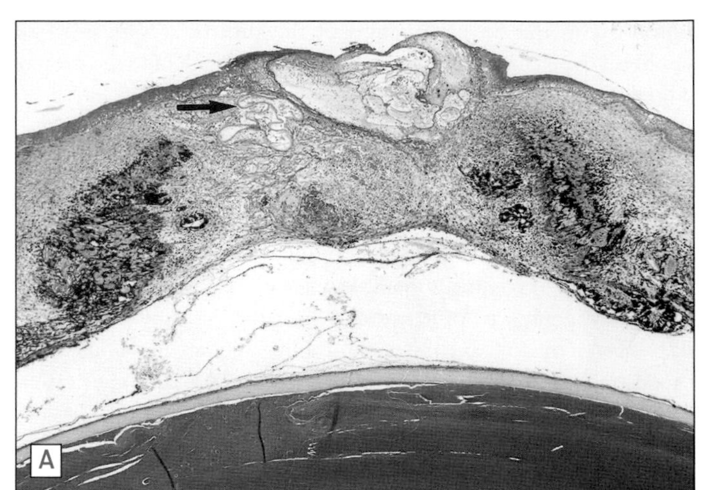

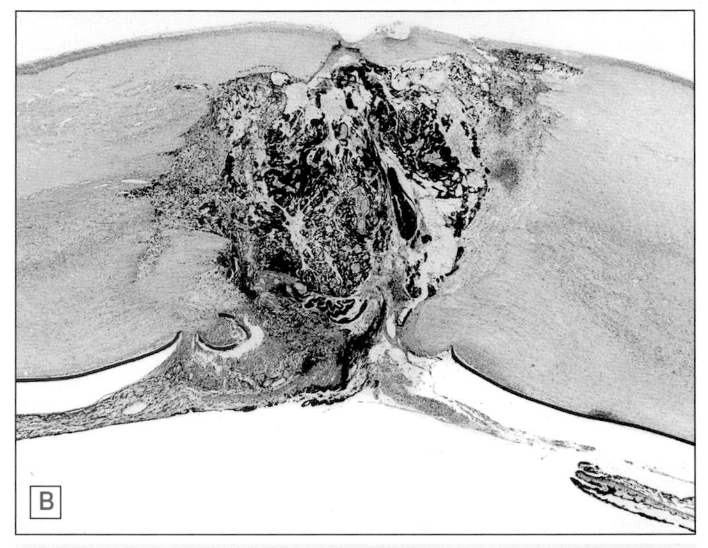

Figure 4.34 A. Healing corneal perforation. Corneal epithelium is attempting to heal across a fibrin mass plugging the defect. Iris is incorporated into the lesion and will form **anterior staphyloma**. Note coiled remnant of Descemet's membrane (arrow). **B.** Iris entrapped within the cornea following perforation of ulcer (**iris prolapse**).

In the case of corneal perforation, the iris flows forward to plug the defect (*iris prolapse*) and may subsequently become incorporated into the corneal scarring. This outcome is usually called **anterior staphyloma**, meaning a focal defect in the ocular fibrous tunic (i.e., cornea) that becomes lined by uvea (Fig. 4.34A, B). The distinction from anterior synechia is of little significance.

The conjunctiva is involved in almost all instances of keratitis, either as a victim of the same injury or as the nearest vascularized tissue to the diseased cornea. Hyperemia, cellular exudation, and lymphofollicular hyperplasia are common as the conjunctiva responds to the diffusion of inflammatory mediators of microbial, leukocytic, and tissue origin from the injured cornea.

There are some instances in which the lesions are found primarily within the stroma. Examples of bacterial or fungal keratitis in which the organisms were implanted into the stroma may cause chronic suppurative keratomalacia with negligible involvement of superficial stroma or epithelium. Alternatively, deep ulcerative septic keratitis may heal superficially, yet persist deep within the stroma. In either of these two situations, the deep lesion is referred to as *stromal abscess*.

Midstromal corneal vascular ingrowth from the limbus is a very common lesion in response to vascular endothelial growth factors elaborated in the course of chronic uveitis of virtually any cause. It appears to be a purely accidental lesion with no obvious purpose, but it does serve as a valuable and permanent histologic marker for previous or ongoing intraocular inflammatory disease. Its liability as a marker for subacute or chronic intraocular inflammation is probably not absolute, because similar midstromal vascularization can probably occur in response to growth factors liberated from detached retina or intraocular neoplasms (see Significance of uveitis).

Pannus keratitis

The only credible candidate for a *genuine stromal keratitis*, in which the primary target for the inflammatory disease is the stroma itself, is **pannus keratitis**. *This is an idiopathic disease seen most frequently in German Shepherds and phenotypically similar breeds.* Its prevalence and severity are directly correlated with altitude, suggesting that *sunlight exposure* is part of the pathogenesis. The clinical disease is distinctive. The early lesion is seen in dogs of either sex, usually in early middle age, as a vascularized opacity growing into the corneal stroma from the limbus. The ingrowth is bilateral although not always of simultaneous onset, and most frequently originates from the ventrolateral limbus. There is no ulceration, but pigmentation is often marked. The untreated lesion eventually infiltrates the entire cornea, converting the superficial stroma to an opaque membrane resembling granulation tissue. At one time, superficial keratectomy was the recommended therapy and so histologic specimens were quite often available. Today, most cases are treated with potent immunosuppressive therapy, and the need to perform a keratectomy to restore vision is rare indeed.

The histologic appearance varies with the duration of the lesion. *The initial lesion is superficial stromal infiltration of mononuclear cells, especially plasma cells.* Subsequently, there is progressive vascularization and fibroplasia in the superficial third of the stroma, accompanied by epithelial hyperplasia and pigmentation that may include the stroma. The deep stroma is never affected.

The pathogenesis of the condition is unknown, but an immune reaction to altered corneal epithelial antigens is hypothesized. Its response to continuous corticosteroid administration supports this hypothesis, as does it striking histologic similarity to discoid lupus and other lupoid dermatoses. Despite the similarity, immunofluorescence tests for intraepithelial or basement membrane immunoglobulin are negative. Infectious agents are not consistently isolated. A histologically similar lesion of the bulbar conjuctiva of third eyelid occurs in the same breed (so-called "*plasmoma*") and may reflect the same mysterious pathogenesis.

Keratoconjunctivitis sicca and desiccation keratitis

The response of the cornea to desiccation depends on the rapidity of onset and the severity of the desiccation. *It is seen as a consequence of inadequacy in the quantity or quality of the tear film* (usually called **keratoconjunctivitis sicca**). It also occurs as a consequence of exophthalmos, improper eyelid closure because of eyelid developmental anomaly, acquired eyelid disease, nerve injury to prevent blinking, profound CNS depression in which the blink reflex is lost, or conditions such as glaucoma or orbital mass that prevent proper eyelid closure because of abnormal ocular size or position. Under such circumstances, the corneal lesion is usually referred to as **desiccation keratitis**, although the effect upon the cornea is exactly the same as in acute keratoconjunctivitis sicca. In those cases in which the desiccation occurs only in a horizontal band not adequately covered by the eyelids for whatever reason, the lesion is sometimes referred to as *band keratopathy*.

If the desiccation is profound and occurs rapidly, the cornea has no time to adapt and the outcome is *acute ulceration*. It can be distinguished from other types of corneal ulceration histologically because *it is the only example of corneal ulceration that occurs in the absence of edema or neutrophilic infiltration* (because there is no tear film to provide either the water or the leukocytes). If the desiccation is only mild, or occurs over a long interval that allows corneal adaptation, the resulting lesion is *corneal cutaneous metaplasia*.

Desiccation keratitis (either acute or chronic) may follow destruction or denervation of lacrimal or accessory lacrimal gland by orbital inflammation, drugs, neoplasia, or trauma. Squamous metaplasia with resultant inadequacy of secretion may be seen with chronic deficiency of vitamin A. Specific lacrimal adenitis with subsequent atrophy is well recognized with coronavirus infection in rats and may be seen in the acute or chronic phases of canine distemper. Similar adenitis probably occurs with other viruses and in other species but such lesions are poorly documented. Transient keratoconjunctivitis sicca may accompany acute herpetic keratoconjunctivitis in cats.

Keratoconjunctivitis sicca, as a specific disease entity, is encountered more commonly in **dogs** than in any other species, with an overall prevalence in North America of about 1%. Most cases are chronic, progressive, and idiopathic. The reason for greater than expected prevalence in certain breeds (English Bulldog, Lhasa Apso, Shih Tzu, West Highland White Terrier, and others) is unknown. Because the disease is amenable to medical or surgical management, few specimens are available for histologic examination until the very chronic stages. At this time, the lacrimal gland is atrophic with interstitial lymphoid infiltration and fibrosis, but provides no clue as to the initial lesion. The ability of certain immune modulators, notably cyclosporine, to reverse the disease, points to some kind of immune-mediated phenomenon, perhaps autoimmunity.

The corneal changes vary with the severity and rapidity of onset of lacrimal deficiency. In acute disease with marked lacrimal deficiency, clinical signs of ulcerative keratitis may occur. The corneal epithelium is thinned, has numerous hydropically degenerate cells, and may suffer full-thickness ulceration. The accompanying stromal changes, including eventual vascularization and fibrosis, are those of ulcerative keratitis. More commonly in dogs, however, the desiccation is not absolute (at least initially) and the epithelial response is protective epidermalization without prior ulceration. Keratinization, marked hyperplasia with rete ridge formation, and pigmentation are commonly seen. Stromal inflammation and vascularization are usually superficial, resulting in a lesion very similar to pannus keratitis. Squamous metaplasia may also occur in the bulbar conjunctiva. The conjunctivitis that clinically is the earliest lesion of keratoconjunctivitis sicca is rarely available for histologic examination.

Herpetic keratitis of cats

Feline herpetic keratitis, caused by *Felid herpesvirus 1,* is seen either as the sole ocular lesion or in concert with conjunctivitis. Clinical signs associated with herpesviral infections in cats include conjunctivitis, keratitis, rhinotracheitis and, in neonates, systemic disease with encephalitis and necrosis in visceral organs. Acquired immunity alters the manifestations of the disease and results in different lesions predominating in different age groups. *Keratitis is commonest in adult cats* and seems to result from activation of latent infection during concurrent immunosuppressive disease or corticosteroid therapy. Concurrent mild respiratory disease may be present, but *in adults the disease is often purely corneal and may even be unilateral.* In contrast, *the infection in adolescent cats causes nonspecific bilateral erosive conjunctivitis without keratitis.* Intranuclear inclusions are numerous within cells prior to sloughing, and leukocytes are sparse until ulceration permits opportunistic contamination. Upper respiratory disease is almost always present.

The corneal lesions fall into two very different categories: *shallow transient erosions and ulcers* that represent the direct cytopathic effect of acute viral infection, and *more severe stromal keratitis* that is probably an immune response to viral antigen in persistent or recurring infections. The typical acute superficial corneal lesions are multifocal minute corneal erosions and ulcers that have a tendency to coalesce into branching dendritic ulcers. Early in the disease, typical herpesviral inclusions may be seen with histology, and herpesviral antigen can be demonstrated with immunofluorescence or other techniques. Severe or recurrent lesions in immunosuppressed cats may result in underlying stromal keratitis with lymphocytic infiltration, persistent edema, and vascularization.

There is much more written about the clinical features and clinical diagnosis of herpesviral keratitis than there it is about its pathology, simply because most cases are never subjected to histologic evaluation. By the time a sample of conjunctiva or cornea is taken for histologic assessment in cases that have been therapeutically resistant, histologic detection of inclusion bodies is futile and immunofluorescence is usually negative. Virus can usually be detected with PCR, but interpretation of that result is almost impossible because of the high prevalence of carriage in asymptomatic, healthy cats. For the same reason, attempts to link persistent herpesviral infection with feline corneal sequestrum or feline eosinophilic keratitis have been less than convincing.

Feline eosinophilic keratitis

Another uniquely feline ocular lesion is seen clinically as unilateral or bilateral proliferative, "fluffy" white stromal keratitis. There is no breed, age, or sex predilection, and no proven association with other ocular or systemic disease. Since the diagnosis is made by cytologic evaluation of superficial scrapings or (occasionally) by histologic examination of surgical keratectomy specimens, this disease is more likely to be seen by pathologists than most other corneal disorders. Scrapings of the surface of the lesion reveal numerous eosinophils and fewer mast cells and other mononuclear leukocytes. Eosinophils may be less conspicuous on histologic examination of keratectomy specimens, perhaps because most seem determined to emigrate through the epithelium and into the tear film rather than remain within the tissue. Instead, the stromal lesion is a *mixture of macrophages, plasma cells, fibroblasts and, unpredictably, mast cells and at least a few eosinophils.* The latter are least frequent in older lesions, either because of time alone or because older lesions are more likely to have received a lot of corticosteroid therapy. A characteristic lesion, not present in every case, is a *dense granular eosinophilic coagulum* along the surface of the keratectomy specimen. It seems to consist of free eosinophil granules. No bacterial or fungal agents have been seen. While there are histologic similarities to cutaneous eosinophilic ulcer and linear granuloma, no statistical association has been proven and the lack of understanding even of the cutaneous eosinophilic lesions makes such attempted comparisons of very limited value. While much speculation exists about the relationship between persistent herpesviral infection and eosinophilic keratitis, there is no proven etiologic link.

Bibliography

Andrew SE. Ocular manifestations of feline herpesvirus. J Feline Med Surg 2001;3:9–16. Erratum in J Feline Med Surg 2001;3:115.

Bedford PGC, Longstaffe JA. Corneal pannus (chronic superficial keratitis) in the German shepherd dog. J Small Anim Pract 1979;20:41–56.

Bellhorn RW, Henkind P. Superficial pigmentary keratitis in the dog. J Am Vet Med Assoc 1966;149:173–175.

Brooks DE, et al. Ulcerative keratitis caused by hemolytic *Streptococcus equi* in eleven horses. Vet Ophthalmol 2000;3:121–125.

Iglewski BH, et al. Pathogenesis of corneal damage from pseudomonas exotoxin A. Invest Ophthalmol 1977;16:73–76.

Kessler E, et al. The corneal response to *Pseudomonas aeruginosa*: histopathological and enzymatic characterization. Invest Ophthalmol 1977;16: 116–125.

Nasisse MP, et al. Detection of feline herpesvirus 1 DNA in corneas of cats with eosinophilic keratitis or corneal sequestration. Am J Vet Res 1998;59:856–858.

Ollivier FJ. Bacterial corneal diseases in dogs and cats. Clin Tech Small Anim Pract 2003;18:193–198.

Panjwani N, et al. Pathogenesis of corneal infection: binding of *Pseudomonas aeruginosa* to specific phospholipids. Infect Immun 1996;64:1819–1825.

Paulsen ME, et al. Feline eosinophilic keratitis: A review of 15 clinical cases. J Am Anim Hosp Assoc 1987;23:63–68.

Rapp E, Kolbl S. Ultrastructural study of unidentified inclusions in the cornea and iridocorneal angle of dogs with pannus. Am J Vet Res 1995;56:779–785.

Steuhl K-P, et al. Relevance of host-derived and bacterial factors in *Pseudomonas aeruginosa* corneal infections. Invest Ophthalmol Vis Sci 1987;28:1559–1568.

Williams DL. Histological and immunohistochemical evaluation of canine chronic superficial keratitis. Res Vet Sci 1999;67:191–195.

Mycotic keratitis

Mycotic keratitis *is a destructive, suppurative, ulcerative and deep stromal keratitis most commonly seen in horses,* but occasionally encountered in all domestic species. The offending fungus is usually a member of the normal conjunctival flora, and its role in the disease is always that of *opportunistic contaminant. Aspergillus* is the most frequent isolate, but cases caused by other common conjunctival fungi like *Alternaria*, *Penicillium*, and *Cladosporium* are not rare. *Most cases are probably iatrogenic,* occurring in animals in which a corneal ulcer, laceration, or penetrating wound had been treated with long-term antibiotics and/or *corticosteroids.* The latter is a particularly common villain in this context. Horses seem particularly prone to mycotic keratitis, perhaps related to the mold-laden, dusty environment in which many horses are housed; only rarely does the lesion occur in dogs or cats. Since virtually all stabled horses have fungi as part of their conjunctival flora, *seeing hyphae within the corneal stroma is required for the diagnosis.* Isolation from a corneal swab or shallow scraping is not adequate.

Because the disease is much more prevalent in horses than any other species, most of the description below is derived from equine cases. The histologic changes in other species, however, are very similar to what occurs in horses. There appears to be a difference in the typical lesion seen in temperate climates and what occurs in horses in very warm and humid environments. In the latter, there are cases in which the fungi are found throughout the cornea and are easily identified by even shallow scraping. That is not the case in those examples of the disease diagnosed in cooler climates, which I will consider the "typical" disease.

The typical early lesion is deep ulcerative keratitis with suppurative keratomalacia. Some chronic lesions are exclusively stromal because of successful epithelial and superficial stromal healing of the initial penetration (or perhaps because therapy eliminated the infection in the superficial stroma). For whatever reason, the typical equine eye enucleated for mycotic keratitis has an intense neutrophil-rich deep stromal keratitis with several characteristic features: neutrophils are karyorrhectic, inflammation is most intense immediately adjacent to Descemet's membrane, and frequently there is lysis of the normally resistant Descemet's membrane with spillage of the corneal inflammation into the anterior chamber. *Fungi are numerous within the malacia of the deep stroma and within Descemet's membrane itself,* but rarely if ever are seen within the anterior chamber (Fig. 4.35A). When they occur within the anterior chamber, they are always anchored to the nearby Descemet's membrane. Despite ample opportunity, there has never been a reported case of disseminated intraocular mycosis as a sequel to mycotic keratitis. Fungi are sparse or absent within the superficial half of the stroma, which explains why corneal scrapings or even keratectomy specimens may fail to reveal the agent. The reason for the apparent targeting of Descemet's membrane is not known, but the presence of the tropism even in untreated eyes suggests that it is a

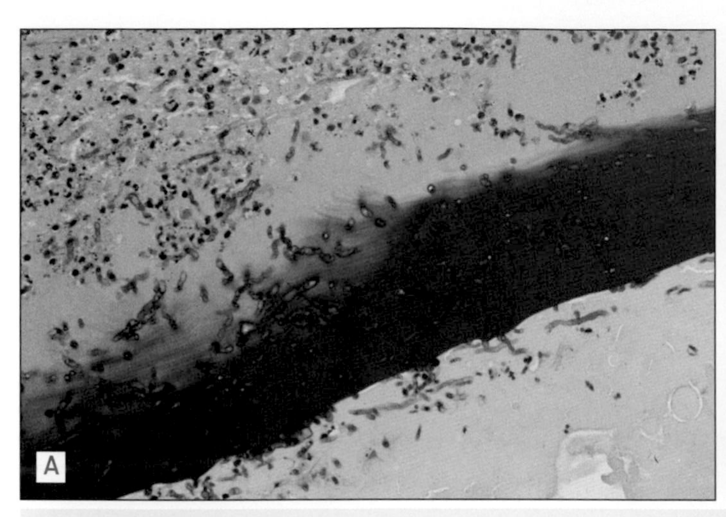

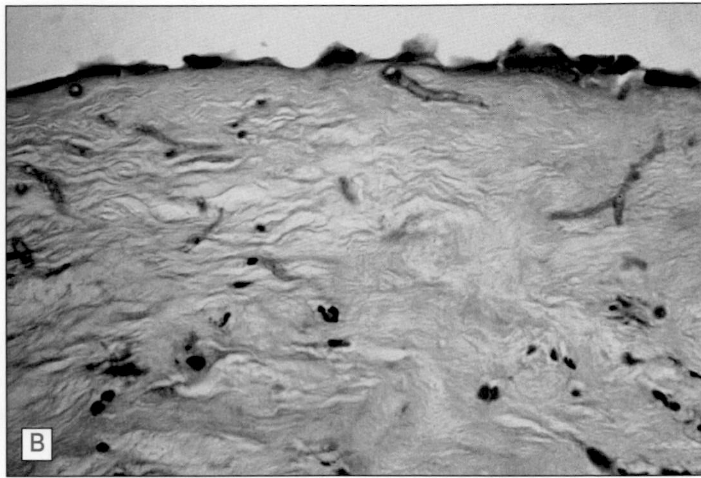

Figure 4.35 A. Equine mycotic keratitis. The fungi typically are found within and adjacent to Descemet's membrane, accompanied by karyorrhectic neutrophils and stromal malacia. **B. Opportunistic fungal contamination** of an equine superficial corneal sequestrum, but distinctly different syndrome from traditional mycotic keratitis. Note the absence of leukocytes.

genuine tropism and not just persistence of a previously generalized stromal infection in the site least likely to be reached by topical fungicides.

In horses in tropical and near-tropical climates (many reports, for example, come from Florida), the fungi are more diffusely distributed within the cornea and are thus more easily captured by routine cytology or culture swabs. While the distribution of the lesion within the cornea is also more diffuse, its fundamental lytic character remains the same.

In horses, cats, and dogs, we will occasionally see *corneal sequestra contaminated with fungal hyphae*; the fungi are easily found on scraping, leading to the mistaken impression that this is true mycotic keratitis (Fig. 4.35B). One could debate the issue, but it seems better to keep this as a separate syndrome quite different from the lesion described above.

Bibliography

Chandler FW, et al. Mycotic keratitis. In: Histopathology of Mycotic Diseases. Chicago, IL:Year Book Medical Publishers, 1980:83–84.

Foley JE, et al. Paecilomycosis in dogs and horses and a review of the literature. J Vet Intern Med 2002;16:238–243.

Gaarder JE, et al. Clinical appearances, healing patterns, risk factors, and outcomes of horses with fungal keratitis: 53 cases (1978–1996). J Am Vet Med Assoc 1998;213:105–112.

Grahn B, et al. Equine keratomycosis: Clinical and laboratory findings in 23 cases. Prog Vet Comp Ophthalmol 1993;3:2–7.

Mendoza L, et al. Canine mycotic keratoconjuntivitis caused by *Acremonium kiliense*. Sabouraudia 1985;23:447–450.

Moore CP, et al. Prevalence of ocular microorganisms in hospitalized and stabled horses. Am J Vet Res 1988;49:773–777.

Infectious bovine keratoconjunctivitis

Infectious bovine keratoconjunctivitis ("pinkeye") vies with squamous cell carcinoma as the most important disease of the bovine eye. It occurs worldwide, is most prevalent in summer due to the increase in fly vectors, and has a clinical expression that ranges from initial conjunctivitis and ulcerative keratitis to iris prolapse, glaucoma, and phthisis bulbi. The prevalence of severe sequelae reflects inadequate management of the disease rather than any special virulence of this agent as compared to other infectious causes of keratitis in other species.

The disease behaves as an infectious epizootic within a susceptible population, frequently affecting over 50% of the cattle at risk within 2 weeks of the initial clinical case. Shedding of virulent organisms by a carrier animal is thought to be the usual route of introduction into a previously unexposed group, although a role for various mechanical or biological vectors is also assumed.

Moraxella bovis has been confirmed as the most important causative agent, and the only one for which Koch's postulates have been fulfilled. Concurrent infection with other agents such as *Mycoplasma bovoculi, Mycoplasma conjunctivae, Acholeplasma laidlawii,* and bovine herpesvirus may contribute to lesion severity. Earlier skepticism about the virulence of *M. bovis,* based upon the unreliability of reproduction of the disease, isolation of the organism from apparently healthy cattle, and failure of isolation from some overtly affected cattle, has been overcome by detailed information on the pathogenesis of the disease. *It is now clear that virulence of M. bovis is associated with hemolytic, leukocytolytic, piliated strains that predominate only in the eyes of affected cattle.* Pathogenic isolates of *M. bovis* express a calcium-dependent transmembrane pore-forming cytotoxin. Nonpiliated, nonhemolytic strains predominate in healthy cattle and are probably part of the normal conjunctival flora. The use of immunofluorescence has demonstrated *M. bovis* in many of the naturally occurring cases for which the results of culture were negative. In naturally occurring outbreaks, the number of isolations of hemolytic *M. bovis* falls to almost zero as the outbreak wanes, but a few chronically affected carriers remain as the most important source of virulent bacteria for outbreaks of disease in the next summer.

In addition to variation in the virulence of different strains of *M. bovis*, sunlight, dust and, perhaps, concurrent infection with infectious bovine rhinotracheitis virus (*Bovine herpesvirus 1)* increase the severity of the disease. Calves are usually affected more severely than cattle over 2 years of age, although absolute resistance to infection seems fragile. The protective effect of serum antibody against the disease is controversial. Specific IgA is found in tears of infected calves, and there is substantial evidence that locally produced IgA is strongly protective.

Following experimental inoculation of virulent *M. bovis* onto the cornea, pilus-mediated adhesion and production of bacterial cytotoxin result in microscopic ulceration in as little as 12 hours. Initial adhesion is to older surface epithelium ("dark cells") and results in the development of microscopic pits in the cell surface. *Moraxella* is found within degenerate epithelial cells, but it is not known whether invasion is necessary for subsequent cellular destruction. *In field epizootics, the earliest lesion is bulbar conjunctival edema and hyperemia, followed in 24–48 hours by the appearance of a shallow central corneal ulcer.* The ulcer is a small (<0.5 cm) focus of epithelial necrosis that may appear as erosion, vesicle, or full-thickness epithelial loss. In untreated animals destined to develop the full clinical expression, the ulcer enlarges, deepens, and frequently attracts enough neutrophils to qualify as a *corneal abscess*. Stromal liquefaction ensues, probably as a result of neutrophil lysis, which is itself initiated by *Moraxella*-derived leukotoxins. By the end of the first week, there is extensive stromal edema and vascularization extending from the limbus. As with any severe ulcerative keratitis, the subsequent progression or regression of the lesion varies with each case as modifications by therapy, opportunistic bacterial and fungal contamination, trauma, inflammation, and immunity interact. Keratomalacia frequently leads to forward coning of the weakened cornea (*keratoconus*). In most instances, whether treated or not, the cornea heals by sloughing of necrotic tissue and filling of the defect by granulation tissue. Re-epithelialization may take up to a month, leaving a cornea that is slightly coned and variably scarred. The scarring often is scant and interferes little with vision in spite of the severity of the primary lesion.

Less satisfactory sequelae, while not common in relation to the overall disease prevalence, are still relatively common. Sterile anterior uveal inflammation may result in focal or generalized adherence of iris to cornea (anterior synechia) or lens (posterior synechia). Descemetocele may progress to corneal rupture, which in turn may lead to phthisis bulbi or resolve by sealing with prolapse of the iris. Synechia and staphyloma may lead to impairment of aqueous drainage and thus to glaucoma.

Infectious keratoconjunctivitis (contagious ophthalmia, pinkeye) of sheep and goats

Epizootics of conjunctivitis and keratitis in sheep and goats share many of the features of the bovine disease: summer prevalence, rapid spread, and exacerbation by dust, sunlight, and flies. Feedlot lambs seem particularly susceptible. Unlike bovine keratoconjunctivitis, the range of clinical signs and proposed causes suggests that there may in fact be several different diseases. Many agents including bacteria, mycoplasmas, chlamydiae and rickettsiae have been suggested as causes, but various mycoplasmas and *Chlamydophila psittaci* may be the most important agents. The lesions caused by *Mycoplasma mycoides* var. *capri* in goats and *Mycoplasma conjunctivae* var. *ovis* in sheep are similar but usually milder than those caused by *Moraxella bovis* in cattle. This is particularly true of goats in which deep corneal ulceration is uncommon.

Keratoconjunctivitis associated with *Chlamydophila psittaci* is usually predominantly conjunctivitis. Initial chemosis and reddening are followed by massive lymphofollicular hyperplasia in bulbar conjunctiva and nictitating membrane. Keratitis may occur but ulceration is seldom prominent. Animals with conjunctivitis may have concurrent polyarthritis from which chlamydiae can be isolated.

Bibliography

Angelos JA, et al. An RTX operon in hemolytic *Moraxella bovis* is absent from nonhemolytic strains. Vet Microbiol 2003;92:363–377.

Brown MH, et al. Infectious bovine keratoconjunctivitis: a review. J Vet Intern Med 1998;12:259–266.

Dagnall GJ. The role of *Branhamella ovis*, *Mycoplasma conjunctivae* and *Chlamydia psittaci* in conjunctivitis of sheep. Br Vet J 1994;150:65–71.

Kagnoyera G, et al. Light and electron microscopic changes in cornea of healthy and immunomodulated calves infected with *Moraxella bovis*. Am J Vet Res 1988;49:386–395.

Rogers DG, et al. Pathogenesis of corneal lesions caused by *Moraxella bovis* in gnotobiotic calves. Vet Pathol 1987;24:287–295.

Vandergaast N, Rosenbusch RF. Infectious bovine keratoconjunctivitis epizootic associated with area-wide emergence of a new *Moraxella bovis* pilus type. Am J Vet Res 1989;50:1438–1441.

Van Halderen A, et al. The identification of *Mycoplasma conjunctivae* as an aetiologic agent of infectious keratoconjunctivitis of sheep in South Africa. Ondeerstepoort J Vet Res 1994;61: 231–237.

Whitley RD, Albert RA. Clinical uveitis and polyarthritis associated with *Mycoplasma* species in young goats. Vet Rec 1984;115:217–218.

Wilt GR, et al. Characterization of the plasmids of *Moraxella bovis*. Am J Vet Res 1989;50:1678–1683.

LENS

The lens is a flattened sphere of epithelial cells suspended in the pupillary aperture by a large number of transparent elastin-like fibers known as *lens zonules*. These originate from the lens capsule near the equator, and fuse with the nonpigmented ciliary epithelium along the lateral surfaces of the ciliary processes or in the valleys between adjacent ciliary processes. *The range of histologic reaction of lens to injury is very limited due to the simplicity of its structure and physiology, and its lack of vascularity.*

The lens is entirely epithelial. Outermost is a *thick, elastic capsule*, which is the basement membrane produced by the underlying germinal epithelial cells. The capsule is thickest at the anterior pole and becomes progressively thinner over the posterior half of the lens. The capsule in the neonate is thin, but it thickens progressively throughout life.

Below the capsule is a layer of simple cuboidal *lens epithelium* that, in all but fetal globes, is found below the capsule of only the anterior half of the lens. The apex of these cells faces inward toward the lens nucleus. At the equator, these germinal cells extend into the lens cortex as the *nuclear bow*, an arc of cells being progressively transformed from cuboidal germinal epithelium to the elongated spindle shape of the mature *lens fibers* (Fig. 4.36). The bulk of the lens is composed of onion-like layers of elongated epithelial cells anchored to each other by interlocking surface ridges, grooves, and ball-and-socket protuberances. These elongated fibers contain no nucleus and few cytoplasmic organelles, relying almost entirely on anaerobic glycolysis for energy. Since the lens cannot shed aging fibers as does skin or intestine, these cells are compacted into *the*

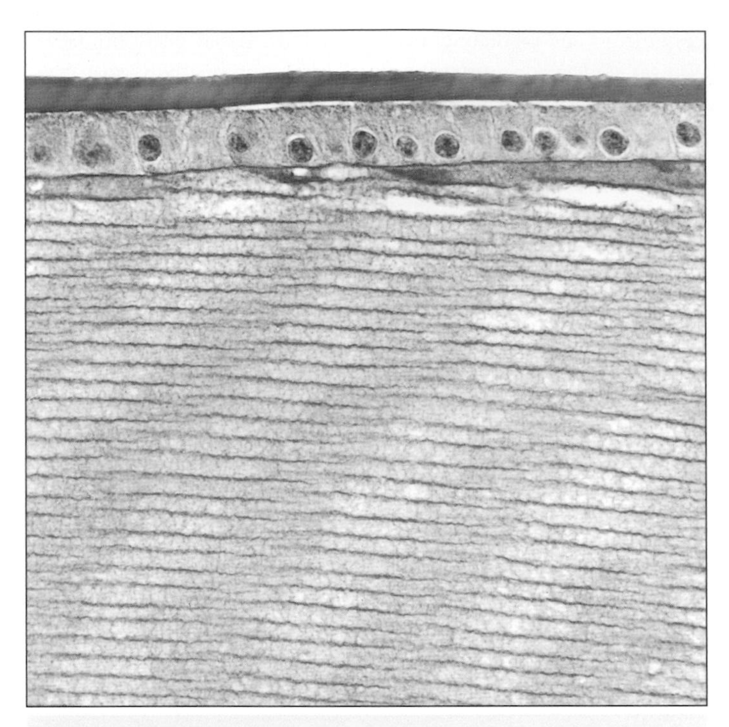

Figure 4.36 Normal canine lens with characteristic regularity of surface epithelium and lens fibers.

oldest central part of the lens, the nucleus. The continuous accumulation of these old desiccated fibers with altered crystalline protein results in the common but visually insignificant *aging change of nuclear sclerosis.*

Although in many ways similar to cornea in structure and function, the optical clarity of lens rests not with the regularity of its fibers but in its high percentage of cytoplasmic soluble crystalline protein and paucity of light-scattering nuclei or mitochondria. The lens is about 35% protein, the highest of any tissue, and over 90% is of the soluble crystalline variety. Insoluble high-molecular-weight protein (albuminoid) is found in the nucleus and cell membranes. Opacity of lens is associated, at least in some cases, with decreasing concentrations of crystalline and increasing albuminoid protein, the latter insoluble in water and optically opaque. *Many of the insults that result in degeneration of lens ultimately interfere with its nutrition.* Since it is avascular in the postnatal animal, *the lens relies entirely upon the aqueous for the delivery of nutrients and removal of metabolic wastes.* Glaucoma, ocular inflammation, metabolic disorders and various toxins share the common feature of altering the amount or quality of lenticular nutrition by altering the flow or composition of the aqueous humor.

Ectopia lentis

The only lenticular defects of importance in domestic animals are those affecting location, configuration, and clarity. Those affecting configuration are usually developmental defects and are discussed earlier. **Dislocations of the lens** may be congenital or acquired, and the latter include spontaneous dislocations and those secondary to trauma and glaucoma. *Apparently spontaneous dislocations* are encountered most frequently in middle-aged (3–8 years) terrier dogs in which an inherited predisposition to bilateral zonular rupture exists. The pathogenesis of the defect has been best studied in the Tibetan Terrier, in which the zonules develop in a dysplastic, reticulate fashion that precedes luxation by several years. *Traumatic dislocation* is usually via blunt trauma, notably automobile accidents. The dislocation may be partial (*subluxation*) or complete (*luxation*), and in the latter instance the free lens may damage corneal endothelium or vitreous causing edema and liquefaction, respectively. Such lenses may be surgically removed but seldom receive histologic examination. Anterior luxation frequently results in glaucoma, perhaps caused by anterior prolapse of the vitreous into the pupil. Lens luxation is inexplicably uncommon in cats. It is seen in middle-aged cats as unilateral and usually anterior luxation. One-third of cases occur in eyes with no other observed lesion, while the remainder occur in eyes with preexistent uveitis or glaucoma, or a history of trauma.

Bibliography

Curtis R. Lens luxation in the dog and cat. Vet Clin North Am: Small Anim Pract 1990;20:755–773.

Martin CL. Zonular defects in the dog: A clinical and scanning electron microscopic study. J Am Anim Hosp Assoc 1978;14:571–579.

Narfstrom K. Hereditary and congenital ocular disease in the cat. J Feline Med Surg 1999;1:135–141.

Cataract

Cataract is the most common and most important disorder of the lens. Cataract means lenticular opacity, and is usually prefixed by adjectives relating to location, maturity, extent, suspected cause, and ophthalmoscopic appearance. Of these adjectives, only those of location and, to some extent, maturity are useful in histologic description. *The simple structure of the lens results in a stereotyped reaction to injury that provides few clues to pathogenesis.* Unless permitted by invasion through a capsular tear, inflammation cannot occur within the avascular and totally epithelial lens.

The main challenge facing the pathologist looking at a histologic section of lens is whether any of the microscopic changes are genuine or not. The lens is difficult to section, and artifacts like fiber disruption and capsular tearing are almost unavoidable. *Histologic changes that distinguish genuine cataract from fixation or sectioning artifact are (in order of overall utility): detection of Morgagnian globules, bladder cells, lens epithelial hyperplasia, posterior migration of lens epithelium, and mineralization* (Fig. 4.37).

Morgagnian globules *are bright pink spherical globules of denatured lens protein.* They are distinguished from artifactual fragmentation of lens fibers because the latter form jagged rectangular fragments, not spheres (Fig. 4.38). With more advanced liquefactive change, fluid lakes appear between fibers, presumably the result of complete liquefaction of fibers. Some of the clefts are probably the result of osmotic fluid imbibition by the cataractous lens. The osmosis results from protein denaturation into more numerous, smaller peptides and from degeneration of the capsular epithelium in which resides the Na–K-dependent ATPase osmotic pump critical to normal lens hydration.

In advanced cataracts, the degenerate fibers may liquefy to the extent that their low-molecular-weight end products diffuse through the semipermeable capsule, resulting in the spontaneous clearing of the opaque lens typical of the *hypermature cataract.* Histologically, such lenses consist of a dense, eccentric residual nucleus in a lake of

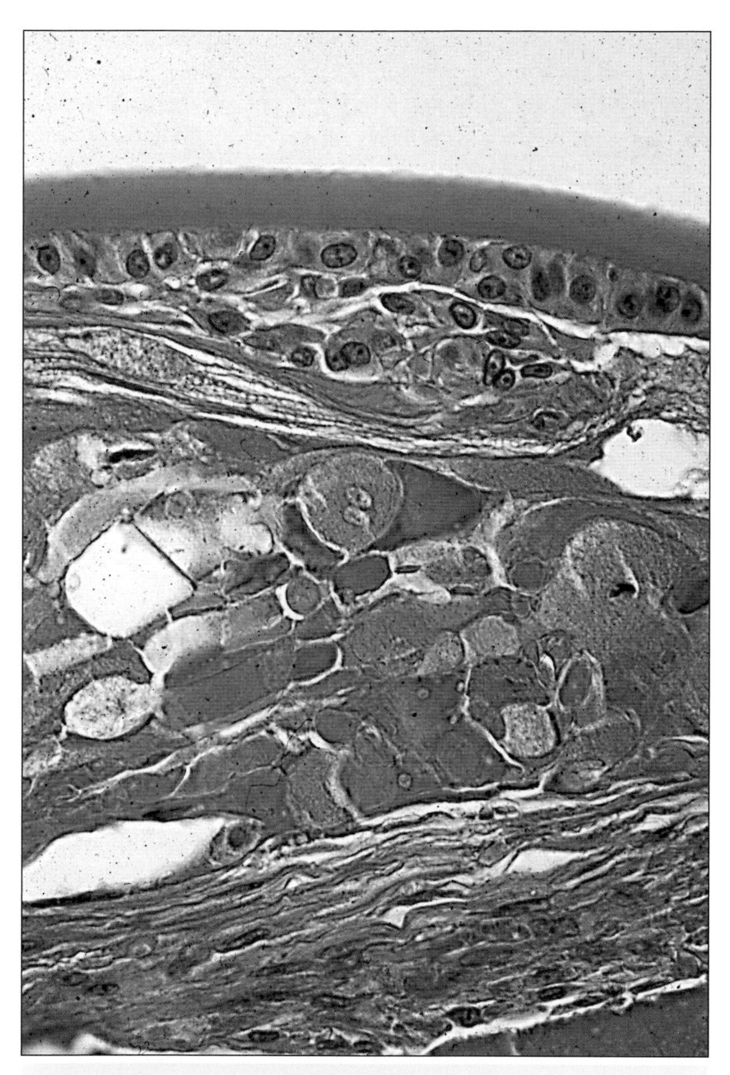

Figure 4.37 The general pathology of **cataract**: fiber liquefaction, reactive hyperplasia of capsular epithelium, and bladder cells.

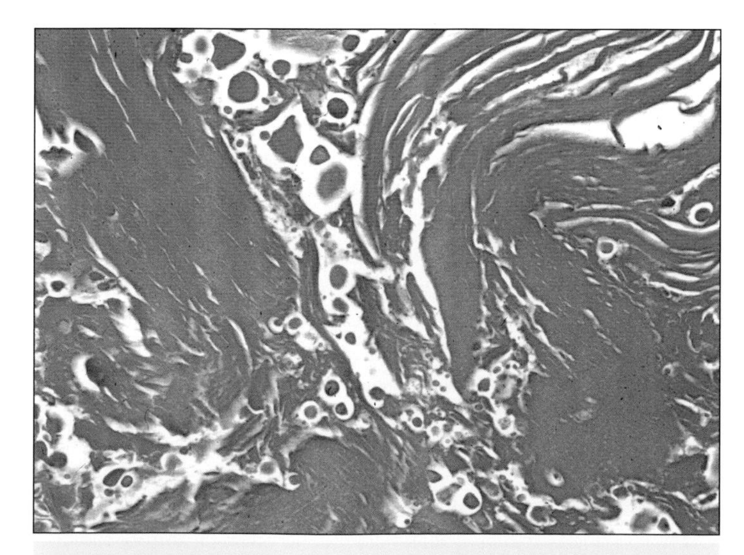

Figure 4.38 Spherical accumulations of denatured lens protein known as **Morgagnian globules**, probably the most reliable histologic criterion for distinguishing cataract from artifactual lens fragmentation.

proteinaceous fluid surrounded by a wrinkled capsule. The adjacent uvea will usually have a moderately severe lymphocytic-plasmacytic infiltration in response to unidentified inflammatory mediators present in that leaking lens fluid. The lesion/process is known as *phacolytic uveitis* (see below).

Bladder cells are claimed to reflect abortive efforts at new fiber formation by lens epithelium. Such efforts are apparently never successful, and the hydropic degeneration of such cells results in the formation of *large foamy nucleated cells called bladder cells* because of their bloated, fusiform shape.

Epithelial hyperplasia or **fibroblastic metaplasia** is the usual histologic counterpart of anterior subcapsular cataract, and is usually seen following focal trauma, or adherence of the iris or of persistent pupillary membranes to the anterior surface of the lens. *Initial epithelial degeneration or necrosis is followed by hyperplasia and sometimes by fibrous metaplasia.* The resultant *epithelial plaque* lies just under the anterior lens capsule. The innermost epithelial layer may remain basilar in type rather than fibroblastic. Each epithelial layer, even if metaplastic, secretes a new basement membrane that separates each layer from the adjacent layers. This characteristic feature is best seen with PAS stains. The end result is a focal plaque formed by multiple, sandwiched layers of flattened epithelium and basement membrane at the anterior pole of the lens. Remnants of adherent iris or pupillary membrane, including pigment, may complicate the histologic appearance.

Posterior migration of lens epithelium is a common change in chronic cataracts. Although it seems to occur more slowly than the changes of Morgagnian globule or bladder cell formation, it is equally reliable (when present) as a histologic indicator of cataract formation. The flattened cuboidal epithelial cells migrate from the equator to line the posterior capsule. Usually, they will also undergo stratification and sometimes fibroblast-like metaplasia. This re-establishment of the fetal morphology is seen most commonly with any chronic cataract in young animals, whose epithelial cells perhaps retain greater migratory ability. Adjacent cortical fibers are usually degenerate (Morgagnian globules, bladder cells, and clefts of granular proteinaceous fluid).

Deposition of calcium salts occurs quite frequently within cataracts of any type, and provides no clue as to pathogenesis.

The sequence of histologic change in cataract is the same regardless of cause, and thus diagnosis of cause can be made only in light of patient data or concurrent disease. In dogs, for example, familial cataracts may be congenital or of later onset. Specific examples may typically occur alone or with other ocular lesions, and occur at an age, in a location and with a progression sufficiently characteristic to allow presumptive diagnosis of a breed-specific syndrome. Cataract also occurs secondary to glaucoma, endophthalmitis, ocular trauma, and anterior segment anomalies, and observation of these latter defects permits presumptive diagnosis of the pathogenesis of the accompanying cataract.

Cataract may result from exposure of the lens to a wide variety of physical and chemical insults such as solar or other irradiation, cold, increased intraocular pressure, toxins, nutritional excesses and deficiencies, nearby inflammation, and direct trauma. The list of potential cataractogenic chemical toxins grows daily and includes food additives, chemotherapeutic agents, and by-products of ocular inflammation. The pathogenesis of the cataract is not determined for more than a few such insults, but a common denominator seems to be the ability to upset the precarious balance between substrate supply and enzymic activity within the almost exclusively anaerobic lens. This imbalance results in degeneration of fibers, accumulation of nonmetabolized substrate or production of abnormal metabolites. The latter two classes of products may be cytotoxic or osmotically active, thus drawing water into the critically dehydrated lens and causing opacity.

Most cataracts in people and animals are not identified as being caused by a single insult, but are assumed to represent the result of years of accumulated and perhaps synergistic cataractogenic activity of environmental, dietary, and inborn insults. *The majority of cataracts seen in veterinary practice fall into one of three categories: inherited, post-inflammatory, and idiopathic.* In reality, the large group of inherited cataracts in dogs is of unknown pathogenesis, although extrapolation from knowledge of similar cataracts in rodents and man suggests that inborn errors of lenticular metabolism are at fault. Postinflammatory cataracts result from injury to lenticular epithelium by adjacent inflammation, interference with aqueous production, composition and flow, and accumulation of toxic bacterial, leukocytic, and plasma by-products in the lenticular environment. Adherence of iris to lens (posterior synechia) inevitably causes a focal subcapsular cataract.

Other than these broad categories, there are a few naturally occurring examples of cataract about which there is some understanding.

Diabetic cataract develops in about 70% of spontaneously diabetic dogs, but is rare in diabetic cats. The opacity is bilateral and begins in the cortex at the equator. Progression to complete cortical opacity usually occurs within a few weeks. The pathogenesis of the cataract has traditionally been ascribed to the excessively high level of glucose within the aqueous. Glucose is normally the major energy source for lens fibers, with most of it used to fuel the Embden–Meyerhof pathway of anaerobic glycolysis. When the rate-limiting enzyme of this pathway, hexokinase, is saturated with glucose, the backup of glucose is shunted to alternative metabolic pathways. Chief among these is the *sorbitol pathway*, activated in the rabbit lens by glucose concentrations of >5 mmol/L (>90 mg/dL). In this pathway, the excess glucose is converted by an aldose reductase to the polyalcohol, sorbitol, which is then slowly reduced to a D-fructose, a ketohexose. Because this second reaction is much slower than the first, *sorbitol may accumulate to very high concentrations within the lens and osmotically attracts water even to the point of hydropic cell rupture.* Under experimental conditions at least, the early cataract may be reversed if aqueous sugar levels are reduced to normal, but the later cataract is irreversible.

However, osmotic events alone are not enough to explain all of the structural and metabolic changes in sugar-induced cataracts. The efficacy of antioxidants in ameliorating such cataracts, the nature of intralenticular biochemical alterations, and detection of increased intralenticular oxidants all point to some kind of oxidative damage as an additional promoter of cataract.

Galactose-induced cataracts probably have the same complex and incompletely understood pathogenesis as the diabetic cataract and are seen in orphaned kangaroos and wallabies raised on cows' milk, as well as in a host of experimental models. Since marsupial milk is much lower in lactose than bovine milk, the enzymically ill-equipped neonate develops osmotic diarrhea from undigested lactose and galactose in the intestine, and some excess galactose enters the aqueous humor. The lens, deficient in the enzymes needed to utilize the galactose by converting it to glucose–6-phosphate for anaerobic glycolysis, shunts the galactose via aldose reductase to its polyalcohol, *dulcitol*, which acts osmotically as does sorbitol to disrupt lens fibers.

Cataract reported in puppies and wolf cubs fed commercial milk replacer, or in kittens on feline milk replacer, has been attributed to *deficiency of arginine*, although in several case reports the specific dietary error was not identified. Cataract due to **dietary deficiency** of any of several sulfur-containing amino acids, zinc, or vitamin C occurs in farmed fish, and many models of nutritional cataract exist in various laboratory animals.

Various forms of **irradiation** cause cataract. The lens absorbs most of the ultraviolet and short-wavelength visible blue light that would otherwise damage the retina. At least in people, the chronic exposure to such irradiation is thought to be important in the pathogenesis of senile cataract. **Sunlight-induced cataract** has been described several times in farmed fish, but not yet for other domestic animals as a naturally occurring phenomenon. Absorption of ultraviolet or near-ultraviolet wavelengths by lens epithelium nucleic acids or lenticular aromatic amino acids results in photochemical generation of free radicals and peroxidative damage to numerous structural components of the lens.

A similar pathogenesis probably explains the development of cataract in animals irradiated as part of cancer therapy. In one study, 28% of dogs receiving **megavoltage X-radiation** for nasal carcinoma developed *diffuse cortical cataract* within 12 months of irradiation. In people, the risk of cataract is dose-related, and reaches virtual certainty with dosages of 800–1500 centigrays or rads, whereas rodents require at least twice that dosage. The dogs in the study cited above received between 3680 and 5000 centagrays. Antioxidants such as vitamin E or C, or hypoxia, are significantly protective against several models of light or other irradiation-induced cataract, providing further support for the common denominator of oxidative stress in the pathogenesis of such cataracts.

The aminoglycoside antibiotic and anthelmintic **hygromycin B** has been shown to induce *posterior cortical and subcapsular cataracts* in sows, but not boars, fed the drug continuously for 10–14 months. The effect is dose-dependent and perhaps even cumulative. Pigs fed the same therapeutic daily dose, but consuming the drug on an 8-week-on/8-week-off basis in accordance with the manufacturer's recommendations, do not develop cataracts. The pathogenesis of the cataract is unknown, but a partial inhibition of hygromycin-induced cataracts in vitro by addition of vitamin E suggests that peroxidative damage to lens fiber membranes may be important. *Deafness* in pigs, and also dogs, caused by hygromycin B is discussed with the Ear.

Traumatic lens rupture results in a spectrum of change much different from the changes of cataract described above. First, massive release of more or less native lens protein at the time of rupture may cause severe perilenticular nonsuppurative endophthalmitis about 10 days after the initial trauma (see **Lens-induced uveitis**). Second, the capsular rent permits leukocytes to enter the lens to speed the dissolution of lens fibers. Fibroblastic metaplasia of lens epithelium may result in cartilage or even bone within the lens. *Even after total destruction of the lens fibers, the durable capsule will be found somewhere in the anterior or posterior chamber as a curled eosinophilic mass*, often encapsulated in fibrous tissue probably derived from surviving lens epithelium or from injured ciliary epithelium. Such remnants distinguish lenticular rupture with subsequent dissolution from true developmental aphakia.

Cataract surgery is nothing more than planned traumatic lens rupture, and it is therefore not surprising that we sometimes encounter the same sequence of events as seen with accidental rupture. The main difference is that, with cataract surgery, the lens is already degenerate and the material that may be released following surgical incision of the capsule is not capable of inducing the same magnitude of inflammatory and proliferative reaction. Nonetheless, *complications of cataract surgery and prosthetic lens implantation are quite common in dogs*, the only species in which the surgery is performed on a regular basis. In most instances, the lens capsule remains within the globe and the degenerate lens material is removed by aspiration. The artificial lens is then implanted within the preexistent capsular "bag." Any lens epithelium left behind after removal of most of the cataractous lens forms the nidus for potential regrowth of lens fibers, usually as a combination of fibroblast-like cells and swollen bladder cells. This postoperative proliferation may use the implanted prosthetic lens (or, in its absence, the lens capsular bag) as the growth substrate, not only causing postoperative opacity but also posing the threat of causing pupillary occlusion. Some degree of postoperative epithelial/fibroblastic proliferation is normal in all such eyes, but the amount can be minimized by religious "vacuuming" of the inner surface of the lens capsule to remove all possible germinal epithelium.

Adhesion of pigmented or nonpigmented cellular material to the anterior lens capsule is a valuable histologic clue. *Pigmented epithelium adherent to the lens capsule is a reliable marker for previous posterior synechia*, even if this synechia has been reversed by surgical or pharmacologic intervention or has been accidentally broken during trimming of the globe. Similarly, fibrous or fibrovascular membranes along the anterior lens capsule most often are derived from previous posterior synechia (but they can represent complications of phacoclastic uveitis, pre-iridal fibrovascular membrane, or persistent pupillary membrane). They are significant causes for pupillary obstruction and secondary glaucoma.

Bibliography

Babizhayev MA. Failure to withstand oxidative stress induced by phospholipid hydroperoxides as a possible cause of the lens opacities in systemic diseases and ageing. Biochim Biophys Acta 1996;1315:87–99.

Clark WL, Peiffer RL. Cellular and tissue response to intraocular lenses. Vet Comp Pathol 1995;5:50–59.

Gelatt KN, et al. Cataracts in the Bichon Frise. Vet Ophthalmol 2003;6:3–9.

Glover TD, Constantinescu GM. Surgery for cataracts. Vet Clin North Am Small Anim Pract 1997;27:1143–1173.

Murata M, et al. The role of aldose reductase in sugar cataract formation: aldose reductase plays a key role in lens epithelial cell death (apoptosis). Chem Biol Interact 2001;130–132(1–3):617–625.

Ranz D, et al. Nutritional lens opacities in two litters of Newfoundland dogs. J Nutr 2002;132(6 Suppl 2):1688S–1689S.

Roberts SM, et al. Ophthalmic complications following megavoltage irradiation of the nasal and paranasal cavities in dogs. J Am Vet Med Assoc 1987;190:43–47.

Salgado D, et al. Diabetic cataracts: different incidence between dogs and cats. Schweiz Arch Tierheilkd 2000;142:349–353.

Williams DL, et al. Prevalence of canine cataract: preliminary results of a cross-sectional study. Vet Ophthalmol 2004;7:29–35.

UVEA

The uvea is the vascular tunic of the eye. It is derived from the primitive neural crest mesenchyme surrounding the primary optic cup (only the vascular endothelium is mesodermal). Its posterior differentiation into *choroid* is guided by the developing retinal pigment epithelium, but its differentiation anteriorly into *iris and ciliary body* is probably orchestrated mostly by lens. The presumptive anterior uveal mesenchyme accompanies the infolding of the neurectoderm at the anterior lip of the optic cup to form the stroma of the iris and ciliary processes. That portion of anterior periorbital mesenchyme not accompanying these neurectodermal ingrowths remains to form the ciliary muscle and trabecular meshwork. Posteriorly it forms the choroid and sclera. In all domestic mammals except the pig, the choroid undergoes further differentiation to produce the *tapetum lucidum* dorsal to the optic disk. Defects in development of the retinal pigment epithelium (including its cranial specialization as iridal and ciliary epithelium) inevitably result in defective induction or differentiation of the adjacent uvea.

The mature uvea includes iris, ciliary body, and choroid, the last divided into vascular portion and tapetum lucidum. The filtration angle is shared by iris, ciliary body, and sclera. Its diseases are discussed in the section Glaucoma.

The **iris** is the most anterior portion of the uveal tract. It is a muscular diaphragm separating anterior from posterior chamber, forming the pupil and resting against the anterior face of the lens. The bulk of the iris is stroma of mesenchymal origin, with melanocytes, fibroblasts, and endothelial cells its major constituents. There is neither epithelium nor basement membrane along its anterior face, but rather a single layer of tightly compacted fibrocytes and melanocytes. *The iris stroma is thus in free communication with the aqueous*, a fact of great importance when we consider the secretion or absorption of inflammatory mediators and growth factors in the anterior half of the globe.

The posterior surface of the iris is formed by the double layer of neurectoderm from the anterior infolding of the optic cup. The two layers are heavily pigmented and are apposed apex to apex, with the basal aspect of the posterior epithelium facing the posterior chamber, and separated from it by a basement membrane. The basilar portion of the anterior epithelium, in contrast, is differentiated to form the smooth muscle fibers of the *dilator muscle* of the iris. These fibers lie along the posterior aspect of the iris stroma immediately adjacent to the epithelium. The *constrictor muscle* is found deeper within iris stroma but only in the pupillary third to quarter of the iris. The iris epithelium is rather loosely adherent between layers and between adjacent cells of the same layer, so that *cystic separation* occurs quite commonly. Numerous spaces reminiscent of bile canaliculi lie between adjacent cells and communicate freely with the aqueous humor of the posterior chamber.

The **ciliary body** extends from the posterior iris root to the origin of the neurosensory retina. Like iris, it consists of an inner double layer of neuroepithelium and an outer mesenchymal stroma. The epithelial cells are oriented apex to apex and are separated from the posterior chamber and vitreous by a basal lamina. Only the outer epithelial layer is pigmented. The ciliary body is divided into an anterior *pars plicata* and a posterior *pars plana*, the latter blending with retina at the *ora ciliaris retinae*. The pars plicata consists of a circumferential ring of villus-like epithelial ingrowths supported by a fibrovascular core, called *ciliary processes*. External to the ciliary processes, the mesenchyme forms a ring of smooth muscle, the *ciliary muscle*, responsible for putting traction on the lens zonules and effecting the changes in lens shape necessary for visual accommodation in mammals (other vertebrates may use different and remarkably effective mechanisms). The muscle in domestic animals, particularly ungulates, is poorly developed and accommodation is thought to be minimal in these species. The lens zonules anchor in the basal lamina of the nonpigmented ciliary epithelium, particularly of the pars plana and within the crypts between ciliary processes. The precise location of this anchoring is highly variable among species.

The **choroid** is the posterior continuation of the stroma of the ciliary body. The posterior continuations of the inner and outer layers of ciliary epithelium are retina and retinal pigment epithelium respectively, with the transition made rather abruptly at the ora ciliaris retinae. *The choroid consists almost entirely of blood vessels and melanocytes*, except for the postnatal metaplasia to tapetum dorsal to the optic disk. The choroid is thinnest peripherally, thickest at the posterior pole, blends indistinctly with sclera externally and is separated from the retinal pigment epithelium internally by a complex basal lamina called *Bruch's membrane*.

Many portions of the uveal tract in carnivores continue to develop for at least several weeks after birth, and many of the uveal anomalies like goniodysgenesis or choroidal hypoplasia probably represent developmental errors in postnatal remodeling and maturation, rather than being truly "congenital."

The **general pathology of uvea** *includes anomalous or incomplete differentiation, degeneration, inflammation, and neoplasia*. Anomalies have been previously discussed, and uveal neoplasms are considered in the section on Ocular neoplasia.

Uveal degenerations, except as a sequel to uveitis, are poorly documented. *Idiopathic atrophy of the iris* is described in Shropshire sheep as a bilateral defect obvious by 1–2 years of age. About 25% of the iris is converted to full- or partial-thickness holes; those of partial thickness are spanned by a posterior bridge of iris epithelium. The eye is otherwise normal except for rudimentary corpora nigra. The pathogenesis of the apparently spontaneous atrophy is unknown. Similar atrophy is extremely common in *old dogs*, particularly those of smaller breeds (Poodles, Chihuahuas, Miniature Schnauzers). It is also seen in *old cats*, although much less frequently than in dogs. In both species, the pathogenesis is unknown and there are no published descriptions of the microscopic lesions.

Uveal cysts probably form as the result of fluid accumulation between the two layers of the posterior iris or ciliary epithelium. Such cyst formation is *common in old dogs* and less common in old cats. These cysts may be seen clinically as one or more translucent black cysts attached to the posterior iris or freely floating in the aqueous. Whether the cysts are truly degenerative, or represent residual lesions of fluid exudation from an undetected anterior uveitis, is unknown. A breed-specific syndrome of *iris cyst formation associated with the development of glaucoma* has been reported in Golden Retrievers and Irish Wolfhounds. In the Retrievers, there is concurrent lymphocytic anterior uveitis, although that uveitis is often barely perceptible when the globe is finally submitted for histologic examination. Whether the subtlety of the inflammation is genuine or just a result of aggressive anti-inflammatory therapy prior to enucleation is unknown. The exact relationship between the uveitis, the cyst formation, and the glaucoma has not been clarified.

Uveitis

Uveal inflammation is common and may result from ocular trauma, noxious chemicals, infectious agents, neoplasia, or immunologic events. In addition, corneal injury may cause hyperemia and increased permeability of anterior uveal vessels either by percolation of bacterial toxins or inflammatory mediators into the aqueous, or by stimulation of a vasoactive sensory reflex via the trigeminal nerve. The uvea may be the initial site of inflammation, as in localization of infectious agents, or may become involved as the nearest vascular tissue capable of responding to injury of the lens, cornea, or ocular chambers. Conversely, the uvea seldom undergoes inflammation without affecting adjacent ocular structures. The pathogenesis of uveitis can be arbitrarily divided into *three broad categories*: those examples associated with the hematogenous localization of infectious agents within the uveal tract, diseases resulting from the uveal response to infectious or noninfectious irritants within the ocular chambers, and "autoimmune" uveitis that results from a failure of immune tolerance or from immune mimicry by some infectious agent.

The vocabulary of uveitis

The vocabulary of uveitis and its sequelae is complex:

- **Anterior uveitis** describes inflammation of iris and ciliary body.
- **Posterior uveitis** involves ciliary body and choroid, with **panuveitis** occasionally used to designate diffuse uveitis.
- **Chorioretinitis** describes inflammation of choroid and, usually less severely, overlying retina.
- **Endophthalmitis** is inflammation of uvea, retina, and ocular cavities, with **panophthalmitis** reserved for inflammation that has spread to involve all ocular structures including sclera.

The usefulness of such terminology is doubtful when one considers the vascular unity of the uvea and its intimate association with other ocular tissues. Disagreement between clinical assessment of the extent of the uveitis and histologic evaluation is common: most cases diagnosed clinically as anterior uveitis would be designated as endophthalmitis by histologic assessment. *By convention, the choice of diagnostic classification is strongly influenced by clinical severity, with anterior uveitis the mildest and panophthalmitis the most severe lesion.*

The significance of uveitis

The major significance of uveitis is its effect on adjacent nonuveal tissues. Some effects result from the accumulation of acute exudates or chemical by-products of inflammation, but most result from the later organization of exudates and proliferative events of wound healing within ocular cavities (Fig. 4.39).

Corneal changes include edema and peripheral stromal hyperemia (*ciliary flush*). The edema results from corneal endothelial damage or from increased permeability of limbic blood vessels responding to inflammatory mediators released from the adjacent uvea. In the former instance, damage may be the direct result of the agent causing uveitis, as occurs in infectious canine hepatitis or feline infectious peritonitis. It may also occur as a result of an immune response to endothelial cells containing antigens of these infectious agents, to cross-reaction between microbial and corneal endothelial antigens (immune mimicry), or as a nonspecific response to the presence of the chemical by-products of inflammation within the anterior chamber. Similar by-products mediate the acute inflammatory response in the nearby limbic and conjunctival vasculature, leading to edema in the peripheral corneal stroma. Hyperemia of this limbic network also results in *the circumferential peripheral corneal stromal hyperemia, resembling*

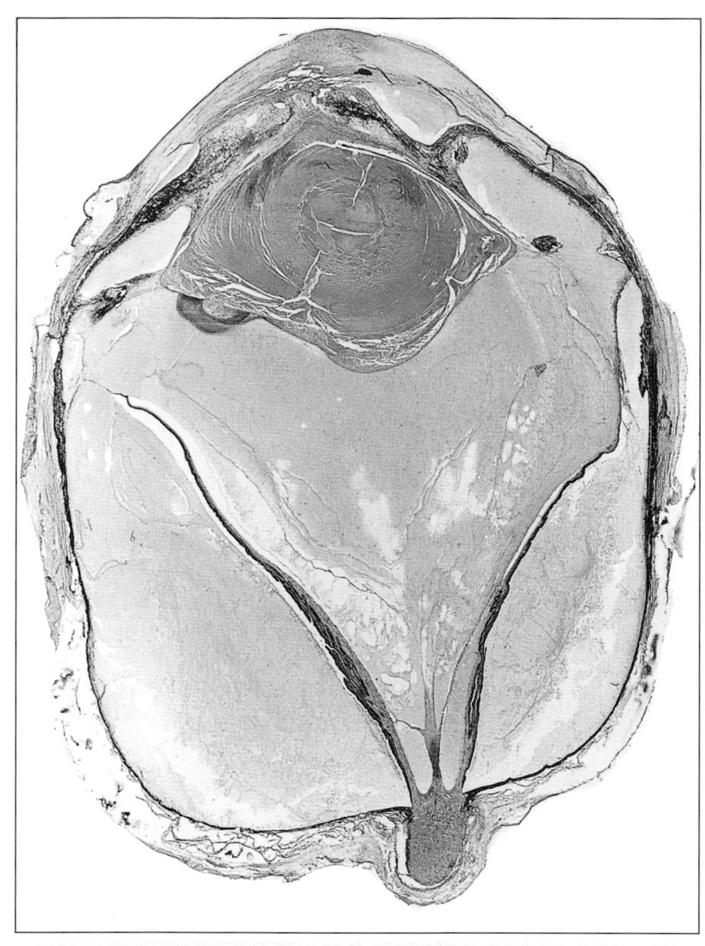

Figure 4.39 Endophthalmitis. Posterior synechia with pupillary block and iris bombé, serous effusion into the aqueous and vitreous humors, and complete serous retinal detachment. Note the healing corneal perforation and the ruptured anterior lens capsule, indicating that this particular example of endophthalmitis is secondary to lens rupture.

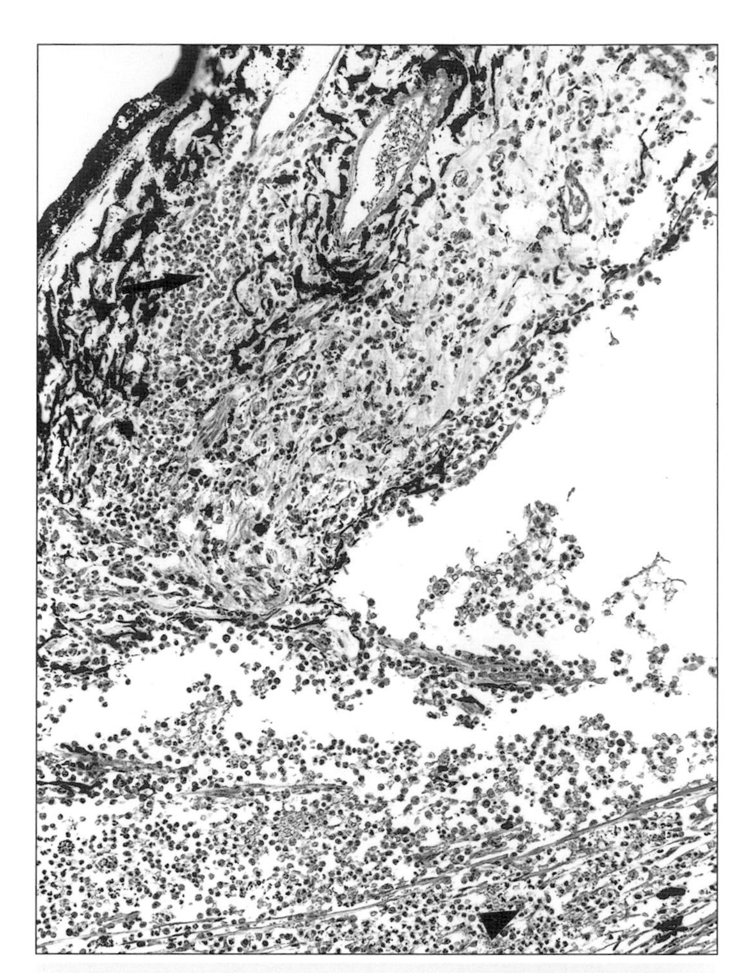

Figure 4.40 Anterior uveitis in a dog. Leukocytes are within the iris stroma and trabecular meshwork. Such exudates rarely if ever obstruct enough of the filtration angle to cause glaucoma. The arrow identifies the pectinate ligament, and the arrowhead is within the corneoscleral portion of the trabecular meshwork.

a brush border, which is a clinical hallmark of anterior uveitis. In eyes with chronic uveitis, corneal edema may also result from glaucoma or from anterior synechia. Persistent edema may lead to stromal fibrosis, vascularization, bullous keratopathy, and the risk of ulceration. *Limbic hyperemia may give way to corneal midstromal vascularization*. This last lesion is extremely common and is a reliable indicator of current or previous uveitis. It is presumed to be an "accidental" and apparently purposeless response to the percolation of angiogenic cytokines from the nearby uveal inflammation.

The accumulation of fibrin, leukocytes, and erythrocytes in the aqueous may result in plugging of the filtration angle and subsequent glaucoma. The infrequent observation of this sequel suggests either unusual potency of the fibrinolytic system within the aqueous, or the inability of exudates to plug more than the most ventral portion of the circumferential angle (Fig. 4.40). Much more common is the organization of inflammatory exudates upon the surface of iris or ciliary body. Adherence of iris to lens (**posterior synechia**) is more common than adherence to cornea (**anterior synechia**) because of the normally intimate association of the lens and iris. If the posterior synechia involves the circumference of the iris, the pupillary flow of aqueous is blocked, posterior chamber pressure rises, and the iris bows forward (**iris bombé**) and may actually adhere anteriorly to the cornea. Glaucoma results from pupillary block, peripheral anterior synechia, or both. In severe and prolonged anterior uveitis, there may be development of a **pre-iridal fibrovascular membrane** on the iris face (Fig. 4.41), which may span the pupil to cause pupillary block. Alternatively, this fibrovascular membrane may extend to cover the face of the pectinate ligament and cause neovascular glaucoma (Fig. 4.42). This membrane may contract on the face of the iris resulting in infolding of the pupillary border to adhere to the anterior (**ectropion uveae**) or posterior (**entropion uveae**) iris surface. Atrophy of iris may follow severe and necrotizing inflammation, and some examples can be distinguished from idiopathic and senile atrophy by the observation of residual lesions of the previous uveitis, such as lymphoid aggregates, focal synechiae, and uveal hyalinization.

The ciliary body suffers the same range of chronic lesions as does the iris. Deposition of PAS-positive hyaline material along the lumenal surface of the ciliary epithelium is particularly frequent in horses. It appears to be deposited in the cytoplasm of the nonpigmented epithelium, and may represent aberrant basement membrane. It is not fibrin; in many instances it has the staining properties of amyloid. Organization of exudate within the posterior chamber or vitreous results in *a retrolental fibrovascular membrane, called a* **cyclitic membrane**, which stretches around the ciliary body and across the back of the lens. Vitreous is almost always liquefied as a result of the severe uveitis, and continued contraction of fibrin in the posterior chamber

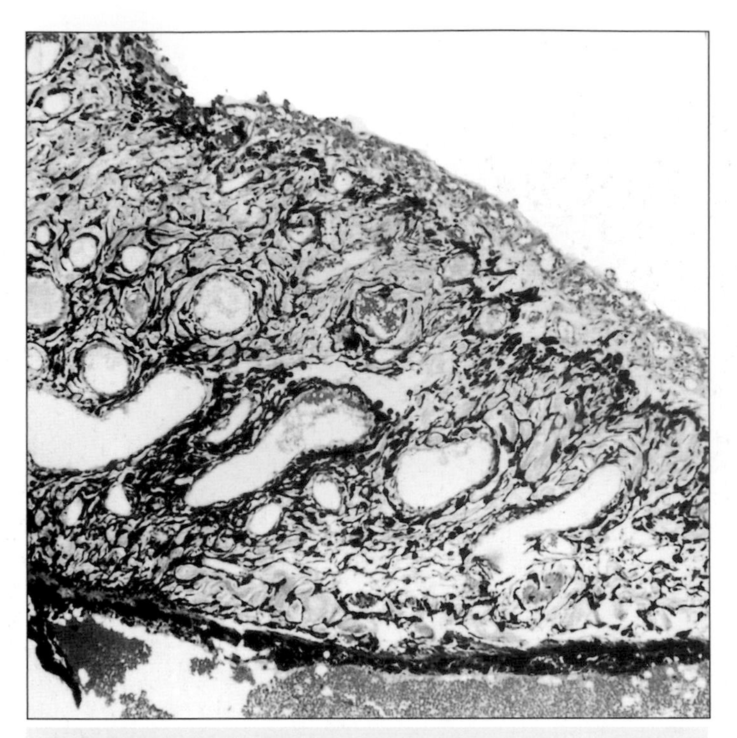

Figure 4.41 Pre-iridal fibrovascular membrane.

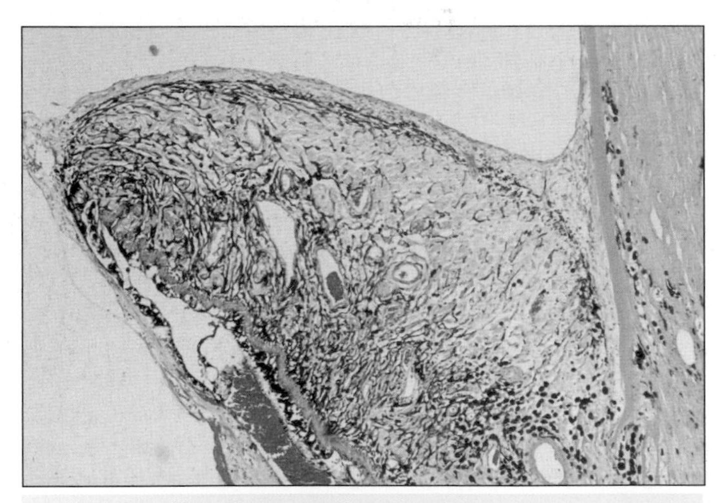

Figure 4.42 Pre-iridal fibrovascular membrane crossing the anterior face of the pectinate ligament, causing secondary glaucoma.

and vitreous causes a **tractional retinal separation**. Histologic examination of most cyclitic membranes reveals a fibrovascular retrolental membrane incorporating lens into its anterior face and a folded, degenerate retina in its posterior surface.

The residual lesions *of chronic choroiditis include focal lymphoid aggregates and scarring.* Tapetum usually remains unaffected. As choroiditis severe enough to evoke these lesions will almost invariably have involved retina and retinal pigment epithelium, the residual scar will involve these structures. *Chorioretinal scars are seen as focal fibrous chorioretinal adhesions* in place of normal retinal pigment epithelium. Because these scars prevent the involved retina from separating as part of processing artifact, they frequently appear as "spot welds" along an otherwise artifactually detached retina. Retinal pigment epithelium may be hypertrophic or hyperplastic, particularly if retina has been chronically separated by choroidal effusion. The fibroblast-like cells forming the scar may be derived from retinal Muller cells, choroidal fibroblasts, or metaplasia of retinal pigment epithelium, the last being the major source.

Cataract *is a common sequel to uveitis*, either as a result of uveal adhesions to lens surface, altered aqueous flow with lenticular malnutrition, exposure to injurious inflammatory by-products or increased aqueous pressure in postinflammatory glaucoma.

Phthisis bulbi *describes a hypotonic, shrunken, structurally disorganized eye that is the end stage of severe ophthalmitis.* Phthisis is seen most commonly as a sequel to severe prolonged suppurative septic ophthalmitis from corneal perforation. Cornea and sclera are thickened by fibrosis and leukocytic infiltration and ocular content is barely recognizable. Mineralization and even ossification may occur, but cartilage is absent (unlike congenitally dysplastic globes). *A shrunken, end-stage eye that contains ocular structures with at least recognizable orientation is properly termed* **atrophia bulbi**. The term is seldom used, but atrophia is much more common than true phthisis bulbi.

Bibliography

Bistner S, et al. Diseases of the uveal tract (part I). Compend Contin Educ Pract Vet 1979;1:868–875, 899–906.

Davidson MG, et al. Feline anterior uveitis: A study of 53 cases. J Am Anim Hosp Assoc 1991;27:77–83.

Massa KL, et al. Causes of uveitis in dogs: 102 cases (1989–2000). Vet Ophthalmol 2002;5:93–98.

Peiffer RL, et al. The pathogenesis and significance of pre-iridal fibrovascular membrane in domestic animals. Vet Pathol 1990;27:41–45.

Sapienza JS, et al. Golden retriever uveitis: 75 cases (1994–1999). Vet Ophthalmol 2000;3:241–246.

Swanson JF. Ocular manifestations of systemic disease in the dog and cat. Vet Clin North Am: Small Anim Pract 1990;20:849–867.

The classification of uveitis

There is no truly satisfactory method for classifying uveitis, or for organizing its presentation in a textbook in a manner suitable for all purposes. It does little good to organize classification based upon the innumerable specific diseases capable of causing uveitis, since that approach suffers from the "catch-22" that you need to know what the disease is before you can read about it! Classification based on pathogenesis suffers from the same problem. The clinical classification as anterior vs. posterior uveitis is essentially irrelevant when looking at histologic sections, because virtually all uveitis would be histologically classified as endophthalmitis. In the end, what seems most practical, at least for an audience of pathologists, is to initially classify uveitis on the basis of exudate type, with subdivision based upon histologic evidence of pathogenesis (lens-induced, traumatic, etc.) or etiology as appropriate.

Uveitis is thus classified as serous, suppurative, granulomatous, or lymphocytic-plasmacytic. The usefulness of such classification in predicting causes decreases as the lesion ages and as the events of host immune response blend with the initial inflammation. Furthermore, the reaction may differ among different compartments within the same globe. In general, the highly mobile neutrophils (if present) will be found mostly within the ocular chambers. The less mobile but longer-lived lymphocytes, plasma cells, or macrophages will usually predominate within the uveal tissue itself. As is true in other tissues such as joint and uterus, this may give rise to conflicting terminology depending upon whether the disease is being diagnosed by aspiration cytology of chamber fluid or histologic assessment of the solid tissue.

Acute serous uveitis involves the usual sequence of protein-rich fluid exudation, sometimes with fibrin, followed by emigration of neutrophils. In the iris, the protein-rich fluid readily percolates through the loose stroma to enter the anterior chamber as the clinically observed **aqueous flare**. The ciliary processes are usually distended by inflammatory stromal edema, perhaps a consequence of the initial inability of the serous exudate to pass through the tight intercellular junctions of the ciliary epithelium. Choroid exhibits the most convincing vascular engorgement as well as edema, with the latter frequently seeping through the retinal pigment epithelium to cause **serous retinal separation**. Since such mild uveitis is not likely to result in removal of the globe, observation of serous uveitis is usually restricted to globes enucleated for other reasons, such as severe ocular trauma, neoplasia, or corneal ulceration.

Suppurative uveitis *usually reflects a bacterial pathogenesis*, such as in the neonatal septicemias of calves, foals, and pigs. Neutrophils also predominate in acute mild neurogenic uveitis associated with corneal epithelial injury and in the acute phase of phacoclastic uveitis. In very mild uveitis, they are found marginated along the endothelium of iris and ciliary venules, in perivascular adventitia, adherent to ciliary processes, and in the filtration angle (see Fig. 4.40). Neutrophils rapidly degenerate within the aqueous to assume an unsegmented globular morphology. Clumps may adhere to the corneal endothelium as **keratic precipitates**, or settle ventrally within the anterior chamber as **hypopyon**. The hypopyon may, in histologic section, seem to be plugging the filtration angle, but only rarely would such exudate cause glaucoma, because only rarely would such exudate be able to occlude a significant part of the circumferential filtration angle. Fibrin exudation may accompany the suppurative inflammation, but fibrinolysis is very efficient within the anterior chamber, and glaucoma rarely results.

Granulomatous uveitis *is characterized by the conspicuous presence of epithelioid macrophages and, occasionally, giant cells*. As is true of granulomatous disease elsewhere, only rarely is the exudate purely granulomatous and most involve substantial participation by neutrophils. Ocular localization of some species of dimorphic fungi or of algae, helminths, or mycobacteria may cause granulomatous endophthalmitis, as may lens rupture and the Vogt–Koyanagi–Harada-like syndrome in dogs.

Lymphocytic-plasmacytic uveitis *is by far the most common histologic type of uveitis encountered in enucleated globes*. The leukocytes resident within the uveal tissue are dominated by lymphocytes and plasma cells, with or without the formation of actual lymphoid aggregates and nodules. It may occur simply as a chronic form of what was initially a suppurative uveitis, but is more frequently seen as the typical manifestation of immune-mediated uveitis, viral infection, phacolytic uveitis, or uveitis secondary to intraocular neoplasia. Inasmuch as the inflammation in most of these examples is probably of immunologic pathogenesis, *it is probably more accurate to consider all lymphocytic-plasmacytic uveitis as immune-mediated*, with the prefix "idiopathic" or the name of the inciting antigen. Dogs, cats, and horses are the species most frequently affected, and in these species the inciting agent is usually unknown.

Specific examples of uveitis/endophthalmitis follow.

Bacterial endophthalmitis

Bacteria may enter the eye hematogenously or via penetrating wounds. Those arriving hematogenously cause their initial lesion in ciliary body or, less frequently, in choroid. Those arising via penetration usually incite the initial reaction in anterior chamber, particularly if the penetration is via perforation of an ulcerated cornea. Most are suppurative, and their extent and severity vary with the size of inoculum, virulence of the agent, and host response and its duration.

The list of organisms capable of causing endophthalmitis is long. *It is probably true that any bacterium capable of bacteremia or septicemia can cause endophthalmitis*. Particularly prominent are the streptococci and coliforms in neonatal septicemia. The failure to detect ocular lesions in such animals is more often the result of the brief, fatal course of the disease than of specific ocular resistance. The ocular lesion may be very mild, better detected by opacification of the plasmoid aqueous in Bouin's or Zenker's fixative than by histologic examination. Histology may reveal only edema of ciliary processes with a few neutrophils along the capillary endothelium or enmeshed in filaments among ciliary processes. The well-known bovine *Histophilus somni* bacteremia, infectious thrombotic meningoencephalitis, is seen as focal rather than diffuse chorioretinitis.

Exceptions to the generalization that bacterial endophthalmitis is suppurative occur if infection is caused by bacteria which, in other tissues, incite lymphocytic or even granulomatous inflammation. *Ocular tuberculosis* is largely of historical interest. It occurred as part of generalized systemic disease and the typical tubercles were most numerous in the choroid. *Mycobacterium tuberculosis* var. *bovis* was the usual isolate except in cats where the human strain was common. In cats, ocular tuberculosis may also occur as keratoconjunctivitis without uveal involvement.

Brucella canis may cause chronic lymphocytic endophthalmitis that is probably immunologically mediated. Agglutinating titers for *B. canis* antigen in aqueous exceed those of serum, and the ocular lesions are similar to those of equine recurrent ophthalmitis.

Listeria monocytogenes often causes endophthalmitis in association with meningoencephalitis in ruminants (see Vol. 1, Nervous system). The condition is unilateral and the pathogenesis is obscure.

Uveitis caused by the rickettsias of *Rocky Mountain spotted fever* and *ehrlichiosis* are discussed under Retinitis.

Mycotic endophthalmitis

Fungi may affect the eye as causes of keratitis, orbital cellulitis, or endophthalmitis. Only rarely do the fungi causing keratitis or orbital infection penetrate the fibrous tunic to cause intraocular disease. However, hematogenous uveal localization is rather common in the course of systemic mycoses caused by *Cryptococcus neoformans* and *Blastomyces dermatitidis* and, less regularly, with *Coccidioides immitis* and *Histoplasma capsulatum*. In immunodeficient animals, one might expect occasionally to detect endophthalmitis as part of generalized disease caused by saprophytic fungi such as *Aspergillus* or *Candida*; these same agents will occasionally cause endophthalmitis in conjunction with penetrating plant foreign bodies. The frequency with which endophthalmitis accompanies systemic mycosis is unknown and probably varies with the specific agent, the species affected, and whether the disease is in an endemic area or is a sporadic occurrence. Hematogenous ocular mycosis is found almost exclusively in dogs, except for cryptococcosis, which is more common in cats. *Blastomyces* and *Cryptococcus* are more likely to invade the eye in the course of generalized infection than are *Coccidioides* or *Histoplasma,* and occurrence in nonendemic areas is strongly linked to prolonged systemic corticosteroid therapy. Involvement is bilateral but not necessarily equal. Blastomycosis, cryptococcosis, and coccidioidomycosis are discussed with the Respiratory system, and histoplasmosis with the Hematopoietic system.

Blastomycosis *is the most frequently reported cause of intraocular mycosis in dogs.* In is rare in cats. Between 20–26% of dogs with the systemic disease are blind or have grossly observed ocular lesions, suggesting that intraocular involvement would be recognized more often if histologic examinations were routinely done. The clinical ocular disease is severe diffuse uveitis, frequently with retinal separation.

The histologic appearance is of diffuse pyogranulomatous or granulomatous endophthalmitis with retinitis, exudative retinal separation and, commonly, granulomatous optic neuritis. Choroiditis is often more pronounced than is the anterior uveitis. The greatest accumulation of leukocytes often is in the subretinal space enlarged by exudative retinal detachment. The causative diagnosis depends upon the demonstration of the spherical-to-oval, thick-walled yeasts in vitreous aspirates or in the histologic section. They are usually most numerous in the subretinal exudate, but are rare in anterior chamber or in retina itself (Fig. 4.43). The organisms are free or within macrophages, are 5–20 μm in diameter, and show occasional *broad-based budding*. Extremes in sizes may result in yeasts from 2–30 μm diameter. The eye may, in addition, have the full spectrum of corneal, lenticular, and glaucomatous sequelae as expected of any severe uveitis. Panophthalmitis with orbital cellulitis is seen in about one-third of enucleated globes.

Cryptococcosis is similar to blastomycosis in that *the lesions are predominantly within retina, choroid, and optic nerve.* However, infection of the eye may arise either hematogenously or by extension from the brain via optic nerves, and lesions are often conspicuously lacking in cellular host reaction. *Large collections of poorly stained pleomorphic yeasts, surrounded by wide capsular halos, impart a typical "soap-bubble" appearance to the histologic lesions* (Fig. 4.44). The yeasts vary in size but most are 4–10 μm in diameter. Round, oval, and crescentic forms are seen. In some animals, however, a granulomatous reaction mimicking that of blastomycosis can be found. In such lesions the organisms typically are scarce.

The frequency with which ***Coccidioides immitis*** infects the eye appears to be low ($\sim$2%), despite the prevalence of generalized infection in endemic areas. The ocular lesion resembles blastomycosis in that *pyogranulomatous reaction occurs around fungal spherules.* The reaction is predominantly purulent around newly ruptured spherules, gradually becoming granulomatous as the released endospores mature. The lesion tends to be more destructive than other mycoses, usually

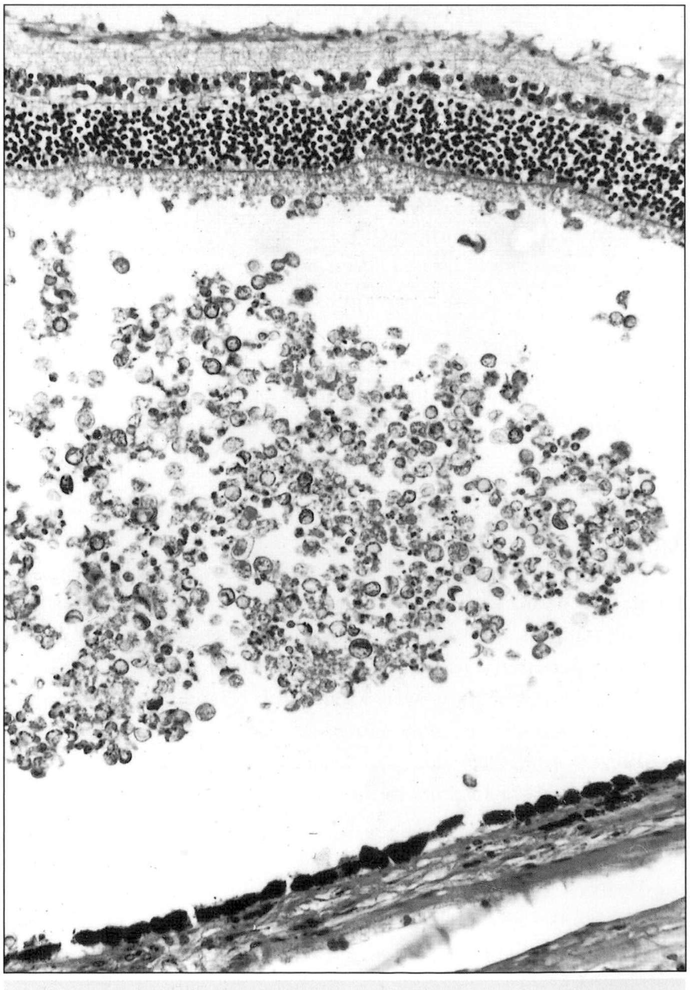

Figure 4.43 Subretinal exudate containing ***Blastomyces dermatitidis***, in a dog receiving long-term corticosteroid therapy.

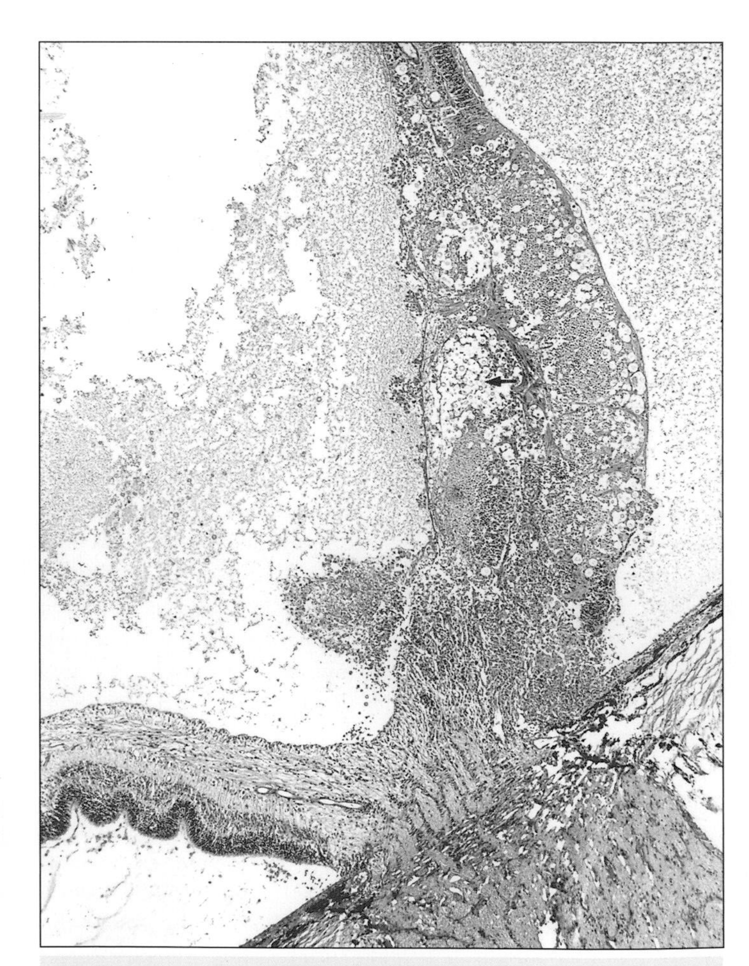

Figure 4.44 Retinal separation and focal necrotic retinitis in a cat with ***Cryptococcus*** infection. Note "soap-bubble" appearance (arrow) and minimal host reaction.

spreading to involve sclera and even episclera in a suppurative panophthalmitis.

Histoplasma capsulatum is a common cause of generalized mycosis in dogs but is rare in other domestic species. It has a predilection for lymphoid tissue and other tissues rich in phagocytes, such as lung and liver, and it is perhaps this preference that accounts for the paucity of ocular involvement in spontaneous disease. In dogs and cats, infiltrative choroiditis or panuveitis occurs and is dominated by plasma cells and by macrophages filled with the organisms. Retinal separation, plasmoid vitreous, and optic neuritis also develop. The reaction tends to target the choroid, and to be less destructive than either blastomycosis or coccidioidomycosis.

Prototheca are not fungi, but they are most easily confused with *Cryptococcus* and *Blastomyces*, and histologic lesions are certainly similar to those occurring in mycotic endophthalmitis. They are *colorless saprophytic algae* capable of causing enteric, cutaneous, mammary, or generalized granulomatous disease in a variety of mammalian species. Ocular lesions have been described only in dogs with the disseminated form of the disease. *The lesions are bilateral and may vary from lymphocytic-plasmacytic to granulomatous panuveitis with optic neuritis and exudative retinal separation.* The host response is usually quite mild. The lesions resemble ocular mycosis, particularly cryptococcosis, and are distinguished only by the observation of the pleomorphic algae. In histologic section, the algae are free or within phagocytes. The organisms are spherical to oval, from 2–20 μm in diameter with a refractile, PAS-positive, and argyrophilic cellulosic cell wall. Each cell consists of granular, weakly basophilic cytoplasm surrounding a central nucleus. *Prototheca* reproduces by asexual multiple fission, so that multiple daughter cells form within a single cell wall. One or two cycles of nuclear division without cytoplasmic cleavage may produce transient multinucleated cells before eventual cytoplasmic division results in up to eight daughter cells. Each daughter cell acquires a capsule, resulting in a parent cell criss-crossed by septations that represent the cell walls of maturing daughter cells. Rupture of the parent cell wall releases the unicellular autospores. Collapsed, crumpled, and seemingly empty cell walls are visible in histologic section. There is no budding as with *Blastomyces* and *Cryptococcus.*

Those canine isolates that were definitively identified were *P. zopfii*. An enteric route of entry is probable inasmuch as necrotic enteritis is a feature of the disease (see Vol. 2, Alimentary system). Immunodeficiency may be a prerequisite for dissemination of the organism. Lesions are found in many visceral organs, skin, and lymph nodes in most cases. The reaction is granulomatous but is usually minimal in comparison to the large number of organisms.

Protozoan endophthalmitis

While ocular lesions have been reported in infections caused by protozoa of the genera *Toxoplasma, Leishmania, Encephalitozoon, Besnoitia,* and *Trypanosoma,* only *Toxoplasma* specifically causes intraocular lesions, although many cases diagnosed as toxoplasmosis were probably caused by *Neospora*. Most of the others cause keratoconjunctivitis that occasionally extends to anterior or generalized uveitis in which the causal agent may be found. The exception is *Encephalitozoon* that may induce periarteritis within the uvea and retina as it does elsewhere.

Toxoplasmosis affecting the eye is, as elsewhere, much more frequently suspected than proven, and clinical diagnoses greatly outnumber those confirmed by histopathology. *The histologic lesion is usually in retina, uvea, or extraocular muscles, and varies from focal, acute coagulative necrosis to granulomatous or lymphocyte-rich inflammation.* The organisms are seen most easily as intracellular pseudocysts during acute disease or as true cysts during remission. The more noxious merozoites are found only with difficulty as 7–9 μm crescentic, basophilic bodies within phagocytes or free amid necrotic debris.

The histologic changes of ocular toxoplasmosis have received various interpretations and valid differences probably exist between species and between individuals of differing immune status. In man, the disseminated disease is usually congenital and the ocular lesion is multifocal necrotic retinitis in which free or encysted *Toxoplasma gondii* are found. There may be lymphocytes and plasma cells in adjacent choroid. In human adults, the ocular lesion is predominantly a lymphocytic-plasmacytic choroiditis, suggesting that the pathogenesis is related more to host immune response to the previously encountered, ubiquitous antigen than it is to local infection.

Lesions analogous to human congenital toxoplasmosis occur in *young cats* as multiple foci of retinal necrosis. Choroiditis may be present and is lymphocytic-plasmacytic, and anterior uveitis is seen in only 20–30% of such cases. *Much more common than this classical retinochoroiditis, however, is lymphocytic-plasmacytic anterior uveitis with serologic evidence of active Toxoplasma infection.* The role of toxoplasmosis in feline anterior uveitis is controversial (see Idiopathic lymphonodular uveitis of cats). Retrospective histologic studies list the majority of such cases as idiopathic and are presumed to be immune-mediated, with antigen or antigens unknown. In the several large published studies, there has not been a single case confirmed by observation of merozoites or cysts in the eye; even serologic evidence in these studies pointed to toxoplasmosis in only 1–2% of cases. In contrast, one study reported evidence of anterior uveal production of toxoplasma-specific antibody in 32 of 69 cats with anterior uveitis, and another report confirmed that anterior uveitis is indeed the most frequent manifestation of toxoplasmosis in cats, seen in 60% of cats with confirmed toxoplasmosis. Nonetheless, evidence remains less than conclusive about the role of *T. gondii* in the prevalent and enigmatic syndrome of anterior uveitis in this species. It may be that the local production of *Toxoplasma* antibody in cats with uveitis is merely the result of nonspecific recruitment of *Toxoplasma*-sensitized lymphocytes into the chronically inflamed uvea, and that lymphoid aggregates in such eyes are producing a whole range of antibody quite irrelevant to the original cause of the uveitis.

The situation in other species is not clear, but the prevalence of ocular lesions seems quite low. Lymphocytic cyclitis and multifocal necrotic retinitis are most frequently described and are usually seen together. *Multifocal choroiditis*, not necessarily adjacent to retinal lesions, is lymphocytic-plasmacytic in most species but granulomatous in sheep. A more common lesion is severe myonecrosis in extraocular muscles associated with free and encysted *Toxoplasma*. Toxoplasmosis is discussed in more detail in Vol. 2, Alimentary system.

Parasitic endophthalmitis

Many parasites are found incidentally in the eye, including: *Echinococcus* in primates and *Cysticercus* in swine, multifocal ischemic chorioretinitis and optic neuritis in elk caused by occlusive vasculitis due to microfilariae of *Elaeophora schneideri*, and uveitis associated with fortuitous localization of larvae of *Toxocara canis* or other ascarids, *Angiostrongylus vasorum, Dirofilaria immitis*, and *Onchocerca cervicalis*. In addition, adults of *Setaria* spp. are occasionally found within the eye of horses. The long threadlike worms are seen floating within the aqueous, and the uveitis that results seems to be the result of mechanical irritation. The only specific intraocular parasitism is seen with the lens fluke of fish (*Diplostomum spathaceum*), which, after penetrating the skin, seeks the lens with remarkable speed and specificity. The principal lesion is cataract induced by the intralenticular presence of hundreds of larvae awaiting ingestion by fish-eating birds for completion of their life cycle, but infected fish may have larvae arrested in many other ocular or extraocular locations.

Chronic mild anterior uveitis is reported to accompany ectopic localization of immature *Dirofilaria immitis* within aqueous and vitreous cavities of canine eyes. Studies of pathology are sparse, but endophthalmitis is reported in which anterior synechiae, subretinal exudate, and early cyclitic membrane may accompany the numerous vitreal and subretinal larval nematodes.

Ocular onchocerciasis affects people and horses. The *human* disease is endemic in Africa and Central America and is one of the most frequent causes of blindness in the world. The microfilariae of the causal agent, *Onchocerca volvulus*, are transmitted by *Simulium* spp. flies, and affect the skin, eyelids, and corneas of children and young adults. The microfilariae are found throughout the eye, but the lesion of greatest visual significance is diffuse sclerosing superficial stromal keratitis complicated by anterior uveitis with synechiae and eventual glaucoma.

Equine onchocerciasis has some similarities. The parasite, *O. cervicalis*, is of worldwide distribution and surveys from the USA document the prevalence of dermal infection in horses as varying from 48 to 96%. About one-half of the infected horses have microfilariae in conjunctiva or sclera. The microfilariae enter the eye only incidentally in the migration from the ligamentum nuchae to the subcutis. The ocular sites of greatest concentration are the peripheral cornea and the lamina propria of the bulbar conjunctiva near the limbus. The microfilariae in the cornea are associated with superficial stromal keratitis resembling the disease of man, albeit much milder. Some of the horses also have anterior uveitis typical of equine recurrent ophthalmitis, prompting theories that *Onchocerca* is one cause of this disease. The microfilariae can be recovered from the conjunctiva and eyelids of horses with uveitis, keratoconjunctivitis, and eyelid depigmentation, but are recovered with equal frequency from horses with no ocular disease and no microscopic reaction to the worms.

Ocular manifestations of **visceral larva migrans** in people are associated with larvae of *Toxocara canis* or, perhaps more frequently, of the raccoon roundworm *Baylisascaris procyonis*. The unilateral granulomatous fundic lesions are caused by a single wandering larva, and are relatively common in children but have rarely been described in nonhuman subjects despite the rather common occurrence of ascarid-induced granulomas in canine kidneys, lungs, or livers. The paucity of reports may not reflect the actual prevalence of disease in specific canine populations. One large survey of working sheepdogs in New Zealand recorded a 39% prevalence of lesions attributed to visceral larva migrans, contrasted to a 6% prevalence in similar dogs living in urban environments. *The active lesions were lymphocytic and granulomatous uveitis, nonsuppurative retinitis, and peripapillary nontapetal retinal necrosis.* Inactive lesions involved choreoretinal scars and multifocal chronic retinal separations in dogs older than 3 years. Larvae most compatible with *Toxocara canis* were seen in sections of some acutely affected eyes. The high prevalence in these dogs was tentatively ascribed to the feeding of uncooked frozen mutton that may have contained *T. canis* larvae as part of a dog–sheep–dog life cycle. A report of similar lesions in Border Collies in the US was associated with the feeding of raw pork.

Ocular disease may also result from the intraocular migration of *fly larvae*. This syndrome, termed *internal ophthalmomyiasis*, is discussed with diseases of conjunctiva.

Bibliography

Bernays ME, Peiffer RL, Jr. Ocular infections with dematiaceous fungi in two cats and a dog. J Am Vet Med Assoc 1998;213:507–509.

Bistner S, et al. Diseases of the uveal tract (part III). Compend Contin Educ Pract Vet 1980;2:46–53.

Bloom JD, et al. Ocular blastomycosis in dogs: 73 cases, 108 eyes (1985–1993). J Am Vet Med Assoc 1996;209:1271–1274.

Callegan MC, et al. Bacterial endophthalmitis: epidemiology, therapeutics, and bacterium-host interactions. Clin Microbiol Rev 2002;15:111–124.

Chandler FW, et al. Histopathology of Mycotic Diseases. Chicago, IL:Year Book Medical Publishers, 1980.

Ciaramella P, et al. A retrospective clinical study of canine leishmaniasis in 150 dogs naturally infected by Leishmania infantum. Vet Rec 1997;141:539–543.

Davidson MG. Toxoplasmosis. Vet Clin North Am Small Anim Pract 2000;30:1051–1062.

Despommier D. Toxocariasis: clinical aspects, epidemiology, medical ecology, and molecular aspects. Clin Microbiol Rev 2003;16:265–272.

Dubey JP, Carpenter JL. Histologically confirmed clinical toxoplasmosis in cats - 100 cases (1952–1990). J Am Vet Med Assoc 1993;203:1556–1566.

Gwin RM, et al. Ocular lesions associated with *Brucella canis* infection in a dog. J Am Anim Hosp Assoc 1980;16:607–610.

Hollingsworth SR. Canine protothecosis. Vet Clin North Am Small Anim Pract 2000;30:1091–1101.

Hughes PL, et al. Multifocal retinitis in New Zealand sheep dogs. Vet Pathol 1987;24:22–27.

Johnson BW, et al. Retinitis and intraocular larval migration in a group of border collies. J Am Anim Hosp Assoc 1989;25:623–629.

Lappin MR, Black JC. *Bartonella* spp infection as a possible cause of uveitis in a cat. J Am Vet Med Assoc 1999;214:1205–1207.

Laus JL, et al. Orbital cellulitis associated with *Toxocara canis* in a dog. Vet Ophthalmol 2003;6:333–336.

Linek J. Mycotic endophthalmitis in a dog caused by *Candida albicans*. Vet Ophthalmol 2004;7:159–162.

Panciera RJ, et al. Ocular histopathology of ehrlichial infections in the dog. Vet Pathol 2001;38:43–46.

Trevino GS. Canine blastomycosis with ocular involvement. Pathol Vet 1966;3:651–658.

Willis AM. Feline leukemia virus and feline immunodeficiency virus. Vet Clin North Am Small Anim Pract 2000;30:971–986.

Viral endophthalmitis

The fuzzy distinction between infectious uveitis/endophthalmitis and immune-mediated disease is most obvious when dealing with viral causes of endophthalmitis, even though it is probably also a major factor in mycotic and parasitic diseases. The distinction is therefore arbitrary, and *discussed below are those diseases that are probably best classified as immune-mediated endophthalmitis for which the antigen is identified as viral.*

Canine adenovirus

Canine adenovirus 1 (infectious canine hepatitis virus) is the best-documented cause of virally induced, immune-mediated uveitis in domestic animals. The systemic disease is discussed in Vol. 2, Liver and biliary system. During the acute viral stage of the disease, viral replication within endothelium and stromal phagocytes of the uvea results in a primary mild nonsuppurative uveitis that usually is clinically undetected. Inoculation of field virus into the anterior chamber of dogs and foxes may result in viral inclusion bodies within corneal endothelium and subsequent edema, but edema is not a feature of the active stage of naturally occurring disease. During the convalescent phase of the disease, or 6–7 days after vaccination with a modified live virus, a small percentage of dogs develops anterior uveitis, endothelial damage, and corneal edema ("*blue eye*") that is a manifestation of type III hypersensitivity to persistent viral antigen in which complement fixation attracts neutrophils. The proteases of neutrophils are responsible for the cell injury.

The histologic lesion is bilateral but not usually of equal intensity, thus clinically apparent disease may be unilateral. *Corneal edema results from diffuse hydropic degeneration of corneal endothelium and secondary stromal edema.* In a small percentage of affected dogs, the damage is so persistent as to cause interstitial keratitis and permanent fibrosis. Whether this sequel results from unusually persistent antigen, unusually severe endothelial damage or age-dependent variation in endothelial regenerative ability is unknown. *Intranuclear inclusion bodies* of adenovirus type may be seen in a few degenerate endothelial cells. There is accompanying anterior uveitis, with lymphocytes and plasma cells around vessels in iris and ciliary body, in the filtration angle and adherent to cornea as keratic precipitates. Choroidal involvement is mild or absent. Sequelae such as synechia or angle obstruction with debris are infrequent, occurring in less than 5% of affected eyes. In most dogs, whether recovering from natural or vaccine-induced infection, the ocular reaction subsides within 3–4 weeks.

Feline infectious peritonitis-associated uveitis

The coronavirus of feline infectious peritonitis causes diffuse uveitis that is probably immune-mediated (see Vol. 2, Alimentary system). The frequency of ocular lesions is unknown because the eyes are not regularly examined in cats with the disease. Estimates based upon clinical examination range from about 10% in an outbreak to 50% of unselected clinical cases. *Most cats that die of the disease have ocular involvement as detected by coagulation of aqueous with acidic fixatives (indicating increased aqueous protein).* The histologic evidence for inflammation in some eyes may be subtle indeed, and such eyes usually reach postmortem without clinically detected uveitis. Conversely, some cats develop severe uveitis attributed to this virus by clinical, serologic, or histologic evaluation, without concurrent evidence of the disease elsewhere.

The typical histologic lesion, as is the case elsewhere in the body, varies with time and location. Leukocytic infiltration is most extensive in ciliary body and adjacent limbic sclera, and is usually a rather even mixture of neutrophils, lymphocytes, plasma cells, and macrophages. In some eyes, the infiltrate is purely histiocytic. The inflammatory cell population often becomes more purely lymphoid in the choroid and more neutrophilic in the anterior chamber. Perivascular lymphocytic-plasmacytic aggregates are common in retrobulbar connective tissue and in the optic nerve sheath, and in the retina. In the retina, the accumulations are larger and are more likely to involve a true phlebitis than is the case with the subtle perivascular retinitis that is a frequent and nonspecific accompaniment to most forms of anterior uveitis. Sequelae to the uveitis are rarely seen, either because the cats are in the late stages of the disease when ocular lesions are examined or because euthanasia halts its progression. Retinal separation with serous subretinal exudate is occasionally observed. The presence of large globular accumulations of macrophages and neutrophils adherent to the corneal endothelium (*keratic precipitates*) is an important clinical hallmark of the disease, and is useful histologically as well. Neutrophilic endothelialitis with severe corneal edema may also occur.

Bovine malignant catarrhal fever-associated uveitis

The presence of severe uveitis is an important clue in the clinical differentiation of malignant catarrhal fever from other bovine systemic disorders, particularly from mucosal disease. The histologic lesions within the eye resemble those elsewhere in the body: arterial necrosis and perivascular and intramural lymphocytic accumulations. The presence of mitotic figures among the lymphoid cells is distinctive. The arteritis usually is most obvious in the iris, but may be seen affecting arterioles or venules in the retina, choroid, meninges of optic nerve, or even peripheral cornea. There is *marked corneal edema with a ring of peripheral corneal stromal vascularization*, clinically seen as a dark red circumferential brush border of straight vessels in the perilimbal cornea. Blood vessels in the conjunctiva and even in the newly vascularized cornea may be targets for the disease, so that the edema and hemorrhage of vessel injury are added to the nonspecific lesions of conjunctivitis and peripheral keratitis that accompany uveitis of any cause in all species.

Infiltration of lymphocytes among corneal endothelial cells is associated with patchy necrosis of that layer, which may also contribute to the corneal edema (Fig. 4.45). A layer of mononuclear leukocytes enmeshed in fibrin often is adherent to the aqueous face of the corneal endothelium.

Even the very early lesions are lymphocytic. In vessels, the first changes involve subendothelial and adventitial lymphocytic and lymphoblastic accumulation, with little necrosis. Despite longstanding speculation for an immune-complex pathogenesis for the vasculitis, proof is lacking. Deposition of immunoglobulin or complement is not a significant feature of the vascular lesion within the eye, and a T-cell-dependent, type IV immune pathogenesis has been suggested.

Immune-mediated uveitis

There is no clear distinction between immune-mediated uveitis and uveitis traditionally ascribed to a specific causative agent. Except for rapidly progressing bacterial uveitis following hematogenous localization or penetrating injury, *virtually all uveitis probably has an immune component superimposed on initial nonspecific inflammation.* Even traumatic uveitis probably permits unusually large amounts of endogenous ocular antigens to enter venous drainage and to reach the spleen and other lymphoid tissue. Types III and IV hypersensitivity have been induced in various laboratory animals using tissue-specific antigens of photoreceptor, uveal, lens, and corneal origin. *Lens-induced uveitis* and an *idiopathic uveitis associated with dermal depigmentation in dogs (the so-called Vogt–Koyanagi–Harada syndrome)* are naturally occurring examples of uveitis induced by endogenous ocular antigens. Recent

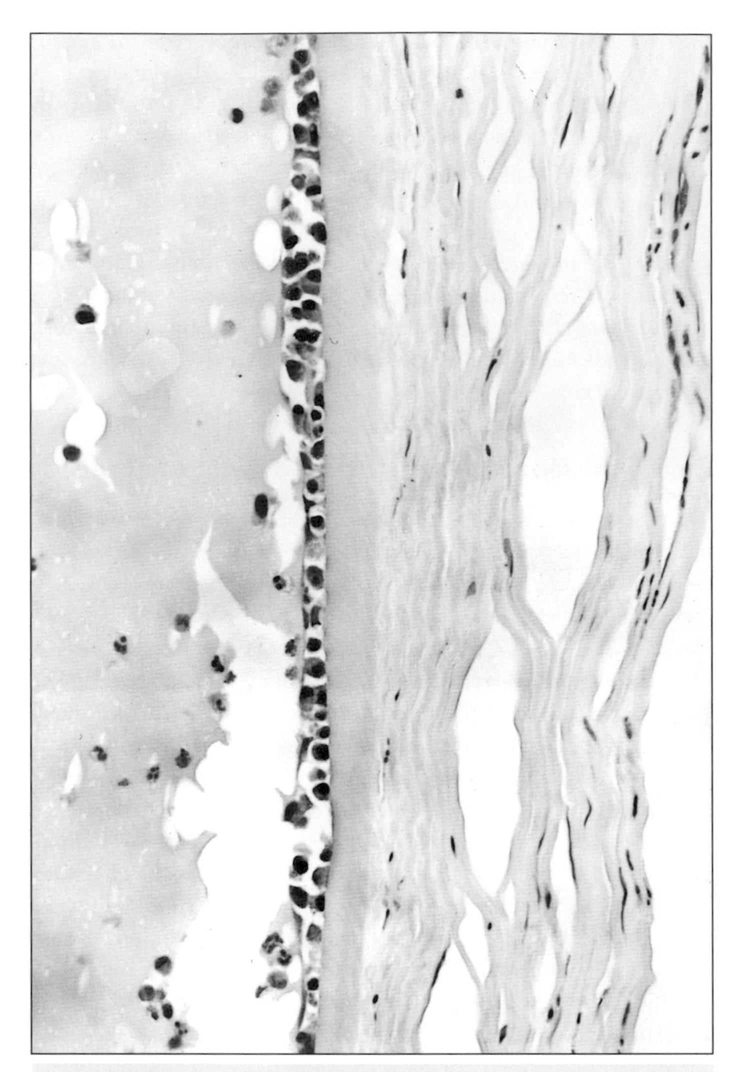

Figure 4.45 Lymphocytes, as part of a presumed **immune-mediated endothelialitis**, obscure the few remaining corneal endothelial cells in bovine malignant catarrhal fever.

demonstration of strong cross-reactivity between *leptospiral antigens* and equine corneal endothelium (immune mimicry) serves to further obscure the distinction between infectious and immune-mediated ocular disease.

Included in this section are those diseases that are exclusively or predominantly immune-mediated, and for which the triggering antigen has not been proven to be an infectious agent. *In general, all are characterized by chronic, lymphocytic-plasmacytic panuveitis, in which the infiltrating leukocytes form lymphoid aggregates and perivascular cuffs.* Clinically, they are either continuously progressive syndromes or subject to periodic irregular clinical exacerbations and remissions.

The normal eye contains almost no lymphoid tissue and, following initial antigenic challenge, must rely on diffusion of antigen to the spleen before effector lymphocytes return to enter the eye. The lymphocytes do so primarily as perivascular aggregates throughout the uvea.

Those examples of uveitis associated with penetrating injury or massive localization of infectious agents cause disruption of the blood–eye barrier. The globe thus responds to the inflammatory stimulus as would any other tissue, and those events will not be further described here.

Hematogenous localization (or experimental inoculation) of less damaging antigen within the ocular chambers that allows the blood–eye barrier to remain intact triggers a remarkable adaptation of the inflammatory and immune response known as anterior segment immune deviation, described below.

The eye was once thought to be an immunologically privileged site, with no resident lymphocytes, no antigen-processing macrophages or dendritic cells, and no lymphatic drainage. These peculiarities, plus the "*blood–eye barrier*" created by the tight intercellular junctions of iris endothelium, ciliary nonpigmented epithelium, and retinal pigment epithelium, fostered the mistaken belief that many intraocular antigens were sufficiently sequestered as to be seen as "non-self" in the event of their release into systemic circulation. The numerous diseases characterized by lymphocytic-plasmacytic uveitis in the absence of an identified infectious agent have thus been incautiously grouped as examples of "autoimmune" reaction to sequestered uveal, lenticular, or retinal antigens.

More recent studies have demonstrated that these supposedly unique and sequestered antigens are neither unique nor completely sequestered, and that antigens of any type introduced into the intraocular environment will trigger a robust immune response. Antigens identical to some of the lenticular or uveal antigens, for example, are found in nonsequestered tissues elsewhere in the body. Antigens inoculated into the anterior chamber induce a systemic humoral and T-cell response, clearly pointing to at least some leakiness in the blood–eye barrier. A variety of experiments have led to the discovery of a carefully regulated system of ocular immunity, termed **anterior chamber-associated immune deviation**. In this system, antigens introduced into the intraocular environment in a relatively controlled fashion are altered by contact with cytokines secreted by trabecular endothelial cells, corneal endothelium, and probably many other resident ocular tissues. The list of specific cytokines and how they alter antigen expression continues to unfold. The first cytokine proven to alter antigen reactivity was TGF-β2, but the list of chemical participants includes TNF-α, vasoactive intestinal peptide, and substance P. These altered antigens are then processed by macrophages and dendritic cells of bone marrow origin that are resident within the uvea. These antigen-presenting cells promote the development, after 5–6 days, of specifically sensitized suppressor T-cells within the spleen. These suppressor cells then return to the uvea where they act to suppress delayed-type hypersensitivity and the production of complement-fixing antibodies. The cells do not blunt the more discriminating noncomplement-fixing antibody production and cytotoxic lymphocytic activation that can destroy unwanted antigen without the messy bystander injury that would be so damaging to the globe.

Whatever their type, the splenic lymphocytes reach the eye about 1 week after experimental introduction of antigen into anterior chamber. Typically the lymphocytes are seen as perivascular aggregates in iris stroma, in the ciliary body and, less obviously, in the choroid and even the retina. In long-standing cases (which are most likely to receive histologic examination) the aggregates may be very large and resemble lymphoid follicles (Fig. 4.46). As in other tissues, amplification of the immune response results in recruitment of lymphocytes that are not necessarily specific for the inciting antigen. The polyclonal nature of these lymphocytes is probably important in the typically recurrent nature of uveitis in all species. Once established in the eye, these cells respond to a diverse range of circulating antigens that enter the eye through a blood–eye barrier disrupted by

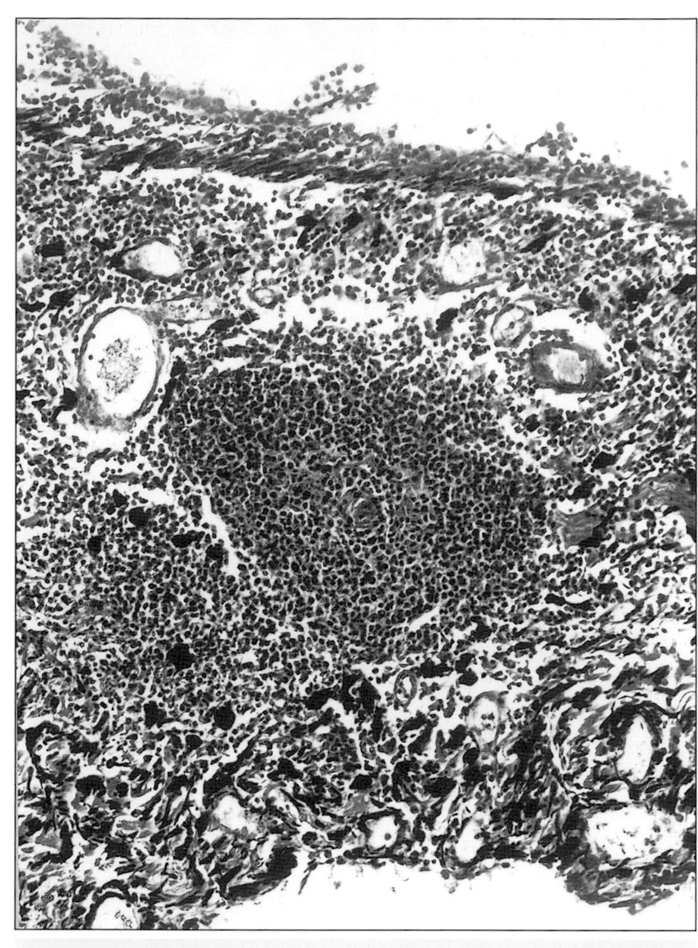

Figure 4.46 Equine recurrent uveitis. Lymphoid nodules in iris stroma.

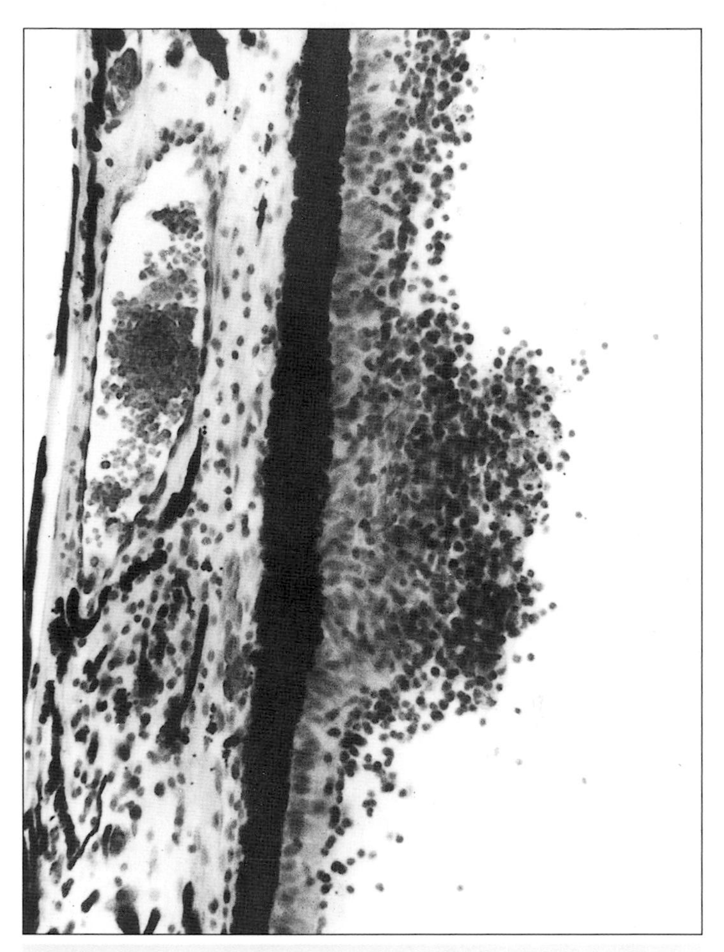

Figure 4.47 Choroiditis and inflammatory infiltrate of pars plana, in **equine recurrent uveitis**.

the previous bout of inflammation. *It is thus possible, or even probable, that chronic, recurrent uveitis results not from persistence of a single antigen, or repeated exposure to the same antigen, but is a stereotyped ocular response to activation of any one of its many acquired lymphoid populations by a variety of circulating antigens or native ocular antigens.*

Specific examples of immune-mediated endophthalmitis are discussed below, and include equine recurrent uveitis, idiopathic lymphonodular uveitis of cats, canine lymphocytic uveitis, canine uveodermatologic syndrome (Vogt–Koyanagi–Harada-like syndrome), and lens-induced uveitis.

Equine recurrent ophthalmitis (periodic ophthalmia)

This is a worldwide and important cause of blindness in horses and mules. The blindness results from repeated attacks of anterior uveitis occurring at unpredictable intervals and with increasing severity. With each attack, there is increasing involvement of the posterior uvea, retina and optic nerve, and increasingly frequent sequelae of cataract, lens luxation, synechiae, retinal separation, and interstitial keratitis. Despite the frequent observation of posterior synechiae, glaucoma is rarely reported. It is speculated that aqueous drainage in horses relies less on the trabecular meshwork and more on uveal resorption than is true of dogs or cats. The disease may initially be unilateral but eventually affects both eyes. Blindness is usually a late sequel, but may occur early in the disease if exudative choroiditis causes retinal separation.

Gross lesions of the acute disease are typical of anterior uveitis in any species: serous conjunctivitis, chemosis, circumcorneal ciliary hyperemia, corneal edema, and plasmoid aqueous and vitreous with fibrin and leukocytes in the aqueous. Clinically, such animals are often systemically ill as detected by fever, decreased appetite, and depression. Lacrimation and photophobia are usually marked. Subsequent attacks tend to become increasingly severe and resolution of the gross lesions between attacks is less complete. Such horses, during the quiescent period, may have one or more of: peripheral corneal vascularization with fibrosis and persistent edema; irregular thickening and pigmentation of iris; multiple posterior synechiae; patchy residual uveal pigment on lens capsule; and peripapillary retinal hyperreflectivity suggesting retinal scarring.

The microscopic lesions depend on the stage of the disease and represent a continuum from anterior uveitis to endophthalmitis with retinal scarring, or even phthisis bulbi. The earliest lesion is anterior uveal inflammation that is transiently neutrophilic but rapidly becomes predominantly lymphocytic. Ciliary processes are most obviously affected. Edema, fibrin, and leukocytes distend the stroma, and leukocytes and fibrin lie in the anterior chamber and in the filtration angle. Neutrophilic-to-lymphocytic pars planitis is fairly common (Fig. 4.47). In the eyes of horses with a history of several attacks of uveitis, the exudate in these acute flare-ups of the disease is almost purely lymphocytic-plasmacytic and is found about vessels of the choroid, retina, and optic nerve as well as the anterior uvea. Peripheral corneal

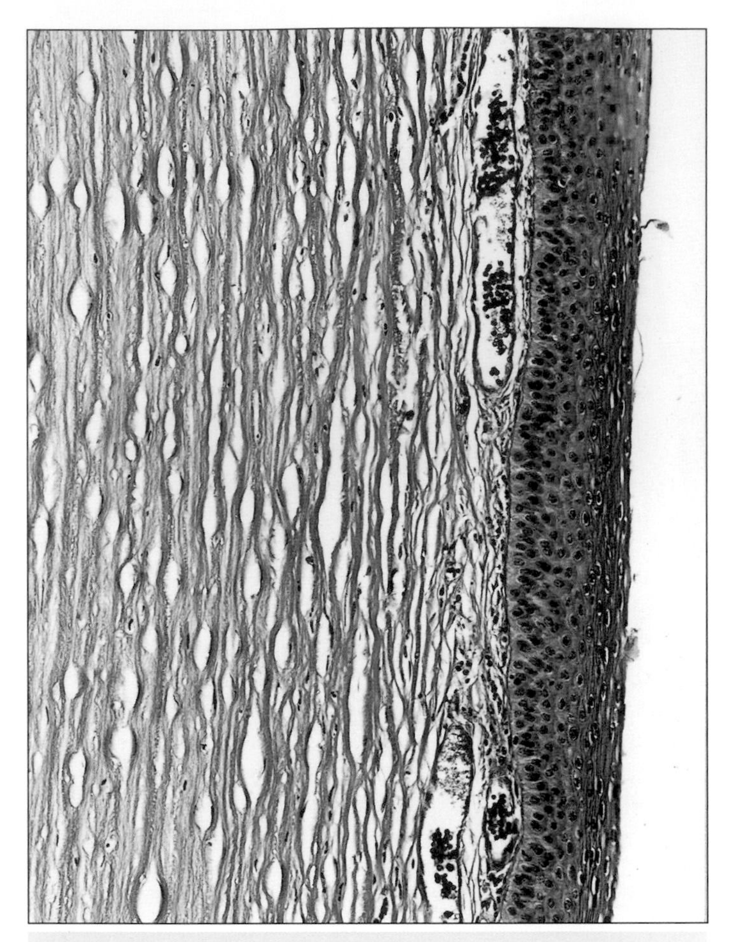

Figure 4.48 Peripheral corneal stromal vascularization and subtle fibrosis in a horse with **equine recurrent uveitis**.

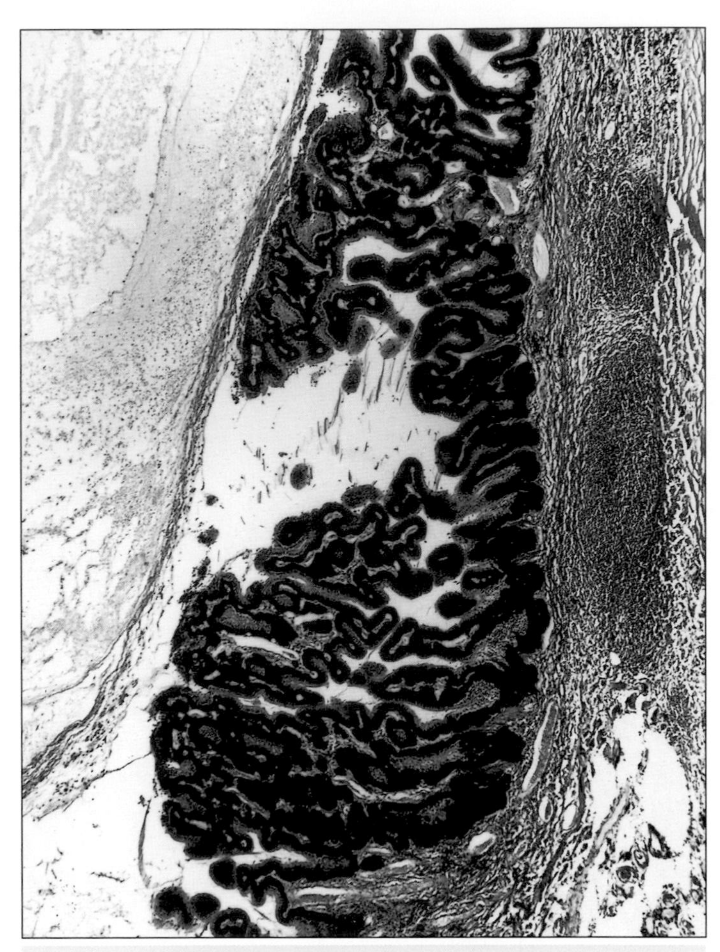

Figure 4.49 Equine recurrent uveitis. Lymphoid nodules may form anywhere in the anterior uvea. Here they coalesce within the stroma just below the ciliary processes.

vascularization, both from conjunctival and limbic ciliary vessels, becomes increasingly prominent and extends further toward the center of the cornea (Fig. 4.48). Edema accompanies the newly formed vessels. The chorioretinitis may be sufficiently exudative to cause multifocal retinal separation. As these severe uveal lesions regress during clinically quiescent periods, they leave behind characteristic residual changes. Relatively early in the disease there is the development of perivascular lymphoid aggregates in the iris and ciliary body that persist and may even form true lymphoid nodules (Fig. 4.49). The ciliary processes may remain thickened by fibrous organization of stromal edema, and a hyaline membrane often seems to cover the ciliary epithelium. This material, in fact, lies within the apical cytoplasm of the nonpigmented ciliary epithelium. In most respects, it resembles amyloid (Fig. 4.50). Small blood vessels persist along corneal stromal lamellae and there is subtle fibrous disorganization of the stroma, the result of previous edema. Peripapillary chorioretinal scarring is seen as focal retinal photoreceptor loss, jumbling of layers and gliosis. Adjacent retinal pigment epithelium may be hypertrophic or hyperplastic, and a focal cluster of lymphocytes in the nearby choroid is common.

Choroidal vessels are unusually thick-walled due to edema or fibrin, the latter probably analogous to the hyalinization described in several reports. Increased vascular permeability persists even in quiescent periods with loss of the blood–aqueous barrier demonstrated by fluorescein angiography. Whether or not this vascular alteration participates in the perpetuation of the uveitis is unknown, but it is known that such alterations predispose to localization of circulating immune complexes and subsequent type III hypersensitivity-induced inflammation.

Focal retinal detachments may reattach by fibrous organization of subretinal exudate or may progress to total separation with a barely recognizable retina adherent to the posterior lens capsule. Gliosis and lymphocytic aggregates may be found within proximal optic nerve. Scarring in optic disk and adjacent retina often is clinically obvious and may occur in horses with no other lesions of uveitis, leading to speculation that it is not really linked to, or at least not specific for, equine recurrent uveitis. Lesions of such sequelae as cataract, chronic conjunctivitis, and glaucoma are described elsewhere.

The *causes and pathogenesis* of recurrent equine ophthalmitis have not been intensively studied, in contrast to the abundance of opinion expressed in reviews or texts. *The almost universal opinion is that the disease is the result of hypersensitivity to exogenous antigen*. The most frequently cited antigens are *Leptospira* and dead microfilariae of *Onchocerca cervicalis*. The demonstration of antigenic cross-reaction between equine corneal endothelium and several common leptospiral serovars suggests that *accidental autoimmunity* may participate in some of the lesions. Cross-reaction with other ocular antigens has not been studied, but the repeated observation that lesion development follows the development of serum or aqueous antibody titers to *Leptospira* makes an immune pathogenesis very likely for this disease syndrome.

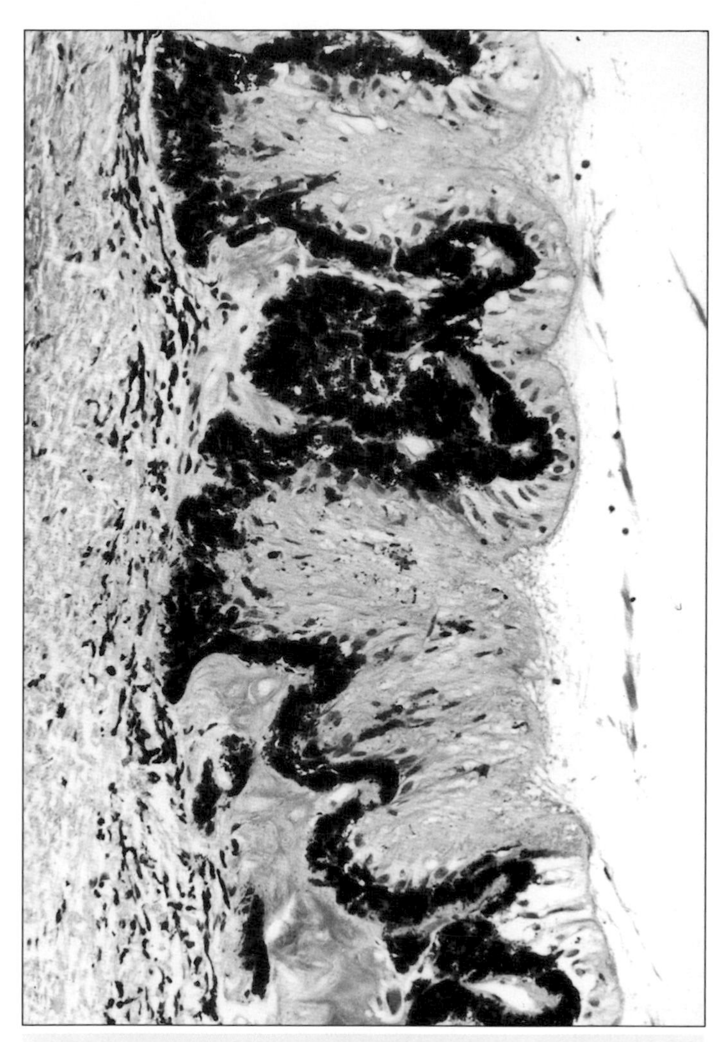

Figure 4.50 Deposition of amyloid-like material within the apical cytoplasm of the inner, nonpigmented ciliary epithelium, unique to **equine recurrent uveitis**.

There seems little doubt that *Leptospira,* particularly *L. pomona*, can initiate uveitis in horses and in man. In both species, the uveitis develops as a sequel to infection, delayed by weeks or years. The initial suspicion of this association was the observation, as early as 1948, that horses with uveitis frequently had very high serum and aqueous humour agglutination titers against *L. pomona*. This observation has since been repeatedly confirmed, and has been supported by the observation of uveitis in 22 of 36 eyes of Shetland ponies inoculated subcutaneously with small numbers of *L. pomona*. All ponies underwent subsequent leptospiremia but none developed ocular lesions until 50 weeks after inoculation. The lesions were typical of anterior uveitis, and six eyes progressed to phthisis bulbi after repeated bouts of uveitis. In 18 eyes, there were central retinal scars typical of the naturally occurring disease. *Although there seems little doubt that hypersensitivity to L. pomona can cause the syndrome of equine recurrent ophthalmitis, it is unlikely to be the only cause.* In a survey in Florida, only one of ten horses with uveitis had a positive microagglutination titer against *L. pomona*. Eight had cutaneous onchocerciasis but that was not significantly different from the overall 60% prevalence of that parasite in the sample population. Typical of the long-standing controversy about this disease is a 1990 survey of horses with uveitis in Virginia and Maryland, in which 52 of 80 affected horses had positive serum titers to one or more leptospiral serovars, and a statistically significant association between uveitis and positive titer was found for the serovars *pomona* and *autumnalis.*

Onchocerca cervicalis infection of the eye is considered briefly with helminthic uveitis. Reaction to dead microfilariae within uveal tissues is considered by some as an important cause of equine recurrent uveitis, although the high prevalence of this parasite in the horse population makes such claims difficult to support statistically. The enthusiasm for this pathogenesis may be generated, in part, by the importance of onchocerciasis as a leading cause of blinding keratitis in people.

Idiopathic lymphonodular uveitis of cats

This is by far the most frequent histologic pattern of the uveitis in cats, and vies with diffuse iris melanoma as the most common cause of glaucoma in this species. It is because of the glaucoma that these eyes are enucleated and thus become available for histologic evaluation. The mechanism by which the uveitis causes the glaucoma is unknown.

Perivascular accumulations of lymphocytes and plasma cells are seen throughout the uvea and, with less regularity, around small vessels in the retina. The iris tends to have the greatest accumulation, and the lymphocytic-plasmacytic perivascular aggregates may become so large as to be clinically visible. Formation of actual lymphoid follicles may occur in chronic and severe cases (Fig. 4.51). The nodules and follicles may also occur within the trabecular meshwork and and within the ciliary body, but choroidal involvement is usually quite subtle.

The syndrome is presumed to be immune-mediated, but the identity of the antigen or antigens is unknown. Its initial clinical presentation is usually unilateral, but the other globe is considered "at risk" for developing subsequent uveitis. There has been no study to document the actual risk. The pattern of serologic reactions in cats with this lymphonodular uveitis is no different than the general population, except perhaps to *Toxoplasma* (see Protozoan endophthalmitis, above). That debate continues, but it seems clear that the syndrome is not associated with the presence of histologically detectable infectious agent within the globe. Studies using immunohistochemistry and PCR to detect infectious agents have been similarly inconclusive.

Idiopathic lymphocytic uveitis in dogs

The histologic lesions are, in general, similar to those described above for cats and horses: *lymphocytic-plasmacytic panuveitis that tends to be more severe in the anterior uvea that in the choroid.* Some cases develop lymphoid nodules and even follicles within the anterior uveal stroma. The disease is bilateral but not necessarily of uniform severity. Unlike the situation in cats, it rarely is associated with glaucoma. The main differential diagnosis is phacolytic uveitis, and indeed in some cases the distinction is impossible.

Uveodermatologic syndrome in dogs (Vogt–Koyanagi–Harada syndrome)

Despite the exotic-sounding name, *this disease is relatively frequent in those areas in which the most susceptible breeds (Akitas, Siberian Huskies, Samoyeds) are popular. The clinical syndrome of facial dermal depigmentation and severe bilateral uveitis is distinctive*, although many dogs examined

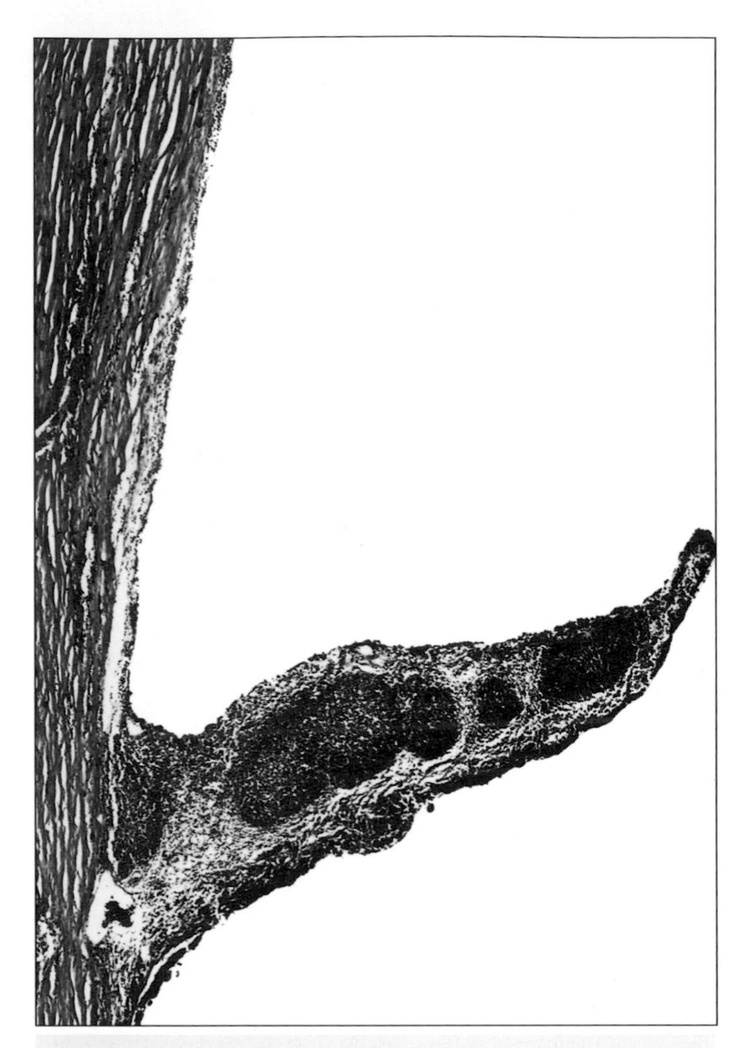

Figure 4.51 Lymphonodular iritis and secondary glaucoma in a cat. The iridocorneal angle has been dislocated far posterior to the termination of Descemet's membrane (angle recession).

for the uveitis are not noted to have skin lesions. The canine syndrome closely parallels the human disease, except for the encephalitis that is the least-frequent part of the human syndrome and has not been confirmed in dogs. The human disease is most prevalent in Orientals; the predilection in dogs for the Japanese Akita is a fascinating but unexplained parallel.

The histologic lesion is a destructive granulomatous endophthalmitis with abundant dispersal of melanin. The melanin-laden retinal pigment epithelium seems to be especially susceptible. Retinal detachment and destructive granulomatous inflammation are seen in advanced cases. The lesion is distinguished from the more prevalent systemic mycotic diseases by the predilection for pigmented tissues within the eye, lack of visceral involvement, and by the distinctive skin lesions if they are present (see Vol. 1, Skin and appendages).

The pathogenesis of the human disease is thought to involve cell-mediated immune reaction to uveal (or epidermal) melanin.

Bibliography

Brem S, et al. 35 leptospira isolated from the vitreous body of 32 horses with recurrent uveitis (ERU). Berl Munch Tierarztl Wochenschr 1999;112:390–393. Erratum in: Berl Munch Tierarztl Wochenschr 2000;113:40.

Cousins SW, et al. Immune privilege and suppression of immunogenic inflammation in the anterior chamber of the eye. Curr Eye Res 1991;10:287.

Curtis R, Barnett KC. The "blue eye" phenomenon. Vet Rec 1983;112:347–353.

Deeg CA, et al. Immunopathology of recurrent uveitis in spontaneously diseased horses. Exp Eye Res 2002;75:127–133.

Dwyer AE, et al. Association of leptospiral seroreactivity and breed with uveitis and blindness in horses: 372 cases (1986–1993). J Am Vet Med Assoc 1995;207:1327–1331.

Gwin RM, et al. Idiopathic uveitis and exudative retinal detachment. J Am Anim Hosp Assoc 1980;16:163–170.

Laus JL, et al. Uveodermatologic syndrome in a Brazilian Fila dog. Vet Ophthalmol 2004;7:193–196.

Lindley DM, et al. Ocular histopathology of Vogt-Koyanagi-Harada-like syndrome in an Akita dog. Vet Pathol 1990;27:294–296.

Lucchesi PM, et al. Serovar distribution of a DNA sequence involved in the antigenic relationship between *Leptospira* and equine cornea. BMC Microbiol 2002;2:3.

Peiffer RL, Jr., Wilcock BP. Histopathologic study of uveitis in cats: 139 cases (1978–1988). J Am Vet Med Assoc 1991;198:135–138.

Schmidt GM, et al. Equine ocular onchocerciasis: Histopathologic study. Am J Vet Res 1982;43: 1371–1375.

Whitely HE, et al. Ocular lesions of bovine malignant catarrhal fever. Vet Pathol 1985;22:219–225.

Lens-induced uveitis

Uveitis in response to leakage of lens material is seen in all species, but is most frequent by far in dogs. The term lens-induced uveitis encompasses two very different syndromes – phacolytic and phacoclastic uveitis – that differ markedly in clinical severity, in histopathology, and in pathogenesis.

Phacolytic uveitis is a *mild lymphocytic-plasmacytic anterior uveitis that occurs in response to the leakage of denatured lens protein through an intact lens capsule, which occurs regularly in the course of maturation of cataracts towards total fiber liquefaction.* The inflammation is readily controlled by routine therapy, so the pathologist is likely to encounter this lesion only as an incidental finding in eyes with hypermature cataracts that were enucleated for reasons unrelated to the uveitis. The lesion is identical to that described for idiopathic ("immune-mediated") uveitis, except it is always mild. Its pathogenesis is unknown. The lens leaks small denatured lens proteins that are not immunogenic but are, perhaps, direct inflammatory stimulants with lymphocytic chemotactic properties.

Phacoclastic uveitis *is, at least histologically, a more complicated disease that follows rupture of a normal lens in an unknown percentage of cases.* The rupture is usually from corneal penetration by a thorn, quill, bullet, or cat claw, and thus usually is of the anterior capsule. The clinical syndrome is distinctive: corneal perforation and mild traumatic uveitis that are successfully managed by conventional therapy, followed by the sudden reappearance of a severe, intractable uveitis 10–14 days after the initial injury. Poor response to medical therapy and the eventual development of glaucoma or phthisis bulbi prompt enucleation, such that *phacoclastic uveitis is one of the most prevalent ocular diseases to be submitted for histologic examination.*

The macroscopic changes in the bisected globe are diagnostic: the lens is flattened in its anteroposterior dimension and there frequently is a wedge of opacification extending from the anterior capsule towards the nucleus. Usually there is posterior synechia, iris

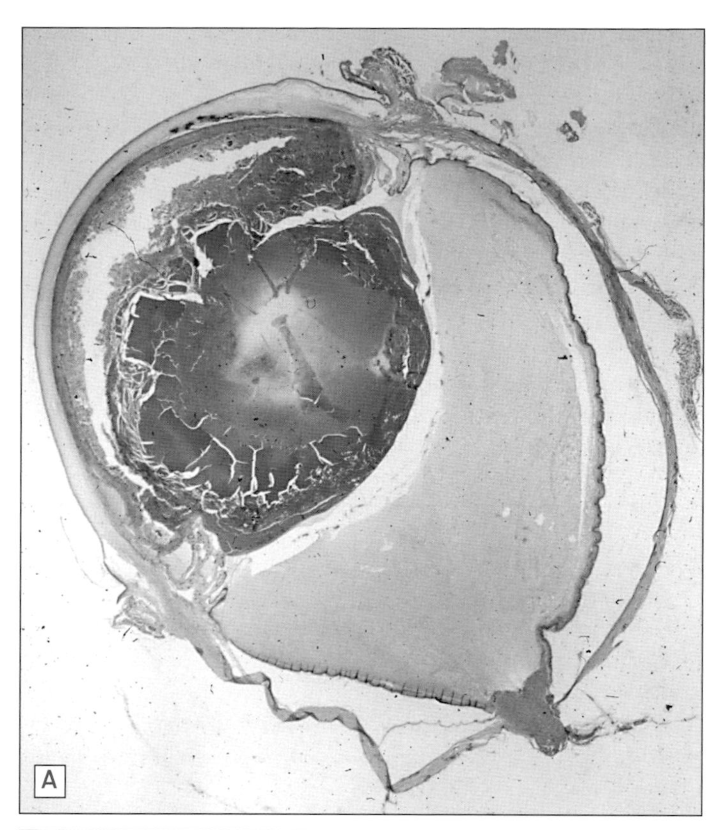

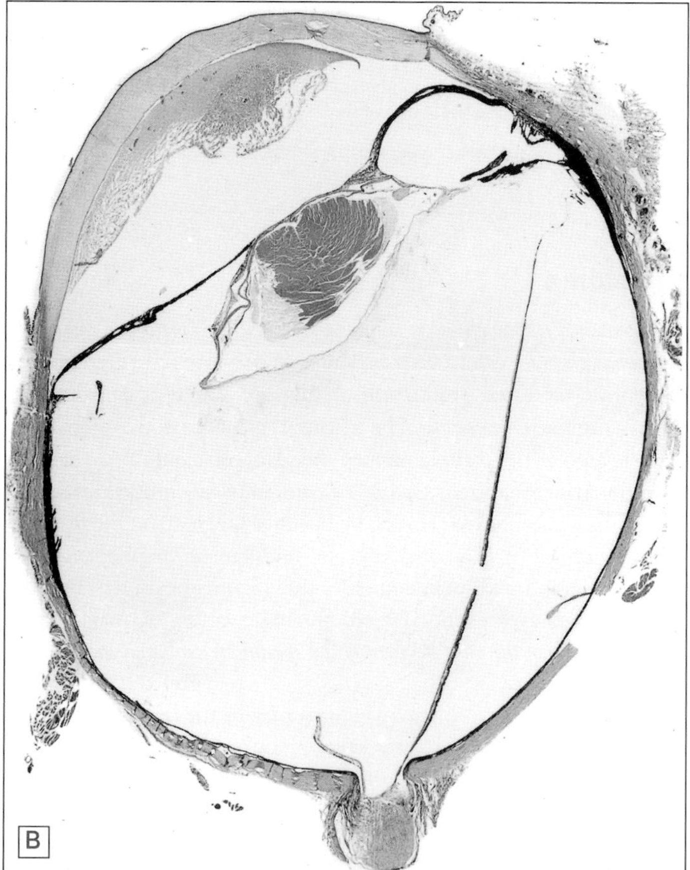

Figure 4.52 A. Acute phacoclastic uveitis following *Encephalitozoon*-induced lens capsule rupture in a rabbit. **B.** Posterior synechia, iris bombé, and glaucomatous cupping of optic disk following **traumatic corneal and lenticular perforation**. The anterior–posterior flattening of the liquified lens is typical.

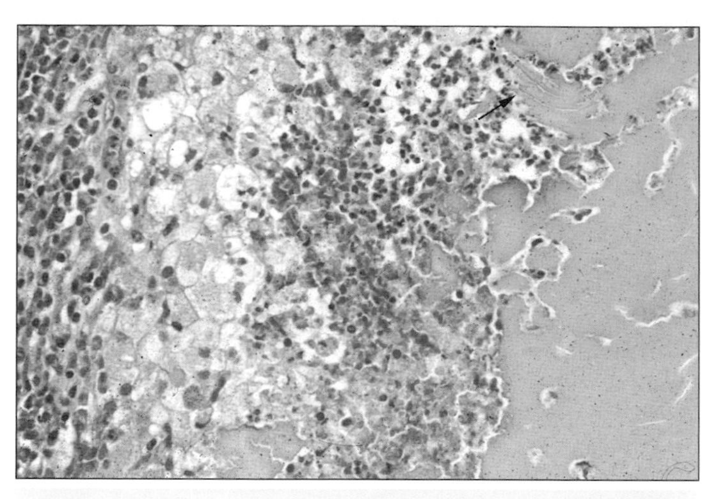

Figure 4.53 Acute phacoclastic uveitis. Laminations of neutrophils, macrophages, and then lymphocytes surround fragments of ruptured lens (arrow).

bombé, and the various other lesions as seen in any severe uveitis (Fig. 4.52A, B).

The histologic lesions vary considerably depending on duration and, probably, on the amount of lens protein that escaped through the rupture site. There are often complex lesions that result from a combination of the direct effects of trauma, immunologic reaction to massive release of lens protein, reparative proliferation of metaplastic lens and/or iridociliary epithelium, and possible contributions by corneal wound healing, sepsis, and glaucoma. It is worth mentioning that some, and perhaps most, of these globes have at least some participation by bacterial infection that occurs concurrently with the original penetrating injury. How much that infection contributes to the histopathology described below remains unknown. Most samples reaching a pathologist are from animals that have been treated extensively with antibiotics, but it is still possible that previous septic inflammation was the significant contributor to the persisting histologic changes.

The simplest and presumably earliest lesion of phacoclastic uveitis occurs at the site of capsular perforation. The edges of the capsule are retracted and coiled outward, and a wedge of neutrophils and liquified lens material extends from the perforation towards the nucleus. The inflammation outside of the lens is usually distinctly perilenticular and involves a mixture of neutrophils and macrophages in the anterior and posterior chambers, and a lymphocyte-dominated reaction within the uveal stroma (Fig. 4.53).

Older lesions (which predominate in most enucleated globes) are dominated by perilenticular proliferative changes of wound repair. There is proliferation and fibroblastic metaplasia of lens epithelium adjacent to the perforation, which escapes from the lens to ramify over the lens surface and frequently incorporates the lens, ciliary processes, and iris leaves into a large fibrous mass that obstructs aqueous outflow. Metaplasia of ciliary epithelium or recruitment of fibroblasts from uveal stroma may contribute to the proliferation (Fig. 4.54). Many such specimens contain little evidence of inflammation other than fibroplasia, probably because of very extensive anti-inflammatory therapy that is, in hindsight, useless against the proliferative events that doom the eye to glaucoma or phthisis.

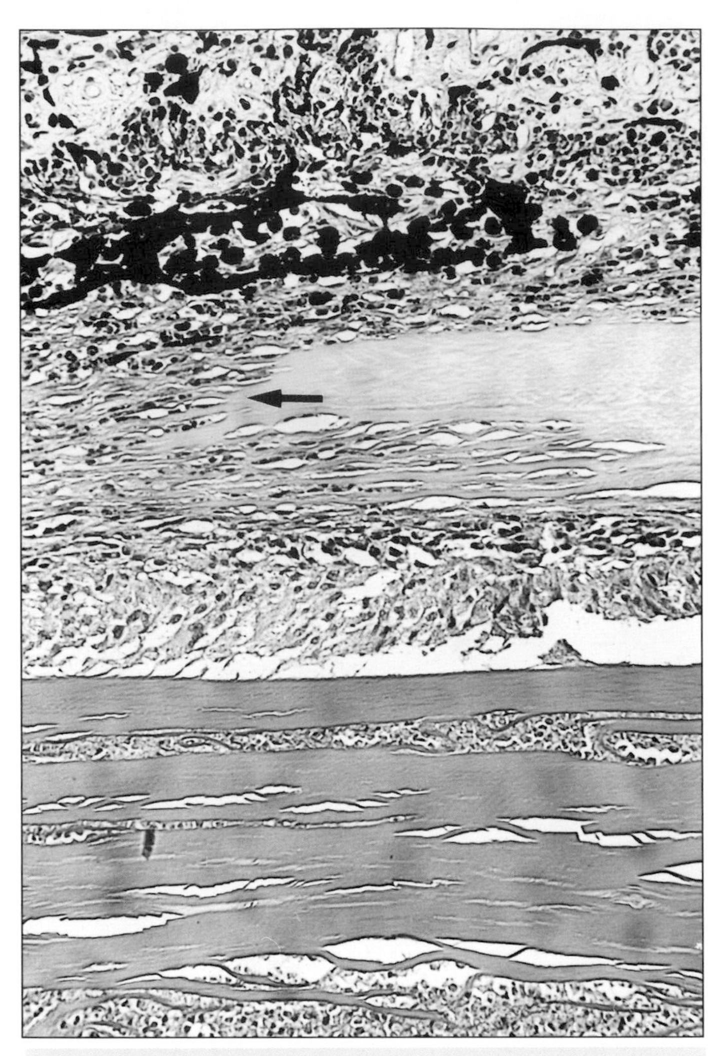

Figure 4.54 Chronic phacoclastic uveitis. Severed ends of anterior lens capsule (arrow) are fimbriated. Typical fibrous proliferation fuses cataractous lens to the (pigmented) iris.

Phacoclastic uveitis is an important complication of cataract surgery in which fragments of lens cortex or epithelium may be left in the eye. These initiate the same inflammatory and proliferative reaction as described above, and the complications are as refractory to conventional anti-inflammatory therapy as is the naturally occurring disease.

The immune pathogenesis of phacoclastic uveitis has been extensively studied, but with no universally accepted conclusion. The current theory is that the release of massive amounts of lens protein antigen overwhelms the splenic T-cell tolerance to small amounts of lens antigen. Recruitment of lens-sensitized lymphocytes into the perilenticular uvea then initiates both the pyogranulomatous perilenticular inflammation and the proliferative events of healing that, unfortunately, doom the eye. This pathogenesis, if true, explains the typical delay between injury and reaction, and why rapid surgical removal of the lens is preventive. It may also explain the unpredictability of phacoclastic uveitis, especially following small perforations in puppies, which seem often to heal uneventfully. Even in adult dogs the disease in unpredictable, so owners' questions about the risk of phacoclastic uveitis as the justification for surgical removal of a perforated lens cannot be answered with certainty. One study found lens removal shortly after perforation prevented serious complications in six of seven dogs thus treated, whereas five of six dogs treated with aggressive medical therapy lost the eye to complications of uveitis.

Two interesting variations on what is basically a canine scheme are seen in rabbits and cats. *Rabbits* suffer what appears to be spontaneous lens capsule rupture of a previously normal lens. The response is well-contained perilenticular granulomatous inflammation very similar to human phacoanaphylactic uveitis. The rupture is associated with the intralenticular presence of *Encephalitiozoon*, and it is assumed that the organisms penetrate and thus weaken the posterior lens capsule. *Cats* occasionally develop lesions similar to those in dogs, but also develop a unique feline primary intraocular pleomorphic sarcoma that may arise from metaplastic lens epithelium or from other transformed epithelial elements in the reparative reaction (see Feline post-traumatic sarcoma).

Bibliography

Davidson MG, et al. Traumatic anterior lens capsule disruption. J Am Anim Hosp Assoc 1991;27:410–414.

Grahn BH, Cullen CL. Equine phacoclastic uveitis: the clinical manifestations, light microscopic findings, and therapy of 7 cases. Can Vet J 2000;41: 376–382.

Paulsen ME, et al. The effect of lens-induced uveitis on the success of extracapsular cataract extraction: a retrospective study of 65 lens removals in the dog. J Am Anim Hosp Assoc 1986;22:49–55.

Peiffer RL, Jr., Wilcock BP. Histopathologic study of uveitis in cats: 139 cases (1978–1988). J Am Vet Med Assoc 1991;198:135–138.

Van der Woerdt A. Lens-induced uveitis. Vet Ophthalmol 2000;3: 227–234.

Wilcock BP, Peiffer RL, Jr. The pathology of lens-induced uveitis in dogs. Vet Pathol 1987;24:549–553.

Wolfer J, et al. Phacoclastic uveitis in the rabbit. Prog Vet Comp Ophthalmol 1993;3:92–97.

Glaucoma

Glaucoma is a pathophysiologic state characterized by a prolonged increase in intraocular pressure. While such increases of pressure may theoretically result from increased production or *decreased removal of aqueous*, only the latter is known to occur. The lesions in glaucomatous eyes include those related to the pathogenesis of the glaucoma and those resulting from the glaucoma itself. *Glaucoma occurs commonly in dogs*, less commonly in cats and horses, and rarely in other species. The medical and surgical control of glaucoma remains problematic despite extensive experimentation with many different therapeutic modalities. Because most affected eyes eventually require enucleation or evisceration, *glaucoma is one of the most frequent ocular conditions submitted for histologic evaluation.*

The lesion predisposing to glaucoma may be the result of *antecedent ocular disease*, particularly intraocular neoplasia and anterior uveal inflammation with posterior or anterior synechiae. Such cases are termed **secondary glaucoma**. **Primary glaucoma** describes those cases without evidence of prior ocular disease and, in practical terms, is *synonymous with malformation of the filtration angle*. Primary glaucoma is seen almost exclusively in dogs, and vies with neoplasia as the most frequent cause of glaucoma in dogs.

Because the pathogenesis of glaucoma so frequently involves developmental or acquired distortion of the filtration angle, a description of that structure is appropriate here.

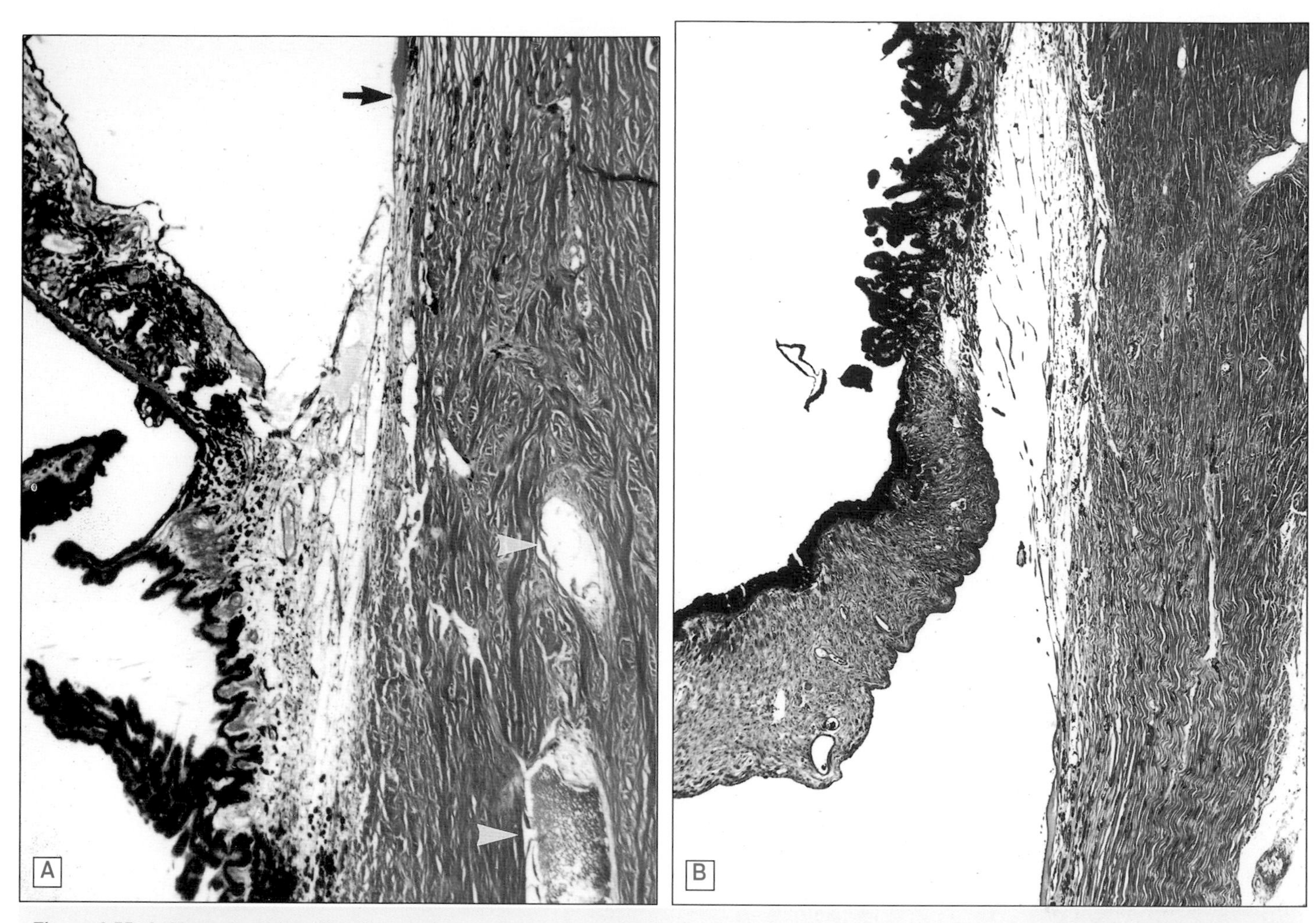

Figure 4.55 A. Normal canine filtration angle showing fenestrated pectinate ligament inserting at the termination of Descemet's membrane (arrow). Large vessels (arrowheads) are part of scleral venous plexus. **B. Normal feline filtration angle**.

The **filtration apparatus** is a series of mesenchymal sieves that occupies the iridocorneal angle, and extends circumferentially around the globe. These sieves appear to form by rarefaction of the same mesenchyme that forms iris stroma, and its rarefaction continues (at least in carnivores) for several weeks after birth. This area of perforated mesenchyme is the **ciliary cleft**, bordered externally by sclera, posteriorly by the muscles of the ciliary body, and internally by the iris stroma. Its anterior border, at least in dogs, extends for about a millimeter into the deep peripheral corneal stroma just external to Descemet's membrane. Its border with the anterior chamber is marked by the **pectinate ligament,** which is visible clinically as a series of cobweb-like branching cords (carnivores) or a fenestrated sheet (ungulates) stretching from the termination of Descemet's membrane to the anterior portion of the iris root. They consist of collagenous cords covered by a very thin endothelium, with a thin intervening layer of basement membrane-like material. The endothelium is continuous with the corneal endothelium, and the collagenous core is continuous with corneal stroma.

Aqueous humor percolating through the pectinate ligament into the ciliary cleft must then pass through mesenchymal sieves consisting of collagenous cords covered by phagocytic and pinocytotic endothelium, called the **trabecular meshwork**. The large, open network of cords occupying most of the ciliary cleft is the uveal trabecular meshwork, while anterior and external to it is a more compressed network called the corneoscleral trabecular meshwork. Ordinarily, aqueous humor produced by the ciliary processes passes through the pupil, through the pectinate ligament, and then through the uveal and corneoscleral trabecular meshworks en route to the *scleral venous plexus* that will return the aqueous to the systemic circulation. Improper development or acquired obstruction of any part of this drainage pathway may result in glaucoma, but one must remember that *the ciliary cleft extends 360° around the iridocorneal angle. Blockage of most of it is required for the development of glaucoma*, and this assessment is virtually impossible with two-dimensional histologic examination. It is quite common to encounter dog eyes with maldeveloped filtration angles in both the dorsal and ventral portions contained in a routine sagittal histologic section, yet with no evidence of glaucoma. Examination of the circumference of the angle with a dissecting microscope or scanning electron microscope in such cases often reveals the maldevelopment to be segmental and thus not a cause for glaucoma.

Differences exist among species in the finer details of angle structure and in the degree to which alternative routes of aqueous outflow are utilized (Fig. 4.55A, B). The horse, for example, has very thick pectinate fibers, and an inconspicuous corneoscleral trabecular meshwork and scleral venous plexus. As implied by these histologic features, *the horse employs alternative routes of aqueous outflow* (into iris stroma and especially posteriorly through ciliary muscle and into choroid) that are much more important than similar routes in dogs or cats. In contrast, the *cat* has extremely delicate pectinate fibers, a very large, open ciliary cleft, a conspicuous scleral venous plexus, and minimal (about 3% of aqueous outflow) reliance on alternative outflow pathways. In dogs, alternative drainage routes account for 15–25% of all outflow. The existence of these alternative routes may explain the absence of glaucoma in some eyes (especially in horses) in which the angle changes would ordinarily have resulted in glaucoma, and may even explain the presence of glaucoma in eyes with apparently normal angles but lesions affecting portions of these other potential drainage routes.

Lesions causing glaucoma

Primary glaucoma is most frequently encountered in dogs. Although theoretically primary glaucoma may have no visible angle lesion (which is frequently the case in people), *in dogs there is almost always a readily detected maldevelopment.* The one exception is primary open-angle glaucoma in Beagle dogs in which there is no visible antecedent lesion. The broad term **goniodysgenesis** encompasses all developmental defects of the filtration angle, of which two types account for most canine cases. *The most prevalent is continuation of mature iris stroma across the trabecular meshwork to insert into the termination of Descemet's membrane.* Some consider this an example of dysplasia of pectinate ligament, and the term **imperforate pectinate ligament** is widely used. The band usually is much thicker than pectinate ligament and lacks the appropriate perforation to allow the drainage of aqueous humor. The trabecular meshwork posterior/exterior to this broad mesenchymal band often seems normal, although that is quite variable (Fig. 4.56A). It is seen as a *breed-related and thus presumably inherited defect* in Bouvier des Flandres, Basset Hounds, American Cocker Spaniels, Dandie Dinmont Terriers, Siberian Huskies, Samoyeds, Chows, and numerous other breeds. The defect, and the resultant glaucoma, is occasionally seen in mixed-breed dogs. The dysplasia is usually bilateral but not necessarily of equal extent, thus the glaucoma is often present initially only in one eye. The prevalence of iridopectinate dysplasia is much higher than the prevalence of glaucoma, and even in dogs with very extensive dysplasia that should seemingly eliminate almost all aqueous drainage, the onset of glaucoma is not until several years of age. It is not unusual to have cases in which clinically detected glaucoma was delayed until 8–10 years of age. Age-related changes in outflow resistance within the alternative routes of aqueous outflow have been postulated as the explanation, as have changes to the angle configuration related to age-related forward movement of the lens. These remain as theories.

Importantly, there appears to be little direct correlation between the severity of the goniodysgenesis and the actual risk of developing glaucoma, its age of onset, or its severity. The extent to which this is true seems to vary by breed, and perhaps the best generalization is that dogs with structurally (i.e., as evaluated by gonioscopy) normal filter angles have no increased risk of glaucoma, while those that have at least some developmental abnormality are at increased risk. *Continuing to breed dogs with abnormal angles increases the prevalence of glaucoma within that line.* It may be that the goniodysgenesis that is visible clinically and histologically is not the direct cause for the glaucoma, but a marker for some other defect in trabecular development that is the real cause of the glaucoma.

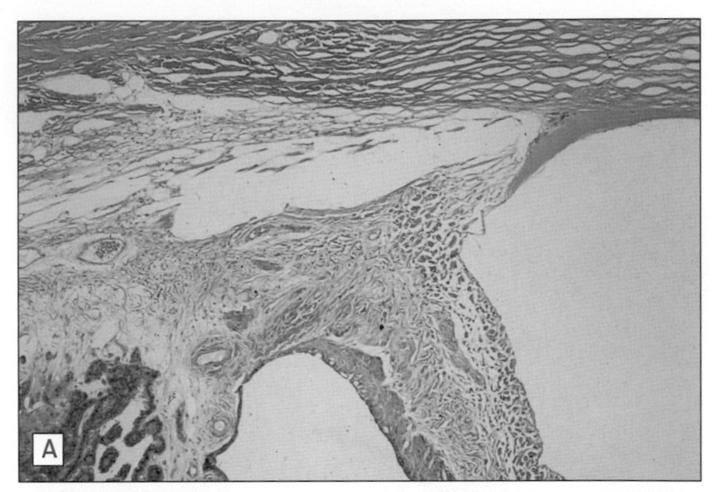

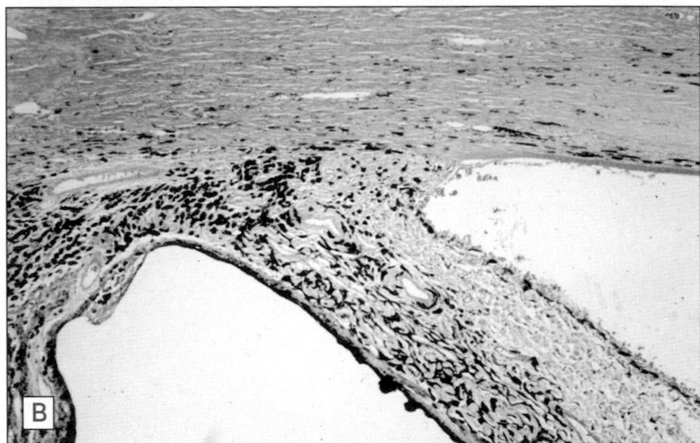

Figure 4.56 A. Goniodysgenesis, with a continuous band of iris-like mesenchyme in place of the normal, perforated pectinate ligament. **B. Trabecular hypoplasia**. This rare, profound arrest in mesenchymal development causes truly congenital glaucoma.

The second major type of goniodysgenesis is seen as a more fundamental arrest in the maturation of the trabecular meshwork such that the ciliary cleft is filled with tissue resembling primitive anterior uveal mesenchyme (Fig. 4.56B). This may occur in conjunction with iris hypoplasia or anterior chamber cleavage syndromes, but it may exist as an isolated defect termed **trabecular hypoplasia**. It has no known familial predilections. Such animals usually have truly congenital glaucoma, in contrast to the adult onset that characterizes the more common breed-associated glaucomas. It is important to note that the remodeling of the trabecular meshwork in dogs and cats continues for several weeks after birth, so that one should avoid overinterpreting apparent angle solidification in very young carnivores.

Secondary glaucoma *occurs most commonly as the result of posterior synechiae as a sequel to anterior uveitis.* The pupillary margin of the iris normally floats along the surface of the lens. Any fibrinous effusion that increases the stickiness of the iris creates a substantial risk of iridocorneal adhesions and resulting pupillary block. Continued production of aqueous humor in the presence of pupillary obstruction results in characteristic forward bowing of the iris known as *iris bombé* (Fig. 4.57). In this condition, the glaucoma is caused not

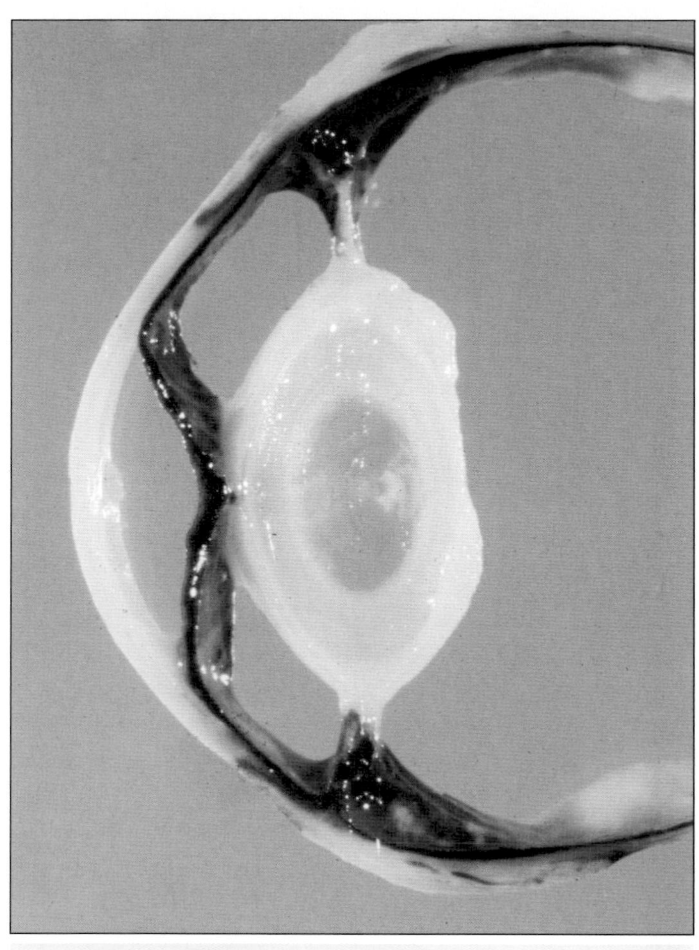

Figure 4.57 Iris bombé, reflecting a combination of posterior synechia, pupillary block, and eventual peripheral anterior synechia.

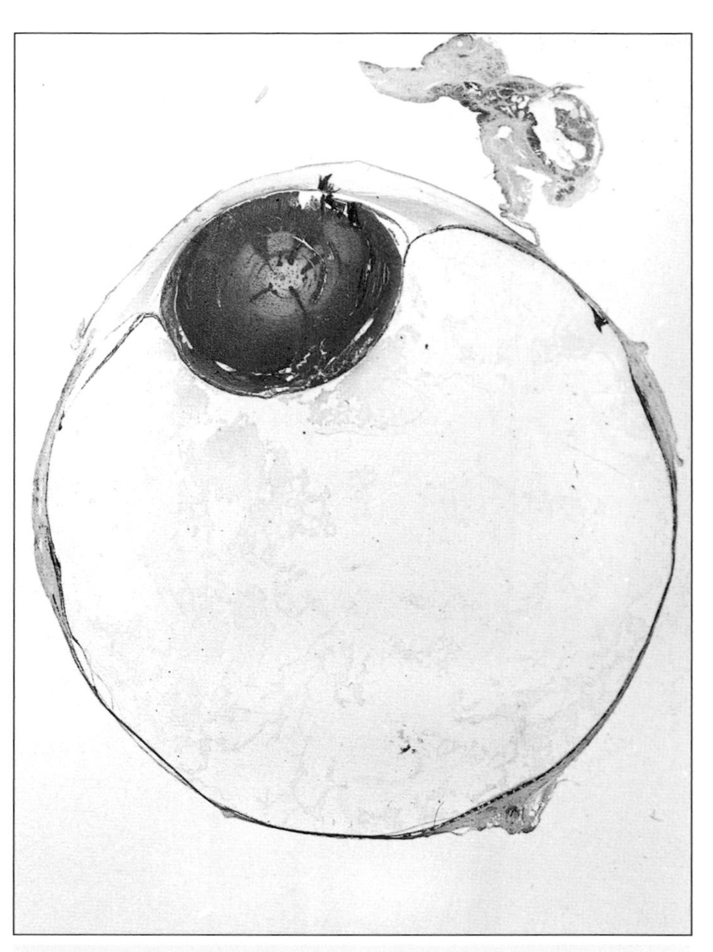

Figure 4.58 Glaucoma caused by swelling of cataractous lens (intumescent cataract) and resultant functional anterior synechia, in a dog. Note thin sclera typical of buphthalmos secondary to glaucoma.

only by pupillary obstruction but by peripheral anterior synechia as the forward bulging of the iris effectively seals the iridocorneal angle. Anterior synechia occurring independently of iris bombé is an occasional cause of secondary glaucoma. Because the iris does not normally contact the cornea, anterior synechia unrelated to iris bombé is frequent only as a consequence of corneal perforation, in which case the iris flows forward as an iris prolapse to seal the defect and may then adhere diffusely to the corneal endothelium (see Fig. 4.34).

Other frequent causes of secondary glaucoma include occlusion of the trabecular meshwork or pupil by pre-iridal fibrovascular membrane or by neoplasia. Posterior migration by corneal endothelium to cover the anterior face of the pectinate ligament and iris is seen quite frequently and may represent an important mechanism for the development of secondary glaucoma, even though the cause for the endothelial migration is usually not obvious. It may be particularly important as a trigger for the still unexplained delayed onset of glaucoma in adult dogs with lifelong goniodysgenesis.

Lens luxation may precipitate glaucoma by allowing vitreous to occlude the pupil, by stimulating anterior uveitis, or by trapping iris against cornea. Rarely, lens swelling with cataract (intumescent cataract) seems to occlude the pupil (Fig. 4.58). In small terrier dogs with an inherited tendency to luxation, there is an unusually high prevalence of glaucoma. Removal of lens prior to the onset of glaucoma prevents the expected glaucoma, seemingly establishing the causal role of the luxation. Posterior synechiae may also occlude the pupil (particularly as part of phacoclastic uveitis), but posterior synechiae usually cause glaucoma via iris bombé and thus a circumferential peripheral anterior synechia.

There are substantial species differences in the prevalence of the mechanisms by which glaucoma may occur. In *dogs*, goniodysgenesis, posterior synechiae with iris bombé, pre-iridal fibrovascular membrane, anterior uveal melanoma, and anterior lens luxation are the leading causes, in approximately that order of prevalence. In *cats*, diffuse iris melanoma and chronic idiopathic lymphonodular uveitis are the only prevalent causes of glaucoma, with posterior synechiae being inexplicably rare. In *horses*, the presence of pre-iridal fibrovascular membranes across the pectinate face is the most frequent cause, although the stimulus for the membrane development is unknown in most reported cases. Many horses with glaucoma have a clinical history of previous uveitis, but histologic assessment of the glaucomatous globe usually reveals very little evidence of that inflammation and no obvious connection between the inflammation and the development of glaucoma. In those horses with glaucoma in which the membrane had not apparently crossed the pectinate ligament, glaucoma may have been caused by obstruction of alternative uveal routes of aqueous outflow, which are more important in horses than in dogs or cats.

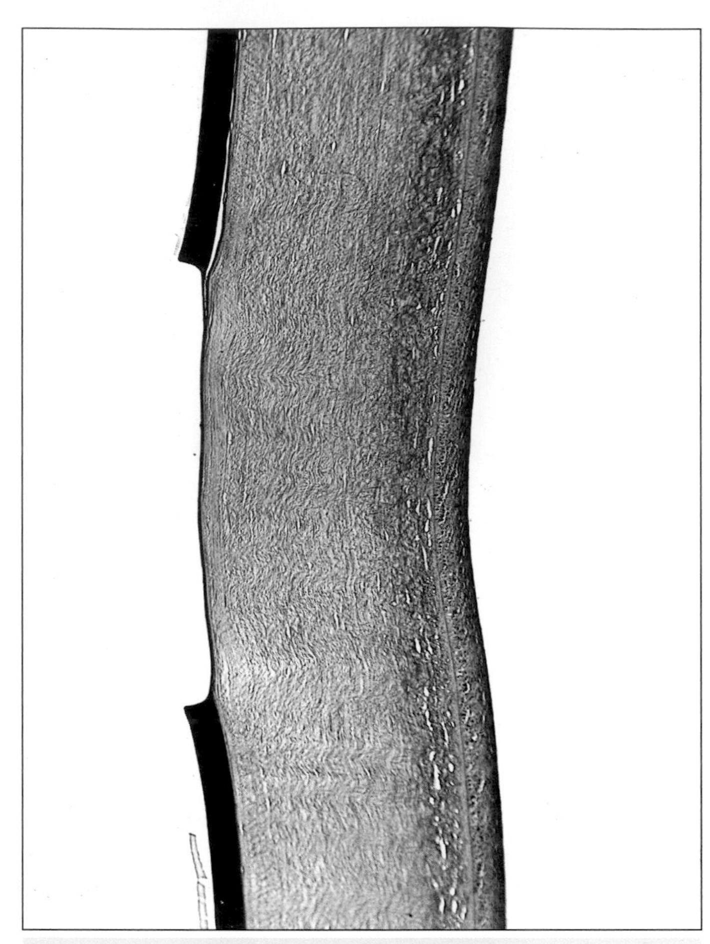

Figure 4.59 Focal break in Descemet's membrane (**corneal stria**) commonly seen in horses and dogs with glaucoma.

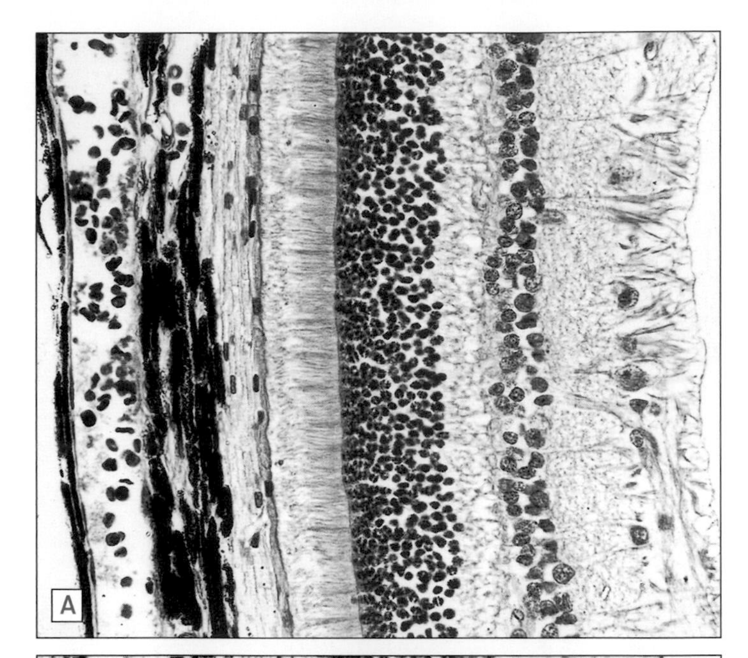

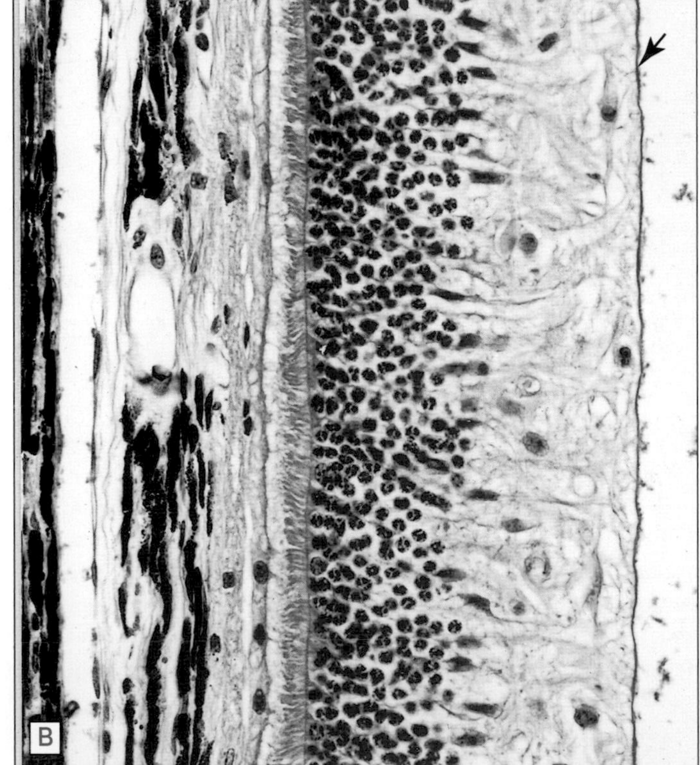

Figure 4.60 A. Normal canine retina overlying tapetum lucidum. **B. Early glaucomatous retinopathy** in a dog. Ganglion cells are absent. Remnant of inner nuclear layer remains. Inner limiting membrane is abnormally prominent (arrow) over atrophic nerve fiber layer.

Lesions resulting from glaucoma

Lesions that develop as a result of glaucoma vary with the duration and severity of the glaucoma and the distensibility of the globe, and affect virtually all parts of the globe. *Enlargement of the globe* (**buphthalmos** or **megaloglobus**) occurs most readily in young animals or in those species with thin scleras such as cats and laboratory animals. In the cornea, increased aqueous pressure injures the corneal endothelium, resulting in *diffuse edema and eventual fibrosis and vascularization*. If buphthalmos occurs, corneal stretching results in rents in Descemet's membrane, visible clinically as **corneal striae** (Fig. 4.59). These are relatively most frequent in horses and least prevalent in cats with glaucoma. Failure of lids to cover the enlarged globe permits *corneal desiccation and eventual ulceration* with all its sequels. If the ocular enlargement has developed only slowly, the cornea may have time to undergo adaptive keratinization and even cutaneous metaplasia. *Cataract is usual*, presumably the result of stagnation of aqueous humor and subsequent lens malnutrition. Iris and ciliary body undergo bland atrophy, most obvious as thinning and flattening of ciliary processes. Collapse of the ciliary cleft and trabecular meshwork itself is frequent and makes evaluation of these structures for possible goniodysgenesis very difficult. *Migration of corneal endothelium across the face of the pectinate ligament and on to the surface of the iris is commonly seen,* but we do not know whether it is part of the pathogenesis of glaucoma, or just a result of that glaucoma.

The retinal lesions are characteristic. Atrophy begins in nerve fiber and ganglion cell layers, making glaucoma the only naturally occurring cause of inner retinal atrophy other than the rare instances of traumatic or neoplastic disruption of optic nerve (Fig. 4.60A, B). *Loss of nerve fibers unmasks the normally inconspicuous Muller fibers*, a lesion that may be more easily seen and more confidently interpreted than the loss of the nerve fibers or ganglion cells themselves (Fig. 4.61). This is

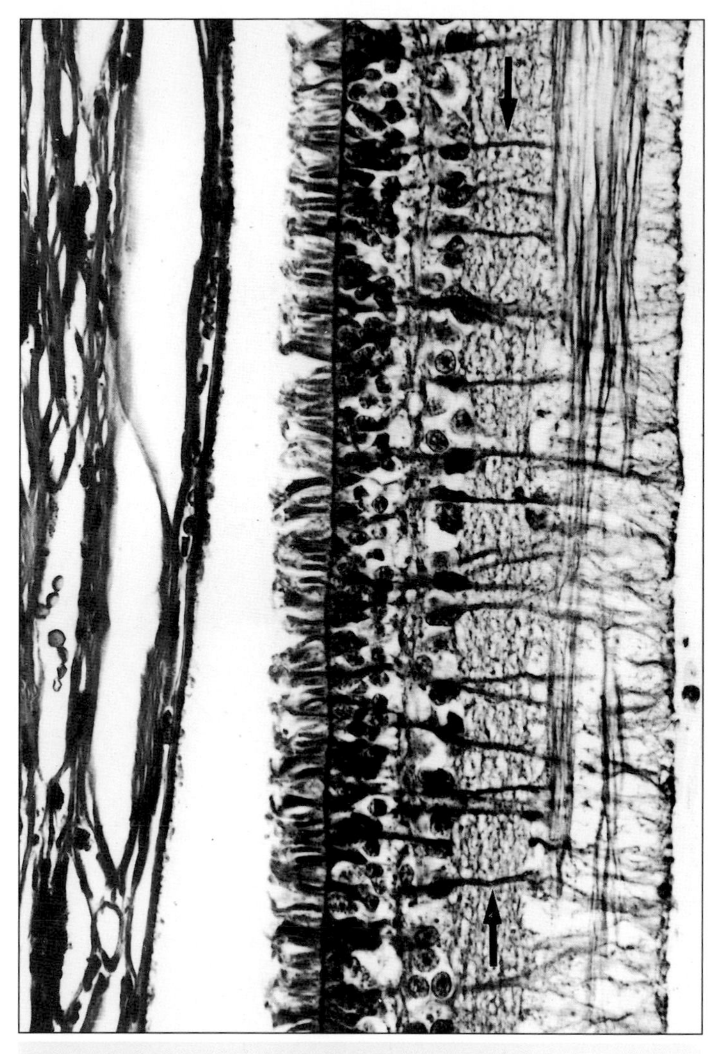

Figure 4.61 Glaucomatous retinal atrophy. Ganglion cells are absent, inner nuclear layer is sparse, and Muller fibers (arrows) unduly obvious due to loss of nerve fiber layer.

particularly true in cats, in which the ganglion cells persist with considerable tenacity under circumstances that would, in dogs, have progressed to a very obvious atrophy. With increasing duration or severity, the inner nuclear layer and its axons and dendrites also atrophy, resulting in thinning of the inner nuclear layer and the blending of this layer with the outer nuclear layer as the plexiform layers (the axons and dendrites of the nuclear layer cells) rarify.

In dogs with high-pressure glaucoma, there is sometimes *full-thickness retinal atrophy* that includes even damage to the RPE. Although the cause is unknown, it may be that the very high pressure causes collapse of choriocapillaris, resulting in ischemic damage to those tissues supplied by this delicate but essential capillary layer. This appears to be a uniquely canine susceptibility, in that the glaucomatous retina of other species rarely if ever shows full-thickness atrophy.

In all species, the dorsal half of the retina is less severely affected than ventral retina. The basis for this sparing remains speculative, but it may be related to the anatomy of the lamina cribrosa and the ease with which increased intraocular pressure compresses axons as they exit through that scleral sieve.

The pathogenesis of the selective ganglion cell loss in glaucoma remains controversial, and there is probably more than one mechanism. The loss may be the result of in situ apoptosis triggered by exposure to elevated retinal and vitreal levels of excitatory amino acids (especially glutamate), a response to pressure-associated ischemic injury, or a result of loss of axoplasmic flow secondary to pressure-induced injury to the optic nerve as it traverses the lamina cribrosa. It is clear that the ganglion cell injury is not directly correlated with the magnitude of the increase in intraocular pressure.

Excavation ("cupping") of the optic disk *is a pathognomonic lesion when present*, but its absence does not rule out the diagnosis. It occurs by at least three mechanisms, any (or all) of which may explain the cupping in an individual eye. Particularly in animals with a thin sclera and lamina cribrosa, the elevation of pressure may cause rapid posterior bowing of the lamina, resulting in visible cupping without apparent nerve atrophy. This is frequently seen in cats and rabbits, but not in ungulates with their thick, rigid lamina. In all species, cupping also occurs by axonal loss from the optic nerve. The pathogenesis for that axonal degeneration is either direct compression of axons or ischemic injury. It has been suggested that the posterior bowing of the lamina cribrosa contributes to the axonal injury by mechanical pinching of axons or blood vessels as they pass through the distorted lamina (Fig. 4.62A, B). This cupping is distinguished from coloboma by the absence of dysplastic neurectoderm lining the defect and by the presence of inner retinal atrophy.

Bibliography

Bjerkas E, et al. Pectinate ligament dysplasia and narrowing of the iridocorneal angle associated with glaucoma in the English Springer Spaniel. Vet Ophthalmol 2002;5:49–54.

Blocker T, Van Der Woerdt A. The feline glaucomas: 82 cases (1995–1999). Vet Ophthalmol 2001;4:81–85.

Brooks DE, et al. Histomorphometry of the optic nerves of normal dogs and dogs with hereditary glaucoma. Exp Eye Res 1995;60:71–89.

Cullen CL, Grahn BH. Equine glaucoma: a retrospective study of 13 cases presented at the Western College of Veterinary Medicine from 1992 to 1999. Can Vet J 2000;41:470–480.

Ekesten, B, Narfstrom K. Correlation of morphologic features of the iridocorneal angle to intraocular pressure in Samoyeds. Am J Vet Res 1991;52: 1875–1878.

Gelatt KN, MacKay EO. Prevalence of the breed-related glaucomas in purebred dogs in North America. Vet Ophthalmol 2004;7:97–111.

Hampson EC, et al. Primary glaucoma in Burmese cats. Aust Vet J 2002;80: 672–680.

Hollander H, et al. Evidence of constriction of optic nerve axons at the lamina cribrosa in the normotensive eye in humans and other mammals. Ophthalmic Res 1995;27:296–309.

Miller PE, et al. Photoreceptor cell death by apoptosis in spontaneous acute glaucoma in dogs. Invest Ophthalmol Vis Scia J 1997;38:163.

Naskar R, Dreyer EB. New horizons in neuroprotection. Surv Ophthalmol 2001;45:250–254.

Smith PJ, et al. Aqueous drainage patterns in the equine eye: scanning electron microscopy of corrosion cast. J Morphol 1988;198:33–42.

van de Sandt RR, et al. Abnormal ocular pigment deposition and glaucoma in the dog. Vet Ophthalmol 2003;6:273–278.

Whiteman AL, et al. Morphologic features of degeneration and cell death in the neurosensory retina in dogs with primary angle-closure glaucoma. Am J Vet Res 2002;63:257–261.

Wilcock BP, et al. Glaucoma in horses. Vet Pathol 1991;28:74–78.

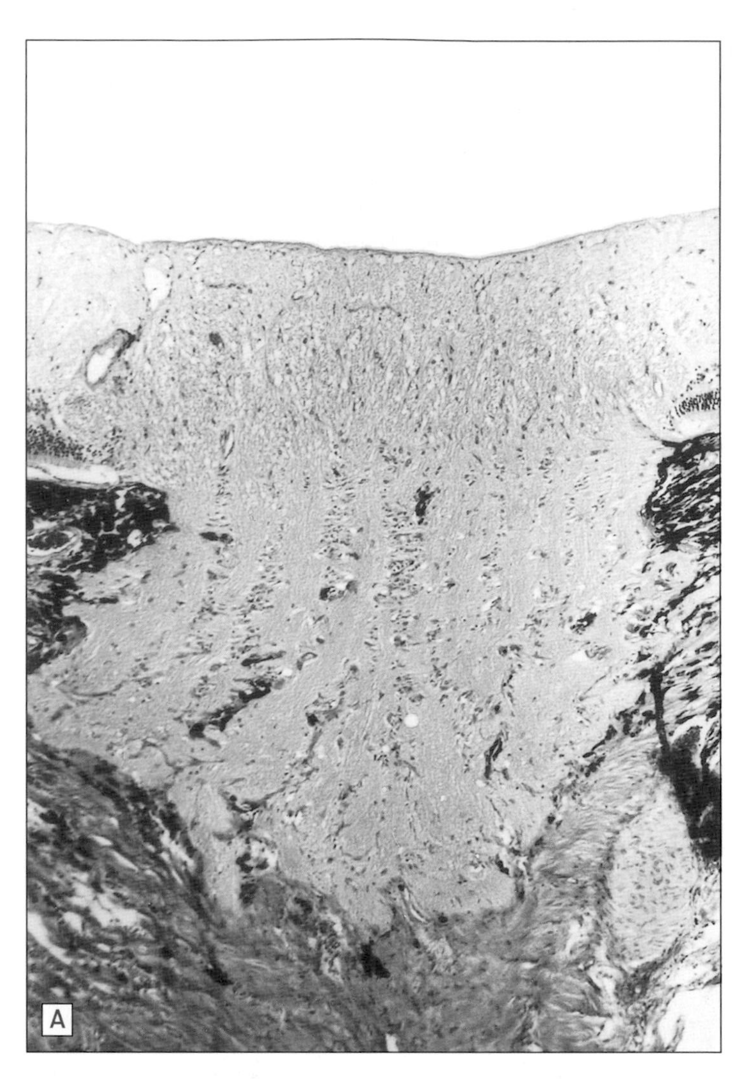

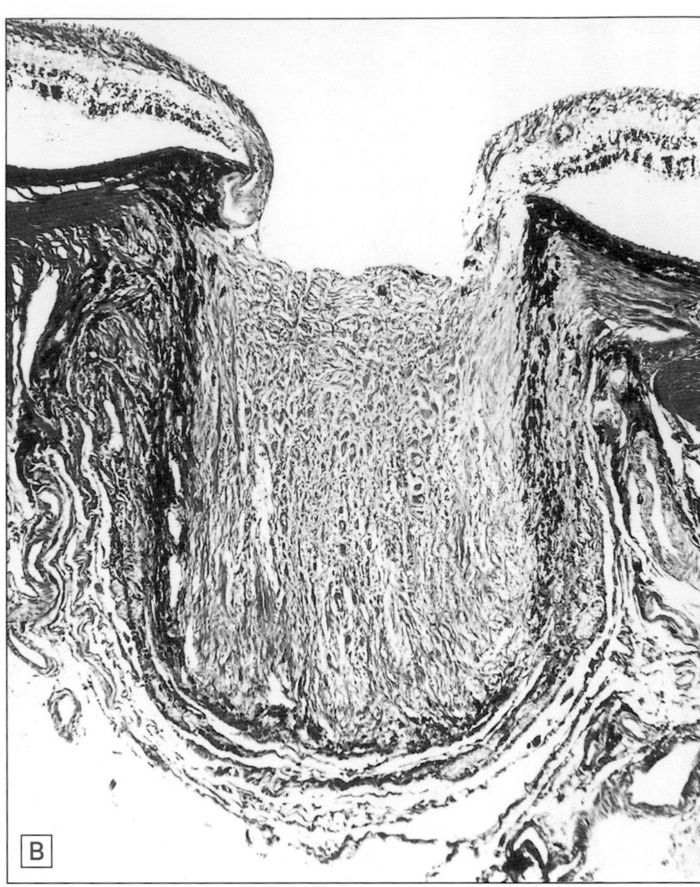

Figure 4.62 A. Normal canine optic disk. **B.** Cupping of optic disk and rarefaction of the nerve in **chronic glaucoma**.

RETINA

When involution of the primary optic vesicle brings into apposition the anterior and posterior poles, the anterior (innermost) neurectodermal layer undergoes mitotic replication and subsequent specialization to form the *nine layers of the neurosensory retina*. The outermost neurectoderm remains as a relatively unspecialized simple cuboidal layer, the *retinal pigment epithelium*. Although it is traditionally considered the tenth retinal layer, its structure, function, and reaction to injury are unlike those of neurosensory retina and it is best discussed separately. *In this discussion, retina refers only to the neurosensory retina.*

In the fixed, bisected globe, the retina is seen as a thin, opaque membrane lining the posterior half of the globe between vitreous and choroid. It joins the darkly pigmented pars plana of the ciliary body at an abrupt transitional point called the *ora ciliaris retinae*. In all but the best-preserved specimens, the retina is separated artifactually from the retinal pigment epithelium and adjacent choroid, remaining adherent only at the ora ciliaris and at the optic disk.

Histologically, the neurosensory retina begins abruptly at the ora ciliaris as a multilayered continuation of the inner layer of the ciliary epithelium. In dogs and sometimes in horses, the layers here are poorly defined and photoreceptors sparse. The peripheral retina is only about half the thickness (100 μm) and has half the photoreceptor density (250 000/mm^2) of the central retina, with fewer nuclear and plexiform elements and a thin innermost nerve fiber layer.

The retina consists of three structural components: neurons, glia, and vasculature. The neurons are the functional elements and transmit the photoactivated electrical impulse from photoreceptor process to occipital cortex. *The photoreceptor is the raison d'etre of the entire globe.* It is a sensory, apical cytoplasmic process of the neurons forming the outer nuclear layer. These processes, called **rods or cones** based upon their shape and ultrastructural composition, extend from the outer nuclear layer toward the choroid. They are enveloped by a glycosaminoglycan interphotoreceptor matrix, and interdigitate with apical processes of the retinal pigment epithelium, but no actual adhesions exist between the two layers. Within the outer segment of the photoreceptors are stacks of collapsed, disk-like spheres that contain the photoactive chemicals. The disks within rod outer segments are constantly produced basally and shed apically at the rate of 80–100 disks per day, with an outer segment turnover time of 6 days in dogs. Effete disk debris is engulfed and degraded by the retinal pigment epithelium. Such turnover has not been demonstrated in the outer segment of cones which have stacks of lamellae formed by infoldings of the plasma membrane. In addition, cones appear to be of many different types within a single retina. It is probably the ratio of different cones sensitive to different wavelengths of light that permits the visual cortex to discriminate color. *In general, fish,* *amphibia, reptiles, and birds have excellent color discrimination. Ungulates can distinguish yellows, blues, and, variably, green and red. Carnivores have very limited color perception, as far as can be determined.*

Other retinal layers are best described in terms of function. The photoelectric stimulus originating in the photoreceptor outer segment is transmitted through the outer nuclear layer and along the axons of the photoreceptor nuclei to the bipolar and horizontal neurons of the *inner nuclear layer.* The accumulation of outer nuclear layer axons and inner nuclear layer dendrites forms the *outer synaptic or plexiform layer.* The inner nuclear layer contains the nuclei of the bipolar, horizontal, amacrine, and glial (Muller) cells. The bipolar cells receive impulses from the photoreceptors and relay them to ganglion cells. The bipolar cells also stimulate the horizontal cells, which transmit the impulse horizontally to excite adjacent bipolar cells. Amacrine cells counterbalance the bipolar cells in that their stimulation releases an inhibitor of ganglion cell excitation. The glial cells are primarily structural support cells, whose processes traverse the retina to form the retinal scaffold and their anterior and posterior terminations fuse to form the inner and outer limiting membranes. The axons of the bipolar and amacrine cells, dendrites of ganglion and horizontal cells, and glial processes form the thick *inner synaptic or plexiform layer.* The *ganglion cell layer* is the thinnest and innermost of the neuronal layers. Large, granular neurons form a single and often sparse layer, supplemented by a few astrocytes, which become bilayered in the area centralis to accommodate the marked increase in photoreceptor density. *The density of ganglion cells predicts, in a general way, visual acuity.* They are most closely packed in animals requiring fine visual discrimination (most birds, predatory fish, many reptiles). In contrast, they are sparse in ungulates who do not feed by sight but who flee at anything that moves. Their axons form the *nerve fiber layer* that gradually increases in thickness towards the optic disk. In most animals, the fibers are not myelinated until they reach the optic disk. The nerve fiber layer is separated from the vitreous by an *internal limiting membrane* formed by the terminations of the Muller fibers and a true basal lamina.

The organization of the **retinal vasculature** is an important variable in ophthalmoscopic examination, both because vascular abnormalities are frequent signposts of disease and because normal species variation can erroneously be diagnosed as disease. Carnivores, ruminants, and swine have large venules and smaller arterioles radiating from the optic disk to the peripheral retina. The horse has about 60 thin, short vessels extending from the disk for about 5 mm into surrounding retina. In dogs and cats, the major vessels lie within the deep half of the nerve fiber layer and the ganglion cell layer. In ruminants and pigs, the vessels are very superficial and bulge into the vitreous, covered only by a thin layer of nerve fibers and basal lamina. The retinal vessels form an end-artery circulation that supplies the inner layers of the retina. The photoreceptors and outer nuclear layers are avascular and receive nutrients primarily by diffusion from choroid. Such dependence cannot be absolute (except in horses) because degeneration of these outer layers is surprisingly slow (weeks to months) following retinal separation. In contrast, occlusion of a retinal vessel results in focal infarction of the inner retina within less than 1 hour.

The blood vessels also participate in the *blood–eye barrier* similar to that already described for the uvea. The tight endothelial junctions and junctions between adjacent retinal pigment epithelial cells conspire to create a retina that is immunologically isolated from nonocular tissues in a manner similar to that described for the uvea. Like the uvea, such a barrier is likely not absolute and the various retinal antigens are likely to be neither totally sequestered nor absolutely unique to the retina. Saline extracts of retina yield the retinal S antigen, and the interphotoreceptor retinoid-binding protein is another antigen that may be important in the initiation or perpetuation of degenerative (see Retinal degeneration) or inflammatory retinopathies.

The **retinal pigment epithelium** extends from the ora ciliaris to the optic disk as the posterior continuation of the outer layer of ciliary epithelium. It forms a simple cuboidal epithelial layer that is separated from the choroid by a complex basal lamina, *Bruch's membrane.* The apical border interdigitates with the photoreceptors, with an average of about 30 photoreceptors contacting a single pigment epithelial cell, but forms no junctional complexes. The inclusion of the adjective "pigmented" is something of a misnomer in domestic species except the pig, inasmuch as the epithelium overlying the tapetum contains no cytoplasmic pigment granules. This seemingly insignificant layer plays a major role in embryologic induction of the eye as previously described, and also plays a crucial role in the nurturing of the photoreceptors throughout life. The pigment epithelium engulfs and degrades obsolete rod and cone outer segments, absorbs light to protect photoreceptors, synthesizes and degrades part of the glycosaminoglycan matrix enveloping photoreceptor outer segments, and participates in the vitamin A–rhodopsin cycle. Which of these functions are most essential for photoreceptor health is still unclear.

The **ocular fundus** *is a clinical term describing those ophthalmoscopically visible portions of the posterior globe excluding vitreous.* The fundus is commonly divided into dorsal tapetal and ventral nontapetal fundus, with the optic disk usually at the junction of the two. The retina, although almost transparent, does absorb some incident and reflected light to dull somewhat the fundus reflection ophthalmoscopically. Areas of retinal atrophy absorb less light and are seen as areas of increased tapetal reflectivity. Pre- or subretinal exudates, conversely, increase light absorption and are seen as focal fundic opacities. Developmental or acquired absence of tapetum allows black choroidal pigment to be seen. More severe choroidal lesions may be seen as red choroidal vasculature or even pink sclera obscured by variable amounts of residual pigment. Particularly in dogs, cats, and horses, selective breeding has made hypoplastic variations in amount and pigmentation of choroid and tapetum normal for particular breed or color varieties.

The **general pathology of retina** is often said to resemble that of brain. While this is undoubtedly true inasmuch as retina is merely an extension of the brain, the prevalence of such lesions as malacia, nonsuppurative perivascular cuffing, and proliferative microgliosis within the retina is very low compared to the brain. While no actual data are published, *most animals with encephalitis do not, in fact, have concurrent retinitis. Retinal inflammation is most often the result of spread from choroid or across the vitreous from anterior uvea.* Degenerations are much more common than inflammations and are not usually accompanied by inflammatory reaction. The mature mammalian retina has no capacity for regeneration of entire neural cells, although photoreceptor outer segments and glia may be replaced if destroyed in the course of degenerative or inflammatory disease. Even the fetal retina has poor regenerative capacity as evidenced by the prevalence of retinal dysplasia following prenatal or neonatal retinal injury. Retinal repair is by proliferation of inner layer astrocytes that eventually form a dense glial scar. Occasionally the astrocytes proliferate along the vitreal face of the retina, forming a preretinal fibroglial membrane. Similar subretinal membranes are seen with chronic detachments and originate from retinal pigment epithelium or Muller cells. The retinal pigment epithelium retains mitotic ability. When injured, these cells respond with hypertrophy, hyperplasia, and fibrous metaplasia. The presence of pigment in the neuroretina is frequent in instances of retinal atrophy, most probably derived from migration of retinal pigment epithelial cells into the adjacent retina.

Autolytic changes are visible within retina within 30 minutes of death, and within a few hours are of sufficient magnitude to interfere with the diagnosis of retinal degenerations. The earliest histologic change is pyknosis of a few nuclei in outer and inner nuclear layers, and loss of uniform density of the photoreceptor layer. Progressive dissolution of the photoreceptor outer segments results in retinal separation. Nuclear layer pyknosis and ganglion cell chromatolysis are widespread within 4–6 hours. *By 12 hours, retinal separation is complete and the extensively folded retina, with autolytic photoreceptors, may mimic genuine retinal separation.* The extensive pyknosis within both nuclear layers distinguishes the two, being absent in antemortem separation (see below for other criteria). By 18 hours after death, the retina is represented by a barely separable bilayer of pyknotic nuclei suspended in a pale, eosinophilic foamy matrix representing fragmented nerve fiber and plexiform layers.

Overview of retinal histopathology

The large amount of information about the causation and clinical features of the various retinal diseases is intimidating and serves to obscure the *fundamental simplicity of retinal histopathology*. The vast majority of retinal lesions fall into three categories: *inflammatory disease* as part of endophthalmitis, *photoreceptor degeneration* from inherited metabolic disease, detachment, or toxicity, and *inner retinal atrophy* (particularly ganglion cells) as a result of glaucoma. The angst over retinal histopathology can be further reduced by recognizing that many diseases of different pathogenesis share the same histologic appearance. For example, there are dozens of inherited photoreceptor diseases of dogs, yet they all look histologically identical. Most are even ultrastructurally identical. Furthermore, photoreceptor degeneration resulting from inherited retinopathy looks histologically identical to atrophy resulting from excessive exposure to light, from chemical toxicity, and even from retinal separation.

Bibliography

Bellhorn RW, et al. Anti-retinal immunoglobulins in canine ocular diseases. Sem Vet Med Surg (Small Anim) 1988;3:28–32.

Buyukmihci N, Aguirre G. Rod disc turnover in the dog. Invest Ophthalmol 1976;15:579–584.

Coli A, Marroni P. Dog retinal ganglion cells: a morphological and morphometrical study in aging. Anat Histol Embryol 1996;25:127–130.

Donovan A. The postnatal development of the cat retina. Exp Eye Res 1966;5:249–254.

Narfstrom K, Ekesten B. Diseases of the canine ocular fundus. In: Gelatt KN, ed. Veterinary Ophthalmology. 3rd edn. Baltimore: Lippincott Williams & Wilkins, 1999:869–933.

Samuelson D. Ophthalmic anatomy. In: Gelatt KN, ed. Veterinary Ophthalmology. 3rd edn. Baltimore: Lippincott Williams & Wilkins, 1999:31–150.

Retinal separation

The retina is firmly attached in the globe only at the ora ciliaris and at the optic disk. *When the retina separates, it does so by cleaving photoreceptors from their interdigitations with the retinal pigment epithelium.* Separation may occur as the result of accumulation of inflammatory exudates, transudates, tumor cells, or helminths between pigment

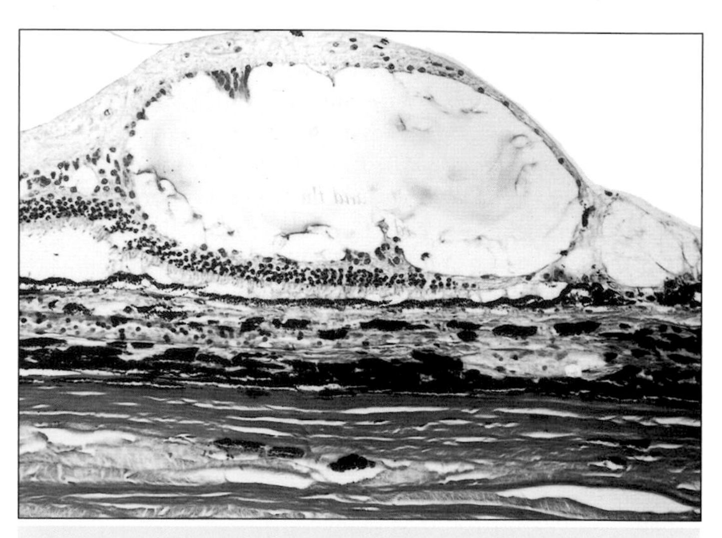

Figure 4.63 Peripheral microcystoid retinal degeneration in a dog. Such change is very common and of no apparent functional significance.

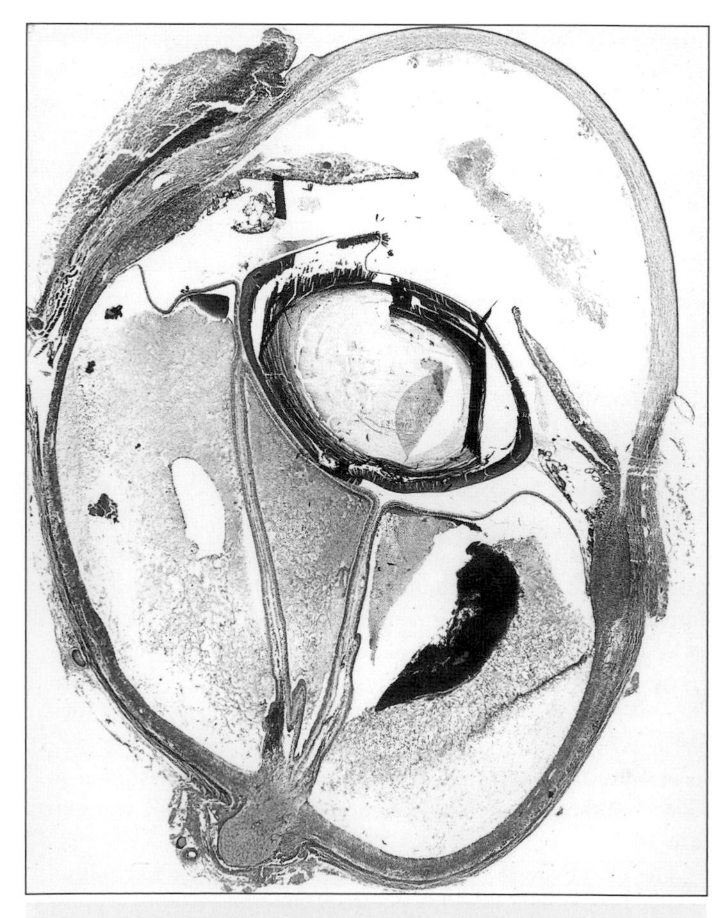

Figure 4.64 Complete retinal exudative separation in a dog with metastatic choroidal melanoma.

epithelium and photoreceptors, by contraction of a cyclitic membrane, or by the subretinal leakage of liquefied vitreous through retinal tears. Such tears may result from orbital trauma or from progression of peripheral cystic retinal degeneration. The latter is relatively common in man but not in domestic animals despite the frequent occurrence of microcystoid retinal degeneration in the peripheral retina of dogs (Fig. 4.63) and, less often, of horses.

The diagnosis of retinal separation in fixed specimens is complicated by the ease with which retinal separation can be induced by delayed fixation or improper handling of globes. *The credibility of the diagnosis is greatly enhanced by the presence of subretinal exudates or cyclitic membranes* (Fig. 4.64), *but in their absence the diagnosis rests upon the observation of photoreceptor outer segment degeneration, hypertrophy and hyperplasia of pigmented epithelium, and the development of marked edema in inner nuclear, ganglion cell and inner plexiform layers* (Fig. 4.65A, B). *Hypertrophy of the retinal pigment epithelium* is the most rapid change, occurring within a few hours of separation. The edematous changes are visible with the light microscope as early as 3 days following experimentally induced separation in owl monkeys. Coalescence of the edema creates a virtual cleavage of inner from outer retina, called **retinoschisis**. The cleavage is spanned by the radial Muller fibers, which seem the only anchor holding retina together. *Photoreceptor degeneration* is slower to appear under the light microscope, with loss of outer segments (probably the most subtle change that can be unequivocally diagnosed with routine light microscopy) visible by about 14 days after experimental saline-induced "exudative" retinal detachment. It is probably much faster than that when the exudate is full of noxious by-products of cell necrosis and inflammation, but no precise figure is available. Inner segments and the cell bodies of the outer nuclear layer are almost unaffected and may remain so for months, suggesting that their maintenance is not so intimately linked to the pigment epithelium as is the case with the outer segments. This temporal hierarchy of change permits reasonably accurate aging of retinal separations, sometimes a necessary or at least interesting assessment in eyes enucleated after numerous clinical examinations or manipulation. The outer retinal lesions are apparently not ischemic inasmuch as there is very little necrosis and no similarity to the lesion induced by retinal artery occlusion. Perhaps the outer layers can survive by diffusion of oxygen and nutrients from the subretinal fluid or from vascularized inner layers, and indeed the speed of photoreceptor atrophy varies with the height of the separation. An exception is seen in horses, inasmuch as the horse retina depends almost entirely on choroidal diffusion for oxygenation. Separation in this species results in rapid, full-thickness retinal infarction. A very

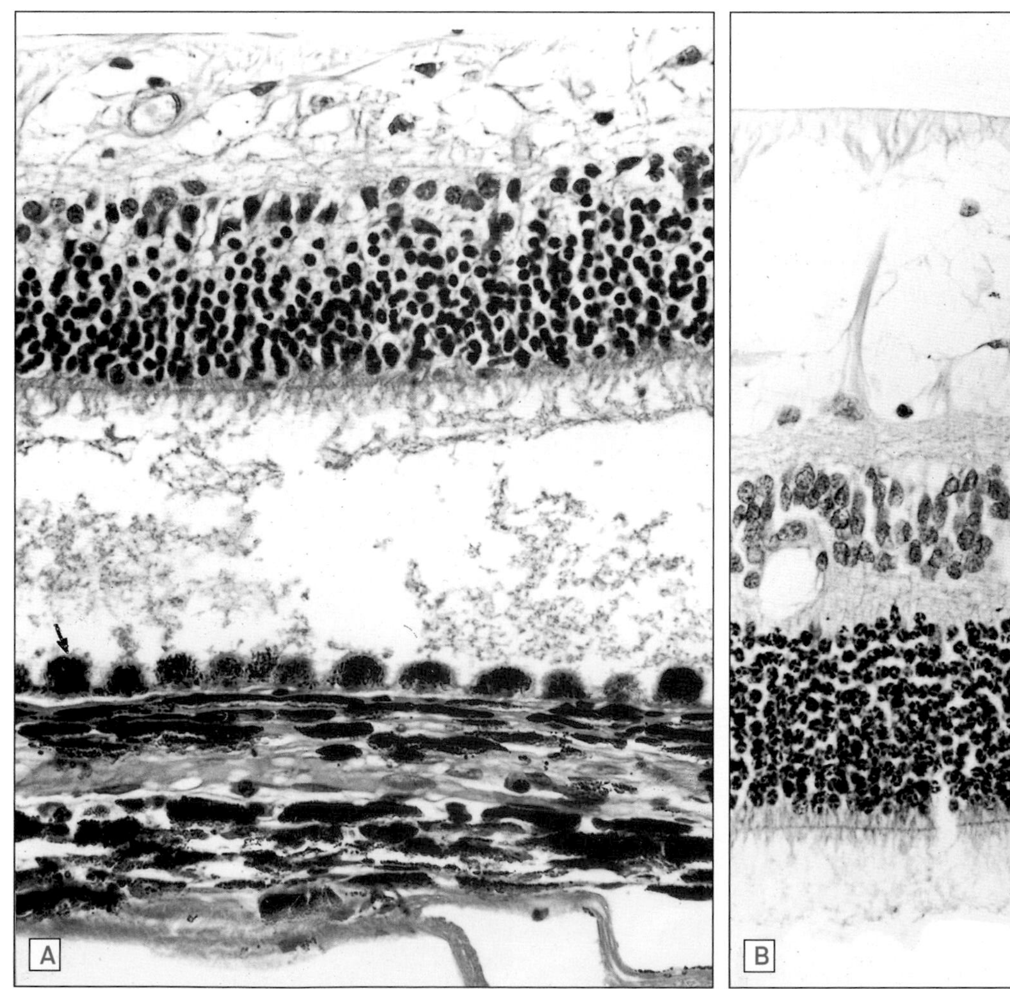

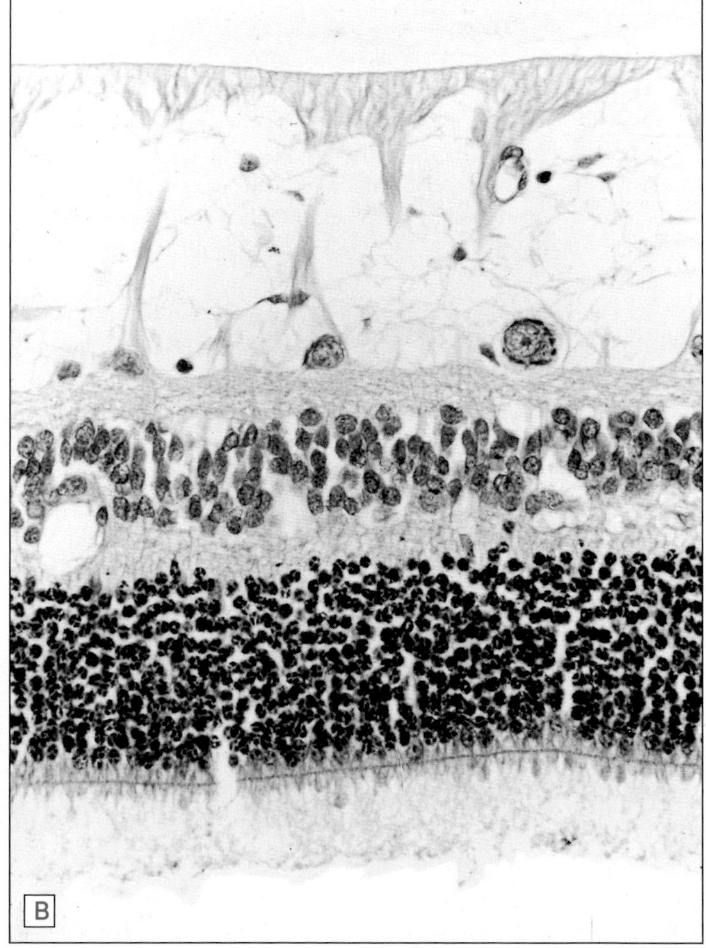

Figure 4.65 A. Serous retinal separation in a dog. Hypertrophic retinal pigment epithelium (arrow); photoreceptors atrophic; loss of nuclei from inner and outer nuclear layers. Blending of nuclear layers due to atrophy of outer plexiform layer. **B. Prolonged retinal separation** with retinal edema and photoreceptor degeneration. Radial Muller cell fibers anchor nerve fiber layer to ganglion cell layer. Retinal outer limiting membrane is prominent because of photoreceptor loss.

frequent lesion in horses is focal, linear, or multifocal chorioretinal glial scarring with pigment migration and fibrous metaplasia of pigment epithelium, a lesion that is probably a healed infarct following traumatic separation or thromboembolic disease.

Bibliography

Aaberg TM, Machemer R. Correlation of naturally occurring detachments with long-term retinal detachment in the owl monkey. Am J Ophthalmol 1970;69:640–650.

Anderson DH, et al. Morphological recovery in the reattached retina. Invest Ophthalmol Vis Sci 1986;27:168–183.

Erickson PA, et al. Retinal detachment in the cat: the outer nuclear and outer plexiform layers. Invest Ophthalmol Vis Sci 1983;24:927–942.

Komaromy AM, et al. Hypertensive retinopathy and choroidopathy in a cat. Vet Ophthalmol 2004;7:3–9.

Lewis GP, et al. Experimental retinal reattachment: a new perspective. Mol Neurobiol 2003;28:159–175.

Linsenmeier RA, Padnick-Silver L. Metabolic dependence of photoreceptors on the choroid in the normal and detached retina. Invest Ophthalmol Vis Sci 2000;41:3117–3123.

Maggio F, et al. Ocular lesions associated with systemic hypertension in cats: 69 cases (1985–1998). J Am Vet Med Assoc 2000;217:695–702.

Matz-Rensing K, et al. Retinal detachment in horses. Equine Vet J 1996;28:111–116.

Retinal degeneration

Retinal degeneration, more commonly called **retinal atrophy**, *may result from senile change, nutritional deficiency, metabolic disorder, or injury caused by infectious, chemical, or physical agents.* With the exception of the previously described glaucomatous retinal atrophy, virtually all are initially degenerations of photoreceptor outer segments or of retinal pigment epithelium, and many retinal atrophies of different pathogenesis have similar histologic appearance. The similarities become even stronger as the lesions progress to the severity usually encountered in enucleated eyes from clinically affected animals. Nonetheless, it is useful to review the subject and to discuss the differences between some of the best-studied examples of naturally occurring retinal atrophies. Most frequent are the inherited retinopathies of dogs grouped under the name, *progressive retinal atrophy*. Less common are retinal degenerations caused by deficiencies of taurine, vitamin E or vitamin A, by excessive visible light, or by several toxic or metabolic diseases.

Inherited retinal atrophies in dogs

Progressive retinal atrophy describes, admittedly with some inaccuracies, *a large group of bilateral retinal diseases in dogs.* They share the clinical features of being bilateral, progressing to blindness and being unassociated with inflammatory or other ocular disease. More than 100 breeds have been identified as affected, although there is little published information as to the prevalence within various breeds. Almost all of the ones thus far studied are inherited as an *autosomal recessive trait.* Some are juvenile-onset degenerations that result from a congenital biochemical defect and are thus properly termed *photoreceptor dysplasias*. Photoreceptors never reach proper ultrastructural or physiologic maturity, and affected dogs may be blind by a year or two of age. Irish Setters, Collies, Norwegian Elkhounds, and Miniature Schnauzers are the best-studied breeds that are affected, each with slightly different clinical expression and biochemical abnormality. Some initially affect only rods, but most affect both rods and cones. Alaskan Malamute dogs have what seems to be a purely cone dysplasia, leaving dogs visually impaired in daylight but with good night (i.e., rod-dependent) vision.

A quite separate group of diseases are currently considered to be *true degenerations* in that photoreceptor development seems normal. It may be, however, that even these inherited atrophies will be shown to have a developmental biochemical defect. *The trend to date has been to reclassify more and more degenerations as biochemical dysplasias*, a consequence of the use of more sensitive investigative techniques.

All of these different diseases may have significant differences in pathogenesis, but by the time the eyes are removed from impaired or totally blind dogs, the histologic and ultrastructural lesions are similar. *At this stage, the old name of progressive retinal atrophy continues to be used as a catchall.* The light microscopic lesion is degeneration of photoreceptors beginning dorsolateral to the optic disk. Over months or years, the photoreceptor loss extends and there is secondary atrophy of nuclear and plexiform layers of retina (Fig. 4.66). Eventually, in dogs permitted to live long enough, the retina remains as a poorly cellular glial scar. Despite the many similarities in clinical and histologic features, the importance of these retinopathies in the study of retinal disease in general warrants some more detailed explanation of the best-described variants.

Retinal atrophy in Irish Setters is described as *rod–cone dysplasia type 1* (rcd1), inherited as a simple autosomal recessive trait. Dogs homozygous for the defect have arrested differentiation of the rod external segments. Cones are less affected. The defect is detected ultrastructurally as early as 16 days after birth, at which time the

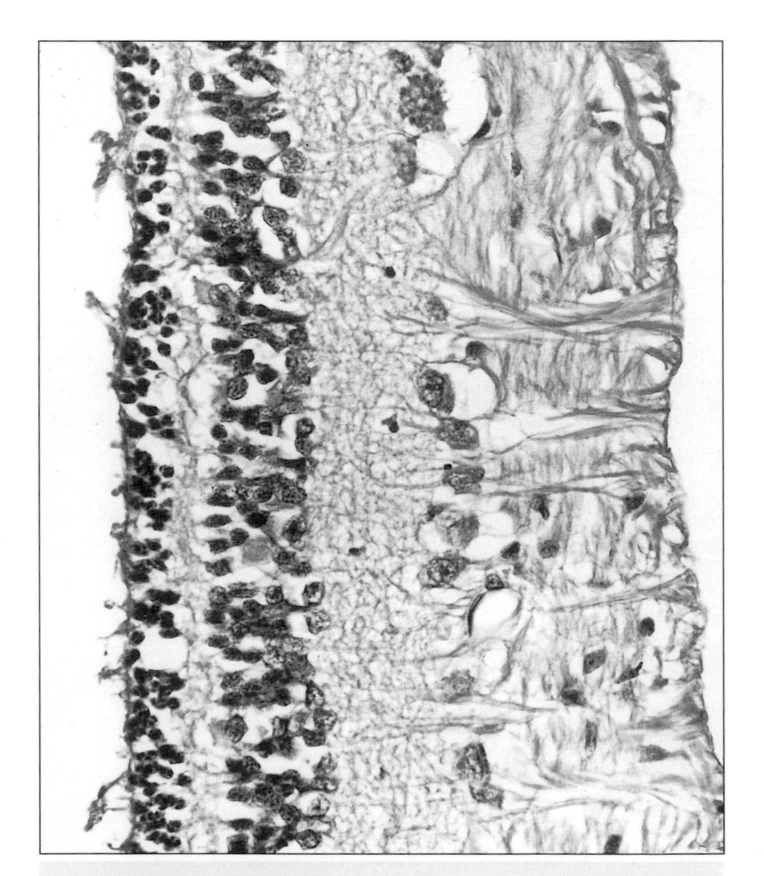

Figure 4.66 Progressive retinal atrophy in an English Cocker Spaniel. Diffuse atrophy of photoreceptors and outer nuclear layer.

outer rod segments should be developing adjacent to the pigment epithelium. Arrested development is followed by degeneration of inner rod segments, so that there is *diffuse loss of all rod photoreceptors by 12 weeks of age*. This is followed by loss of cones and of outer nuclear layer. The central retina is affected earlier and more severely than is peripheral retina. By the time the dog is about 1 year of age, there is diffuse atrophy of the outer nuclear layer, and the inner nuclear layer is in direct contact with the pigment epithelium. The inner retinal layers are unaffected. Dogs show visual deficits in dim light as early as 6 weeks of age and are usually blind by 1 year. *The biochemical defect is a marked deficiency of the phosphodiesterase responsible for the continuous hydrolysis of cyclic guanine monophosphate within outer segments.* While the function of the enzyme in this site is not fully understood, the resultant excess of cGMP is toxic to photoreceptors in vitro, and is known to cause arrested development or degeneration of rod outer segments in vivo. In the Irish Setter, the substrate levels are about ten times higher in affected than in control dogs, and the elevation precedes morphologic change in the photoreceptors. There are other biochemical retinal abnormalities (in rhodopsin and in membrane lipids), but it is not known whether they are primary abnormalities or merely effects of the cGMP phosphodiesterase deficiency. *The basic defect in rcd1 in Irish Setters is a nonsense mutation in the cGMP phosphodiesterase beta-subunit gene (PDE6B).* Also in the Irish Setter breed, there is a late-onset, progressive retinal atrophy that is likely hereditary, and that is distinct from rcd1.

Rough Collies have a *virtually identical photoreceptor dysplasia*, also inherited as an autosomal recessive trait. The progression of the lesion is slightly slower than in Irish Setters, but the biochemical defects are virtually identical. It appears that the defect results from a mutation of different genes than are involved with the Irish Setter dysplasia. In neither instance is it clear how photoreceptor death leads to death of all the outer nuclear layer neurons.

Retinal atrophy in Norwegian Elkhounds *is a historical disease, now eliminated*, that resembled the Collie and Irish Setter diseases in most clinical respects, but the biochemical defect was never identified. It was apparently not related to elevated cGMP. Onset of visual deficits in dim light was early; progression to blindness was only slightly less rapid than that in Setters. Ultrastructurally and biochemically, however, the two diseases were distinct. In Elkhounds, the primary lesion was restricted to rods. The rods were not arrested in their development but developed imperfectly. Light microscopic lesions appeared at about 6 months of age and progressed to complete photoreceptor loss by 1–2 years.

A *second type of rod–cone dysplasia* exists in this breed, with rapid progression to blindness by 12–18 months of age. Photoreceptor growth is erratic and apparently uncoordinated, but there is also dysplasia of rod and cone axonal synaptic junctions in the outer plexiform layer, which results in greatly reduced transmission of impulses from the photoreceptors. Ultrastructural changes are present in both the rod and cone outer segments as early as a few weeks after birth, but progression to complete retinal degeneration takes many years.

Cone degeneration (dysplasia) in Alaskan Malamute dogs *is a progressive and highly selective cone dysplasia*, inherited as a simple recessive trait. Although now rare because of elimination by selective breeding, it remains an interesting example of specific cone dysfunction. Affected dogs are noticed to have poor vision in bright light as early as 8 weeks of age. Night vision is, and remains, clinically normal, as does the ophthalmoscopic appearance of affected eyes. The ultrastructural lesion is disorganization and loss of cones, with rods normal. Adult dogs have no cone outer segments, and atrophic inner segments, but no change in rods or outer nuclear layer.

Rod–cone degeneration in Miniature Poodles *is classified as a true degeneration in that photoreceptor differentiation seems to be normal until 6–9 weeks of age*. After this time, and progressing at an unpredictable rate, there is disk disorganization and plasma membrane fragmentation in rod outer segments, visible as early as 15 weeks of age in the retina adjacent to the optic nerve. Peripheral retina is unaffected at this early stage, but by several years of age, the entire retina is affected. Cones are affected in a similar but milder fashion later in the disease course. The reason for the fragmentation is unknown, but it is known that affected dogs have abnormally slow outer segment turnover (about 40% of normal) prior to any observed structural change. Affected Poodles have evidence for a decreased rate of incorporation of docosahexanoic acid, the major long-chain structural membrane fatty acid, into rod outer segments. It may be that the decreased disk turnover permits older membranes to unduly persist and to be peroxidatively damaged in situ. The histologic lesion is identical to that of Irish Setters or Norwegian Elkhounds. Cataracts are present in many Poodles with retinal atrophy. Because of wide variation in disease progression, dogs may not be noticed to have dim-light deficiencies until middle, or even old, age.

An *almost identical disease* occurs in English and American Cocker Spaniels, Labrador Retrievers and Portuguese Waterdogs, resulting from a *mutation at the same genetic locus*. The diseases differ from breed to breed in the age of clinical onset and geographic distribution within the retina as seen ophthalmoscopically. The list of breeds reported to have some type of progressive retinal dysplasia/degeneration grows daily, and it is hard to determine how many of these represent a purely local phenomenon related to one or two specific lines of dogs, and which ones are truly global problems.

Central progressive retinal atrophy of dogs (pigmented epithelial dystrophy) denotes *a peculiar lesion in retinal pigment epithelium of dogs that apparently results from defective intracellular phagocytosis of shed photoreceptor outer segments*. Normal pigment epithelium engulfs and enzymatically degrades this material, resulting in a gradual buildup of intracellular lipopigments throughout life. In dogs with this pigment epithelial dystrophy, membrane peroxidation is excessive, and lipopigments accumulate to excess. Associated with the pigmentary accumulation, the epithelial cells hypertrophy. Photoreceptor outer segments adjacent to hypertrophic pigment epithelium degenerate. As the lesion progresses, hypertrophy and hyperplasia of epithelium give rise to dysplastic pigmented cell clumps. Within such clusters there may be an eosinophilic, hyaline, periodic acid-Schiff positive concretion resembling drusen. This material, rather frequent in ophthalmic specimens from people with a variety of degenerative retinal or choroidal diseases, is a concretion of excess basal lamina produced by the pigment epithelium. The eventual histologic lesion in affected dogs is a *monolayer of hypertrophic, lipochrome-rich pigment epithelial cells with multifocal hyperplastic clumps*. Retina has atrophy of photoreceptors and outer nuclear layer, and some irregular gliosis. Pigment-laden cells may invade the retina.

The disease is sporadic and of unpredictable clinical progression. The prevalence is, for example, much higher in Great Britain than in

North America, where it is rare. Retrieving and herding dogs are most frequently affected, with particularly high prevalence in Briards. The prevalence seems to vary dramatically from region to region, and over time. The ophthalmoscopic lesion of irregular black mottling begins near the optic disk and may progress to generalized pigment mottling interspersed with the increased reflectivity of atrophic retina. The mode of transmission is autosomal recessive in those breeds for which it is known. An interesting speculation, based upon morphologic similarities, is that the disease represents a defect in vitamin E metabolism within pigment epithelium. In Briards, the disease has been termed congenital stationary (i.e., nonprogressive) night blindness, although in many cases the disease does undergo slow clinical progression so the designation as "stationary" may not be appropriate. The *genetic defect (deletion of RPE65)* allows injurious accumulation of phospholipid esters of photoreceptor origin within the RPE, which eventually can be seen histologically as accumulation of lipid vacuoles.

Sudden acquired retinal degeneration is *an enigmatic, rapidly progressing photoreceptor degeneration that is histologically identical to the inherited progressive retinal atrophies. Blindness occurs very rapidly (over a period of a few days to a few weeks). Affected dogs are adult or even elderly, and the disease can affect any breed or crossbreed.* The fundoscopic lesion is bilaterally symmetrical and diffuse across the retina, but histologic studies of the early lesions are very few. The cause is unknown, but the presence of the retinal disease is linked to systemic signs of polyuria, polydipsia, and elevated serum cholesterol and alkaline phosphatase. Some, but not even the majority, of the affected dogs have adrenal cortical hyperfunction. How this malfunction causes the irreversible retinopathy, if indeed it does, is unknown. One small study demonstrated circulating, complement-fixing antibody to retinal S-antigen and interphotoreceptor retinoid-binding protein, raising the possibility that the disease is a cytotoxic autoimmune phenomenon.

Photoreceptor degenerations and dysplasias in cats

Photoreceptor degeneration is much less commonly observed in cats than in dogs. In the past, the great majority of cases have probably been examples of dietary taurine deficiency causing so-called *feline central retinal degeneration.* This once common disease has now become rare because of changes to virtually all commercial feline diets, but it will still occur in animals fed homemade diets and in those cats habitually eating some types of dog food. It is discussed in greater detail under nutritional retinopathies below.

Inherited retinal dysplasias and degenerations have been reported as sporadic occurrences in a variety of cat breeds, but only in the *Abyssinian breed* has the syndrome been adequately studied. In this breed there are two different diseases: *early-onset rod–cone dysplasia* and *late-onset retinal degeneration* affecting rods much sooner than cones. The early-onset dysplasia is inherited as an autosomal dominant trait. It is histologically and ultrastructurally similar to the disease in Irish Setter dogs, and a similar defect in the activity of cGMP phosphodiesterase has been reported. Affected cats are blind by a few months of age.

The late-onset retinal degeneration is inherited as an autosomal recessive, and affected cats progress slowly to blindness by 5–10 years of age. The earliest structural changes are in rod outer segments in peripheral retina, with jumbling of the rod disks and patchy blunting of the photoreceptors themselves. Only after many years is there histologically detected diffuse photoreceptor loss. A much more prevalent feline retinopathy, caused by deficiency of dietary taurine, is discussed later.

Inherited night blindness in horses

This poorly documented disease affects the *Appaloosa breed* and is probably inherited, and is seen as night blindness with daylight vision that is usually, but not always, normal. No structural lesion is seen in retinas of affected horses, and functional studies point to a defect in intraretinal synaptic transmission in outer plexiform or inner nuclear layers rather than a defect in photoreceptors.

Bibliography

Aguirre GD, et al. Frequency of the codon 807 mutation in the cGMP phosphodiesterase beta-subunit gene in Irish setters and other dog breeds with hereditary retinal degeneration. J Hered 1999;90:143–147.

Chaudieu G, Molon-Noblot S. Early retinopathy in the Bernese Mountain Dog in France: preliminary observations. Vet Ophthalmol 2004;7:175–184.

Dekomien G, Epplen JT. The canine Recoverin (RCV1) gene: a candidate gene for generalized progressive retinal atrophy. Mol Vis 2002;8:436–441.

Djajadiningrat-Laanen SC, et al. Familial non-rcd1 generalised retinal degeneration in Irish setters. J Small Anim Pract 2003;44:113–116.

Giuliano EA, van der Woerdt A. Feline retinal degeneration: clinical experience and new findings (1994–1997). J Am Anim Hosp Assoc 1999;35:511–514.

Grahn BH, Cullen CL. Retinopathy of Great Pyrenees dogs: fluorescein angiography, light microscopy and transmitting and scanning electron microscopy. Vet Ophthalmol 2001;4:191–199.

Kemp CM, Jacobson SG. Rhodopsin levels in the central retinas of normal miniature poodles and those with progressive rod-cone degeneration. Exp Eye Res 1992;54:947–956.

Kukekova AV, et al. Cloning and characterization of canine SHARP1 and its evaluation as a positional candidate for canine early retinal degeneration (erd). Gene 2003;312:335–343.

Lin CT, et al. Canine inherited retinal degenerations: update on molecular genetic research and its clinical application. J Small Anim Pract 2002;43:426–432.

Millichamp NJ. Retinal degeneration in the dog and cat. Vet Clin North Am: Small Anim Pract 1990;20:799–836.

McLellan GJ, et al. Vitamin E deficiency in dogs with retinal pigment epithelial dystrophy. Vet Rec 2002;151:663–667.

Petersen-Jones SM, et al. cGMP phosphodiesterase-alpha mutation causes progressive retinal atrophy in the Cardigan Welsh corgi dog. Invest Ophthalmol Vis Sci 1999;40:1637–1644.

Sidjanin DJ, et al. Canine CNGB3 mutations establish cone degeneration as orthologous to the human achromatopsia locus ACHM3. Hum Mol Genet 2002;11:1823–1833.

Veske A, et al. Retinal dystrophy of Swedish briard/briard-beagle dogs is due to a 4-bp deletion in RPE65. Genomics 1999;57:57–61.

Witzel DA, et al. Night blindness in the appaloosa: sibling occurrence. J Am Anim Hosp Assoc 1977;13:383–386.

Wrigstad A, et al. Slowly progressive changes of the retina and the retinal pigment epithelium in Briard dogs with hereditary retinal dystrophy. Doc Ophthalmol 1994;87:337–354.

Light-induced retinal degeneration

Light of various wavelengths has a variety of injurious effects on cornea, lens, or retina that vary with the wavelength, duration, and intensity of the light.

The effects also vary with a large but poorly understood group of animal variables that include ocular pigmentation, habitat, previous experience with photoperiod, nutrition, body temperature, age and, most obviously, species. The wavelength of light has the greatest effect; short wavelengths in the *ultraviolet and blue range* (up to about 475 nm) have the greatest energy per photon and are the most damaging. Fortunately, most of these wavelengths are absorbed by cornea and lens, so that their lethal effects on retina are seldom seen. They may cause corneal epithelial injury or cataract, although these effects are apparently rare in domestic animals (see Cataract).

In people, accidental exposure to light from arc welding, solar eclipses, or ophthalmic examination or operating equipment (including lasers) creates the potential for rapid injury from mechanical disruption or heat. While such damage is certainly possible in other animals, most naturally occurring lesions result from the additive effects of much less intense ultraviolet and short wavelength visible light because of unnatural photoperiods. Animals with poorly pigmented eyes, and those adapted for nocturnal vision, are most susceptible. Susceptibility also increases with age and with temperature.

The initial lesion is disruption of rod outer segment disks, with eventual destruction of all photoreceptors and their nuclei. Because the lesion is identical to most inherited, nutritional, and toxic retinopathies, *the diagnosis is made on the circumstantial evidence of abnormally bright light, abnormally long light photoperiod, or a rapid change in photoperiod.* Most instances occur with rodents or fish kept in continuous fluorescent light. Albino rodents or deepwater fish are, predictably, the most susceptible.

The mechanism by which visible light of moderate intensity damages the retina is still incompletely understood, and different experimental models give rise to different theories. Most studies use blue light in the 400–475 nm range, which, unlike shorter ultraviolet wavelengths, is not filtered out by the cornea or lens. The most popular theory is that of light-induced oxidation of the very abundant polyunsaturated long chain fatty acids of the rod disks, with the generation of free radicals to then cause cell membrane damage. This theory gains support from studies showing a protective effect by vitamin C or E, and enhanced injury under conditions of retinal hyperoxia.

Nutritional retinopathy

Nutritional causes of retinal degeneration include deficiencies of *vitamins C, A, or E,* and the amino acid, *taurine.* Retinal atrophy and cataracts have been seen in fish with a dietary deficiency of vitamin C. The lesions were thought to be light induced, with the fish unusually susceptible because of the deficiency in the antioxidant effects of the vitamin. The ocular lesions of vitamin E deficiency resemble those of retinal pigment epithelial dystrophy and were referred to briefly under that heading. Pups fed severely deficient diets develop night blindness within about 6 weeks, and an extinguished electroretinogram suggestive of diffuse photoreceptor damage. These last two effects are not seen in naturally occurring central retinal atrophy. Retinopathy has been described in primates and dogs fed rations deliberately and severely deficient in vitamin E. *Lipofuscin*, seen as eosinophilic cytoplasmic inclusions, accumulated to excess in the pigment epithelium, and was followed by hypertrophy of the pigment epithelium and degeneration of photoreceptor outer segments. Eventually there was full-thickness central retinal atrophy and some small foci of retinal separation. Retinal degeneration with ceroid-lipofuscin accumulation in the retinal pigment epithelium has also been noted in vitamin E-deficient horses, but did not appear to cause visual impairment.

Hypovitaminosis A

Retinopathy caused by hypovitaminosis A is seldom encountered except in growing cattle or swine kept in confinement and fed a ration deficient in the vitamin over months or years. Grains other than corn (maize) are very poor sources of vitamin A, and the level in corn falls markedly with prolonged storage. Green pasture is very rich in carotene, which is converted to vitamin A by intestinal epithelium. Hay that is excessively dry, leached by rain, cut late in the year, or stored for prolonged periods is a much less adequate source. In most pastured animals, the liver reserves are sufficient to prevent clinical signs of deficiency for at least 6 months and often up to 2 years. Young, rapidly growing animals have greater requirements and smaller stores of the vitamin and are thus more susceptible than adults.

Hypovitaminosis A affects bone remodeling and causes epithelial cell atrophy and defects in synthesis of rhodopsin. Ocular lesions can result from each of these three defects.

As previously discussed, *maternal deficiency of vitamin A causes blindness in offspring due to defective remodeling of optic nerve foraminae and subsequent ischemic or pressure atrophy of the nerve.* In piglets, there may be massive ocular dysplasia and such anomalies as cleft palate, skeletal deformities, hydrocephalus, epidermal cysts, genital hypoplasia, and anomalous hearts. *Optic nerve atrophy is preceded by optic disk swelling (papilledema),* and followed by atrophy of nerve fiber and ganglion cell layers. This sequence of events may occur if very young animals are on deficient diets, with the optic nerve changes being caused in part by stenosis of optic foramen and in part by increased cerebrospinal fluid pressure that itself results from atrophy and metaplasia of arachnoid villi. The papilledema precedes optic nerve necrosis and is reversible. The corneal lesions of hypovitaminosis A have received scant attention and are seldom seen in natural outbreaks.

The acquired ocular effect of hypovitaminosis A involves photoreceptor outer segments. The ophthalmoscopic lesion is multifocal retinal atrophy and scarring in animals with slow or absent pupillary light reflex and apparent blindness. The histologic lesion is patchy-to-diffuse photoreceptor atrophy which first affects the rod outer segments. Night blindness is thus the initial complaint and is often the chief complaint about a deficient herd. Eventually the atrophy affects all photoreceptors and their nuclei, and may progress to full-thickness atrophy with scarring. The lesions have been produced in all domestic species on specially formulated diets, but naturally occurring retinal lesions are almost restricted to cattle with chronic deficiencies.

The pathogenesis of the photoreceptor atrophy demonstrates the structure–function interdependence of retinal cells. Vitamin A is converted to retinene and then to the glycoprotein rhodopsin. Rhodopsin is stored as a component of the lamellar disks of the outer segment. Light initiates a physicochemical change in rhodopsin, resulting in a cascade of events culminating in the hyperpolarization of the outer segment membrane. The resultant electrical impulse is transmitted to bipolar cells, ganglion cells and then to brain. *Deficiency of vitamin A necessarily results in a deficiency of rhodopsin.* The corresponding ultrastructural lesion is swelling, then fragmentation of lamellar disks that can be reversed by therapy with vitamin A, unless inner segments have also been affected. Regeneration simulates normal development and requires about 2 weeks to rebuild outer segments completely. Vitamin A is discussed further in Vol. 1, Bones and joints.

Taurine-deficiency retinopathy

Retinal degeneration caused by taurine deficiency is seen only in cats, although taurine is the predominant free amino acid in the retina of other species. Among domestic mammals, only the cat seems unable to synthesize taurine from cysteine in amounts adequate for retinal function. Taurine is considered a dietary essential for cats, and its deficiency results in *characteristic central retinal atrophy* and in *myocardial failure* (see Vol. 3, Cardiovascular system). Changes in commercial diets, and better recognition of the risk of diseases related to taurine deficiency, have almost eliminated this disease.

The ocular lesion of taurine deficiency was first detected in cats fed semi-purified diets in which casein was the only protein. After several months, such cats developed focal retinal atrophy adjacent to the optic disk, which progressed to generalized retinal atrophy. Supplementation with taurine halted but did not reverse the lesion, presumably because photoreceptor nuclei or inner segments already had been damaged. The clinical and histologic features of this newly recognized nutritional retinopathy were virtually identical to those that had already been recognized in an idiopathic, naturally occurring disease of cats called "*feline central retinal degeneration*." It is assumed that the two diseases are actually the same, although that may not be true in every single instance. At least some of the cases of idiopathic central atrophy were associated with the feeding of dry dog food, which (for a cat) is deficient in taurine.

The clinical lesion is a *focal lesion of tapetal hyperreflectivity* that is bilateral, dorsolateral to the optic disk and is usually unassociated with visual impairment. *The histologic lesion is photoreceptor degeneration,* initially targeting cone outer segments but eventually affecting rods as well. The rods of the peripheral retina are the last to degenerate. Taurine also seems essential for membrane integrity of the tapetal reflective rodlets, so that dissolution of the membrane surrounding these crystalline intracytoplasmic inclusions is another characteristic lesion. Less clear is the association of taurine deficiency with diffuse retinal atrophy in cats (Fig. 4.67).

Familial atrophy occurs in Abyssinian and Persian cats, but most cases are of unknown cause. Continued deficiency of taurine leads to diffuse retinal atrophy and thus might be responsible.

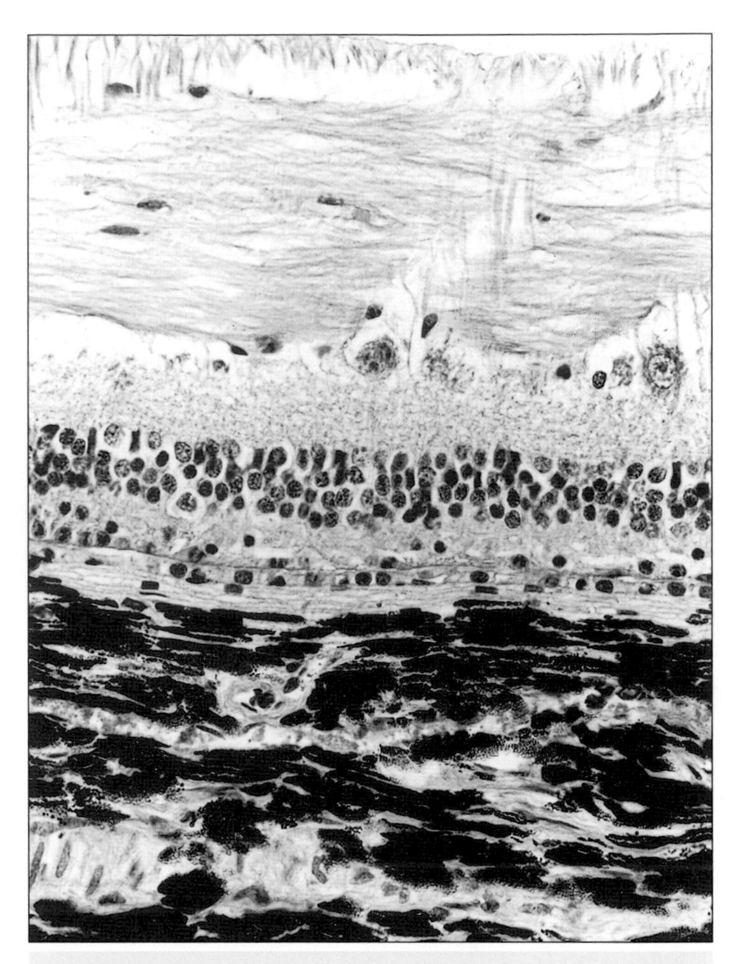

Figure 4.67 Idiopathic diffuse retinal atrophy in a cat. Note complete atrophy of photoreceptors and depletion of outer nuclear layer.

Toxic retinopathies

Experimental toxic retinopathies have been caused by many chemicals and toxic plants, but only a few toxic plants cause important diseases of domestic animals.

Bracken fern (*Pteris aquilinum*) causes progressive retinal degeneration in sheep in several areas of Great Britain. The common name "bright blindness" refers to pupillary dilation and tapetal hyperreflectivity of the severely affected sheep. The disease has been seen only in flocks grazing hills rich in bracken fern, and has been reproduced by prolonged feeding of the fern to sheep. A similar syndrome has been noted in cattle during long-term exposure to the fern. The lesion is usually seen in middle-aged or older sheep as bilateral and initially central tapetal hyperreflectivity. Diffuse involvement follows. *The histologic lesion is nonspecific, consisting of photoreceptor outer segment degeneration progressing to depletion of all retinal layers.*

Blindness is one of the features of intoxication with **locoweed,** *Astragalus* and *Oxytropis* spp., in the USA, **darling pea** (*Swainsona* spp.), **blind grass** (*Stypandra* spp.) in Australia, and **selenium indicator plants** worldwide.

Astragalus and *Swainsona* cause a *neurovisceral lysosomal storage disease* analogous to genetically transmitted mannosidosis (see Vol. 1, Nervous system). All members of the genus *Swainsona* contain an indolizidine alkaloid, swainsonine, which is a potent inhibitor of lysosomal mannosidase. At least some *Astragalus* spp. contain a similar alkaloid. Chronic ingestion of the plant occurs in cattle, sheep, and horses forced to eat the plants on dry pastures where nothing more palatable is available. Affected animals develop behavioral abnormalities and defects of gait and vision. The histologic lesion consists of widespread cytoplasmic vacuolation in most organs due to the intralysosomal accumulation of mannose-rich oligosaccharides. Onset of clinical signs may require several months of heavy *Swainsona* ingestion, but ultrastructural vacuolation is seen within a few days. The ocular lesion is, as elsewhere in the central nervous system, vacuolation of neuronal cytoplasm and, later, axonal degeneration. The vacuolation is readily reversible upon cessation of ingestion of the plant and seems not to be the lesion responsible for clinical signs. The axonal degeneration is not reversible and is probably the more important lesion. Whether blindness is retinal or central in origin is unknown.

Poisoning with *Stypandra* spp. occurs in sheep and goats on dry pastures in southwestern Australia. The plant is among the first to reappear after autumn rains end the drought, and is eaten if nothing better is available. Acute intoxication is frequently fatal. Animals surviving the acute stage become blind and ataxic. In retina, there is diffuse photoreceptor atrophy and patchy hyperplasia of retinal pigment epithelium. Axonal degeneration is found within the optic nerve and elsewhere within the central nervous system.

The colloquial term *"blind staggers" refers to chronic intoxication of sheep and cattle with plants known to accumulate organic selenium selectively*. Affected animals wander aimlessly, become weak and ataxic and are finally paralyzed prior to death. There is some question as to whether blindness is genuine or merely the result of stupor. Ocular lesions are not described. The syndrome of blind staggers does not occur in experimental selenium toxicity, and it is possible that the syndrome is of much more complex pathogenesis than simple selenium toxicity. Plants of the genera *Astragalus* and *Oxytropis* are selenium accumulators as well as sources of swainsonine-like alkaloids.

Mycotoxicosis associated with the consumption of *Corallocytostroma* sp. fungus on Mitchell grass is reported to cause "black soil blindness" in cattle in Australia. The disease presents as rapidly progressive blindness and death. The histologic lesion is not described.

Photoreceptor degeneration has been described in cats treated with the antibiotic **enrofloxacin**. Initial reports suggested that this was an idiosyncratic reaction since the toxicity occurred after administration of the drug at recommended dosages. Subsequent analysis suggests that this is a direct toxicity that occurs when the retina is exposed to unusually high levels of this widely used antibiotic, even when administered at the daily recommended dosages (subsequently revised). Retinotoxic levels are likely to be reached when the drug is given by rapid intravenous infusion or when given to cats with impaired renal or liver function that may not properly metabolize and eliminate the drug. *Toxicity is thus most likely to be seen in old cats receiving prolonged therapy*. Similar retinal toxicity is likely to be shared by other fluoroquinolone antibiotics. Most cats had clinically obvious visual impairment within a few weeks of drug administration, and the blindness was permanent in most cases.

Miscellaneous retinopathies

Retinal lesions are found in a number of metabolic disorders and systemic states. Best known among these is diabetes mellitus, but retinal lesions are found also in any of the neuronal storage diseases, coagulation disorders, anemia, disseminated intravascular coagulation, hyperviscosity syndrome, hypertension, and following excessive exposure to oxygen or light.

Diabetes mellitus is *the major cause of blindness in people in North America. The cause of the blindness is chorioretinal vascular disease with subsequent retinal degeneration*. The characteristic lesions are seen only in patients with diabetes of 10–15 years duration. Even though virtually all chronic diabetics develop some retinal lesions, fewer than 10% become blind. Blindness is strongly predictive of the development of fatal diabetic nephropathy. Lesion development is not prevented by insulin replacement. Other ocular lesions include cataract, rubeosis iridis, glycogen-induced vacuolation of iris epithelium, and massive thickening of the ciliary basal lamina. The corneal epithelium may be unduly fragile, and tear production may be reduced.

The retinal lesion in people is mostly the result of microvascular disease. Loss of retinal pericytes, development of microaneurysms, thickening of capillary basal lamina and retinal hemorrhages constitute the early, degenerative phase of the retinopathy. This is followed by a proliferative phase in which more capillary aneurysms, arteriolar–venular shunts and neovascularization occur as the presumed responses to retinal ischemia. The neovascularization is initially bland and confined to the retina, but later there is extension into preretinal vitreous with accompanying fibroplasia (retinitis proliferans). Hemorrhages and hyalinized collections of leaked plasma are common in the retina.

In nonprimates, the naturally occurring retinopathy is seen only in dogs and, even then, infrequently. This low frequency may be due to the fact that affected dogs do not live long enough for the retinal disease to develop. In dogs deliberately made diabetic and kept for up to 6 years, microvascular lesions typical of human diabetes occur. Pericyte loss is accompanied by capillary aneurysms, reactive endothelial proliferation, and perivascular plasmoid exudates or hemorrhages.

Other types of **ischemic retinal injury** are much more frequent in domestic animals than is diabetic retinopathy. *Undoubtedly the most frequent examples are associated with vascular hypertension in cats and, less frequently, in dogs*. Ischemic retinopathy as a consequence of *DIC*, of *tumor metastasis*, or of *bacteremia* is fairly common, with the prevalence varying greatly with species. *Perhaps the most common example of ischemic retinal injury is that resulting from retinal detachment*. The blood vessels of the choriocapillaris supply oxygen and other nutrients to the photoreceptors and outer nuclear layer, hence retinal detachment inevitably results in gradual outer retinal ischemic/malnutritive atrophy.

Hypertensive retinopathy *is in most cases associated with chronic renal failure*. At least 60% of dogs with chronic renal failure are hypertensive. Dogs and cats are most frequently affected. In cats, hypertensive retinopathy is also claimed to be associated with hyperthyroidism, but a study of 100 hyperthyroid cats did not provide any evidence for that anecdotal association.

The macroscopic ocular lesions include retinal or preretinal hemorrhage, retinal edema, and retinal detachment because of serous effusion from injured choroidal blood vessels. *The histologic lesions are primarily in retinal and choroidal vessels*, which have lesions varying from fibrinoid necrosis of tunica media to medial hypertrophy with adventitial fibrosis. Changes that are probably secondary to vessel damage include localized retinal necrosis, exudative retinal separation with resultant atrophy of photoreceptors and hypertrophy of retinal pigment epithelium, and intraretinal hemosiderin deposition (Fig. 4.68). Usually there is ischemic necrosis of RPE, which allows for the leakage of hypertensive edema fluid from the choroid into the subretinal space (which would normally be prevented by the tight junctions between adjacent RPE cells). Vascular lesions and associated necrosis may also occur in anterior uvea. Eyes that are eventually enucleated or obtained at necropsy may have a variety of other lesions that probably occur secondary to chronic retinal detachment and chronic intraocular hemorrhage. Most notable among these is pre-iridal fibrovascular membrane and its resultant hyphema or neovascular glaucoma.

The early lesions, likely to be seen only under experimental conditions, are the result of exaggerated autoregulatory vasoconstriction in response to systemic hypertension. Sustained vasoconstriction leads to ischemic necrosis of the deprived retina, RPE or choroid, as well as necrosis of vascular endothelium distal to the constricted precapillary sphincters. The histologic consequences are focal retinal necrosis, and leakage of

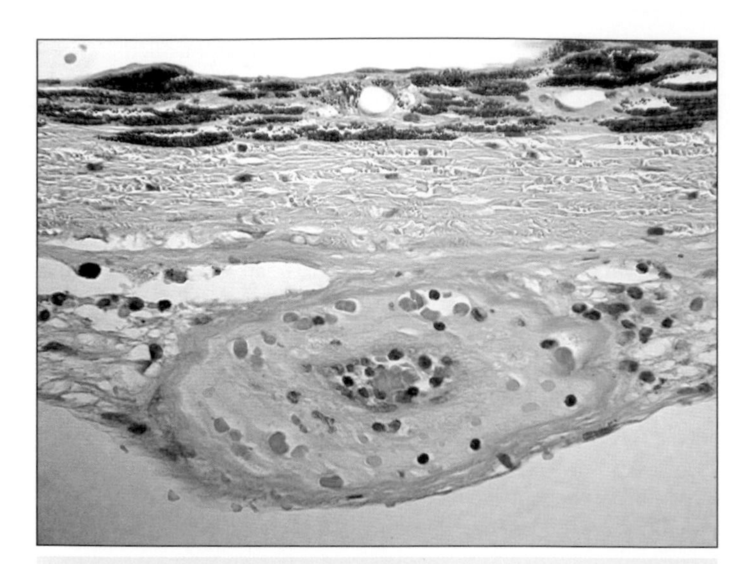

Figure 4.68 Hypertensive retinopathy.

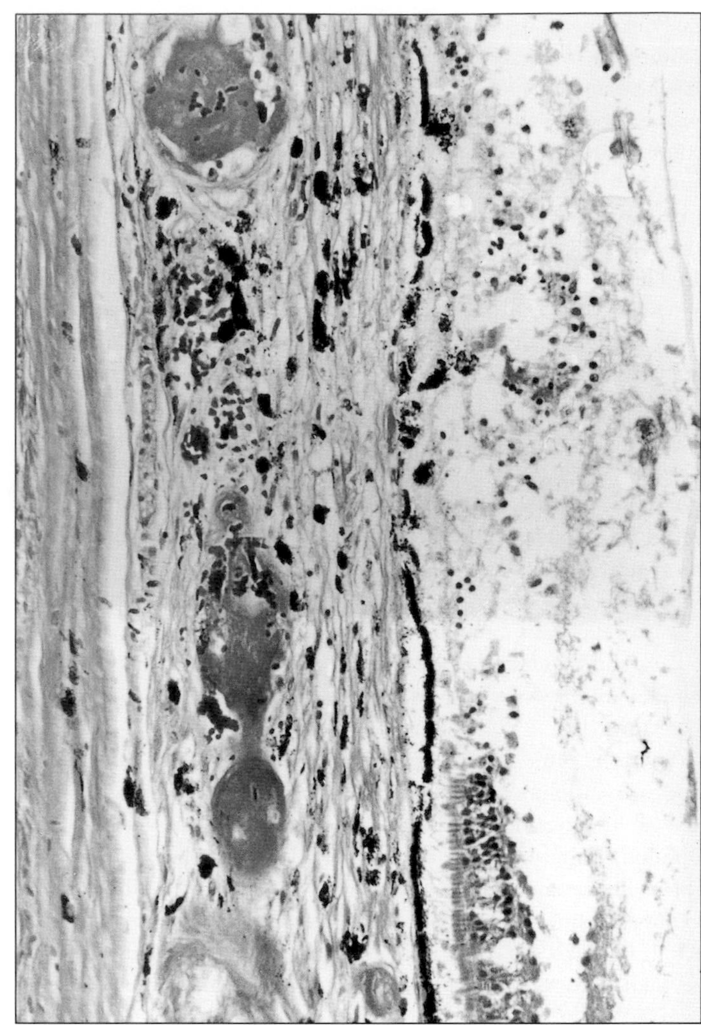

Figure 4.69 Choroidal thrombosis and vasculitis in a horse with idiopathic purpura hemorrhagica. Note **infarction** of adjacent retina.

plasma or even erythrocytes through damaged endothelium. This leakage causes intramural fibrinoid change in the vessels and edema or hemorrhage in adjacent retina.

Retinal infarction, usually seen as a combination of hemorrhage and liquefaction, occurs subsequent to retinal vessel thrombosis, occlusion by tumor emboli, or vasculitis associated with immune disease or a few infectious diseases (Fig. 4.69). The most likely to be encountered are thrombotic meningoencephalitis of cattle, and Rocky Mountain spotted fever or ehrlichiosis in dogs. In addition to the vascular lesions themselves, which may have specific characteristics associated with the individual diseases, the retinal lesions vary from focal hemorrhage to areas of hemorrhagic liquefactive necrosis or healed lesions of chorioretinal scarring.

Similar retinal scarring has been seen in horses following massive but sublethal blood loss, as in surgery or from nasal hemorrhage subsequent to severe cranial trauma. Affected eyes have multifocal retinal atrophy and hyperpigmentation. Similar lesions may also result from focal retinal separation. In horses, such separation carries a high risk of causing focal retinal infarction because they have such limited intrinsic retinal vasculature (see Fig. 4.69).

Retinal hemorrhages are seen in a variety of primary clotting disorders, in thrombocytopenia of any cause, and in degenerative or inflammatory vascular disorders. Retinal hemorrhages also recur in cats with profound anemia of any cause; the mechanism is unknown. The lesions heal with scarring if the cat survives the anemia, suggesting that the hemorrhage is only the most visible manifestation of multifocal and probably ischemic retinopathy.

Many of the **neuronal storage diseases** cause retinal lesions identical to those in the brain. The list of those with described ocular lesions probably reflects those in which the eyes have been examined rather than a true reflection of those diseases in which ocular lesions do, or do not, occur. Those interested should consult a useful, referenced table in the text by Slatter.

Senile retinopathy *is characterized by microcystoid degeneration*, which is very common in dogs from middle age onwards (see Fig. 4.63). A similar lesion is found occasionally in horses. The lesion affects peripheral retina adjacent to ora ciliaris and for a variable distance medially. There is formation of small cystic spaces within inner nuclear and plexiform layers, fusion of inner and outer nuclear layers, pigment cell accumulation and haphazard atrophy and mingling of nuclei in a manner simulating peripheral retinal dysplasia. If the cysts rupture to the vitreal face, the retina external to the cyst is seen as an atrophic hole. Such holes are foci of extreme retinal thinning, and only the external limiting membrane separates vitreous from pigment epithelium. The pigment epithelium and choroid are usually normal but they too may show atrophy and fibrosis. Intermingling of cysts and holes in peripheral retina is common. Complete breaks are uncommon and do not usually lead to retinal separation, as occurs in people.

Multifocal coalescing peripheral retinal atrophy is very frequent in very old dogs and horses, but is of no apparent visual importance.

Bibliography

Andersen AC, Hart GH. Histological changes in the retina of the vitamin A deficient horse. Am J Vet Res 1943;4:307–317.

Bradley R, et al. The pathology of a retinal degeneration in Friesian cows. J Comp Pathol 1982;92:69–83.

Crispin SM, Mould JRB. Systemic hypertensive disease and the feline fundus. Vet Ophthalmol 2001;4:131–140.

Davidson MG, et al. Retinal degeneration associated with vitamin E deficiency in hunting dogs. J Am Vet Med Assoc 1998;213:645–651.

Djajadiningrat-Laanen SC, et al. Progressive retinal atrophy in Abyssinian and Somali cats in the Netherlands (1981–2001). Tijdschr Diergeneeskd 2002;127:508–514.

Goss-Sampson MA, et al. Retinal abnormalities in experimental vitamin E deficiency. Free Radic Biol Med 1998;25:457–462.

Gwin RM, et al. Hypertensive retinopathy associated with hypothyroidism, hypercholesterolemia, and renal failure in a dog. J Am Anim Hosp Assoc 1978;14:200–209.

Huxtable CR, Dorling PR. Swainsonine-induced mannosidosis. Am J Pathol 1982;107:124–126.

Jubb TF, et al. Black soil blindness: a new mycotoxicosis of cattle grazing *Corallocytostroma*-infected Mitchell grass (*Astrebla* spp.). Aust Vet J 1996;73:49–51.

Kremer I, et al. Oxygen-induced retinopathy in newborn kittens. Invest Ophthalmol Vis Sci 1987;28:126–130.

Leon A, et al. Lesion topography and new histological features in feline taurine deficiency retinopathy. Exp Eye Res 1995;61:731–741.

Lerman S. Light-induced changes in ocular tissues. In: Miller D, ed. Clinical Light Damage to the Eye. New York: Springer-Verlag, 1987:Chapter 10:183–215.

Maggio F, et al. Ocular lesions associated with systemic hypertension in cats: 69 cases (1985–1998). J Am Vet Med Assoc 2000;217:695–702.

Mason CS, et al. Congenital ocular abnormalities in calves associated with maternal hypovitaminosis A. Vet Rec 2003;153:213–214.

McLellan GJ, et al. Clinical and pathological observations in English cocker spaniels with primary metabolic vitamin E deficiency and retinal pigment epithelial dystrophy. Vet Rec 2003;153:287–292.

Michels M, Sternberg P, Jr. Operating microscope-induced retinal phototoxicity: pathophysiology, clinical manifestations and prevention. Surv Ophthalmol 1990;34:237–252.

Riis RC, et al. Ocular manifestations of equine motor neuron disease. Equine Vet J 1999;31:99–110.

Schaller JP, et al. Induction of retinal degeneration in cats by methylnitrosourea and ketamine hydrochloride. Vet Pathol 1981;18:239–247.

Slatter D. Retina. In: Slatter D, ed. Fundamentals of Veterinary Ophthalmology. 3rd ed. Philadelphia, PA: WB Saunders, 2001:419–456.

Stiles J, et al. The prevalence of retinopathy in cats with systemic hypertension and chronic renal failure or hyperthyroidism. J Am Anim Hosp Assoc 1994;30:564–572.

Toole DO, et al. Bilateral retinal microangiopathy in a dog with diabetes mellitus and hypoadrenocorticism. Vet Pathol 1984;21:120–121.

Tulsiani DRP, et al. Swainsonine inhibits the biosynthesis of complex glycoproteins by inhibition of Golgi mannosidase II. J Biol Chem 1982;257:7936–7939.

Van der Woerdt A, Peterson ME. Prevalence of ocular abnormalities in cats with hyperthyroidism. J Vet Intern Med 2000;14:202–203.

Van Donkersgoed J, Clark EG. Blindness caused by hypovitaminosis A in feedlot cattle. Can Vet J 1988;29:925–927.

Van Kampen KR, James LR. Ophthalmic lesions in locoweed poisoning of cattle, sheep and horses. Am J Vet Res 1971;32:1293–1295.

Wiebe V, Hamilton P. Fluoroquinolone-induced retinal degeneration in cats. J Am Vet Med Assoc 2002;221:1568–1571.

Zuclich JA. Ultraviolet induced damage in the primate cornea and retina. Curr Eye Res 1984;3:27–34.

Retinitis

Retinitis as the sole ocular lesion is rare, but may occur in animals with neurotropic virus infections, with toxoplasmosis, and with thrombotic meningoencephalitis of cattle (Fig. 4.70). In the latter disease, however, it is more usual to find the typical thrombotic, inflammatory lesions in choroid as well as retina. Their character is identical to the lesions in the brain. The multifocal chorioretinal scars expected as sequelae are seldom seen, perhaps because cattle with neurologic and ocular lesions almost inevitably die. The prevalence of the ocular lesion, useful as an aid in the clinical diagnosis, is estimated at 30–50% in animals with the septicemic form of the disease, and as high as 65% in experimentally infected calves.

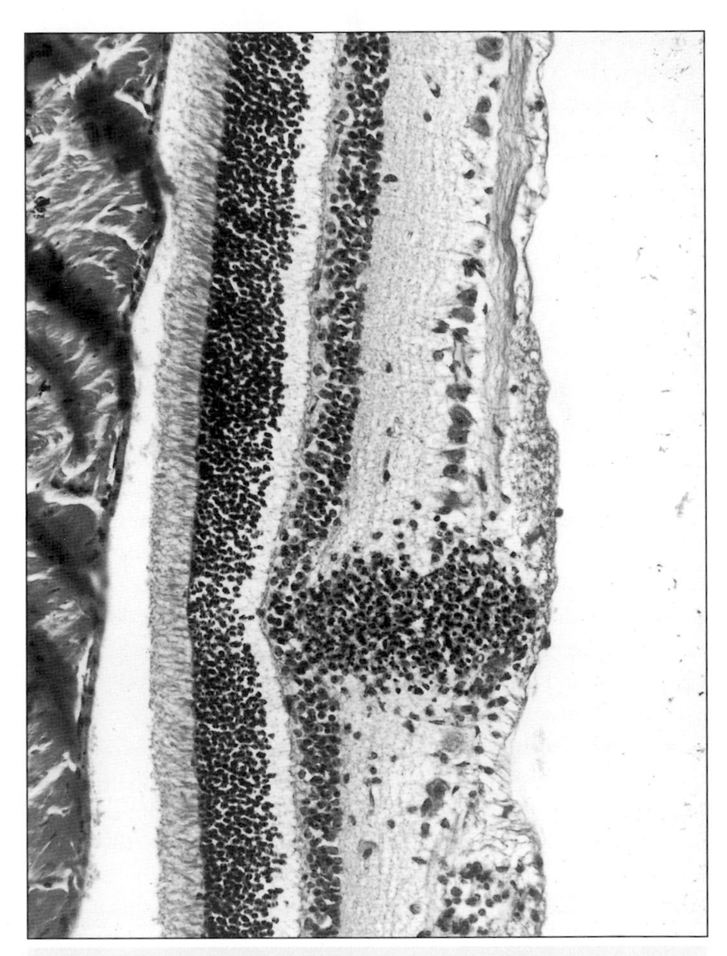

Figure 4.70 Focal destructive retinitis due to *Histophilus somni* infection in a steer.

Multifocal viral retinitis with the same histologic features as the respective brain lesions occurs in animals with classical swine fever, rabies, Teschen disease, Borna disease, pseudorabies in pigs, canine distemper, and scrapie (a prion disease). Undoubtedly the list is incomplete, and is probably limited only by the rarity with which retinas receive histologic evaluation in animals dying with systemic viral, bacterial, and protozoal diseases. *The ocular lesions associated with canine distemper will be described here in some detail as the archetypal example of viral retinopathy* (other aspects of canine distemper are discussed in Vol. 2, Respiratory system).

Retinal and optic nerve lesions occur in most dogs with naturally occurring **canine distemper.** The lesions most often are degenerative rather than inflammatory, although some of the degenerative changes may have been sites of inflammation earlier in the disease course.

Acute lymphocytic-plasmacytic chorioretinitis and optic neuritis are found in about 25% of dogs submitted for laboratory confirmation of the disease. Random perivascular cuffing, edema, focal exudative retinal separation, and hypertrophy of retinal pigment epithelium are present. Eosinophilic intranuclear inclusion bodies occur in ganglion cells or astrocytes in 30–40% of the cases, which is the only etiologically specific change in what is an otherwise nonspecific picture shared by many systemic infections.

The more prevalent lesions are multiple random foci of retinal degeneration and scarring. These usually affect the full thickness of retina, and are most likely sequelae to the previous undetected retinitis. Such foci often contain numerous melanin-laden cells, probably derived from migration of adjacent, injured retinal pigment epithelium. Occasionally only the outer nuclear layer and photoreceptors are missing, probably a sequel to focal exudative retinal detachment.

Optic nerve lesions of one type or another are present in all dogs with ocular lesions. Nonsuppurative neuritis, astrocytic scarring and demyelination similar to that in brain are the three most frequent changes. In those dogs suffering only the demyelinating disease, the ocular lesions may be inapparent, or there may be demyelination of optic nerve and ganglion cell degeneration.

Other infectious examples of retinitis in dogs include **Rocky Mountain spotted fever** (RMSF, *Rickettsia rickettsii*) and **canine ehrlichiosis** (*Ehrlichia canis*). The clinical and histologic ocular lesions are virtually identical and occur in a high percentage (80% for RMSF) of dogs with active infection. Most of the lesions result from injury to vascular endothelium parasitized by the rickettsiae; multifocal hemorrhage, edema, and vascular necrosis occur in all parts of the eye. *Multifocal retinal hemorrhage, perivascular retinal edema, and necrosis of endothelium in retinal venules and arterioles are the characteristic retinal changes.* While often listed along with other agents as a cause of anterior uveitis or endophthalmitis, most naturally occurring infections have clinical signs attributable only to the vascular injury rather than a genuine uveal inflammation. There is one report of unusually severe uveitis occurring 14–28 days after experimental infection with *Rickettsia rickettsii*, following the disappearance of all other signs of the acute systemic disease. Dogs thus affected had neutrophilic and lymphocytic destructive vasculitis, assumed to represent a type III immune reaction to parasitized endothelium.

Viscera larva migrans from *Toxocara canis* has been linked to granulomatous endophthalmitis and chorioretinitis in dogs. It is likely that many of these cases were actually caused by the raccoon roundworm *Baylisascaris procyonis* (see Parasitic endophthalmitis).

Bibliography

Barnett KC, Palmer AC. Retinopathy in sheep affected with natural scrapie. Res Vet Sci 1971;12:383–385.

Davidson MG, et al. Vascular permeability and coagulation during *Rickettsia rickettsii* infection in dogs. Am J Vet Res 1990;51:165–170.

Dukes TW. The ocular lesions in thromboembolic meningoencephalitis (ITEME) of cattle. Can Vet J 1971;12:180–182.

Fischer CA. Retinal and retinochoroidal lesions in early neuropathic canine distemper. J Am Vet Med Assoc 1971;158:740–752.

Panciera RJ, et al. Ocular histopathology of ehrlichial infections in the dog. Vet Pathol 2001;38:43–46.

OPTIC NERVE

The optic nerve is a white fiber tract of brain formed by the outgrowth of ganglion cell axons from the eye through sieve-like perforations in posterior polar sclera, called the *lamina cribrosa*. The axons travel within a preformed neurectodermal tube formed by the primary optic stalk to reach the optic chiasm and then the lateral geniculate body. The neurectoderm lining the optic stalk induces the surrounding mesenchyme to form the three meningeal layers, similar to and continuous with those of brain itself. Later differentiation of neurectoderm produces astrocytes and oligodendroglia that, together with the ganglion cell, axons, and fibrovascular septa from pia mater, form the substance of the optic nerve. The *optic disk* is the intraocular portion of the nerve and is the only portion available to ophthalmoscopic examination. It is formed by the convergence of ganglion cell axons prior to their exit via the lamina cribrosa. The axons of the nerve fiber layer are unmyelinated, and at what point (relative to lamina cribrosa) the axons become myelinated determines the ophthalmoscopic appearance of the optic disk. Histologically, the disk is unmyelinated in most domestic species except the dog, contains abundant glia and may have a small paracentral excavation – *the physiologic cup* – from which Bergmeister's papilla originates. A few pigmented cells are commonly seen, as are small neuroblastic clusters, both probably minor anomalies of retinal differentiation but of no significance.

There is considerable variation in the normal histology of the optic nerve among animals of different species and ages. Optic disk myelination has already been mentioned. The lamina cribrosa is formed by heavy fibrous trabeculae in horses, dogs, and cattle and is therefore more obvious than in cats and laboratory animals. Fibrous septa within the nerve are prominent in cattle and horses, and their similarity to the axons in hematoxylin and eosin sections may mask a pathologic paucity of nerve fibers. The fibrous tissue reportedly increases with age.

The general pathology of optic nerve shares features of both retinal and neural disease. Because it is in direct continuity with both structures via its axons, and with brain via the perineural cerebrospinal fluid, it is common for optic nerve to be affected by diseases of either retina or brain. Thus optic neuritis is expected in at least a proportion of animals suffering with inflammation of retina or neural white matter, and optic nerve atrophy inevitably follows loss of ganglion cells. Fortuitous hematogenous localization of infectious agents or tumor cells may occur in optic nerve as anywhere else.

Papilledema *is hydropic swelling of the optic disk.* It may result from extraocular events that cause an increase in cerebrospinal fluid pressure within the optic nerve or from local vascular leakage. The former is usually associated with retrobulbar tissue masses, but is also seen with intracranial neoplasms and with hypovitaminosis A. Ocular hypotony may cause optic disk edema as a result of decreased tissue hydrostatic pressure. Serous inflammation within the nerve also results in papilledema. Papilledema is a common clinical diagnosis that rarely is available for histologic examination.

Optic neuritis *is a term sometimes used rather broadly to describe both inflammatory and degenerative diseases of the nerve.* Optic neuritis is seen clinically as swelling, hyperemia, and focal hemorrhage within the optic disk. Affected animals, usually dogs or horses, are blind when the lesion is bilateral. Although described as a clinical entity not associated with other ocular lesions, histopathologic confirmation is lacking. Optic neuritis may, of course, accompany any case of retinitis or endophthalmitis.

The pattern of inflammation within the nerve may provide clues to the pathogenesis of the neuritis. Perineuritis, or optic nerve leptomeningitis, is typical of meningeal spread of bacterial meningitis from the brain. Toxoplasmosis and cryptococcosis frequently cause multifocal and nonselective lesions within the extraocular nerve, as does canine distemper. Optic neuritis originating as endophthalmitis is usually restricted to the optic disk. Feline infectious peritonitis is frequently associated with perineuritis and optic neuritis in which the mononuclear aggregates are around blood vessels in the meninges and in the extensions of the meninges into the nerve.

Chronic optic neuritis, like its counterpart in the brain, is characterized by focal gliosis, astrocytic scarring, and secondary axonal degeneration. The loss of axons may be partially masked by the increased prominence of glia and pial septa.

Degeneration of the optic nerve *is part of optic neuritis, glaucoma, and chronic, severe retinal atrophy of any cause.* Initiation of gliosis and fibrosis may eventually make the chronic degenerative lesion indistinguishable from that of chronic inflammation. The most frequently diagnosed example is that following *trauma* to one or both nerves in dogs or cats struck by cars (Fig. 4.71). The gross lesion may be avulsion or contusion. Injury to the nerve may be instantaneous as caused by tearing or complete severance, or may result from vascular injury with slightly delayed ischemic necrosis. In severed nerves, there is disintegration of the distal axons back to the lateral geniculate body. The proximal portion of each affected axon dies back to the ganglion cell, which eventually also dies. The inner nuclear layer remains unaffected, a useful criterion to distinguish traumatic, "die back," ganglion cell atrophy from that of glaucoma.

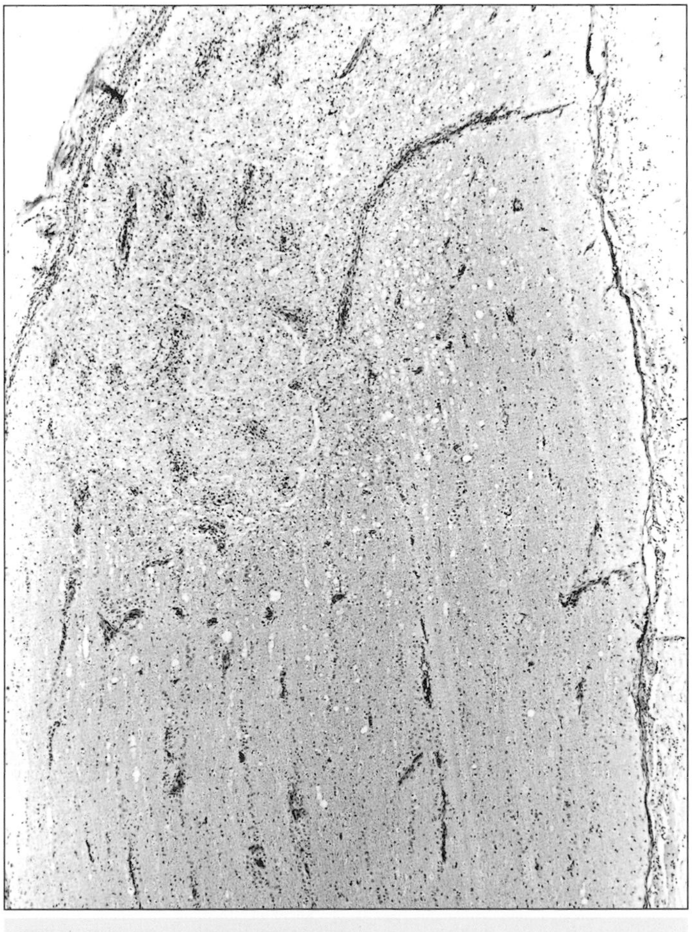

Degeneration of optic nerve also occurs in calves *deficient in vitamin A*, and in ruminants ingesting *male fern* or *hexachlorophene*. Ingestion of male fern, *Dryopteris*, on pasture or as a taenicidal extract causes papilledema and subsequent optic nerve demyelination when ingested in large amounts. Retina may be unaffected early, but ganglion cell atrophy occurs eventually. Hexachlorophene administered to calves or sheep as an anthelmintic causes edema and then atrophy and gliosis of optic nerve.

Proliferative optic neuropathy is an unusual lesion of horses. Anecdotal descriptions are numerous, but histologic descriptions are few. The lesion is a raised, gray mass on the surface of the optic disk, unassociated with visual deficit. *The mass is composed of spherical mononuclear cells with hyperchromatic, eccentric nuclei and foamy eosinophilic cytoplasm* (Fig. 4.72). Some of these cells are also found within extraocular optic nerve. The cytoplasmic content may be stored lipid, but its origin is not known. The described lesion bears much resemblance to the proliferation of myelin-laden macrophages that occurs

Figure 4.71 Axonal degeneration in the retrobulbar, intraorbital optic nerve in a dog, 11 days after being struck by a car.

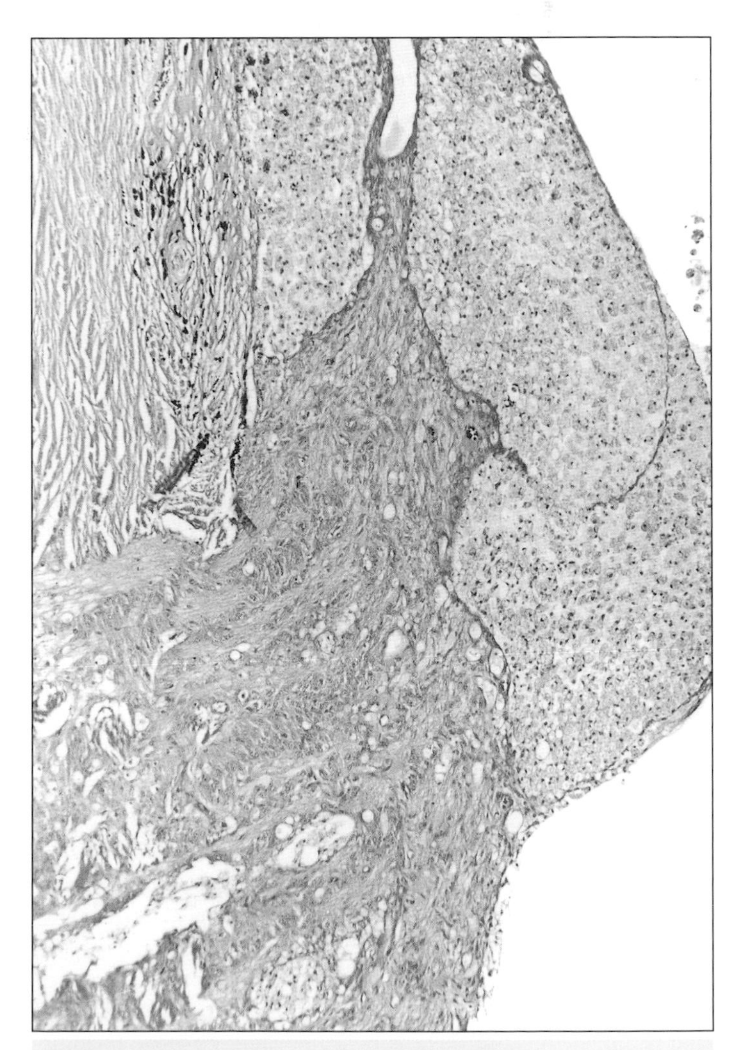

Figure 4.72 Equine proliferative optic neuropathy. The identity of the foamy cells is much debated, but they are probably reactive macrophages full of lipid.

in and on optic nerves injured by trauma or ischemia. Also, the distinction between the proliferative optic neuropathy and gliomas or granular cell tumors described in various reports is unclear.

Bibliography

Bistner S, et al. Neuroepithelial tumor of the optic nerve in a horse. Cornell Vet 1983;73:30–40.

Gelatt KN, et al. Optic disc astrocytoma in a horse. Can Vet J 1971;12:53–55.

Nafe LA, Carter JD. Canine optic neuritis. Compend Cont Ed 1981;3:978–984.

Riis RC, Rebhun WC. Proliferative optic neuropathy in a horse caused by a granular cell tumour. Equine Vet J Suppl 1990;10:69–72.

Saunders LZ, Rubin LF. Ophthalmic Pathology of Animals. Basel: Karger, 1975:152–157.

SCLERA

The **limbus** *marks the transition from the avascular, nonpigmented and very orderly cornea to the vascularized, pigmented and interwoven fibrous tissue that identifies sclera.* The sclera forms the posterior two-thirds of the fibrous tunic of the eye, blending with choroid on its inner aspect and orbital fascia exteriorly. Its thickness increases with age and varies considerably among domestic species. In cattle and horses, it is thickest at the posterior pole (2.2 mm in cattle and 1.3 mm in horses) and thinnest at the orbital equator (1.0 mm in cattle, about 0.5 mm in horses). In dogs and cats, it is much thinner, about 0.3 mm at the posterior pole and 0.1 mm at the equator, varying somewhat with age and globe size. In carnivores, however, there is a circumferential ring of thickened (1 mm) sclera at the limbus in which is buried the venous plexus receiving aqueous drainage. The sclera is perforated by numerous vessels and nerves, the most notable of which are the optic nerve and limbic scleral venous plexus.

The optic nerve fibers exit the globe through extensive scleral fenestrations called the **lamina cribrosa**. Diseases of the sclera are few in comparison to diseases of other ocular structures. Most are inflammatory and arise by extension from within the globe or from orbital cellulitis. *The efficiency with which the sclera resists inflammatory spread is evidenced by the infrequency of panophthalmitis as opposed to endophthalmitis, and the even greater infrequency of intraocular involvement resulting from orbital inflammation.* When the sclera is involved in inflammatory disease originating within the eye, its initial involvement is seen histologically as leukocytes in perivascular adventitia that is in direct communication with the choroid. A similar phenomenon is seen in scleral extension of choroidal neoplasms, in which collars of tumor cells surround scleral vessels but show little inclination to infiltrate directly into scleral connective tissue.

Nodular granulomatous episcleritis (ocular nodular fasciitis) *is the most prevalent disease of dogs that is primarily scleral.* It occurs rarely in cats. It is the proliferative, nodular lesion of the limbus that has been variously termed nodular fasciitis, nodular scleritis or episcleritis, fibrous histiocytoma, proliferative keratoconjunctivitis, conjunctival granuloma, and Collie granuloma. The various names reflect the spectrum of clinical presentations of this lesion. The variations are treated as a single entity, nodular granulomatous episcleritis (NGE), in this discussion. My decision to do so is purely for the sake of simplicity, since there is no compelling evidence to justify splitting this histologic entity into multiple diseases simply because the lesions may occur in various locations within and below the conjunctiva, and clinical management is similar for all.

The usual macroscopic lesion is a firm, painless, moveable, nodular swelling, 0.5–1.0 cm in diameter, below the bulbar conjunctiva at, or just posterior to, the limbus. Infiltrative extension of the mass into the peripheral corneal stroma is accompanied by edema and vascularization (Fig. 4.73A). Although the temporal limbus unilaterally is the most frequent site for initial occurrence, other common locations include the third eyelid and elsewhere along the limbus. Third eyelid involvement is often bilateral, and occurs almost exclusively in rough Collies. Limbic and nictitans involvement may occur in the same dog and even in the same eye.

Ocular nodular fasciitis behaves as would a locally infiltrative neoplasm. Extension is usually into peripheral corneal stroma and posteriorly into sclera, episclera, and Tenon's capsule. The tissue of origin of this lesion is unresolved. Fibrous tissue of sclera, episclera, and Tenon's capsule have all been suggested. Lesions involving the third eyelid, or the rare case of palpebral subconjunctival origin, probably originate from the fascia native to those structures. Histologic examination distinguishes this lesion from extension of intraocular tumors or the rare scleral sarcomas. Occasionally, infiltration of therapeutically refractory fasciitis is so extensive, both into cornea and sclera, as to require enucleation.

Histologically, the lesion is a proliferative, nonencapsulated mixture of histiocytic cells, spindle cells, and mononuclear leukocytes (Fig. 4.73B). The spindle cells may be fibroblasts, histiocytes, or a mixture of both. The spindle cells are haphazardly arranged and, despite a fibrous appearance to the section, surprisingly little collagen is demonstrated by special stains, except in coarse septa that may dissect the mass into irregular lobules. Reticulin, however, is abundant. The mononuclear leukocytes are found loosely throughout the mass but are usually most numerous near the periphery. *Important histologic features are the absence of collagenolysis and the absence of discrete granulomas.* While the lesion may be quite granulomatous, the macrophages are uniformly intermingled with the other cellular elements. When present in peripheral cornea, the above cell mixture affects stroma but spares the epithelium and an adjacent zone of subepithelial stroma.

Necrotizing scleritis *is a rare lesion seen in dogs as a poorly delineated inflammatory and proliferative lesion of the anterior sclera.* The disease incites much more inflammatory reaction, as measured by clinical criteria, than does nodular fasciitis. *The lesion consists of coalescing scleral granulomas centered on remnants of denatured, refractile collagen.* Eosinophils sometimes are seen in the centers as well. The formation of true granulomas may not be prominent, but at least a few are required to distinguish this lesion from nodular granulomatous episcleritis described above. The lesion tends to slowly spread circumferentially and posteriorly to involve the entire sclera, and involvement of uvea and even retina with granulomas eventually occurs. Bilateral involvement is usual, but not necessarily at the same time. Response to anti-inflammatory therapy is poor unless that therapy is very aggressive, and so an unusually high percentage of eyes with this disease eventually become available for histologic assessment. No etiologic agent has been seen.

ORBIT

Diseases of the orbit are few and relatively uncommon in domestic animals except for those resulting from trauma and, in dogs, from neoplasia. Systemic diseases of bone, muscle, blood vessels, and nerves may incidentally

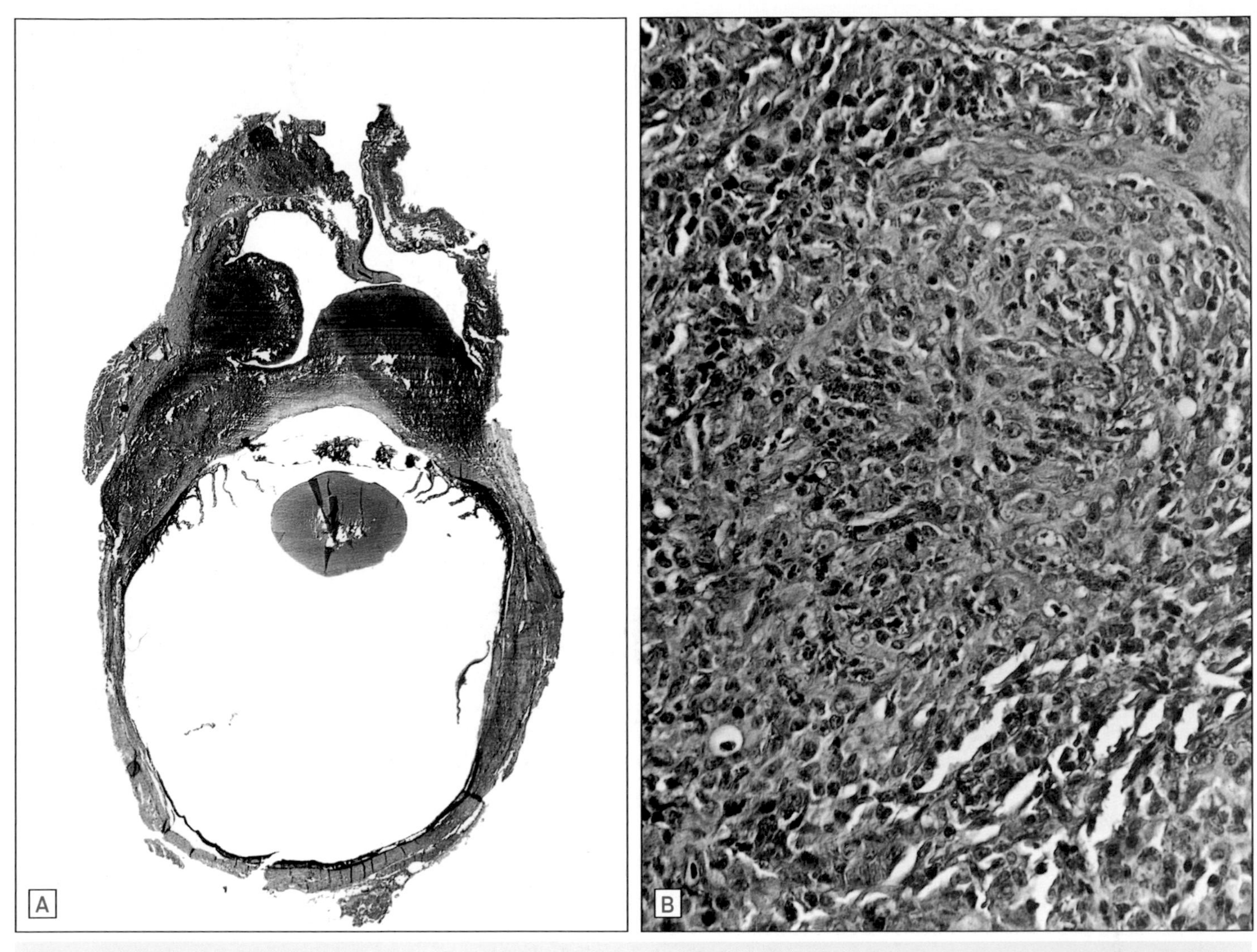

Figure 4.73 Nodular granulomatous episcleritis syndrome. A. Unusually extensive lesion, which progressed for 2 years without adequate therapy. **B.** Higher magnification, demonstrating the characteristic intermingling of lymphocytes, macrophages, and fibroblasts without actual granuloma formation.

affect orbital components. Orbital fat fluctuates with nutritional status contributing to the enophthalmos of malnourished animals. Ordinarily, however, orbital disease arises by extension of inflammatory lesions from the mouth, paranasal sinuses, or from penetrating wounds through periorbital soft tissue. Extension from intraocular inflammation is surprisingly rare, a tribute to the barrier offered by the sclera. Conversely, orbital disease rarely invades the globe. Metastatic orbital neoplasia is rare except for lymphoma of cattle and cats. Direct invasion by malignancies arising in the mouth, facial bone, nasal cavity, or sinus is more common. While theoretically the orbit may suffer from primary neoplasia of any of the bony or soft tissues within it, such occurrences are infrequent. Of these, optic nerve meningiomas, ill-defined spindle-cell sarcomas, and lacrimal gland tumors in dogs are the most common (see Ocular neoplasia).

Orbital cellulitis *is the term commonly used to describe pyogenic orbital inflammation*. The cause is usually bacterial and the pathogenesis involves extension from nearby inflammation of paranasal sinuses, molar tooth socket, or periorbital soft tissue. Only rarely does uncontrolled endophthalmitis spread through the sclera into the orbit. Bacteremic localization within the orbit, while presumably occurring as do such localizations elsewhere, is seldom detected except perhaps for *Streptococcus equi* infection in young horses.

Orbital myositis *occurs as a specific syndrome in dogs, affecting the extraocular muscles.* It affects primarily young dogs of large breeds, and is not associated with masticatory or generalized myositis. The histologic changes are identical to immune-mediated masticatory myositis, with multifocal random interstitial lymphocytic myositis, muscle fiber necrosis, and subsequent fibrosis. Antibodies against type 2M muscle fibers have been demonstrated in affected dogs.

Orbital inflammation most frequently results from *penetrating foreign bodies*, whether by direct penetration or particle migration from conjunctival sac or pharynx. Horses seem particularly prone. Aberrant localization by nematode parasites (*Dirofilaria immitis*, *Ancylostoma caninum*) or *Diptera* larvae is reported.

Bibliography

Allgoewer I, et al. Extraocular muscle myositis and restrictive strabismus in ten dogs. Vet Ophthalmol 2000;3:21–26.

Baptiste KE, Grahn BH. Equine orbital neoplasia: a review of 10 cases (1983–1998). Can Vet J 2000;41:291–295.

Carpenter JL, et al. Canine bilateral extraocular polymyositis. Vet Pathol 1989;26:510–512.

Gwin RM, et al. Ophthalmic nodular fasciitis in the dog. J Am Vet Med Assoc 1977;170:611–614.

Moore CP, et al. Equine pseudotumors. Vet Ophthalmol 2000;3:57–63.

Paulsen ME, et al. Nodular granulomatous episclerokeratitis in dogs: 19 cases (1973–1985). J Am Vet Med Assoc 1987;190:1581–1587.

Smith JS, et al. Infiltrative corneal lesions resembling fibrous histiocytoma: clinical and pathologic findings in six dogs and one cat. J Am Vet Med Assoc 1976;169:722–726.

OCULAR NEOPLASIA

Although the eye is the site of a wide range of primary and metastatic neoplasms, only a few are of sufficient prevalence or importance to justify discussion here. This is not to say that neoplasia is unimportant, and in fact exactly the opposite is true. *At least in dogs and cats, which are the species from which we are most likely to receive histologic specimens for assessment, neoplasia is second only to glaucoma as a cause for enucleation.*

Primary ocular tumors may arise from the eyelids and adnexa, from optic nerve, or from within the globe. Those arising within the globe may originate from any of the tissues, but only those from uveal melanoblasts and iridociliary neurectoderm are anything other than rare. *Most primary intraocular tumors have negligible potential for metastasis.* Dogs and cats are most frequently affected; primary intraocular neoplasms are inexplicably rare in other domestic species.

Metastatic ocular neoplasia is reported rather infrequently but it is common when sought. Multicentric lymphoma in cats, dogs, and cattle regularly involves the eye, although in cattle the retrobulbar tissue is preferred over the eye itself. *With the exception of malignant lymphoma, carcinomas are reported more frequently than sarcomas.* This probably reflects the greater metastatic potential of carcinomas in general rather than any specific difference in ocular tropism. Uveal vessels are the usual sites of lodgement, and ocular disease may result from vessel occlusion, or from inflammation in response to tumor antigen, or to necrosis of either tumor or damaged host tissue. *Hyphema is more common in eyes with tumor-induced uveitis than with uveitis of other causes and is therefore a diagnostically useful sign.*

Bibliography

Dubielzig RR. Ocular neoplasia in small animals. Vet Clin North Am: Small Anim Pract 1990;20:837–848.

Dugan SJ. Ocular neoplasia. Vet Clin North Am 1992;8:609–626.

Miller PE, Dubielzig RR. Ocular Tumors. In: Withrow SJ, MacEwen EG, eds. A Small Animal Clinical Oncology. 3rd edn. Philadelphia, PA: W.B.Saunders, 2001:532–545.

Wilcock BP, et al. Histological Classification of Ocular and Otic Tumors of Domestic Animals. WHO International Histologic Classification of Tumors of Domestic Animals. Second Series. Washington, DC: AFIP, 2002.

Eyelid and conjunctival neoplasms

Squamous cell carcinoma

Squamous cell carcinoma arises from the conjunctival epithelium of the limbus, third eyelid, or eyelid in cattle, horses, cats, and dogs, in that order of frequency. **Bovine** *ocular squamous cell carcinoma is one of the most common and most economically significant neoplasms of domestic animals.* Its relative rarity in dogs is peculiar and unexplained.

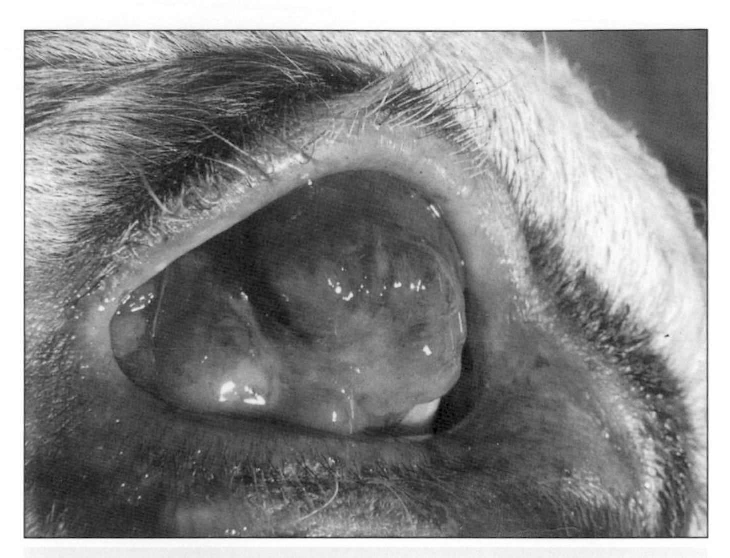

Figure 4.74 Squamous cell carcinoma in an ox.

The prevalence of the disease in all species is related to exposure to ultraviolet radiation and to lack of pigment in lids and conjunctiva. Its geographic prevalence is therefore directly correlated with altitude and inversely correlated with latitude, as well as with the prevalence of animals with poor periocular pigmentation. In cattle, in which this disease is of greatest significance, the prevalence is highest in the "white-faced" Hereford breed and in the high altitude regions of the Canadian and American West. It also occurs in other breeds of cattle, as well as Indian water buffalo, sheep, and cattalo (Fig. 4.74). Variation in prevalence in different lines of Herefords even in the same region has led to speculation that other genetic factors within the breed, other than facial pigmentation, may influence susceptibility. The question of etiology has been further widened by demonstration of papillomaviruses in some of the papillomatous precursor lesions that eventually transform into squamous cell carcinoma. Similar papillomaviruses, as well as being the causative agents of cutaneous warts, have been demonstrated in bovine alimentary papillomas in Scotland, and viral DNA persists in the squamous-cell carcinomas that arise from these papillomas in cattle grazing pastures that contain bracken fern. It remains to be determined whether or not there is any relationship between a viral component of the ocular carcinoma and the fact that in many cases the tumor regresses after immunotherapy. *At least at the moment, no viral particle or viral genome has been consistently demonstrated in ocular squamous cell carcinomas in any species.* Environmental co-carcinogens such as those in bracken fern have not yet been implicated in the induction of ocular tumors.

The tumor in all species develops through a series of premalignant stages, called epidermal plaques and papillomas, before proceeding over months or years to carcinoma in-situ and to invasive carcinoma (Fig. 4.75). Spontaneous regression of the precancerous lesions may occur with an estimated frequency of 25–50%. At least in cattle, plaques are much more common (about 6:1) than papillomas or outright carcinomas. The *epidermal plaque* is characterized by marked acanthosis, with variable presence of keratinization, dyskeratosis, and epidermal downgrowth into the subconjuctival connective tissue. Invasion through basal layer or basement membrane is not seen. *Papilloma* also involves acanthosis but, in addition, there is marked para- and hyperkeratosis with

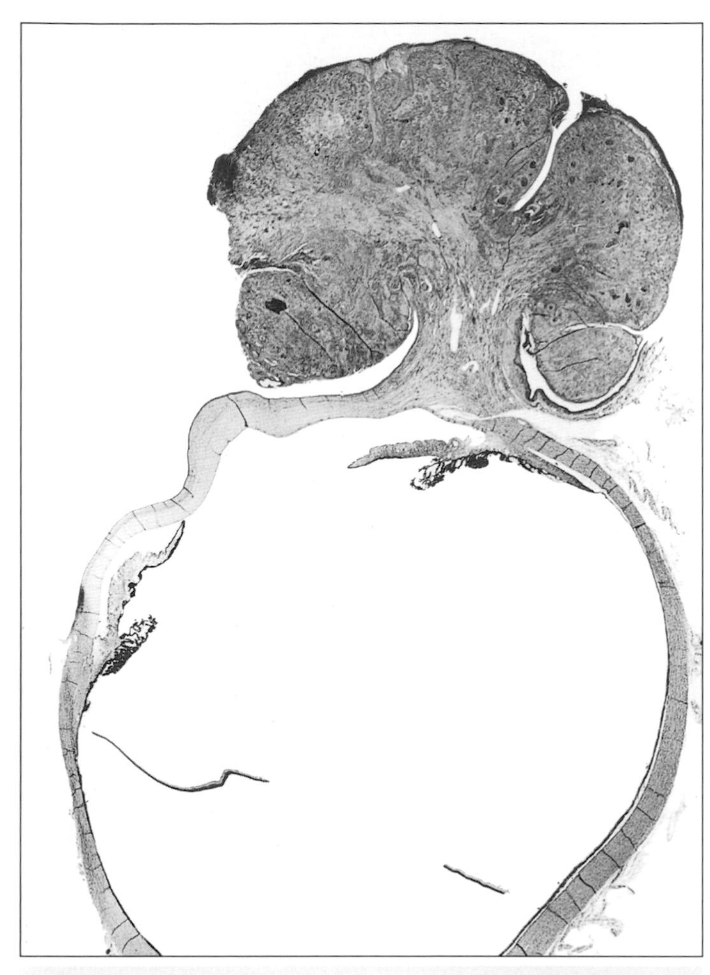

Figure 4.75 Squamous papilloma of corneoscleral junction in an ox.

papillary projections supported by a vascularized connective tissue core. Papillomas may be up to 3.0 cm in diameter, pedunculated or sessile, and are often ulcerated. *Carcinoma in situ* arises by focal or multifocal transformation of increasingly dysplastic cell nests in the deep layers of plaques or papillomas. *Fully developed carcinoma* has squamous cell invasion across the basement membrane. Tumor invasion is almost always accompanied by *intense lymphocytic-plasmacytic infiltration*, presumably the host response to tumor antigen. It is assumed that it is this response that is responsible for regression of some of the precursor lesions, although spontaneous regression of fully developed carcinoma is rare. Stimulation of immune-mediated rejection by intralesional inoculation of antigenic tumor extracts or nonspecific lymphocyte stimulants induces partial or total regression of small tumors.

Histologically, ocular squamous cell carcinoma resembles similar tumors in other sites and ranges from well-differentiated carcinomas with keratin pearl formation to anaplastic carcinomas with marked nuclear size variation and mononuclear tumor giant cells (Fig. 4.76A, B). *Metastatic or invasive potential has not been correlated with histologic criteria, but there is a correlation between site of origin and subsequent behavior.* Most surveys in cattle identify the bulbar conjunctiva of the limbus as the most frequent site of origin, estimated at about 70% of all occurrences. Some surveys consider nictitating membrane as next most frequent, with palpebral conjunctiva of the true eyelid as third. Other reports claim nictitans origin to be uncommon, and eyelid tumors to be as common as those of limbic origin. Tumors arise only very rarely from the cornea because of the limited mitotic capability of that tissue. Apparent corneal tumors are almost always extensions from tumors arising at the limbus. Tumors arising at the limbus are confronted by the dense and poorly vascularized connective tissue of sclera and peripheral cornea, which retards metastasis to extraocular sites. Invasion of corneal stroma and sclera occurs slowly, but intraocular invasion is very uncommon (Fig. 4.77). Tumors arising from the nictitans extend to the root of the membrane and then to the cartilage and bone of the orbit and internal nares. *Metastasis probably will eventually occur in all instances*, with parotid lymph node the initial site. Wide dissemination to thoracic and abdominal organs has been reported and is probably limited only by the limited longevity of the target animals.

Squamous cell carcinoma of the **equine** eye is much less thoroughly documented, but is quite common. In contrast to cattle, *the preferred site is the edge of the third eyelid, followed by limbic bulbar conjunctiva.* This targeting is, again, inversely correlated with the presence of protective melanin pigmentation, and is positively correlated with those factors causing increased exposure to ultraviolet radiation. In some reports, heavy draft horses are predisposed, but all breeds may be affected. The mean age of affected horses is about 9 years. Bilateral involvement is seen in 15–20%. The same range of precancerous lesions occurs in horses as in cattle. Prognosis is strongly influenced by therapy, but even the untreated neoplasm is slow to metastasize and even then it is usually only to local lymph nodes. Retrospective studies document 10–15% of equine ocular squamous cell carcinomas to have regional or distant spread, but the data do not consider duration of the disease prior to therapy.

In **cats,** *ocular squamous cell carcinoma most frequently affects the skin or palpebral conjunctiva of the eyelids.* White cats are particularly susceptible, and squamous cell carcinomas in these animals may occur simultaneously or sequentially on eyelids, ear pinnae, nose, and lips. The early lesion is one of sunlight-induced epithelial necrosis, and even the early neoplasm may be ulcerated and inflamed to a degree that may mask its neoplastic character and delay appropriate therapy. Growth tends to be circumferential around the lid margins, resulting in a palpebral fissure bordered by a thickened, red, and ulcerated tumor. Metastasis to local lymph nodes occurs late in the course of the disease.

In **dogs,** *squamous cell carcinoma infrequently involves the eye.* Proliferative eyelid or conjunctival growths in dogs are much more likely to be Meibomian adenomas, viral and nonviral papillomas, or nodular granulomatous episcleritis. In one study of 202 canine eyelid neoplasms, squamous cell carcinoma accounted for only 2% of lesions. Precancerous changes probably occur but, in contrast to cattle and horses, eyelid papillomas in dogs are usually benign and nonprogressive lesions.

Bibliography

Anderson DE, Badzioch M. Association between solar radiation and ocular squamous cell carcinoma in cattle. Am J Vet Res 1991;52:784–787.

Anson MA, et al. Bovine herpesvirus-5 (DN-599) antigens in cells derived from bovine ocular squamous cell carcinoma. Can J Comp Med 1982;46:334–337.

Atluru D, et al. Tumor-associated antigens of bovine cancer eye. Vet Immun Immunopathol 1982;3:279–286.

Dugan SJ, et al. Prognostic factors and survival of horses with ocular/adnexal squamous cell carcinoma: 147 cases (1978–1988). J Am Vet Med Assoc 1991;198:298–303.

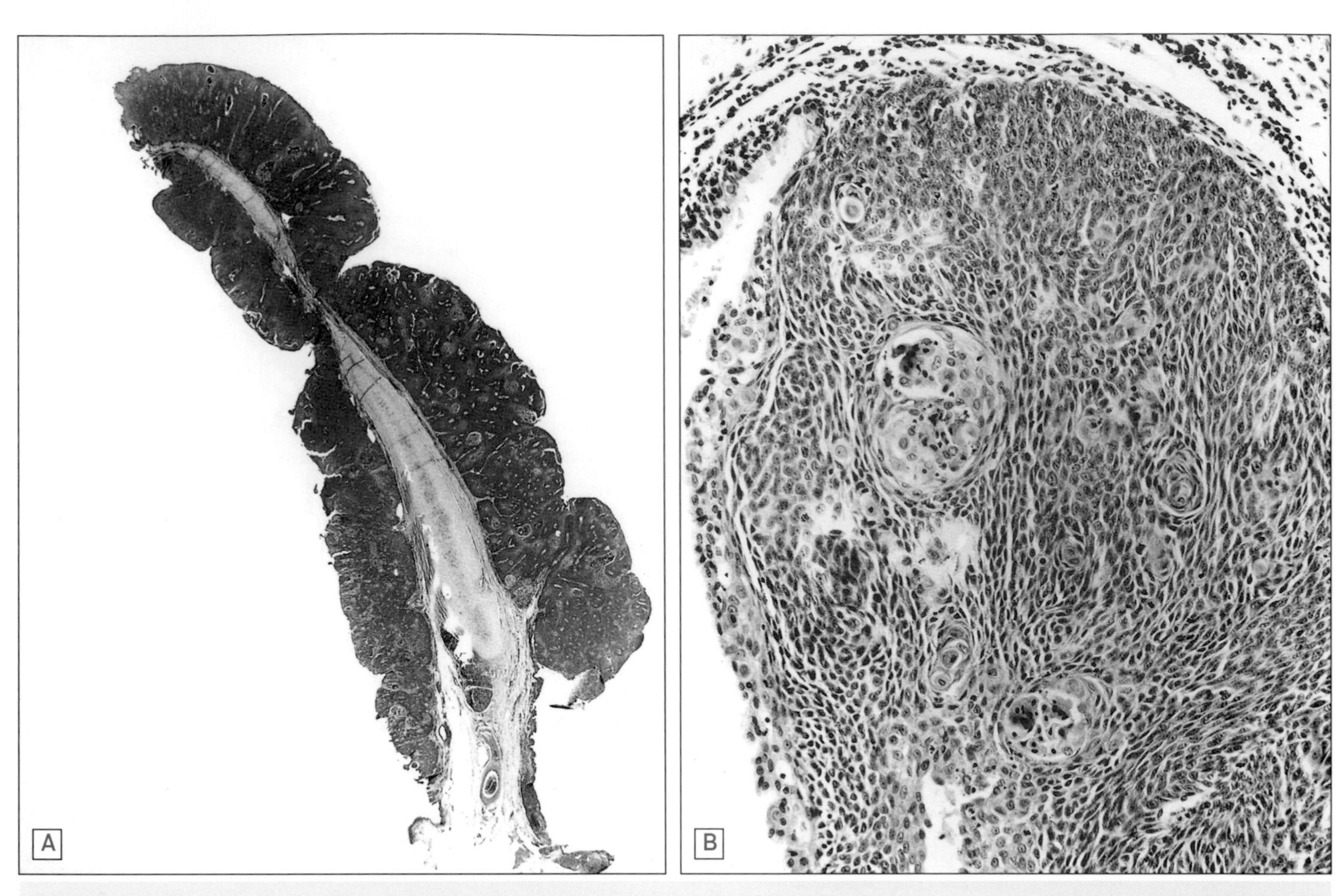

Figure 4.76 A. Early squamous cell carcinoma involving conjunctiva of nictitating membrane in a horse. **B.** Histology of **A**; disorderly and defective maturation, premature keratinization, and invasion across the basement membrane.

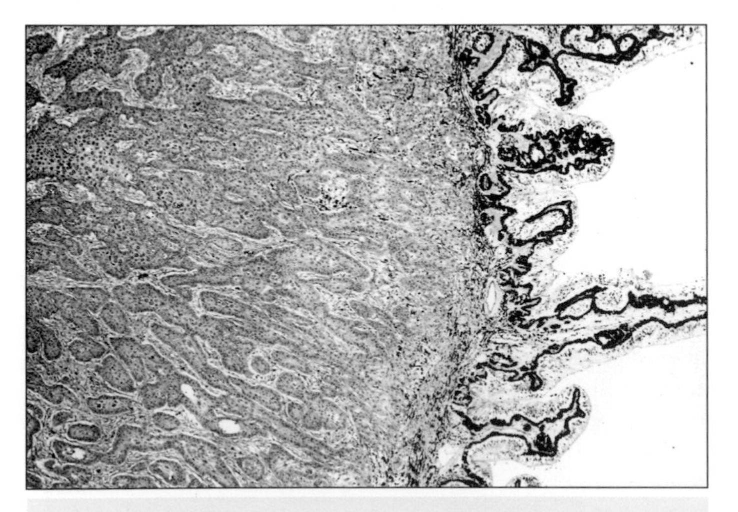

Figure 4.77 Scleral squamous cell carcinoma in a horse has grown inward to approach ciliary processes, an unusual behavior for these normally exophytic tumors.

Rutten VP, et al. Search for bovine papilloma virus DNA in bovine ocular squamous cell carcinomas (BOSCC) and BOSCC-derived cell lines. Am J Vet Res 1992;53:1477–1481.

Teifke JP, Lohr CV. Immunohistochemical detection of P53 overexpression in paraffin wax-embedded squamous cell carcinomas of cattle, horses, cats and dogs. J Comp Pathol 1996;114:205–210.

Williams LW, Gelatt KN. Ocular squamous cell carcinoma. In: Gelatt KN, ed. Veterinary Ophthalmology. Philadelphia, PA: Lea and Febiger, 1981:622–632.

Meibomian adenoma

Meibomian adenoma is the most common ocular neoplasm of dogs, accounting for at least 70% of eyelid tumors. It is comparable in many respects to sebaceous adenomas found elsewhere in the skin. However, these tumors originate specifically from Meibomian gland and not from other eyelid sebaceous glands, and they regularly have at least some histologic features that are infrequently seen in their cutaneous sebaceous counterparts. In the eyelid tumors, *the lobules of foamy, eosinophilic sebaceous cells are intermingled with a prominent population of basal (reserve) cells.* The basal cells often account for 50% or more of the tumor cells. In many instances, the basal cell component is so prominent as to cause diagnosis to be made of basal cell tumor with sebaceous differentiation (comparable to cutaneous sebaceous epithelioma) or even Meibomian adenocarcinoma. Many have substantial melanin within the basal cells. None metastasize, and even the so-called carcinomas show little inclination for invasive growth. Other distinctive but not invariable features are papillary hyperplasia of the overlying epithelium of the eyelid margin, a marked lymphocytic-plasmacytic infiltrate among tumor lobules and around the tumor margins, and a localized granulomatous response (chalazion) to leaking secretion (Fig. 4.78A, B).

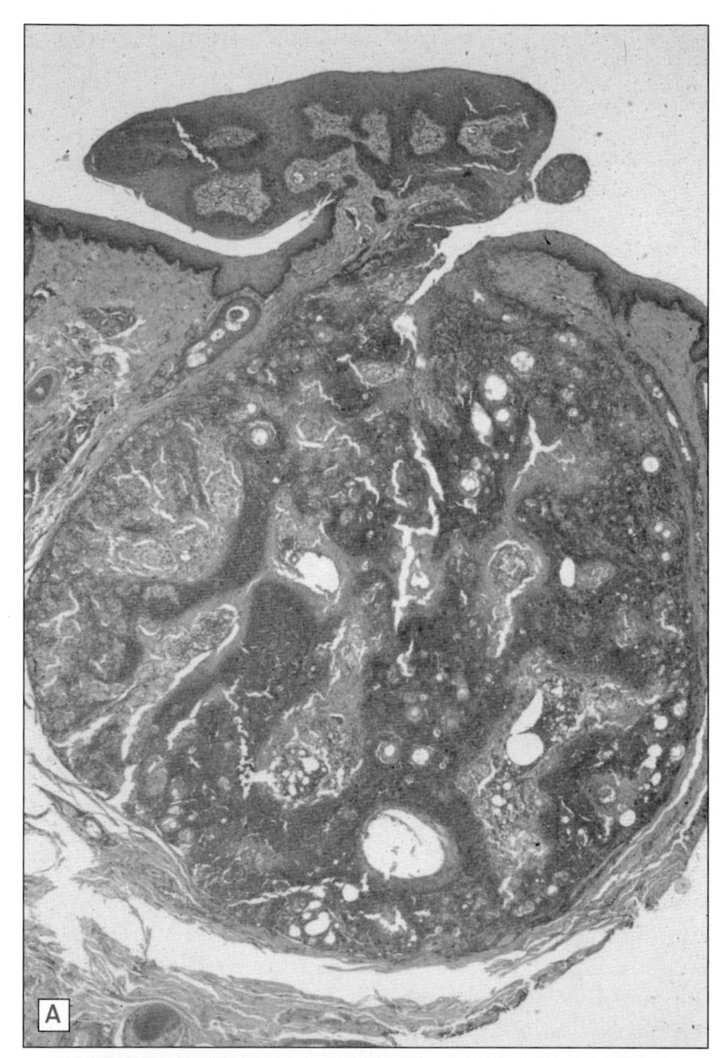

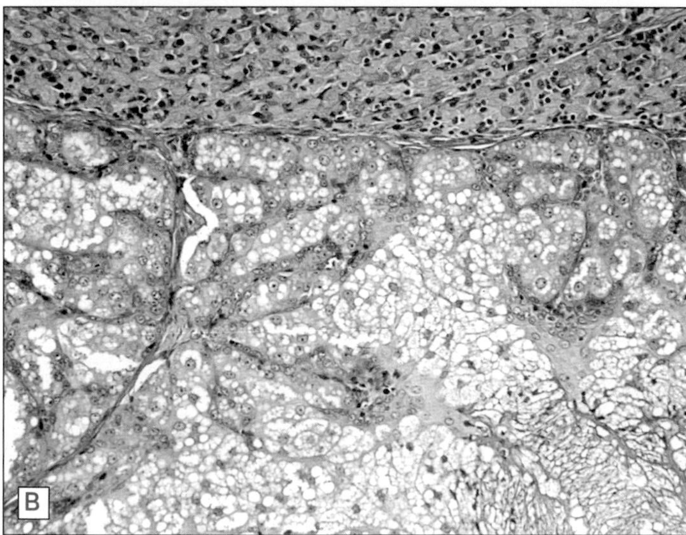

Figure 4.78 Meibomian adenoma. A. The relative proportions of germinal basal cells and mature sebaceous cells vary widely, but without any apparent prognostic significance. Papillary hyperplasia of the overlying eyelid marginal skin is frequently seen. **B.** Meibomian adenoma (below) with a surrounding zone of foamy macrophages (above) typical of chalazion.

Other adnexal and conjunctival tumors

A wide range of neoplasms has been reported to occasionally affect the conjunctiva or adnexa of domestic animals. Most examples are reported primarily in dogs, and they are listed below in order of overall prevalence in that species.

Melanocytoma *is probably the second most common tumor of the eyelid in dogs*. It will occasionally occur in cats and in gray horses. In dogs it is a typical cutaneous benign melanoma, identical to what occur so frequently anywhere else in skin. In cats, they are also similar to those tumors occurring elsewhere in skin, and more than half are both histologically and behaviorally malignant. It is important to note that the behavior of melanocytic tumors associated with the eye is greatly influenced by exact anatomic location, so these comments are applicable only to those melanomas arising in the haired skin of the eyelid.

Other melanomas arising from conjunctiva are described below in the section on Melanotic tumors of the eye. In brief, **limbal (epibulbar) melanocytoma** arises from the melanocytes that inhabit the stroma of the corneoscleral junction. It is benign. In contrast, **primary conjunctival melanoma** arises from the melanocytes of the palpebral or bulbar conjunctiva itself, and most examples are behaviorally aggressive.

Conjunctival papilloma usually arises from bulbar conjunctiva as a series of slender protruding stalks of conjunctival lamina propria covered by bland, often pigmented, stratified squamous epithelium with no cytologic atypia and no ballooning degeneration as is typical of viral papillomas. Viral papillomas associated with *Canine oral papillomavirus*, identical to those affecting the mouth, will occasionally occur in any portion of conjunctiva.

Conjunctival vascular tumors *represent a continuum from telangiectasia to hemangioma and hemangiosarcoma*. They arise with equal frequency in the temporal (lateral) bulbar conjunctiva and along the leading edge of the third eyelid, suggesting that sunlight is important in their pathogenesis. They usually arise in the very superficial subepithelial vascular plexus. *Surgical excision is invariably curative*, with virtually no metastatic risk regardless of cytologic and histologic criteria of malignancy. Some examples are associated with *marked dysplastic pseudocarcinomatous hyperplasia of the overlying conjunctival epithelium that divides the vascular tumor into lobules*, and some use the term **angiokeratoma** to describe this variant. It behaves as do the other conjunctival vascular tumors. Behaviorally malignant examples seem more prevalent in horses, where more than half of the reported cases are solid hemangiosarcomas with very aggressive local infiltration and, usually, distant metastasis. They are easily mistaken for fibrosarcomas because they have such poor channel formation and so little blood. Indeed, some of these might arise from lymphatic endothelium. There is much speculation, but no proof, that sunlight is important in their causation.

Nodular granulomatous episcleritis (also known as ocular nodular fasciitis, ocular fibrous histiocytoma) *is not a neoplasm*, but its clinical appearance is easily confused with neoplasia and samples will be submitted as probable neoplasms. It is more fully discussed under Diseases of the sclera.

Mast cell tumors, with the same histologic range as those rising elsewhere in skin, may occur in the conjunctiva of dogs. Their biological behavior has not been documented. In cats, mast cell tumors more commonly arise within the haired skin of the eyelid.

Adenocarcinoma of the gland of the third eyelid occurs as a nodular swelling in very old dogs (mean age 11.5 years). They occur, albeit very rarely, in cats. *They are locally infiltrative, recur after attempted resection, but are cured by complete removal of the third eyelid.* Only chronically neglected cases metastasize to lung after a very protracted local expansion. Histologically, these are tubular carcinomas with abundant squamous metaplasia. They should not be confused with the prominence of the gland that occurs with prolapse of the gland ("cherry eye") or with lymphocytic interstitial adenitis.

Lymphoma may have several ocular manifestations, the most frequent of which are diffuse uveal metastases as part of generalized lymphoma in dogs or cats, or as retrobulbar tumor in cattle. It may occasionally occur as a conjunctival disease as part of generalized lymphoma or as a mucocutaneous manifestation of epitheliotropic lymphoma. There are several reports of conjunctival or third eyelid lymphoma occurring in horses and in cats as an apparently isolated lesion that can be cured by local excision, suggesting that they have actually arisen in those locations.

Bibliography

Collins BK, et al. Biologic behavior and histologic characteristics of canine conjunctival melanoma. Prog Vet Comp Ophthalmol 1993;3:135–140.

George C, Summers BA. Angiokeratoma: a benign vascular tumor of the dog. J Small Anim Pract 1990;31:390–392.

Glaze MB, et al. A case of equine adnexal lymphosarcoma. Eq Vet J 1990; 10:83–84.

Håkanson N, et al. Granuloma formation following subconjunctival injection of triamcinolone in two dogs. J Am Anim Hosp Assoc 1991;27:89–92.

Hargis AM, et al. Tumor and tumor-like lesions of perilimbal conjunctiva in laboratory dogs. J Am Vet Med Assoc 1978;173:1185–1190.

Krehbiel JD, Langham RF. Eyelid neoplasms of dogs. Am J Vet Res 1975;36:115–119.

Martin CL. Canine epibulbar melanomas and their management. J Am Anim Hosp Assoc 1981;17:83–90.

Moore PF, et al. Ocular angiosarcoma in the horse: morphological and immunohistochemical studies. Vet Pathol 1988;23:240–244.

Mughannam AJ, et al. Conjunctival vascular tumors in six dogs. Comp Vet Pathol 1997;7:56–59.

Paulsen ME, et al. Nodular granulomatous episcleritokeratitis in dogs: 19 cases (1973–1985). J Am Vet Med Assoc 1987;190:1581–1587.

Roberts SM, et al. Prevalence and treatment of palpebral neoplasms in the dog: 200 cases (1975–1983). J Am Vet Med Assoc 1986;189:1355–1359.

Wilcock BP, Peiffer RL. Adenocarcinoma of the gland of the third eyelid in seven dogs. J Am Vet Med Assoc 1988;193:1549–1550.

Melanotic tumors of the eye

Our understanding of the biology of primary ocular melanomas in animals has suffered greatly from the premature assumption that they were similar to the much-studied human ocular melanomas. Perhaps because of this error, a great many enucleated globes were available for histologic evaluation, inadvertently allowing the flurry of retrospective studies that eventually established ocular melanomas in dogs and cats as distinct entities quite different in structure and behavior from the human neoplasms.

Primary melanocytic tumors of the eye or adnexa are common in dogs and cats, rare in horses, and almost nonexistent in other domestic species. Even in dogs and cats, the prevalence and behavior of the various types of ocular melanomas and melanocytomas differ markedly, so that generalizations must be studiously avoided.

In **dogs**, this list of distinct clinical/histologic entities includes benign eyelid melanocytoma, malignant conjunctival melanoma, limbal melanocytoma, anterior uveal melanocytoma, and choroidal melanocytoma. In **cats**, the list is the same but it is dominated by diffuse iris melanoma. Malignant cutaneous melanomas occasionally affect the eyelid or arise within the conjunctiva, and there are a few reports of limbal and anterior uveal melanocytomas similar to those occurring in dogs. In **horses**, one encounters cutaneous melanocytomas in the skin of the eyelids, primarily in gray horses. There are a few reports of benign anterior uveal melanocytomas, and one report of a locally invasive, histologically malignant conjunctival melanoma.

Melanocytomas and malignant melanomas arising within the haired skin of canine and feline eyelid, respectively, are identical to those arising elsewhere in the skin and they will not be further discussed here.

Melanomas arising in the conjunctiva are very infrequent compared to most other ocular melanocytic tumors. The few case reports do not allow for generalizations about behavior, but *they often are histologically and behaviorally malignant.* Their relationship to eyelid melanoma seems analogous to those of the lip, where melanomas of the haired exterior lip are benign like most skin melanomas, while those of the mucous membrane of the inside of the lip are malignant like those elsewhere in the mouth. Conjunctival melanomas may appear as well-pigmented tumors of bland, plump melanocytes with little anisokaryosis or mitotic activity, or as cytologically malignant tumors with marked anisocytosis, anisokaryosis, hyperchromasia, and even multinucleation. Primary conjunctival melanomas often are poorly melanotic. The most reliable histologic criterion in such cases is the observation of intraepithelial nests of tumor cells. Local recurrence and spread after excision is frequent, and metastasis to lung has been reported.

Limbal (epibulbar) melanocytoma *is a histologically and behaviorally benign tumor* of the melanocytes normally found in an oblique line that demarcates the junction of corneal stroma with sclera at the limbus. The tumor is composed of large plump melanocytes with a central nucleus and abundant cytoplasmic pigment. Mitotic figures are absent and nuclear variation is minimal. The tumor grows outwardly as a protruding spherical nodule, hence the alternative name of *epibulbar melanoma*. There may be nodular expansion into peripheral cornea, but virtually never into the uvea or anterior chamber. *Except for location, these tumors are identical to anterior uveal melanocytomas.* This creates a problem when one encounters the tumor that occupies both the anterior uvea and the limbus. These should be assumed to be anterior uveal melanocytomas extending outwardly, since it appears that primary limbal melanocytomas have essentially no ability to invade the globe.

Anterior uveal melanocytoma *is the most frequent intraocular tumor in dogs*. It is topographically, histologically, and behaviorally unrelated to human epithelioid ocular melanomas to which it was long compared. The typical tumor arises from melanocytes of the iris root or adjacent ciliary body, and is composed of variable proportions of lightly pigmented spindle cells and heavily pigmented plump melanocytes identical to those of limbal melanomas. The spindle cells are assumed to be the proliferative population, and the plump cells probably represent the mature, end-stage melanocytes with a storehouse of cytoplasmic pigment (Fig. 4.79A, B, C).

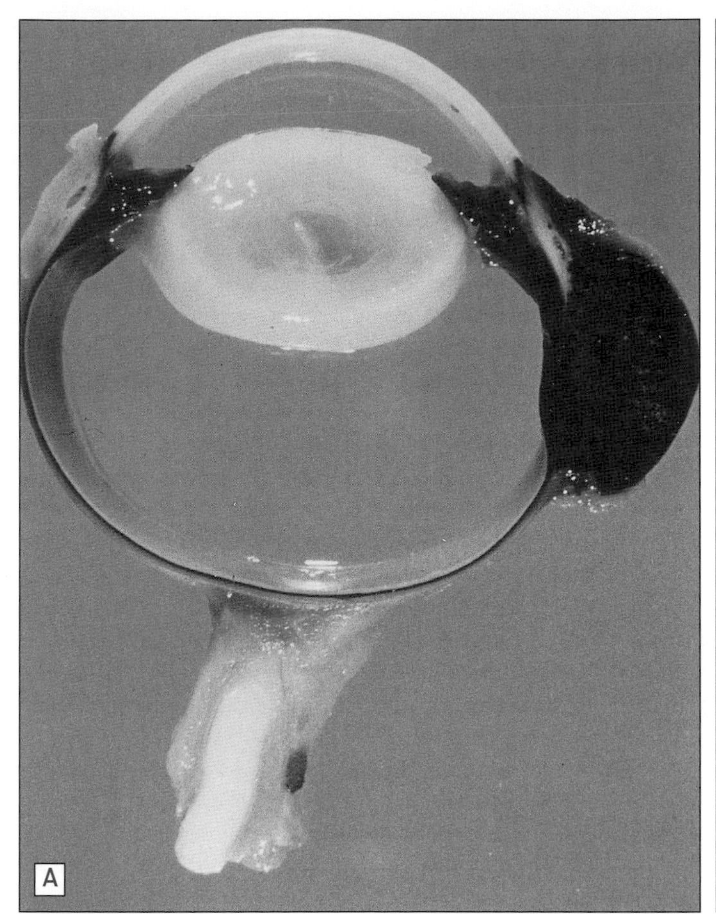

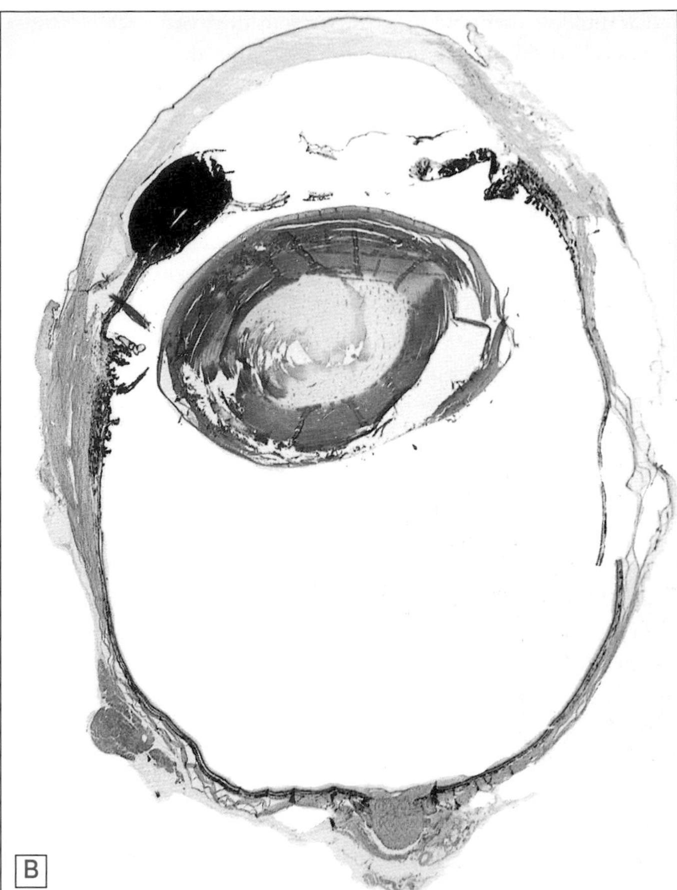

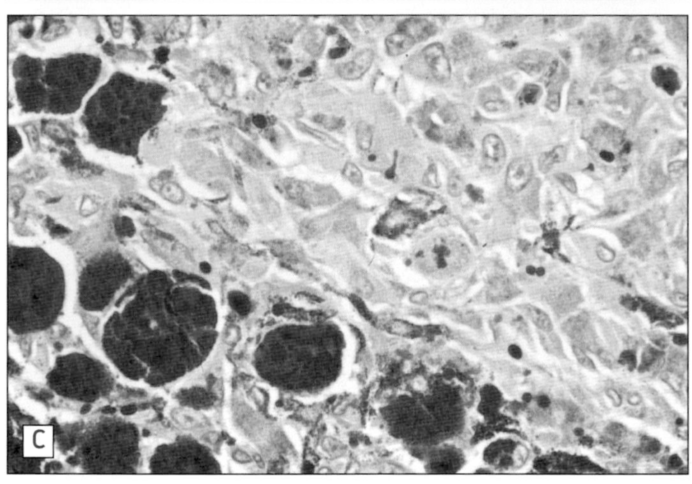

Figure 4.79 Anterior uveal melanocytoma. **A.** Tumor with extension through the trabecular meshwork to grow as a **subconjunctival nodule**. Distinguishing this tumor, clinically, from primary limbal melanoma can be difficult. **B.** Unusually **discrete** example. **C.** Example, dominated by heavily pigmented endstage **"plump cells"** with just a few poorly pigmented, spindle-to-polygonal-shaped germinal cells.

The diagnosis itself presents no problem, but offering an accurate prognosis is more complex. About 15% of all canine anterior uveal melanocytomas are histologically malignant, and one-third of these (or about 5% of all uveal melanocytomas) have been confirmed to be behaviorally malignant by virtue of extraocular metastases. *This small group of genuine malignancies can be predicted by mitotic index*. Histologically malignant tumors are dominated by the spindle cells rather than the plump cells, are more lightly pigmented, have much more anisokaryosis and more mitotic figures than the benign tumors. Of these, mitotic index is the most reliable predictor of behavior. Benign tumors have virtually no mitotic figures. Those confirmed as behaviorally malignant have three or more (usually many more!) mitoses in ten high-power (40×) microscopic fields; conversely, not all tumors with high mitotic index are destined for metastasis.

Even these benign melanocytomas are eventually significant to the eye, spreading transsclerally and circumferentially within the globe. *Glaucoma* from occlusion of ciliary cleft is probably the eventual fate of all eyes with this neoplasm. *Uveitis* from tumor necrosis or *hyphema* from tumor-induced uveal neovascularization are other frequent accompaniments.

Feline multifocal uveal melanocytoma *is a rare tumor of cats* that looks histologically identical to the canine uveal melanocytomas. They are sufficiently different from the much more common diffuse iris melanoma of cats to justify a separate classification. There is no published information about metastatic risk. They seem to arise as multiple foci randomly throughout the uveal tract, expanding inwardly to create multiple nodules within the ocular cavities, and sometimes outwardly as space-occupying scleral nodules.

Equine anterior uveal melancytomas occur most often in gray horses, many quite young (less than 8 years). Most involve anterior uvea and are histologically similar to the benign uveal melanocytomas of dogs. None has metastasized. Although almost all intraocular melanocytic tumors of cats are diffuse iris melanomas, one will occasionally encounter focal or **multifocal melanocytomas** similar to those of dogs. Other than having a more unpredictable site of origin within the uveal tract, they seem histologically and behaviorally identical to their more common canine counterparts.

Choroidal melanocytomas account for about 80% of all human ocular melanomas, but are rare in other species. The few cases described in dogs were discovered as incidental findings on fundoscopic examination, and grew very slowly. They seem very similar to the benign melanocytomas of limbus or anterior uvea: well pigmented, cytologically bland, and cause clinical signs only by their slow expansion to cause retinal detachment or compression of optic nerve. There is a single report of systemic metastasis from a tumor that looked histologically benign.

Clinically insignificant **iris nevi** or **freckles** occur in dogs as nonprogressive pigmented spots. Their only significance is to cause unnecessary enucleation. Histologically, the lesions are well-circumscribed clusters of bland melanocytes adjacent to the anterior border layer of the iris.

Feline diffuse iris melanomas are unique. The usual clinical presentation is of patchy iris hyperpigmentation that very slowly progresses to diffuse iris hyperpigmentation and thickening over several years. *The eventual outcome is virtually always glaucoma* (Fig. 4.80A).

It was at first considered an interesting but benign lesion. Subsequent retrospective studies have been unanimous in documenting a *moderate metastatic risk*. Because cats seem even more elusive than dogs in terms of follow-up studies, the actual number of cases with good postoperative data is small, and considerable debate persists among ophthalmologists about the real risk of metastasis by these tumors. It seems clear that the probability that a cat will die from metastatic disease is low, but the prevalence of clinically silent visceral metastasis is quite high. This contrast is probably related to the very slow growth rate of the metastatic tumor foci, which is exactly what happens within the globe itself.

Histologically, these tumors diffusely infiltrate the stroma of the iris and the ciliary cleft, and then the overlying sclera, peripheral cornea, and ciliary body. They are notoriously pleomorphic, and are apt to be misdiagnosed by those pathologists not aware of this disease as malignant lymphoma or anaplastic metastatic malignancy. Tumor cells vary from spindle-shaped cells to multinucleated epithelioid cells (Fig. 4.80B, C). Pigmentation often is light and the cytoplasm may be foamy and eosinophilic. Balloon cells with foamy cytoplasm and very distinct cell boundaries are frequent in some tumors. The accurate prediction of tumor behavior is compromised, in all published studies, by the low percentage of affected cats available for follow-up. Metastasis has been correlated with large tumor size, intrascleral spread, and mitotic index.

It remains unclear whether cats also can have focal-to-coalescing hyperpigmentation of the anterior iris stroma that is not precancerous. Some cases, as in dogs, seem nonprogressive and harmless (although follow-up information is anecdotal). Others slowly coalesce and thicken, at which time they are indistinguishable from diffuse iris melanoma. When sampled for histology, virtually all such lesions look like early melanomas, but of course, most of these apparently harmless, nonprogressive lesions do not receive histologic evaluation!

Pigmentary (melanocytic) glaucoma *is included here because it is histologically indistinguishable from a diffuse uveal melanocytoma.* The syndrome was originally described as a bilateral but asymmetrical massive pigmentation of the uveal tract of Cairn Terrier dogs that seemed to be causing glaucoma. Histologically, the anterior uvea and even the choroid are thickened by a heavy, diffuse accumulation of large plump cells histologically indistinguishable from those of ordinary canine anterior uveal melanocytoma. The syndrome has been described in a few other breeds in association with glaucoma, but the syndrome remains controversial because one can encounter equally heavy pigmentation in clinically normal globes from breeds that typically have very heavy pigmentation, such as Kerry Blue Terriers, Scottish Terriers, black Labradors, and others. *The causal relationship between the pigmentation and glaucoma therefore remains somewhat controversial.* Some would prefer to refer to the disease as "canine diffuse uveal melanosis," or even as diffuse uveal melanocytoma. Original claims that these accumulating cells are abnormal melanocytes have been challenged by recent electron microscopy indicating that the majority of the accumulating cells are melanin-laden macrophages. That is perhaps not surprising and it does not rule out the possibility that this is indeed a melanocytic proliferative disorder that, over time, has had a lot of leakage of melanin and thus a lot of macrophage recruitment.

Bibliography

Acland GM, et al. Diffuse iris melanoma in cats. J Am Vet Med Assoc 1980;176:52–56.

Barnett KC, Platt H. Intraocular melanomata in the horse. Eq Vet J 1990;10:76–82.

Belkin PV. Malignant melanoma of the bulbar conjunctiva in a dog. Vet Med Small Anim Clin 1975;70:957–958.

Cook CS, et al. Malignant melanoma of the conjunctiva in a cat. J Am Vet Med Assoc 1985;5:505–506.

Dubielzig RR, et al. Choroidal melanomas in dogs. Vet Pathol 1985;22:582–585.

Duncan DE, Peiffer RL. Morphology and prognostic indicators of anterior uveal melanomas in cats. Prog Vet Comp Ophthalmol 1991;1:25–32.

Gelatt KN, et al. Primary iridal pigmented masses in three dogs. J Am Anim Hosp Assoc 1979;15:339–344.

Giuliano EA, et al. A matched observational study of canine survival with primary intraocular melanocytic neoplasia. Vet Ophthalmol 1999;2:185–190.

Harling DE, et al. Feline limbal melanoma: four cases. J Am Anim Hosp Assoc 1986;22:795–802.

Harris BP, Dubielzig RR. Atypical primary ocular melanoma in cats. Vet Ophthal 1999;2:121–124.

Hirst LW, Jabs DA. Benign epibulbar melanocytoma in a horse. J Am Vet Med Assoc 1983;183:333–334.

Kalishman JB, et al. A matched observational study of survival in cats with enucleation due to diffuse iris melanoma. Vet Ophthalmol 1998;1:25–29.

Martin CL. Canine epibulbar melanomas and their management. J Am Anim Hosp Assoc 1981;17:83–90.

Moore CP, et al. Conjunctival malignant melanoma in a horse. Vet Ophthalmol 2000;3:201–208.

Patnaik AK, Mooney S. Feline melanoma: a comparative study of ocular, oral, and dermal neoplasms. Vet Pathol 1988;25:105–112.

Roels S, Ducatelle R. Malignant melanoma of the nictitating membrane in a cat (*Felis vulgaris*). J Comp Pathol 1998;119:189–193.

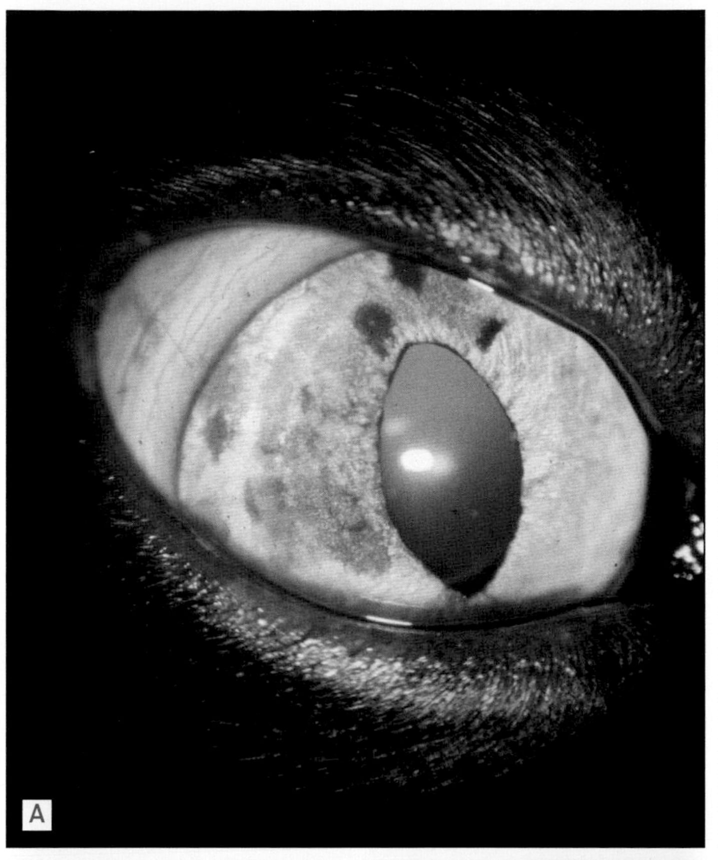

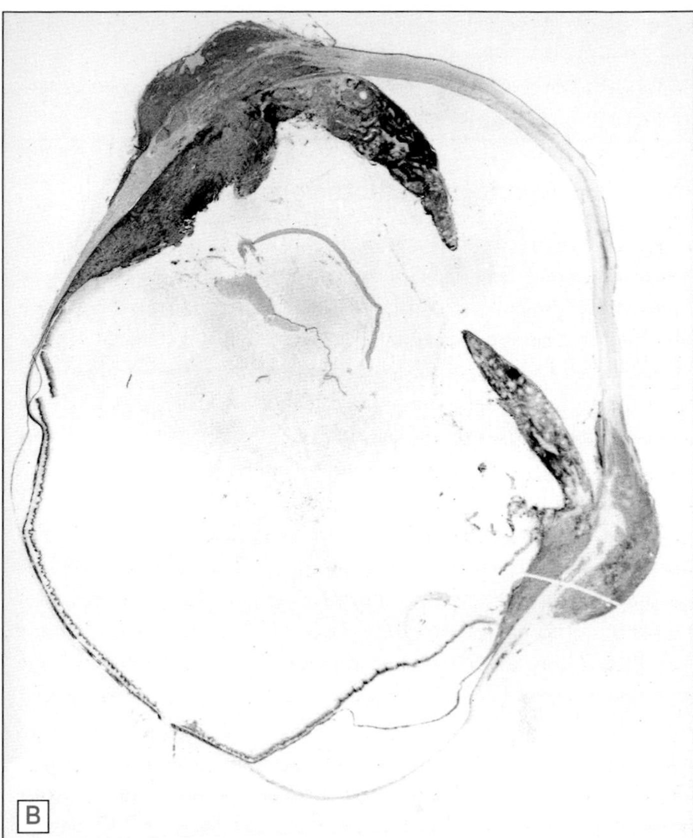

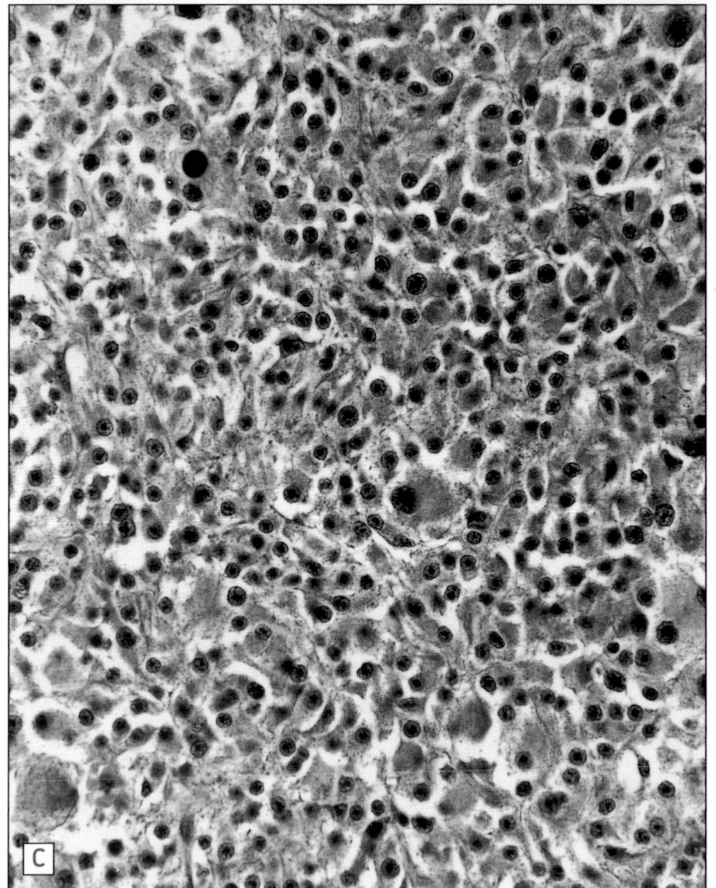

Figure 4.80 Feline diffuse iris melanoma. **A.** Gross presentation. **B.** Low magnification illustrating the typical, diffuse growth habit and scleral invasion. **C.** Pleomorphic round cells; pigmentation is light and mononuclear giant cells are conspicuous.

Roswitha ROM, et al. Abnormal ocular pigmented deposition and glaucoma in the dog. Vet Ophthalmol 2003;6:273–278.

Wilcock BP, Peiffer RL, Jr. Morphology and behavior of primary ocular melanomas in 91 dogs. Vet Pathol 1986;23:418–424.

Tumors of ocular neurectoderm

These tumors include iridociliary epithelial tumors from mature anterior uveal neurectoderm, and medulloepithelioma and retinoblastoma from embryonic neurectoderm. The prevalence of these neoplasms is second to anterior uveal melanomas and melanocytomas, although it is perhaps underestimated because the most common examples are small, slowly expansive tumors within the posterior chamber that are unlikely to cause clinical signs. They are relatively common in dogs, uncommon in cats, and virtually unknown in other species except for medulloepitheliomas in horses.

Iridociliary epithelial tumor (iridociliary adenoma, iridociliary carcinoma) is the most common of this group. Most examples are well-differentiated papillary or tubular adenomas arising from the nonpigmented inner layer of ciliary or iris epithelium (Fig. 4.81). There are certainly examples in which the histologic and cytologic character is more primitive, but metastasis is so rare (if indeed it exists at all) that there is *no justification for diagnosing any of these tumors as iridociliary carcinomas.* Most originate from the pars plicata, but occasionally the histologic evidence points to origin from posterior iris epithelium. The tumor cells usually resemble mature ciliary epithelium and usually have very little associated stroma. Nuclei are basilar, regular, and are surrounded by eosinophilic cytoplasm (Fig. 4.82A). The tumor cells are not pigmented, although melanophages are occasionally seen within tumor stroma. *They make an abundance of basal lamina* oriented, as in normal ciliary epithelium, toward the inside of the eye. Its abundance, easily seen with periodic acid-Schiff reagent, is useful in distinguishing ciliary tumors from carcinomas metastatic to the eye. Examples that have little tubular or papillary organization, or a more primitive cytologic character, may be difficult to recognize as being of iridociliary epithelial origin. They almost always retain abundant basement membrane production that can be accentuated with PAS staining. *The cells also stain for vimentin, S-100, and neuron-specific enolase, which makes them unique among tumors that otherwise look epithelial.* Such additional staining may occasionally be necessary to distinguish primitive iridociliary epithelial tumors from metastatic carcinomas.

Even small iridociliary epithelial tumors may cause hyphema or glaucoma, attributed to this tumor's strong propensity to induce pre-iridal fibrovascular membranes (Fig. 4.82B). This is, presumably, the result of absorption through the porous anterior border layer of the iris of fibrovascular growth factors produced by the tumor cells in an effort to ensure their own survival. Iridociliary tumors are more likely to induce such neovascularization than is any other ocular disease.

Medulloepitheliomas and retinoblastomas *arise from the primitive neurectoderm of the optic cup.* Retinoblastoma is the second most frequent neoplasm of children, yet a critical review of the veterinary literature reveals only a single acceptable diagnosis of this tumor. Conversely, *medulloepitheliomas* are rare in children but many examples have been observed in animals, mainly in the *horse* in which these are probably the *most common primary intraocular tumor.* The neoplasm may originate from any portion of embryonic neurectoderm and may show differentiation into any neurectodermal derivative, i.e., retina, ciliary epithelium, vitreous, or neuroglia (Fig. 4.83A, B). The typical neoplasm is a loose network of branching cords of small basophilic neuroblasts resembling those of embryonic retina. Mitotic figures are numerous. The cords have definite polarity; they rest upon a basement membrane analogous to the inner limiting membrane of retina and some have adjoining apical terminal bars analogous to outer limiting membrane. A typical feature is the clustering of neuroblasts around an empty central lumen defined by the terminal bars, creating a true rosette (Fig. 4.84). The basilar portion of the rosette or cord faces a hyaluronic acid-rich myxoid matrix analogous to the vitreous. This histologic feature may be found in only a few foci within a huge mass that is otherwise composed of poorly differentiated, neuroblast-like cells. Many tumors also contain foci of cartilage, skeletal muscle, or brain tissue and are classified as *teratoid medulloepitheliomas.* Metastases are not recorded, despite many of these being classified histologically as "malignant."

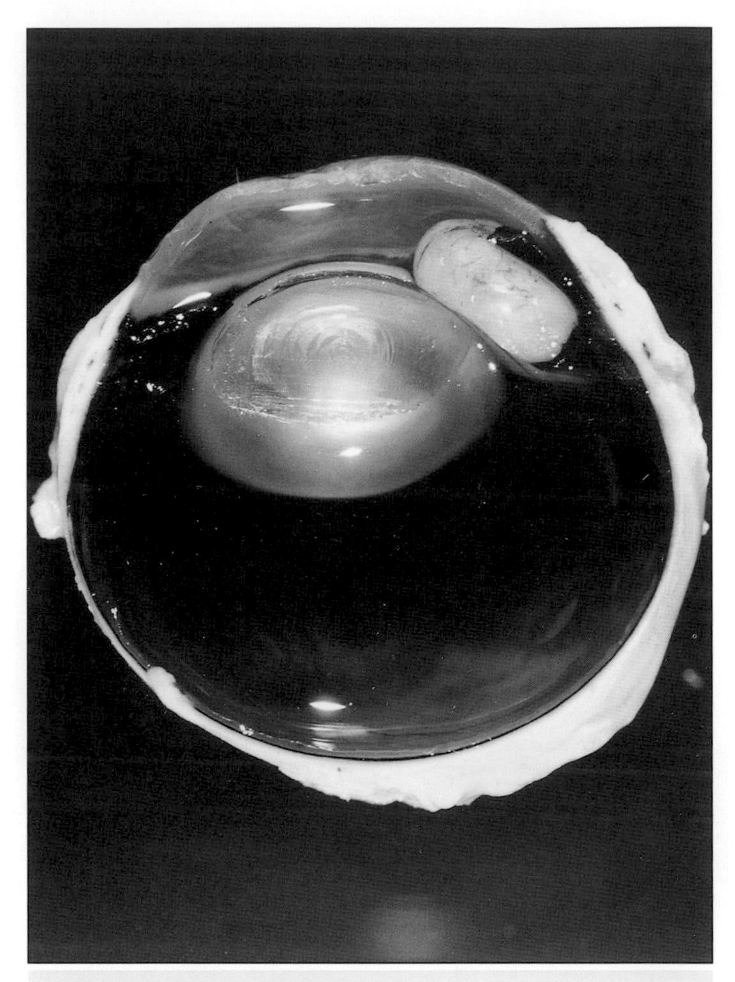

Figure 4.81 Iridociliary adenoma in a dog.

Bibliography

Dubielzig RR, et al. Iridociliary epithelial tumors in 100 dogs and 17 cats: a morphological study. Vet Ophthalmol 1998;1:223–231.

Eagle RC, et al. Malignant medulloepithelioma of the optic nerve in a horse. Vet Pathol 1978;15:488–494.

Hogan RN, Albert DM. Does retinoblastoma occur in animals? Prog Vet Comp Opthalmol 1991;1:73–82.

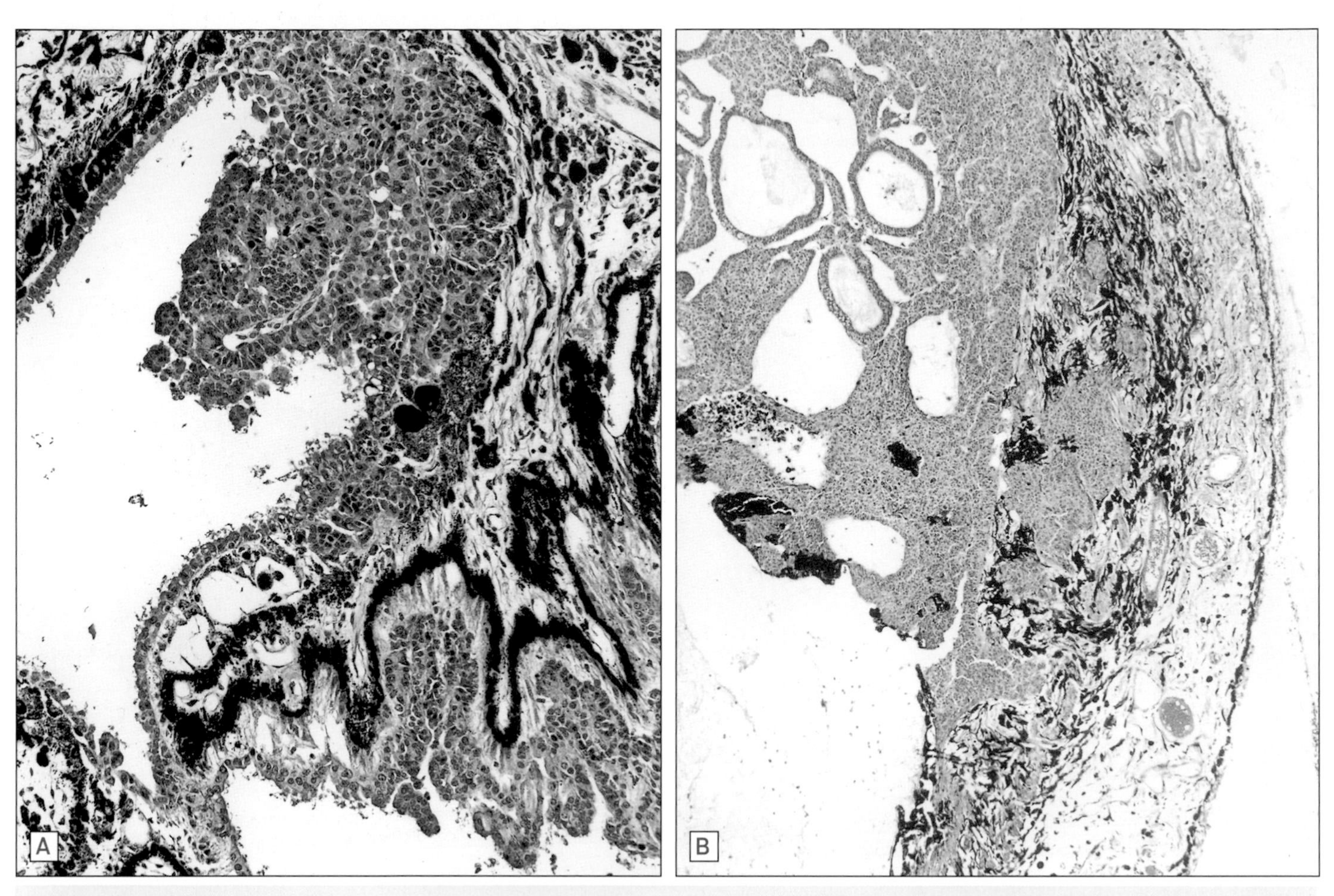

Figure 4.82 Iridociliary adenoma in a dog. **A.** Note well-differentiated tubular proliferation. **B.** Note the presence of tumor within the posterior iris stroma as well as in the posterior chamber, and the preiridal fibrovascular membrane.

Jensen OA, et al. Neuroepithelial tumor of the retina in a dog. Vet Ophthalmol 2003;6:57–60.

Langloss JM, et al. Malignant intraocular teratoid medulloepithelioma in three dogs. Vet Pathol 1976;13:343–352.

Peiffer RL. Ciliary body epithelial tumors in the dog and cat: a report of 13 cases. J Small Anim Pract 1983;24:347–370.

Wilcock B, Williams MM. Malignant intraocular medulloepithelioma in a dog. J Am Anim Hosp Assoc 1980;16:617–619.

Feline post-traumatic sarcoma

This syndrome seems unique to cats. As the name implies, eyes subjected to *trauma, especially penetrating injury*, are prone to develop pleomorphic spindle-cell sarcomas that destroy the globe and have substantial risk of metastasis. The interval between injury and observed tumor varies from 5 months to 11 years. Those skeptical about claiming such neoplasia to be the result of an injury 10 years previously prefer to call these tumors "primary ocular sarcomas," although such lag times are common in experimental models of carcinogenesis. The risk for injured eyes to develop sarcoma is unknown. Almost all recorded cases have perforated lenses. Most of these tumors appear to be fibrosarcomas, but some have a mixed epithelial–mesenchymal phenotype, and elaborate basement membrane-type matrix as well as express vimentin strongly. Based on immunopositivity for collagen type IV and crystallin alpha A, at least some of these tumors are of lens epithelial origin. Of relevance to ocular surgeons is the development of sarcomas in cat eyes receiving prosthetic lens implants, presumably viewed by the eye as just another form of unwanted lenticular trauma.

The tumor itself varies from fibrosarcoma to osteosarcoma to giant cell tumor, varying even within the same eye. The tumor tends to first surround the lens, then to line the inside of the eye, and finally to extend via scleral venous plexus or optic nerve to involve the orbit (Fig. 4.85). *The inclination to "line the globe" is a repeatable feature that is useful in distinguishing primary ocular sarcoma from rare metastatic sarcomas.* Most cases are presented with advanced disease, and follow-up data to document the prevalence of metastasis are scant. Available evidence documents a metastatic risk of at least 60%, and in many cases there is remarkably rapid development of post-enucleation neurologic signs attributable to invasion of brain via the optic foramen.

Bibliography

Dubielzig RR, et al. Morphologic features of feline ocular sarcomas in 10 cats: light microscopy, ultrastructure, and immunohistochemistry. Prog Vet Comp Ophthalmol 1994;4:7–12.

Peiffer RL, et al. Primary ocular sarcomas in the cat. J Small Anim Pract 1988;29:105–116.

Zeiss CJ, et al. Feline intraocular tumors may arise from transformation of lens epithelium. Vet Pathol 2003;40:355–362.

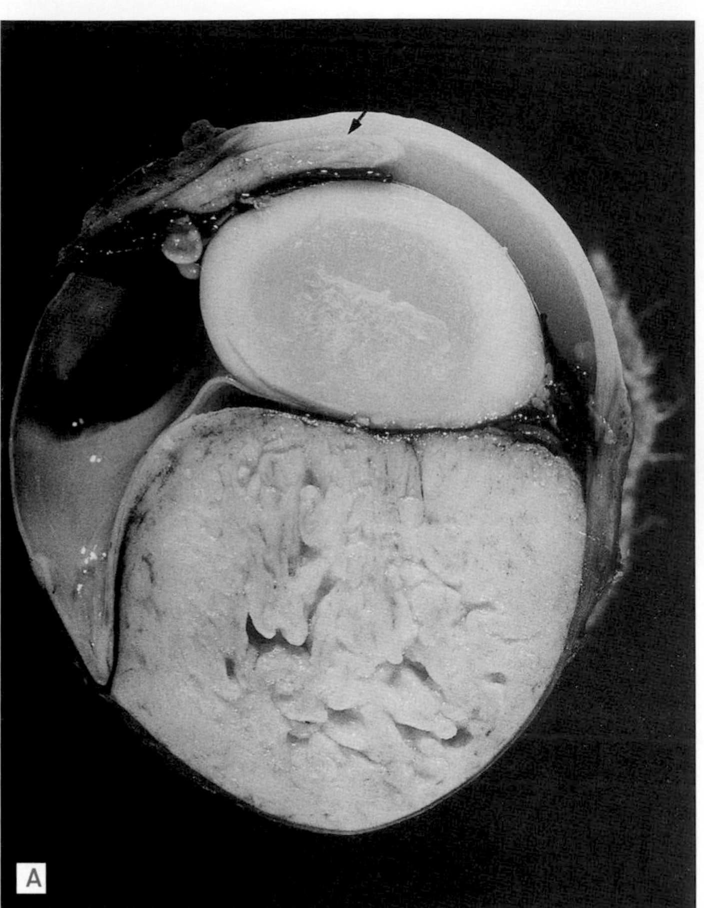

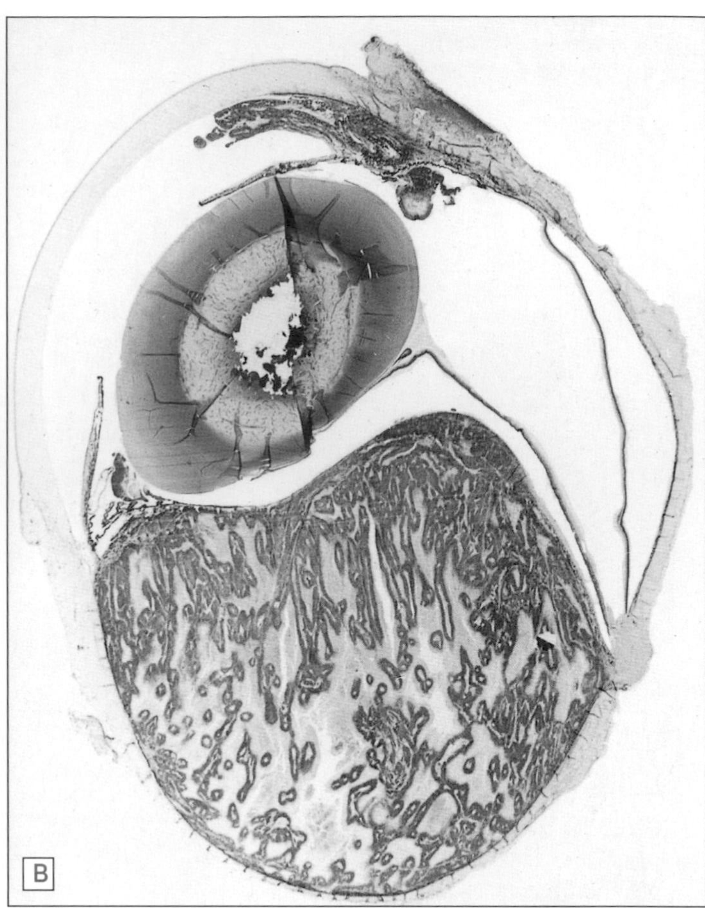

Figure 4.83 Medulloepithelioma in a dog. **A.** The main tumor lies between choroid and retinal pigment epithelium. There is also tumor in anterior chamber (arrow). **B.** Histologic section of (**A**). Note tubular latticework of the tumor.

Optic nerve tumors

While the optic nerve and adjacent retina can presumably develop all of the neoplasms of the central nervous system (excepting those from tissues such as ependyma that are not present in the eye), documented examples are few indeed. Most are reported as individual case reports prior to the era of immunohistochemical markers that would have permitted more precise classification.

Optic nerve meningioma *has a distinctive macroscopic and histologic appearance*. It has been described only in dogs, although it will probably be seen in other species as we begin to look. The tumor probably arises from meningial rests of arachnoid cells that project through the dura mater of the optic nerve into the orbital connective tissue. Tumors arising from these cells create a conical soft tissue mass that surrounds the optic nerve, but usually remains within the cone created by the extraocular muscles. Limited extension into the choroid or posterior vitreous through the optic nerve occurs only occasionally; more often, there is infiltration into the muscle and fat of the orbit. Most often, *the histologic appearance is of large stellate mesenchymal cells that can be confused with epithelial cells*. They have abundant glassy eosinophilic cytoplasm, and may or may not form the *characteristic swirling pattern* typical of central nervous system meningiomas in general (Fig. 4.86). Myxoid, chondroid, or even osseous metaplasia is quite common. Metastasis appears to be extremely infrequent.

Tumors published as **optic nerve astrocytomas** or as less specific "gliomas" were, in retrospect, *more likely to be examples of proliferative optic neuropathy* with the accumulation of reactive astrocytes and macrophages.

Primary orbital neoplasms

Tumors may be primary within the orbit, or arise by extension from adjacent structures or by hematogenous localization. They usually produce deviation or protrusion of the globe with secondary desiccation keratitis. Only those arising as primary tumors within the orbit are considered here. After saying that, *it is not always easy to decide whether the tumor is indeed primary or not*, and the decision is often made only after failure to find any credible primary tumor elsewhere. Of the primary orbital tumors reported in dogs and in horses, *sarcomas are much more prevalent than epithelial tumors*. The sarcomas are a bewildering array of locally infiltrative spindle cell tumors of unknown origin, with the abundance of diagnoses probably reflecting the diversity of pathologists' opinions rather than actual proof of histologic identity. Metastasis is rare but their infiltrative growth habit in this difficult site makes eventual elective euthanasia a frequent outcome.

Among the primary sarcomas, the only ones deserving specific consideration because of a distinctive histologic appearance are

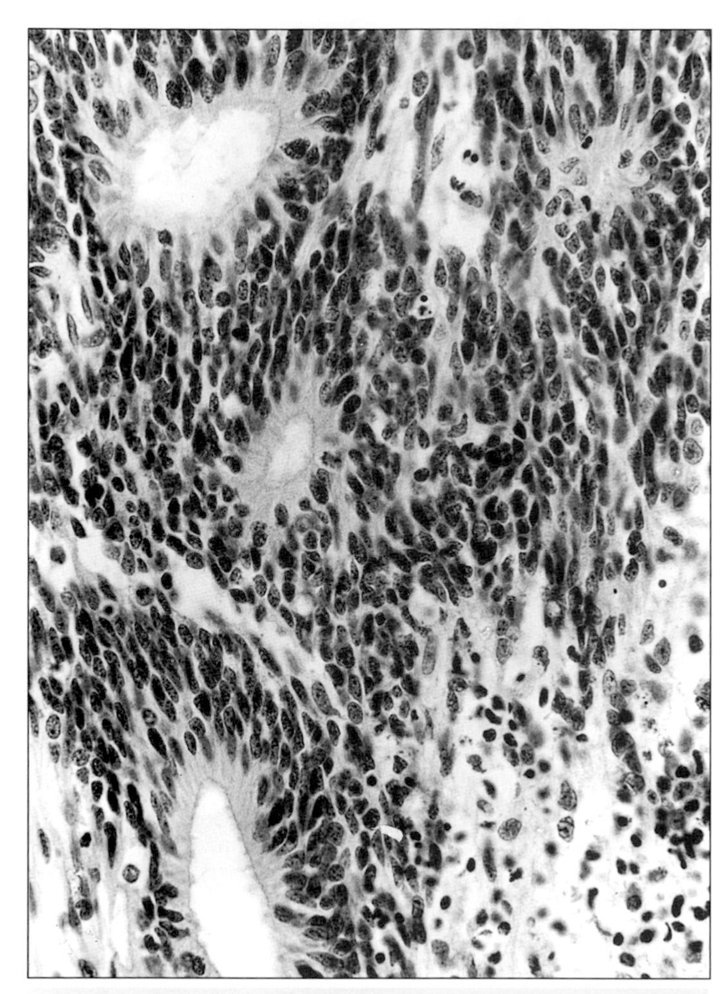

Figure 4.84 Medulloepithelioma in a dog. Note rosette with rudimentary formation of retinal outer limiting membrane and photoreceptors.

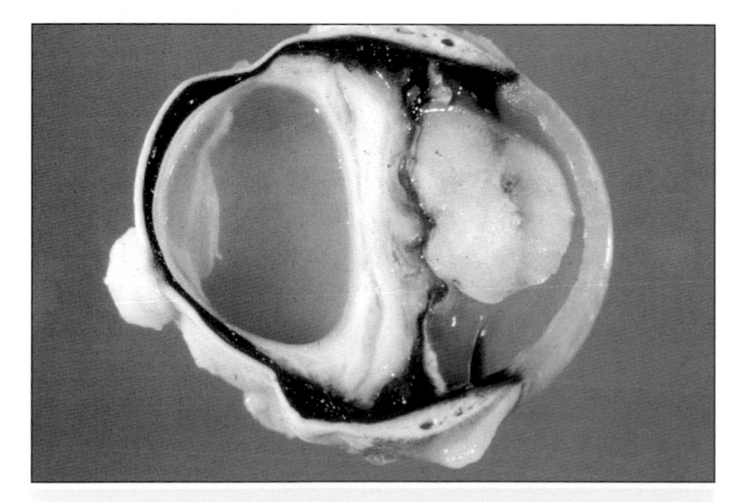

Figure 4.85 Primary feline ocular sarcoma arising from the lens and growing to "line" the posterior half of the globe.

multilobular osteochondrosarcomas and *optic nerve meningiomas*. The latter were described in the preceding section. The **multilobular osteochondrosarcomas** arise from the aponeuroses between adjacent bones of the orbit, and are identical in appearance and behavior to this tumor arising elsewhere in the canine skull.

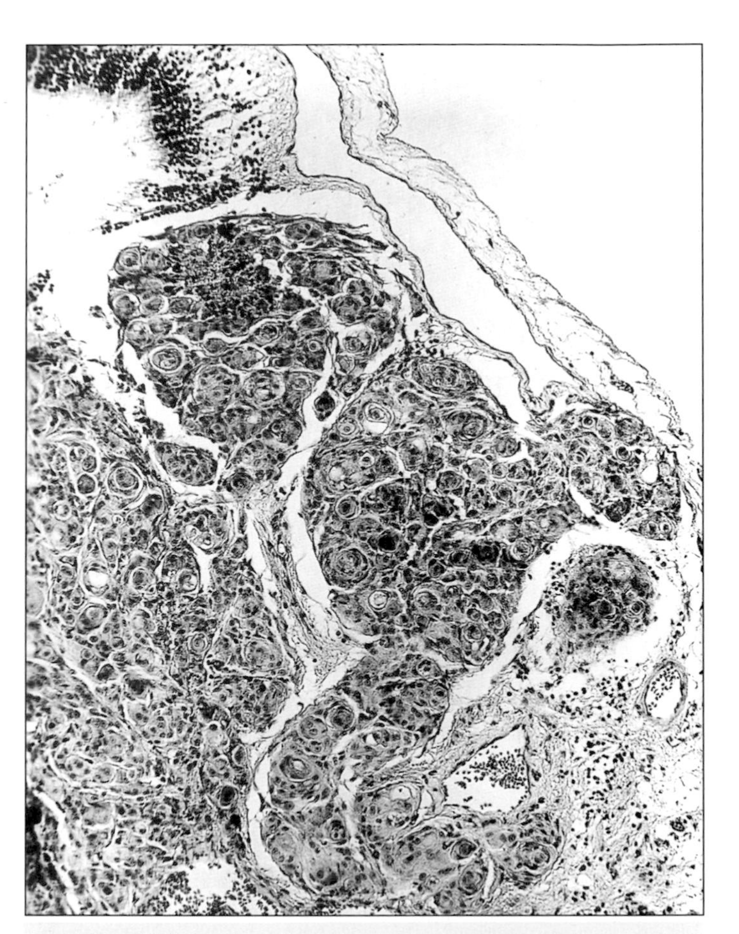

Figure 4.86 Meningioma of optic nerve invading eye in a dog.

Most primary epithelial tumors of the canine orbit are **lacrimal adenocarcinomas**, *which are locally invasive, recur after attempted resection, but which apparently have little metastatic potential.* In truth, there is so little follow-up information about these uncommon tumors that any statement about metastatic risk is premature. Both adenoma and nodular hyperplasia occur, but seem much less frequent than the malignant tumors. Tumors infiltrating the orbit from the nearby *zygomatic salivary gland* are similar histologically and behaviorally to lacrimal adenocarcinomas. They can sometimes be distinguished on the basis of location alone, but it is also helpful that the zygomatic gland is a mixed salivary gland with a prominent mucinous component that may be retained in well-differentiated tumors. The lacrimal gland is purely serous.

Primitive neuroepithelial tumors of unknown origin are occasionally seen in young dogs and in horses. They are composed of nests, cords, and rosette-like structures formed by small hyperchromatic neuroblastic cells with a very high mitotic index. Very rapid spread throughout the orbit and into brain occurs in affected dogs, but the extremely sparse information on these tumors in horses (four cases in two reports) suggest that they may be much less aggressive in horses than in dogs.

Tumors metastatic within the globe and orbit

The list of tumors that may be found as metastatic localizations within the globe or orbit is the same as any list of metastatic neoplasms in general. Any estimates of prevalence are unreliable because the globe is not routinely investigated in animals dying from disseminated malignancy. *Most of the reported cases are carcinomas*, simply because carcinomas are more likely to undergo hematogenous dissemination than are sarcomas (with the round cell "lymphoreticular" malignancies being a notable exception). In dogs, the most common are probably transitional cell carcinomas and mammary carcinomas, whereas in cats mammary adenocarcinoma and bronchial adenocarcinomas are probably the most prevalent. Across all species, however, *malignant lymphoma* is undoubtedly at the top of the list both as an intraocular and as an orbital metastatic tumor.

Bibliography

Attali-Soussay K, et al. Retrobulbar tumors in dogs and cats: 25 cases. Vet Ophthalmol 2001;4:19–27.

Baptiste KE, Grahn BH. Equine orbital neoplasia: a review of 10 cases (1983–1998). Can Vet J 41:291–295.

Basher AWP, et al. Orbital neuroendocrine tumors in three horses. J Am Vet Med Assoc 1997;210:668–671.

Headrick JF, et al. Canine lobular orbital adenoma: a report of 15 cases with distinctive features. Vet Ophthalmol 2004;7:47–51.

Hendrix DV, Gelatt KN. Diagnosis, treatment and outcome of orbital neoplasia in dogs: a retrospective study of 44 cases. J Small Anim Pract 2000;41:105–108.

Mauldin EA, et al. Canine orbital meningiomas: a review of 22 cases. Vet Ophthalmol 2000;3:11–16.

Ear

GENERAL CONSIDERATIONS

Diseases of the ear of domestic animals are of limited interest to most veterinary pathologists. Of the three broad categories – *defects of hearing, otitis media, and otitis externa* – only otitis media in farm animals regularly receives some attention, but even that is usually restricted to macroscopic examination at necropsy. Otitis externa is almost exclusively the realm of the clinical practitioner and microbiologist, although hyperplasia of chronically inflamed epithelium within the external ear canal may simulate neoplasia and be submitted for histologic interpretation. Disorders of hearing certainly occur in domestic animals, but their prominence in the medical literature is the result more of their usefulness as models for human deafness than of their intrinsic importance in animals. The growing availability of equipment for evaluation of hearing may, however, see a resurgence of interest in deafness in specific breeds or colors of dogs and cats. The tedious task of preparing adequate sections of the cochlea and labyrinth when related to the relative importance or prevalence of the diseases makes examination of the inner ear a rare event in most veterinary institutions. The gross and microscopic anatomy of the ear in the various species is reviewed in specialized texts and the appropriate references are included in the bibliography.

EXTERNAL EAR

Diseases of the external ear may be a local manifestation of generalized skin disease or may specifically affect the ear because of some anatomic or physiologic peculiarity. Disorders of skin that only incidentally affect the ear are discussed in Vol. 1, Skin and appendages.

Ear tip necrosis *may result from frostbite, cold-agglutinin disease, ergot poisoning, thrombosis during the course of septicemia, or from trauma inflicted by the animal itself or by cannibalistic herdmates.* Particularly in pigs, the prevalence of atrophic and misshapen ears may be quite high in individual herds. This usually results from septicemia, sarcoptic mange, or cannibalism. In some instances, however, no such history can be elicited, and a syndrome of infectious ear necrosis has been proposed. Culture of ears showing marginal lesions results in isolation of a variety of bacterial agents, and claims for a primary bacterial etiology are not convincing. The one that comes closest is the spirochete *Borrelia suilla*. It usually acts as an opportunistic contaminant of abraded skin in pigs, giving rise to localized (usually ear margins) or generalized ulcerative dermatitis.

Auricular hematoma *occurs as a consequence of trauma, usually from excessive head shaking by dogs with otitis externa.* Dogs and pigs with *pendulous ears* are particularly prone to hematoma formation, but cats are occasionally affected as well. Hematomas usually develop on the concave side of the pinna and are initially fluctuant but become firm as the hematoma (or blood-contaminated seroma) organizes. As it is converted to granulation tissue by fibroblastic and capillary ingrowth, the lesions become hard. Subsequent fibroblastic contraction may result in disfigurement of the pinna.

The location of the initial damage is unclear. Subcutaneous and subperichondrial sites are suggested, but a predominantly intrachondral location seems most likely. The cartilage plate of the pinna is cleaved by a longitudinal fracture and then by the hemorrhage. Granulation tissue forms at the interface of blood and cartilage, and the lesion is eventually converted to a fibrous scar. Late in the reparative process, regeneration of cartilage occurs adjacent to perichondrium or the ruptured edge of the cartilage. The intrachondral location of the hematomas is thought to be the result of rupture of vessels as they pass through minute foraminae in the cartilage plate. The conventional view that the initial lesion results from shear forces or outright trauma caused by head shaking has recently been challenged by one study of 40 dogs and 20 cats with auricular hematoma. No association with ear configuration or otitis externa was found, but most affected animals had serum and local tissue changes interpreted as *evidence for a lupus-like autoimmune disease.* The link between this proposed pathogenesis and the observation of the early cartilaginous fractures and hemorrhages was not made.

Dermatologic disease of the ear pinna may be part of a generalized skin disorder, but a few diseases seem unique to the ear. *Pigs with chronic sarcoptic mange* may have gross lesions only on the ears, consisting of reddening, crusting, and thickening of the pinna. *Short-haired* *dogs with pendulous ears* (Dachshunds, Pointers, Bloodhounds) are predisposed to chronic dermatitis of the ear margin, variously termed *marginal auricular dermatosis* or *ear margin seborrhea*. The gross lesion is a multifocal, greasy, gray, nodular encrustation that may coalesce to cause thickening of the entire ear margin. The histologic lesion resembles that of seborrhea elsewhere, with hyperkeratosis, acanthosis, and mild superficial perivascular dermatitis in which mononuclear leukocytes predominate.

Chronic ulcerative dermatitis of the ear margin of white cats (*feline solar dermatitis*) is discussed below as a premalignant lesion under squamous cell carcinoma, as is a similar disease of sheep.

Alopecia of the pinna occurs in dogs and in Siamese cats. In dogs, the alopecia appears gradually and progresses slowly. There is a strong *breed predilection* for Dachshunds, but it can be seen in other breeds including Italian Greyhounds and Whippets. The cause is unknown. The microscopic lesion is miniaturization of anagen follicles, without follicular destruction and without inflammation. In cats the lesion may wax and wane at irregular intervals throughout life. The histologic changes, in cats, have not been described.

Pinnal vasculitis is surprisingly frequent and resembles the lesion of cutaneous vasculitis elsewhere. In its mildest form, it may cause only pilosebaceous atrophy and thus may mimic the lesions of idiopathic pinnal alopecia when examined clinically.

Otitis externa

Otitis externa is a very common disorder in dogs and cats, and is probably equally common in many other species if they were to be examined. It may involve predisposing, primary, and perpetuating factors. In dogs, the pathogenesis is complex, while in cats, cattle, and goats, the *ear mite* is by far the major initiating factor. In tropical climates, infestation with rhabditiform nematodes (*Rhabditis* spp.) can be an important cause of otitis externa in cattle. *Otitis externa in dogs is most prevalent in breeds with pendulous ears or with abundant hair within the ear canal*, which implies that inadequate circulation of air and entrapment of moisture are important predispositions to the disease. *Foreign bodies*, usually foxtail or grass awns, may be important mechanical irritants, creating a breach for microbial infection, but since otitis is common in city dogs, other factors apparently are involved. The role of microorganisms in the pathogenesis of otitis externa is, as elsewhere, intimately linked to environmental circumstances that permit their uncontrolled proliferation. The bacteria and fungi cultured from diseased ears almost invariably are members of the normal aural flora. *Staphylococcus* spp., *Pseudomonas* spp., *Proteus* spp., and the yeast *Malassezia pachydermatis* are cultured much more frequently or in greater numbers from ears with otitis than from normal ears, but this may be related as much to their resistance to antimicrobial treatment as to their causative role. The lipid-rich environment of the ear canal favors the lipophilic *Malassezia*, which is the best candidate for a primary pathogen in the causation of canine otitis externa inasmuch as it frequently is the only pathogen isolated, and affected ears improve dramatically with antifungal therapy.

Otitis externa in species other than dogs is closely correlated to infestation with ear mites, and even in dogs acariasis can be an important contributor.

Otodectes cynotis *is the ear mite of carnivores*. The importance of the mite in initiating otitis externa is not entirely clear because the ear canal, once inflamed, becomes an environment unsuitable for the mites and thus gives rise to misleadingly low estimates of the prevalence of ear mites in dogs with otitis. As few as five mites can initiate otitis externa in dogs, with bacterial and mycotic opportunists rapidly masking the role of mites in the development of the lesion. Estimates vary from 2–50% prevalence of mites in dogs with otitis externa.

In cats, the role of mites is firmly established. In contrast to dogs, all cats have erect and sparsely haired pinnae and the role of ear carriage and hair is negligible. There is a poor correlation between the number of mites, the severity of inflammation in the external meatus, and clinical signs.

The mites are obligate parasites, spending their entire 3–4-week life cycle on the host. Transmission between animals of the same or different species readily occurs, and spread of the mites from their preferred aural niche to paws as the animal scratches, or tail as it sleeps with tail curled to touch the ear, is occasionally seen.

The mechanism by which the mites initiate otitis is controversial. Some maintain that the mites feed only on epithelial debris, while others claim that the mites pierce the epithelium and ingest blood and lymph. The latter claim is supported by the demonstration of host-specific serum components within the mites, but such components could exist in exudates, and should not be considered proof of penetrating feeding behavior.

The variation in the number of mites necessary to cause clinically obvious otitis, the species variation and some tenuous age resistance to disease (if not infection) suggest an allergic basis for the otitis. Most cats, and perhaps dogs, probably are infected with mites at some time. They may react to subsequent minor infection with immune-mediated inflammation of a severity not predicted by the small number of mites within the ear canal.

Psoroptes cuniculi, *the ear mite of rabbits*, also affects goats, horses, and deer. Its prevalence among domestic animals seems to be greatest in *goats*, ranging from about 20–80%. Careful examination may be required to find the mites. Clinical signs in goats, if present at all, are usually mild, consisting of ear twitching and head shaking. The ear canal of goats is the best site for isolation of several pathogenic *Mycoplasma* species in clinically normal animals. The same mycoplasmas were isolated from ear mites (*P. cuniculi* or *Raillietia caprae*) of infected goats, fuelling speculation that the mites are important vectors of the mycoplasmas in endemic herds. Similar coexistence of ear mites and mycoplasmas has been observed in cattle, but identification of the bacteria within the mites was not reported.

Psoroptes cuniculi may be quite common in horses (20% of horses in one Australian report) but it is unclear how frequently it causes clinical signs. Head shaking and resentment of handling of the ears are the usual signs.

Raillietia auris, *the ear mite of cattle*, occurs in most areas of the world. Infection seems to be common but is rarely of clinical significance. Manifestations of disease may follow extension of the otitis externa through the tympanum, and affected animals show head tilt and circling due to otitis interna. As with so many other agents observed or isolated from the external ear canal, it is difficult to prove a direct causal association between the presence of the mites and lesions or clinical signs of otitis.

Otobius megnini, *the spinose ear tick*, is parasitic on domestic ruminants, pigs, horses, and dogs and cats in restricted geographic areas. Infestation may be so heavy that the ear canals are full of ticks, making diagnosis easy. In light infestations, they occur deep in the folds of the ear, at the bottom of the external meatus. Only the larvae and nymphs are parasitic. The larvae attach themselves to the skin below the hairline and, biting through the skin, suck lymph until they are engorged. The parasites irritate the external auditory meatus and the ensuing exudate may completely fill it. In addition, secondary bacterial infection may occur in the inflamed areas around the bite wounds, and this infection may extend downward and cause otitis media. The microscopic appearance of the ear in this infestation has not been described.

The lesions of **otitis externa** *are nonspecific.* The relationship between type of exudate and causative agent has not been critically evaluated. The initial macroscopic lesion is hyperemia of the external auditory meatus followed by accumulation of serum, cerumen, leukocytes, and epithelial debris. A predominance of leukocytes tends to produce a suppurative exudate whereas cerumen yields a dry, dark-brown crumbly accumulation.

The histopathology of otitis externa varies with the duration of the inflammation and is rather typical inflammation of any epithelial surface. Only chronic lesions are likely to be seen by the pathologist. Such specimens show epidermal hyperplasia with acanthosis, atrophy of hair follicles, hyperkeratosis, and parakeratosis. Crusts of inflammatory debris adhere to the epithelial surface. Ulceration may be present, particularly if *Pseudomonas* is predominant, and *Malassezia* yeasts may be seen in the surface keratin or debris. The dermis contains numerous lymphocytes, plasma cells, mast cells, and neutrophils, the latter usually within dilated venules or adjacent to ulcers. Neutrophils are very sparse in mite-induced otitis. In very chronic and severe examples, dermal fibrosis is marked and ossification may occur. A feature of chronic otitis externa is *increased production of cerumen.* Histologically, there is hyperplasia of the normally very large sebaceous glands and cystic hyperplasia of the coiled tubular apocrine ceruminous glands, which are distended by eosinophilic cerumen. The combination of epithelial hyperplasia, glandular hyperplasia, and stromal fibroplasia may create proliferative lesions that occlude the ear canal and simulate neoplasia.

Bibliography

Cook, R.W. Ear mites (*Raillietia manfredi and Psoroptes cuniculi*) in goats in New South Wales. Aust Vet J 1981;57:72–75.

Cottew GS. Mycoplasmas in ears. Aust Vet J 1985;62:420.

Duarte ER, Hamdan JS. Otitis in cattle, an aetiological review. J Vet Med B Infect Dis Vet Public Health 2004;51:1–7.

Dubielzig RR, et al. Pathogenesis of canine aural hematomas. J Am Vet Med Assoc 1984;8:873–876.

Faccini JL, Costa AL. Subclinical psoroptic otocariasis in Brazilian sheep with comments on a technique for mite collection. Exp Appl Acarol 1992;13:227–229.

Jacobson LS. Diagnosis and medical treatment of otitis externa in the dog and cat. J S Afr Vet Assoc 2002;73:162–170.

Jubb TF, et al. Suppurative otitis in cattle associated with ear mites (*Raillietia auris*). Aust Vet J 1993;70:354–355.

Kuwahara J. Canine and feline aural hematoma: Clinical, experimental and clinicopathologic observations. Am J Vet Res 1986;47:2300–2308.

Littlejohn AI. Psoroptic mange in the goat. Vet Rec 1968;82:148–155.

Morris DO. *Malassezia* dermatitis and otitis. Vet Clin N Amer Small Anim Pract 1999;29:1303–1310.

Powell MB, et al. Reaginic hypersensitivity in *Otodectes cynotis* infection of cats and mode of mite feeding. Am J Vet Res 1980;41:877–882.

Rosser EJ Jr. Causes of otitis externa. Vet Clin North Am Small Anim Pract 2004;34:459–468.

van der Gaag, I. The pathology of the external ear canal in dogs and cats. Vet Q 1986;8:307–327.

MIDDLE EAR

Otitis media

Otitis media *is inflammation of the tympanic cavity within the temporal bone. Its cause is almost always bacterial, the organisms reaching the poorly drained cavity via the Eustachian tube or following perforation of the tympanum.* In swine and lambs, the infection usually ascends from the pharynx via the Eustachian tube. In calves, the pathogenesis may depend on the age of the calves and a variety of management factors. In young dairy calves, *Mycoplasma bovis* causes unilateral or bilateral fibrinopurulent otitis media, sometimes even with bone lysis and remodeling. Affected animals may have no other lesions of *M. bovis* infection, or may have concurrent polyarthritis and/or necrotizing bronchopneumonia. In feedlot cattle, outbreaks of otitis media have been associated with isolation of *Pasteurella multocida*. Those organisms are normal inhabitants of the bovine ear canal, so the significance of these isolates is hard to evaluate: mycoplasma was not sought.

In dogs and cats, chronic otitis externa is the major predisposition, although the tympanum is quite resistant to inflammatory lysis. There are insufficient cases recorded in other species to permit generalization. *In all species, there is circumstantial evidence for hematogenous localization of infection in the middle and inner ear,* perhaps occurring most often in pigs. Otitis media with subsequent vestibular disease can be the presenting clinical complaint in cats with cryptococcosis.

Otitis media as a clinically obvious entity is most frequent in *feeder pigs*. The infection is usually unilateral and associated with hemolytic streptococci, but may involve *Actinobacillus pleuropneumoniae* or *Mycoplasma hyorhinis*. The clinical signs of head tilt, circling, and ataxia suggest involvement of the inner ear in most instances. Otitis media in swine may occur as small epizootics involving a dozen or more pigs. The basis for the clustering of the disease is unproven, but its sporadic association with atrophic rhinitis suggests spread from the upper respiratory tract. In *lambs*, the lesion is usually clinically undetected and unilateral, and often occurs in association with pneumonia. *Mannheimia haemolytica* is the usual isolate from both ear and lung. Bottle-feeding also increases the prevalence of otitis media in lambs. Otitis media/interna is uncommon in *horses*, but can occur as a chronic, insidious infection with the unique sequel of temporohyoid osteoarthropathy in some horses. Head shaking may be the only presenting clinical sign.

Regardless of the route of entry, the lesion and its progression are similar. The epithelium lining the tympanic cavity is hyperemic, edematous, and may be ulcerated. Neutrophils exuding from the reactive vessels under the epithelium enter the tympanic cavity, joining the initially serous or serofibrinous exudate to make it progressively more purulent. Exudate may temporarily drain into the pharynx via the Eustachian tube, which is soon sealed by inflammatory swelling of its epithelium. In severe infections, the exudate escapes via inflammatory lysis of the tympanum or, rarely, the bone on the ventral floor of the tympanic bulla. Chronic inflammation is characterized by inspissation of exudate, lysis of the ossicles and, occasionally, the tympanum, and spread to inner ear and brainstem. Another sequel noted in dogs with otitis media is mineralization of necrotic material within the tympanic bullae to form **otoliths**. Otolithiasis may cause signs of vestibular disease.

The presence of **inflammatory polyps**, either unilateral or bilateral, of the middle ear in dogs is an unusual association with, and possible cause of, otitis externa/media. Surgical removal of aural polyps has resulted in a good prognosis. Nasopharyngeal polyps have also been noted in this location in cats (see Neoplasms and like lesions below).

Primary secretory otitis media (PSOM) has been diagnosed in Cavalier King Charles Spaniels with signs of moderate-to-severe pain in the head or neck, and/or neurological signs. A highly viscous mucus plug filled the middle ear and caused the tympanic membrane to bulge outwards. The prognosis was good following removal of the mucus plug, flushing of the middle ear, and local and systemic medical therapy.

Bibliography

Beatty JA, et al. Peripheral vestibular disease associated with cryptococcosis in three cats. J Feline Med Surg 2000;2:29–34.

Blythe LL. Otitis media and interna and temporohyoid osteoarthropathy. Vet Clin North Am Equine Pract 1997;13:21–42.

Duff JP, et al. Otitis in a weaned pig: a new pathological role for *Actinobacillus* (*Haemophilus*) *pleuropneumoniae*. Vet Rec 1996;139:561–563.

Friis NF, et al. *Mycoplasma hyorhinis* isolation from cases of otitis media in piglets. Acta Vet Scand 2002;43:191–193.

Jensen R, et al. Middle ear infection in feedlot lambs. J Am Vet Med Assoc 1982;181:805–807.

Kudnig ST. Nasopharyngeal polyps in cats. Clin Tech Small Anim Pract 2002;17:174–177.

Maeda T, et al. *Mycoplasma bovis*-associated suppurative otitis media and pneumonia in bull calves. J Comp Pathol 2003;129:100–110.

Olson LD. Gross and microscopic lesions of middle and inner ear infections in swine. Am J Vet Res 1982;42:1433–1440.

Pratschke KM. Inflammatory polyps of the middle ear in 5 dogs. Vet Surg 2003;32:292–296.

Spangler EA, Dewey CW. Meningoencephalitis secondary to bacterial otitis media/interna in a dog. J Am Anim Hosp Assoc 2000;36:239–243.

Stern-Bertholtz W, et al. Primary secretory otitis media in the Cavalier King Charles spaniel: a review of 61 cases. J Small Anim Pract 2003;44: 253–256.

Walz PH, et al. Otitis media in preweaned Holstein dairy calves in Michigan due to *Mycoplasma bovis*. J Vet Diag Invest 1997;9:250–254.

Ziemer LS, et al. Otolithiasis in three dogs. Vet Radiol Ultrasound 2003; 44:28–31.

INNER EAR

Otitis interna

Otitis interna *is almost always the result of infection spreading from the middle ear.* The inflammation is usually of bacterial origin and thus suppurative. Ascension via the eighth cranial nerve is relatively frequent, and results in focal suppurative meningitis or encephalitis in the region of the pons. *The usual clinical syndrome is vestibular dysfunction*, described in a subsequent section.

Deafness

Deafness is difficult to assess in animals, and its diagnosis by simply observing behavioral abnormalities is almost impossible unless the animal is totally and bilaterally deaf. The recent introduction of electrodiagnostic tests has identified a higher prevalence of deafness, especially in dogs, than was suspected. **Conductive deafness** results from interference with the conduction of sound to the sensory end organ (of Corti) by diseases of external or middle ear. Alternatively, **sensorineural deafness** results from maldevelopment or degeneration of the sensory organ, eighth nerve, or auditory pathways within the brain. The last is very unusual and, because of the multitude of possible pathways, is seen only in massive destructive lesions with their neurologic signs overshadowing the hearing loss. *Nerve deafness usually involves the organ of Corti, and is by far the most prevalent type of deafness encountered in animals by virtue of hereditary deafness in several breeds of dogs, and in dogs or cats with color dilution anomalies.* Conductive deafness may result from obliteration of the external auditory meatus by chronic proliferative inflammation or tumor, from inflammatory or traumatic rupture of the tympanum, or from entrapment of the ossicles in exudates or granulation tissue. Rarely there is destruction of the middle or inner ears by osteomyelitis or neoplasia.

The anatomy of the auditory apparatus is complex. The sensory fibers of the eighth cranial nerve terminate at the base of sensory hair cells within the organ of Corti, the latter a sensory specialization of the epithelium lining the cochlear duct. Excitation of the hair cells results from pulsations within the endolymph fluid that fills the entire membranous labyrinth including the cochlear duct. The precise mechanism of such excitation remains unknown. Sound waves in the environment reach the endolymph via the tympanum and ossicles. Vibration of the tympanum is transmitted to the ossicles, and vibration of the ossicles causes vibration of the oval window that separates the footplate of the stapes from the endolymph. Any lesion that interferes with vibration of the tympanum or ossicle interferes with the establishment of fluid waves within the endolymph. Traumatic fracture of ossicles, rupture of tympanum, or dampening of vibration by exudates within the middle ear can do this.

Hereditary cochleosaccular degeneration

Hereditary deafness *in association with incomplete pigmentation of the hair coat and uvea is seen in cats, dogs, mink, and mice. Incompletely documented examples exist in other domestic species.* The pigmentary defect is not true albinism but is white spotting or merling, the distinction being the absence of melanocytes in white areas in the latter instance and functionally defective melanocytes in the former. In some instances, the hearing defect is associated with inheritance of the merling gene. All homozygotes and many of the heterozygotes are deaf and have some degree of iris heterochromia. In other instances there is heterochromia iridis but no apparent coat color dilution (Dalmatian dogs), while in others both eyes and coat are phenotypically normal. Even when the coat color is white, as in deaf Bull Terriers, the genetic basis for the white coat and the associated deafness need not be the merling gene. Out of this confusing picture one should rescue the concept that *color-dilute animals have ocular heterochromia and deafness much more frequently than normal animals, but that other genetic bases for deafness also exist.* Ocular anomalies and deafness commonly are encountered in the same animal, probably the result of the inductive influence of pigmentation on both organs. For example, all white cats with blue irises are deaf as are many Dalmatian dogs with iris heterochromia. Several dog breeds, particularly Dalmatians and English Setters, have a prevalence of early-onset deafness in excess of that predictable from their prevalence in the overall canine population. Prominent also are merle dogs such as Australian Shepherds, Australian Blue Heelers, Old English Sheepdogs and Great Danes.

The fully developed lesion of **cochleosaccular degeneration** *is atrophy of the sensory and supporting cells of the organ of Corti and the saccular macula, collapse of the dorsal or lateral walls of the cochlear and saccular membranous labyrinth, and secondary degeneration of the neurons within the spiral ganglion.* The osseous portion of the labyrinth is unaffected as is the vestibular portion of the inner ear. With minor variations, all cases in dogs and cats are similar. Initial structure and function are normal, but there is failure to achieve normal maturation and, subsequently, degeneration occurs.

The carnivore ear is completely developed at birth and continues to mature for 2 (organ of Corti) to 4 (stria vascularis) weeks. Thereafter, the epithelial lining of the cochlear duct is incapable of mitotic regeneration. In white kittens, the ear is morphologically and physiologically normal at birth but shows arrested development as early as 1 week of age. At this time there is inward sagging of the free dorsolateral wall of the cochlear duct (Reissner's membrane) and saccule, and hydropic change in the stria vascularis. The degeneration within the organ of Corti and adjacent nutritive stria vascularis is so rapid that there is no consensus as to the initial or causal lesion. It may be that degeneration of the stria vascularis results in ischemic degeneration of the avascular organ of Corti, or there may be a primary defect within the sensory cells themselves resulting from an inborn metabolic error.

Senile deafness

Many animals become hard of hearing as they reach old age. This phenomenon, called **presbycusis**, is more frequently observed in old dogs because dogs tend to be kept well into their advanced years and because hearing loss is more readily noticed in them than in other species. In humans, the loss of hearing is progressive from about the fortieth year of life and particularly affects hearing of high tones. The cause seems to be inherent age-related degeneration of the epithelial tissues within the cochlea and of the spiral ganglion, a process that may be accelerated by excessive noise, arteriosclerosis, and nutritional factors. The essential lesions are atrophy of all epithelial structures within the cochlear duct and the associated auditory nerves, as well as neuronal atrophy within the spiral ganglion. Occasionally, the major lesion is atrophy within the stria vascularis or the basal membrane supporting the organ of Corti.

Presbycusis in animals has been studied in guinea pigs, rats, mice, dogs, and cats. *Degeneration of the hair cells in the organ of Corti and loss of neurons from the spiral ganglion are the common denominators in all such instances, and presumably is the aging change common to all mammalian species.* Stria vascularis atrophy has not been seen in these animals.

Acoustic and chemical ototoxicity

Noise, *either as a sudden loud noise or as moderate but prolonged environmental background, causes degeneration of the sensory hair cells within the organ of Corti.* Loud noise causes hair cell necrosis and even outright disruption of the organ of Corti or Reissner's membrane by mechanical trauma mediated via fluid waves within the endolymph, which must be the otic equivalent of tidal waves. Environmental noise is frequently an occupational hazard. The eventual lesion is hair cell necrosis, but whether this results from repeated sublethal microtrauma by noise peaks or by interference with hair cell metabolism is not known. That animals are susceptible to such trauma is well established in experimental models, but investigation of naturally occurring examples is not reported.

The list of chemicals that are ototoxic is very long, and is even longer if idiosyncratic drug injury is included. Only a few major examples likely to be encountered in veterinary practice are included here.

Aminoglycoside antibiotics *(gentamicin, streptomycin, kanamycin, neomycin, and others) are all nephrotoxic and ototoxic in proportion to their blood levels and duration of administration.* Overdosing, or administration to animals with decreased renal function, markedly increases the risk of toxic injury to the inner ear. Clinical signs of vestibular dysfunction precede evidence of hearing impairment. The initial lesion affecting hearing is degeneration of the apical portion of cochlear hair cells. The earliest visible lesion is mitochondrial swelling and increased number of myelin figures. The early lesion is reversible but later becomes permanent, presumably as mitochondrial swelling leads to structural disintegration of cellular respiratory enzymes and cell death. Cats are particularly susceptible and vestibular toxicity (defects of posture, balance, and gait) precedes clinical evidence of hearing loss. Ordinarily, these signs appear only after several weeks of aminoglycoside therapy.

The **diuretics** *furosemide, bumetanide, and ethacrynic acid are chemically related and all are ototoxic to dogs and cats.* Other domestic species have not been tested. Electrophysiologic evidence of hearing impairment occurs within a few hours of even a single high dose but is unaccompanied by structural changes within the cochlea. The exception is ethacrynic acid intoxication in which edema of the stria vascularis is seen ultrastructurally. There is a corresponding alteration in the composition of the endolymph produced by the stria. The hearing impairment, which occurs frequently in people receiving therapeutic doses of the drugs, is assumed to result from structural or physiologic lesions in the hair cells nourished by this abnormal endolymph.

Acetylsalicylic acid (aspirin) and its derivatives are ototoxic for man and several laboratory animal models, but no structural lesion has yet been detected.

The antibacterial-anthelmintic agent, **hygromycin B**, as well as causing cataracts in swine (see Eye) also causes permanent deafness in dogs if therapeutic dosages are given. The drug is not approved for use in dogs. Deafness is reported occasionally in swine receiving the medication in excess of recommended levels. Histologic descriptions of cochlear lesions are not available.

The antiseptic combination of **chlorhexidine and cetrimide** (Savlon7) is a widely used antiseptic that occasionally is used to cleanse the external ear canal. If used in dogs or cats with a ruptured typanic membrane, this solution is *toxic to both vestibular and cochlear cells*, although the clinical signs in affected animals are primarily vestibular.

Other causes of deafness

Deafness is reported in people with various *storage diseases*, but few animal counterparts have been studied for this specific defect.

Goats with β-mannosidosis have deformed ear pinnae, bony exostoses within the tympanic cavity, and deforming accumulation of oligosaccharides within lysosomes of many tissues of middle and inner ear. Epithelial and mesothelial cells of Reissner's membrane, most structural cells of the organ of Corti, and cochlear neurons of the spiral ganglion are all affected, even at a few days of age.

Vestibular dysfunction

Vestibular dysfunction is characterized by head tilt and falling towards the affected side, ataxia without weakness, and nystagmus. Clinical signs are most obvious with unilateral disease. The lesion may be in brain or in the vestibular apparatus, or both. Animals with vestibular dysfunction caused by brain lesions, as in listeriosis or canine distemper, usually show other signs of neurologic dysfunction. Since vestibular signs are more readily detected than is partial hearing loss, *mild lesions of the inner ear are more frequently associated with vestibular abnormalities than with hearing deficits.*

The causes of peripheral vestibular disease are the same as those causing deafness: uncontrolled otitis media, trauma, invasive neoplasia, and a number of drugs. Congenital vestibular disease has been reported in several dog breeds, but no morphologic observations were given. *Nonspecific destruction of part or all of the vestibular apparatus as a sequel to otitis media is by far the most common cause of labyrinthitis in all species.*

Idiopathic vestibular disease occurs in old dogs and in cats of any age. In old dogs, it is often mistakenly diagnosed as an acute cerebrovascular accident (stroke), but there is no demonstrable brain lesion in such dogs, and most have rapid, spontaneous remission of clinical signs unless prevented by premature euthanasia. No histologic examination of the labyrinth has been reported. An equally mysterious acute vestibular dysfunction affects cats of any age. Recovery usually occurs over a few days to weeks. No lesions are reported.

Bibliography

Branišaks M, Burda H. Inner ear structure in the deaf and normally hearing dalmatian dog. J Comp Pathol 1985;95:295–299.

Coppens AG, et al. Inner ear morphology in a bilaterally deaf Dogo Argentino pup. J Comp Pathol 2003;128:67–70.

Knowles K, et al. Reduction of spiral ganglion neurons in the aging canine with hearing loss. J Vet Med Assoc 1989;36:188–199.

Liberman MC, Kiang NYS. Acoustic trauma in cats. Cochlear pathology and auditory-nerve activity. Acta Otolaryngol 1978;[Suppl]358:1–63.

Merchant SR. Ototoxicity. Vet Clin North Am Small Anim Pract 1994;24:971–980.

Render JA, et al. Otic pathology of caprine β-mannosidosis. Vet Pathol 1988;25:437–442.

Ryugo DK, et al. Separate forms of pathology in the cochlea of congenitally deaf white cats. Hear Res 2003;181:73–84.

Strain GM. Deafness prevalence and pigmentation and gender associations in dog breeds at risk. Vet J 2004;167:23–32.

Thomas WB. Vestibular dysfunction. Vet Clin North Am Small Anim Pract 2000;30:227–249.

Wilkes MK, Palmer AC. Congenital deafness in dobermans. Vet Rec 1986;118:218–219.

Wright Ch.G. Neural damage in the guinea pig cochlea after noise exposure. A light microscopic study. Acta Otolaryngol 1976;82:82–94.

Neoplasms and like lesions

Neoplasms of the ear include those capable of affecting skin elsewhere, as well as primary tumors of ceruminous glands and, very rarely, tumors of Eustachian or auditory epithelium and of cranial nerves. Inflammatory polyps are included in this section because of their gross resemblance to neoplasia.

Squamous cell carcinoma *is by far the most important skin tumor affecting the ear*, although the predilection of *canine histiocytoma* for the ear pinna probably makes it the most frequent tumor affecting the pinna. Squamous cell carcinoma of the ear occurs commonly in *white cats*, with a frequency more than ten times that of nonwhite cats, and in *sheep* in sunny climates. In cats, the tumor has a long precancerous phase consisting of erythematous, ulcerative dermatitis of the ear margin known as *feline solar, or actinic, dermatitis* because of its association with exposure to sunlight. Other sparsely haired areas, such as the nose, lips, and eyelids, may be affected. Histologically, the lesion consists of multifocal coalescing epidermal necrosis overlying a diffuse superficial dermal infiltrate of lymphocytes and plasma cells. The lesion waxes and wanes with the intensity of sunlight. *Epidermal hyperplasia proceeds to dysplasia, carcinoma in situ and invasive squamous cell carcinoma in a manner analogous to bovine ocular squamous cell carcinoma.* The lesion is bilateral but not necessarily of synchronous progression. The progression to invasive neoplasia usually occurs over 3 or 4 years. Metastasis is a late occurrence and prevented (at least in the case of ears) by amputation. Rarely, squamous cell carcinoma occurs within the external ear canal or even within the tympanic cavity of the middle ear. Local infiltration results in damage to cranial nerves VII and VIII with resultant signs of vestibular dysfunction and facial paralysis.

Ceruminous adenomas and adenocarcinomas *occur in dogs and cats.* The tumors represent a continuum from histologically benign to histologically malignant, and are thus very similar to tumors of apocrine sweat glands elsewhere in skin. The ceruminous glands are modified sweat glands within the deep portion of the external auditory meatus. Tumors are relatively more prevalent in cats than in dogs, and in both species they tend to occur in very old animals. In dogs most are benign, but in cats about half are histologically malignant. The adenomas are smooth nodular or pedunculated masses seldom exceeding 1 cm in diameter. The epithelium overlying the tumor is intact unless there is concurrent otitis externa. Ceruminous gland tumors cannot be distinguished in the live animal from cystic dilation with epithelial hyperplasia typical of chronic otitis externa. Carcinomas may occasionally invade from the auditory meatus into the region of the parotid salivary gland or into bone, and when very anaplastic may be confused with salivary carcinoma. The diagnosis of carcinoma usually is based on histologic criteria of anaplasia and local invasiveness rather than on behavioral evidence of metastasis.

Histologically, adenomas are well-differentiated tubular and cystic growths. The epithelial cells are cuboidal and eosinophilic. They may be flattened when the tubular or acinar lumen is dilated. *The most typical feature is the presence within lumina of deeply eosinophilic or orange, colloid-like secretion typical of cerumen.* Mixed ceruminous tumors analogous to mixed apocrine sweat glands or mammary tumors occur infrequently. Carcinomas do not differ markedly from adenomas but have less secretion and more cellular anaplasia, and show invasion by tumor cells into an abundant fibrous stroma rich in mononuclear leukocytes. Mixed tumors with cartilage and bone are described.

Benign cutaneous plasmacytoma occurs with unexplained frequency in the external ear canal of dogs. It has the same histologic appearance here as it does in other locations such as the larynx and skin.

As expected, *various other neoplasms* have been described in the external ear canal or tympanic cavity of dogs and cats. All would seem to be rare, and no prognostic statements are justified by the small numbers. In one small series in dogs, eight of 11 middle ear neoplasms originated in the external ear and perforated the tympanic membrane. Two were papillary adenomas formed by ciliated columnar epithelium and goblet cells, thought to have arisen from the epithelium of the dorsal portion of the tympanic cavity. The final case was an anaplastic carcinoma of unknown origin involving oropharynx and ear.

Nasopharyngeal polyps *occur quite frequently in cats*. The distinctive histologic lesion is a loose mass of connective tissue containing numerous small blood vessels and mononuclear leukocytes, covered by epithelium that may be either stratified, nonkeratinized squamous, or simple-to-bilayered ciliated columnar. *The detection of ciliated epithelium is a prerequisite for the histologic confirmation of nasopharyngeal polyp*. Often the ciliated epithelium is found only focally in protected subepithelial glands, but nonetheless it is the characteristic feature distinguishing this lesion from nonspecific proliferations of glands and connective tissue seen in many cases of chronic otitis externa. The presence of this ciliated epithelium is used to support theories that such polyps originate from the Eustachian tube, but in fact the only proven origin is from ciliated epithelium of the tympanic cavity itself. Some of these polyps are grotesque, protruding from outer ear, hanging into the oropharynx, or even protruding through the nose. A familial occurrence has been seen in Abyssinian and Himalayan kittens, further confusing the debate about the cause of these distinctive lesions.

Under the umbrella of **inflammatory polyp** fall many of the tumor-like proliferations excised from the external ear canal of dogs (rarely cats) with chronic otitis externa. The lesion consists of variable proportions of hyperplastic surface epithelium, hyperplastic or dysplastic sebaceous and ceruminous glands, fibroplasia, and leukocytes. The rupture of the glands often adds the lesions of sterile foreign body periadenitis to the chronic inflammation associated with the bacteria, yeast, or foreign bodies causing the initial otitis itself. Such masses are macroscopically indistinguishable from genuine ceruminous neoplasms; *the histologic distinction is made by observing a mixture of inflammation, fibrosis, and hyperplasia of both sebaceous and apocrine glands within the hyperplastic polyps, whereas the tumor is represented by the proliferation of a single cell type.*

Another nodular lesion, clinically resembling neoplasia, is the **dentigerous cyst** of heterotopic polydontia in foals, seen as a draining nodule on the rostral aspect of the base of the pinna.

Bibliography

de Lorimier LP, et al. T-cell lymphoma of the tympanic bulla in a feline leukemia virus-negative cat. Can Vet J 2003;44:987–989.

Indrieri RJ, Taylor RF. Vestibular dysfunction caused by squamous cell carcinoma involving the middle ear and inner ear in two cats. J Am Vet Med Assoc 1984;184:471–473.

Little CJL, et al. Neoplasia involving the middle ear cavity of dogs. Vet Rec 1989;124:54–57.

Muilenburg RK, Fry TR. Feline nasopharyngeal polyps. Vet Clin North Am Small Anim Pract 2002;32:839–849.

Pratschke KM. Inflammatory polyps of the middle ear in 5 dogs. Vet Surg 2003;32:292–296.

Rogers KS. Tumors of the ear canal. Vet Clin North Am: Small Anim Pract 1988;18:859–868.

Veir JK, et al. Feline inflammatory polyps: historical, clinical, and PCR findings for feline calici virus and feline herpes virus-1 in 28 cases. J Feline Med Surg 2002;4:195–199.

Venker-van Haagen AJ, van der Gaag I. Tumors of the external ear. Vet Q 1998;20(Suppl 1):S7.

Wilcock BP, et al. Histological Classification of Ocular and Otic Tumors of Domestic Animals. WHO International Histologic Classification of Tumors of Domestic Animals, Second Series, Washington, DC: AFIP, 2002.

5 Skin and appendages

Pamela E. Ginn, Joanne E. K. L. Mansell, and Pauline M. Rakich

GENERAL CONSIDERATIONS

The skin is the largest organ of the body and, because of its visibility, it is familiar to all, veterinarians as well as laymen. Consequently, any change in the skin or hair is noticeable and may be a cause for concern. While serious internal organic conditions may be ignored or overlooked because of their covert nature, even mild dermatologic diseases are likely to be brought to veterinary attention. In many veterinary practices, dermatologic cases constitute a major component of the caseload. The diseases range from minor, esthetic problems to life-threatening conditions. Many diseases produce severe economic losses because of damage to wool, hides, and meat or from decreased milk production or growth rates. Even apparently mild hair and skin changes may affect the health of the animal and have serious consequences.

The skin serves numerous functions but one of the most important is protection of the individual from the external environment. The hair and stratum corneum, composed of tightly packed keratinized cells permeated by an emulsion of sebum and sweat, form a physical barrier against potential physical, chemical, or microbial damage. The skin also has a protective chemical barrier composed of inorganic salts, proteins, and fatty acids. A number of proteins have been identified in skin washings from various species and some of these include immunoglobulins of various classes, interferon, albumin, transferrin, and complement. Fatty acids, such as linoleic acid, have antibacterial and antifungal properties. The skin also has *normal microflora* that contribute to skin defense. A mixed population of symbiotic bacteria lives and multiplies permanently on the skin surface and thereby inhibits invading microorganisms. Occasional yeasts and fungal hyphae may also comprise the resident microflora. The skin is also a major sense organ and it protects the organism from desiccation. It is involved in photoprotection, immunosurveillance, nutrient and fat metabolism, and water balance. The skin is involved in temperature regulation by virtue of the hair coat, blood flow, and, in some species, sweating. Lastly, the skin can serve as a window to internal diseases.

As dermatologic cases are more commonly presented to veterinary clinicians for examination, skin biopsies have become a routine diagnostic procedure. An understanding of the pathologic processes in skin, as in any tissue, requires a thorough understanding of the normal structure and function of skin. *As a general rule, the clinician is more familiar with the gross pathology than is the pathologist because the majority of the cases are examined by the pathologist only in the form of a limited number of very small skin biopsies.* This fact underscores the importance of the inclusion of the gross findings in the surgical pathology request. The pathologist must be aware of normal variations in skin components from different body regions and from different species to correctly interpret deviations from normal. The basic architecture is similar in all mammals but skin thickness varies between species and region of the body within the same species. The dermis contributes most to the difference in skin thickness. The epidermis varies less markedly, but tends to be thinner in areas with thick hair and thicker in those areas without hair, such as mucocutaneous junctions. In general, skin thickness decreases dorsally to ventrally on the trunk and proximally to distally on the limbs. The skin is thickest over the dorsal surface of the body and lateral aspect of the limbs and thinnest on the ventral aspect of the trunk and medial limbs.

The integument is composed of epidermis, dermis, hair follicles, adnexal glands, and the subcutis. The appendages include nails, hooves, and claws.

Epidermis

The epidermis is a continually renewing tissue in which keratinocytes move from the basal layer outward to the skin surface where they are ultimately shed. During their migration through the epidermis, cells undergo changes in shape, structure, and composition until they are shed as dead, cornified husks of cells. Protection of an individual from the environment is largely dependent on the structural integrity of the epidermis. *To maintain uniform epidermal thickness and normal barrier function, basal cell proliferation, orderly cell differentiation through the various layers, and cell death must be balanced.* Knowledge of the regulation of this complex, dynamic process is incomplete and primarily based on cultured keratinocytes. Epidermal growth factor, insulin-like growth factor-I, keratinocyte growth factor, basic fibroblast growth factor, interleukin-1, interleukin-6, transforming growth factor-α, vitamin D_3, and retinoids are some of the factors thought to be involved in the growth and differentiation of keratinocytes.

One of the most important and abundant products of keratinocytes is *keratin*. It forms the cytoskeleton of keratinocytes and is thus responsible for the shape of the cells. It is also responsible for structural stability and it contributes to the impervious nature of the stratum corneum. Keratin is composed of acidic and basic pairs of subunits that are differentially expressed by keratinocytes of various layers of the epidermis. Basal cells express keratins K5 and K14, while commitment to differentiation in suprabasal keratinocytes is associated with induction of differentiation-specific keratins K1 and K10.

The epidermis is divided into four layers:

- The **stratum basale** (*basal layer*) is the deep germinative layer of the epidermis and is composed of a single layer of cuboidal to low columnar cells resting on the basement membrane. These cells are mitotically active and their daughter cells continually migrate upward to replenish cells in overlying layers. The basal layer is thought to be *composed of two populations of cells*: (1) *stem cells*, which have a long lifespan, long cycling phase, and short S period; and (2) *transit amplifying cells*, which undergo only a limited number of divisions before terminally differentiating. Mitotic figures and apoptotic cells are occasionally evident. The basal cells are attached to the underlying basement membrane by *hemidesmosomes* and to adjacent and overlying keratinocytes by *desmosomes*. Desmosomes are anchoring structures that mediate adhesion between cells. They have a complex structure that includes *cadherin proteins* of two types, desmocollins and desmogleins. These proteins have different isoforms and they are differentially expressed in different layers of the epidermis. While basal cells express a pair of desmogleins and desmocollins of simple epithelia, desmosomes of the spinous layer express a more varied array of isoforms. These adhesion molecules have been identified as the target in several blistering autoimmune diseases.
- The **stratum spinosum** (*prickle cell layer*) is characterized by *prominent intercellular bridges that are the desmosomal attachments between cells*. The spinous appearance is due to shrinkage artifact that occurs during tissue processing. The cells are polyhedral to

slightly flattened and are arranged in one or two layers in haired skin of dogs and cats and up to four layers in large animals. This layer is much thicker in lightly haired or nonhaired skin and may be up to 20 cells thick in the footpads and nasal planum. Cells of the upper spinous layer synthesize the protein *involucrin*, which is a constituent of the cornified envelope of the stratum corneum.

- The **stratum granulosum** is variably present in haired skin and is one or two cells thick when present. It is usually four to eight cell layers thick in nonhaired skin or at the infundibulum of hair follicles. The stratum granulosum is composed of flattened cells with shrunken nuclei and deeply basophilic keratohyaline granules of variable size and shape. The granules are composed of the precursor of *filaggrin*, a histidine-rich interfibrillary matrix protein that *functions as a biologic glue* that aggregates and aligns keratin filaments together. Stratum granulosum cells also contain *laminar granules* (membrane-coating granules, Odland bodies, keratinosomes), small organelles containing a mixture of lipids that are released to the intercellular space where they coat the cells and contribute to the hydrophobic barrier of the stratum corneum. The cells also synthesize the cysteine-rich protein *loricrin*, a major precursor of the cornified envelope. Dissolution of the nucleus and other organelles begins in upper layers of the stratum granulosum, probably through the action of lysosomal enzymes.
- The **stratum corneum** is the *impermeable, insoluble, highly protective layer* that keeps microorganisms out and essential body fluids in. It is composed of anucleate, dead, flattened eosinophilic cells (*squames*) that are continually shed. Thickness varies greatly according to body region and species. It is thickest in nonhaired areas such as footpads and nasal planum. Routine fixation and processing usually result in loss of approximately 50% of this layer. The cells are arranged in vertical interlocking columns in which intercellular spaces are filled with lipids derived from the laminar granules. The *basket-weave pattern* commonly visible in formalin-fixed sections is an artifact caused by loss of soluble intracellular constituents during routine processing. Structural support for these cells is provided by the cornified cell envelope. The cornified envelope is a complex structure composed of a number of proteins, including involucrin, loricrin, and keratolinin. The proteins are deposited on the inner membrane of the keratinocytes and are cross-linked by transglutaminases to form a highly insoluble, electron-dense band. The keratin in these cells is organized into large macrofilaments that confer mechanical resistance to the cells. The structural stability of the horny layer is derived from the association of the keratinized cells and insoluble extracellular lipids, a structure likened to a wall in which the cells represent the bricks and the lipids the mortar.

Epidermal non-keratinocytes

In addition to keratinocytes, which comprise approximately 85–90% of the cells of the epidermis, *small numbers of dendritic cells also reside in the epidermis*. These include *melanocytes, Langerhans cells, and Merkel cells*. **Melanocytes** are located in the basal layer of the epidermis and outer root sheath of hair follicles; and in HE sections they appear as clear cells with a small dark-staining nucleus due to shrinkage artifact. There is ~1 melanocyte per 10–20 keratinocytes. They can be visualized more specifically with silver stains, which demonstrate their dendritic processes. Derived from the neural crest, melanocytes migrate into the epidermis during early fetal life. Their processes are intertwined between the surrounding keratinocytes to which they transfer melanin pigment. A melanocyte and its surrounding constellation of keratinocytes is termed the "*epidermal melanin unit*." Melanogenesis occurs in membrane-bound organelles called *melanosomes*, which originate from the Golgi. The melanosomes migrate to the tips of the dendrites and are phagocytosed by adjacent keratinocytes. Most melanin pigment in skin is in the basal layer; but in dark-skinned animals, melanin may be present throughout the epidermis. Melanin is photoprotective and exposure to ultraviolet light increases melanin production, often resulting in a cap of pigment granules over the nucleus. Skin pigmentation is affected by local inflammation because melanocytes respond to inflammatory mediators by increasing or decreasing melanogenesis and by altering melanin transfer to keratinocytes.

Langerhans cells *are bone marrow-derived dendritic cells that are functionally and immunologically related to monocyte-macrophage cells*. They appear as clear cells on routine HE sections and may be distributed from the stratum basale to the stratum spinosum, depending on species and region of the skin. They are usually less numerous than melanocytes, however. Langerhans cells are characterized ultrastructurally by rod- or racket-shaped cytoplasmic granules called *Birbeck granules*. Birbeck granules have been identified in Langerhans cells of the pig, cat, cattle, sheep, goat, horse, and human, but not in the epidermal dendritic cells of the dog. Histochemical markers expressed by Langerhans cells include CD1, class II MHC (major histocompatibility) antigens, CD45, vimentin, and S-100. The long dendritic processes of Langerhans cells traverse the intercellular space to the granular cell layer where *they function in immunosurveillance as antigen-presenting cells*. Langerhans cells trap antigens in the epidermis and migrate via afferent lymphatics to draining lymph nodes where they present antigen to T cells in paracortical areas, resulting in proliferation of a population of sensitized T cells. Exposure to UVB radiation decreases Langerhans cell numbers in the epidermis and interferes with their antigen-presenting capacity. Langerhans cells are involved in development of contact hypersensitivity, and increased numbers of epidermal Langerhans cells have been found in horses with insect hypersensitivity and dogs with discoid lupus erythematosus, hypersensitivities, and deep pyodermas.

A second type of clear cell in the basal layer is the **Merkel cell** whose *origin is unknown*. Unlike melanocytes, Merkel cells are connected to adjacent keratinocytes by desmosomes. Merkel cells are also located in the external root sheath of hair follicles. They are identified ultrastructurally by characteristic *dense-core cytoplasmic granules*. Immunohistochemical markers include cytokeratin, neurofilaments, neuron-specific enolase, and desmosomal proteins. Merkel cells have been identified in the dog, cat, sheep, pig, monkey, various laboratory animals, birds, reptiles, and amphibians. Their density in the epidermis is variable and they are in highest numbers in areas involved with sensory perception. Merkel cells form *Merkel cell–neurite complexes* with axons in tylotrich pads that are thought to function as slow-adapting mechanoreceptors and in sinus hairs. Their exact function in these structures is uncertain but they are thought not to act as sensory cells but rather to function as abutments for deformation of the mechanosensitive nerve endings. Merkel cells are also thought to have various neuroendocrine effects and to be involved in control of the hair cycle.

Basement membrane zone

The basement membrane zone (BMZ) is the structurally and biochemically complex junction between the epidermis and dermis. Both the epidermis and dermis contribute to production of the various components of the BMZ. The area is indistinct in HE sections but visible as a thin, homogeneous band with PAS stain. It varies in thickness in different sites and is most prominent in nonhaired areas of skin and mucocutaneous junctions. In all animals but the pig, the dermal–epidermal junction is straight and the BMZ parallels the skin surface; while in pigs and humans, the dermal–epidermal junction is thrown into undulating folds called rete ridges. *The BMZ has a crucial role in anchoring the epidermis to the dermis; and abnormalities of the BMZ result in serious and potentially fatal bullous diseases.* The BMZ also influences growth and differentiation of keratinocytes and acts as a selective barrier for passage of molecules between the epidermis and dermis.

Ultrastructurally, the BMZ is composed of: (1) the **plasma membrane** of basal keratinocytes with their specialized attachment structures, *hemidesmosomes*; (2) the electron-lucent **lamina lucida**; (3) the electron-dense **lamina densa**; and (4) the subbasal **lamina fibrous zone**. Hemidesmosomes are located on the basal aspect of basal keratinocytes and they consist of a cytoplasmic plaque that connects to the cytoskeleton and a transmembrane portion that binds to the underlying basement membrane. The *cytoplasmic plaque* is composed of a number of proteins, including bullous pemphigoid antigen 230 (bullous pemphigoid antigen 1) and plectin, which connect keratin 5 and 14 intermediate filaments to the plasma membrane. Hemidesmosomes also have a transmembrane portion that includes $\alpha6\beta4$ integrin and bullous pemphigoid antigen 2 (type XVII collagen). The proposed ligand for $\alpha6\beta4$ integrin is laminin 5, which is a component of the anchoring filaments of the lamina lucida, and this binding mediates the stable adhesion of keratinocytes to components of the BMZ. *Anchoring filaments* are 2–4 nm diameter filaments composed of laminin 5 (also called epiligrin, kalinin, and BM600). They pass from the plasma membrane through the lamina lucida to attach to the lamina densa. The lamina densa is composed of multiple molecules, including collagen type IV, laminin, nidogen, and several glycoproteins. The lamina densa is connected to anchoring plaques of the underlying dermis by anchoring fibrils. The subbasal lamina fibrous zone of the superficial dermis is composed of anchoring fibrils, anchoring plaques, and microfibrils. Anchoring fibrils are composed of collagen type VII and form looping arrays with one or both ends of the fibrils attached to the lamina densa, thereby anchoring the BMZ to the dermis.

Dermis

The dermis is involved in maintenance and repair of the skin and is the major component responsible for the tensile strength and elasticity of the skin. In addition, the thickness of the dermis largely determines the thickness of the skin. *The dermis is composed of collagen and elastic fibers embedded in a ground substance, blood and lymphatic vessels, nerves, and low numbers of mixed cells.* Except for pigs, domestic animals have no dermal papillae as occur in human skin. Thus, instead of papillary and reticular dermis, the dermis is divided somewhat arbitrarily into *superficial and deep dermis* in domestic animals.

The **dermal fibers** include collagen, reticulum fibers, and elastic fibers, all of which are synthesized by dermal fibroblasts. Collagen fibers are the most abundant constituent of the dermis and they confer tensile strength to skin. The majority of *dermal collagen is types I and III.* The superficial dermis is composed of fine, loosely arranged collagen fibers. The deep dermis consists of thick, densely arranged collagen fibers that roughly parallel the skin surface. Reticulum fibers represent a special thin type of collagen. *Elastic fibers* are inconspicuous in routine HE sections. They can be visualized with special stains such as orcein stain or Verhoeff–van Gieson elastin stain. They are thicker and less numerous in the deep dermis and arranged parallel to the skin surface. The elastic fibers become progressively thinner near the epidermis.

The **ground or interstitial substance** is an amorphous gel-sol that fills the space between dermal structures but allows electrolytes, nutrients, growth factors, and cells to pass through. It consists of *proteoglycans and glycoproteins*. Proteoglycans are high-molecular-weight complexes composed of glycosaminoglycans linked to proteins and those most abundant in the dermis include hyaluronic acid and various chondroitin sulfates. Proteoglycans bind various chemical mediators and thereby function as storage matrix as well as provide lubrication and structural support. *Fibronectins* are a family of glycoproteins involved in mediating cell–cell and cell–matrix interactions that are required for various cell functions including cell adhesion, phagocytosis, and cell migration. The ground substance is usually not visible in normal HE sections; however, a fine granular to fibrillar basophilic material is occasionally evident between collagen fibers. This material is especially abundant in the dermis of Chinese Shar-Peis as a normal variant for this breed.

The **dermal vasculature** is arranged in three intercommunicating plexuses. The *deep plexus* is located at the junction of the dermis and subcutis and it supplies branches to the *middle plexus*, which is located at the level of the sebaceous glands. It, in turn, supplies branches to the *superficial plexus*. The capillary loops parallel to the skin surface immediately beneath the epidermis arise from the superficial plexus. An unusual vascular arrangement is present in the dermis of the llama. It consists of clusters of capillary-size, thick-walled vessels lined by plump endothelial cells distributed throughout the superficial and middle dermis. Dermal lymphatic vessels are inconspicuous in normal skin and only become visible when they become dilated because of increased lymphatic drainage. The skin is supplied with sensory and autonomic nerves that are usually associated with blood vessels.

The dermis is normally **sparsely cellular**. *Fibroblasts* are distributed in low numbers throughout the dermis. They synthesize most of the fibrillar and ground substance proteins of the dermis as well as various growth factors and cytokines. *Melanocytes* in the dermis are usually located near superficial dermal vessels. In contrast to melanocytes of the epidermis and hair follicles ("secretory melanocytes"), dermal melanocytes do not transfer their melanin to surrounding cells ("continent melanocytes"). Normal dermis also contains small numbers of perivascular *monocytes and lymphocytes,* which are indistinguishable from each other. Dermal lymphocytes are T cells of the helper subtype primarily.

Mast cells are tissue-dwelling cells that are most numerous in sites, such as the skin, that interface with the environment. Mast cell numbers in skin vary greatly depending on body location, with numbers ranging from 0–60 per high-power field in cats, and 0–40 per high-power field in dogs. They are in highest numbers in the skin of the caudal pinna in both dogs and cats. They are concentrated around blood vessels, especially postcapillary venules. Mast cells are not present in normal epidermis. Although mast cells are evident in routine HE sections, they are better visualized with Giemsa and toluidine blue, which stain mast cell granules metachromatically.

Mast cells originate in the bone marrow and are released as unidentifiable precursors into the blood. These *immature mast cell precursors are thought to home to the skin* because of mast cell growth factor expression by dermal endothelial cells. Their final differentiation and maturation is controlled by the local microenvironment, including stem cell factor, which is a fibroblast-derived growth factor, and various T-cell-derived cytokines (IL-3, 4, 9, 10). Mast cells have laminin receptors that mediate their adhesion to the extracellular matrix. The perivascular space is rich in laminin, which contributes to the localization of mast cells to this site. Mast cells are a heterogeneous population based on differences in histochemical, biochemical, and functional characteristics that vary between species and different tissues within a single species. Mast cell heterogeneity has been demonstrated in the skin of cattle, dogs, and sheep. A subpopulation of mast cells that does not exhibit metachromasia following formalin fixation has been demonstrated in the skin of dogs and cattle, and heterogeneity of protein content has been identified in dermal mast cells of sheep.

Mast cell granules contain an array of *preformed mediators*; but they are also capable of *synthesizing mediators* such as leukotrienes (LTC_4) and prostaglandins (PGD_2) following stimulation. Tumor necrosis factor-α, a potent pro-inflammatory cytokine, is both preformed and newly synthesized upon activation of mast cells. Mast cells have long been known to be the *critical effector cell* in initiation of acute type I hypersensitivity reactions and in protection against parasitic infections with helminths and ectoparasitic arthropods. More recently, however, it has become apparent that mast cells also function in persistent chronic inflammatory reactions, tissue repair and remodeling, pathologic fibrosis, angiogenesis, hemostasis, hematopoiesis, antibody production, protection against bacterial infections, response to neoplasms, and possibly in control of the hair cycle.

Dermal muscles

Arrector pili muscles are smooth muscles present in all haired skin. They arise in the connective tissue of the superficial dermis and attach to the connective tissue sheath of the hair follicle below the level of the sebaceous gland duct. They are situated on the obtuse angle of the hair follicle and when the muscles contract, the hair follicles are pulled into a vertical position (*piloerection*). This results in formation of air pockets in the hair coat, which provides insulation. Contraction of arrector pili muscles may also be involved in emptying of sebaceous glands. These muscles are largest in skin of the dorsal midline from the neck to the tail. They may be vacuolated in normal animals, especially aged dogs. In addition to arrector pili muscles, pigs also have **interfollicular smooth muscles**. These muscles span the triad of hair follicles at a level midway between the sebaceous and apocrine glands. Their contraction draws the hair follicles together and rotates the outer follicle of the triad. The functional significance of this muscle is uncertain.

Skeletal muscles may be present in the muzzle, forehead, eyelid, and perianal regions. These muscle fibers originate from cutaneous trunci muscle that penetrates into the dermis to allow voluntary movement of the skin. Skeletal muscle fibers also are associated with the large sinus hairs of the face.

Immunologic function

The skin has been proposed to function as an immunosurveillance organ and the term skin-associated lymphoid tissue (SALT), analogous to gut and bronchial-associated lymphoid tissues (GALT, BALT), has been suggested to describe those cellular elements of the skin that deal with antigenic challenges at the skin surface. However, this concept has been disputed because of presumed differences in immune function between the common mucosal immune system and normal skin. The alternative name, **skin immune system (SIS)**, has been suggested as a more appropriate term to encompass the skin-specific immune response-associated cells and humoral factors present in normal skin. Key components of this system *include keratinocytes, Langerhans cells, the dermal perivascular unit, and skin-homing T cells*.

- **Keratinocytes** produce multiple inflammatory cytokines, adhesion molecules, and chemotactic factors following nonspecific stimulation, and thereby have a nonspecific proinflammatory and up-regulating effect.
- **Langerhans cells** are thought to trap antigens in the epidermis, migrate out to regional lymph nodes via lymphatics, and present the antigen to T cells. Thus, induction of the immune response does not normally occur within the skin itself but rather in the skin-draining lymph nodes.
- The **dermal perivascular unit** consists of the mast cells, monocytes and macrophages, tissue dendritic cells, and T cells situated around postcapillary venules. As a result of cytokines such as IL-1 and TNF-α released by injured keratinocytes, endothelial cells increase their expression of addressins ICAM-1 and E-selectin and vascular cell adhesion molecule (VCAM-1). These vascular endothelial molecules promote adhesion of circulating leukocytes, especially granulocytes and memory T cells.
- E-selectin is thought to act as an adhesion molecule or vascular addressin for a specific subset of **skin-homing memory T cells**, which have the ligand cutaneous lymphocyte antigen (CLA) on their surface. A circulating pool of such skin-homing T lymphocytes, identified by CLA antigen, represents the cellular basis of immunologic memory of skin.

Thus, it appears that the proinflammatory, up-regulating effects of keratinocytes prepare the dermis for specific immunologic activity, while migrating antigen-presenting Langerhans cells induce expansion of specific lymphocytes in skin-draining lymph nodes. T cells are then recruited to the skin because of binding of skin-specific adhesion molecules to the vascular addressins of dermal endothelial cells.

Hair follicles

Hair serves a number of functions including protection, thermal insulation, social communication, and sensory perception. Arrangement and type of hair follicles vary with species, breed, individual, and body region. In general, however, hair follicle density is greatest over the dorsolateral aspect of the body and least on the ventral aspect. Hair follicles are classified as *primary or secondary*, and *simple or compound*. **Primary hairs** have a large diameter, are rooted more deeply in the dermis, and are associated with sebaceous and sweat glands and an arrector pili muscle. **Secondary hair follicles** are smaller in diameter, are more superficially rooted, and may be accompanied by a sebaceous gland but lack a sweat gland and arrector pili muscle. Follicles in which a single hair emerges from the follicular orifice are termed **simple follicles**; while those in which multiple hairs emerge from a single opening are called **compound follicles**. Each hair of the compound follicle has its own *papilla*; but at the level of the sebaceous gland opening, the follicles unite to exit from a single external follicular orifice. Horses and cattle have simple hair follicles that are evenly distributed. Pigs have simple follicles that are grouped in clusters of two to four surrounded by dense connective tissue. In sheep, the hair-growing areas consist predominantly of simple follicles whereas the wool-growing areas have many compound follicles and consist of clusters of three primary follicles and a number of secondary follicles. Goats have primary follicles in groups of three with three to six secondary follicles associated with each group. Follicular arrangement in dogs and cats consists of two to five large primary hairs surrounded by groups of smaller secondary hairs. The primary hairs tend to be simple while the secondary hairs are compound. As many as 15 hairs may emerge from a single follicular orifice. In cats, secondary hairs far outnumber primary hairs (10–24 secondary hairs : one primary hair).

The hair follicle is formed by a downward invasion of the surface ectoderm (*primary hair germ*) into the underlying mesoderm of the embryo. As they grow down, the epithelial cells envelop a small group of mesenchymal cells in the underlying dermis. These mesodermal cells eventually become the **follicular papilla** that repeatedly induces and maintains growth of the hair follicle throughout the life of the individual. If the papilla is somehow damaged or destroyed, the hair follicle fails to regrow. The epithelial downgrowth eventually becomes canalized to form the hair follicle. In longitudinal section, the fully developed hair follicle consists of three segments:

- the **lower or inferior portion**, from the base of the follicle to the point of insertion of the arrector pili muscle;
- the **isthmus**, the short section from the attachment of the arrector pili muscle to the entrance of the sebaceous duct; and
- the **infundibulum**, extending from the entrance of the sebaceous duct to the follicular orifice.

The entire hair follicle beneath the isthmus, i.e., the inferior segment, can be considered temporary because it disappears during the involution stage of the hair cycle and reforms again during the active phase. In contrast, *the isthmus and infundibular portions of the hair follicle are permanent.*

The **base of the hair follicle** consists of a terminal bulbous expansion of epithelial cells, the hair bulb, with a concavity at its bottom that is occupied by the connective tissue papilla. The *bulb* is composed of the highly proliferative matrix cells and melanocytes and they are separated from the papilla by a thin extension of the basement membrane. The *matrix cells* give rise to six different cell types arranged in concentric layers. *The three innermost layers form the medulla, cortex, and cuticle of the emerging hair.* The next three layers form the *cuticle, Huxley layer, and Henle layer of the inner root sheath.* These layers are further surrounded by the outer root sheath, which is an extension of the epidermis and becomes continuous with the epidermis in the upper portion of the follicle. *External to the outer root sheath* are the *glassy membrane*, corresponding to the basement membrane of the epidermis, and finally the *connective tissue sheath.* All three layers of the inner root sheath keratinize by means of eosinophilic trichohyaline granules and become fully keratinized and disintegrate at the level of the isthmus. The inner root sheath is responsible for providing the rigid support for the developing hair and its final shape, e.g., twisted hair follicles produce curly hairs. From the base of the hair follicle to the isthmus, the outer root sheath is covered by the inner root sheath and it does not keratinize. In the isthmus, where the inner root sheath is no longer present, the outer root sheath undergoes trichilemmal keratinization, i.e., without keratohyaline granules. In the infundibulum, the outer root sheath is identical to surface epidermis and undergoes keratinization with formation of keratohyaline granules.

Hair does not grow continuously but rather in *cycles* consisting of a growth phase, **anagen**; a transitional or involuting phase, **catagen**; and a resting phase, **telogen**. This cyclic activity is thought to be an adaptive response to seasonal variation in ambient temperature. The hair growth cycle varies between different species, breeds, body sites, and hair follicle type. In domestic animals, *neighboring hairs cycle independently of each other and are in different stages of the hair cycle at any one time.* Hair shaft length is directly related to the duration of anagen phase, which is preordained according to body region and genetics. At the onset of catagen, mitotic activity of matrix cells and melanin production by melanocytes of the hair bulb cease. The keratinocytes of the inferior segment of the follicle undergo a controlled process of involution via a burst of apoptosis. This results in the upward migration of the hair follicle and the lower follicle becoming a thin cord of epithelial cells surrounded by a fibrous root sheath. Growth of the inner root sheath stops so that the lower end of the hair shaft is surrounded by thick trichilemmal keratin. The thin cord of epithelial cells is surrounded by a thickened, corrugated glassy membrane; and as it retracts upward, it is followed by the shrunken, contracted papilla. In telogen phase, the base of the bulb is located at the level of attachment of the arrector pili muscle and is approximately one-third of its former length. The base of the hair is encased in trichilemmal keratin and surrounded completely by outer root sheath (*club hair*). A population of stem cells (secondary hair germ) remains somewhere in the permanent portion of the hair follicle. These cells eventually reform the hair follicle during the next growth cycle. In rodents, the *bulge region of the follicle* appears to be the site that contains slow-cycling relatively undifferentiated cells from which arise a population of transient amplifying cells that become the matrix keratinocytes of the new hair bulb. *The bulge region is an area on the outer root sheath at the base of the permanent portion of the hair follicle to which the arrector pili muscle attaches.* It is not yet clear whether or not hair follicles of other domestic species have a similar bulge region of the hair follicle.

Hair growth in many animals has been shown to be regulated by photoperiod, ambient temperature, various hormones, nutritional status, and general health. However, the exact mechanisms that control the cycle are incompletely understood. Growth and development of hair are influenced by many growth factors; these include fibroblast growth factor (FGF), epidermal growth factor (EGF), insulin-like growth factor-1 (IGF-1), transforming growth factor-β (TGF-β), and keratinocyte growth factor (KGF, same as FGF-7). Both IGF-1 and KGF are produced by the dermal papilla and their receptors are found in the overlying anagen hair follicle matrix cells. Factors from the papilla mesenchymal cells are thought to act on a stem cell population in the permanent upper portion of the hair follicle. These competent cells respond to the signals from the papilla by growing deep into the dermis to form the full-length anagen hair follicle. Transition between anagen and catagen appears to be regulated by FGF-5.

The *histologic appearance* of the hair follicle changes considerably during the hair cycle. The **anagen** stage is characterized by a well-developed flame-shaped plump dermal papilla that is capped completely by the hair bulb. The bulb is located in the deep dermis or subcutis and even bulbs of secondary hairs are surrounded by fat because tracts of fatty tissue extend upward from the subcutaneous fat. A layer of columnar matrix cells lines the papilla and melanocytes are dispersed among the matrix cells in pigmented hair follicles. **Catagen** stage is characterized by a thick glassy membrane that is irregular and undulating above the bulb of the hair follicle. The basement membrane between the dermal papilla and matrix is also thickened. The papilla is smaller, more compact because of decreased extracellular matrix and loss of capillary loops, and it is ovoid or round rather than spindle-shaped. The overlying matrix cells are no longer columnar and they appear disorganized. **Telogen** phase is distinguished by the club hair that has a brush-like appearance produced by keratinized fibers extending between the base of the club hair and the cells of the outer root sheath. The dermal papilla is a condensed ball of cells separated from the matrix cells and surrounded by its basement membrane.

Sinus hairs *(tactile hairs, vibrissae) are highly specialized mechanoreceptors that respond to vibratory stimuli as well as static hair displacements.* They are located on the muzzle (whiskers, vibrissae), face, throat, and palmar aspect of the carpus. They are thick, stiff hairs which are tapered distally. Histologically, they are composed of large single follicles surrounded by an endothelial cell-lined blood-filled sinus situated within the dermal connective tissue sheath. The sinus is supplied with numerous nerves; and skeletal muscles attach to the outer sheath of the follicle to confer some voluntary control of the hairs.

Sebaceous glands

Sebaceous glands are distributed throughout the haired skin and are essential for maintaining normal skin and hair. *Sebaceous glands produce sebum, an oily secretion composed of triglycerides, phospholipids, and cholesterol.* This material combines with sweat to form an emulsion that coats the skin to act as a physical barrier to retain moisture and maintain normal hydration, and as a chemical barrier against microbial pathogens. In addition, the oily film coats the hair shafts to give them a glossy sheen; it also acts as a *pheromone.* Lastly, sebaceous glands also appear to be involved with normal hair development, because, in the absence of sebaceous glands, the hair shaft fails to separate normally from the sheath.

Sebaceous glands consist of a solid mass of epithelial cells surrounded by a connective tissue sheath. The periphery of the gland consists of a single layer of cuboidal mitotically active cells resting on a basal lamina, analogous to basal cells of the epidermis. As the cells move inward toward the duct, they enlarge and accumulate lipid that is lost during routine processing. Sebaceous glands are *holocrine glands* and their secretion is formed by decomposition of cells. This is brought about by release of lysosomal enzymes in cells nearest the duct causing them to disintegrate and form sebum, which empties via a squamous epithelium-lined duct into the upper portion of the hair canal. All primary hairs and some secondary hairs have sebaceous glands. They are usually largest in areas with lowest hair follicle density such as mucocutaneous junctions, interdigital spaces, coronet, and dorsal neck and rump. Sebaceous glands are especially numerous and well developed in the chin of cats (*submental organ*), dorsal surface of the tail in dogs and cats (*tail gland*), base of the horn in goats, and infraorbital, inguinal, and interdigital regions of sheep. The footpads and nasal planum are devoid of sebaceous glands, and they are rare in glabrous skin where they empty directly to the skin surface.

Perianal glands

These are specialized secretory glands in the perianal regions, and they are commonly sites for the development of lesions.

- *Anal glands.* These are *specialized apocrine glands* that open directly onto anal skin and into specialized cystic structures on the lateral aspects of the anal canal, the anal sacs. The anal sacs are usually flaccid cystic cavities containing odoriferous secretions, presumably with some territorial marking function. They are present in many species, including domestic and wild felids, ferrets, raccoons, mink, rodents, pigs, and canids.
- *Perianal glands.* These glands are presumed to be *modified sebaceous glands* based on their typical histology, and are comprised of small glands and nests of cells without a prominent ductular network. Islands of these glands are concentrated in the subcutis around the perimeter of the anus, but foci are commonly present over lateral and ventral aspects of the base of the tail, less commonly on the dorsum of the tail, and in the skin of the prepuce and rump. The glands are distinctive, comprised of lobules of large eosinophilic epithelial cells (*hepatoid cells*) surrounded by low numbers of small basal reserve cells. Larger ducts are often lined by stratified squamous epithelium. *Perianal (circumanal) glands are best described in the dog*, and are most developed in entire males. Their function is uncertain, but they may have a role in steroid metabolism, in production of pheromones, and in territorial marking. Similar glands are also present in cats and in pericloacal glands of reptiles, where they probably have similar roles in territorial marking.

Sweat glands

Two types of sweat glands are present in the skin of mammals; they differ in origin, distribution, and possibly in the mode of secretion. These glands have been called apocrine and eccrine glands; but because of questions concerning the mechanism of the secretory process of these glands, the names *epitrichial and atrichial glands have been proposed for apocrine and eccrine glands, respectively.* **Apocrine (epitrichial) sweat glands** develop embryologically from primary hair germ and they are distributed throughout all haired skin, usually deep to the sebaceous glands. *Apocrine glands are associated with primary hair follicles only* and they tend to be largest in areas with lower hair follicle density, such as mucocutaneous junctions, interdigital spaces, coronet, and dorsal midline. Sweat mixes with sebum to form the protective skin surface film. Apocrine sweat glands function in thermoregulation only in horses and cattle. In other species, the secretion may contribute to scent that is involved in social communication. Apocrine secretion may also provide a means of excreting waste products and secreting immunoglobulins that are present on the skin surface. They are *simple saccular or tubular glands* with a coiled secretory portion and straight duct. The secretory portion is composed of a single row of flat cuboidal to columnar epithelial cells surrounded by a single layer of myoepithelial cells situated between the secretory cells and basal lamina. *The duct empties into the pilary canal usually above the entrance of the sebaceous duct or, rarely, directly to the skin surface.* The name apocrine refers to the mode of secretion, which was originally thought to involve pinching off (apo = off) of a portion of the cell. The existence of an apocrine secretory process has been questioned; however, ultrastructural examination of these glands in humans, pigs, horses, and dogs indicates that *several modes of secretion are involved*, including the apocrine type.

In contrast to apocrine glands, **eccrine (atrichial) sweat glands** are derived from the embryonal epidermis rather then from the primary hair germ and they are located only in specialized areas. They occur in the *footpad of dogs and cats, frog of ungulates, snout of pigs, planum nasolabiale of cattle, and medial surface of the carpus of pigs (carpal glands)*. The function of eccrine glands is uncertain. The secretion may be involved with scent signaling and in the footpad of cats it may improve frictional capacity of the paw. Eccrine glands are histologically similar to apocrine glands but their ducts open directly to the skin surface. There is no recent detailed examination of eccrine gland secretion to identify the mode of secretion conclusively.

Subcutis

The deepest layer of the skin is the subcutis. It is composed of lipocytes subdivided into lobules by thin bands of collagen and small vessels. The collagenous septa provide structural support by compartmentalizing the subcutis and anchoring the dermis to the fascial planes deep to the subcutis.

Bibliography

Al-Bagdadi FK, et al. Histology of the hair cycle in male beagle dogs. Am J Vet Res 1979;40:11734–1741.

Atoji Y, et al. Circumanal glands of the dog: a new classification and cell degeneration. Anat Rec 1998;250:251–267.

Becker AB, et al. Mast cell heterogeneity in dog skin. Anat Rec 1985;213:477–480.

Borradori L, Sonnenberg A. Structure and function of hemidesmosomes: More than simple adhesion complexes. J Invest Dermatol 1999;112:411–418.

Bos JD, Kapsenberg ML. The skin immune system: progress in cutaneous biology. Immunol Today 1993;14:75–78.

Danilenko DM, et al. Keratinocyte growth factor is an important endogenous mediator of hair follicle growth, development, and differentiation. Normalization of the nu/nu follicular differentiation defect and amelioration of chemotherapy-induced alopecia. Am J Pathol 1995;147:145–154.

Foster AP. A study of the number and distribution of cutaneous mast cells in cats with disease not affecting the skin. Vet Dermatol 1994;5:17–20.

Galli SJ. New concepts about the mast cell. New Engl J Med 1993;328:257–265.

Gargiulo AM, et al. The process of secretion in swine apocrine sweat glands. Anat Histol Embryol 1990;19:264–268.

Hill PB, Martin RJ. A review of mast cell biology. Vet Dermatol 1998;9:145–166.

Iwasaki T. An electron microscopic study on secretory process in canine apocrine sweat gland. Jpn J Vet Sci 1981;43:733–740.

Kube P, et al. Distribution, density and heterogeneity of canine mast cells and influence of fixation techniques. Histochem Cell Biol 1998;110:129–135.

Lavker RM, et al. Hair follicle stem cells: Their location, role in hair cycle, and involvement in skin tumor formation. J Invest Dermatol 1993;101:16s–26s.

Marinkovich MP. The molecular genetics of basement membrane diseases. Arch Dermatol 1993;129:1557–1565.

Messenger AG. The control of hair growth: An overview. J Invest Dermatol 1993;101:4s–9s.

Meyer W, et al. Cytological and lectin histochemical characterization of secretion production and secretion composition in the tubular glands of the canine anal sacs. Cells Tissues Organs 2001;168:203–219.

Paus R, Cotsarelis G. The biology of hair follicles. New Engl J Med 1999; 341:491–497.

Robert C, Kupper TS. Inflammatory skin diseases, T cells, and immune surveillance. New Engl J Med 1999;341:1817–1827.

Stenn KS, et al. Hair follicle growth controls. Dermatol Clin 1996;14:543–558.

Sture GH, et al. Ovine mast cell heterogeneity is defined by the distribution of sheep mast cell proteinase. Vet Immunol Immunopathol 1995;48:275–285.

Suter MM, et al. Review article. Keratinocyte biology and pathology. Vet Dermatol 1997;8:67–100.

Uitto J, Christiano AM. Molecular genetics of the cutaneous basement membrane zone. Perspectives on epidermolysis bullosa and other blistering skin diseases. J Clin Invest 1992;90:687–692.

White SD, Yager JA. Resident dendritic cells in the epidermis: Langerhans cells, Merkel cells and melanocytes. Vet Dermatol 1995;6:1–8.

DERMATOHISTOPATHOLOGY

The pathology of the skin, more than that of any other organ, has a specialized vocabulary because many histopathologic changes are unique to the skin. The following is a glossary of terms used in dermatopathology.

Glossary

Acantholysis is a *loss of cohesion between epidermal cells* resulting in intraepidermal clefts, vesicles and bullae (Fig. 5.1). This process may also involve the outer root sheath of hair follicles. Acantholysis is caused by the breakdown of desmosomes between keratinocytes and is characteristic of the *pemphigus complex*. It can also be the result of the action of proteolytic enzymes released by neutrophils or eosinophils in an inflammatory process.

Acanthosis specifically indicates an *increased thickness of the stratum spinosum*, and is due to hyperplasia and occasionally to hypertrophy of cells of the stratum spinosum. Acanthosis, however, is *often used synonymously with hyperplasia* when referring to the epidermis.

Apoptosis refers to *individual programmed cell death*. It is usually seen in the basal layer but can be seen in any layer of the epidermis. Apoptotic keratinocytes histologically resemble dyskeratotic keratinocytes and are eosinophilic and shrunken. They are sometimes referred to as *apoptotic bodies* (colloid bodies, hyaline bodies, Civatte bodies).

Atrophy, in regard to the epidermis, is decreased thickness of the epidermis due to *decreased thickness of the stratum spinosum*. An early sign of epidermal atrophy is the loss of the rete ridges in areas of skin where they are normally present. *The extremely thin normal epidermis of domestic animals makes atrophy very difficult to detect.* It is

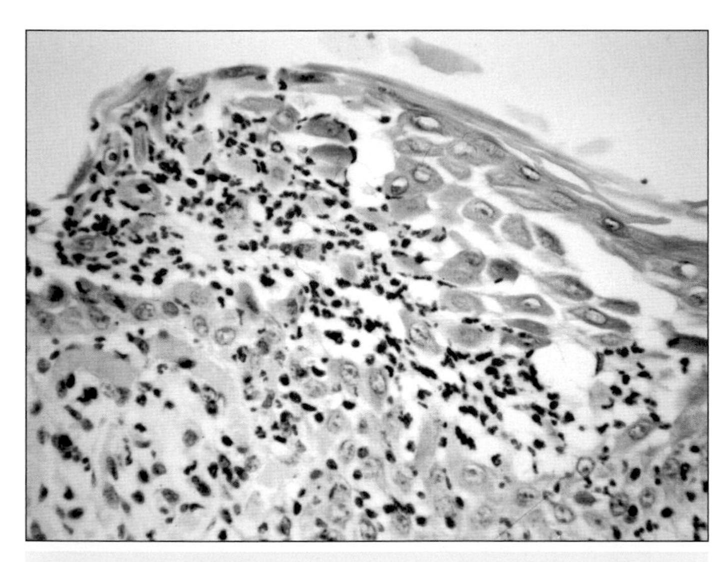

Figure 5.1 Acantholysis in pemphigus foliaceus. Loss of cohesion between keratinocytes leads to individualization of cells. Note cells have normal nuclear morphology.

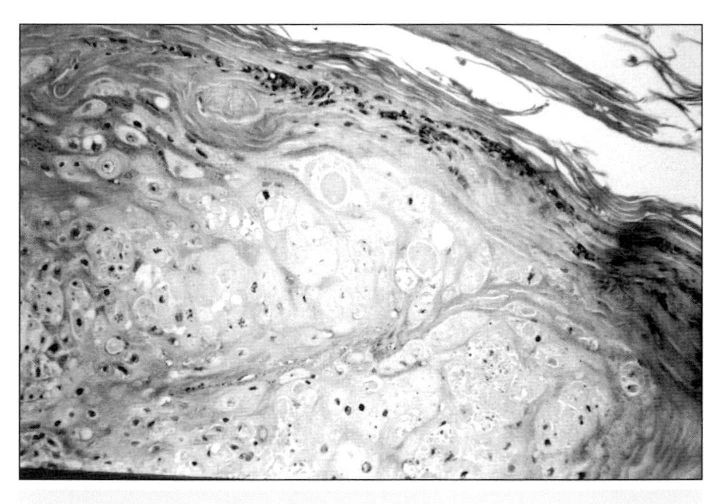

Figure 5.2 Ballooning degeneration in viral dermatitis. Keratinocytes are enlarged and pale due to marked intracellular edema.

seen with endocrine, some immune-mediated dermatoses, and as a result of ischemia. *Dermal atrophy* is thinning of dermal collagen fibrils resulting in decreased dermal thickness, as is seen in some endocrine dermatoses.

Ballooning degeneration of the epidermis is due to *intracellular edema* (Fig. 5.2). It is characterized by swollen eosinophilic cytoplasm, enlarged or condensed nuclei, and a loss of cohesion resulting in acantholysis and sometimes vesicle formation. Ballooning degeneration is a *characteristic feature of viral infections*, particularly of herpesviruses and poxviruses.

Bullae are *collections of fluid* within or below the epidermis greater than 1.0 cm in diameter. They may be caused by severe intercellular or intracellular edema, ballooning degeneration, acantholysis, hydropic degeneration of basal cells, subepidermal edema or other factors resulting in dermoepidermal separation such as the autoantibodies in bullous pemphigoid. Bullae may be *subcorneal, intragranular, suprabasilar or intrabasal, or subepidermal in location.*

Clefts are *slit-like spaces*, which do not contain fluid, within the epidermis or at the dermoepidermal junction. Clefts may be caused by acantholysis or hydropic degeneration of basal cells. However, clefts may also result from handling artifacts.

Collagen degeneration is a *structural and tinctorial change* characterized by slight basophilia, a granular appearance and frayed edges of collagen fibrils, seen with feline, canine and equine eosinophilic granuloma, or other eosinophil-rich conditions, such as mast cell tumors.

Comedo *is a cystically dilated, keratin-filled hair follicle.* Comedones are characteristically seen in Schnauzer comedo syndrome, some endocrine dermatopathies, and actinic dermatitis.

Crusts are consolidated, desiccated surface masses composed of various combinations of keratin, serum, cellular debris and often microorganisms. Crusts are further described on the basis of their composition: *serous* (mostly serum), *hemorrhagic* (mostly blood), *cellular* (mostly inflammatory cells), and *serocellular* (a mixture of serum and inflammatory cells). Crusts should be examined closely for dermatophyte spores and hyphae, *Dermatophilus congolensis*, or large numbers of acantholytic keratinocytes which can be indicators of pemphigus complex. Bacteria are commonly seen in crusts and are not necessarily of diagnostic importance.

Dells are *small depressions or hollows* in the surface of the epidermis independent of adnexal structures. They are usually associated with focal epidermal atrophy and orthokeratotic hyperkeratosis.

Dermal edema is recognized by *dilated lymphatics* (not visible in normal skin), widened spaces between blood vessels and perivascular collagen (*perivascular edema*) or widened spaces between dermal collagen fibers (*interstitial edema*). The dilated lymphatics and widened perivascular and interstitial spaces may or may not contain lightly eosinophilic, homogeneous, proteinaceous fluid. Dermal edema is a common feature of any *inflammatory dermatosis*. Severe edema of the superficial dermis may result in subepidermal vesicles and bullae, necrosis of the overlying epidermis, and predisposition to artifactual dermoepidermal separation during handling and processing of biopsy specimens. Severe edema of the superficial dermis may result in vertical orientation and stretching of collagen fibers, producing the "gossamer" (web-like) collagen effect seen in severe urticaria.

Desmoplasia usually refers to *fibroplasia and collagenous stroma induced by neoplastic processes.*

Dyskeratosis is *premature or abnormal keratinization of individual keratinocytes* in the epidermis or follicular epithelium. Histologically, dyskeratotic cells are eosinophilic and shrunken with condensed, dark-staining nuclei (Fig. 5.3). Dyskeratosis may be seen in a number of dermatoses including lupus erythematosus, erythema multiforme, and graft versus host disease. It can also occur in neoplastic dermatoses, especially papillomas. Dyskeratosis is a feature of the severe epidermal dysplasia that precedes the development of some squamous cell carcinomas.

Dysplasia refers to *faulty or abnormal development* of the epidermis, hair follicles, or any component of the skin. It is an abnormal but non-neoplastic change, however it can accompany neoplastic changes.

Dystrophic mineralization is the deposition of *calcium salts as basophilic, amorphous, granular material along collagen fibrils* as in hyperglucocorticism. Dystrophic mineralization of the hair follicle basement membrane can be seen in hyperglucocorticism, and as a senile change in dogs, especially poodles.

Epidermolytic hyperkeratosis (*granular cell degeneration*) is a change in the stratum granulosum characterized by perinuclear

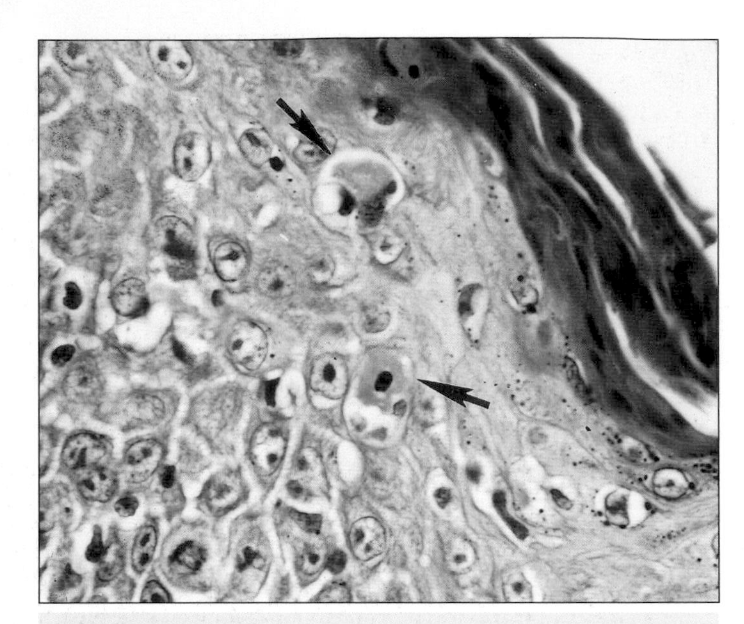

Figure 5.3 Dyskeratosis. Individual keratinocytes have premature or abnormal keratinization. They are shrunken, dark-staining, and have pyknotic nuclei (arrows).

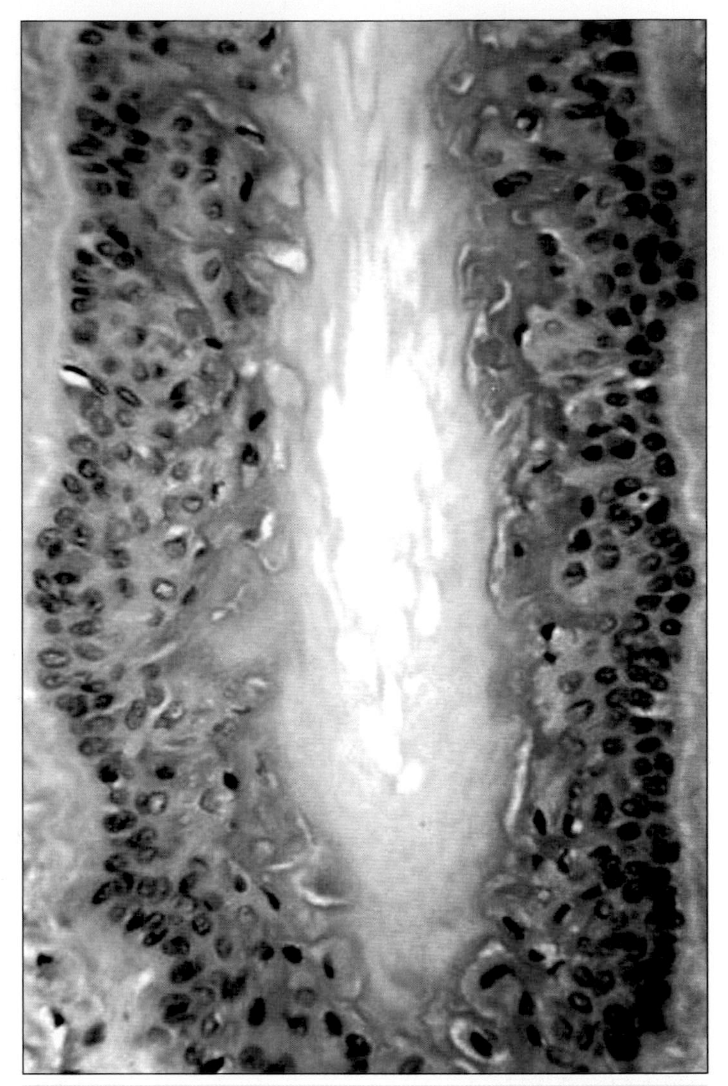

Figure 5.4 Flame follicle. Follicle with pronounced eosinophilic tricholemmal keratinization. The keratin has a serrated border resembling a flickering flame. (Courtesy of B Dunstan.)

clear halos, large irregular keratohyaline granules, a markedly thickened stratum granulosum, and orthokeratotic hyperkeratosis. It may be seen in certain types of ichthyosis, linear epidermal nevi, or can be an incidental finding in a variety of conditions.

Epidermal mast cells are frequently seen in biopsies from cats with inflammatory dermatoses. They are found within the epidermis as well as the hair follicle outer root sheath, and are most commonly found in diseases associated with tissue eosinophilia, such as feline eosinophilic plaque and feline eosinophilic granuloma.

Exocytosis *is the migration of inflammatory cells and/or erythrocytes through the intercellular spaces of the epidermis*. Exocytosis of inflammatory cells is a common feature of any inflammatory dermatosis. Exocytosis of neutrophils implies an infectious process, whereas exocytosis of eosinophils suggests a hypersensitivity, such as ectoparasitism and feline eosinophilic plaque. Exocytosis of erythrocytes implies purpura, severe vasodilation, or trauma.

Festoons are *dermal papillae, devoid of attached epidermal cells, which project into a vesicle or bulla*. Festoons can be seen in porphyria, bullous pemphigoid and epidermolysis bullosa.

Fibrinoid degeneration is the deposition of fibrin in vessel walls, or in dermal collagen.

Fibroplasia is a reactive process and is the formation and development of fibrous tissue due to increased number of fibroblasts.

Flame figures *are areas of refractile collagen surrounded by eosinophils and eosinophil degranulation products*. In chronic lesions, the eosinophil content decreases, histiocytes increase in number and *palisading granulomas* may be formed. Flame figures may be seen in eosinophilic granuloma, sterile eosinophilic pustulosis, insect/arthropod bite reactions, and other eosinophil-rich conditions.

Flame follicles *are catagen and telogen follicles with pronounced eosinophilic trichilemmal keratin* (Fig. 5.4). These can be seen in endocrinopathies, and are also prominent in normal haired skin of plush-coated breeds of dog, such as the Nordic breeds and Pomeranians.

Follicular atrophy refers to the *gradual involution and disappearance of hair follicles* characteristic of hormonal dermatoses, follicular dystrophies and ischemia.

Follicular dystrophy indicates *abnormally formed hair follicles*.

Follicular keratosis refers to *keratin-filled hair follicles*. This is a common feature of diverse conditions such as endocrine and many inflammatory dermatoses.

Folliculitis is inflammation of the hair follicle. It can further be divided into *mural folliculitis* (inflammation of the follicular epithelium) (Fig. 5.5A), *luminal folliculitis* (inflammation in the follicular lumen) (Fig. 5.5B), and *perifolliculitis* (inflammation around but not significantly impinging on the follicle) (Fig. 5.5C).

Furunculosis is *inflammation of the hair follicle that has resulted in destruction of the follicular epithelium and release of the luminal contents into the dermis, causing dermal inflammation* (Fig. 5.6). This can be seen in any process that is destructive to hair follicles, such as bacterial infection, dermatophytosis, demodicosis, and trauma.

Granulation tissue formation is a reparative process that is characterized by the presence of fibroblasts, edema, inflammatory cells, and neocapillaries. The blood vessels have plump endothelial cells and

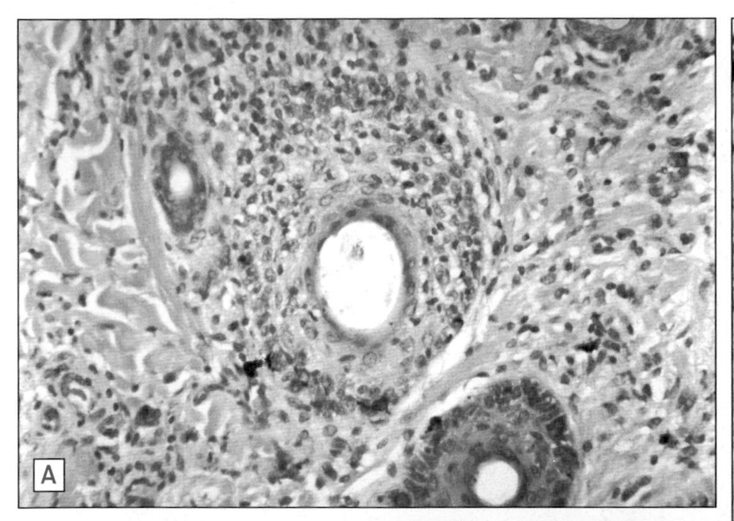

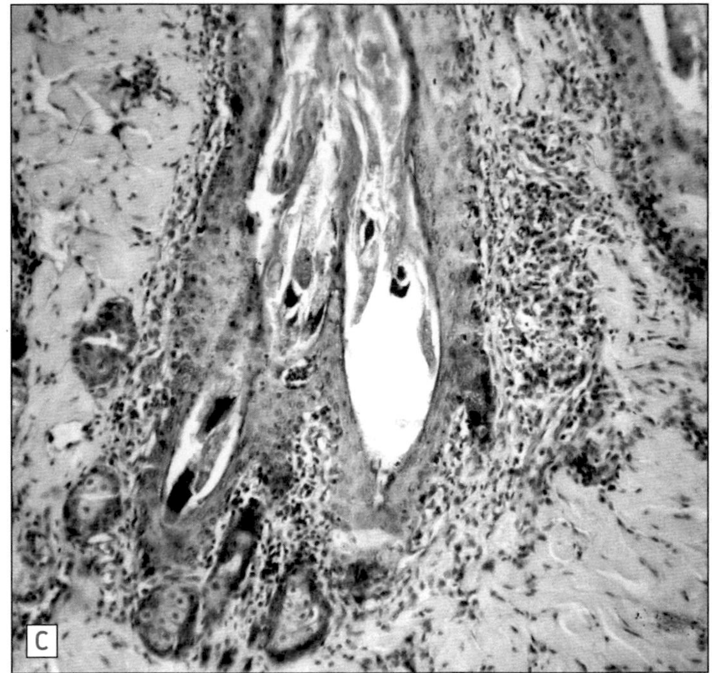

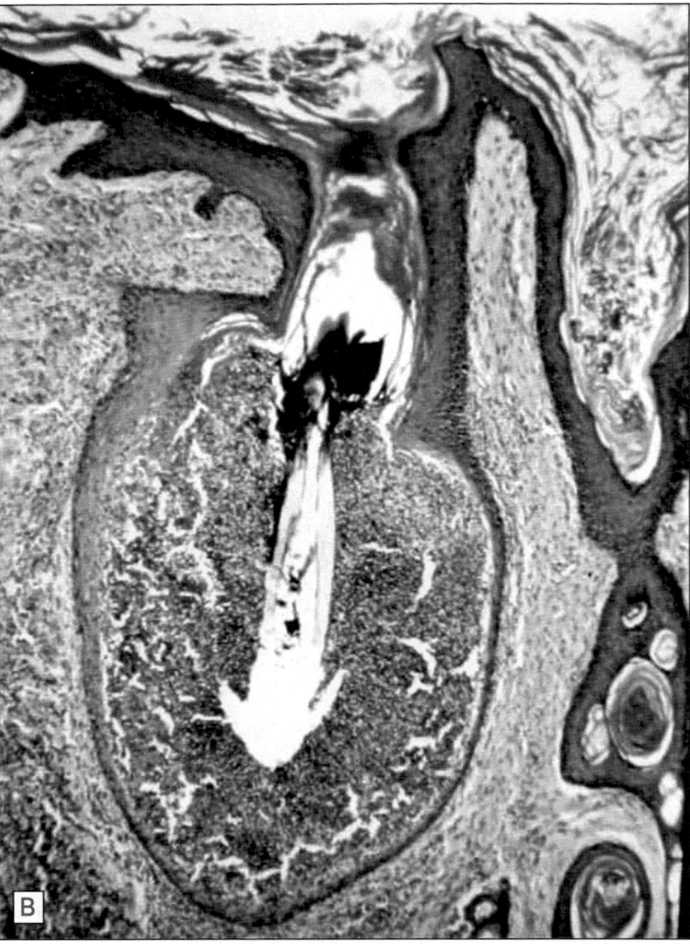

Figure 5.5 Folliculitis A. Mural folliculitis in equine linear alopecia. Note the wall of the hair follicle is infiltrated by mononuclear leukocytes. **B. Luminal folliculitis** in pyoderma. Note the follicular lumen is distended with leukocytes and debris. (Courtesy of B Dunstan.) **C. Perifolliculitis** in demodicosis. Note the leukocytes infiltrating the dermis adjacent to the follicular wall without significantly disrupting the follicular wall.

are oriented perpendicular to the surface of the skin. Fibroblasts and collagen fibrils are oriented parallel to the surface of the skin.

Grenz zone is a *zone of relatively normal collagen that separates the epidermis from an underlying dermal alteration*. A Grenz zone may be seen in neoplastic conditions, such as plasma cell tumors, and granulomatous disorders.

Hamartoma is *a tumor-like malformation composed of an abnormal mixture of normal tissue elements or an abnormal proportion of a single element*. Unlike a **choristoma**, the components of a hamartoma are normal to the location. By definition, hamartomas are congenital lesions, however they may not be detected until later in life and the term is often used interchangeably with nevus, which can be congenital or tardive in onset.

Hidradenitis *is inflammation of apocrine (peritrichial) sweat glands*. These glands commonly become involved secondarily in suppurative and granulomatous dermatoses. Periglandular accumulation of plasma cells is commonly seen in chronic infections, lichenoid dermatoses, and acral lick dermatitis.

Horn cysts (keratin cysts) are circular cystic structures surrounded by flattened epidermal cells. *They contain concentrically arranged lamellar keratin*. Horn cysts are features of a number of follicular and epithelial tumors. **Pseudo-horn cysts** are keratin-filled, cyst-like structures formed by the *irregular invagination of a hyperplastic, hyperkeratotic epidermis*. They are seen in numerous hyperplastic or neoplastic epidermal dermatoses.

Horn pearls (squamous pearls, keratin pearls) are focal, circular, *concentric layers of squamous cells showing gradual keratinization toward the center*, often accompanied by cellular atypia and dyskeratosis. Horn pearls are features of squamous cell carcinoma, keratoacanthoma and pseudocarcinomatous hyperplasia.

Hyalin is an eosinophilic, glassy, homogeneous, refractile material composed of *type IV collagen*. The term is often used as an adjective in descriptions (**hyaline**).

Hypergranulosis indicates *increased thickness of the stratum granulosum*, often accompanied by larger, more intensely stained granules. Hypergranulosis may be seen in any dermatosis in which there is epidermal hyperplasia.

Hyperkeratosis, *increased thickness of the stratum corneum*, is a common finding in many chronic dermatoses. It can be either **orthokeratotic** (without nuclei) (Fig. 5.7A), or **parakeratotic** (nuclei

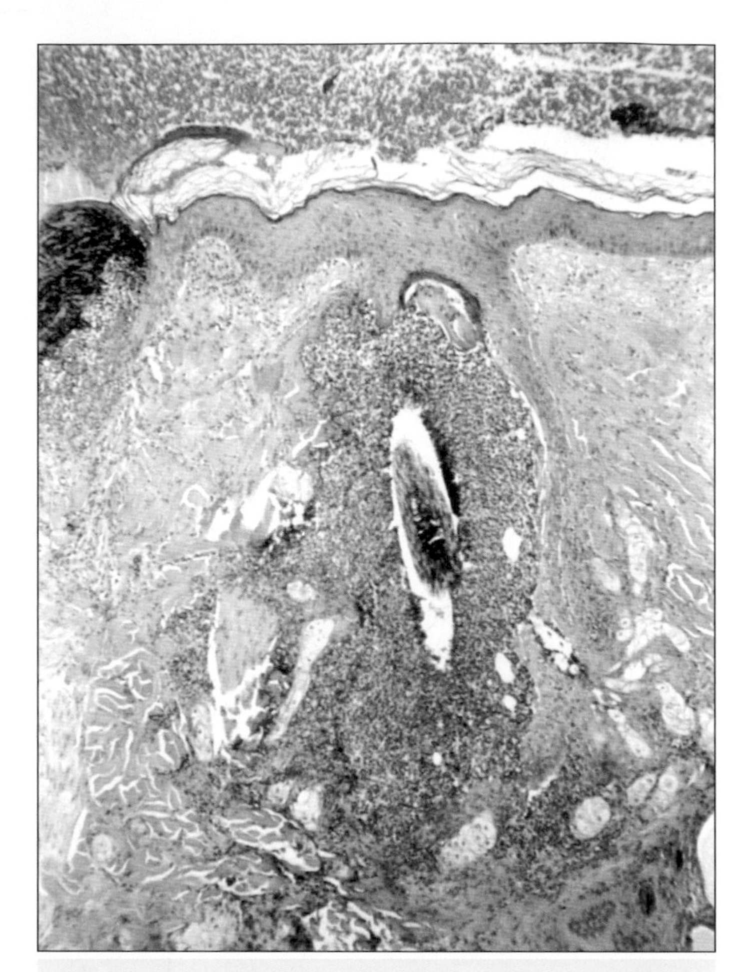

Figure 5.6 Furunculosis in bacterial folliculitis. The wall of the follicle has been perforated and follicular contents are in the dermis.

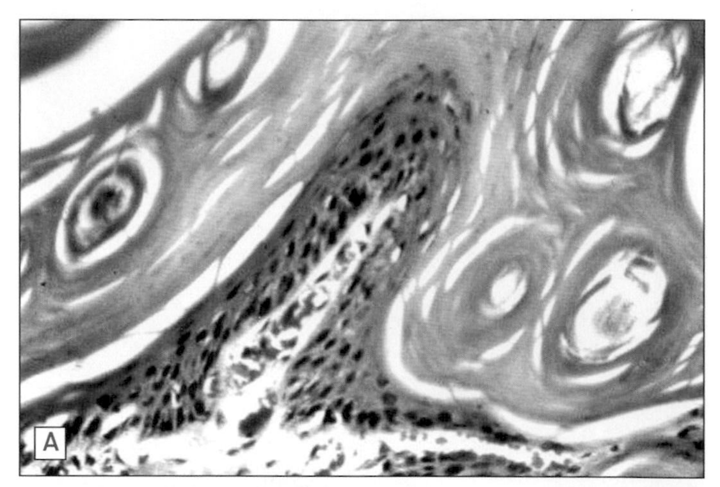

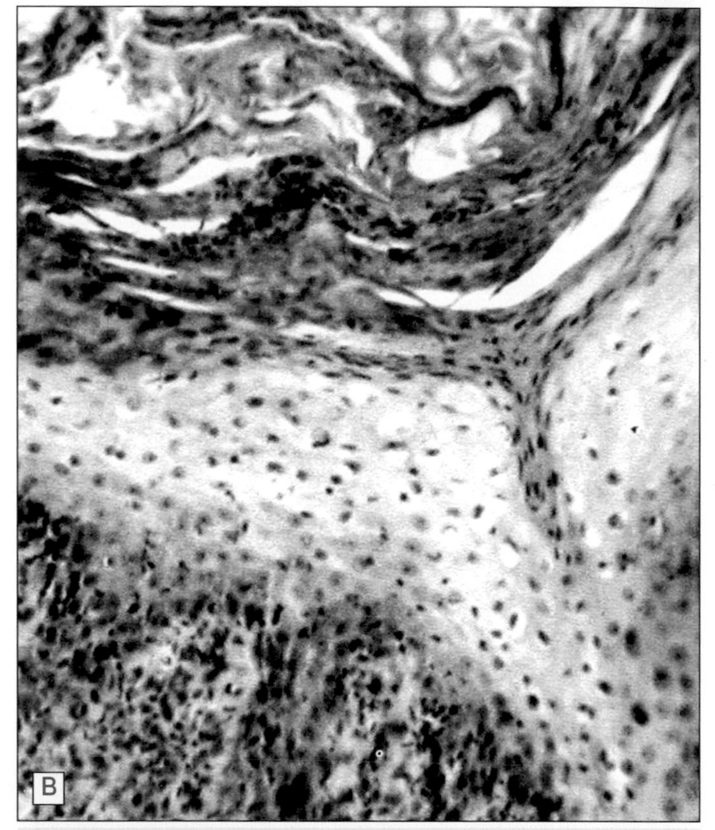

Figure 5.7 A. Orthokeratosis in ichthyosis. Laminated layers of compact anuclear keratin cover the epidermal surface. (Courtesy of B Dunstan.) **B. Parakeratosis** in zinc-responsive dermatosis. A thick layer of keratin with nucleated keratinocytes covers the epidermal surface.

retained) (Fig. 5.7B). *Hyperkeratosis and orthokeratosis are sometimes used synonymously*. Orthokeratosis can be divided into basket weave (the normal pattern in the stratum corneum), compact, and laminated. *Basket weave orthokeratosis* is the most common form, present not only in normal stratum corneum, but also in orthokeratotic disorders such as disorders of keratinization, endocrinopathies and hypersensitivities. *Compact orthokeratosis* can be seen in lichenoid dermatoses, cutaneous horns, and chronic trauma. *Laminated orthokeratosis* characterizes ichthyosis. Orthokeratosis and parakeratosis are not mutually exclusive and are often seen in the same section of hyperkeratotic skin. *Diffuse parakeratosis* can be seen in many chronic dermatoses, especially chronic ectoparasitism, zinc-responsive dermatosis, dermatophilosis, dermatophytosis, or thallotoxicosis. Multifocal parakeratotic caps over the shoulders of follicular ostia is a feature of idiopathic seborrheic dermatitis. Diffuse orthokeratotic hyperkeratosis suggests endocrinopathies, nutritional deficiencies, seborrhea, and ichthyosis. Marked orthokeratotic hyperkeratosis involving the hair follicles suggests vitamin A-responsive dermatosis, acne, Schnauzer comedo syndrome, or endocrine dermatopathies such as hyperadrenocorticism.

Hyperpigmentation refers to *increased melanin within the epidermis and, often, concurrently in dermal melanophages*. Hyperpigmentation may be focal or diffuse, and confined to the stratum basale or present throughout all epidermal layers. It is a common nondiagnostic finding in chronic inflammatory and hormonal dermatoses, as well as in some developmental and neoplastic disorders. Hyperpigmentation must always be cautiously assessed with regard to the animal's normal pigmentation.

Hyperplasia is an increase in the number of cells. In reference to the epidermis, it means an increased thickness due to an increased number of keratinocytes. *Epidermal hyperplasia is a common feature of almost all chronic inflammatory conditions*. *Acanthosis* is a term often used synonymously with epidermal hyperplasia. Epidermal hyperplasia may be further specified as *irregular* (in which the hyperplastic rete ridges are uneven in shape and height); *regular or psoriasiform* (in which the hyperplastic rete ridges are of even thickness and length); *papillated* (digitate projections of the epidermis above the skin surface); and *pseudocarcinomatous* (extreme, irregular hyperplasia that may

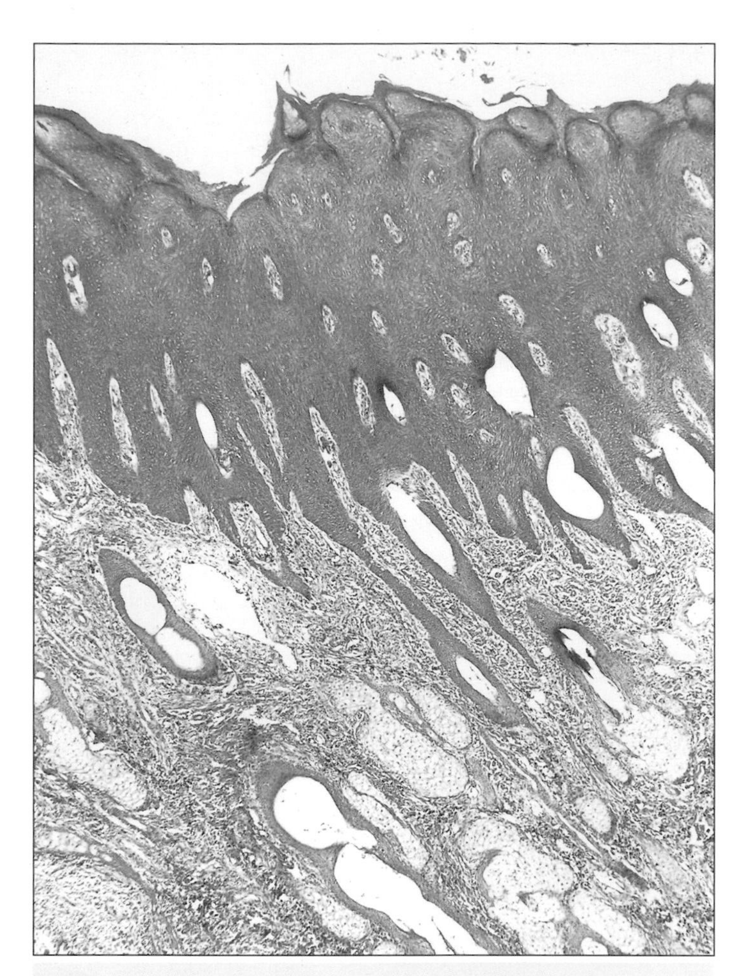

Figure 5.8 Pseudocarcinomatous epidermal hyperplasia. The epidermis has marked, irregular hyperplasia with branched or fused rete pegs. The basement membrane is intact and there is no cellular atypia.

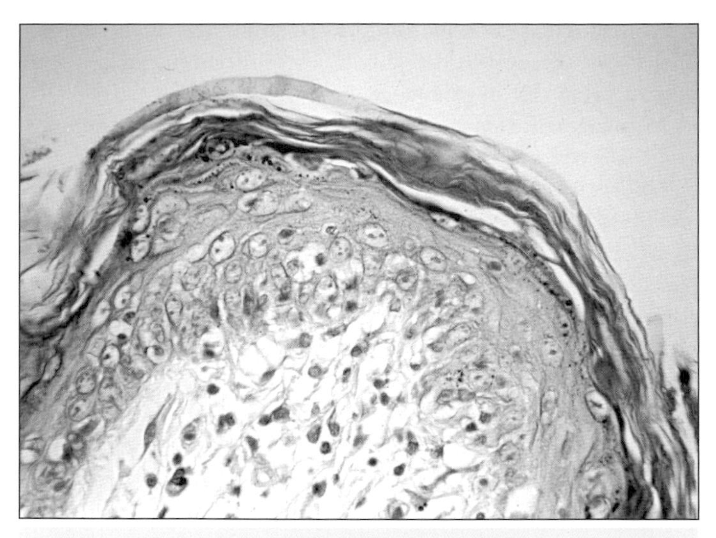

Figure 5.9 Hydropic degeneration. Clear vacuoles are present within and below basal keratinocytes.

demonstrate increased mitotic activity and branched or fused rete pegs) (Fig. 5.8). The process may resemble squamous cell carcinoma; however, there is no cellular atypia, and the basement membrane remains intact. *Irregular epidermal hyperplasia is nonspecific and is the most common type*. Regular epidermal hyperplasia is fairly uncommon and may indicate specific dermatoses, such as lichenoid psoriasiform dermatosis of the Springer Spaniel. Papillated hyperplasia is most commonly seen in seborrheic dermatitis, and in papillomas. Pseudocarcinomatous hyperplasia is most often seen at the margin of a chronic ulcer, or may be associated with underlying chronic dermal suppurative, granulomatous or neoplastic processes.

Hypopigmentation refers to *decreased melanin in the epidermis*. It may be associated with congenital or acquired idiopathic defects in melanization (leukoderma, vitiligo), toxic effects of certain chemicals on melanocytes (e.g., monobenzyl ether of dihydroquinone in rubbers and plastics), inflammatory disorders that affect melanization or destroy melanocytes, hormonal disorders, and dermatoses featuring hydropic degeneration of basal cells (e.g., lupus erythematosus). In those hypopigmented dermatoses associated with hydropic degeneration of basal cells, the underlying superficial dermis usually reveals pigmentary incontinence.

Intracellular edema of the epidermis is characterized by increased size, cytoplasmic pallor, and, sometimes, displacement of the nucleus to the periphery of the affected cell. Intracellular edema of the epidermis may affect cells in a laminar fashion, leading to horizontal layers of edematous keratinocytes. Severe intracellular edema may result in reticular degeneration and intraepidermal vesicles. *Intracellular edema is a common feature of any acute or subacute inflammatory dermatosis*. **Hydropic degeneration** is a specific type of intracellular edema restricted to the basal layer and sometimes the basal cells of the outer root sheath of hair follicles. Hydropic degeneration may result in intrabasal clefts or vesicles, or subepidermal clefts or vesicles due to dermoepidermal separation. It is characterized by clear vacuoles within basal keratinocytes, sometimes accompanied by individual keratinocyte necrosis (Fig. 5.9). **Vacuolar degeneration** is sometimes seen in conjunction with hydropic degeneration and refers to vacuoles above and below the basement membrane zone. Hydropic degeneration of basal cells can be seen in lichenoid dermatitides, drug eruptions, lupoid dermatoses, and dermatomyositis. Caution must be exercised not to confuse freezing artifact or delayed fixation artifact with intracellular edema.

Lymphoid nodules are well-circumscribed, rounded, dense, sometimes perivascular accumulations of predominantly mature lymphocytes in the deep dermis and/or subcutis. They are uncommon and *seen primarily in the cat*. They are seen most frequently in conjunction with immune-mediated dermatoses, dermatoses associated with tissue eosinophilia, and in panniculitis such as injection site panniculitis. They can also be seen in insect-bite granuloma (pseudolymphoma).

Mucinosis (myxedema, myxoid degeneration, mucoid degeneration) is characterized by increased amounts of an amorphous, granular, basophilic material that separates, thins or replaces dermal collagen fibers and surrounds blood vessels and appendages in hematoxylin and eosin-stained sections. Only small amounts of mucin are visible in normal skin, mostly around appendages and blood vessels. Mucin is more easily demonstrated with stains for acid mucopolysaccharides such as Alcian blue and colloidal iron. Mucinous degeneration may be seen as a focal process in numerous inflammatory, neoplastic and developmental dermatoses. Diffuse mucinosis is a feature of normal skin of the Chinese Shar-Pei dog, is occasionally seen in idiopathic mucinosis, and has rarely been reported in hypothyroidism and acromegaly.

Multinucleated keratinocyte. Keratinocytes with multiple nuclei can occasionally be seen in viral infections, such as herpesvirus and FeLV infections.

Munro's microabscess is a small, desiccated accumulation of *neutrophils* within the stratum corneum.

Necrosis is the death of cells or tissues. *Necrotic keratinocytes* are identified by loss of intercellular bridges with resultant rounding-up of the cell, and a normal-sized or swollen eosinophilic cytoplasm. The nucleus becomes pyknotic and cytoplasm becomes eosinophilic and homogeneous, and the cell loses its normal shape. Individual keratinocyte necrosis can occur in drug eruptions, graft-versus-host disease, and interface dermatoses. Necrosis of the epidermis or dermis may be more extensive due to physical and chemical injury, or to interference with vascular supply.

Nests (theques) are well-circumscribed clusters or groups of cells within the epidermis and/or the dermis. Nests are seen in some neoplastic and hamartomatous dermatoses such as melanocytic nevi and melanomas.

Nevus is a focal malformation of the skin, congenital or tardive in onset, consisting of *local excess of one or several of the normal mature constituents of the skin.* The term nevus should always be used with a modifier such as *melanocytic, epidermal, vascular, collagenous, organoid,* etc. The term nevus and hamartoma are often used interchangeably, as, although hamartomas are by definition congenital lesions, they are often not noticed until later in life.

Panniculitis (steatitis) refers to *inflammation of subcutaneous fat.* It can occur without significant involvement of the overlying dermis and epidermis (sterile nodular panniculitis, feline nutritional steatitis, bacterial or fungal panniculitis, lupus erythematosus panniculitis, subcutaneous fat sclerosis), or can be involved by extension of inflammation of the dermis. Fat micropseudocyst formation and lipocytes containing radially arranged needle-shaped clefts can be seen with subcutaneous fat sclerosis and idiopathic sterile panniculitis.

Papillomatosis refers to the projection of dermal papillae and epidermis above the surface of the skin resulting in an irregular undulating configuration of the epidermis. Papillomatosis is often associated with epidermal hyperplasia and is seen with chronic inflammatory and neoplastic dermatoses.

Pautrier's microabscess is a small, focal accumulation of *abnormal lymphoid cells* in the epidermis or follicular epithelium, typical of epitheliotropic lymphoma (Fig. 5.10).

Pigmentary incontinence *refers to the presence of melanin granules free within the subepidermal dermis and within dermal macrophages (melanophages).* It can result from any process that damages the stratum basale, especially hydropic degeneration of basal cells (lichenoid dermatoses, lupus erythematosus, dermatomyositis and erythema multiforme).

Pustules are cavities in the epidermis or follicular epithelium filled with inflammatory cells, usually neutrophils or eosinophils.

Reticular degeneration is caused by severe intracellular edema of epidermal cells. *These cells burst, resulting in multilocular intraepidermal vesicles whose septa are formed by resistant cell walls.* It may be seen with any acute or subacute inflammatory dermatosis, such as acute contact dermatitis.

Satellitosis *refers to individual necrotic keratinocytes in the epidermis surrounded by lymphoid cells (satellite cells)* (Fig. 5.11). It is a characteristic finding in erythema multiforme and occasionally is seen in other interface dermatoses.

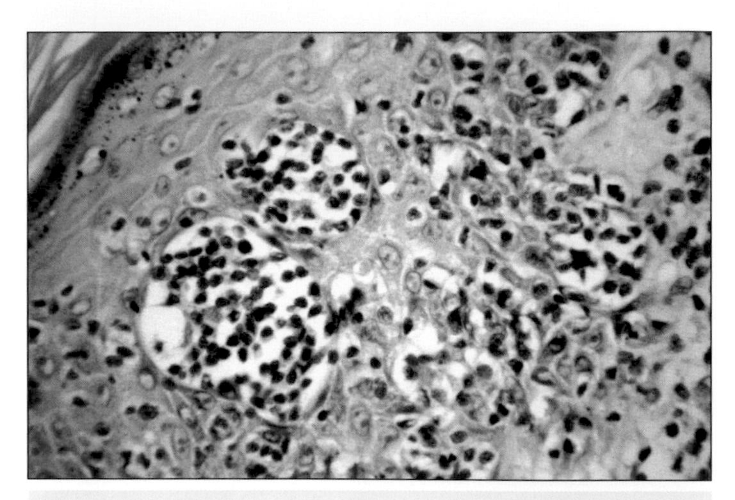

Figure 5.10 Pautrier's microabscess in epidermotropic lymphoma. Nests of neoplastic lymphocytes reside in clear spaces within the epidermis.

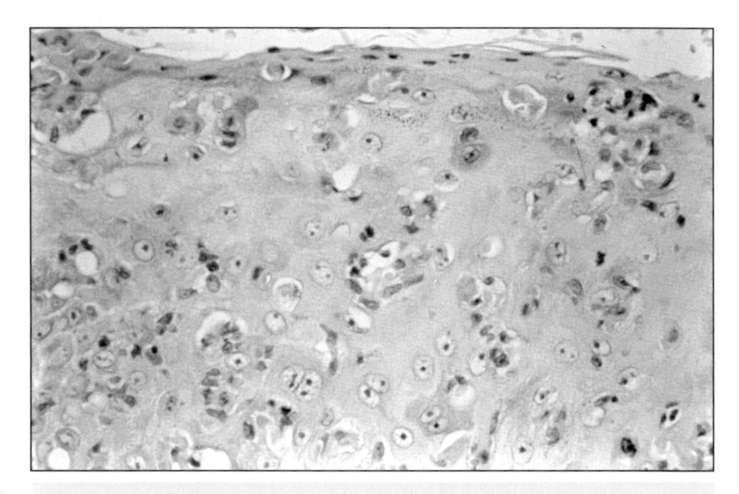

Figure 5.11 Satellitosis in erythema multiforme. Lymphocytes cluster around dyskeratotic, necrotic or apoptotic keratinocytes.

Sclerosis (scar) is the end point of fibrosis. *Increased numbers of collagen fibers* have a thick, eosinophilic, hyalinized appearance and the number of fibroblasts is greatly reduced.

Sebaceous gland hyperplasia refers to increased numbers of sebaceous glands and is common in chronic inflammatory conditions. Nodular aggregates of hyperplastic sebaceous glands are a common senile finding and are frequently multifocal.

Spongiform pustule of Kogoj is *multilocular accumulation of neutrophils within a sponge-like area of the stratum granulosum and stratum spinosum.*

Spongiosis (intercellular edema) of the epidermis is characterized by widening of the intercellular spaces with accentuation of the intercellular bridges, giving the involved epidermis a "spongy" appearance (Fig. 5.12A). Severe intercellular edema may lead to rupture of the intercellular bridges and the formation of *intraepidermal vesicles* (Fig. 5.12B). Severe spongiotic vesicle formation may disrupt the basement membrane zone in some areas, giving the appearance of subepidermal vesicles. Intercellular edema is a common feature of acute or subacute inflammatory dermatoses. Diffuse spongiosis, which also involves the hair follicle outer root sheath, may be seen in

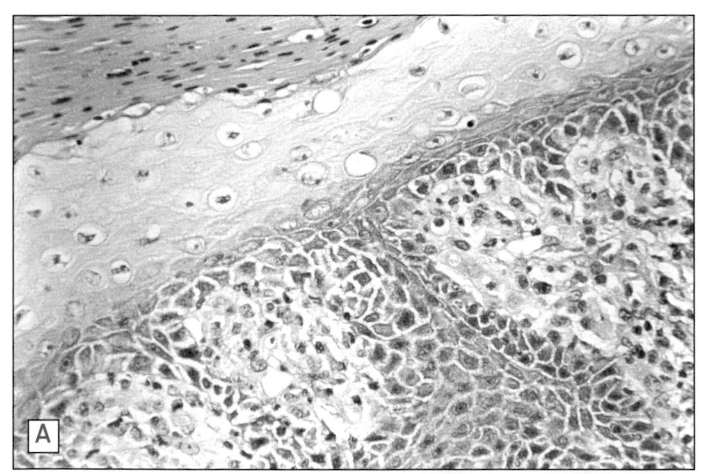

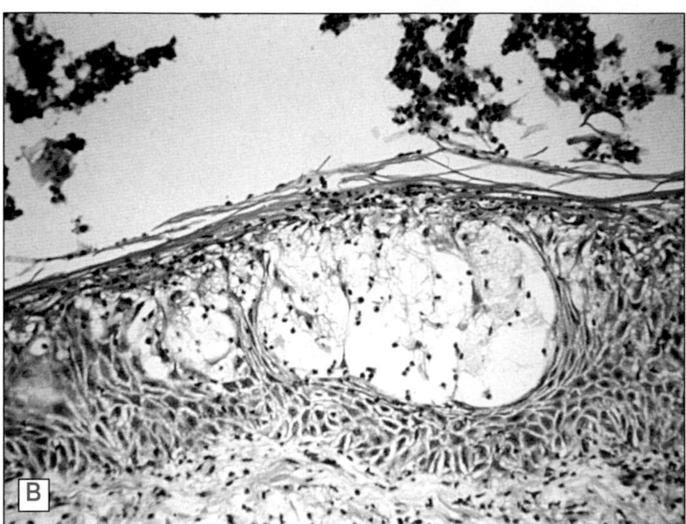

Figure 5.12 A. Spongiosis and laminar intracellular edema in superficial necrolytic dermatitis. Extracellular edema resulting in widening of intercellular spaces between keratinocytes of the deeper epidermis and a linear distribution of pale-staining keratinocytes affected by intracellular edema in the mid-epidermis. **B. Spongiosis with vesicle formation**. Marked intercellular edema has led to breakdown of intercellular bridges and vesicle formation. (Courtesy of B Dunstan.)

other inflammatory disorders including feline eosinophilic plaque or granuloma. Spongiosis of the upper one-half of the epidermis, which is overlaid by marked diffuse parakeratotic hyperkeratosis, is seen in superficial necrolytic dermatitis (hepatocutaneous syndrome).

Squamous eddies *are whorl-like patterns of squamous cells with no atypia, dyskeratosis or central keratinization*. Squamous eddies are features of numerous neoplastic and hyperplastic epidermal disorders.

Transepidermal elimination *is a mechanism by which foreign or altered constituents can be removed from the dermis*. This can be illustrated by the elimination of mineralized collagen across the epidermis and follicular epithelium in calcinosis cutis.

Vesicle is a *fluid filled blister less than 1.0 cm in diameter* in, or immediately below, the epidermis. They may be *subcorneal, suprabasilar, or subepidermal*. When these lesions contain large numbers of inflammatory cells, they may be referred to as **vesicopustules**.

Villus is a dermal papilla covered by one or two layers of epidermal cells that projects into the base of a vesicle or bulla. Villi are seen in pemphigus vulgaris and warty dyskeratoma.

Pattern analysis

The pattern of cell distribution in the skin and the cell types present are extremely important diagnostic clues to many dermatoses. *Pattern analysis is based on recognition of ten different non-neoplastic reaction patterns in the skin at scanning magnification*. At higher magnification, the predominant cell type can be identified and described as *lymphocytic, histiocytic, neutrophilic, eosinophilic, or plasmacytic*. Pattern analysis frequently allows a pathologist to generate a list of differential diagnoses. It is far more efficient to use pattern recognition, and then differentiate between the diseases that demonstrate that pattern, than to learn the histologic features of each disease. It is not unusual to see more than one pattern of inflammation in a biopsy. This can be due to the presence of more than one dermatosis, or due to the presence of both a primary and secondary condition, such as perivascular dermatitis due to a hypersensitivity with a secondary pustular pattern due to pyoderma. Another common combination of patterns would be an overall pattern of perivascular dermatitis (due to hypersensitivity reactions or ectoparasitism) or atrophic dermatosis (due to endocrinopathy) with a subordinate, focal pattern of folliculitis, furunculosis, or intraepidermal pustular dermatitis (due to secondary bacterial infection). It can be difficult to assess the importance of each pattern within the biopsy, and *it becomes very important to recognize which patterns are more specific than others in order to identify the primary condition*. An example would be an interface dermatitis, which is more specific for certain dermatoses than is a perivascular pattern (the least specific).

Perivascular dermatitis

Perivascular dermatitis is the *least specific of the patterns of inflammation*, and it is necessary to observe the type of leukocyte involved and the epidermal changes, in order to create a differential list. In perivascular dermatitis, *the predominant inflammatory reaction is centered around the superficial or deep dermal blood vessels, or both*. Most perivascular dermatitides involve predominantly the superficial dermal blood vessels. Concurrent involvement of the deep dermal blood vessels suggests a systemic disease (infection, immune-mediated). In the horse, most perivascular dermatitides are both superficial and deep. *The primary cause of superficial perivascular dermatitis is a hypersensitivity reaction*, although chronic bacterial infections, viral infections, diseases of altered keratinization, and nutritional deficiencies can all demonstrate this pattern at some point during evolution of the condition. Any perivascular dermatitis containing significant numbers of *eosinophils* should first be suspected of representing an allergic dermatitis such as ectoparasitism, food allergic dermatitis, or atopy. Focal areas of eosinophilic exocytosis and necrosis ("*epidermal nibbles*") are suggestive of ectoparasitism. Other perivascular dermatitides that may contain eosinophils include zinc-responsive dermatosis, equine multisystemic eosinophilic epitheliotropic disease, and chronic pyoderma. Perivascular dermatitis is subdivided on the basis of accompanying epidermal changes into four types:

- In **pure perivascular dermatitis**, there are few or no epidermal changes. The most common dermatoses in this category include acute hypersensitivity reactions and urticaria (Fig. 5.13).
- **Perivascular dermatitis with spongiosis** is characterized by various degrees of spongiosis and spongiotic vesicle formation. Severe spongiotic vesiculation may disrupt the basement

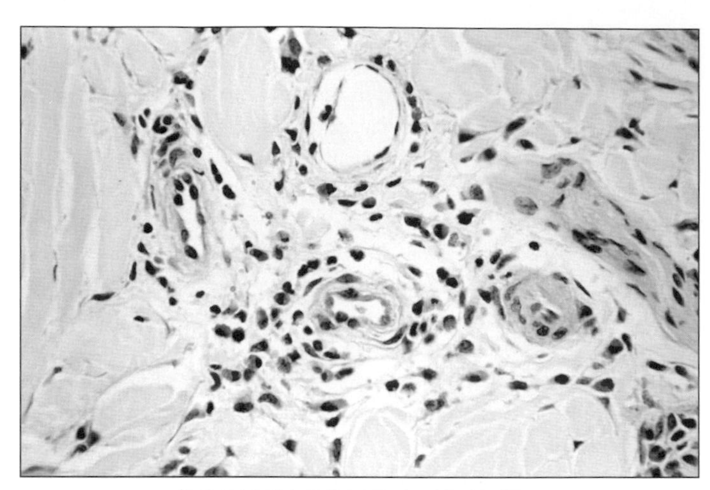

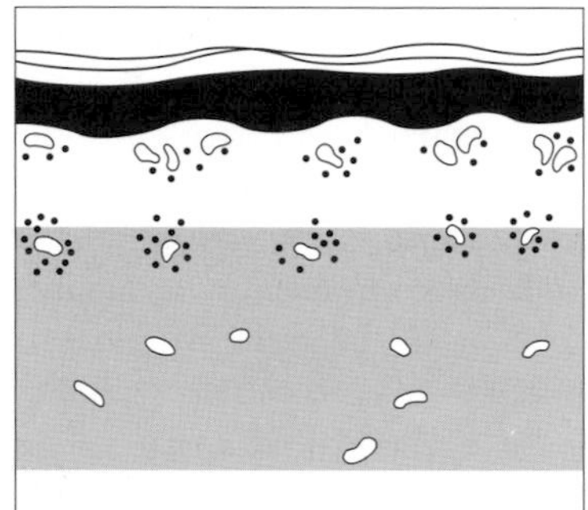

Figure 5.13 Histologic and schematic appearance of **superficial perivascular dermatitis**. *Culicoides* insect bite hypersensitivity. Note leukocytes, in this case eosinophils, surrounding dermal vessels.

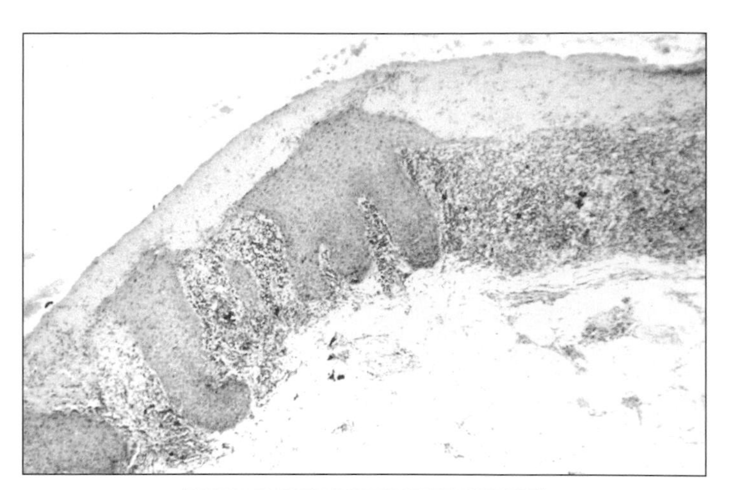

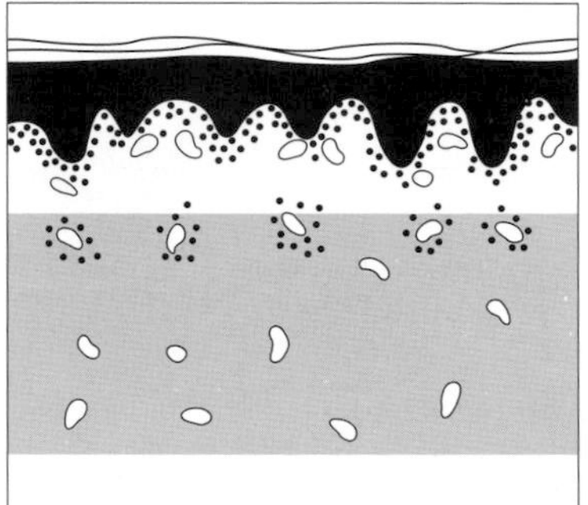

Figure 5.14 Histologic and schematic appearance of **lichenoid interface dermatitis** in discoid lupus erythematosus. Large numbers of lymphocytes and plasma cells abut the epidermal-dermal junction. The basal layer of the epidermis demonstrates apoptosis and vacuolar degeneration of keratinocytes.

membrane zone resulting in subepidermal vesicles. The epidermis usually shows various degrees of hyperkeratosis and hyperplasia. The most common dermatoses in this category include hypersensitivity reactions, acute contact or irritant dermatitis, ectoparasitism, feline eosinophilic plaque, feline miliary dermatitis, and viral infections. When the hair follicle outer root sheath is also involved, feline allergic dermatitides, such as feline eosinophilic plaque and feline eosinophilic granuloma, are suggested.

- **Perivascular dermatitis with epidermal hyperplasia** is characterized by various degrees of epidermal hyperplasia and hyperkeratosis with little or no spongiosis. This is a common, nondiagnostic, chronic reaction pattern. The most common dermatoses in this category are chronic hypersensitivity reactions, diseases of altered keratinization, acral lick dermatitis, and any dermatitis that has undergone chronic irritation and trauma.
- **Perivascular dermatitis with hyperkeratosis** is characterized by various degrees of either orthokeratosis or parakeratosis. The presence of orthokeratosis suggests diseases of altered keratinization (seborrhea) or ichthyosis, and the presence of parakeratosis suggests zinc-responsive dermatosis, chronic ectoparasite hypersensitivity, or *Malassezia* dermatitis.

Interface dermatitis

Interface dermatitis is characterized by damage to the basal layer of keratinocytes, such as basal cell degeneration or necrosis of keratinocytes, that obscures the dermoepidermal junction. This pattern can be divided into interface cell-poor (interface changes with minimal superficial dermal inflammation) or interface lichenoid (interface changes with a lichenoid band of mononuclear inflammation). Pigmentary incontinence and apoptotic bodies are commonly seen in both types.

- The **cell-poor interface pattern** can be seen in diseases such as dermatomyositis, systemic lupus erythematosus, erythema multiforme, drug eruptions, graft-versus-host reactions, bovine viral diarrhea, rinderpest, and bovine pseudo-lumpy skin disease.
- The **lichenoid interface pattern** can be seen with discoid lupus erythematosus, idiopathic lichenoid dermatoses, lichenoid keratoses, Vogt–Koyanagi–Harada-like syndrome (uveodermatologic syndrome), panepidermal pustular pemphigus, lichenoid psoriasiform dermatosis of Springer Spaniels, malignant catarrhal fever, and drug eruptions (Fig. 5.14). The lichenoid band of inflammation is usually lymphocytic and plasmacytic, except in VKH-like syndrome where it is primarily composed of lymphocytes and histiocytes that contain fine melanin granules.

Caution should be exercised in differentiating interface lichenoid *inflammation from* lichenoid *inflammation.* The latter refers to a lichenoid band of inflammation, commonly heavily plasmacytic, closely apposed to the dermoepidermal junction, that does not necessarily involve damage to the basal cell layer, such as chronic pyoderma, mucocutaneous pyoderma, and ectoparasitism (scabies or *Cheyletiella*) in dogs. In these cases, the lichenoid band of inflammation can also include neutrophils or eosinophils.

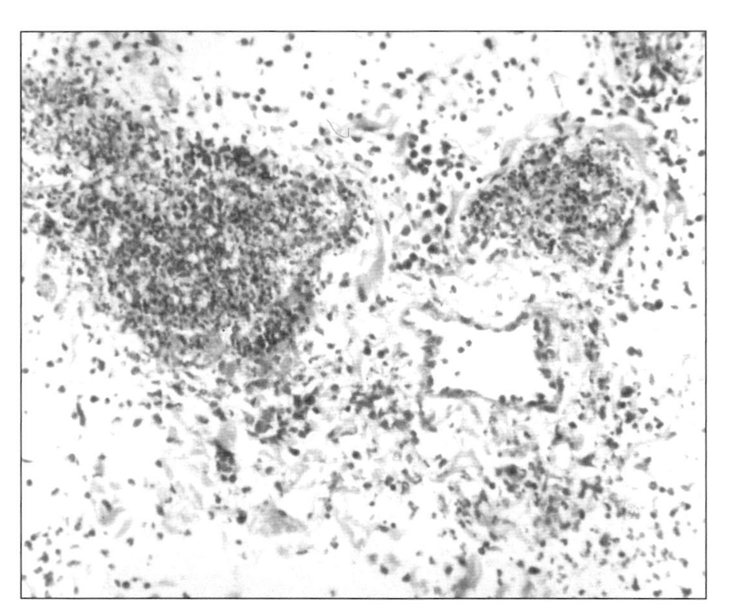
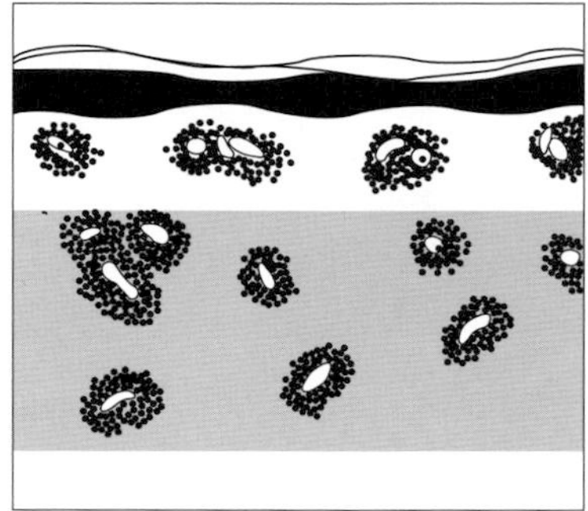

Figure 5.15 Histologic and schematic appearance of **vasculitis**. Leukocytes target vessel walls. Fibrin, erythrocytes and leukocytic debris are in the dermis and vessel walls.

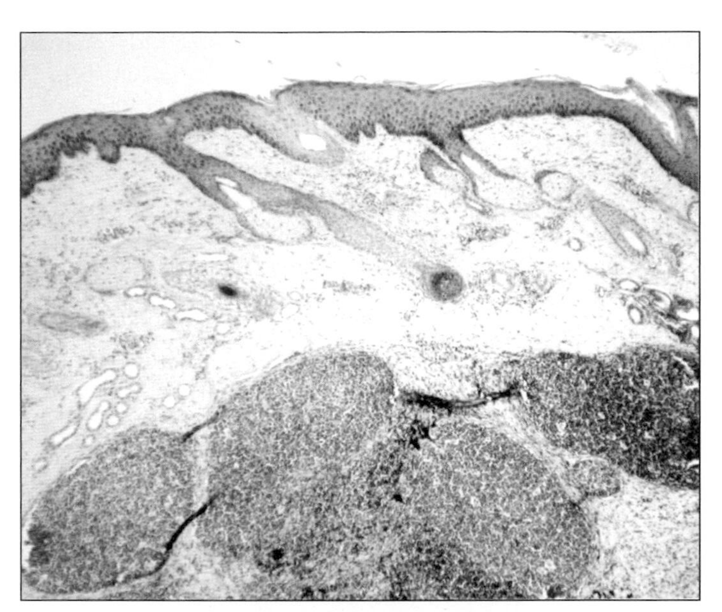
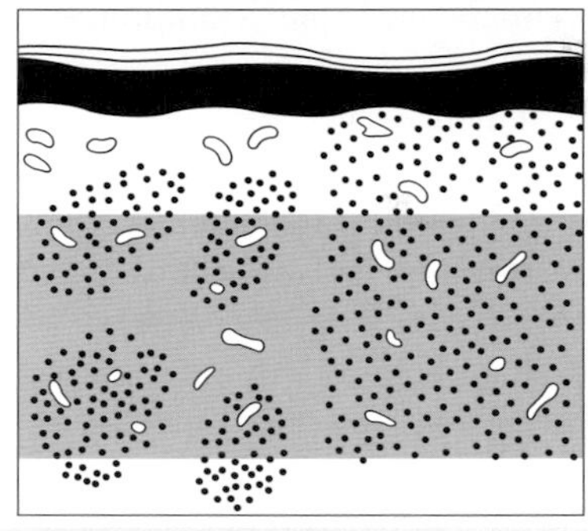

Figure 5.16 Histologic and schematic appearance of **nodular-to-diffuse dermatitis** in fungal dermatitis. Coalescing nodules of lymphocytes, plasma cells, and macrophages obscure the deep dermis.

Vasculitis

Vasculitis is characterized by *inflammation targeting the walls of venules or arterioles*, resulting in at least partial destruction of the vessel wall, sometimes with fibrin deposition (Fig. 5.15). It can be accompanied by fibrinoid necrosis, thrombosis, hemorrhage, and evidence of ischemia. Vasculitis can be immune mediated or septic. *Immune-mediated vasculitis* is due to type III hypersensitivity. The deposition of antigen–antibody complexes in vessel walls activates complement, which results in generation of factors chemotactic for neutrophils. Activation of neutrophils with release of reactive oxygen species and lysosomal enzymes then directly damages vessel walls. *Septic vasculitis* is caused by systemic infection with agents that have a predilection for endothelial cells, resulting in endothelial damage. Vasculitis can also be locally induced by bacterial antigens deposited in vessel walls.

Vasculitis can further be classified on the basis of the *dominant inflammatory cell* within vessel walls. There are neutrophilic, eosinophilic, lymphocytic and mixed types. It should be noted that the inflammatory cell involved often reflects the stage of the disease rather than characterizing a specific disease.

- **Neutrophilic vasculitis** is by far the most common type and may be *leukocytoclastic* (associated with karyorrhexis of neutrophils resulting in "nuclear dust") or *nonleukocytoclastic*. It is seen with connective tissue disorders, hypersensitivity reactions, septicemia, equine purpura hemorrhagica, Rocky Mountain spotted fever, classical swine fever, thrombophlebitis, and as an idiopathic disorder.
- **Lymphocytic vasculitis** may be seen with dermatomyositis, malignant catarrhal fever, vaccine-induced panniculitis, lymphomatoid granulomatosis, and rarely in cutaneous lymphoma. It can also reflect a chronic stage of a vasculitis that was originally neutrophilic.
- **Eosinophilic vasculitis** is rare. It is seen most commonly in lesions induced by arthropod insult, feline eosinophilic granulomas, and rarely in mast cell tumors.

Nodular and diffuse dermatitis

Nodular and diffuse dermatitis is characterized by nodules, or diffuse sheet-like infiltrates of inflammatory cells, in the dermis or subcutis (Fig. 5.16). Nodular and diffuse dermatitis may be characterized by the predominant cell type present (neutrophils, macrophages, lymphocytes, eosinophils, or mixed). The inciting antigen may be an infectious agent, noninfectious material, or the inflammation may be idiopathic. **Neutrophils** predominate in dermal abscesses associated with infectious agents such as bacteria, fungi, algae, and protozoa. They can also be present in sterile lesions, as in foreign body reactions and the sterile pyogranuloma syndrome. **Histiocytes** predominate in *granulomatous inflammation*, which is typically chronic. Granulomatous infiltrates containing large numbers of neutrophils are frequently called *pyogranulomas*. While all granulomatous dermatitis is nodular or diffuse in pattern, not all nodular and diffuse dermatitides are granulomatous.

Granulomas are nodular masses of granulomatous inflammation. They may be subclassified as "tuberculoid" (a central zone of neutrophils and necrosis surrounded by histiocytes, epithelioid macrophages, and giant cells, in turn surrounded by lymphocytes and an outer layer of fibroblasts) or "sarcoidal" (consisting of epithelioid macrophages). *Tuberculoid granulomas* may be seen in tuberculosis, feline leprosy, atypical mycobacterial infection, and *Corynebacterium pseudotuberculosis* infections. *Sarcoidal granulomas* may be seen in sterile sarcoidal granulomas and foreign body reactions. *"Palisading" granulomas* are characterized by the alignment of histiocytes like staves around a central focus of collagen degeneration (feline, canine, and equine eosinophilic granuloma, equine mastocytoma), parasite or fungus (habronemiasis, pythiosis, conidiobolomycosis, basidiobolomycosis, demodicosis), lipids (xanthoma), or other foreign material (e.g., calcium as in dystrophic calcinosis cutis and calcinosis circumscripta). Granulomas and pyogranulomas that track hair follicles resulting in large, vertically oriented ("sausage-shaped") lesions are seen in sterile granuloma/pyogranuloma syndrome of dogs and cats, or can be seen together with folliculitis due to the presence of intrafollicular antigens such as dermatophytes.

Nodular and diffuse dermatitis is often associated with certain unusual inflammatory cell types. **Foam cells** are histiocytes with vacuolated cytoplasm due to their contents (lipid, debris, microorganisms). **Epithelioid macrophages** are histiocytes with elongated or oval vesicular nuclei and abundant finely granular, eosinophilic cytoplasm with ill-defined cell borders. **Multinucleated giant cells** are histiocytic variants that assume three morphologic forms: *Langhans* (nuclei form a circle or semicircle at the periphery of the cell), *foreign-body* (nuclei are scattered throughout the cytoplasm), and *Touton* (nuclei form a wreath which surrounds a central, homogeneous, amphophilic core of cytoplasm that is, in turn, surrounded by abundant foamy cytoplasm). In general, these three forms of giant cells have little diagnostic specificity, although the Touton variety is strongly indicative of xanthomas, and the Langhans type suggests the need for an acid-fast stain. **Eosinophils** may predominate in feline, canine, and equine eosinophilic granuloma, in certain parasitic dermatoses (habronemiasis, elaeophoriasis, parafilariasis, dirofilariasis, dracunculiasis), furunculosis, and in hairy vetch toxicosis. Mixed cellular infiltrates are most commonly neutrophils and macrophages (pyogranuloma), or eosinophils and macrophages (eosinophilic granuloma), or a combination of the three cell types. **Plasma cells** are common components of nodular and diffuse dermatitis in domestic animals and are of no particular diagnostic significance. They may contain eosinophilic, intracytoplasmic inclusions, which are called *Russell bodies*. These accumulations of glycoprotein are largely globulin and may be large enough to displace the cell nucleus. Reactions to ruptured hair follicles are a common cause of nodular and diffuse pyogranulomatous dermatitis in domestic animals, and any such lesion should be examined for keratinous and epithelial debris. All other nodular and diffuse dermatitides should be cultured, examined in polarized light for foreign material and stained for bacteria and fungi. In general, microorganisms are most likely to be found near areas of suppuration and necrosis.

Intraepidermal vesicular and pustular dermatitis

Intraepidermal vesicles and pustules can be caused by intercellular edema which can be seen in any acute or subacute dermatosis, viral infections, hydropic degeneration of keratinocytes, and by acantholysis (Fig. 5.17). It can be useful to subdivide this category on the basis of the site of the vesicle or pustule within the epidermis.

- *Subcorneal pustules and vesicles* are most commonly seen in pemphigus foliaceus, pustules associated with superficial pyoderma, and eosinophilic pustules due to hypersensitivities.
- *Pustules and vesicles in the stratum spinosum* are most commonly seen in the pemphigus complex, viral diseases, and occasionally in hepatocutaneous syndrome.
- *Suprabasilar pustules and vesicles* are a feature of pemphigus vulgaris.

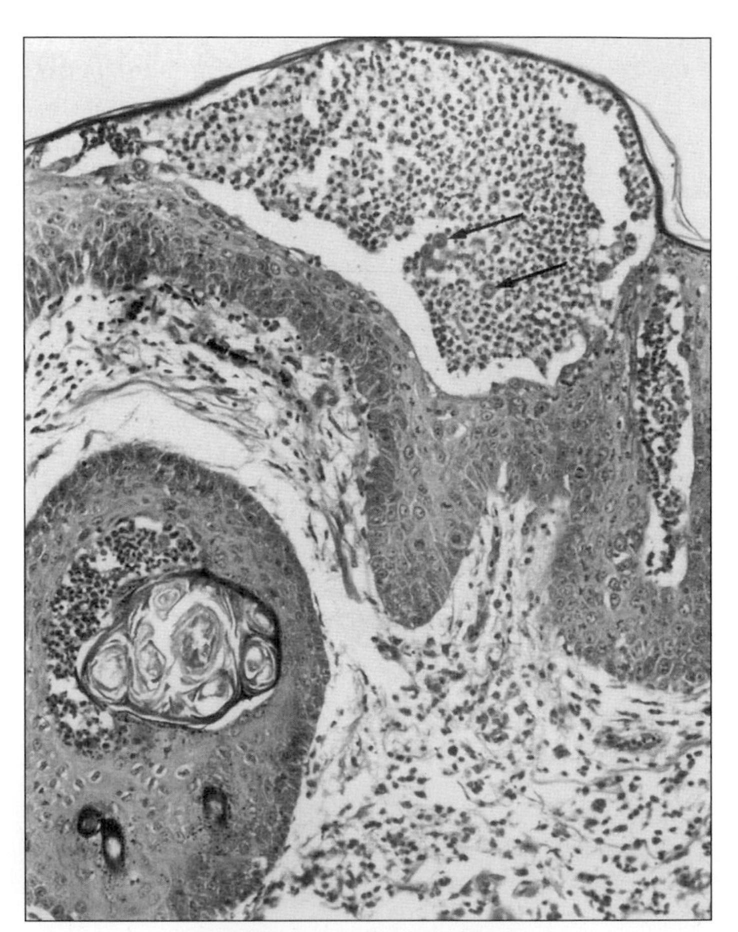

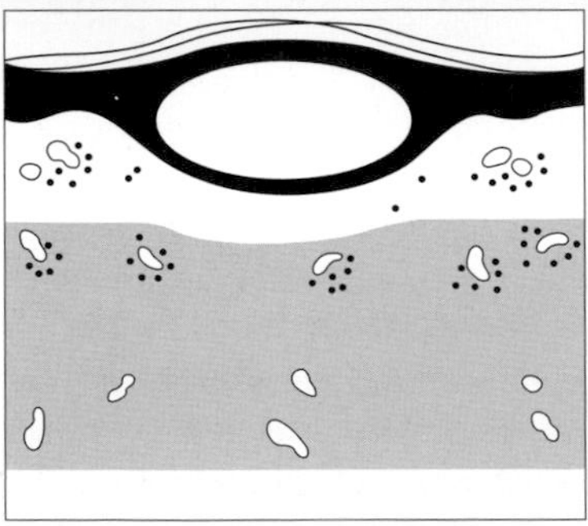

Figure 5.17 Histologic and schematic appearance of **intra-epidermal vesicular/pustular dermatitis** in pemphigus foliaceus. A collection of leukocytes and acantholytic keratinocytes (arrows) are within a subcorneal pustule. The follicular epithelium is also involved.

- *Intrabasilar vesicles* can be seen in lupus erythematosus, dermatomyositis, erythema multiforme, graft-versus-host disease, and toxic epidermal necrolysis.

Subepidermal vesicular and pustular dermatitis

This pattern is characterized by separation of the epidermis from the dermis (Fig. 5.18). Subepidermal vesicles and pustules may be formed through hydropic degeneration of basal cells, dermoepidermal separation, severe subepidermal edema and/or cellular infiltration, and severe intercellular edema with disruption of the basement membrane zone. Caution is warranted when examining older lesions, as re-epithelialization may result in subepidermal vesicles and pustules assuming an intraepidermal location as re-epithelialization forms a pseudo-base to a vesicle. Such re-epithelialization is usually recognized as a single layer of flattened, elongated basal epidermal cells at the base of the vesicle or pustule.

Perifolliculitis, folliculitis, and furunculosis

Perifolliculitis (see Fig. 5.5C) means accumulation of inflammatory cells around a hair follicle in which the inflammation does not significantly impinge on the follicular epithelium. It can be accompanied by mild follicular spongiosis**. Mural folliculitis** (see Fig. 5.5A) is characterized by inflammation which targets the wall of the follicle. **Luminal folliculitis** (see Fig. 5.5B) implies the accumulation of inflammatory cells within follicular lumina. **Furunculosis** (see Fig. 5.6) occurs when the hair follicle ruptures releasing the contents into the dermis. *Perifolliculitis, mural and luminal folliculitis, and furunculosis usually represent a pathologic continuum and all may be present in the same specimen.* Follicular inflammation is a common gross and microscopic finding in dogs, and is less common in other species. It can be caused by intrafollicular bacteria, dermatophytes, and parasites such as *Demodex* spp., *Pelodera strongyloides, and Stephanofilaria* spp. It can also be secondary to pruritus caused by atopy, food allergic dermatitis, ectoparasites, and keratinization disorders such as seborrhea. The folliculitides associated with bacteria, fungi and parasites are usually suppurative initially, whereas those associated with atopy, food allergy, and seborrheic dermatitis are usually predominantly initially spongiotic (small numbers of exocytosing mononuclear cells and/or neutrophils). Any chronic folliculitis, particularly where there is furunculosis, can become pyogranulomatous or granulomatous.

Furunculosis, regardless of the initiating cause, is frequently associated with locally large numbers of eosinophils presumably due to a reaction to released keratin. Idiopathic sterile eosinophilic folliculitides may be seen in cattle and dogs (sterile eosinophilic pustulosis). Insect stings are postulated as the cause of eosinophilic folliculitides affecting the nose of dogs. In cats and horses, sterile eosinophilic folliculitis may be seen in conjunction with hypersensitivity reactions (mosquito bite hypersensitivity, atopy, food allergy, onchocerciasis, equine eosinophilic granuloma, *Culicoides* hypersensitivity, flea bite hypersensitivity). Feline herpesviral dermatitis can also result in eosinophilic folliculitis and furunculosis.

Mural folliculitis can be seen in the pemphigus complex, and these disorders should be considered if there is marked acantholysis. The hair follicle outer root sheath may be involved in hydropic degeneration and lichenoid cellular infiltrates of lupus erythematosus, drug eruptions, erythema multiforme and idiopathic lichenoid dermatoses.

Lymphocytic peribulbitis directed at the bulb of anagen hair follicles is characteristic of alopecia areata. Perifollicular fibrosis is commonly seen in chronic folliculitides, dermatomyositis and chronic granulomatous sebaceous adenitis.

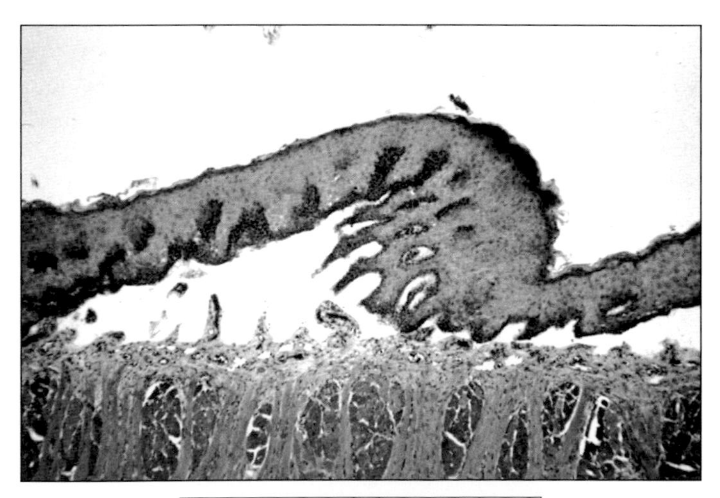

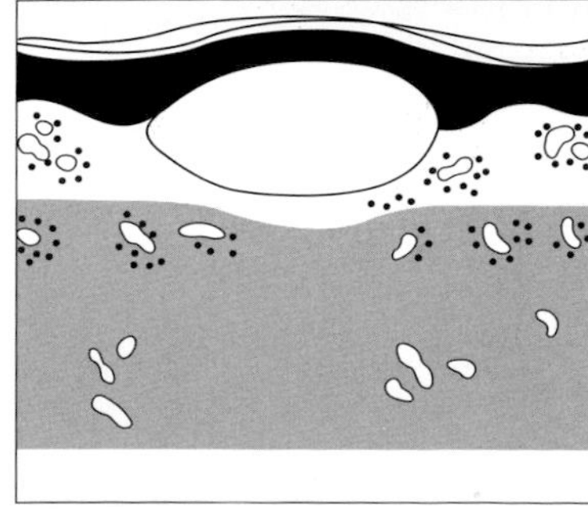

Figure 5.18 Histologic and schematic appearance of **sub-epidermal vesicular dermatitis** in epidermolysis bullosa. The epidermis is separated at the dermal–epidermal junction. (Courtesy of B Dunstan.)

Fibrosing dermatitis

Fibrosis marks the resolving stage of an intense, destructive inflammatory reaction or signifies an ongoing, more insidious, inflammatory process. Fibrosis which is recognizable histologically does not necessarily produce a visible clinical scar. Ulcers limited to the upper portion of the superficial dermis do not usually result in scarring, whereas virtually all ulcers that extend into the deep dermis result in fibrosis and clinical signs of scarring. *Fibrosing dermatitis follows many severe insults to the dermis and is often of minimal diagnostic value.* Common causes of fibrosing dermatitis include furunculosis, equine exuberant granulation tissue, actinic dermatitis, acral lick dermatitis, scleroderma, and morphea (localized scleroderma).

Panniculitis

Panniculitis is inflammation of subcutaneous fat (Fig. 5.19). This inflammation often also secondarily involves the deep dermis. Likewise, the panniculus can be secondarily involved in deep dermal inflammation. Panniculitis may be caused by infectious agents, foreign bodies, vitamin E deficiency, trauma, pancreatic disease, vasculitis, drug eruption, and lupus erythematosus. However, it is often sterile and idiopathic.

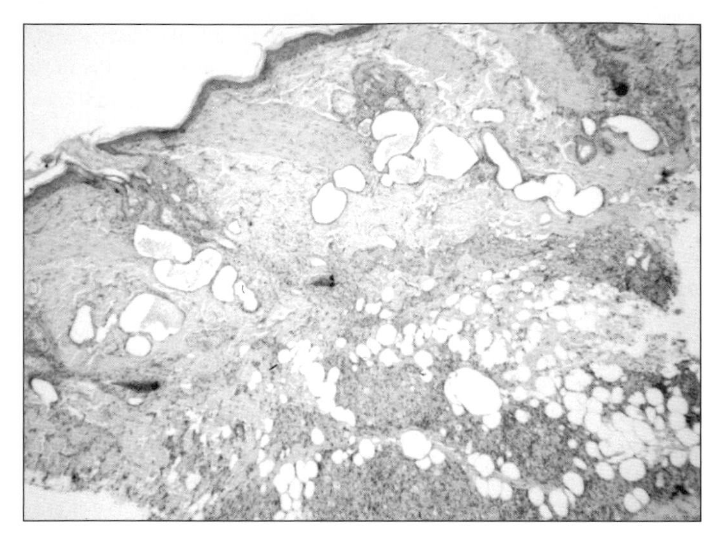

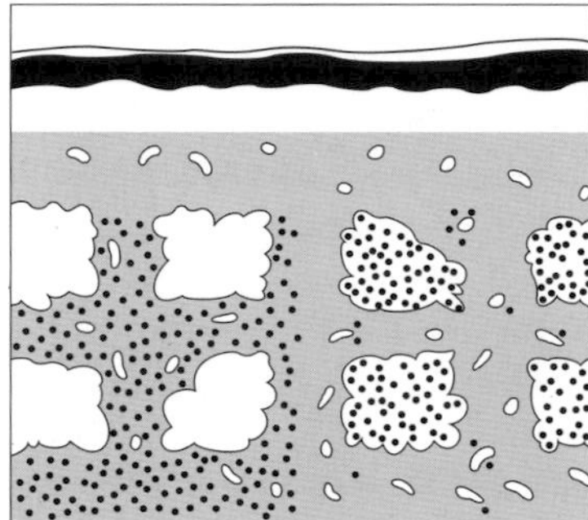

Figure 5.19 Histologic and schematic appearance of **panniculitis**. Inflammation targets the subcutaneous tissues. Note replacement of the adipose tissue with leukocytic aggregates.

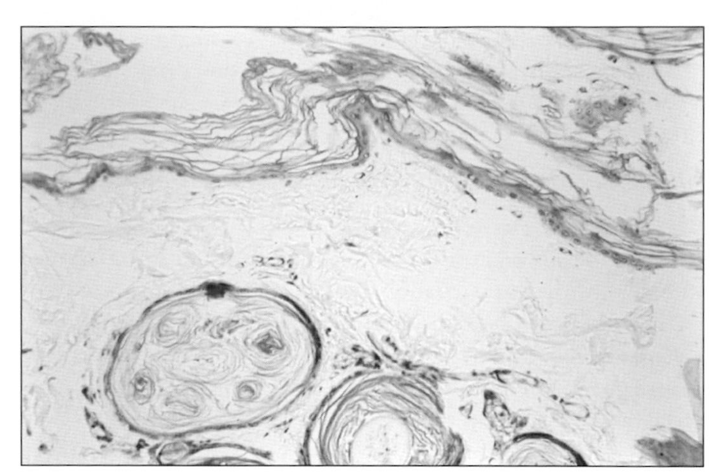

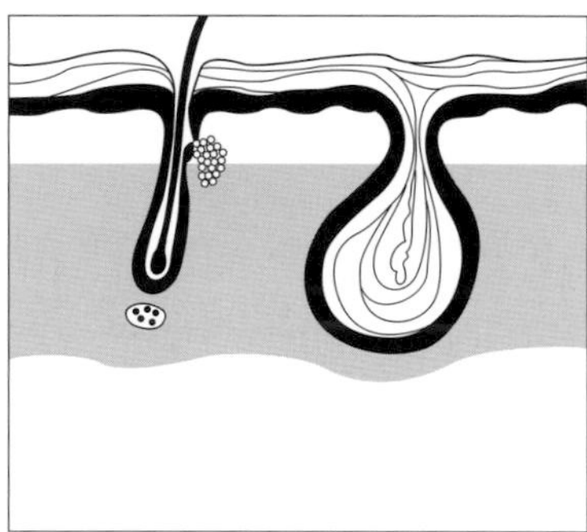

Figure 5.20 Histologic and schematic appearance of **atrophic dermatosis**. The epidermis is 1–2 cells thick, follicles are reduced to small epithelial cell clusters, the dermis has sparse collagen fibers, and sebaceous glands are inconspicuous. In the schematic, note the thin dermis, hyperkeratosis, pilosebaceous atrophy, follicular keratosis and plugging.

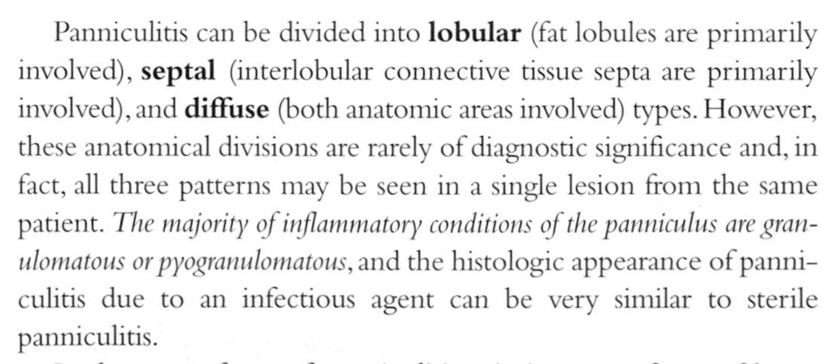

Panniculitis can be divided into **lobular** (fat lobules are primarily involved), **septal** (interlobular connective tissue septa are primarily involved), and **diffuse** (both anatomic areas involved) types. However, these anatomical divisions are rarely of diagnostic significance and, in fact, all three patterns may be seen in a single lesion from the same patient. *The majority of inflammatory conditions of the panniculus are granulomatous or pyogranulomatous*, and the histologic appearance of panniculitis due to an infectious agent can be very similar to sterile panniculitis.

In dogs, one form of panniculitis mimics a rare form of lupus erythematosus (lupus erythematosus panniculitis or lupus profundus). It is characterized by lobular hyaline degeneration of fat, lymphocytic vasculitis, lymphoid nodules, and sometimes mucinous degeneration. A similar microscopic lesion occurs in dogs at sites of previous rabies vaccination.

Atrophic dermatosis

Atrophic dermatosis is usually characterized by atrophic changes in the hair follicles and adnexal structures (Fig. 5.20). *It can also refer to atrophy of the epidermis or the dermis. Evaluation of atrophy of the epidermis and dermis should always take into account the site from which the biopsy was taken.* Epidermis is normally thicker on the dorsum than the ventrum, and hair follicles and shafts are larger and closer together on the dorsum than on the ventral or glabrous skin. In addition, familiarity with the various stages of the hair follicle cycle is essential if atrophy of the follicle is to be evaluated. Atrophic dermatosis is often accompanied by some, or all, of the following features: atrophic hair follicles (telogen and catagen follicles are usually predominant), orthokeratotic hyperkeratosis, follicular keratosis, decreased numbers of hair shafts in follicular infundibula, epidermal atrophy, sebaceous gland atrophy, and dermal atrophy (this can be difficult to assess without site-matched controls). Atrophic dermatosis is rarely diagnostic for a specific condition but can suggest a group of diseases such as the *endocrine dermatoses, the most common cause of atrophic dermatosis*. It will almost always be necessary to confirm the identity of the endocrinopathy with endocrinological function tests. Other less common causes of atrophic dermatoses include ischemia, heritable dysplasias such as dermal atrophy in cutaneous asthenia (dermatosparaxis), and paraneoplastic alopecia. Atrophic dermatosis is not an inflammatory pattern, but can be secondarily affected with inflammation, for example, pyoderma superimposed on an endocrine dermatopathy.

Follicular and adnexal atrophy can also be secondary, rather than the primary disease process. An example would be follicular atrophy as a result of a chronic inflammatory process, such as chronic allergic dermatitis, or sebaceous adenitis. In this case there would be histologic evidence of the chronic inflammation previously present, such as scarring.

Bibliography

Claudy A. Pathogenesis of leukocytoclastic vasculitis. Eur J Dermatol 1998; 8:75–79.

Fitzpatrick JE. Patterns in dermatopathology. In: Farmer ER, Hood AF, eds. Pathology of the Skin. 2nd ed. USA: McGraw-Hill, 2000:113–130.
Foster AP. A study of the number and distribution of cutaneous mast cells in cats with disease not affecting the skin. Vet Dermatol 1994;5:17–20.
Gross TL, et al. An anatomical classification of folliculitis. Vet Dermatol 1997;8:147–156.
Noli C, et al. Apoptosis in selected skin diseases. Vet Dermatol 1998;9:221–229.
Scott DW. Lymphoid nodules in skin biopsies from dogs, cats, and horses with nonneoplastic dermatoses. Cornell Vet 1989;79:267–272.
Seaman WJ, Chang SH. Dermal perifollicular mineralization of toy poodle bitches. Vet Pathol 1984;21:122–123.
Shiohara T, et al. Induction and control of lichenoid tissue reactions. Springer Semin Immunopathol 1992;13:369–385.
Steffen C. Dyskeratosis and the dyskeratoses. Am J Dermatopathol 1988;10:356–363.
Trump BF, et al. The pathways of cell death: Oncosis, apoptosis, and necrosis. Toxicol Pathol 1997;25:82–87.
Weedon D. An approach to the interpretation of skin biopsies. In: Weedon D, ed. Skin Pathology. New York: Churchill Livingstone, 1997:3–26.
Yager JA. Introduction to histological interpretation of inflammatory and degenerative lesions of the skin. In: Yager JA, Wilcock BP, eds.Color Atlas and Text of Surgical Pathology of the Dog and Cat. London: Mosby-Year Book, 1994:11–50.

CONGENITAL AND HEREDITARY DISEASES OF SKIN

Congenital diseases are those that are present at birth. They may be hereditary or result from other factors that were present during development in utero. Various environmental influences, such as infectious agents, nutrient imbalances, toxic chemicals and plants, and ambient temperature, present during gestation can bring about abnormalities in the skin and hair that are present at birth but are not hereditary. Some congenital diseases are incompatible with life and result in death at birth or shortly thereafter. Congenital abnormalities of the skin may be associated with abnormalities of other tissues or organs. In contrast, although they are genetically determined, some hereditary abnormalities of skin (*genodermatoses*) are not apparent at birth and may instead be manifested later in life, i.e., tardive onset. For example, color dilution alopecia may not be evident until early adulthood. These conditions will be covered elsewhere in the chapter under the appropriate section.

As developments in medical science have reduced the incidence of preventable diseases, an increasing awareness of genetic diseases has developed. New genetic disorders are being recognized at an increasing rate as the degree of diagnostic sophistication of veterinary medicine has grown. This is happening, at least in part, because knowledge from genetic disorders in humans often leads to recognition of similar diseases in animals. Once an analogous genetic disease is identified in animals, affected animals may be used to gain new knowledge regarding the genetics, pathogenesis, or treatment of the condition, thereby producing reciprocal benefits for both human and animal health.

Epitheliogenesis imperfecta

Epitheliogenesis imperfecta (EI) is a congenital condition in which localized or widespread areas of the squamous epithelium of the skin and mucous membranes are absent. It is an uncommon to rare anomaly of calves, piglets, foals, lambs, puppies, and kittens. Lesions consist of sharply demarcated, variably sized defects in the epidermis or mucosa, resulting in exposure of a glistening, red, moist, hairless dermis, or oral or esophageal submucosa (Fig. 5.21). Hooves and nails may be absent or poorly developed; teeth may be malformed; and pinnae may be absent. Congenital defects involving other systems are also present in some affected animals. Fetuses with extensive lesions are generally born dead. Affected animals born live may die in early postnatal life because of infection or septicemia, or secondary to dehydration and electrolyte abnormalities resulting from loss of large amounts of water from the nonepithelialized surfaces. Small lesions heal with cicatrization and may be compatible with life. In all species, *histologic lesions are an abrupt absence of epithelium and a lack of adnexal structures in the dermis or rare rudimentary hair follicles devoid of apocrine and sebaceous glands.*

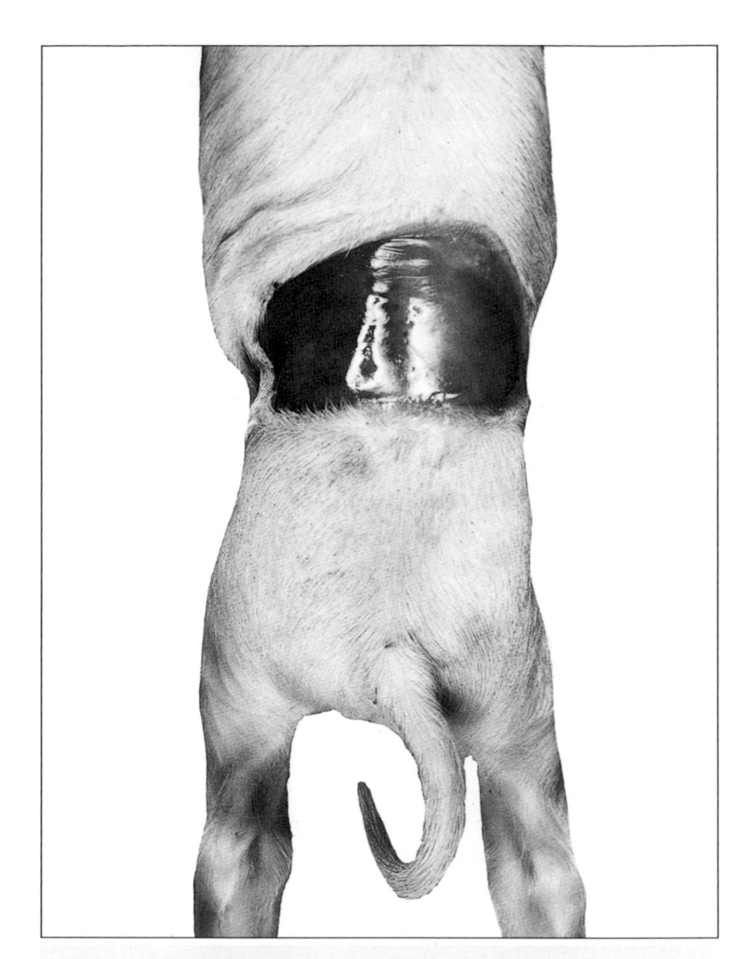

Figure 5.21 Epitheliogenesis imperfecta in a pig.

Epitheliogenesis imperfecta has been reported most often in **calves** and it occurs in many breeds. The condition appears to be an *autosomal recessive trait* and it is seen most often in herds in which there is extensive inbreeding. Both male and female calves are affected. Lesions are usually extensive and involve the extremities most commonly; however, any portion of the body may be affected as well as the squamous epithelium of the muzzle, lips, and oral cavity. Hooves and dewclaws may be missing or incompletely formed. Some affected calves also have deformed teeth and lack pinnae. Brachygnathia and atresia ani have accompanied the cutaneous abnormalities in some calves. Defects in collagen and lipid biosynthesis by dermal fibroblasts have been reported in a calf with epitheliogenesis imperfecta. However, the histologic abnormality seen in this calf was dermal–epidermal clefting; and ultrastructural examination indicated ballooning degeneration and confluent vacuole formation of the basal cells, changes suggestive of epidermolytic epidermolysis bullosa rather than of epitheliogenesis imperfecta.

Epitheliogenesis imperfecta appears to be a recessively inherited trait in **piglets**. Only male piglets were affected in one report and it was thus speculated that the condition is sex-linked. Most piglets have extensive lesions and die shortly after birth. Piglets with small focal lesions may survive but are smaller than normal littermates. At least some affected piglets also have hydroureter and hydronephrosis. Lesions in **foals** usually involve the legs and oral cavity. The proximal esophagus may also be affected and hooves may be lacking. In some instances, teeth are malformed. EI is hereditary in newborn American Saddlebred foals, and is linked to mutation in a gene coding for a laminin subunit protein on equine chromosome 8q. It is unknown, but likely, that EI is genetic in lambs, puppies, and kittens. In **lambs**, epitheliogenesis imperfecta is similar grossly to "red foot," a colloquial term for epidermolysis bullosa, with sloughing of hooves and ulceration of the tongue and hard palate. EI is very rare in **dogs**. In a closed colony of Beagle dogs in which 1500 puppies were born during a 4-year period, only one case occurred, suggesting a spontaneous mutation rather than an inherited anomaly. EI was reported in a litter of Siamese **kittens** with linear ulcers on the tongue.

Bibliography

Agerholm JS, et al. Investigations on the occurrence of hereditary diseases in the Danish cattle population 1989–1991. Acta Vet Scand 1993;34:245–253.

Bentinck-Smith J. A congenital epithelial defect in a herd of Berkshire swine. Cornell Vet 1951;41:47–51.

Dalir-Naghadeh B, et al. Congenital bovine epitheliogenesis imperfecta: a report of three cases from Iran. J Vet Med A Physiol Pathol Clin Med 2004;51:409–412.

Dubielzig RR, et al. Dental dysplasia and epitheliogenesis imperfecta in a foal. Vet Pathol 1986;23:325–327.

Frey J, et al. Collagen and lipid biosynthesis in a case of epitheliogenesis imperfecta in cattle. J Invest Dermatol 1989;93:83–86.

Hewitt MP, et al. Epitheliogenesis imperfecta in a black Labrador puppy. Can Vet J 1975;16:371–374.

Lieto LD, Cothran EG. The epitheliogenesis imperfecta locus maps to equine chromosome 8 in American Saddlebred horses. Cytogenet Genome Res 2003;102:207–210.

Munday BL. Epitheliogenesis imperfecta in lambs and kittens. Br Vet J 1970;126:47.

Tontis A, Hofstetter H. Epitheliogenesis imperfecta in lambs. Schweiz Arch Tierheilkd 1991;133:287–289.

Wattles

Wattles (tassels), similar to those seen in goats, occur occasionally in pigs and rarely in sheep. They occur in many breeds of **pigs** with no apparent sex predilection and are inherited as an autosomal dominant trait. Wattles are asymptomatic, cylindrical, teat-like structures that hang from the ventral mandibular region. They are 5–7 cm long and may be unilateral or bilateral. Histologically, they are composed of a core of fibrocartilage, surrounded by fibrous and adipose connective tissue, and covered by haired skin. Wattles have also been reported in Dorset Down, Merino, and Karakul **sheep**. The structures in sheep are smaller than those of pigs and they lack the fibrocartilaginous core seen in wattles of goats and pigs.

Bibliography

Lancaster MJ, Medwell WD. Neck wattles in lambs. Aust Vet J 1991;68:75–76.

Roberts E, Morrill CC. Inheritance and histology of wattles in swine. J Hered 1944;35:149–151.

Ichthyosis (congenital disorders of cornification)

Ichthyosis is a heterogeneous group of disorders of cornification that are all characterized by hyperkeratosis and accumulations of scales (Fig. 5.22). The name is derived from the Greek word for fish because of the fish scale-like appearance of the hyperkeratotic skin. Ichthyosis in animals is a rare congenital condition that has been reported in cattle, dogs, pigs, chickens, laboratory mice, and a llama. The disease in humans is classified into four major and several minor forms based on clinical, histologic, cell kinetic, and genetic characteristics. Kinetic studies have shown that two of the major forms, lamellar ichthyosis and epidermolytic hyperkeratosis, are proliferation keratoses resulting from accelerated cell turnover causing abnormal cell maturation and excessive keratin. In contrast, icthyosis vulgaris and X-linked ichthyosis, the other two major forms, are retention hyperkeratoses related to increased cohesiveness between stratum corneum cells resulting in decreased loss of keratin. The biochemical defects in the various types of ichthyosis are still being investigated.

Ichthyosis vulgaris, the most common form in humans, is an autosomal dominant disease characterized histologically by orthokeratotic hyperkeratosis and a decreased or absent granular layer, and ultrastructurally by a delay in dissolution of desmosomes in the stratum corneum and small, abnormal keratohyaline granules. It is produced by a defect in synthesis of filaggrin. **X-linked ichthyosis**, a recessive form in which males have more severe disease than female heterozygotes, is caused by an absence of steroid sulfatase activity. Steroid sulfatase acts on cholesteryl sulfate, a product of lamellar granules or Odland bodies, which is discharged into the intercellular space and is involved in cell cohesion in the lower stratum

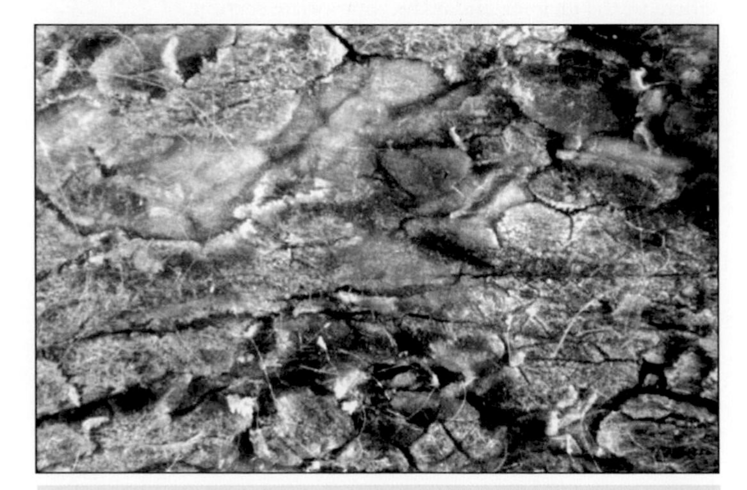

Figure 5.22 Ichthyosis. Note adherent plaques of keratin. (Courtesy of B Dunstan.)

corneum. Failure of the enzyme to inactivate cholesteryl sulfate results in persistent cell cohesion and interferes with the normal process of desquamation. The histologic features of X-linked recessive ichthyosis are orthokeratotic hyperkeratosis with a normal or hyperplastic granular layer. Keratohyaline granules are ultrastructurally normal. **Epidermolytic hyperkeratosis**, also called bullous congenital ichthyosiform erythroderma or bullous ichthyosis, is an autosomal dominant form characterized histologically by orthokeratotic and parakeratotic hyperkeratosis, vacuolation of keratinocytes in the upper stratum spinosum and stratum granulosum, and a markedly thickened granular layer with increased numbers of irregularly shaped keratohyaline granules. Ultrastructural changes consist of increased numbers and clumping of tonofilaments, premature formation of keratohyaline granules, and abnormal association of desmosomes and tonofilaments resulting in acantholysis. The biochemical basis is a defect in the K1 and K10 genes. **Lamellar ichthyosis** is an autosomal recessive ichthyosis characterized histologically by compact orthokeratotic hyperkeratosis and mild acanthosis. It is thought to be caused by a defect of keratinocyte transglutaminase which results in decreased cross-linking of loricrin and involucrin and thus interferes with formation of the cornified cell envelope. **Harlequin ichthyosis** is a rare autosomal recessive, usually fatal form to which some cases of ichthyosis in calves have been compared. In this form of ichthyosis, there is a thick compact stratum corneum with follicular hyperkeratosis and variable appearance of the stratum granulosum. The exact biochemical defect is uncertain but abnormal lamellar granule formation and secretion and a defect in protein phosphatase, which may be involved in processing of filaggrin, have been demonstrated. The majority of cases of ichthyosis in animals have been compared to lamellar ichthyosis of humans based on the clinical and light microscopic features (Fig. 5.23). However, *cases that have been characterized more completely do not correlate well with the human classification system*. The biochemical defect has not been determined in any of the cases of ichthyosis reported in animals thus far.

Ichthyosis has been reported in many breeds of **cattle** and the mode of inheritance appears to be *autosomal recessive*. Both males and females are affected. Two forms of ichthyosis have been described in cattle, *ichthyosis fetalis* and *ichthyosis congenita*. However, the underlying molecular defect(s) is unknown, and it is uncertain whether the forms are distinct diseases or merely represent variations in expression of a single abnormality. *Ichthyosis fetalis* is the more severe form and it has been compared to the harlequin fetus form of ichthyosis in humans. Affected calves are dead at birth or die shortly after birth. The skin is hairless and covered by thick scales divided into plates by deep fissures which represent normal cleavage planes of the skin. The tight, inelastic skin is everted at the mucocutaneous junctions and the ears are usually smaller than normal. *Ichthyosis congenita* is a less severe form compatible with life in which the limbs, abdomen, and muzzle are primarily involved. The skin is dry, hard, and inflexible like old leather and may be prominently folded. There are flat plates of hyperkeratosis in which dense mats of hairs are entrapped. The keratin plaques are separated by shallow hyperemic fissures. The condition is characterized histologically by *prominent laminated orthokeratotic hyperkeratosis of the epidermis and superficial portion of hair follicles*. The epidermal surface is wrinkled or folded and acanthosis is variable.

Ichthyosis has been reported rarely in various purebred and mixed-breed **dogs**. In all cases, parents of affected animals have been clinically normal and thus a *recessive mode of inheritance was suspected*; however, the pattern of inheritance has not been documented by breeding studies. The biochemical abnormality has not been identified in any of the cases, but ultrastructural findings and cell kinetic studies performed in a few dogs with ichthyosis suggested a *proliferative mechanism* for the condition. Lesions are evident at birth; and both male and female pups are affected. The entire body is usually involved but in some cases lesions are limited to the sparsely haired portions of the body. Tightly adherent light tan-gray or parchment-like scales or thick plaques are frequently widely distributed. The skin is variably thickened and may be greasy; and the hair is thin and dull or absent in patches. Some affected dogs are smaller than their normal littermates. Footpads are frequently also hyperkeratotic and appear to be painful. Histologically, there is *marked orthokeratotic hyperkeratosis that includes the infundibular portion of hair follicles*. The epidermal surface is frequently irregular and the epidermis is mildly to moderately hyperplastic. In many of the cases, the granular layer contains an increased number of enlarged and irregular keratohyaline granules and many cells are vacuolated and degenerated leading to microvesicle formation. The dermis is usually normal or has nonspecific inflammation.

Several familial disorders of cornification have been described in dogs. An unusual hereditary condition has been reported in five related *female*

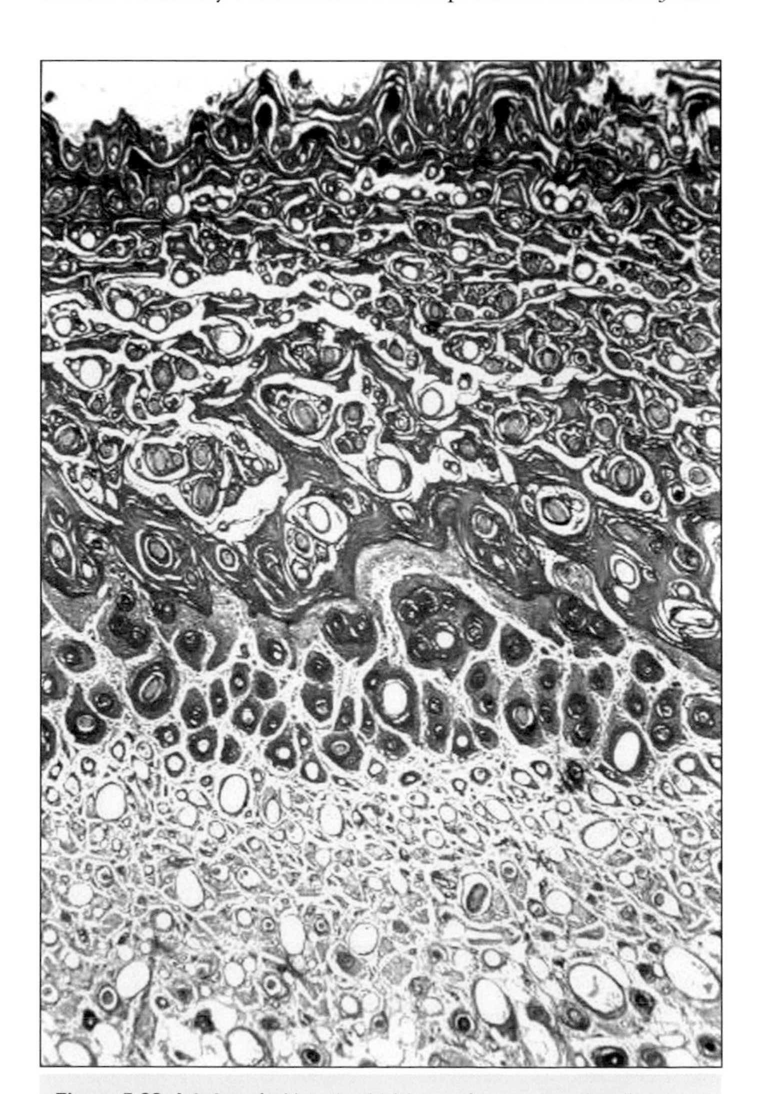

Figure 5.23 Ichthyosis. Note the thick layer of excess keratin adherent to the epidermal surface. (Courtesy of B Dunstan.)

Rottweiler dogs. Since no related males were affected, an X-linked mode of inheritance was suspected. Cutaneous lesions consisted of generalized scaling and hyperkeratotic pigmented plaques. Three dogs also had multiple noncutaneous congenital anomalies. Histologic findings in these dogs included intracellular keratinocyte edema, epidermal vacuoles, and primarily parakeratotic hyperkeratosis of the surface and follicular epidermis. Ultrastructural changes in two of the dogs included large keratohyaline granules, tonofilament clumps, and numerous lipid vacuoles in the stratum corneum and granulosum. The clinical, histologic, and ultrastructural features of this disorder cannot be classified into any single disorder of cornification in humans. *Hereditary footpad hyperkeratosis* has been reported in Irish Terriers and in a family of Dogues de Bordeaux. All footpads become progressively hyperkeratotic, fissured, and painful. Both males and females are affected and lesions are evident by six months of age. The mode of inheritance has not been determined. The histologic features are mild to moderate papillated epidermal hyperplasia and diffuse orthokeratotic hyperkeratosis.

Bibliography

Alhaidari Z, et al. Congenital ichthyosis in two cavalier King Charles spaniel littermates. Vet Dermatol 1994;5:117–121.

Ammirati CT, Mallory SB. The major inherited disorders of cornification. New advances in pathogenesis. Dermatol Clinics 1998;16:497–508.

Baker JR, Ward WR. Ichthyosis in domestic animals: A review of the literature and a case report. Br Vet J 1985;141:1–8.

Helman RG, et al. Ichthyosiform dermatosis in a soft-coated wheaten terrier. Vet Dermatol 1997;8:53–58.

Julian RJ. Ichthyosis congenita in cattle. Vet Med 1960;55:35–41.

Lewis DT, et al. A hereditary disorder of cornification and multiple congenital defects in five Rottweiler dogs. Vet Dermatol 1998;9:61–72.

Lewis DT, et al. Characterization and management of a Jack Russell terrier with congenital ichthyosis. Vet Dermatol 1998;9:111–118.

Mecklenburg L, et al. Epidermolytic ichthyosis in a dog: clinical, histopathological, immunohistochemical and ultrastructural findings. J Comp Pathol 2000; 122:307–311.

Paradis M. Footpad hyperkeratosis in a family of Dogues de Bordeaux. Vet Dermatol 1992;3:75–78.

Hereditary zinc deficiency

Hereditary zinc deficiency occurs in cattle and Bull Terrier dogs and results in multisystemic disease that includes skin lesions. Animals are normal at birth and usually begin developing skin lesions at approximately one to two months of age at which time growth retardation also becomes evident. Skin lesions consist of crusting which is most prominent on the face and distal extremities, dry flaky skin, and hair color fading. A decrease in serum zinc concentration precedes clinical signs; and alkaline phosphatase, a zinc-dependent enzyme, frequently decreases in parallel with the zinc concentration. Affected animals also commonly have diarrhea. Animals with hereditary zinc deficiency have a hypoplastic thymus; and, consequently, secondary infections are common because of associated immune system dysfunction involving both humoral and cell-mediated immunity. The condition is an *autosomal recessive trait* in both cattle and dogs; and it is considered analogous to acrodermatitis enteropathica of humans. *The characteristic histologic lesion is marked diffuse parakeratotic hyperkeratosis*.

Hereditary zinc deficiency in cattle is also called *lethal trait A 46, hereditary parakeratosis, hereditary thymic aplasia*, and *Adema disease*. It affects Friesian cattle and Black Pied Danish cattle of Friesian descent in Europe, and has been reported in Shorthorn cattle in the United States. The condition normally begins with depression, diarrhea, and skin lesions when calves are 4–8 weeks of age. The skin becomes dry and flaky and the hair coat is rough. Patches of erythema, scaling, oozing, crusting, and alopecia begin on the muzzle and then appear around the eyes, ears, and intermandibular space. Similar lesions develop later on the legs; and the skin around the stifles, fetlocks, and coronary bands becomes particularly crusty, fissured, and painful. The flanks, perianal area, and ventral abdomen may also be affected. The hair may lighten in color, a change that may be especially prominent around the eyes and resemble the spectacle lesion of copper deficiency. Affected calves are lethargic, drool, and may have difficulty suckling. They are smaller than unaffected calves of the same age. Conjunctivitis, rhinitis, bronchopneumonia, and other infections are common because of *immune dysfunction*. Untreated calves usually die 4–8 weeks after the onset of clinical disease.

Oral zinc supplementation effects a complete reversal of clinical signs and may restore thymic morphology if instituted early enough. *Intestinal malabsorption of zinc is the cause of the disorder in cattle*. Zinc is absorbed from the intestine by two separate pathways, i.e., a transporter-dependent active system and passive diffusion, and it is the zinc-binding ligand system which is suspected to be defective. A cysteine-rich intestinal protein (CRIP) has been identified in the ligand-dependent pathway and has been suggested as being defective in this condition.

The most striking and consistent gross abnormality is *marked thymic hypoplasia*. Histologic abnormalities include *depletion of small lymphocytes* of the thymus, especially in the cortical region, and hypoplasia of the spleen, lymph nodes, and Peyer's patches. The skin lesions are characterized histologically by *perivascular dermatitis, acanthosis, pallor and vacuolation of the upper spinous and granular layers, and marked diffuse parakeratosis*. Neutrophilic exocytosis and superficial bacterial cocci may be prominent.

Lethal acrodermatitis of Bull Terrier dogs is also thought to be caused by an abnormality in zinc absorption or metabolism; however, zinc supplementation fails to produce clinical improvement. The concentrations of both serum zinc and copper have been found to be lower in affected bull terriers as compared to control dogs, raising the question of the role of copper deficiency in the pathogenesis of the canine disease. The condition is characterized by growth retardation, progressive skin lesions, paronychia, diarrhea, abnormal behavior, bronchopneumonia, and death usually by 18 months. Some affected puppies have lighter pigmentation than their normal littermates and this difference becomes more pronounced with age. By 2 months of age, they are obviously smaller than their normal littermates. Skin lesions usually begin by 6–8 weeks of age and consist of crusty exfoliative lesions involving the distal extremities, footpads, and mucocutaneous junctions, particularly around the eyes and mouth. Digits are prominently splayed and footpads develop cracks and frond-like masses of keratin. The skin is erythematous and moist under the crusts. Interdigital pyoderma and paronychia are common. Many affected dogs also have diarrhea and exhibit abnormal behavior consisting of increased aggressiveness initially, and lethargy and decreased responsiveness later in the course of disease. Respiratory tract infections are common and bronchopneumonia is a common cause of death.

Extracutaneous necropsy lesions consist of a *small or absent thymus* and may also include a high, arched palate and brachygnathia inferior. Histologic changes in the skin are *mild to moderate perivascular dermatitis, moderate to marked acanthosis which may be accompanied by pallor of the superficial epidermis, and marked diffuse parakeratotic hyperkeratosis.* There may also be neutrophilic exocytosis, intraepidermal neutrophilic pustules, and serocellular crusts containing bacterial cocci and/or yeasts. Diagnosis is straightforward if signalment and clinical history are known. If this information is not available, differential diagnoses include superficial necrolytic dermatitis, zinc-responsive dermatosis, and generic dog food dermatosis. However, parakeratosis is less severe in these diseases and superficial epidermal necrolysis is not a feature of lethal acrodermatitis.

Bibliography

Machen M, et al. Bovine hereditary zinc deficiency: lethal trait A 46. J Vet Diagn Invest 1996;8:219–227.

Perafan-Riveros C, et al. Acrodermatitis enteropathica: case report and review of the literature. Pediatr Dermatol 2002;19:426–431.

Perryman LE, et al. Lymphocyte alterations in zinc-deficient calves with lethal trait A 46. Vet Immunol Immunopathol 1989;21:239–248.

Smits B, et al. Lethal acrodermatitis in Bull Terriers: A problem of defective zinc metabolism. Vet Dermatol 1991;2:91–96.

Uchida Y, et al. Serum concentrations of zinc and copper in Bull Terriers with lethal acrodermatitis and tail chasing behavior. Am J Vet Res 1997;58:808–810.

Vogt DW, et al. Hereditary parakeratosis in Shorthorn beef calves. Am J Vet Res 1988;49:120–121.

Epidermolysis bullosa

Epidermolysis bullosa is a heterogeneous group of mechanobullous genodermatoses which are all characterized by skin and mucous membrane blistering and ulceration in response to minor mechanical trauma (Fig. 5.24). Lesions are a result of insufficient coherence of the dermal–epidermal junction because of structural defects in the basement membrane zone. The molecular bases for the various forms of epidermolysis bullosa have been discovered only in recent years. The condition is divided into three broad groups based on the ultrastructural level of the skin cleavage, i.e., epidermolysis bullosa simplex (epidermolytic epidermolysis bullosa), junctional epidermolysis bullosa, and dystrophic epidermolysis bullosa (dermolytic epidermolysis bullosa). Epidermolysis bullosa is further classified into more than 20 subtypes in humans based on clinical manifestations of skin lesions, mode of inheritance, and presence or absence of extracutaneous abnormalities, as well as ultrastructural features. The clinical presentation may range from minimal localized involvement of hands and feet to severe, life-threatening generalized blistering with extracutaneous involvement. Corneal erosions, tooth, nail, and hair abnormalities, and tracheal, gastrointestinal, genitourinary, and musculoskeletal involvement occur in various subtypes of epidermolysis bullosa in humans. In animals, epidermolysis bullosa has been reported rarely and, in most instances, has led to the death of affected individuals.

Epidermolysis bullosa simplex is characterized by *cytolysis of the basal keratinocytes,* which produces intraepidermal clefting. This form of the disease is caused by fragility of the epidermal basal cells because of mutations in basal cell-specific keratins 5 and 14. These

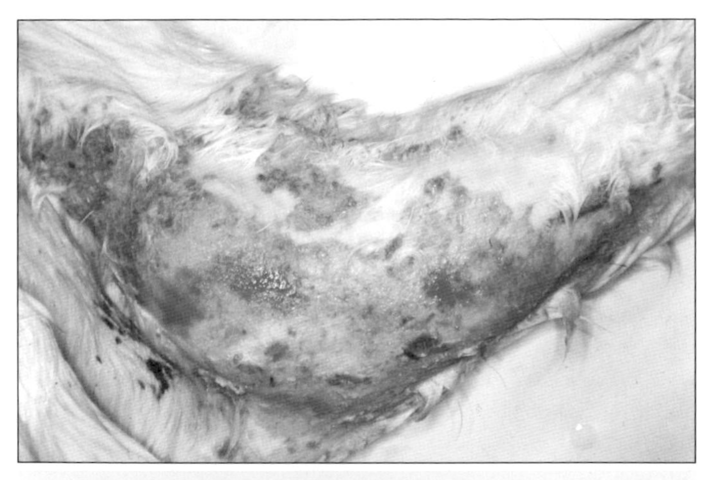

Figure 5.24 Epidermolysis bullosa. An easily detached epidermis led to extensive ulceration in areas exposed to minor mechanical trauma. (Courtesy of B Dunstan.)

mutations result in disruption of the assembly, structure, and/or function of the keratin intermediate filaments that act as the skeleton of basal keratinocytes. Ultrastructurally, cytolysis of the basal cells is seen as intra-epidermal clefting. In some forms, cytolysis is preceded by aggregation and clumping of the keratin tonofilaments which are attached to hemidesmosomes. In **junctional epidermolysis bullosa**, clefting occurs within the lamina lucida because of abnormalities of the anchoring filament-hemidesmosome complexes, which may be reduced in number and poorly formed or may be completely absent. Most cases of junctional epidermolysis bullosa are due to a deficiency or abnormality in one of the hemidesmosome-associated proteins laminin-5, collagen XVII (also called BPAG 2 and BP180), or integrin $\alpha 6\beta 4$, or the extracellular protein LAD-1, which is secreted by epidermal cells and localizes to the upper aspect of the anchoring filaments. **Dystrophic epidermolysis bullosa** is characterized by a split in the superficial dermis below the lamina densa in the region of the anchoring fibrils, which are fewer in number and distorted or completely absent. The molecular cause of dystrophic epidermolysis bullosa is a mutation in the anchoring fibril protein, type VII collagen.

Affected animals usually develop lesions shortly after birth; however, in some cases, the disease is not evident until the animal is several months old. *Initial lesions consist of vesicles and bullae, but they quickly rupture and only ulcers may be evident clinically.* Lesions are located in areas of the skin and mucous membranes which are most prone to frictional trauma such as *over bony prominences of the distal extremities, foot pads, lips, tongue, palate, and gingiva.* Hoof sloughing and nail dystrophy and shedding accompany skin lesions in some forms of the disease. Lesions may be induced accidentally by rough handling of an affected animal or intentionally for diagnostic purposes by gentle frictional trauma.

Histologically, most forms of epidermolysis bullosa are characterized by subepidermal clefts and vesicles with minimal inflammation (see Fig. 5.18), changes which are indistinguishable from bullous pemphigoid. Even in the epidermolytic form of epidermolysis bullosa, the cleavage is usually so low in the epidermis that the vesicle appears subepidermal in routine sections. PAS staining to visualize the basement membrane zone may be helpful in determining the level of cleavage, but definitive diagnosis requires ultrastructural examination. Basement membrane antigen mapping by immunofluorescence or immunohistochemistry may be a diagnostic adjunct or alternative to electron microscopy to establish the diagnosis. In epidermolysis bullosa simplex, the PAS-positive basement membrane is at the base of the blister as are type IV collagen, laminin, and BP (bullous pemphigoid) antigen. In junctional epidermolysis bullosa, the PAS-positive basement membrane, type IV collagen, and laminin are at the base of the blister, whereas the BP antigen is primarily on the blister roof. The PAS-positive basement membrane as well as all three basement membrane proteins, i.e., type IV collagen, laminin, and BP antigen, are at the roof of the blister in dystrophic epidermolysis bullosa.

Cattle

A congenital mechanobullous disease, identified as *epidermolysis bullosa simplex*, was described in 25 of 72 calves sired by a single Simmental bull. The condition appeared to be inherited as an *autosomal dominant trait* with high mortality. Lesions were evident in newborn calves and consisted of ulcers of the muzzle, lips, gingiva, dorsum of the tongue, and around joints of distal limbs. Calves were unthrifty, became emaciated after weaning, and developed areas of alopecia, hyperkeratosis, ulcers, and exfoliative dermatitis. Three animals kept under laboratory conditions showed a gradual improvement in severity of lesions but rough handling could still elicit lesions. Histologic changes were typical of epidermolysis bullosa and consisted of *dermal-epidermal separation unassociated with any significant inflammation*. PAS-positive basement membrane was evident on the dermal side of the cleft. In thin sections of skin, cytolysis of the basal keratinocytes was seen but no ultrastructural examination was done to confirm the diagnosis.

A mechanobullous disease suspected to be *dystrophic epidermolysis bullosa* has been reported in Texas Brangus calves with a common bull in their pedigree. The calves developed ulceration of distal limbs and oral mucosa, nasolabial mucosal sloughing, and sloughing of hooves within the first few days of life. The mode of inheritance was suspected to be recessive because of extensive inbreeding. Histologically, the lesions were dermal-epidermal clefts with the PAS-positive basement membrane remaining attached to the basal cell layer, i.e., forming the roof of the bullae. Ultrastructural examination revealed that the lamina densa was attached to the basal layer of the epidermis; inadequate fixation prevented accurate evaluation of the anchoring fibrils.

A *congenital mechanobullous dermatosis of uncertain type* has been described in Angus calves in New Zealand and Murrah buffalo (*Bubalus bubalis*) calves in Brazil. In both reports, skin lesions developed in newborn calves in sites prone to trauma or were induced by trauma. Hoof separation and sloughing were also observed; and in buffalo calves, horns were frequently deformed and partially or completely separated from the underlying corium. Mucous membrane and mucocutaneous involvement was seen in the Angus calves but not in the buffalo calves. The histologic changes seen in the Angus calves were separation of prickle cells and basal cells from each other and sometimes basal cells from the underlying dermis, resulting in *suprabasilar to sub-basilar vesicles* and subsequent shedding of the epithelium. Many basal and prickle cells contained large eosinophilic cytoplasmic bodies. In the Murrah buffalo calves, the characteristic histologic alteration was *suprabasilar clefting* with detachment of the stratum spinosum from the underlying basal layer. Ultrastructural changes in affected areas of skin in the buffalo calves consisted of a loss of desmosomal adhesion between the basal and prickle cell layers. The basal lamina, hemidesmosomes, anchoring fibrils, and anchoring filaments appeared normal. In the Angus calves, desmosomes were lacking or fewer than normal, and many keratinocytes contained a mass of tonofilaments arranged in whorls. Hemidesmosomes were normal. Although the clinical presentation of these cases was typical of epidermolysis bullosa, the histologic and ultrastructural features were unlike those of the common forms of epidermolysis bullosa. However, some variants of epidermolysis bullosa simplex in humans are characterized by cleft formation with acantholysis in the middle or upper epidermis, and in some instances cells contain round clumps within their cytoplasm produced by aggregation of tonofilaments. In both reports, the condition in the calves was suspected to be inherited as an *autosomal recessive* trait.

Sheep

A congenital bullous disease suggestive of *dystrophic epidermolysis bullosa* has been described in Suffolk and South Dorset Down lambs in New Zealand, Scottish Blackface lambs, and Weisses Alpenschaf lambs in Switzerland. Blisters which evolved into ulcers were seen at birth or within the first few weeks of life. Lesions occurred in areas with sparse hair and those prone to frictional trauma such as the muzzle, ears, groin, coronary band, lips, tongue, gums, dental pad, and palate. Lameness and hoof separation and sloughing were common and gave rise to the colloquial name "red foot disease" in Scotland. The lambs grew poorly and were underdeveloped, changes attributed to oral ulceration and reluctance to nurse. Histologic changes were typical of epidermolysis bullosa and consisted of *dermal–epidermal separation with minimal inflammation*. The PAS-positive basement membrane zone remained attached to the epithelium and formed the roof of the vesicle, suggestive of dystrophic epidermolysis bullosa. Only in the Swiss Weisses Alpenschaf has the condition been characterized. Ultrastructural examination of skin from the Swiss lambs indicated that the splitting was below the lamina densa and that anchoring fibrils were absent or rare and rudimentary. Antigen mapping of the lesion identified laminin and type IV collagen at the roof of the cleft, which *confirms sub-lamina densa blistering*; and no type VII collagen, the major structural component of anchoring fibrils, could be identified. These findings are consistent with the dystrophic form of epidermolysis bullosa. The disease was found to have a *recessive mode of inheritance*.

Horses

Junctional epidermolysis bullosa (JEB) has been described in both male and female Belgian foals within the first week or two of life, corresponding to the severe Herlitz form of JEB in humans. Lesions consist of skin and oral mucosal ulceration, most often of the carpi, stifles, hocks, fetlocks, tongue, gingiva, and hard palate. Hoof separation and sloughing (exungulation) are common features. Extracutaneous lesions are rare, and included ocular lesions in one foal and dental dysplasia in another. The histologic lesions consist of *subepidermal clefting with minimal inflammation and PAS-positive basement membrane material evident at the base of the cleft*. Ultrastructurally, the separation is located within the lamina lucida, indicating that hemidesmosomes are underdeveloped. The trait is inherited as an autosomal recessive. The mutation responsible – a cytosine insertion in exon 10 of the LAMC2 gene – has also been identified in JEB phenotype horses in two French draft breeds, the Breton and Comtois.

Dogs

All three forms of epidermolysis bullosa have been reported in dogs. However, the initial cases reported as epidermolysis bullosa simplex in young collies are now thought to represent a mild form of dermatomyositis with unrecognized myositis. *Junctional epidermolysis bullosa* has been described in a newborn Toy Poodle and in three puppies less than 1 month of age from a litter of seven German Shorthaired Pointers. Vesicles, bullae, and ulcers were present on multiple foot pads, in haired skin of frictional sites, and the oral cavity. The lateral hocks, elbows, stifles, and carpi were most commonly involved. No onychodystrophy or dental enamel dysplasia were evident. All of the puppies were euthanized because of the severity of the lesions. A case of *nonlethal junctional epidermolysis bullosa* has been reported in a 4-year-old female mixed-breed dog with a history of vesicles, erosions, crusts, and alopecia since birth. Lesions initially occurred on the lips and ventral abdomen and eventually progressed to involve the face, trunk, tail, and acral regions. Cutaneous atrophy and hyperpigmentation, alopecia, and nail dystrophy developed later. Histologic changes in all affected dogs consisted of subepidermal clefts and vesicles with minimal inflammation and no basal keratinocyte degeneration. The earliest changes seen in sections from the newborn poodle puppy were individual vacuoles in the basement membrane zone. Coalescence of vacuoles led to formation of subepidermal clefts. PAS staining demonstrated the basement membrane at the base of the cleft. Ultrastructural examination in all dogs revealed the separation to be within the lamina lucida. However, changes in hemidesmosomes were variable in the three reports. In the poodle, hemidesmosomes appeared rudimentary in comparison to a normal dog; whereas in the adult mixed-breed dog, hemidesmosomal attachment plaques were hypoplastic and no sub-basal dense plate was apparent. No hemidesmosomal abnormalities were evident in skin sections from the German Shorthaired Pointers. Immunostaining for hemidesmosomal-anchoring filament proteins in the German Shorthaired Pointer puppies indicated that expression of laminin-5 and integrin $\alpha 6 \beta 4$ was normal but collagen XVII (BPAG2, BP180) was undetectable. In skin sections from the adult mixed-breed dog, expression of laminin-5, BPAG2, the $\alpha 6$ subunit of integrin $\alpha 6 \beta 4$, and type VII collagen was similar to that of normal canine skin.

Dystrophic epidermolysis bullosa has been reported in a 4-year-old female Akita with a life-long history of trauma-induced ulcers and scars over pressure points of limbs and on foot pads. Nail dystrophy was apparent from 1 year of age. The lesions had periodic exacerbations and remissions. The histologic changes were *dermal–epidermal clefting* with minimal inflammation and PAS-positive basement membrane visible at the roof of the cleft. Ultrastructural examination indicated that the separation was beneath the lamina densa and anchoring fibrils were in reduced numbers. Expression of type VII collagen, the major structural protein of anchoring fibrils, was normal. A *dominant mode of inheritance* was speculated in this nonlethal case of epidermolysis bullosa because the dominant form of dystrophic epidermolysis bullosa in humans is typically relatively mild.

Cats

Epidermolysis bullosa appears to be *very rare in cats*. Two cases of dystrophic epidermolysis bullosa have been reported in unrelated cats. The cats were a male domestic shorthair and a Persian female cat. Skin lesions were evident in both cats by the age of 3 months. Lesions consisted of ulceration of multiple foot pads, the palate, oropharynx, gums, tongue, and dorsal spinous skin. Most claws had sloughed and suppurative, ulcerative paronychia affected all four feet. Histologic examination of skin biopsies showed dermal–epidermal separation progressing to ulceration. Type IV collagen was shown by immunohistochemistry to be present at the roof of the blisters. *Sub-lamina densa clefting* was confirmed by electron microscopic examination; and anchoring fibrils were markedly reduced in number and appeared rudimentary and filamentous in skin sections from the Persian cat. Immunofluorescent staining for collagen VII, the primary component of anchoring fibrils, was markedly reduced. *A mutation in the collagen VII encoding gene, COL7A1, was suggested as the cause,* since this gene is mutated in all subsets of dystrophic epidermolysis bullosa in affected human patients.

An undetermined type of epidermolysis bullosa was reported in a 3-year-old male domestic longhaired cat in the United Kingdom. The skin condition had been evident since the cat was 3 months old; a female littermate obtained at the same time showed no skin abnormalities. The affected cat had widespread skin lesions that consisted of scarring, alopecia, crusting, seborrhea, blistering, and ulceration. Several nails had been shed and very few whiskers were present. No lesions were evident in the oral cavity. Histologically, lesions were characterized by dermal–epidermal separation. Ultrastructural examination indicated the cleavage to be above the lamina densa and that hemidesmosomes and anchoring fibrils were fewer and less distinct when compared to skin from a normal cat.

Bibliography

Bassett H. A congenital bovine epidermolysis resembling epidermolysis bullosa simplex of man. Vet Rec 1987:121:8–11.

Bruckner-Tuderman L, et al. Animal model for dermolytic mechanobullous disease: Sheep with recessive dystrophic epidermolysis bullosa lack collagen VII. J Invest Dermatol 1991;96:452–458.

Frame SR, et al. Hereditary junctional mechanobullous disease in a foal. J Am Vet Med Assoc 1988;193:1420–1424.

Johnson GC, et al. Ultrastructure of junctional epidermolysis bullosa in Belgian foals. J Comp Pathol 1988;98:329–336.

Jolly RD, et al. Familial acantholysis of Angus calves. Vet Pathol 1973;10:473–483.

McTaggart HS, et al. Red foot disease of lambs. Vet Rec 1974;94:153–159.

Milenkovic D, et al. A mutation in the LAMC2 gene causes the Herlitz junctional epidermolysis bullosa (H-JEB) in two French draft horse breeds. Genet Sel Evol 2003;35:249–256.

Nagata M, et al. Dystrophic form of inherited epidermolysis bullosa in a dog (Akita Inu). Br J Dermatol 1995;133:1000–1003.

Nagata M, et al. Non-lethal junctional epidermolysis bullosa in a dog. Br J Dermatol 1997;137:445–449.

O'Dair HA, Henderson JP. Suspected mechanobullous skin disease in a cat. J Small Anim Pract 1994;35:24–27.

Olivry T, et al. Absent expression of collagen XVII (BPAG2, BP180) in canine familial localized junctional epidermolysis bullosa. Vet Dermatol 1997;8:203–212.

Olivry T, et al. Reduced anchoring fibril formation and collagen VII immunoreactivity in feline dystrophic epidermolysis bullosa. Vet Pathol 1999;36:616–618.

Palazzi X, et al. Inherited dystrophic epidermolysis bullosa in inbred dogs: A spontaneous animal model for somatic gene therapy. J Invest Dermatol 2000;115:135–137.

Paller AS. Lessons from skin blistering: Molecular mechanisms and unusual patterns of inheritance. Am J Pathol 1996;148:1727–1731.

Riet-Correa F, et al. Hereditary suprabasilar acantholytic mechanobullous dermatosis in buffaloes (*Bubalus bubalis*). Vet Pathol 1994;31:450–454.

Spirito F, et al. Animal models for skin blistering conditions: absence of laminin 5 causes hereditary junctional mechanobullous disease in the Belgian horse. J Invest Dermatol 2002;119:684–691.

Thompson KG, et al. A mechanobullous disease with sub-basilar separation in Brangus calves. Vet Pathol 1985;22:283–285.

Weedon D. Epidermolysis bullosa. In: Skin Pathology. Edinburgh: Churchill Livingstone, 1997:124–129.

White SD, et al. Dystrophic (dermolytic) epidermolysis bullosa in a cat. Vet Dermatol 1993;4:91–95.

Canine inherited epidermal acantholysis

A dominantly inherited epidermal acantholytic disease resembling human Hailey–Hailey disease/benign familial chronic pemphigus has been described in English Setters. Hailey–Hailey disease is an autosomal dominant hereditary skin disorder of cellular cohesion characterized by dissociation of epidermal keratinocytes that are subjected to frictional trauma. Lesions in people consist of vesicles and bullae usually located in large skin folds and regions exposed to chronic frictional trauma; mucosal involvement is rare. The histologic characteristics of the condition include *suprabasal clefting and extensive separation of keratinocytes which remain loosely in place*, giving the appearance of a "dilapidated brick wall." Because of the resemblance to autoimmune pemphigus, Hailey–Hailey disease is also called benign familial chronic pemphigus. A widespread intrinsic weakness in keratinocyte adhesion appears to be present but the molecular defect responsible for the disorder is unknown. Desmosomes appear normal in intact skin; structural proteins of desmosomes, adherens junctions, and gap junctions studied so far appear to be expressed normally.

The condition was seen in a 7-month-old male dog and in two of his female offspring, at the ages of 1 and 2 months. Lesions consisted of well-demarcated, alopecic, erythematous, markedly hyperplastic plaques with a rough surface, occasional serous crusting, and peripheral scaling. They occurred on the ventral thorax, head, and stifle. The clinical appearance of the lesions and their location were not typical of the human disease, but the *histologic and ultrastructural features were similar to benign familial chronic pemphigus*. Microscopically, the epidermis was markedly hyperplastic and suprabasal keratinocytes were much larger than those in the perilesional epidermis. Extensive acantholysis resulted in lacuna formation in the suprabasal and upper epidermis and the follicular epithelium. Ultrastructural changes included increased intercellular spaces, perinuclear tonofilament aggregation, and intact desmosome-tonofilament complexes and actin filament in early lesions. Immunohistochemical examination of various desmosomal proteins failed to demonstrate any abnormalities and the molecular defect in these dogs was not identified.

Bibliography

Cooley JE, et al. Hailey-Hailey disease keratinocytes: Normal assembly of cell-cell junctions *in vitro*. J Invest Dermatol 1996;107:877–881.

Haftek M, et al. Internalization of gap junctions in benign familial pemphigus (Hailey-Hailey disease) and keratosis follicularis (Darier's disease). Br J Dermatol 1999;141:224–230.

Sueki H, et al. Dominantly inherited epidermal acantholysis in dogs, simulating human benign familial chronic pemphigus (Hailey-Hailey disease). Br J Dermatol 1997;136:190–196.

Congenital hypotrichosis

Congenital hypotrichosis has been described in all domestic species but it occurs most frequently in calves. The hairlessness may be associated with congenital anomalies of other systems such as brachygnathism, dental defects, and thymic or genital abnormalities. Many affected animals are otherwise completely healthy, but some forms of congenital hypotrichosis are associated with ill-thrift and early death. Deliberate propagation of spontaneous mutations producing hairlessness has resulted in development of *specific hairless breeds* such as the Chinese Crested dog, Mexican Hairless dog, American Hairless Terrier, Sphinx cat, and Mexican Hairless pig, among others. The hair coat is an important protective barrier for animals and when it is compromised, as in congenital hypotrichosis, *affected animals are predisposed to sunburn, less tolerant to temperature extremes, and more susceptible to bacterial and fungal infection.*

Hairlessness varies from partial to complete. Partial hypotrichosis is frequently bilaterally symmetrical and the hair that is present is frequently abnormal. It is usually sparse, short and fine, or coarse and wiry, brittle, and easily broken or epilated. Histologic changes are variable, likely a reflection of the different mutations responsible for the hypotrichosis. Some affected animals have only follicular disease; while others have involvement of other skin appendages, in which case the condition is called ectodermal dysplasia.

Genetic hypotrichosis must be differentiated from various causes of non-genetic hypotrichosis. Iodine deficiency can cause goiter and hypotrichosis in piglets, lambs, and calves. Adenohypophyseal hypoplasia in Guernseys and Jerseys, and maternal ingestion of *Veratrum album* by Japanese cattle, have been associated with hairlessness in calves. In addition, alopecia of various degrees has been associated with intrauterine infection with *Bovine viral diarrhea virus* in calves and *Classical swine fever virus* in piglets.

Cattle

Various types of inherited hypotrichosis occur in cattle. Many breeds of cattle are affected and the mode of inheritance varies with the particular form of hypotrichosis. Histologic features are not well characterized for all forms of hypotrichosis in cattle.

A form of **lethal hypotrichosis** occurs in Holstein-Friesian and Japanese native cattle. Calves are born almost hairless and have only small amounts of hair on the muzzle, eyelids, ears, tail, and pasterns. The condition is inherited as a simple autosomal recessive trait, and homozygous calves die within hours after birth. Histologically the skin contains normal numbers of follicles but they are shallow, rudimentary in appearance and do not form hairs. Sebaceous glands and arrector pili muscles appear normal while sweat glands undergo cystic degeneration.

A condition called **semihairlessness** has been reported in polled and horned Hereford calves. Calves have a thin coat of short fine, curly hair at birth and progressively develop a patchy sparse coat of coarse wiry hair which is thicker and longer on legs than elsewhere. The skin is wrinkled and scaly. Animals may not grow well and may have a wild temperament. The condition is a simple autosomal recessive trait. The histologic changes described are dysplastic hair follicles that do not produce hairs. Similar histologic features have been described in **viable hypotrichosis** reported in various breeds of cattle, including Guernseys, Jerseys, Holsteins, Ayrshires, and Herefords. Calves are born with variable degrees of hairlessness. The condition appears to be inherited as a simple autosomal recessive trait in all breeds affected.

Hypotrichosis and anodontia (hypotrichosis anodontia defect, HAD) has been described in male mixed Maine-Anjou-Normandy cross calves and suspected to be a sex-linked recessive trait. Calves are born hairless and toothless and develop a fine, downy hair coat and partial dentition after several months. Affected calves also have a thick protruding tongue, defective horns, and hypoplastic testicles, and they usually do not survive beyond 6 months of age. Histologic changes include small, inactive hair follicles, deformed dermal papillae lacking a vascular network, and degenerative sweat glands. An HAD syndrome, with hypotrichosis, almost complete lack of teeth, and complete absence of eccrine nasolabial glands, has been observed in a family of German Holsteins; similar anomalies in humans are known as X-linked anhidrotic ectodermal dysplasia (ED1). This Holstein phenotype was inherited as a monogenic X-linked recessive trait, and was caused by a deletion in the bovine *ED1* gene.

Hypotrichosis and incisor anodontia (hypotrichosis incisor defect, HID) has been described in Holstein-Friesian cross calves, and inheritance is suspected to be an X-linked incompletely dominant gene. Affected calves have variable areas of thin coat of fine short silky hairs usually involving the face, neck, ears, back, and inner thighs. Eyelashes, vibrissae, and tail brush are usually normal. Calves may become normal with age. Histologically, there are numerous small hairs but large medullated hairs are absent and only telogen follicles are evident in severely affected HID calves.

Inherited epidermal dysplasia, also called **baldy calf syndrome**, is a lethal disease of Holstein- Friesian calves that is likely inherited as a single autosomal recessive trait. The disease causes loss of condition and skin, horn, and hoof lesions that can be confused with inherited zinc deficiency. Calves appear normal at birth; but at one to two months they begin to lose condition despite normal appetite, and develop generalized hair loss and patchy areas of scaly, wrinkled, thickened skin over the neck, shoulders, flanks, and on pressure points. Hooves are elongated, narrow, and pointed and frequently have horizontal rippling. Horns fail to develop and ear tips are curled backwards. Calves have fine slender limbs and drool. They become emaciated and usually die at 6–8 months of age. Histologic examination indicates variable atrophy of adnexa, remnants of hair follicles and sebaceous glands incorporated into the basal layer, and scattered atrophic remnants of apocrine sweat glands.

Congenital hypotrichosis of Hereford cattle is thought to be due to a simple autosomal dominant gene. Alopecia is variable and nonprogressive. Calves have thin, pliable skin, extremely curly facial hair, and may have sparse pellage of thin soft curly, easily broken and epilated hairs, or they may be completely hairless. Some calves also have impaired hoof development. The condition is characterized histologically by hypoplastic or degenerate hair follicles with vacuolation and necrosis of Huxley's and Henle's layers and abnormally large trichohyaline granules in Huxley's layer. Most follicles contain fragmented hair shafts. Arrector pili muscles are reduced in number and frequently not associated with hair shafts. Ultrastructural examination indicates that the giant trichohyaline granules lack normal micro- and macrofilament structures.

A condition consisting of **congenital anemia, dyskeratosis, and progressive alopecia** has also been described in polled Hereford calves in Canada and the USA. Affected calves are often small at birth and have a prominent forehead. They have a hyperkeratotic muzzle with a dirty-faced appearance, and their hair is wiry and kinked or tightly curled and easily epilated. Alopecia is evident initially on the bridge of the nose and ears and it becomes generalized but is most severe on the head, lateral neck, shoulders, and back. The skin of the face and neck is wrinkled and hairless skin is hyperkeratotic. Affected calves also have nonregenerative anemia and fail to grow despite a normal appetite. Histologic abnormalities in the skin consist of orthokeratotic hyperkeratosis and hypergranulosis extending into the infundibular portion of hair follicles and prominent dyskeratosis (apoptosis) of individual epidermal and follicular keratinocytes. Hair follicles are in normal number but many follicles are in telogen phase. There is degeneration of the internal root sheath and atrophy of sebaceous glands. The bone marrow is hyperplastic and characterized by ineffective erythropoiesis with maturation arrest in the late rubricyte stage.

The "**rat-tail syndrome**" is a form of hereditary congenital hypotrichosis that occurs in a small percentage of calves produced by crossing some Continental cattle breeds, e.g., Simmental, with black Angus or Holsteins. The calves have short, curly, malformed, sometimes sparse hair and a lack of normal tail switch development.

Dogs

Congenital hypotrichosis has been reported in *many breeds of dogs*. In most cases, a single puppy of a litter is affected but in some reports several puppies in a litter have been affected. The majority of cases of hypotrichosis in dogs have been in males, and may be referred to as *X-linked ectodermal dysplasia*. Hairlessness may be virtually complete or involve discrete areas that are typically distributed symmetrically. In such cases, areas most commonly affected include the top of the head, ears, ventrum, medial aspect of the legs, and the lumbosacral area. The skin is initially normal but frequently becomes hyperpigmented, hyperkeratotic, and greasy as affected dogs age. Some affected dogs also have sparse, short, wiry whiskers or they may be altogether absent. Eyelashes may also be absent. Some dogs also have missing or misshapen teeth or conjunctivitis. Most cases of hypotrichosis in a single puppy are assumed to be a spontaneous mutation; but X-linked recessive mode of inheritance has been confirmed in a family of Miniature Poodles and German Shepherd Dogs with hypotrichosis. *Histologic changes are variable*, no doubt reflecting differences in underlying abnormalities. In some cases, there are decreased numbers of hair follicles that contain poorly formed or no hair shafts but with normal sebaceous and sweat glands. In other cases, all follicles and associated appendages are absent. These dogs usually also have dental abnormalities and are considered to have a more general abnormality termed a *congenital ectodermal defect*. Footpad biopsies of such dogs also demonstrate a lack of eccrine sweat glands. The underlying molecular defect is unknown in all cases but an abnormality in the epidermal growth factor (EGF) signaling pathway was speculated in the German Shepherd Dogs with hypotrichosis since fibroblasts from these dogs had decreased expression of EGF receptor on their plasma membranes.

Cats

An autosomal recessive form of congenital hypotrichosis has been described in *Siamese and Birman kittens*. The Birman kittens were born virtually hairless and had short fragile wrinkled whiskers or lacked whiskers altogether. Both males and females were affected. Although initially healthy, all affected kittens in one report died by 13 weeks of age from various infections. Necropsy examination of some of the affected Birman kittens revealed *thymic aplasia and lymphoid depletion* of paracortical regions of lymph nodes, spleen, and Peyer's patches, suggesting an immunologic deficiency. Histologic examination of skin indicated reduced numbers of primary hair follicles, which were hypoplastic and devoid of hairs. Sebaceous glands were normal but sweat glands were hypoplastic and in decreased number, and arrector pili muscles were rare.

Hereditary hypotrichosis is recognized in **piglets** and there may be both dominant and recessive forms. The dominant form is thought to be lethal in homozygotes; it is characterized histologically by a decreased number of hair follicles and most appear atrophic. Congenital hypotrichosis is thought to be a simple autosomal recessive trait in polled Dorset **sheep**. Alopecia is most pronounced on the face and legs. Histologic abnormalities consist of hypoplastic hair follicles containing keratosebaceous material but no hairs. Congenital hypotrichosis has been described in a Percheron, but is rare in **horses**. Congenital hypotrichosis is rare in **goats**.

Bibliography

Bracho GA, et al. Further studies of congenital hypotrichosis in Hereford cattle. Zbl Vet Med A 1984;31:72–80.

Casal ML, et al. Congenital hypotrichosis with thymic aplasia in nine Birman kittens. J Am Anim Hosp Assoc 1994;30:600–602.

Casal ML, et al. X-linked ectodermal dysplasia in the dog. J Hered 1997;88:513–517.

Drogemuller C, et al. Congenital hypotrichosis with anodontia in cattle: a genetic, clinical and histological analysis. Vet Dermatol 2002;13:307–313.

Hanna PE, Ogilvie TH. Congenital hypotrichosis in an Ayrshire calf. Can Vet J 1989;30:249–250.

Hendy-Ibbs PM. Hairless cats in Great Britain. J Hered 1984;75:506–507.

Ihrke PJ, et al. Generalized congenital hypotrichosis in a female Rottweiler. Vet Dermatol 1993;4:65–69.

Jubb TF, et al. Inherited epidermal dysplasia in Holstein-Friesian calves. Aust Vet J 1990;67:16–18.

Mackie JT, McIntyre B. Congenital hypotrichosis in Poll Dorset sheep. Aust Vet J 1992;69:146–147.

Moura E, Cirio SM. Clinical and genetic aspects of X-linked ectodermal dysplasia in the dog – a review including three new spontaneous cases. Vet Dermatol 2004;15:269–277.

Schalles RR, Cundiff LV. Inheritance of the "rat-tail" syndrome and its effect on calf performance. J Anim Sci 1999;77:1144–1147.

Steffen DJ, et al. Ultrastructural findings in congenital anemia, dyskeratosis, and progressive alopecia in Polled Hereford calves. Vet Pathol 1992;29:203–209.

Valentine BA, et al. Congenital hypotrichosis in a Percheron draught horse. Vet Dermatol 2001;12:215–217.

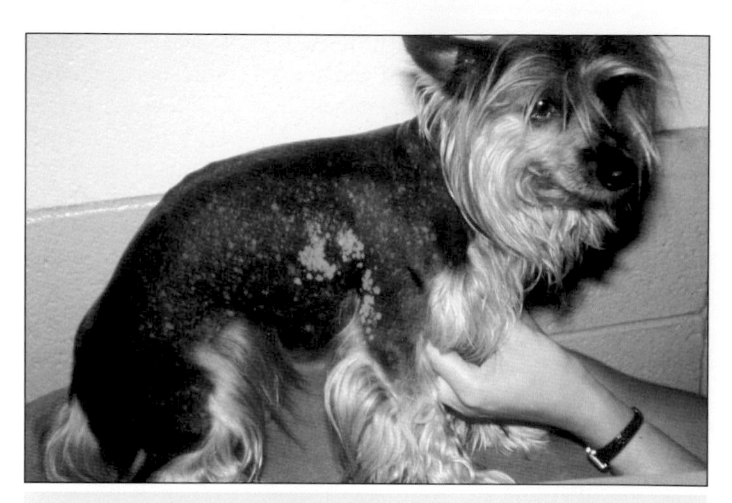

Figure 5.25 Color dilution alopecia in a Yorkshire Terrier. Note thin hair coat and patchy alopecia. (Courtesy of B Dunstan.)

Hypotrichosis associated with pigmentary alterations

Generalized or regional alopecia attributed to follicular dysplasias that include histologic evidence of pigment abnormalities have been frequently described in dogs and less frequently in other species. They have arbitrarily been divided into two categories.

The first of these two categories is **color-dilution alopecia** described in color-dilute animals of breeds such as the Doberman Pinscher, Irish Setter, Dachshund, Chow Chow, Poodle, Whippet, Italian Greyhound, Boston Terrier, Chihuahua, Saluki, Yorkshire Terriers, and mongrels in which the onset of alopecia can be tardive, generally ranging from four months to three years. Puppies are born with normal hair, but develop slowly progressive alopecia (Fig. 5.25). Pedigree analysis in color-dilute Dachshunds suggests this disorder may be inherited as an autosomal recessive trait. The histologic lesions include *misshapen, fragmented anagen hair follicles with pigment clumping in follicular epithelium, hair bulb matrix cells, hair shafts, infundibular keratin, and epidermis* (Fig. 5.26). *Melanin-containing macrophages are frequently present in the dermis around hair bulbs*. There can be some hair follicle atrophy in chronic cases, however this is a secondary change. A condition similar to color dilution-alopecia in dogs has been described in cattle as **cross-related congenital hypotrichosis.** This has been reported in crosses involving Simmental, Gelbvieh and Charolais cattle, most common in the Simmental-Angus and Simmental-Holstein crosses. The condition appears in calves that have color-dilute (gray or chocolate) coats. The affected hair is short, curly and sparsely haired leaving the white haired areas of the coat unaffected. The histologic lesions are virtually identical to canine color-dilution alopecia. **Coat-color-linked hair follicle dysplasia** has also been described in buckskin Holstein cows (color-dilute tan-and-white Holsteins). These animals have short and clinically abnormal hair in the tan areas of the coat.

The second traditional category is **black hair follicular dysplasia**, seen in bi- or tri-color black and white dogs, such as Bassett Hounds, Beagles, Bearded Collies, and mongrels, and in Holstein cattle, in which the alopecia affects only the black-haired areas of the coat, and in which onset is generally in the first few weeks or

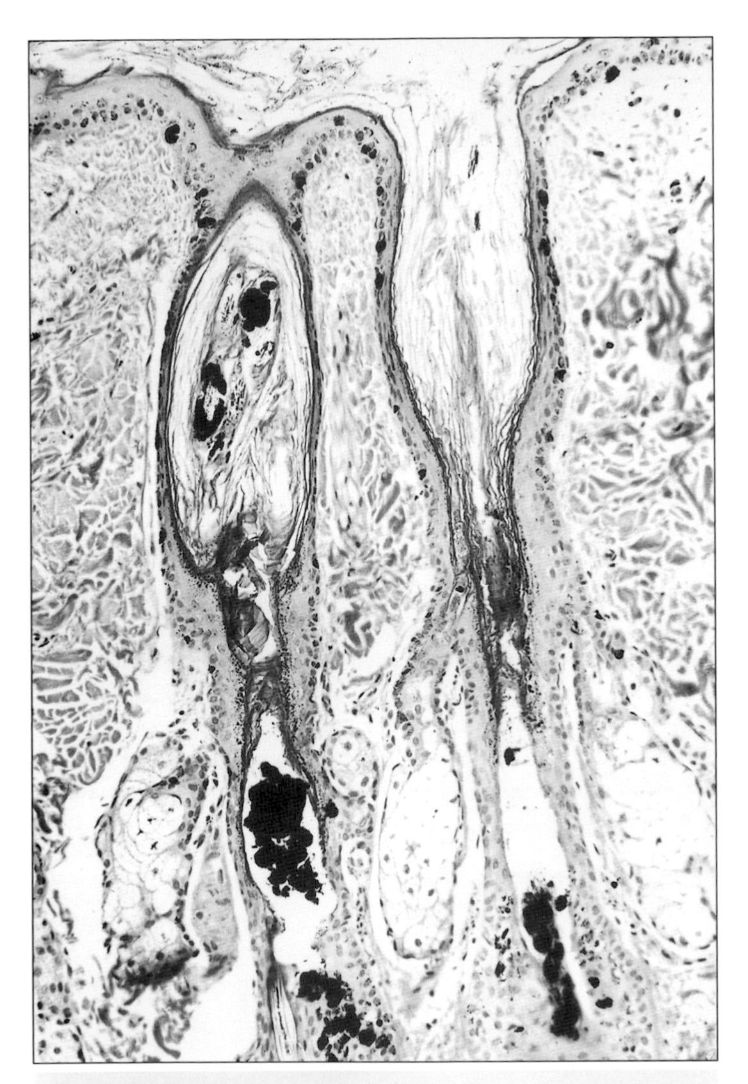

Figure 5.26 Color dilution alopecia in a dog. Note the clumped melanin in the fractured, misshapen hair shafts, follicular hyperkeratosis, and prominent melanocytes in the overlying epidermis.

months of life. Black hair follicular dysplasia is thought to be an autosomal inherited disorder in mongrel puppies, and is thought to have a genetic component in some purebred animals such as Bearded Collies. *The histologic lesions in black hair follicular dysplasias are virtually identical to those of color-dilution alopecia.* A difference in the appearance of the melanin clumps in whole mounts of hair shafts has been suggested.

There are *other follicular dysplasias associated with pigment abnormalities* that do not fall easily into these two categories, but have similar histologic changes. These include follicular dysplasia in the **Portuguese Water Dog** which occurs in the black or red color phase of this breed. These are not color-dilute dogs and the onset can be tardive, generally between 3 months and 5 years. **Black-and-red Doberman Pinschers** that are not phenotypically color dilute, are also reported to have a follicular dysplasia that is generally confined to the caudal dorsum and that has an adult onset. Follicular dysplasia has been described in **Weimaraners**, in which affected young adults had progressive alopecia of the trunk with recurrent folliculitis/furunculosis. In **cattle**, follicular dysplasia has been reported in black Angus and black Angus-Brahman cross; the histologic changes are similar to those in dogs. These cattle are all black animals that are not phenotypically color dilute, however there is adult onset of alopecia that is more commonly associated with color-dilution alopecia. In view of the dysplasias in Portuguese Water Dogs, black-and-red Doberman Pinschers, and black Angus and their crosses that occur in animals not phenotypically color dilute but that can have adult onset, *it is quite possible that separation of follicular dysplasias with pigmentary alteration into color-dilution alopecia and black-hair follicular dysplasia is artificial.* It is likely that these histologically similar follicular dysplasias are subtypes of a single process, however until the mechanism underlying follicular dysplasia is characterized the classification is somewhat arbitrary.

Bibliography

Ayers JR, et al. Pathological studies of cross-related congenital hypotrichosis in cattle. J Vet Med 1989;36:447–456.

Beco L, et al. Color dilution alopecia in seven Dachshunds. A clinical study and the hereditary, microscopical and ultrastructural aspect of the disease. Vet Dermatol 1996;7:91–97.

Carlotti DN. Canine hereditary black hair follicular dysplasia and colour mutant alopecia: clinical and histopathological aspects. In: von Tscharner C, Halliwell REW, eds. Advances in Veterinary Dermatology. Vol 1. London: Baillière Tindall, 1990:395–396.

Hargis AM, et al. Black hair follicular dysplasia in black and white Saluki dogs: Differentiation from color mutant alopecia in the Doberman Pinscher by microscopic examination of hairs. Vet Dermatol 1991;2:69–83.

Laffort-Dassot C, et al. Follicular dysplasia in five Weimaraners. Vet Dermatol 2002;13:253–260.

Mansell JL. Follicular dysplasia in two cows. Vet Dermatol 1999;10:143–147.

Miller WH. Color dilution alopecia in Doberman Pinschers with blue or fawn coat colors: A study on the incidence and histopathology of this disorder. Vet Dermatol 1990;1:113–122.

Miller WH. Follicular dysplasia in adult black and red Doberman Pinschers. Vet Dermatol 1990;1:181–187.

Miller WH. Alopecia associated with coat color dilution in two Yorkshire terriers, one saluki and one mix-breed dog. J Am Anim Hosp Assoc 1991;27:39–43.

Miller WH, Scott DW. Follicular dysplasia of the Portuguese water dog. Vet Dermatol 1995;6:67–74.

Ostrowski S, Evans A. Coat-color-linked hair follicle dysplasia in "buckskin" Holstein cows in central California. Agri Pract 1989;10:12–13.

Hypertrichosis

Congenital hypertrichosis, a condition characterized by an *excessive amount of hair*, is rare. In some instances, the abnormality involves a change in the character of the hair rather than an absolute increase in amount. Excessively long hair is inherited as an autosomal dominant trait in **Friesian cattle** in Europe. The condition results in discomfort during hot weather and decreased productivity. High environmental temperature during gestation has been associated with an unusual hairy appearance of newborn **lambs**. The lambs are small and most do not survive to weaning; the histologic appearance of this abnormality has not been described. *Border disease* is a congenital pestiviral infection of sheep in which lambs are born weak and small, have an abnormal haircoat, and exhibit tonic-clonic spasms (*hairy shaker disease*). Instead of the normal short, fine, closely crimped birthcoat, affected lambs have a long straight coarse coat. The coat abnormality is due to aberrant differentiation of hair follicles that develops only when infection occurs prior to 80 days of gestation. The histologic changes include enlargement of primary hair follicles with an increased degree of medullation and a decreased number and retarded development of secondary follicles.

Bibliography

Derbyshire MB, Barlow RM. Experiments in Border disease. IX. The pathogenesis of the skin lesion. J Comp Pathol 1976;86:557–570.

Shelton M. Relation of environmental temperature during gestation to birth weight and mortality of lambs. J Anim Sci 1964;23:360–364.

Canine dermatomyositis

Dermatomyositis is an idiopathic inflammatory condition of skin, muscle, and occasionally blood vessels of humans and dogs. A familial pattern of occurrence has been found in Collies, Shetland Sheepdogs (Shelties), and their crosses. Dermatomyositis in collies is an autosomal dominant trait with variable expressivity; and it appears to be widespread in Collies in the USA. The disease in Collies has been proposed as a model for a non-fatal form of childhood dermatomyositis, although familial cases are uncommon in humans. The condition in Shelties is assumed to be inherited in a similar manner but the mode of inheritance has not been confirmed by breeding studies. Dermatomyositis has been identified in Shelties in the United Kingdom. The disease has not been characterized as well in this breed; but it appears that myositis is a less prominent feature of the disease in Shelties. Occasional cases of dermatomyositis have been reported in other breeds of dogs; nothing is known regarding the nature of inheritance of the disease in these dogs.

The cause and pathogenesis of dermatomyositis are unknown. Variation in expression of dermatomyositis in dogs suggests that factors other than simple autosomal dominant inheritance are involved in the etiopathogenesis of the disease. Immunologic mechanisms are thought to be involved in this disease in humans and both cell-mediated and humoral immunity have been implicated in the pathogenesis. In Collies with dermatomyositis, serum levels of circulating immune complexes were found to be increased above normal before clinical disease was evident, the onset and severity of dermatitis and myositis correlated with the serum levels of circulating immune complexes and IgG, and circulating immune complex levels decreased to normal as disease resolved. These findings suggest that the immune complexes initiated inflammation rather than resulted from it. IgG was identified as the immunoglobulin component of the immune complexes but the identity of the antigen component was not determined. Dermatomyositis has been associated with viral, bacterial, and *Toxoplasma* infections but infectious agents are generally not isolated from tissues of affected people. Crystalline structures, suggestive of picornaviruses, have been seen in endothelial cells of muscle from severely affected collies. Cases in humans have also occurred following immunization, therapy with various drugs, during pregnancy, and in association with neoplasia.

Skin lesions usually develop in juvenile dogs 7 weeks to 6 months of age. *Earliest lesions consist of small pustules, vesicles, papules, and nodules which evolve into erythematous, crusty, ulcerated, alopecic areas with hypo- or hyperpigmentation* (Fig. 5.27). Lesions are most common on the pinnae, bridge of the nose, lips, periocular skin, over bony prominences of the distal extremities, sternum, and tip of the tail. Mucous membranes and mucocutaneous junctions may be transiently involved early in the course of disease. Footpad ulceration is rare. The disease exhibits a *waxing and waning course* over weeks to months with a variable outcome. In mildly to moderately affected dogs, lesions may resolve spontaneously in 6–12 months; while in severely affected dogs, lesions may regress but do not usually resolve completely and disease may be lifelong and extensive. Lesions heal with no residual scarring in mildly affected dogs; permanent alopecic, hypo- or hyperpigmented disfiguring scars develop, especially on the face, in severely affected dogs. Lesions may be exacerbated by estrus, parturition, or exposure to sunlight. Although cases of adult-onset dermatomyositis have been reported, it is likely that at least some of these dogs had mild transient lesions that were overlooked when they were pups and subsequently developed more obvious disease as adults.

Myositis usually develops several weeks after dermatitis and is proportional in severity to the dermatitis. It is usually first recognized as a bilaterally symmetrical decrease in temporal muscle mass. However, because of the dolichocephalic shape of the collie head, mild temporal or masseter muscle atrophy may be missed. *Myositis principally involves muscles of mastication and extremities below the elbow and stifle*, but it is more generalized in more severely affected dogs. Over time, active myositis is succeeded by muscle atrophy and fibrosis. Generalized symmetrical muscle atrophy, weakness, and exercise intolerance may develop in moderately and severely affected dogs.

Various additional abnormalities may accompany skin and muscle lesions in more severely affected dogs. Peripheral lymph nodes are

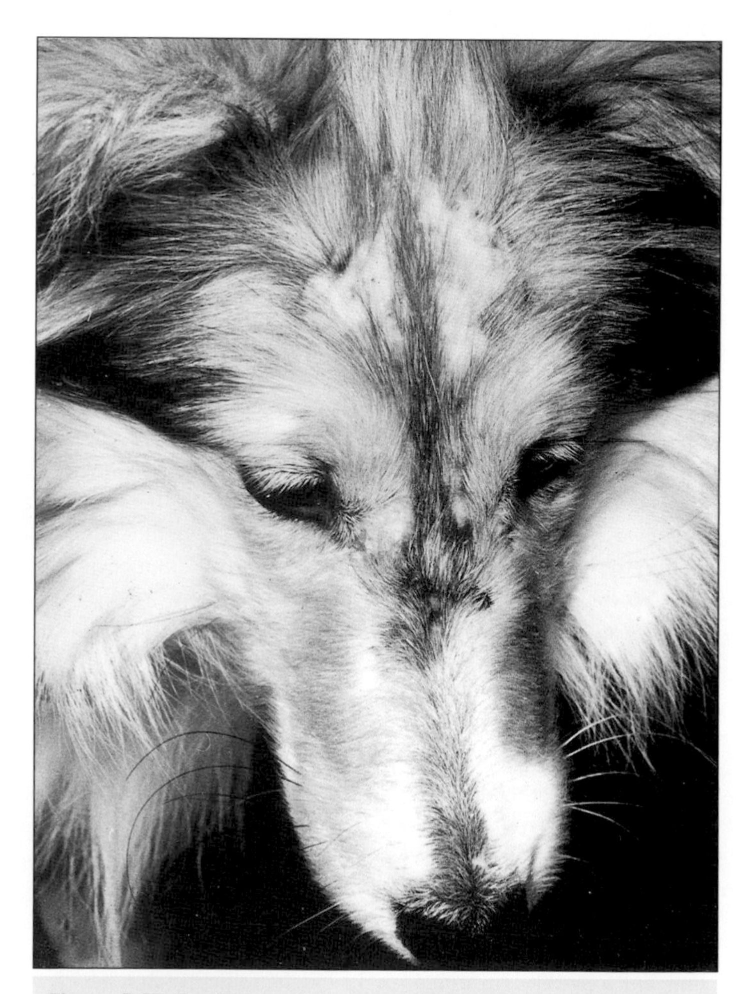

Figure 5.27 Familial canine dermatomyositis in a puppy. Alopecia and crusting of the face.

enlarged because of reactive hyperplasia. Conjunctivitis may develop in dogs with severe periocular skin lesions or because of facial palsy and inability to blink. More severely affected dogs are small and unthrifty in comparison to normal or mildly affected dogs. Fever and joint swelling are noted in some dogs. Secondary bacterial pyoderma, septicemia, or megaesophagus with secondary aspiration pneumonia may develop in more severely affected dogs. Demodicosis may also be present and complicate diagnosis. Severe secondary amyloidosis with resultant renal failure has been described in one affected Collie.

Affected dogs have variable and usually nonspecific *clinicopathologic abnormalities*. Moderately and severely affected dogs commonly have inflammatory leukogram changes which include neutrophilia, with or without a left shift, and monocytosis. Nonregenerative anemia typical of chronic inflammation may develop in severely affected dogs. Serum creatine kinase levels in collies with dermatomyositis were normal or only slightly increased; however, most serum muscle enzyme determinations were done in later stages of disease when active myositis may have been waning. Mild to moderate elevations in serum creatine kinase concentrations were present in several young Shelties with the disease. Occasionally, dogs have positive Coombs' tests, and rarely rheumatoid factor (RF) tests are positive.

The histologic changes in the skin are variable and may be quite subtle or nonspecific. Early lesions consist of scattered individual vacuolated or shrunken, brightly eosinophilic necrotic keratinocytes in the epidermis and infundibular portion of hair follicles. Hydropic degeneration of basal keratinocytes is often present and leads to *dermal-epidermal clefts* that develop into vesicles that contain proteinaceous fluid, erythrocytes, and inflammatory cells. Diagnostically useful artifactual dermal-epidermal separation may be induced at the margins of the section by the shearing action of the punch biopsy. Ulceration and crusting result from lesions with extensive dermal-epidermal separation. Intra-epidermal pustules are uncommon. Hyperkeratosis and acanthosis are variable. In the absence of ulceration, dermal inflammation tends to be mild and consists of mixed cells either surrounding superficial dermal vessels, hair follicles, and glands or distributed in an interface pattern or in some cases diffusely distributed. The infiltrate includes mononuclear cells primarily, fewer neutrophils, and occasional eosinophils and mast cells. *The most consistently present histologic abnormalities are follicular atrophy and perifollicular inflammation that may be accompanied by perifollicular fibrosis* (Fig. 5.28A, B). Variable

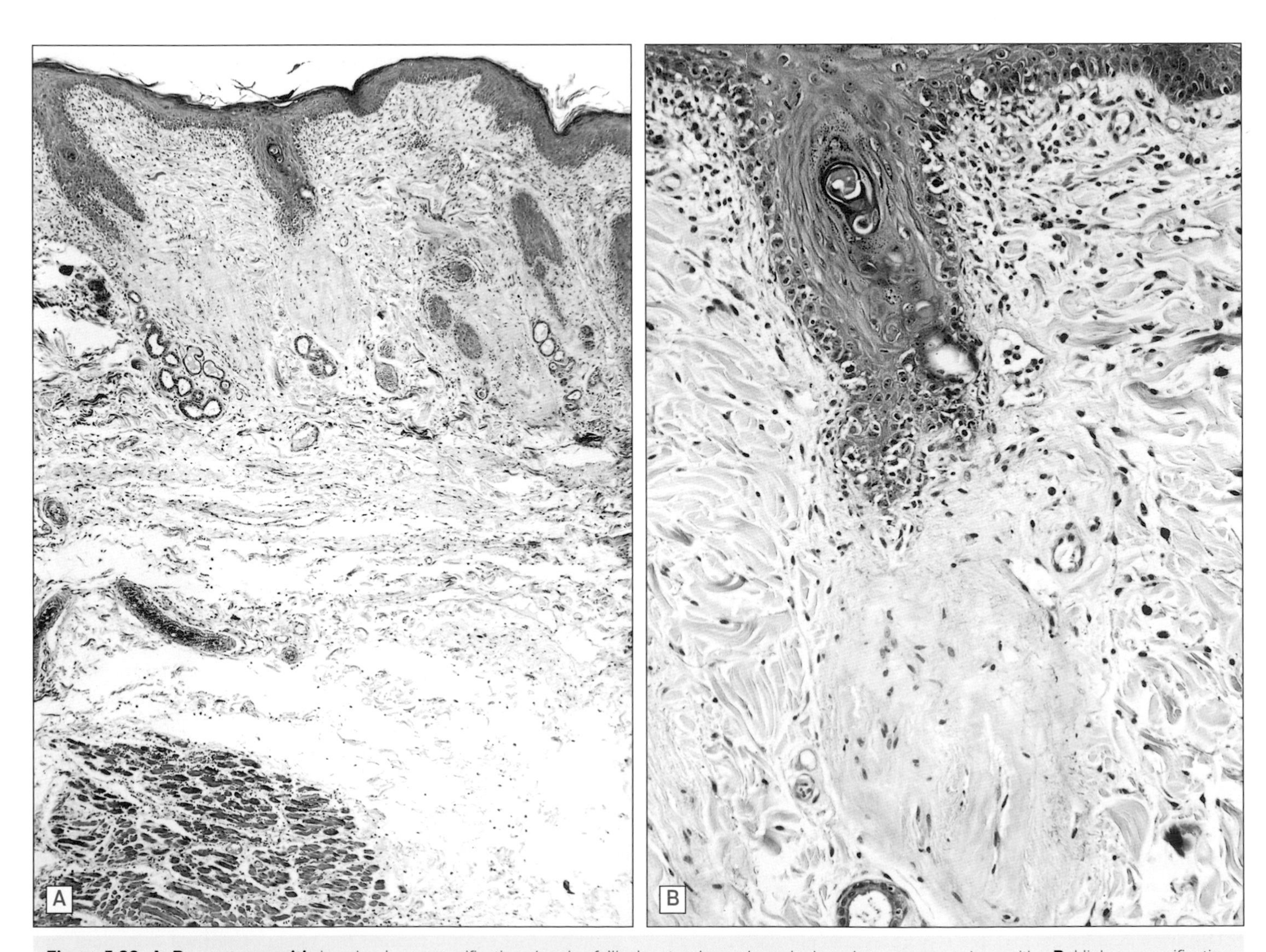

Figure 5.28 A. Dermatomyositis in a dog. Low magnification showing follicular atrophy, orphaned adnexal structures, and myositis. **B.** Higher magnification showing cell-poor hydropic, interface dermatitis and marked follicular atrophy and perifollicular fibrosis.

dermal fibrosis is usually evident in biopsies from dogs older than 6 months. *Muscle lesions* include multifocal interstitial and perivascular infiltrations with mixed cells; myofiber degeneration, regeneration, and atrophy; and fibrosis. *Vasculitis* is an infrequent and subtle finding in the skin, muscle, and occasionally in other tissues.

The principal differential diagnosis is lupus erythematosus and the two diseases may be indistinguishable on individual biopsies. However, lichenoid dermal inflammation is usually prominent in discoid and some cases of systemic lupus erythematosus but is not characteristic of dermatomyositis. Follicular atrophy, a common feature of dermatomyositis, is not usually present in lupus erythematosus. Lupus erythematosus is not typically a disease of young dogs. In some cases, immunologic tests may be required to differentiate the two diseases. Direct immunofluorescent antibody examination, antinuclear antibody test (ANA), and lupus erythematosus test (LE) are frequently positive in lupus erythematosus but negative in dermatomyositis.

Bibliography

Ferguson EA, et al. Dermatomyositis in five Shetland sheepdogs in the United Kingdom. Vet Rec 2000;146:214–217.

Hargis AM, et al. Severe secondary amyloidosis in a dog with dermatomyositis. J Comp Pathol 1989;100:427–433.

Hargis AM, Mundell AC. Familial canine dermatomyositis. Compend Contin Educ Pract Vet 1992;14:855–862, 864–865.

White SD, et al. Dermatomyositis in an adult Pembroke Welsh corgi. J Am Anim Hosp Assoc 1992;28:398–401.

Hereditary connective tissue disorders

The connective tissue components of the skin include collagen (primarily types I and III), elastic fibers, and ground substance composed of glycoproteins and proteoglycans. A defect in any one of these skin molecules can result in structural and functional abnormalities of the entire tissue. Inherited connective tissue disorders of skin may consist of abnormalities involving only one of these components or there may be concurrent alterations in several components. Hereditary collagen dysplasia, the most commonly recognized connective tissue disease, is a complex group of disorders of collagen that results in decreased tensile strength of the skin and may also affect other connective tissues. Alterations in elastic fibers and ground substance may accompany some forms of collagen dysplasia but there are also diseases in which an abnormality of the elastic fibers or ground substance appears to be primary. *Diagnosis of many of these conditions requires ultrastructural examination and biochemical analysis to confirm the presence of structural abnormalities and to identify the molecular defect.*

Hereditary collagen dysplasia

Collagen dysplasia (dermatosparaxis, Ehlers–Danlos syndrome, cutaneous asthenia, cutis hyperelastica) has been reported in humans, cattle, sheep, horses, dogs, cats, mink, and rabbits. Collagen is the major structural protein in skin and other connective tissues and abnormalities in its structure result in skin that is fragile, easily torn, and frequently hyperextensible and loose. In humans, Ehlers–Danlos syndrome (EDS) is divided into at least ten types based on clinical, biochemical, and molecular genetic studies. The natural history of clinical disease and mode of inheritance vary among the different types of EDS. Joint laxity, vascular abnormalities, bowel or uterine rupture, bone abnormalities, ocular abnormalities, and periodontal disease occur in addition to the fragile skin in the various forms of human EDS. Inheritance may be autosomal dominant, autosomal recessive, or X-linked recessive. In animals, clinical disease has been restricted almost exclusively to skin abnormalities and has been characterized in only a few breeding colonies or herd outbreaks. Most instances of collagen dysplasia occur in single animals and the molecular defect and mode of inheritance are usually not determined.

Individuals with inherited collagen dysplasia typically have a *history of frequent skin lacerations following routine handling*, such as shearing or manual restraint, normal activities such as scratching or playing with littermates, or minor trauma. The skin wounds commonly *develop into wide gaping wounds with minimal hemorrhage.* Healing usually proceeds normally but results in *characteristic thin, pale wrinkled scars* resembling cigarette or tissue paper. Extracutaneous signs, such as joint laxity and ocular abnormalities, have been reported in animals only rarely. The skin is usually soft and velvety, hyperextensible, and may hang in loose folds. In some affected animals, the skin laxity becomes progressively more pronounced with age. Severity of clinical signs is variable, even among animals with the same biochemical abnormality. This variability in clinical severity is most pronounced in sheep. One form of the disease described in sheep exhibits such severe manifestations that all lambs die or require euthanasia within the first day or two of life. A second milder form of collagen dysplasia is usually not recognized until later in life when sheep are handled for shearing. *In general, the disease tends to be most severe in sheep, less severe in cattle, followed by dogs and cats, and least severe in horses.*

Diagnosis of collagen dysplasia is based on typical clinical signs and demonstration of morphologic or biochemical abnormalities of the dermal collagen. In some cases, abnormalities are evident at the light microscopic level but frequently none are found or the differences are subtle and difficult to determine except by comparison to a breed- and age-matched control. The dermis may be normal, thinner than normal, or thicker than normal because of an increased amount of ground substance. Collagen fibers may be widely separated, finer and paler than normal, and haphazardly arranged. Rarely, increased numbers of elastic fibers are seen with elastic stains. Fibroblasts are in increased numbers in the dermis of some affected animals. Abnormal collagen fibers may stain unevenly with collagen stains such as Masson's trichrome. Instead of the uniform blue staining of normal collagen, the abnormal collagen may have a red core. This staining feature is not unique to collagen dysplasia, however, as uneven collagen staining also occurs with degenerative disorders of collagen.

In most cases, ultrastructural examination is required to confirm the collagen abnormality. A variety of alterations of collagen fibrils have been found. In longitudinal sections, collagen fibrils may be loosely wound and flat or helical. In cross-section, they may have several irregular thin projecting arms that give them a "hieroglyphic" appearance. This appearance is typical of dermatosparaxis of sheep and cattle and has also been described in a Himalayan cat and a dog. In other forms of the disease, the collagen fibrils are shaped normally but vary markedly in diameter from the normal range. They may all be uniformly larger or smaller or there is a mixed population of fibrils that extend beyond the range of normal minimum and maximum diameter sizes. The fibrils frequently are loose and disorganized rather than being arranged in uniform, compact bundles.

The ultrastructural abnormalities are not specific and biochemical analysis is necessary to determine the particular molecular defect. Collagen synthesis is a multi-step process that includes extensive post-translational processing involving multiple intracellular and extracellular enzymes. Abnormalities in several of these enzymes as well as structural mutations involving the collagen chains have been identified in the various forms of collagen dysplasia in humans and animals. For unknown reasons, the same biochemical defect may produce different clinical abnormalities in different individuals and in different species.

Cattle

Collagen dysplasia in cattle is usually referred to as *dermatosparaxis,* which means "torn skin." The condition is *caused by a mutation in the gene for procollagen I N-proteinase* (also called procollagen aminopeptidase), the enzyme that excises the amino-propeptide of type I and type II procollagens. Each of the three polypeptide chains making up a collagen molecule have short extensions at the amino and carboxy termini. These additional propeptides make the molecules soluble to aid in their transport out of the cell. Subsequent extracellular conversion of the procollagen to collagen requires two enzymes to cleave the amino and carboxy terminal extensions. Following cleavage of the procollagen peptides, the collagen molecules spontaneously assemble into collagen fibrils. *The defect in processing of type I procollagen to collagen results in abnormal precursor molecules with peptide extensions which inhibit formation of uniform fibers and fibers capable of producing normal cross-links.* They assemble instead into abnormal ribbon-shaped collagen fibrils lacking normal tensile strength. Dermatosparaxis in cattle is recessively inherited as is the biochemically analogous condition in humans, EDS type VII C, although clinical signs are not identical.

Most affected calves have thick, wet skin that tears easily and sometimes hangs in loose folds. Associated joint laxity and soft bones have been reported rarely. Light microscopic changes consist of a thicker than normal dermis composed of sparse bundles of fine pale collagen distributed in abundant Alcian-blue-positive ground substance (proteoglycans). Individual collagen fibers are smaller in diameter than in normal skin and their arrangement appears disorganized. There may be an increase in dermal elastin and number of fibroblasts. Ultrastructural examination reveals the collagen to be arranged in loose, twisted flat or helical ribbons rather than being organized in compact parallel arrays. In cross-section, these fibrils have irregular projecting arms which confer a "hieroglyphic" appearance.

Sheep

At least two forms of collagen dysplasia, called *dermatosparaxis*, have been described in sheep, i.e., a *severe form in lambs* noted shortly after birth, and a *milder form* not apparent until sheep are handled as adults. The severe form has been described in Norwegian Dala sheep, Border-Leicester-Southdown crossbred sheep in Australia, and white Dorper sheep in South Africa. The condition is inherited as a simple autosomal recessive trait. Only in the Dala breed has the biochemical defect been identified and it consists of a deficiency in procollagen aminopeptidase activity, as in bovine dermatosparaxis. In Border-Leicester-Southdown crossbred lambs the biochemical abnormality was not determined but it did not appear to be a procollagen peptidase deficiency since there was no increase in dermal procollagen detected. Affected lambs develop skin lacerations during birth or shortly thereafter. The skin is soft and edematous. Lambs frequently die within a few days as a consequence of wound infection and septicemia. Gross examination of the skin indicates that the dermis is moist and thicker than normal with a jelly-like consistency. In some instances, increased friability of internal organs and joint capsules was observed. The histologic and ultrastructural abnormalities are similar to those in cattle with dermatosparaxis.

The *less severe form of dermatosparaxis* has been found in Merino sheep in Australia when adult sheep were handled for shearing. No skin hyperelasticity or joint hypermobility are associated with the skin fragility. The skin lacerations predispose affected individuals to infections and fly-strike. This form is also caused by a deficiency of procollagen aminopeptidase activity. Light microscopic examination reveals a loose, more open appearance to the dermis and a significant increase in the number of dermal fibroblasts in comparison to normal skin. Most collagen fiber bundles are smaller and more lightly stained than those in normal skin. The collagen in some areas is arranged in prominent layers. Transmission electron microscopic examination shows a combination of distorted, hieroglyphic-type fibrils mixed with normal collagen fibrils.

Horses

Collagen dysplasia has been reported in Quarter Horses, a Thoroughbred gelding, and an Arabian-cross filly. An *autosomal recessive* mode of inheritance has been suggested but not proven in the Quarter Horses; *the biochemical defect has not been identified in any of the equine cases.* The condition is not usually recognized until the animal is 6–12 months old and develops frequent skin wounds and scarring on the legs, shoulders, and saddle area. The skin is hyperextensible; but in some cases, the abnormal skin involves sharply delineated areas interspersed among large areas of normal skin. This unusual feature has not been described in other species.

Histologic examination of affected skin may not indicate any dermal abnormalities or the dermis may be thinner than normal and collagen fibers may appear smaller than normal when compared to a control. In some cases, the collagen fibers have abnormal red cores when stained with Masson's trichrome. Ultrastructural changes in two Quarter Horses included disorganized and nonparallel collagen fibril arrangement, increased space between collagen fibrils, and irregular outlines and increased variation in the diameter of collagen fibrils. In contrast, ultrastructural changes in an Arabian-cross filly were suggestive of collagen degeneration. Collagen fibrils were uniform and densely packed in parallel arrays in unaffected areas of skin from this horse; but in sections from abnormal, fragile skin, collagen fibrils were fragmented, widely separated by granular material, disorganized, and associated with phagocytic fibroblasts. These ultrastructural abnormalities are unlike those described in other horses or species.

Dogs

Collagen dysplasia has been described in many purebred and mixed-breed dogs. Affected dogs typically have *soft, easily torn, hyperextensible skin* (Fig. 5.29). In some cases, the skin hangs in loose pendulous folds, a feature that frequently becomes more prominent with age. Thin, white scars are typically the sequelae to skin wounds. Ocular

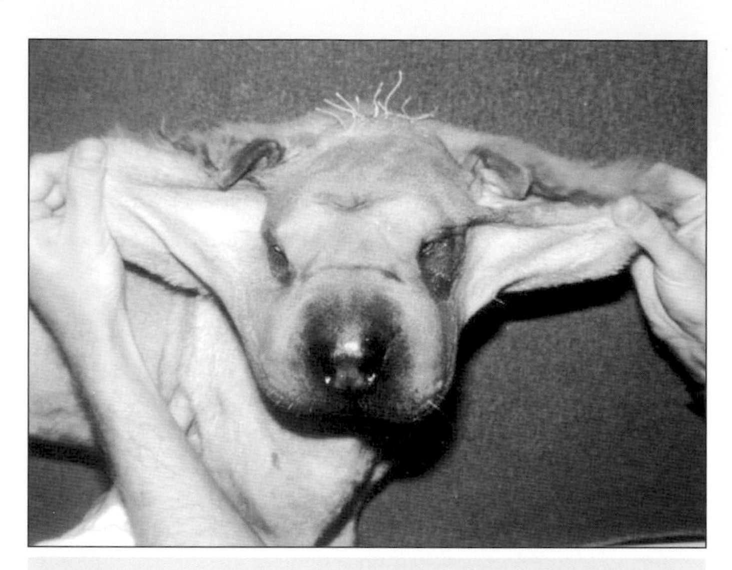

Figure 5.29 Collagen dysplasia in a dog. Note hyperextensible facial skin. (Courtesy of B Dunstan.)

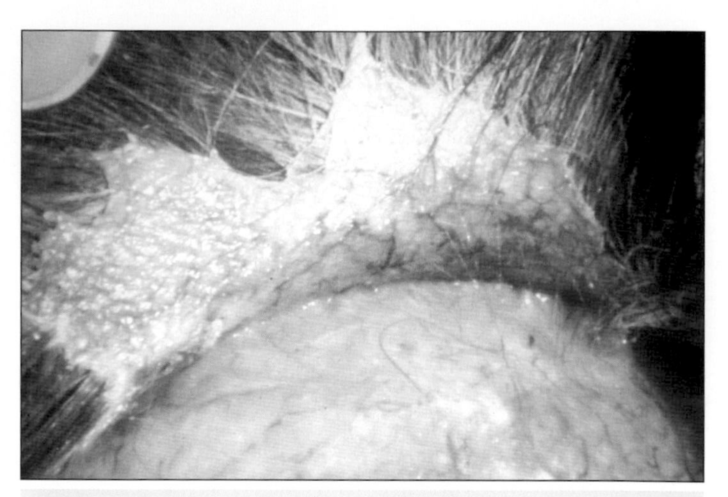

Figure 5.30 Feline cutaneous asthenia. Note tearing of fragile skin with minimal hemorrhage. (Courtesy of R Rosychuk.)

abnormalities and joint laxity, associated problems commonly seen in humans with EDS, have been reported infrequently in dogs, and bone abnormalities are rare. Several breeding studies have shown collagen dysplasia to be inherited in a simple autosomal dominant manner with complete penetrance. *The biochemical abnormality has not been identified in any cases of collagen dysplasia in dogs*; but the skin of Springer Spaniels with collagen dysplasia has been found to have more uncross-linked α-chains than collagen from normal dogs.

Histologic changes may be subtle and consist of dermal thinning evident only in comparison to a section from a normal control. In other cases, a decreased amount of dermal collagen, collagen disorganization, variation in collagen staining, increased number of elastic fibers, or increased amount of extracellular matrix may be seen. The abnormal collagen fibers may stain red with trichrome stain. Ultrastructural abnormalities of the collagen consist of variation in the fibril diameter, shape abnormalities, fibril disorganization, and loose fibril packing. A mixture of normal and abnormal collagen fibers may be present.

Cats

Collagen dysplasia in cats is usually referred to as *cutaneous asthenia*, although in early cases reported it was called dermatosparaxis. The condition has been reported in a number of breeds; *in the majority of the cases, neither the biochemical defect nor the mode of inheritance has been identified*. In a single Himalayan cat with collagen dysplasia, the abnormality was determined to be a defect of the amino-terminal procollagen peptidase, as in dermatosparaxis of cattle and sheep. This cat could not be bred, however, and the mode of inheritance was not determined. A breeding study based on an affected male domestic shorthair cat indicated that the condition is inherited as an autosomal dominant trait and heterozygous individuals synthesize both normal and abnormal collagen molecules.

Cats with cutaneous asthenia have thin, soft, velvety skin that tears easily but with minimal hemorrhage (Fig. 5.30). Lacerations heal to form typical white, tissue paper-like scars. In some cats, loose folds of skin develop as the cats age. No joint laxity has been described in cats with cutaneous asthenia. Histologic examination of the skin yields variable results. No dermal changes are evident in some cases; while in others, the dermis is thinner and collagen fibers are finer and separated by an increased amount of ground substance when compared to skin from an unaffected cat. Normal collagen fibers stain uniformly blue with Masson's trichrome stain while abnormal fibers exhibit segmental red staining areas that are birefringent under polarized light. Ultrastructural examination indicates that normal and abnormal collagen fibers may be present in varying proportions. Abnormal fibers are characterized by disorganized, tangled, nonparallel packing of fibrils. Abnormal "hieroglyphic" fibrils were a feature of the affected Himalayan cat.

Skin fragility in cats has also been reported as an acquired condition associated with a number of conditions including spontaneous and iatrogenic hyperglucocorticism, diabetes mellitus, hepatic lipidosis, cholangiocarcinoma, and administration of various drugs. The histologic and ultrastructural changes of collagen in cats with acquired skin fragility may be similar or indistinguishable from those seen in cats with cutaneous asthenia.

Abnormalities of elastic fibers

An *excess of elastic fibers* was reported in several piglets of a litter of Large White X Essex pigs with multiple circular to oval shallow depressed skin lesions. The skin was abnormally elastic in these areas and seemed to be bound less tightly to the underlying subcutis. The increase in thick elastic fibers was present only in those areas in which the skin was hyperextensible and the condition was termed **cutis hyperelastica**.

Congenital abnormalities of ground substance

Proteoglycan deficiency

An abnormality of dermal proteoglycan is a rarely documented cause of fragile skin in humans and animals. Proteoglycan is composed of a core protein and glycosaminoglycan (mucopolysaccharide) side chains, and it is the major component of the extracellular ground substance of the dermis. A 4-month-old female Holstein calf with skin fragility, soft and hyperextensible skin, and poor wound healing typical of dermatosparaxis was found to have normal collagen fibers. However, levels of dermatan sulfate proteoglycan in the dermal connective tissue were undetectable. The defect was identified as a mutation involving the gene that codes for the proteoglycan core protein. The mode of inheritance was not determined.

Cutaneous mucinosis of Chinese Shar-Pei dogs

Cutaneous mucinosis is a dermal connective tissue disorder in which *excessive mucin accumulates in the skin*. Mucin is a gel-like substance comprised primarily of acid glycosaminoglycan, hyaluronic acid, and water. *The inherited form of cutaneous mucinosis is considered normal in the Chinese Shar-Pei dog* and is responsible for the thick, wrinkled skin characteristic of the breed. The degree of mucin accumulation is variable. In some dogs, large lakes of mucin form nodules or cysts that may rupture and drip clear, stringy fluid.

Histologically, cutaneous mucinosis is characterized by a variable increase in dermal thickness because of excessive mucin separating collagen fibers. Mucin has great water-binding capacity and thus contains a substantial amount of water, the majority of which is removed during processing of the tissue. What remains in HE-stained tissue sections is fine basophilic granular to fibrillar material separating dermal collagen fibers. Special stains can be used to better visualize the mucin; these include Alcian blue at pH 2.5, which stains mucin blue-green, and mucicarmine, which stains it red. Mucin stains metachromatically with toluidine blue and methylene blue. PAS stain, which stains neutral mucopolysaccharides, does not stain dermal mucin.

Bibliography

Atroshi F, et al. A heritable disorder of collagen tissue in Finnish crossbred sheep. Zbl Vet Med A 1983;30:233–241.

Barnett KC, Cottrell BD. Ehlers-Danlos syndrome in a dog: ocular, cutaneous and articular abnormalities. J Small Anim Pract 1987;28:941–946.

Bavinton JH, et al. A morphologic study of a mild form of ovine dermatosparaxis. J Invest Dermatol 1985;84:391–395.

Benitah N, et al. Diaphragmatic and perineal hernias associated with cutaneous asthenia in a cat. J Am Vet Med Assoc 2004;224:706–709.

Byers PH. Ehlers-Danlos syndrome: Recent advances and current understanding of the clinical and genetic heterogeneity. J Invest Dermatol 1994;103:47s–52s.

Colige A, et al. Human Ehlers-Danlos syndrome type VII C and bovine dermatosparaxis are caused by mutations in the procollagen I N-proteinase gene. Am J Hum Genet 1999;65:308–317.

Dillberger JE, Altman NH. Focal mucinosis in dogs: Seven cases and review of cutaneous mucinoses of man and animals. Vet Pathol 1986;23:132–139.

Fernandez CJ, et al. Staining abnormalities of dermal collagen in cats with cutaneous asthenia or acquired skin fragility as demonstrated with Masson's trichrome stain. Vet Dermatol 1998;9:49–54.

Gunson DE, et al. Dermal collagen degradation and phagocytosis. Occurrence in a horse with hyperextensible fragile skin. Arch Dermatol 1984;120:599–604.

Hardy MH, et al. An inherited connective tissue disease in the horse. Lab Invest 1988;59:253–262.

Lopez A, et al. Cutaneous mucinosis and mastocytosis in a shar-pei. Can Vet J 1999;40:881–883.

Paciello O, et al. Ehlers-Danlos-like syndrome in 2 dogs: clinical, histologic, and ultrastructural findings. Vet Clin Pathol 2003;32:13–18.

Parish WE, Done JT. Seven apparently congenital non-infectious conditions of the skin of the pig, resembling congenital defects in man. J Comp Pathol 1962;72:286–298.

Rodriguez F, et al. Collagen dysplasia in a litter of Garafiano shepherd dogs. J Vet Med A 1996;43:509–512.

Sequeira JL, et al. Collagen dysplasia (cutaneous asthenia) in a cat. Vet Pathol 1999;36:603–606.

Tajima M, et al. Gene defect of dermatan sulfate proteoglycan of cattle affected with a variant form of Ehlers-Danlos syndrome. J Vet Intern Med 1999;13:202–205.

van Halderen A, Green JR. Dermatosparaxis in White Dorper sheep. J S Afr Vet Assoc 1988;59:45.

Wick G, et al. Immunohistologic analysis of fetal and dermatosparactic calf and sheep skin with antisera to procollagen and collagen type I. Lab Invest 1978;39:151–156.

Dermatosis vegetans

Dermatosis vegetans is an inherited disorder of young pigs characterized by vegetating skin lesions, hoof malformation, and giant cell pneumonia. The condition is a simple autosomal recessive trait of Landrace swine in Europe, Canada, and Australia. Clinically affected pigs grow slowly, become emaciated and unkempt, and usually die by 2 months of life. The economic impact of the disease may be considerable since virtually all homozygotes die before reaching slaughter age.

Skin lesions may be present at birth, but more commonly they develop during the first 3 weeks of life, and in rare cases may not arise until 2–3 months of age. *Lesions begin as erythematous papules*, 0.5–2.0 cm in diameter, usually on the ventral abdomen and medial aspect of the thighs. They may extend up the sides and back but do not affect the head. The papules enlarge peripherally over the course of 2 or 3 days and the center becomes depressed. At this stage, the lesions are clinically similar to pityriasis rosea. The papules enlarge to form *plaques* with a depressed center filled with characteristic gray to brown-black granular brittle material. Over a period of weeks, the lesions continue to expand and develop a dry, horny, papilloma-like appearance. They become dark brown to black and *each crusty plaque is surrounded by a hyperemic raised border that sharply demarcates the lesions from the surrounding normal skin* (Fig. 5.31A). As lesions spread peripherally, they coalesce to form extensive areas covered by black crusts. Affected piglets frequently die when lesions reach the typical papilloma-like appearance at 5–8 weeks of age. Skin lesions then begin to resolve if the pig survives.

When they occur, *foot and hoof lesions* are always present at birth (Fig. 5.31B). Usually more than 1 limb is affected and typically all digits, including accessory digits, of an affected foot are involved. The coronary region is markedly swollen and erythematous; and the skin is covered by yellow-brown greasy material. The wall of the hoof is thickened by ridges and furrows parallel to the coronary band. Affected hooves become progressively enlarged, wider, and flatter than normal if pigs survive to 5 or 6 months. Coronary band changes, however, diminish as the pig ages.

At birth, affected piglets seem otherwise normal but over a period of weeks they gradually decline in growth and vitality. Except for animals that die perinatally, virtually all affected pigs show signs of *respiratory dysfunction*, typically increased respiratory rate and labored respiration, several days prior to death. Affected pigs commonly develop anemia and secondary infections, especially bacterial pneumonia.

The *histologic lesions* in the skin vary according to the stage of the condition. Initially, there is superficial dermal edema, vascular congestion, and dermal infiltration with numerous granulocytes, many

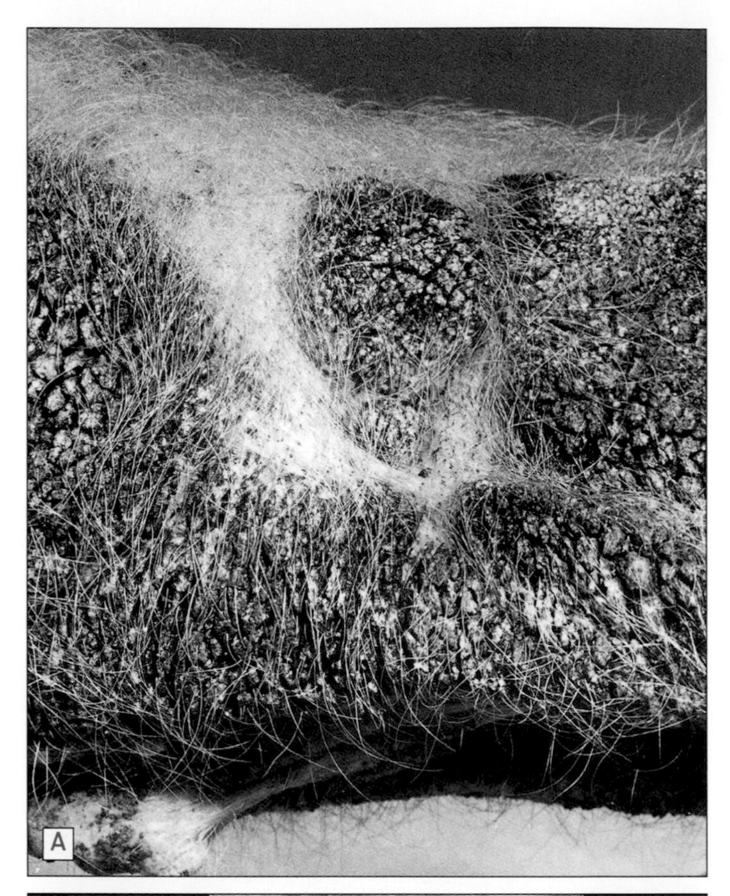

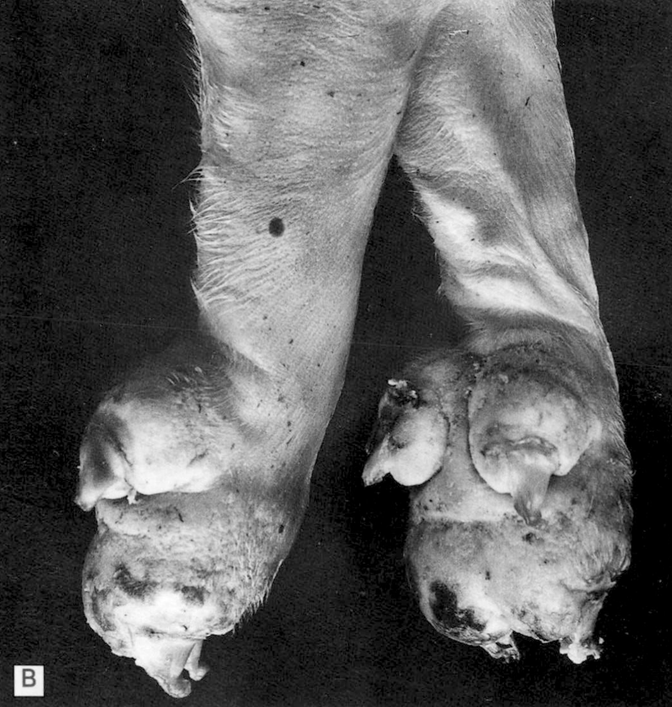

Figure 5.31. Dermatosis vegetans in a pig. **A.** Coalesced, crusted lesions on the abdominal wall. (Courtesy of DH Percy.) **B.** Congenital lesions of the feet. (Courtesy of JA Flatla.)

of which are eosinophils. Fully developed lesions are characterized by *marked orthokeratotic and parakeratotic hyperkeratosis, prominent irregular epidermal hyperplasia, intercellular edema, and intraepidermal pustules and microabscesses containing eosinophils and neutrophils.* The characteristic histologic lesion in the lung is *giant cells in alveoli.* The giant cells have been identified immunohistochemically as originating from monocytes/macrophages. In chronic cases, epithelialization and interstitial fibrosis are evident and multinucleated giant cells may be infrequent when the condition has lasted several months. Typical pulmonary changes may be obscured by secondary infections.

Bibliography

Evensen O. An immunohistochemical study on the cytogenetic origin of pulmonary multinucleate giant cells in porcine dermatosis vegetans. Vet Pathol 1993;30:162–170.

Percy DH, Hulland TJ. The histopathological changes in the skin of pigs with dermatosis vegetans. Can J Comp Med 1969;33:48–54.

Dermoid cyst

The dermoid cyst (dermoid sinus) is an uncommon developmental anomaly that has been reported in dogs, cats, horses, and cattle. It is caused by defective epidermal closure along embryonic fissures, which isolates an island of ectoderm in the dermis or subcutis. The majority of dermoid cysts occur on the dorsal midline because of incomplete separation of skin and neural tube during embryonic development; but they also occur in other locations. Although present at birth, dermoid cysts are usually asymptomatic and may not be noticed until they become distended or infected in an older animal. The cyst usually *contains hair, keratin, and sebum* and this material may produce progressive enlargement of the structure so that it becomes clinically apparent. Cysts frequently become infected, producing clinical signs such as purulent discharge, local swelling from cellulitis, or neurologic signs secondary to meningomyelitis.

In **dogs**, dermoid cysts have been reported most commonly in the *Rhodesian Ridgeback*, a breed in which the lesion appears to be inherited as a simple recessive trait. Dermoid cysts have also been reported in a Siberian Husky, Yorkshire Terrier, Shih Tzu, and Boxer. It is unknown whether the lesion is an inherited condition in other breeds of dogs. Dermoid cysts have been associated with multiple vertebral and spinal malformations and hindlimb neurologic deficits in several dogs. The rare condition of *nasal dermoid sinus cyst* results in a discharging sinus over the external nares in dogs; the cyst may extend into the cranial vault and cause cerebral abscessation or recurrent meningitis. In one survey, all cases in *horses* were in Thoroughbreds. Several cases reported in *cattle* all involved Angus. Dermoid cysts are rare in *cats*, and both cases reported were in domestic shorthairs.

Dermoid cysts may be single or multiple. They consist of a well-circumscribed circular or tubular structure in the skin or subcutis and frequently connect to the skin surface by a small pore. A tuft of hair may protrude through this pore and it may be surrounded by a whorl of hair. The cyst may end blindly in the subcutis, it may connect to the dorsal spinous process of vertebrae directly or by a fibrous cord, or rarely it extends down to be continuous with the dura mater of the spinal cord. *Microscopically*, the dermoid cyst is a circular or tubular structure lined by a wall of well differentiated, keratinizing squamous epithelium with associated small but well developed hair follicles, sebaceous glands, and occasional apocrine sweat glands. The hair shafts project into the cyst cavity which also contains keratin and variable amounts of sebum. Bacterial infection results in neutrophilic infiltration into the cyst. Pyogranulomatous dermatitis or cellulitis ensues when the cyst ruptures because of infection, trauma, or obstruction of the pore.

Bibliography

Anderson DM, White RA. Nasal dermoid sinus cysts in the dog. Vet Surg 2002;31:303–308.

Baird AN, et al. Dermoid cyst in a bull. J Am Vet Med Assoc 1993;202:298.

Cornegliani L, Ghibaudo G. A dermoid sinus in a Siberian Husky. Vet Dermatol 1999;10:47–49.

Fatone G, et al. Dermoid sinus and spinal malformations in a Yorkshire terrier: Diagnosis and follow-up. J Small Anim Pract 1995;36:178–180.

Hillyer LL, et al. Epidermal (infundibular) and dermoid cysts in the dorsal midline of a three-year-old thoroughbred-cross gelding. Vet Dermatol 2003;14: 205–209.

Rochat MC, et al. Dermoid cysts in cats: two cases and a review of the literature. J Vet Diagn Invest 1996;8:505–507.

Tshamala M, Moens Y. True dermoid cyst in a Rhodesian ridgeback. J Small Anim Pract 2000; 41:352–353.

DISORDERS OF EPIDERMAL DIFFERENTIATION

The epidermis is stratified squamous epithelium that forms a continuously regenerating protective sheet around the body. Basal keratinocytes proliferate, then differentiate, become keratinized and are then sloughed. *In normal canine skin, the migration from the basal to the cornified layer requires 22 days*, as measured by tritiated thymidine incorporation studies. This turnover rate is shortened in some skin diseases; for example, in seborrheic skin disease it is 7–8 days. The basement membrane separates the epidermis from the dermis and basal keratinocytes rest on this membrane anchored by hemidesmosomes and focal adhesions. Basal keratinocytes are the only cells in the epidermis that can undergo mitosis, and once mitosis occurs, the basal cell proceeds to undergo terminal differentiation. These post-mitotic cells enter the stratum spinosum, develop intercellular attachments, desmosomes and adherens junctions, and change the keratin composition of the cytoplasmic keratin filaments. In the basal layer, keratins K5 and K14 are expressed, whereas in the suprabasal cells, K1 and K10 are expressed. The intercellular and cell substrate adhesions are complex. *Hemidesmosomes* and *desmosomes* are stable junctions that associate with cytoplasmic keratin filaments, whereas *focal adhesions* and *adherens junctions* connect to actin filaments and are transitory adhesions. *Integrins* are receptors that mediate cell–substrate adhesion, whereas *cadherins* mediate cell–cell adhesion. As the cells are pushed outwards they move into the stratum granulosum. Here they start to make proteins that make up *keratohyaline granules*. As the cells move into the stratum corneum, the cytoplasmic organelles are lost and they become metabolically inactive. These flattened inactive keratinocytes are compacted into a keratin layer that eventually exfoliates. In this way, *the epidermis is continuously regenerating and degenerating by proliferation, differentiation, and keratinization*.

While the cells are moving outward, keratin polypeptides form and polymerize into *keratin intermediate filaments* that are epithelial specific and the major component of the cytoskeleton of epithelial cells. The keratin intermediate filaments aggregate into *tonofilaments* which connect with desmosomes, and therefore indirectly with adjacent cells. The molecular structure of keratin is very important, and genetic mutation can affect keratin filament formation. There are at least 30 keratins in epithelium; K9–20 are acidic (type I), and K1–8 are basic (type II). Two different keratins (one acidic and one basic) pair to form *heterodimers*, for example K1 and K10 in suprabasal cells, and K5 and K14 in basal cells. Hyperproliferative epidermis in skin diseases expresses keratins K6 and K16, not seen in normal skin.

When the cells reach the stratum granulosum they start to synthesize proteins, stored in keratohyaline granules, necessary to form the mechanically strong *macrokeratins* in the stratum corneum. One of these, profilaggrin, dephosphorylates to form *filaggrin*, the major molecule responsible for the glue-like aggregation of intermediate filaments. *Loricrin* is also stored in keratohyaline granules, and this polypeptide contributes to the cell envelope; an insoluble intracytoplasmic barrier. *Other proteins* involved in cell envelope formation include involucrin, cystatin A, CREP (cystine-rich envelope protein), trichohyaline, SPRR (small proline-rich proteins), sciellin, and filaggrin. All of these serve as substrates for *transglutaminases* that polymerize and crosslink these proteins in the formation of the cell envelope. Three different transglutaminases have been identified in the skin. The granular layer also contains small lipid-rich granules – *submembranous lamellar bodies* (Odland bodies, membrane-coating granules) – that contain lipids necessary to form a permeability barrier between cells when they are secreted into the intercellular space. Keratinocytes forming the stratum corneum are dead and can be sloughed when desmosomes are broken down. Hydrolytic enzymes such as cathepsin B-like, carboxypeptidase, and acid phosphatase are thought to be responsible for this desmosomal degradation and subsequent keratinocyte desquamation.

In various epidermal diseases, this orderly epidermal turnover is altered. For instance, increased proliferation and/or decreased dyshesion of epithelial cells will lead to thickening of the epidermis. Nutritional factors such as amino acids, vitamins A or B, zinc, fatty acids, and copper influence proper differentiation and maintenance of the epidermis. Altered expression of different molecules and keratin mutations are the focus of much research.

Bibliography

Borradori L, Sonnenberg A. Structure and function of hemidesmosomes: more than simple adhesion complexes. J Invest Dermatol 1999;112:411–418.

Boyer B, Thiery JP. Epithelial cell adhesion mechanisms. J Membrane Biol 1989;112:97–108.

Eckert RL, et al. The epidermal keratinocyte as a model for the study of gene regulation and cell differentiation. Physiol Rev 1997;77:397–424.

Fuchs E. Epidermal differentiation: The bare essentials. J Cell Biol 1990;111:2807–2814.

HogenEsch H, et al. Changes in keratin and filaggrin expression in the skin of chronic proliferative dermatitis (cpdm) mutant mice. Pathobiol 1999;67:45–50.

Hohl D. Cornified cell envelope. Dermatologica 1990;180:201–211.

Kwochka KW. The structure and function of epidermal lipids. Vet Dermatol 1993;4:151–159.

Mehrel T, et al. Identification of a major keratinocyte cell envelope protein, loricrin. Cell 1990;61:1103–1112.

Suter MM, et al. Keratinocyte biology and pathology. Vet Dermatol 1997;8:67–100.

Suter MM, et al. Differential expression of cell surface antigens on canine keratinocytes defined by monoclonal antibodies. J Histochem Cytochem 1990;38:541–549.

Smack DP, et al. Keratin and keratinization. J Am Acad Dermatol 1994;30:85–102.

Thacher SM. Purification of keratinocyte transglutaminase and its expression during squamous differentiation. J Invest Dermatol 1989;92:578–584.

Seborrhea

Seborrhea is a term used to describe a broad range of conditions ranging from dry flaky skin to severe oily or scaling, crusty lesions with alopecia. Seborrhea literally means "abnormal flow of sebum," however, the major clinical abnormality in seborrheic skin diseases is *altered keratinization*. Current terminology favors the use of the term *cornification defect* to cover all hyperkeratotic conditions from ichthyosis to flaky skin. The seborrheas can be divided into *primary idiopathic seborrhea* or *secondary seborrhea* where there is an underlying primary dermatosis.

The majority of seborrheic skin diseases are secondary. They can be secondary to disorders such as hormonal imbalances (especially hypothyroidism, hyperadrenocorticism and sex hormone imbalances), ectoparasitism (especially cheyletiellosis, pediculosis and demodicosis), endoparasitism, dermatophytosis, hypersensitivities (inhalant, dietary, drug), abnormal lipid metabolism (malabsorption, liver or pancreatic disease, diabetes mellitus), dietary deficiencies (fatty acids, protein, vitamin A, zinc), chronic catabolic states, environmental factors (especially hot, dry conditions), autoimmune disease (systemic lupus erythematosus, pemphigus foliaceus), and neoplasia (epitheliotropic lymphoma and internal malignancy).

Whatever the underlying cause, seborrheic skin is characterized by certain abnormalities. The first is *altered keratinization with or without altered glandular function*. This is reflected grossly by various degrees of scaling and crusting, with or without greasiness. Second, the surface lipids, whether the seborrheic skin is dry or greasy, have an *increased percentage of free fatty acids and cholesterol, and a decreased percentage of diester waxes*. Third, the altered keratinization and lipid film are accompanied by *a marked increase in the number of surface bacteria per unit of skin*. In addition, the bacterial flora usually switches from the normally nonpathogenic resident micrococci, corynebacteria and coagulase-negative and coagulase-positive staphylococci to a pure, heavy potentially pathogenic population of *coagulase-positive staphylococci*. Thus seborrheic skin, regardless of the underlying cause, is *often complicated by secondary bacterial disease*.

Clinically, seborrheic skin disease is often separated into three morphologic types:

- **Seborrhea sicca** is characterized by dry skin with focal or diffuse flaking and accumulations of white-to-gray nonadherent scales.
- **Seborrhea oleosa** is characterized by focal or diffuse scaling associated with excessive lipid production that produces yellowish to brownish material that adheres to the skin and hair.
- **Seborrheic dermatitis** is characterized by scaling and greasiness with gross evidence of local or diffuse inflammation. Pruritus and/or secondary bacterial infection is often present with all three forms. This clinical categorization has little significance in terms of differential diagnosis, and animals may be dry in one area of the body and greasy in another.

Seborrheic skin disease is reported most commonly in the dog, but also occurs in horses, cats, goats, sheep, cattle, rodents, and primates.

Primary idiopathic seborrhea

Seborrheic skin disease is common in **dogs**. Primary idiopathic seborrheic skin disease occurs in many breeds. The association with particular breeds and also an early age of onset suggest that primary canine seborrhea *may have an inherited basis*. Cocker Spaniels and Springer Spaniels tend to have a greasy, inflammatory form of seborrhea with numerous hyperkeratotic plaques, comedones and follicular casts. *Inflammatory ceruminous otitis externa* is also a constant finding. In Cocker Spaniels, cell proliferation kinetics indicate that seborrheic individuals have increased epithelial cell proliferation of the epidermis, hair follicle infundibulum and sebaceous gland. In addition, recombinant grafting studies have shown that the hyperproliferative epidermis from seborrheic Cocker Spaniels remains hyperproliferative, suggesting that the abnormality may be in the keratinocyte itself. *Other breeds with primary, greasy seborrhea* include the Basset Hound, West Highland White Terrier, German Shepherd, Dachshund, and Chinese Shar-Pei. Breeds having a *dry form of primary seborrhea* include the Irish Setter, Doberman Pinscher, Dachshund, and West Highland White Terrier. Primary seborrhea in German Shepherds, West Highland White Terriers, and Labrador Retrievers is often very inflammatory, lichenified, and pruritic. Seborrheic skin disease is typically more pronounced on the face, pinnae, trunk, pressure points, intertriginous areas, mucocutaneous areas, and paws. In Labrador Retrievers, the distribution is often strikingly ventral ("water-line disease").

Primary seborrhea is uncommon in cats and horses. Primary seborrhea oleosa, presumably of autosomal recessive inheritance, has been described in Persian **cats**. Severely affected kittens show lesions at 3–4 days of age, and develop progressively severe, generalized greasiness, matting of the haircoat, rancid odor, comedones, alopecia, and ceruminous otitis externa. Pruritus is absent. A milder form of the disease is recognized in 6–8-week-old kittens, with mild to moderate greasiness of the skin and haircoat. Primary seborrhea in the **horse** occurs in both dry and greasy forms, and tends to be restricted to the mane and tail. Pruritus is absent. Generalized primary seborrhea is rare in the horse.

Primary idiopathic seborrhea is usually characterized histologically by *superficial perivascular dermatitis*. *Epidermal hyperplasia* is usually mild to moderate and papillated in configuration. A pronounced keratinization defect is present, typified by *alternating vertical tiers of orthokeratotic and parakeratotic hyperkeratosis*. The parakeratosis is typically found overlying the shoulders of follicular ostia (*parakeratotic "caps"*). The underlying dermal papillae are often edematous, leading to spongiosis and *leukocytic exocytosis of the overlying epidermis ("papillary squirting"*) (Fig. 5.32). Spongiform or Munro's microabscesses may be seen in conjunction with the parakeratosis. The perivascular inflammatory cells include variable combinations of lymphocytes, neutrophils, plasma cells, macrophages, and mast cells. Since *secondary bacterial infection is common*, subordinate patterns of suppurative folliculitis, furunculosis, perifolliculitis and intraepidermal pustular dermatitis are frequently seen.

Secondary seborrhea

Secondary seborrheic skin disease is also characterized by a *pronounced keratinization defect, orthokeratotic and/or parakeratotic in nature*. The overlying histologic reaction pattern, however, reflects the underlying disease process (hypersensitivity, ectoparasitism, endocrinopathy, etc.). Occasionally, in predisposed breeds, it is necessary to attempt to eliminate coexisting dermatoses to determine if a primary seborrhea is also present.

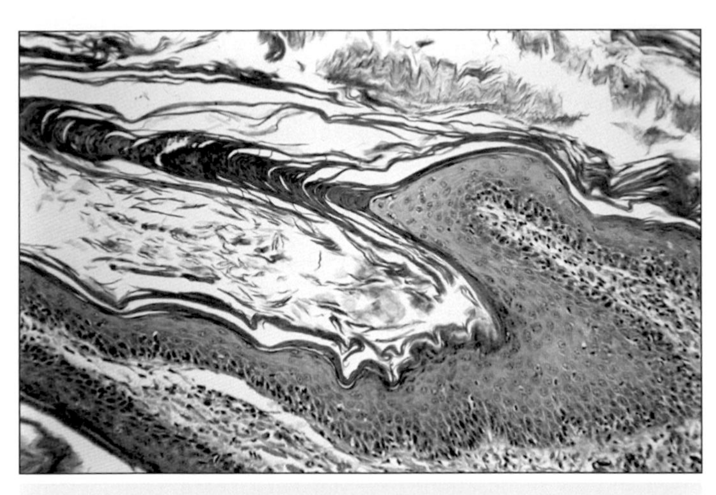

Figure 5.32 Primary idiopathic seborrhea in a dog. Papillated epidermal hyperplasia with vertical tiers of orthokeratotic and parakeratotic hyperkeratosis. (Courtesy of B Dunstan.)

Bibliography

Jefferies AR, et al. Seborrhoeic dermatitis in pigmy goats. Vet Dermatol 1991;2:109–117.

Kwochka KW, Rademakers AM. Cell proliferation kinetics of epidermis, hair follicles, and sebaceous glands of cocker spaniels with idiopathic seborrhea. Am J Vet Res 1989;50:1918–1922.

Paradis M, Scott DW. Hereditary primary seborrhea oleosa in Persian cats. Feline Pract 1990;18:17–20.

Pin D. Seborrhoeic dermatitis in a goat due to *Malassezia pachydermatis*. Vet Dermatol 2004;15:53–56.

Power HT, et al. Use of Etretinate for treatment of primary keratinization disorders (idiopathic seborrhea) in cocker spaniels, West Highland white terriers, and basset hounds. J Am Vet Med Assoc 1992;201:419–429.

Scott DW, Miller WH. Primary seborrhea in English Springer spaniels: a retrospective study of 14 cases. J Small Anim Pract 1996;37:173–178.

Acne

Acne is seen in *short-coated breeds of* **dogs**, especially English Bulldogs, Boxers, German Shorthaired Pointers, Great Danes, and Doberman Pinschers. It usually occurs between 3–12 months of age with no sex predilection and occasionally persists into adult life. The *etiology and pathogenesis are unknown*, but, since this is a disease seen in association with puberty in dogs, may be similar to that in humans, involving increased circulating levels of androgens and "acne-prone" skin. The lesions of canine acne are *asymptomatic papules and pustules, which arise from comedones*. Typically, the *chin and lips* are involved. Secondary bacterial folliculitis and furunculosis may occur. Histologically, there is marked orthokeratotic hyperkeratosis, dilation and plugging of hair follicles, and variable inflammation.

Acne is common in **cats** and has no sex or breed predilections. It usually occurs in mature cats, is asymptomatic, and persists for life. It is therefore unlike acne in the dog or humans as it is not associated with puberty. The cause is unknown. The lesions of feline acne are *asymptomatic comedones on the chin and lips*. Occasionally, secondary bacterial folliculitis and furunculosis develop. Histologically, marked orthokeratotic hyperkeratosis, dilation and plugging of hair follicles with variable inflammation are seen.

Schnauzer comedo syndrome

This condition occurs only in the Miniature Schnauzer breed. Either sex may be affected, and the condition usually develops early in life. The exclusive occurrence in Schnauzers and the early onset suggest that this syndrome *may be a developmental dysplasia of hair follicles with an inherited basis*. Clinically, the condition is characterized by multiple asymptomatic comedones over the *dorsal midline*. Occasionally, secondary bacterial folliculitis and furunculosis may develop. Histologically, there is marked orthokeratotic hyperkeratosis, dilation and plugging of hair follicles (comedones), and variable inflammation.

Tail gland hyperplasia

Many **dogs** have an oval area of skin on the dorsal surface of the tail above the fifth to seventh coccygeal vertebrae referred to as the *tail (supracaudal, preen) gland*. Microscopically, large, densely packed *perianal ("hepatoid") and sebaceous glands* characterize this area. In some dogs, especially adult to aged males, this area enlarges. The enlargement is usually firm to slightly spongy, and associated with partial alopecia, scaling and greasiness. At this stage, the lesion is asymptomatic. Occasionally, the lesions become cystic and/or secondarily infected, or neoplastic.

In most instances, canine tail gland hyperplasia is associated with *hormonal imbalances*, especially elevated levels of blood testosterone. Histologically, the lesions are characterized by *marked hyperplasia of the perianal gland component, with a variable inflammatory response*.

The entire dorsal surface of the tail in **cats** is replete with large, densely packed sebaceous glands, recently proposed to be embryonal hepatoid glands. In some cats, especially sexually active males of the Persian, Siamese and Rex breeds, this area becomes clinically seborrheic, whereupon a brown to black, greasy keratosebaceous material accumulates on the hairs of the skin surface. Unless secondarily infected, the condition is asymptomatic. The cause of feline tail gland hyperplasia is unknown, and the colloquialism "stud tail" is misleading, as the condition is also seen in intact females and neutered males and females. Histologically, the condition is characterized by *marked hyperplasia of sebaceous glands, with variable orthokeratotic hyperkeratosis and inflammation*.

Bibliography

Scott DW, Reimers TJ. Tail gland and perianal gland hyperplasia associated with testicular neoplasia and hypertestosteronemia in a dog. Canine Pract 1986;13:15–17.

Shabadash SA, Zelinkina TI. Cat caudal gland is hepatoid. Izv Akad Nauk Ser Biol. 1997;5:556–570.

Canine nasodigital hyperkeratosis

Canine nasodigital hyperkeratosis is characterized by *increased amounts of horny keratin on the nasal planum and/or footpads*. This disorder may be seen in association with canine distemper (hard pad disease), pemphigus foliaceus, pemphigus erythematosus, systemic or discoid lupus erythematosus, zinc-responsive dermatoses, superficial necrolytic dermatitis, and as an idiopathic senile change. Digital hyperkeratosis occurs as an hereditary disorder in Irish Terriers and dogues de Bordeaux; nasal hyperkeratosis may occur as a hereditary disorder in young Labrador Retrievers. Histologically, *marked orthokeratotic and/or parakeratotic hyperkeratosis and irregular to papillated epidermal hyperplasia* characterize nasodigital hyperkeratosis. Age, breed, and other histopathologic findings reflect those of the underlying diseases.

Keratoses

Keratoses are firm, elevated, circumscribed areas of excessive keratin production. In humans, keratoses are common and of numerous types. *Keratoses are uncommonly reported in domestic animals.* Actinic keratoses are discussed elsewhere.

Equine linear alopecia (linear keratosis) is a characteristic clinical entity. It occurs in many breeds, however Quarter Horses seem to be predisposed. The age of onset is usually at 1–5 years. The clinical lesions are characterized by one or more *vertically oriented linear areas of alopecia, with variable crusting and scaling*. They are usually unilateral and occur most commonly on the *neck, shoulder and lateral thorax*. The lesions are usually asymptomatic, and may be persistent or permanent. The *etiology of the condition is unknown* but may involve an immune-mediated attack on the wall of the hair follicle. The reason for the linearity is unknown. Histologically the lesion is characterized by *lymphocytic or lymphohistiocytic mural folliculitis*, sometimes with follicular destruction (Fig. 5.33A, B). Multinucleated giant cells are variably present. Sebaceous glands can be secondarily effaced, and there is a variable amount of orthokeratotic or parakeratotic hyperkeratosis, with or without superficial perivascular nonsuppurative inflammation. Linear keratoses with a similar gross and histologic appearance have also been described in *cattle*.

Equine cannon keratosis is a clinically recognizable disease of the horse. It represents a localized form of seborrheic dermatosis, can occur at any age, and has no breed predilection. The colloquial term, "stud crud," is inappropriate as it also occurs in mares. The lesions consist of *vertically oriented, moderately well demarcated areas of alopecia, scaling and crusting on the cranial surface of the rear cannon bones*. The lesions are usually bilateral and persist for life. Pruritus and pain are absent. Histopathologic findings include orthokeratotic and/or parakeratotic hyperkeratosis, irregular to papillated epidermal hyperplasia, and mild superficial perivascular dermatitis featuring lymphocytes and macrophages.

Seborrheic keratoses have been recognized in dogs. They are of unknown cause, and have nothing to do with seborrhea. They may be single or multiple and have no apparent age, breed, sex or site predilections. The lesions are elevated plaques or nodules with a hyperkeratotic, often greasy surface. They are frequently hyperpigmented. Pruritus and pain are usually absent. Histologically, seborrheic keratoses are characterized by orthokeratotic hyperkeratosis, epidermal hyperplasia (basaloid and squamoid), and papillomatosis. In humans, the sudden appearance or enlargement of multiple lesions can be associated with an internal malignancy. This association has not been made in domestic animals.

Lichenoid keratoses have been reported as single or occasionally multiple wart-like papules or hyperkeratotic plaques that may be hyperpigmented on the *inner surface of the pinna in dogs*. Age, breed and sex predilections have not been noted. Histologically, irregular to papillated epidermal hyperplasia, moderate to marked orthokeratotic and/or parakeratotic hyperkeratosis, and a lichenoid inflammatory infiltrate predominantly consisting of lymphocytes and plasma cells characterizes lichenoid keratosis.

Lichenoid dermatoses are rare skin disorders of dogs and cats. There is no apparent age, breed, or sex predilection. The dermatoses are characterized by the usually asymptomatic, *symmetric, grouped, flat-topped papules and plaques that are variably distributed, and that develop a scaly to markedly hyperkeratotic surface*. The lesions are *self-limiting* although resolution may take several years. Histologically these dermatoses are characterized by lichenoid interface dermatitis composed of plasma cells and lymphocytes, marked orthokeratotic hyperkeratosis and follicular keratosis, and moderate epidermal hyperplasia. Apoptotic keratinocytes can be seen primarily, although not exclusively, in the basal layer and there is often hydropic degeneration of basal keratinocytes. If focal areas of suppurative epidermitis and/or suppurative folliculitis are present, a lichenoid tissue reaction in response to staphylococcal infection should be suspected.

Cutaneous horns are recognized occasionally in all domestic species. Some are of unknown cause; *others originate from papillomas, basal cell tumors, squamous cell carcinomas or other keratoses*. In cattle, sheep, and goats, cutaneous horns may arise in lesions of dermatophilosis. In the cat, multiple cutaneous horns on the footpads have been reported in association with *Feline leukemia virus* (FeLV) infection; FeLV was

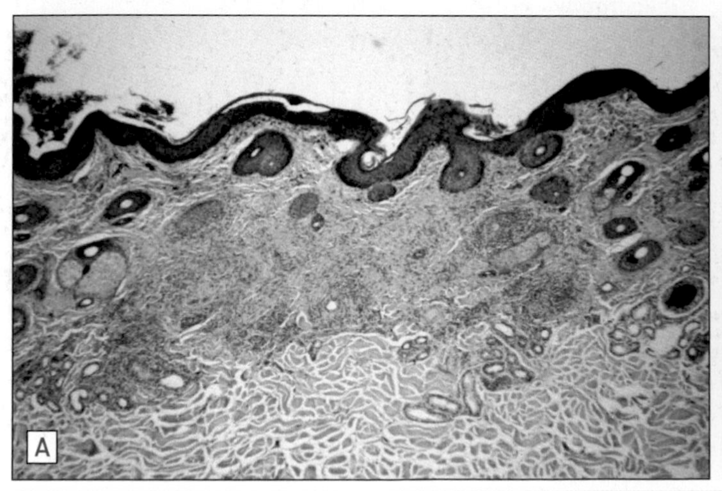

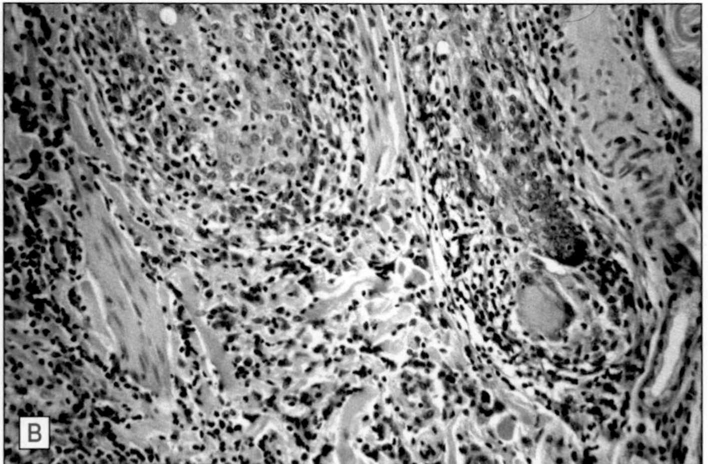

Figure 5.33 Equine linear alopecia. A. Low magnification showing a follicular orientation of the inflammatory infiltrate. **B.** Lymphohistiocytic to granulomatous mural folliculitis disrupts hair follicles.

cultured from the horns, and type C viral particles were seen in the lesions with the electron microscope.

Cutaneous horns may be single or multiple, and have no apparent age, breed, sex or site predilections. The lesions are *firm, well-circumscribed horn-like projections from the skin*. They may be small (1 mm diameter × 5 mm length) or quite large (3 cm diameter × 12 cm length). Histologically, cutaneous horns are characterized by *extensive, compact, laminated, orthokeratotic, and/or parakeratotic hyperkeratosis*. The base of the horn must be inspected for the possible underlying cause.

Linear epidermal nevi are characterized histologically by *linear hyperkeratosis with epidermal hyperplasia*. They have been reported in several species. These include linear epidermal nevi in Belgian horses, inflammatory linear verrucous epidermal nevus in dogs, and a hereditary disorder of cornification in Rottweiler dogs (see Congenital and hereditary diseases of skin). The term nevus implies a lesion present at birth and composed of mature elements, and therefore since these linear hyperkeratotic lesions have in common an early age of onset, *they may represent linear epidermal nevi that have tardive onset*. Equine cannon keratosis is grossly and histologically similar to linear epidermal nevi but differs from the linear epidermal nevi of Belgian horses as it can occur at any age and is restricted to the skin of the cannon area.

Bibliography

Anderson WI, et al. Idiopathic benign lichenoid keratosis on the pinna of the ear in four dogs. Cornell Vet 1989;79:179–184.

Deprez P, et al. A case of bovine linear keratosis. Vet Dermatol 1995;6:45–49.

Gill PA, Purvis-Smith G. Idiopathic lichenoid dermatosis in a Doberman bitch. Aust Vet Pract 1995;25:144–146.

Page N, et al. Hereditary nasal hyperkeratosis in Labrador Retrievers. Proc Am Acad Vet Dermatol – Am Coll Vet Dermatol 1999:41–42.

Paradis M, et al. Linear epidermal nevi in a family of Belgian horses. Equine Practice 1993;15:10–14.

Rees CA, Goldschmidt MH. Cutaneous horn and squamous cell carcinoma in situ (Bowen's disease) in a cat. J Am Anim Hosp Assoc 1998;34:485–486.

White SD, et al. Inflammatory linear verrucous epidermal nevus in four dogs. Vet Dermatol 1993;3:107–114.

von Tscharner C, et al. Disorders of cornification. Vet Dermatol 2000;11:187–189.

Yager JA, Wilcock BP. Perivascular dermatitis. In: Surgical Pathology of the Dog and Cat – Dermatopathology and Skin Tumors. London:Wolfe Publishing, 1994:69–70.

Yager JA, Wilcock BP. Interface dermatitis. In: Surgical Pathology of the Dog and Cat – Dermatopathology and Skin Tumors. London: Wolfe Publishing, 1994: 85–105.

Sebaceous adenitis

Sebaceous adenitis is an *uncommon skin disease of dogs* that has also been reported in the cat and rabbit. The condition has been reported in numerous breeds of dog and in mongrels, however there *is breed predilection* for Standard Poodles, Akitas, Samoyeds, and Vizslas, suggesting a genetic basis. In Standard Poodles and Akitas, an autosomal recessive trait is proposed. Onset of the disorder is usually in young adults to middle-aged animals and there is no sex predilection.

The early lesions consist of patches of scaling and alopecia that tend to appear on the *ears and dorsum*. In short-coated dogs, these progress to annular areas of alopecia and scaling on the trunk and head. Longer-coated animals initially develop a thin coat due to loss of the undercoat, and then develop symmetrical multifocal to generalized areas of patchy alopecia and brittle to broken hairs encircled by yellow to brown follicular casts. Secondary bacterial infection is common. Early histopathologic changes are characterized by *granulomatous or pyogranulomatous inflammation targeted on the sebaceous glands and eventually destroying the gland* (Fig. 5.34A). Inflammation can occasionally impinge secondarily on the follicular epithelium causing folliculitis. Orthokeratotic and/or parakeratotic hyperkeratosis together with follicular keratosis can be marked. In the chronic stages, both active inflammation and sebaceous glands may be absent, and there may be perifollicular fibrosis (Fig. 5.34B). After the disappearance of the glands, the hair follicles frequently assume a "stretched out" configuration and are keratin filled. Regeneration of sebaceous glands after variable amounts of time has been reported in occasional cases.

The pathogenesis of this disease has not been fully characterized. Several possibilities include: (1) destruction of the gland due to immune-mediated mechanisms leading to secondary hyperkeratosis; (2) a

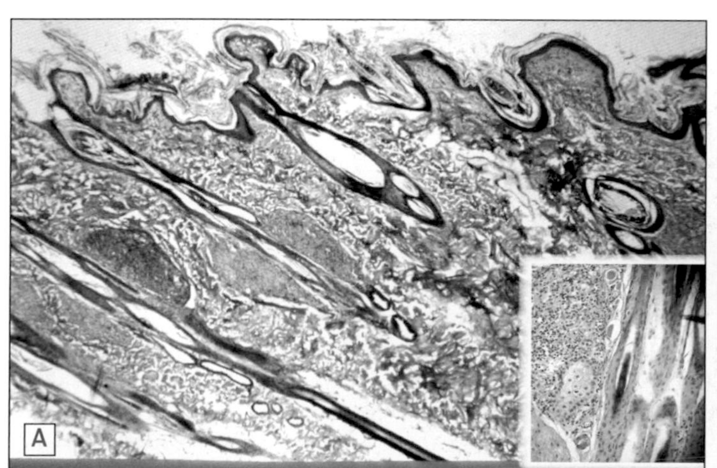

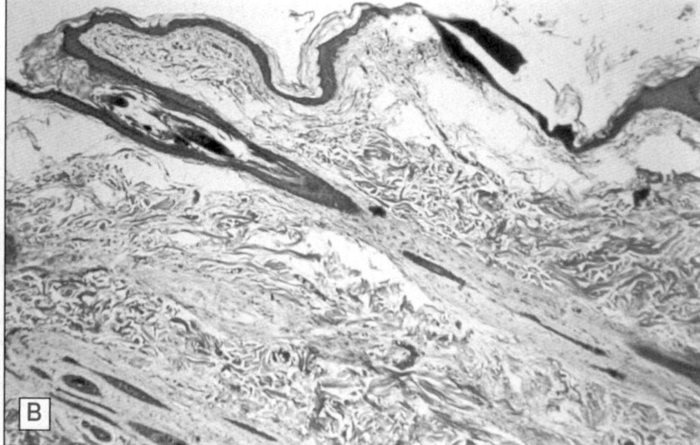

Figure 5.34 Sebaceous adenitis in a dog. **A.** Early lesions. Mononuclear leukocytes target sebaceous glands. Sebocytes are destroyed by the inflammation (see inset). **B.** Late lesions. Inflammation is minimal and areas of fibrosis have replaced sebaceous glands. There is epidermal and follicular hyperkeratosis. (Courtesy of B Dunstan.)

primary keratinization defect resulting in increased amounts of follicular keratin blocking the sebaceous duct and causing inflammation of the gland; or (3) a defect in the structure of the sebaceous duct or gland resulting in inflammation directed at free sebum. In the predisposed breeds such as Standard Poodles and Akita, a genetic basis seems probable together with other factors that would explain the variation in onset and progression of the disease.

Bibliography

Dunstan RW, Hargis AM. The diagnosis of sebaceous adenitis in standard poodle dogs. In: Kirk RW, ed. Current Vet Therapy XII. Philadelphia, PA: WB Saunders, 1995;619–622.

Reichler IM, et al. Sebaceous adenitis in the Akita: clinical observations, histopathology and heredity. Vet Dermatol 2001;12:243–253.

Scarff DH. Sebaceous adenitis in standard poodles. Vet Rec 2000;146:476.

Spaterna A, et al. Sebaceous adenitis in the dog: three cases. Vet Res Commun 2003;27(Suppl 1):441–443.

von Tscharner C, et al. Disorders of cornification. Vet Dermatol 2000;11:187–189.

Wendlberger U. Sebaceous adenitis in a cat. Kleintierpraxis 1999;44:293.

White SD, et al. Sebaceous adenitis in four domestic rabbits (*Oryctalagus cuniculus*). Vet Dermatol 2000;11:53–60.

Vitamin A-responsive dermatosis

Vitamin A-responsive seborrheic dermatoses occur most commonly in Cocker Spaniels, but can occur in other breeds (see Nutritional diseases of skin). There is, however, no clinicopathologic evidence to suggest that these animals have vitamin A deficiency.

Lichenoid-psoriasiform dermatosis of Springer Spaniels

This is an uncommon dermatosis that affects young English Springer Spaniels of either sex. Asymptomatic, generally symmetric, hyperkeratotic, erythematous papules usually begin on the pinnae and groin, coalesce to plaques, and progressively involve large areas of the body, especially the ventral abdomen and prepuce. Secondary bacterial infection is common.

Histopathologic findings include *lichenoid dermatitis* composed predominantly of plasma cells, with areas of *psoriasiform epidermal hyperplasia*, occasional apoptotic basal keratinocytes, intraepidermal microabscesses (containing eosinophils and neutrophils), and Munro's microabscesses. Chronic lesions frequently show papillated epidermal hyperplasia, papillomatosis, and moderate to marked orthokeratotic and/or parakeratotic hyperkeratosis. *The histologic findings are very similar to lichenoid keratosis and must be differentiated clinically by knowledge of distribution of lesions and knowledge of the breed.*

Bibliography

Gross TL, et al. Psoriasiform lichenoid dermatitis in the Springer spaniel. Vet Pathol 1986;23:76–78.

Mason KV, et al. Characterization of lichenoid-psoriasiform dermatosis of Springer spaniels. J Am Vet Med Assoc 1986;189:897–901.

Ear margin dermatosis

This is an idiopathic seborrheic disorder that is localized to the margins of the pinnae. It occurs primarily in the Dachshund, although it can be seen in other breeds with pendulous ears. It may represent a localized primary seborrhea. There is no sex predilection, and the disorder usually begins in young adults. Waxy keratosebaceous accumulations and alopecia follow initial scaling of the ear margins. The disease is symmetrical and asymptomatic. The dermatosis may be complicated by secondary bacterial infection and fissures, at which point ulceration, oozing, crusting, pain and pruritus may be seen. Histopathologic findings are characterized by *marked orthokeratotic and/or parakeratotic hyperkeratosis with follicular keratosis and variable mild superficial perivascular dermatitis.*

Exfoliative dermatoses (exfoliative erythroderma)

This refers to a cutaneous reaction pattern that can be associated with many diseases. Clinically it is characterized by scaling and erythema that can be localized or generalized. Most cases of exfoliative dermatosis have been reported *in association with thymoma, cutaneous lymphoma, visceral malignant neoplasms, drug reactions, or are idiopathic.* Histopathologic findings can reflect the underlying condition and can include parakeratosis, epidermal acanthosis, variable psoriasiform epidermal hyperplasia, variable lymphocytic exocytosis, and perivascular to lichenoid dermal inflammation.

Exfoliative dermatosis resembling human large plaque parapsoriasis has been reported in a dog and a cat. The human disease, to which these cases were compared, is frequently a precursor to mycosis fungoides.

Bibliography

Rottenberg S, et al. Thymoma-associated exfoliative dermatitis in cats. Vet Pathol 2004;41:429–433.

Schick RO, et al. Cutaneous lymphosarcoma and leukemia in a cat. J Am Vet Med Assoc 1993;203:1155–1158.

Scott DW. Exfoliative dermatoses in a dog and a cat resembling large plaque parapsoriasis in humans. Compan Anim Pract 1988;2:22–29.

Turek MM. Cutaneous paraneoplastic syndromes in dogs and cats: a review of the literature. Vet Dermatol 2003;14:279–296.

Hyperplastic dermatosis of West Highland White Terriers

This is a *severe chronic seborrheic disorder* in which there is a marked breed association with West Highland White Terriers. It was previously referred to as "epidermal dysplasia of West Highland White Terriers;" however epidermal hyperplasia is a more common finding. Epidermal disorganization or keratinocyte abnormalities characteristic of dysplasia are not present. Clinical signs begin at <1 year to middle age, with severely affected dogs tending to have an earlier age of onset.

Erythema and scaling with pruritus develop on the trunk, especially axillary and inguinal regions, and progress to involve the whole body. In chronic cases, the skin becomes lichenified, alopecic, hyperpigmented, and greasy. This combination of gross lesions has led to this condition being referred to as the "armadillo Westie syndrome." Histologic epidermal lesions are characterized by *acanthosis with mild to marked orthokeratosis or parakeratosis.* The base of the hyperplastic epithelium can have a scalloped appearance, and there is multifocal spongiosis with lymphocytic exocytosis. *There is commonly secondary pyoderma and/or infection with Malassezia*. The absence of *Malassezia* organisms in histologic sections does not necessarily exclude their presence as the organisms may be lost in tissue processing. Cytological evaluation for yeasts is a more reliable indicator of the presence and numbers of yeasts. *The lesions of hyperplastic dermatosis of West Highland White Terriers can be very similar histologically to lesions of chronic allergic dermatitis,* and the two conditions can frequently coexist in this breed. The condition may actually be a tissue reaction secondary to an allergic dermatitis or infectious condition and not a primary disease entity.

Bibliography

Gross TL, et al. Hyperplastic dermatosis of the West Highland White Terrier. In: Gross TL, et al., eds. Veterinary Dermatopathology: A Macroscopic and Microscopic Evaluation of Canine and Feline Skin Disease. St. Louis, MO: Mosby-Year Book, 1992:81–83.

Nett CS, et al. Epidermal dysplasia and *Malassezia* infection in two West Highland White Terrier siblings: an inherited skin disorder or reaction to severe *Malassezia* infection? Vet Dermatol 2001;12:285–290.

Equine coronary band dystrophy

Equine coronary band dystrophy is a condition of *unknown etiology and pathogenesis*. The condition affects adult horses of any breed, but draft breeds are considered predisposed. Equine coronary band dystrophy is characterized by *marked proliferation and hyperkeratosis of the epidermis of the coronary band and in some cases the chestnuts and ergots*. Usually all four limbs are affected; however the lesion may not encompass the entire coronary band. Clinically, the coronary band is thickened, crusty and scaly. Cracks and fissures may develop and lead to lameness. The chestnuts and ergots are similarly affected and may be ulcerated. Histologically, the epidermis of affected areas is characterized by marked papillary hyperplasia and marked ortho- to parakeratotic hyperkeratosis. In some areas, there is ballooning degeneration of keratinocytes. Dermal inflammation is minimal unless secondary infection is present. *The diagnosis is made by ruling out other differential diagnoses that include pemphigus foliaceus, the hepatocutaneous syndrome, bacterial or fungal infection, selenium toxicosis, and eosinophilic exfoliative dermatitis*. The condition is chronic and treatment palliative.

Bibliography

Menzies-Gow NJ, et al. Coronary band dystrophy in two horses. Vet Rec 2002;150:665–668.

Von Tscharner C, et al. Stannard's illustrated equine dermatology notes – an introduction. Vet Dermatol 2000;11:187–189.

Ichthyosis

The ichthyoses are rare disorders of cornification that result in severe generalized scaling. These disorders are congenital and heritable (see Congenital and hereditary diseases of skin).

DISORDERS OF PIGMENTATION

Melanin pigments are responsible for the coloration of the hair, skin, and eyes, and also play an important role in photoprotection. Melanin is synthesized by melanocytes, which are dendritic cells originating as melanoblasts in the neural crest. Melanoblasts develop in the neural crest, migrate to peripheral sites such as skin, hair follicles, and dermis, differentiate into melanocytes, and synthesize melanosomes and melanin. Genetic mutations affecting any of these steps can lead to hereditary hypopigmentation. Many such mutations have been characterized in the murine model but this area has been little studied in domestic animals. Many types of exogenous influences, such as inflammation, UV radiation, endocrinopathies, autoimmune diseases, and nutritional status can affect melanocytes in the skin resulting in acquired hypopigmentation or hyperpigmentation.

Melanin synthesis in melanocytes takes place in *melanosomes*, which are round or elliptic membrane-bound organelles thought to be derived from endoplasmic reticulum and containing enzymes from the Golgi and lysosomal system. Melanosomes are designated type I through type IV, according to their stage of maturation. Type I melanosomes contain no melanin and are electron-lucent, whereas type IV are mature melanosomes that are electron-dense and migrate to the tips of the dendritic processes to be transferred to adjacent epithelial cells. Melanogenesis in round melanosomes produces *eumelanins, the black pigments*, and in elliptic melanosomes produces *pheomelanins, red and yellow pigments*. Pigment types in horses, sheep, goats, and llamas have been analyzed. These melanin pigments arise from the common metabolic pathway of conversion of tyrosine to DOPA and then oxidation to DOPAquinone. *Tyrosinase*, a copper-containing enzyme, is the critical and rate-limiting enzyme in this pathway, catalyzing tyrosine to DOPA. Many gene products are sequentially important to the melanoblast and melanocyte during their development and maturation. Apart from tyrosinase, the molecular role of these gene products has not been completely characterized, but it appears that platelet-derived growth factor (PDGF), and receptors for fibroblast growth factor (FGF-2), endothelin-B, and the Steel factor (cKIT) are crucial.

Cutaneous pigmentary disorders can be divided into disorders of *hyperpigmentation* and *hypopigmentation*.

Bibliography

Alhaidari Z, et al. Melanocytogenesis and melanogenesis: genetic regulation and comparative clinical diseases. Vet Dermatol 1999;10:3–16.

Boissy RE, Norlund JJ. Molecular basis of congenital hypopigmentary disorders in humans: A review. Pigm Cell Res 1997;10:12–24.

Sponenberg DP, et al. Pigment types of various color genotypes of horses. Pigm Cell Res 1988;1:410–413.

Sponenberg DP, et al. Pigment types in sheep, goats, and llamas. Pigm Cell Res 1988;1:414–418.

Disorders of hyperpigmentation

Acquired hyperpigmentation

Acquired hyperpigmentation of the skin (**melanoderma**) is encountered frequently. It is usually post inflammatory, a result of minor or chronic irritation, and may be accompanied by mild hyperkeratosis. *Both melanosis and hyperkeratosis are common responses to mild injuries by agents as diverse as mites and irradiation*. Hypermelanosis results from an increased rate of melanosome production, an increase in melanosome size, or an increase in the degree of melanization of the melanosome. It is usually associated with an accelerated melanocyte turnover with an increased number of melanosomes, as occurs following trauma and ultraviolet light exposure. Inflammatory mediators likely play a role in stimulating melanocyte production. Activation of pre-existing immature melanocytes by sunlight, estrogen, and progesterone is thought to occur. Endothelin-1, which is produced and secreted by keratinocytes after UV-irradiation, has been shown to accelerate melanogenesis. Basic fibroblast growth factor (bFGF) has been shown to be a mitogen for human melanocytes. Proliferating human epidermal cells in culture produce bFGF, perhaps illustrating the mechanism behind the hyperplastic and hyperpigmented lesions that typify many chronic dermatoses.

Acquired hyperpigmentation may also involve hair (**melanotrichia**). This is usually seen as a result of inflammatory skin disorders, especially those caused by biting insects in the horse and also has been described in white Merino sheep exposed to ultraviolet light.

Bibliography

Forrest JW, Fleet MR. Pigmented spots in the wool-bearing skin of white Merino sheep induced by ultraviolet light. Aust J Biol Sci 1986;39:125–136.

Guaguère E, et al. Troubles de la pigmentation mélanique en dermatologie des carnivores. 3. Hypermélanoses. Point Vét 1987;18:699–709.

Halaban R, et al. Basic fibroblast growth factor from human keratinocytes is a natural mitogen for melanocytes. J Cell Biol 1988;107:1611–1619.

Mizoguchi M, et al. Clinical, pathological, and etiologic aspects of acquired dermal melanocytosis. Pigm Cell Res 1997;10:176–183.

Focal macular melanosis

Lentigo simplex has been reported in *cats and dogs*, and is most common in cats with orange, cream, or tricolored coats. The lesions are flat, or minimally raised, pigmented macules and usually occur on the mucocutaneous junctions of the mouth, eye, and nose, and the footpads. Lesions tend to start at less than one year of age and may increase in size and number with age. *The lesions are of no significance except that they can be confused clinically with melanoma or pigmented nevus.* Histologically, lentigines are characterized by minimal to mild epidermal hyperplasia with formation of elongated rete ridges. There are increased numbers of melanocytes, particularly in the stratum basale, and usually increased melanin in basal keratinocytes. Low numbers of melanophages may be present in the underlying dermis. Papillated epidermal hyperplasia and hyperkeratosis are not present. Generalized lesions have been reported in a silver cat.

Merino **sheep** may acquire pigmented macules, particularly after shearing. *Lesions are concentrated on the back suggesting a role for sunlight exposure.* Experimental exposure to ultraviolet light induced lesions as early as 10 days post-irradiation. Histologically, these lesions are characterized by increased numbers of epidermal melanocytes at the dermoepidermal junction and in the normally non-pigmented outer root sheath epithelium.

Bibliography

Ber Rahman S, Bhawan J. Lentigo. Int J Dermatol 1996;35:229–238.

Gross TL, et al. Lentigo. In: Gross TL, et al., eds. Veterinary Dermatopathology. St Louis, MO: Mosby-Year Book, 1992:456–458.

Nash S, Paulsen D. Generalized lentigines in a silver cat. J Am Vet Med Assoc 1990;196:1500–1501.

Scott DW. Lentigo simplex in orange cats. Compan Anim Pract 1987;1:23–25.

Canine acanthosis nigricans

Canine acanthosis nigricans *is an idiopathic dermatitis, characterized by progressive hyperpigmentation, alopecia, and lichenification.* The lesions are roughly bilaterally symmetrical and typically start in the axillae, spreading to involve proximal limbs, ventral abdomen, neck, and inguinal area. Seborrhea, *Malassezia* infection, and bacterial pyoderma are frequent complications. Histologic examination reveals a hyperplastic dermatitis with orthokeratotic and parakeratotic hyperkeratosis, acanthosis and rete ridge formation. All layers of the epidermis are heavily melanized. Spongiosis, neutrophilic exocytosis, and serous crusts may also be present. The dermal inflammatory reaction is mild, pleomorphic in cell type, and superficial perivascular in location.

The primary or idiopathic form of acanthosis nigricans occurs predominantly in Dachshunds. In view of the early age of onset (usually <1 year old) and the strong predilection for dachshunds, it is probable that canine idiopathic acanthosis nigricans is a *heritable disorder.* In man, some forms of acanthosis nigricans are associated with internal malignancies, hyperinsulinemia, insulin resistance, drug administration, endocrine dysfunction, and concurrent autoimmune disease; a similar correlation has not been demonstrated in dogs. The histologic lesions of primary acanthosis nigricans are virtually identical to the common histologic changes associated with chronic pruritic dermatitides (sometimes referred to as pseudo-acanthosis nigricans or secondary acanthosis nigricans) due to several causes, including chronic pyoderma, atopy and seborrheic dermatitis, and some endocrine disorders. *The diagnosis of primary acanthosis nigricans requires clinical correlation together with the histologic findings to support the diagnosis in a young Dachshund with compatible distribution of lesions.*

Bibliography

Anderson RK. Canine acanthosis nigricans. Compend Contin Educ Pract Vet 1979;1:466–471.

Yager J, Wilcock B. Color Atlas and Text of Surgical Pathology of the Dog and Cat. St. Louis, MO: Mosby, 1994:64.

Acromelanism

Acromelanism is seen in Siamese and Himalayan cats, rabbits, and mice. It is a condition in which coat color can be influenced by external temperature (high temperatures producing light hairs, low temperatures producing dark hairs) and factors affecting heat production and loss (alopecia, inflammation). *The coat color changes are usually temporary*, and the hair returns to the normal color with the next hair cycle. *These phenomena are due to a missense nucleotide substitution in tyrosinase making the enzyme thermally unstable.*

Bibliography

Giebel LB, et al. A tyrosinase gene missense mutation in temperature-sensitive type I oculocutaneous albinism. A human homologue to the Siamese cat and Himalayan mouse. J Clin Invest 1991;87:1119–1122.

Iljin NA, Iljin VN. Temperature effects on the color of the Siamese cat. J Hered 1930;21:309–318.

Disorders of hypopigmentation

Leukoderma and leukotrichia

Reduction in pigmentation of the skin is **leukoderma**, and of the hair is **leukotrichia**. Leukoderma and leukotrichia may occur independently. They can result from a decrease in melanin (**hypomelanosis**), a complete absence of melanin (**amelanosis**), or from a loss of existing melanin (**depigmentation**). These events result from either an absence of the pigment-synthesizing melanocytes or from a failure of melanocytes to produce normal amounts of melanin or to transfer it to adjacent keratinocytes.

Hereditary hypopigmentation

Hereditary hypopigmentation can be divided into *melanocytopenic hypomelanosis* characterized by the absence of melanocytes in affected areas, and *melanopenic hypomelanosis* in which melanocytes are present but defective. The condition can be localized, focally extensive, or generalized. Melanocytopenic hypomelanosis can be extensive, as is seen in animals with Waardenburg syndromes and in piebaldism. In these cases, there is failure of melanoblasts to migrate from the neural crest into the skin, or failure to survive in the skin. Melanocytopenic hypomelanosis can also be localized, as in vitiligo, in which there is genetically programmed destruction of melanocytes. Melanopenic hypomelanosis is seen in the various forms of albinism.

Melanocytopenic hypomelanosis

Syndromes analogous to the human **Waardenburg syndrome** have been reported in cats, dogs, horses, and rabbits. *Affected animals typically have white coats and blue or heterochromatic irides, and are deaf.* In *cats*, this has been shown to be due to an autosomal dominant mutation with complete penetrance for loss of pigmentation and incomplete penetrance for deafness. In *dogs*, this syndrome has been described in breeds such as the Dalmatian, Bull Terrier, Sealyham Terrier, Collie, and Great Dane. A syndrome analogous to human Waardenburg type-4 (Hirschsprung disease) has been reported in mice with lethal spotting mutation, and in American Paint horses in which white foals from overo mares are born with aganglionic colons. These foals develop colic and die shortly after birth.

Piebaldism is also a form of genetic melanocytopenic hypomelanosis resulting in *multifocal white patches* in which there is absence of melanocytes due to a congenital failure of melanoblasts to migrate from the neural crest to the skin, or by their inability to survive and proliferate in the skin. Piebaldism has been *seen in many species* including horses, dogs such as the Dalmatian, cats, cattle, and rodents. The defect has been shown to be a mutation in the gene encoding c-kit tyrosine kinase receptor, or a mutation in the gene for stem cell factor, which is the receptor ligand. The c-kit tyrosine kinase receptor is associated with proliferation and survival of melanoblasts.

Literally meaning, "blemish," **vitiligo** is a melanocytopenic hypomelanosis of humans and animals, which is characterized by *gradually expanding pale macules that are often symmetrical or segmental in distribution* (Fig. 5.35). Vitiligo has been described in the dog, cat, horse, cattle, and the Smyth chicken (DAM chicken) which has been used as an animal model of the human disease. The immediate cause of vitiligo is the destruction of melanocytes. It is considered to be a *genetic amelanosis inherited as an autosomal recessive trait in animals*. It is thought to be a polygenic disease necessitating simultaneous mutations in several genes resulting in melanocyte destruction or increased risk of immune-mediated destruction of melanocytes. Theories regarding the pathogenesis of this disease include autoimmune destruction of melanocytes, a neurogenic theory involving release of a neurochemical from peripheral nerves that inhibits melanogenesis, a self-destruction theory that involves failure of protection of melanocytes against the toxic effects of melanin precursors, or a combination of factors. Circulating antimelanocytic antibodies have been detected in some studies, lending support to an immune-mediated pathogenesis.

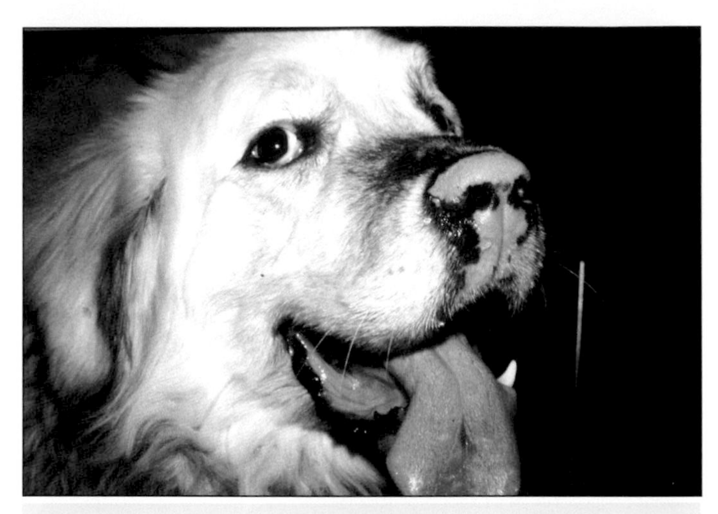

Figure 5.35 Vitiligo in a dog. Coalescing pale macules on the skin of the nasal planum and lips. (Courtesy of B Dunstan.)

Vitiligo in the **dog** has been described in Belgian Tervuren, Doberman Pinscher, Newfoundland, Rottweiler, German Shepherd, Dachshund, German Shorthaired Pointer, and Old English Sheepdogs. Vitiligo in a Dachshund developed concurrently with juvenile-onset diabetes mellitus. The condition best characterized is seen in Belgian Tervurens. The depigmentation in this breed occurs chiefly on the pigmented skin and mucous membranes of the face and mouth in young adult dogs. Histologic examination of affected skin shows an epithelium devoid of both pigment granules and DOPA-positive cells. Electron microscopy confirms the lack of melanocytes in the lesions; their place is taken by Langerhans or indeterminate dendritic cells. Antimelanocytic antibodies have been demonstrated in affected dogs but not in normal animals.

Vitiligo has also been described in **horses**. In one form, the "**Arabian fading syndrome**," affected animals develop round, depigmented macules on the lips, muzzle, around the eyes, and occasionally the anus, vulva, prepuce, and hooves. The disease can start at any age, but is more common in horses under 2 years of age. Circulating antimelanocytic antibodies have been detected in some cases.

In **cattle**, vitiligo-like lesions have been described in Holstein-Friesians, in black Japanese cattle, and in water buffalo.

Siamese cats may develop vitiligo. Antibodies to an 85-kDa surface antigen of melanocytes were demonstrated in four cats with vitiligo. No antibodies were detected in three normal Siamese cats tested.

Bibliography

Alhaidari Z, et al. Melanocytogenesis and melanogenesis: genetic regulation and comparative clinical diseases. Vet Dermatol 1999;10:3–16.

Boissy RE, Norlund JJ. Molecular basis of congenital hypopigmentary disorders in humans: A review. Pigm Cell Res 1997;10:12–24.

Cerundolo R, et al. Vitiligo in two water buffaloes: histological, histochemical, and ultrastructural investigations. Pigm Cell Res 1993;6:23–28.

Kemp EH, et al. Immunological pathomechanisms in vitiligo. Expert Rev Mol Med 2001;2001:1–22.

Lopez R, et al. A clinical, pathological and immunopathological study of vitiligo in a Siamese cat. Vet Dermatol 1994;5:27–32.

Mahaffey MB, et al. Focal loss of pigment in the Belgian tervuren dog. J Am Vet Med Assoc 1978;173:390–396.

Naughton GK, et al. Antibodies to surface antigens of pigmented cells in animals with vitiligo. Proc Soc Exper Biol Med 1986;181:423–426.

Scott DW. Large Animal Dermatology. Philadelphia: WB Saunders, 1988:387–392.

Spritz RA. Piebaldism, Waardenburg syndrome, and related disorders of melanocyte development. Sem Cutaneous Med Surg 1997;16:15–23.

Melanopenic hypomelanosis

The various forms of **albinism** are examples of melanopenic hypomelanosis. In albino animals and people, melanocytes are present and normally distributed but are defective in function and fail to synthesize melanin. The extent of the biochemical defect varies, so that *albinism covers a spectrum from amelanosis, oculocutaneous albinism (OCA), through graded pigmentary dilution*. Oculocutaneous albinisms and pigment dilutions are inherited as autosomal recessive traits. In albino animals with white hair and skin, and translucent irides, there is a mutation in the tyrosinase gene resulting in no residual enzyme activity. A mutation resulting in residual enzyme activity produces animals born with white hair but producing blond or pigmented hair as juveniles. The skin remains white but can develop pigmented nevi. This form has been reported in a gorilla.

Chediak-Higashi syndrome in humans, Hereford, Brangus and Japanese Black cattle, Persian cats, mink, blue and silver fox, and various other animal species is an example of *partial albinism and is inherited as an autosomal recessive trait*. While melanin is produced, there is a mutation of the *beige* gene, which plays a major role in generating cellular organelles. This results in a membrane defect leading to the formation of giant melanosomes that are passed with difficulty to the keratinocytes. The clumping of these giant melanosomes produces the color dilution effect. Chediak–Higashi syndrome is discussed with the Hematopoietic system.

Cyclic hematopoiesis (cyclic neutropenia), a lethal hereditary disease of Collie dogs, is caused by an autosomal recessive gene with a pleiotropic effect on coat color dilution. Affected dogs are silver-gray. The abnormal hair pigmentation results from the diminished formation of melanin from its precursor tyrosine rather than from pigment clumping. The normal collie coat color is restored in animals receiving bone marrow transplants to correct cyclic hematopoiesis. The hematological aspects of this disease are considered with the Hematopoietic system.

Coat color dilution has been reported in many species. It occurs in many breeds of dog, in cats, particularly Siamese cats, horses, and cattle. The pale coat coloration is due to clumping of large melanin granules in hair follicles and sometimes in the epidermis. In cats, dilute coat color is thought to be due to an autosomal recessive trait (*Maltese dilution*). **Color-dilution alopecia**, a tardive-onset hypotrichosis associated with color dilution traits in the dog, is discussed under Congenital and hereditary diseases of the skin.

Bibliography

Adalsteinsson S. Albinism in Icelandic sheep. J Hered 1977;68:347–349.

Ogawa H, et al. Clinical, morphologic, and biochemical characteristics of Chediak-Higashi syndrome in fifty-six Japanese Black cattle. Am J Vet Res 1997;58:1221–1226.

Prieur DJ, Collier LL. Maltese dilution of domestic cats. A generalized cutaneous albinism lacking ocular involvement. J Hered 1984;75:41–44.

Schmutz SM, et al. A form of albinism in cattle is caused by a tyrosinase frameshift mutation. Mamm Genome 2004;15:62–67.

Yang TJ. Recovery of hair coat color in gray collie (cyclic neutropenia) – normal bone marrow transplant chimeras. Am J Pathol 1978;91:149–152.

Acquired hypopigmentation

This follows damage to the epidermal melanin unit by various insults, including trauma, inflammation, radiation, contactants, endocrinopathies, infections and nutritional deficiencies. In general, the severity of the injury determines whether an insult will result in hypo- or hyperpigmentation. *Mild injury results in pigmentary incontinence and epidermal hypopigmentation*; however a mild injury allows accelerated keratinocyte turnover and a subsequent increase in production of melanosomes. *Severe injury results in the death of melanocytes and no subsequent repigmentation.*

Examples of depigmenting diseases in **horses** include onchocerciasis, *Culicoides* hypersensitivity, ventral midline dermatitis, and coital vesicular exanthema. Depigmenting lesions in horses may result from contact with equipment such as rubber bit guards or crupper straps or with feed buckets. Monobenzene ether of hydroquinone, a common ingredient in rubber, inhibits melanogenesis.

In **dogs**, hypopigmentation can occur in immune-mediated diseases such as lupus erythematosus, drug eruptions, bullous pemphigoid, and the various forms of pemphigus. Acquired depigmentation of the lips and/or nose also occurs in dogs as a result of contact with rubber dishes or toys containing dihydroquinone monobenzene ethers. Microbial lesions, such as deep pyoderma, may heal with depigmentation. Depigmenting lesions have been noted also in canine leishmaniasis and in dermatophytosis caused by *Microsporum persicolor*. Epitheliotropic lymphoma often presents with depigmenting, ulcerative lesions of skin and mucocutaneous junctions. Transient depigmentation has been reported in drug eruptions. Subcutaneous injection of corticosteroid or progesterone hormones may lead to focal hypopigmentation in the dog.

Uveodermatologic syndrome (Vogt–Koyanagi–Harada-like syndrome)

A depigmenting condition in dogs, partially resembles an extremely rare condition in humans, the Vogt–Koyanagi–Harada syndrome. *The arctic breeds such as the Akita, Siberian Husky, Samoyed, and Malamute are predisposed to this condition*, however it has been reported in many breeds. The cause is unknown, although an immune-mediated attack on melanocytes, as in the human disease, is presumed. The canine

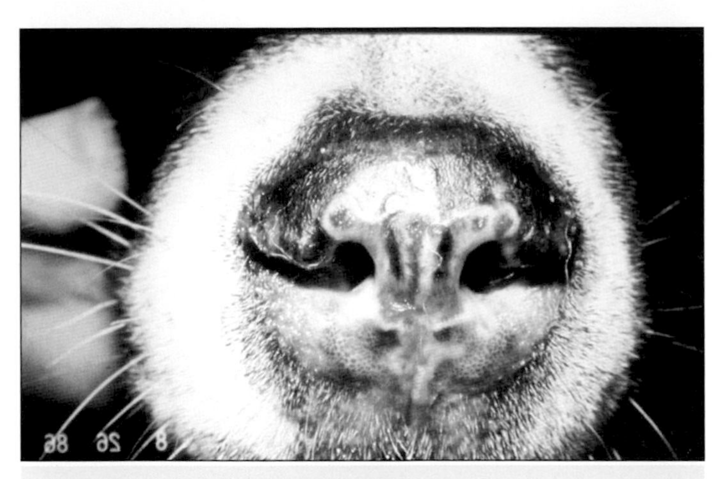

Figure 5.36 Uveodermatologic syndrome in a dog. Note depigmentation of the nose. (Courtesy of K Campbell.)

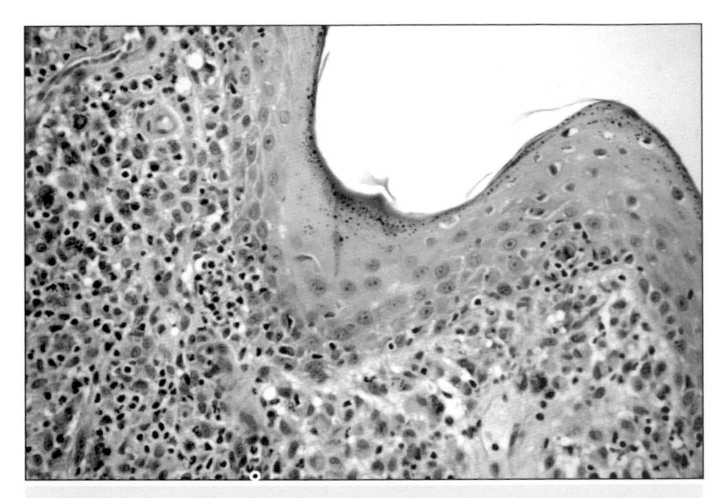

Figure 5.37 Uveodermatologic syndrome in a dog. Lichenoid interface, predominantly histiocytic, dermatitis with rare degeneration of basal keratinocytes and pigmentary incontinence.

lesions comprise *bilateral panuveitis* (see Vol. 1, Eye and ear) and *bilateral cutaneous depigmentation*, chiefly of the lips, nose, and periorbital skin (Fig. 5.36). Ocular lesions most often precede onset of cutaneous lesions. The scrotum, vulva, perianal skin, and footpads are less often affected. Leukotrichia is a common finding around the areas of leukoderma. Occasionally, depigmented lesions become ulcerated, erythematous or crusted. The histologic pattern of the cutaneous lesion is an *interface dermatitis with uncommon degeneration of basal keratinocytes, and a lichenoid inflammatory cell infiltrate in which large histiocytic cells usually predominate* (Fig. 5.37). Pigmentary incontinence is a common finding in areas of depigmentation but vacuolar change of the basal keratinocytes is not. This, and the histiocytic nature of the inflammatory infiltrate, are *major features of differentiation from discoid and systemic lupus.*

Bibliography

Morgan RV. Vogt-Koyanagi-Harada syndrome in humans and dogs. Compend Contin Educ Pract Vet 1989;11:1211–1218.

Warmoes T. Canine model of Vogt-Koyanagi-Harada syndrome. Le Point Veterinaire 1999;30:249–254.

Leukotrichia

Reticulated leukotrichia, colloquially known as "tiger stripe," is recognized in the Standardbred, Thoroughbred, and Quarter Horse breeds. The lesions occur predominantly in yearlings and comprise linear crusts arranged in a cross-hatch pattern on the dorsal midline from the withers to the tail. Transient alopecia and a regrowth of permanently white hair follow crusting. The underlying skin has normal pigmentation. Well-documented precise descriptions of the expected histologic lesions are lacking. Some reports indicate an interface lichenoid dermatitis may be present, while others suggest that a mild superficial dermal mononuclear cell infiltrate and pigmentary incontinence are to be expected. The etiology and pathogenesis are unknown. **Spotted leukotrichia** occurs in the horse as multiple, often somewhat symmetrical, small circular areas of white hair. The spots occur most commonly on the rump and thorax, and Arabians have a predilection. The etiology and pathogenesis are unknown. **Hyperesthetic leukotrichia**, so-called because the lesions are extremely painful, has been reported only in Californian horses. Single or multiple crusted lesions occur on the dorsal midline and heal leaving permanently white hairs. Leukotrichia, also termed *poliosis*, has been reported in **dogs** in association with Vogt–Koyanagi–Harada syndrome, tyrosinase deficiency in Chow Chows, and as an idiopathic, possibly heritable condition in a litter of Labrador Retrievers. In the last example, the condition resolved.

Bibliography

Fadok VA. Update on four unusual equine dermatoses. Vet Clin North Am Eq Pract 1995;11:105–110.

Von Tsharner C. Pigmentary disorders. Vet Dermatol 2000;11:205–210.

White SD, Batch S. Leukotrichia in a litter of Labrador retrievers. J Am Anim Hosp Assoc 1990;26:319–321.

Alopecia areata and universalis

Leukotrichia can be associated with alopecia areata. These disorders are discussed in more detail under Other immune-mediated dermatoses.

Copper deficiency

This pigmentary disorder is seen primarily in *cattle and sheep*. It has also been reported in *moose*, and experimentally in *dogs*. Copper deficiency may be simple or conditioned by other dietary substances, particularly sulfate and molybdenum. Since copper is an essential constituent of tyrosinase, there is *depressed tyrosinase activity*, and deficient animals show depigmentation of hair or wool. Affected cattle with normally black coats become rusty-brown and develop "spectacle" lesions round the eyes. Black sheep develop intermittent bands of light-colored wool corresponding to periods of restricted availability of copper (Fig. 5.38). The deficiency of copper also affects the physical nature of the wool or hair. In sheep, *the wool has less crimp*, prompting the colloquial name of "string" or "steely" wool. The straightness of the wool is due to inadequate keratinization, probably caused by imperfect oxidation of sulfhydryl groups in prekeratin, a process that involves copper (Fig. 5.39).

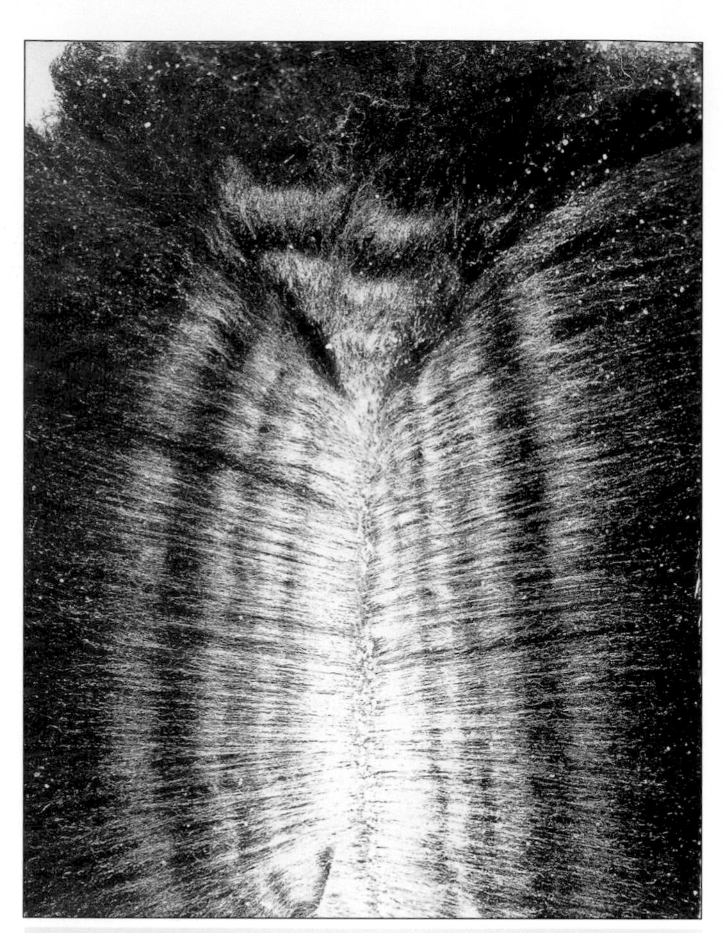

Figure 5.38 Copper deficiency. Black-wooled sheep with bands of achromotrichia corresponding to periods of molybdenum administration. (Courtesy of WJ Hartley.)

PHYSICOCHEMICAL DISEASES OF SKIN

The integument has a large surface area in direct contact with the environment and is hence extremely vulnerable to chemical and physical injuries. *Physical stresses* include friction, pressure, vibration, electricity, high and low ambient temperatures, humidity, visible light, and ultraviolet, infrared and ionizing radiation. Cutaneous reactions to visible light are discussed separately. *Chemical toxins* may exert their effect directly as in irritant contact dermatitis or envenomation or indirectly, as in thallium poisoning.

Physical injury to skin

Mechanical, frictional, and traumatic injury

The hair coat of most domestic animals protects from "blisters" that so commonly develop in human skin subjected to prolonged pressure or frictional contact with a hard surface. The following examples tend to occur in heavy animals with skin exposed to repeated or constant pressure such as in animals immobilized by paralysis, or in those exposed to a physically harsh environment.

Dogs

Calluses occur when continual or repetitive pressure or friction is applied to a localized area of skin and represent a protective response of the integument to the physical injury. They tend to occur over bony prominences, particularly the hocks, elbows, lateral surfaces of the digits and on the sternum. Callosities can develop in all domestic animal species, but are most common in dogs, particularly the giant breeds, and in pigs housed on concrete floors with inadequate bedding. They are characterized by epidermal proliferation with prominent epidermal and follicular hyperkeratosis. Dilated hair follicles may lead to furunculosis with

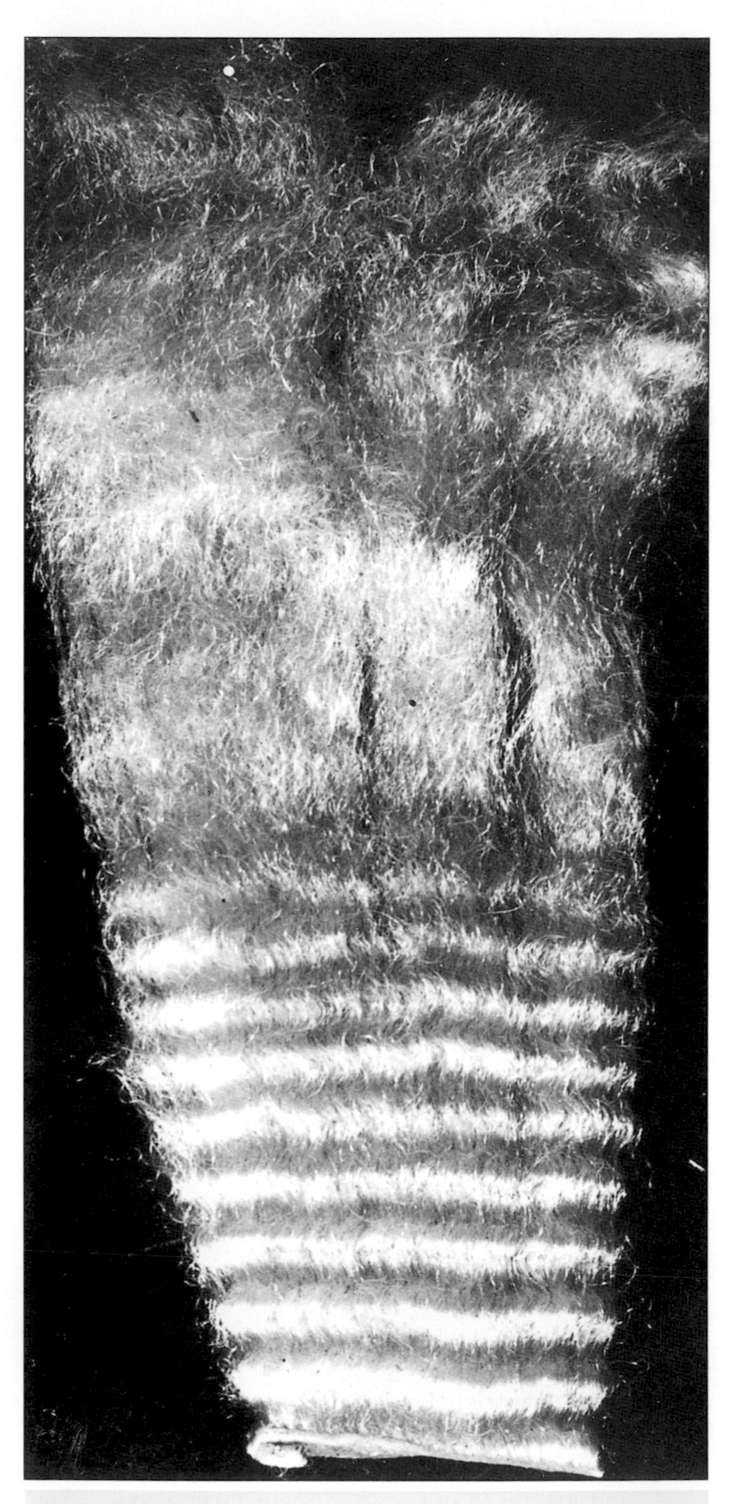

Figure 5.39 Staple from sheep that received 1.0 mg of copper per day, then 10 mg per day. Note stringiness and lack of crimp on deficient regime. (Courtesy of WJ Hartley.)

secondary pyoderma, severe suppurative to pyogranulomatous dermatitis and eventual fibrosis. Grossly, callosities are *well-circumscribed, lichenified, raised, alopecic, gray, keratinous plaques*. Ulceration may occur. The pig may also develop bursitis.

A **hygroma** *is a false or acquired bursa, which develops subcutaneously over bony prominences*. Hygromas are most common in the giant breeds of dogs at pressure points such as the lateral aspect of the elbow, the greater trochanter of the femur and the tuber coxae. Hip dysplasia in dogs can lead to elbow hygromas as dogs develop an abnormal method of lying down that relies upon dropping to the olecranons to spare the hips. Usually pressure induces a protective callus, but in some animals persistent decubitus ulcers or recurrent hematoma formation eventually lead to the induction of a hygroma. The gross lesion is a variably sized cystic cavity separated from the skin by loose connective tissue. The wall of the hygroma is dense connective tissue that may have a smooth or a villus inner lining. The contents are mucinous and yellow to red, depending on the degree of hemorrhage. *Histologically, the wall is composed of granulation tissue of variable maturity*. A flattened layer of fibroblasts may give the appearance of an epithelial lining. The cavity may contain clumps of fibrin. Organization of fibrin deposits at the margin of the cavity gives rise to the grossly apparent villus projections that occasionally undergo cartilaginous metaplasia.

Decubitus ulcers *are the result of ischemic necrosis that follows application of constant pressure to a localized area of skin*. Studies in Greyhounds suggest that intermittent repeated focal vascular occlusion leads to increased tissue damage from *reperfusion injury*. Thromboxane A_2 and its metabolite, thromboxane B_2, are thought to contribute to vasoconstriction and platelet aggregation. Predisposing conditions include prolonged recumbency, lack of proper bedding, improperly applied bandages or casts, poorly fitting tack, atrophy of muscle, loss of fat, malnutrition associated with systemic disease, contusions, irritation from feces or urine, and body types with large bones, thin skin and low body fat. In large animals, post-anesthetic myopathies, laminitis, and neurologic diseases are predisposing conditions. The "downer" cow is particularly prone to decubitus ulcers. *Decubitus ulcers are graded from I to IV*. In grade I, the lesion consists of focal erythema. In grade II, an ulcer extends into the subcutis. In grade III, the ulcer extends into the deep fascia and the wound edges may be undermined. Grade IV ulcers extend to bone, have undermined edges, and possibly underlying osteomyelitis and septic arthritis.

Intertrigo *refers to localized dermatitis affecting folded areas of skin*. The combined effect of friction, heat, maceration, bacterial or yeast proliferation and irritation by retained secretions leads to superficial inflammation. Examples in dogs include *facial, lip, vulvar and tail fold dermatitis*. Obesity is a predisposing factor. Body fold dermatitis is particularly common in Chinese Shar-Pei puppies. Udder-thigh dermatitis occurs predominantly in first-calf *dairy heifers*. Udder edema is a predisposing factor. Lesions are erythematous and swollen, sometimes ulcerated and often have an unpleasant odor. Histologically, the epidermis is hyperplastic, spongiotic and possibly eroded or ulcerated. Surface pustules, neutrophilic exocytosis, and pigmentary incontinence may be present. The dermis has a dense band of lymphocytes and plasma cells at the dermoepidermal junction. Mucocutaneous pyoderma is the primary differential.

Traumatic injury to the skin is quite common in dogs and is often associated with *compound fractures* sustained in motor vehicle accidents. *Dogfight wounds* tend to be tears rather than punctures, as occur in cats; consequently abscesses are a less common sequel. A plethora of **foreign bodies** may penetrate the canine integument, two of the more dramatic examples being *foxtails* and *porcupine quills*. The external ear canal and interdigital webs are favored sites for grass awn entry and subsequent migration. Retrievers or other animals wounded with *steel shot* may develop fistulous tracts or abscesses as steel shot corrodes when embedded in tissues.

Myospherulosis is a rare form of foreign body reaction in which endogenous erythrocytes interact with an exogenous substance, such as antibiotics or ointments, or with endogenous fat. *The lesions are subcutaneous nodules composed of sheets of large macrophages in which the cytoplasm is filled with homogeneous eosinophilic spherules*. These structures may resemble fungal organisms but are negative with fungal special stains such as periodic acid-Schiff. The spherules stain for endogenous peroxidase, thus establishing their identity as erythrocytes.

Traction alopecia has been reported in dogs. It results from low-grade local ischemia induced by traction on hairs. The traction force is applied by elastic ties or hair barrettes applied to pull the forelock hair into a topknot. The lesions are focal patches of cutaneous atrophy and alopecia that may become eroded and crusted. Histologically, the lesion is an *atrophic dermatosis*. The epidermis is thin and may occasionally show single cell necrosis, erosion or ulceration. The hair follicles are inactive and atrophic, pale staining and appear "faded." Inflammation is minimal and is restricted to areas of surface ulceration.

Pyotraumatic dermatitis or "hot spot" is a common complication of allergic dermatitis or any pruritic dermatosis that leads to an *itch–scratch cycle*. It occurs most often in times of warm, humid weather. Breeds with a thick undercoat, such as German Shepherds, Golden Retrievers, Labradors, and Saint Bernards, are particularly susceptible. Lesions are extremely painful and occur at sites of *self-trauma*, such as the dorsal rump in a flea-infested animal. Grossly, the initial lesions are erythematous, exudative, sharply demarcated patches, spreading extensively if not treated. The surface may be colonized by gram-positive cocci. Alopecia and hyperpigmentation are the typical sequelae. Pyotraumatic dermatitis is characterized histologically by *epidermal ulceration*. A thick serocellular inflammatory crust covers the denuded dermis. The predominantly neutrophilic reaction tends to be restricted to the area beneath the ulcer. Folliculitis and furunculosis are not features of classical pyotraumatic dermatitis but occasionally are concurrent conditions as indicated clinically by scattered papules at the periphery of the lesion. Eosinophils and/or folliculitis were common in one series of cases.

Cats

This species is particularly prone to develop subcutaneous abscesses or cellulitis as a result of fight wounds. The cat bite produces a puncture-type wound that seals over and enables the introduced bacteria (chiefly oral flora) to multiply in the damaged tissue.

Cattle

Tail tip necrosis of feedlot beef cattle is a disease in which slatted-floor housing has been shown to be an important causal factor. The pathogenesis is presumed to be *ischemia*, secondary to compression of, or blunt trauma to, the more proximal parts of the tail. Clinically, there is alopecia, scaling and crusting. Ulceration and suppuration are frequent sequelae. In early lesions, histologic examination reveals only perivascular edema and hemorrhage. Fully developed lesions are characterized by dermal scarring, follicular atrophy, vascular wall hypertrophy, and fragmentation of extravasated erythrocytes.

Pigs

Intensive rearing systems for swine production have increased the occurrence of a variety of traumatic lesions. Those in piglets probably result from contact with *concrete floors* in farrowing crates. The knees are the most common site affected, followed by the fetlocks and hocks. The nipples, particularly the cranial pair, are often involved, as is the tail. The lesions occur within a few hours of birth as circumscribed red macules followed by necrosis, ulceration and crusting. The ulcers heal over 3–4 weeks leaving no permanent defect. The supernumerary digits of the hind legs are subject to trauma in sows housed on concrete slats. Trauma resulting from *vices* such as tail biting, ear biting and flank biting are increasingly common in growing pigs under intensive rearing systems of management. Wounds from a variety of causes, including fight wounds, often develop into subcutaneous abscesses in pigs.

Horses

Cutaneous wounds are common in horses and can be largely attributed to the flighty temperament of the species. *Exuberant granulation tissue, "proud flesh,"* is a relatively frequent and serious sequel to wounds of the distal limbs. Poor circulation, minimal soft tissue, lack of adequate drainage and a tendency for excessive movement predisposes the distal limbs to the development of excess granulation tissue. The gross lesion, *a tumor-like mass of red-brown tissue, must be distinguished from equine sarcoid, cutaneous habronemiasis, mycoses, pythiosis, and squamous cell carcinoma.* Histologically, immature capillaries and capillary loops arranged perpendicularly to the elongated fibroblasts and newly synthesized collagen are distinctive features. A superficial layer of granulation tissue may form in association with any of the above-mentioned conditions, and the entire lesion should be examined before a diagnosis is made.

Injection site reactions are not uncommon in domestic animals. Subcutaneously administered vaccines and therapeutic drugs may be responsible. The nodules may ulcerate or fistulate and are often suspected to be neoplasms. *Histologically, the classic injection site reaction is composed predominantly of nodular aggregates of lymphocytes arranged around a central core of caseous necrosis.* Lymphocytes may form follicles. Irregular refractile or faintly basophilic granular material is often embedded in the eosinophilic debris or found within phagocytic cells. Plasma cells, macrophages and multinucleated giant cells are also present, but in lesser numbers than the lymphocytes. The strong antigenic stimulus provided by the exogenous antigen sometimes results in the formation of germinal centers. The heterogeneity of the cell population and the lack of anaplastic characteristics in the lymphoid cells may differentiate these lesions, sometimes termed *pseudolymphoma*, from genuine lymphoma. Vaccine administration in **cats** has been linked to the development of a variety of sarcomas, including fibrosarcomas, osteosarcomas, malignant fibrous histiocytomas, chondrosarcomas, and rhabdomyosarcomas. **Vaccine-associated sarcomas** have the unique features of a *subcutaneous location, concurrent lymphocytic infiltrates, and possibly macrophages containing granular foreign material.* The proposed mechanism involves an over-zealous reparative response followed by malignant transformation of mesenchymal cells. Antigen load and degree of inflammation present at the vaccination site are possible influencing factors. Aluminum adjuvant particles have been identified in tumor associated macrophages, however, vaccine-associated sarcomas have also been documented to arise from the use of non-adjuvanted vaccines. Injection of killed **rabies vaccine** in **dogs** can lead to focal mononuclear vasculitis and ischemic atrophy of surrounding follicles resulting in a focal area of alopecia and is further discussed under Immune-mediated dermatoses. **Injection site eosinophilic granulomas** with necrotic centers developed in some **horses** within 1–3 days as a response to the use of silicone coated hypodermic needles. The lesion is suspected to be a form of delayed hypersensitivity.

Bibliography

Bartels KE, et al. Corrosion potential of steel bird shot in dogs. J Am Vet Med Assoc 1991;199:856–863.

Brennan KE, Ihrke PJ. Grass awn migration in dogs and cats. A retrospective study of 182 cases. J Am Vet Med Assoc 1983;182:1201–1204.

Gross TL, et al. Atrophic diseases of the hair follicle. In: Veterinary Dermatopathology A Macroscopic and Microscopic Evaluation of Canine and Feline Skin Disease. St Louis, Mo: Mosby Year Book, 1992:295–297.

Hargis AM, et al. Myospherulosis in the subcutis of a dog. Vet Pathol 1984;21:248–251.

Hendrick MJ, Dunagan CA. Focal necrotizing granulomatous panniculitis associated with subcutaneous injection of rabies vaccine in cats and dogs: 10 cases (1988–1989). J Am Vet Med Assoc 1991;198:304–305.

Hershey AE, et al. Prognosis for presumed feline vaccine-associated sarcoma after excision: 61 cases (1986–1996). J Am Vet Med Assoc 2000;216:58–61.

Holm BR, et al. A prospective study of the clinical findings, treatment and histopathology of 44 cases of pyotraumatic dermatitis. Vet Dermatol 2004;15:369–376.

Jelinek F. Postinflammatory sarcoma in cats. Exp Toxicol Pathol 2003;55:167–172.

Madsen EB, Nielsen K. A study of tail tip necrosis in young fattening bulls on slatted floors. Nord Vet Med 1985;37:349–357.

O'Dair HA, Foster AP. Focal and generalized alopecia. Vet Clin North Am 1995;25:858–861.

Ordeix L, et al. Traction alopecia with vasculitis in an Old English sheepdog. J Small Anim Pract 2001;42:304–305.

Penny RHC, et al. Clinical observations of necrosis of the skin of suckling piglets. Aust Vet J 1971;47:529–537.

Sigmund von HM, et al. Udder-thigh dermatitis of cattle: epidemiological, clinical and bacteriological investigations. Bov Pract 1983;18:18–23.

Slovis NM, et al. Injection site eosinophilic granulomas and collagenolysis in 3 horses. J Vet Intern Med 1999;13:606–612.

Swaim SF, et al. Pressure wounds in animals. Compend Contin Educ Pract Vet 1996;18:203–218.

Vitale CB, et al. Vaccine-induced ischemic dermatopathy in the dog. Vet Dermatol 1999;10:131–141.

Psychogenic injury

Several conditions in animals are considered to be similar to **obsessive-compulsive disorders** in humans. In theory, stress causes an increase in the production of endorphins creating reinforcement of the stereotypic behavior characterizing each syndrome.

Psychogenic alopecia in **cats**, a self-induced form of alopecia precipitated or exacerbated by environmental stress, is similar to the obsessive-compulsive disorder of humans, trichotillomania. The condition can occur in any cat but is most common in oriental breeds. Clinically, cats groom excessively, licking and pulling at the haircoat. Psychogenic alopecia/dermatitis has *two clinical forms*. In one, *psychogenic dermatitis*, affected cats lick and chew at a single site creating a well-demarcated erythematous, ulcerated lesion of variable size, which usually is located on an extremity, the abdomen or flank. The lesion grossly resembles those of eosinophilic plaque. The second, or *alopecic form*, is characterized by partial alopecia, broken hairs and normal skin. The lesions often occur as a "stripe" along the dorsal mid-line but may involve perineal, genital, caudomedial thigh, medial elbow, or abdominal areas. This distribution pattern is usually symmetrical resembling feline endocrine alopecia but *the hairs in psychogenic alopecia are broken off rather than easily epilated as occurs in endocrine alopecia*. Diagnosis is largely dependent on history and clinical signs. A trichogram examination of epilated hairs reveals a normal anagen to telogen ratio and fractured tips of hairs rather than tapered ends. *Microscopic examination of skin in the alopecic form is usually normal*, although wrinkling of the outer root sheath and intra- and perifollicular hemorrhage may reflect the trauma applied to the hairs. The inflammatory form has no distinctive histologic features, as it is a nonspecific, ulcerative, hyperplastic, superficial perivascular dermatitis. *Differentials for the alopecic form include endocrine dermatopathy and pruritic skin conditions such as atopy, flea allergic dermatitis, and cheyletiellosis.* As pruritus in the cat is manifest in part by excessive grooming, any degree of perivascular eosinophilic dermatitis should be considered indicative of an underlying hypersensitivity disorder. The condition must also be differentiated from **feline acquired hair shaft abnormality**, a condition resembling *trichorrhexis nodosa* in humans. In this condition, cats with an underlying pruritic skin disease such as flea allergic dermatitis groom excessively. Weakened hair shafts break easily and lead to alopecia. A trichogram reveals white nodes on the hair shafts corresponding to foci of frayed cortical fibers. A biopsy should show evidence of the underlying hypersensitivity condition.

Dogs also develop *psychogenic dermatitis including foot chewing and licking, tail-biting, and flank-sucking*. The gross lesions may be slight but the superficial excoriations often develop into pyoderma. **Acral lick dermatitis**, otherwise known as "lick granuloma" or neurodermatitis, is a relatively common psychogenic dermatitis of dogs, particularly in large active breeds younger than 5 years. Males are affected twice as frequently as females. The areas traumatized by persistent licking and chewing are most commonly the cranial carpus and metacarpus, followed by the radius, tibia and metatarsus. Erythema and epidermal excoriations give rise to a single well-circumscribed, eroded or ulcerated, oval plaque. Occasionally, lesions are multiple. Secondary bacterial infection may result. Re-epithelialization of the lesion leaves a well-circumscribed alopecic plaque often with peripheral hyperpigmentation. Histologically, acral lick dermatitis is a *hyperplastic superficial perivascular dermatitis with marked orthokeratotic and parakeratotic hyperkeratosis, acanthosis and rete ridge formation* (Fig. 5.40). There is a sharp transition between the hyperplastic and ulcerated epidermis, which is covered by a thick scale-crust. Superficial dermal fibrosis is usually marked and collagen fibers in dermal papillae are often arranged perpendicular to the surface epithelium (Fig. 5.41). *This "vertical streaking" of collagen is thought to result from chronic irritation.*

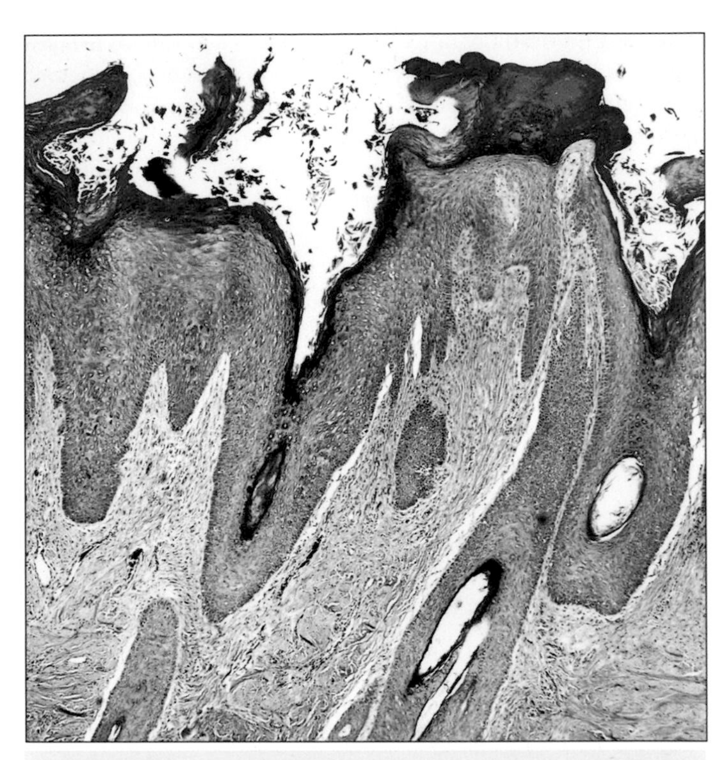

Figure 5.40 Acral lick dermatitis in a dog. Hyperplastic superficial perivascular dermatitis with marked orthokeratotic and parakeratotic hyperkeratosis, acanthosis and rete ridge formation.

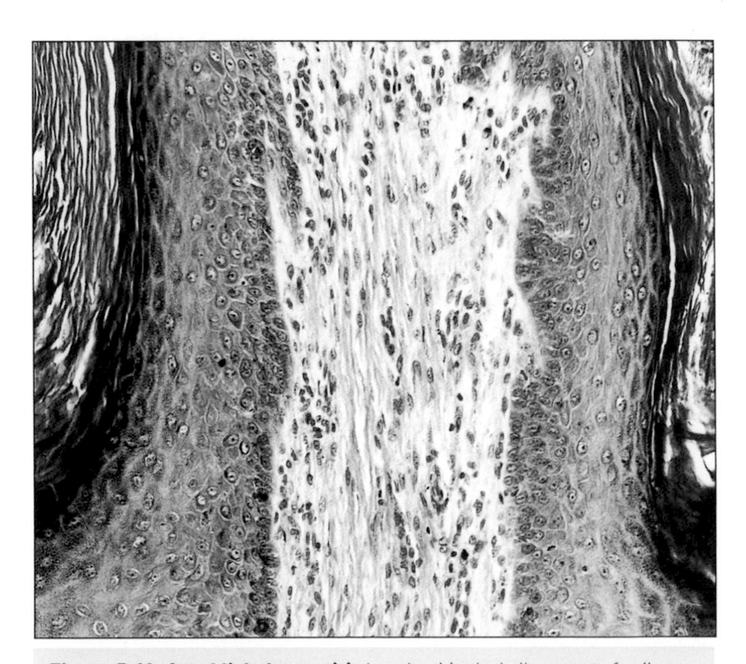

Figure 5.41 Acral lick dermatitis in a dog. Vertical alignment of collagen.

Perifolliculitis, folliculitis and sometimes furunculosis are often present. Plasmacytic infiltrates often surround the sweat glands. Sebaceous glands and hair follicles appear hyperplastic. *The primary differential is self trauma due to a pre-existing localized bacterial infection.*

In **horses**, the **equine self-mutilation syndrome** can be misinterpreted as a possible cutaneous disorder as horses bite, kick, or rub the flank or pectoral areas. The behavior is usually accompanied by vocalization, spinning or rolling and is most common in *stallions*.

The condition is thought to be *stress related.* There are no primary cutaneous lesions, however secondary excoriations may be present.

A **self-destructive behavioral condition** primarily affecting **first-calf heifers** is characterized by *excessive licking of the udder and teats* sometimes leading to teat necrosis and culling. The condition is associated with udder edema and increased levels of histamine in the udder tissue leading to pruritus.

Bibliography

Alhaidari Z, et al. Acquired feline hair shaft abnormality resembling trichorrhexis nodosa in humans. Vet Dermatol 1996;7:235–238.

Dodman NH, et al. Equine self-mutilation syndrome (57 cases) J Am Vet Med Assoc 1994;204:1219–1223.

Goldberger E, Rapoport JL. Canine acral lick dermatitis: response to the antiobsessional drug clomipramine. J Am Anim Hosp Assoc 1991;27:179–182.

Sawyer LS, et al. Psychogenic alopecia in cats: 11 cases (1993–1996). J Am Vet Med Assoc 1999;214:71–74.

Virga V. Behavioral dermatology. Vet Clin North Am Small Anim Pract 2003;33:231–251.

Yeruham I, Markusfeld O. Self destructive behavior in dairy cattle. Vet Rec 1996;138:308.

Mineral deposition in cutaneous tissues

Deposition of insoluble calcium salts within cutaneous tissues can occur as a result of injury or degeneration of skin components (**dystrophic mineralization** or calcification), secondary to calcium/phosphorus metabolic alterations (**metastatic mineralization** or calcification), as an idiopathic condition, or may occur iatrogenically. Mechanisms leading to calcium salt deposition are complex and involve such factors as the lower pH of injured tissue, mitochondrial concentration of calcium and phosphorus, and the influx of calcium into injured cells in dystrophic forms. In metastatic forms, loss of mineralization inhibitors, changing of ions into a solid phase, and phosphate ion initiation of crystal formation are implicated in salt formation. Mineralization can be *localized*, as in inflammatory foci (granulomas), in degenerative lesions (follicular cysts), or in neoplasms (pilomatricomas), or may be *generalized* as in the tissue mineralization associated with chronic renal failure.

The most well-known form of cutaneous mineralization is the classic form of **calcinosis cutis** associated with hyperadrenocorticism, which is discussed in Endocrine diseases of skin. For ease of comparison, other known types of cutaneous mineralization are discussed here. **Calcinosis universalis** *refers to widespread areas of calcinosis cutis* and can be seen with hypercortisolism, percutaneous absorption of calcium-containing products, or from the iatrogenic administration of calcium-containing solutions. Some forms of calcinosis cutis can be indistinguishable histologically from calcinosis cutis associated with hyperadrenocorticism. The clinical presentation, concurrent abnormalities, signalment and history should allow distinction of the various forms of calcinosis cutis.

Percutaneous absorption of products containing **calcium chloride or calcium carbonate** has occurred naturally in *dogs*. Multifocal, flat-topped and centrally ulcerated papules and small nodules affected glabrous skin, such as the lips, axilla, inguinal and interdigital skin. Histologically, the lesions comprised granulomas centered on degenerate, mineralized collagen fibers. Ultrastructural examination of experimental lesions indicated that mineral was deposited within the collagen bundles within 24 hours of initial skin contact. The main differential diagnosis was *calcinosis cutis of hyperadrenocorticism*, to which the lesions are histologically identical.

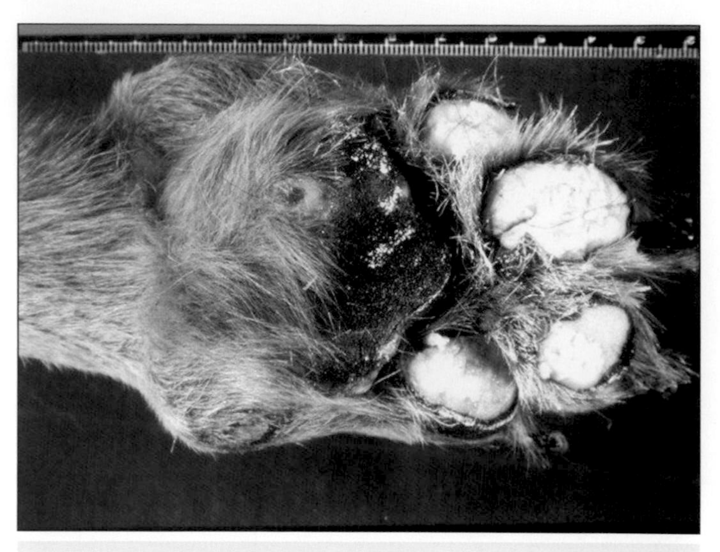

Figure 5.42 Calcinosis circumscripta in a dog. Note chalky material exuding from footpads. (Courtesy of B Dunstan.)

A chemically induced, iatrogenic form of calcinosis cutis has been reported in humans and a dog as a consequence of the subcutaneous administration of a **10% calcium gluconate** solution for treatment of hypoparathyroidism. In the dog, calcium salts formed on basement membranes, dermal collagen, vessel walls and adipocyte membranes. Dermoepidermal separation, pyogranulomatous dermatitis, panniculitis and vasculopathy ensued, leading to marked necrosis and sloughing of the skin. Concurrent hyperphosphatemia was thought to predispose to precipitation of calcium salts.

Dogs with systemic blastomycosis treated with **amphotericin B** developed lesions that resolved over time and were *indistinguishable from calcinosis cutis of hypercortisolism*. Dogs had severe granulomatous cutaneous lesions that may have been predisposed to dystrophic mineralization, but mineralizing lesions were more extensive or separate from primary inflammatory lesions. The dogs had no clinically significant serum calcium/phosphorus abnormalities. Additional factors suspected to contribute to mineralization included mild intermittent serum calcium fluctuations, mononuclear cell production of factors leading to increased osteoclast-mediated bone resorption, and alteration of vitamin D metabolism.

Calcinosis circumscripta (tumoral calcinosis) occurs most often in *dogs, horses* and occasionally *cats* (see also Ectopic mineralization and ossification, in Vol. 1, Bones and joints). Lesions in dogs are most often solitary but can be multiple and occur most often in large breeds <2 years of age. German Shepherd Dogs are predisposed. The *skin over bony prominences of the limbs* is most often affected. The tongue and paravertebral soft tissues, footpads, edges of the pinna in dogs with cropped ears, and cheeks of Boston Terriers are other reported sites. Calcinosis circumscripta of the dorsal thoracolumbar region at a site of previous progestogen injection has been reported in a cat.

The gross and histologic features of the lesion evolve over time. Initially, the lesion may be bulging, fluctuant or cystic, variably ulcerated and contains chalky white material (Fig. 5.42). Histologically,

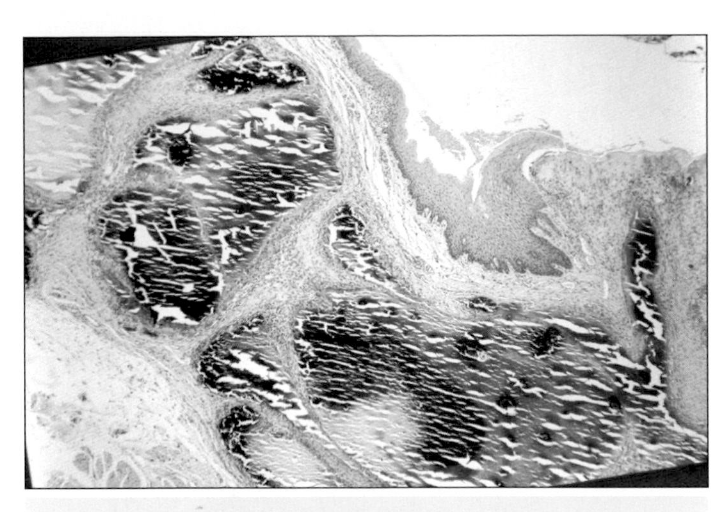

Figure 5.43 Calcinosis circumscripta in a dog. Dermal lakes of basophilic granular material are surrounded by mild fibrosis and giant cells, macrophages and fewer lymphocytes and plasma cells.

subcutaneous to deep dermal lakes of basophilic granular material that stain with von Kossa are surrounded by mild fibrosis and a cellular zone of variable width with giant cells, large macrophages and fewer lymphocytes and plasma cells (Fig. 5.43). Over time, the lesions become firm, progressively more mineralized, and associated with dense fibrous connective tissue bands. Inflammation may subside to some degree over time and osseous or cartilaginous metaplasia may take place. Epidermal sequestration or transepidermal elimination of mineralized material may lead to ulceration.

The pathogenesis of calcinosis circumscripta is not known. Dystrophic mineralization secondary to previous tissue trauma has been proposed based on the predilection for skin covering bony prominences. This explanation is not entirely satisfactory as the lesions do not recur after surgical excision, and trauma to these sites in large dogs would be expected to be repetitive. The name "apocrine cystic calcinosis" was previously applied to calcinosis circumscripta since it has been documented to arise from degenerating, cystic apocrine glands. A relationship to apocrine glands is not evident in most cases. Lesions have also developed at sites of previous injections, or in association with surgical sites sutured with polydioxanone sutures. Cases of calcinosis circumscripta have also been reported to occur in the footpads of dogs and cats with chronic renal failure, and in the footpads of an otherwise healthy German Shepherd Dog and in another German Shepherd Dog with pododermatitis. Symmetrical cases that resolved spontaneously have been reported in young dogs with underlying skeletal disease such as hypertrophic osteodystrophy. It is likely that multiple factors are involved in the pathogenesis of calcinosis circumscripta.

Bibliography

Davidson EB, et al. Calcinosis circumscripta of the thoracic wall in a German shepherd dog. J Am Anim Hosp Assoc 1998;34:153–156.

Frazier KS, et al. Multiple cutaneous metaplastic ossification associated with iatrogenic hyperglucocorticism. J Vet Diag Invest 1998;10:303–307.

Gortel K, et al. Calcinosis cutis associated with systemic blastomycosis in three dogs. J Am Anim Hosp Assoc 1999;35:368–374.

Gross TL. Calcinosis circumscripta and renal dysplasia in a dog. Vet Dermatol 1997;8:27–32.

O'Brien CR, Wilkie JS. Calcinosis circumscripta following an injection of proligesterone in a Burmese cat. Aust Vet J 2001;79:187–189.

Paradis M, Scott DW. Calcinosis cutis secondary to percutaneous penetration of calcium carbonate in a Dalmatian. Can Vet J 1989;30:57–59.

Schaer M, et al. Severe calcinosis cutis associated with treatment of hypoparathyroidism in a dog. J Am Anim Hosp Assoc 2001;37:364–369.

Scott DW, Bueger RG. Idiopathic calcinosis circumscripta in the dog: A retrospective analysis of 130 cases. J Am Anim Hosp Assoc 1987;24:651–658.

Stone WC, et al. The pathologic mineralization of soft tissue: Calcinosis circumscripta in horses. Compend Contin Educ Pract Vet 1990;12:1643–1648.

Cold injury

Most cold-induced cutaneous lesions (frostbite) result not only from direct freezing and disruption of the cells, but more importantly from vascular injury and resultant tissue anoxia. In experimental frostbite lesions in Hanford miniature swine, vacuolation of keratinocytes was the earliest change in the epidermis followed by spongiosis, epidermal necrosis, and separation of the necrotic epithelium from the dermis. Hyperemia and hemorrhage were also early lesions. Inflammatory changes, comprising neutrophilic infiltration and necrotizing vasculitis, occurred 6–46 h postinjury. Thrombosis of small arterioles increased in severity up to 1 week postinjury. By 2 weeks, considerable epithelial regeneration had taken place, either as a complete replacement or as crescents beneath the necrotic epidermis.

Cutaneous injury resulting from cold is uncommon in well-nourished, healthy domestic animals. Well-acclimatized long-haired animals can tolerate temperatures of –50°C for indefinite periods. Cold injury occurs most commonly on the tips of the ears and tail of cats, the scrotum of male dogs and bulls, and the tips of the ears, tail and teats in cattle. The teats are particularly vulnerable if cows are turned out into the cold with wet udders. Affected skin is cool, pale and hypoesthetic. The gross lesions include alopecia, scaling and pigmentary alterations of the skin, hair or both. In severe cases, the ischemic necrosis results in dry gangrene and sloughing of the affected part.

Bibliography

Arvesen A, et al. Early and late functional and histopathological perturbations in the rabbit ear-artery following local cold injury. Vasa 1999;28:85–94.

Schoning P, Hamlet MP. Experimental frostbite in Hanford miniature swine. I. Epithelial changes. II. Vascular changes. Br J Exp Pathol 1989;70:41–49, 51–57.

Thermal injury

Heat may be applied to the skin in a variety of forms and, depending on duration and intensity, will produce *mild to severe necrotizing lesions*. Longer exposure to lower temperatures is more damaging than short exposure to higher temperatures. The lowest temperature at which skin can burn is 44°C (111°F). *Dry heat causes desiccation and carbonization, whereas moist heat causes "boiling" or coagulation.* Thermal injury in domestic animals may be caused by hot liquids, steam, heating pads, hair dryers, drying cages, hot metals such as wood stoves or car engines, fires, friction from rope "scalds," electrical burns from chewing electrical wires, improperly grounded electrocautery units, or lightning strikes. Animals struck by lightning may show a jagged line of singed hair running down a shoulder or flank (Fig. 5.44). This finding is valuable in establishing an otherwise difficult diagnosis. Rarely, small animals incur microwave burns.

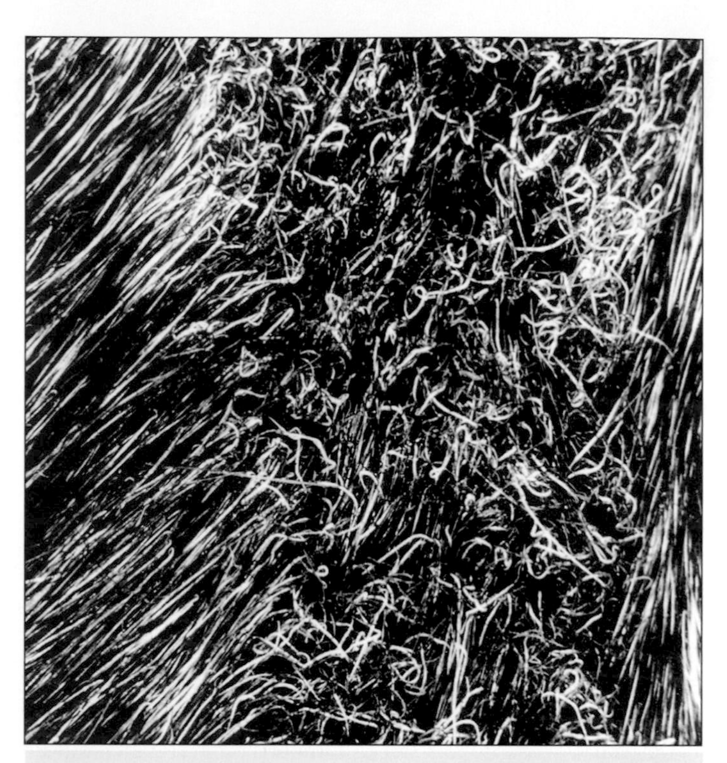

Figure 5.44 Lightning strike. A linear arrangement of singed hairs. (Courtesy of MA Hayes.)

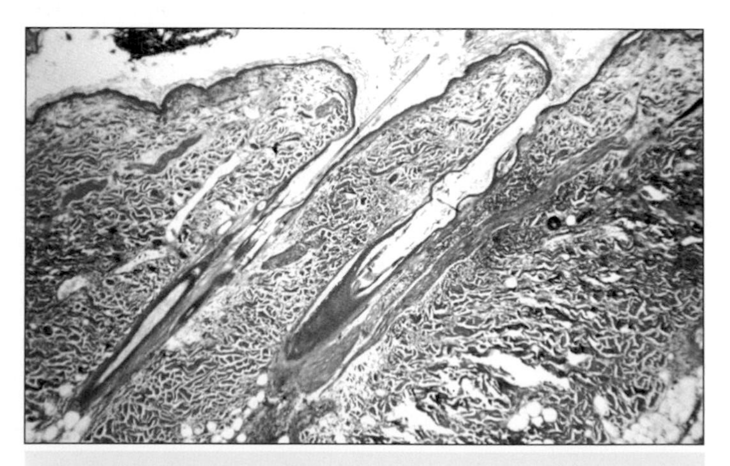

Figure 5.45 Burn. Note diffuse coagulative necrosis of the epidermis. (Courtesy of B Dunstan.)

Burns are classified into four degrees according to depth of injury.

- **First-degree burns** *involve only the epidermis*. The heated areas are erythematous and edematous as a result of vascular reaction in the dermis, but vesicles do not form. The epithelial cells show no morphological sign of injury although there may be surface desquamation after a few days.
- *In* **second-degree burns**, *the epidermis and part of the dermis are damaged*. The cytoplasm of the epithelial cells is hypereosinophilic, and the nuclei are shrunken or karyorrhexic. Coagulative necrosis of the epidermis (Fig. 5.45) can occur in the absence of substantial dermal injury and often "wicks" down to involve the follicular epithelium (Fig. 5.46). The vascular changes are more prominent than in lesser burns, with marked dermal edema and spongiosis. Vesicles and bullae form in the epidermis, often at the dermoepidermal junction. The bullae contain serum, granular debris, and leukocytes. Healing can be complete if secondary infection does not lead to deeper injury.

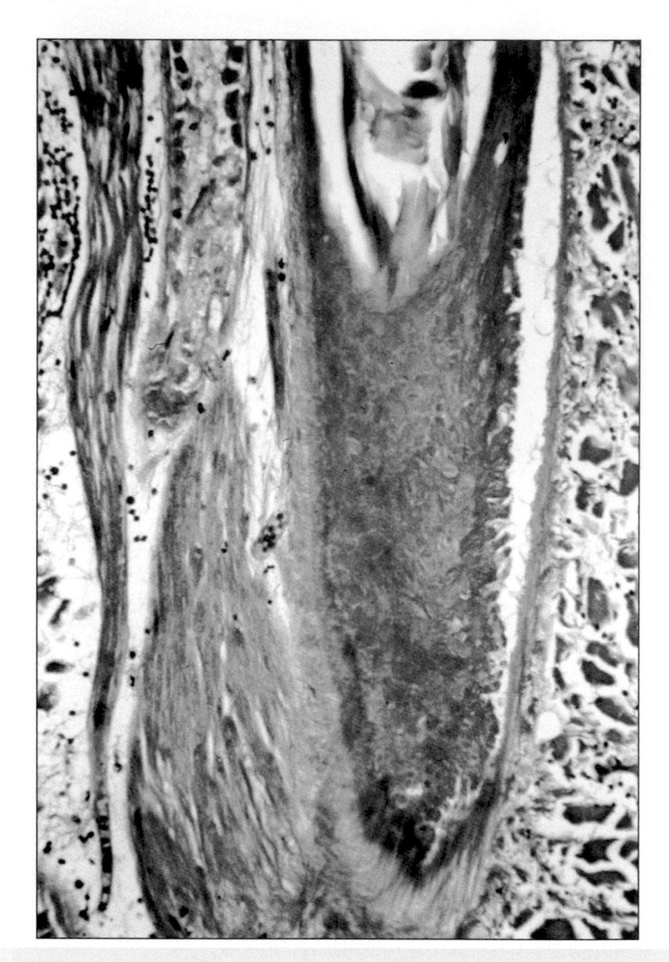

Figure 5.46 Burn. Coagulative necrosis of the epidermis can often "wick" down to involve the follicular epithelium. (Courtesy of B Dunstan.)

- *In* **third-degree burns**, *the destructive effect of the heat extends full thickness through the epidermis and dermis*, causing coagulation necrosis of connective tissues, blood vessels and adnexa. Thermal injury causes thrombosis of blood vessels and vascular leakage leading to the coagulative necrosis of more superficial tissues. Heat of sufficient intensity or duration to penetrate this deeply usually desiccates and chars the outer epidermis. Coagulation necrosis of the dermis produces a swollen amorphous accretion of the connective tissues accompanied by an acute inflammatory reaction. Over time, histiocytes infiltrate the subcutis and fibrosis ensues. Subcutaneous vasculitis may be present. The necrotic tissue sloughs, and the defect is filled in by granulation tissue. Permanent scarring with loss of adnexa results.
- **Fourth-degree burns** *are similar in character to those of third degree but penetrate below the dermis to and beyond the subcutaneous fascia*; their local consequences depend on what lies underneath. Heat in surface tissue is conducted to deeper tissues via the blood and lymph. The degree of injury may not be evident for several days after the insult occurred. Follicular and sweat gland damage continues for 24–48 hours. Once lesions fully develop, the progress of injury should cease, which is helpful in making the diagnosis. Histologically, thermally induced tissue damage is not sharply demarcated and should dissipate gradually with increasing depth of the biopsy. *Clinical differentials* include toxic epidermal necrolysis, erythema

multiforme major, bullous pemphigoid, pemphigus vulgaris, vasculitis, trauma, and other causes of ischemia. Lesions from thermal injury sometimes have an abnormal anatomical distribution or pattern such as drips, angles, lines, or areas of contact that may be helpful in the differential diagnosis.

Microwave burns are unique in that the lesions are sharply delineated histologically without a tapering of the degree of coagulative necrosis in the deeper tissues. The degree of injury is uniform throughout the tissue and inflammation is minimal. The depth of damage depends on the frequency of the microwaves with some frequencies sparing the superficial tissues and coagulating the deeper tissues. Pain perception may not occur until the damage is done and lesions may not be evident for up to 6 days. There is no surface charring, blister formation, or edema. There is thrombosis of vessels and the tissue is mummified. Injury is due to ionizing radiation leading to heat generated from the vibration of molecules in the tissue.

Full-thickness cutaneous burns have been reported to occur in black-haired spots of Dalmatians as a result of **solar radiation**. Normally, cutaneous injury from solar radiation affects lightly pigmented sparsely haired skin rather than areas protected by pigment. *Black skin absorbs approximately 45% more solar radiation than white skin.* The absorption of visible light (400–700 nm) can result in the production of thermal energy resulting in a burn. UV light (100–400 nm) does not penetrate into the dermis and does not produce substantial thermal energy, but has other deleterious effects (see Actinic diseases of skin). Pain, prompting moving to the shade, was likely not perceived by the dogs as the burns were multifocal involving only black-haired areas and Dalmatians are primarily white.

Another unique type of thermal injury, **radiant heat dermatitis**, is similar to *erythema ab igne* in humans. Tissue damage occurs from repeated exposure to moderate heat. Radiant heat dermatitis has been reported as an asymptomatic condition in dogs sleeping next to wood burning stoves or fires, or chronically exposed to heat lamps. The lesions were on the dorsolateral trunk and had a drip-like configuration. Grossly, irregular areas of alopecia were erythematous and hyperpigmented peripherally. Centrally, the lesions are scaly and depigmented. In the acute form, lesions resemble actinic dermatosis with epidermal thinning, basal cell vacuolation, and possible epidermal dysplasia. The dermis has thin fragmented collagen, increased elastin fibers, and melanin and hemosiderin deposits. Over time, epidermal and infundibular hyperplasia, hyperkeratosis and dyskeratosis develop with focal spongiosis and cell necrosis. Karyomegaly of basal cells, dermal edema and mucinosis, hyperplastic sebaceous glands, dilated apocrine glands, and mixed perivascular dermatitis may be present.

Radiation injury

Advances in the treatment of cancer in companion animals have made the possibility of **radiation-induced skin injury** more likely. Clinicians and pathologists need to be able to recognize these lesions in order to provide the best management options and accurate prognosis for resolution of the lesions. *The varieties of radiation modalities available have variable degrees of tissue penetration and potential for tissue injury.* Some forms of radiotherapy penetrate deeper tissues while sparing the skin and others are more concentrated in the superficial tissues or are preferentially absorbed by specific tissues. The type of radiation therapy, source, dose, intensity, and duration of exposure dictate the range of possible side effects. Ionizing photons disrupt chemical bonds in cells leading to injury or cell death. Some cells are not lethally damaged but sustain DNA damage to the extent that replication/replacement are not possible. The effects of radiation damage can be divided into acute and chronic forms.

Acute radiation injury to the skin is a result of damage to rapidly dividing cells. Damage is self-limiting and recovery is associated with rapid cell turnover. Clinical lesions of radiation dermatitis appear 2–4 weeks after exposure. Initially, there is erythema, pain, edema, and heat, followed several weeks later by dry or moist desquamation depending on the degree of injury. Histologically, the lesions resemble a second-degree burn, with suprabasilar or subepidermal bullae formation, dermal edema with fibrin exudation, and a marked leukocytic infiltrate. Re-epithelialization occurs over a period of 10–60 days. The damage sustained to germinal epithelium of hair follicles and sebaceous glands leads to *alopecia* within 2–4 weeks after exposure. Hair re-growth will follow over the next several months but damage to sebaceous glands is not reversible and leads to *permanent scaling*.

The *chronic lesions of radiation injury* are evident months to years after treatment and are primarily *due to damage to the microvasculature*. The epidermis is thin, friable, and in some areas hyperplastic, and may become neoplastic. There is hyperpigmentation and hyperkeratosis. Chronic exudative ulcers may develop but granulation tissue does not form. The dermis is fibrotic with atypical fibroblasts, telangiectasia, and possibly deep arteriolar changes. Endothelial swelling, necrosis and thrombosis lead to occlusion and excessive endothelial proliferation, that when combined with the effects of vascular leakage, leads to vascular collapse. This condition of progressive vessel abnormalities is referred to as *obliterative endoarteritis* and is known to form a "histohematic" barrier to surrounding tissue, leading to continued anoxia and nutrient shortage.

Bibliography

Coyne BE, et al. Thermoelectric burns from improper grounding of electrocautery units: two case reports. J Am Anim Hosp Assoc 1993;29:7–9.
Dernell WS, Wheaton LG. Surgical management of radiation injury-part I. Compend Contin Educ Pract Vet 1995;17:181–190.
Gieser DR, Walker RD. Management of large animal thermal injuries. Compend Contin Educ Pract Vet 1985;7:S69–S78.
Gross TL, Ihrke PJ. Necrotizing diseases of the epidermis. In: Gross TL, et al. eds. Veterinary Dermatopathology. A Macroscopic and Microscopic Evaluation of Canine and Feline Skin Disease. St Louis, Mo: Mosby Year Book, 1992:41–50.
Hargis AM, Lewis TP. Full-thickness cutaneous burn in black-haired skin on the dorsum of the body of a Dalmatian puppy. Vet Dermatol 1999;10:39–42.
Reedy LM, Clubb FJ. Microwave burn in a toy poodle: A case report. J Am Anim Hosp Assoc 1991;27:497–500.
Scarratt WK, et al. Cutaneous thermal injury in a horse. Eq Pract 1984;6:13–17.
Swaim SF, et al. Heating pads and thermal burns in small animals. J Am Anim Hosp Assoc 1989;25:156–162.
Walder EJ, Hargis AM. Chronic moderate heat dermatitis (erythema ab igne) in five dogs, three cats and one silvered langur. Vet Dermatol 2002;13:283–292.

Chemical injury to skin

Primary irritant contact dermatitis

One of the important functions of the skin is to provide protection against external noxious agents. *The stratum corneum is the major protective barrier*. Its integrity is highly dependent on its water content, which in turn is protected by the lipids of the stratum corneum.

Penetration of the skin is enhanced by physical damage to the stratum corneum, chemical alteration of the barrier components, overhydration of the stratum corneum by excess moisture, increased temperature, or alterations of the skin pH. Irritant substances may induce damage by altering the water-holding capacity of the keratin layer or by penetrating the epidermis and directly damaging the cells. Irritant substances vary markedly in their potency. Some, such as strong acids or alkalis, induce immediate and severe tissue damage; others, such as mild detergents or soaps, may require repetitive applications and covering of the area to assist penetration before lesions develop.

Primary irritant contact dermatitis must be distinguished from allergic contact dermatitis (discussed under Hypersensitivity dermatoses). *Irritant contact dermatitis is the more common condition in animals and does not involve prior sensitization.* It may occur in any species, but is most frequent in the horse, cow and dog. The types of agents capable of causing direct cutaneous damage include acids, such as carbolic or sulfuric, alkalis, cresol tars, paints, kerosene, turpentine, antiseptics, and insecticides. An example of the last-mentioned is "flea collar dermatitis" of dogs and cats. Feces and urine are also potential irritants.

The distribution of gross lesions of contact irritant dermatitis in the dog and cat typically involves the glabrous skin of the ventral abdomen, axilla, medial thigh, perianal and perineal areas, footpads (Fig. 5.47A), ventral tail, chin, and inner aspect of the pinnae. The hairy skin is only involved if the irritant substance is in an aerosol or liquid form. Flea collar dermatitis lesions occur as a band around the neck corresponding to the position of the offending collar. In horses, lesions occur most commonly on the muzzle, lower limbs and in areas of contact with the riding tack. Horses with diarrhea may develop severe irritant dermatitis on the soiled perineum.

The *gross lesions*, which typically have a sudden onset, are marked erythema, swelling, and a transient papular-vesicular stage that leads to ulceration and, in severe cases, sloughing of the affected skin. The sequelae include alopecia, scarring, and alteration in skin and hair pigmentation. Hyperpigmentation occurs in most species of domestic animals, but in horses, leukoderma or leukotrichia may be a permanent result of irritant contact dermatitis. Severe lesions can be considered a chemical burn. Differentials include thermal injury and allergic contact dermatitis.

The histologic lesions of irritant contact dermatitis are not pathognomonic, nor can they be distinguished from those of allergic contact dermatitis (Fig. 5.47B). Superficial spongiotic or hyperplastic perivascular dermatitis characterizes both, and vesicles may form. The inflammatory infiltrate is variable in nature, probably reflecting such factors as chronicity, self-trauma and secondary infection. *The diagnosis of irritant contact dermatitis depends largely on the history and the clinical signs, particularly the distribution of the lesions.*

In **swine**, cutaneous erythema and pruritus have been observed within 48 hours of *tiamulin* administration. The most severely affected pigs were recumbent and developed *fatal necrolytic dermatitis*. The areas most severely affected were those in contact with feces and urine. Histologic lesions included full-thickness epidermal necrosis, intraepidermal pustules, and serocellular crusting. It was hypothesized that the lesions represent a severe form of contact

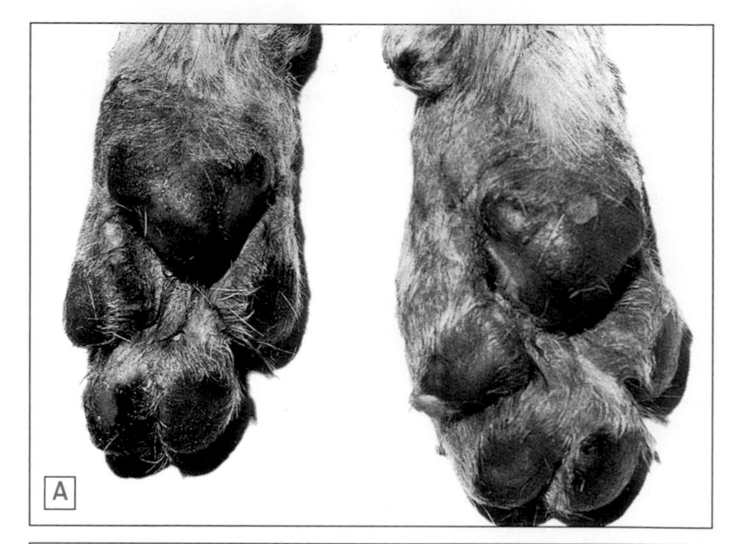

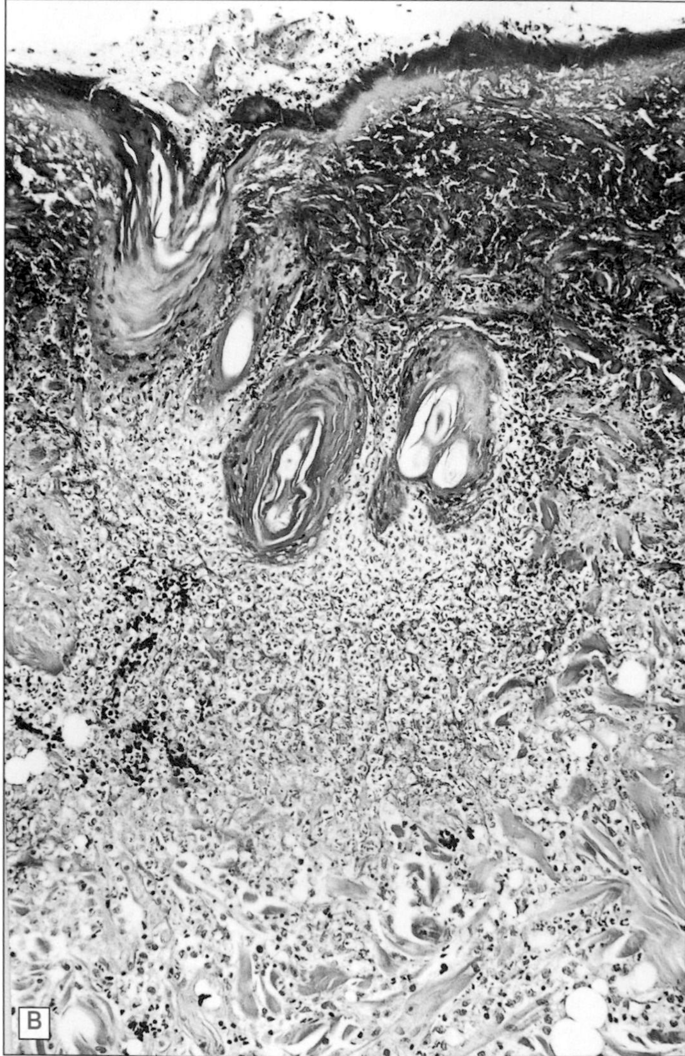

Figure 5.47 Irritant contact dermatitis in a dog. **A.** Footpad swelling and erythema, due to alkali exposure. (Courtesy of RP Johnson.) **B.** Coagulative necrosis of the epidermis and superficial to mid dermis, due to Varsol burn.

irritant dermatitis to tiamulin or one of its metabolites in the excreta. Skin lesions regressed when the drug was withdrawn.

An eosinophilic dermatitis was observed in pigs following heavy salting of pen floors. Lesions were present on the feet.

Bibliography

Andersson P, Petaja E. Profound eosinophilic dermatitis in swine caused by sodium chloride. Nord Vet Med 1968;20:706–707.

Gross TL, Ihrke PJ. Spongiotic diseases of the epidermis. In: Gross TL, et al., eds. Veterinary Dermatopathology. St. Louis, MO: Mosby Year Book, 1992:52–57.

Lapèrle A. Dermatite aigue chez des porcs traités à la tiamuline. Med Vét Quebec 1990;20:20–22.

Nesbitt GH, Schmitz JA. Contact dermatitis in the dog: A review of 35 cases. J Am Anim Hosp Assoc 1977;13:155–163.

Scott DW, et al. Small Animal Dermatology. 5th ed. Philadelphia, PA: WB Saunders, 1995:867–869.

Envenomation

The venom of insects, spiders, other arthropods and snakes can cause mild or severe skin lesions with or without systemic signs. Effects are dependent upon composition of the venom, individual victim response, anatomic location of the envenomation, and specific characteristics of the offending organism which may be influenced by season of the year, geographic location, time since last inflicted bite or sting, depth of injury, etc. Different species of animals respond differently to the same venom.

Stings from *Solenopsis invicta*, the **imported fire ant** are common in humans in South America and in most of the southern United States. The ants swarm by the hundreds, covering objects or parts of victims and simultaneously inflict numerous painful stings. The fire ant venom is primarily comprised of an insoluble alkaloid (solenopsin A), shown to be cytotoxic, bactericidal, fungicidal, insecticidal, and hemolytic. Lesions in dogs have been documented and consist of initial swelling progressing to erythematous nodules within 10–20 minutes. Histologically, the sting in dogs produces a vertically oriented zone of coagulative dermal necrosis with variable epidermal necrosis. Necrosis includes the adnexa and may extend into the subcutis. Lesions resolve quickly. Severe type I hypersensitivity (anaphylaxis) reactions are possible.

Stings from **hymenopteran insects** such as *bees, wasps, and hornets* produce effects of a local (angioedema) or possibly systemic type I hypersensitivity reaction due to the histamine, serotonin, and kinins in the venom (see Hypersensitivity dermatoses). Multiple stings dermatoses lead to toxic reactions that can be fatal.

Spider bites are rarely documented definitively in animal or human patients as the initial bite goes unnoticed and the spider is no longer recoverable by the time lesions develop. Bites occur most often on the face and extremities. Most spider bites produce localized pain, erythema and swelling and are not of further consequence. Spiders of importance to the study of the integumentary system are those with venoms leading to *dermonecrosis and eschar formation, a condition referred to as "necrotic arachnidism."* The **brown recluse spider** (*Loxosceles reclusus*) is the spider most well-known to induce dermal necrosis, although there are a number of others. Brown recluse venom contains hyaluronidase and sphingomyelinase-D, which degrade tissues. A blister with a surrounding pale halo and more peripheral erythema characterizes initial reactions documented in humans and some experimental animals. Necrosis and eschar formation occur within 5–7 days. Ulceration may be extensive. Histologically, there is hemorrhage and edema, neutrophilic vasculitis and arterial wall necrosis. The epidermis and dermis undergo necrosis that may extend into the subcutis and underlying muscle. Panniculitis may be present. Eventually, there is dermal scarring and replacement of the subcutis and muscle by hypocellular connective tissue. Brown recluse spider bites in humans can also lead to massive hemolysis. *Differentials include other venomous bites, vasculitis, slough due to iatrogenic injection of irritating substances, thermal burns, necrotizing fasciitis or other cutaneous infection, septic embolization, or trauma.* Compatible lesions, environmental history, and ruling out other conditions producing similar lesions can lead to the presumptive diagnosis of a spider bite.

Snakebite envenomation produces local tissue necrosis and variable systemic effects. Snake venom contains various enzymes, proteins, peptides, and kinins. Systemic effects of snake venom include paralysis, coagulation disturbances, shock, increased capillary permeability, myocardial damage, rhabdomyolysis, and renal failure. Of the five genera of venomous snakes, *crotaline* (rattlesnake, copperhead, cottonmouth and others) *venom* contains the highest concentration of proteolytic enzymes. Local effects include pain, edema, hemorrhage, bullae formation, necrosis, and sloughing of tissue. Bites inflicted in the head or neck region may lead to swelling that interferes with respiration. Bites of pit vipers also introduce potentially dangerous bacteria such as *Clostridial* sp. into the puncture wound. Bites are common in the dog, horse, and, to a lesser degree, cats, and most often are inflicted on the head or legs. The differential diagnoses are similar to those for necrotic arachnidism.

Bibliography

Cowell AK, et al. Severe systemic reactions to *Hymenoptera* stings in three dogs. J Am Vet Med Assoc 1991;198:1014–1016.

da Silva PH, et al. Brown spiders and loxoscelism. Toxicon 2004;44:693–709.

Dickinson CE, et al. Rattlesnake venom poisoning in horses: 32 cases (1973–1993). J Am Vet Med Assoc 1996;208:1866–1871.

Friberg CA, Lewis DT. Insect hypersensitivity in small animals. Compend Contin Educ Pract Vet 1998;20:1121–1131.

Hudelson S, Hudelson P. Pathophysiology of snake envenomation and evaluation of treatments - Part I. Compend Contin Educ Pract Vet 1995;17:889–896.

Rakich PM, et al. Clinical and histologic characterization of cutaneous reactions to stings of the imported fire ant (*Solenopsis invicta*) in dogs. Vet Pathol 1993;30:555–559.

Sams HH, et al. Necrotic arachnidism. J Am Acad Dermatol 2001;44:561–573.

Thallotoxicosis

The heavy metal thallium is a potent toxin with pharmacological actions similar to lead and mercury. Thallium salts are odorless, tasteless, colorless, and water soluble. Thallium was used extensively as a rodenticide and insecticide prior to 1963 when its sale to the general public in the United States and some other countries was banned. It continued to be used by government agencies as a pesticide and in various industries, such as the manufacture of optical lenses, jewelry, and scintillation counters, until the US Environmental Protection Agency banned thallium manufacture in 1972. Thallium is still used in some parts of the world, and its use may increase as pests develop resistance to more selective poisons.

Accidental or malicious thallium poisoning is rare and is due to the use of undestroyed supplies of old, but newly exposed baits. *It occurs chiefly in dogs*, less often in cats and is reported in sheep, cattle and pigs. The LD_{50} for the dog is 10–15 mg/kg, and the toxin is cumulative. Absorption occurs rapidly from the gastrointestinal and respiratory tracts and skin. The toxin is disseminated widely in the body and is persistent, being very slowly excreted in bile and urine.

The mechanism of toxicity is not fully understood. There are two main hypotheses. The first holds that thallium exerts its toxic effect by combining with sulfhydryl groups, a mechanism common to many heavy metals and leading to disruption of mitochondrial respiratory chain enzymes. The second, which is based on the similarity of ionic radii between thallium and potassium, suggests that thallium may replace potassium in many critical biochemical functions, thus acting as a general cellular poison. The toxic effect may be, in part, due to thallium interacting adversely with derivatives of riboflavin. Thallium can depolarize nerve cell membranes and antagonize effects of calcium on the heart.

The clinical effects depend on the dose and rapidity of administration. Signs of *acute thallotoxicosis* are evident within 12 hours of exposure and are characterized by severe gastrointestinal irritation and neurological signs, including motor paralysis. Glossitis, stomatitis, rhinitis, and bronchitis develop. Death by respiratory failure may occur. Animals may survive the acute episode to develop the chronic syndrome or may bypass the acute disease altogether. Cutaneous, renal and neurological abnormalities, progressive debilitation, and death characterize the *chronic syndrome*.

The *cutaneous lesions* develop 7–10 days after ingestion of thallium and principally affect frictional areas. The pattern of skin involvement in cats and dogs is characteristic, beginning at the commissures of the lips or nasal cleft, occasionally on the ear margins and expanding over the face and head. The mucous membranes are characteristically "brick-red" and may be ulcerated. Lesions also develop on the interdigital skin, footpads, axillae, inguinal areas, perineum and lateral extensor surfaces. The lesions are *marked erythema, scaling, alopecia, exudation, and crusting*. The layers of scale-crust exfoliate with attached hairs to leave a raw, oozing surface. The paws often become very swollen. In more chronic cases, thick scales on the footpads resemble "hard pad" disease conventionally associated with canine distemper. In less severely affected animals, *ease of depilation may be the only clinical indication of thallium poisoning*. The pathogenesis of the alopecia is not fully understood. While thallium enters the hair, as do other heavy metals, by binding to sulfhydryl groups in the keratin, this is unlikely to be destructive to the hair follicle. Thallium may interfere with the energy metabolism of the rapidly dividing matrix cells of anagen follicles. In experimental intoxication of rats, a rapid decline in the mitotic rate is followed by necrosis of the matrix cells within 48 hours. The follicle passes into an abnormal catagen phase followed by complete involution (telogen). However, no club attachment is formed and the hairs are rapidly shed. If the animal survives, hair growth is resumed. Thallium also severely alters the keratinization process and both the surface and external root sheath epithelium demonstrate marked parakeratotic hyperkeratosis.

The *microscopic lesions* in the skin are dominated by *massive, diffuse parakeratotic hyperkeratosis*, which affects both surface and external root sheath epithelia. There is accompanying follicular plugging, hypogranulosis and epidermal hyperplasia (Fig. 5.48). Neutrophil exocytosis and spongiform pustules develop in both surface and follicular epithelia. Partial or full thickness necrosis of the surface epithelium may also occur. The dermal lesions include marked hyperemia, edema, erythrocytic exocytosis and infiltration of neutrophils and mononuclear cells. There may be focal necrosis of sweat and sebaceous glands. Hair follicles are mostly in catagen or telogen. Degenerative changes are noted in anagen follicles.

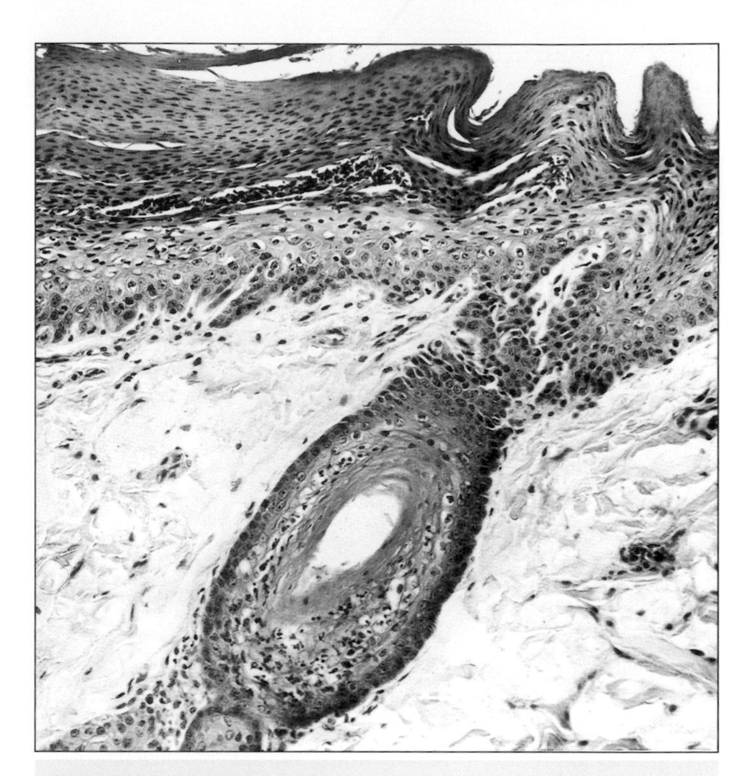
Figure 5.48 Thallium toxicity in a dog. Marked parakeratosis.

Histologic lesions in *other tissues* include multifocal necrosis of myocardial and skeletal muscle fibers, nephrosis, pulmonary edema, reticuloendothelial hyperplasia and lymphoid depletion of spleen and lymph nodes. Secondary bacterial bronchopneumonia may occur as a result of the damage to ciliated epithelia and resultant disturbance of the mucociliary apparatus. Hemorrhagic gastroenteritis occurs in acute thallotoxicosis. Focal suppurative pancreatitis has been described in several animals, but its causal relationship to thallium is not established. Ulcerative esophagitis follows dilation secondary to neuronal damage. Lesions in the central nervous system include neuronal chromatolysis, neuronophagia, and severe edema with little glial reaction. Myelinated peripheral nerves have degenerative lesions including focal distension of myelin sheaths and swelling and occasional fragmentation of axons.

The *differential diagnoses* of acute thallium toxicity include other heavy metal toxicoses, infectious and noninfectious causes of hemorrhagic gastroenteritis, and pancreatitis. Differentials for the clinical lesions include superficial necrolytic dermatitis, zinc-responsive dermatosis, generic dog food dermatosis, toxic epidermal necrolysis, mucocutaneous candidiasis, epitheliotropic lymphoma, and autoimmune diseases such as pemphigus vulgaris and bullous pemphigoid. The *microscopic lesions of thallium toxicosis, zinc-responsive dermatosis, and superficial necrolytic dermatitis are similar* and confirmation requires a compatible history and demonstration of thallium in the urine by the Gabriel–Dubin colorimetric assay or in the stomach contents, suspected bait, urine, liver or kidneys by atomic absorption spectroscopy.

Bibliography

Arbiser JL, et al. Effects of thallium ion on cellular components of the skin. J Dermatol 1997;24:147–155.

Galvan-Arzate S, Santamaria A. Thallium toxicity. Toxicol Lett 1998;99:1–13.

Mulkey JP, Oehme FW. A review of thallium toxicity. Vet Hum Toxicol 1993;35:445–453.

Thomas ML, McKeever PJ. Chronic thallium toxicosis in a dog. J Am Anim Hosp Assoc 1993;29:211–215.

Zook BC, et al. Thallium poisoning in cats. J Am Vet Med Assoc 1968;153:285–299.

Arsenic toxicosis

Arsenic is the metal most toxic to the skin and is found as a component of wood preservatives, herbicides, insecticides, insulation materials, paint pigments, feed additives, and some medications, and is a by-product of some mining activities. It is a water supply contaminant in some parts of Mexico, Argentina, Chile, Taiwan, India, the UK, and the USA. Safe standards for levels of arsenic in drinking water have not been established. Arsenic is absorbed by the gastrointestinal tract and skin and is excreted in urine, bile, milk, hair, nails, and exfoliated epidermal cells. Its presence in the skin increases the skin's susceptibility to damage by UV light. Chronic arsenic exposure in humans occurs in environmental (water contamination) and industrial settings and is associated with increased incidence of visceral and cutaneous malignancies, Bowen's disease, palmar and solar hyperkeratoses, and cutaneous pigmentary disturbances. The generation of free radicals with resultant nucleic acid damage is suspected to be involved in arsenic-related carcinogenesis. Arsenic may lead to cellular proliferation through increased production of keratinocyte-derived growth factors. *Urine, hair, and liver are the tissues of choice for establishing arsenic exposure.*

Acute arsenic poisoning is an important toxicosis in domestic animals, particularly cattle and dogs, and is due to sulfhydryl group binding and inhibition of cellular metabolism. Signs and lesions are referable to the gastrointestinal tract, liver, and kidneys. Skin lesions are the result of chronic systemic low-level arsenic exposure or to direct contact. *Arsenic is an established low-grade corrosive that produces irritant contact dermatitis.* Contact lesions occur in animals sprayed or dipped in a concentrated arsenic solution or in dogs lying on heavily contaminated ground. Lesions include erythema and epidermal necrosis leading to the formation of non-healing ulcers. Lesions may affect oral cavity, lips, other mucocutaneous junctions and the feet. Less is known about the effects of chronic systemic exposure of arsenic on the skin in animals, however, chronic arsenic poisoning in farm animals is associated with ill thrift and a dry, seborrheic, alopecic coat.

Bibliography

Col M, et al. Arsenic-related Bowen's disease, palmar keratoses, and skin cancer. Environ Health Perspect 1999;107:687–689.

Evinger JV, Blakemore JC. Dermatitis in a dog associated with exposure to an arsenic compound. J Am Vet Med Assoc 1984;184:1281–1282.

Germolec DR, et al. Arsenic enhancement of skin neoplasia by chronic stimulation of growth factors. Am J Pathol 1998;153:1775–1785.

Lansdown ABG. Physiological and toxicological changes in the skin resulting from the action and interaction of metal ions. Crit Rev Toxicol 1995;25:397–462.

Pace LW, et al. Acute arsenic toxicosis in five horses. Vet Pathol 1997;34:160–164.

Thomas DJ, et al. The cellular metabolism and systemic toxicity of arsenic. Toxicol Appl Pharmacol 2001;176:127–144.

Mercury toxicosis

Organomercurial toxicosis in domestic animals is associated chiefly with neurologic and renal disorders and is discussed in Vol. 1, Nervous system and Vol. 2, Urinary system, respectively. In chronic poisoning in **cattle**, skin manifestations including *pustules, ulcers, hyperkeratosis and alopecia* at the tail head are described, but their pathogenesis is poorly understood. **Horses** ingesting mercury-treated seed grain develop *total body alopecia*, followed by loss of the long hairs of mane, tail and forelock. The hooves are not affected and the cutaneous lesion is mild scaling. Experimental chronic methylmercury intoxication in horses produces *exudative dermatitis*, but histologic lesions are not described. Local toxic contact dermatitis follows application of mercurial-containing counterirritants to the legs in horses.

Bibliography

Irving F, Butler DG. Ammoniated mercury toxicity in cattle. Can Vet J 1975;16:260–264.

Seawright AA, et al. Chronic methylmercurialism in a horse. Vet Hum Toxicol 1978;20:6–9.

Cutaneous iodism

Iodides have widespread use as antiseptics, expectorants, intravenous contrast agents, bronchodilators, antithyrotoxicants, and as salt or feed additives. Iodine is readily absorbed from the skin. The majority of reports of adverse effects of iodine occur as hypersensitivity reactions and not toxicoses. *Generalized seborrhea sicca* is reported in horses and cattle accidentally overdosed with iodine-containing drugs or medicated feed. In experimental toxicosis of calves, the cutaneous lesions were limited to scaly patches without alopecia. Conversely, suspected iodism in a horse produced generalized alopecia, sparing only the face, mane and tail.

Bibliography

Fadok VA, Wild S. Suspected cutaneous iodism in a horse. J Am Vet Med Assoc 1983;10:1104–1106.

Ginn PE, et al. Self-limiting subepidermal bullous disease in a neonatal foal. Vet Dermatol 1998;9:249–256.

Mangkoewidjojo S, et al. Pathologic features of iodide toxicosis in calves. Am J Vet Res 1980;41:1057–1061.

Selenium toxicosis

Selenium is a metalloid that acts as an antioxidant with toxic potential. It has chemical properties similar to sulfur. It is excreted from the body in urine, feces, and sweat and integumentary structures. Experimental studies in rodents suggest that selenium may diminish UV radiation-induced skin damage when applied topically. However, some forms are strong contact irritants and vesiculants. The toxic potential of selenium in the diet varies by the chemical form present, nature of the diet, rate of consumption, and by the species and individual animal. The mechanism by which selenium might exert its effects on the integument and appendages is not known, but conceivably, being competitive with sulfur, it modifies the structure of keratin.

Selenium is widely distributed in soils at concentrations ranging from 0.01 parts per million (ppm) or less to 500 ppm or more. Areas of high soil concentration are particularly extensive in parts of the USA (Wyoming, Montana, Utah, Colorado, North and South Dakota, Arizona, Kansas, and Nebraska) and in western Canada, but also occur in parts of Australia, New Zealand, China, Ireland, Mexico, and Israel, among other countries.

Selenium toxicosis occurs in *horses, cattle, sheep, and pigs*, chiefly as a result of the ingestion of plants that have accumulated toxic levels of selenium, but occasionally as a result of accidental overdose of selenium supplements. Plants are divisible into seleniferous and nonseleniferous species. **Seleniferous plants** can selectively concentrate selenium in their foliage and seeds as compared with nonseleniferous species grown under the same conditions. The seleniferous species are subdivided into obligate accumulators, which require high levels of selenium for survival and facultative accumulators. The former, which include members of the genus *Astragalus*, *Machaeranthera* and *Stanleya,* may accumulate over 1000 ppm selenium. Because of their high requirement for selenium, they are known as "indicator" species. Facultative or secondary selenium accumulators such as *Aster, Atriplex, Castilleja,* and *Gutierrezia* take up lesser amounts of selenium. Many nonseleniferous weeds, crop plants, and grasses are capable of passively accumulating selenium if growing on soils with high selenium content. Also, indicator plants increase the availability of selenium to nonseleniferous plants by converting insoluble selenites to soluble selenates and returning these to the soil. Selenium poisoning can occur whenever seleniferous plants are eaten irrespective of levels of selenium in the soil, and it can occur whenever the levels of water-soluble selenium in the soil are high, irrespective of the botanical composition.

Seleniferous plants are not palatable and indigenous stock learns to avoid them. Selenium poisoning occurs chiefly in newly introduced or traveling animals and in indigenous animals forced to eat the seleniferous plants in times of scarcity. Clinically, there are acute and chronic syndromes associated with the ingestion of seleniferous plants such as *Astragalus* and *Oxytropis*. *Acute toxicity* causes severe gastrointestinal and cardiovascular signs with mortality in some instances approaching 100%. Two different syndromes have been described as *chronic selenium poisoning*. "**Blind staggers**," characterized by neurological signs, is probably not due to selenium alone but to other toxic principles in the seleniferous plants. The second syndrome is named "**alkali disease**" because it was originally believed that the pH of the selenium-rich soils was a factor in its pathogenesis. Unlike blind staggers, alkali disease is reproducible in ungulates fed sublethal concentrations of selenium. The presence of internal lesions such as nephrosis, myocardial degeneration, and hepatic fibrosis in chronically poisoned livestock is not found in experimentally reproduced disease, suggesting other factors are involved.

Horses and cattle chronically intoxicated with selenium become emaciated and develop partial alopecia and a general roughness of coat. Foals delivered from affected mares may have lesions. Initially, there is loss of the long hairs in the mane, forelock, and tail of horses (leading to the name "bobtail" disease), and loss of the long tail hairs in cattle. Sheep do not show cutaneous lesions, although in Australia fleece shedding has been attributed to selenium toxicity on some properties.

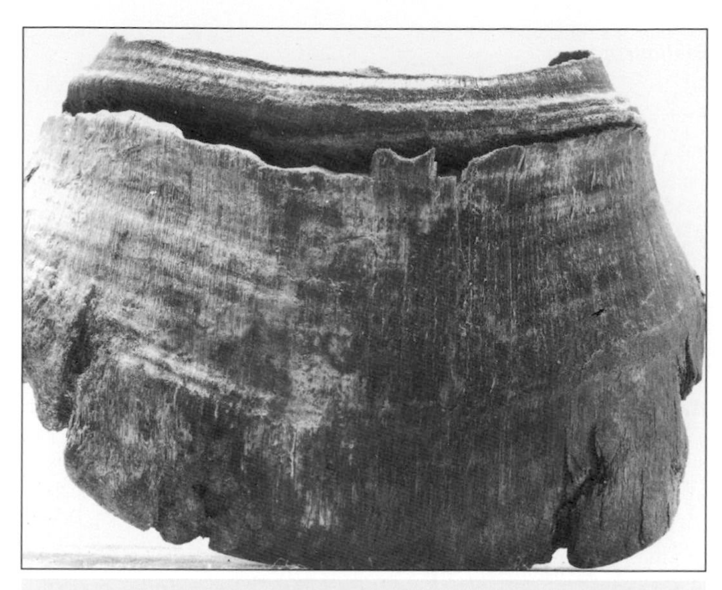

Figure 5.49 Selenium toxicosis in a horse. Hoof wall deformed by rings and grooves. (Courtesy of Queensland Department of Agriculture.)

Selenium toxicity is also suspected in alopecias of the beard and flanks of goats in the western United States. In all species, lesions commencing at the coronary band may lead to separation and shedding of the hoof or to the formation of dystrophic grooves, cracks, or corrugations that parallel the coronary band resulting in lameness (Fig. 5.49). Lesions take months to develop. *Histologic lesions* of experimental chronic selenium toxicosis in cattle showed extensive separation of the stratum medium of the hoof with replacement by parakeratotic cellular debris. The germinal epithelium of the hoof wall was disorganized, parakeratotic and hyperplastic. Hair follicles from the tail were atrophic with dyskeratosis and mild hyperkeratosis.

Diagnosis requires the demonstration of compatible clinical signs, progression of lesions, and identification of a dietary source of selenium with a concentration in the air-dried feed sample of >5 ppm selenium. High levels of selenium in the blood (>2 ppm) or integumentary tissues such as hair, hoofwall or sole (>10 ppm) should also be present. Individual animals have a variable response to selenium exposure and some animals with high levels of selenium may not show signs of toxicosis.

Bibliography

Burke KE, et al. The effects of topical and oral L-selenomethionine on pigmentation and skin cancer induced by ultraviolet irradiation. Nutr Cancer 1992; 17:123–137.

Davidson-York D, et al. Selenium elimination in pigs after an outbreak of selenium toxicosis. J Vet Diagn Invest 1999;11:352–357.

O'Toole D, Raisbeck MF. Pathology of experimentally induced chronic selenosis (alkali disease) in yearling cattle. J Vet Diagn Invest 1995;7:364–373.

Raisbeck MF. Selenosis. Vet Clin North Am Food Anim Pract 2000;16:465–480.

Stowe HD, et al. Selenium toxicosis in feeder pigs. J Am Vet Med Assoc 1992;201:292–295.

Tinggi U. Essentiality and toxicity of selenium and its status in Australia: a review. Toxicol Lett 2003;137:103–110.

Traub-Dargatz JL, Hamar DW. Selenium toxicity in horses. Compend Contin Educ Pract Vet 1986;8:771–776.

Van Kampen KR, James LF. Manifestations of intoxication by selenium-accumulating plants. In: Keeler RF, et al., eds. Effects of Poisonous Plants on Livestock. New York: Academic Press, 1978:135–138.

Witte ST, et al. Chronic selenosis in horses fed locally produced alfalfa hay. J Am Vet Med Assoc 1993;202:406–409.

Organochlorine and organobromine toxicoses

Organochlorine and organobromine compounds implicated in toxicities causing, among others, cutaneous lesions, include the *highly chlorinated naphthalenes (HCN)*, *polybrominated biphenyls (PBBs)*, and *dibenzofurans*. *Polychlorinated biphenyls (PCBs)* are the cause of an important industrial dermatitis of humans known as *chloracne*.

Highly chlorinated naphthalene (HCN) toxicosis (X-disease, bovine hyperkeratosis), the result of exposure to tetra-, penta-, hexa-, hepta-, or octachloronaphthalenes, is largely of *historical interest*. HCNs were found to be responsible for high mortality and large economic losses in the cattle industry within the United States, Australia, New Zealand, and Germany during the 1940s and early 1950s. HCN was a common additive in many petroleum products including those used as lubricants for farm machinery such as feed pelleting equipment, wood preservatives, roofing paper and building board. HCNs were a frequent feed contaminant. *These chemicals have not been used in lubricants since 1953*. Recent reports are the result of animals exposed to dumps with stores of old lubricant or abandoned machinery lubricated years ago with HCN containing products. Percutaneous exposure produces cutaneous lesions, whereas parenteral exposure results in both cutaneous and visceral lesions. The poison is cumulative and the disease is chronic. Lesions of HCN toxicity result from interference with the conversion of carotene to vitamin A and resemble the lesions of vitamin A deficiency. The first sign of poisoning is a fall in vitamin A levels in the plasma.

Cattle are the most susceptible species. Initial signs are increased lacrimation and drooling, depression, decreased appetite, and weight loss. Within the first few months, *hallmark cutaneous lesions of marked alopecia with nonpruritic, lichenified, deeply fissured plaques of hyperkeratotic scale are evident on the skin of the neck, shoulders and perineum*. Lesions gradually generalize, sparing only the legs. Marked involvement of the skin of the medial thighs is characteristic. Horn growth may be delayed. The animal may die before the skin lesions are severe, if exposure is high. Concurrent severe secondary infections with *Bovine papular stomatitis virus*, papilloma virus or dermatophytes may be present. The histologic lesions are marked hyperkeratosis of surface and follicular epithelia. Internal lesions are the result of hyperplasia and squamous metaplasia of the epithelial lining of ducts and glands of the body including liver, pancreas, kidneys, and reproductive tract. Bulls may present with epididymal enlargement early in the disease process from hyperplasia and squamous metaplasia of ducts.

Differential diagnoses include other markedly hyperkeratotic dermatopathies such as zinc or vitamin A deficiency, dermatophilosis, dermatophytosis, or toxicosis due to other polyhalogenated aromatic compounds. Definitive diagnosis is dependent upon identification of a source of HCN and extraction of the toxin by capillary gas chromatography and mass spectrometry. Vitamin A levels in the plasma and liver are low, but toxicosis cannot be reversed by vitamin A therapy and the prognosis is poor.

Cutaneous lesions in **cats** exposed to wood preservatives have been ascribed to chlorinated naphthalene toxicity. The lesions include bilateral alopecia and encrustations on the eyelid and around the nostrils.

Pentachlorophenol (PCP)-contaminated wood shavings used as bedding led to chronic toxicity characterized by a *proliferative dermatitis* with crusting, scaling and alopecia accompanied by a *multitude of systemic signs* including peripheral edema, bone marrow hypoplasia, liver disease and wasting in a group of horses. Gross and histologic cutaneous lesions resembled those of HCN toxicity. Wood shavings containing four times the maximal allowable levels of PCP/kg were traced to a lumber company using improper processing techniques. Toxicity was attributed to dibenzofuran and chlorinated dibenzo-p-dioxin isomers found as contaminants of the PCP. *Contaminants of PCP products include a large group of dioxin isomers with a wide range of toxicity that can vary by species exposed and among animals within the species*. PCP compounds are used as antiseptics, disinfectants, herbicides, fungicides, and wood and hide preservatives. The toxicity of the herbicide, agent Orange, widely sprayed in Vietnam, is attributed to *dioxin contaminants*. The compounds enter the body via oral, dermal, or respiratory routes. High exposure leads to rapid death due to uncoupling of mitochondrial oxidative phosphorylation. Chronic toxicity is more common. The contaminants in the PCP compounds are thought to bind to aromatic hydrocarbon receptors in the cell nucleus and influence gene expression. The response may be proliferative or suppressive. Elevated levels of the compounds can be demonstrated in the liver and adipose tissue years after exposure, whereas serum levels are cleared quickly. Similar cases of dioxin isomer toxicity have been reported in *horses* exposed to riding arenas sprayed with contaminated waste oil used for dust control.

Bibliography

Carter CD, et al. Tetrachlorodibenzodioxin: an accidental poisoning episode in horse arenas. Science 1975;188:738–740.

Fries GF. The PBB episode in Michigan: an overall appraisal. CRC Crit Rev Toxicol 1985;16:105–156.

Kerkvliet NI, et al. Dioxin intoxication from chronic exposure of horses to pentachlorophenol-contaminated wood shavings. J Am Vet Med Assoc 1992;201:296–302.

Panciera RJ, et al. Bovine hyperkeratosis: Historical review and report of an outbreak. Compend Contin Educ Pract Vet 1993;15:1287–1294.

Mimosine toxicosis

Mimosine is a *toxic amino acid* found as a main constituent in the tropical to subtropical, cultivated *leguminous shrubs*, *Mimosa pudica* and *Leucaena leucocephala* (formerly *L. glauca*). Mimosine and its metabolite, 3-hydroxy-4-(1H)-pyridone (DHP), are toxic. In ruminants, mimosine is a depilatory, whereas DHP is a goitrogen. Poisoning can be acute or chronic and is characterized by *alopecia*, *poor growth*, *oral ulcerations*, and *goiter* not prevented by iodine supplementation. Toxicity occurs in a number of countries and goes by a variety of local names: *jumbey* in the West Indies, *lamtoro* in Indonesia, and *koa haole* in Hawaii. A variation of animal susceptibility to mimosine toxicity in different parts of the world is due to the geographic distribution of ruminal bacteria capable of degrading DHP. In vitro antemortem assays for detection of DHP-degrading bacteria can be performed on feces or ruminal contents. A group of bacteria, *Synergistes jonesii*, can be inoculated into the rumen of livestock to prevent toxicity. Mimosine has been shown to reduce DNA synthesis and to block the progression of the cell cycle by chelating iron. DHP prevents iodine binding in the thyroid gland. *Mimosine toxicity occurs in horses, cattle, pigs, and sheep* and has been experimentally reproduced in cattle and laboratory animals.

Horses appear to be most susceptible and lose their hair, especially the long hair of the mane and tail. In severe cases, there is patchy loss of hair above and below the hocks and knees and on the flanks and neck. Disturbed growth at the coronet and periople may produce dystrophic rings on the hooves. There is loss of condition and weakness that perhaps is attributable to malnutrition rather than to mimosine.

Mimosine has a marked depilatory action on the fleece of **sheep**. The fleece becomes easily epilated 14 days after a single oral dose of 400–650 mg/kg body weight. DNA synthesis in the wool follicles is reduced. Mimosine toxicity causing depilation in **pigs** is reported from Indonesia and the Bahamas.

Bibliography

Hammond AC. *Leucaena* toxicosis and its control in ruminants. Review. J Anim Sci 1995;73:1487–1492.

Kulp KS, Vulliet PR. Mimosine blocks cell cycle progression by chelating iron in asynchronous human breast cancer cells. Toxicol Appl Pharmacol 1996;139:356–364.

Mladenov E, Anachkova B. DNA breaks induction by mimosine. Z Naturforsch [C] 2003;58:732–735.

Reis PJ, et al. Fate of mimosine administered orally to sheep and its effectiveness as a defleecing agent. Aust J Biol Sci 1975;28:495–501.

Gangrenous ergotism and fescue toxicosis

These two conditions can be considered together because the cutaneous lesions of chronic ergotism caused by *Claviceps purpurea* and those of poisoning by tall fescue, *Festuca arundinacea* or *F. eliator*, are identical.

Ergotism is the oldest known mycotoxicosis. The ergot of *Claviceps* spp. fungi is a *compacted mass of hyphae, the sclerotium*, which develops in the seed heads of many species of grasses and cereal grains and completely replaces the ovary. *Ergotism is the disease that results from ingestion of toxic alkaloids produced by the fungi*. The alkaloids are derivatives of lysergic acid and include *ergotamine, ergometrine and ergotoxine*, which is a composite of three alkaloids. The quantity and spectrum of alkaloids in the ergots vary considerably with the strain of fungus, type of plant, season of the year, climatic conditions and other regional factors. The ergots also produce a *variety of amines*, such as histamine, acetylcholine and other nitrogenous compounds with physiological activity.

Of the various pharmacological effects exerted by the ergot alkaloids, the most important in the pathogenesis of gangrenous ergotism is direct stimulation of adrenergic nerves supplying arteriolar smooth muscle. This produces *marked peripheral vasoconstriction*. Arteriolar spasm and damage to capillary endothelium leads to thrombosis and ischemic necrosis of tissues.

Gangrenous ergotism caused by *C. purpurea* is a disease mainly of cattle. It may occur in animals at pasture but is more common in housed animals fed infected grain. Gangrenous ergotism represents the chronic form of intoxication by ergot-producing fungi. Chronic ergotism develops after a week of feeding contaminated grain and begins with *acute lameness with redness and swelling of the extremities*. The hindlegs are more frequently affected than the forelegs. Lesions seldom extend above the fetlock (Fig. 5.50), but ischemic necrosis may extend to the mid-metatarsus. The feet become cold and insensitive with dry necrosis and a prominent line of separation between viable and dead tissue. The necrotic tissue may slough. Ergotism also causes *dry gangrene of the tips of the ears and tail*. Gangrenous ergotism has been described in goats feeding on ergot-infected pasture. The toxicosis can be produced experimentally in sheep, but the syndrome is quite different from that in cattle, being characterized by ulceration of the tongue and of the alimentary mucosae. Sows are relatively resistant but may develop agalactia as a result of central inhibition of prolactin secretion.

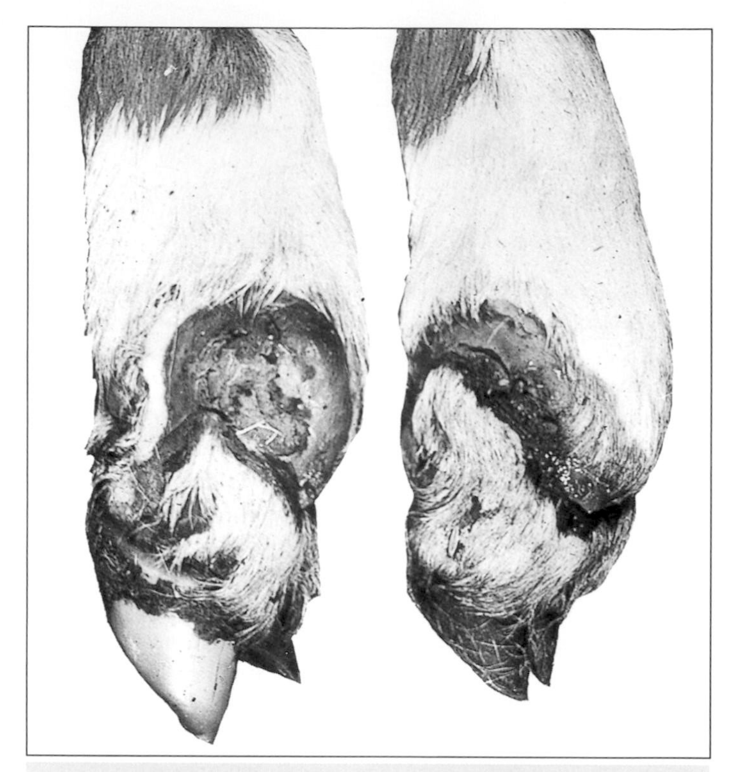

Figure 5.50 Ergotism in a calf. Sharply demarcated ischemic necrosis of distal extremities.

Fescue toxicosis has a variable presentation depending upon the animal species exposed. The most common manifestation, "*fescue foot*," is a disease of *cattle* characterized in the acute form by *dry gangrene of the extremities* commencing 2 weeks after ingestion of the tall fescue grass, *Festuca arundinacea*. This perennial grass is the most common pasture plant in the United States and is usually harmless. The endophytic fungus *Neotyphodium (Acremonium) coenophialum* infects approximately 75% of fescue pastures and imparts increased resistance of the plant to insects and extreme environmental temperatures. Under certain poorly understood conditions, the endophyte-infected plant is toxic. Fescue foot tends to occur with the onset of colder weather indicating that low ambient temperatures may contribute to its development. The alkaloids, *ergonovine, ergotamine, and N-acetyl loline* are responsible for toxicity and act as *peripheral vasoconstrictors*. The acute syndrome in cattle is virtually identical to ergotism.

A chronic disease in **cattle**, known as "summer slump," refers to an increased susceptibility to heat stress seen in certain breeds of cattle in conditions of high environmental temperature combined with intake of endophyte-infected fescue. Cattle have decreased skin temperature and open-mouth breathing suggesting defective thermoregulation. Experimental intravenous injection of alkaloids found in fescue produced lowered skin temperature, heart rate, and prolactin levels, and elevated blood pressure and respiratory rates in heifers. Ingestion of endophyte-infected fescue in **horses** does not lead to the visibly evident effects of peripheral vasoconstriction as in cattle, but experimental studies have demonstrated peripheral vasoconstriction does occur suggesting exposure could lead to foot or leg problems. The more commonly recognized manifestations of fescue toxicosis in the horse are *prolonged gestation, agalactia, thickened placentas, and possible abortion*. Abdominal lipomatosis associated with marked necrosis of abdominal fat and severe weight loss occurs in *domestic ruminants* and some species of wildlife consuming endophyte-infected fescue. A heritable predisposition exists in cattle.

Bibliography

Abney KL, et al. Vasoconstrictive effects of tall fescue alkaloids on equine vasculature. J Eq Vet Sci 1993;13:334–340.

Botha CJ, et al. Gangrenous ergotism in cattle grazing fescue (*Festuca elatior* L.) in South Africa. J S Afr Vet Assoc 2004;75:45–48.

Browning R, Browning ML. Effect of ergotamine and ergonovine on thermal regulation and cardiovascular function in cattle. J Anim Sci 1997;75:176–181.

Smith GW, et al. Abdominal fat necrosis in a pygmy goat associated with fescue toxicosis. J Vet Diagn Invest 2004;16:356–359.

Tor-Agbidye J, et al. Correlation of endophyte toxins (ergovaline and lolitrem B) with clinical disease: fescue foot and perennial ryegrass staggers. Vet Hum Toxicol 2001;43:140–146.

Wallace LL, et al. Effects on environmental heat and intake of tall fescue seed infested with *Acremonium coenophialum* on the acid-base status of young bulls. J Vet Diagn Invest 1996;8:233–237.

Tricothecene toxicoses

Macrocyclic trichothecene toxins produced by the fungus *Stachybotrys* spp. cause **stachybotryotoxicosis**. *Ulcerative and necrotizing lesions of the skin and mucous membranes* have been reported in horses, cattle, sheep, and pigs, chiefly from Russia and Eastern Europe. Initial lesions affect the lips, buccal commissures and nostrils. Marked edema of the face may follow. Death follows development of *hemorrhagic diathesis, enteritis, and septicemia*. At necropsy, lesions in addition to the hemorrhagic diathesis include alimentary ulceration, pneumonia, renal infarcts, multifocal hepatic necrosis, and lymphadenitis. In many instances, these lesions may represent secondary mycotic or bacterial involvement.

T-2 toxin is a highly irritant trichothecene mycotoxin from *Fusarium* molds on grain, and causes cutaneous ulceration when applied locally to the skin of pigs. Experimental feeding of T-2 toxin contaminated feed, in combination with aflatoxin, induces crusting and ulceration of the lips, snout, buccal commissures and prepuce. The pathogenesis of the lesion is thought to be *contact irritant dermatitis* due directly to the T-2 toxin or to a urinary metabolite, HT-2 toxin.

Various other trichothecene mycotoxins are also cutaneous irritants and may cause vomition or feed refusal.

Bibliography

Harvey RB. Cutaneous ulceration and necrosis in pigs fed aflatoxin and T-2 toxin containing diets. J Vet Diagn Invest 1990:227–229.

Hintikka EL. Stachybotryotoxicosis in cattle and captive animals: Stachybotryotoxicosis in horses: Stachybotryotoxicosis in sheep: Stachybotryotoxicosis in swine. In: Wyllie TD, Morehouse LG, eds. Mycotoxic Fungi, Mycotoxins and Mycotoxicoses. New York: Dekker, 1978:152–161, 181–185, 203–207, 268–273.

Le Bars J, Le Bars P. Recent acute and subacute mycotoxicoses recognized in France. Vet Res 1996;27:383–394.

Vetch toxicosis and vetch-like diseases

Hairy vetch (*Vicia villosa* Roth) is a cultivated legume used as pasture, hay and silage in most of the United States, and in other countries such as Argentina, Australia, and South Africa. Hairy vetch toxicosis in **cattle** is seen as three unique syndromes: (1) acute neurological disease and hemolysis, followed by death after consumption of seeds; (2) swelling of the upper body accompanied by herpetiform eruptions of the oral mucous membranes, respiratory distress and death after consuming vetch pasture; and, (3) a syndrome characterized by *dermatitis, conjunctivitis, diarrhea, and granulomatous inflammation of many organs*. This third syndrome is the most common form of hairy vetch toxicosis and occurs in cattle and, to a lesser extent, *horses* after consumption of vetch-containing pastures. The clinical syndrome begins two or more weeks after consumption and consists of pruritic dermatitis, diarrhea (possibly bloody), and wasting. Morbidity is low and mortality is high. Holsteins, Angus and cattle 3 years or older are more often affected. Death in cattle occurs approximately 10–20 days after illness begins.

Initial lesions consist of a rough coat with papules and crusts affecting the skin of the udder, teats, escutcheon and neck, followed by involvement of the trunk, face and limbs. The skin becomes less pliable, alopecic, and lichenified. Marked pruritus leads to excoriations. At necropsy, *yellow nodular infiltrates disrupt the architecture of a wide range of organs*, but are most severe in myocardium, kidney, lymph nodes, thyroid and adrenal glands. The kidney may have radially oriented cortical infiltrates that follow the vasculature. Other affected organs may include the mammary and salivary glands, liver, urinary bladder, meninges, and spleen. Histologically, *the infiltrates consist of monocytes, lymphocytes, plasma cells, multinucleated giant cells, and in the cow, eosinophils*. The skin has similar perivascular to diffuse infiltrates, marked hyperkeratosis, and dermal and epidermal edema. This form of the disease has been induced experimentally in an Angus cow that had recovered from vetch toxicosis the previous year. Lesions were evident 11 days after feeding vetch. Death occurred even though vetch was removed from the diet at 12 days. Experimental lesions mirrored those of naturally occurring disease with the additional finding of necrosis of cutaneous apocrine glands.

Other species of *Vicia* and additional compounds are capable of inducing disease indistinguishable from vetch toxicity.

Pyrexia with dermatitis in dairy cows is a syndrome with similarities to hairy vetch toxicity. It has been reported in the United States, England, Wales, France, and the Netherlands. Friesian dairy cows developed pruritic papular eruptions affecting the head and neck, tail head and udder. Secondary lesions were due to self-trauma. In another outbreak, hemorrhages were a prominent clinical sign. The episode in Wales was associated with the introduction of a new silage additive on several farms. The outbreak in the Netherlands was associated with the feeding of *di-ureido-isobutane*

(DUIB) in the seed cake. This condition was reproduced in two cows by feeding a DUIB-containing diet for one month. Histologically, *the lesions of the Dutch outbreak also resembled those of the putative hairy vetch toxicity*. Visceral lesions resembling hairy vetch toxicity occur in dairy cows fed a diet containing *citrus pulp;* the syndrome resolves after removal of citrus pulp from the diet.

Hairy vetch toxicosis in **horses** resembles that in cattle except for the infrequent finding of eosinophils in the infiltrate and lack of heart involvement. Conditions very similar to vetch toxicosis have been reported in horses with no vetch exposure. These cases have been variably referred to as "idiopathic granulomatous disease involving the skin," "systemic granulomatous disease," "generalized granulomatous disease" or "equine sarcoidosis." Organ involvement is variable. Skin lesions include scaling, crusting and alopecia on the face or limbs that progress to a generalized exfoliative dermatitis. Histologically, *the skin has multifocal, sometimes perifollicular to deep dermal nodules of granulomatous inflammation*. Sarcoidosis in man has a genetic basis and is thought to represent a hypersensitivity response to a persistent antigen. These idiopathic conditions in the horse are fairly indistinguishable and should be considered "*vetch- like disease*" until more information is available.

Toxicity from vetch seeds is known to be due to the presence of *prussic acid*. The cause of the granulomatous diseases listed above remains unclear. Nor is it certain whether they represent one entity or a common tissue reaction to a variety of insults. One proposed pathogenesis is that ingestion of vetch or another substance leads to antigen formation in the form of a hapten or a complete antigen that sensitizes lymphocytes and evokes the cell-mediated response upon repeat exposure. Factors that support this hypothesis are the resemblance of the histologic lesions to a type IV hypersensitivity response, age incidence, low morbidity, genetic influence and possible need for repeat exposure. Lymphocyte blastogenesis and cutaneous hypersensitivity studies have not substantiated this hypothesis, however, only a few vetch antigens have been studied.

The diagnosis of vetch toxicity or vetch-like disease is a *diagnosis by exclusion*. It is made after review of the herd history, and character and distribution of the lesions. The combination of lesions is fairly distinctive.

Bibliography

Dyson DA, Reed JBH. Haemorrhagic syndrome of cattle of suspected mycotoxic origin. Vet Rec 1977;100:400–402.

Fighera RA, Barros CS. Systemic granulomatous disease in Brazilian cattle grazing pasture containing vetch (*Vicia* spp). Vet Hum Toxicol 2004;46:62–66.

Green JR, Kleynhans R. Suspected vetch (*Vicia benghalensis* L) poisoning in a Friesland cow in the Republic of South Africa. J S Afr Vet Assoc 1989: 60:109–110.

Panciera RJ, et al. Hairy vetch (*Vicia villosa* Roth) poisoning of cattle, update and experimental induction of disease. J Vet Diagn Invest 1992;4:318–325.

Saunders GK, et al. Suspected citrus pulp toxicosis in dairy cattle. J Vet Diagn Invest 2000;12:269–271.

Thomas GW. Pyrexia with dermatitis in dairy cows. In Pract 1979;1:16–18.

Woods LW, et al. Systemic granulomatous disease in a horse grazing pasture containing vetch (*Vicia* sp.) J Vet Diagn Invest 1992;4:356–360.

Wood PR, et al. Granulomatous enteritis and cutaneous arteritis in a horse. J Am Vet Med Assoc 1993;203:1573–1575.

Quassinoid toxicosis

Quassinoid compounds, such as neoquassin and quassin found in hardwood trees of the genus *Quassia (Simarouba amara)* in the family Simaroubaceae, have been reported to be associated with a *vesiculobullous dermatitis of the skin* around the eyes, nose, ears, anus and lips of horses. *Wood shavings* from these plants have been incorporated in bedding and the outbreaks have occurred in large numbers of exposed horses. Gross lesions develop within the first few days of exposure and most often resolve within a week. Systemic signs such as anorexia and icterus accompany cutaneous lesions in some cases. Hepatopathy and nephrosis have been reported. Similar symmetrical lesions of the oral mucosa, mucocutaneous junctions, and pressure points have been reported in dogs exposed to *Simarouba* shavings.

Quassinoids have been shown experimentally to have insecticidal and anthelmintic properties while their derivatives have antitumor, antiulcer, and cytotoxic activity in vitro. The mechanisms leading to toxicity are not known. Definitive diagnosis is dependent upon a compatible history, exclusion of viral diseases such as vesicular stomatitis and exposure to other toxins, and the positive identification of plants of the *Quassia* genus in the bedding material.

Bibliography

Campagnolo ER, et al. Outbreak of vesicular dermatitis among horses at a Midwestern horse show. J Am Vet Med Assoc 1995;207:211–213.

Declercq J. Suspected wood poisoning caused by *Simarouba amara* (marupa/caixeta) shavings in two dogs with erosive stomatitis and dermatitis. Vet Dermatol 2004;15:188–193.

Matsumura T. *Simarouba* poisoning in horses - Japan. Eq Dis Q 2002;10:2.

ACTINIC DISEASES OF SKIN

The radiant energy of the sun includes components that are potentially harmful to mammalian skin. This radiation is known as **actinic radiation** and its acute effect is the well-known *sunburn* reaction. **Photosensitization** is essentially an *exacerbated form of sunburn*, caused by the activation of photodynamic chemicals in the skin by radiation of an appropriate wavelength and is discussed under the heading Photosensitization dermatitis. **Photoallergy** is distinct from phototoxicity; *it occurs when the photoproduct of an exogenous chemical acts as an antigen*. Photoallergic reactions require prior sensitization to the drug or chemical and are more clinically diverse. Photoallergies have not been documented conclusively in animals. **Skin cancers** induced or exacerbated by actinic radiation are considered with Tumors of the epidermis.

Direct effect of solar radiation

Solar energy is a form of non-ionizing radiation comprised of ultraviolet light (100–400 nm), visible light (400–700 nm), and infrared light (700–20 000 nm) rays. *Most of the direct photobiologic reactions in the skin are induced by high energy light in the ultraviolet radiation UVB range (290–320 nm)*. Longer wavelengths of 320–400 nm constitute UVA and may augment UVB-mediated damage. The integument is normally protected against the deleterious effects of ultraviolet radiation by the hair coat, the stratum corneum and melanin pigmentation. The quantity of ozone, smog, altitude, latitude, season of the year and time of day also strongly influence the amount of UV rays reaching the skin. The greatest potential for solar-induced skin damage occurs at high altitudes and temperate latitudes during mid-summer days, and in thin, lightly pigmented, sparsely haired, sun-exposed skin. An increasing prevalence of sun-induced dermatoses and tumors has been noted in humans, coincident with *the depletion of the ozone layer and a consequent increase in the intensity of ultraviolet radiation reaching the earth's surface*. This trend may also become evident in animals. Potentially, all animals are susceptible to the acute and chronic effects of actinic radiation, but the protection afforded by the hair coat, and to a lesser extent stratum corneum and skin pigmentation, is normally sufficient to prevent solar-induced damage. The conditions described below typically affect animals whose anatomical defenses are poor, either by lacking skin pigmentation or hair cover.

UVB radiation stimulates light-absorbing molecules in the skin referred to as chromophores. *Chromophores include keratin proteins, melanin, carotene, nucleic acids, peptide bonds and some amino acids*, to name a few. Light absorbed by chromophores results in electron transfers and free radical production. *Free radical mediated cellular damage* is discussed elsewhere. Energy dissipated from electron transfers induces chemical reactions to form altered cell components referred to as *photoproducts* that include altered DNA molecules, enzymes, and hydrogen and disulfide bonds within proteins. Nucleoprotein is susceptible to ultraviolet radiation damage resulting in mitotic inhibition and, if extensive enough, cell death. Sublethal damage may promote mutagenesis or carcinogenesis by the formation of thymidine dimers between pyrimidine base pairs of DNA. Pyrimidine dimer repair mechanisms normally correct DNA damage prior to cell replication, however repeated or extensive damage may lead to failure of repair mechanisms and cell transformation. The "*sunburn cell*" associated with UV damage is a keratinocyte that has undergone apoptosis. UVB-induced keratinocyte apoptosis is a complex event that involves cytokines such as TNFα and probable p53-mediated induction of apoptosis in cells sustaining substantial DNA damage. Studies in mice have shown that UVB radiation-induced apoptotic keratinocytes are replaced by hyperproliferative keratinocytes leading to epidermal hyperplasia, suggesting apoptosis and hyperplasia are related events. Ultraviolet light also induces mutations of the p53 tumor suppressor gene in keratinocytes contributing to a proliferative advantage to mutated cells that is found in solar-induced actinic keratoses and squamous cell carcinomas in humans. These findings indicate ultraviolet radiation can serve as both a tumor initiator and promoter. UV radiation may also alter immunologic reactivity in favor of the growth of the tumor, through the induction of suppressor T cells and possible impairment of natural killer cell function. UVB radiation exposure reduces the number of Langerhans cells and impairs their antigen-presenting functions. Contact hypersensitivity responses in experimental animals are reduced following UVB irradiation.

Apoptotic keratinocytes, "sunburn cells," arranged singly or in clusters or bands in the outer stratum spinosum are a characteristic microscopic feature of acute sun-induced epithelial damage. These may be induced within 30 minutes of sun exposure. Other lesions include spongiosis, vacuolation of keratinocytes, loss of the granular layer, and, in severe burns, vesiculation. Dermal hyperemia and edema are prominent features. In mild lesions, there is a slight increase in mononuclear cells; in severe burns, there is marked vascular damage, erythrocyte extravasation and neutrophilic exocytosis. The initial lesion of UV-irradiation induced injury consists of transient erythema, probably due to a direct heating effect and the photobiologic effects of UVB acting directly on dermal capillaries. The delayed erythema reaction may be due to direct damage to endothelial cells or the release of cytokines from the radiation-damaged keratinocytes. Ultraviolet radiation has been shown to increase the production of keratinocyte-derived cytokines. Ultraviolet light also induces adaptive responses in the epidermis, in particular epidermal hyperplasia and alterations in melanin pigmentation. An immediate pigment darkening is due to changes in existing melanin, and the delayed or "tanning" reaction to stimulation of melanogenesis and proliferation of melanocytes. *Melanin both absorbs and scatters UV radiation and, being able to trap free radicals, is important in minimizing the deleterious effects of incident photons*. Basal keratinocytes with melanin granules forming protective caps over the nucleus have an increased distribution in sun-exposed skin. In chronically sun-damaged skin, pigment distribution can become irregular due to impaired transfer of melanin from melanocytes to keratinocytes, thereby weakening host defenses. *Long-term effects* of ultraviolet irradiation include variable degenerative changes in the dermis (solar elastosis and fibrosis), adnexa (comedones, cysts), and epidermis (solar keratosis). Lesions vary by species and among individuals within the species.

Solar dermatitis, or *sunburn*, occurs most frequently in *cats, dogs, pigs, cows, and goats*. The lesions in *cats* typically affect the tips of the ears, nose, eyelids, and lips of white, blue-eyed animals. The initial lesion is erythema followed by alopecia, scaling and crusting (Fig. 5.51). The ear tip may curl over. Lesions are exacerbated each summer, often eventuating in malignant transformation into squamous cell carcinoma. Primary phototoxicity in swine occurs in white or light-colored *pigs*. While any age group may be affected, the condition is most severe in suckling and weaner pigs. Occasionally, severely affected ears may slough. Light-colored *goats* and *cows* are also prone to solar dermatitis. The udders are particularly susceptible when does are turned out into strong sunlight after a winter indoors.

Solar dermatitis occurs most often in *short-haired dogs with light pigmentation*. Breeds most often affected include Bull Terriers, Whippets, Beagles, and Dalmatians. Lesions are most often present on the ventrolateral abdomen and thorax, lateral flank, hocks, and bridge of nose in nonpigmented skin. Such lesions are probably related to the basking behavior exhibited by the animals. *Early lesions of erythema and scaling evolve into thick, lichenified, erythematous, crusted patches and plaques*. Hemorrhagic bullae may develop. The most consistent histologic finding in dogs with chronic solar dermatitis is a *narrow, hypocellular, pale-staining band of collagen along the dermoepidermal junction*. This change may be present prior to clinical signs of actinic dermatitis and may be used as an indicator of solar damage if the history, anatomical site, and breed are supportive. Other changes noted in canine sun-damaged skin include epidermal acanthosis, apocrine gland ectasia, and follicular keratosis resulting in follicular cyst formation and possible furunculosis, particularly over pressure points (Fig. 5.52A). A layer of fibrosis often surrounds cystic follicles. A superficial perivascular mixed infiltrate of lymphocytes, plasma cells, monocytes, neutrophils, and rare eosinophils is usually present. Furunculosis leads to a marked foreign-body response. Follicular changes are thought to be due to loss of support of follicles, however elastin studies in dogs have not demonstrated degeneration of elastin fibers supporting the follicular wall. Advanced lesions may have epidermal dysplasia (Fig. 5.52B) or concurrent UV-light induced neoplasms such as a squamous cell carcinoma, hemangioma, or hemangiosarcoma. It is important to note that UV light-induced neoplasms may arise in skin devoid of other changes suggestive of actinic damage. *Actinic comedones* may also be present without lesions suggestive of actinic epidermal damage. *Differentials* are many and include other conditions resulting in comedone formation, acne, various allergies, bacterial or fungal infections, neoplasia or a primary keratinization disorder. Restriction of lesions to nonpigmented, sparsely haired skin and a history of sun exposure should be helpful in differentiation.

Solar elastosis, a hallmark of chronic sun exposure in humans, has been described only rarely in *dogs, cats, sheep and horses* and essentially represents *disorganization of dermal components due to*

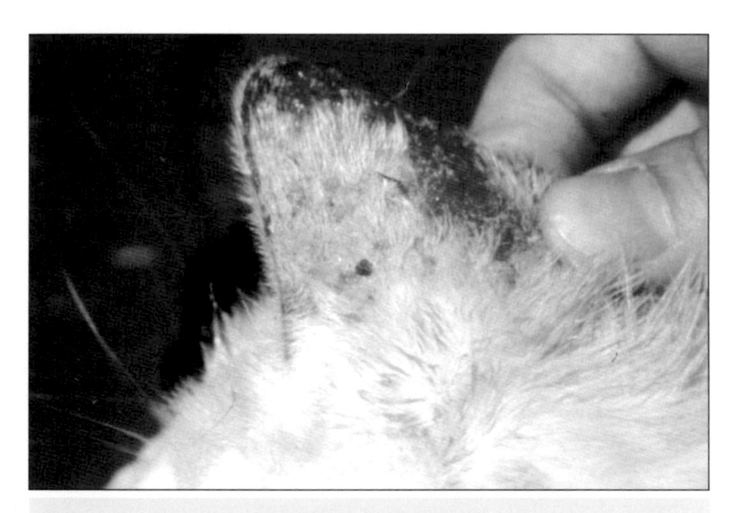

Figure 5.51 Solar dermatitis in a white cat, with erythematous, crusted patches and plaques on the pinnae.

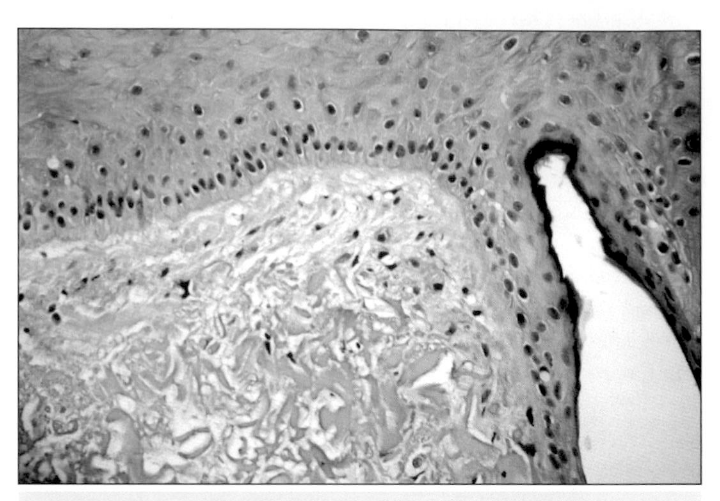

Figure 5.53 Solar elastosis. The dermis is filled with agglomerated, thick, irregular, basophilic degenerate elastic fibers.

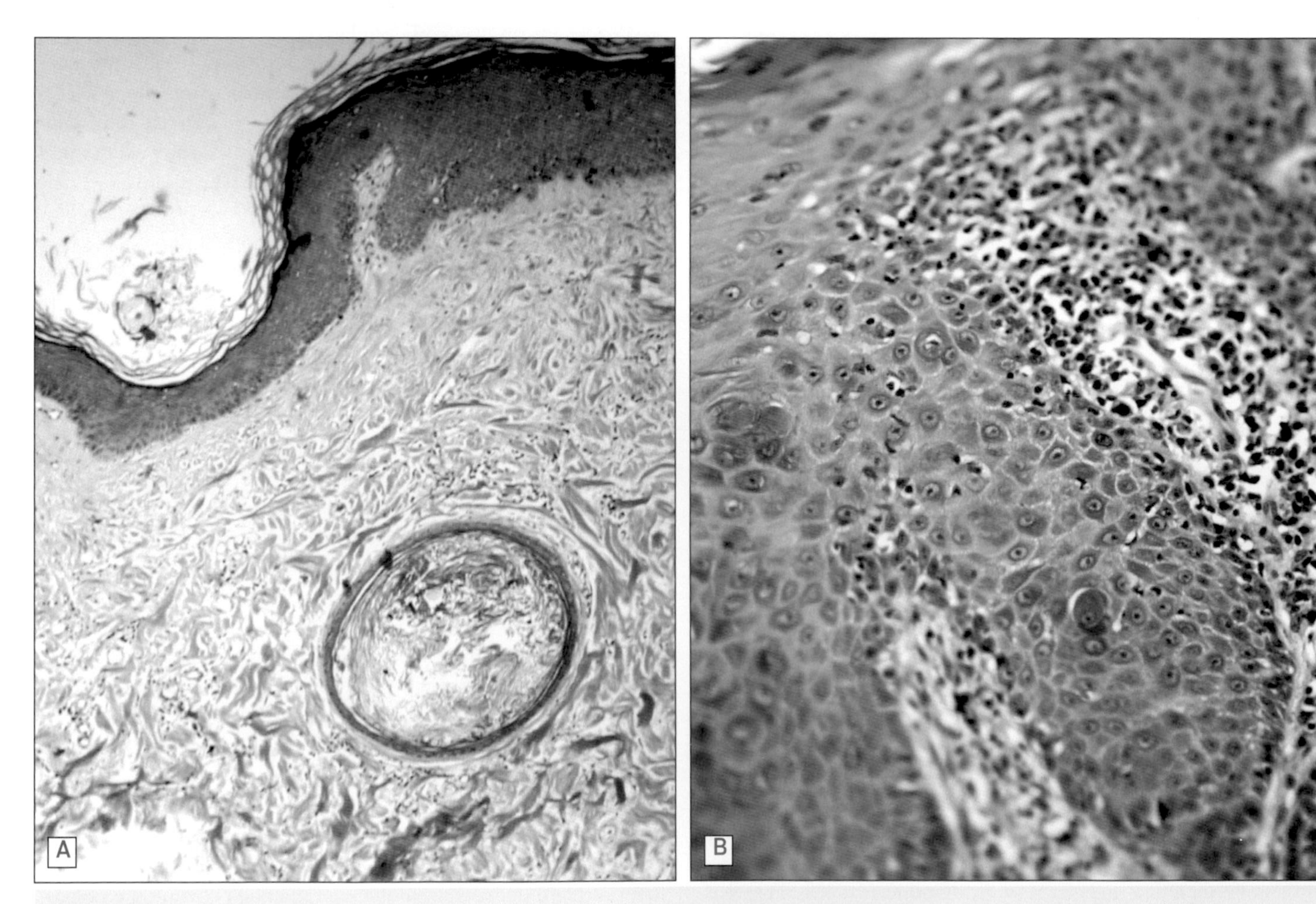

Figure 5.52 Solar dermatitis. **A.** Note hyperplastic epidermis, superficial layer of pale dermal collagen, and comedone formation. **B.** Hyperplastic epidermis with "**sunburn cells**" and other evidence of dysplasia.

altered fibroblast function. The lesions usually occur in conjunction with solar radiation-associated neoplasms, particularly squamous cell carcinomas. Solar elastosis appears in hematoxylin and eosin-stained sections as *scattered or agglomerated, thick, irregular, basophilic degenerate elastic fibers* (Fig. 5.53). Silver impregnation staining techniques may be needed to demonstrate elastin changes in animals. Solar dermatitis is often present without evidence of elastosis.

Solar keratoses, common *precancerous skin lesions* in humans, occur in cats, dogs and horses. The conjunctiva of horses with white eyelids is a common site. Histologically, the early lesions have many of the features of sunburn, including epidermal hyperplasia, spongiosis, acute dermal inflammation and focal necrotic keratinocytes. More chronic lesions show pronounced epidermal hyperplasia with *dysplasia*, ortho- and parakeratotic hyperkeratosis, perivascular mononuclear cell infiltrates and dermal scarring, but seldom develop significant solar elastosis, as typifies human solar keratoses. *Lesions frequently progress to invasive squamous cell carcinoma*. Solar keratoses may also develop cutaneous horns.

Bibliography

Baba T, et al. The study of ultraviolet B-induced apoptosis in cultured mouse keratinocytes and in mouse skin. J Dermatol Sci 1996;12:18–23.

Campbell GA, et al. Solar elastosis with squamous cell carcinoma in two horses. Vet Pathol 1987;24:463–464.

Frank LA, et al. Distribution and appearance of elastic fibers in the dermis of clinically normal dogs and dogs with solar dermatitis and other dermatoses. Am J Vet Res 1996;57:178–181.

Irving RA, et al. Porphyrin values and treatment of feline solar dermatitis. Am J Vet Res 1982;43:2067–2069.

Kimura T, Kunio D. Responses of the skin over the dorsum to sunlight in hairless descendants of Mexican hairless dogs. Am J Vet Res 1994;55:199–203.

Leffell DJ. The scientific basis of skin cancer. J Am Acad Dermatol 2000;42(1 Pt 2):18–22.

Miyauchi-Hashimoto H, et al. Ultraviolet radiation-induced suppression of natural killer cell activity is enhanced in xeroderma pigmentosum group A (XPA) model mice. J Invest Dermatol 1999;12:965–970.

Montagna W, et al. Histology of sun-damaged human skin. J Am Acad Dermatol 1989;21:907–918.

Ouhtit A, et al. Temporal events in skin injury and the early adaptive responses in ultraviolet-irradiated mouse skin. Am J Pathol 2000;156:201–207.

Roberts LK, et al. Ultraviolet light and modulation of the immune response. In: Norris DA, ed. Immune Mechanisms in Cutaneous Disease. New York: Marcel Dekker, 1989:167–218.

Ziegler A, et al. Sunburn and p53 in the onset of skin cancer. Nature 1994;372:773–776.

Photosensitization dermatitis

Photosensitization dermatitis occurs in animals when photodynamic or fluorescent pigments are deposited in sunlight exposed skin. Photodynamic pigments absorb ultraviolet light or visible light in the action spectrum and convert it to light of a longer wavelength, usually beyond the UVB range. The energy from the absorbed light leads to tissue injury by reacting directly with molecular oxygen, producing reactive oxygen intermediates such as superoxide anion, singlet oxygen and hydroxyl radical. Oxygen free radicals may also be formed indirectly, as the result of a calcium-dependent, protease-mediated activation of xanthine-oxidase in the skin. Release of reactive oxygen species initiates chain reactions which lead to mast cell degranulation and damage to cell membranes, nucleic acids, proteins and subcellular organelles, particularly lysosomes and mitochondria.

The photodynamic agent usually reaches the skin via the *systemic circulation*, although *percutaneous absorption* of some photodynamic agents can cause local contact photosensitization. The agent may originate externally or it may be an endogenous substance that has accumulated to an abnormal degree as a result of metabolic dysfunction. Sources include *plant pigments and drugs* or, in the case of metabolic dysfunction, the *by-products of hemoglobin metabolism or chlorophyll degradation products*. The three categories of photosensitization are classified according to the source of the agents.

- In *type I, or primary photosensitization*, the animal *ingests plants or drugs* containing photoreactive substances that are deposited in the skin. Most exogenous sources of photoreactive pigments are found in plants, and therefore foraging animals such as horses, sheep, cattle and goats are most frequently affected.
- In *type II photosensitization*, an inherent inability to properly metabolize heme pigments necessary for erythrocyte production leads to the build up of the photoreactive pigments, *hematoporphyrins*.
- An abnormal build up of *phylloerythrin*, a degradation product of chlorophyll, induces *type III photosensitization*. This is known also as *hepatogenous photosensitization* because it depends upon the failure of a damaged or immature liver to eliminate phylloerythrin. Type III photosensitization occurs most often in animals ingesting large amounts of green forage.
- A fourth group contains those examples of photosensitization for which the pathogenesis is presently undetermined.

The **gross lesions** are similar for all forms of photosensitization. They occur on those areas of the body most exposed to sunlight and which lack protective fleece, hair coat or skin pigmentation. In *cattle*, any area of light-colored skin is susceptible. This is best demonstrated in broken-colored animals such as Holsteins, in which the white skin is affected but the black is spared. The relatively hairless skin of the teats, udder, perineum and muzzle is also affected. The ventral surface of the tongue is frequently affected in cattle if constantly exposed during licking. In *sheep*, the susceptible sites are the ears, eyelids, face, muzzle and coronets, although the back may be affected in animals with an open fleece or which have been shorn closely. The udders and teats of dairy *goats* are predisposed. In *horses*, lesions are most common on the face, perineum, and distal extremities but may affect any white skin. Lesions in *pigs* are uncommon, and have a predilection for the ears, eyelids, udder, and back. Photosensitization is rare in *dogs* and *cats* and causative agents remain obscure.

The initial reaction in photosensitization is erythema, followed by edema, which is more prominent in sheep than in cattle. The very marked edema of the ears in sheep causes them to droop and swelling of the muzzle may cause dyspnea. The disease in sheep is appropriately known as "bighead" or geeldikkop, a South African term meaning "thick, yellow head;" the equivalent term in New Zealand is "facial eczema." The lesions are *intensely pruritic*, causing rubbing, scratching and kicking at affected parts. Vesicles or bullae may develop. There is marked exudation and extensive necrosis. Affected skin becomes dry and sloughs in desiccated sheets (Fig. 5.54). Necrosis is frequently seen on the upper surfaces of the ears

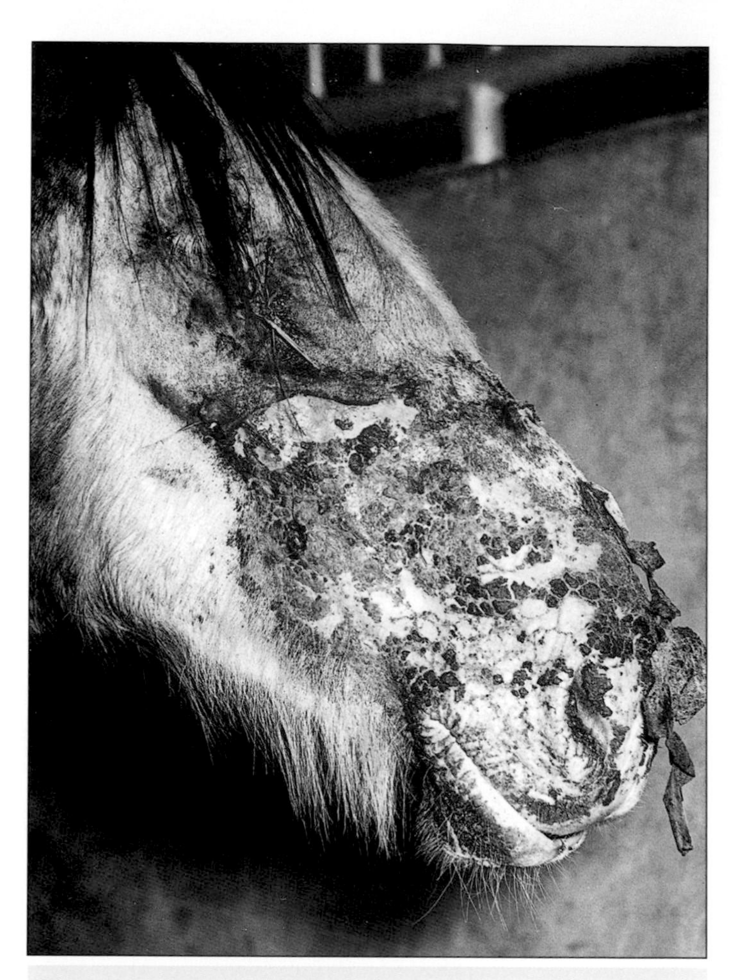

Figure 5.54 Photosensitization in a horse. Note necrosis and sloughing of skin from white areas of the face.

of sheep; the tips typically curl upwards as a result of mummification or may slough entirely. There is swelling of the eyelids and excessive lacrimation. Among the more obscure manifestations of photosensitization is the convulsive reaction of some sheep and cattle, photosensitized by ingestion of St. John's wort, on contact with cold water. *Icterus* typically is associated with hepatogenous photosensitization, but hepatogenous photosensitization may occur in its absence. Economic losses in livestock can be severe due to damaged hides, weight loss, fly-strikes, secondary infections, and reluctance of animals to let the young nurse damaged udders. In severe episodes of photosensitization, animals may die. This is more often the result of concomitant damage to other organs, particularly the liver, than to cutaneous damage alone. Injury to erythrocytes in cutaneous circulation may produce severe hemolysis.

Histologic lesions mirror the gross lesions with *coagulative necrosis of the epidermis* and possibly the follicular epithelium, adnexal glands, and superficial dermis. Subepidermal clefts or vesicles form and the *dermis is edematous*. Endothelial cells of the superficial, mid, and occasionally deep dermal vessels are often swollen or necrotic. Fibrinoid degeneration of vessel walls and thrombosis may be present. Initially, inflammation is sparse but soon the lesions are infiltrated by neutrophils. Secondary bacterial colonization is common.

Differential diagnosis should include other vesicular or necrotizing dermatopathies, including chemical or thermal burns. *Establishing the diagnosis is dependent upon anatomic distribution of lesions in nonpigmented, poorly haired, sun-exposed regions*. Lesions limited to areas of contact such as the extremities, ventrum or muzzle suggests the presence of a contact photosensitizing agent. Multiple affected animals in a herd suggest exposure to a photosensitizing agent rather than a photoallergic reaction. Types I, II, and III photosensitivities can be differentiated by signalment and concurrent clinical signs, such as evidence of liver disease combined with examination of pastures and feedstuffs, and investigating photodynamic drug or chemical exposure. The *Candida albicans* inhibition assay is a simple, inexpensive, quantitative, and relatively rapid assay for screening plants and feedstuffs for potential primary contact or systemic photosensitizers. The test does not detect all phototoxins. Thin-layer chromatography techniques may be useful in identifying phototoxic compounds. Analysis of suspect vegetation for the identification and quantification of fungal spores may be needed to establish fungal organisms and associated mycotoxins as contributing factors.

Primary photosensitization (type I photosensitization)

Plants are the most common cause of primary photosensitization; hence herbivores are most commonly affected. Additional sources include *mycotoxins, molds, chemicals and drugs. The majority of photosensitizing plants contain pigments belonging to either the helianthrone or furocoumarin family of pigments.*

The **helianthrones** include the red fluorescent pigments, *hypericin and fagopyrin*. Some of the most commonly implicated plants include St. John's wort (*Hypericum perforatum*) and buckwheat (*Fagopyrum* spp.), and the resulting diseases are referred to as *hypericism* and *fagopyrism*, respectively. Photosensitization induced by St. John's wort affects horses, cattle, sheep and goats. Hypericin is present at all stages of plant growth but significant amounts are consumed by livestock only when the plant is prolific or other feed is scarce. Other related plants that can lead to hypericism include goatweed, Tipton weed, amber, cammock, and Klamath weed. Photosensitization induced by buckwheat affects sheep, pigs, cattle, goats, and horses.

The **furocoumarin** family of pigments contains the photodynamic agents, *psoralens*. Photosensitization occurs in cattle, sheep, white chickens, and ducks as a result of ingestion of plants such as spring parsley (*Cymopterus watsonii*), bishop's weed *(Ammi majus)* and Dutchman's breeches *(Thamnosma texana)*. The furocoumarins differ from the helianthrone photosensitizing pigments by inducing, additionally, *corneal edema and keratoconjunctivitis*. Primary photodermatitis of pigs in Argentina occurred after consumption of feed contaminated with *Ammi majus* seeds containing the furocoumarin, xanthotoxin. Furocoumarins have also been documented to form *phytoallexins* in fungus-infected parsnips (*Pastinaca sativa*) and celery (*Apium graveolens*), leading to **phytophotocontact dermatitis**. *Psoralens adsorbed onto the skin react with UV light*. These have been associated with phytophotocontact dermatitis in pigs in New Zealand. Lesions were vesicular, affecting only the dorsal aspect of the snout. Rubbing the snouts and feet of white pigs with the leaves of the fungus-infected celery and parsnips before exposing the areas to UV light reproduced the lesions. *Cymopterus watsoni* causes phytophotodermatitis in sheep in Utah and Nevada. Lesions principally affected the non-wooled areas, such as the muzzle, lips and udder. High lamb mortality may be incurred from mismothering. Contact photodermatitis suspected to be caused by giant hogweed (*Heracleum* *mantegazzianum*) occurred in dogs. Giant hogweed contains psoralens and has been documented to cause photodermatitis in man, ducks, and goats.

Texas cattle and deer develop primary photosensitization after consuming moldy leaves of *Cooperia pedunculata*. In addition to skin lesions, keratitis occurs frequently and may lead to blindness.

Ingestion of alsike clover (*Trifolium hybridum*), also known as red clover hay, results in a primary photodermatitis referred to as *trifoliosis* in cattle, sheep, hogs, and some horses. Trifoliosis has been reported in the USA, Canada, Australia, and England. A second syndrome, referred to as *alsike clover poisoning*, is characterized by hepatic dysfunction and photodermatitis and has only been reported in the horse. The toxic mechanism is not known but is thought to be due to a toxin within the plant itself or to the presence of a mycotoxin. The variable presentations are speculated to be related to seasonal changes, stage of plant growth, soil and environmental conditions.

A condition clinically and histologically compatible with a primary photodermatitis occurred in 12 of 30 Harrier Hounds in a kennel in New Zealand. Lesions were limited to the nonpigmented, sun-exposed skin of the tri-colored hounds and resolved within a short period of time with supportive care. The hounds were fed a diet of horse and cattle meat. Although an ingested compound was suspected as the cause, no phototoxin could be identified. Similar cases have been reported in Foxhounds in England and Border Collie dogs in New Zealand.

Phenothiazine photosensitization is characterized by typical cutaneous lesions and in ruminants by the additional lesions of corneal edema and keratoconjunctivitis. The secretion of the ruminal metabolite, phenothiazine sulfoxide, in tears and aqueous humor, has explained the unusual location of the lesions. Phenothiazine photosensitization occurs most commonly in *calves* but also in *sheep, swine, and birds*. Pigs develop cutaneous lesions more frequently than sheep or cattle, probably because the activating radiation is more able to penetrate the integument. The greater susceptibility of calves has been ascribed to a relatively inefficient conversion of the photodynamic sulfoxide metabolite back to phenothiazine in the liver. This conversion depends on effective mixed-function oxidase enzyme activity in the liver.

Photosensitization due to defective pigment synthesis (type II photosensitization)

Photosensitization due to *endogenous pigment accumulation* is the result of a congenital enzyme deficiency causing abnormal heme synthesis with the resultant blood and tissue accumulation of photodynamic agents such as *uroporphyrin I, coproporphyrin I and protoporphyrin III*.

Bovine congenital hematopoietic porphyria *is the result of a deficiency in uroporphyrinogen III cosynthetase*, a key enzyme in heme biosynthesis. The condition is inherited as a simple recessive trait affecting many breeds including Shorthorn, Ayrshire, Holstein and Jamaican cattle. It has also been reported in crossbred cattle. The disease is known as "osteohemochromatosis" and "pink tooth," both suggested by the *red-brown coloration of porphyrin pigments in dentin and bone*. The pigment is also deposited in other tissues but the discoloration may be obvious only in lungs, spleen, and kidney in which it is deposited in the interstitial tissue and tubular epithelium. The pigments are *excreted in the urine*; hence the alternative names "porphyrinuria" and "hematoporphyrinuria." Affected urine is amber to brown, darkens on exposure to light, and fluoresces bright red on exposure to ultraviolet radiation. *Affected teeth and bones also fluoresce.* The anemia of bovine congenital erythropoietic porphyria is discussed in Vol. 3, Hematopoietic system.

The cutaneous lesions result from the photodynamic properties of the accumulated porphyrins, in particular the *uroporphyrins* that absorb UVA radiation. Reactive oxygen species directly induced by the porphyrins or, possibly, via activation of xanthine oxidase in the skin are responsible for the cell membrane damage. The gross cutaneous lesions are typical of photosensitization. The microscopic lesions closely resemble those of erythropoietic porphyrias in man. The chief lesions are subepidermal clefts, hyalinization of dermal capillary walls, and a minimal infiltrate of inflammatory cells. The basement membrane zone lines the base of the subepidermal cleft, in some instances covering small projections of dermal papillae (festoons). Festoons are a more prominent feature of the human lesion since dermal papillae are better developed in human skin.

Bovine erythropoietic protoporphyria is inherited as a *recessive trait in Limousin cattle* in the United States. It differs from bovine congenital porphyria in that photodermatitis is the sole clinical manifestation of the disease. Animals do not have discolored teeth, anemia or urine porphyrin excretion. The enzyme defect is a *deficiency of ferrochelatase*, which allows protoporphyrin IX to accumulate in blood and tissues. Heterozygotes have reduced (50%) ferrochelatase activity and are clinically normal.

Porphyria of **swine** is inherited as a *dominant characteristic*. Although it mimics certain aspects of bovine erythropoietic porphyria, *photosensitization does not occur*, even in white-skinned animals. The defect in porcine porphyria is not known.

Photosensitization occurs in Siamese **cats** with excessive accumulation of uroporphyrinogen I, coproporphyrinogen I and protoporphyrins in blood, urine, feces and tissues. The defect is presumably a *deficiency of uroporphyrinogen cosynthetase III*, as has been established in humans and cattle.

Hepatogenous photosensitization (type III photosensitization)

The most common form of photosensitization in domestic animals occurs in conjunction with primary hepatocellular damage or, less commonly, bile duct obstruction and is due to impaired capacity of the liver to excrete the potent photodynamic agent, **phylloerythrin**. Phylloerythrin is a chlorophyll catabolite formed by microbial action in the intestinal tract and transported to the liver via the portal circulation. Hepatocytes assimilate the phylloerythrin and excrete it into the bile. One of the earliest signs of liver cell damage is a reduced ability to transport and excrete phylloerythrin. Mild renal tubular damage caused by some toxins may further inhibit the excretion of phylloerythrin. The circulating phylloerythrin accumulates in tissues including the skin. *Photodermatitis occurs provided the animal is on a chlorophyll-rich diet and is exposed to sufficient solar radiation of the appropriate wavelength*. High ambient solar radiation and lack of shade are contributing factors. Photosensitization tends to occur most often when the hepatic damage is generalized, even if mild. Severe focal necrotizing lesions of the liver generally do not cause photosensitization because there is enough hepatic reserve to remove the phylloerythrin from the circulation. The cause of hepatic damage may be a plant toxin, mycotoxin, infectious agent, or chemical.

Toxic plants and mycotoxins account for most cases of hepatogenous photosensitization. A few of the many plants implicated in hepatotoxic photosensitization include lantana (*Lantana camara*), bog asphodel (*Narthecium ossifragum*), *Tribulus terrestris*, *Agave lecheguilla*, *Nolina texana*, *Cymadothea trifolii*-infested clover, *Trifolium hybridum* ("alsike clover poisoning"), and *Panicum* spp. grasses such as kleingrass (*Panicum coloratum*). Kleingrass is a perennial grass forage crop with a toxic principle suspected to be a saponin. Cases of kleingrass induced-photosensitization are sporadic, potentially related to environmental conditions and have been reported in Australia, Africa, and Texas. Some plants work in combination; black sagebrush appears to precondition sheep to photosensitization caused ultimately by *Tetradymia* spp.

A number of reports of hepatogenous photosensitization in livestock cite a variety of common forage crops such as alfalfa hay or silage, winter wheat, Bermuda grass pasture, crab grass, oat stubble, or various clover pastures. In the majority of cases, the toxicity was preceded by unusual climatic conditions of drought, increased rainfall, or temperature variations. In many cases, a specific toxic compound cannot be identified. A plausible explanation is the establishment of optimum conditions for the production of mycotoxins, hepatotoxins or photodynamic agents in the damaged plant material.

Forages containing the mycotoxin, *sporidesmin*, from spores of *Pithomyces chartarum* cause **facial eczema**, an economically important hepatogenous photosensitization of sheep and cattle in Australia, New Zealand, South Africa, and the northwestern United States. *Geeldikkop*, a disease characterized by hepatogenous photosensitization, is associated with extensive losses among sheep and goats in South Africa. A hepatogenous photosensitization, secondary to a presumed genetic defect in phylloerythrin transport, has been reported in Corriedale lambs. Hepatogenous photosensitization is discussed in more detail in Vol. 2, Liver and biliary system.

Bibliography

Ames T, et al. Secondary photosensitivity in horses eating *Cymadothea trifolii*-infested clover. Proc Am Assoc Vet Lab Diagn 1994;37:45.

Athar M, et al. A novel mechanism for the generation of superoxide anions in hematoporphyrin derivative-mediated cutaneous photosensitization. J Clin Invest 1989;83:1137–1143.

Betty RC, Trikojus VM. Hypericin and a non-fluorescent photosensitive pigment from St. John's wort (*Hypericum perforatum*). Aust J Exp Biol Med Sci 1943;21:175–182.

Binns W, et al. *Cymopterus watsonii*: a photosensitizing plant for sheep. Vet Med Small Anim Clin 1964;59:375–379.

Casteel SW, et al. Photosensitization outbreak in Shorthorn calves in Missouri. J Vet Diagn Invest 1991;3:180–182.

Colon JL, et al. Hepatic dysfunction and photodermatitis secondary to alsike clover poisoning. Compend Contin Educ Pract Vet 1996;18:1022–1026.

Cornelius CE, et al. Hepatic pigmentation with photosensitivity. A syndrome in Corriedale sheep resembling Dubin-Johnson syndrome in man. J Am Vet Med Assoc 1965;146:709–713.

Cornick JL, et al. Kleingrass-associated hepatotoxicosis in horses. J Am Vet Med Assoc 1988;193:932–935.

De Vries H, et al. Photochemical reactions of quindoxin, olaquindox, carbadox and cyadox with protein, indicating photoallergic properties. Toxicol 1990; 63:85–95.

Dickie CW, Berryman JR. Polioencephalomalacia and photosensitization associated with *Kochia scoparia* consumption in range cattle. J Am Vet Med Assoc 1979;175:463–465.

Dollahite JW, et al. Photosensitization in cattle and sheep caused by feeding *Ammi majus* (greater Ammi; bishop's weed). Am J Vet Res 1978;39:193–197.

Dolowy WC. Giant hogweed photodermatitis in two dogs in Bellevue, Washington. J Am Vet Med Assoc 1996;209:722.

Enzie FD, Whitmore GE. Photosensitization keratitis in young goats following treatment with phenothiazine. J Am Vet Med Assoc 1953;123:237–238.

Fairley RA, Mackenzie IS. Photosensitivity in a kennel of harrier hounds. Vet Dermatol 1994;5:1–7.

Fourie PJJ. The occurrence of congenital porphyrinuria (pink tooth) in cattle in South Africa (Swaziland). Onderstepoort J Vet Sci 1936;7:535–566.

Glastonbury JRW, Boal GK. Geeldikkop in goats. Aust Vet J 1985;62:62.

Hansen DE, et al. Photosensitization associated with exposure to *Pithomyces chartarum* in lambs. J Am Vet Med Assoc 1994;204:1668–1671.

House JK, et al. Primary photosensitization related to ingestion of alfalfa silage by cattle. J Am Vet Med Assoc 1996;209:1604–1607.

Laksevela B, Dishington IW. Bog asphodel (*Northecium ossifragum*) as a cause of photosensitization of lambs in Norway. Vet Rec 1983;112:375–378.

Lopez TA, et al. Ergotism and photosensitization in swine produced by the combined ingestion of *Claviceps purpurea* sclerotia and *Ammi majus* seeds. J Vet Diagn Invest 1997;9:68–71.

Montgomery JF, et al. A vesiculo-bullous disease in pigs resembling foot and mouth disease. II. Experimental reproduction of the lesion. N Z Vet J 1987;35:27–30.

Morison WL, et al. Photoimmunology. Arch Dermatol 1979;115:350–355.

Oertli EH, et al. Phototoxic effect of *Thamnosma texana* (Dutchman's breeches) in sheep. Am J Vet Res 1983;44:1126–1129.

Pearson EG. Photosensitivity in horses. Compend Contin Educ Pract Vet 1996;18:1026–1029.

Rowe LD. Photosensitization problems in livestock. Vet Clin N Am 1989;5:301–323.

Sassa S, et al. Accumulation of protoporphyria IX from D-aminolevulinic acid in bovine skin fibroblasts with hereditary erythropoietic protoporphyria. J Exp Med 1981;153:1094–1101.

Scott DW, et al. Dermatohistopathologic changes in bovine congenital porphyria. Cornell Vet 1979;69:145–158.

With TK. A short history of porphyrins and the porphyrias. Int J Biochem 1980;11:189–200.

With TK. Porphyria in animals. Clin Hematol 1980;9:345–370.

Witte ST, Curry SL. Hepatogenous photosensitization in cattle fed a grass hay. J Vet Diagn Invest 1993;5:133–136.

Yamashita C, et al. Congenital porphyria in swine. Nippon Juigaku Zasshi 1980;42:353–359.

Photoaggravated dermatoses

In humans, several autoimmune dermatoses are exacerbated by exposure to UV light. These include pemphigus, lupus erythematosus, and bullous pemphigoid. A similar relationship has been proposed in the analogous canine diseases.

A poorly understood disease in the *horse*, **photoactivated vasculitis** affects only the white-haired extremities. The pathogenesis is not currently known. An immune-mediated vasculitis, in which immune complexes may be acting as photodynamic agents has been proposed. Percutaneous absorption of initiating agents has not been ruled out. Affected horses have normal liver function and no known exposure to photosensitizing compounds. In addition, lesions may be restricted to one white extremity, other white areas on the horse are unaffected and the lesions do not always regress with cessation of exposure to sunlight, all indicating the lesions are *not a form of photosensitization*. The lesions often affect the heels and must be differentiated from the other manifestations of the "greasy heel" complex. The acute lesions are well demarcated, erythematous, oozing and crusted; erosion and ulceration may occur and the affected limb may be edematous and painful. The chronic lesions are hyperkeratotic plaques. Histologically, there is intense dermal edema, vascular dilation and subtle small vessel leukocytoclastic vasculitis, affecting only the superficial plexus. Thrombi may be seen occasionally. The epidermis may be eroded or ulcerated but undergoes papillary hyperplasia over time.

Bibliography

Stannard AA. Photoactivated vasculitis. In: Robinson NE, ed. Current Therapy in Equine Medicine II. Philadelphia, PA: WB Saunders, 1987:647.

von Tscharner C, et al. Stannard's illustrated equine dermatology notes. Vet Dermatol 2000;11:161–215.

NUTRITIONAL DISEASES OF SKIN

The elasticity of the skin, the orderly maturation of the epidermis and the quality and luster of the horny appendages are an indication of the state of the health of the animal as a whole. This applies equally to nutritional diseases and to diseases of other causes. Many systemic diseases result in cutaneous changes. The general metabolic transformations that take place in the skin are not qualitatively different from those in other tissues but there are some quantitative differences, such as the high requirements and turnover of sulfur-containing amino acids in the elaboration of keratin. *In most metabolic disturbances and deficiencies of essential nutrients, whether from dietary lack, malabsorption, the action of antimetabolites, or the body's inability to properly absorb or utilize nutrients, changes will be reflected in the skin*. The molecular basis for these skin lesions is, however, poorly understood. There are only a few syndromes that occur naturally and are sufficiently clearly defined to warrant discussion here. A larger number can be produced experimentally. Cutaneous manifestations of systemic disease not known to be a result of a nutritional derangement are discussed in other, more appropriate sections of this chapter such as Endocrine diseases of skin and Cutaneous paraneoplastic syndromes.

Protein–calorie deficiency

Starvation or protein–calorie malnutrition results in changes in the skin, the first being the *disappearance of subcutaneous fat*. Even though water intake may not be restricted, there is reduced hydration of the connective tissues of the subcutis and dermis, and the skin wrinkles and loses its elasticity. As hair is 95% protein, *hair growth and keratinization can require up to 25–30% of an animal's daily protein requirement*. Protein deficiencies are rare but can occur in cats fed primarily food formulated for dogs, in young dogs fed a low-protein diet, or in animals with increased nutrient requirements.

An early sign of starvation is the development of a *dull, dry and often brittle hair coat*. Hypotrichosis develops as a thinning of the hair rather than baldness, and seasonal shedding may cease or be prolonged. Lesions may be symmetrical on the head and trunk and spread to the limbs. The skin may atrophy, or hyperkeratosis, hyperpigmentation, and possibly loss of hair pigmentation develop. In pigs, the skin often becomes hyperkeratotic and assumes a dirty, dry appearance and the hair becomes long and shaggy. The skin of a malnourished animal has an increased susceptibility to bacterial infection and parasitic infestations and their effects. Under-nutrition of the pregnant ewe, between 115–135 days of gestation, decreases the number of secondary wool follicles in the developing fetus. Most experimental work on the effects of nutrition on hair growth have been performed in sheep, the purpose being either to improve wool production or to investigate chemical methods of shearing. Changing sheep from a low-protein to a high-protein diet led to a 33% increase in fleece production, due mostly to an increase in the rate of mitosis in the hair bulb. Specific amino acid deficiencies have been investigated as potential replacements for mechanical shearing as wool production is highly dependant upon levels of certain amino acids, specifically cysteine.

The effects of starvation on other organs such as liver, pancreas, bone, and bone marrow are discussed elsewhere.

Fatty acid deficiency

Fatty acid deficiency may occur in all domestic species in association with general dietary deficiency, malabsorption or liver disease. Deficiencies may be evident in animals when the fat has either leached from a diet, has become rancid from improper or prolonged storage, or when the diet was formulated with low fat content to save cost. Animals on specially formulated low-fat diets for therapeutic reasons may develop signs of fatty acid deficiency and require specific types of supplementation. Animals on antioxidant-deficient diets may also develop signs of fatty acid deficiency. Cutaneous lesions take months to develop and begin with *diffuse scaling, loss of haircoat sheen, and alopecia*. The scaliness is initially dry but over months progresses to an oily, often pruritic stage. Otitis externa may be an accompanying lesion and the skin is susceptible to secondary bacterial and yeast infection. Histologic lesions include *epidermal hyperplasia, orthokeratotic or parakeratotic hyperkeratosis and hypergranulosis*. The pathologic mechanisms underlying the epidermal hyperproliferation are not well understood. Experimental studies demonstrated an increase in epidermal DNA synthesis and a decrease in prostaglandin E and F levels in the skin of essential fatty acid-deficient mice. The lower prostaglandin levels likely reflect a lack of precursor arachidonic acid. Deficiency of prostaglandin E_2 could influence epidermal cell kinetics through its effect on ratios of cyclic AMP to GMP. Supplementation of animal diets with balanced omega-6 and omega-3 fatty acids is thought to modulate arachidonic acid metabolism and subsequent production of leukotrienes and prostaglandins that in turn may influence epidermal turnover kinetics and the inflammatory response.

A seborrheic dermatosis in **cats** characterized by dry scaly skin and alopecia is responsive to fatty acid supplementation but is not likely to be the result of a true deficiency. Experimental essential fatty acid deprivation in cats produces dry, scaly coats. Diets containing linoleic acid and linolenic acids as the sole source of essential fatty acids also induce a seborrheic dermatosis. Cats are obligate carnivores, as they lack delta-6-desaturase, the enzyme responsible for converting these 18-carbon fatty acids to longer chain fatty acids. Arachidonic acid is an essential fatty acid for the cat.

Hypovitaminoses and vitamin-responsive dermatoses

Cutaneous lesions may occur as manifestations of deficiencies of *vitamins A, C, and E, riboflavin, pantothenic acid, biotin, and niacin*. Most of these are described in experimentally induced deficiencies. Many of the naturally occurring hypovitaminoses are probably not the result of a single vitamin deficiency but represent the cumulative effect of several inadequacies of the diet.

Vitamin A deficiency

Vitamin A is a fat-soluble vitamin belonging to a group of compounds referred to as *retinoids*.Vitamin A is involved in cellular growth and differentiation, as well as in visual processes and reproduction. Vitamin A has a controlling effect on epithelial differentiation. *Cutaneous lesions of vitamin A deficiency are squamous epithelial hyperkeratosis and squamous metaplasia of secretory epithelia.*Vitamin A oversupplementation is teratogenic and can lead to toxicity if liver storage capacity is exceeded. Signs are manifest primarily in the skeletal system and liver, or as malformations of the fetus in pregnant animals.

Hypovitaminosis A has been reported in all species of domestic animals, although many accounts are anecdotal. It may be secondary to dietary deficiency, decreased intestinal absorption, liver disease or toxicities such as chlorinated naphthalene toxicity of cattle. Bile and pancreatic enzymes are needed for dietary absorption of vitamin A. The cutaneous lesions of hypovitaminosis A in *cattle* are a marked scaling and crusting dermatitis; in the *pig*, follicular hyperkeratosis; and, in *cats*, scaling, follicular plugging and alopecia. A report in the *dog* indicated thickened, hyperpigmented skin with alopecia and follicular hyperkeratosis.

Vitamin A-responsive dermatoses occur in **dogs** and almost exclusively in the Cocker Spaniel. In one syndrome, Cocker Spaniels are predisposed, probably because of a congenital abnormality of epidermopoiesis and keratinization (see Seborrhea). The lesions include hyperkeratotic plaques, follicular plugging and the formation of keratin fronds. Ventral and lateral chest and abdomen are sites of predilection. There may be accompanying otitis externa and pyoderma. Histologically, *the predominant lesion is marked follicular keratosis* (Fig. 5.55). Vertically oriented keratin casts protrude from the follicular ostia. There is mild to moderate epidermal hyperplasia and surface hyperkeratosis of the basket weave type. Dermal inflammation is mild, mononuclear and perivascular, unless secondary bacterial infection intervenes to produce neutrophilic folliculitis and/or furunculosis. There are rare reports of vitamin A-responsive dermatoses in other breeds of dogs. These diseases are not vitamin A deficiencies per se, in that plasma levels of vitamin A are within the normal range. The fact that therapy is effective can be attributed more to the "normalizing" effect of vitamin A (and retinoids) on cellular differentiation in the epidermis. Differentials include primary or secondary seborrhea and late-stage sebaceous adenitis. Oral supplementation with vitamin A may be needed to confirm the diagnosis.

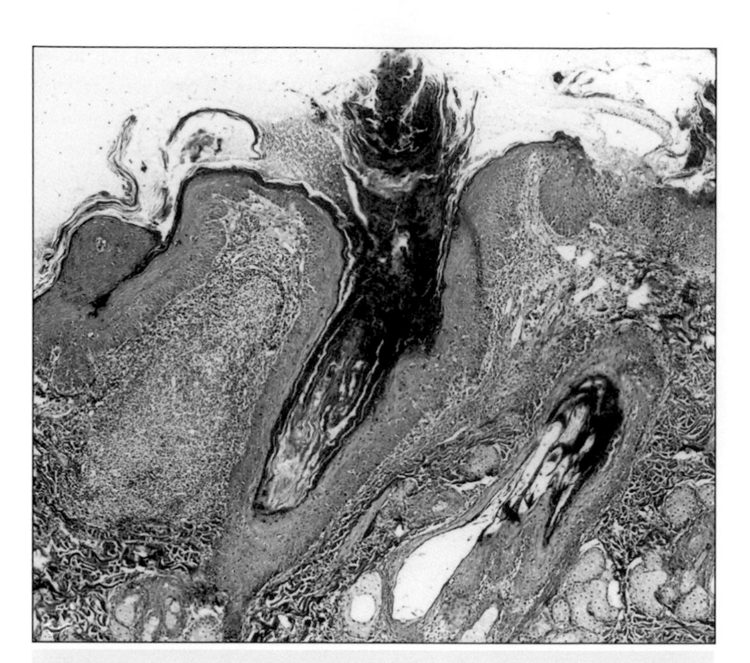

Figure 5.55 Vitamin A-responsive dermatosis. Note the marked follicular hyperkeratosis. (Courtesy of Parker WM, Hardy MH, and J Am Anim Hosp Assoc.)

Vitamin B deficiencies

The **B-vitamin complex** is essential to the maintenance and proper functioning of many important metabolic pathways. B vitamins are water soluble and not stored within the body, necessitating a constant dietary supply. These vitamins interact with each other, with vitamin C, and with fat-soluble vitamins. Single deficiencies of these vitamins are rare. *Deficiencies result in dry, flaky seborrhea with alopecia, anorexia, and weight loss.*

Riboflavin (vitamin B2) deficiency is mostly a problem in *swine and chickens* fed grain rations with borderline concentrations of the vitamin. Ruminants do not become deficient because of rumen synthesis of the B-complex vitamins. Young calves, however, may develop deficiency if deprived of milk or an appropriate replacer. Animals develop hyperemia around the lips, nose and buccal mucosa, diarrhea, weight loss and generalized alopecia. Cutaneous lesions described in hyporiboflavinosis include scaling and ulcerative dermatitis in the pig, erythema, scaling and dry hair coat on the ventral abdomen and hindlegs in the dog, and alopecia in the cat.

Pantothenic acid is a component of coenzyme A, an essential factor for entrance of acetic acid into the Krebs' cycle. Deficiency is documented in *pigs*, but may occur in dogs and calves. Pantothenic acid deficiency in pigs produces progressive alopecia with dermatitis and ulceration, in addition to the general effects of weight loss, diarrhea and neurologic signs. Young pre-ruminant calves may show dermatologic signs that include alopecia, a roughened coat and dermatitis. Leukotrichia has been described in dogs.

Biotin deficiency rarely occurs spontaneously, except in intensively reared *swine*, as the vitamin is widely distributed in feeds. Biotin is essential for proper utilization of fats, glucose, and amino acids. Feeding raw egg whites that contain avidin, a substance that renders biotin unavailable, may induce deficiencies. Cutaneous lesions reported in biotin-deficient pigs include *alopecia, pustular dermatitis and cracked hooves*, causing lameness and significant economic loss. Microscopic lesions include epidermal hyperplasia, orthokeratotic and parakeratotic hyperkeratosis, epidermal necrosis and pustules, and folliculitis. A deficiency attributed, in part, to a lack of vitamin B, probably biotin, was reported in *lambs* reared artificially on reconstituted cow's milk. Alopecia was largely due to a fleece in which individual fibers were thin, weak and straight. Histologically and ultrastructurally, the wool fibers had reduced numbers of cortical cells. Histochemical stains showed a delay in the incorporation and oxidation of sulfhydryl groups. Supplementation with B-group vitamins partially restored the fleece. Biotin deficiency reportedly causes a dry, brittle, hair coat, scaling and leukotrichia in *dogs*. Dogs deficient in biotin may develop periocular and facial alopecia resembling the clinical lesions of systemic lupus erythematosus, discoid lupus, or other dermatoses affecting the face.

Niacin is a component of the pyridine nucleotides NAD+ and NADP+ needed for the function of a number of enzymes involved in nutrient metabolism. Deficiency occurs spontaneously in animals fed diets low in pyridoxine (vitamin B6) and tryptophan as all of these components are needed for pyridine nucleotide synthesis. *Pigs* fed a low animal protein diet that is also high in corn renders niacin unavailable to the animal due to low tryptophan levels. Cutaneous lesions include alopecia and a crusting dermatitis. Niacin deficiency in *dogs* induces reddening and ulceration of the oral mucous membranes, resembling human hyponiacinosis, known as "*pellagra*." Reports of canine cases from the first quarter of the 20th century indicate severe necrotizing glossitis and stomatitis leading to the term "*black tongue*."

Pyridoxine (vitamin B_6) serves as coenzyme in amino acid and protein metabolism. Deficiency produced experimentally in *cats* resulted in a dull, unkempt coat with scaliness and alopecia of the head and extremities. Histologically, hair follicles were in telogen and there was epidermal and follicular hyperkeratosis. Since pyridoxine may be indirectly involved in zinc transport, through its effect on tryptophan metabolism, these effects might be due to alteration in the levels of zinc. Isoniazid has been reported to inactivate pyridoxine.

Vitamin C deficiency

Vitamin C (ascorbic acid) is required for the proper synthesis and structural maintenance of collagen and as a component of a number of essential enzymes. Almost all mammals synthesize vitamin C with the exception of humans, nonhuman primates, guinea pigs, Indian fruit bats, and Indian pipistrels. Insects, invertebrates, and fish also cannot synthesize vitamin C. *Deficiencies (scurvy or scorbutus) are limited to these species of animals*, and signs are related to the inability of fibroblasts to form collagen or osteoid and are discussed in Vol. 1, Bones and joints.

Vitamin E deficiency

Vitamin E deficiency is discussed primarily in Vol. 1, Bones and joints and Vol. 2, Liver and biliary system. Steatitis or "*yellow-fat disease*" involves subcutaneous fat and may be seen clinically as a skin disease. The yellowness of the fat is due to the *deposition of ceroid*. Vitamin E acts as an antioxidant to prevent lipid peroxidation. Dietary requirements vary by species and individual and with the other components of the diet. Naturally occurring vitamin E deficiency has not been reported in the dog.

Nutritional panniculitis occurs in *cats, mink, foals and swine*. The disease is associated with the feeding of *fishmeal, fish offal or other products with a high concentration of unsaturated fatty acids*. Diets with a high content of oily fish such as tuna, white fish and sardines are most often implicated, however, the condition in cats also has been associated with diets containing primarily liver, diets with only a small fish content, or improperly stored or outdated commercial cat food. The practice of feeding high-fish diets to cats is reported to be common in Greece. Destruction of vitamin E also occurs in food that, through improper processing or storage, becomes rancid. The disease is not, however, the result of a simple deficiency, since cats fed diets deficient in vitamin E but also lacking in unsaturated fatty acids, do not develop panniculitis. In *mink and foals*, it may be associated with degeneration of muscles, and in *swine* it may occur alone or be associated with any one or combination of ulceration of the squamous mucosa of the stomach, muscle degeneration, and hepatosis dietetica. The disease has variable mortality in *cats* after a short clinical course in which there is progressive depression, possible fever, hyperesthesia, reluctance to move, palpable thickening and increased firmness of the subcutaneous fat, easiest to detect in the inguinal region. The changes are not confined to the subcutaneous tissues but affect all fat depots. Biopsy reveals fat that varies from gray to lemon yellow to orange and is indurated and sometimes edematous. Hematological changes may include neutrophilic leukocytosis and anemia.

The initial histologic change is deposition of globules of ceroid in the interstitial tissue. This, together with a fishy odor, may be all that is observed in swine in which the fat is soft and gray rather than yellow. In most affected cats, *fat necrosis stimulates inflammation, which is initially neutrophilic but becomes granulomatous*. Numerous macrophages, and occasionally giant cells, ingest the ceroid pigment. Mineralization may be present. Ceroid may be found also in macrophages of the liver, spleen and lymph nodes. In cats, the initial differential should include infectious steatitis, sterile nodular panniculitis, lupus panniculitis, or other noncutaneous diseases such as feline infectious peritonitis, ascites of various causes, and other causes of hyperesthesia. *The clinical signs and the demonstration of ceroid, a variant of lipofuscin, which is acid fast and autofluorescent, should establish the diagnosis*.

Vitamin E-responsive dermatosis has been described in **goats**. Kids and adults, on a selenium-deficient diet, developed periorbital alopecia and generalized seborrhea. The haircoat was dull and brittle. Histologically, the lesions were orthokeratotic hyperkeratosis and mild superficial perivascular dermatitis, in which mononuclear cells predominated.

In **dogs**, a variety of conditions including dermatomyositis, acanthosis nigricans, demodicosis, and discoid lupus erythematosus are variably responsive to topical or systemic vitamin E therapy. Improvement in condition is thought to be due to the antioxidant properties of vitamin E leading to the stabilization of cell membranes and modulation of the inflammatory response through arachidonic acid and prostaglandin metabolism and actions on leukocytes.

Alopecia in **calves** associated with the feeding of milk substitute was attributed, in part, to vitamin E deficiency. The calves had low levels of serum vitamin E and the hair regrew after vitamin E therapy was initiated for concurrent nutritional myopathy.

Bibliography

Blanchard PC, et al. Pathology associated with vitamin B-6 deficiency in growing kittens. J Nutr 1991;121:S77–S78.

Carey CJ, Morris JG. Biotin deficiency in the cat and the effect on hepatic propionyl CoA carboxylase. J Nutr 1977;107:330–334.

Chapman RE, Black JL. Abnormal wool growth and alopecia of artificially reared lambs. Aust J Biol Sci 1981;34:11–26.

Codner EC, Thatcher CD. Nutritional management of skin disease. Compend Contin Educ Pract Vet 1993;15:411–423.

De Jong MF, Sytsema JR. Field experience with d-biotin supplementation to gilt and sowfeeds. Vet Q 1983;5:58–67.

Elias PM, et al. Retinoid effects on epidermal structure, differentiation, and permeability. Lab Invest 1981;44:531–540.

Frigg M, et al. Clinical study on the effect of biotin on skin conditions in dogs. Schweizer Arch Tierheilkunde 1989;131:621–625.

Hutchison G, Mellor DJ. Effects of maternal nutrition on the initiation of secondary wool follicles in foetal sheep. J Comp Pathol 1983;93:577–583.

Hynd PI. Effects of nutrition on wool follicle cell kinetics in sheep differing in efficiency of wool production. Aust J Agric Res 1989;40:409–417.

Ihrke PJ, Goldschmidt MH. Vitamin A-responsive dermatosis in the dog. J Am Vet Med Assoc 1983;182:687–690.

Niza MM, et al. Feline pansteatitis revisited: hazards of unbalanced home-made diets. J Feline Med Surg 2003;5:271–277.

Pritchard GC. Alopecia in calves associated with milk substitute feeding. Vet Rec 1983;112:435–436.

Scott DW, et al., eds. Nutritional skin diseases. In: Small Animal Dermatology. 5th ed. Philadelphia, PA: WB Saunders, 1995:890–901.

Ward KA, et al. The regulation of wool growth in transgenic animals. In: von Tscharner C, Halliwell REW, eds. Advances in Veterinary Dermatology. Vol 1. London: Baillière Tindall, 1990:70–76.

Watson TD. Diet and skin disease in dogs and cats. J Nutr 1998;128(12 Suppl):2783S–2789S.

Mineral deficiency and mineral-responsive dermatoses

Iodine, cobalt, copper, and zinc deficiencies may lead to integumentary lesions. Iodine deficiency is discussed in Vol. 3, Endocrine glands. The effects of copper deficiency on wool and hair are referred to under Disorders of pigmentation. Cobalt deficiency causes a progressive, wasting disease in ruminants. There are nonspecific changes in the wool or hair coat including lack of growth and increased fragility.

Zinc deficiency

Zinc is an essential trace element. Zinc is a component of many important metalloenzymes and is a cofactor for many others. It exerts its primary effect through zinc-dependent enzymes that regulate RNA and DNA metabolism. Zinc thus plays a role in all metabolic processes involved with tissue growth, maturation and repair, and is involved in vitamin A metabolism and in enzymes needed for free radical scavenging. Zinc also modulates many aspects of the immune and inflammatory responses. The relationship between the changes in particular tissue enzyme activities brought about by zinc deficiency and clinical manifestations of the deficiency syndrome are not, however, well understood. In the integument, a substantial proportion of zinc is in the wool or the hair coat. Naturally occurring true zinc deficiency is extremely rare in cats, and not reported in horses, or dogs. On the other hand, zinc-responsive dermatoses are described in the dog in the following sections.

Zinc deficiency causes anorexia, alterations in food utilization, growth retardation, reproductive disorders, depression of the immune response, hematologic abnormalities, depression of central nervous system development, decreased wound healing, and keratinization defects in epidermis, hair, wool, and horny appendages. True zinc deficiency is of most significance in the pig.

Parakeratosis in swine

Zinc-responsive dermatosis in swine (parakeratosis) became an important clinical entity in the 1950s, coincident with and related to the widespread introduction of dry meal feeding. *The cause is not a simple deficiency.* The availability of dietary zinc is adversely affected by the presence of phytic acid in plant protein rations, a high concentration of calcium, a low concentration of free fatty acids, alterations in intestinal flora, and the presence of bacterial and viral enteric pathogens such as transmissible gastroenteritis virus. Zinc deficiency may induce secondary vitamin A deficiency as a result of its effect on appetite and food utilization. Economic losses are due to depression of growth rate, but, with improved management techniques, *parakeratosis is no longer a major problem.* Parakeratosis occurs in young, growing pigs, 2–4 months of age. The initial gross lesions are erythematous macules on the ventral abdomen and medial surface of the thigh. The lesions develop into papules, which become covered with a gray-brown, dry, roughened scale-crust that may reach 5–7 mm in thickness. Deep fissures penetrate the crust and are filled with brown-black detritus, which is composed of sebum, sweat, soil and other debris. These areas are susceptible to secondary bacterial infection, often leading to pyoderma or subcutaneous abscessation. *Lesions are roughly symmetrical and have a predilection for the lower limbs, particularly over the joints, around the eyes, ears, snout, scrotum and tail.* In severely affected animals, lesions may become generalized. Pruritus is not a feature of parakeratosis. The dorsal surface of the tongue is "furred" and the esophageal mucosa loses its normal smooth sheen and becomes dull and white.

The microscopic lesion in the skin is marked hyperplastic dermatitis with diffuse parakeratotic hyperkeratosis (Fig. 5.56A, B). The oral mucous membranes also demonstrate hyperplastic epithelium. Acanthosis, elongation of rete ridges, and mitotic figures in the basal keratinocytes are regular features of the hyperplastic response of the epidermis. The dermal lesions in uncomplicated parakeratosis include variable vasodilation and a mild to moderate, predominantly mononuclear cell, perivascular infiltrate. With bacterial infection, there may be nodular or diffuse neutrophilic dermatitis, folliculitis, perifolliculitis or furunculosis.

Parakeratosis in swine must be differentiated grossly from sarcoptic mange and exudative epidermitis. The former is usually intensely pruritic, and the latter usually occurs in a younger age group and the scale-crust is greasy rather than dry. Parakeratosis is rarely fatal unless toxemia or septicemia secondary to cutaneous bacterial infection develops or because of exacerbation of intercurrent infections such as pneumonia. Affected pigs recover rapidly upon zinc supplementation.

Zinc deficiency in ruminants

The clinical signs and gross lesions of zinc deficiency in ruminants are similar to those described in pigs. Hyperkeratosis also affects the forestomachs. Naturally occurring zinc-deficiency dermatoses are uncommon in **cattle**, but have been reported, for example, in grazing cattle from Guyana and housed dairy cows in Finland. The

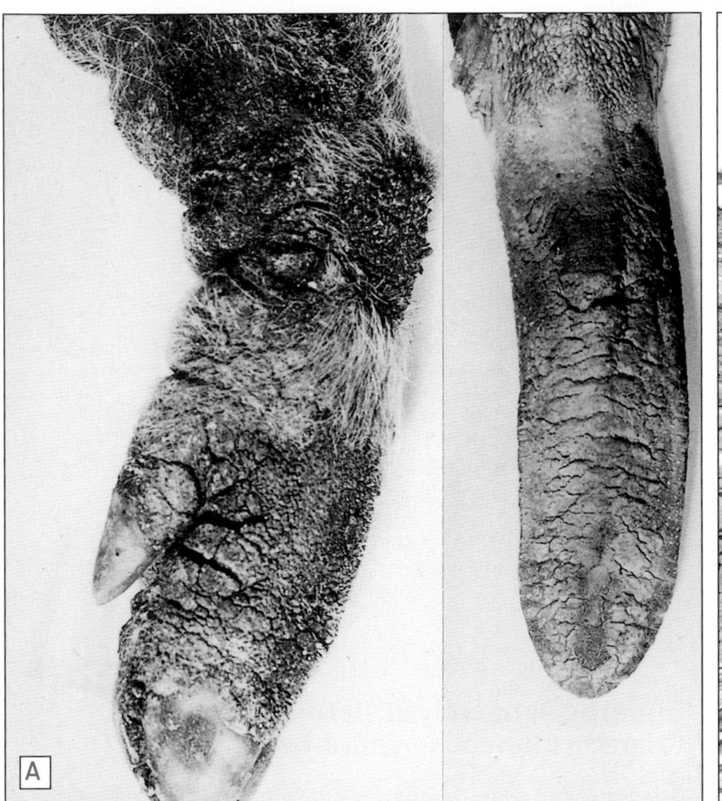

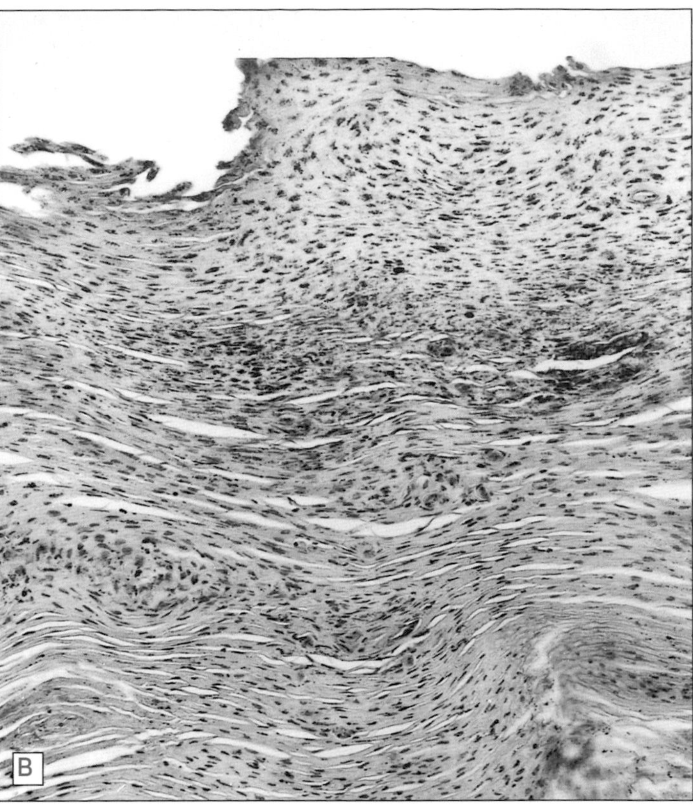

Figure 5.56 Zinc-responsive dermatosis in a pig. **A.** Marked hyperkeratosis of the skin of the foreleg and tongue epithelium. **B.** Marked parakeratotic hyperkeratosis.

hereditary zinc deficiencies of cattle are discussed under Congenital and hereditary diseases of skin.

In **sheep** with naturally occurring deficiency, histologically the hyperkeratosis is predominantly of the orthokeratotic rather than the parakeratotic type. Sheep also have thin, easily epilated, red-brown stained wool and loss of fleece. Wool eating and drooling are prominent clinical signs. Crusting and scaling lesions develop around the eyes, nose, hooves, and scrotum and on pressure points. The normal ringed structure of the horns is lost and the horns are shed. Abnormal growth of the hooves may lead to soreness and the adoption of a kyphotic stance.

Zinc-responsive dermatoses in **goats** are reported from the USA, Europe and Australia, sometimes associated with depressed reproductive efficiency. Experimental zinc deficiency of goats produces the typical weight loss, alopecia and parakeratotic scaling dermatosis described in other ruminant species.

Bibliography

Luecke RW, et al. Calcium and zinc in parakeratosis of swine. J Anim Sci 1957;16:3–11.

Singer LJ, et al. Zinc responsive dermatopathy in goats: two field cases. Contemp Top Lab Anim Sci 2000;39:32–35.

Suttle NF. Problems in the diagnosis and anticipation of trace element deficiencies in grazing livestock. Vet Rec 1986;119:148–152.

White CL, et al. The effect of zinc deficiency on wool growth and skin and wool follicle histology of male Merino lambs. Br J Nutr 1994;71:425–435.

Whitenack DL, et al. Influence of enteric infection on zinc utilization and clinical signs and lesions of zinc deficiency in young swine. Am J Vet Res 1978;39:1447–1454.

Canine zinc-responsive dermatoses

Naturally occurring zinc-responsive dermatoses in the dog fall under two syndromes:

- **Syndrome 1** *affects primarily Siberian Huskies and Alaskan Malamutes*, and rarely other breeds not of Arctic origin, such as Great Danes. The cutaneous lesions usually become manifest before the dogs are 1 yr of age. Older dogs may develop lesions during times of stress such as pregnancy, lactation or intercurrent disease. Lesions comprise *scaling and crusting dermatitis* with a predilection for the face, particularly around the eyes, lips and nose, pressure points and footpads (Fig. 5.57A). Lesions may be unilateral initially and progress to a bilateral distribution. Pruritus may be present. Secondary pyoderma is not uncommon. *The pathogenesis of the syndrome is not well established*. Alaskan Malamutes with chondrodysplasia have zinc-responsive spermatozoal defects and reduced zinc absorption from the intestinal tract; possibly malabsorption is responsible for the dermatological disease. Lifetime supplementation of zinc is necessary to alleviate signs.
- **Syndrome 2** *occurs in puppies of any breed and is associated with a relative deficiency of zinc, probably secondary to excessively high levels of calcium and/or phytates in the diet in rapidly growing animals*. In the USA, this disease has been associated with the feeding of *generic dog food*, in Britain and Sweden with the feeding of soy- and/or cereal-based diets. Recovery quickly follows restoration of a diet meeting the National Research Council standards for canine nutrition or zinc supplementation of cereal diets. Now that dog food manufacturers are aware of the problem, *the disease is less common*. The gross

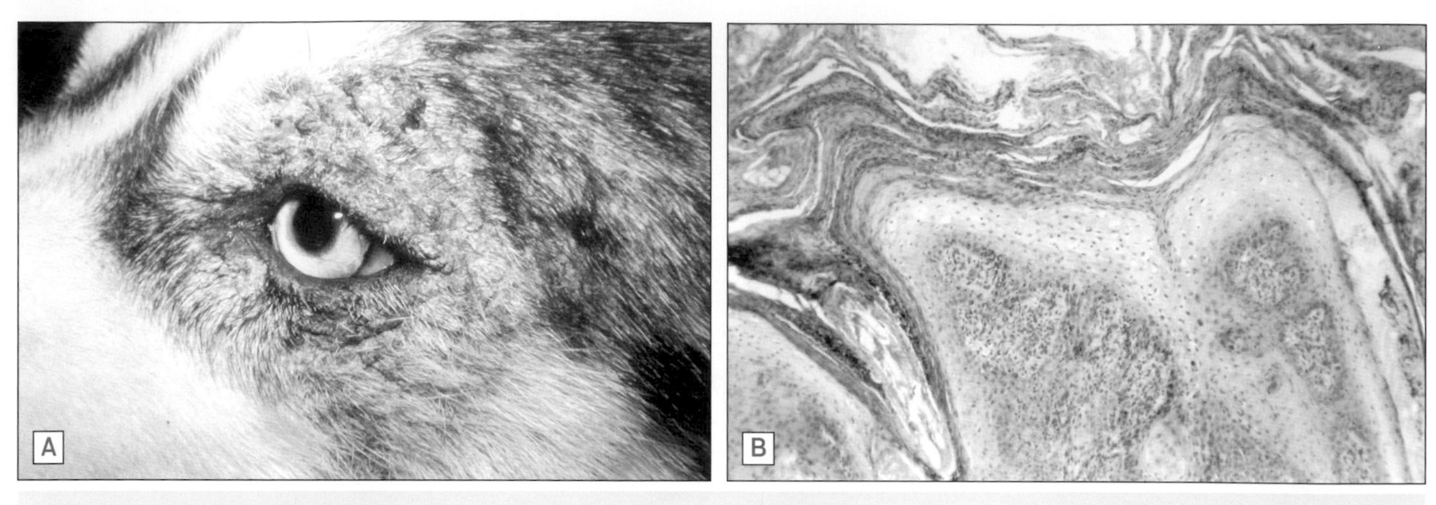

Figure 5.57 Zinc-responsive dermatitis in a dog. **A.** Scaling and crusting dermatitis of the face. (Courtesy of B Dunstan.) **B.** Papillary epidermal hyperplasia, marked epidermal edema and parakeratotic hyperkeratosis affecting the epithelium of the skin surface and follicular ostia.

lesions are multiple, scaling and crusted plaques, particularly affecting the muzzle, pressure points, distal extremities and trunk. There is extreme thickening and fissuring of the footpads and, sometimes, the planum nasale. Secondary pyoderma may develop and puppies often show a local lymphadenopathy.

The histologic lesions of both syndromes are usually typical of zinc deficiency, with papillary epidermal hyperplasia, marked spongiotic parakeratotic hyperkeratosis affecting the epithelium of the skin surface and follicular ostia, and multifocal neutrophilic crusts (Fig. 5.57B). Mild to moderate superficial perivascular mononuclear or eosinophil-rich dermatitis is present. Some reports indicate that the keratinization defect was sufficiently severe to induce dyskeratotic changes at all levels of the epidermis, while in others orthokeratotic hyperkeratosis alone was found.

Differential diagnoses include superficial necrolytic dermatitis, thallium toxicity and chronic hypersensitivity dermatitis that may look very similar histologically. Dermatophytosis, demodicosis, and pyoderma should be considered based upon gross lesions. *The signalment, history, lesion distribution, and pathologic changes should help to establish the diagnosis.* In some cases, response to dietary changes and/or zinc supplementation may be needed for confirmation of the suspected diagnosis. Serum and plasma zinc levels are not an accurate method of assessing zinc status. Values, even in a normal animal, are subject to marked variation according to sex, age, stress, concurrent disease, and collection methods. It is possible that dietary factors other than zinc are involved in some of these diseases, particularly those responding to dietary changes and not just to zinc supplementation.

Bibliography

Colombini S. Canine zinc-responsive dermatosis. Vet Clin North Am: Small Anim Pract 1999;29:1373–1383.

Thoday KL. Diet-related zinc-responsive skin disease in dogs: a dying dermatosis? J Small Anim Pract 1989;30:213–215.

White SD, et al. Zinc-responsive dermatosis in dogs: 41 cases and literature review. Vet Dermatol 2001;12:101–109.

Superficial necrolytic dermatitis (hepatocutaneous syndrome)

A histologically distinct cutaneous reaction pattern characterized by the so called "red, white, and blue" *epidermal changes of parakeratosis, epidermal necrolysis or laminar intra-epidermal edema, and basilar hyperplasia* has been recognized most often in the *dog*, and occasionally in the *cat*. The condition resembles necrolytic migratory erythema, a human paraneoplastic syndrome most often associated with alpha cell neoplasms of the pancreas. *The pathogenesis of superficial necrolytic dermatitis (SND) is unknown, but hepatic dysfunction and derangement of glucose and amino acid metabolism are clearly involved.* Elevated glucagon levels alone are unlikely to be directly responsible for the skin lesions, as both dogs and humans may develop the disease in their absence and dermatitis is not an inevitable result of the hyperglucagonemic state. Hypoaminoacidemia, due to sustained gluconeogenesis and increased hepatic catabolism, is documented in both canine and human patients and it has been postulated that it may deplete epidermal proteins and induce epidermal necrosis. Zinc and fatty acid metabolism may also be deranged. *The most likely pathogenesis of abnormal or impaired ability to properly utilize nutrients and the clinical and histologic similarities of this entity to zinc-responsive dermatoses* warrant discussion of SND in this section.

In dogs, SND has been reported to occur in association with a variety of systemic diseases including *glucagon-secreting tumors of the pancreas, hyperglucagonemia, diabetes mellitus, and liver disease.* Over 90% of the reported canine cases are associated with *severe hepatopathy*. The variety of concurrent diseases and the histologic appearance have led to terms for the characteristic cutaneous reaction pattern in dogs. These include superficial necrolytic dermatitis, hepatocutaneous syndrome, diabetic dermatopathy, metabolic epidermal necrosis, and necrolytic migratory erythema. Diabetes and hyperglucagonemia in some cases could be secondary to the hepatic degeneration. A feline case was associated with a pancreatic carcinoma presumably of endocrine origin.

Lesions have a roughly bilaterally symmetrical distribution. The muzzle, lips, periocular skin, edges of the pinnae, distal extremities,

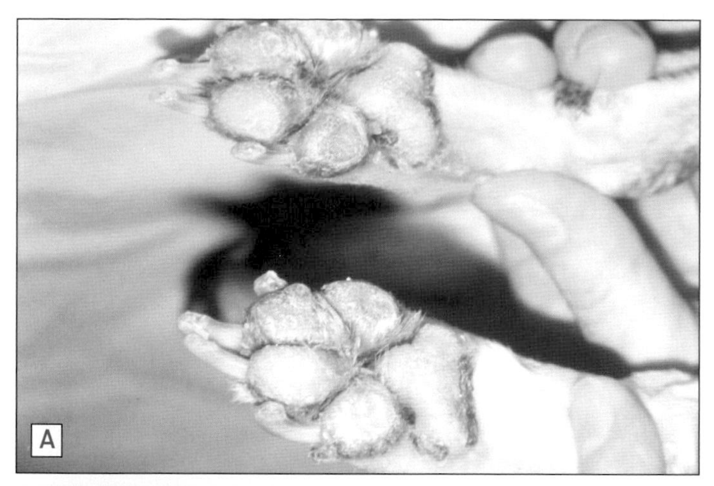

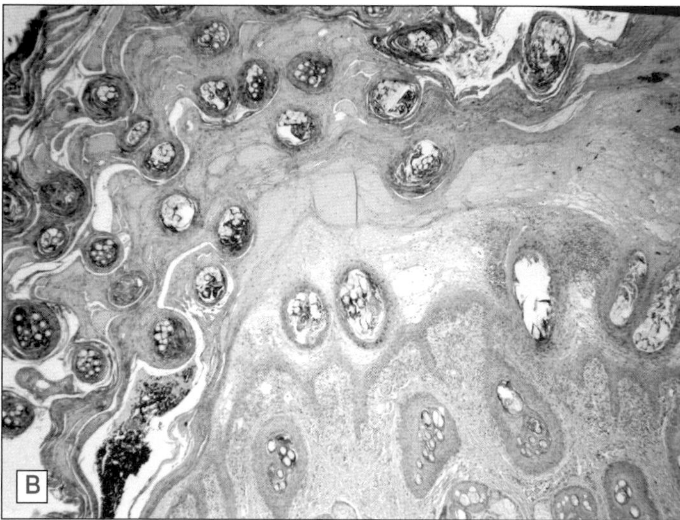

Figure 5.58 Superficial necrolytic dermatitis in a dog. **A.** Marked hyperkeratosis of the footpads. **B.** The histologic changes of the epidermis make a characteristic "red (parakeratosis), white (epidermal edema), and blue (basilar hyperplasia)" pattern.

ventrum and points of pressure or friction, such as the hocks, and the external genitalia are typically affected. Oral and mucocutaneous lesions are occasionally reported. Lesions are erythematous, erosive, ulcerative and crusted. The footpads are markedly hyperkeratotic (Fig. 5.58A). Footpad lesions were not a feature of SND in the cat. *The histologic lesions of the "red, white and blue" epidermis are virtually pathognomonic - the distinctive feature is a band of hydropic, pale-staining keratinocytes in the upper half of a usually acanthotic stratum spinosum* (Fig. 5.58B). Both intra- and intercellular edema contribute to the epidermal pallor. As these cells degenerate, clefts and vesicles may form in the outer stratum spinosum. Neutrophils may accumulate to form subcorneal pustules. The stratum corneum is diffusely and markedly parakeratotic and appears hypereosinophilic in comparison to the subjacent pale-staining stratum spinosum of the epidermis. The epithelium of the follicular infundibulum can also be affected. The basal cell layer is basophilic and hyperplastic, forming small rete ridges. Dermal inflammation is minimal, and predominantly mononuclear and perivascular. In eroded lesions, neutrophilic exocytosis is prominent and inflammatory crust covers the surface.

In cases associated with liver disease, the most commonly associated gross lesion is a *nodular liver with intervening firm, collapsed parenchyma*. Histologically, there is loss of parenchyma and minimal inflammation. Hepatocytes are markedly vacuolated due partially to fatty degeneration. The nodules have been interpreted in some cases to represent regeneration and in others to be comprised of nodular remnants of atrophic hepatic parenchyma.

The diagnosis is based on typical histologic findings. However, the pathognomonic epidermal edema may not be present in every biopsy. *Differential diagnoses* include other parakeratotic, hyperplastic dermatitides, such as the zinc-responsive dermatoses, lethal acrodermatitis of bull terriers, and thallium toxicity. The clinical differential is the same as listed for zinc-responsive dermatoses. The prognosis is generally considered poor since most cases have advanced liver disease. Cases associated with a pancreatic neoplasm may have resolution of skin lesions following tumor excision.

Bibliography

Allenspach K, et al. Glucagon-producing neuroendocrine tumour associated with hypoaminoacidaemia and skin lesions. J Small Anim Pract 2000;41:402–406.

Byrne KP. Metabolic epidermal necrosis-hepatocutaneous syndrome. Vet Clin North Am Small Anim Pract 1999;29:1337–1355.

Hill PB, et al. Resolution of skin lesions and long-term survival in a dog with superficial necrolytic dermatitis and liver cirrhosis. J Small Anim Pract 2000;41:519–523.

Kimmel SE, et al. Clinicopathological, ultrasonographic, and histopathological findings of superficial necrolytic dermatitis with hepatopathy in a cat. J Am Anim Hosp Assoc 2003;39:23–27.

Outerbridge CA, et al. Plasma amino acid concentrations in 36 dogs with histologically confirmed superficial necrolytic dermatitis. Vet Dermatol 2002; 13:177–186.

Turek MM. Cutaneous paraneoplastic syndromes in dogs and cats: a review of the literature. Vet Dermatol 2003;14:279–296.

ENDOCRINE DISEASES OF SKIN

Endocrine disorders frequently manifest clinically as skin disease, but these dermatoses are rarely specific for any one endocrinopathy. While these dermatopathies are more common in dogs, they can occur in any species. **Clinical features** of many endocrine dermatoses include *a dry, coarse, brittle, dull, easily epilated haircoat that fails to regrow after clipping, hypotrichosis and hyperpigmentation, and alopecia that is frequently bilaterally symmetrical.* Secondary pyoderma and seborrhea are common. In addition, endocrine dermatoses share many **histologic features**, *including orthokeratotic hyperkeratosis, follicular keratosis, dilation of follicular ostia and infundibula, hair follicle atrophy, absence of hair shafts in follicles, increased numbers of telogen follicles, variably increased trichilemmal keratinization (flame follicles) of follicles, and epidermal hyperpigmentation.* These histologic changes suggest an endocrine dermatosis but frequently are not pathognomonic for a specific endocrinopathy. *A combination of clinical and histologic features together with clinical testing to demonstrate hormonal deficiency or excess is required for confirmation.*

Hypothyroidism

Hypothyroidism is the most common endocrine dermatopathy in **dogs**, and almost all cases are due to primary hypothyroidism. The most common cause is thought to be *lymphocytic thyroiditis*, an immune-mediated condition similar to Hashimoto's thyroiditis in humans. *Idiopathic thyroid atrophy* is also a common cause and may represent the end stage of lymphocytic thyroiditis. *Other causes* include developmental defects of the thyroid gland and rarely iodine deficiency. Pituitary neoplasia, or hypopituitarism, resulting in decreased secretion of TSH can cause secondary hypothyroidism. It is a disease of middle-aged dogs and there is no sex predilection, although the incidence is increased in neutered males and ovariohysterectomized females. Breeds that are predisposed include the Doberman Pinscher, Golden Retriever, Chow Chow, Great Dane, Irish Wolfhound, Boxer, English Bulldog, Dachshund, Afghan Hound, Newfoundland, Alaskan Malamute, Brittany Spaniel, Poodle, Irish Setter, and Miniature Schnauzer. *Clinical cutaneous changes* include secondary seborrhea, dry, coarse, brittle hair, hair that does not regrow after clipping, hypotrichosis with fine retained hairs, hyperpigmentation and alopecia that tends to develop first in areas of friction and can progress to become bilaterally symmetrical. Pruritus is not a feature unless there is secondary pyoderma or seborrhea. Histologic changes can be nonspecific and simply suggest an endocrinopathy. The most common changes are orthokeratotic hyperkeratosis with follicular keratosis, epidermal hyperplasia, and hair follicles in telogen or atrophied. Changes that are more specific but less common are myxedema, and dermal thickening.

Hypothyroidism occurs less frequently in other domestic animals, and usually in association with iodine deficiency and goiter. In **Merino sheep** and **Afrikander cattle**, a hereditary defect in the biosynthesis of thyroid hormone produces symmetric hypotrichosis and thick, myxedematous, wrinkled skin. In **goats**, hypothyroidism occurs in a mixed strain of Saanen and dwarf goats in association with a hereditary congenital thyroglobulin deficiency. Gross cutaneous changes include bilaterally symmetrical hypotrichosis and thick, myxedematous, scaly skin. Histologic findings include orthokeratotic hyperkeratosis, follicular keratosis, diffuse dermal mucinous degeneration (myxedema) and dermal thickening.

Hyperadrenocorticism

Hyperadrenocorticism is common in **dogs** and can be caused by bilateral adrenocortical hyperplasia resulting from a *pituitary tumor* (pituitary-dependent hyperadrenocorticism), a *neoplasm of the adrenal cortex* (usually unilateral), or exogenously administered glucocorticoids resulting in *iatrogenic hyperglucocorticism*. Of the naturally occurring forms, the pituitary-dependent form is considerably more common. The disease is seen most commonly in middle-aged or older dogs, and the Boxer, Boston Terrier, Dachshund, and Poodle are predisposed. Clinical cutaneous changes can include *bilaterally symmetric hypotrichosis or alopecia affecting primarily skin of the trunk, pendulous abdomen, thin skin that has decreased elasticity, slow wound healing, hyperpigmentation, telangiectasia, scaling, comedones, and calcinosis cutis* (Figs 5.59, 5.60A). Lesions of calcinosis cutis occur most commonly in the axilla, groin, or dorsal neck region and appear as erythematous papules that frequently ulcerate and exude a white, chalky material. Calcinosis cutis is almost always the result of iatrogenic hyperadrenocorticism. Other causes of mineral deposits in the skin are discussed under Physical injury to skin.

Histologically, canine hyperadrenocorticism is characterized by thin epidermal and follicular epithelium, which can be between 1–3 cell layers (Fig. 5.60B). If calcinosis cutis is present, the epidermis is frequently hyperplastic and can be ulcerated. Other changes can include orthokeratotic hyperkeratosis, marked follicular keratosis sometimes with comedone formation, thin dermis, hair follicles

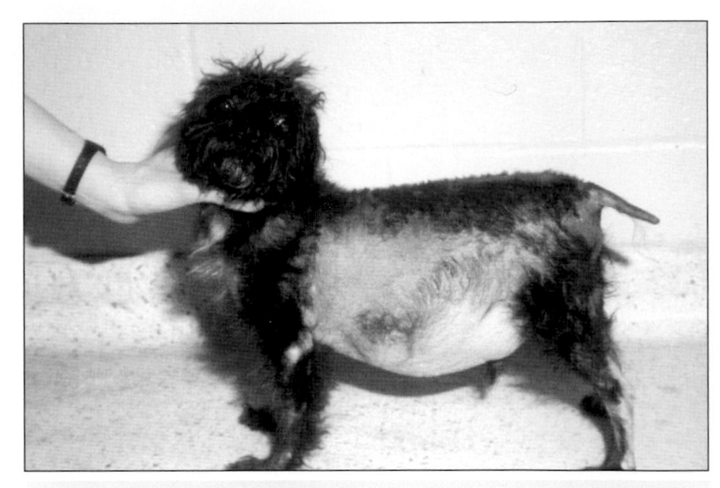

Figure 5.59 Hyperadrenocorticism in a dog. Note pendulous abdomen, truncal alopecia, and redistribution of adipose tissue. (Courtesy of B Dunstan.)

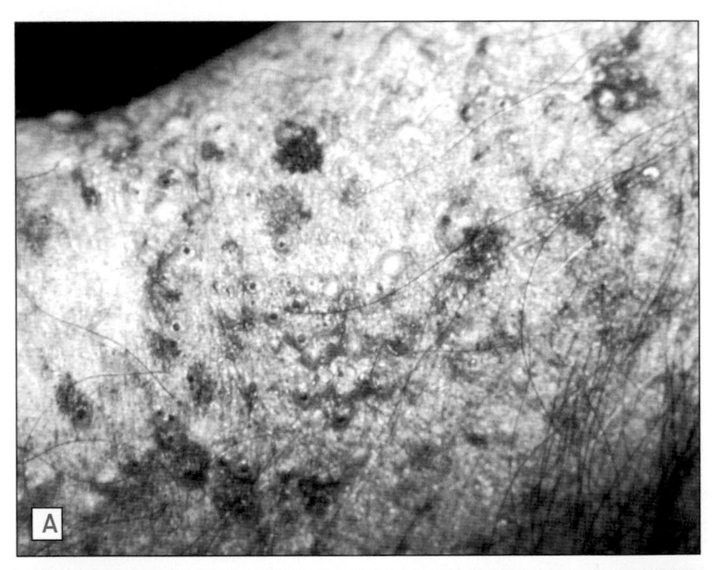

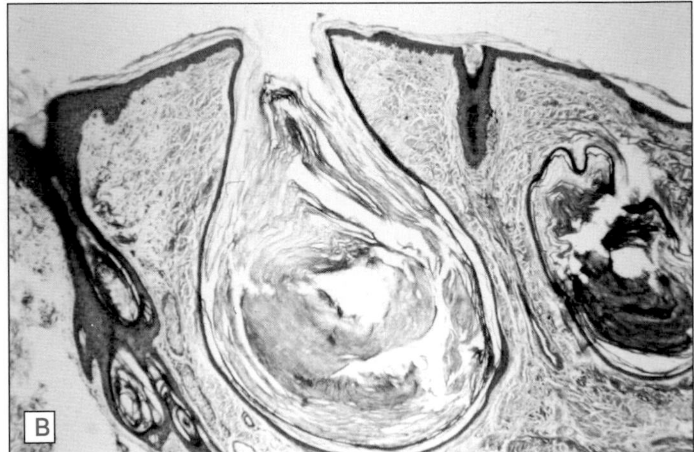

Figure 5.60 A. Comedones in a dog. Note gross appearance of distended follicles. (Courtesy of B Dunstan.) **B. Hyperadrenocorticism** in a dog. Note thin epidermis and hair follicles distended with keratin. (Courtesy of B Dunstan.)

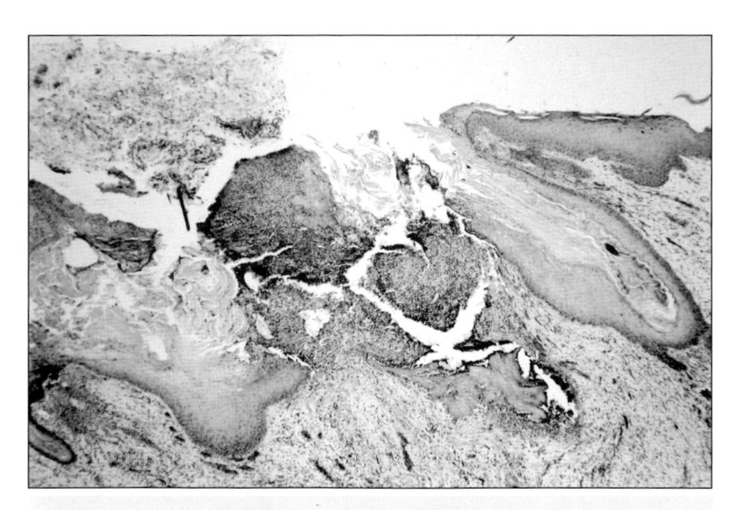

Figure 5.61 Calcinosis cutis in hyperadrenocorticism in a dog. The epidermis is hyperplastic. A large area of mineralized dermal collagen accompanied by granulomatous inflammation is undergoing transepidermal elimination.

that are frequently in telogen or catagen, sebaceous gland atrophy, and variable hyperpigmentation. Phlebectasia has been reported in dogs. *The presence of calcinosis cutis* (Fig. 5.61), *which can occasionally result in osseous metaplasia, is virtually pathognomonic for hyperadrenocorticism*, bearing in mind that mineralization of the external root sheath can be seen in normal old dogs, and in Poodles. Cutaneous histologic lesions of hyperadrenocorticism can occur focally at the site of topical glucocorticoid application.

Hyperadrenocorticism is considerably less common in **cats**. As in dogs, the condition is more commonly pituitary dependent than adrenal dependent or iatrogenic. The clinical presentation in cats is similar to that in the dog, however in addition there is often concurrent diabetes mellitus, and marked skin fragility and friability in which dermal collagen is reduced. This can result in tearing and lacerations of the skin (*feline skin fragility syndrome*). Histologic lesions in the cat are similar to those in the dog, however calcinosis cutis and telangiectasia have not been reported.

Hyperadrenocorticism occurs in **horses** and is almost always seen in association with *hypertrophy, adenomatous hyperplasia, or functional neoplasms of the pars intermedia of the pituitary*. The disease affects primarily aged horses and has no breed or sex predilection. Gross cutaneous changes may include a coarse, brittle, long, shaggy hair coat (hirsutism), an abnormal shedding pattern, episodic hyperhidrosis, poor wound healing, decreased muscle tone, weight loss, and susceptibility to secondary skin infections.

Hyposomatotropism and hypersomatotropism

Hyposomatotropism occurs in young **dogs** with *congenital pituitary dwarfism usually due to pituitary cysts*. In the German Shepherd Dog and Carnelian Bear Dog, pituitary dwarfism is thought to be inherited as a simple autosomal recessive condition and is usually associated with a cystic Rathke's cleft. The pituitary deficiency is often accompanied by deficiencies in thyroid, adrenal and sex hormones. The growth retardation due to the pituitary defect can be accompanied by a puppy coat that fails to shed and the development of endocrine alopecia with typical histologic changes.

Hypersomatotropism (*acromegaly*) is very rare in **dogs**. Excessive somatotropin (growth hormone) production is associated with administration of progestins or with the metestrus (luteal) phase of the estrous cycle in intact female dogs. Cutaneous changes include thick, folded, myxedematous skin, especially on the head, neck and distal extremities. The haircoat may be long and thick and the nails may exhibit rapid overgrowth. Histologic findings in canine hypersomatotropism include thickened dermis due to increased production of glycosaminoglycans and collagen by dermal fibroblasts. Myxedema is present in about a third of cases.

Hyperestrogenism

Hyperestrogenism can occur in male or female **dogs**. In middle-aged to older intact male dogs it is associated with *functional testicular neoplasms*, primarily Sertoli cell neoplasms, and occasionally functional interstitial cell tumors and seminomas. The Boxer, Shetland Sheepdog, Cairn Terrier, Pekingese, Collie and Weimaraners are predisposed. Hyperestrogenism is also seen in middle-aged to older intact female dogs with *polycystic ovaries or functional ovarian neoplasms*. It can also occur in male or female dogs following estrogen administration.

Gross cutaneous changes include *symmetrical hypotrichosis or alopecia*, which typically originates at the perineum and genital region and progresses cranially on the trunk. The hair is dry and dull, is easily epilated, can fail to regrow after clipping, and can be accompanied by hyperpigmentation, especially macular pigmentation. Male dogs may develop a pendulous prepuce, gynecomastia, or prostatomegaly with squamous metaplasia of the prostatic ducts. Females may develop an enlarged vulva. Histologic changes include hair follicles that are primarily in telogen, orthokeratotic hyperkeratosis, and follicular keratosis.

Alopecia X

Growth hormone/castration-responsive dermatosis has many synonyms, including hyposomatotropism of the adult dog, sex-hormone alopecia, pseudo-Cushing's syndrome, testosterone-responsive dermatosis, estrogen-responsive dermatosis, congenital adrenal hyperplasia like-syndrome. This diversity in nomenclature reflects the differences in endocrine values and responses to various treatments and the fact that the pathogenesis of this condition has not been fully characterized. *To simplify the nomenclature, the condition is now being referred to as* **alopecia X**. These dogs have normal thyroid function and adrenal function, and most theories involve a deficiency or imbalance in sex hormones and/or growth hormone deficiency. There may be partial deficiency of 21-hydroxylase or other adrenocortical enzymes necessary for adrenal steroidogenesis.

Alopecia X occurs most often in *plush-coated Nordic breeds*, such as the Pomeranian, Keeshond, Chow Chow, Samoyed, Siberian Husky, Alaskan Malamute, Norwegian Elkhound, American Eskimo Dog, and occasionally in other breeds. Affected dogs have *symmetrical alopecia* of the trunk, perineum, caudal thighs, and neck, sparing the head and distal extremities (Fig. 5.62). Hyperpigmentation is common. Alopecia X usually develops between one and two years of age and either sex can be affected. Initial histologic changes are characterized by *follicular atrophy*; trichilemmal keratinization in primary hairs can be quite prominent. Caution is warranted in making the diagnosis of

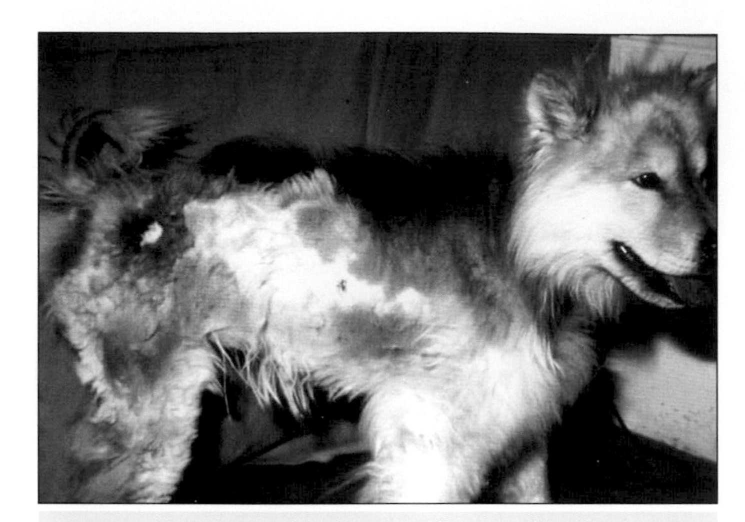

Figure 5.62 Alopecia X in a dog. (Courtesy of B Dunstan.)

Alopecia X based exclusively on this feature as normal primary hair follicles of Nordic breeds can have increased trichilemmal keratinization.

Canine recurrent flank alopecia

Canine recurrent flank alopecia (seasonal flank alopecia, cyclical flank alopecia) is a condition seen most commonly in the Boxer, English Bulldog, Airedale Terrier, Schnauzer, and Griffon Korthal, but can occur in many breeds. It is characterized by alopecia of the skin of the flank that is usually bilaterally symmetrical, rarely unilateral, and occurs recurrently or seasonally. The first episode occurs at approximately 4 years of age but can be variable. In the northern hemisphere, the onset of alopecia is usually between November and March. There is spontaneous hair regrowth after 3–8 months, however occasional dogs have progressively less hair regrowth after each episode. Rare dogs fail to regrow hair after the first episode; and some dogs have one episode of alopecia that never recurs.

Clinically, the bilaterally symmetrical lesions are usually confined to the thoracolumbar regions, have well demarcated margins with abrupt transition from affected to unaffected skin, and are usually hyperpigmented. Histologic changes are those of *non-inflammatory, non-scarring follicular atrophy*. Follicular infundibula are dilated and filled with keratin that can extend into the openings of the primary and secondary atrophic follicles, giving the appearance of an inverted footprint over the remnants of the follicular epithelium (Fig. 5.63).

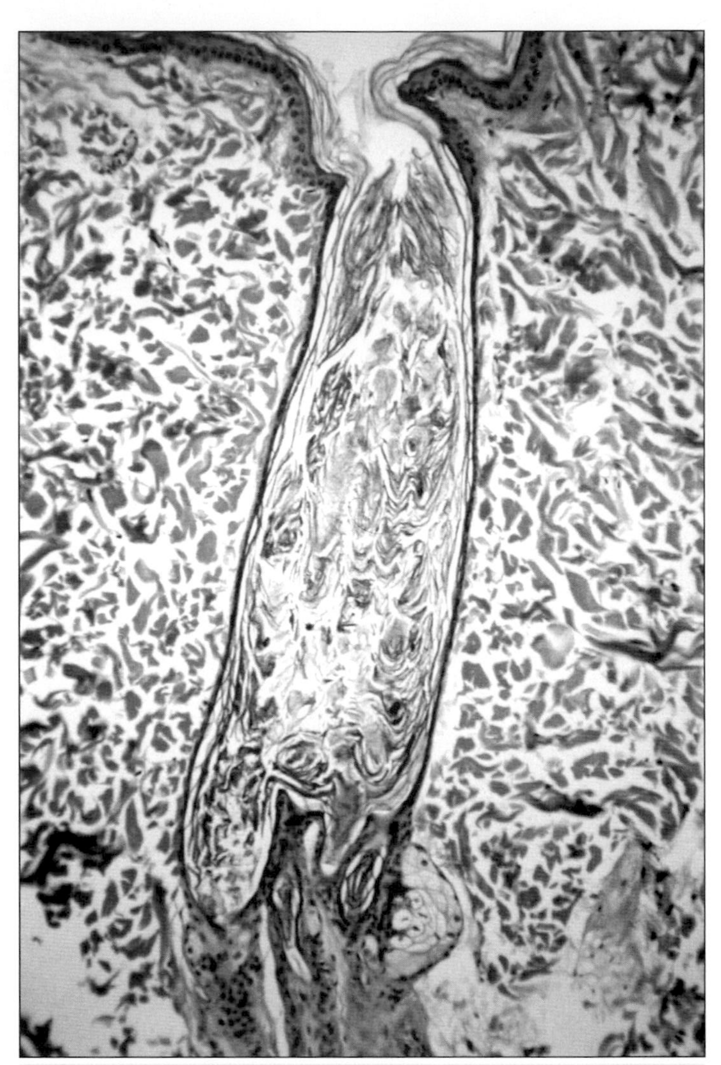

Figure 5.63 Recurrent flank alopecia in a dog. Follicular infundibula are dilated and filled with keratin that extends into the openings of the primary and secondary atrophic follicles, giving the appearance of an inverted footprint. (Courtesy of B Dunstan.)

Bibliography

Barsanti JA, et al. Diethylstilbestrol-induced alopecia in a dog. J Am Vet Med Assoc 1983:182:63–64.

Credille KM, et al. The effects of thyroid hormones on the skin of beagle dogs. J Vet Intern Med 2001;15:539–546.

Daminet S, Paradis M. Evaluation of thyroid function in dogs suffering from recurrent flank alopecia. Can Vet J 2000;41:699–703.

Doliger S, et al. Histochemical study of cutaneous mucins in hypothyroid dogs. Vet Pathol 1995;32:628–634.

Frank LA, et al. Adrenal steroid hormone concentrations in dogs with hair cycle arrest (Alopecia X) before and during treatment with melatonin and mitotane. Vet Dermatol 2004;15:278–284.

Frazier KS, et al. Multiple cutaneous ossification associated with iatrogenic hyperglucocorticism. J Vet Diagn Invest 1998;10:303–307.

Gross TL, Ihrke PJ. The histologic analysis of endocrine-related alopecia in the dog. In: von Tscharner C, Halliwell REW, eds. Advances in Veterinary Dermatology. London: Baillière Tindall, 1990:75–88.

Helton-Rhodes K, et al. Cutaneous manifestations of feline hyperadrenocorticism. In: Ihrke PJ, et al. eds. Advances in Veterinary Dermatology. Vol. 2. Oxford: Pergamon Press. 1993:391–396.

Levy M, et al. Diagnosis and treatment of equine Cushing's disease. Compend Contin Educ Pract Vet 1999;21:766–769.

Miller MA, Dunstan RW. Seasonal flank alopecia in Boxers and Airedale Terriers: 24 cases (1985–1992). J Am Vet Med Assoc 1993;203:1567–1572.

Panciera DL. Hypothyroidism in dogs – 66 cases (1987–1992). J Am Vet Med Assoc 1994;204:761–767.

Rac R, et al. Congenital goitre in Merino sheep due to an inherited defect in the biosynthesis of thyroid hormone. Res Vet Sci 1968;9:209–223.

Rosser EJ. Castration responsive dermatosis in the dog. In: von Tscharner C, Halliwell REW, eds. Advances in Veterinary Dermatology. London: Baillière Tindall, 1990:75–88.

Rosychuk RAW. Dermatologic manifestations of canine hypothyroidism and the usefulness of dermatohistopathology in establishing a diagnosis. Canine Pract 1997;22:25–26.

Scott DW. Cutaneous phlebectasias in cushingoid dogs. J Am Anim Hosp Assoc 1985;21:35–354.

Scott DW, Concannon PW. Gross and microscopic changes in the skin of dogs with progestogen-induced acromegaly and elevated growth hormone levels. J Am Anim Hosp Assoc 1983;19:523–527.

Seaman WJ, Chang SH. Dermal perifollicular mineralization of toy poodle bitches. Vet Pathol 1984;21:122–123.

Watson PJ, Herrtage ME. Hyperadrenocorticism in six cats. J Small Anim Pract 1998;39:175–184.

White SD, et al. Cutaneous markers of canine hyperadrenocorticism. Compend Contin Educ Pract Vet 1989;11:446–463.

IMMUNE-MEDIATED DERMATOSES

Hypersensitivity dermatoses

Contact with exogenous antigens usually leads to induction of a protective response, but when the immune response causes damage to tissues, it is called *hypersensitivity or allergy*. Compounds such as dust, pollens, food, drugs, microbiologic agents, insect components, and various chemicals contain antigens that are normally innocuous but may induce allergic reactions in predisposed individuals. Most cutaneous hypersensitivity reactions are mediated by type I (immediate) hypersensitivity, type IV (cell-mediated or delayed) hypersensitivity, or by a combination of the two types. Hypersensitivity reactions cause a variety of dermatoses that range from annoying and uncomfortable to severely debilitating or life-threatening. Allergic dermatoses are common and important in dogs, cats, and horses and are rarely reported in food animals.

Urticaria and angioedema

Urticaria (hives, heat bumps) and **angioedema** (angioneurotic edema) *are variably pruritic, edematous skin lesions produced by mediators released by basophils and dermal mast cells.* Urticaria and angioedema are most common in horses, uncommon in dogs, and rare in ruminants, pigs, and cats. A wide variety of immunologic and nonimmunologic causes have been implicated, but frequently the specific causative agent cannot be determined for a particular individual. Immunologic causes of urticaria/angioedema are thought to involve type I hypersensitivity reactions primarily; type III hypersensitivity is involved occasionally. *Recognized initiators* in all species include foods and food additives, drugs, biologic agents, stinging and biting arthropods, intestinal parasites, inhalant and contact allergens, and bacterial, fungal, and viral infections. *Nonimmunologic factors* associated with urticaria/angioedema include physical factors such as heat, cold, or pressure; mast cell degranulating agents such as radiocontrast media; and agents that result in perturbation of arachidonic acid metabolism. Deficiency of C1 esterase inhibitor is a genetic cause of chronic urticaria in humans. Aspirin and other nonsteroidal anti-inflammatory drugs, psychological stress, and concurrent febrile illness may be *exacerbating factors*, if not causative ones, in humans with chronic urticaria. Another cause of chronic urticaria identified in humans is IgG autoantibody directed against the IgE receptor of cutaneous mast cells and circulating basophils. Binding of the autoantibody to this receptor induces release of histamine. Irrespective of cause, the *final common pathway is increased vascular permeability and resultant edema produced by histamine, the major mediator, and possibly also by kinins, eicosanoids, and neuropeptides.*

Drugs are probably the most frequent cause of urticaria in **horses**. A wide variety of systemic drugs and biological products have been implicated in initiating urticaria. *Wheals* frequently develop in minutes to hours after exposure to the offending drug and usually subside within several hours. *Cholinergic or heat-reflex urticaria*, induced by exercise or a hot bath, has been reported in a horse. Pruritus in this horse appeared to be exacerbated by pelleted feed. An unusual form of urticaria called *dermatographism*, which is induced by blunt pressure to the skin, has also been described in the horse. In some instances, urticaria is thought to be caused by *overfeeding of grains*, especially those high in protein content ("protein bumps," "feed bumps"). Lesions occur anywhere on the body but are most common on the face, neck, and thorax. In **cattle**, a unique form of urticaria has been described in high-producing dairy cows, especially Jerseys and Guernseys, that become sensitized to casein in their own milk (*milk allergy*). Foods, drugs, biologic agents, and venomous stings are reported most frequently as causes of urticaria and angioedema in **dogs** and **cats**.

Urticaria is characterized by *wheals (hives), which are discrete, well-circumscribed, erythematous, edematous plaques with a flat-top and steep sides* (Fig. 5.64). They are cool and pit upon digital pressure. They vary in size and may coalesce to measure many centimeters in diameter. Wheals are usually round; but in some instances they assume bizarre and irregular serpentine shapes. The overlying hair may stand erect, giving the impression of a follicular disease. The lesions may be localized to a single body region, e.g., lateral neck, head, or thorax, or they may involve the entire body. The individual lesions usually last less than 12–24 hours and disappear leaving no residual skin changes unless pruritus results in self-mutilation. Although individual lesions are transient, new ones may erupt over a period of days or weeks. *Angioedema consists of larger, less well demarcated swellings* that originate subcutaneously. With time, the swellings may gravitate ventrally. Angioedema is a potentially serious condition since involvement of perilaryngeal tissues may cause asphyxiation. Approximately 50% of affected humans develop both lesions concurrently but development of both wheals and angioedema does not seem to be as common in animals.

Microscopic lesions are variable and nonspecific. The epidermis is usually normal in nontraumatized lesions. Urticaria is characterized by *dermal edema,* which is visualized as widening of spaces between collagen fibers in the superficial and middle dermis. The change may be very subtle and can be missed. Edema is typically more severe and involves the deep dermis and subcutaneous tissue in angioedema. Small vessels are congested and lymphatics are dilated. Inflammation is inconsistent. When present, it usually consists of perivascular granulocytes, mast cells, and fewer lymphocytes and macrophages. The reaction involves the upper and middle dermis in urticaria and the deep dermis and subcutis in angioedema. Vasculitis is not a typical feature of urticaria and angioedema.

Diagnosis is usually based on the history and appearance and transitory nature of the clinical lesions. Biopsy is performed to rule out other conditions when the lesions are recurrent or chronic and the diagnosis is uncertain. Identification of a particular inciting

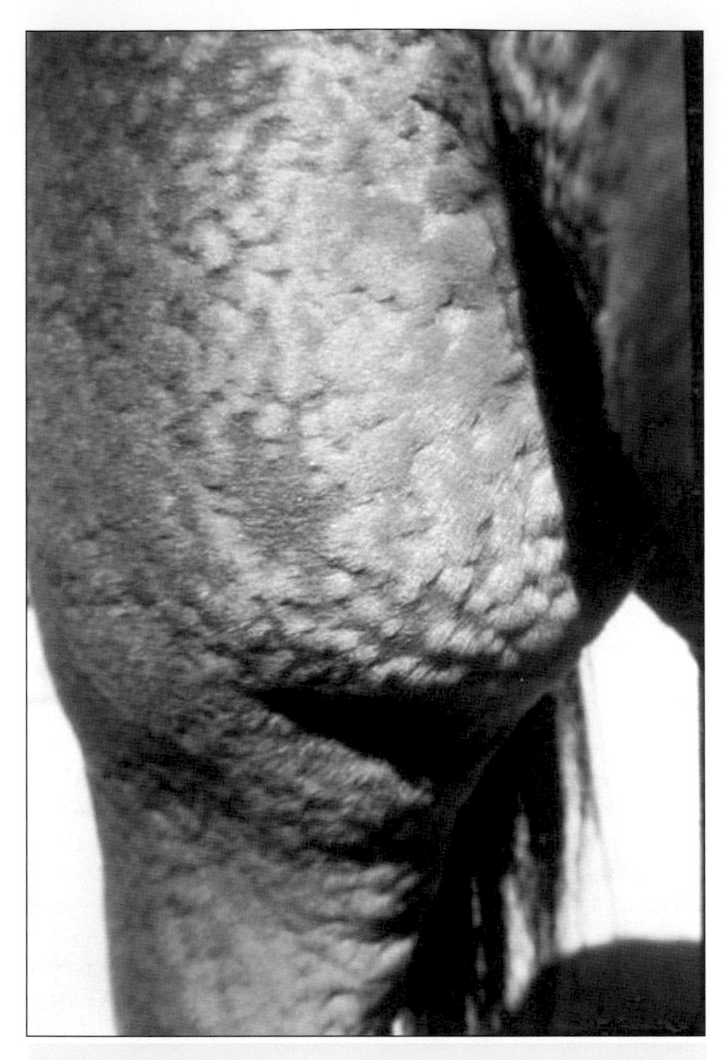

Figure 5.64 Urticaria in a horse. Discrete, well-circumscribed, erythematous, edematous plaques with a flat-top and steep sides. (Courtesy of B Dunstan.)

cause relies on history and a combination of elimination trials, environmental alterations, intradermal skin testing, and insect control measures.

Bibliography

Dibbern DA Jr, Dreskin SC. Urticaria and angioedema: an overview. Immunol Allergy Clin North Am 2004;24:141–162.

Evans AG. Urticaria in horses. Compend Contin Educ Pract Vet 1993;15:626–632.

Jose-Cunilleras E, et al. Intradermal testing in healthy horses and horses with chronic obstructive pulmonary disease, recurrent urticaria, or allergic dermatitis. J Am Vet Med Assoc 2001;219:1115–1121.

Kaplan AP. Chronic urticaria: pathogenesis and treatment. J Allergy Clin Immunol 2004;114:465–474.

Logas D, et al. Cholinergic pruritus in a horse. J Am Vet Med Assoc 1992;201:90–91.

Matthews NS, et al. Urticarial response during anesthesia in a horse. Eq Vet J 1994;25:555–556.

Atopic dermatitis

Atopy is an inherited tendency to produce IgE antibodies and develop clinical allergy to pollens and other innocuous environmental antigens. Clinical disease can involve the respiratory tract, and consist of allergic rhinitis and asthma, or the skin, and manifest as atopic dermatitis. In animals, atopic dermatitis is much more common than the respiratory manifestations of atopy. Allergic rhinitis occurs in cattle, however.

Atopic dermatitis is a multifactorial skin disease in which there is a complex interrelationship between genetic, environmental, skin barrier, pharmacologic, psychologic, and immunologic factors that contribute to the development and severity of the disease. Although clearly a *genetic disorder*, the genetic mapping of atopic dermatitis is not simple and more than one gene appears to be involved. The *pathogenesis* of atopic dermatitis is incompletely understood but it is thought to be caused by an *underlying immunoregulatory imbalance* producing activation of a subpopulation of T helper type 2 lymphocytes (Th2 cells) that release cytokines important to the pathogenesis of atopic dermatitis. Th2 cells produce IL-4, IL-5, and IL-13 and are associated with IgE-mediated reactions. IL-4 is a critical cytokine in the development of allergic diseases. It signals T cells to become Th2 cells, which are the major source of IL-4 production, thereby initiating a self-amplifying process. IL-4 induces expression of IgE receptors on Langerhans cells, resulting in enhanced antigen presentation capability. IL-4 and IL-13 induce the antibody isotype switch from IgM to IgE. They also up-regulate expression of vascular cell adhesion molecule–1 (VCAM-1), an adhesion molecule expressed by cutaneous endothelial cells and involved in migration of eosinophils and mononuclear cells into sites of allergic inflammation. IL-5 promotes differentiation, vascular endothelial adhesion, and survival of eosinophils. In contrast, Th1 cells produce IFN-γ, which inhibits IgE synthesis and differentiation of Th2 cells. The balance between Th1 and Th2 cells may be modulated by biochemical defects in monocytes. Peripheral blood mononuclear cells of individuals with atopic dermatitis have been shown to have increased activity of phosphodiesterase, which results in increased monocyte prostaglandin E_2 (PGE_2) production. PGE_2 tends to inhibit Th1 production of IFN-γ and accentuate IL-4 secretion by Th2 cells.

IgE appears to have a multifunctional role in the pathogenesis of atopic dermatitis. An immediate type hypersensitivity reaction develops within minutes of allergen exposure when mast cells bearing allergen-specific IgE bind allergen and release a variety of preformed mediators, most notably histamine. The skin histamine content has been found to be increased in humans and dogs with atopic dermatitis. *Activated mast cells* also release cytokines such as IL-4, IL-5, IL-6, TNF-α, and platelet activating factor (PAF) that further promote inflammation. An IgE-dependent late-phase reaction develops subsequently when expression of leukocyte adhesion molecules on postcapillary venule endothelium promotes influx of eosinophils, neutrophils, and mononuclear cells into the skin. Eosinophils release various mediators including PAF, eosinophil major basic protein (MBP), eosinophil cationic protein (ECP), and cytokines that promote inflammation and cause tissue damage. Antigen-specific IgE antibodies also appear to be involved in a non-classical role in antigen uptake and processing. IgE-bearing antigen-presenting cells (APCs), particularly Langerhans cells and dermal dendritic cells, bind, process, and present specific antigen locally to allergen-specific indeterminate T cells (Th0) thereby directing them to the Th2 cell phenotype. Moreover, IgE-mediated antigen presentation increases the presenting capacity of these APCs up to 100-fold, a mechanism known as "*facilitated antigen presentation*." Ultimately, B cells are stimulated to produce more allergen-specific IgE, which is bound to antigen-presenting cells, and a vicious cycle of facilitated antigen presentation is perpetuated.

Atopic dermatitis traditionally has been thought to be triggered by inhaled aeroallergens, hence the synonym **allergic inhalant dermatitis**. However, there is evidence both in humans and animals suggesting that *a transepidermal route of exposure may be involved instead or as well.* In the dog, such a route of antigen presentation is suggested by the typical distribution of skin lesions primarily to ventral, sparsely haired areas. Immunohistochemical studies of lesional skin from humans, dogs, and cats with atopic dermatitis have found increased numbers and focal aggregation of activated Langerhans cells within the epidermis. *These findings are interpreted to represent antigen capture within the epidermis.* Increased numbers of T cells are also seen in the epidermis. Clustering of dendritic cells is also evident in the superficial dermis, suggesting increased local antigen capture and/or antigen presentation to T cells. Furthermore, both the aggregated epidermal Langerhans cells and dermal dendritic cells are positive for surface IgE, findings consistent with the theory that cutaneous allergen capture or presentation is mediated by IgE. In lesional skin of atopic dogs, epidermal eosinophil exocytosis, subcorneal eosinophilic micropustule formation, and eosinophil degranulation have been observed and interpreted to indicate that the interaction between allergen and immunocompetent cells occurs in the epidermis and results in the release of eosinophil chemotactic factors by keratinocytes or epidermal Langerhans cells. In addition, increased expression of adhesion molecules by dermal endothelial cells has been found. Increased numbers of CD4+ and CD8+ T cells are seen in lesional atopic skin of humans, cats, and dogs. Tissue-selective homing of T cells is thought to be regulated at the level of T cell recognition of vascular endothelial cells via interaction of differentially expressed T lymphocyte homing receptors, such as cutaneous lymphocyte antigen (CLA), and their endothelial cell ligands. Therefore, *increased expression of endothelial adhesion molecules promotes migration of increased numbers of CLA+ T cells into the skin.* The tendency to develop atopic dermatitis as opposed to asthma or allergic rhinitis may depend on differences in skin-versus lung-seeking propensity of the memory/effector T lymphocytes.

The characteristic feature of atopic dermatitis is intense pruritus but the pathogenesis is not well understood. It is thought to be driven by local release of pharmacologic mediators, including histamine, neuropeptides, and eicosanoids; however, it does not appear that histamine is a major pruritogen in atopic dermatitis. Of the various chemical mediators, *neuropeptides* may be particularly important in the pathophysiology of itching in the atopic individual. In addition, atopic dermatitis appears to be associated with a decreased threshold for pruritus. The development of clinical lesions is also partially dependent on skin trauma caused by scratching. Once the itch-scratch cycle is initiated, mechanical trauma to the keratinocytes results in release of various proinflammatory cytokines that can maintain and promote inflammation. These include IL-1, TNF-α, and IL-4. It is unclear whether there is also an intrinsic keratinocyte defect. Keratinocytes from humans with atopic dermatitis exhibit enhanced production of GM-CSF in response to IL-1, which can contribute to increased numbers and enhanced antigen-presenting function of dendritic cells.

Atopic dermatitis is associated with a cell-mediated immunodeficiency that appears to be confined to the skin. Consequently, patients with atopic dermatitis have an increased tendency to develop skin infections, which are generally superficial. Superficial infection with *Malassezia* is common in humans and dogs with atopic dermatitis. Lesional skin of humans and dogs with atopic dermatitis has a high incidence of colonization with pathogenic strains of staphylococci. Besides causing superficial pyoderma, *S. aureus* in humans is believed to augment allergen-induced skin inflammation in atopic dermatitis by secreting exotoxins that act as *superantigens*. Superantigens have the capacity to activate large classes of T cells nonspecifically by virtue of their ability to bridge the linkage between the class II major histocompatibility complex molecule on the APC and the T cell receptor without having to be processed and presented by the APC. IgE antibodies directed against these exotoxins have been identified in individuals with atopic dermatitis and the severity of disease correlates with these IgE antibodies, presumably because the locally produced exotoxins are absorbed through the skin surface and cause IgE-dependent mast cell degranulation within the dermis. Other toxins secreted by *S. aureus* organisms have been found to induce release of TNF-α by keratinocytes and cause inflammation by nonspecific mechanisms.

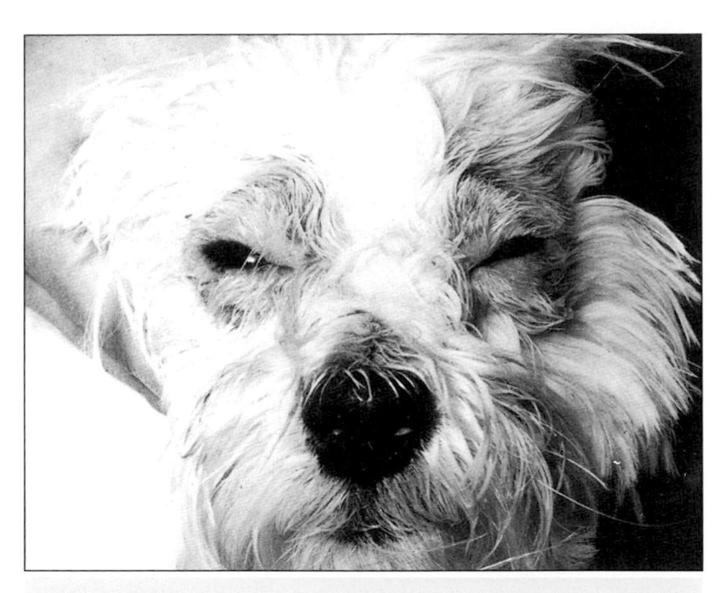

Figure 5.65 Atopy in a dog.

Atopic dermatitis is a common condition in **dogs** and is estimated to affect 10–15% of the population. It is second only to flea-bite hypersensitivity in those geographical areas with fleas. It has a *familial pattern* but the mode of inheritance is unknown. No relationship between dog leukocyte-antigen (DL-A) and canine atopy could be found. Breeds thought to be predisposed include the Chinese Shar-Pei, Cairn Terrier, West Highland White Terrier, Scottish Terrier, Lhasa Apso, Shih Tzu, Wire-haired Fox Terrier, Dalmatian, Pug, Irish Setter, Boston Terrier, Golden Retriever, Boxer, English Setter, Labrador Retriever, Miniature Schnauzer, Belgian Tervuren, and Beauceron. Females are affected more commonly in some studies, while in others no sex predilection has been found. The age of onset is variable but disease usually is apparent between 1 and 3 years of age. It is rare in dogs less than 6 months, except in Chinese Shar-Peis which may develop disease as early as 3 months of age; and, unless there is a change in the environment, most dogs develop clinical signs by 6 years.

The *primary clinical sign is pruritus,* which frequently begins seasonally but eventually becomes perennial. Pruritus most commonly affects the face (Fig. 5.65), paws, distal extremities, and ventrum and is manifested typically as face-rubbing and foot-chewing and licking. Skin lesions are usually due to self-trauma, secondary bacterial pyoderma, *Malassezia*-dermatitis, and secondary seborrhea. Secondary skin changes include variable alopecia, salivary staining of the hair, excoriations, papules, pustules, crusts, hyperpigmentation, lichenification, and pyotraumatic dermatitis. Eventually cutaneous involvement may become generalized. Atopic dogs characteristically have an unpleasant odor that results from a combination of seborrhea, secondary bacterial or yeast infection, and hyperhidrosis. Atopic otitis externa is common. Noncutaneous clinical signs are rare and may include conjunctivitis, rhinitis, asthma, and gastrointestinal disorders.

No breed or sex predilection is apparent in **cats** with atopic dermatitis; and it is uncertain whether there is an inherited predisposition. Clinical signs usually develop at 6 months to 2 years of age. *Pruritus* is the primary clinical sign but it may not be obvious because of the secretive nature of cats. Instead, hair loss, secondary to covert licking and chewing, may be the only abnormality and the skin may appear normal. *Clinical lesions of atopic dermatitis in cats are extremely variable*. They may include, in addition to self-induced alopecia, eosinophilic granuloma complex lesions, miliary dermatitis, recurrent swelling of the lower lip, otitis externa, and pruritus of the face, pinnae, and neck. *Miliary dermatitis is a clinical reaction pattern of cats* that consists of numerous small erythematous crust-covered papules. It is not specific for atopic dermatitis and may also occur in ectoparasite, food, and drug hypersensitivities. Noncutaneous signs associated with atopy in cats include sneezing, conjunctivitis, coughing, and asthma. Lymphadenopathy may be present in cats with miliary dermatitis or eosinophilic granulomas.

Pruritus is the primary clinical sign in **horses** with atopy. Some cases are manifested as recurrent pruritic urticaria. Onset is usually between 1.5 and 4 years of age. Skin lesions usually develop secondarily in response to self-trauma and include alopecia, excoriations, lichenification, and hyperpigmentation. The face, ears, ventrum, and legs are most commonly affected. Arabians and Thoroughbreds may be predisposed. A seasonal pruritic dermatosis typical of atopic dermatitis has been described in two **Suffolk ewes**.

Microscopic changes associated with atopic dermatitis have been considered nonspecific and usually consist of perivascular to interstitial dermatitis. In *dogs*, the epidermis is variably hyperplastic and may have mild, patchy intercellular edema, focal parakeratosis, and crusting. Erosion and ulceration may be present from self-trauma. Exocytosis of lymphocytes or eosinophils and small subcorneal accumulations of eosinophils may be seen. Dermal inflammation is superficial perivascular to interstitial, and consists of lymphocytes and macrophages primarily. Mast cells are in increased numbers and may be numerous. Eosinophils and neutrophils are usually in low numbers, but eosinophils may be missed because of degranulation. Sebaceous glands are hyperplastic and apocrine sweat glands may be dilated in chronic lesions. Superficial dermal blood vessels may be congested and the superficial dermis may be mildly edematous.

Histologic changes in the skin of *cats* with atopic dermatitis vary according to the lesions biopsied. The epidermis varies from normal to variably hyperplastic. Serocellular crusts, foci of intercellular edema and epidermal necrosis, and exocytosis of small numbers of eosinophils are usually present in lesions of miliary dermatitis. The dermis contains a superficial perivascular to interstitial infiltrate of mixed cells. Mast cells, eosinophils, lymphocytes, and neutrophils are typically present but vary in their proportions. Neutrophils are most numerous in areas of erosion or ulceration. In some cases, the lesions are those of an eosinophilic plaque. The microscopic lesion in *atopic horses and sheep* is hyperplastic perivascular dermatitis with a predominance of eosinophils.

Diagnosis of atopic dermatitis is based on compatible history and physical examination findings coupled with demonstration of allergen-specific IgE antibodies. In dogs, measurement of total serum IgE has not been found to be useful because there is no significant difference in IgE concentrations between atopic and clinically normal dogs. *Intradermal skin testing* (IDST) has been considered to be the most reliable method of identifying clinically relevant allergens. In vitro tests that measure concentrations of allergen-specific IgE are commercially available but generally have been found to correlate poorly with IDST results. However, newer procedures for measurement of allergen-specific IgE may be more accurate in identifying clinically relevant allergens. Diagnosis may be complicated by the presence of concurrent hypersensitivity conditions such as flea-bite allergy or food allergy.

Bibliography

DeBoer DJ. Canine atopic dermatitis: new targets, new therapies. J Nutr 2004;134(8 Suppl):2056S–2061S.

DeBoer DJ, Hillier A. The ACVD task force on canine atopic dermatitis (XVI): laboratory evaluation of dogs with atopic dermatitis with serum-based "allergy" tests. Vet Immunol Immunopathol 2001;81:277–287.

Gross TL, et al. Correlation of histologic and immunologic findings in cats with miliary dermatitis. J Am Vet Med Assoc 1986;189:1322–1325.

Halliwell REW. Efficacy of hyposensitization in feline allergic diseases based upon results of *in vitro* testing for allergen-specific immunoglobulin E. J Am Anim Hosp Assoc 1997;33:282–288.

Hämmerling R, DeWeck AL. Comparison of two diagnostic tests for canine atopy using monoclonal anti-IgE antibodies. Vet Dermatol 1998;9:191–199.

Hanifin JM, Chan SC. Monocyte phosphodiesterase abnormalities and dysregulation of lymphocyte function in atopic dermatitis. J Invest Dermatol 1995;105:84S–88S.

Hill PB, et al. Concentrations of total serum IgE, IgA, and IgG in atopic and parasitized dogs. Vet Immunol Immunopathol 1995;44:105–113.

Leung DYM. Pathogenesis of atopic dermatitis. J Allergy Clin Immunol 1999;104:S99–108.

Nimmo-Wilkie JS, et al. Morphometric analyses of the skin of dogs with atopic dermatitis and correlations with cutaneous and plasma histamine and total serum IgE. Vet Pathol 1990;27:179–186.

O'Dair HA, et al. An open prospective investigation into aetiology in a group of cats with suspected allergic skin disease. Vet Dermatol 1996;7:193–202.

Olivry T, Hill PB. The ACVD task force on canine atopic dermatitis (XVIII): histopathology of skin lesions. Vet Immunol Immunopathol 2001;81:305–309.

Rees CA. Canine and feline atopic dermatitis: a review of the diagnostic options. Clin Tech Small Anim Pract 2001;16:230–232.

Roosje PJ, et al. Increased numbers of CD4+ and CD8+ T cells in lesional skin of cats with allergic dermatitis. Vet Pathol 1998;35:268–273.

Sinke JD, et al. Immunophenotyping of skin-infiltrating T-cell subsets in dogs with atopic dermatitis. Vet Immunol Immunopathol 1997;57:13–23.

Zunic M. Comparison between IMMUNODOT tests and the intradermal skin test in atopic dogs. Vet Dermatol 1998;9:201–205.

Food hypersensitivity (allergy)

Food hypersensitivity refers to an exaggerated, immunologically mediated reaction to specific food allergens resulting in disease. This hypersensitivity reaction may be mediated by IgE (type I hypersensitivity) and by non-IgE-mediated mechanisms. Food-induced allergic reactions are responsible for a variety of signs involving the skin, gastrointestinal tract, and respiratory tract. The skin may represent the second most frequent target organ, after the gastrointestinal tract, in food hypersensitivity reactions.

Food allergy in humans is thought to develop as a consequence of physiologic and immunologic immaturity resulting in increased absorption of food antigens during the first few months to years of life in association with the inherited tendency for increased production of IgE antibody. Absorption of intact food proteins appears to be limited normally by the intestinal mucosal barrier and by combination of the proteins with food allergen-specific IgA secreted into the gut. However, adult levels of IgA are not generally produced until puberty and this relative IgA deficiency may contribute to increased permeability of the gastrointestinal barrier during childhood. Gastrointestinal infections and parasitism may also contribute to disruption of the mucosal barrier to increase absorption of food antigens. The majority of food allergens are *glycoproteins* with molecular weight between 10 000 and 80 000 daltons, which tend to be resistant to proteolysis and are heat-stable and water-soluble. Even in the mature intestine, approximately 2% of ingested food antigens are absorbed into the circulation in an immunologic form. However, these immunologically recognizable proteins do not normally cause adverse reactions despite being transported throughout the body because tolerance develops in most individuals. Tolerance is thought to involve activation of CD8+ T suppressor cells in GALT to suppress an immune response. The development of tolerance to food appears to have little effect on B cells since antibody production to food proteins is a universal phenomenon; although low concentrations of serum IgG, IgM, and IgA food-specific antibodies are found in normal individuals, they are of no clinical consequence. In genetically predisposed infants, however, ingested antigens result in excessive production of IgE antibodies. These food-specific antibodies bind high affinity receptors on mast cells, dendritic cells, and macrophages in tissues and basophils in circulation. When food allergens penetrate mucosal barriers and reach the IgE bound to mast cells and basophils, mediators are released that induce the signs of immediate hypersensitivity. Activated mast cells also generate various mediators (such as IL-4, tumor necrosis factor α, and platelet activating factor) that may induce an IgE-mediated late-phase response in which eosinophils, lymphocytes, and monocytes are attracted to the site of reaction and release additional inflammatory mediators and cytokines. Mononuclear cells can be induced to secrete "histamine-releasing factors" that interact with IgE bound to basophils and possibly other cells to increase releasibility of these cells. In addition, IgE antibodies bound to Langerhans cells lead to more efficient capture of antigens and preferential activation of Th2 lymphocytes that promote allergic inflammatory reactions. The development of dermatitis rather than respiratory signs in individuals with food allergy may relate to homing of allergen-specific T cells to the skin by way of cutaneous lymphocyte-associated antigen (CLA), a homing molecule that directs these cells to the skin.

The pathomechanism of food hypersensitivity in animals is unknown, but it is assumed to be an IgE-mediated hypersensitivity reaction as in humans. It is not known when the gastrointestinal tract of companion animals becomes mature. Since gastrointestinal parasitism and viral enteritides are relatively common in animals, disruption of the intestinal mucosal barrier may be an important factor in the development of food hypersensitivity. Food allergy, as recognized in animals, is clinically different from the condition in humans, however. In humans, food hypersensitivity is most commonly seen in infants and young children; and in many cases, a loss of clinical sensitivity develops after 1–3 years of an appropriate food elimination diet. Although signs may initially develop in young animals, food hypersensitivity is typically a disease of adult animals and no loss of clinical sensitivity has been observed in affected animals. Furthermore, laboratory and clinical evidence suggests that food-specific IgE antibody directly contributes to the pathogenesis of atopic dermatitis in humans. In animals, food allergy is currently considered a separate entity from atopic dermatitis, although the two conditions may coexist.

Food allergy is thought to be the third most common hypersensitivity in **dogs** after flea-bite allergy and atopic dermatitis. The prevalence is unknown but food hypersensitivity has been suggested to account for 10–15% of canine allergic dermatoses. A significant number of dogs with food allergy, ranging from 23% to 45% in various studies, have concurrent hypersensitivity conditions such as atopic dermatitis, flea-bite allergy, or both. The most common allergens identified are *beef, wheat, dairy products, chicken, eggs, corn, and soy*. Some dogs, up to 64% in one study of 25 dogs with food allergy, react to two or more dog food ingredients, suggesting that multiple food hypersensitivities are not uncommon. Signs of food allergy may develop at any age; but in approximately 50% of dogs, signs are seen before 1 year of age and may occur as early as 4 months. No sex predisposition has been found. Breed predilection is uncertain. None has been found in some studies, while different breeds have been found to be at increased risk in various studies, no doubt reflecting regional differences in genetic pools.

Clinical signs in dogs are extremely variable. *The most consistent sign is pruritus* that is usually nonseasonal and may be generalized or localized to the feet, face and ears; inguinal and axillary regions; or lumbosacral and perineal area. Depending on the location of the pruritus, food allergy may mimic sarcoptic mange, flea allergy dermatitis, or atopic dermatitis. The pruritus may be unresponsive or poorly responsive to glucocorticoid therapy. Primary skin lesions may include erythema, papules, or pruritic urticaria-angioedema but they are frequently obscured by self-trauma as a consequence of chronic pruritus. More commonly, only secondary lesions are seen and these typically include excoriation, alopecia, hyperpigmentation, lichenification, scales, crusts, ulceration, and seborrhea. In a small number of cases, pruritic otitis externa or recurrent superficial pyoderma may occur in the absence of any other clinical signs of food allergy. Bacterial pyoderma and *Malassezia* infection are common secondary complications. Some dogs also exhibit *concurrent gastrointestinal signs*, which include increased frequency of defecation most commonly, and mucus and/or blood in feces, tenesmus, vomiting, or diarrhea less frequently. Neurologic signs, such as malaise and seizures, and respiratory signs have been reported rarely in conjunction with skin lesions in dogs with food allergy.

The prevalence of food allergy in **cats** is unknown. No breed or sex predilection is apparent. Most cases are recognized in young adult cats. The major complaint is *severe pruritus* that is usually nonseasonal and frequently poorly responsive to glucocorticoid therapy. The face, ears, and neck are most commonly involved but pruritus may be generalized (Fig. 5.66). Allergens identified include

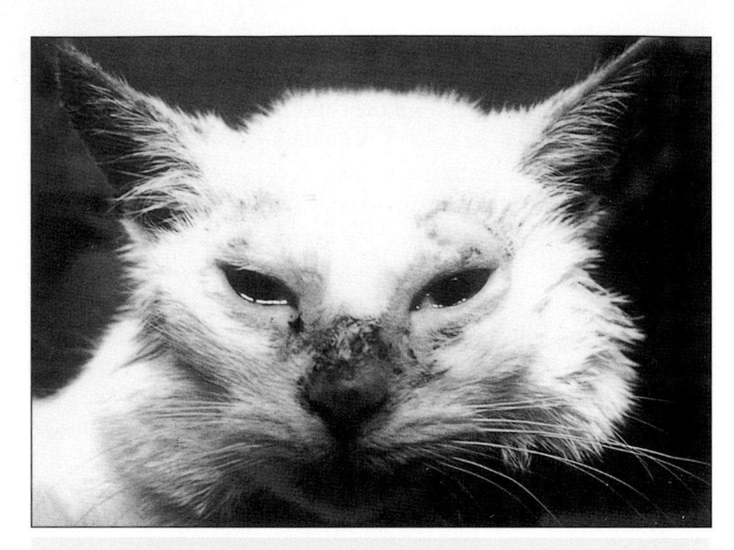

Figure 5.66 Food allergy in a kitten. Periocular and nasal alopecia, crusting, and erythema.

fish, lamb, milk, whale meat, beef, chicken, rabbit, eggs, and pork. Food allergic cats may also have other hypersensitivity conditions such as atopic dermatitis or flea-bite allergy. Skin lesions are extremely variable and include erythema, angioedema-urticaria, self-induced alopecia and excoriations, crusting, seborrhea, or miliary dermatitis. They may be localized to the face and head or generalized in distribution. Eosinophilic granuloma complex lesions may be a manifestation of food allergy. Concurrent gastrointestinal or respiratory signs are uncommon.

Food hypersensitivity has been reported rarely in **horses**, **cattle**, and **pigs**. Substances that have been incriminated include wheat, barley, bran, oats, concentrates, and tonics in horses; wheat, bran, corn, clover hay, rice bran, and soybeans in cattle; and clover pasture in pigs. Clinical signs in horses and cattle are pruritic papular eruptions, pruritic urticaria, and tail rubbing. A condition described as food allergy in white hogs on new clover pasture consisted of generalized erythema and skin pain, depression, and reluctance to move. The description of this condition is more suggestive of an adverse food reaction, such as photosensitization, than of food hypersensitivity, however.

The microscopic lesions associated with food allergy are variable and are not diagnostic. The epidermis is variably acanthotic and may be multifocally spongiotic. Crusting, erosion, and ulceration may be present. The superficial dermis is mildly to moderately edematous and inflammation is variable. In dogs, inflammation may be perivascular, interstitial, or diffuse. The cells are mixed and include lymphocytes, macrophages, eosinophils, and mast cells. Neutrophils and plasma cells are present in numbers proportional to the degree of self-trauma. Sebaceous and apocrine glands may be hyperplastic in chronic lesions. In cats, dermal inflammation may be a superficial perivascular mononuclear dermatitis but more commonly is characterized by eosinophilic inflammation that is perivascular to diffuse and extends into the subcutis. Mast cell numbers are commonly moderately to markedly increased throughout the dermis. Collagen degeneration may occur in areas of intense eosinophilic inflammation. Eosinophilic folliculitis and furunculosis and lesions of eosinophilic plaque are present in some cases of food allergy in cats. The microscopic lesion ascribed to food allergy in large animals is superficial perivascular dermatitis, with eosinophils comprising a significant proportion of the inflammatory cells.

The *diagnosis* of food allergy is made by a combination of appropriate clinical history, exclusion of other pruritic conditions, and resolution of pruritus with feeding of a hypoallergenic diet. Intradermal skin testing and measurement of serum allergen-specific IgE levels have been found to be unreliable for diagnosis of food allergy in animals.

Bibliography

Chesney CJ. Food sensitivity in the dog: a quantitative study. J Small Anim Pract 2002;43:203–207.

Guilford WG, et al. Food sensitivity in cats with chronic idiopathic gastrointestinal problems. J Vet Intern Med 2001;15:7–13.

Harvey RG. Food allergy and dietary intolerance in dogs: A report of 25 cases. J Small Anim Pract 1993;34:175–179.

Ishida R, et al. Antigen-specific histamine release in dogs with food hypersensitivity. J Vet Med Sci 2003;65:435–438.

Jackson HA. Diagnostic techniques in dermatology: the investigation and diagnosis of adverse food reactions in dogs and cats. Clin Tech Small Anim Pract 2001;16:233–235.

Jeffers JG, et al. Diagnostic testing of dogs for food hypersensitivity. J Am Vet Med Assoc 1991;198:245–250.

Kunkle G, Horner S. Validity of skin testing for diagnosis of food allergy in dogs. J Am Vet Med Assoc 1992;200:677–680.

Mueller R, Tsohalis J. Evaluation of serum allergen-specific IgE for the diagnosis of food adverse reactions in the dog. Vet Dermatol 1998;9:167–171.

Paterson S. Food hypersensitivity in 20 dogs with skin and gastrointestinal signs. J Small Anim Pract 1995;36:529–534.

Sampson HA. Food allergy. Part I: Immunopathogenesis and clinical disorders. J Allergy Clin Immunol 1999;103:717–728.

Sicherer SH, Sampson HA. Food hypersensitivity and atopic dermatitis: Pathophysiology, epidemiology, diagnosis, and management. J Allergy Clin Immunol 1999;104:S114–S122.

Allergic contact dermatitis

Allergic contact dermatitis is an uncommon hypersensitivity condition in domestic animals. Although considered a typical delayed (type IV) hypersensitivity reaction, *there is considerable overlap in pathogenesis between allergic contact dermatitis and primary irritant dermatitis and the rigid distinction between the two conditions is becoming blurred.* It has been estimated to account for 1–10% of dermatoses in dogs. The low incidence, as compared to that in humans, is thought to be due to the natural protection afforded by the hair coat of most animals and by the decreased exposure to potential allergens in cosmetics and industrial chemicals.

Allergic contact dermatitis is caused by contact with a nonirritating concentration of a substance to which an individual has previously become sensitized. The compounds involved are usually lipid-soluble haptens (low-molecular-weight substances) that become immunogenic only after penetrating the epidermis and binding covalently to an autologous structural or cell surface protein to form a complete antigen. This antigen is subsequently internalized and processed by Langerhans cells and presented to CD4+ T cells. Langerhans cells are crucial to development of allergic contact dermatitis as depletion of these cells results in a decreased ability to induce contact sensitization. During the induction phase of the reaction, Langerhans cells present antigen to CD4+ cells in the paracortical region of regional lymph nodes where the specifically sensitized T cells undergo clonal expansion and then circulate as memory cells in blood and home to skin by virtue of adhesion molecules that bind to addressins on endothelial cells. Development of allergic contact dermatitis depends on the nature of the allergen, frequency of contact, and state of the skin. *Factors that damage the integrity of the protective barrier of the skin predispose to development of allergic contact dermatitis.* The induction phase is typically a prolonged process, estimated to require 6 months to 2 years to develop. While strong immunogens can elicit sensitivity after as short a period of contact as 7 to 21 days, most contact allergens are weaker immunogens and require chronic repeated exposure for sensitization to develop. Upon subsequent exposure to the contact allergen, specifically sensitized T cells in skin and circulation are presented the antigen by Langerhans cells (*elicitation phase*), become activated, and elaborate various cytokines that attract and activate other inflammatory cells and stimulate proliferation of the epidermis. Only a very small fraction (<1%) of the infiltrating T cells are specific for a relevant antigen. Thus, various amplification and recruitment mechanisms are involved in induction of the reactions. The activated T cells secrete a Th1 profile of cytokines, including IFNγ and TNFβ, which recruit and activate a wide variety of inflammatory cells, affect keratinocyte function and differentiation, and induce expression of adhesion molecules on endothelial cells and keratinocytes. TNFβ and IFNγ induce expression of ICAM-1 on keratinocytes and endothelium, which promotes homing of T cells to the dermis and epidermis. Unlike the delayed-type hypersensitivity reaction that develops in response to antigen injected into the dermis which primarily involves CD4+ cells, the response to hapten painted on the epidermis involves both CD4+ and CD8+ T cells. Local production of cytokines induces arrival of more T cells and further amplification of proinflammatory mechanisms. Irritated keratinocytes also release a variety of cytokines that induce or augment the inflammatory response.

Allergic contact dermatitis has been reported most frequently in *dogs and horses*, although most cases have not been confirmed by patch testing. Numerous *plants and chemicals* have been suspected or shown to cause allergic contact dermatitis in animals. In dogs, wandering Jew (*Tradescantia fluminensis*), spreading dayflower (*Cornelina diffusa*), doveweed (*Murdannia nudiflora*), leaves and bulbs of plants in the family Amaryllidaceae, dandelion leaves, cedar wood, and Asian jasmine have been implicated in cases of allergic contact dermatitis. Cobalt and nickel ions, pine oil resin found in cleaning products, topical medications such as neomycin, rubber, cement, and various fragrances such as those in shampoos and carpet deodorizers are a few of the chemical causes of allergic contact dermatitis in dogs and cats. In horses, pasture plants, insecticides, various dyes and preservatives of tack items, soaps, and bedding materials have been suggested as causes of allergic contact dermatitis.

The *clinical course* is typically prolonged and lesions in dogs are usually confined to sparsely haired areas of the body such as the lips, chin, ventral cervical and thoracic areas, abdomen, scrotum, perineum, and ventral interdigital skin. Foot pads are usually protected by the thick stratum corneum; however, cracking of foot pads of all four feet was a feature described in a cat with suspected allergic contact dermatitis to carpet deodorizer. Lesion distribution is also dependent on the contactant involved. *Primary lesions include erythema, papules, plaques, and vesicles*, but these are very transient and thus rarely seen. *Pruritus is variable*, ranging from mild to severe. *Chronic secondary lesions are more commonly seen and include alopecia, lichenification, scaling, crusting, excoriations, and pigmentary changes.* Secondary bacterial or fungal infection may complicate lesions.

Microscopic changes described in various reports of allergic contact dermatitis in animals have been conflicting. *Differences in histologic lesions no doubt reflect, at least in part, differences in stage of the reaction.* While neutrophils have been the predominant cell type seen in some cases, lymphocytes or eosinophils predominated in others. The epidermis may be variably spongiotic and may develop vesicles in some areas. In allergic contact dermatitis produced experimentally in dogs by topical application of 1-chloro-2,4-dinitrochlorobenzene (DNCB), histologic changes at 48 and 72 hours post-challenge included mild acanthosis, mild dermal edema, and perivascular and perifollicular infiltrations of lymphocytes and macrophages. Mild and focal to widespread and marked epidermal necrosis may occur, both in patch test reaction sites as well as in spontaneous lesions. Exocytosis of inflammatory cells is a common feature but the cells vary and may be neutrophils, lymphocytes, eosinophils or a combination thereof. The superficial dermis may be edematous and the predominant inflammatory cells may be lymphocytes, neutrophils, or eosinophils. Inflammation may be perivascular, diffuse interstitial, or lichenoid and frequently perifollicular. *The histologic changes of allergic contact dermatitis are frequently indistinguishable from those caused by irritant contact dermatitis.*

The list of *differential diagnoses* is extensive and includes a wide variety of allergic and parasitic conditions, bacterial and fungal infections, and irritant contact dermatitis. When a single animal of a group is affected, allergic contact dermatitis is considered more likely than irritant dermatitis. *Diagnosis is based on history, physical examination findings, exclusion of other dermatoses, and is confirmed by restriction followed by provocative exposure to the suspected allergen or patch testing.*

Bibliography

Jörundsson E, et al. Prominence of γδ T cells in the elicitation phase of dinitrochlorobenzene-induced contact hypersensitivity in lambs. Vet Pathol 1999;36:42–50.

Leung DYM, et al. Allergic and immunologic skin disorders. J Am Med Assoc 1997;278:1914–1923.

Marchal I S-A, et al. Feline Langerhans cells migrate from skin and vaginal mucosa to regional lymph nodes during experimental contact sensitization with fluorescein isothiocyanate. Vet Dermatol 1998;9:9–17.

Marsella R, et al. Use of pentoxifylline in the treatment of allergic contact reactions to plants of the Commelinceae family in dogs. Vet Dermatol 1997;8:121–126.

Thomsen MK, Thomsen HK. Histopathological changes in canine allergic contact dermatitis patch test reactions. A study on spontaneously hypersensitive dogs. Acta Vet Scand 1989;30:379–384.

Walder EJ, Conroy JD. Contact dermatitis in dogs and cats: Pathogenesis, histopathology, experimental induction and case reports. Vet Dermatol 1994;5:149–162.

Willemse T, Vroom MA. Allergic dermatitis in a great Dane due to contact with hippeastrum. Vet Rec 1988;122:490–491.

Insect hypersensitivity

Insects are cosmopolitan in their distribution and virtually all animals are exposed to them. Many insects are capable of inducing allergic reactions, including various dermatoses. *Antigens of insect origin that produce hypersensitivity are usually proteins and sources include venom, saliva, whole bodies, shed skins, egg capsules, feces, and insect hemoglobin.* These antigens can be introduced via the bite or sting of insects or by inhalation, ingestion, or percutaneous absorption. In general, lesions associated with insect hypersensitivity are *seasonal* or seasonally more severe and *involve short- or sparsely haired regions*, such as the nose, muzzle, pinnae, inguinal area, and distal extremities. *Lesions typically consist of pruritic crusted papules and are characterized histologically by eosinophilic inflammation.*

The most well known insect hypersensitivities of veterinary significance are those caused by an allergic reaction to salivary antigens and these are *flea-bite hypersensitivity of dogs and cats* and *Culicoides hypersensitivity of horses*. More recently, a *hypersensitivity to mosquito bites has been recognized in cats* and an *eosinophilic furunculosis of the face of dogs* is suspected to be a hypersensitivity response to the sting or bite of various insects. The first three of these conditions will be discussed in this section. Canine eosinophilic furunculosis of the face is discussed under Eosinophilic and collagenolytic dermatitides.

Flea-bite hypersensitivity is a pruritic dermatitis caused by hypersensitivity to allergens in the saliva of fleas. *It is the most common allergic dermatosis of dogs and cats in flea-endemic regions.* The cat flea, *Ctenocephalides felis felis*, is the major initiator of the condition. Since many animals harbor large numbers of fleas without any apparent skin abnormalities, it is likely that animals develop skin disease as a result of flea infestation only if they are allergic to fleas.

Both type I and type IV hypersensitivity reactions are believed to be involved in the pathogenesis of flea-bite hypersensitivity. Participation of immediate hypersensitivity is supported by the fact that clinically allergic animals develop immediate skin reactions in response to intradermal injection of flea antigen and that IgE antibodies to flea antigen are demonstrable in sera from allergic animals. Histologic evidence also supports a role for immediate hypersensitivity and suggests that cell mediated/delayed hypersensitivity is involved in the pathogenesis of flea allergy as well. Many flea allergic animals also have delayed skin test reactions, further support for a type IV hypersensitivity component. Upregulation of mast cell proteases has been demonstrated during sensitization, with selective release of mast cell tryptase after exposure to flea antigen.

No breed or sex predilections have been reported in flea-bite hypersensitivity; and in cats, no age predilection has been recognized. In dogs, disease occurs most commonly between 3 and 5 years, unless naive dogs are moved to a flea-endemic area at a later age. Disease is rare prior to 6 months. Signs tend to be more severe in summer and fall in animals living in areas with cold winters but are year-round in those living in warm regions or where indoor infestation persists. Affected individuals may have other hypersensitivity conditions, such as atopic dermatitis or food allergy.

Flea-bite hypersensitivity in **dogs** is characterized by pruritus, erythema, wheals, and papules that may become crusted. *Primary lesions are usually obscured by secondary lesions that develop in response to chronic pruritus.* These may include hyperkeratosis, lichenification, hyperpigmentation, alopecia, excoriations, redundant skin folds on the rump and caudal thighs, and seborrhea. Lesions typically involve the dorsal lumbosacral area, flanks, caudal and medial aspect of the thighs, and ventral abdomen. In severely hypersensitive dogs, lesions may become generalized. Pyotraumatic dermatitis ("hot spots") and bacterial pyoderma are common secondary complications. Firm alopecic nodules ("fibropruritic nodules") may develop on the dorsal lumbosacral region secondary to self-trauma in chronically affected dogs. Differential diagnoses include other hypersensitivity conditions (atopic dermatitis, food allergy), sarcoptic mange, cheyletiellosis, and bacterial or yeast infection.

The lesions of flea-bite hypersensitivity in **cats** are extremely variable. The most common manifestation is multiple erythematous pruritic papules covered by brown crust ("*miliary dermatitis*") on the dorsal lumbosacral area, flanks, caudal and medial aspect of the thighs, ventral abdomen, and neck. In some cats, the condition may be manifested as over-zealous grooming rather than scratching, producing alopecia that may be ventral abdominal, bilaterally symmetrical along the lateral aspect of the trunk, or dorsal lumbosacral. The skin may appear completely normal grossly or excoriations, crusts, scales, and hyperpigmented macules may be seen. Fleas or flea dirt may not be evident because of the fastidious grooming behavior typical of most cats. Eosinophilic granuloma complex lesions have also been associated with flea-bite hypersensitivity in cats. Secondary bacterial pyoderma is uncommon. Differential diagnosis is extensive because the manifestations of flea allergy are so varied in cats. *The most common differentials for miliary dermatitis include other hypersensitivity conditions (atopic dermatitis, food hypersensitivity), dermatophytosis, and cheyletiellosis.* Cases characterized by self-induced alopecia with normal appearing skin may resemble an endocrinopathy.

Histopathology is useful in confirming the suspected diagnosis of a hypersensitivity condition, but *the microscopic changes associated with flea-bite hypersensitivity are similar to those seen in other hypersensitivities and the specific diagnosis cannot be made histologically.* The epidermis is variably acanthotic and foci of spongiosis and serocellular crusting are commonly seen. Mixed orthokeratotic and parakeratotic hyperkeratosis and self-induced erosion or ulceration may be present. Foci of epidermal necrosis and intraepidermal eosinophilic pustules may be evident. The superficial dermis is mildly to moderately edematous and a perivascular to interstitial infiltration of eosinophils, lymphocytes, fewer macrophages, and mast cells is present in the superficial to mid-dermis in dogs and may extend into the subcutis in cats. The proportion of eosinophils in relation to mononuclear cells varies, with eosinophils being most numerous in early lesions and mononuclear cells predominating in more chronic reactions. Melanophages are in variable numbers and may be numerous in chronic cases with prominent lichenification. Sebaceous and apocrine glands may be hyperplastic in chronic lesions. Neutrophils are numerous in association with ulceration or bacterial infection. In cats, eosinophilic mural folliculitis and furunculosis have been seen in flea bites as have histologic lesions of eosinophilic granuloma complex.

***Culicoides* (insect) hypersensitivity** *is the most common allergic dermatosis of horses.* It occurs worldwide and *Culicoides* spp. gnats are the most common cause. The condition is known by a variety of colloquial names worldwide, including Queensland itch, kasen, dhobie itch, sweet itch, muck itch, summer itch, and summer eczema. It is a major annoyance to horse and owner and substantial economic losses can be incurred from treatment, prevention, and damage caused by scratching horses. *Culicoides* hypersensitivity is an *intensely pruritic dermatosis* that can render affected animals too restless and anxious to perform.

The insects are also called biting midges, punkies, and "no-see-ums." Hundreds of different species exist throughout the world and they vary in their favored feeding sites and time of activity. They are most active when the ambient temperature is greater than

10°C (50°F), when humidity is high, and when there is no breeze since they are weak fliers. The insects are in highest numbers in wetlands and swampy areas.

The hypersensitivity to salivary antigens of *Culicoides* gnats is thought to be mediated by *both type I and type IV hypersensitivity reactions*. Support for immediate hypersensitivity is provided by immediate skin test reactivity to *Culicoides* antigens, presence of specific IgE in affected horses, and peripheral eosinophilia and increased blood histamine concentrations during periods of insect activity. The presence of increased numbers of primarily CD4+ T lymphocytes and eosinophils in skin test reactions is also consistent with immediate hypersensitivity. Also, sulfidoleukotriene generation from peripheral blood leukocytes in response to *Culicoides* extract was increased in horses with insect hypersensitivity, indicating involvement of IgE-mediated hypersensitivity in the pathogenesis of *Culicoides* hypersensitivity. Delayed reactions (up to 48 hr) to intradermal skin tests suggest that type IV hypersensitivity may also be involved in the pathogenesis of the condition.

Culicoides hypersensitivity is typically a seasonal disease but in warm climates it may be a problem virtually year-round. Horses of any breed and either sex are affected; pedigree studies suggest there may be a genetic basis. Lesions are uncommon in horses less than 2 years old; however, in tropical and subtropical climates with a long insect season, sensitization and mild clinical disease may develop within the first year of exposure. The favored feeding sites vary with the species of *Culicoides* endemic to a particular environment, accounting for the varied distribution of skin lesions. Distribution may be dorsal and involve the head, ears, neck, withers, back, and tailhead; or it may be primarily ventral and involve the intermandibular space, legs, and ventral midline. In some areas, such as Florida in the USA, multiple species of *Culicoides* are active at different times and have different favored feeding sites such that disease may be generalized. The *primary lesions are pruritic papules* that may be recognized initially by clusters of erect hairs and commonly become encrusted. Because of severe pruritus, however, self-mutilation obscures the primary lesions and results in *more commonly observed secondary lesions such as excoriations, crusts, lichenification, pigmentary changes, broken hairs, alopecia, and a short stubbled tail ("rat tail")* (Fig. 5.67). The mane may be rubbed off and the skin over the neck and withers may become thickened and rugose. Lesions typically heal during winter and recur in spring or summer and commonly worsen with age. Affected horses may scratch and bite themselves and rub objects in their environment, thereby causing damage to themselves, their riders, and environmental objects. Constant anxiety and restlessness may prevent severely affected animals from performing as riding or show animals. Also, since sweating exacerbates pruritus, affected horses cannot be worked vigorously. The differential diagnoses include ectoparasitism and other hypersensitivity dermatoses. The *diagnosis* is based on seasonality of the condition, location and appearance of lesions, sporadic occurrence of the condition in a group, eliminating other diseases, and response to therapy.

The *histologic lesions* of *Culicoides* hypersensitivity are typically *superficial or superficial and deep perivascular dermatitis consisting of eosinophils and lymphocytes primarily*. The epidermis is variably acanthotic, spongiotic, and hyperkeratotic with foci of parakeratosis, and may be focally necrotic. Increased numbers of T lymphocytes and Langerhans cells are present in the basal portion of the epidermis. Erosions and ulceration may be present as a result of self-trauma and are associated with neutrophilic inflammation. The dermis is variably edematous and increased numbers of mast cells, which may be degranulated, are present. In some cases, eosinophilic inflammation is diffuse and collagen degeneration or eosinophilic folliculitis may also be seen.

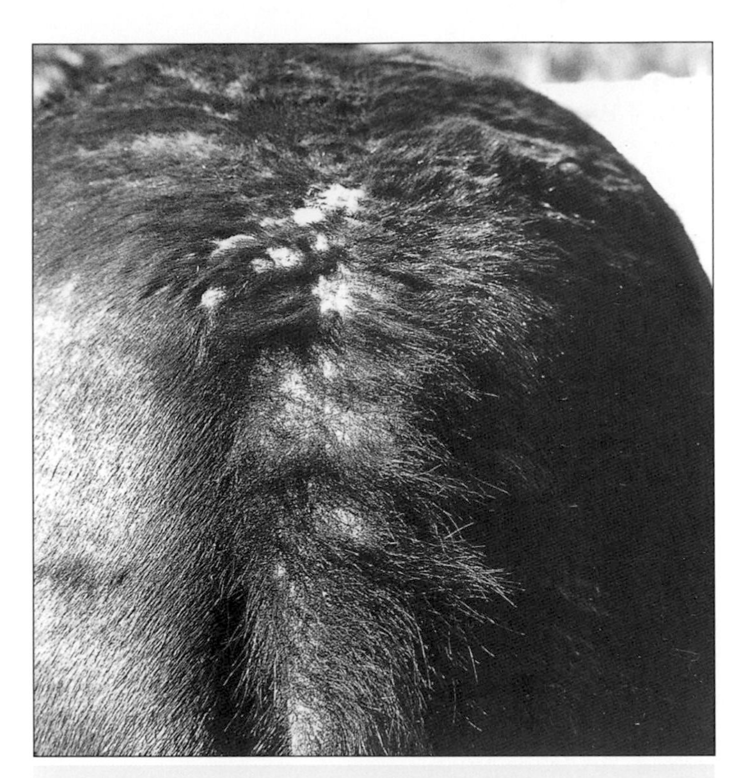

Figure 5.67 *Culicoides* hypersensitivity in a horse. Alopecia, crusting and scaling at the tail head ("rat tail").

A seasonal pruritic dermatosis attributed to *Culicoides* hypersensitivity has also been described in *cattle, sheep, and donkeys*. Affected sheep were 2–5 years of age and had an intensely pruritic, exudative dermatitis with loss of wool and marked skin thickening of the abdomen, udder, teats, and legs. Lesions in adult dairy cattle consisted of marked thickening and folding of the skin of the head, ears, and neck. Donkeys developed exudative dermatitis, alopecia, crusting, and skin thickening of the legs and head. Affected animals were restless and often bit at themselves, suggesting that they were intensely pruritic. Histologic examination of biopsies from affected sheep and cows showed primarily an eosinophilic dermal infiltrate.

Mosquito-bite hypersensitivity dermatitis has been documented in the Mosquito-bite dermatitis section.

Bibliography

Benarafa C, et al. Role of the chemokine eotaxin in the pathogenesis of equine sweet itch. Vet Rec 2002;151:691–693.

Bevier DE. Insect and arachnid hypersensitivity. Vet Clin North Am: Small Anim Pract 1999;29:1385–1405.

Friberg CA, Lewis DT. Insect hypersensitivity in small animals. Compend Contin Educ Pract Vet 1998;20:1121–1131.

Greiner EC. Entomologic evaluation of insect hypersensitivity in horses. Vet Clin North Am: Eq Pract 1995;11:29–41.

Gross TL, Halliwell REW. Lesions of experimental flea bite hypersensitivity in the dog. Vet Pathol 1985;22:78–81.

Kunkle GA, et al. Pilot study to assess the effects of early flea exposure on the development of flea hypersensitivity in cats. J Feline Med Surg 2003;5:287–294.
Kurotaki T, et al. Immunopathological study on equine insect hypersensitivity ("Kasen") in Japan. J Comp Pathol 1994;110:145–152.
Lee SE, et al. Putative salivary allergens of the cat flea, *Ctenocephalides felis felis*. Vet Immunol Immunopathol 1999;69:229–237.
Lewis DT, et al. Clinical and histological evaluation of immediate and delayed flea antigen intradermal skin test and flea bite sites in normal and flea-allergic cats. Vet Dermatol 1999;10:29–37.
Marti E, et al. On the genetic basis of equine allergic diseases: II. Insect bite dermal hypersensitivity. Eq Vet J 1992;24:113–117.
Marti E, et al. Sulfidoleukotriene generation from peripheral blood leukocytes of horses affected with insect bite dermal hypersensitivity. Vet Immunol Immunopathol 1999;71:307–320.
McKelvie J, et al. Characterisation of lymphocyte subpopulations in the skin and circulation of horses with sweet itch (*Culicoides* hypersensitivity). Eq Vet J 1999;31:466–472.
von Ruedorffer U, et al. Flea bite hypersensitivity: new aspects on the involvement of mast cells. Vet J 2003;165:149–156.
Wilson AD, et al. Detection of IgG and IgE serum antibodies to *Culicoides* salivary gland antigens in horses with insect dermal hypersensitivity (sweet itch). Equine Vet J 2001;33:707–713.
Yeruham I, et al. Field observations in Israel on hypersensitivity in cattle, sheep and donkeys caused by *Culicoides*. Aust Vet J 1993;70:348–352.

Hormonal hypersensitivity

Pruritic dermatitis resulting from hypersensitivity to endogenous sex hormones is recognized in women ("autoimmune progesterone dermatitis") and is *very rare in dogs*. Results of intradermal skin tests with aqueous progesterone in women indicate that type I (immediate) and/or type IV hypersensitivity are involved. *Most canine cases are in intact females, frequently with a history of irregular estrus or recurrent pseudopregnancy*. The condition is characterized by *intense pruritus* that develops or is exacerbated near the time of estrus or pseudopregnancy but tends to become more severe and protracted with each episode; pruritus is generally perennial in male dogs. Bilaterally symmetric erythema and crusted papules typically begin in the dorsal lumbosacral, perineal, genital, and caudomedial thigh areas and progress cranially. In chronic cases the condition is generalized and the skin becomes alopecic and lichenified. Pruritus is usually unresponsive to glucocorticoid treatment. Differential diagnoses include other allergic conditions and sarcoptic mange. The microscopic lesion is a hyperplastic superficial perivascular dermatitis in which neutrophils, mononuclear cells, or eosinophils may predominate. *Diagnostic clues include poor response to glucocorticoid therapy and development or exacerbation of cutaneous signs coincident with estrus or pseudopregnancy*. Gonadectomy is curative.

Bibliography

Scott DW, Miller WH. Probable hormonal hypersensitivity in two male dogs. Canine Pract 1999;17:14–17, 20.

Intestinal parasite hypersensitivity

Hypersensitivity to intestinal parasites has been suspected of causing pruritic dermatoses in *dogs, cats, horses, and humans*. The pathomechanism is unknown but a type I hypersensitivity reaction has been proposed. *Ascarids, coccidia, hookworms, tapeworms, and whipworms have rarely been associated with pruritic dermatoses that resolve with elimination of the intestinal parasites*. Lesions that have been attributed to intestinal parasite hypersensitivity include multifocal or generalized papulocrustous eruptions, pruritic seborrheic disease, pruritic urticaria, and pruritus without skin lesions. The histologic changes described are superficial perivascular dermatitis with variable numbers of eosinophils, ranging from few to many. Diagnosis is based on fecal examination and resolution of the skin lesions following appropriate parasiticidal therapy.

Bibliography

Cooper PJ. Intestinal worms and human allergy. Parasite Immunol 2004;26:455–467.
Scott DW, et al. Muller & Kirk's Small Animal Dermatology. 6th ed. Philadelphia, PA: WB Saunders, 2000.

Autoimmune dermatoses

The autoimmune skin diseases are *uncommon to rare* but merit detailed consideration as many are debilitating to life-threatening and require specific therapy. *Their characteristic microscopic lesions combined with clinical information and careful interpretation of ancillary studies often enables a specific diagnosis to be made*. In the vast majority of cases, the stimulus triggering the aberrant T or B cell responses against self-antigens is unknown. Drug therapy, underlying neoplasia (see Paraneoplastic pemphigus, p. 652), tissue injury, infectious diseases, other autoimmune diseases, and genetic makeup are all factors known to be associated with the occurrence of autoimmune diseases. Penicillinamine, for example, may precipitate clinically, histologically and immunologically classical cases of pemphigus in humans, which regress when the drug is withdrawn. Drug-induced forms of pemphigus are thought to be the result of haptenization of keratinocyte antigens rendering them immunogenic. One theory suggests environmental agents, such as drugs, influence T cells by causing DNA methylation abnormalities that, in turn, alter gene expression. Exposure to ultraviolet light is known to exacerbate cutaneous autoimmune disease perhaps by inducing keratinocyte ICAM-1 expression and keratinocyte production of pro-inflammatory cytokines. Still another theory suggests that the structural similarities of peptide fragments of some infectious agents to host proteins may trigger post-infectious autosensitization.

The recognition that one autoimmune disease, tissue injury, inflammatory or neoplastic process in an individual may precede the onset of cutaneous autoimmune disease led to investigation of the phenomenon termed "*epitope spreading*." Epitope spreading refers to the process by which the targets of the autoimmune response do not remain fixed but drift to include other epitopes on the same protein or nearby proteins of the same tissue. This may account for regional variations in pemphigus antigen expression and the clinical variation of cutaneous autoimmune diseases. Epitope spreading may also account for aberrant immune responses developing to tissue antigens after the tissue has been injured, possibly leading to the release or exposure of a previously sequestered antigen.

Selection of fresh lesions is crucial to diagnosis. Demonstration of tissue-bound or circulating autoantibody using appropriate immunological tests may be helpful in confirming the diagnosis of an autoimmune skin disease. However, such tests (e.g., direct and indirect immunofluorescence testing, immunohistochemistry) are fraught with interpretation pitfalls (false-positive or false-negative test results) and should

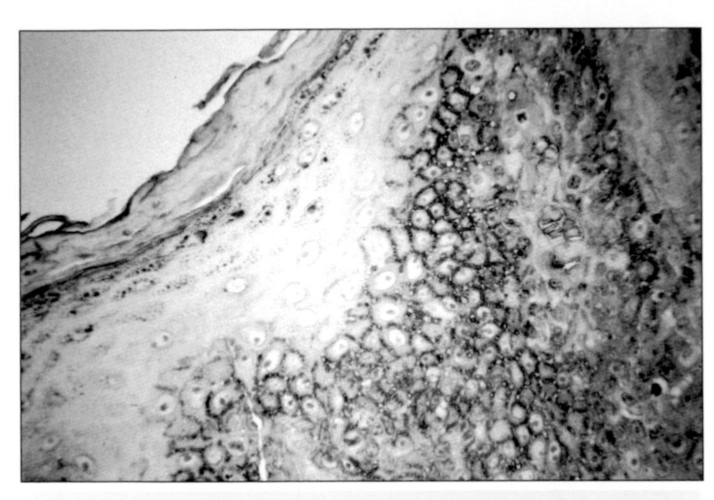

Figure 5.68 Immunoperoxidase stain of **pemphigus complex**. Note diffuse intense labeling of intercellular bridges.

never be interpreted in the absence of histologic examination. Demonstration of autoantibodies does not necessarily confirm causative roles for these antibodies, just as negative results do not necessarily exclude the diagnosis of a cutaneous autoimmune disease. For example, the various entities of the pemphigus complex are characterized by the deposition of immunoglobulin, with or without complement, on the surface of keratinocytes or at the basement membrane zone using the techniques of direct immunofluorescence (IF) testing or immunohistochemistry (IHC) (Fig. 5.68). Unfortunately, false-negative (poor lesion selection, prior glucocorticoid therapy) and false positive (any dermatosis in which spongiosis or numerous lymphocytes and plasma cells are present) reactions are frequent. In addition, normal epithelium of the canine nasal planum and footpad often label nonspecifically. Hence, *these immunopathological tests can only be interpreted in the light of clinical and histopathological findings*. Indirect immunofluorescence testing has variable usefulness in domestic animals with pemphigus as results may be falsely negative or "pemphigus-like" antibodies can be occasionally found in non-pemphigus diseases. Recent studies indicate indirect IF testing for canine PF is useful provided the appropriate substrate (bovine esophagus) is used. In many of the putative cases of autoimmune skin disease in animals, the criteria for autoimmunity have not been met fully.

Bibliography

Bradley GA, Calderwood Mays MB. Immunoperoxidase staining for the detection of autoantibodies in canine autoimmune skin disease: Comparison to immunofluorescence results. Vet Immunol Immunopathol 1990;26:105–113.

Chan LS, et al. Epitope spreading: Lessons from autoimmune skin diseases. J Invest Dermatol 1998;110:103–109.

Day MJ, et al. Immune-mediated skin disease in the dog and cat. J Comp Pathol 1993;109:395–407.

Iwasaki T, et al. Effect of substrate on indirect immunofluorescence tests for canine pemphigus foliaceus. Vet Pathol 1996;33:332–336.

Kalaher KM, et al. Direct immunofluorescence testing of normal feline nasal planum and footpad. Cornell Vet 1990;80:105–109.

Rose NR. The role of infection in the pathogenesis of autoimmune diseases. Semin Immunol 1998;10:5–13.

Rubin RL. Etiology and mechanisms of drug-induced lupus. Curr Opin Rheumatol 1999;11:357–363.

White SD, et al. Putative drug-related pemphigus foliaceus in four dogs. Vet Dermatol 2002;13:195–202.

Zipfel W, et al. Demonstration of immunoglobulins and complement in canine and feline autoimmune and non-autoimmune skin diseases with the direct immunofluorescence and indirect immunoperoxidase method. J Vet Med 1992;39:494–501.

Autoimmune diseases characterized by vesicles, pustules, or bullae as the primary lesion

The pemphigus complex

Pemphigus refers to *a group of autoimmune skin diseases characterized clinically by pustules, vesicles, bullae, erosions and ulcers and histologically by loss of adhesion between cells (acantholysis)*. Autoantibodies directed against antigens within various stratified squamous epithelia, including skin, mucocutaneous junctions, oral mucosa, esophagus, and vagina, develop and can be detected via immunologic assays. *Different types of pemphigus are recognized based on the level at which acantholysis occurs within the epidermis, and the clinical and immunological findings*. Autoantibodies are directed against components of keratinocyte transmembrane glycoproteins responsible for keratinocyte cell-to-cell adhesion (desmosomes) or cell-to-substrate adhesion (hemidesmosomes). Desmosomes are more numerous in the more superficial layers of the epidermis and vary in protein subunit composition. Hemidesmosomes are present on the basal surface of the basal layer of the epidermis. Vesicles, pustules, or bullae form within the various layers of the epidermis or at the basement membrane zone according to the location of the target antigen. Severity of clinical disease is related to the depth of vesicle or bullae formation, with the more severe lesions associated with separations deep within or below the epidermis. The mechanisms leading to acantholysis are not completely understood. Antigen-antibody binding may result in a type II immune reaction or promote proinflammatory cytokine release from keratinocytes. The binding of pemphigus autoantibodies to keratinocyte antigens is associated with the synthesis and secretion of urokinase-type plasminogen activator (uPA), a serine protease that activates plasminogen. Activation of plasminogen may indirectly induce the cleaving of intercellular contacts. Anti-uPA antibodies or the specific inhibitor of uPA, plasminogen activator inhibitor type-2, inhibit lesion formation in vitro. Another hypothesis proposes that the binding of autoantibodies to keratinocyte antigens may disrupt the structural integrity of the adhesion molecule. Experimental studies in mice have demonstrated that acantholysis in pemphigus foliaceus (PF) can occur with passive transfer of PF IgG autoantibody as well as with transfer of Fab fragments and $F(ab')_2$ fragments in both complement-sufficient and complement-deficient mice.

Pemphigus foliaceus (PF) is the *most common form of pemphigus in domestic animals* and has been reported in the *dog, cat, horse, and goat*. In humans, PF autoantibodies recognize the desmosomal protein, *desmoglein 1*. Desmoglein 1 autoantibodies have also been identified in dogs, but autoantibodies to other keratinocyte antigens and to the basement membrane have also been identified, indicating that PF, at least in the dog, may be an immunologically heterogeneous disease. Desmoglein 1 belongs to the cadherin family of cell-adhesion molecules, and is found primarily in the upper layers of the epidermis and in only small amounts in the oral mucosa. In PF, the acantholytic process occurs at a superficial level in the epidermis producing clinical lesions that are *typically exfoliative rather than obviously erosive or ulcerative*. There is no sex predilection in **dogs**, but Akitas, Chow Chows, Bearded Collies, Collies, Chinese Shar-Peis, Dachshunds, Newfoundlands, Doberman Pinschers, Schipperkes, English Springer Spaniels, and Appaloosa horses appear predisposed. In dogs, most cases occur prior to 5 years of age. The gross lesions are similar in all species and are usually cutaneous and involve mucosa only rarely, as mucosal epithelium has desmoglein 3 as a prominent superficial adhesion molecule rather than desmoglein 1. Lesions may wax and wane. Erythematous macules give rise to transient pustules that rupture to form very shallow erosions that become covered by thick crust and scale. Alopecia is often marked. *Lesions in the dog and cat tend to appear first on the nose and spread to periorbital areas, the ears, neck and ventral abdomen.* Involvement of the feet may produce marked papillary hyperkeratosis and crusting of the footpads, and there is a *predilection for the nail beds*, occasionally leading to sloughing of nails. In **cats**, lesions are often seen around the nipples in addition to lesions on the face and ears (Fig. 5.69A). PF is the most common autoimmune skin disease in **horses;** lesions often begin on the face or distal extremities, or may be localized to coronets. In any species, the lesions may become generalized (Fig. 5.69B, C). Foals may also be affected with a benign form of PF that responds rapidly to treatment or may resolve spontaneously. Pain and pruritus may be present.

The histologic pattern of pemphigus foliaceus is an acantholytic subcorneal (see Figs. 5.1 and 5.17) *or intragranular pustular dermatitis.* Either neutrophils or eosinophils may predominate. At the base of the pustule, acantholytic keratinocytes continue to detach and enter the pustule. Ruptured pustules form a thick inflammatory crust in which acantholytic cells are prominent. The external root sheath of the hair follicle undergoes a similar acantholytic process. Dermal infiltrates consist of mild perivascular to interstitial neutrophils or eosinophils. There is dermal edema, vascular congestion and occasionally, hemorrhage. Rarely, a lichenoid inflammatory infiltrate is seen. *Deposition of IgG at intercellular bridges in all layers of the suprabasilar epidermis or in the superficial epidermis demonstrated by IF or IHC is characteristic, but not specific, for PF.* Secondary bacterial infection may complicate lesions. *The primary differential for PF is superficial bacterial folliculitis.* Acantholytic cells are more numerous and can more often be found in rafts in PF than in superficial folliculitis. *The "cling-on" stratum granulosum cells are only present in PF.* In PF, pustules also span the interfollicular epidermis encompassing multiple follicles whereas in superficial folliculitis pustules are more likely to be centered on single follicles. Evidence of recornification and reformation of pustules is often prominent in PF. Dermatophytosis and superficial pyoderma (impetigo) can also have similar gross and histologic lesions. Careful examination of skin sections with fungal and bacterial stains and possibly cultures may be needed for differentiation. Impetigo does not involve hair follicles whereas PF may.

Panepidermal pustular pemphigus (PPP) refers to a form of pemphigus in the dog that encompasses some of the features of **pemphigus foliaceus**, **pemphigus vegetans**, and **pemphigus erythematosus**, previously thought to be distinct entities. It is similar to pemphigus foliaceus in that lesions develop in the superficial epidermis, however, lesions are not restricted to the superficial layers of the epidermis so it does not neatly fit the same criteria as PF. Immunological studies have not definitively documented the presence of autoantibodies to desmosomal or hemidesmosomal proteins

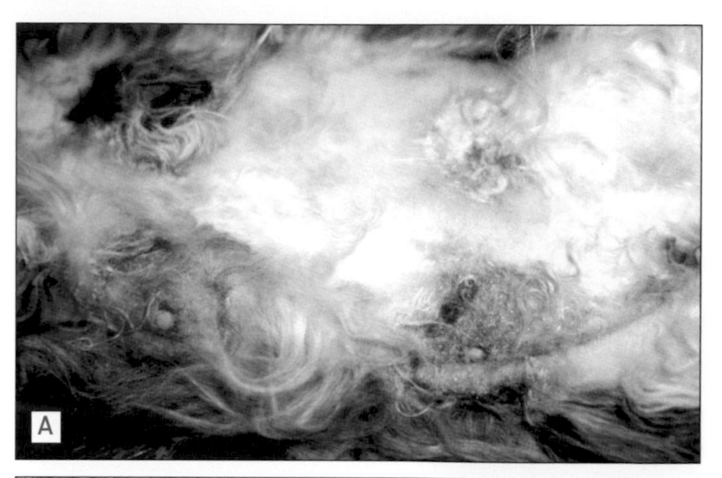
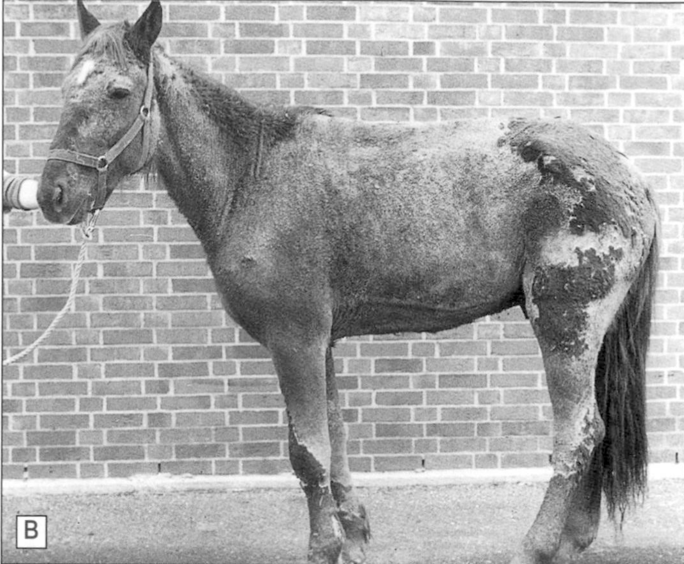
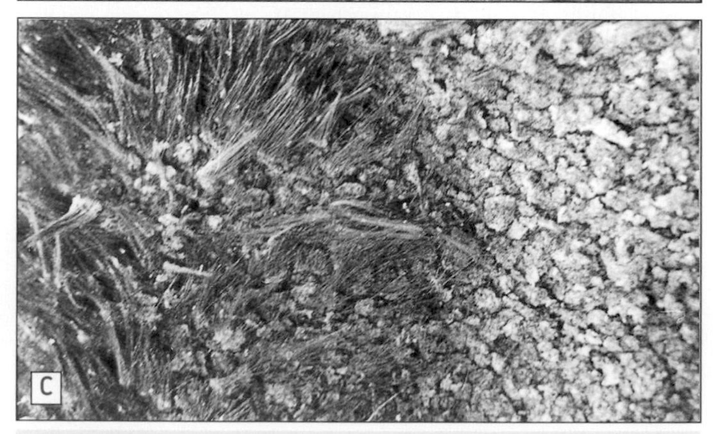

Figure 5.69 Pemphigus foliaceus. **A.** Note alopecia and crusts of the skin around the nipples in a cat. (Courtesy of K Beale.) **B.** Generalized exfoliative dermatitis and alopecia in a horse. **C.** Detail of skin from (**B**) showing massive build up of scales and crusts.

in PPP, but studies evaluating autoantibody epidermal binding patterns in dogs with PF have identified four main IgG intercellular epidermal patterns. One pattern indicates that antibodies to desmoglein 1 are present as they are in PF. Other IgG autoantibodies have been detected against intracellular keratinocyte antigens in

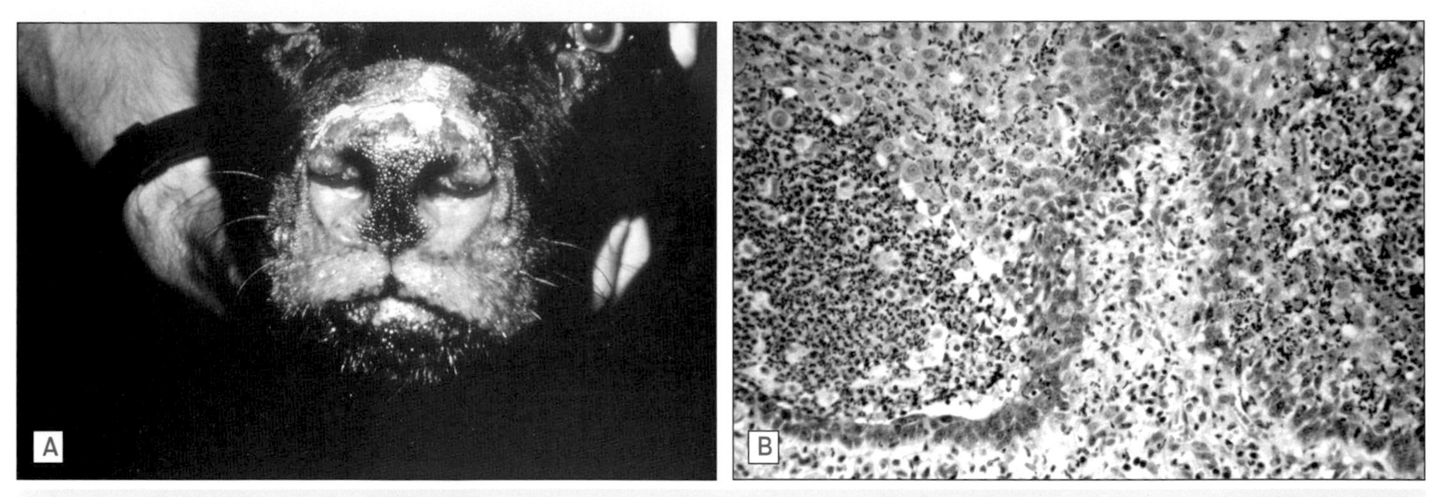

Figure 5.70 Panepidermal pustular pemphigus. (Courtesy of B Dunstan.) **A.** Scaly and crusted plaques and papules of the skin of the face and nasal planum. **B.** Pustules are present at several levels of the surface epithelium, including the suprabasal layers.

the stratum basale, spinosum, granulosum, and corneum, and basement membrane, substantiating the immunologically heterogeneous characteristics of pemphigus subtypes in the dog. These autoantibody binding patterns help to explain the variable location of epidermal pustules in subtypes of canine PF. *Original designations of pemphigus vegetans and pemphigus erythematosus in animals were based on similarities to the human conditions. Further studies suggest the conditions are not directly comparable.* Pemphigus erythematosus was considered to be a variant of PF with a facial or "lupus" lesion distribution occurring in dogs and cats. Criteria for diagnosis and differentiation from PF were dependant upon the immunological demonstration of both a diffuse cell surface IF or IHC pattern typical of the pemphigus group and a linear band of immunoglobulin, with or without complement, deposited at the basement membrane zone. For reasons previously stated, IF and IHC are not dependable. Reported cases of pemphigus vegetans in veterinary patients are very limited and originally thought to be benign variants of pemphigus vulgaris. The lack of clear clinical or histologic distinction between pemphigus vegetans and pemphigus erythematosus in the dog has led to the new inclusive entity of PPP by some veterinary dermatopathologists; however, *classification is controversial.* Some veterinary dermatopathologists also consider PPP to be a subtype of PF. Differentiation of PPP from typical cases of PF is discussed below.

PPP is less common than PF, but more common than PV. Akitas and Chow Chows are predisposed to develop both PPP and PF. In most cases, lesions first appear on the head in a symmetrical distribution involving the medial canthi of the eyes ("lupus distribution") and inner surfaces of the pinnae and nasal planum (Fig. 5.70A). The condition may remain localized to the head or proceed to the prepuce, abdomen, nail beds, and footpads. Some cases become generalized. *Gross lesions* are characterized initially by *erythematous macules* leading to *vesiculopustular lesions* resembling those of PF. Over time however, *the lesions progress to proliferative, scaly and crusted plaques or papules. Verrucous vegetations studded with small pustules are characteristic.* Depigmentation of the nasal planum may develop. The predominant *histologic lesions* are *numerous large, intraepithelial pustules composed of eosinophils, neutrophils and a few to large numbers of acantholytic epithelial cells.* These pustules occur at several levels through the surface epithelium, down to the suprabasal layers and also involve the infundibular outer root sheath (Fig. 5.70B). An eosinophilic to neutrophilic intra-infundibular mural folliculitis may be present. In mature lesions, there is papillated epidermal hyperplasia. The dermis has a perivascular to interstitial mixed infiltrate with eosinophils. Biopsies from the mucocutaneous junction or the nasal planum may be intensely plasmacytic and lichenoid. IFA or IHC may demonstrate immunoglobulin at intercellular bridges and/or the basement membrane zone, however results can be variable. *Histologic differentials* include *predominantly facial PF, discoid or systemic lupus, mycosis fungoides, pyoderma or bacterial folliculitis, dermatophytosis, and the uveodermatologic syndrome.* In PF, pustules are restricted to the stratum granulosum and stratum spinosum; in PPP, they occur in the deeper layers of the epidermis. PPP is also very proliferative compared to PF.

Pemphigus vulgaris *is the most severe and the more rare form of pemphigus in animals.* This life-threatening disease has been reported in the *dog, cat, horse, goat, monkey, and llama.* There are no apparent breed or sex predilections. Middle-aged **dogs** are most commonly affected. In humans and dogs, pemphigus vulgaris autoantibodies recognize the desmosomal protein, desmoglein 3. Desmoglein 3 also belongs to the cadherin family of cell-adhesion molecules and is most prominent in the area of the basal layer of keratinocytes of the epidermis and mucosal epithelium, hence lesions occur deeper in the epidermis and in the oral mucosa.. Desmoglein 3 is not a component of hemidesmosomes. The *fragile vesicles or bullae in the epidermis are extremely transient and readily rupture* to leave the more common presenting lesion of a roughly circular, shallow, flat-based erosion or ulcer. The margins often develop epidermal collarettes. Firm sliding pressure to adjacent unaffected skin may induce fresh vesicle formation or dislodge the skin (*the Nikolsky sign*). Lesions involve mucous membranes (Fig. 5.71A), mucocutaneous junctions and skin in the mechanically stressed areas such as the inguinal and axillary regions. Oral involvement is present in 90% of cases, and in 50% of cases the lesions commence in the mouth. Involvement of the nailbeds occurs also and corneal ulceration may be present. Animals may be febrile, depressed, and anorectic and have leukocytosis. Drooling is often a presenting complaint.

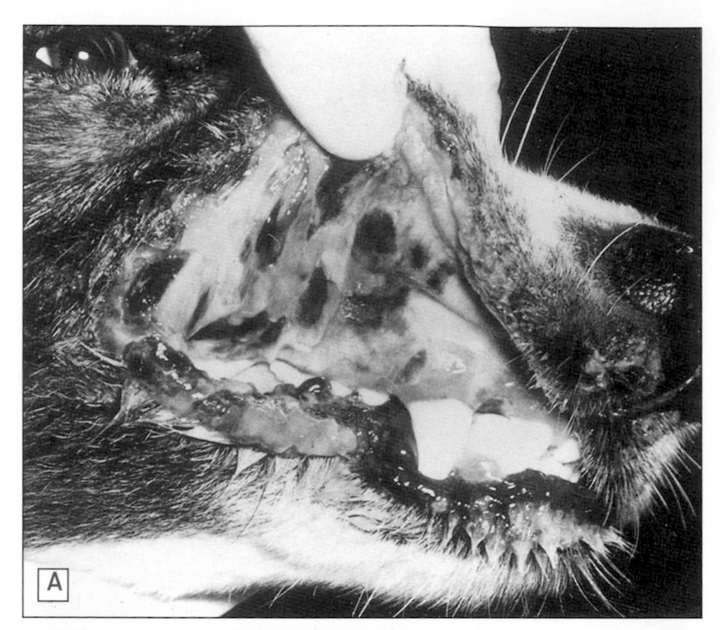

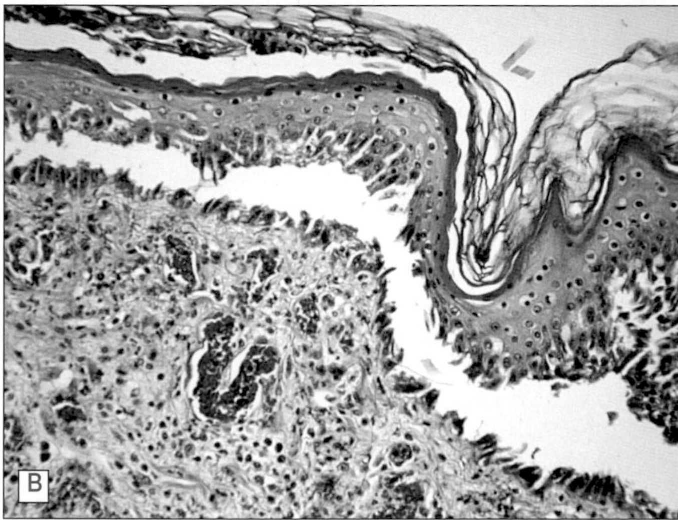

Figure 5.71 Pemphigus vulgaris. A. Flaccid bullae in oral mucosa. (Courtesy of Parker WM, and Can Vet J.) **B.** Separation of the epidermis occurs between the stratum spinosum and stratum basale. Basal keratinocytes also lose intercellular contact leaving the basal layer arranged to resemble a "row of tombstones." (Courtesy of B Dunstan.)

Microscopically, *the earliest lesions consist of spongiosis and vacuolation of the suprabasilar epidermis progressing to suprabasilar acantholysis with intraepidermal clefts, vesicles or bullae between the stratum basale and the stratum spinosum* (Fig. 5.71B). The basal keratinocytes, although separated from each other following disruption of intercellular contacts, are anchored to the basal lamina resembling a "row of tombstones." The outer layers of the epidermis form the roof of the vesicle that may contain a few acantholytic keratinocytes, singly or in clumps, but few or no inflammatory cells. The process may extend into the hair follicle epithelium. The dermal reaction in haired skin varies from a mild superficial perivascular to interstitial accumulation of mononuclear cells and eosinophils. A moderately intense lymphocytic-plasmacytic interface infiltrate may be present in mucosal lesions. The immunological pattern of labeling for autoantibodies with IFA or IHC is similar as that for PF. Recently, a variant of PV with IgG autoantibodies directed against plakin proteins and desmogleins 1 and 3 has been documented in the dog. Previously, autoantibodies to plakin proteins were thought to be unique to pemphigus associated with occult neoplasia (see Paraneoplastic pemphigus, p. 652).

Clinical differentials include bullous pemphigoid, erythema multiforme, toxic epidermal necrolysis, systemic lupus erythematosus, idiopathic ulcerative dermatosis of Collies and Shetland Sheepdogs, mycosis fungoides, and other diseases resulting in oral ulcers. Histopathologic findings of primary lesions in PV are diagnostic.

Bibliography

Espana A, et al. Mechanisms of acantholysis in pemphigus foliaceus. Clin Immunol Immunopathol 1997;85:83–89.

Eversole LR. Immunopathology of oral mucosal ulcerative, desquamative, and bullous diseases. Oral Surg Oral Med Oral Pathol 1994;77:555–571.

Gross TL, et al., eds. Bullous and vesicular diseases of the epidermis and dermal-epidermal junction. In: Veterinary Dermatopathology, A Macroscopic and Microscopic Evaluation of Canine and Feline Skin Disease. St. Louis, MO: Mosby Year Book, 1992:22–40.

Kuhl KA, et al. Comparative histopathology of pemphigus foliaceus and superficial folliculitis in the dog. Vet Pathol 1994;31:19–27.

Mattise AW. Canine pemphigus vegetans: A report of 16 cases. Proc Ann Meeting Am Acad Vet Dermatol – Am Coll Vet Dermatol 1991;7:28.

Olivry T, et al. Desmoglein-3 is a target autoantigen in spontaneous canine pemphigus vulgaris. Exp Dermatol 2003;12:198–203.

Olivry T, Chan LS. Autoimmune blistering dermatoses in domestic animals. Clin Dermatol 2001;19:750–760.

Preziosi DE, et al. Feline pemphigus foliaceus: a retrospective analysis of 57 cases. Vet Dermatol 2003;14:313–321.

Scott DW, et al., eds. Immunologic skin diseases. In: Muller and Kirk's Small Animal Dermatology. Philadelphia, PA: WB Saunders, 1995:856–606.

Suter MM, et al. Ultrastructural localization of pemphigus vulgaris antigen on canine keratinocytes *in vivo* and *in vitro*. Am J Vet Res 1990;51:507–511.

Suter MM, et al. Bullous autoimmune skin diseases in animals. 13th Proc Am Acad Vet Dermatol – Am Coll Vet Dermatol Meeting, 1997:100–103.

Valdez RA, et al. Use of corticosteroids and aurothioglucose in a pygmy goat with pemphigus foliaceus. J Am Vet Med Assoc 1995;207:761–765.

Vandenabeele SI, et al. Pemphigus foliaceus in the horse: a retrospective study of 20 cases. Vet Dermatol 2004;15:381–388.

Wurm S, et al. Comparative pathology of pemphigus in dogs and humans. Clin Dermatol 1994;12:515–524.

Bullous pemphigoid

Bullous pemphigoid is *a chronic, autoimmune skin disease characterized clinically by vesicles, bullae and ulcers, and histologically by subepidermal vesicles/bullae containing eosinophils or other leukocytes*. In humans, the autoantibodies are directed against bullous pemphigoid antigen 1 (BPAG1, a 230-kDa intercellular antigen) and bullous pemphigoid antigen 2 (BPAG2, also called type XVII collagen, a 180-kDa hemidesmosomal transmembrane molecule). In animals, only BPAG2 has been identified. The mechanism of dermoepidermal separation is thought to be the result of the release of proinflammatory cytokines IL-1, IL-5, IL-6, IL-8 and others by keratinocytes altered by antigen-antibody interactions. Cytokines recruit neutrophils and eosinophils leading to the release of damaging proteases. Separation of basal cells from the underlying dermis may also be the direct result of

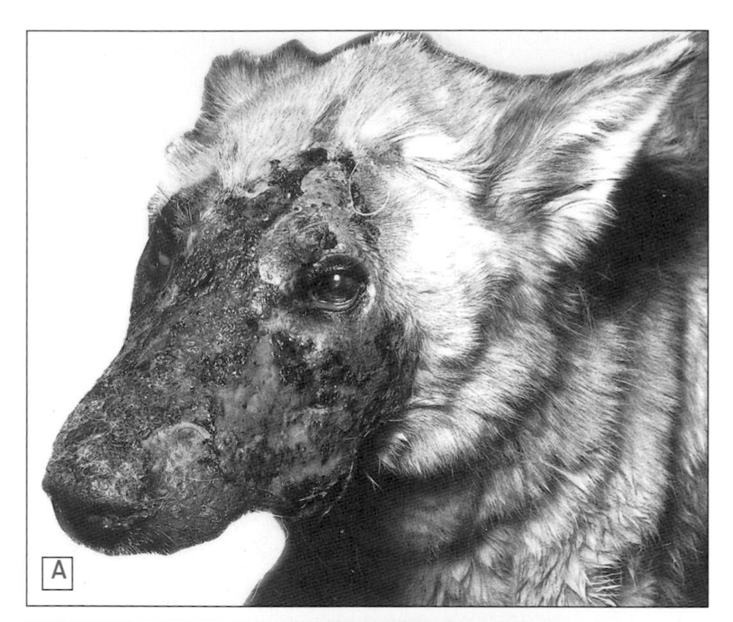

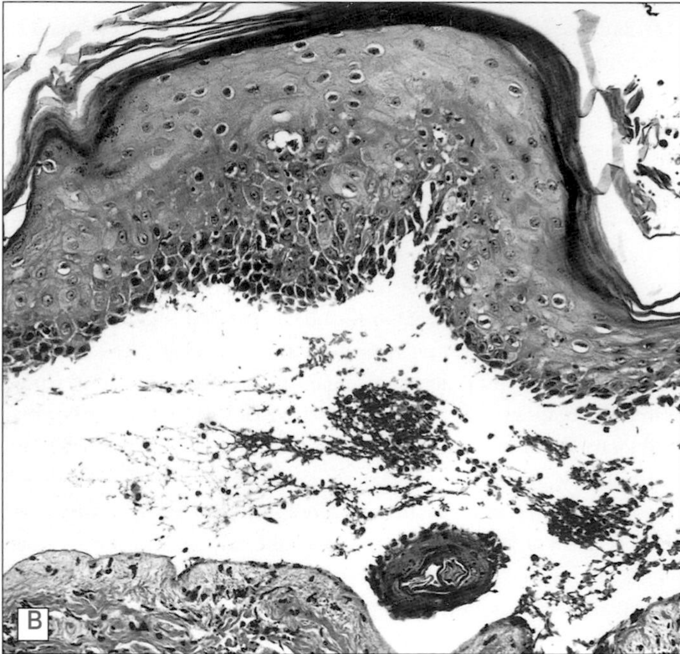

Figure 5.72 Bullous pemphigoid in a dog. **A.** Severe ulcerative facial lesion. **B.** Subepidermal vesiculation. The basement membrane zone forms the floor of the vesicle. Note the lack of acantholysis.

disorganization or internalization of components of the hemidesmosomes. In almost all cases, the stimulus triggering the immune response is unknown, although drugs may precipitate clinically, histologically and immunopathologically classical cases of pemphigoid that regress when the drug is withdrawn. Exposure to ultraviolet light is known to exacerbate bullous pemphigoid.

Bullous pemphigoid occurs in *dogs, cats, pigs, and horses*, with no apparent age or sex predilection. *Collies* appear predisposed. The gross lesions are vesiculobullous, ulcerative and crusted in nature. Grossly, bullous pemphigoid is usually indistinguishable from pemphigus vulgaris. In **dogs**, the lesions affect mucous membranes, particularly of the oral cavity, mucocutaneous junctions, and skin of the face, ears, axilla, groin, and paws (Fig. 5.72A). In **cats**, lesions may be more commonly present on the commissures of the lips, oral mucosa, and hairless regions of the concave aspect of the pinnae. In **horses**, the lesions are often generalized with marked sloughing of the oral mucosa and signs of systemic illness. Lesions on the rump and back characterize the disease in **Yucatan mini-pigs**. Mucosal lesions in pigs have not been described.

Histologically, there is *a subepidermal bulla filled with fibrin and variable numbers of neutrophils, eosinophils and mononuclear cells* (Fig. 5.72B). Eosinophils are not always present as they are in lesions of humans. *Acantholytic keratinocytes are not present.* The basal cells that line the roof of the bulla are not initially degenerate. The basement membrane zone lines the floor of the bulla as separation occurs within the lamina lucida. There is often marked subepidermal vacuolar alteration. The dermis is usually markedly edematous, capillaries are dilated and lined with swollen endothelial cells, and there is perivascular accumulation of neutrophils, eosinophils and mononuclear cells. Mild to moderate lichenoid interface dermatitis may be present, particularly in mucocutaneous regions. *Histologic differential diagnoses* include pemphigus vulgaris, systemic lupus erythematosus, epidermolysis bullosa, toxic epidermal necrolysis, and thermal burns.

Classically, bullous pemphigoid is characterized by the presence of *immunoglobulin (IgG, M, or A) and/or complement deposited at the basement membrane zone* within skin lesions. The BP180 antigen extends to the lateral and apical aspects of basal keratinocytes and labeling may extend to these areas. Serum autoantibodies may be detected in some cases.

Bibliography

Iwasaki T, et al. Canine bullous pemphigoid (BP): Identification of the 180-kD canine BP antigen by circulating autoantibodies. Vet Pathol 1995;32:387–393.

Olivry T, et al. A spontaneously arising porcine model of bullous pemphigoid. Arch Dermatol Res 2000;292:37–45.

Olivry T, et al. Equine bullous pemphigoid IgG autoantibodies target linear epitopes in the NC16A ectodomain of collagen XVII (BP180, BPAG2). Vet Immunol Immunopathol 2000;73:45–52.

Olivry T, Jackson HA. Diagnosing new autoimmune blistering skin diseases of dogs and cats. Clin Tech Small Anim Pract 2001;16:225–229.

Tanaka T, et al. cDNA cloning of bullous pemphigoid (BP) antigen reveals structural and sequence homology with desmoplakin (DP) I. J Invest Dermatol 1990; 94:583.

Linear IgA disease in dogs

Linear IgA disease (LAD) *is an acquired autoimmune subepidermal blistering disease occurring in humans and recently characterized in the dog.* IgG and/or IgA autoantibodies against LAD-1, defined as the processed extracellular domain of type XVII collagen, are demonstrable at the basement membrane zone of lesional skin and in the serum of affected dogs and humans. It is interesting to note the bullous pemphigoid (BP) antigen is also type XVII collagen, however in BP, antibodies recognize the transmembrane form of type XVII collagen. Clinically, LAD is characterized by erosions, ulcers, and crusts on the face, extremities, and in the oral cavity. Histologically, dermoepidermal clefting with little or no neutrophilic infiltration is present. *Differential diagnoses are similar to those listed for BP and TEN.* Differentiation of LAD from other subepidermal blistering diseases requires demonstration of linear IgA deposits at the basement membrane zone of skin lesions as well as identification of circulating autoantibodies against the target antigen, LAD-1. Too few cases have been documented in the dog to define the prognosis.

Bibliography

Olivry T, et al. Autoantibodies against the processed ectodomain of collagen XVII (BPAG2, BP180) define a canine homologue of linear IgA disease of humans. Vet Pathol 2000;37: 302–309.

Epidermolysis bullosa acquisita in the dog

Epidermolysis bullosa acquisita (EBA) is a subepidermal blistering disease characterized by vesicle formation in areas of concurrent neutrophilic superficial dermatitis. The condition has been reported in dogs and humans. Circulating and tissue-bound autoantibodies targeting the distal end of anchoring fibrils in the sub-lamina densa of the lower basement membrane zone have been demonstrated using immunofluorescence and immunoelectron microscopy. The actual target antigen has been shown to be the amino-terminal globular non-collagenous domain of type VII collagen. Clinical lesions in the dog are characterized by erythematous and urticarial eruption with vesicles, bullae, or ulcerations arising in areas subject to friction, including oral ulcerations. Histologically, dermoepidermal separation is present in association with marked neutrophilic inflammation in the superficial dermis and within the vesicles and bullae. Too few cases have been documented to provide information regarding triggering events or clinical outcome. Differentials include those listed for BP.

Bibliography

Olivry T, et al. Canine epidermolysis bullosa acquisita: circulating autoantibodies target the aminoterminal non-collagenous (NC1) domain of collagen VII in anchoring fibrils. Vet Dermatol 1998;9:19–31.

Olivry T, et al. Novel localized variant of canine epidermolysis bullosa acquisita. Vet Rec 2000;146:193–194.

Paraneoplastic pemphigus

Paraneoplastic pemphigus (PNP) is an aggressive form of pemphigus most often associated with solid or hematopoietic neoplasia. One case in a dog could not be associated with an underlying neoplasm, so it is possible for the condition to occur in the absence of underlying neoplasia. PNP has been documented in *humans and dogs*. Cutaneous lesions may precede detection of the neoplastic process. The condition is resistant to treatment.

Lesions consist of *severe mucosal and mucocutaneous blistering and erosions*. Histologically, lesions have a combined pattern of erythema multiforme and suprabasilar acantholysis characteristic of pemphigus vulgaris. Lymphohistiocytic, lichenoid interface dermatitis and apoptosis of keratinocytes with lymphocytic satellitosis throughout the epidermis are characteristic. Immunologically, labeling of intercellular bridges and/or basement membrane is detected by IHC or IFA staining. Direct immunofluorescence studies implicate autoantibodies to a 190 kDa protein, the 210 and 250 kDa desmoplakin proteins, and to the 230 kDa BPAGI, one of the bullous pemphigoid antigens. Not all cases with the above described lesions and autoantibodies have underlying neoplasia. Histologic differentials include PPP and those listed for PV and BP.

Bibliography

Lemmens P, et al. Paraneoplastic pemphigus in a dog. Vet Dermatol 1998;9:127–134.

Turek MM. Cutaneous paraneoplastic syndromes in dogs and cats: a review of the literature. Vet Dermatol 2003;14:279–296.

Lupus erythematosus

Lupus erythematosus occurs in two forms: *systemic lupus erythematosus*, affecting multiple tissues including the skin, and *discoid lupus erythematosus* that is localized to the skin. While the two conditions share cutaneous lesions and certain immunological abnormalities, it is not certain that the one is a localized form of the other. Progression of discoid lupus to systemic lupus rarely, if ever, occurs.

Systemic lupus erythematosus (SLE) is a multisystem disease characterized by abnormalities in both the humoral and cellular immune systems. In the active state in the dog, lymphopenia with a marked decrease in percentage and absolute numbers of CD8+ cells and a decrease in absolute numbers of CD4+ cells occurs. The resulting CD4+:CD8+ ratio is increased from approximately 2.3 in the normal dog to almost 6 in dogs with active SLE. This ratio corrects with response to appropriate therapy. T-cell subset imbalances result in altered immune regulation and B cell hyperactivity. General failure of immune autoregulation, including defects of suppressor T-cell function and dysregulation of endogenous cytokines such as IL-6, results in the *production of antibodies against a variety of membrane and soluble antigens*. The most characteristic of these are the antinuclear antibodies directed against double-stranded DNA, RNA, nucleoprotein and histone-related antigens. Antibodies are also detected against erythrocytes, leukocytes, platelets, organ-specific antigens, clotting factors and IgG (rheumatoid factor). While some of these antibodies may be responsible for tissue injury, *the main tissue damage is effected by the antigen-antibody complexes that deposit at various sites throughout the body and incite a type III hypersensitivity reaction*. In the skin, the antigen-antibody complexes are located under the basement membrane zone of the epidermis and to a lesser extent in the walls of the dermal blood vessels. *Ultraviolet light exacerbates lesions* presumably by inducing the translocation of antigens normally expressed only intracellularly, such as extractable nuclear antigens, to the keratinocyte cell membrane. Specific autoantibodies to these antigens attach to keratinocytes and induce keratinocyte death by antibody-dependent cellular cytotoxicity mediated by lymphocytes or monocytes. Injured keratinocytes then release a plethora of cytokines including IL-1, IL-2, IL-6, and TNFβ with the resultant localization of the lymphohistiocytic infiltrate and increased B-cell activity. Other studies suggest ultraviolet radiation induces ICAM-1 expression, which in turn promotes release of TNFα. ICAM-1 is the major ligand for LFA-1, an adhesion molecule found on all leukocytes.

Canine and **feline** SLE occurs without clear age or sex predilections. Most dogs are middle-aged at the time of diagnosis. In humans, there is a clear preponderance of SLE in females, whereas one canine study found male dogs were more commonly affected. Collies, Shetland Sheepdogs, German Shepherd Dogs, and Siamese, Persian, and Himalayan cats appear predisposed. SLE is a chronic condition that *may wax and wane*, and clinical signs may appear sequentially rather than simultaneously, confounding the diagnosis. Sex hormones and nutrition are known to modulate disease activity. Drug administration, pregnancy, prolonged exposure to extreme heat or cold, and excessive exposures to UV radiation have been known to trigger onset of SLE. *Polyarthritis, fever of unknown origin, anemia, thrombocytopenia, stomatitis, glomerulonephritis, and dermatitis are the most common manifestations.* Polymyositis, lymphedema, and neurological signs may also be present. Dermatological signs occur in ~1/3 of affected dogs and cats. Skin lesions tend to occur in areas exposed to sunlight such as the face, ears, nose, lips, and sparsely haired, lightly pigmented, thin skin of other body regions (Fig. 5.73A). Footpads may be hyperkeratotic or ulcerated. Nail beds may be involved. *Gross skin lesions are extremely variable*, from a mucocutaneous, ulcerative dermatitis resembling pemphigus vulgaris and bullous pemphigoid to erythema, scaling and alopecia of little specificity. A bullous form of SLE with IgG autoantibody against collagen VII has been reported in the dog and found to be similar to the condition in humans. Secondary bacterial pyodermas are common. Occasionally, dogs develop a symmetrical scaling, erythematous and alopecic maculopapular lesion extending over the bridge of the nose onto the cheeks, resembling in distribution the classical malar rash of human systemic lupus.

The most common presenting sign in **horses** with SLE is *a sharply demarcated zone of depigmentation of the skin around the eyes, lips, nostrils, genitalia and skin of the perianal and perineal regions.* Depigmentation may be gradual or rapid and may be accompanied by erythema and scaling. Additional lesions reported have included lymphedema of the extremities, panniculitis, alopecia, and scaling of the face, neck, and trunk, and generalized exfoliative dermatitis. Systemic signs such as polyarthritis, anemia, thrombocytopenia, proteinuria, fever and weight loss may also occur in the horse, but are not common.

The microscopic lesions of SLE are variable. The critical diagnostic pattern is lichenoid interface dermatitis with hydropic degeneration of basal cells and a lymphohistiocytic to plasmacytic infiltrate at the dermoepidermal junction (Fig. 5.73B). Lymphocytes predominate. *Apoptosis of basal keratinocytes and pigmentary incontinence, a consequence of the basal cell degeneration, are diagnostically helpful histologic lesions, as is marked subepidermal vacuolar change* (Fig. 5.73C). Occasionally, this change or a leukocytoclastic vasculitis may lead to cleft or bulla formation between the dermis and epidermis. The same changes often affect follicular epithelia. A *subepidermal bullous form of SLE* with documented circulating IgG autoantibodies to type VII collagen as well as IgG deposits at the basement membrane zone has also been reported in a dog. In the acute cutaneous lesions of SLE, there is moderate to marked dermal edema, capillary dilation, extravasation of leukocytes and erythrocytes and variable lymphohistiocytic infiltrates around vessels of superficial and deep capillary plexuses. Mucinous degeneration may be prominent. As the lesion becomes chronic, there is focal thickening of the basement membrane zone reflecting accumulation of antigen-antibody complexes. Fibrinoid deposits may also occur around superficial blood vessels. Occasionally leukocytoclastic vasculitis develops. Other lesions include ortho- or parakeratotic hyperkeratosis, epidermal hyperplasia, dyskeratosis, adnexal atrophy and dermal fibrosis. Although some follicles may atrophy over time, other follicles in anagen are typically present. Immunoglobulin and complement deposition at the basement membrane zone may be detectable by IF or IHC staining. An ANA titer of >256 is present in 97–100% of dogs with SLE but is not

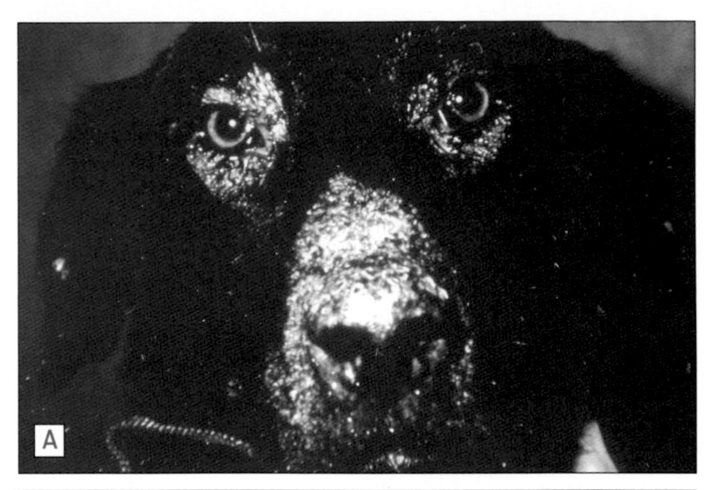

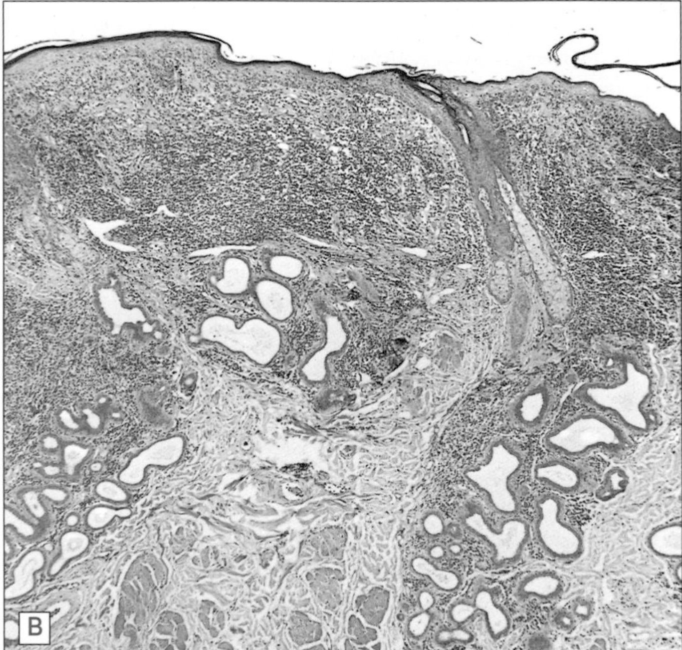

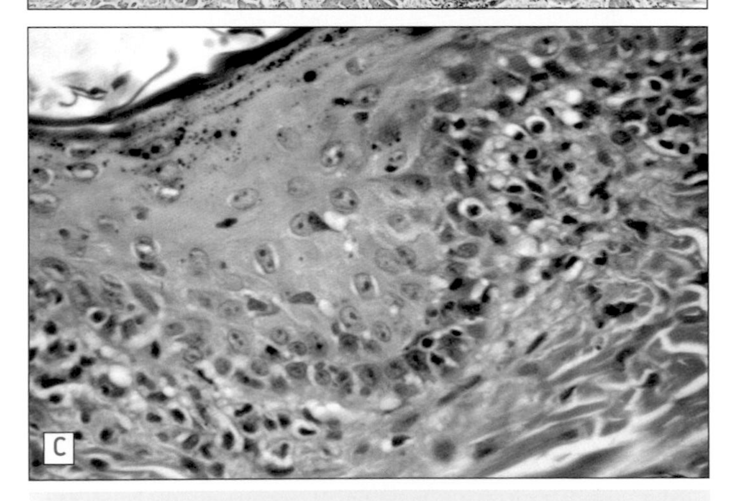

Figure 5.73 Systemic lupus erythematosus (SLE). **A. Symmetrical facial lesions** in SLE. (Courtesy of K Beale.) **B. Lichenoid interface dermatitis** in SLE. **C.** Hydropic degeneration of basal cells, apoptosis, and a lymphohistiocytic-to-plasmacytic infiltrate at the dermoepidermal junction in SLE.

entirely specific for the disease. *Differential diagnoses* vary with the type of lesions present but may include other autoimmune skin diseases, drug eruption, vasculitis, mycosis fungoides, dermatomyositis, demodicosis, dermatophytosis, and seborrhea. In the horse, other depigmenting conditions such as idiopathic leukoderma and the breed-specific, juvenile Arabian leukoderma should be considered.

The localized cutaneous form or **discoid** form of **lupus erythematosus** (DLE) is described most commonly in the *dog*, and rarely in *horses and cats*. DLE as a distinct entity in animals is currently under close scrutiny, and terminology for this clinicopathologic condition is likely to change as the pathogenesis becomes understood and may be found to be different from SLE. The relationship of DLE to SLE is obscure, as DLE does not progress to SLE. The human form of DLE is not comparable to the current condition referred to as DLE in animals. **Photosensitive nasal dermatitis** *is a more general term proposed for use for these conditions in animals until the pathogenesis can be determined.* In **dogs**, the disease is more prevalent in bitches and there is a marked breed predilection in Collies, Shetland Sheepdogs, Siberian Huskies, and German Shepherds. *Sunlight exacerbates the lesions*, which typically affect the nasal planum in dogs and cats, and the face and neck in horses. In the dog, perioral, periocular, and pinnal skin may also be affected. The lesions include erythema, depigmentation, scaling, crusting, alopecia and occasionally ulceration. Rarely, dogs are presented with only nasodigital hyperkeratosis. *Histologic findings are very similar as previously described for systemic lupus.* The epidermis may be more hyperplastic and the infiltrate is predominantly comprised of lymphocytes and macrophages with fewer plasma cells, and is often denser than in SLE. If a secondary mucocutaneous pyoderma is present, plasma cells may be more numerous. IF or IHC staining may reveal IgM, IgG, IgA, and/or complement at the basement membrane zone, however false-positives of the nasal planum are common. *Clinical differential diagnoses* include nasal solar dermatitis, PF, PPP, uveodermatologic syndrome, contact dermatitis, SLE, trauma, mycosis fungoides, drug eruption, dermatomyositis, and vitiligo. *A major histologic differential is a mucocutaneous pyoderma.* Mucocutaneous pyodermas lack evidence of basal cell damage and are predominantly plasmacytic. Both conditions may be present simultaneously.

Vesicular cutaneous lupus erythematosus is a disorder formerly known as *ulcerative dermatosis of the Collie and Shetland Sheepdog*. This condition was originally thought to be a variant of dermatomyositis, but recent immunological studies indicate the presence of autoantibodies that target nuclear antigens similar to that seen in cutaneous lupus erythematosus. Antinuclear antibody testing is negative. Lesions develop in middle-aged to older dogs. The Shetland Sheepdog and Collie appear predisposed to lesion development. Clinical lesions consist of vesicles and bullae that evolve into erosions and ulcers. The inguinal and axillary regions are most commonly involved, but lesions may also occur on mucocutaneous junctions. Histologic changes consist of interface lymphocytic dermatitis with hydropic degeneration of basal cells, keratinocyte apoptosis, and extensive vesicles and bullae at the epidermal–dermal junction.

Exfoliative cutaneous lupus erythematosus, formerly known as *lupoid dermatosis of the German shorthair pointer*, occurs in young (3 months to 3 years) German Shorthair Pointers. Gross lesions consist of scaling and crusting commencing on the head and back but becoming generalized. The most severe lesions are often present at pressure points and the scrotum. Pyrexia, peripheral lymphadenopathy and lethargy may be present. Histologic changes mimic cutaneous lesions of systemic lupus erythematosus. Some affected dogs may have a positive antinuclear antibody test.

Lupus panniculitis (lupus profundus) is *characterized by well-circumscribed subcutaneous nodules over the trunk and proximal extremities.* It is reported rarely in dogs. Histologically, it is initially a septal panniculitis with dense nodular infiltrates of lymphocytes and plasma cells and fewer macrophages. The fat lobules may undergo necrosis, often represented by hyalinization without mineralization. Usually *the dermis and epidermis show the typical microscopic features of lupus*, including hydropic degeneration of basal cells, pigmentary incontinence, thickened basement membrane zone and sclerosis of the dermis. Abundant mucinous degeneration is usually prominent. Leukocytoclastic vasculitis may be present in the interlobular septa. Histologically, lupus panniculitis is distinctive, but a rabies vaccine-induced lymphocytic panniculitis, that is virtually indistinguishable histologically, occurs in dogs.

Bibliography

Bennion SD, et al. In three patterns of interface dermatitis, different patterns of expression of intercellular adhesion molecule-1 (ICAM-1) indicate different triggers of disease. J Invest Dermatol 1995;105:71S–79S.

Chabanne L, et al. Canine systemic lupus erythematosus. Part I. Clinical and biologic aspects. Compend Contin Educ Pract Vet 1999;21:135–141.

Geor RJ, et al. Systemic lupus erythematosus in a filly. J Am Vet Med Assoc 1990;197:1489–1492.

Goldman M. Cytokines in the pathophysiology of systemic lupus erythematosus. Autoimmunity 1990;8:175–179.

Fournel C, et al. Canine systemic lupus erythematosus. I. A study of 75 cases. Lupus 1992;1:133–139.

Jackson HA, Olivry T. Ulcerative dermatosis of the Shetland sheepdog and rough collie dog may represent a novel vesicular variant of cutaneous lupus erythematosus. Vet Dermatol 2001;12:19–27.

Linker-Israeli M, et al. Elevated levels of endogenous IL-6 in systemic lupus erythematosus. A putative role in pathogenesis. J Immunol 1991;147:117–123.

Olivry T. Cutaneous manifestations of lupus in humans and dogs. Proc Eur Soc Vet Dermatol Workshop on Skin Immunol Le Mas D' Artigny Stain-Paul de Venice , France 2000.

Olivry T, et al. Bullous systemic lupus erythematosus (type 1) in a dog. Vet Rec 1999;145:165–169.

Scott DW, et al. Immunologic Skin Diseases. In: Scott DW, et al., eds. Muller and Kirk's Small Animal Dermatology. 5th ed. Philadelphia, PA: WB Saunders, 1995:578–588.

Sontheimer RD. The lexicon of cutaneous lupus erythematosus – A review and personal perspective on the nomenclature and classification of the cutaneous manifestations of lupus erythematosus. Lupus 1997;6:84–95.

Soulard M, et al. Autoimmune antibodies to hnRNPG protein in dogs with systemic lupus erythematosus: epitope mapping of the antigen. J Autoimmun 2002;18:221–229.

Vitale CB, et al. Systemic lupus erythematosus in a cat: fulfillment of the American Rheumatism Association criteria with supportive skin histopathology. Vet Dermatol 1997;8:133–138.

vonTscharner C, et al. Stannard's illustrated equine dermatology notes. Vet Dermatol 2000;11:163–178.

Yager JA, Wilcock BP. Part II.5: Interface dermatitis. In: Color Atlas and Text of Surgical Pathology of the Dog and Cat: Dermatopathology and Skin Tumors. London: Mosby-Year Book, 1994:93–96.

Yung RL, et al. New concepts in the pathogenesis of drug-induced lupus. Lab Invest 1996;73:746–759.

Other immune-mediated dermatoses

Drug eruptions

Drug eruptions are occasionally reported in *dogs, cats, and horses* and rarely in other domestic animals. Drugs responsible for skin eruptions may be administered *orally, topically, or by injection or inhalation*. Any drug may cause an eruption, and any one drug consistently produces no specific type of reaction. Thus, *drug eruption can mimic virtually any dermatosis. Erythema multiforme, toxic epidermal necrolysis, and vasculitis are well-recognized dermatoses that can be manifestations of cutaneous drug eruptions* and are described individually later in this section. *Criteria* for establishing a cutaneous reaction as a confirmed drug eruption include: (1) elimination of other causes of the skin lesions, (2) timing of onset of reaction with administration of a suspect drug, (3) improvement upon drug withdrawal, (4) recognition that the suspect drug has been associated with similar reactions in other animals or species in the past, and (5) recurrence of lesions upon rechallenge of the patient with the drug. Understandably, all five of these criteria are not often met, particularly rechallenge as this can be associated with high morbidity or mortality. Time period between drug administration and onset of an adverse reaction varies widely from hours to months and lesions can result from a single or repeated administration. *Drug-induced gross and histologic lesions are not pathognomonic* for an adverse cutaneous drug eruption although histopathological changes may often point to a limited list of differentials. *Histologic patterns that have been recognized as forms of adverse drug reactions include: urticaria; perivascular dermatitis (allergy-like); hydropic and/or lichenoid interface dermatitis (erythema multiforme, toxic epidermal necrolysis, lupus erythematosus-like); perforating folliculitis; vasculitis; intraepidermal vesiculopustular dermatitis (pemphigus-like); and subepidermal bullous reactions (pemphigoid-like)*. The pathogenesis of lesion formation in many types of drug eruptions is not known with certainty. Drug hypersensitivities are believed to involve all four types of hypersensitivity reactions, and in some cases are not thought to be immunologically mediated.

The most common drugs recognized to produce hypersensitivity reactions in domestic animals are the *sulfonamides (especially trimethoprim-potentiated) and penicillins*. Erythema multiforme and toxic epidermal necrolysis (discussed later in this section) have been seen most commonly with trimethoprim-potentiated *sulfonamides, cephalosporins and levamisole. Diethylcarbamazine* and *5-fluorocytosine* have been associated with fixed drug eruption on the scrotum of dogs. The ulcerative lesions healed with hyperpigmentation when the drug was withdrawn but recrudescence at the same site, with vesiculation, occurred when the dog was rechallenged. *The mechanism underlying fixed drug eruption is unknown*. In people, the epidermal invasion of T cells in fixed drug eruptions is associated with the expression of the intracellular adhesion molecule ICAM-1 on the surface of lesional keratinocytes. *Cyclosporin* has been reported to cause a lymphoplasmacytoid dermatitis with malignant features, usually manifest as a solitary plaque or nodule. *Urticaria and angioedema* have been associated with levamisole, barbiturates and some antibiotics. Drug eruptions manifesting as *exfoliative erythroderma* have been seen in dogs treated with levamisole and lincomycin. Drug eruptions resembling bullous pemphigoid clinically, histologically and immunohistochemically have been associated with *triamcinolone*. It is quite possible that some cases described as bullous pemphigoid actually represent drug eruptions. Pemphigus foliaceus-like drug eruptions have been described in cats treated with ampicillin or cimetidine and dogs receiving trimethoprim-sulfonamide. Lesions consisted of classical subcorneal pustules with acantholytic cells, with an additional feature of vasculitis in some cases. Systemic lupus-like drug reactions have been reported in dogs and in cats. Cutaneous vasculitis caused by immune complex deposition may be initiated by drug administration. Sulfadiazine administration in Doberman Pinschers causes a poorly defined skin rash as well as ocular, joint, kidney, and hematological abnormalities suggestive of systemic vasculitis.

Bibliography

Affolter VK, von Tscharner C. Cutaneous drug reactions: a retrospective study of histopathological changes and their correlation with the clinical disease. Vet Dermatol 1993;4:79–86.

Evans AG, Stannard AA. Idiopathic multiple cutaneous seromas in a horse: a possible manifestation of drug eruption. Eq Pract 1990;12:27–34.

Ginn PE, et al. Self-limiting subepidermal bullous disease in a neonatal foal. Vet Dermatol 1998;9:249–256.

Ihrke PJ. Cutaneous adverse drug reactions. Compend Contin Educ Pract Vet 1997;19:87–92.

Mason KV. Blistering drug eruptions in animals. Clin Dermatol 1993;11:567–574.

McEwan NA, et al. Drug eruption in a cat resembling pemphigus foliaceus. J Small Anim Pract 1987;28:713–720.

McKenna JK, Leiferman KM. Dermatologic drug reactions. Immunol Allergy Clin North Am 2004;24:399–423.

Noli C, et al. A retrospective evaluation of adverse reactions to trimethoprim-sulphonamide combinations in dogs and cats. Vet Q 1995;17:123–128.

Ruocco V, Sacerdoti G. Pemphigus and bullous pemphigoid due to drugs. Int J Dermatol 1991;30:307–312.

Scott DW, Miller WH. Idiosyncratic cutaneous adverse drug reactions in the cat: Literature review and report of 14 cases (1990–1996). Feline Pract 1998; 26:10–15.

Shiohara T, et al. Fixed drug eruption. Expression of epidermal keratinocyte adhesion molecule-1 (ICAM-1). Arch Dermatol 1989;125:1371–1376.

Cryopathies

Cryopathies are cold-related hypersensitivity syndromes that include **cold agglutinin disease**, *a condition in which erythrocyte autoantibodies react at lower temperatures to produce microvascular thrombosis in superficial dermal vessels*. Other cryopathies are small vessel vasculopathies associated with abnormal serum proteins (paraproteins) that precipitate out of the serum at cooler temperatures and redissolve upon warming. *Paraproteins include cryofibrinogens, cryoglobulins, macroglobulins, and gamma heavy chains*. Cryoglobulins may be monoclonal IgG or IgM (type I cryoglobulinemia), or mixed mono- and polyclonal with one antibody directed against the other, in which case, immune complexes are in the circulation (type II cryoglobulinemia). In type III cryoglobulinemia, the immunoglobulins are polyclonal. Type I cryoglobulinemia is often associated with underlying disease such as multiple myeloma, leukemia, or lymphoma where as in type II or III, connective tissue disease such as SLE, or a systemic infection is present. Type II and III may also be idiopathic. *Most cases reported in* *dogs and cats are the result of cold-reacting anti-erythrocyte antibodies*. Cold agglutinin disease has been reported rarely to cause skin disease in dogs and cats. Cold agglutinin disease as a post-infectious event has been reported in sheep, horses, and pigs. One report in Birman cats occurred in association with neonatal isoerythrolysis and suggested that group B blood group cats may be predisposed. Lead exposure and hemobartonellosis have also been implicated as predisposing factors in dogs and cats. Cryopathy due to cryofibrinogens and cryoglobulins has also been reported in the dog. A monoclonal cryoglobulinemia associated with multiple myeloma has been reported in a cat.

Cutaneous signs associated with cryopathies result from vascular insufficiency (obstruction, stasis, spasm, and thrombosis). Lesions include erythema, purpura, cyanosis, necrosis, ulceration, and occasionally sloughing of extremities, and are precipitated or exacerbated by exposure to cold. The paws, pinnae, nose and tip of the tail are typically involved. Skin biopsy usually reveals necrosis, ulceration and often secondary suppurative changes. *Microvascular thrombosis* may be evident in cold agglutinin disease. In other types of cryopathies, paraproteins are precipitated out and deposited throughout vessel walls and within vascular lumens. The proteins stain pink with HE and bright red with PAS. *Hemorrhage* may be present. In type I cryopathies, inflammation is usually absent, whereas a leukocytoclastic vasculitis is often present in types II and III. *Diagnosis requires a test for cryoprecipitates and analysis of serum proteins*. Erythrocyte agglutination on a cooled slide that reverses upon warming and a positive Coombs' test at 4°C should be present in cases of cold agglutinating anti-erythrocyte antibodies. *Differential diagnoses include frostbites, disseminated intravascular coagulation, SLE, dermatomyositis, and other causes of vasculitis.*

Bibliography

Barnhill RL, Busam KJ. Vascular Diseases. In: Elder D, et al., eds. Lever's Histopathology of the Skin. 8th ed. Philadelphia, PA: Lippincott-Raven, 1997:196–197.

Bridle KH, Littlewood JD. Tail tip necrosis in two litters of Birman kittens. J Small Anim Pract 1998;39:88–89.

Dickson NJ. Cold agglutinin disease in a puppy associated with lead intoxication. J Small Anim Pract 1990;31:105–108.

Godfrey DR, Anderson M. Cold agglutinin disease in a cat. J Small Anim Pract 1994;35:267–270.

Hickford FH, et al. Monoclonal immunoglobulin G cryoglobulinemia and multiple myeloma in a domestic shorthair. J Am Vet Med Assoc 2000;217:1029–1033.

Nagata M, et al. Cryoglobulinaemia and cryfibrinogenaemia: a comparison of canine and human cases. Vet Dermatol 1998;9:277–281.

Zulty JC, Kociba GJ. Cold agglutinins in cats with haemobartonellosis. J Am Vet Med Assoc 1990;196:907–910.

Graft-versus-host disease

Graft-versus-host disease (GVH) occurs as a complication of bone marrow transplantation. It has been recorded in *humans, dogs, cats, and horses*. The disease results from donor T-lymphocyte responses to recipient histocompatibility antigens in the *acute phase*, and from immunocompetent recipient lymphocyte responses to transplantation antigens in the *chronic phase*. Principal target organs are the *skin, liver and intestinal tract*. GVH is considered the *classic example of cell-mediated attack upon the epidermis*. Proposed target cells in the skin include basal keratinocytes, follicular stem cells, and/or Langerhans cells. Studies indicate both CD8+ and CD4+ lymphocytes are active in the disease process, with CD8+ T cells found more often in the epidermis and CD4+ T cells in the dermal infiltrate. NK cells may also play a role. T cell production of IFNγ results in keratinocyte expression of ICAM-1, the binding molecule for LFA-1 found on infiltrating T cells. TNFα production by activated keratinocytes and Langerhans cells and IFNγ lead to keratinocyte production of IL-8 attracting more lymphocytes.

Skin lesions in the acute phase include generalized erythematous macules, multifocal alopecia, and ulcerative dermatitis. Oral lesions, epidermal detachment and follicular papules may be present. In the chronic phase, erythema, irregular hyperpigmentation, dermal fibrosis, cutaneous atrophy, and cicatricial alopecia from chronic ulceration may occur. *Histologic findings* include various degrees of hydropic and/or lichenoid interface dermatitis with marked lymphocytic satellitosis of necrotic keratinocytes in all layers of the epidermis and the follicular epithelium. There are lymphocytic exocytosis and spongiosis. Dermal lymphocytic infiltrate is variable. Dermal–epidermal cleft or ulceration may also be present. Over time, epidermal atrophy and dermal sclerosis with loss of adnexa may occur. Basal layer vacuolation and inflammation persist. *Differential diagnoses* include erythema multiforme, toxic epidermal necrolysis or other drug eruption, alopecia areata, and radiation dermatitis. *The history and the triad of cutaneous, hepatic and intestinal signs should lead to the proper diagnosis of GVH.*

Erythema multiforme

Erythema multiforme (EM) is an uncommon cutaneous reaction reported in the *dog, cat, horse, and cow*. EM is *usually triggered by drug therapy or infection* (viral, fungal, or bacterial), but may also occur in conjunction with underlying *neoplasia*, or may be *idiopathic*, particularly in older dogs. A few of the drugs reported to trigger EM in animals include *d-limonene-based dips, levamisole, cephalexin, trimethoprim-sulfa, gentamicin, and penicillin*. The pathogenesis is not completely understood, however studies support a *combined type III and IV immune reaction* as the mechanism of lesion formation. The possibility also exists that a drug or infectious agent may induce keratinocytes to undergo apoptosis without involvement of the immune system. The *histologic lesions*, cellular infiltrates and types of lymphocytes present mirror that of GVH disease, lending further support for a cell-mediated immune response. IF or IHC results are variable but may show deposits of immunoglobulin and/or complement in the dermal microvasculature or at the dermoepidermal junction. Circulating immune-complexes may also be present. It is unclear whether these findings indicate a role for humoral immunity in skin lesions or are epiphenomena. Antibodies to the desmosomal proteins, desmoplakin I and II have been documented in cases of EM major (see below) in humans but it is not yet determined whether antibodies formed secondary to keratinocyte damage and antigen exposure or as a primary event.

EM occurs in *two forms* that may overlap one another and with toxic epidermal necrolysis. **EM minor** *is characterized chiefly by an acute onset of symmetric erythematous macules and papules* (Fig. 5.74A). These spread peripherally and clear centrally to produce annular, serpiginous to arciform and polycyclic patterns (Fig. 5.74B). *Classic "target" lesions may be present* (5.74C).

Urticarial plaques with similar configurations and vesiculobullous lesions also occur. Lesions tend to involve mucocutaneous junctions,

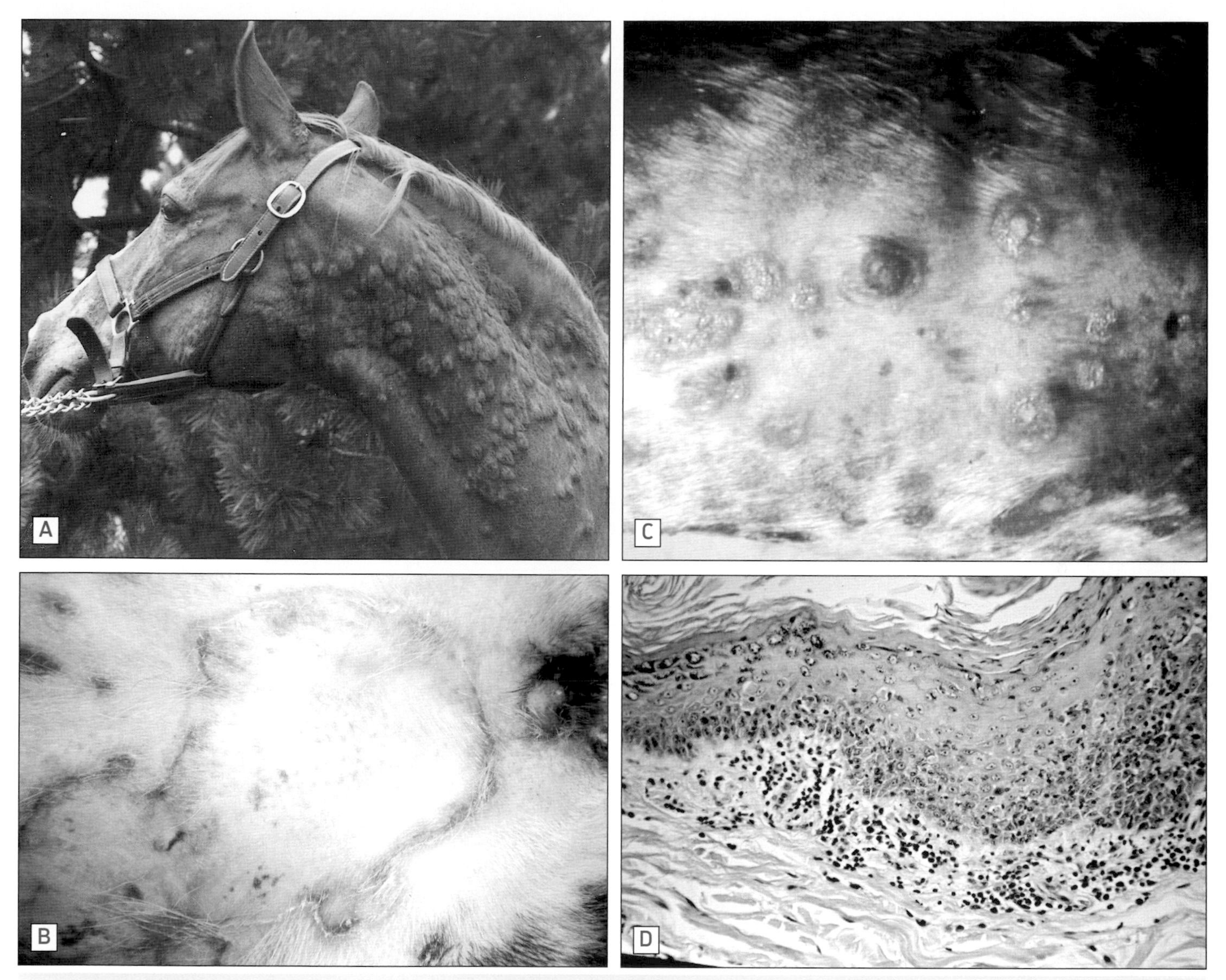

Figure 5.74 Erythema multiforme (EM). **A.** In a horse, **multiple irregular plaques** that are not transient as they are in urticaria (see Fig. 5.64). **B.** Erythematous and erosive **serpiginous to arciform lesions** in EM in a dog. (Courtesy of University of Florida Clinical Dermatology Service.) **C. Classical target lesions** with central clearing in EM in a dog. (Courtesy of University of Florida Clinical Dermatology Service.) **D.** Characteristic **interface dermatitis** with necrotic keratinocytes, often with lymphocytic satellitosis, scattered throughout the epidermis in EM in a dog.

the ventral trunk, proximal limbs and occasionally the nose and footpads. Pruritus is usually not a feature and there are no systemic signs, other than those attributable to the underlying cause. In **EM major** (Stevens–Johnson syndrome), *widespread mucosal lesions, extensive necrotizing and vesiculobullous skin lesions and signs of systemic illness such as pain, lethargy, pyrexia, and anorexia are present*. Histologically, the lesions of EM show the *characteristic interface dermatitis* (Fig. 5.74D). Necrotic keratinocytes, often with lymphocytic satellitosis, are scattered throughout the epidermis and the adnexal epithelia (see Fig. 5.11). A sparse lymphohistiocytic infiltrate occurs at the dermoepidermal junction and around superficial blood vessels. Vasculitis is not a feature. As the lesion ages, the infiltrate may become more dense, subepidermal bullae may develop and the epidermal necrosis may become confluent. Secondary exudation follows necrosis. *Clinical differentials* include TEN, burns, SLE, urticaria, vasculitis, other immune-mediated dermatoses, mycosis fungoides, superficial necrolytic dermatitis, and necrotic arachnidism. The *histologic pattern* is shared by GVH disease, acute lupus erythematosus, and less severe forms of toxic epidermal necrolysis. Occasionally, lesions may histologically resemble mycosis fungoides (MF). Important distinguishing features are atypical lymphocytes (MF) and apoptosis accompanied by lymphocytic satellitosis in all levels of the epidermis (EM). A less common finding in erythema multiforme is severe dermal edema with vertical orientation of dermal collagen and subepidermal vesiculation. *EM may be self-limiting, resolve with elimination of underlying triggering event, or as in some idiopathic cases, become chronic or recurrent.* Chronic EM is more commonly seen in older dogs and is characterized by the additional changes of a proliferative epidermis with marked parakeratosis and extensive lymphocytic exocytosis.

Toxic epidermal necrolysis

Toxic epidermal necrolysis (TEN) is characterized by disseminated erythema, widespread bullous necrosis of epidermis and mucous membranes,

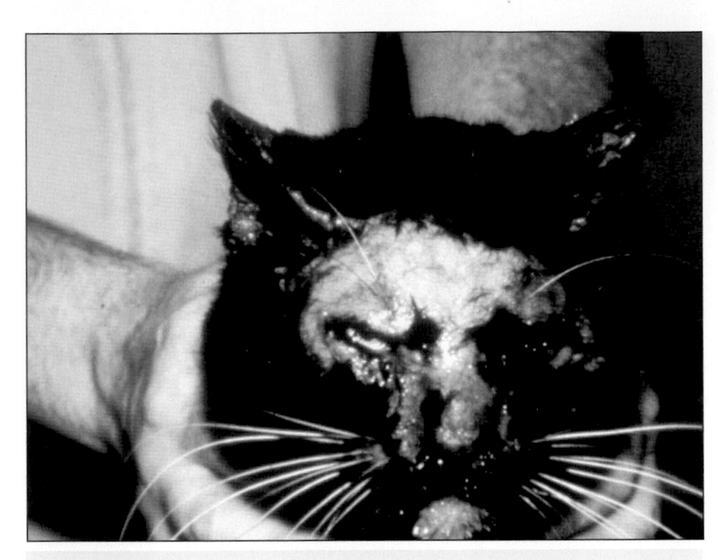

Figure 5.75 Complete loss of the epidermis of the skin of the face in **toxic epidermal necrolysis.** (Courtesy of University of Florida Clinical Dermatology Service.)

and severe toxicity. It is most often associated with drug intake or concurrent infections, but many cases are idiopathic. TEN and EM major (Stevens–Johnson syndrome) are very similar in clinical presentation, and one may be the extension of the other. The lesions of erythema multiforme major show areas of full-thickness epidermal necrosis as in TEN, but differences in the clinical course, response to therapy, and fatality rate suggest that they are separate entities.

The pathogenesis of TEN is not known. Cell-mediated immune mechanisms have been postulated as the basis for necrosis. Lymphopenia and alterations in the T-helper and T-suppressor lymphocyte ratios occur in human patients. Drugs associated with TEN, however, do not induce lymphocyte transformation in vitro. Furthermore, the widespread confluent epidermal necrosis, in the virtual absence of infiltrating inflammatory cells, argues against an effector role for cytotoxic lymphocytes. As in EM, lesional deposition of antibody and complement may represent epiphenomena.

Toxic epidermal necrolysis is a serious, acute-onset and life-threatening disease in dogs and cats. It has been associated with concurrent infectious disease or neoplasia, and *is a form of drug eruption*. Drugs implicated include penicillins, cephalosporins, levamisole, and 5-fluorocytosine. Affected animals are painful, anorectic, febrile, depressed and lethargic. Mortality is high. Lesions are usually generalized and involve mucous membranes, mucocutaneous junctions, and haired skin (Fig. 5.75). There is ulceration, often with an epidermal collarette, crusting, scaling and secondary pyoderma. The skin is extremely painful and fragile and may slough with routine handling. A *positive Nikolsky sign* is often present and large sheets of epidermis may detach. Vesiculation may occur but is often transient. Lesions may also involve the respiratory and digestive tracts. *Grossly*, toxic epidermal necrolysis may be difficult to distinguish from EM major, superficial burns, pemphigus vulgaris, bullous pemphigoid, systemic lupus erythematosus, thallium poisoning, mycosis fungoides, necrotic arachnidism and candidiasis.

Histologically, *TEN is characterized by full thickness coagulative necrosis of the epidermis, which may extend into the external root sheath of the hair follicle*. Separation of the necrotic epidermis occurs at the dermoepidermal junction and leads to subepidermal vesiculation. Dermal inflammation is minimal until the epidermis becomes detached. The reaction, when present, is perivascular or rarely lichenoid and chiefly lymphohistiocytic. Lesions with less than full-thickness epidermal necrosis and more intense dermal inflammation may be indistinguishable from cases of erythema multiforme with confluent zones of keratinocyte necrosis.

Bibliography

Bennion SD, et al. In three different types of interface dermatitis, different patterns of expression of intercellular adhesion molecule-1 (ICAM-1) indicate different triggers of disease. J Invest Dermatol 1995;105: Supplement 71S–79S.

Cohen LM, et al. Noninfectious vesiculobullous and vesiculopustular diseases. In: Elder D, et al., eds. Lever's Histopathology of the Skin. 8th ed. Philadelphia, PA: Lippincott-Raven, 1997:239–244.

Favrot C, et al. Parvovirus infection of keratinocytes as a cause of canine erythema multiforme. Vet Pathol 2000;37:647–649.

Foedinger D, et al. Autoantibodies to desmoplakin I and II in patients with erythema multiforme. J Exp Med 1995;181:169–179.

Gross TL, et al., eds. Necrotizing diseases of the epidermis. In: Veterinary Dermatopathology. A Macroscopic and Microscopic Evaluation of Canine and Feline Skin Disease. St. Louis, MO: Mosby Year Book, 1992:41–46.

Hinn AC, et al. Erythema multiforme, Stevens-Johnson syndrome and toxic epidermal necrolysis in the dog: clinical classification, drug exposure, and histopathological correlations. J Vet Allergy Clin Immunol 1998;6:13–20.

March PA, et al. Superficial necrolytic dermatitis in 11 dogs with a history of phenobarbital administration (1995–2002). J Vet Intern Med 2004;18:65–74.

Nuttall TJ, Malham T. Successful intravenous human immunoglobulin treatment of drug-induced Stevens-Johnson syndrome in a dog. J Small Anim Pract 2004;45:357–361.

Paquet P, Pierard GE. Erythema multiforme and toxic epidermal necrolysis: A comparative study. Am J Dermatopathol 1997;19:127–132.

Rosenbaum MR, Kerlin RL. Erythema multiforme major and disseminated intravascular coagulation in a dog following application of d-limonene-based insecticidal dip. J Amer Vet Med Assoc 1995;207:1315–1319.

Yager JA, Wilcock BP. Part II.5: Interface dermatitis. In: Color Atlas and Text of Surgical Pathology of the Dog and Cat: Dermatopathology and Skin Tumors. London: Mosby-Year Book, 1994:86–89.

Vasculitis

Cutaneous vasculitis, a condition in which dermal vessels are the principal target of injury, can be associated with a primary immunopathogenic event, or may be secondary to drug therapy, infectious agents, systemic connective tissue disease, underlying malignancy, toxins, or, often may be idiopathic. Classic examples include infection with an endotheliotropic organism (*Rickettsia rickettsii*), immune-complex vasculitis (systemic lupus erythematosus) and septicemia (*Erysipelothrix rhusiopathiae*). Although cutaneous vasculitis has many causes, many cases fall into the category of type III hypersensitivity reactions. Cutaneous vasculitis may be a secondary event associated with cutaneous diseases such as staphylococcal infections. Drug-induced vasculitis is thought to be the result of haptenization of host proteins, direct drug toxicity against vessel walls, autoantibodies against endothelial cells, or possibly cell-mediated cytotoxic reactions against vessels.

Cutaneous vasculitis is seen most often in the *dog and horse* and is considered to be rare in cats, pigs and cattle. Approximately 50% of cases of vasculitis in dogs and horses are idiopathic. *Gross lesions suggestive of vasculitis include erythematous plaques or macules, palpable*

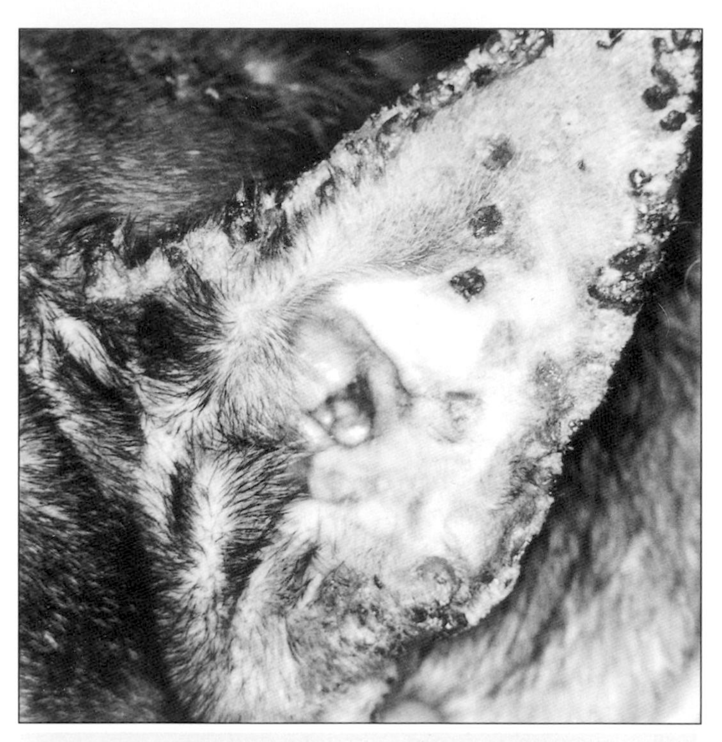

Figure 5.76 Typical punched-out ulcers on the margins of the ears, due to **vasculitis** in a dog.

purpura, hemorrhagic bullae, edema, necrosis, and well-demarcated ulcers (Fig. 5.76). Ischemic necrosis may occur leading to eschar formation and sloughing of the skin or distal extremities. Paws, pinnae, lips, tail, and oral mucosa are most commonly affected. Ischemic atrophy of folliculosebaceous units may lead to areas of alopecia and scaling in long standing lesions of more subtle vasculitis.

Small arterioles, capillaries and post-capillary venules are most often affected in cutaneous vasculitis. Histologic lesions in the classic case feature evidence of damage to the vessel wall such as *necrotic cell debris and fibrinoid necrosis within the vessel wall, mural infiltrates of either neutrophils or lymphocytes, and intramural or perivascular edema, hemorrhage or fibrin exudation* (see Fig. 5.15). Subtle cases of vasculitis may be characterized by edema, rare necrotic cells in the vicinity of vessels and a mild interstitial mononuclear cell infiltrate. Microscopic evidence of vasculitis in the dog is often subtle and may lead to underdiagnosis of the condition. Some pathologists prefer to refer to very cell-poor cases of vasculitis as a *vasculopathy* rather than true vasculitis when degenerative lesions of vessel wall and evidence of ischemia are detected in the absence of inflammation of vessel walls. Edema, hemorrhage, and evidence of ischemia and homogenization of dermal collagen are helpful changes. *A preponderance of leukocytes in vessels walls rather than in the dermis suggests that vessels are the primary target of inflammation and not just serving to deliver leukocytes.* Vessels will stand out in the section due to the attraction of leukocytes to vessel walls.

Some generalizations regarding the pathogenesis of the vasculitis can be made from types of leukocytes present within vessel walls; however, the types of leukocytes present does not necessarily point to a particular etiology and may simply reflect the stage of the disease process.

- *Neutrophilic vasculitis* is most suggestive of a type III immune-complex hypersensitivity reaction and is often referred to as *leukocytoclastic vasculitis* if neutrophil degeneration and nuclear karyorrhexis are evident. Examples include the vasculitis associated with staphylococcal dermatitis in dogs, immune-mediated vasculitis as in SLE, some drug eruptions, and septicemia.
- *Lymphocytic vasculitis* may suggest a cell-mediated immune basis, such as rabies vaccine-induced cutaneous vasculitis and some drug eruptions.
- *Eosinophilic vascular infiltrates* are most suggestive of a type I hypersensitivity reaction. Eosinophils may be the predominant cells in some cases of equine vasculitis and in association with the markedly eosinophilic dermatitis seen in some arthropod bite lesions, mast cell tumors, or in lesions of the eosinophilic granuloma complex in the cat.

Involvement of deep dermal blood vessels in all cases may suggest systemic disease.

In **dogs**, cutaneous vasculitis has been associated with drugs, systemic or localized infections (Rocky Mountain spotted fever, staphylococcal pyoderma), malignancies and connective tissue diseases. Familial or inherited forms of vasculitis have also been recognized.

- A syndrome of cutaneous ulceration in conjunction with limb edema and/or acute renal failure, referred to as *cutaneous and renal glomerular vasculopathy (CRGV) of Greyhounds* or in layman's terms "Alabama rot" has been reported sporadically in young greyhounds throughout the United States. Multifocal cutaneous ulcers, renal afferent arteriolar and dermal arterial thrombosis, azotemia, microangiopathic hemolytic anemia and thrombocytopenia with normal coagulation times characterize CRGV. Cutaneous lesions may occur in the absence of renal or other systemic disease. The syndrome has many features in common with the hemolytic-uremic syndrome in people caused by a Shiga-like toxin induced endothelial cell necrosis. *Studies have failed to identify infectious agents, toxins, or evidence of an immune-mediated reaction in CRGV.* Exposure to Shiga-like toxin-producing *E. coli* has not been completely ruled out. Affected dogs may be genetically predisposed to develop CRGV as outbreaks have occurred in related groups of dogs. Hemorrhage, fibrinoid arteritis, thrombosis with infarction and ulceration characterize the skin lesions which are most often found on the limbs. Renal glomerular necrosis and tubular necrosis are present in the kidneys.
- A genodermatosis affecting *German Shepherd Dog puppies* characterized by swelling, depigmentation and frequent ulceration of footpads, ear and tail tips and nasal planum depigmentation has been reported in Canada. A neutrophilic to mononuclear nodular dermatitis, dermal collagenolysis, and subtle vasculitis are present histologically. Nasal lesions correspond to an hydropic interface dermatitis. The cause is unknown but presumed to be immunologically mediated as lesions are temporally related to vaccination dates. Dogs recover by 5–6 months of age. The condition may also be related to an underlying collagen disorder, as musculoskeletal abnormalities are also present.
- Familial vasculitis has been reported in a litter of *Scottish Terriers*. Lesions were limited to the nasal epithelium and mucosa and were characterized by leukocytoclastic vasculitis and pyogranulomatous inflammation leading to ulceration and destruction of the nasal planum.
- Cutaneous vasculitis leading to alopecia and ulcerative lesions of the extremities and bony prominences with histologic lesions

virtually indistinguishable from dermatomyositis of Collies and Shetland Sheepdogs (see Congenital and hereditary diseases of skin) has been reported in *Jack Russell Terriers*.
- Lymphocytic to mixed mononuclear vasculitis, often associated with cutaneous infarction, has been noted in dogs with the systemic lymphoproliferative disorder, *lymphomatoid granulomatosis*.

In **horses**, cutaneous vasculitis has been seen with or following numerous infections, such as *Streptococcus, Influenza A virus, Equine arteritis virus, Equine infectious anemia virus, Ehrlichia, Rhodococcus equi*, and *Corynebacterium pseudotuberculosis*.

- *Equine purpura hemorrhagica* is an acute, usually streptococcal infection (strangles)-associated, leukocytoclastic vasculitis characterized clinically by urticaria and extensive edema of the distal limbs, ventrum and head. These swellings may progress to exudation and sloughing.
- *Pastern leukocytoclastic vasculitis* is a syndrome unique to the horse that affects the unpigmented, sun-exposed skin of distal extremities, hence ultraviolet radiation is thought to play a role in the pathogenesis. Adult horses are most often affected. There is no evidence of liver disease or exposure to photosensitizing compounds. Interestingly, a single limb may be affected although other limbs lack pigment as well. Lesions are crusty, eroded or ulcerated, sharply demarcated and may be associated with extensive edema and pain. Histologically, a leukocytoclastic vasculitis of the superficial dermal vessels is present. Chronic cases develop papillary hyperplasia of the epidermis giving the lesion a verrucous appearance.

Cutaneous vasculitis in **pigs** is most commonly associated with *Erysipelothrix rhusiopathiae* infection. Systemic vasculitis affecting primarily the skin and kidneys has been reported recently in pigs and has been called the *dermatitis/nephropathy syndrome*. Skin lesions consisted of irregularly enlarging hemorrhagic macules and papules on the ears, limbs, abdomen, thorax and perineum. *Leukocytoclastic vasculitis* was present in the dermis, panniculus, synovium, and renal pelvis. Pigs had concurrent pneumonia and immunological studies suggested *Porcine reproductive and respiratory syndrome virus* might be associated with the condition. Direct immunofluorescence testing or immunohistochemistry may demonstrate immunoglobulin and/or complement in vessel walls and occasionally at the basement membrane zone in suspected cases of vasculitis. Positive tests are most likely in lesions less than 24 hours old. False positives occur also. Adverse drug reactions, infection, familial vasculopathies, cryopathies, and systemic autoimmune diseases such as SLE should be ruled as possible causes. In many cases, a specific cause cannot be determined.

Bibliography

Affolter VK, von Tscharner C. Cutaneous drug reactions: a retrospective study of histopathological changes and their correlation with the clinical disease. Vet Dermatol 1992;3:157–163.

Cowan LA, et al. Clinical and clinicopathologic abnormalities in greyhounds with cutaneous and renal glomerular vasculopathy: 18 cases (1992–1994). J Am Vet Med Assoc 1997;210:789–793.

Ihrke PJ. Cutaneous adverse drug reactions. Compend Contin Educ Pract Vet 1997;Suppl 19:87–92.

Malik R, et al. Acute febrile neutrophilic vasculitis of the skin of young Shar-Pei dogs. Aust Vet J 2002;80:200–206.

Morris DD. Cutaneous vasculitis in horses: 19 cases (1978–1985). J Am Vet Med Assoc 1987;191:460–464.

Nichols PR, et al. A retrospective study of canine and feline cutaneous vasculitis. Vet Dermatol 2001;12:255–264.

Parker WM, Foster RA. Cutaneous vasculitis in five Jack Russell Terriers. Vet Dermatol 1996;7:109–115.

Pedersen K, Scott DW. Idiopathic pyogranulomatous inflammation and leukoclastic vasculitis of the nasal planum, nostrils, and nasal mucosa in Scottish Terriers in Denmark. Vet Dermatol 1991;2:85–89.

Segaes J, et al. Porcine dermatitis and nephropathy syndrome in Spain. Vet Rec 1998;142:483–486.

Thibault S, et al. Cutaneous and systemic necrotizing vasculitis in swine. Vet Pathol 1998;35:108–116.

von Tscharner C, et al. Stannard's illustrated equine dermatology notes. Vet Dermatol 2000;11:163–178.

Weir JAM, et al. Familial cutaneous vasculopathy of German shepherds: Clinical, genetic, and preliminary pathological and immunological studies. Can Vet J 1994;35:763–769.

Yager JA, Wilcock BP. Vasculitis. In: Surgical Pathology of the Dog and Cat: Dermatopathology and Skin Tumors. London: Mosby Year Book, 1994:107–118.

Rabies vaccine-induced vasculitis and alopecia in dogs

An ischemic dermatopathy leading to alopecic, hyperpigmented patches of atrophic skin (Fig. 5.77A) is a recognized form of injection-site reaction associated with the subcutaneous administration of rabies vaccines in dogs. All breeds are affected, but Poodles, Yorkshire and Silky Terriers are predisposed. Lesions most often develop at sites of previous vaccination, but occasionally multifocal lesions may occur. Lesions may appear months after the vaccine was administered. The *histologic appearance is highly characteristic*, although the vascular lesions are subtle. Venules, arterioles and small arteries develop a *very mild chronic lymphocytic vasculitis*, characterized by thickening of the vessel wall, a few intramural mononuclear inflammatory cells, scattered nuclear debris and variable perivascular mononuclear infiltrates (Fig. 5.77B). Occasionally a more florid leukocytoclastic vasculitis is seen. A cell-poor interface dermatitis with vacuolar change in the basal epithelial layer and pigmentary incontinence and mural folliculitis may be present in some cases. The dermis is atrophic and hyalinized, sometimes mucinous and hair follicles are in telogen and pale staining ("faded") (Fig. 5.77C). A diffuse increase in mononuclear cells throughout the dermis is accompanied by lymphocytic panniculitis. The additional lesions of erosions and ulcers of the oral mucosa and skin of the extremities and bony prominences and ischemic myopathy in subjacent musculature have been reported in cases with multicentric involvement. Immunofluorescence staining has identified rabies antigen in the vessels and epithelium of the hair follicles. A low-grade immune-mediated vasculitis with resultant tissue anoxia leading to the atrophic changes in the overlying skin has been suggested as the pathogenesis. Lesions may remain for months to years. Differential diagnoses include dermatomyositis, traction alopecia, idiopathic vasculopathy, and lupus profundus.

Bibliography

Nichols PR, et al. A retrospective study of canine and feline cutaneous vasculitis. Vet Dermatol 2001;12:255–264.

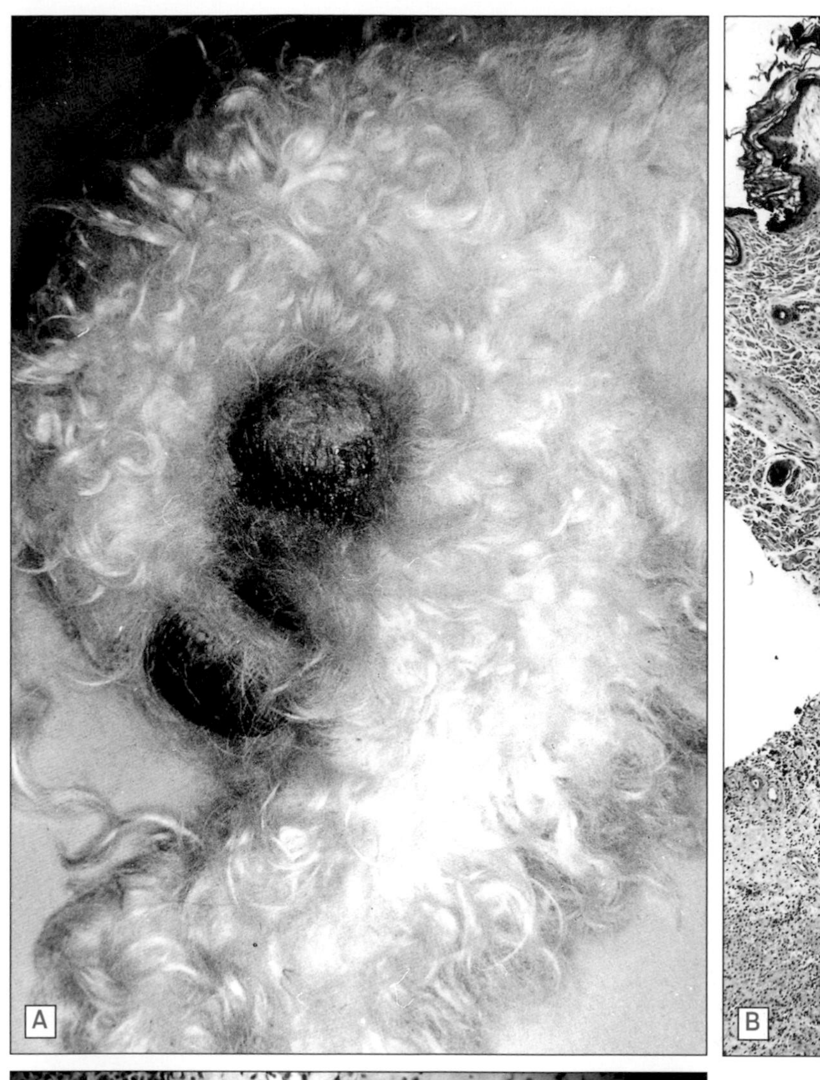

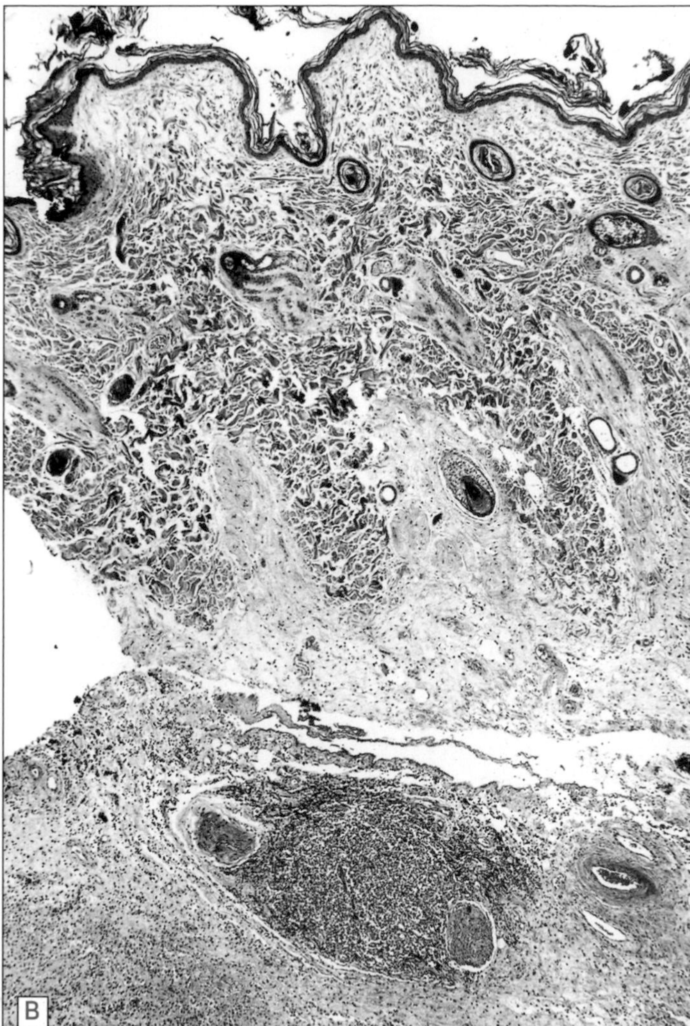

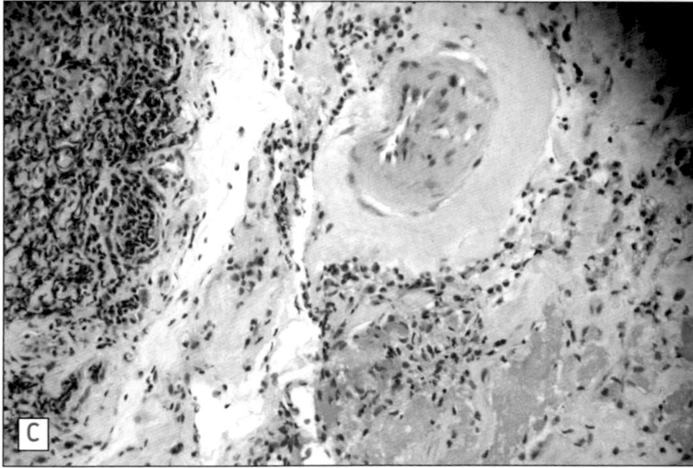

Figure 5.77 Rabies vaccine-associated vasculitis. A. Focal area of **hyperpigmentation and alopecia** on the caudal thigh in a Poodle. (Courtesy of L Schmeitzel.) **B. Marked atrophy** of the overlying epidermis and follicles, and **lymphocytic panniculitis**. **C. Fibrinoid degeneration** of vessel wall, intimal proliferation and perivascular aggregates of large macrophages containing granular material, as well as extracellular deposits of granular material.

Vitale CB, et al. Vaccine-induced ischemic dermatopathy in the dog. Vet Dermatol 1999;10:131–142.

Wilcock BP, Yager JA. Focal cutaneous vasculitis and alopecia at sites of rabies vaccination in dogs. J Am Vet Med Assoc 1986;188:1174–1177.

Canine uveodermatologic syndrome (Vogt–Koyanagi–Harada (VKH) syndrome)

This syndrome, seen only in dogs and humans, is characterized by the concurrent *acute onset of bilateral uveitis and depigmentation of the nose, lips, eyelids and occasionally the footpads and anus.* Although the cause of the disorder is unknown, a cell-mediated hypersensitivity to melanin has been hypothesized. It is discussed further under Disorders of pigmentation.

Plasma cell pododermatitis

This is a *rare disorder of cats* of all breeds, ages and sexes. A recent study found 50% of cases were positive for feline immunodeficiency virus. Although the pathogenesis is unknown, the tissue plasmacytosis, hypergammaglobulinemia, and beneficial response to immunomodulating drugs *suggest an immune-mediated basis*. In addition, occasional cats have other abnormalities, such as renal amyloidosis, plasmacytic stomatitis, positive anti-nuclear antibody tests, Coombs-positive anemia, polyclonal gammopathy, or glomerulonephritis with positive direct immunofluorescence testing (immunoglobulin deposited at the basement membrane zone). Clinically, plasma cell pododermatitis begins as soft, nonpainful swelling of multiple footpads on multiple paws. The central metacarpal or metatarsal pads are usually most severely affected. Affected pads feel soft due to collapse of the underlying fatpad. Footpad surfaces are crosshatched with white scaly striae but may become ulcerated or develop fleshy granulomatous proliferations which may hemorrhage. Lameness develops with progression of the lesions. Some cases spontaneously resolve or may recur seasonally.

Histologically, early lesions are characterized by *superficial and deep perivascular dermatitis with plasma cells predominating*. Later, there is a diffuse plasmacytic dermatitis. Russell bodies can be numerous. Leukocytoclastic vasculitis is rarely seen. Ulcerated or proliferative lesions show various degrees of superimposed suppurative-to-pyogranulomatous inflammation. The gross and histologic features are diagnostic.

Bibliography

Dias Pereira P, Faustino AM. Feline plasma cell pododermatitis: a study of 8 cases. Vet Dermatol 2003;14:333–337.

Guaguere E, et al. Feline pododermatitis. Vet Dermatol 1992;3:1–12.

Cutaneous amyloidosis

The physical structure of amyloid gives it special properties, such as apple green birefringence when Congo red-stained sections are polarized. The amyloid fibrils (AL amyloid) are derived from monoclonal immunoglobulin light chains. Cutaneous amyloidosis occurs rarely in *horses and dogs*. The cutaneous lesions are not usually associated with known triggering factors in horses; but in dogs, cutaneous amyloidosis has been associated with monoclonal gammopathy, dermatomyositis, and is seen occasionally in the stroma of plasmacytomas of skin and oral cavity (see Cutaneous plasmacytoma). In **dogs** with monoclonal gammopathy, purpuric lesions are seen, and cutaneous hemorrhage is easily induced by minor external trauma. The superficial dermis contains an amorphous, homogeneous, eosinophilic substance, and the walls of blood vessels in the involved area are thickened by deposition of the same substance.

In **horses**, the lesions are multiple, asymptomatic papules, nodules, and plaques that are most commonly seen on the head, neck, shoulders and pectoral region. There is no established breed, age, or sex predisposition. The lesions are firm, well-circumscribed and 0.5–10 cm in diameter. The overlying skin and haircoat are normal. The initial lesions may be urticarial in type. The cutaneous lesions may be accompanied by similar nodules in the respiratory mucosa and regional lymph nodes but are seldom associated with systemic amyloidosis. Lesions may regress, become recurrent or progressively enlarge. Histologic findings include *nodular-to-diffuse granulomatous dermatitis and panniculitis. Large extracellular deposits of amyloid appear as variably sized areas of homogeneous, amorphous, hyaline, eosinophilic material, which may contain clefts or fractures*. Multinucleated histiocytic giant cells are usually numerous. *Clinical differentials* include infectious and non-infectious granulomas, cutaneous neoplasms, and eosinophilic granulomas.

Bibliography

Gliatto JM, Alroy J. Cutaneous amyloidosis in a horse with lymphoma. Vet Rec 1995;137:68–69.

Gross TL, Ihrke PJ. Cutaneous amyloidosis. In: Gross TL, et al., eds. Veterinary Dermatopathology. A Macroscopic and Microscopic Evaluation of Canine and Feline Skin Disease. St. Louis, MO: Mosby Year Book, 1992:229–232.

Mathison PT. Eosinophilic nodular dermatoses. Vet Clin North Am: Eq Pract 1995;11:81–83.

Alopecia areata

Alopecia areata (AA) is a non-scarring, asymptomatic, inflammatory alopecia occurring in humans, nonhuman primates, dogs, cats, horses and cattle. Alopecia areata may be focal, multifocal or generalized (alopecia universalis). Lesions occur most commonly on the face, neck and trunk. Leukotrichia may be seen in some animals initially. Areas of alopecia are usually hyperpigmented and areas of alopecia may exhibit sparse numbers of short, dystrophic hairs (Fig. 5.78A). Lesions may be bilaterally symmetrical. There is no apparent age, breed, or sex predilection. In horses, the mane and tail are often affected. Currently, there are two rodent models available to study the condition, the C3H/HeJ mouse and the Dundee experimental bald rat.

Early, clinically active lesions are characterized histologically by an accumulation of lymphocytes ("swarm of bees") in and around the inferior segment of anagen hair follicles – the classic example of *peribulbar lymphocytic folliculitis* (Fig. 5.78B). Unfortunately, the classic lesion is not always evident and more subtle bulbar inflammation is the rule. Bulbar keratinocytes are frequently vacuolated, apoptotic or karyorrhectic. Pigmentary incontinence and melanophagia in the peribulbar region are also typical findings. Telogen follicles are unaffected and dystrophic hair follicles may be present. Demonstration of the lymphocytic peribulbitis may be difficult and require examination of multiple sections from different levels of the paraffin-embedded biopsy specimen. Biopsies from the periphery of early, expanding lesions are most rewarding. *Histologic findings in chronic, clinically static lesions are nondiagnostic*, revealing a predominance of telogen hair follicles and follicular atrophy, that may be misdiagnosed as an endocrine skin disorder. Immunologic studies in dogs and horses have indicated that the intrabulbar lymphocytes are primarily cytotoxic CD8+ lymphocytes. CD1+ dendritic antigen-presenting cells and both CD8+ and CD4+ lymphocytes are found in the peribulbar infiltrate. In addition, various autoantibodies targeting trichohyaline, hair keratins, and other components of the hair follicle have been demonstrated in various species, indicating a role for humoral immunity. In dogs and horses, *AA frequently spontaneously reverses itself*, however sometimes the hair regrowth is white. *Clinical differentials* include telogen effluvium and many other causes of lymphocytic mural folliculitis such as EM, SLE, GVH, ischemia, and demodicosis, to name a few. *The distinguishing feature of AA is the fact that the hair bulb and inferior segment of anagen hairs are the primary*

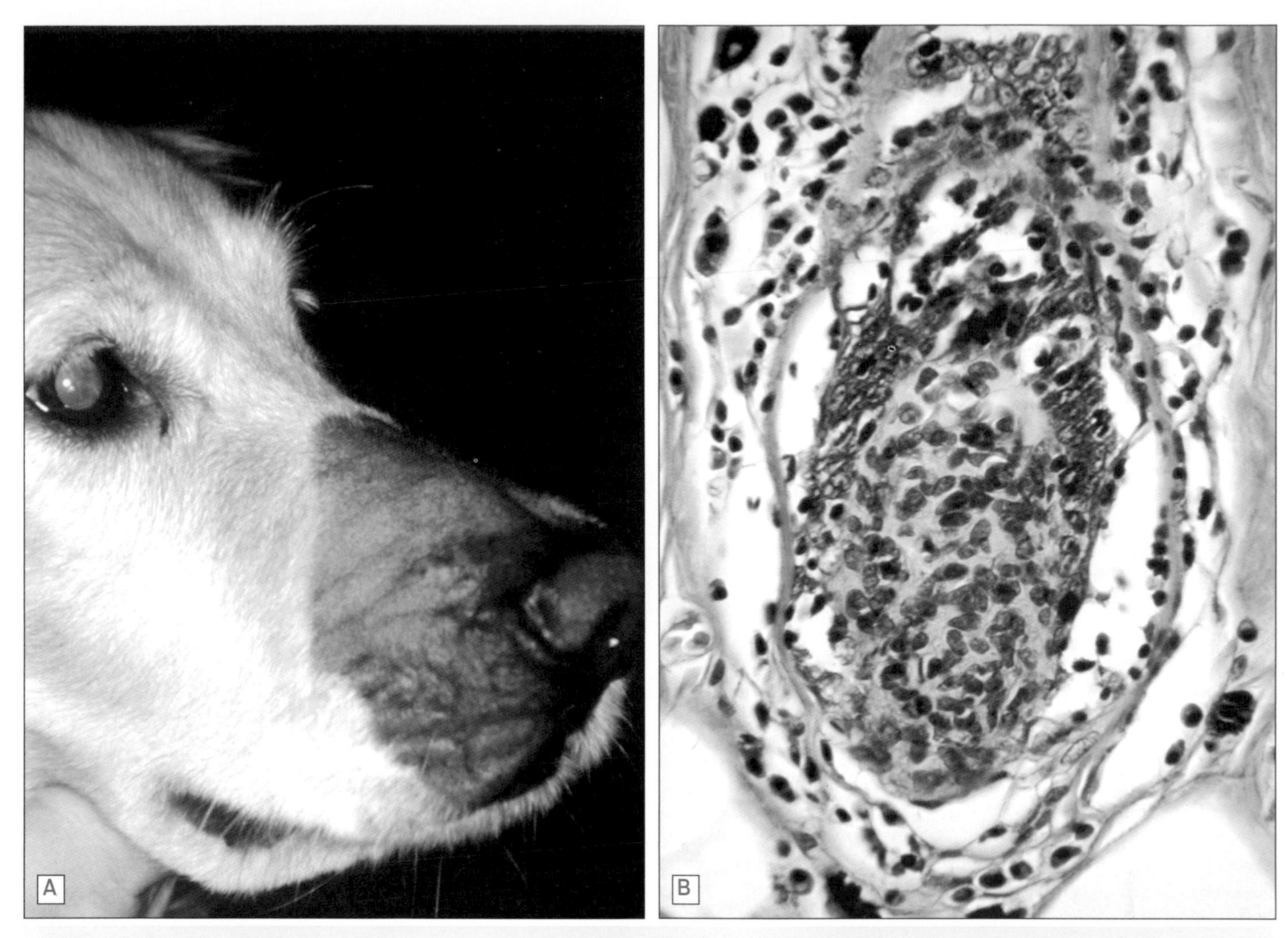

Figure 5.78 Alopecia areata in a dog. **A.** Note discrete area of non-inflamed, **hyperpigmented alopecic skin.** (Courtesy of K Beale.) **B. Peribulbar lymphocytic folliculitis.** Lymphocytes are in and around the hair bulb. (Courtesy of B Dunstan.)

targets of inflammation rather than the infundibulum or the isthmus, although the isthmus has been reported to be affected in a horse.

Bibliography

Colombo S, et al. Alopecia areata with lymphocytic mural folliculitis affecting the isthmus in a thoroughbred mare. Vet Dermatol 2004;15:260–265.

De Jonghe SR, et al. Trachyonychia associated with alopecia areata in a Rhodesian Ridgeback. Vet Dermatol 1999;10:123–126.

Gross TL, et al. Anatomical classification of folliculitis. Vet Dermatol 1997;8:147–156.

McElwee KJ, et al. Comparison of alopecia areata in humans and nonhuman mammalian species. Pathobiol 1998;66:368–376.

Olivry T. Autoimmune diseases of the hair follicles. Proc Eur Soc Vet Dermatol Workshop on Skin Immunol, Le Mas D'Artigny Stain-Paul de Vence, France, 2000.

Olivry T, et al. Antifollicular cell-mediated and humoral immunity in canine alopecia areata. Vet Dermatol 1996;7:67–79.

Scott DW, Gourreau JM. Alopecia areata (pelade) chez les bovins. Point Vét 1990;22:671–674.

Tobin DJ, et al. A natural canine homologue of alopecia areata in humans. Br J Dermatol 2003;149:938–950.

VIRAL DISEASES OF SKIN

Cutaneous lesions occur in the course of a number of viral diseases in domestic animals. Viruses may induce skin lesions upon *local infection*, but the intact integument is resistant to viral penetration; injection via an arthropod bite or introduction through a cutaneous wound is a prerequisite for infection. Examples of local viral infection include papillomas induced by the Papovaviridae, bovine mammillitis induced by a herpesvirus, and the so-called milker's nodule in humans caused by a parapoxvirus. More often, viruses localize in the skin during the viremic phase of a *systemic infection*. Examples include some poxvirus infections, malignant catarrhal fever and the vesicular diseases, such as vesicular stomatitis, and foot and mouth disease. Pantropic viruses, such as *Canine distemper virus* and *Classical swine fever virus*, may cause cutaneous lesions; but *most viruses causing cutaneous lesions are epitheliotropic*. Some epitheliotropic viruses, in particular the Poxviridae, have a predilection for the epithelium of the skin. Others, including the viruses associated with the mucosal diseases, cause primary lesions in the alimentary tract with lesser involvement of the skin.

A "rash," comprising erythematous macules due to long-lasting dilation of dermal blood vessels, is often associated with systemic viral disease in humans. Such lesions are uncommon in animals, but may be hidden by the haircoat. Exceptions are the *cutaneous erythema* occurring in classical swine fever and African swine fever, and hemorrhagic diathesis of skin occurring with disseminated *Porcine adenovirus* infection. In addition, a condition known as *dermatitis/nephropathy syndrome of pigs*, seen clinically as erythematous macules, papules, and plaques, due to cutaneous and systemic necrotizing vasculitis, may be associated with *Porcine circovirus 2* (PCV2) infection, with possible roles for *Porcine reproductive and respiratory syndrome virus* (PRRSV) and *Pasteurella multocida*.

Cutaneous viral diseases are *more common in food-producing animals than in pets*. Some of these diseases, notably sheeppox, cause significant mortality. Others have an economic impact because of their deleterious effect on production. Herpes mammillitis and pseudocowpox, for example, reduce milk yield in dairy cattle; contagious pustular dermatitis affects the growth rate of lambs by interfering with their ability to suckle. A few of the large animal viral dermatoses are extremely mild, for example molluscum contagiosum in the horse. Systemic viral diseases with cutaneous manifestations are rare in dogs and cats. *Canine distemper virus* is associated with nasodigital hyperkeratosis, so-called "hard pad" disease, and pustular dermatitis. In cats, rare occurrences of cutaneous disease occur with *Feline calicivirus* infection. Cutaneous lesions caused by *Felid herpesvirus 1* can occur in the absence of respiratory disease, a presumed recrudescence of a latent herpesvirus infection.

Traditionally, viral diseases have been *diagnosed* by light and electron microscopy, serology, and viral culture. However, the development of monoclonal antibodies to specific viruses for use with immunofluorescence and immunoperoxidase techniques is increasingly being used for specific and rapid diagnosis.

Bibliography

Choi C, Chae C. Colocalization of porcine reproductive and respiratory syndrome virus and porcine circovirus 2 in porcine dermatitis and nephropathy syndrome by double-labeling technique. Vet Pathol 2001;38:436–441.

Fenner F, et al. Veterinary Virology. 2nd ed. San Diego, CA: Academic Press, 1993.

Haines DM, et al. Immunohistochemical detection of canine distemper virus in haired skin, nasal mucosa, and footpad epithelium: a method for antemortem diagnosis of infection. J Vet Diagn Invest 1999;11:396–399.

Maeda H, et al. Distemper skin lesions in a dog. J Vet Med 1994;41:247–250.

Tang KN, et al. Disseminated adenovirus infection associated with cutaneous and visceral hemorrhages in a nursing piglet. Vet Pathol 1995;32:433–437.

Thibault S, et al. Cutaneous and systemic necrotizing vasculitis in swine. Vet Pathol 1998;35:108–116.

Timoney JF, et al. Hagan and Bruner's Microbiology and Infectious Diseases of Domestic Animals. 8th ed. Ithaca: Comstock Publishing, 1988.

Poxviral infections

The Poxviridae is a large family of complex DNA viruses. *Highly epitheliotropic, they cause cutaneous and systemic disease in birds, wild and domestic mammals and humans. Some members of the Poxviridae, including Sheeppox virus, Ectromelia virus, Monkeypox virus, and the now eradicated Variola virus (human smallpox), cause severe systemic disease.* Others cause mild, localized disease, for example pseudocowpox that chiefly affects the teats of milking cows. A few poxviruses are associated with hyperplastic or neoplastic conditions, such as molluscum contagiosum in horses and Shope fibroma of rabbits.

The Poxviridae share group-specific nucleoprotein antigens. Animal poxviruses are in the subfamily Chordopoxvirinae. The genera (*species names italicized*) include:

- *Orthopoxvirus* – *Camelpox virus, Cowpox virus, Ectromelia virus* (mousepox virus), *Monkeypox virus, Vaccinia virus* (buffalopox virus, rabbitpox virus). Unassigned member of the genus: Uasin Gishu disease virus.
- *Parapoxvirus* – *Bovine papular stomatitis virus, Orf virus* (contagious pustular dermatitis virus, contagious ecthyma virus), *Parapox virus of red deer, Pseudocowpox virus* (milker's nodule virus). Unassigned members in the genus: Auzduk disease virus (Camel contagious ecthyma virus), Chamois contagious ecthyma virus, Sealpox virus, and a virus that causes papillomatous dermatitis and pododermatitis in cattle.
- *Avipoxvirus* – *Fowlpox virus, Pigeonpox virus*, and many other avian poxviruses.
- *Capripoxvirus* – *Goatpox virus, Lumpy skin disease virus, Sheeppox virus.*
- *Leporipoxvirus* – *Myxoma virus; Rabbit fibroma virus* (Shope fibroma virus).
- *Suipoxvirus* – *Swinepox virus.*
- *Molluscipoxvirus* – *Molluscum contagiosum virus.*
- *Yatapoxvirus* – *Tanapox virus,* Yaba monkey tumor virus.

Many of the poxviruses are host-specific; but the orthopoxviruses, such as *Cowpox virus* and *Vaccinia virus*, affect a wide range of species. Some poxviruses, for example *Pseudocowpox virus*, are zoonotic. *Infection is usually achieved by cutaneous or respiratory routes.* Poxviruses, whether acquired by the subcutaneous or respiratory routes, usually gain access to the systemic circulation via the lymphatic system, although multiplication at the site of injection in the skin may lead to direct entry into the blood and primary viremia. Secondary viremia disseminates the virus back to the skin and to other target organs.

Poxviruses induce lesions by a variety of mechanisms. Degenerative changes in the epithelium are caused by virus replication and induce *vesicular lesions* typical of many poxvirus infections. Degenerative lesions in the dermal or submucosal tissues sometimes result from ischemia secondary to vascular damage caused by viral multiplication in endothelial cells. Poxvirus infections also *induce proliferative lesions*. Poxviruses, such as *Orf virus*, replicating in the epidermis typically induce hyperplasia along with degenerative changes. Host cell DNA synthesis is stimulated before the onset of cytoplasmic virus-related DNA replication. Proliferative changes may be explained by a gene, present in several poxviruses including *Molluscum contagiosum virus*, whose product has significant homology with epidermal growth factor. Poxviruses also encode for functions that may counteract host defenses. These include genes related to those encoding the SERPINs (a superfamily of related proteins important in regulating serine protease enzymes that mediate kinin, complement, fibrinolytic and coagulation pathways) and genes encoding anti-interferon activities.

Pox lesions have a typical developmental sequence. They commence as erythematous macules, become papular, and then vesicular. The vesicular stage is well developed in some pox infections, such as sheeppox, and is transient or non-existent in others, such as contagious pustular dermatitis. Vesicles develop into *umbilicated pustules with a depressed center and a raised, often erythematous border.* This lesion is the so-called "*pock*." The pustules rupture and a crust forms on the surface. This crust may become very thick, as in lesions of contagious pustular dermatitis. Lesions heal and often leave a residual scar. The mucosal lesions are briefly vesicular and develop into ulcers rather than pustules.

Histologically, pox lesions begin as epidermal cytoplasmic swelling and vacuolation, usually first affecting the cells of the outer stratum spinosum. There is evidence, from experimental studies with the virus of contagious pustular dermatitis, that post-injury proliferating keratinocytes are the target for viral replication. Rupture of the damaged keratinocytes produces multiloculated vesicles, so-called *reticular degeneration*. The early dermal lesions include edema, vascular dilation, a perivascular mononuclear cell infiltrate and a variable neutrophilic infiltrate. Neutrophils migrate into the epidermis and aggregate in vesicles to form microabscesses. Large intraepidermal pustules may form and sometimes extend into the superficial dermis. There is usually marked epithelial hyperplasia and sometimes pseudocarcinomatous hyperplasia of the adjacent epithelium. This contributes to the raised border of the umbilicated pustule. Rupture of the pustule produces an inflammatory crust, often colonized on its surface by bacteria.

Poxvirus lesions often contain *characteristic intracytoplasmic inclusion bodies*. These are single or multiple and of varying size and duration. The more prominent inclusions are designated *type A*. They are eosinophilic, reflecting their high protein content, and weakly Feulgen-positive. *Smaller, basophilic Feulgen-positive type B* bodies also occur and represent the site of virus replication.

Diagnosis of poxvirus infections is usually based on *typical clinical appearance* and may be supported by *characteristic histologic lesions*. Parapoxviruses are ultrastructurally distinct from the other poxviruses that are morphologically similar to each other when viewed by electron microscopy.

Bibliography

Buller RM, Palumbo GJ. Poxvirus pathogenesis. Microbiol Rev 1991;55:80–122.

Fenner F, et al. The Orthopoxviruses. New York: Academic Press, 1989.

Lewis-Jones S. Zoonotic poxvirus infections in humans. Curr Opin Infect Dis 2004;17:81–89.

Parapoxviral diseases

Contagious pustular dermatitis

Contagious pustular dermatitis is a poxviral disease of *sheep and goats*, with incidental infections occurring in humans, camels, cows, and many wild ruminants, and very rarely dogs. The disease is caused by *Orf virus*, a *Parapoxvirus* closely related to *Pseudocowpox virus* and *Bovine papular stomatitis virus*. Synonyms for contagious pustular dermatitis include contagious ecthyma, orf, infectious labial dermatitis, soremouth, and scabby mouth.

The disease is geographically widespread and occurs wherever sheep or goats are raised. The virus can repeatedly infect sheep and goats; and while live-virus vaccines control the disease and decrease the severity of the disease, they also ensure its continuance by perpetuating infection in the environment. The economic significance of contagious pustular dermatitis results chiefly from loss of condition, since *affected animals neither suckle nor graze*. Morbidity in a susceptible population may reach 90%, but mortality rarely exceeds 1% unless secondary infection intervenes, or unless the animals are immunosuppressed or stressed in which case mortality can be high. Mortality often results from the invasion of primary lesions by the larvae of the screwworm fly (*Cochliomyia hominivorax*) or by bacteria such as *Fusobacterium necrophorum* and occasionally *Dermatophilus congolensis*. Cellulitis may complicate pedal lesions, mastitis may complicate mammary lesions, and necrotizing stomatitis and aspiration pneumonia may complicate oral lesions.

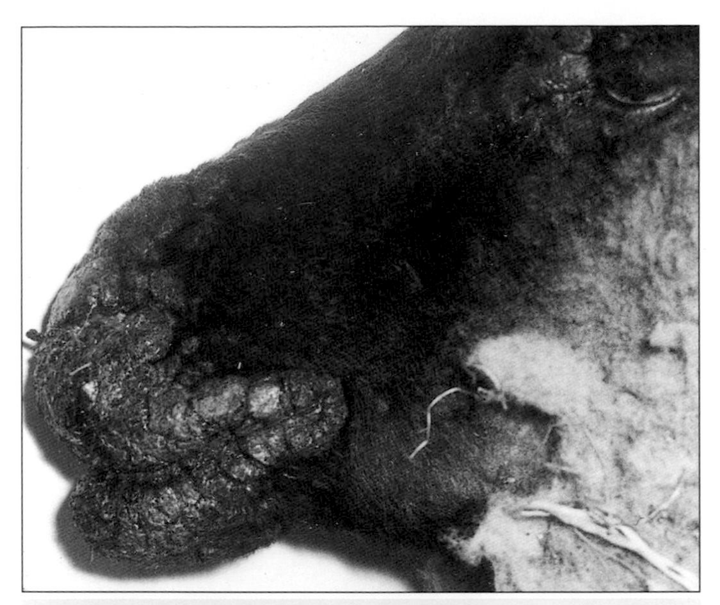

Figure 5.79 Contagious pustular dermatitis (orf) in a sheep. Scabby lesions at the margins of the lips.

Contagious pustular dermatitis affects sheep and goats of all breeds. *It is predominantly a disease of lambs and kids*. Infection is established through cutaneous abrasions, particularly those associated with dry and prickly pasture or forage. Clinically affected lambs may transmit the virus to the udder of the ewe. The virus is hardy and probably persists in a dry environment indefinitely in crust material shed from affected animals. Chronically infected, reinfected or, possibly, latently infected carrier animals may allow the virus to persist in a flock for several years.

Gross lesions usually commence at the commissures of the lips and spread around the lip margins to the muzzle (Fig. 5.79). Primary lesions sometimes occur on the face about the eyes. In severe cases, lesions may develop on the gingiva, dental pad, palate and tongue (Fig. 5.80A). Lesions mainly confined to the tongue must be differentiated from those of foot and mouth disease. The buccal lesions are raised, red or gray foci with a surrounding zone of hyperemia. Very rarely, lesions extend to the esophagus, rumen and omasum in the lower alimentary canal, causing ulcerative gastroenteritis, and in lungs and heart. Lesions on the limbs are less common than on the lips and tend to involve the coronet, interdigital cleft, and bulb of the heels. They may extend, in severe cases, to the knee or hock on the caudal aspect of the leg. Lesions of the mammary gland affect the teats and adjacent skin of the udder. Lesions may develop in other areas of sparsely wooled skin such as the inner thigh, axilla, and the edge of wounds in recently earmarked lambs, or tail-dock sites. Proliferative lesions affecting predominantly the head, neck and body have been described in Nubian goats.

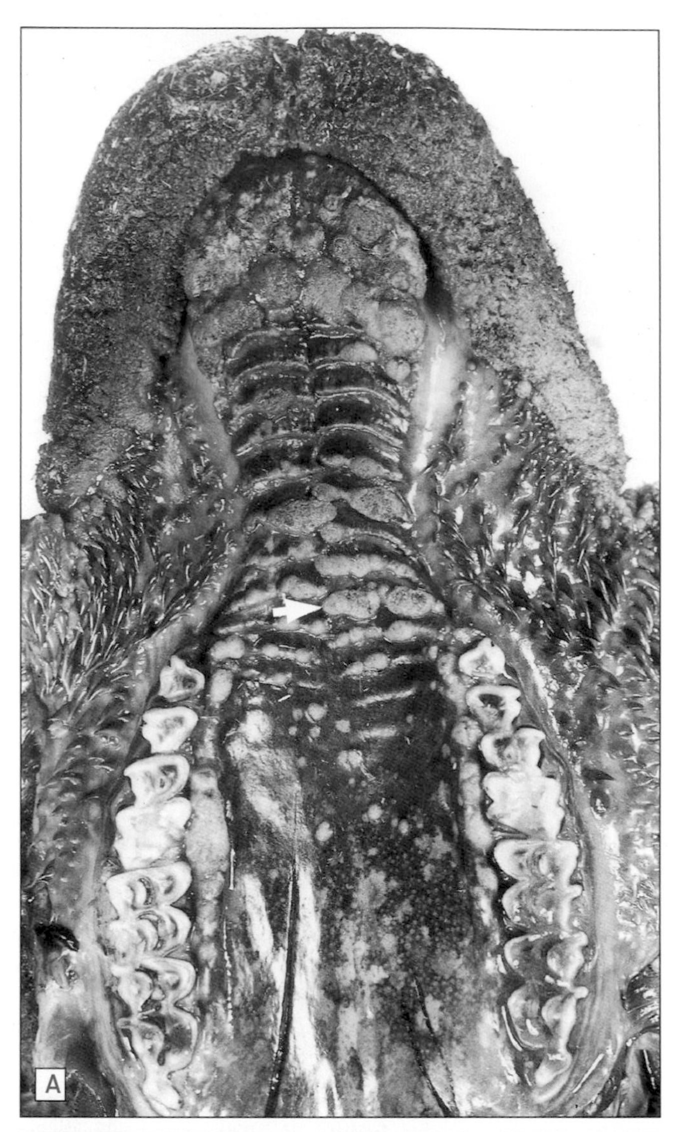

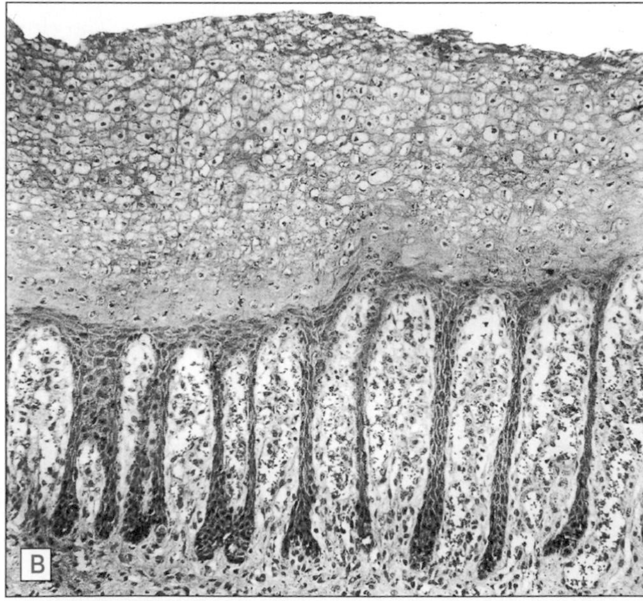

Figure 5.80 Contagious pustular dermatitis in a sheep. **A.** Crusty, proliferative lesions on the lips, dental pad, and palate (arrow). **B.** Note marked epithelial proliferation and increased vascularity and intracellular edema of keratinocytes.

The lesions develop through the typical pox phases but are much more proliferative. The vesicular stage is transient and pustules are flat rather than umbilicated. The most significant feature of the gross lesion is the layer of thick brown-gray crust that may be elevated 2–4 mm above the skin surface. Depending on the degree of secondary infection, regression is usually complete by 4 weeks. Papillomatous growths, resulting from continued epidermal proliferation, sometimes occur.

The microscopic lesions of contagious pustular dermatitis are characterized by vacuolation and swelling of keratinocytes in the stratum spinosum, reticular degeneration, marked epidermal proliferation, intraepidermal microabscesses, and accumulation of scale-crust. In experimentally abraded sheep skin, the active site of viral replication was found to be the newly proliferative keratinocyte population, growing up under the superficial necrotic layer. By ~30 hours postinfection, keratinocyte swelling and vacuolation commences in the outer stratum spinosum. It is accompanied by cytoplasmic basophilia, which corresponds ultrastructurally to an increased number of polyribosomes presumably active in viral protein synthesis. Basophilic intracytoplasmic inclusion bodies are reported as early as 31 hr post-infection. By 72 hours postinfection, the keratinocytes show nuclear pyknosis and marked hydropic change, leading to reticular degeneration. The term ballooning degeneration is often used, but the keratinocytes do not have the homogeneous eosinophilic cytoplasm typical of this condition. At this time intracytoplasmic eosinophilic inclusion bodies appear. The inclusion bodies persist for 3–4 days, as long as the hydropic cells are found. The proliferative reaction in the epidermis is underway by 55 hours postinfection with mitotic figures numerous in the stratum basale. By 3 days postinfection, the epithelium is 3–4 times normal thickness and rete ridges are markedly elongated (Fig. 5.80B). Pseudocarcinomatous hyperplasia is common.

Dermal lesions include superficial edema, marked capillary dilation, and an early influx of neutrophils, followed by a marked accumulation of MHC class II dendritic cells, with CD4+ T cells, CD8+ T cells, and B cells. A thick layer of scale-crust is built up, composed of ortho- and parakeratotic hyperkeratosis, proteinaceous fluid, degenerating neutrophils, cellular debris and bacterial colonies. The subsequent microscopic appearance of the lesions depends on the degree of secondary bacterial infection.

Contagious pustular dermatitis occurs in camels and a variety of wild and captive ungulates. Dogs may acquire infection by eating infected lamb carcasses. Lesions resemble those in sheep. It is a *zoonotic disease* and is a recognized occupational hazard amongst goat and sheep handlers.

Bibliography

de la Concha-Bermejillo A, et al. Severe persistent orf in young goats. J Vet Diagn Invest 2003;15:423–431.

Gumbrell RC, McGregor DA. Outbreak of severe fatal orf in lambs. Vet Rec 1997;141:150–151.

Haig DM, Mercer AA. Ovine diseases. Orf Vet Res 1998;29:311–326.

Mercer A, et al. Molecular genetic analyses of parapox pathogenic for humans. Arch Virol Suppl 1997;13:25–34.

Ulcerative dermatosis of sheep

Ulcerative dermatosis is a disease of the epidermis of sheep that has been reported in the literature as being caused by an *unclassified poxvirus*, which is similar to *Orf virus*, but the viruses do not cross-protect. The disease has been reported in South Africa where it is known as "pisgoed" or "pisgras," in the United Kingdom as a contagious venereal infection, and in the USA where it is known as "lip and leg ulceration," "anovulvitis," "infectious balanoposthitis" and "ulcerative vulvitis." The various names indicate the *essential features of the disease, which are ulcerative papules on the lips, face, legs, feet, vulva, prepuce and, occasionally, the glans penis.* The genital lesions are transmissible by coitus.

Presumably, infection results from viral contact with damaged skin. *The pathologic process is primarily ulcerative*, with ulcers of up to 4–5 cm in diameter and 3–5 mm deep. Pus covers the granulation tissue at the base of the ulcer and underlies a scab that is thin, brown and bloody, and unlike the thick parakeratotic crusts that develop in contagious pustular dermatitis. The underlying dermis is diffusely swollen, especially in distensible parts such as the vulva and prepuce. The lesions on the hairy parts of the face tend to be fairly well circumscribed, but those of the feet tend to spread, especially on the interdigital skin. The vulval lesions usually begin on the tip and spread around the margins of the lips. An ulcerative ring tends to form around the preputial orifice, but the preputial mucosa is spared. Lesions on the glans penis remain moist. The urethral process may become necrotic. The labial and pedal lesions must be distinguished from those of contagious pustular dermatitis and foot-and-mouth disease, and the preputial lesions must be distinguished from noncontagious forms of balanoposthitis. *Detailed descriptions of the histopathology of ulcerative dermatitis are lacking*; the lesions are supposedly distinguishable from those of contagious pustular dermatitis by the *lack of epithelial hyperplasia*.

Bibliography

Steyn DG. Pisgoed or pisgras (ulcerative dermatosis). 16th Rep Direct Vet Services Anim Indust Union S Afr 1930:417–420.

Trueblood MS. Relationship of ovine contagious ecthyma and ulcerative dermatosis. Cornell Vet 1966;56:521–526.

Vestweber JG, Milleret RJ. Ulcerative dermatosis in sheep (a case report). Vet Med Small Anim Clin 1972;67:672–674.

Pseudocowpox

Pseudocowpox is caused by *Pseudocowpox virus*, a *Parapoxvirus*. The virus is closely related to *Bovine papular stomatitis virus* and *Orf virus*. *It is a common endemic infection in cattle throughout most of the world.* It affects chiefly milking herds and occasionally beef herds. Morbidity in a herd approaches 100% but only 10–15% of cows are affected at any one time. The economic significance lies in the effect on milk production, either as a result of sore teats or because of secondary bacterial mastitis. Lesions, which affect the teats (Fig. 5.81), udder, and perineum, commence as erythematous macules and papules, but do not form the umbilicated pustules seen in cowpox and vaccinia infections. Instead, a characteristic ring or horseshoe-shaped crust forms that may become umbilicated as it expands, but infrequently ulcerates. *The histologic appearance of lesions is typical of other poxviral infections.* The lesions usually heal within 6 weeks. Occasionally, lesions develop in the mouth and on the muzzle of suckling calves, and the infection can be spread by cross-suckling as well as poor hygiene in milking sheds. Transmission to people induces "milker's nodule."

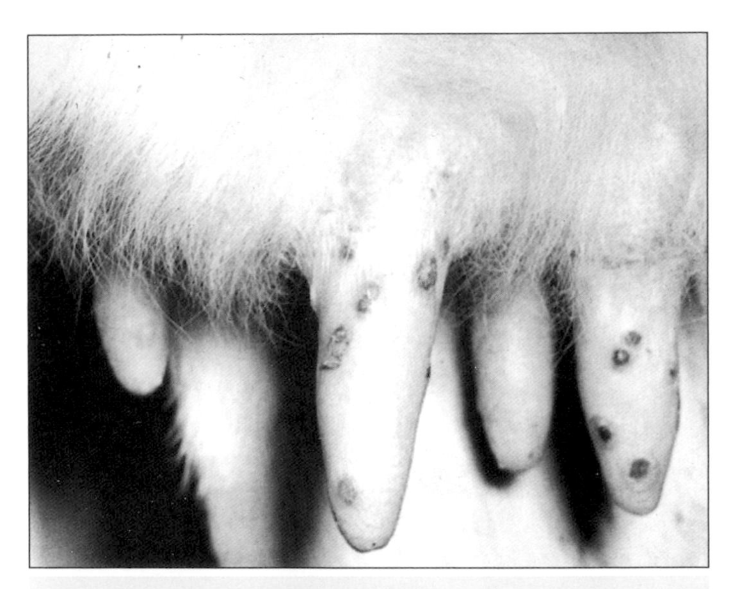

Figure 5.81 Pseudocowpox on the teats of a cow.

Bovine papular stomatitis

Bovine papular stomatitis virus is distributed worldwide, and although it causes disease more commonly in *cattle <2 years old* it can occur at any age and in any breed. Lesions occur on the *muzzle, nostrils, lips, and mouth* (see Vol. 2, Alimentary system), and cows with suckling calves can develop *teat and udder lesions*. The development and appearance of the lesions are similar to pseudocowpox, with resolution of lesions in days to weeks. A chronic form has been described in which exudative necrotic dermatitis involved the trunk as well as the mouth, and in which the animals died in 4–6 weeks. *Transmission to humans induces lesions identical to "milker's nodule"* caused by *Pseudocowpox virus* infection. The histologic appearance of lesions is typical of other poxviral infections.

Bibliography

Bowman KF, et al. Cutaneous form of bovine papular stomatitis in man. J Am Med Assoc 1981;246:2813–2818.

Gibbs EPJ. Viral diseases of the skin of the bovine teat and udder. Vet Clin North Am 1984;6:187–202.

Nagington J, et al. Bovine papular stomatitis, pseudocowpox and milker's nodules. Vet Rec 1967;81:306–313.

Yeruham I, et al. Clinical and pathological description of a chronic form of bovine papular stomatitis. J Comp Pathol 1994;111:279–286.

Parapox of red deer

A new addition to the genus *Parapox* is the *Parapox virus of red deer*, first noted in 1986 in farmed red deer in New Zealand. Morbidity is high, but mortality is low unless secondary infections are present. The virus causes crusty lesions on the lips, muzzle, face, ears, and neck, and on the antler velvet in stags. Removal of the crusts leaves a red raw ulcer. Histologic lesions are characterized by *epithelial hyperplasia with ballooning degeneration, dyskeratosis, and eosinophilic cytoplasmic viral inclusions*.

Bibliography

Horner GW, et al. Parapox infections in New Zealand farmed red deer (*Cervus elaphus*). NZ Vet J 1987;35:41–45.

Robinson AJ, Mercer AA. Parapoxvirus of red deer: evidence for its inclusion as a new member in the genus parapoxvirus. Virology 1995;208:812–815.

Orthopoxviral diseases

Cowpox

Cowpox virus and cowpox-like viruses belong to the genus *Orthopoxvirus*. They are closely related to, but antigenically different from, *Vaccinia virus*. Cowpox affects a range of species including *wild and domestic Felidae, cattle, dogs*, rodents, humans, and several zoo and circus animals including elephants and rhinoceros. Cowpox occurs in the *UK and Europe*. Outbreaks reported from other geographical locations can be ascribed to *Vaccinia virus* infection; the lesions induced by the two orthopoxviruses are clinically indistinguishable. In cattle, *Cowpox virus* infection is manifested by poxvirus lesions that develop on the *teats and udder*, and occasionally at other sites such as the muzzle of suckling calves. *Cowpox virus* is not endemic in cattle and *infections in cattle are uncommon*. Re-evaluation of the epidemiology of *Cowpox virus* relegates cattle to a minor role, and it has become increasingly clear from serologic surveys that *small wild rodents, such as voles and mice, are the virus reservoir*, and it is from this reservoir that other mammals can become infected accidentally. Domestic cats, and rarely dogs, in UK and Europe, can be infected by hunting wild rodents, and cats occasionally have been shown to be able to transmit the infection to humans. The evidence suggests, however, that the virus is of low infectivity for humans. Since the first report in 1978, *Cowpox virus* infection has been documented with increasing frequency within its geographical range of the UK and Europe. Epidemiological studies show a higher prevalence in free-ranging country-dwelling cats and a seasonal incidence in the autumn, a time when the small mammal population is at its highest. These features further support the serologic evidence of a wild rodent reservoir of virus.

Domestic cats develop *cutaneous* and, occasionally, *respiratory lesions*. The primary lesions in cats have a predilection for the *face and forepaws*. Approximately 50% of cats show a single primary cutaneous lesion, usually on the head, neck, forelimbs, or paws. The initial lesion is ulcerative and has been described as "bite-like." Lesions heal by granulation, but may occasionally develop into abscesses or cellulitis. The secondary cutaneous lesions develop 4–16 days after the onset of the primary lesion. Generalization from primary inoculation sites in the skin has also been demonstrated in experimentally infected cats. Mucocutaneous junctions, oral mucosa and the tongue may also be involved. *Secondary lesions* are multiple (usually more than ten lesions). They commence as firm 2–3 mm nodules, enlarging over 2–3 days to form 0.5–2 cm, circular, ulcerated papules or plaques. Lesions are rarely vesicular except on the oral mucosa and inner aspect of the pinna. The ulcers heal with thick gray crusts over 2–3 weeks. Cellulitis may develop but generally secondary bacterial infection is not a significant complication. Corticosteroid or progesterone therapy may be responsible for converting a local infection into a generalized one or exacerbating the secondary lesions in some animals. Although fatal *Cowpox virus* infection has been seen in cats with concurrent *Feline immunodeficiency virus* (FIV) infection, there is no convincing evidence to show a direct relationship. Approximately 30% of *Cowpox virus*-infected cats concurrently infected with FIV have uneventful recoveries.

The disease is rarely fatal. Approximately 20% of cats show some signs of malaise in the acute stage of secondary lesion development, presumably associated with a viremic phase, and a few exhibit clinical signs of upper respiratory tract disease. Lower respiratory tract lesions, which are rare in domestic cats, include pleural effusion and localized areas of cream-colored consolidation in the ventral lung lobes. They are thought to develop from systemic spread rather than from primary respiratory infection.

The *microscopic lesions* in naturally infected cats are *focal, sharply demarcated ulcers covered by fibrinonecrotic exudate*. The ulcers may extend to the deep dermis, subcutis or even muscle. An intense dermal inflammatory cell infiltrate of neutrophils and mononuclear cells may be associated with the base of the ulcers. *Eosinophilic, homogeneous, intracytoplasmic inclusion bodies*, 3–7 μm in diameter, occur in keratinocytes in the hyperplastic epithelium at the margin of the ulcers and in the epithelium of the external root sheath and sebaceous gland. Epidermal lesions typical of poxvirus infections develop in cats experimentally infected intravenously or by skin scarification. These lesions include focal hyperplasia, with reticular degeneration and multilocular vesiculation. Epidermal cells bordering the vesicles contain eosinophilic intracytoplasmic inclusion bodies. Viral inclusions also occur in macrophages, fibroblasts and endothelial cells. The extensive necrosis is probably ischemic in origin following viral damage to endothelial cells. The pulmonary lesion is a necrotizing alveolitis in which eosinophilic inclusion bodies are present in the degenerating cells.

Electron microscopic examination of scabs reveals typical orthopox virions. *Cowpox virus* infection may be confirmed by immunohistochemical staining of lesions, PCR, or virus isolation. Serological tests may be helpful in establishing retrospective diagnoses, as virus neutralizing antibodies are persistent for several years.

There have been outbreaks of severe orthopox infections in several species of **nondomestic Felidae** in English and Russian zoos. Lions, cheetahs, pumas, jaguars, and ocelots have been affected. Rats were implicated as the source of infection in the Russian outbreaks. Two forms of the disease are recognized. The cutaneous form is rarely fatal. The lesions are ulcerative and crusted as described for domestic cats. The respiratory form is uniformly fatal and consist of severe fibrinous and necrotizing bronchopneumonia and pleuritis. A virus closely resembling *Cowpox virus* is responsible.

Bibliography

Baxby D, Bennett M. Cowpox: a re-evaluation of the risks of human cowpox based on new epidemiological information. Arch Virol Suppl 1997;13:1–12.

Baxby D, et al. An outbreak of cowpox in captive cheetahs: virological and epidemiological studies. J Hyg (Camb) 1982;89:365–372.

Chantrey J, et al. Cowpox: reservoir hosts and geographical range. Epidemiol Infect 1999;122:455–460.

Godfrey DR, et al. Unusual presentations of cowpox infection in cats. J Small Anim Pract 2004;45:202–205.

Marennikova SS, et al. Outbreak of pox disease among Carnivora (Felidae) and Edentata. J Infect Dis 1977;135:358–366.

Meyer H, et al. Characterization of orthopoxviruses isolated from man and animals in Germany. Arch Virol 1999;144:491–501.

Smith KC, et al. Skin lesions caused by orthopoxvirus infection in a dog. J Small An Pract 1999;40:495–497.

Vaccinia

Vaccinia virus, the type species for the *Orthopoxvirus* genus, *does not cause natural infection in domestic animals. The origin of the virus is controversial.* One theory is that it represents the laboratory survival of horsepoxvirus, which is now extinct in nature, and that horse-derived material was the source of vaccine material used by Edward Jenner in 1817 to protect against variola or smallpox. Another theory is that *Vaccinia virus* was derived from *Cowpox virus* by repeated passage on the skin of cows, sheep, and other animals, and that "horsepox" was due to the infection of horses with *Cowpox virus*. Incidental infections in cattle, horses and pigs were transferred from vaccinated people. The lesions in cattle are indistinguishable from those of cowpox and in swine are indistinguishable from those of swinepox. When vaccinia is inoculated onto scarified skin of horses, papular lesions resembling a naturally occurring poxvirus infection described in horses in the USA result. Furthermore, inoculation of the skin of the flexor surface of the pastern produces lesions resembling the classical "grease heel" form of horsepox. *Vaccinia virus infections of animals are rare* now that smallpox has been eradicated and routine vaccination has been discontinued.

Bibliography

Baxby D. Edward Jenner's inquiry: a bicentenary analysis. Vaccine 1999;17:301–307.
Patel DD, et al. Isolation of cowpoxvirus A-type inclusions and characterization of their major protein component. Virology 1986;149:174–189.
Studdert MJ. Experimental vaccinia virus infection of horses. Aust Vet J 1989;66:157–159.

Buffalopox

Buffalopox virus, an *Orthopoxvirus* closely related to *Vaccinia virus*, is the cause of buffalopox, an economically important disease of domestic buffaloes. It is thought that Buffalopox virus is a subspecies of *Vaccinia virus* resident in the water buffalo population. In India it is considered to be an emerging enzootic virus and can occur in epidemic form, with significant economic impact. It has been reported in Pakistan, Indonesia, Egypt, Italy, and Russia. Zebu cattle are apparently refractory to infection. The lesions predominantly affect the teats, udder, medial aspects of the thighs, lips and muzzle but may be generalized, especially in calves. *Buffalopox virus can be zoonotic*, causing lesions primarily on the hands. Human-to-human transmission has been postulated following the occurrence of disease in children who had had no contact with infected animals. Experimentally, the virus can be transmitted to cattle, rabbits, guinea pigs, and mice.

Bibliography

Anand Kumar P, Butchaiah G. Partial antigenic characterization of buffalopox virus. Vet Res Commun 2004;28:543–552.
Fenner F, et al. The Orthopoxviruses. New York: Academic Press, 1989.
Kolhapure RM, et al. Investigation of buffalopox outbreaks in Maharashtra state during 1992–1996. Indian J Med Res 1997;106:441–446.
Singh M, et al. Biological transmissibility of buffalopoxvirus. J Appl An Res 1996;9:79–88.

Camelpox

Camelpox virus, a distinct species of *Orthopoxvirus*, causes severe disease in *dromedary camels*. It is characterized by *high morbidity and a relatively high mortality rate* in young animals. A major effect is a fall in milk production and loss of condition. The disease is widespread in northern and eastern Africa and mid-eastern Asia but has not been reported in Australia. Lesions affect both *skin and mucous membranes* and follow the usual pattern of pox lesions. Lesions tend to be most concentrated around the mucocutaneous junctions of the face but may be found on the neck and forelegs. Rarely, the infection can involve the respiratory system or become systemic. Generalized skin lesions occur more typically in calves. Fatalities are usually associated with *secondary bacterial infection leading to septicemia*, a phenomenon more prevalent in the rainy season. Clinically, *the lesions can be identical to parapox* (camel contagious ecthyma) and laboratory tests such as ELISA, PCR, and immunohistochemistry, as well as electron microscopy, can be used to differentiate the infections.

Bibliography

Afonso CL, et al. The genome of camelpox virus. Virology 2002;295:1–9.
Kinne J, et al. Pathological studies on camelpox lesions of the respiratory system in the United Arab Emirates (UAE). J Comp Pathol 1998;118:257–266.
Pfeffer M, et al. Fatal form of camelpox virus infection. Vet J 1998;155:107–109.
Pfeffer M, et al. Diagnostic procedures for poxvirus infections in camelids. J Camel Pract Res 1998;5:189–195.

"Horsepox" and Uasin Gishu disease

Horsepox was a common disease of horses in the 18th and 19th centuries; however, *it became naturally extinct at the end of the 19th century*. It is thought that Jenner, in his "cowpox" vaccination experiments to protect humans from smallpox, was actually using horse-derived material as a source of the vaccine, and that *Vaccinia virus* may be the long-lost agent of horsepox. Experimental infection of horses with *Vaccinia virus* reproduces the "grease heel" lesions of Jenner's horsepox and the more generalized form known as *equine papular dermatitis*. Orthopoxviruses have been isolated from equine papular dermatitis; however, the virus has not been fully characterized. *Orthopoxvirus* has also been isolated from Uasin Gishu disease in Kenya, and Uasin Gishu disease virus is closely related to *Vaccinia virus* and *Cowpox virus*.

Poxviral lesions in the horse take *several clinical forms*. Jenner originally described an exudative dermatitis of the flexor aspects of the hind pasterns. The condition is colloquially named "*grease heel*" because thick, yellow grease-like exudate mats the hair. Unfortunately, poxvirus infection is only one manifestation of this clinical entity, sparking considerable controversy as to the true nature of equine pox.

A second form has a predilection for the *muzzle and buccal cavity*. The lesions, which develop in the typical sequence of a pock, affect the inner surface of the lips and cheeks, the gums, and the ventral surface of the tongue. Following the development of the buccal eruptions, crops of pocks may appear in the rostral nares, on the face and on other parts of the body. It is a benign infection, sometimes seriously complicated by bacterial contamination.

Another manifestation takes the form of generalized papular eruptions. In the USA and Australia, the disease is known as

equine papular dermatitis. This is a highly contagious disorder, spreading by direct contact and through infected harness, bedding and grooming tools. The lesions are firm papules, up to 0.5 cm diameter, which tend to develop on the lateral neck and shoulder and thorax but become generalized. The papules become crusted and the crusts slough to leave circular alopecic patches. Resolution may take 6 weeks.

Uasin Gishu disease from Kenya is also characterized by generalized skin lesions but the disease differs clinically from equine papular dermatitis. Lesions begin similarly as small papules but develop into crusted papillomatous proliferations, up to 2 cm diameter. Lesions eventually resolve but the disease may continue for 2 years. The histologic lesions of Uasin Gishu are identical to molluscum contagiosum.

Bibliography

Baxby D. Edward Jenner's inquiry; a bicentenary analysis. Vaccine 1999; 17:301–307.

Eby CH. A note on the history of horsepox. J Am Vet Med Assoc 1958;132:420–422.

Kaminjolo JS, Winqvist G. Histopathology of skin lesions in Uasin Gishu skin disease of horses. J Comp Pathol 1975;85:391–395.

McIntyre RW. Virus papular dermatitis of the horse. Am J Vet Res 1949;10:229–232.

Tizard I. Grease, anthraxgate, and kennel cough: a revisionist history of early veterinary vaccines. Adv Vet Med 1999;41:7–24.

Equine molluscum contagiosum

Equine molluscum contagiosum is another proliferative poxvirus infection in the horse, and *the causal virus is now thought to be identical to, or closely related to, human Molluscum contagiosum virus.* In horses this is a mildly contagious, self-limiting cutaneous infection. In situ hybridization experiments indicate there is very close homology between the equine and human *Molluscum contagiosum virus.* Attempts to grow both the human and equine *Molluscum contagiosum virus* in culture have failed, and this can help differentiate the virus from the orthopoxvirus of Uasin Gishu, which produces histologically and clinically similar lesions, but which can be grown in culture. Cutaneous lesions resembling the human and equine condition clinically, microscopically and ultrastructurally occur in macropods (kangaroos and quokkas) and chimpanzees. The small, self-limiting lesions are easily overlooked and usually are found incidentally at autopsy or surgery. The equine lesions may be localized to the *penis, prepuce, axillary and inguinal areas, and muzzle.* Concurrent systemic disease, such as granulomatous enteritis, may predispose to more widespread distribution. Commencing as multiple, circular, smooth-surfaced, gray-white 1–2 mm papules, the lesions become umbilicated and develop a central pore from which a tiny caseous plug is extruded.

The microscopic lesions of molluscum contagiosum are highly characteristic. *Well-demarcated foci of epidermal hyperplasia and hypertrophy form pear-shaped lobules in the superficial dermis.* The individual keratinocytes are markedly swollen and contain *large intracytoplasmic inclusions known as "molluscum bodies"* (Fig. 5.82). These occur initially as eosinophilic, floccular aggregates in the cells of the inner stratum spinosum. As the keratinocytes move towards the surface, the inclusions grow in size and density, compressing the nucleus against the cytoplasmic membrane until it is a thin crescent. The inclusion becomes increasingly basophilic so that cells of the stratum corneum contain deep-purple molluscum bodies. These exfoliate through a pore that forms in the stratum corneum and enlarges into a central crater. There is usually no dermal reaction. Molluscum bodies are easily identified in cytological preparations. The inclusions contain myriads of poxvirus particles at various developmental stages, but to date no attempts have been made to culture these viruses, presumably because the diagnosis has been post-mortem.

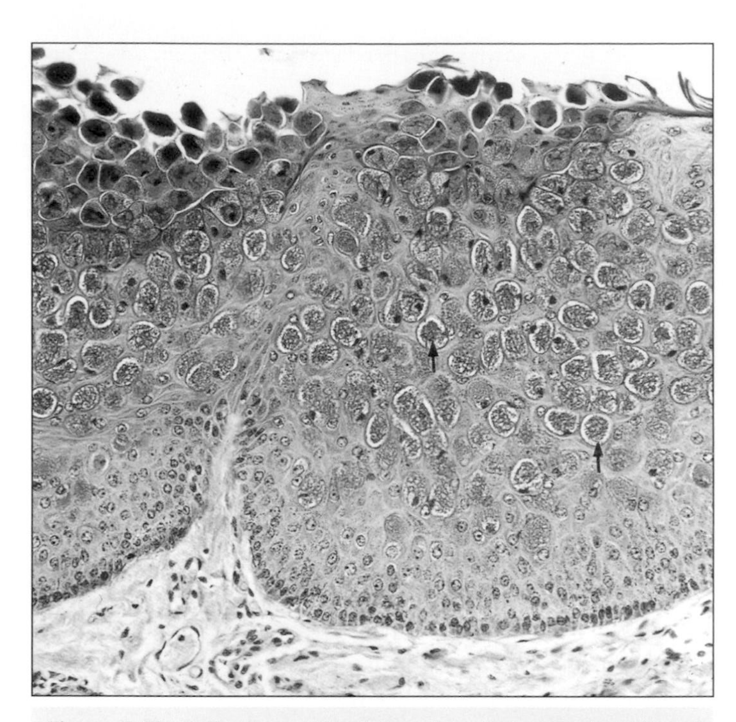

Figure 5.82 Molluscum contagiosum in a horse. Focal epidermal hyperplasia. Note large intracytoplasmic inclusion bodies referred to as "molluscum bodies" (arrows).

Bibliography

Lange L, et al. Molluscum contagiosum in three horses. J S Afr Vet Assoc 1991;62:68–71.

Porter CD, Archard LC. Characterization and physical mapping of molluscum contagiosum virus DNA and location of a sequence capable of encoding a conserved domain of epidermal growth factor. J Gen Virol 1987;68:673–682.

Thompson CH, Yager JA. Close relationship between equine and human molluscum contagiosum virus demonstrated by in situ hybridization. Res Vet Sci 1998;64:157–161.

Capripoxviral diseases

Sheeppox, goatpox and lumpy skin disease of cattle are caused by viruses of the genus *Capripoxvirus* and cause significant economic losses in countries where they are endemic. The exact relationship between these viruses has been controversial. *It is believed that they represent strains of a single virus.* The evidence includes antigenic and biochemical similarity, a high degree of nucleotide sequence homology, lack of absolute host specificity in most strains, evidence of recombination in the field, and demonstration of cross-infection and cross-protection. The viruses are indistinguishable by conventional serology; nevertheless the geographic distributions of the

3 are different indicating the viruses are distinct, and most strains of *Capripoxvirus* show definite host preferences. PCR methods of diagnosis of capripoxvirus have been developed so that classical virology methods based on live virus need not be used in areas of the world where the virus is exotic.

Bibliography

Gerson PD, Black DN. A comparison of the genomes of capripoxvirus isolates from sheep, goats and cattle. Virology 1988;164:341–349.

Heine HG, et al. A capripoxvirus detection PCR and antibody ELISA based on the major antigen p32, the homologue of the vaccinia virus H3L gene. J Immunol Methods 1999;227:187–196.

Kitching RP, et al. The characterisation of African strains of capripoxvirus. Epidem Infect 1989;102:335–343.

Sheeppox

Sheeppox is the most serious of the pox diseases of domestic animals. It exists in Africa, Asia, and the Middle East where, despite attempts at vaccination, it is responsible for cycles of epidemic disease followed by periods of endemic maintenance with low morbidity. The disease is exotic to the Americas, Australia, and New Zealand. Eradication measures eliminated the disease from Britain in the mid-19th century but have only recently been successful in Eastern European countries. *Sheeppox causes extensive economic loss* through high mortality, reduced meat, milk or wool yields, commercial inhibitions from quarantine requirements, and the cost of disease prevention programs.

Transmission of infection is by direct contact with diseased sheep or indirect contact via contaminated environment. Insect transmission has been demonstrated experimentally. *Sheeppox virus* is resistant to desiccation and remains viable for up to 2 months on wool or 6 months in dried crust. There are breed differences in disease susceptibility. Fine-wooled Merino sheep are particularly sensitive whereas breeds native to endemic areas, such as Algerian sheep, are comparatively resistant. Sheeppox occurs in all ages of sheep with high morbidity, and mortality as high as 50%; but the disease is most severe in lambs, with mortality reaching 80–100%. A high level of background immunity, such as occurs in endemic areas of Kenya, is associated with low mortality, even in the young.

Sheeppox is a *systemic disease*. Infection is usually by the respiratory route but may occur through skin abrasions. The incubation period is 4–7 days and is followed by a leukocyte-associated viremia. The virus localizes in many organs including the skin where the virus concentration is highest 10–14 days postinfection. The initial clinical signs are fever, lacrimation, drooling, serous nasal discharge, and hyperesthesia. Skin lesions, which develop 1–2 days later, have a predilection for the sparsely wooled areas and typically involve eyelids, cheeks, nostrils, vulva, udder, scrotum, prepuce, ventral surface of the tail, and medial thigh.

The macroscopic lesions follow the typical pattern for pox infections. *Sheeppox lesions have a prominent vesicular stage* (Fig. 5.83A, B). The vesicles are umbilicated and, being multilocular, yield only a small amount of fluid if punctured. Occasionally a large vesicle forms as a result of cleavage of necrotic epidermis from underlying dermis. The *pustule stage* is characterized by the formation of a thin crust. In severely affected animals, the lesions coalesce.

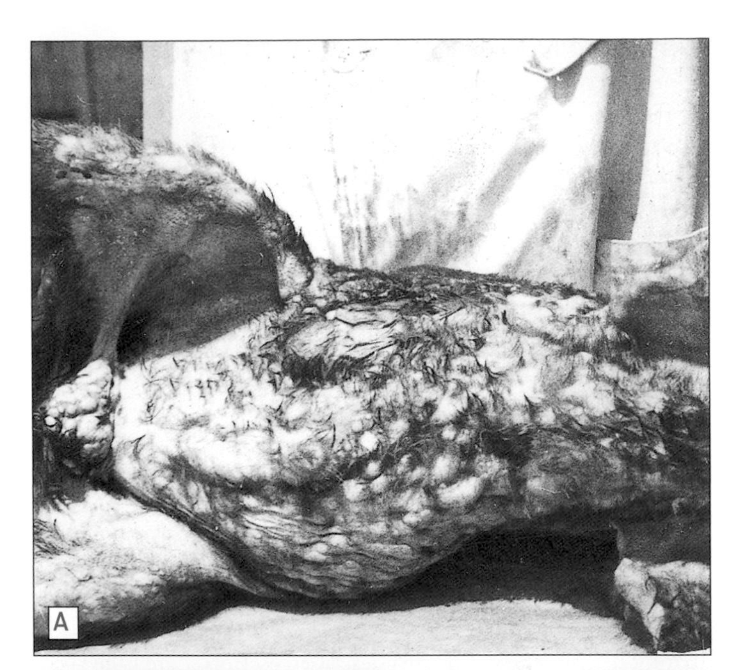

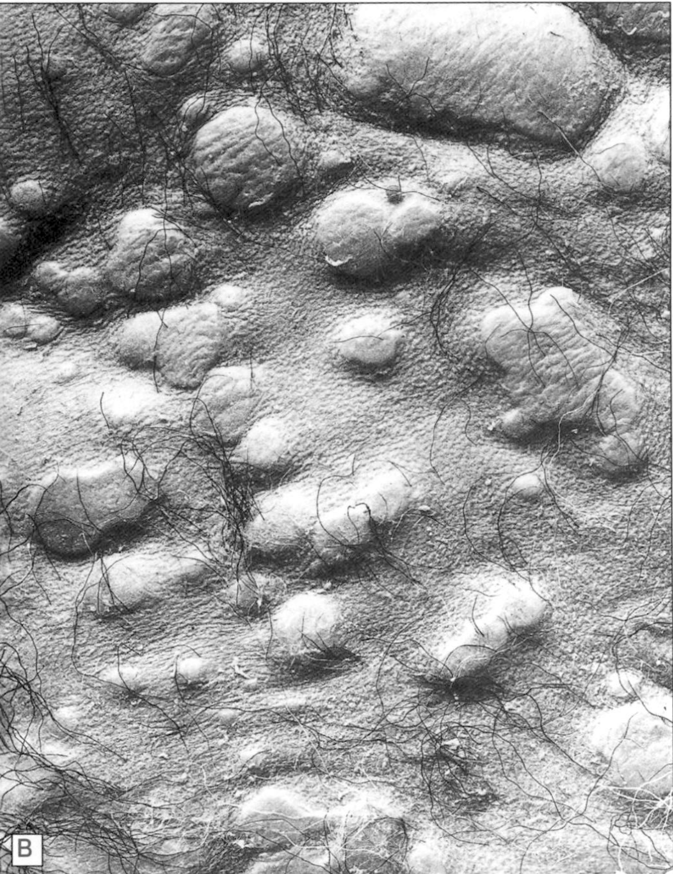

Figure 5.83 Sheeppox. (Courtesy of X Ivanov). **A.** Disseminated irregular swellings involving ventral abdomen and scrotum **B.** Close-up of papules.

There may be marked, gelatinous dermal edema. Highly susceptible animals often develop hemorrhagic papules early in the course of the disease and, later, ulcerative lesions in the gastrointestinal and respiratory tracts. Approximately one-third of animals develop multiple pulmonary lesions that comprise *foci of pulmonary consolidation*.

The kidneys have multifocal, circular, fleshy nodules throughout the renal cortices.

Healing of the skin lesions is slow, taking up to 6 weeks and a scar may remain. In the milder form of the disease, seen in endemic areas, the full range of pox lesions does not develop. Instead, epidermal proliferation produces papules covered by scale-crust, which heal with desquamation in a few days. Such lesions often occur on the ventral surface of the tail.

Sheeppox lesions have the typical epithelial changes for the group, including marked vacuolar degeneration of stratum spinosum keratinocytes, microvesiculation, eosinophilic intracytoplasmic inclusion bodies, and epidermal hyperplasia. The lesions affect both surface epithelium and that of the hair follicles. There are, in addition, *marked dermal lesions* reflecting the systemic route of cutaneous involvement and possibly implicating immune-mediated lesions in addition to those caused by direct viral damage. The initial dermal lesions, corresponding to the macroscopic erythematous macule, are marked edema, hyperemia and neutrophilic exocytosis. During the papular stage, large numbers of mononuclear cells accumulate in the increasingly edematous dermis. These cells, first described by Borrel, are called "cellules claveleuses" or "*sheeppox cells*" and are characteristic of the disease. The nuclei of sheeppox cells are vacuolated and have marginated chromatin. The vacuolated cytoplasm contains single, occasionally multiple, *eosinophilic intracytoplasmic inclusion bodies*. Sheeppox cells are virus-infected monocytes, macrophages and fibroblasts, but not endothelial cells. Approximately 10 days post-infection and corresponding with the most prominent epithelial lesions and peak of skin infectivity, severe necrotizing vasculitis develops in arterioles and post-capillary venules. Virus particles have not been identified in endothelial cells, and the vasculitis may be due to immune-complex deposition. Ischemic necrosis of the dermis and overlying epidermis follows.

The pulmonary lesions are proliferative alveolitis and bronchiolitis with focal areas of caseous necrosis. Alveolar septal cells contain intracytoplasmic inclusion bodies. Additional histologic lesions, characterized by the accumulation of sheeppox cells, may involve heart, kidney, liver, adrenals, thyroid and pancreas.

The course and outcome of sheeppox depend not only on the usual host-virus relationship but also on the nature and location of secondary infections. The virus itself may cause death during the febrile, eruptive phase of the disease. Of great importance, however, are the secondary bacterial infections that rapidly develop in the necrotic tissue of the pocks. Death is often due to bacterial septicemia or pneumonia.

Goatpox

Goatpox, caused by *Goatpox virus*, occurs in North Africa and the Middle East. A benign form of goatpox occurs in California and Sweden. The clinical signs of goatpox vary in different geographic areas. The disease has *many parallels with sheeppox, but is generally milder* with a low mortality rate (5%), although generalized eruption with mortality rates approaching 100% may occur. The cutaneous lesions have a predilection for the same areas as for sheeppox. In nursing kids, lesions may appear on the buccal mucosa or rostral nares. In animals with higher levels of resistance, the lesions may be confined to the udder, teats, inner aspects of thighs or ventral surface of the tail.

Bibliography

Garner MG, et al. The extent and impact of sheep pox and goat pox in the state of Maharashtra, India. Trop Anim Health Prod 2000;32:205–223.

Gulbahar MY, et al. Immunohistochemical detection of antigen in lamb tissues naturally infected with sheeppox virus. J Vet Med B Infect Dis Vet Public Health 2000;47:173–181.

Kitching RP, Mellor PS. Insect transmission of capripoxvirus. Res Vet Sci 1986;40:255–258.

Rao TV, Bandyopadhyay SK. A comprehensive review of goat pox and sheep pox and their diagnosis. Anim Health Res Rev 2000;1:127–136.

Lumpy skin disease

Lumpy skin disease, caused by *Lumpy skin disease virus* of the *Capripoxvirus* genus, is a disease of cattle, buffalo, and occasionally other wild species of hoofstock, characterized by the *eruption of multiple, well-circumscribed skin nodules, accompanied by fever, ventral edema, and generalized lymphadenopathy*. Lumpy-skin disease is found throughout the African continent and Madagascar, with sporadic reports from the Middle East and Israel.

Cattle of all ages, sex and breeds are affected, although the disease is more severe in Channel Island breeds. Both *Bos indicus* and *Bos taurus* cattle are susceptible, however the disease can be less clinically severe in Zebu breeds. The disease occurs in epidemics – a notable one in 1944 affected 8 million cattle. Infection is transmitted mechanically by a variety of biting insects. Epidemics tend to follow periods of prolonged rainfall, which favor population increases in vector species. A forest maintenance cycle, probably involving Cape buffalo, is thought to be the reservoir of infection in the inter-epidemic periods. No reservoir host apart from cattle has been identified.

The morbidity is extremely variable and inapparent infection is not uncommon. *Mortality is usually low*; around 1% but may be >50%. Economic losses are due to debilitation, loss of milk and meat production, damage to hides, and reproductive wastage due to fever-associated abortions and temporary sterility in bulls.

The natural incubation period of lumpy-skin disease is 2–4 weeks, but this may be halved in experimental infection. In severely affected animals, the development of large numbers of cutaneous lesions over most of the body is preceded by fever, marked weight loss, profuse drooling, oculonasal discharge, ventral edema and generalized lymphadenopathy. In the mild disease, there may be few isolated nodules and no prodromal fever. *The cutaneous lesions are firm, circumscribed, flat-topped nodules 0.5–5.0 cm in diameter* (Fig. 5.84). They may coalesce. The nodules have a creamy-gray color on cut section and involve the full width of the cutis, extending into the subcutis and occasionally adjacent muscles. Nodules affecting the scrotum, perineum, udder, vulva, glans penis, eyelids and conjunctiva are usually flatter, and in non-pigmented tissue are surrounded by a zone of intense hyperemia. *The fate of the nodules varies. Typically, they undergo central necrosis and sequestration, but some may resolve rapidly and completely, and others may fail to separate but, instead, become indurated and persist as hard intradermal lumps for many months.* Sequestration is preceded by central necrosis in the nodule and occurs rapidly. Separation of the epidermis around the margin of the nodule exposes a rim of dermal granulation tissue. As the process of separation extends into the dermis, the nodule comes to contain a *core or sequestrum of*

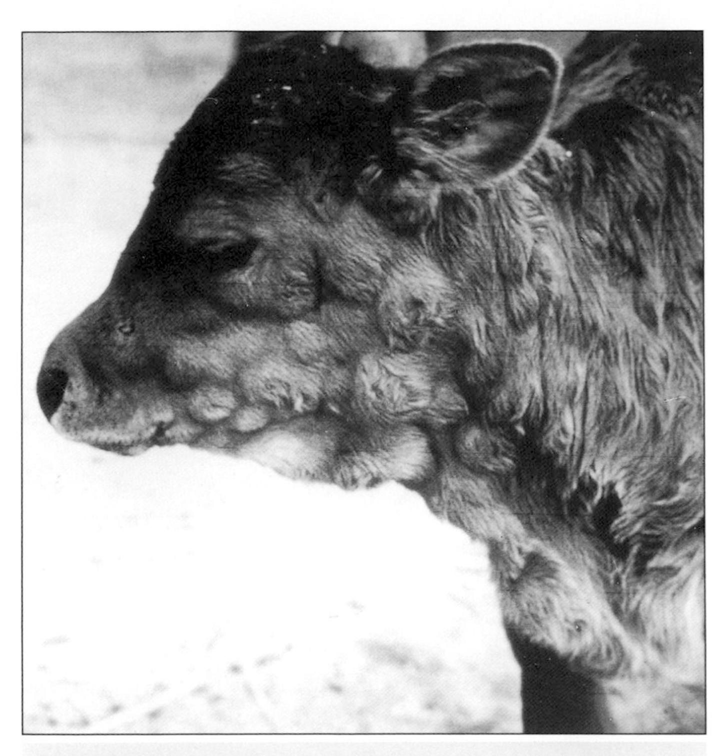

Figure 5.84 Circumscribed, nodular lesions of the skin in **lumpy skin disease** in a calf. (Courtesy of CC Brown.)

necrotic material ("sit-fast"), which is cone-shaped and flat-topped. When the sequestrum is removed, a deep ulcer remains which is slowly filled with granulation tissue. *Secondary bacterial infections* develop in the necrotic cores of the nodules and contribute very significantly to the seriousness of the disease. Large craterous ulcers develop which lead to lymphangitis and lymphadenitis. Local extension of lesions causes blindness, tenosynovitis, arthritis or mastitis.

The mucous membranes of the upper respiratory and upper alimentary tracts often develop multiple, discrete ulcerative lesions, irrespective of the number of cutaneous nodules. Those in the respiratory tract may cause swelling sufficient to result in severe dyspnea and asphyxia. Aspiration may lead to pneumonia or, if the animal recovers, scarring may cause stenosis of the cranial portion of the trachea. Nodules occasionally occur in parenchymal organs including kidneys, lungs and testes.

Although the virus is introduced percutaneously, *the infection is systemic*. A leukocyte-associated viremia disseminates the virus to various tissues, including the skin where greatest virus concentration occurs 9–12 days postinfection. The virus infects a wide range of cells, including keratinocytes, mucous and serous glandular epithelium, fibrocytes, skeletal muscle, macrophages, pericytes, and endothelial cells. *Damage to endothelial cells causes vasculitis that is central to the pathogenesis of the lumpy-skin disease lesions.*

Acute lesions consist of vasculitis, lymphangitis, thrombosis, marked dermal edema that sometimes induces dermoepidermal separation, and infarction. The epidermis shows the typical vacuolar changes associated with poxvirus infection. *Intracytoplasmic, eosinophilic, homogeneous, and occasionally granular, inclusion bodies* occur in endothelial cells, pericytes, keratinocytes, macrophages and fibroblasts. Virions in various stages of development are present in these inclusion-containing cells and in peripheral nerves. Neutrophils, macrophages and occasionally eosinophils migrate into the dermis in the acute lesions to be replaced as the lesion ages by a predominantly mononuclear cell population. The infarcted tissue is sequestered and surrounded by granulation tissue. Inclusion bodies are absent from the resolving lesions but may be present in adjacent skin or sebaceous glands. Lymph nodes are edematous and hyperplastic.

The chief differential diagnosis is **pseudo-lumpy skin disease** *caused by a herpesvirus identical to the bovine herpes mammillitis virus but originally known as the Allerton virus.* Pseudo-lumpy skin disease is a milder condition clinically and the nodules are superficial, resembling only the early stage of lumpy-skin disease. Confirmation of the latter is best achieved by demonstration of poxvirus particles in fresh or formalin fixed tissue.

Bibliography

Greth A, et al. Capripoxvirus disease in an Arabian oryx (*Oryx leucoryx*) from Saudi Arabia. J Wildl Dis 1992;28:295–300.

Hunter P, Wallace D. Lumpy skin disease in southern Africa: a review of the disease and aspects of control. J S Afr Vet Assoc 2001;72:68–71.

Tulman ER, et al. Genome of lumpy skin disease virus. J Virol 2001;75:7122–7130.

Yeruham I, et al. Spread of lumpy skin disease in Israeli dairy herds. Vet Rec 1995;137:91–93.

Suipoxviral disease

Swinepox

The host-specific *Swinepox virus*, the sole member of genus *Suipoxvirus*, is the chief cause of pox lesions in swine. In the past, *Vaccinia virus* was also responsible. The disease occurs worldwide and is endemic in areas of intensive swine production. The disease has received relatively little attention as it is *usually mild and mortality is negligible. It chiefly affects young, growing piglets* but occurs in neonates promoting speculation that transplacental infection may be possible. Normally, *swinepox virus* is transmitted by contact. The virus is resistant and persists in dried crust from infected animals. The sucking louse *Haematopinus suis* often acts as a mechanical vector and also assists infection by causing skin trauma. *The gross lesions typically affect the ventral and lateral abdomen, lateral thorax, and medial foreleg and thigh* (Fig. 5.85A). Occasionally, lesions on the dorsum predominate. In severe infection, lesions may be generalized and rarely involve the oral cavity, pharynx, esophagus, stomach, trachea and bronchi. The morphology of the gross lesions follows the typical pattern of pox infection. The erythematous papules usually transform into umbilicated pustules without a significant vesicular stage. The inflammatory crust eventually sheds to leave a white macule. *Grossly, swinepox must be differentiated from the vesicular diseases, classical swine fever, pityriasis rosea, dermatosis vegetans, and sunburn.*

The histologic lesions also follow the pattern for pox infections (Fig. 5.85B). The eosinophilic, intracytoplasmic inclusion bodies are quite transient and are not found in older lesions. Vacuoles develop in the nuclei of infected stratum spinosum keratinocytes early in the course of swinepox infection.

Vaccinia virus causes lesions in swine that are clinically difficult to differentiate from *Swinepox virus* infection. However with the eradication of smallpox and the cessation of smallpox vaccination, swinepox is now the primary poxviral disease of swine. Vaccinia viral infections have a shorter incubation period and smaller, more

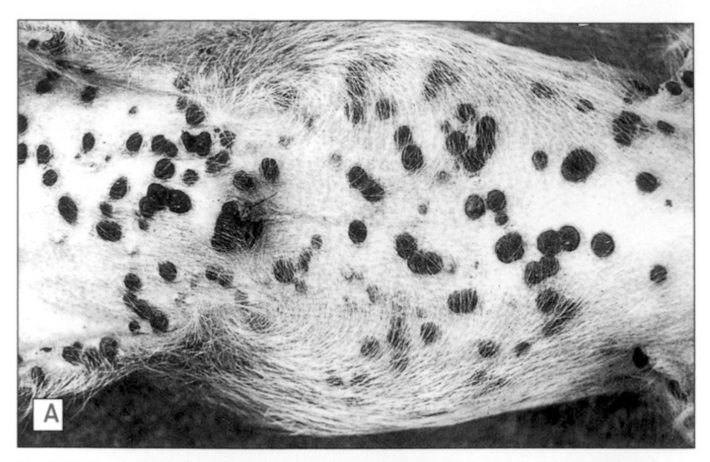

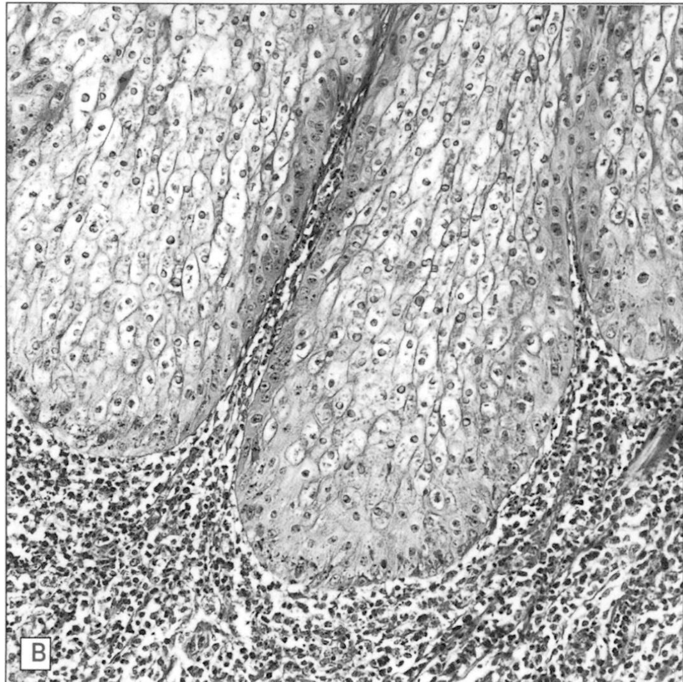

Figure 5.85 Swinepox. A. Gross lesions on ventral body. **B.** Marked acanthosis and intracellular edema and diffuse dermatitis.

transient lesions. Histologically the lesions are very similar except that nuclear vacuoles are not observed. The diseases are definitively differentiated only by virological examination.

Bibliography

Afonso CL, et al. The genome of swinepox virus. J Virol 2002;76:783–790.

Garg SK, et al. Swinepox. Vet Bull 1989;59:441–448.

Massung RF, Moyer RW. The molecular biology of swinepox. II. The infectious cycle. Virology 1991;180:355–364.

Thibault S, et al. Congenital swinepox: a sporadic skin disorder in nursing piglets. Swine Health Production 1998;6:276–278.

Herpesviral infections

The Herpesviridae is a large family of *enveloped DNA viruses* responsible for important animal diseases, of which relatively few are primary skin diseases. *Bovine herpesvirus 2* causes primary cutaneous infections and is widespread in many parts of the world. It is responsible for 2 distinct clinical forms of skin disease; *bovine mammillitis of cattle*, which is the major cutaneous infection, and *pseudo-lumpy skin disease*. Skin lesions occur in systemic herpesvirus infections such as *malignant catarrhal fever*, and *infectious bovine rhinotracheitis* in cattle, and *pseudorabies* in pigs. Skin lesions associated with *Felid herpesvirus 1* infection are also recognized, usually in the absence of respiratory lesions. Vesicles, pustules, ulcers and depigmentation are seen on the genital organs and occasionally the lips and nostrils of horses with *Equid herpesvirus 3* infection (equine coital exanthema), and in *Bovine herpesvirus 1* infectious vulvovaginitis and balanoposthitis.

Bibliography

Ezura K. Gastrointestinal and skin lesions in piglets naturally infected with pseudorabies virus. J Vet Diagn Invest 1995;7:451–455.

Fenner F, et al. Veterinary Virology. 2nd ed. San Diego, CA: Academic Press, 1993.

Bovine herpesvirus 2 diseases

Pseudo-lumpy skin disease

Bovine herpesvirus 2 (BoHV2) is a member of the Alphaherpesvirinae subfamily and is antigenically related to human Herpes simplex virus 1. First isolated in Africa in 1957 from lesions resembling lumpy-skin disease, it was named the *Allerton virus*. The associated disease was subsequently named "pseudo-lumpy skin disease" to differentiate it from the more serious disease caused by *Lumpy skin disease virus*. Pseudo-lumpy skin disease is widespread in southern Africa with sporadic reports from Australia, the UK, and the USA. It is characterized by a generalized eruption of superficial cutaneous nodules that develop a central depression but that heal without scar formation and do not produce the deep necrotic sequestra of true lumpy skin disease.

Bibliography

d'Offay JM, et al. Use of a polymerase chain reaction assay to detect bovine herpesvirus type 2 DNA in skin lesions from cattle suspected to have pseudo-lumpy skin disease. J Am Vet Med Assoc 2003;222:1404–1407.

Woods JA, et al. Isolation of bovine herpesvirus-2 (BHV-2) from a case of pseudo-lumpy skin disease in the United Kingdom. Vet Rec 1996;138:113–114.

Bovine herpes mammillitis

Bovine herpes mammillitis, or ulcerative mammillitis, is a localized form of BoHV2 infection seen sporadically in the USA, Canada, Great Britain, Europe, Africa, and Australia. Serological surveys indicate that *infection is much more common than disease*. In Africa and Asia, several species of wild animals have antibody titers to the virus, although clinical disease is not seen.

Herpes mammillitis is *chiefly a disease of lactating dairy cows* but occurs in heifers about to calve and in beef animals. The incidence is usually sporadic with occasional local epidemics in fully susceptible herds. In previously exposed herds, the disease affects only the recently introduced nonimmune, first-calf heifers. There is no mortality. The economic significance of teat lesions lies in the effect on milk production or secondary bacterial mastitis, which complicate ~20% of cases.

Intact teat skin is refractory to virus penetration, indicating that *some form of teat trauma precedes infection*. Transmission of the virus is presumed to involve mechanical vectors, particularly the milking machine, but biting flies, such as *Stomoxys calcitrans*, have also been implicated. In the latter instance, it is difficult to explain the localization of lesions to the teat and mammary gland. Local tissue temperature has, however, been shown to be critical in the pathogenesis, and environmental conditions have been associated with the incidence of outbreaks. Experimental cutaneous inoculation of BoHV2 results in higher virus titers and larger and more persistent lesions when the site is kept cold. The increased prevalence of disease in the autumn months may also relate to the temperature sensitivity of the virus. The source of infection within a herd is not known, but latency, a characteristic of the Herpesviridae, is likely important. Latency has been demonstrated in experimental BoHV2 infections.

The macroscopic lesions affect the teats, less frequently the udder and occasionally the perineum of lactating cows. Transmission of infection to nursing calves may result in ulcerative lesions of the muzzle, chin, lips, and occasionally the oral cavity. Teat lesions develop after a 3–7-day incubation period. *The teat becomes very swollen and painful and develops 1–2 cm diameter plaques.* Vesicles are rare. The epidermis in the center of the plaque becomes necrotic and sloughs to expose an erythematous, irregularly shaped ulcer. Exuded serum mixed with blood forms a thin brown crust, which is easily displaced by the teat cups. The lesions heal beneath the crust and there is no residual scar. Lesions on the udder are often diffuse, giving rise to the term "gangrene of the udder." Regional lymph nodes are swollen in the early stages.

The microscopic lesions are characterized by the formation of epithelial syncytia containing prominent intranuclear eosinophilic inclusion bodies. The inclusion bodies are typical Cowdry type A. The nuclear chromatin is marginated and the eosinophilic inclusions are surrounded by a clear halo. The inclusions are numerous from the time of the first macroscopic lesion until the fifth day. Thereafter, they are very difficult to find. Syncytial cell formation commences early in groups of cells in the stratum basale and inner stratum spinosum. The process extends to involve the full thickness of the epidermis, the outer root sheath of the hair follicle infundibulum, and the sebaceous gland. By day 5 after macroscopic lesions develop, the epidermis is necrotic, although the outlines of syncytial cells are apparent. The inclusion bodies lose their sharp outline and fill the entire nucleus. Some are free in the necrotic epidermis, released from fragmenting nuclei. The necrotic epidermis and adnexa are infiltrated with large numbers of neutrophils. Loss of the necrotic epithelium leaves an ulcer, which is covered by hemorrhagic and fibrinous exudate and a band of degenerating neutrophils. Deeper, there is dermal edema and a predominantly mononuclear cell infiltrate. In the healed lesion, the epithelium is re-established; there is superficial dermal fibrosis, and a perivascular infiltrate of predominantly mononuclear cells.

The diagnosis of herpes mammillitis is confirmed by isolation of the virus. A rapid provisional diagnosis may be made by examining clinical material by electron microscopy. Biopsy is diagnostic if lesions are collected before the fifth day. Cytology smears prepared from an early lesion are diagnostic if syncytial cells containing eosinophilic intranuclear inclusion bodies are found. Serological tests allow a retrospective diagnosis provided paired samples are collected and a rising titer identified.

Experimental intravenous inoculation of **sheep** with BoHV2 results in lesions resembling those of similarly inoculated cattle. Naturally occurring outbreaks of dermatitis of the pasterns caused by BoHV2 have been described in captive Dahl sheep. Goats will only develop skin lesions following intravenous inoculation.

Bibliography

Bhat MN, et al. Serological evidence of bovine herpesvirus 1 and 2 in Asian elephants. J Wildl Dis 1997;33:919–920.

Gibbs EPJ, et al. Experimental study of the epidemiology of bovine herpes mammillitis. Res Vet Sci 1973;14:139–144.

Janett F, et al. Bovine herpes mammillitis: clinical symptoms and serologic course. Schweiz Arch Tierheilkd 2000;142:375–380.

Letchworth GJ, Carmichael LE. Local tissue temperature: a critical factor in the pathogenesis of bovine herpesvirus 2. Infect Immun 1984;43:1072–1079.

O'Connor M. Meteorological features associated with outbreaks of bovine herpes mammillitis in Ireland. Irish Vet J 1995;48:71–80.

Westbury HA. Infection of sheep and goats with bovid herpesvirus 2. Res Vet Sci 1981;31:353–357.

Bovine herpesvirus 4 diseases

A strain of *Bovine herpesvirus 4* (BoHV-4) can cause udder lesions on dairy cows (**mammary pustular dermatitis**); the teats are not involved. The macroscopic lesions are *vesicles, pustules, ulcers and crusts*, originally 2–4 mm in diameter, becoming larger with coalescence. The microscopic lesion is *intraepidermal pustular dermatitis*. The etiologic association between BoHV-4 and the cutaneous disease is controversial however, as the virus is an ubiquitous herpesvirus of cattle that can produce no disease when experimentally inoculated into susceptible cattle and can be isolated from cell cultures prepared from clinically normal cattle. While not a primary mastitis pathogen, BoHV-4 may prolong cases of bacterial mastitis. BoHV-4 infection is considered a risk factor for abortion in cows, and is reported as a cause of endometritis in postparturient dairy cows.

Bibliography

Frazier K, et al. Endometritis in postparturient cattle associated with bovine herpesvirus-4 infection: 15 cases. J Vet Diagn Invest 2001;13:502–508.

Kalman D, et al. Role of bovine herpesvirus 4 in bacterial bovine mastitis. Microb Pathog 2004;37:125–129.

Osorio FA, Reed DE. Experimental inoculation of cattle with bovine herpesvirus-4: evidence for a lymphoid-associated persistent infection. Am J Vet Res 1983; 44:980.

Thiry E, et al. The biology of bovine herpesvirus-4. Ann Med Vet 1992;136:617–624.

Felid herpesvirus 1

Felid herpesvirus 1 (FeHV-1, Feline viral rhinotracheitis virus), a well recognized pathogen of the upper respiratory tract, is commonly associated with oral ulceration. It can also be associated with *focal ulcerative lesions primarily on the haired skin of the face or on the nasal planum*, with rare reports of lesions on the feet and trunk. The lesions generally occur in the absence of clinical respiratory signs. In common with other herpesviruses, FeHV-1 can establish latency in the trigeminal ganglion. As affected cats often have a history of previous respiratory disease or recent stress, recrudescence of a latent herpesvirus infection is likely. *The macroscopic lesions consist of crusts, ulcers, and vesicles, frequently on the face or nasal planum, which can be persistent or recurrent* (Fig. 5.86A). Microscopically, the lesions are

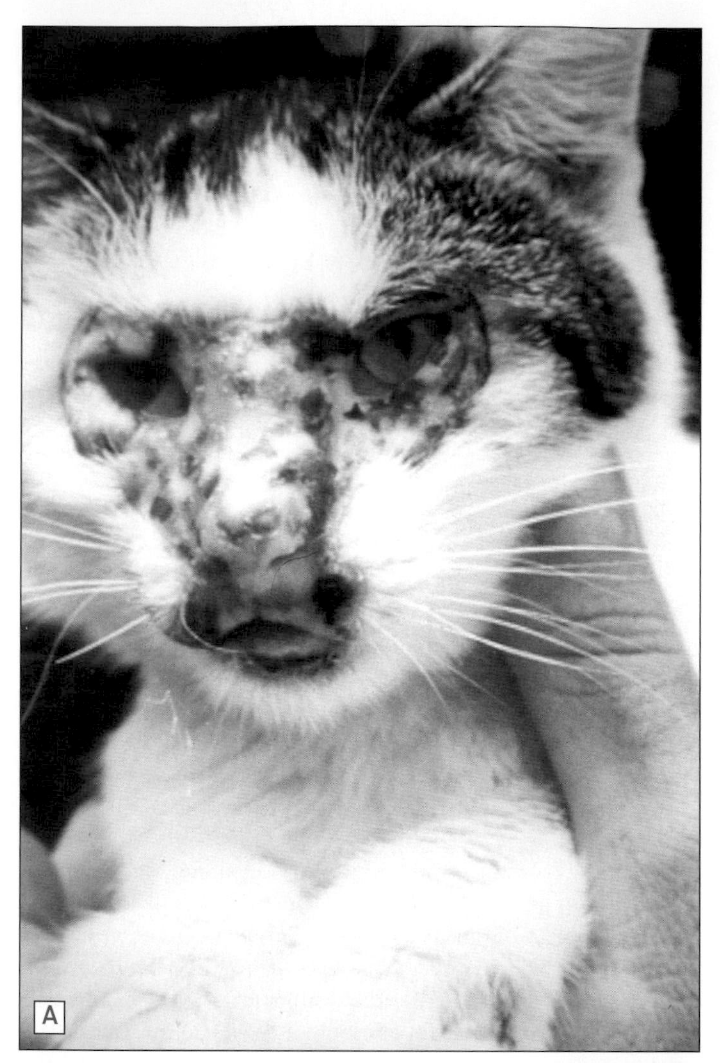

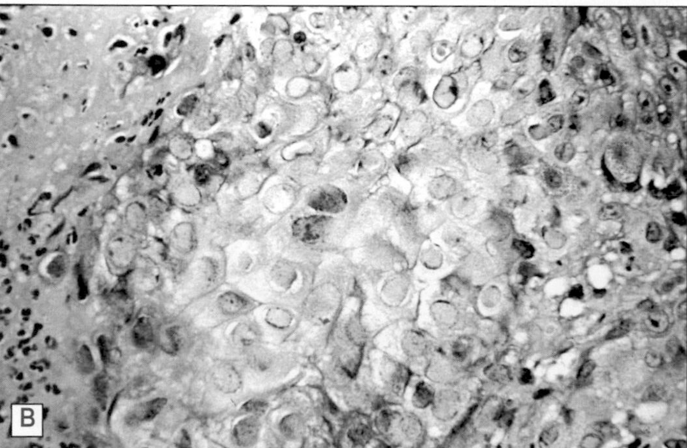

Figure 5.86 Feline herpesvirus dermatitis. A. Marked ulceration and crusting lesions of the face. (Courtesy of University of Florida Clinical Dermatology Service.) **B.** Note marked intracellular edema and **intranuclear inclusions** within keratinocytes.

ulcerative and necrotizing, and the mixed dermal inflammation frequently includes numerous eosinophils. Adnexae can be destroyed and free keratin in the dermis is associated with eosinophils and foci of collagen degeneration. *Large amphophilic or glassy intranuclear inclusions* are present in the surface and adnexal epithelium (Fig. 5.86B). They are variable in number and sometimes hard to find in small rafts of epithelial cells surrounded by necrotic debris. The similarity of the inflammatory component in this condition with that of the feline hypersensitivity conditions, such as mosquito bite hypersensitivity or feline eosinophilic ulcer, warrants close scrutiny of eosinophilic necrotizing cutaneous lesions for intranuclear inclusions or examination by molecular techniques.

Bibliography

Hargis AM, et al. Ulcerative facial and nasal dermatitis and stomatitis in cats associated with feline herpesvirus 1. Vet Dermatol 1999;10:267–274.

Nasisse MP, et al. Isolation of feline herpesvirus 1 from the trigeminal ganglia of acutely and chronically infected cats. J Vet Intern Med 1992;6:102–103.

Suchy A, et al. Diagnosis of feline herpesvirus infection by immunohistochemistry, polymerase chain reaction, and in situ hybridization. J Vet Diagn Invest 2000;12:186–191.

Retroviral infections

Several skin disorders have been associated with retroviral infections caused by ***Feline leukemia virus*** (FeLV) and ***Feline immunodeficiency virus*** (FIV) in **cats**. Since both viruses are immunosuppressive, *most dermatological conditions are considered secondary*. However, primary viral infection of keratinocytes has been reported. Scaling, crusting and alopecic lesions affecting primarily the head and face with occasional involvement of trunk and extremities is seen uncommonly in FeLV-infected cats. Histologically, syncytial keratinocytes are seen in the epidermis and superficial follicular epithelium, accompanied by dyskeratosis, pustules, and ulcers. Immunohistochemical staining demonstrates FeLV antigen in epithelial cells and giant cells. In addition, cutaneous keratin horns seen in FeLV-infected cats have been represented as a primary effect of viral infection of keratinocytes. Recurrent pyoderma and paronychia have been attributed to the immunosuppressive effects of FeLV. Bacterial skin disease affecting the face and cellulitis associated with ear tags are described in the acute stage of experimental FIV infection in specific-pathogen-free kittens. Dermatological diseases associated with naturally occurring chronic FIV infection include generalized demodectic mange, notoedric mange, cowpoxvirus infections, pustular pyoderma, atypical mycobacteriosis, miliary dermatitis and abscesses. Cats that are FIV-positive are more frequently diagnosed as having subcutaneous abscesses and cellulitis than are noninfected cats. Since the virus is shed in high titer in the saliva, and bite wounds are thought to be an important mode of transmission, this finding may simply reflect a greater tendency for cats that fight to become FIV-positive. Many of the associations made between retroviral infection and specific diseases are anecdotal.

Bibliography

Fleming EJ, et al. Clinical, hematologic, and survival data from cats infected with feline immunodeficiency virus (1983–1988). J Am Vet Med Assoc 1991; 199:913–916.

Gross TL, et al. Giant cell dermatosis in FeLV-positive cats. Vet Dermatol 1993;4:117–122.

Merchant SR, Taboada J. Systemic diseases with cutaneous manifestations. Vet Clin North Am Small Anim Pract 1995;25:945–959.

Parvoviral infections

More typically associated with reproductive problems, ***Porcine parvovirus*** (PPV) has been implicated in outbreaks of vesicular and ulcerative dermatitis and glossitis in 1–4-week-old piglets in the midwestern USA. Various clinical signs, including diarrhea and sneezing, accompanied the skin lesions. *Small slit-like erosions, ruptured vesicles, and extensive ulceration were seen on the tongue, lips, snout, coronary band and interdigital spaces.* Severe lesions sometimes led to separation and sloughing of the hoof wall. Intact vesicles were seen rarely. Sporadic cases have been reported in which the lesions were exudative rather than ulcerative. They were grossly indistinguishable from those of exudative epidermitis. PPV has been cultured from skin and internal organs of affected piglets and PPV antigen has been detected in hair follicles of lesional skin. Skin lesions were reproduced with tissue culture-origin PPV, but were not as severe as those induced with crude suspensions prepared from the skin lesions. In the sporadic cases, *Staphylococcus* spp. and *Swinepox virus* were also recovered. It is likely that the severe clinical disease results from dual bacterial and viral infection.

Bibliography

Lager KM, Mengeling WL. Porcine parvovirus associated with cutaneous lesions in piglets. J Vet Diagn Invest 1994;6:357–359.

Whitaker HK, et al. Parvovirus infection in pigs with exudative skin disease. J Vet Diagn Invest 1990;2:244–246.

Papillomaviral infections

Papillomaviruses are associated with a variety of proliferative skin lesions, typically benign epithelial neoplasms, although they have also been shown to be associated with proliferative cutaneous plaques and papules. Although these lesions are almost always benign and often self-limiting, there is evidence that in some cases, both in humans and animals, the virus can be a factor in the development of malignant tumors. Papillomaviruses tend to be species-specific viruses that affect stratified squamous epithelium in all domestic, and numerous wildlife, species. Papillomavirus-associated lesions are discussed under Tumors of the epidermis.

BACTERIAL DISEASES OF SKIN

Normal skin of healthy individuals is highly resistant to invasion by bacteria due to natural defense mechanisms, consisting of physical, chemical, and microbial components. The stratum corneum is composed of tightly packed keratinized cells and intercellular substance derived from lamellar granules that form an impermeable physical barrier. Furthermore, this layer continually desquamates and any adherent bacteria are lost as the outer cells are shed. The sebum-sweat emulsion, which spreads along the skin surface, contains a variety of antibacterial substances including fatty acids, inorganic salts, and proteins such as complement components, transferrin, and immunoglobulins. Finally, the normal skin microflora prevents pathogenic bacteria from multiplying and becoming established on the skin. These normal resident bacteria are a mixture of organisms that live in symbiosis and maintain static, consistent populations restricted to the superficial layers of the stratum corneum and hair follicle infundibula. They inhibit colonization of invading organisms by competition for limited nutrients and production of antibacterial substances. The protective effect of bacterial interference is well documented. For example, the development of exudative epidermitis has been prevented by exposing piglets to avirulent strains of *Staphylococcus hyicus*.

The normal skin flora is established shortly after birth and it is difficult subsequently to introduce other bacteria. The normal resident flora of skin has been investigated most extensively in dogs. Coagulase-negative staphylococci, *Micrococcus* spp, some aerobic gram-negative species, and *Clostridium* spp. are most numerous and are probably residents of canine skin. The presence of coagulase-positive staphylococci in the normal canine microflora is controversial. *Staphylococcus intermedius*, the most common canine skin pathogen, is commonly isolated from the anus and nares and less frequently from the skin and hair of dogs. The mucous membrane sites may act as carrier sites for seeding of the skin, where *S. intermedius* may be a transient organism taking advantage of temporary changes in local microenvironment that permit its short-term proliferation. In all species, skin surface humidity and temperature are important factors in determining the composition and density of skin microflora, with hot humid conditions being associated with increased numbers of skin bacteria. Regional variation in numbers and types of bacteria occurs, and moist intertriginous areas and oily skin have the highest numbers of bacteria.

Cutaneous bacterial infections are typically pyogenic and are thus commonly called **pyodermas**. They can be categorized as *primary and secondary* or *superficial and deep*. Primary pyodermas are those in which no underlying cause can be found. However, *it is now thought that the vast majority of pyodermas are secondary to underlying cutaneous, endocrine, or immunologic abnormalities*. Localized disruption of normal host defenses may be produced by maceration, biting ectoparasites, scratching, abrasions and other skin wounds, or introduction of foreign bodies such as plant thorns or awns; such disruption promotes development of clinical infection. Allergic, seborrheic, and follicular disorders are the most common predisposing causes of bacterial skin infection in dogs. Hypothyroidism and spontaneous and iatrogenic hyperadrenocorticism are common metabolic conditions associated with pyoderma. Primary immunologic abnormalities are uncommon predisposing factors.

Bacterial skin disease is seen much more frequently in dogs than in any other mammalian species, and pyoderma is one of the most common skin diseases in dogs. This apparent increased susceptibility of dogs to pyoderma has been attributed to the relatively thin, compact stratum corneum, the small amount of intercellular lipids in the stratum corneum, lack of a protective lipid seal at the entrance of canine hair follicles, and the relatively high pH of canine skin. *S. intermedius* is the predominant bacterial isolate from canine pyodermas. The factors that promote proliferation of *S. intermedius* on the skin and development of pyoderma are poorly understood. Pathogenicity of staphylococci in humans correlates with various proteins and toxins thought to act as virulence factors. Similarly, a role has been suggested for *S. intermedius* exotoxins (superantigens) in the pathogenesis of canine pyoderma.

Coagulase-positive staphylococci are also the most common bacteria isolated from pyoderma in horses (*S. aureus*, *S. intermedius*), in goats (*S. intermedius*, *S. aureus*), and in cattle and sheep (*S. aureus*). *Staphylococcus hyicus* causes exudative epidermitis in piglets and has been associated with superficial pyoderma in several other species.

Many other bacteria cause skin infections. *Dermatophilus congolensis* is responsible for superficial pyoderma in many species. Many gram-negative bacteria are opportunistic pathogens that can invade already diseased or compromised skin. Organisms that are typically associated with infections of other organ systems occasionally cause skin disease. *Listeria monocytogenes* has been found to be the cause of pyoderma in a small number of humans and a dog. Although bacterial infections are typically associated with neutrophilic inflammation, certain bacteria such as mycobacteria, *Actinomyces,* and *Nocardia* typically produce *granulomatous dermatitis or panniculitis*.

Bibliography

Burkett G, Frank LA. Comparison of production of *Staphylococcus intermedius* exotoxin among clinically normal dogs, atopic dogs with recurrent pyoderma, and dogs with a single episode of pyoderma. J Am Vet Med Assoc 1998;213:232–234.

Harvey RG, Lloyd DH. The distribution of bacteria (other than staphylococci and *Propionibacterium acnes*) on the hair, at the skin surface and within hair follicles of dogs. Vet Dermatol 1995;6:79–84.

Hendricks A, et al. Frequency of superantigen-producing *Staphylococcus intermedius* isolates from canine pyoderma and proliferation-inducing potential of superantigens in dogs. Res Vet Sci 2002;73:273–277.

Hill PB, Moriello KA. Canine pyoderma. J Am Vet Med Assoc 1994;204:334–340.

Lloyd D. Ecology of the skin: Balance and disruption. Compend Contin Educ Pract Vet 1997;19(suppl):97–100.

Lloyd DH, et al. Location of the microflora in the skin of cattle. Br Vet J 1979;135:519–526.

Loncarevic S, et al. A case of canine cutaneous listeriosis. Vet Dermatol 1999;10:69–71.

Mason IS, et al. A review of the biology of canine skin with respect to the commensals *Staphylococcus intermedius, Demodex canis* and *Malassezia pachydermatis*. Vet Dermatol 1996;7:119–132.

Saijonmaa-Koulumies LE, Lloyd DH. Colonization of neonatal puppies by *Staphylococcus intermedius*. Vet Dermatol 2002;13:123–130.

Superficial bacterial pyoderma

Superficial pyodermas involve the epidermis and/or superficial portion of hair follicles. They occur more commonly than deep pyodermas. Superficial pyodermas usually are of short duration, heal without scarring, and are not usually associated with systemic illness. *Gross lesions are extremely variable* and include papules, pustules, crusts, circular scaling areas of alopecia (**epidermal collarettes**) (Fig. 5.87), hyperpigmented or erythematous macules, a moth-eaten appearance to the hair coat, diffuse erythroderma, and hyperpigmented lichenified plaques. *Microscopic lesions* consist of subcorneal or loosely organized, spongiotic superficial epidermal pustules, superficial folliculitis, and crusts. Neutrophils are the predominant inflammatory cell. Bacteria are not always visible histologically and culture may be necessary to confirm the etiology.

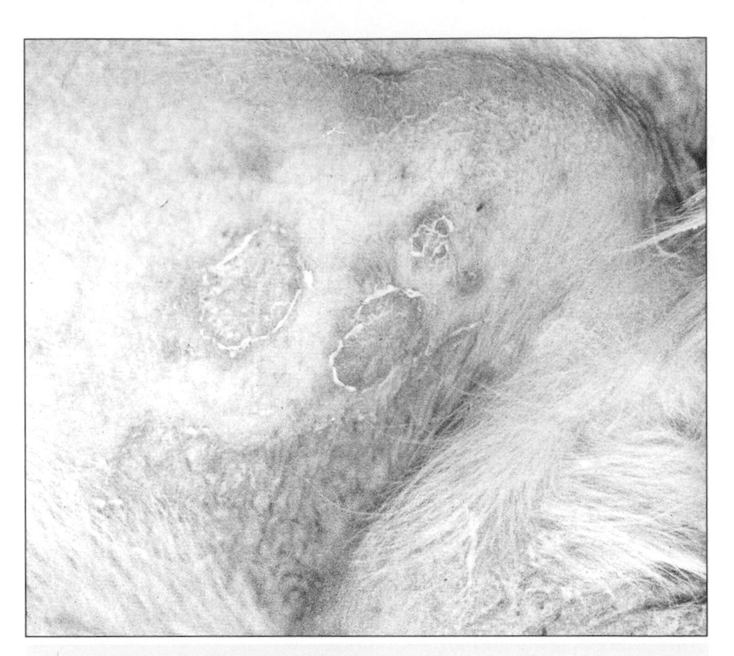

Figure 5.87 Superficial pyoderma. Annular erythematous lesions with epidermal collarette.

Impetigo

Impetigo is a superficial pustular dermatitis that does not involve hair follicles. It is most common in dogs but also occurs in kittens, piglets, cows, sheep, and goats. Impetigo is usually caused by *coagulase-positive staphylococci in association with predisposing causes*. Moist and dirty environments, cutaneous abrasions, parasitism, stress, and poor nutrition are common predisposing factors in most species. Impetigo in adult dogs is frequently seen in conjunction with diabetes mellitus, hypothyroidism, and natural or iatrogenic hyperglucocorticism. Lesions develop in young kittens as a result of excessive wetting of the skin by the queen as she transports the kittens.

The lesions begin as small erythematous papules that develop into superficial pustules (Fig. 5.88A). They are fragile and rupture easily, leaving a honey-colored crust adherent to a shallow erosion. A *bullous form of impetigo*, consisting of large flaccid pustules, is more common in adult dogs. In *puppies*, the lesions are most common on the glabrous skin of the inguinal and axillary areas. In *kittens*, the lesions are usually confined to sites which are most commonly in contact with the queen's mouth; these include the back of the neck, head, and shoulder areas. Lesions in *cows and does* are usually on the udder, especially at the base of the teats and the intermammary sulcus. Occasionally, the infection extends to involve the teats, ventral abdomen, medial thighs, perineum, and ventral surface of the tail. The lesions are infectious and may be spread by the milker to other cows or does and to the hands of milkers. One outbreak of contagious impetigo in a herd of dairy cattle was associated with crowding and intensive showering of the cows to decrease heat stress during the heat of summer.

The microscopic lesion of impetigo is a subcorneal pustule composed of neutrophils primarily (Fig. 5.88B). The pustules usually extend above the skin surface and are located between hair follicles. Bullous impetigo consists of larger pustules that span several hair follicles. Acantholysis may be mild. Gram-positive cocci are present within intact pustules. The epidermis is mildly to moderately acanthotic and variable intercellular edema is common beneath pustules. The superficial dermis is edematous and superficial perivascular to interstitial inflammation is composed of neutrophils primarily. *The principal differential diagnosis is pemphigus foliaceus.* However, in contrast to pemphigus, acantholysis is absent or minimal in impetigo and bacteria are present in intact pustules of impetigo.

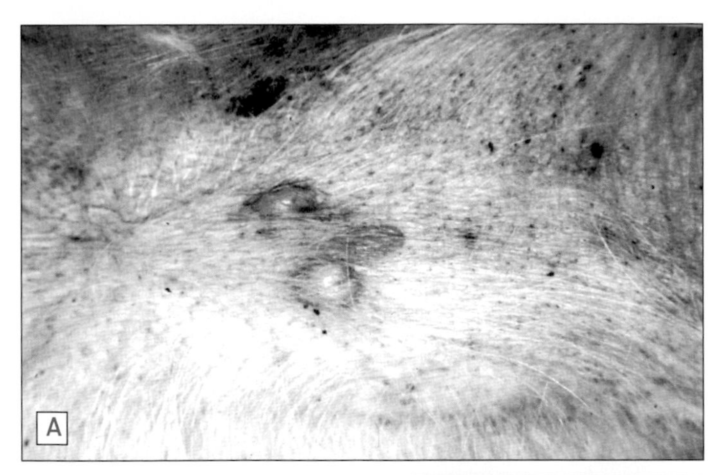

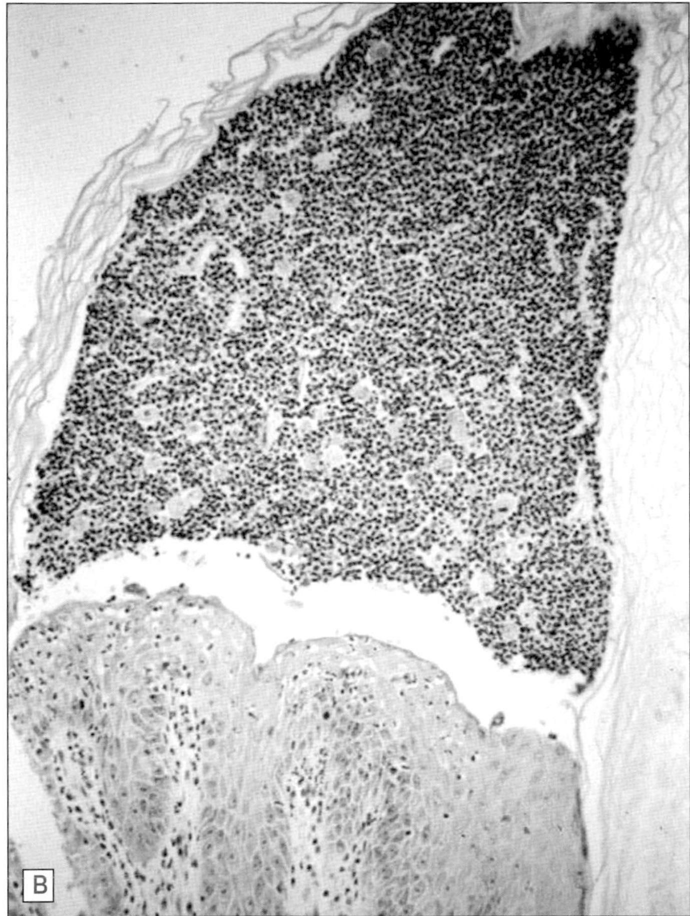

Figure 5.88 Superficial pyoderma (impetigo) in a puppy. **A.** Note pustules. (Courtesy of University of Florida Clinical Dermatology Service.) **B. Subcorneal pustule** in superficial pyoderma (impetigo).

Exudative epidermitis of pigs

Exudative epidermitis is an acute, exudative, superficial pyoderma of young pigs caused by Staphylococcus hyicus. The disease has also been called **greasy-pig disease**, impetigo contagiosa suis, and seborrhea oleosa. The infection occurs worldwide wherever intensive pig production is carried out. It is most common in *piglets 5–35 days of age*, but mild cases occur in older pigs also. The morbidity ranges from 10–90% and mortality from 5–90%. Mortality is higher in young pigs with lower resistance. Usually, when a litter is affected, all piglets develop the disease. *The infection may cause significant economic loss*; and in some countries, such as Denmark, the incidence appears to be increasing. Autogenous vaccines prepared from toxigenic strains of bacteria are used to prevent infection.

The *pathogenesis* of exudative epidermitis is incompletely understood. Both virulent and nonvirulent strains of *S. hyicus* are part of the normal skin flora of healthy pigs. The highest rates of carriage of the organism are found in the youngest piglets, suggesting that the organisms are acquired at birth. However, the presence of virulent organisms is not sufficient to produce disease. It is thought that infection develops as a result of *trauma* that breaches the skin barrier. Other factors that may predispose piglets to developing clinical disease include *agalactia of the sow, concurrent infections, and nutritional deficiencies*. *S. hyicus* strains are virulent by virtue of their ability to produce an *exotoxin* which, when injected in purified form or in cell-free extracts, is capable of producing exfoliative skin lesions in pigs which are typical of exudative epidermitis. Initial characterization of the exotoxin indicated that it has a molecular weight of approximately 27 kDa, is heat labile, appears to target epidermal cells of the stratum granulosum, and thereby produces intra-epidermal cleavage between the stratum corneum and stratum granulosum. More recent studies have identified at least three, and possibly four, antigenically distinct exfoliative toxins and shown them to be *metalloproteases*.

Exudative epidermitis has been compared to staphylococcal scalded skin syndrome of humans, which is also caused by several serologically distinct types of exfoliative toxins (epidermolysins). However, the presence of cocci in the lesions of piglets makes exudative epidermitis *more comparable to human bullous impetigo*, a superficial vesiculopustular infection that is also caused by staphylococcal exfoliative toxins and which contains gram-positive cocci within intact pustules. In contrast, staphylococci are present at a distant, usually extra-cutaneous, site in staphylococcal scalded skin syndrome rather than in the skin lesions. The toxins in both of these human conditions cause separation at the interface between the stratum spinosum and stratum granulosum by an unknown mechanism. However, it appears that the toxin acts primarily on intercellular substance, and binding to filaggrin may be involved in the pathogenesis. The disease affects children primarily, because the exfoliative toxin is excreted more slowly by the immature kidneys of young children. In addition, most adults are protected by anti-toxin antibody which young children do not have. Less rapid toxin excretion and lack of protective antibodies may also explain the greater incidence and severity of exudative epidermitis in the youngest piglets.

The disease can be divided into peracute, acute, and subacute forms.

- In the *peracute form*, most common in piglets only a few days old, there is abrupt onset of lesions around the eyes, snout, chin, and on the ears with extension to the medial aspect of the legs. Lesions then rapidly spread to the thorax, abdomen, entire legs, and hooves. Lesions begin as peeling of small areas of the stratum corneum leaving red, glistening, moist areas. These areas are quickly covered by *greasy, dark brown exudate*. Lesions become generalized in 24 to 48 hours and the entire body is erythematous and covered with brown, greasy, malodorous exudate (Fig. 5.89). Erosions of the coronary bands and heels commonly develop. Conjunctivitis also occurs frequently and typically causes matting together of the eyelids and results in an inability to see.

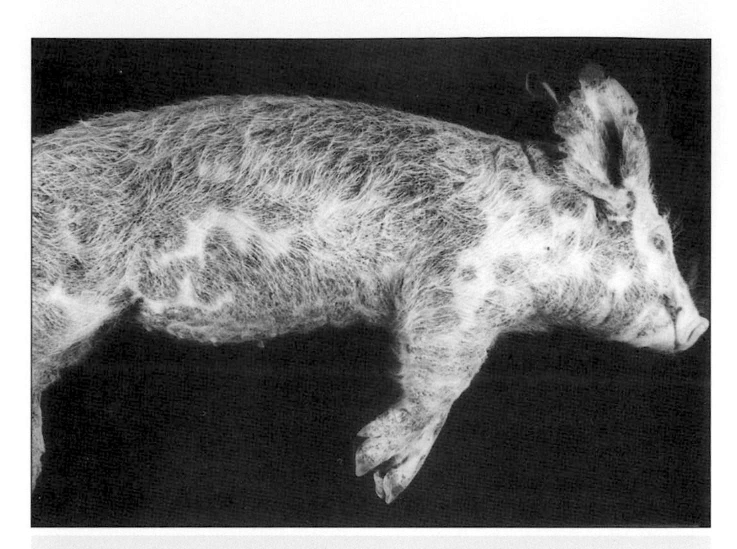

Figure 5.89 Exudative epidermitis ("greasy-pig disease").

Death occurs within 3–5 days as a result of dehydration, electrolyte imbalance, negative energy balance, and septicemia.

- In the *acute form*, the course is more protracted. The skin becomes thick and wrinkled and the exudate covering the entire body becomes dry, hard, and cracked, producing a generalized furrowed appearance. The underlying skin visible in the furrows is red.
- The *subacute form* occurs in older piglets and skin lesions are milder and usually confined to the head and ears. The subacute disease may appear as a dandruff-like scaling or as red-brown macules. Older piglets with less severe forms of disease frequently survive, however recovery is slow and the piglets are severely stunted. Additional lesions that may also occur in affected piglets are subcutaneous abscesses, necrosis of the ears and tail, and polyarthritis.

The earliest *microscopic lesion* is a subcorneal vesicular to pustular dermatitis. Extension of infection to hair follicles results in a superficial purulent folliculitis. In fully developed lesions, the skin is covered with a thick crust composed of ortho- and parakeratotic keratin, lakes of serum, accumulations of neutrophils, necrotic debris, and microcolonies of gram-positive cocci. The epidermis is variably acanthotic and rete ridges are elongated. Cells in the outer stratum spinosum exhibit variable intracellular edema. Neutrophilic exocytosis, intercellular edema, and spongiotic pustules may be seen in the epidermis and infundibular portion of hair follicles. The dermis is edematous, dermal vessels are congested, and there is a perivascular to interstitial neutrophilic infiltrate. Dermal inflammation is more intense and diffuse in areas of ulceration. In subacute cases, exudation is less severe and there is more marked epidermal hyperplasia, hyperkeratosis, and parakeratosis. Inflammation in the dermis becomes primarily mononuclear.

Microscopic lesions may also be seen in *other tissues*. Lymph nodes draining severely affected areas of skin contain foci of hemorrhage, purulent inflammation, and occasional microcolonies of bacterial cocci. Renal lesions are common and bacteremia is not required for them to be present. The lesions are distinctive, with early vacuolation of the epithelium of collecting ducts and renal pelvis progressing to epithelial degeneration and exfoliation. Intratubular casts of desquamated epithelium may be sufficiently severe to be evident macroscopically, leading to linear striations of the renal pelvis, and accumulation of cellular sediment in the pelvis and ureters. The process may be sufficiently severe to occlude the ureters. In cases in which bacteremia is present, purulent pyelonephritis is common. Animals with greasy pig disease may also have lesions in the oral cavity and conjunctiva, and the causative organism has been associated with abortion in sows.

The *differential diagnoses* for exudative epidermitis include zinc deficiency/ parakeratosis, sarcoptic mange, streptococcal pyoderma, and viral infections. In young pigs, the lesions are sufficiently distinctive that the disease is not confused with other conditions.

Staphylococcus hyicus has also been proposed as the cause of the so-called *flank-biting and necrotic ear syndromes of pigs*. Both conditions are characterized by large erosive to ulcerative crusty skin lesions in early weaned pigs. *S. hyicus* has been associated with skin lesions in *other species*. The organism is not uncommon in cattle and is frequently secondary to parasitic skin disease. The organism was isolated from skin lesions of a young pygmy goat with chronic generalized seborrheic dermatitis and alopecia. The microscopic lesion was a purulent exudative epidermitis similar to that in pigs. *S. hyicus* has been cultured from a number of horses with exudative crusty alopecic skin lesions on the distal limbs that resembled "grease heel" clinically.

Bibliography

Andresen LO. Differentiation and distribution of three types of exfoliative toxin produced by *Staphylococcus hyicus* from pigs with exudative epidermitis. FEMS Immunol Med Microbiol 1998;20:301–310.

Devriese LA, et al. *Staphylococcus hyicus* in skin lesions of horses. Eq Vet J 1983;15:263–265.

Hardwick N, et al. Staphylococcal scalded skin syndrome in an adult. Influence of immune and renal factors. Br J Dermatol 1995;132:468–471.

Hazarika RA, et al. Cutaneous infection associated with *Staphylococcus hyicus* in cattle. Res Vet Sci 1991;50:374–375.

Mirt D. Lesions of so-called flank biting and necrotic ear syndrome in pigs. Vet Rec 1999;144:92–96.

Prevost G, et al. Staphylococcal epidermolysins. Curr Opin Infect Dis 2003;16:71–76.

Sato H, et al. Isolation of exfoliative toxin from *Staphylococcus hyicus subsp. hyicus* and its exfoliative activity in the piglet. Vet Microbiol 1991;27:263–275.

Schamber G, Alstad AD. Isolation of *Staphylococcus hyicus* from seborrheic dermatitis in a pygmy goat. J Vet Diagn Invest 1989;1:276–277.

Takeuchi S, et al. A metalloprotease is common to swine, avian and bovine isolates of *Staphylococcus hyicus*. Vet Microbiol 2000;71:169–174.

Tanabe T, et al. Correlation between occurrence of exudative epidermitis and exfoliative toxin-producing ability of *Staphylococcus hyicus*. Vet Microbiol 1996;48:9–17.

Terauchi R, et al. Isolation of exfoliative toxin from *Staphylococcus intermedius* and its local toxicity in dogs. Vet Microbiol 2003;94:19–29.

Yeruham I, et al. Contagious impetigo in a dairy cattle herd. Vet Dermatol 1996;7:239–242.

Dermatophilosis

Dermatophilosis (cutaneous streptothricosis, mycotic dermatitis, cutaneous actinomycosis, lumpy wool, strawberry foot rot, rain scald, rain rot, Kirchi, Gasin-Gishu, Senkobo disease, Drodo-Boka, Savi, Ambarr-Madow) is an *acute, subacute, or chronic superficial exudative dermatitis caused by the actinomycete Dermatophilus congolensis*. The disease occurs worldwide and has a wide host range but it is *most common in the hot humid tropics and subtropics and in areas with heavy prolonged rains.* In hot monsoon climates, cattle are the primary animals affected and the disease is endemic in some portions of Africa. In more temperate climates, sheep and goats are involved primarily. The disease is occasional in horses and it is rare in dogs, cats, pigs, and humans. Cases of dermatophilosis have also been reported in camels, mules, donkeys, zebras, giraffes, Thompson's gazelles, woodchucks, striped skunks, raccoons, hedgehogs, gerbils, foxes, ground squirrels, seals, owl monkeys, captive polar bears, chamois, tortoises, and Australian bearded lizards. There is no apparent sex or age predilection; and congenital infections have been reported in calves and lambs.

In cattle and sheep, dermatophilosis causes important economic losses by virtue of decreased meat and milk production, damaged hides, wool loss, and devaluation, infertility, and early culling. Severe udder and teat lesions may interfere with suckling by calves and result in decreased growth rate. Affected animals are predisposed to secondary infections and cutaneous myiasis. Severely affected animals of any species may become emaciated and die.

Dermatophilus congolensis is a gram-positive pleomorphic bacterium whose natural habitat is unknown. The organism is probably not free-living since attempts to culture it from soil have been unsuccessful. Clinically normal carrier animals and crusts from infected animals probably serve as sources of infection. *D. congolensis* has a distinctive life cycle in which *coccoid bodies germinate to produce branching filaments* (Fig. 5.90A). These filaments undergo transverse and longitudinal septation to *form parallel rows of coccoid bodies.* The cocci are resistant to unfavorable conditions and are reproductively dormant until the appropriate wet conditions occur and they are activated to become motile zoospores.

Dermatophilosis cannot be reproduced experimentally to resemble natural disease, even with large doses of the organism. *Multiple factors* appear to be involved in pathogenesis of the natural disease. Two factors that appear to be most important are trauma to the skin and prolonged wetting. Zoospores are unable to overcome the protective barriers of the hair, surface lipid film, and stratum corneum, and their entry is facilitated by breaks in the skin surface. Trauma from ectoparasites, shearing, dipping, barb wire injuries, sharp stones, and scratches from sharp vegetation can act as portals of entry for the organisms. Besides producing skin trauma, external parasites such as flies, mites, lice, ticks, and mosquitoes also act as mechanical vectors. *In addition to skin trauma, prolonged moisture is needed for the activation, proliferation, and spread of the zoospores.* Wetting may also act to breach skin barriers by dissolving the surface lipid film and softening the stratum corneum. Outbreaks of dermatophilosis are frequently associated with periods of unusually heavy rainfall, housing in pastures or paddocks with standing water or mud, or after intensive high-pressure washing of animals.

Other factors involved in development of disease are less well understood. Genetic factors may be involved, since some breeds of cattle appear to be more resistant to disease than are others. Skin color appears to have an effect because some light-skinned breeds or light-skinned areas may be more susceptible to infection. A definite association between infestation with the tick *Amblyomma variegatum* and occurrence of dermatophilosis in cattle has been found. In herds with effective tick prevention, there is a much lower incidence or diminished severity of the disease. Since the lesions of dermatophilosis do not correspond to sites of tick attachment, a systemic effect on the animal's immune system has been suspected. Experimental support for tick-induced immunosuppression has been found in studies comparing in vitro lymphocyte stimulation responses wherein tick-infested cattle had lower mitogen-induced lymphoblast transformation responses than tick-free cattle, and addition of their serum to lymphocytes from tick-free cattle had an inhibitory effect on the response. In addition, concurrent diseases or stresses may contribute to the development of dermatophilosis by compromising the host's immune system. Intestinal parasitism, nutritional deficiencies, stress of pregnancy or migration, viral infections, and other infectious diseases may increase susceptibility to the condition.

Once the normal skin surface has been disrupted and activated zoospores gain access to the epidermis, infection can develop. The zoospores are apparently attracted to the low carbon dioxide concentration of the normal epidermis and there they germinate to *form mycelia that invade the viable epidermis and outer root sheaths of hair follicles.* Only rarely do the bacteria proliferate in the dermis or deeper tissues. The means by which *D. congolensis* invades the epidermis is unknown but recent investigations have found a variety of enzymes released into the culture fluid of the bacteria suggesting that *the ability of the organism to produce exoenzymes may be the pathogenetic mechanism.* As the filaments invade the epidermis, keratinocytes at sites of penetration begin to cornify and numerous neutrophils accumulate beneath and migrate into the epidermis, which subsequently separates from the underlying dermis. The neutrophils inhibit further invasion by the organism, and the epidermis reforms from cells in adjacent external hair follicle sheaths. This new epidermis is again invaded by organisms arising from the hair follicles to initiate another cycle of epidermal penetration, neutrophilic exocytosis, and epidermal detachment. *These repeated sequences of bacterial invasion, inflammation, and epidermal regeneration produce the thick laminar and parakeratotic crusts characteristic of dermatophilosis.*

Why some animals develop mild localized disease that resolves rapidly and spontaneously while others develop chronic widespread and debilitating disease is unknown. Skin commensal bacteria, primarily *Bacillus spp.*, have been shown to produce substances inhibitory to growth of *D. congolensis* in culture. It has been suggested that if a similar effect is present in vitro, bacteria normally present on skin produce substances that are bacteriostatic or bactericidal and thus prevent *D. congolensis* from proliferating. Differences in microflora of different individuals or breeds of animals could explain differences in response to infection. Furthermore, during the rainy season these bacterial inhibitors could be leached out or diluted to ineffective concentrations, permitting proliferation of *D. congolensis.* Differences in individual immune function or responses have been sought to explain why some animals recover quickly while others develop chronic infections. Chronically infected sheep have been found to have decreased numbers of dendritic cells in the dermis, to produce lower antibody titers in response to a novel antigen injected subcutaneously, and to have differences in an allele of a molecule which forms a portion of the T-cell receptor complex when compared to sheep which recovered spontaneously. The conclusions drawn from these studies were that poorer antigen presentation, differences in T-cell function, and a less vigorous antibody response to bacterial cell surface antigens may have allowed more widespread establishment of lesions and decreased ability to resolve lesions by chronically infected sheep. However, in other studies no correlation between serum antibody level and resistance

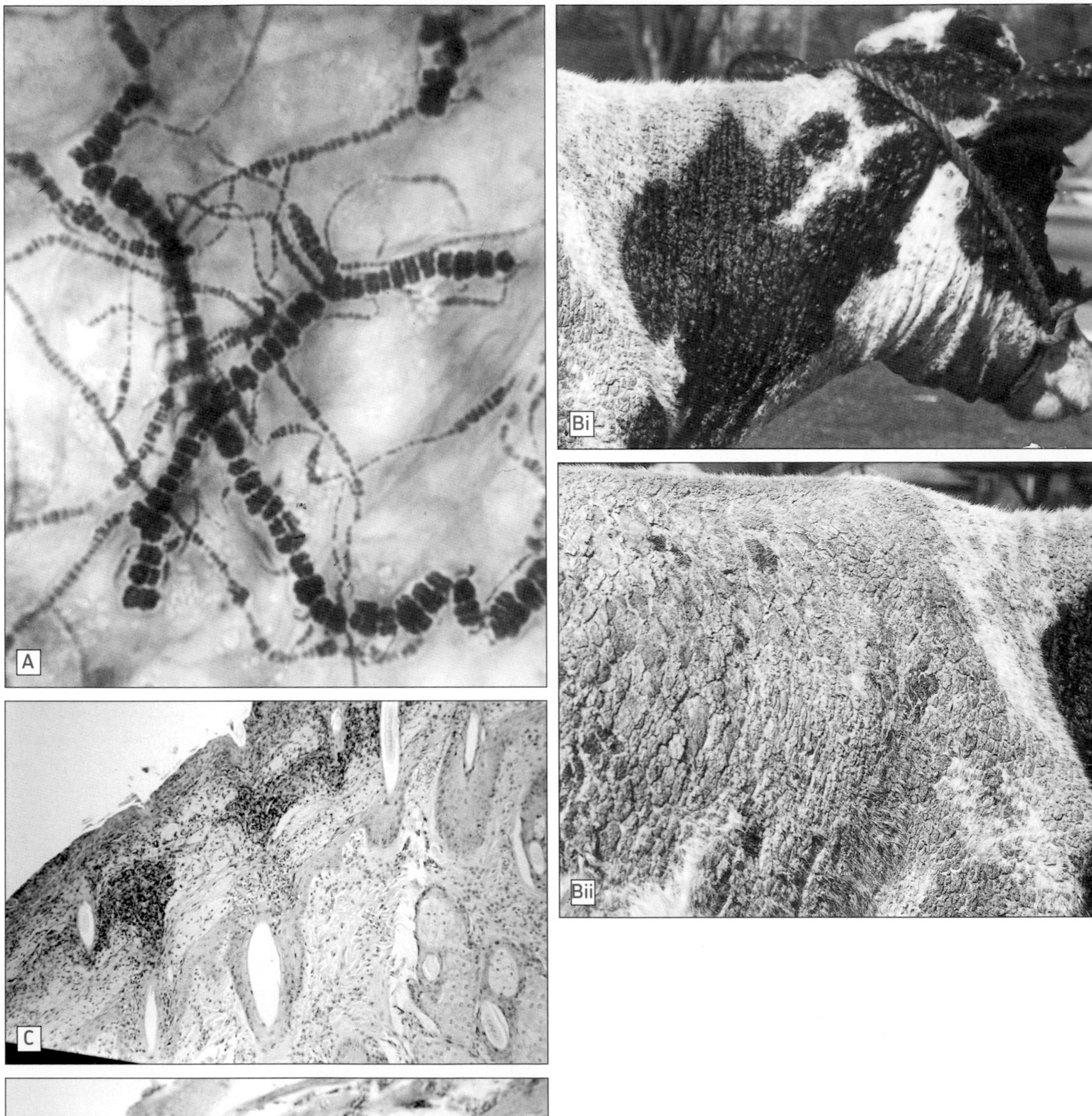

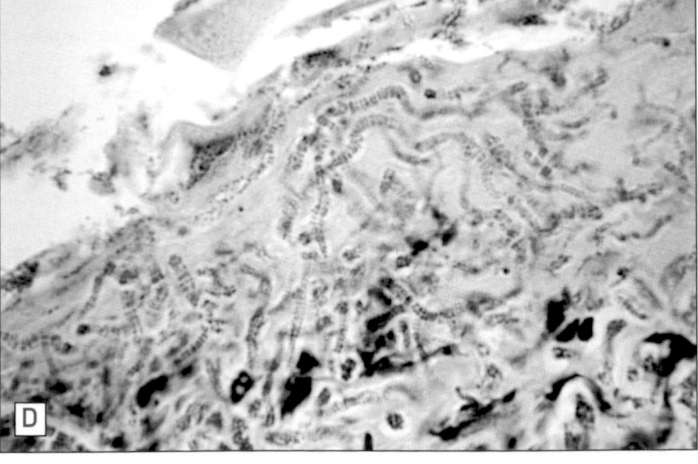

Figure 5.90 Dermatophilosis (*Dermatophilus congolensis* infection) **A.** Branching filaments with transverse and longitudinal septation in smear of *Dermatophilus congolensis*. **Bi/Bii. Extensive crusting** of the skin in dermatophilosis in a cow. **C.** Dermatophilosis in a horse. Note thick **crusts** composed of alternating layers of parakeratotic and orthokeratotic keratin. **D.** Higher magnification of (**C**). Crusts are composed of serous fluid, degenerative inflammatory cells, and **bacterial filaments** composed of multiple parallel rows of cocci.

to infection was found. Specific antibodies of various classes have also been detected on the skin surface but their role is unknown. Studies of vaccines against *D. congolensis* in sheep have shown that vaccines based on one strain of *D. congolensis* gave some protection against homologous challenge but were ineffective against challenge with a different strain of the bacterium. The involvement of antibody in resolution of disease is supported by histologic observations in which a chronological correlation was shown between lesion resolution and the presence of increased numbers of dermal plasma cells, many of which contained IgA, suggesting a role for this immunoglobulin in humoral immunity at the skin surface.

The *earliest lesions* of dermatophilosis consist of patches of slight erythema that are visible only in unpigmented areas. Very small papules and pustules develop next and are more evident by palpation than by visual inspection. As the lesions become covered by exudate and hairs become entrapped within the developing crust, they form small tufts that resemble paintbrushes. *As these small lesions coalesce, they form the typical large oval to circular domed yellow-brown adherent scabs which when removed leave a moist hyperemic base that may bleed.* The lesions are painful and nonpruritic. In chronic cases, lesions progress to form thick layers of dry spongy material involving extensive areas of long hair or hard wart-like crusts that protrude above the hair surface, usually in areas with a short haircoat (Fig. 5.90B). *Differential diagnoses include dermatophytosis, staphylococcal dermatitis, mite infestation, various viral infections, zinc-responsive dermatosis, and pemphigus foliaceus.*

The distribution of lesions in **cattle** is variable. Lesions confined to the face and ears are most often seen in young suckling calves. In other forms of the disease, lesions occur on the brisket, axillae, and inguinal areas or on the udder and teats of cows and scrotum and prepuce of bulls. Cattle standing in deep water or mud develop lesions on the legs. Lesions located in the perineum and tail are assumed to result from trauma caused by mounting by other animals. In many cases, lesions are diffusely distributed over the head, topline of the neck and body to the tail, and dorsal sides. *Animals with greater than 50% of body involvement often show weight loss, dehydration, and death.* Rare instances of subcutaneous abscesses, lymphadenitis, and oral lesions have been reported.

In **sheep**, infection of the wooled areas is frequently missed in early stages and some animals recover spontaneously during the acute stage of infection. If the disease continues to progress, the wool of the neck, back, and flank becomes matted with exudate to form dense pyramidal masses (lumpy wool, mycotic dermatitis) which may last for months to years in some individuals. *Strawberry foot rot* is an infection that begins at the coronet regions and may progress to involve the skin to the carpi and/or tarsi. In some cases, crusts may be confined to the ears, nose, and face, a clinical form common in lambs. Concurrent infection with contagious ecthyma has been reported.

Dermatophilosis in **goats** frequently consists of 2–3-mm crusty lesions on the pinnae and tail of kids and large pyramidal crusts on the dorsal midline, sides, caudal thighs, and scrotum of adults. Lesions involving the distal limbs resemble strawberry foot rot of sheep. Concurrent infection with contagious ecthyma may occur and secondary infections with staphylococci, streptococci, or corynebacteria may develop.

In **horses**, lesions of dermatophilosis are frequently located on the dorsal aspect of the body and look as if large drops of liquid have scalded the skin (*rain scald*). Horses kept in wet, marshy, or muddy enclosures, and undergoing trauma to the legs develop lesions of the distal extremities primarily (grease heel, scratches, mud fever). Lesions on the legs may be associated with swelling, pain, and lameness. In some instances, only the head is affected. Unpigmented skin may be more susceptible to infection and lesions on these areas are typically very erythematous. Outbreaks in show horses have been associated with frequent high-pressure washing.

Dermatophilosis cases reported in **cats** are notable in that they have all been subcutaneous or extracutaneous infections. The lesions consisted of draining nodules involving or in the area of the popliteal lymph nodes or the subcutaneous tissue of a paw and masses on the tongue and serosal surface of the urinary bladder. In at least one of the cats with subcutaneous infection, superficial wounds suggestive of a recent cat fight were seen, prompting speculation that the infection was traumatically introduced.

The earliest *histologic lesions* of dermatophilosis are superficial dermal congestion, edema, and neutrophil infiltration of the superficial dermis. Exocytosis of neutrophils becomes more pronounced as lesions progress and intraepidermal or subcorneal pustules may develop. Eventually, repeated cycles of bacterial invasion and inflammation result in *thick crusts composed of alternating layers of parakeratotic and orthokeratotic keratin, serous fluid, degenerate inflammatory cells, and bacterial filaments composed of multiple parallel rows of cocci* (Fig. 5.90C, D). The epidermis is acanthotic with orthokeratotic and parakeratotic hyperkeratosis. Purulent folliculitis with intralesional bacterial filaments is also usually present. Dermal inflammation is usually mild and superficial perivascular. In cases of dermatophilosis in cats and rare instances of subcutaneous and lymph node infection in cattle, the lesions consist of granulomas or pyogranulomas with scattered necrotic foci which contain typical *D. congolensis* filaments.

Bibliography

Ambrose N, et al. Immune responses to *Dermatophilus congolensis* infections. Parasitol Today 1999;15:295–300.

Ambrose NC, et al. Preliminary characterization of extracellular serine proteases of *Dermatophilus congolensis* isolates from cattle, sheep and horses. Vet Microbiol 1998;62:321–335.

Ellis TM, et al. Variation in cultural, morphological, biochemical properties and infectivity of Australian isolates of *Dermatophilus congolensis*. Vet Microbiol 1993;38:81–102.

Gitao CG, et al. An outbreak of a mixed infection of *Dermatophilus congolensis* and *Microsporum gypseum* in camels (*Camelus dromedarius*) in Saudi Arabia. Rev Sci Tech 1998;17:749–755.

Hermoso de Mendoza J, et al. Enzymatic activities of *Dermatophilus congolensis* measured by APIZYM. Vet Microbiol 1993;37:175–179.

Kaya O, et al. Isolation of *Dermatophilus congolensis* from a cat. J Vet Med B Infect Dis Vet Public Health 2000;47:155–157.

Kingali JM, et al. Inhibition of *Dermatophilus congolensis* by substances produced by bacteria found on the skin. Vet Microbiol 1990;22:237–240.

Koney EB, et al. The association between *Amblyomma variegatum* and dermatophilosis: Epidemiology and immunology. Trop Anim Hlth Prod 1996;28:18S–25S.

Masters AA, et al. Difference between lambs with chronic and mild dermatophilosis in frequency of alleles of CD3γ. Vet Microbiol 1997;57:337–345.

Msami HM, et al. *Dermatophilus congolensis* infection in goats in Tanzania. Trop Anim Health Prod 2001;33:367–377.

Scott DW. Large Animal Dermatology. Philadelphia, PA: WB Saunders, 1988.

Yeruham I, et al. Outbreak of dermatophilosis in a horse herd in Israel. J Vet Med 1996;43:393–398.
Zaria LT. *Dermatophilus congolensis* infection (dermatophilosis) in animals and man! An update. Comp Immunol Microbiol Infect Dis 1993;16:179–222.

Deep bacterial pyoderma

Deep pyodermas are serious bacterial infections that involve the hair follicle, dermis, and/or subcutis. They are usually chronic or recurrent, heal with scarring, and are commonly associated with regional or generalized lymphadenopathy and systemic signs. The clinical appearance of deep pyoderma is tremendously diverse. Lesions commonly seen in deep pyodermas include dark red or violaceous raised nodules, poorly demarcated areas of tissue swelling, hemorrhagic bullae, fistulous tracts, abscesses, purulent or serosanguineous exudate that dries to form crusts, and necrotic or ulcerated skin covered by crusts. Pain may be severe. Microscopic changes associated with deep pyodermas include folliculitis, furunculosis, nodular to diffuse dermatitis or panniculitis, and variable fibrosis. Bacteria may not be seen microscopically even with special stains.

Staphylococcal folliculitis and furunculosis

Staphylococcus spp. are the most common cause of folliculitis in domestic animals. Other organisms less frequently or rarely associated with folliculitis include *Streptococcus* spp., *Corynebacterium* spp., *Pseudomonas* spp., *Bacillus* spp., and *Pasteurella multocida*. Inflammation of the deep portion of hair follicles frequently results in rupture of the follicular wall (furunculosis) and extension of infection to the surrounding dermis and panniculus. *Staphylococcal folliculitis and furunculosis are very common in the dog, common in horses, goats, and sheep, and uncommon in cats, cattle, and pigs.* Skin lesions associated with folliculitis and furunculosis are extremely variable. The earliest skin lesion is a follicular papule with one or several hairs protruding from the center. The papule develops into a pustule but these are very fragile, break easily, and are thus very transient. Consequently, crusted papules are seen more commonly than are pustules. In short-haired dogs, horses, and cattle, the earliest clinical sign is a dishevelment of the haircoat produced by small groups of hairs tufting together above the skin surface, an appearance that can be confused with urticaria. As the hairs fall out of infected follicles, multiple small foci of alopecia and scaling develop. The hair coat develops a moth-eaten appearance as the areas of alopecia become progressively larger. Lesions often enlarge and develop a central ulcer that discharges purulent or serosanguineous exudate that dries to form a crust. When furunculosis occurs, dark red to violaceous nodules, draining fistulae, ulcers, and extensive tissue swelling develop (Fig. 5.91). Hemorrhagic bullae may be prominent in some cases. Scarring, alterations in pigmentation of the hair and skin, and lichenification may result. Regional and generalized lymphadenopathy are common. Constitutional signs, such as fever and anorexia, may occur when infection is severe or extensive.

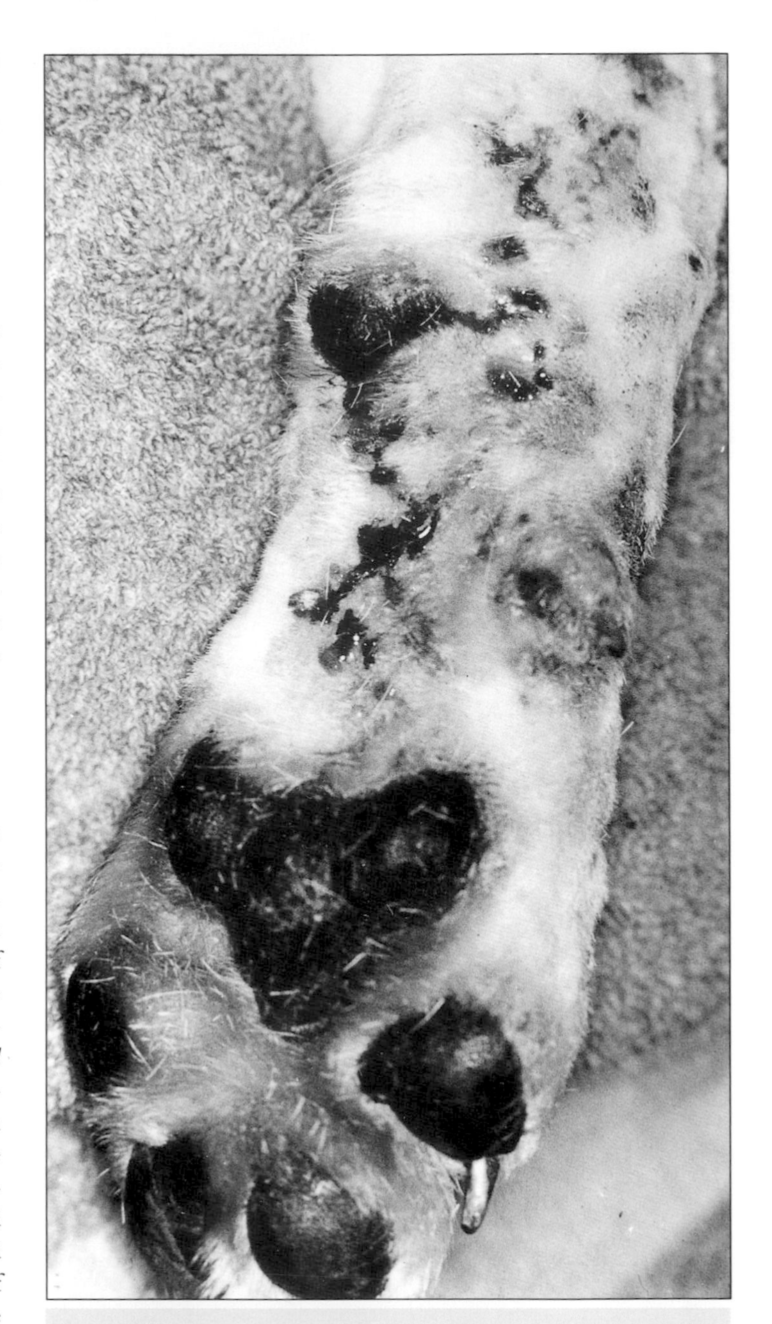

Figure 5.91 Deep pyoderma in a dog. Swollen paw with multiple draining tracts.

The *microscopic changes* of staphylococcal folliculitis and furunculosis are as varied as the gross lesions. The epidermis is variably acanthotic and may be ulcerated. Serocellular crusting is common. Staphylococcal folliculitis is characterized by *neutrophilic inflammation* but the relative number of neutrophils is extremely variable, depending on the duration of the infection and presence of furunculosis. Pustules composed of neutrophils and variable numbers of eosinophils may be seen within the infundibulum or ostium of hair follicles. Neutrophils accumulate within the lumen of hair follicles, distending the lumen and frequently causing rupture of the hair follicle wall (see Fig. 5.5B). Neutrophils, eosinophils, macrophages, and plasma cells form dense sheets in the dermis and may extend to the panniculus. Hemorrhagic bullae consist of large pustules with hemorrhage in the interfollicular dermis. Large dermal pustules may form cavitary lesions. Release of hair and keratin into the dermis or panniculus induces an *intense foreign body reaction* that may completely efface the follicle (see Fig. 5.6). Fragments of hair or keratin may be surrounded by discrete granulomas composed of multinucleated giant cells, epithelioid macrophages, and neutrophils (*trichogranuloma*). Eosinophils may be numerous around the fragments of hair and keratin. Inflammation may become diffuse as adjacent furuncles coalesce and replace normal dermal structures completely. Hemorrhage and fibroplasia are variable. Bacteria may not be evident even with special stains such as tissue Gram stain or Giemsa stain.

Deep pyoderma is not as common as superficial pyoderma but is still a relatively common disease in **dogs**. *Staphylococcus intermedius* is usually the primary pathogen in bacterial folliculitis and furunculosis in dogs. However, gram-negative bacteria such as *Proteus*, *Pseudomonas*, and *E. coli* are not uncommon secondary invaders. Infection may be localized or widespread. *Localized forms* of staphylococcal deep pyoderma commonly involve the bridge of the nose, the chin ("canine acne"), feet (pedal folliculitis-furunculosis), and pressure points. A particularly refractory form of staphylococcal pyoderma has been recognized in German Shepherd Dogs. *German Shepherd pyoderma* is poorly understood; but because of the breed predilection, an inherited component has been suggested. The condition typically begins as pruritus involving the lumbosacral, caudal abdominal, and medial thigh regions. Lesions initially resemble pyotraumatic dermatitis and the lesion distribution is suggestive of flea allergy dermatitis. As the condition progresses, lesions assume an appearance typical of chronic pyoderma and frequently become more widespread. An underlying predisposing cause is frequently not apparent, and an immunologic abnormality is suspected. Neutrophil chemotaxis and killing capacity appear to be normal. Limited studies in a small number of affected German Shepherd Dogs have found a cell-mediated immunodeficiency by the lymphocyte transformation test and a marked increase in the CD8+ T lymphocytes in peripheral blood. Whether these changes are a cause or effect of the disease is unknown. Examination of T and B lymphocytes in histologic sections found a marked paucity of T lymphocytes in lesions of deep pyoderma of German Shepherd Dogs as compared to similar lesions from dogs of other breeds.

Staphylococcal pyoderma in **horses** most often involves the harness, saddle (saddle scab, saddle boils), neck, and dorsal lumbosacral regions. *Friction from tack* is considered an important initiating factor. It is most common in the summer, coincident with excessive sweating, higher environmental temperature and humidity, and increased numbers of biting insects. Lesions are usually painful rather than pruritic. *Staphylococcal pyoderma may be one of many causes of "grease heel,"* in which lesions involve the caudal aspect of the pastern and fetlock areas of one or more legs. In tail pyoderma, the dorsal surface of the tail is particularly affected and infection is usually secondary to skin abrasions caused by tail rubbing associated with insect bites, mange, biting lice, pinworms, or vice. Although much less common, *Corynebacterium pseudotuberculosis* can cause folliculitis and clinical lesions ("contagious acne") similar to those with staphylococcal folliculitis.

Staphylococcal pyoderma is common in **goats** and frequently begins on the udder and spreads to the ventral abdomen, medial thighs, perineal area, face, pinnae, and distal limbs. Severe infections, particularly those with secondary mastitis, may produce pyrexia, anorexia, depression, and septicemia. In **sheep**, staphylococcal pyoderma may occur as a benign pustular dermatitis on the lips and perineum in otherwise healthy 3- to 4-week-old lambs. Lesions usually regress spontaneously within 3 weeks. A more severe form of infection involves the face (facial eczema, eye scab), particularly of adult ewes just prior to lambing. Facial dermatitis appears to be contagious, and spread is thought to result from head abrasions sustained while feeding at troughs or by fighting.

Staphylococcal pyoderma occurs occasionally in cattle, pigs, and cats. Infection in **cattle** is seen most commonly in young bulls on the tail, perineum, scrotum, and face. Trauma and poor hygiene may be initiating factors. Staphylococcal pyoderma in **pigs** usually occurs on the hindquarters, abdomen, and chest of piglets less than 8 weeks of age and spontaneously regresses. Pyoderma is uncommon in **cats** and may be mistaken for other diseases. Lesions may consist of a crusted papular eruption on the face, head, or over the dorsum that clinically resembles miliary dermatitis associated with various hypersensitivity conditions. Scaling, crusting, or ulceration of footpads or nailbeds may be confused with pemphigus foliaceus or dermatophytosis.

Bibliography

Chabanne L, et al. Lymphocyte subset abnormalities in German shepherd dog pyoderma (GSP). Vet Immunol Immunopathol 1995;49:189–198.

Day MJ. An immunopathological study of deep pyoderma in the dog. Res Vet Sci 1994;56:18–23.

Denerolle P, et al. German shepherd dog pyoderma: a prospective study of 23 cases. Vet Dermatol 1998;9:243–248.

Rosser EJ. German shepherd dog pyoderma: A prospective study of 12 dogs. J Am Anim Hosp Assoc 1997;33:355–363.

White SD. Pyoderma in five cats. J Am Anim Hosp Assoc 1991;27:141–146.

Wisselink MA, et al. Leukocyte mobilization to skin lesions, determination of cell surface receptors (CD11b/CD18) and phagocytic capacities of neutrophils in dogs with chronic deep pyoderma. Vet Immunol Immunopathol 1997;57:179–186.

Abscesses and cellulitis

Abscesses *are well-circumscribed accumulations of pus.* **Cellulitis** *is a severe, deep, suppurative infection that is poorly defined and tends to dissect through tissue planes. The lesions are usually painful and overlying skin is often friable, dark, devitalized, and may be sloughed.* The wounds frequently have a putrid smell and may be emphysematous if the organism is a gas-producer (*Clostridium* spp., *Bacteroides* spp.). Pyrexia and regional lymphadenopathy may be present. Abscesses and cellulitis are fairly common in large animals and are *one of the most common disorders in cats*, where they are a frequent sequel to fight wounds. Other predisposing causes include traumatic puncture wounds, foreign bodies, injections, and shearing and clipping wounds. Microscopically, abscesses consist of central accumulations of neutrophils and/or necrotic debris, frequently surrounded by a wall of granulation tissue or dense collagenous connective tissue, depending on duration. In contrast, cellulitis is poorly circumscribed and consists of extensive purulent to pyogranulomatous dermal and subcutaneous inflammation that may be accompanied by hemorrhage, necrosis, and thrombosis. Bacteria may or may not be visible histologically.

A wide variety of aerobic and anaerobic bacteria have been associated with abscesses and cellulitis. The most common organisms include staphylococci (dogs, Thoroughbred horses, cattle), *Clostridium* spp. (malignant edema, gas gangrene, and big head in horses, cattle, sheep, goats, pigs, and dogs), *Pasteurella multocida* (cats), and *Corynebacterium pseudotuberculosis* (abscesses in horses, goats, cattle, and sheep; ulcerative lymphangitis in horses, cattle, sheep, and goats; caseous lymphadenitis in sheep and goats). *Rhodococcus equi,* most commonly associated with pneumonia in young horses, has been isolated from cutaneous abscesses and cellulitis in young horses and rarely in cats. *Pasteurella granulomatis* has been associated with a disease in southern Brazil called *lechiguana* which is characterized by large subcutaneous fibrosing eosinophilic abscesses. Lesions are most commonly located in the scapular region and the condition is frequently fatal if untreated. Various *mycoplasmas* and mycoplasma-like organisms have been recovered from abscesses in cats and from decubital abscesses in calves.

Streptococcus canis has been isolated from dogs with an intensely painful **necrotizing fasciitis**. The infection begins as cellulitis, frequently 12–48 hours after minor trauma, that rapidly progresses to shock and necrotizing fasciitis. The condition is similar to streptococcal toxic shock syndrome of humans caused by *S. pyogenes.* The condition is characterized grossly by *extensive exudation along fascial planes and necrosis of subcutaneous fat and fascia*, resulting in extensive sloughing of necrotic skin. The microscopic lesions of necrotizing fasciitis include severe necrosis, suppuration, fibrinous exudation, and hemorrhage of the dermis and subcutaneous fat, fascia, and muscle. In some instances, the epidermis and superficial dermis are infarcted as a result of thrombosis of dermal and subcutaneous blood vessels. Colonies of bacterial cocci may be evident in the inflamed subcutaneous tissue.

Conditions that resemble **toxic shock syndrome** in humans have been described in dogs. *Streptococcus canis* has been documented as the cause in most dogs; however, other bacteria, especially *Staphylococcus intermedius*, that produce exotoxins – including toxic shock syndrome toxin-1 – could potentially play a role. The site of infection can be the skin, as seen with necrotizing fasciitis; however, the primary site of infection in some dogs has been the lung or urinary tract. In dogs with toxic shock-like syndrome, but without necrotizing fasciitis, clinical skin lesions include multicentric to generalized cutaneous erythema. Some dogs also have edema and vesicles or pustules that progress to ulcers. The ears, extremities, and ventrum are frequently affected, and dogs can be depressed and have fever, anemia, thrombocytopenia, and neutrophilia. Histologically, these dogs have superficial dermatitis with apoptotic keratinocytes bordered by neutrophils. The lesions can progress to full-thickness necrosis and ulceration of the epidermis. As in necrotizing fasciitis, lesions can be fatal without early therapy with appropriate antibiotics. The cause of the skin lesions in the dogs with toxic shock-like syndrome, but without necrotizing fasciitis, has not been determined. In humans, the skin lesion is thought to result from nonspecific stimulation of lymphocytes by exotoxins with superantigen activity and the release of cytokines, including TNF-α.

Bibliography

DeWinter LM, et al. Virulence of *Streptococcus canis* from canine streptococcal toxic shock syndrome and necrotizing fasciitis. Vet Microbiol 1999;70:95–110.

Fairley RA, Fairley NM. *Rhodococcus equi* infection of cats. Vet Dermatol 1999;10:43–46.

Kinde H, et al. *Mycoplasma bovis* associated with decubital abscesses in Holstein calves. J Vet Diagn Invest 1993;5:194–197.

Miller CW, et al. Streptococcal toxic shock syndrome in dogs. J Am Vet Med Assoc 1996;209:1421–1426.

Nguhiu-Mwangi JA, et al. Necrosis and sloughing of skin associated with limb cellulitis in four cows and a calf: predisposing causes, treatment and prognosis. Vet Rec 1991;129:192–195.

Riet-Correa F, et al. Lechiguana (focal proliferative fibrogranulomatous panniculitis) in cattle. Vet Res Commun 2000;24:557–572.

Walker RD, et al. Recovery of two mycoplasma species from abscesses in a cat following bite wounds from a dog. J Vet Diagn Invest 1995;7:154–156.

Yager JA, et al. Streptococcal necrotizing fasciitis and toxic shock syndrome in dogs. Proc 13th AAVD/ACVD meeting. 1997:122–123.

Cutaneous bacterial granulomas

A wide variety of bacteria are capable of producing granulomatous inflammation of the skin. The organisms are frequently of *low virulence* and are introduced by *traumatic implantation*. These infections are typically *slowly progressive* and produce *cutaneous or subcutaneous nodules*. Inflammation is nodular or diffuse, granulomatous or pyogranulomatous, and involves the dermis, panniculus, or both. *Diagnosis commonly requires special stains such as tissue Gram stain and routine or modified acid-fast stains*. Staining frozen sections of formalin-fixed tissue may be necessary to demonstrate the bacteria in some atypical mycobacterial infections. Organisms are so infrequent in some cases that confirmation of the bacterial etiology cannot be made histologically and depends instead on cultural isolation of the agent.

Actinomycosis and nocardiosis

Actinomycosis and nocardiosis are uncommon subacute-to-chronic opportunistic cutaneous, pulmonary, and disseminated infections that develop secondary to wound contamination, inhalation, or ingestion. The diseases are discussed together because of their clinical and histologic similarities. *Actinomyces* and *Nocardia* are the most common actinomycetes, so-called higher bacteria, which cause disease, but occasional reports of infections in animals by other actinomycetes include *Streptomyces* and *Actinomadura*. The infections occur sporadically and are worldwide in distribution. They are not considered of public health significance.

Actinomyces species are gram-positive, non-acid fast, filamentous anaerobic or microaerophilic rods that are *commensal inhabitants of the oral cavity, intestine, and upper respiratory tract*. Cutaneous infection is usually secondary to bites, penetrating wounds caused by foreign bodies such as quills or grass awns, and wounds contaminated by licking. Cutaneous actinomycosis occurs in dogs, cats, horses, and cattle. Infection in pigs usually involves the mammary gland. Several retrospective studies in dogs indicate that young, large breed, male dogs that are used or housed outdoors are most commonly affected. *Actinomyces viscosus* is cultured most commonly from animal infections; but the organism is fastidious and difficult to culture and frequently it is not speciated even when cultured.

Nocardia species are common *soil saprophytes* that are ubiquitous in the soil and water and on plants. They cause infection by wound contamination, inhalation, or ingestion. They are aerobic, gram-positive, filamentous organisms that may be acid fast. There appears to be considerable variation in the degree of pathogenicity among various strains of the organism. Experimental infections suggest that defense against nocardial infections involves both neutrophils, which may have an immediate role in inhibiting the growth of the organisms, and cell-mediated immunity, which is responsible for the ultimate clearance of infection. Cutaneous nocardiosis is reported most frequently in dogs, cats, horses, and cattle. The most common isolate is *Nocardia asteroides*. Cutaneous nocardiosis in cattle, called *bovine farcy*, is caused by an organism originally called *N. farcinica* but is now thought to be *N. asteroides*. Farcy occurs in Africa, Asia, and South America.

The *gross lesions* of actinomycosis and nocardiosis are usually indistinguishable. They consist of abscesses, cellulitis, ulcerated nodules, draining fistulous tracts, and dense fibrous masses. *When the triad of clinical signs consisting of tumefaction, draining sinuses, and tissue grains is present, the lesion can be termed an* **actinomycotic mycetoma**. Lesions progress slowly by local extension. They occur most commonly on the head, neck, and extremities. Pleural and retroperitoneal infections may extend to involve the subcutaneous tissues of the lateral thoracic wall and flank area, respectively. The exudate is variable and ranges from thin serosanguineous to thick purulohemorrhagic. It may be odorless or foul-smelling and contain white, yellow, tan, or gray "**sulfur granules**." Sulfur granules are more common in actinomycosis than in nocardiosis. Regional lymphadenopathy frequently accompanies skin lesions. In cats, lesions on the ventral abdomen resemble mycobacterial infections. Actinomycosis in cattle usually involves the mandible or maxilla causing proliferative osteitis ("*lumpy jaw*"); the infection may extend from the bone to the overlying skin to form firm nodules, abscesses, and draining sinus tracts with extensive fibrosis. The cutaneous lesions of bovine farcy are typically associated with lymphangitis and lymphadenitis and are clinically similar to those caused by tuberculosis.

Microscopically, actinomycosis and nocardiosis are characterized by *pyogranulomatous dermatitis and panniculitis*. The epidermis is variably acanthotic and may be ulcerated. The dermis and subcutis contain central accumulations of neutrophils surrounded by a wall of epithelioid macrophages and variable numbers of multinucleated giant cells. Necrosis may be prominent within the central abscess. The pyogranulomas are separated by granulation tissue or dense fibrous connective tissue containing lymphocytes and plasma cells. Fibrosis tends to be more common and severe in actinomycosis than in nocardiosis. Organized masses, measuring 30–3000 μm or more in diameter, of basophilic or amphophilic-staining organisms, may be seen in the centers of the abscesses (Fig. 5.92). They are commonly bordered by a clubbed corona of brightly eosinophilic *Splendore-Hoeppli material. These structures correspond to the sulfur granules seen grossly in the exudate.* Granule formation is a more common feature of actinomycosis; in nocardiosis, the bacteria tend to be distributed singly among the neutrophils or within the macrophages and are difficult or impossible to see in HE-stained sections. However, *Nocardia* species may form granules in cutaneous lesions that are morphologically indistinguishable from those of *Actinomyces*. In Gram-stained sections, the bacteria are evident as delicate, branched, and beaded filaments, from 10–30 μm or more long and 0.5–1.0 μm wide. Fragmentation of filaments produces coccobacillary forms. The filamentous nature of the bacteria is most apparent at the periphery of granules; while coccobacillary forms constitute the centers of granules. The beaded appearance is due to alternating gram-positive and gram-negative regions within the filament and is less prominent with *Actinomyces* than with *Nocardia* species. *Actinomyces* are acid-fast negative with most acid-fast stains. Some, but not all, filaments of *Nocardia* may stain strongly acid-fast with modified acid-fast stain. However, *Nocardia* species are not invariably acid-fast and, if negative, cannot be differentiated from *Actinomyces*. Thus culture must be done to identify the organism. *Nocardia* species may resemble opportunistic mycobacteria but they do not stain with routine acid-fast stain as do mycobacteria. A single random section may not contain granules and serial sections may be necessary to find organisms. However, small biopsies may not contain organisms at all. Since granules or individual organisms may be rare, a wide *wedge biopsy* including deep subcutaneous tissue is more likely to contain organisms than are punch biopsies.

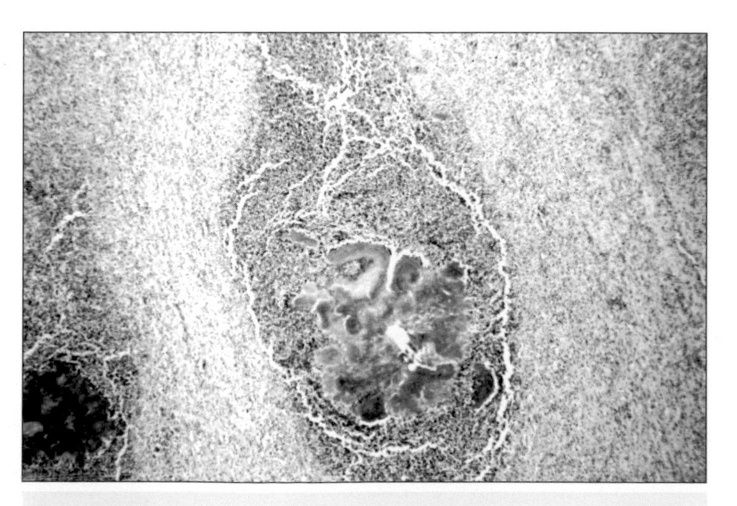

Figure 5.92 Abscess with clusters of organisms in the center in **actinomycosis** in a cow.

Bibliography

Biberstein EL, et al. *Nocardia asteroides* infection in horses: A review. J Am Vet Med Assoc 1985;186:273–277.

Davenport DJ, Johnson GC. Cutaneous nocardiosis in a cat. J Am Vet Med Assoc 1986;188:728–729.

Filice GA, Niewoehner DE. Contribution of neutrophils and cell-mediated immunity to control of *Nocardia asteroides* in murine lungs. J Infect Dis 1987;156:113–121.

Kirpensteijn J, Fingland RB. Cutaneous actinomycosis and nocardiosis in dogs: 48 cases (1980–1990). J Am Vet Med Assoc 1992;201:917–920.

Specht TE, et al. Skin pustules and nodules caused by *Actinomyces viscosus* in a horse. J Am Vet Med Assoc 1991;198:457–459.

Mycobacterial infections

The genus *Mycobacterium* is a large group of acid-fast organisms that includes both obligate pathogens and many saprophytic organisms that are occasionally opportunistic pathogens. They cause chronic infections of various organ systems, including the skin. The members of the *tuberculosis complex*, *M. tuberculosis,* and *M. bovis*, are obligate pathogens that cause tuberculosis in humans and a wide range of domestic animals worldwide. Pulmonary and gastrointestinal lesions are most common in tuberculosis, *but the skin can become involved in disseminated infections* and, rarely, infection may be confined to the skin. In contrast, *infections with saprophytic mycobacteria frequently involve the skin and they are usually acquired by wound contamination or traumatic implantation.* Cutaneous mycobacterial infections are reported most frequently in cats and less often in dogs. *Mycobacterial lesions are all characterized by granulomatous or pyogranulomatous dermatitis and/or panniculitis with variable necrosis.* These infections can be diagnosed by cytologic or histologic examination and organisms are best visualized with acid-fast or modified acid-fast stain. The organisms may be rare to numerous and the number of acid-fast bacilli seen within the lesion cannot be used to identify the specific organism involved.

Culture is necessary for definitive identification of the organism so that appropriate therapy and the zoonotic potential of the infection may be determined. *Many of the organisms are extremely fastidious and difficult to culture and isolation may require many weeks to months.* The need for culture is becoming increasingly obviated by molecular-based techniques which can identify the organisms in tissue section and can be completed within a few days.

Feline leprosy

Feline leprosy is a rare localized cutaneous infection caused by acid-fast bacilli that are not culturable by standard mycobacteriological methods. The infection has a widespread distribution, with cases reported in New Zealand, Australia, North America, and Europe. Cases are frequently associated with temperate maritime regions. Feline leprosy has no zoonotic potential.

Based on successful transmission to rats and mice and comparison of delayed type hypersensitivity skin reactions in cats, the causative agent of feline leprosy has been speculated to be *Mycobacterium lepraemurium*. This is the organism that causes rodent leprosy; it is a slow-growing organism that is isolated only with difficulty using enrichment techniques. The means of transmission is unknown, but *bites of cats or rodents, contact with rodents, and soil contamination of cutaneous wounds are thought to be involved.* Since the agent of human leprosy, or Hansen's disease, has been found in viable form in mosquitoes, bed bugs, ticks, and fleas, it has been suggested that transmission of feline leprosy may involve similar vectors. *Immunosuppression* has been suggested as contributing to development of infection, but such factors have not been identified in the vast majority of reported cases. Recently, the organism was identified by molecular analysis as *M. lepraemurium* in tissue specimens from four of eight cases of feline leprosy examined. However, two cases were found to be infected with a mycobacterium that had 16S ribosomal RNA gene sequence sharing closest nucleotide sequence identity with that of *M. malmoense*. These findings suggest that *feline leprosy may not be caused by a single agent.*

Feline leprosy occurs most commonly in young adult cats 1–3 years old; no breed or sex predilection is evident. Several studies have found an increased incidence of disease in the winter. Lesions may be located anywhere but are most frequent on the head and limbs. They consist of single or multiple, nonpainful cutaneous or subcutaneous nodules which are haired, alopecic, or ulcerated. They may be soft and fleshy or firm and measure up to 3–4 cm diameter. *The nodules are frequently mistaken for neoplasms.* Affected cats may also have regional lymphadenopathy but they are usually otherwise healthy. A second syndrome has been identified in cats >9 years old, with generalized skin involvement and a slowly progressive clinical course, caused by a novel mycobacterial species that is present in large to enormous numbers.

The *histologic changes* consist of granulomatous inflammation involving the dermis and frequently the subcutis. The epidermis is variably acanthotic or ulcerated. The predominant cells are *large, pale, foamy epithelioid macrophages* arranged in focal aggregates or diffuse sheets that replace normal architecture (Fig. 5.93). Lymphocytes, plasma cells, and neutrophils are in variable numbers. Multinucleated giant cells and small foci of caseous necrosis are present in some lesions. *Acid-fast organisms are demonstrable by routine acid-fast stains, such as Ziehl–Neelsen and Kinyoun's,* and are usually in moderate

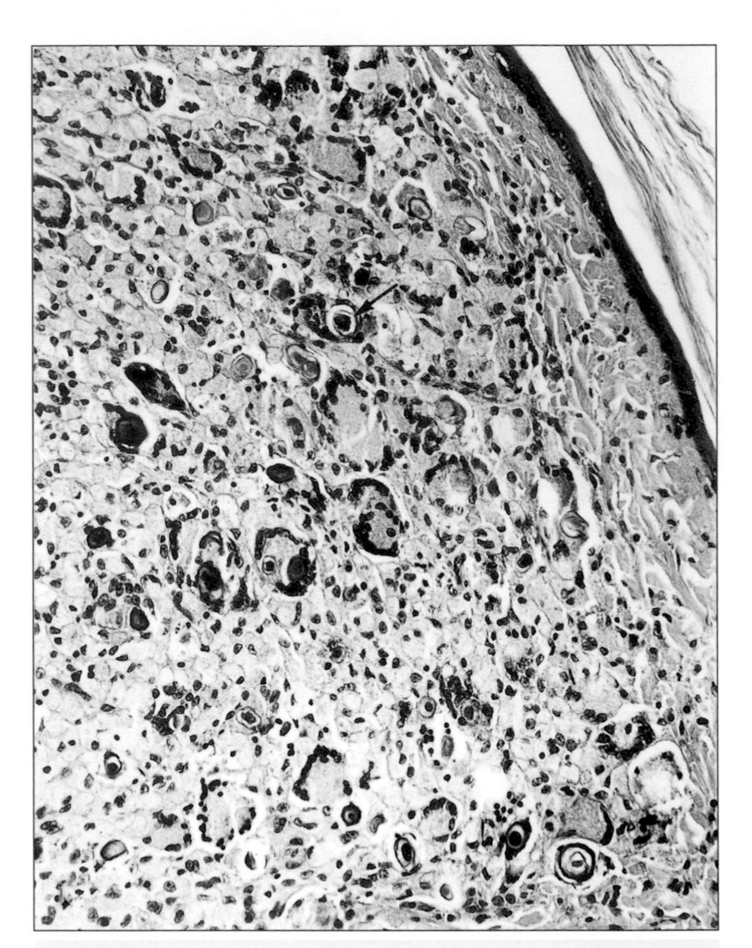

Figure 5.93 Macrophages, concretions (arrow), and multinucleate giant cells in **feline leprosy**.

numbers within macrophages or in necrotic foci. However, acid-fast bacilli may be in massive numbers in some cases or only rare in others. Mineralization and encapsulation are not typical of feline leprosy. The *histologic features* of feline leprosy have been compared to human leprosy, in which the particular histologic reaction is associated with the host's resistance. Whether this is also true for feline leprosy has not been determined. Reactions consisting of epithelioid granulomas with central caseous necrosis surrounded by a zone of lymphocytes usually contain numerous organisms within the necrotic foci. These lesions are compared to the *tuberculoid response* of human Hansen's disease, which is considered a *high-resistance form.* A second type of reaction in cats consists of solid sheets of large foamy macrophages and many multinucleated giant cells, with acid-fast bacilli being numerous in both cell types. Perivascular lymphocytes and plasma cells vary from few to many. This latter type of reaction has been compared to the *lepromatous form* of human leprosy which is considered to be the *low-resistance form* associated with a deficit in cell-mediated immunity. Neutrophils are present in both types of lesions but are most numerous in the lepromatous form, often resulting in a pyogranulomatous reaction. Nerve involvement, the most important histologic feature of Hansen's disease, is only sporadically observed in feline leprosy. Regional lymph nodes are characterized by variable architectural disruption by infiltrates of macrophages. Acid-fast bacteria are rare within lymph nodes.

Differential diagnoses include other mycobacterial infections, mycotic infections, and cutaneous xanthoma/xanthogranuloma. Xanthomas are sterile granulomatous lesions composed of foamy macrophages, which resemble the lepromatous form of feline leprosy. However, this form of feline leprosy is usually associated with numerous acid-fast bacteria and acid-fast staining will allow differentiation from xanthomas. Mycotic infections can usually be differentiated by demonstration of fungal elements with special stains and culture of a compatible fungal agent. Diagnosis of feline leprosy is complicated by the fact that it cannot be reliably differentiated from other mycobacterial infections histologically. Traditionally, feline leprosy has been diagnosed when acid-fast bacteria were identified in a granulomatous skin lesion from which mycobacteria could not be cultured. However, failure to culture mycobacteria does not confirm a diagnosis of feline leprosy since there are other mycobacterial species that are difficult to culture, organisms may not be cultured because of technical difficulties, or because organisms may be rare or unevenly distributed within the tissue and the sample may not be representative. As molecular-based diagnostic tests become more common, the diagnosis of feline leprosy as well as other mycobacterial infections will become more rapid and accurate than when based on histologic examination and culture.

Opportunistic, or atypical, mycobacteria

Opportunistic, or atypical, mycobacteria are widespread saprophytes commonly found in *water, soil, and decaying vegetation*. They include rapidly growing and slow-growing organisms. Human and animal infections caused by opportunistic mycobacteria are being reported with increasing frequency. Cutaneous lesions with rapidly growing opportunistic mycobacteria have been reported primarily in cats and less frequently in dogs. Isolates associated with skin infections include *Mycobacterium chelonae, M. fortuitum, M. phlei, M. smegmatis, M. thermoresistible*, and *M. xenopi*. Although cutaneous disease has also been caused by slow-growing atypical mycobacteria, these organisms are more commonly associated with disseminated disease that is indistinguishable from tuberculosis. *M. avium-intracellulare* complex (MAC) is the most common slow-growing opportunistic mycobacterium isolated from cutaneous disease in cats and dogs. *M. kansasii* has been cultured from skin lesions in cattle. Cutaneous infections are thought to be acquired from the environment following trauma such as bite or fight wounds, abrasions, and puncture wounds. Cutaneous disease occurs most commonly in adult cats that hunt or fight frequently and may be more common in obese individuals. After inoculation of organisms into a wound, the lesion develops slowly over a period of weeks to months. Experimental evidence indicates that introduction of acid-fast bacilli into oil or adipose tissue enhances their pathogenicity, possibly by providing nutrients for their growth or by protecting them from the host immune response. Animal-to-animal transmission is not thought to occur. Underlying predisposing diseases or immunologic compromise are often present in humans with these infections but are usually not identified in animals. Affected cats tested for feline leukemia virus and feline immunodeficiency virus infections have been negative.

The clinical course of opportunistic mycobacterial infection is typically prolonged. *Lesions include single or multiple cutaneous and subcutaneous nodules, plaques, purpuric macules, or diffuse swellings*. Multiple punctate ulcers or large fistulous tracts frequently develop and discharge serous, serosanguineous, or purulent exudate that is not usually malodorous. Lesions in cats caused by rapidly growing opportunistic organisms are characteristically located in the subcutaneous fat of the inguinal area. The tissue becomes progressively thickened, board-like, and firmly attached to the body wall. Lesions slowly enlarge and may involve the entire ventrum or extend up the lateral aspect of the trunk. Regional lymph nodes may become enlarged. Despite extensive cutaneous involvement, affected animals usually remain active and normal and exhibit no systemic signs. Skin lesions in cattle are frequently located on the distal limbs.

The *microscopic lesions* of atypical cutaneous mycobacteriosis are usually *multinodular-to-diffuse pyogranulomatous dermatitis and panniculitis*. Since inflammation is generally most intense in the subcutaneous fat, a *deep wedge biopsy* is preferable to a punch biopsy for diagnosis. Infections caused by rapidly growing mycobacteria typically contain circular clear vacuoles surrounded by a rim of neutrophils and a wider outer zone of epithelioid macrophages and variable numbers of neutrophils among more diffuse inflammation composed of macrophages, neutrophils, and lymphoid cells (Fig. 5.94A). Multinucleated giant cells are infrequent. *Organisms are characteristically rare and difficult to find but are usually located in small clumps within the clear vacuoles* (Fig. 5.94B). Small numbers of organisms may also be found within macrophages. The bacilli may stain more intensely with modified acid-fast stain than with routine acid-fast stain. In some instances, staining frozen sections of formalin-fixed tissue may result in enhanced acid-fast staining. The organisms are long rods to short filamentous bacilli. Intracellular bacteria tend to be shorter rods. The organisms stain unevenly positive with tissue Gram stains, resulting in a beaded appearance to the bacilli. *Because of the scarcity of organisms, any single section may lack organisms and the diagnosis will be missed.* The clear vacuoles characteristically seen among inflammatory cells in lesions with rapidly growing opportunistic mycobacteria are not typical of lesions caused by MAC organisms. Moreover, acid-fast bacilli are frequently numerous and are demonstrable by routine acid-fast stains in MAC infections. Lesions in cats caused by MAC organisms may be indistinguishable from feline leprosy. In rare instances, fibroplasia may be marked and the lesion may be confused for a spindle cell tumor. *The specific diagnosis of opportunistic mycobacterial infection requires identification by culture or molecular-based techniques.* Because of the scarcity of organisms in some lesions, diagnosis may require multiple attempts at biopsy and culture.

Miscellaneous mycobacterial infections

Although tuberculosis caused by *M. bovis* typically produces pulmonary or alimentary lesions, in some cases the skin may be the only apparent site of infection. In a survey of 57 cats with *M. bovis* infection in New Zealand, *nonhealing skin lesions* were the most common clinical sign and no evidence of internal disease was evident in the cats with skin disease. Lesions occurred in various body locations, including the legs, shoulder, flank, and inguinal area. The majority of cases occurred in regions in which *M. bovis* is endemic in the Australian brush-tailed possum and it was speculated that skin infections were more common than the classical forms of tuberculosis because they were acquired from *bite or scratch wounds from infected possums*. The histologic features consisted of poorly circumscribed pyogranulomatous inflammation extending along fascial

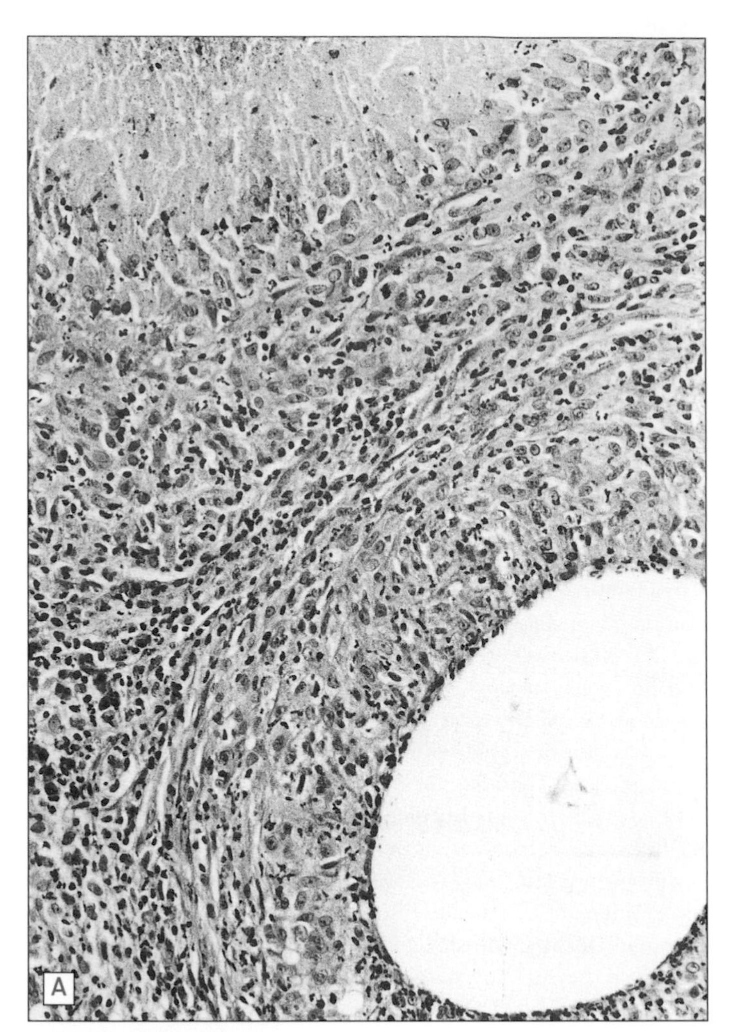

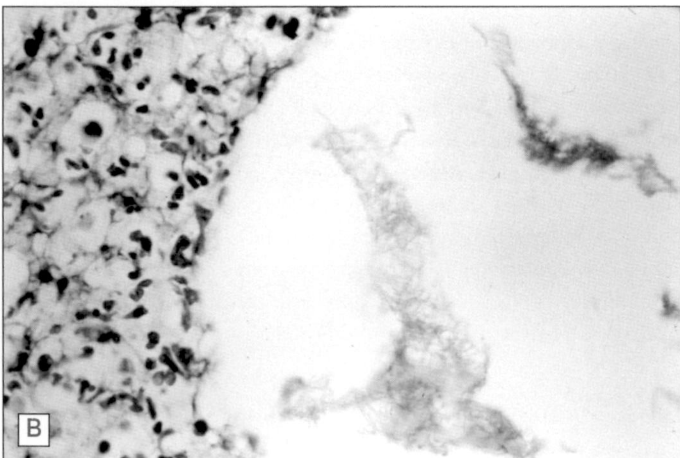

Figure 5.94 Atypical mycobacteriosis in a cat. **A.** Accumulations of mixed leukocytes with neutrophils, bordering a fat globule. **B.** High magnification of fat globule containing **filamentous organisms**.

planes. Coagulative necrosis was moderate to extensive. Acid-fast bacilli varied from rare to innumerable. Without cultural identification of the organisms, the histologic lesions could be confused for feline leprosy and other mycobacterial infections. No evidence of a zoonotic risk was found, since no pet owners became infected despite the presence of large numbers of organisms in some of the skin lesions.

Infection with an as yet unidentified mycobacterium with characteristics intermediate between *M. tuberculosis* and *M. bovis* has been described in cats in the United Kingdom and Channel Islands and termed **feline tuberculosis syndrome**. Adult cats with a history of hunting may be predisposed to the infection. All cats tested for feline leukemia virus and feline immunodeficiency virus were negative and no evidence of immunosuppression was found. *The primary clinical signs were cutaneous lesions*; while lesions more typical of classical tuberculosis, such as generalized lymphadenopathy and respiratory signs, were evident in only a few of the cats. *Skin lesions included swellings, firm raised nodules, and draining sinuses*. Some of the lesions arose in sites of previous bite wounds. Regional lymphadenopathy was frequently present. Microscopic lesions consisted of *discrete and coalescing pyogranulomatous dermatitis and panniculitis*. Granulomas composed of epithelioid macrophages and fewer neutrophils were surrounded by more diffuse infiltrates of macrophages, neutrophils, plasma cells, and lymphocytes in a proliferating granulation tissue stroma. Necrosis was variable and ranged from a few scattered foci located within some of the granulomas to extensive coalescing foci. Organisms were visible with routine acid-fast stain and were usually in low numbers but were numerous in a few cases. The zoonotic potential of this mycobacterial infection is unknown.

A condition referred to as **canine leproid granuloma syndrome** has been described in dogs in Australia, Africa, and North America. The disease is characterized by *cutaneous lesions in which acid-fast bacteria are visible histologically but cannot be cultured*. Short-coated breeds, particularly Boxers and their crosses as well as Doberman Pinschers and Bullmastiffs, appear to have a predilection for the infection. Lesions consist of *single or multiple, firm, painless nodules primarily on the head and especially on the dorsal surface of the pinnae*. The frequent location on the head led to speculation that transmission involves biting flies or insects. In some cases, lesions spontaneously resolved after weeks to months. In other cases, lesions persisted indefinitely and progressively enlarged or additional lesions developed and became ulcerated. Lymph node and internal organ involvement was not seen. The microscopic features of the condition were not described but acid-fast bacteria were reported to vary from numerous to infrequent, widely scattered, and very difficult to find in tissue sections. Preliminary molecular-based identification of the organisms suggests that the etiological agent(s) is *a new mycobacterial species grouped within the saprophytic mycobacteria*.

Bibliography

Aranaz A, et al. Use of polymerase chain reaction in the diagnosis of tuberculosis in cats and dogs. Vet Rec 1996;138:276–280.

Bercovier H, Vincent V. Mycobacterial infections in domestic and wild animals due to *Mycobacterium marinum, M. fortuitum, M. chelonae, M. porcinum, M. farcinogenes, M. smegmatis, M. scrofulaceum, M. xenopi, M. kansasii, M. simiae* and *M. genavense*. Rev Sci Tech 2001;20:265–290.

de Lisle GW, et al. A report of tuberculosis in cats in New Zealand, and the examination of strains of *Mycobacterium bovis* by DNA restriction endonuclease analysis. N Z Vet J 1990;38:10–13.

Foley JE, et al. Clinical, microscopic, and molecular aspects of canine leproid granuloma in the United States. Vet Pathol 2002;39:234–239.

Foster ES, et al. Cutaneous lesion caused by *Mycobacterium tuberculosis* in a dog. J Am Vet Med Assoc 1986;188:1188–1190.

Fox LE, et al. Disseminated subcutaneous *Mycobacterium fortuitum* infection in a dog. J Am Vet Med Assoc 1995;206:53–55.
Gunn-Moore DA, et al. Feline tuberculosis: a literature review and discussion of 19 cases caused by an unusual mycobacterial variant. Vet Rec 1996;138:53–58.
Hughes MS, et al. Determination of the etiology of presumptive feline leprosy by 16S rRNA gene analysis. J Clin Microbiol 1997;35:2464–2471.
Lemarie SL. Mycobacterial dermatitis. Vet Clin North Am Small Anim Pract 1999;29:1291–1301.
Lewis DT, et al. Experimental reproduction of feline *Mycobacterium fortuitum* panniculitis. Vet Dermatol 1994;5:189–195.
Malik R, et al. Subcutaneous granuloma caused by *Mycobacterium avium* complex infection in a cat. Aust Vet J 1998;76:604–607.
Malik R, et al. Feline leprosy: two different clinical syndromes. J Feline Med Surg 2002;4:43–59.
Miller MA, et al. Inflammatory pseudotumor in a cat with cutaneous mycobacteriosis. Vet Pathol 1999;36:161–163.
Roccabianca P, et al. Feline leprosy: Spontaneous remission in a cat. J Am Anim Hosp Assoc 1996;32:189–193.
Stevenson K, et al. Feline skin granuloma associated with *Mycobacterium avium*. Vet Rec 1998;143:109–110.

Botryomycosis

Botryomycosis (bacterial pseudomycosis, bacterial granuloma) is *a chronic infection caused by nonfilamentous bacteria that form colonies visible as tissue grains or granules within lesions*. Clinically and histologically, the condition resembles actinomycotic and eumycotic mycetomas. The disease occurs in humans and all domestic animals. Although reported rarely, the condition is probably not uncommon. Lesions are usually localized in the skin and subcutis but may extend deep to involve underlying bone and muscle. Disseminated infection with visceral involvement is rare. Coagulase-positive staphylococci are involved most commonly; but streptococci, *Pseudomonas, Actinobacillus, Pasteurella, Proteus, Escherichia*, and other organisms have also been isolated from lesions. Infection is thought to develop as a result of wound contamination or trauma such as bites, lacerations, or puncture wounds with foreign bodies.

Lesions typically consist of *firm, nonpruritic single or multiple nodules that ulcerate and develop draining fistulae*. They discharge purulent material which frequently contains *white to yellow sand-like grains*. The microscopic lesion is characterized by the presence of *basophilic granules within the center of neutrophilic abscesses or pyogranulomas in the dermis or subcutis*. These granules correspond to the grains seen grossly in the discharge. They are surrounded and separated by fibrous tissue which may be quite extensive. Plant debris or other foreign material may also be seen in the lesions and indicate the means of infection. The granules consist of compact bacterial colonies which are usually surrounded by amorphous, deeply eosinophilic, radially arranged Splendore-Hoeppli material. The name of the condition is, in part, derived from the appearance of the granules which was thought to be suggestive of a *bunch of grapes*. The bacteria are not well delineated in H&E-stained sections, thus *special stains are usually necessary to distinguish the organisms from actinomycotic bacteria and fungi*. Individual cocci or bacilli within the granules are seen most clearly in sections stained with tissue Gram or Giemsa stains. The GMS procedure also stains bacteria and allows differentiation from fungi.

Bibliography

Donovan GA, Gross TL. Cutaneous botryomycosis (bacterial granulomas) in dairy cows caused by *Pseudomonas aeruginosa*. J Am Vet Med Assoc 1984;184:197–199.
Scott DW. Bacterial pseudomycosis (botryomycosis) in the horse. Eq Pract 1988;10:15–19.
Walton DK, et al. Cutaneous bacterial granuloma (botryomycosis) in a dog and cat. J Am Anim Hosp Assoc 1983;19:537–541.

Bacterial pododermatitis of ruminants

Footrot

Footrot is a highly contagious bacterial infection of the digits of *sheep, cattle, and goats*. It has also been reported in *pigs*. The multistrain, gram-negative, obligate anaerobe *Dichelobacter* (formerly *Bacteroides*) *nodosus* is the essential causal pathogen. *Footrot should not be confused with necrobacillosis of the ruminant foot*, which is a noncontagious, mixed bacterial infection in which *Fusobacterium necrophorum* is the principal pathogen. Footrot occurs worldwide in areas with temperate climate and moderate to high rainfall. The condition is particularly important in sheep because of the economic impact it has on both the wool and meat industries. *Footrot is a major disease in high rainfall areas*, such as Australia and New Zealand, and *can produce severe lameness* because of necrosis of the sensitive laminae and separation of the hoof. The reduced mobility and reluctance of affected animals to eat results in weight loss and decreased wool quality and growth rate, which correlate in a linear manner with the number of feet infected. In addition to the production losses, the cost of treatment and control contribute to significant economic losses.

The pathogenesis of footrot is complex and has been studied most extensively in sheep. The disease is initiated by *maceration of the interdigital skin* brought about commonly by extended exposure to lush, continually wet pasture. Disease is thus most common in rainy seasons. Minor wounds, abrasions from stones, sharp plants, or long coarse grasses, and damage caused by migrating *Strongyloides* larvae are additional factors that can predispose to development of clinical footrot. The damaged epidermis then becomes colonized by *Fusobacterium necrophorum*, aerobic diphtheroids, coliforms, and other common bacteria originating from the soil, skin, and feces. *Footrot develops if the dermatitis is subsequently complicated by infection with D. nodosus*. The bacterium is an obligate parasite of the ruminant hoof and carrier animals serve as the source for uninfected stock. Transmission of infection requires adequate moisture and a mean ambient temperature greater than 10°C. Direct contact between susceptible and infected sheep is not required for transmission of infection. Contact with contaminated substrate for less than 1 hour has been shown to be adequate for transmission; and outbreaks have been associated with contact with environment contaminated by affected animals as long as 4 days previously. *F. necrophorum* and *D. nodosus* act synergistically to produce clinical disease. *D. nodosus* produces a variety of *extracellular proteases* that are thought to digest the horn and allow bacterial invasion of the epidermal matrix of the horn. It also produces a *heat-stable soluble factor* that enhances the growth and invasiveness of *F. necrophorum*. *F. necrophorum* produces a *leukocidal exotoxin* that reduces phagocytosis.

The separation of horn is caused by lysis of the epidermal matrix as a result of the local inflammatory response rather than from direct bacterial attack. *Arcanobacterium pyogenes* and other aerobic bacteria are usually located superficially in the lesion where they remove oxygen, destroy hydrogen peroxide, and create the anaerobic environment necessary for the growth of the two anaerobic pathogens.

Footrot in sheep is a complex clinical disease syndrome. The spectrum of clinical disease is divided into three major forms: *virulent, intermediate, and benign*. Factors associated with severity and persistence of infection include virulence of the particular strain of *D. nodosus*, the environment, and host resistance. Considerable variation exists in the natural resistance to the disease and there is evidence to suggest a genetic basis for the variation in resistance. A possible association between alleles of the major histocompatibility complex (MHC) class II region and resistance to footrot has been found. Most Merino flocks are considered to have a high proportion of susceptible animals. Virulence of *D. nodosus* varies widely from strain to strain. Virulent strains of the bacterium produce more extracellular proteases, including elastase; and proteases from virulent strains tend to be more thermostable than those from benign strains. Two genomic regions of *D. nodosus* are preferentially associated with more virulent isolates of the bacterium. These regions have been named *vap*, for virulence-associated protein, and *vrl*, for virulence-related locus. Although useful as indicators of virulence, the function of these two regions has not been determined. The *virulent form of footrot in sheep* is the serious, persistent form of the disease characterized by severe necrotic damage to the hoof and extensive separation of hoof horn in more than one foot in a high percentage of the sheep. The infection may persist for more than 1 year if not treated, and chronically infected sheep may die of emaciation as a result of severe pain and lameness. Affected animals are also predisposed to flystrike. *Benign footrot*, also called "*foot-scald*," is a milder, less persistent form of the condition. It is typically characterized by moderate interdigital dermatitis which causes mild lameness and minimal production loss. The benign form has a greater propensity for self-cure.

Footrot in sheep develops approximately 10–20 days after exposure and *begins as interdigital dermatitis in the axial bulbar notch*. At this early stage, the interdigital skin is pale, swollen, and moist. Inflammation progressively extends forward and caudad around the bulb of the heel. Separation of the horn usually occurs 7 days later, beginning at the skin-horn junction and spreading to the bulb and sole. The animal is severely lame at this stage. From the sole, the process spreads to the hoof wall to involve the axial and abaxial surfaces of the digits. Exudation is minimal and consists of a small amount of gray, greasy malodorous material in the cleft beneath the underrun horn. Since the infection does not destroy the germinative layers of the horn, new horn is continually being regenerated but is rapidly destroyed as long as the infection continues. Chronically infected feet become long and misshapen.

Benign footrot is indistinguishable from the early stages of virulent footrot. However, *in benign footrot the erosions usually remain confined to the caudal aspect of the interdigital cleft*. Occasionally there is separation of the soft horn of the heel and caudal portion of the sole but there is no separation of the hard horn. Affected sheep may appear normal or exhibit mild, temporary lameness. The effect of benign footrot on production is minimal.

Diagnosis of footrot in sheep is based on clinical signs, demonstration of D. nodosus in smears from lesional material, and culture and biochemical characterization of isolates to identify antigenic and virulence variants. Because the organism is slow to grow, culture and biochemical testing is time-consuming and may require up to 10–14 days. Gene probes have been developed to identify the virulence-associated loci vap and vrl in lesional material. This testing can be completed within 48–72 hours.

Footrot of **cattle and goats** is typically a *less severe disease* and resembles the benign form of footrot of sheep. Infection with *D. nodosus* is more common than is clinical disease. Direct transmission can occur between sheep and goats in the same environment but the innate resistance of goats appears to be greater than that of sheep. The lesions in goats tend to stay confined to the interdigital skin. Underrunning lesions are not common in goats and are usually restricted to a portion of the soft horn. *D. nodosus* isolates from *cattle* with footrot tend to be relatively benign strains. Footrot in cattle usually begins at the caudal aspect of the interdigital space, spreads laterally on the bulbs of the heels, and eventually involves the entire interdigital space. *Lesions usually remain confined to the interdigital skin* which may be eroded, ulcerated, or become deeply fissured. The fissures are covered with necrotic material with a characteristic fetid odor. Lesions may extend to the heels and mild separation of the soft horn may develop. Extensive undermining of the horn, as occurs in sheep, does not typically occur in cattle. Affected animals stand on their toes. In rare severe cases, fever, anorexia, recumbency, and decreased milk production may develop.

Bibliography

Billington SJ, et al. Virulence regions and virulence factors of the ovine footrot pathogen, *Dichelobacter nodosus*. FEMS Microbiol Lett 1996;145:147–156.

Escayg AP, et al. Association between alleles of the ovine major histocompatibility complex and resistance to footrot. Res Vet Sci 1997;63:283–287.

Ghimire SC, et al. Transmission of virulent footrot between sheep and goats. Aust Vet J 1999;77:450–453.

Kennan RM, et al. The type IV fimbrial subunit gene (fimA) of *Dichelobacter nodosus* is essential for virulence, protease secretion, and natural competence. J Bacteriol 2001;183:4451–4458.

Marshall DJ, et al. The effect of footrot on body weight and wool growth of sheep. Aust Vet J 1991;68:45–49.

Piriz S, et al. Bacteriological study of footrot in pigs: a preliminary note. Vet Rec 1996;139:17–19.

Whittington RJ. Observations on the indirect transmission of virulent ovine footrot in sheep yards and its spread in sheep on unimproved pasture. Aust Vet J 1995;72:132–134.

Zhou H, et al. Rapid and accurate typing of *Dichelobacter nodosus* using PCR amplification and reverse dot-blot hybridisation. Vet Microbiol 2001;80:149–162.

Papillomatous digital dermatitis

Papillomatous digital dermatitis is a painful, contagious dermatitis of the feet of *cattle* that occurs worldwide. The condition is also called *footwarts* and *hairy heelwarts*; and clinically and histologically, it appears to be the same disease as *digital dermatitis, interdigital papillomatosis, verrucose dermatitis, and digital papillomatosis*. Papillomatous digital dermatitis is economically important because it frequently *causes moderate-to-severe lameness* that results in weight loss, decreased milk production, and poor reproductive performance. A similar condition has been reported in *sheep and a horse*. The condition in horses is not as rare as might be supposed from the literature, and is recognized in diagnostic laboratories where horses are commonly submitted for disease investigations.

The *vast majority of cases are in dairy cows* but it has also been reported in beef cattle. Although the disease occurs in all ages, the highest incidence appears to be in *replacement heifers*. The etiology of papillomatous digital dermatitis is unknown but it is *suspected to be bacterial* based on the favorable response to antibacterial therapy, presence of numerous *intralesional spirochetes*, lack of demonstrable viruses and other known pathogens, and evidence of a specific humoral response in affected animals to spirochetes isolated from lesions of papillomatous digital dermatitis. The spirochetes have been identified as *Treponema phagedenis*-like. Genetic analysis indicates that the organisms are related to pathogenic human treponemes associated with periodontitis. The condition is also usually associated with management conditions in which the feet of cattle remain wet for prolonged periods, such as following a rainy season, during indoor confined housing in the winter, or in muddy corrals. The condition tends to disappear when cattle are on pasture, but some outbreaks are unassociated with any apparent predisposing factors.

Papillomatous digital dermatitis most commonly affects the skin proximal and adjacent to the interdigital space at the back of the hindfeet. The front feet are less frequently involved and usually only one foot is affected. The cranial aspect of the foot and the interdigital skin are rarely involved. Lesions are painful, forcing the animal to shift its weight to the toe of the foot and resulting in clubbing of the affected foot and atrophy of the bulbs of the heels. Early lesions are well-circumscribed, round-to-oval, red plaques up to 6 cm in diameter with a moist granular surface prone to bleeding and with a very strong, pungent odor. They are partially to completely alopecic and may be bordered by hypertrophied hairs two to three times longer than normal. The lesions become progressively more proliferative and less painful with time. Mature lesions are irregular wart-like growths or filamentous papillae which measure 0.5–1.0 mm in diameter and 1 mm to 3 cm in length and are pale yellow, gray, or brown.

The early *microscopic changes* of papillomatous digital dermatitis consist of mild epidermal hyperplasia with foci of erosion, necrosis, ballooning degeneration, and microabscesses. The basal layer exhibits an increased mitotic index. The dermis contains minimal perivascular inflammation. Mixed bacteria may be present in the outer necrotic debris but only spirochetes are present in the deeper viable epidermis. Two morphologically distinct spirochetes have been demonstrated to be in large numbers in early lesions. One is a long thin type with few twists and the other is a short, thick spirochete with many twists. The spirochetes are oriented perpendicular to the epidermis and appear to invade the keratinocytes. The older lesions are composed of frond-like projections or plaques of markedly hyperplastic epidermis with parakeratosis and hyperkeratosis. Foci of necrosis and hemorrhage, ballooning degeneration, and aggregates of neutrophils are scattered throughout the hyperplastic epidermis. At this later stage, inflammation is more intense in the dermis and plasma cells may be numerous.

Bibliography

Choi B-K, et al. Spirochetes from digital dermatitis lesions in cattle are closely related to treponemes associated with human periodontitis. Int J Sys Bacteriol 1997;47:175–181.

Demirkan I, et al. The frequent detection of a treponeme in bovine digital dermatitis by immunocytochemistry and polymerase chain reaction. Vet Microbiol 1998;60:285–292.

Döpfer D, et al. Histological and bacteriological evaluation of digital dermatitis in cattle, with special reference to spirochaetes and *Campylobacter faecalis*. Vet Rec 1997;140:620–623.

Naylor RD, et al. Isolation of spirochaetes from an incident of severe virulent ovine footrot. Vet Rec 1998;143:690–691.

Rashmir-Raven AM, et al. Papillomatous pastern dermatitis with spirochetes and *Pelodera strongyloides* in a Tennessee Walking horse. J Vet Diagn Invest 2000;12:287–291.

Read DH, Walker RL. Papillomatous digital dermatitis (footwarts) in California dairy cattle: clinical and gross pathologic findings. J Vet Diagn Invest 1998;10:67–76.

Rijpkema SGT, et al. Partial identification of spirochaetes from two dairy cows with digital dermatitis by polymerase chain reaction analysis of the 16S ribosomal RNA gene. Vet Rec 1997;140:257–259.

Trott DJ, et al. Characterization of *Treponema phagedenis*-like spirochetes isolated from papillomatous digital dermatitis lesions in dairy cattle. J Clin Microbiol 2003;41:2522–2529.

Skin lesions in systemic bacterial disease

Skin lesions may develop during the course of systemic bacterial infection. They frequently arise *as a result of vasculitis and/or thrombosis*. This occurs most commonly in **pigs**. Swine erysipelas, caused by *Erysipelothrix rhusiopathiae*, is a generalized septicemia that is commonly associated with *blue-purple rhomboidal plaques (diamond skin lesions)* (Fig. 5.95). These lesions are obvious on light-skinned pigs but may require palpation for detection on pigmented animals. The lesions either regress spontaneously or undergo necrosis,

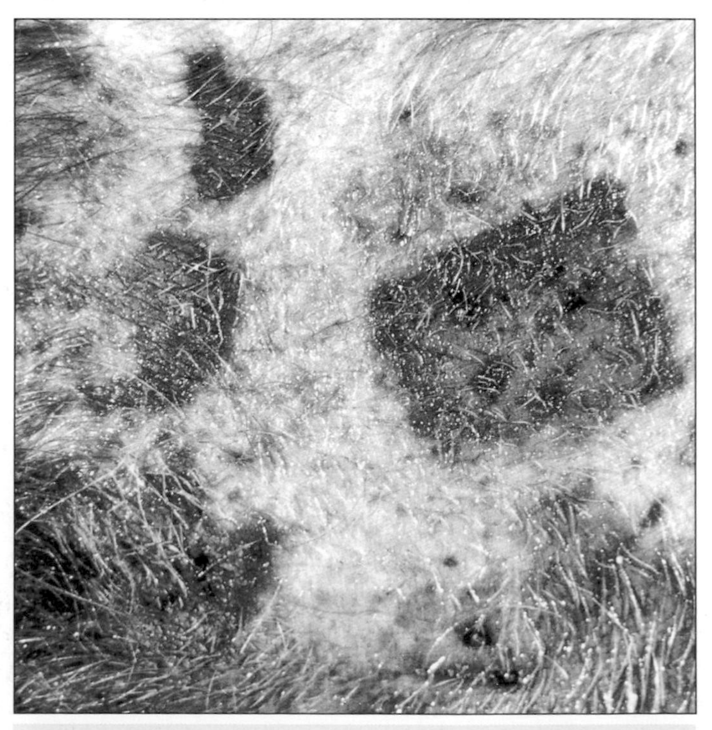

Figure 5.95 Classical "diamond skin" lesions in ***Erysipelothrix rhusiopathiae*** infection in a pig.

become hard and dry, and eventually slough. Severely affected ears and tail may also be sloughed. Microscopic findings include marked dermal congestion, neutrophilic vasculitis, cutaneous necrosis, and suppurative hidradenitis. Various gram-negative septicemias, in particular septicemic salmonellosis caused by *S. choleraesuis*, may produce blue-purple discoloration of the skin of the ears, ventral abdomen, snout, and tail primarily as a result of *endotoxin-induced venous thrombosis*. *Pasteurella multocida* may cause similar skin lesions in pigs. *Edema disease*, caused by a hemolytic *E. coli* may be associated with subcutaneous edema secondary to vascular hyaline degeneration, fibrinoid necrosis, and mural edema.

Skin lesions occur less commonly in other domestic species with systemic bacterial infection. *Salmonella dublin* infections in **cattle** may produce gangrene of distal extremities, tail, and pinnae as a consequence of vascular thrombosis. Cutaneous lesions are uncommon in **dogs** with systemic infections. Rocky Mountain spotted fever, caused by *Rickettsia rickettsii*, is most often associated with skin lesions. These consist primarily of edema and hyperemia; petechial and ecchymotic hemorrhages may also occur but typically involve mucous membranes rather than the skin. Acral dermal necrosis occurs rarely. Microscopic findings consist of necrotizing vasculitis, which may result in cutaneous necrosis. Dogs with Lyme borreliosis, caused by *Borrelia burgdorferi*, may develop a small, reddened skin lesion at the site of tick attachment. This lesion usually disappears within a week and is very inconspicuous as compared to the striking expanding, annular erythematous rash (erythema chronicum migrans) typical of the infection in humans.

FUNGAL DISEASES OF SKIN

Fungi are ubiquitous in the environment but, of the thousands present, only a few are capable of causing infection in animals. *The vast majority of fungi in nature are incapable of causing infection because they are unable to breach two major physiologic barriers to fungal growth in tissue: temperature and oxidation-reduction potential.* Many fungi have an optimal growth range considerably below the temperature of the body and cannot survive the relatively high temperature of the body. Other fungi, even if thermotolerant, cannot survive in the reduced state of living tissue. The propensity of fungi to cause infection is dependent not only on their ability to adapt to the tissue environment and temperature, but also to withstand the lytic activity of the host's cellular defenses. Some fungi are *true pathogens* with the ability to cause disease in normal individuals while many more organisms are *opportunistic pathogens* that infect individuals who have become immunologically or otherwise compromised and are unable to resist and suppress the fungal invasion. Immunocompromise by various infectious agents, such as *Human immunodeficiency virus, Feline leukemia virus, Feline immunodeficiency virus,* and *Canine distemper virus,* as well as pharmacologic immunosuppression, are important predisposing factors in development of some fungal infections. However, many mycotic infections occur in individuals without any clinically overt immune impairment. These infections are likely a consequence of an overwhelming exposure to the infectious propagules or mild immunologic defects that are not readily apparent. Mycotic infections are commonly divided into three categories: cutaneous, subcutaneous, and systemic.

- **Cutaneous mycoses** are the most common fungal diseases in veterinary medicine. The infections are generally confined to the nonliving cornified layers of the skin, hair, and claws.
- The **subcutaneous mycoses** are fungal infections that involve the skin and subcutaneous tissues. They are caused by a wide variety of saprophytic fungi that gain entry by traumatic implantation. Infection is a very indolent process and usually remains localized to the site of entry with slow spread to surrounding tissue.
- The **systemic mycoses** are infections of the internal organs. Cutaneous involvement usually occurs as a result of hematogenous dissemination. Skin lesions from direct cutaneous inoculation in systemic mycoses are rare. These infections include blastomycosis, cryptococcosis, coccidioidomycosis, and histoplasmosis. Occasionally the diagnosis of a systemic fungal infection/mycosis, particularly blastomycosis in dogs and cryptococcosis in cats, is made by biopsy of skin lesions.

Histopathology is an important diagnostic tool for fungal infections. It is a relatively rapid and inexpensive means to make a definitive or presumptive diagnosis of mycotic infection. In many cases, fungal infections are mistaken for neoplasms and the entire lesion is fixed and submitted for histologic examination. Consequently, only fixed tissue is available and the pathologist has the responsibility for the final diagnosis because the organism cannot be cultured. Some fungal organisms have distinctive enough morphologic features that, if present in sufficient numbers, they can be identified with a high degree of certainty, e.g., *Blastomyces, Cryptococcus,* and *Coccidioides*. Other mycotic infections are caused by a variety of fungi that are similar in appearance in tissues and cannot be specifically identified, although the disease can be named, e.g., dermatophytosis, phaeohyphomycosis, and eumycotic mycetoma. In some cases, fungi may be detectable in tissues but may be impossible to identify and only the conclusion that mycotic infection exists can be made. Although immunofluorescence and immunohistochemical methods for identification of fungi in formalin-fixed, paraffin-embedded tissue sections have been developed, the specific antisera are not readily available, and *culture remains the mainstay for identification of fungal pathogens.* Some fungi stain with H&E but many fungi do not stain or stain very poorly with H&E. However, even in these cases, fungal infection can be suspected because of the presence of clear circular or linear structures, representing unstained fungal hyphae, within the lesion. *Special fungal stains*, such as Gomori methenamine silver (GMS), which stains fungi black, and periodic acid-Schiff (PAS), which stains fungi pink-red, delineate the fungi so their morphology can be examined. In general, GMS is better for screening tissue because some fungal-like organisms (e.g., *Pythium*) stain poorly with PAS. Fungal stains may mask the natural color of fungi, however. To determine whether a fungus is pigmented, it can be examined in unstained cleared and mounted sections or a melanin stain, such as Fontana-Masson, can be applied to the tissue.

Bibliography

Chandler FW, et al. Color Atlas and Text of the Histopathology of Mycotic Diseases. Chicago, IL: Year Book Medical Publishers, Inc., 1980.

Matsumoto T, et al. Developments in hyalohyphomycosis and phaeohyphomycosis. J Med Vet Mycol 1994;32,(suppl 1):329–349.

Rippon JW. Medical Mycology. The Pathogenic Fungi and the Pathogenic Actinomycetes. 3rd ed. Philadelphia, PA: WB Saunders, 1988.

Cutaneous fungal infections

Cutaneous mycoses are infections in which the fungal organisms are generally confined to the nonliving keratinized tissues, i.e., *stratum corneum, hair, claw, and horn*. Pathologic changes, which occur in response to the infectious agent and its metabolic products, involve the epidermis and dermis and may vary from minimal to severe and extensive. These infections include candidiasis, *Malassezia* dermatitis, and dermatophytosis.

Candidiasis

Candidiasis (candidosis, moniliasis, thrush) is a rare opportunistic infection of skin, mucocutaneous junctions, external ear canal, and the claw bed. *Candida* spp. yeasts are normal inhabitants of the upper respiratory, alimentary, and genital tracts but are not normally present on the skin except at mucocutaneous junctions of body orifices. Factors which alter the superficial keratin barrier (such as maceration, chronic trauma, or burns), upset normal flora (such as prolonged broad spectrum antibiotic therapy), or produce immunosuppression (such as diabetes mellitus, hyperadrenocorticism, neoplasia, viral infections, cytotoxic chemotherapy, or prolonged glucocorticoid treatment) predispose to infection with the organism. Since neutrophils are a major defense mechanism against *Candida*, prolonged neutropenia renders an individual more susceptible to candidiasis. The other major mechanism for eliminating *Candida* from the skin surface is T-cell-mediated immunity.

Infections have been described in *dogs, cats, pigs, horses, and goats*. Lesions are variable and may begin as papules, pustules, and vesicles which evolve into characteristic *sharply delineated ulcers with erythematous borders and a malodorous surface with moist gray-white exudate*. Chronic lesions consist of thickened alopecic hyperkeratotic skin with prominent folds. Histologic changes include hyperkeratosis, parakeratosis, serocellular crusts, subcorneal or superficial epidermal neutrophilic pustules, and spongiosis. The dermis is edematous and contains a superficial perivascular to interstitial mixed infiltrate. *Yeasts, pseudohyphae, and hyphae may be numerous but are best visualized with PAS or GMS stains.* Generally, yeasts are most numerous on the surface of the lesions, while hyphae and pseudohyphae extend into the epidermis.

Bibliography

Ihrke PJ, et al. Cutaneous fungal flora in twenty horses free of skin or ocular disease. Am J Vet Res 1988;49:770–772.

Lehmann PF. Immunology of fungal infections in animals. Vet Immunol Immunopathol 1985;10:33–69.

Lloyd D. Ecology of skin: Balance and disruption. Compend Conti Educ Pract Vet Suppl 1997;19:97–100.

Pichler ME, et al. Cutaneous and mucocutaneous candidiasis in a dog. Compend Contin Educ Pract Vet 1985;7:225–230.

Reynolds IM, et al. Cutaneous candidiasis in swine. J Am Vet Med Assoc 1968;152:182–186.

Malassezia dermatitis

Malassezia pachydermatis (formerly Pityrosporum canis) is a constituent of the normal resident flora of the skin and mucous membranes of dogs and cats and a common cause of ceruminous otitis. Its role as a cause of dermatitis has been controversial. Evidence that the organism is capable of acting as an opportunistic pathogen is provided by cases of chronic dermatitis in which large numbers of yeasts are evident on the skin surface and lesions resolve following antifungal therapy. Predisposing factors are thought to be required for the yeast to cause clinical disease. Excessive surface lipid or cerumen, high humidity, or failure of host defense mechanisms to control overgrowth of the yeast may predispose an animal to develop clinical disease. Many dogs with *Malassezia* dermatitis also have allergic skin disease, seborrhea, or bacterial pyoderma as well as a history of long-term corticosteroid or antibiotic treatment; it is unclear whether these concurrent disorders are involved in development of yeast infection or are merely coincidental. Humans with atopic dermatitis have an increased incidence of *Malassezia* skin infections. Dogs with *Malassezia* dermatitis develop high serum titers of specific IgG antibody and exhibit significantly greater skin test reactions in response to intradermal injection of *M. pachydermatis* extracts than dogs without evidence of *Malassezia* dermatitis, suggesting that *hypersensitivity may be involved in the pathogenesis of clinical disease*. Various breeds of dogs have been found to be at increased risk for *Malassezia* dermatitis in different reports. These differences in affected breeds may reflect regional variation in breed popularity or differences in regional gene pool. In several reports, however, the Basset Hound has been found to have a predilection for this disorder. When numbers of *M. pachydermatis* yeasts on the skin were examined, normal Basset Hounds were found to have higher carriage levels of the yeast as compared to normal mixed-breed dogs, a fact that may contribute to the increased incidence of the disorder in this breed. No sex predilection is evident and most cases are in adult dogs. *Malassezia* dermatitis is reported rarely in cats and has been associated with various neoplasms and other conditions that could alter the host immune response.

Lesions associated with Malassezia dermatitis include erythema, alopecia, greasiness, yellow-gray scaly plaques, lichenification, and hyperpigmentation (Fig. 5.96A). A rancid offensive odor is typical; and moderate to severe pruritus is a common feature. The face, ears, ventral neck, axilla, inguinal area, cranial aspect of the legs, caudal thighs, and feet are most commonly involved. Involvement of one or several of these areas is more common than generalized disease. *Malassezia* dermatitis in cats is seen as black ceruminous otitis externa, chronic chin acne, or generalized erythematous scaly dermatitis.

Histologic features of *Malassezia* dermatitis consist of variable hyperkeratosis, parakeratosis, scale-crusts, and irregular epidermal hyperplasia with intercellular edema (Fig. 5.96B). Exocytosis of lymphocytes, neutrophils, or eosinophils has been found in various reports. Rarely, intra-epidermal eosinophilic pustules were found in dogs without any apparent concurrent dermatosis. There is variable edema and perivascular to interstitial infiltration of mixed cells in the superficial dermis. *Malassezia* organisms are *oval to footprint- or peanut-shaped yeasts located in the stratum corneum or in crusts.* They are usually seen in focal aggregates rather than diffusely distributed and they can best be visualized with PAS or GMS stains. The organism will be missed if the skin surface was scrubbed prior to obtaining the biopsy or if the surface debris is lost during processing.

Bibliography

Bond R, Lloyd DG. Skin and mucosal populations of *Malassezia pachydermatis* in healthy and seborrhoeic Basset Hounds. Vet Dermatol 1997;8:101–106.

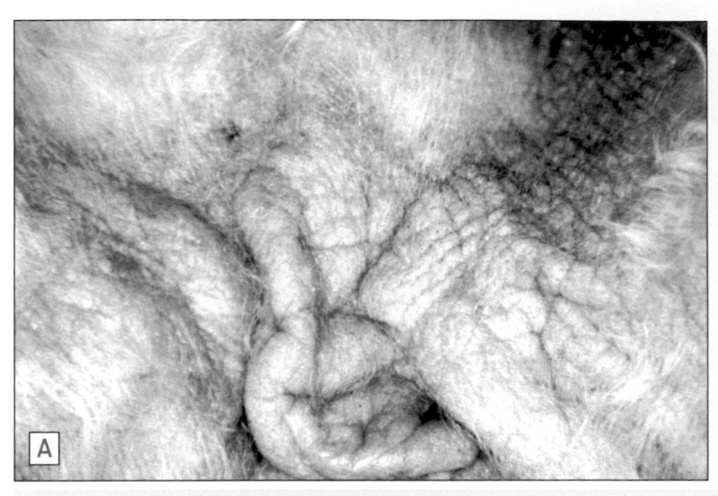

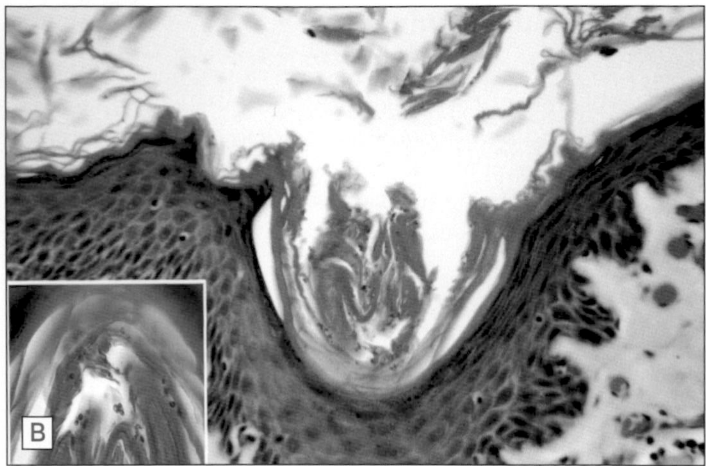

Figure 5.96 ***Malassezia*** **dermatitis** in a dog. **A.** The skin is erythematous, alopecic, greasy, lichenified, and hyperpigmented. (Courtesy of K Beale.) **B.** The epidermis is irregularly hyperplastic with moderate parakeratosis. Yeasts can be seen within the keratin (see inset). (Courtesy of B Dunstan.)

Bond R, et al. Humoral and cell-mediated responses to *Malassezia pachydermatis* in healthy dogs and dogs with *Malassezia* dermatitis. Vet Rec 1998;143:381–384.

Forster-Van Hufte MA, et al. Resolution of exfoliative dermatitis and *Malassezia pachydermatis* overgrowth in a cat after surgical thymoma resection. J Small Anim Pract 1997;38:451–454.

Godfrey DR. A case of feline paraneoplastic alopecia with secondary *Malassezia*-associated dermatitis. J Small Anim Pract 1998;39:394–396.

Mauldin EA, et al. *Malassezia* dermatitis in the dog: a retrospective histopathological and immunopathological study of 86 cases (1990–95). Vet Dermatol 1997;8:191–202.

Morris DO, et al. Type-1 hypersensitivity reactions to *Malassezia pachydermatis* extracts in atopic dogs. Am J Vet Res 1998;59:836–841.

Dermatophytosis

Dermatophytosis ("**ringworm**") *is a superficial fungal infection generally confined to the keratin layers of the skin, hair, and nails.* In rare instances, deeper tissues are involved. The infection is caused by a group of fungi that are capable of using keratin as a source of nutrients and are among the few fungi that cause communicable disease. Infection can vary from mild to severe as a consequence of the host's reactions to metabolic products of the fungus, virulence of the particular species or strain, location of the infection, and local environmental factors. In general, the infection has no effect on growth rate or other measures of productivity, but economic losses may result from hide damage or inability to show infected animals.

The infection is caused by fungi of the genera *Microsporum*, *Trichophyton*, and *Epidermophyton,* which are cosmopolitan in distribution. They are commonly divided according to the host preference and natural habitat of the fungus. The **anthropophilic** dermatophytes are primarily adapted to humans and rarely infect other animals (e.g., *T. rubrum*, *T. mentagrophytes* var. *interdigitale*). Animals occasionally develop infections with these organisms as a reverse zoonosis from infected humans. The **zoophilic** species are those dermatophytes that have become adapted to animals and typically cause less inflammation in their adapted hosts than do geophilic or anthropophilic dermatophytes (e.g., *M. canis* in cats, *T. equinum* in horses). They occasionally infect humans. **Geophilic** species (e.g., *M. gypseum*) normally inhabit the soil in association with keratinous debris in the process of decomposition but they may cause human and animal infection. *M. canis*, *M. gypseum*, and *T. mentagrophytes cause the majority of infections in animals.*

Incidence and prevalence of dermatophytosis vary with individual host factors, health status, climate, season, natural reservoirs, and local environment. A variety of local and systemic factors may predispose an individual to infection. Areas of chronically warm, moist skin are more likely to become clinically infected. Long-term corticosteroid administration, cytotoxic drugs, diabetes mellitus, hematologic malignancies, and other causes of natural or iatrogenic immunosuppression are associated with susceptibility to dermatophytosis. Incidence of infection is increased with hot, humid weather and when populations of stable flies and mosquitoes are large. In confined animals, infection is common in fall and winter when animals are crowded together in wet, poorly ventilated, unsanitary conditions with decreased exposure to sunlight. Young animals appear to be more susceptible to infection than adults. Reasons for this apparent predisposition include immaturity of host immunity, lack of previous exposure, and age-related differences in biochemical properties of the skin, such as qualitative or quantitative differences in antifungal fatty acids in sebum secretions. Transmission of dermatophytosis occurs by direct contact with infected animals or indirectly by exposure to infective hair and scales in the environment (contaminated grooming equipment, bedding, saddles, cages, etc.). *Hair fragments containing infectious arthrospores are the most effective means of transmission.* They can remain infectious for more than 18 months if protected from the deleterious effects of ultraviolet light. This material is the major source of persistent environmental contamination. Certain dermatophytes are associated with specific sources. *M. canis*, despite its name, is most commonly associated with cats, and the cat is considered the reservoir for this dermatophyte. *T. mentagrophytes* dermatophytosis is typically acquired from small rodents; infection with *M. gypseum*, a geophilic dermatophyte, is assumed to be acquired from digging or rooting in contaminated soil. An animal's habitat is an important factor in the incidence and type of infection contracted. In a survey of dermatophytosis in Madras, India, a predominance of *M. gypseum* was cultured from stray dogs, which would be expected to have frequent contact with soil. In contrast, pet dogs were infected primarily with zoophilic (*T. mentagrophytes*) and anthropophilic (*T. rubrum*) dermatophytes, the latter infections suspected to be reverse zoonoses since there was a history of exposure to people known to be infected with *T. rubrum* in most of the cases.

Normal skin is relatively inhospitable to fungal growth because of low moisture conditions, antifungal substances in the surface film, and normal resident flora. Sebum contains fatty acids which are fungistatic and play an important role in resistance to infection. The process by which the stratum corneum is continually renewed may also present a form of defense against organisms because the process results in continuous shedding of the stratum corneum and thus removes infecting organisms with the sloughed keratin. Disruption of the stratum corneum, either by microabrasions or maceration, appears to be important in facilitating invasion by the fungus. Fungal cells adhere to keratinocytes and migrate to the follicular orifice. Dermatophytes produce keratinolytic enzymes, keratinases, which hydrolyze keratin and enable them to penetrate and invade the hair shaft. They grow downward within the hair shaft toward the hair bulb until they reach the keratogenous zone where they stop since they cannot grow in viable tissue. Infection continues as long as the downward growth of the fungus is in equilibrium with keratin production; if not, the fungus is sloughed and the hair is cleared of infection. When the hair enters telogen phase, keratin production stops and fungal growth ceases. Hair shafts are weakened as a result of penetration by the fungi and they become brittle and easily broken.

Dermatophytosis in healthy individuals is *usually self-limiting*, with lesions resolving in several weeks to two or three months. An inverse relationship appears to exist between the degree of inflammation produced by the fungal pathogen and chronicity of infection. Defense against infection involves both immune and non-immune mechanisms. The epidermis represents more than just a passive barrier against entry of invading microorganisms, because keratinocytes produce a variety of eicosanoids, growth factors, chemotactic cytokines, interleukins, and colony stimulating factors that can mediate inflammation. In addition, increased epidermal proliferation occurs early in infection, even before an immunologic response develops, and helps expel the organisms by desquamation. Cell wall components of the organisms activate complement via the alternative pathway. Chemotactic factors generated in the complement cascade as well as those produced by keratinocytes attract neutrophils, which are the chief effector cells. They can kill fungi with products generated in the oxidative burst and also by nonoxidative microbicidal substances within their granules. Neutrophils also have fungistatic activity via *calprotectin*, a calcium- and zinc-binding protein. Macrophages are involved to a lesser extent and produce nitric oxide, which inhibits fungal growth. Nonspecific mechanisms prevent invasion into deeper tissues even in the absence of immunity. Substances in the dermis may prevent growth of organisms. Some of these include unsaturated transferrin, which may interfere with fungal growth in the dermis by competition for iron, and α_2-macroglobulin which inhibits keratinases. Both humoral and cell-mediated immunity develop in response to infection with dermatophytes. Antibodies develop against keratinase as well as fungal glycoproteins but they apparently do not help eliminate infection since the highest titers are found in patients with chronic infections. In contrast, development of cell-mediated immunity is associated with clinical cure and elimination of the organism. In experimental *M. canis* infections in cats, there was no relationship between antibody titers and recovery; but a close temporal relationship was found between the development of increased lymphocyte proliferative responses and regression of lesions. Cell-mediated immunity is the major immunologic defense in clearing dermatophyte infections. Immunity post-infection is relative, so re-infection is possible; however, lesions are smaller and resolve more quickly when an animal is re-infected with the same organism.

Impaired T-cell function has been associated with chronic or recurrent dermatophyte infections. An increased incidence of dermatophyte carriage has been found in cats infected with feline immunodeficiency virus (FIV), and severe dermatophyte infections are common in people with AIDS. However, even apparently healthy individuals can have persistent infections. *Inhibitory factors*, which can interfere with lymphocyte blastogenesis in vitro, have been found in serum of people with chronic dermatophyte infection. In addition, *T. rubrum* cell wall mannan has been shown to inhibit lymphoproliferation in vitro and is thought to be involved in the pathogenesis of chronic infections. Chronic dermatophyte infections have also been reported in dogs. *Trichophyton* spp. and *M. persicolor* dermatophyte infections, lasting up to 5 years in some cases, have been described in dogs without any other evidence of an immunodeficiency disorder, suggesting that these organisms may also produce inhibitory substances which prevent development of an effective immune response and elimination of the organism.

The *clinical signs* of dermatophytosis are highly variable and depend on the host-fungus interaction. Well-adapted species, such as *M. canis* infection in cats, produce minimal inflammation while less-adapted species, such as the zoophilic dermatophyte *M. gypseum*, produce more significant inflammation and more prominent lesions. *Expanding circular patches of scaling and alopecia or stubbled hairs are considered the classical lesion of dermatophytosis but these are frequently the exception rather than the rule* (Fig. 5.97A, B). Follicular papules and pustules, more extensive inflammation caused by furunculosis, and crusting are prominent in many cases. Lesions are typically non-pruritic, but occasionally pruritus is intense. *Infection of nails is called* **onychomycosis** and is characterized by misshapen, crumbly or easily broken, and split nails that may be sloughed. **Kerions** are rapidly developing tender erythematous alopecic nodules that may ulcerate. They are usually solitary and most common on the face and forelimbs of dogs that dig in the dirt. These lesions result from *severe furunculosis* producing locally extensive inflammation that may be confused for a tumor. A rare form, the **dermatophyte pseudomycetoma** seen almost exclusively in Persian cats, occurs as *subcutaneous nodules* (Fig. 5.98A, B).

The microscopic lesions of dermatophytosis are as variable as the clinical lesions. *Histopathology is not considered as sensitive as culture for diagnosis*; but it can be used to confirm infection when the significance of a cultured organism is in question. It is most useful in the nodular forms, such as kerion and pseudomycetoma, which are frequently negative when superficial material is cultured. Biopsies should be taken within the outer border of expanding alopecia as this is the most active site of infection and organisms are most likely to be present. In some cases, fungal organisms are evident in HE-stained sections, but *in many instances, fungal stains (PAS, GMS) are necessary to demonstrate infection*. Dermatophytes occur as septate hyphae that

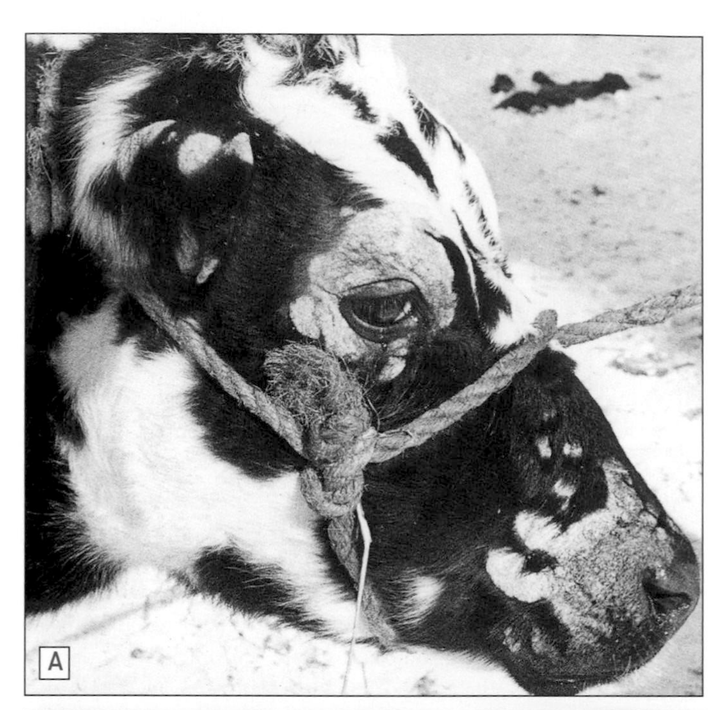

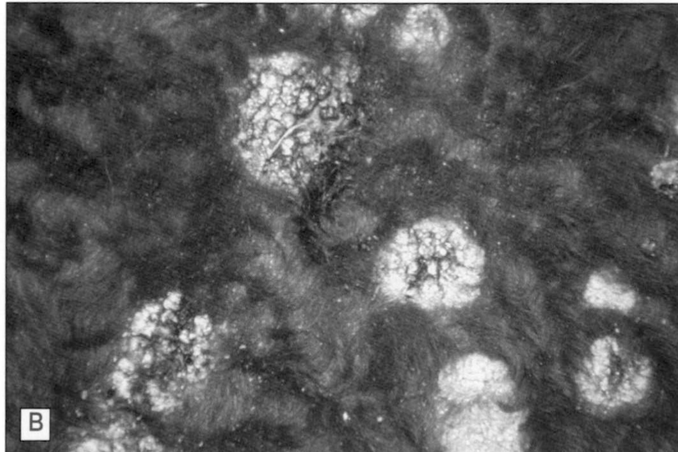

Figure 5.97 Dermatophytosis in a calf. **A.** Gray-white, rough, hairless lesions on the ear, muzzle, and periorbital skin. **B.** Classical "ringworm" lesions of expanding circular patches of scaling and alopecia.

break up into chains of round-to-oval arthrospores in the surface and follicular keratin. *Hyphae are also usually present in the hair shafts and arthrospores are formed on the outside of the hairs (ectothrix) or within the hairs (endothrix).* In rare cases, fungal organisms are present only in the surface keratin; if this material was removed in preparing the skin for obtaining the biopsy or is lost during tissue processing, the diagnosis will be missed. *Ortho- and parakeratotic hyperkeratosis* is a typical feature, and acanthosis is variable, ranging from mild to marked (Fig. 5.99A). Inflammation may be very mild and consist of low numbers of perivascular and perifollicular lymphocytes and macrophages. This is the case when infection is caused by a species of dermatophyte that is well adapted to its host (Fig. 5.99B). *Neutrophilic luminal folliculitis* is a common lesion in dermatophytosis and may result in *follicular rupture and development of discrete granulomas* surrounding fragments of hair at the base of the follicles (Fig. 5.99C). *Eosinophils* may be numerous in these trichogranulomas.

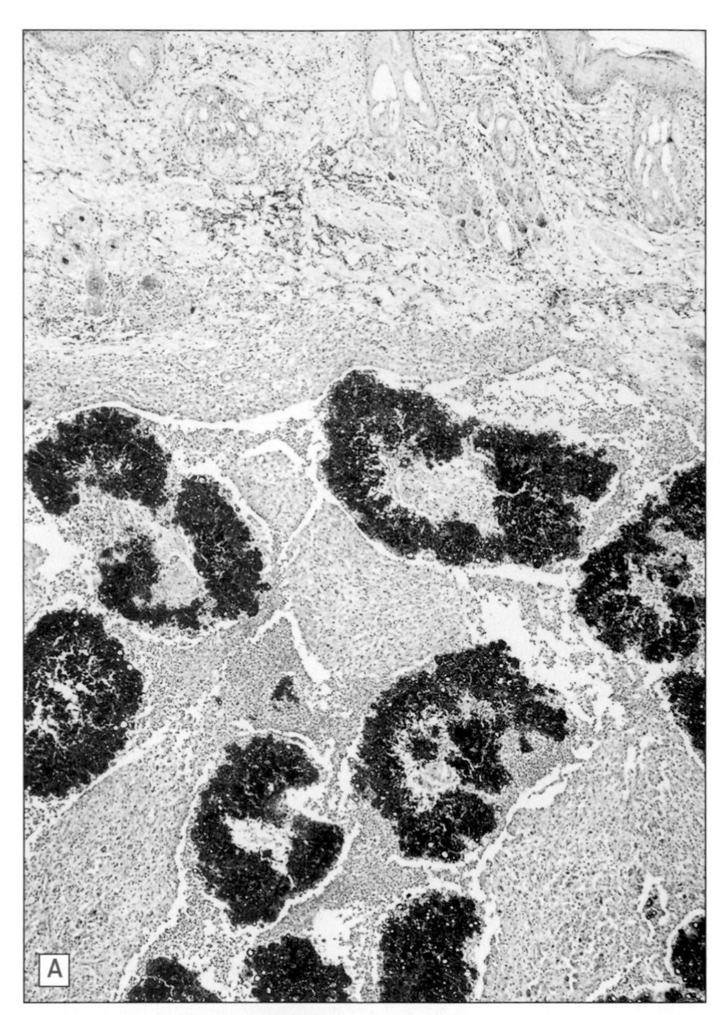

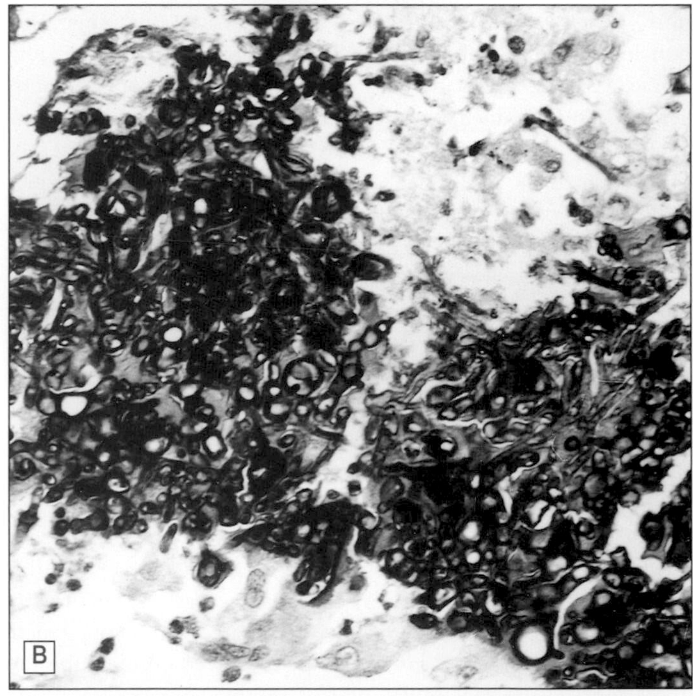

Figure 5.98 ***Microsporum canis*** **pseudomycetoma** in a Persian cat. **A.** Myriads of fungal hyphae (PAS-positive) in the panniculus surrounded by granulomatous inflammation. **B.** Higher magnification of (**A**) showing the appearance of the **hyphae**.

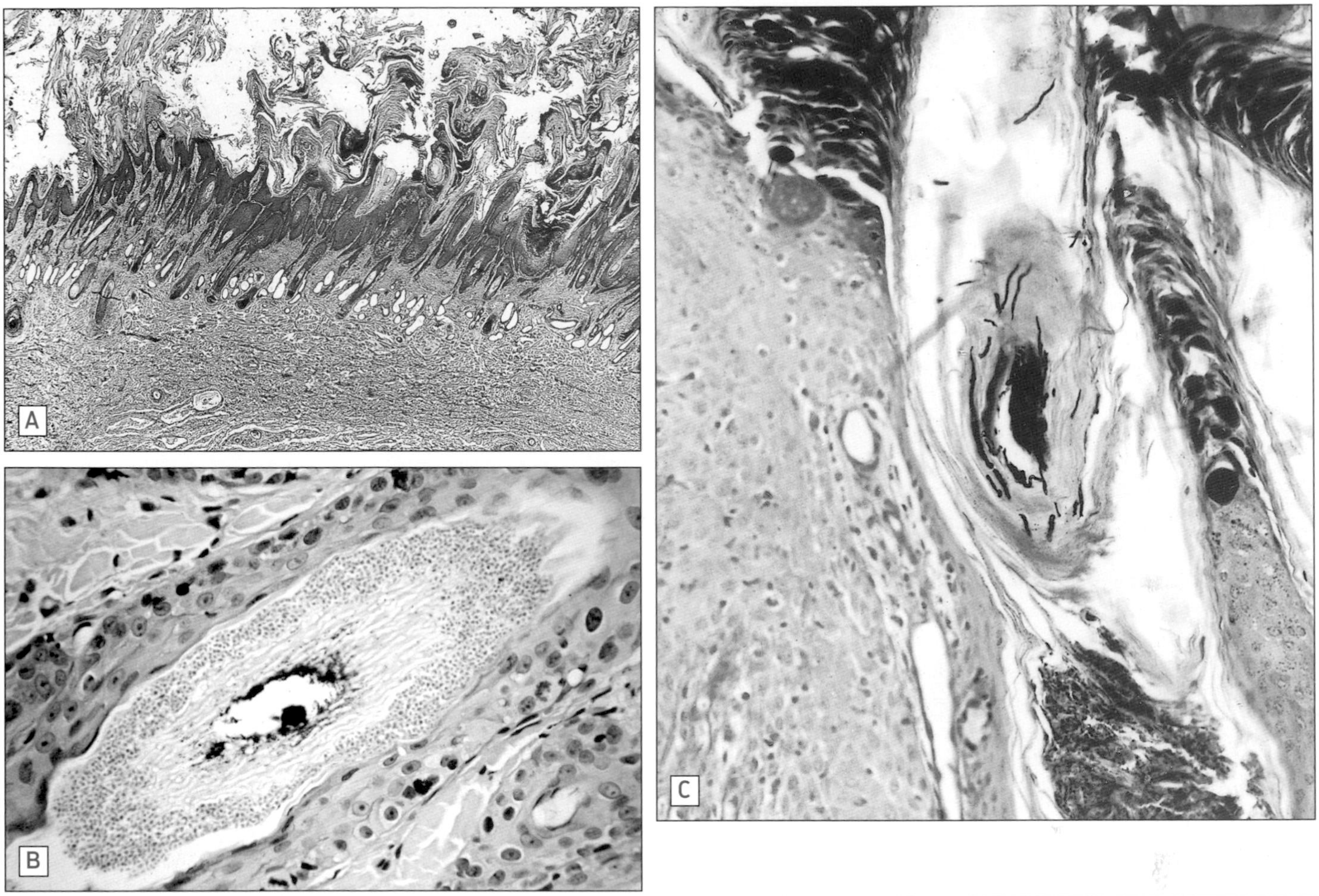

Figure 5.99 **Dermatophytosis**. **A.** Acanthosis and hyperkeratosis in a calf. **B.** Hair follicle heavily colonized by **fungal spores**, with minimal inflammation. **C. Filamentous organisms** in a follicle accompanied by leukocytes, in dermatophytosis in a calf; silver impregnation.

Kerions consist of diffuse pyogranulomatous inflammation in the deep dermis produced by extensive furunculosis. This form of inflammation is most commonly caused by poorly adapted organisms, such as the geophilic dermatophyte *M. gypseum*. Hair fragments containing hyphae and arthrospores are frequently present among the inflammatory cells but may be destroyed by the intense inflammatory reaction. *In some cases, the pattern of inflammation may be confused with autoimmune diseases.* Lymphocytic lichenoid interface dermatitis and subcorneal pustules containing neutrophils and acantholytic cells have been reported in several cases of dermatophytosis in dogs and horses; however, organisms were evident with fungal stains. The *dermatophyte pseudomycetoma* is characterized by masses of fungal elements surrounded by granulomatous or pyogranulomatous inflammation in the deep dermis and subcutis.

Cattle

Dermatophytosis is *common* in cattle and is most prevalent in calves. *T. verrucosum* is the most frequent isolate; others include *T. mentagrophytes, T. equinum, M. gypseum, M. nanum*, and *M. canis*. Outbreaks are associated with *crowding and confinement indoors during fall and winter.* Lesions occur on the *neck, head and ears, and pelvic area* most commonly. The intermaxillary space and dewlap are common sites for lesions in bulls. Lesions consist of *circular areas of alopecia with variable crusting or scaling*. In calves, the entire neck may become alopecic, crusty, thickened, and corrugated and lesions may be intensely pruritic. The disease may be of some economic significance because of damage to hides or restrictions on showing or marketing of infected animals. In very severe cases, loss of condition and decreased milk production or weight gain may result. A live attenuated vaccine for *T. verrucosum* has been effective in control of bovine dermatophytosis in Europe.

Sheep and goats

Dermatophytosis is *rare* in goats and sheep. *T. verrucosum* is the most common isolate. Lesions are usually on the *face, ears, neck, and limbs* in goats. In sheep, lesions are usually on the haired areas of the face and ears and may be intensely pruritic. *M. gypseum* infection in show lambs in the United States, called "*club lamb fungus*" by laypersons, involves wooled skin anywhere on the body but lesions are especially common on the lateral thorax. This condition is of zoonotic significance since, in approximately 50% of families with affected lambs, at least one family member had skin lesions consistent with ringworm. Outbreaks of *M. canis* dermatophytosis in sheep also involve the wooled parts of the body. In infections involving the fleece, lesions consist of circular areas of matted, discolored wool, several millimeters to up to 6 cm in diameter. Pruritus is variable.

Pigs

Dermatophytosis is *rare* in pigs. *M. nanum* is the most common isolate and infection produces little effect on the general health of the animal. *T. verrucosum* occurs in pigs housed in premises previously occupied by cattle. Infections also are also caused by *T. mentagrophytes, M. canis,* and *M. gypseum*. The lesions of *M. nanum* are especially common behind the ears and on the trunk, and consist of irregular dark patches with fine brown scales or crusts. No alopecia or pruritus occurs. Lesions may resolve spontaneously or spread slowly to involve extensive areas. An outbreak of dermatophytosis caused by *M. canis* in pigs was characterized by red alopecic patches of variable size on the backs and flanks. Pruritus was mild. The source of the infection was suspected to be rabbits, which had skin lesions clinically consistent with ringworm, or possibly from cats on the farm.

Horses

Dermatophytosis in the horse (*girth itch, tinea*) is caused by a variety of organisms but most commonly by *T. equinum*. Infections with *T. mentagrophytes* and *M. gypseum* are also common; *T. verrucosum* and *M. canis* infections are less frequent. Lesions occur most often in *areas in contact with the saddle and tack* when infection is spread by contaminated equipment or riders. In some cases, the caudal aspect of the pastern may be the only site affected and resemble "grease heel" or "scratches." Outbreaks of dermatophytosis caused by *M. gypseum* have been associated with periods of humid weather and a high incidence of mosquitoes and stable flies. In some training establishments, over 30% of the horses have ringworm and the causative agent is *M. gypseum*. The mane and tail areas are not usually affected. Initial lesions may be papular and resemble fly bites or urticaria but within several days they become the more typical scaly or crusty circular alopecic foci. The lesions of *M. gypseum* tend to be smaller than those of *T. equinum*. Pruritus varies from severe to absent. Lesions may continue to expand for one or two months and then regress as an immune response develops. Several horses with *T. equinum* dermatophytosis that resembled pemphigus foliaceus have been described. Two adult horses developed rapidly progressive painful widespread dermatitis consisting of papules, pustules, crusting, scaling, and erosions. Microscopically, lesions were characterized by prominent acantholysis. However, fungal arthrospores and hyphae were also evident and lesions resolved with antifungal therapy.

Dogs

M. canis is considered the most common cause of dermatophytosis in dogs; but in some areas, infections caused by *M. gypseum* predominate. *T. mentagrophytes* infection is less frequent. Infections with anthropophilic species *Epidermophyton floccosum* and *T. rubrum* have been reported and suspected to have been acquired from infected humans. Initial lesions are frequently on the face and forelegs. The lesions of dermatophytosis are grossly indistinguishable from demodicosis or pyoderma. Dogs with dermatophytosis frequently exhibit classic expanding annular patches of alopecia, scaling or crusting with an erythematous border. Scaling and crusting vary from mild to severe. Follicular papules and pustules are also common. Severe folliculitis and furunculosis may result in permanent alopecia and scarring. In some cases the lesions consist of generalized greasy scaling resembling seborrhea. Pruritus is usually absent but may be severe in some cases. Cases of dermatophytosis caused by *T. mentagrophytes, T. terrestre*, and *M. persicolor* with a very long duration (1–5 years) have been reported. These infections suggest that there is *little tendency for spontaneous resolution in some infections*, a situation analogous to chronic dermatophytosis in humans. Kerions are often associated with *M. gypseum* or *T. mentagrophytes* infections. Infection by *M. persicolor*, a rare zoophilic dermatophyte associated with voles, may produce lesions characterized by prominent scaling but minimal alopecia. This dermatophyte does not invade hair and thus fungal organisms are seen only in the surface keratin. *Onychomycosis is rare* and may consist of chronic inflammation of the ungual fold or infection of the claw alone, producing deformity or fragility of the claw. *Several cases of Trichophyton dermatophytosis with clinical and histologic features resembling pemphigus erythematosus have been reported.* These dogs had scaling, crusting facial dermatitis and alopecia. Microscopically, lesions included interface dermatitis accompanied by intraepidermal pustules with acantholytic cells, suggestive of an immune-mediated disease. However, fungal elements were demonstrable with fungal stains.

Cats

Dermatophytosis is a *common* disease in cats and infection may be endemic in large catteries, with up to 35% of cats being culture positive. The vast majority of cases (greater than 90%) are caused by *M. canis*, which is of considerable public health significance because of its zoonotic potential. Despite the name, this dermatophyte is well adapted to the cat and induces minimal host response. In some surveys, long-haired cats have a higher incidence of positive cultures than do short-haired cats. Geographic differences may influence the prevalence of various dermatophytes. A survey of dermatophytes isolated from cats in shelters in the United States found *M. canis* isolates to predominate in the southeastern United States; while in cats from the northern United States, anthropophilic organisms were cultured and *M. canis* was not isolated from any cat. An *M. canis* fungal cell wall vaccine developed for use in cats has been shown to induce both humoral and cell-mediated immune responses, but it does not appear to be protective against challenge exposure with a large number of fungal spores.

Lesions are extremely variable. They frequently begin on the face, ears, and forelegs and may become generalized. Pruritus is uncommon but may be moderate. Classical circular foci of alopecia and crusting or scaling are more common in kittens. In adult cats, lesions may be extremely subtle and consist of patchy mild alopecia or broken hairs with little skin change. Scaling and crusting may be absent or severe. Some cases appear as papulocrustous miliary dermatitis or as feline acne. Folliculitis with alopecia is uncommon. Microscopic findings are variable. In some cases, organisms are infrequent and only a single infected hair may be found in a biopsy, while in other cases organisms may be numerous. Pseudomycetomas are subcutaneous nodules that occur in Persian cats. They are an atypical form of dermatophytosis caused by *M. canis* in which the deep dermis and subcutis are involved. There is frequently also a history of previous or concurrent superficial dermatophyte infection. Lesions are usually focal and measure 2–3 cm in diameter; but in some instances, they are multiple and involve extensive areas. They consist of discrete masses of bizarre distorted septate fungal hyphae, larger thick-walled fungal cells resembling *chlamydospores*, and chains of round structures surrounded by a hyaline eosinophilic Splendore-Hoeppli reaction. These granules are surrounded by granulomatous or pyogranulomatous inflammation. Fungal organisms are not necessarily present in the hair and keratin of the overlying skin.

Bibliography

Blake JS, et al. An immunoinhibitory cell wall glycoprotein (mannan) from *Trichophyton rubrum*. J Invest Dermatol 1991;96:657–661.

Carlotti DN, Bensignor E. Dermatophytosis due to *Microsporum persicolor* (13 cases) or *Microsporum gypseum* (20 cases) in dogs. Vet Dermatol 1999;10:17–27.

Chandler FW, et al. Color Atlas and Text of the Histopathology of Mycotic Diseases. Chicago, IL: Year Book Medical Publishers, Inc, 1980.

Connole MD, Baynes ID. Ringworm caused by *Microsporum nanum* in pigs in Queensland. Austr Vet J 1966;42:19–24.

DeBoer DJ, Moriello KA. Humoral and cellular immune responses to *Microsporum canis* in naturally occurring feline dermatophytosis. J Med Vet Mycol 1993;31:121–132.

DeBoer DJ, Moriello KA. The immune response to *Microsporum canis* induced by a fungal cell wall vaccine. Vet Dermatol 1994;5:47–55.

Gambale W, et al. Dermatophytes and other fungi of the haircoat of cats without dermatophytosis in the city of Sao Paulo, Brazil. Fel Pract 1993;21:29–33.

González Cabo JF, et al. An outbreak of dermatophytosis in pigs caused by *Microsporum canis*. Mycopathologia 1995;129:79–80.

Gordon PJ, Bond R. Efficacy of a live attenuated *Trichophyton verrucosum* vaccine for control of bovine dermatophytosis. Vet Rec 1996;139:395–396.

Hullinger GA, et al. Dermatophytosis in show lambs in the United States. Vet Dermatol 1999;10:73–76.

Kushida T, Watanabe S. Canine ringworm caused by *Trichophyton rubrum*: Probable transmission from man to animal. Sabouraudia 1975;13:30–32.

Mancianti F, et al. Mycological findings in feline immunodeficiency virus-infected cats. J Med Vet Mycol 1992;30:257–259.

Medleau L, Rakich PM. *Microsporum canis* pseudomycetomas in a cat. J Am Anim Hosp Assoc 1994;30:573–576.

Moriello KA, et al. Isolation of dermatophytes from the haircoats of stray cats from selected animal shelters in two different geographic regions in the United States. Vet Dermatol 1994;5:57–62.

Parker WM, Yager JA. *Trichophyton* dermatophytosis – A disease easily confused with pemphigus erythematosus. Can Vet J 1997;38:502–505.

Pascoe RR. Studies on the prevalence of ringworm among horses in racing and breeding stables. Austr Vet J 1976;52:419–421.

Pier AC, et al. Animal ringworm – its aetiology, public health significance and control. J Med Vet Mycol 1994;32(suppl 1):133–150.

Ranganathan S, et al. A survey of dermatophytosis in animals in Madras, India. Mycopathologia 1998;140:137–140.

Scott DW. Marked acantholysis associated with dermatophytosis due to *Trichophyton equinum* in two horses. Vet Dermatol 1994;5:105–110.

Sharp MW, et al. *Microsporum canis* infection in sheep. Vet Rec 1993;132:388.

Sparkes AH, et al. *Microsporum canis*: Inapparent carriage by cats and the viability of arthrospores. J Small Anim Pract 1994;35:397–401.

Sparkes AH, et al. Epidemiological and diagnostic features of canine and feline dermatophytosis in the United Kingdom from 1956–1991. Vet Rec 1993;133:57–61.

Sparkes AH, et al. Experimental *Microsporum canis* infection in cats: correlation between immunological and clinical observations. J Med Vet Mycol 1995;33:177–184.

Terreni AA, et al. *Epidermophyton floccosum* infection in a dog from the United States. J Med Vet Mycol 1985;23:141–142.

Wagner DK, Sohnle PG. Cutaneous defenses against dermatophytes and yeasts. Clin Microbiol Rev 1995;8:317–335.

Weitzman I, Summerbell RC. The dermatophytes. Clin Microbiol Rev 1995;8:240–259.

Subcutaneous fungal infections

The subcutaneous mycoses are a heterogeneous group of infections caused by a wide variety of fungi of low virulence that require mechanical introduction into tissue before they can cause disease. The organisms are common saprophytes that normally exist in soil, vegetation, or on normal skin and hair. Their ability to adapt to the tissue environment and elicit disease is variable. The clinical course is usually insidiously progressive over a period of months to years. Infection usually remains localized to the site of entry and surrounding tissues. Slow extension by way of lymphatics occurs in some diseases; but widespread dissemination is rare. Granulocytes are involved in control of many subcutaneous fungi, and granulocytopenia may render an individual more susceptible to subcutaneous mycoses.

Eumycotic mycetoma

Mycetomas are tumor-like infections of skin and subcutaneous tissues caused by two different types of organisms: actinomycetes (**actinomycotic mycetoma**) and fungi (**eumycotic mycetoma**). They are caused by a diverse group of organisms, many totally unrelated to each other, all of which elicit similar clinical disease. *Mycetomas are characterized clinically by the triad of tumefaction (swelling), draining tracts, and grains in the discharge.* Eumycotic mycetomas are those caused by fungi and they have been reported worldwide in humans, occasionally in dogs and horses, and rarely in cattle and cats. A wide variety of fungi that exist as saprophytes in the soil or on plants have been associated with mycetomas. The organisms involved may also cause other clinical diseases, e.g., phaeohyphomycosis and mycotic granulomas, when the three criteria are not present for a diagnosis of a mycetoma. Some cases reported in the veterinary literature as mycetomas are actually phaeohyphomycosis. Mycetomas usually involve skin and subcutaneous tissues and sometimes extend to involve underlying bone. *Curvularia* spp. and *Scedosporium apiospermum* (*Pseudallescheria boydii*) are most commonly involved in mycetomas in animals; *Cladophialophora bantiana* was identified as the cause of eumycetoma in one dog. These organisms are introduced by *wound contamination or implantation* by thorns and other plant material. Lesions often do not develop for many months after inoculation of the fungus. This long incubation period is thought to represent the time needed by the organism to adapt to the environment of the host tissues. All cases have become infected from sources in nature and thus *the condition is not contagious.*

Lesions in animals are widely distributed on the body but they frequently occur on the extremities and the face. In rare cases, subcutaneous lesions develop in dogs as extensions of abdominal infection. Disseminated infections have been reported rarely. Lesions are usually solitary and begin as small dermal or subcutaneous papules or nodules that enlarge gradually over a period of months to years. As the lesion slowly enlarges, deeper tissues such as muscle and bone may become involved. The reaction to the fungus is suppurative and inflammation is accompanied by prominent fibrosis that produces progressive swelling. Abscesses evolve into fistulas that emerge to the surface and give rise to the characteristic appearance of a mycetoma. The fistulas discharge serous, purulent, or hemorrhagic exudate containing grains. *The grains or granules are composed of aggregates of fungal organisms* and vary in size from 0.1 mm to several millimeters in size and may be white, yellow, pink-red, brown, or black. The color, size, shape, and texture of the grains may be sufficiently characteristic to suggest the etiologic agent, but *definitive identification of the fungus requires culture. Curvularia* spp. and *Madurella* spp. have been associated with black-grained mycetomas, while *P. boydii* is usually associated with white grains.

Microscopically, the lesions are similar regardless of the etiologic agent. *The salient histologic feature is the presence of granules in a tumor-like mass of chronically inflamed tissue.* Granules are spherical, lobular, or scroll-shaped masses of fungal hyphae that are 2–6 μm in diameter, septate, and branching. They are pigmented or nonpigmented. Chlamydospores are also frequently present, especially at the periphery of the mass. The fungal hyphae may be embedded in an amorphous eosinophilic "cement-like" substance. The granules of some mycetomas are surrounded by an amorphous eosinophilic radially arranged or smoothly contoured Splendore-Hoeppli reaction. The granules are located within abscesses composed of neutrophils and necrotic debris. *Fragments of plant material* may be seen within the lesion adjacent to the granules and are suspected to be the vehicle of infection. The abscesses vary in size and are present in the dermis and subcutis. Abscesses are surrounded by a chronic inflammatory reaction consisting of epithelioid macrophages, multinucleated giant cells, and fewer plasma cells and lymphocytes. Fibrous connective tissue of variable maturity separates the inflammatory foci. In some cases, *special stains may be needed to determine if the grains are composed of bacteria or fungi*. If the grains are hard, they may be displaced or removed altogether from the tissue because of drag on the microtome blade during sectioning. Multiple sections may be needed to find granules. The internal configuration of a granule may be suggestive of a specific fungus or group of fungi. Definitive identification of the organism can be made on tissue sections by immunofluorescence techniques but the specific antisera are not readily available and *culture is the usual means of identification.*

Bibliography

Allison N, et al. Eumycotic mycetoma caused by *Pseudallescheria boydii* in a dog. J Am Vet Med Assoc 1989;194:797–799.

Boomke J, et al. Black grain mycetoma (maduromycosis) in horses. Onderstepoort J Vet Res 1977;44:249–252.

Elad D, et al. Eumycetoma caused by *Curvularia lunata* in a dog. Mycopathologia 1991;116:113–118.

Guillot J, et al. Eumycetoma caused by *Cladophialophora bantiana* in a dog. J Clin Microbiol 2004;42:4901–4903.

Lambrechts N, et al. Black grain eumycetoma (*Madurella mycetomatis*) in the abdominal cavity of a dog. J Med Vet Mycol 1991;29:211–214.

Phaeohyphomycosis

Phaeohyphomycosis is an uncommon opportunistic subcutaneous, cerebral, or systemic infection caused by a wide variety of fungi that are all characterized by formation of dematiaceous, or pigmented, hyphae in tissue. The pigmentation is due to the presence of melanin and results of experimental studies suggest that the pigment may act as a virulence factor in development of infection. The organisms responsible for these infections are worldwide in distribution and are widespread in the soil, on wood, and in vegetation. Some of the organisms can also be cultured from the skin of healthy people and animals. Subcutaneous infection is thought to result from wound contamination or traumatic implantation of wood slivers, thorns, sticks, and the like. The taxonomy of the organisms as well as their names and the diseases they cause have been changed frequently, causing confusion in the literature. The list of organisms identified as causative agents of phaeohyphomycosis is continually increasing. Some of the fungi that have been associated with phaeohyphomycosis in animals include *Alternaria alternata, Bipolaris* (Drechslera) *spicifera, Xylohypha bantiana (Torula bantiana, Cladosporium bantianum, Cladosporium trichoides), Curvularia geniculata, C. lunata, Exophiala jeanselmei, Ochroconis* (Dactylaria) spp., *Phialophora verrucosa*, and *Wangiella* spp.

Phaeohyphomycosis has been reported most frequently in *cats* and occasionally in *horses, dogs, cattle, and goats*. The disease also occurs in humans. Some of the cases reported in the veterinary literature as mycetomas, in which small groups of dematiaceous fungi are present within tissues but which do not otherwise fulfill the clinical criteria of mycetomas, are actually cases of phaeohyphomycosis. No underlying immune deficiency is apparent in most cases of subcutaneous phaeohyphomycosis; whereas disseminated infections have been associated with immunologic compromise or debilitating disease. Subcutaneous infection with *Staphylotrichum coccosporum*, a fungus previously thought to be nonpathogenic was described in a cat positive for *Feline leukemia virus*. Subcutaneous infection is insidiously progressive and evolves over months to years.

Lesions of pheohyphomycosis consist of *single or multiple subcutaneous nodules*. The *fungal pigmentation may be grossly visible in the tissue* and, in some cases, the nodule is so dark it may be mistaken for a melanoma. In *cats*, lesions are usually single and occur most commonly on the face and feet. Firm to fluctuant subcutaneous nodules grow slowly and may be ulcerated or have draining tracts. Multiple recurrences following surgical excision are common. The clinical course in some reported cases has been several years. Lesions in *horses* are frequently multiple and located on several different parts of the body. Occasionally nodules may be generalized. Multiple ulcerated cutaneous nodules are the usual form of the infection described in *cattle*, and lesions may also be present in the nasal mucosa. Lesions in *dogs* are also frequently multiple and may be extensive. They consist of poorly circumscribed ulcerated or fistulating nodules or plaques on the feet and legs. In one affected dog, lesions consisted of multiple nodules in the area of ascending lymphatics of a leg and an enlarged regional lymph node, a clinical appearance similar to the cutaneous-lymphatic form of sporotrichosis.

The histologic diagnosis of phaeohyphomycosis is made by demonstrating pigmented hyphae within the tissue. The lesions consist of multifocal-to-diffuse pyogranulomatous dermatitis and panniculitis. The overlying epidermis is acanthotic or multifocally to diffusely ulcerated. Microabscesses with foci of necrosis are frequently prominent. Necrosis may be extensive. Fungi are distributed throughout the lesion as scattered small aggregates and individual hyphae. *The hyphae are septate, 2–6 μm wide, and branched or unbranched.* They are often constricted at their prominent thick septations and may contain single or chains of thick-walled vesicular swellings, 25 μm or more in diameter, that resemble chlamydospores. *The innate brown pigment may not be readily apparent,* but at least some pale yellow-brown to black hyphae will be found in unstained (cleared and mounted) or HE-stained tissue sections.

If pigmentation is not readily apparent, a melanin stain , such as Fontana-Masson, has been suggested to confirm the presence of melanin in the hyphae. However, some nondematiaceous fungi have been found to be Fontana-Masson positive, calling into question the usefulness of the procedure. Fungal stains demonstrate the organisms well but can mask the natural color. The etiologic agents are so similar in appearance within tissues that they cannot be identified on the basis of their morphology. Culture is always needed for specific identification of the fungi. Phaeohyphomycosis has been confused with eumycotic mycetomas caused by dematiaceous fungi. *The fungi in mycetomas form discrete organized granules, whereas those of phaeohyphomycosis appear as individual hyphae and small aggregates scattered throughout the lesion.* The aggregates of hyphae in phaeohyphomycosis may be surrounded by Splendore-Hoeppli material but this does not constitute a granule. The fungal elements of pheohyphomycosis are frequently intracellular within epithelioid macrophages and multinucleated giant cells; granules of mycetomas are nearly always extracellular.

Bibliography

Abramo F, et al. Feline cutaneous phaeohyphomycosis due to *Cladophyalophora bantiana*. J Feline Med Surg 2002;4:157–163.

Chermette R, et al. *Exophiala spinifera* nasal infection in a cat and a literature review of feline phaeohyphomycosis. J Mycol Med 1997;7:149–158.

Fondati A, et al. A case of feline phaeohyphomycosis due to *Fonsecaea pedrosoi*. Vet Dermatol 2001;12:297–301.

Fuchs A, et al. Subcutaneous mycosis in a cat due to *Staphylotrichum coccosporum*. Mycoses 1996;39:381–385.

Genovese LM, et al. Cutaneous nodular phaeohyphomycosis in five horses associated with *Alternaria alternata* infection. Vet Rec 2001;148:55–56.

Herraez P, et al. Invasive phaeohyphomycosis caused by *Curvularia* species in a dog. Vet Pathol 2001;38:456–459.

Kimura M, McGinnis MR. Fontana-Masson-stained tissue from culture-proven mycoses. Arch Pathol Lab Med 1998;122:1107–1111.

Matsumoto T, et al. Developments in hyalohyphomycosis and phaeohyphomycosis. J Med Vet Mycol 1994;32(suppl):329–349.

McKay JS, et al. Cutaneous alternariosis in a cat. J Small Anim Pract 2001;42:75–78.

Waurzyniak BJ, et al. Dual systemic mycosis caused by *Bipolaris spicifera* and *Torulopsis glabrata* in a dog. Vet Pathol 1992;29:566–569.

Whitford HW, et al. *Exserohilum* dermal granulomas in a bovine. J Vet Diagn Invest 1989;1:78–81.

Sporotrichosis

Sporotrichosis is an uncommon chronic infection usually limited to skin and subcutaneous tissue caused by the opportunist fungal pathogen Sporothrix schenckii. The organism is a dimorphic fungus, growing as hyphae at environmental temperatures and in yeast form in tissue. *S. schenckii* exists as a saprophyte distributed worldwide in the soil, on plants, and on various plant materials. The organism is considered only weakly pathogenic and a great deal of variability occurs in virulence of strains isolated from soil. Disease is most common in temperate and tropical zones. Sporotrichosis has been reported in horses, mules, donkeys, cattle, goats, swine, dogs, cats, rats, mice, hamsters, domestic fowl, camels, dolphins, armadillos, chimpanzees, and humans. The infection has been *reported most often in horses, cats, and dogs*. Infection is usually acquired by wound contamination or inoculation of the organism into tissue by puncture wounds caused by thorns, wood splinters, or contaminated claws. Pulmonary infection is acquired by inhalation of spores. In humans, the disease is considered an occupational hazard for those who work with the soil, plants, or plant materials.

Sporotrichosis is subdivided into *three clinical forms*.

- The **primary cutaneous form** consists of multiple scattered raised alopecic, ulcerated, crusted nodules or plaques that remain confined to the point(s) of entry of the organism. It is thought that this form results from a *high degree of host immunity*, preventing spread of infection. Nodules may become ulcerated and associated with seropurulent exudate and crust formation. The normal grooming behavior of cats may result in autoinoculation and spread of lesions to distant sites. The cutaneous form may have a very chronic course. An unusual case of sporotrichosis in a dog consisted of otitis externa characterized by multiple cutaneous nodules which persisted for more than 5 years. A donkey with sporotrichosis had multiple slowly progressive facial lesions for 2 years before the disease was diagnosed.
- The **cutaneous-lymphatic form** involves the skin, subcutaneous tissue, and associated lymphatics. Lesions begin as firm round nodules at the site of entry, usually on an extremity, and spread proximally along lymphatics. Lymphatic vessels become thick and corded and a series of secondary nodules forms as the infection progresses. The nodules may break open and discharge seropurulent material. Lesions may cavitate and expose extensive areas of underlying muscle and bone. Regional lymphadenopathy is common. This is the most common form in *horses*. Lesions generally involve the proximal forelimbs, chest, and thigh but usually no regional lymph node involvement is evident. *Dogs* usually have the cutaneous or cutaneous-lymphatic form. The head, pinnae, and trunk are involved most frequently. In *cats*, lesions are usually located on the head, distal limbs, and base of the tail. The initial draining puncture wounds may be indistinguishable from cat-inflicted fight wound infections.
- The **extracutaneous/disseminated form** may involve a single extracutaneous tissue, such as osteoarticular sporotrichosis, or multiple internal organs. It develops as a sequela to cutaneous-lymphatic infection or following inhalation of the fungus. The disseminated form of sporotrichosis *occurs most frequently in cats*, and no immunosuppressive factors are usually identified. In experimentally induced sporotrichosis in cats, organisms were shown by culture to have disseminated to viscera in 50% of the cases. Cats with disseminated sporotrichosis are often febrile, depressed, and anorexic.

Microscopically, sporotrichosis is usually a *nodular to diffuse pyogranulomatous or granulomatous inflammatory reaction involving the dermis and subcutaneous fat*. The epidermis is acanthotic or ulcerated. Neutrophils, epithelioid macrophages, multinucleated giant cells, and fewer lymphocytes and plasma cells form discrete granulomas or extensive sheets of inflammation replacing dermal and subcutaneous tissues. Fibrosis is variable; and necrosis may be extensive. *Yeast(s) surrounded by a stellate radial corona of brightly eosinophilic material (asteroid body/Splendore-Hoeppli reaction) are seen in some cases.* The yeasts appear as round, oval, or elongated ("cigar"-shaped) single or budding cells which measure 2–6 μm or more in diameter for the round and oval forms and 2×3 to 3×10 μm for the cigar form

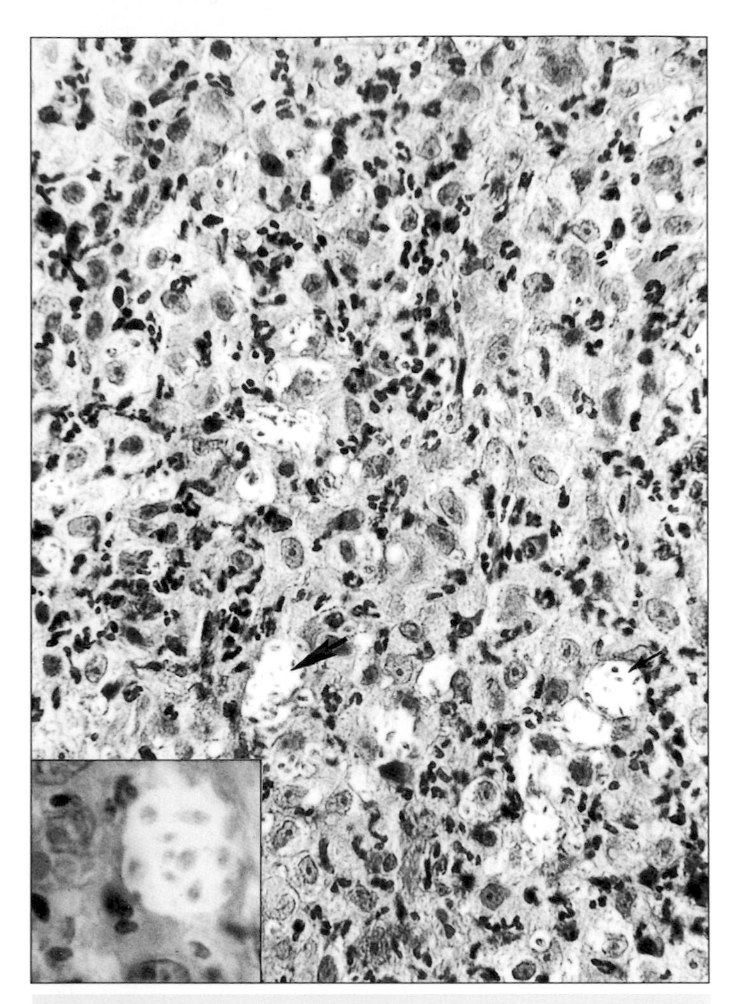

Figure 5.100 Pyogranulomatous inflammation with organisms in vacuoles (see inset) in **sporotrichosis**.

(Fig. 5.100). The cigar forms are considered characteristic of *Sporothrix* but they may not be found regularly. *In general, organisms are numerous in lesions from cats and rare in tissues from dogs and horses.* However, in immunosuppressed dogs, yeasts may be numerous. The yeasts may be extracellular or within neutrophils and macrophages. The yeasts have a refractile cell wall from which the cytoplasm may shrink during processing and give the appearance of a capsule. In such instances and when no cigar forms are evident, the organism may be mistaken for *Cryptococcus neoformans* or *Histoplasma capsulatum*. Yeasts stand out clearly with fungal stains, but serial sections may be needed to demonstrate even a single organism. Without a significant number of cigar-shaped forms, identification may not be possible. In these cases, *immunoperoxidase or fluorescent antibody staining* using specific *S. schenckii* antiserum is necessary for definitive identification of the organism. Organisms may not be found despite the use of serial sections and special stains, and diagnosis in such cases requires culture. The yeast can usually be cultured from tissue obtained from areas of active inflammation even in dogs and horses, which typically have very few organisms in tissue. In cats, cytologic examination of exudates and material obtained by fine needle aspiration of nodules is frequently diagnostic because sufficient numbers of yeasts are usually present to identify the organism.

Sporotrichosis is considered a zoonotic disease. Transmission of the infection from cats to humans has been reported many times and *infected cats pose a significant public health danger*. Veterinarians, other veterinary professionals and students, and owners exposed to ulcerated wounds or exudates from infected cats have developed infections. The organism may be able to penetrate intact skin since not all patients who develop lesions can recall having wounds or being bitten or scratched by infected cats. The large number of organisms typically present in lesions from cats is thought to be the reason for the transmission of disease from cats to humans. However, even when the lesions in cats had few organisms, transmission to humans has occurred. In contrast, infection was not transmitted from a dog with multiple cutaneous lesions containing relatively numerous organisms to several adults and children with whom the dog had had frequent contact for the 2 year duration of infection. These cases suggest that factors in addition to absolute numbers of yeasts are involved in the apparent ease of cat-to-human transmission.

Bibliography

Barros MB, et al. Cat-transmitted sporotrichosis epidemic in Rio de Janeiro, Brazil: description of a series of cases. Clin Infect Dis 2004;38:529–535.

Irizarry-Rovira AR, et al. Diagnosis of sporotrichosis in a donkey using direct fluorescein-labeled antibody testing. J Vet Diagn Invest 2000;12:180–183.

Schubach TM, et al. Evaluation of an epidemic of sporotrichosis in cats: 347 cases (1998–2001). J Am Vet Med Assoc 2004;224:1623–1629.

Shany M. A mixed fungal infection in a dog: sporotrichosis and cryptococcosis. Can Vet J 2000;41:799–800.

Welsh RD. Sporotrichosis. J Am Vet Med Assoc 2003;223:1123–1126.

Cutaneous oomycosis (pythiosis and lagenidiosis)

Oomycosis refers to infection by *Pythium insidiosum* (formerly *Hyphomyces destruens*) or *Lagenidium* sp. organisms, both of which are aquatic dimorphic water molds and members of the Oomycetes in the kingdom Protista. These opportunistic pathogens live in warm stagnant water and are most often reported in regions with tropical to subtropical environments. The organisms are thought to enter the skin through cutaneous wounds, and infection may involve the dermis, subcutis or distant tissue as described below.

Pythiosis (leeches, swamp cancer, bursattee, phycomycosis) is *a chronic cutaneous-subcutaneous, gastrointestinal, or multisystemic granulomatous infection of horses, dogs, cattle, cats, and humans living in tropical, subtropical, and temperate regions* throughout the world. *Pythium* spp. occur in the soil and aquatic environments worldwide, and some are important plant pathogens. *P. insidiosum* is unique in that it has adapted to colonize mammalian tissues. The organisms require warm weather and moisture for reproduction and thus the majority of cases occur in late summer and fall in tropical and subtropical areas. Water lilies, grasses, and debris of plants found in aquatic or humid habitats appear to support the propagation of *Pythium* spp. The infective stage of the organism is a biflagellate aquatic zoospore that is released seasonally in association with warm weather and moisture. Infection is thought to be acquired from prolonged contact with stagnant fresh water containing the newly emerged zoospores that are motile and are attracted chemotactically to injured tissue. The zoospores produce a substance that enables them to attach to host tissues during initial stages of infection and they appear to play an important role in producing infection. However, the zoospore stage is not known to form in tissue and the infection is thus not considered to have zoonotic potential.

Not all animals with pythiosis have a history of contact with permanent bodies of water, suggesting that the organism may proliferate in temporary stands of water or even on wet grasses.

Cutaneous pythiosis has been reported most frequently in **horses**. No age, breed, or sex predilection is recognized. Lesions occur most commonly on the *limbs, distal to the carpus and hock*, and on the ventral aspect of the thorax and abdomen, sites that are most likely to be in contact with stagnant water and would be traumatized by aquatic plants or vegetation (Fig. 5.101A). Affected horses frequently have a history of prolonged contact with water in lakes, ponds, swamps, or flooded areas. Lesions are usually single but occasional horses develop lesions in several separate sites. Lesions begin as nodules that enlarge very rapidly to become circular masses of granulation tissue. The masses ulcerate or develop multiple fistulous tracts that drain thick purulohemorrhagic material. The sinuses also contain characteristic gray-white to pale yellow coral-like concretions (called *leeches* or *kunkers*) that may be extruded at the skin surface (Fig. 5.101B). The colloquial name leeches is based on the initial misidentification of the masses. *These structures are unique to the horse* and are not seen in other animals with pythiosis. Lesions are frequently extremely pruritic, and biting or rubbing the lesion contributes to tissue damage. The largest lesions usually develop on the thorax and abdomen and may attain a size of 45 cm or more in diameter. In chronic cases, underlying bone may be invaded. Regional lymph nodes may be involved but visceral spread is rare. *The clinical appearance of the lesions may resemble basidiobolomycosis, cutaneous habronemiasis, excessive granulation tissue, and neoplasia (particularly sarcoid and squamous cell carcinoma).*

Cutaneous pythiosis has been reported less frequently in **dogs** than has the gastrointestinal form. The disease occurs most often in young adult, large breed dogs, and German Shepherd Dogs may be predisposed. The disease in dogs is relentlessly progressive with no proven medical treatment. Most lesions are on the extremities but they may also occur on the face, ventral abdomen and chest, and in the perineal area. In most cases, a single body region is involved. *The initial lesion is a poorly circumscribed dermal nodule that rapidly expands peripherally and extends into the subcutis to form multiple secondary nodules* (Fig. 5.101C). The nodules develop into spongy masses that ulcerate, become necrotic, and develop multiple fistulous tracts that drain purulohemorrhagic exudate. Early lesions on the legs may resemble acral lick granulomas. Pruritus is not as constant a feature in dogs as it is in horses with pythiosis. A common clinicopathologic abnormality is absolute eosinophilia.

Pythiosis has been reported infrequently in **cattle**. Most cases have been in beef calves <12 months of age. Calves of both sexes have been affected. The majority of the lesions are located on the distal extremities. They consist of irregular swellings with ulceration and multiple draining tracts. Although no concretions have been present, the tissue contains numerous yellow punctate foci. Reports of pythiosis in **cats** are rare. As in other species, lesions usually are located on the extremities. In at least two cats, the lesions progressed very slowly and the clinical course was much more protracted than is typical of the disease in dogs and horses. Moreover, nodules remained confined to the subcutaneous tissues and there was no involvement of the overlying skin.

Microscopically, the lesions consist of *granulomatous inflammation with foci of liquefactive necrosis and extensive fibrosis* involving the dermis and subcutis. The epidermis is acanthotic or focally to diffusely ulcerated. The necrotic foci consist of eosinophilic coagula containing necrotic eosinophils and sometimes degenerate collagen and small necrotic blood vessels. Necrotic foci are most expansive in lesions from horses and they correspond to the concretions seen grossly (Fig. 5.101D). The necrotic material is surrounded by viable eosinophils, epithelioid macrophages, and occasional multinucleated giant cells. The organism is located in the necrotic foci but it does not stain with H&E. However, the presence of hyphae may be detected by occasional clear, unstained circular or linear spaces within the necrotic debris. Pythium stains poorly or not at all with PAS, but it is readily stained with GMS and appears as *thick-walled, sparsely septate hyphae, 4–10 μm in diameter, with occasional branching* (Fig. 5.101E). Organisms are usually most numerous in necrotic foci and may also be seen in walls of small arterioles. They are rare in areas of granulomatous inflammation and they are not usually present in intervening connective tissue. The hyphae are similar to those of the zygomycetes *Basidiobolus* and *Conidiobolus*. The hyphae of these organisms tend to be broader, ranging from 5–15 μm in diameter, however the differentiation of *Pythium* sp. from the zygomycetes in tissue is frequently impossible.

Diagnosis of pythiosis is based on the appearance of the gross lesions, microscopic lesions, and culture of the organism. Pythium is readily cultured in most instances; but in some cases, it cannot be grown. Failure to culture the organism may be related to sample handling because refrigeration decreases its survival and freezing kills the organism. Definitive identification of the oomycete, however, requires that the cultured organism be induced to produce the diagnostic zoospores, a process that is complicated, time-consuming, and not always successful. Because of the rapidly progressive course of the disease in many animals, a more rapid means of diagnosis is preferable so that an accurate prognosis may be made and specific therapy instituted. To this end, PCR assays, immunohistochemistry, and immunoblot analyses have been developed for identification and differentiation of *Pythium insidiosum, Lagenidium* and the zygomycetes. Not all assays are available for each organism, but a combination of assays and evaluation of the clinical information and laboratory results can lead to a definitive diagnosis.

Cutaneous lagenidiosis is remarkably similar to cutaneous pythiosis in geographic occurrence and clinical and histologic lesions. Lagenidiosis has been reported only in dogs. Gross lesions consist of nodular and necrotizing lesions of the limbs and trunk that drain and may be accompanied by lymphadenitis. The disease is also very aggressive, and affected dogs frequently develop lesions of the great vessels, mediastinum, lungs, and esophagus. *Histologic lesions are indistinguishable from those of pythiosis and zygomycosis.* Again, clinical presentation, PCR assays, immunohistochemistry and immunoblot analyses are needed to differentiate these infections.

Bibliography

Chaffin MK, et al. Multicentric cutaneous pythiosis in a foal. J Am Vet Med Assoc 1992;201:310–312.

Dykstra MJ, et al. A description of cutaneous-subcutaneous pythiosis in fifteen dogs. Med Mycol 1999;37:427–433.

Grooters AM. Pythiosis, lagenidiosis, and zygomycosis in small animals. Vet Clin North Am Small Anim Pract 2003;33:695–720.

Grooters AM, et al. Clinicopathologic findings associated with *Lagenidium* sp. Infection in 6 dogs: initial description of an emerging oomycosis. J Vet Intern Med 2003;17:637–646.

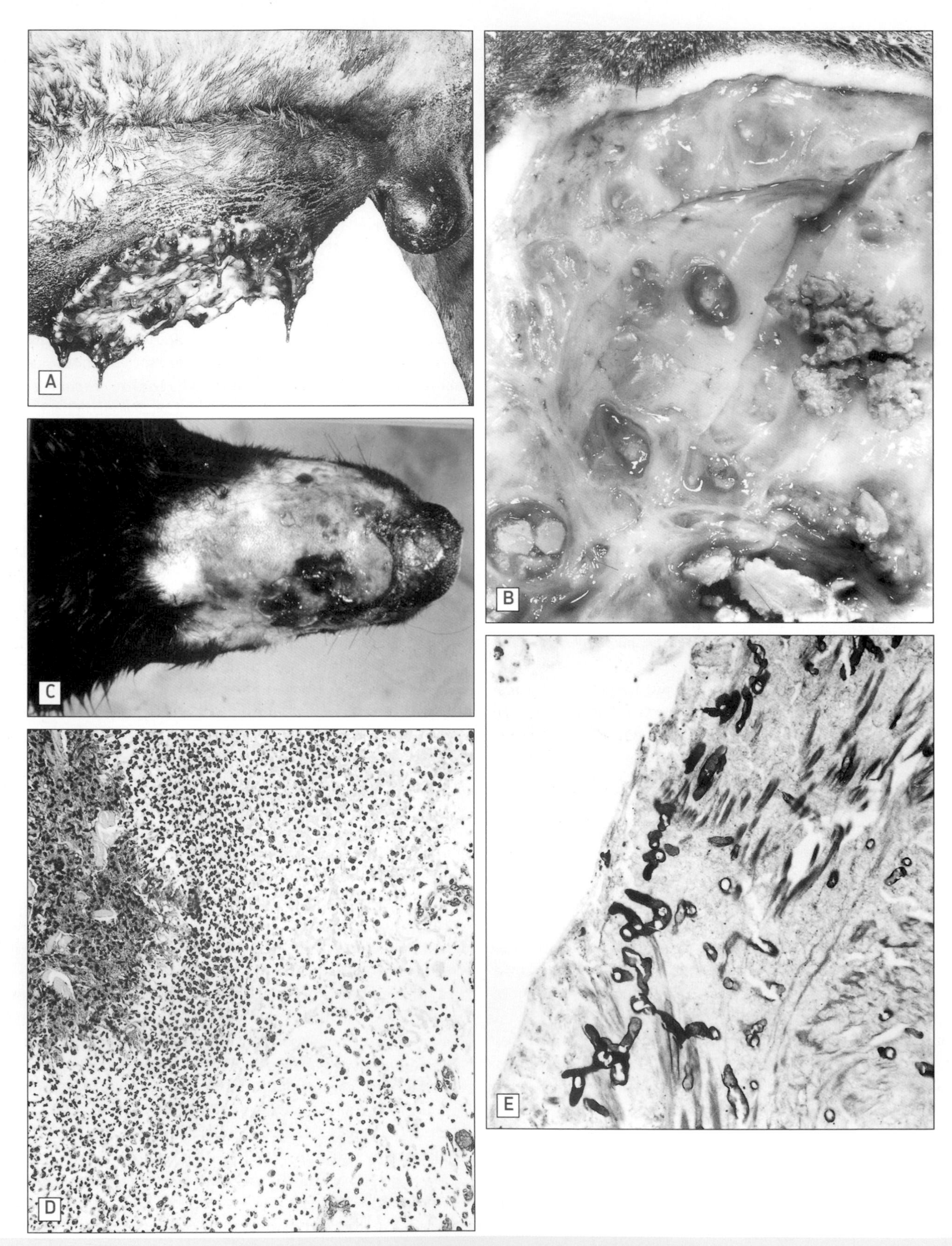

Figure 5.101 Pythiosis. **A.** Ulcerated, draining lesion on the ventral abdominal skin in a horse. **B.** Cut surface reveals granulation tissue and multiple, light-colored cores of necrotic debris ("**kunkers**") in equine pythiosis. **C.** Multiple, ulcerated and draining tracts on the skin of the face in pythiosis in a dog. **D.** Section through edge of necrotic core (above, left) in equine pythiosis. **E. Hyphae-like structures** of organism at the edge of the lesion in equine pythiosis.

Mendoza L, et al. Infections caused by the oomycetous pathogen *Pythium insidiosum*. J Mycol Méd 1996;6:151–164.
Miller RI, Campbell RSF. The comparative pathology of equine cutaneous phycomycosis. Vet Pathol 1984;21:325–332.
Santurio JM, et al. Cutaneous pythiosis insidiosi in calves from the Pantanal region of Brazil. Mycopathologia 1998;141:123–125.
Schurko AM, et al. Development of a species-specific probe for *Pythium insidiosum* and the diagnosis of pythiosis. J Clin Microbiol 2004;42:2411–2418.

Zygomycosis

Zygomycosis refers to subcutaneous, systemic, or rhinocerebral infections caused by a wide variety of zygomycete fungi. The unifying diagnostic feature of zygomycosis is that the organisms all form infrequently septate hyphae that are typically significantly broader than other fungi with filamentous tissue forms, such as *Aspergillus* or the agents of phaeohyphomycosis. The hyphae are unpigmented and commonly range from 6–25 µm in diameter. The class Zygomycetes is composed of two orders. The order Mucorales includes *Rhizopus*, *Mucor*, *Absidia*, *Mortierella*, *Rhizomucor*, among other genera; and diseases caused by these organisms have been called **mucormycosis**. The order Entomophthorales contains the genera *Basidiobolus* and *Conidiobolus* and disease caused by these fungi is called **entomophthoromycosis**. The term phycomycosis was used when zygomycetes and oomycetes, such as *Pythium* spp., were grouped together in a single division. However, as the oomycetes have been determined not to be true fungi and their taxonomy has been reclassified, the term has become obsolete because the taxonomic equivalent no longer exists. The diseases should be referred to as zygomycosis or pythiosis. Zygomycetes are cosmopolitan in distribution and they are widespread in nature. They all occur as soil saprophytes, agents of decay, insect pathogens, or as components of normal skin and hair flora. They are common laboratory contaminants and are thus sometimes ignored when cultured from clinical specimens. The portal of entry may be cutaneous, gastrointestinal, or respiratory. Zygomycosis is not a contagious disease, the environment being the source of all infections.

Zygomycosis is a *rare disease of humans and animals*, including dogs, cats, horses, llamas, sheep, and pigs. The disease in humans usually occurs in debilitated or immunocompromised individuals. In animals, however, immune compromise is usually not evident and disease may be the result of exposure to a large number of organisms. *Traumatic implantation* is thought to be the portal of entry for the subcutaneous form. Inoculation by biting insects has also been suspected to be a means of entry for the organisms. Members of the order Mucorales usually cause disseminated disease, and *angioinvasion by hyphae is a characteristic feature*. Zygomycosis in dogs and cats is usually in the form of *fatal gastrointestinal mucormycosis*. Zygomycosis caused by *Rhizopus oryzae* has been reported in pigs in which the disease consisted of subcutaneous granulomas with draining tracts as well as lesions in the stomach, liver, and lymph nodes. *In general, fungi of the order Entomophthorales cause localized subcutaneous granulomas*. These infections occur most often in tropical and subtropical regions. The fungus *Conidiobolus* is distinguished by its predilection for the nasal mucosa, nares, and surrounding skin. Infections by various species of this organism have been reported in dogs, horses, llamas, and sheep.

Zygomycosis occurs most frequently in **horses** and infections are usually caused by *Basidiobolus haptosporus* (basidiobolomycosis) and *Conidiobolus coronatus* (conidiobolomycosis). The lesions consist of circular ulcerated nodules or swellings with serosanguineous exudate. Small irregular gritty masses of yellow-white material (kunkers, leeches) may be discharged to the surface along with the exudate. Basidiobolomycosis usually involves the chest, trunk, head, or neck. Solitary lesions are the rule and they may grow rapidly and become very large. Pruritus is a common feature. *A discontinuous undulating band of yellow-white material that sharply demarcates the superficial hemorrhagic, edematous tissue from the underlying fibrogranulation tissue characterizes the cut surface of granulomas.* The clinical lesions are similar to those of pythiosis but may sometimes be differentiated in the horse by differences in anatomic location, number and appearance of kunkers, and epidemiology. The granulomas of zygomycosis usually affect the lateral aspects of the trunk, neck, and head, and the kunkers are less numerous, smaller, and of no particular shape. In contrast, lesions of pythiosis are commonly located on the lower limbs and contain numerous, large, coral-shaped kunkers. Furthermore, pythiosis is typically associated with access to standing water. *No such association with water exists for basidiobolomycosis or conidiobolomycosis*, which are caused by agents found in soil and decaying vegetation.

Unlike the protracted clinical course typical of most cases of zygomycosis, nasal zygomycosis in **sheep** caused by *C. incongruus* results in loss of condition and death within a period of 7–10 days after initial clinical signs. This infection produces prominent asymmetrical swelling of the face, extending from the nostrils to the eyes, and marked thickening of the skin and subcutaneous tissue. In advanced cases, the nasal skin is alopecic and necrotic.

Subcutaneous zygomycosis caused by *Conidiobolus* of unknown species has been reported in a young adult **dog**. Lesions involved the skin of a hind leg and the thoracic wall but not the nasal mucosa or skin surrounding the nose. The lesions on the leg began as an ulcerated mass that progressed to circumferential swelling and induration with numerous coalescing ulcers draining serosanguineous fluid. The condition exhibited some waxing and waning, but new lesions continued to develop. No immunologic compromise or predisposing factors were apparent.

Microscopically, zygomycosis is characterized by *multifocal-to-diffuse eosinophilic and granulomatous dermatitis and panniculitis with multifocal necrosis*. Necrotic foci consist of eosinophilic coagulated material corresponding to the kunkers seen grossly. Eosinophils, neutrophils, epithelioid macrophages, and multinucleated giant cells surround the eosinophilic coagula and are separated by fibrovascular connective tissue. Fungi are usually located in necrotic foci and may be seen as clear linear or circular hyphal "ghosts" often surrounded by Splendore-Hoeppli material (Fig. 5.102). Basophilic granular protoplasm may be visible with H&E stain, but the organisms are usually better visualized with GMS stain. They frequently stain poorly with PAS. The hyphae range from 5–20.5 µm diameter for *B. haptosporus* and 5–12.8 µm for *C. coronatus*. Hyphae are thin-walled, vary moderately in diameter, and have occasional septations and uncommon branching. Folded, twisted, or compressed hyphae may be seen. The lesions of nasal zygomycosis caused by *C. incongruus* in sheep are characterized by segmental necrosis and thrombosis of subcutaneous blood vessels. Many fungal hyphae are visible in necrotic foci, in thrombi, and within vessel walls. This propensity to invade blood vessels is common with Mucorales but is an unusual feature for the Entomophthorales.

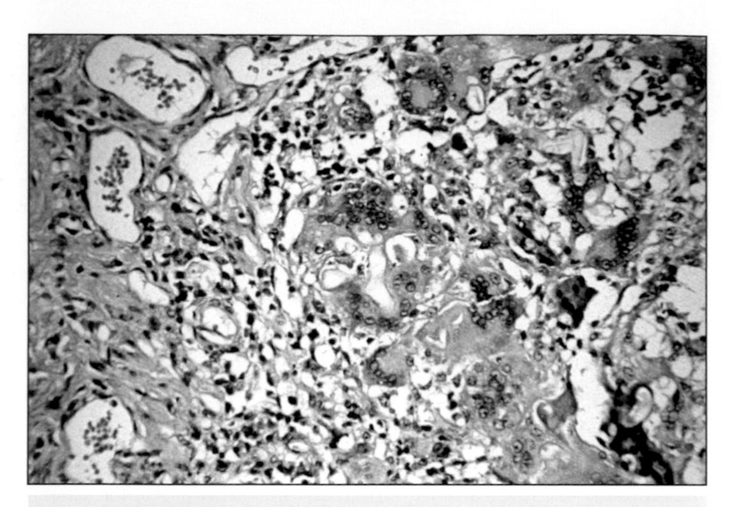

Figure 5.102 Zygomycosis. *Conidiobolus* sp. dermatitis in a dog. Note clear linear and circular hyphal "ghosts" amid granulomatous inflammation.

The microscopic lesions of basidiobolomycosis and conidiobolomycosis are similar to those of pythiosis and the diseases may be histologically indistinguishable, especially when the width of hyphae is at the narrow end of the range. All members of the zygomycetes are morphologically similar in tissue, and consequently culture is necessary for specific identification. Although immunohistochemical identification of fungi in tissue sections has been reported, the specific antisera are not readily available and culture remains the usual means of identification.

Bibliography

Carrigan MJ, et al. Ovine nasal zygomycosis caused by *Conidiobolus incongruus*. Aust Vet J 1992;69:237–240.

French RA, Ashworth CD. Zygomycosis caused by *Conidiobolus coronatus* in a llama (*Lama glama*). Vet Pathol 1994;31:120–122.

Greene CE, et al. Infection with *Basidiobolus ranarum* in two dogs. J Am Vet Med Assoc 2002;221:528–532.

Grooters AM. Pythiosis, lagenidiosis, and zygomycosis in small animals. Vet Clin North Am Small Anim Pract 2003;33:695–720.

Hillier A, et al. Canine subcutaneous zygomycosis caused by *Conidiobolus* sp.: A case report and review of *Conidiobolus* infections in other species. Vet Dermatol 1994;5:205–213.

Jensen HE, et al. Immunohistochemical diagnosis of systemic bovine zygomycosis by murine monoclonal antibodies. Vet Pathol 1996;33:176–183.

Miller RI, Campbell RSF. The comparative pathology of equine cutaneous phycomycosis. Vet Pathol 1984;21:325–332.

Miscellaneous fungal infections of skin

Infections with various opportunist fungi are reported sporadically in animals. These organisms are ubiquitous in the environment, common contaminants of laboratory cultures, and frequently also a component of skin and hair flora of normal animals. Thus, *diagnosis of infection is difficult to make by culture alone and requires histologic demonstration of tissue invasion by morphologically compatible organisms.* In humans, these infections are usually associated with immunosuppression and neutropenia, but predisposing factors are not usually identified in animals. A convenient means of classifying opportunistic subcutaneous mycotic infections is based on the presence or absence of pigment in mycelia. Those caused by *pigmented ("phaeoid") fungi are called phaeohyphomycosis* and have already been discussed. *Infections caused by colorless or hyaline fungi are called* hyalohyphomycosis. Organisms that cause infection with some regularity or have some particularly distinctive feature are assigned to a separate category, e.g., aspergillosis, pythiosis, etc. Reports of infection with dematiaceous fungi and the number of fungi causing phaeohyphomycosis are more numerous than those caused by unpigmented fungi. The system is artificial in that completely unrelated organisms fall into the same category. However, most of these organisms have similar tissue morphology and elicit the same pathologic response, i.e., (pyo)granulomatous dermatitis and panniculitis. Culture or immunofluorescence or immunohistochemical staining of tissue sections is necessary for specific identification of these organisms.

Cutaneous **hyalohyphomycosis** caused by *Acremonium* and *Fusarium* has been described in dogs and cats. *Aspergillus* species are not commonly associated with skin infections. Subcutaneous infection with *Aspergillus versicolor* producing a nodular mass on the upper lip was reported in an adult Saddlebred mare. The lesion recurred once following surgical excision but had not recurred one year after the second surgical excision. *A. terreus* has been associated with subcutaneous granulomas in an adult Holstein cow without any lesions elsewhere. Dogs with disseminated aspergillosis may rarely develop cutaneous lesions secondarily.

Geotrichosis is a *rare* disseminated, bronchopulmonary, oral, vaginal, cutaneous, or alimentary infection caused by *Geotrichum candidum*. Cutaneous infections have been reported in dogs, snakes, humans, flamingos, horses, and a giant tortoise. *G. candidum* is a ubiquitous soil saprophyte and is also part of normal flora of the oral cavity, intestine, skin and hair. Lesions were on the head and back in dogs and on the head and neck in horses. Gross lesions varied from well-circumscribed ulcers covered by exudate to nonulcerated nodular masses with variable alopecia and desquamation. Infection appeared to be pruritic in several affected horses. Geotrichosis has also been associated with paronychia and onychodystrophy in several dogs. Microscopically, branching septate hyphae were present in the surface keratin and exudate, necrotic epidermis, and extended into the dermis. The organism may be confused histologically with *Candida*, *Aspergillus*, and *Trichosporon*.

Paecilomycosis is a *rare* subcutaneous or disseminated infection of cats and dogs caused by *Paecilomyces* fungi. The organism is a common airborne contaminant that may be resistant to many sterilizing techniques. Skin lesions typically consist of focal masses or edematous swellings, frequently on the feet and legs. Lesions have also been described on the face and nasal cavity. One disseminated infection in a young adult German Shepherd was thought to originate from an external ear infection.

Trichosporon yeasts cause white piedra, cutaneous infections, systemic infections, pneumonitis, valvular endocarditis, and have been associated with abortions. In humans, disseminated systemic infections usually occur in immunocompromised patients with granulocytopenia. White piedra is a mycotic infection of hair shafts caused by *T. beigellii* (*T. cutaneum*) in humans, monkeys, and horses in temperate to tropical climates. The infection is characterized by *firm, irregular white or pale brown nodules on hair shafts*. In horses, the long hairs of the mane, tail, and forelock are affected. *The nodules consist of tightly packed septate hyphae that are held together by a cement-like substance.* Cutaneous trichosporonosis is *rare* and has been reported only in cats. One cat also had multicentric lymphosarcoma that may have caused immunosuppression. Lesions reported in cats consisted of a nodule in a nostril and an ulcerated mass on the distal leg at the site of a previous cat bite wound. Microscopically, the organisms consist of budding yeast cells and hyaline, branched septate hyphae.

Bibliography

Doster AR, et al. Trichosporonosis in two cats. J Am Vet Med Assoc 1987;190:1184–1186.

Fleming RV, et al. Emerging and less common fungal pathogens. Infect Dis Clin North Am 2002;16:915–933.

Foley JE, et al. Paecilomycosis in dogs and horses and a review of the literature. J Vet Intern Med 2002;16:238–243.

Keegan KG, et al. Subcutaneous mycetoma-like granuloma in a horse caused by *Aspergillus versicolor*. J Vet Diagn Invest 1995;7:564–567.

Keller M, et al. Keratinopathogenic mould fungi and dermatophytes in healthy and diseased hooves of horses. Vet Rec 2000;147:619–622.

March PA, et al. Diagnosis, treatment, and temporary remission of disseminated paecilomycosis in a Vizsla. J Am Anim Hosp Assoc 1996;32:509–514.

Matsumoto T, et al. Developments in hyalohyphomycosis and phaeohyphomycosis. J Med Vet Mycol 1994;32(suppl 1):329–349.

Reppas GP, Snoeck TD. Cutaneous geotrichosis in a dog. Aust Vet J 1999;77:567–569.

PROTOZOAL DISEASES OF SKIN

Cutaneous lesions occur in several **systemic or localized protozoal** infections. Differentials for protozoal dermatitis should include *Besnoitia* sp., *Leishmania* sp., *Caryospora* sp., *Neospora* sp., *Toxoplasma* sp., and *Sarcocystis* sp. The majority of these cutaneous protozoal infections have been reported in **dogs**, however some cause serious disease in other domestic species as described below. *Toxoplasma* sp. is considered an opportunistic pathogen most often seen in dogs concurrently infected with canine distemper virus. Cutaneous infection with toxoplasma organisms has not been reported, however the morphological similarities to other protozoal organisms reported to cause dermatitis in animals warrant considering it in the differential of protozoal dermatitis. Cytologic, histologic, immunohistologic and ultrastructural studies can be used to differentiate organisms that are histologically similar. Cutaneous lesions have also been associated with *Theileria* and *Babesia* infections (see Vol. 3, Hematopoietic system). *Trypanosoma equiperdum* and dourine are discussed in Vol. 3, Female genital system.

Besnoitiosis

Members of the genus *Besnoitia* are responsible for a serious disease of *cattle and horses* and, more rarely, donkeys, goats, and sheep. In North America, opossums, caribou, reindeer, and mule deer may serve as intermediate hosts. The genus is currently classified under the family Sarcocystidae, in the subfamily Toxoplasmatinae.

Besnoitia have a *two-host life cycle*. The *definitive hosts are felids* and the intermediate hosts vary with the parasitic species. For *B. besnoiti*, the intermediate host is the ox and for *B. bennetti* it is the horse. These two organisms are morphologically identical by light microscopy and are distinguished only by their host range. Sexual reproduction occurs in the intestinal tract of the definitive host and the sporulated oocysts are passed in the feces. *The exact mode of infection of the intermediate hosts is not known*, but contamination of watering places and mechanical transmission by blood sucking insects may be involved. The life cycle in the intermediate host is characterized by release of sporozoites from sporulated oocysts and the subsequent dissemination of tachyzoites that lead to bradyzoite cyst formation. Cysts occur mostly in the dermis, subcutis, fascia, muscle, mucosa of the upper respiratory tract, pharynx, and conjunctiva. Infection, however, may be generalized and is typically so in some infections in rodents and wild animals. *The tissue cysts represent parasitized host cells* – the fibroblast in *B. wallacei* infection of rodents and the histiocyte in *B. besnoiti* experimental infection of rabbits. The bradyzoites multiply in cellular vacuoles and induce hyperplastic and hypertrophic changes in the host cells. These often divide to form multinucleated cells. The enlarging mass of crescent-shaped bradyzoites compresses the cell cytoplasm and nuclei into a thin rim forming an inner coat to the cyst. A hyalinized collagenous cyst wall is laid down around the parasitized cell. The cysts, which measure up to 500 μm with a 10–30 μm thick wall, are visible to the naked eye. Ingesting parasitized tissue from the intermediate host infects the definitive host.

Bovine besnoitiosis is a serious disease in South Africa and is associated with severe loss of condition in affected cattle, mortality up to 10% and marked damage to the hide. The disease also occurs in central and northern Africa, southern Europe, Asia, South America, and Russia. After an incubation period of ~1 week, a *pyrexic phase* develops in which animals become anorexic, depressed and reluctant to move. Approximately 1–4 weeks after the onset of the pyrexic phase and corresponding with cutaneous cyst formation, generalized lymphadenopathy, edematous swellings of the extremities and severe systemic signs develop. Pregnant cows may abort at this time. The second stage is known as the *depilatory stage* since it is characterized by marked alopecia, thickening of the skin, exudation and fissuring. *The cysts may be visible macroscopically in the scleral conjunctiva or nasal mucosa as small, round, white foci*. Animals lose condition and up to 10% mortality may occur at this point. The third phase is characterized by *dry seborrhea*. Animals remain unthrifty for an extended period and rarely regrow a normal hair coat. The skin remains alopecic, lichenified and scaly.

Histologically, epidermal hyperplasia, marked hyperemia, dermal edema and perivascular accumulations of lymphocytes, plasma cells and large histiocytes that will become hosts to the parasites accompany the acute febrile stage. *Crescent-shaped trophozoites occur in arterioles and lymphatics and free in tissue spaces*. Occasionally they may be detected in macrophages. As the parasites become encysted, inflammation and edema diminish. *The mature cysts incite little or no cellular reaction unless they rupture*; a necrotizing or granulomatous response ensues around the collapsed hyaline capsule. Numerous eosinophils are present in these reactions. The mature cyst wall has *four distinct layers*. Outermost is a condensed, hyalinized, laminated, birefringent layer of collagen fibers. Next is a very thin homogeneous intermediate zone. The third layer is the cytoplasm of the host cell and in this layer lie the several giant, vesicular but compressed host cell nuclei. A thin inner membrane, probably condensed cell cytoplasm, encloses the dense mass of 5–7 μm crescentic bradyzoites. These may be separated from the wall by an artifactual shrinkage space. *Lesions in other tissues* include focal disseminated myositis, keratitis, periostitis, endosteitis, lymphadenitis, pneumonia, periorchitis, orchitis, epididymitis, arteritis, and perineuritis.

Besnoitiosis in **horses, donkeys**, and **burros** has cutaneous lesions similar to those described in cattle. **Caprine** besnoitiosis occurs in Iran in both wild and domestic species. The *Besnoitia* cysts are observed in the skin, blood vessels, epididymis and testes. The pathological changes are comparable to those of *B. besnoiti* infection in cattle. In an outbreak affecting more than 500 domestic goats in Kenya, ocular cysts were the most common finding, but cysts were found in many body systems. Dorper **sheep** were also affected in that outbreak. A disease resembling besnoitiosis was reported in New Zealand lambs.

Bibliography

Davis WP, et al. Besnoitiosis in a miniature donkey. Vet Dermatol 1997;8:139–143.

Dubey JP, et al. Ultrastructure of *Besnoitia besnoiti* tissue cysts and bradyzoites. J Eukaryot Microbiol 2003;50:240–244.

Ellis JT, et al. Molecular phylogeny of *Besnoitia* and the genetic relationships among *Besnoitia* of cattle, wildebeest and goats. Protist 2000;151:329–336.

Njagi ON, et al. An epidemic of besnoitiosis in cattle in Kenya. Onderstepoort J Vet Res 1998;65:133–136.

Oryan A, Sadeghi MJ. An epizootic of besnoitiosis in goats in Fars province of Iran. Vet Res Commun 1997;21:559–570.

Leishmaniasis

Members of the genus *Leishmania* are responsible for systemic disease in man, dogs, cats, horses, and other mammals. Members of the *L. donovani* complex cause most infections. This intracellular parasite of the mononuclear-phagocytic system is *transmitted to animals and man by blood sucking sandflies.* The parasite's life cycle and manifestations of visceral disease are discussed in Vol. 3, Hematopoietic system. This zoonotic disease is endemic in Mediterranean countries and in parts of Africa, India, and Central and South America. Past reports of the disease in North America primarily involved animals with a history of foreign travel, however endemic foci of leishmaniasis now exist in Texas, Oklahoma, and Ohio. Recent reports indicate cases of canine visceral leishmaniasis have been confirmed in 21 of the United States and in southern Canada. The geographic distribution of the disease can be expected to continue to rise with the advent of increased international travel and the existence of immunosuppressive viral infections and therapeutics.

Studies in mice and dogs indicate that resistance to infection is dependent upon a Th1-type of immune response, while susceptibility is associated with a Th2-type of immune response. The alopecic form of the cutaneous disease as described below in the dog has been shown to be associated with fewer organisms and a more appropriate cellular immune response in terms of number of antigen-presenting Langerhans cells, MHCII-positive keratinocytes and infiltrating T cells. In contrast, dogs with the nodular form lacked antigen-presenting cells and had more numerous macrophages containing large numbers of organisms. It has been suggested that the clinical and histologic lesions may be useful in establishing a prognosis for remission in that the character of the lesions that develops reflects epidermal immunocompetence. Leishmaniasis is often associated with concurrent dermatoses such as opportunistic infections, parasitism, autoimmune disease, or neoplasia. This association and documented peripheral blood lymphocyte subset abnormalities *suggest that leishmaniasis may induce immune dysfunction. Cytology, immunohistochemistry, PCR, and serologic testing can help confirm diagnosis of the disease.* Currently, there is no cure for canine leishmaniasis, however, remission is possible.

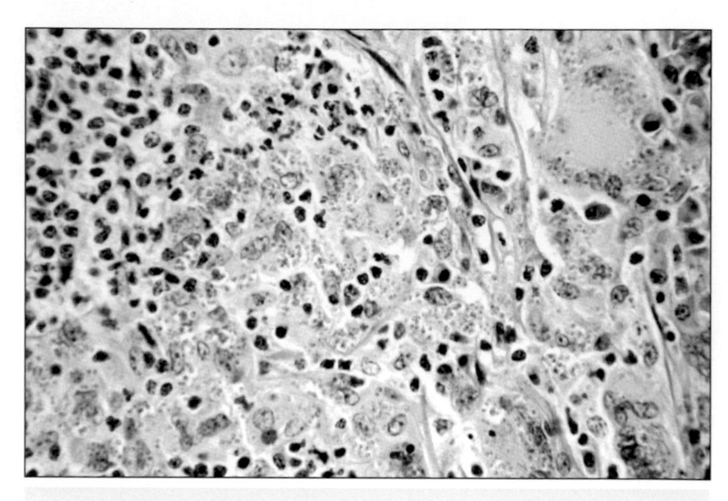

Figure 5.103 Leishmaniasis in a horse. Granulomatous inflammation. Macrophages and many multinucleate giant cells contain multiple *Leishmania* amastigotes.

The *skin* is one of the main organs affected in systemic leishmaniasis in **dogs**. Gross and histologic lesions are highly variable depending on host response and concurrent disease. Gross lesions may be alopecic, ulcerative, nodular or pustular. Onychogryposis and paronychia have also been reported. Alopecia with dry scaling on the head or entire body and multiple areas of ulceration of the skin of the head and limbs are seen most frequently. Initial lesions of alopecia are often periocular and referred to as "*lunettes*." Nonpainful, nonpruritic, variably ulcerated nodules varying from <1.0 cm to several cm in size may also be present but are less common. Nodules are most common on the ears, eyelids, and face but can be anywhere on the body. *Nodular mucosal leishmaniasis* affecting the oral cavity, tongue, nose, and penis has been reported in the dog. Unusual cases of leishmaniasis may present as a *generalized subcorneal pustular dermatitis.* Histologically, *the more common lesions consist of hyperkeratotic, nodular to diffuse superficial and deep, granulomatous dermatitis* (Fig. 5.103). Foci of inflammation may be perivascular, perifollicular, or interstitial in orientation. Perifollicular lesions frequently replace sebaceous glands. Some animals have infiltrates consisting primarily of large, foamy macrophages with numerous organisms and fewer plasma cells and lymphocytes while other animals have larger numbers of lymphocytes and plasma cells, indicating a more effective cellular immune response. Multinucleated giant cells may be present. The infiltrate in areas of ulceration includes neutrophils. *Leishmania* amastigotes are most commonly identified within macrophages, however they can occasionally be found within other leukocytes, endothelial cells or fibroblasts. In areas of necrosis, amastigotes may be free within the interstitium.

Clinical differentials for the skin lesions are numerous and vary with the types of lesions and include sarcoptic and demodectic mange, seborrhea, pemphigus foliaceus, systemic lupus erythematosus, bacterial infections, and superficial necrolytic dermatitis and zinc-responsive dermatitis, to name a few. The nodular form must be differentiated grossly from various cutaneous neoplasms, and grossly and histologically from infectious or sterile granulomas. *Leishmania* sp. *can be distinguished from other protozoa via light microscopy by recognition of the kinetoplast oriented perpendicular to the nucleus.*

Cutaneous leishmaniasis has been reported in **cats** in Europe and South America, and in a cat living in Texas; the cat was presented repeatedly with progressive, multiple, non-ulcerated cutaneous nodules on the ears, face, and nasal mucosa. Histologic lesions were described as dermal infiltrates of macrophages containing *Leishmania* amastigotes. No evidence of systemic infection was found at necropsy 7 years after the initial cutaneous lesions containing amastigotes were identified.

Cutaneous leishmaniasis has been reported in **horses, mules, and donkeys** in Europe, South America, and in a horse in North America and another in Puerto Rico. Lesions consist of crusted or ulcerated nodules on the pinna, head, and neck or less commonly the legs, scrotum and penis. Histologically, the dermis contains nodular to diffuse infiltrates of macrophages and lymphocytes or distinct granulomas with organisms identified in macrophages or free within the interstitium. Cutaneous lesions may not be associated with systemic infection.

Bibliography

Barnes JC, et al. Diffuse cutaneous leishmaniasis in a cat. J Am Vet Med Assoc 1993;202:416–418.

Bourdoiseau G, et al. Lymphocyte subset abnormalities in canine leishmaniasis. Vet Immunol Immunopathol 1997;56:345–351.

Bourdoiseau G, et al. Immunohistochemical detection of *Leishmania infantum* in formalin-fixed, paraffin-embedded sections of canine skin and lymph nodes. J Vet Diagn Invest 1997;9:439–440.

Ciaramella P, et al. A retrospective clinical study of canine leishmaniasis in 150 dogs naturally infected by *Leishmania infantum*. Vet Rec 1997;141:539–543.

Fondevila D, et al. Epidermal immunocompetence in canine leishmaniasis. Vet Immunol Immunopathol 1997;56:319–327.

Font A, et al. Canine mucosal leishmaniasis. J Am Anim Hosp Assoc 1996; 32:131–137.

Hervas J, et al. Two cases of feline visceral and cutaneous leishmaniosis in Spain. J Feline Med Surg 1999;1:101–105.

Koutinas AF, et al. Clinical considerations on canine visceral leishmaniasis in Greece: A retrospective study of 158 cases (1989–1996). J Am Anim Hosp Assoc 1999;35:376–383.

Mozos E, et al. Leishmaniasis and generalized demodicosis in three dogs: a clinicopathological and immunohistochemical study. J Comp Pathol 1999;120:257–268.

Ramos-Vara JA, et al. Cutaneous leishmaniasis in two horses. Vet Pathol 1996;33:731–743.

Roura X, et al. Detection of *Leishmania* infection in paraffin-embedded skin biopsies of dogs using polymerase chain reaction. J Vet Diag Invest 1999;11:385–387.

Schubach TM, et al. American cutaneous leishmaniasis in two cats from Rio de Janeiro, Brazil: first report of natural infection with *Leishmania (Viannia) braziliensis*. Trans R Soc Trop Med Hyg 2004;98:165–167.

Solano-Gallego L, et al. Cutaneous leishmaniosis in three horses in Spain. Equine Vet J 2003;35:320–323.

Miscellaneous coccidian parasites

Caryospora spp., apicomplexan parasites whose primary hosts are reptiles and raptors, rarely cause *pyogranulomatous dermatitis in puppies*. Immunosuppression and concurrent disease, such as canine distemper, likely play a facilitatory role. Lesions involve skin and draining lymph nodes and comprise diffuse pyogranulomatous dermatitis. Macrophages contain large numbers of intracellular organisms, including schizonts, gamonts, oocysts, and caryocysts. Caryocysts have a thin cyst wall enclosing the host cell nucleus and contain up to three sporozoites. Not all stages of the life cycle may be present in the tissue sections, precluding a microscopic diagnosis in some cases. Immunohistochemical studies identified the agent in one case as *C. bigenetica*. Experimental oral infection of immunosuppressed puppies with *C. bigenetica* induced typical skin lesions affecting muzzle, periocular skin, footpads, ears and abdomen within 10 days of inoculation.

Neospora caninum is a cyst-forming protozoal parasite of *dogs, cattle, sheep, goats, horses, and deer*. It is best known as a cause of bovine abortion capable of transplacental transmission. It typically causes systemic and neurologic disease. *N. caninum* is considered a primary pathogen in dogs with the majority of cases occurring as neurological disease in puppies. Cutaneous lesions occur in mature dogs often with underlying immunosuppression from drug therapy or concurrent disease. It is not known whether the disease in adult dogs results from a reactivated congenital infection or from a recently acquired infection. Lesions have been described as *multifocal-to-generalized, ulcerative and nodular dermatitis*. Histologically, there is pyogranulomatous and eosinophilic, to necrotizing and hemorrhagic, dermatitis. Numerous tachyzoites, 4–7 μm × 1.5–5 μm, may be seen in macrophages, keratinocytes, and neutrophils, and rarely in endothelial cells and fibroblasts. Tissue cysts are not present in the cutaneous lesions. Identification of *N. caninum* can be confirmed by immunohistochemistry.

An unidentified ***Sarcocystis*-like protozoan** was associated with *multiple cutaneous abscesses and disseminated visceral lesions in a dog*. The skin lesions were diffuse, necrotizing, hemorrhagic and suppurative. Large numbers of protozoa were present, primarily in macrophages and neutrophils, and occasionally in fibroblasts and endothelial cells. Some vessels contained thrombi and there was associated dermal and epidermal infarction. The organism did not stain with antisera to the other apicomplexan parasites so far identified as causing dermatitis in dogs, namely *Neospora caninum* and *Caryospora* sp.

Bibliography

Dubey JP, et al. *Caryospora*-associated dermatitis in dogs. J Parasitol 1990; 76:552–556.

Dubey JP, et al. Fatal cutaneous and visceral infection in a Rottweiler dog associated with a *Sarcocystis*-like protozoon. J Vet Diagn Invest 1991;3:72–75.

La Perle KMD, et al. Cutaneous neosporosis in two adult dogs on chronic immunosuppressive therapy. J Vet Diagn Invest 2001;13:252–255.

Ordeix L, et al. Cutaneous neosporosis during treatment of pemphigus foliaceus in a dog. J Am Anim Hosp Assoc 2002;38:415–419.

ALGAL DISEASES OF SKIN: PROTOTHECOSIS

Protothecosis is an uncommon disease caused by *Prototheca* spp. organisms, which are thought to be *colorless, nonphotosynthetic variants of the green alga Chlorella*. The organism is ubiquitous in organic matter and in fresh and marine waters. Reports of infection in humans and domestic and wild animals are worldwide, but the majority of cases are from the southeastern United States. The two most common species associated with infection are *Prototheca wickerhamii* and *P. zopfii*. *Mastitis in cows and disseminated disease in dogs are more common than cutaneous-subcutaneous infection*. In humans, the cutaneous form is the most common and is thought to be initiated by traumatic implantation, resulting in a protracted and indolent clinical course. *Cutaneous protothecosis has been reported in dogs and cats* from the USA, Australia, England, and Spain. In those cases in which the organism was speciated, *P. zopfii* is most often associated with disseminated disease, whereas the cutaneous form has been caused by *P. wickerhamii*.

Despite widespread distribution of *Prototheca* spp., *the prevalence of infection is very low* and attempts to reproduce infection experimentally have met with mixed success. This has led to speculation that the organism is an *opportunist with low pathogenicity* that requires an underlying immunologic dysfunction for the development of disease. Most humans with cutaneous protothecosis have a concurrent disease condition that may alter the immune response to the organism. Except in one dog with disseminated protothecosis, no immunologic deficit has been identified in animals with cutaneous or disseminated disease. However, there is evidence to suggest that infection may become established in an individual with minor immunosuppression and that the algae may further compromise the host immune response.

The cutaneous lesions are variable and consist of small crusty ulcerative lesions, multiple miliary nodules, firm raised nodules, or poorly demarcated subcutaneous swellings anywhere on the body. The tissue is soft and uniformly pale tan or white. Histologically, the masses consist of *diffuse infiltrates of primarily epithelioid macrophages* in the dermis and subcutis. Multinucleated giant cells, neutrophils, and lymphoid cells are in variable numbers, and foci of necrosis may be present. *Organisms are typically numerous but they are only lightly stained with H&E and therefore are poorly visualized.* The cell wall and internal contents are readily stained with fungal stains, e.g., Gridley (GF), Gomori methenamine silver (GMS), and periodic acid-Schiff (PAS). The organisms vary from 1.3–25 μm in diameter and consist of cells called *sporangia* that divide by internal cleavage to form multiple *endospores*. Identification of *Prototheca* can be made reliably by examination of tissue sections, but species identification usually requires culture or immunofluorescence methods because differences in the two species are subtle. *P. wickerhamii* sporangia are smaller and round in comparison to the larger and oval or cylindrical shape of most *P. zopfii*. *Protothecae must be differentiated from Chlorella algae*, whose natural green pigmentation is removed in fixation and routine tissue processing. In contrast to *Prototheca* cells, *Chlorella* sporangia contain many large starch granules that are stained by GF, GMS, and PAS.

Bibliography

Dillberger JE, et al. Protothecosis in two cats. J Am Vet Med Assoc 1988;192:1557–1559.

Ginel PJ, et al. Cutaneous protothecosis in a dog. Vet Rec 1997;140:651–653.

Hollingsworth SR. Canine protothecosis. Vet Clin North Am Small Anim Pract 2000;30:1091–1101.

Perez J, et al. Canine cutaneous protothecosis: an immunohistochemical analysis of the inflammatory cellular infiltrate. J Comp Pathol 1997;117:83–89.

Rakich PM, Latimer KS. Altered immune function in a dog with disseminated protothecosis. J Am Vet Med Assoc 1984;185:681–683.

ARTHROPOD ECTOPARASITES

Of the parasitic arthropods, only small a fraction are parasites of domestic animals, but the harmfulness of these is quite out of proportion to their number. Some, such as the mites, are pathogens in their own right, but *the majority of them owe their immense importance to their ability to act as mechanical or biological transmitters for many pathogenic viruses, bacteria, protozoa and helminths.* Their role as vectors is discussed in relation to the specific diseases throughout these volumes.

The parasites of concern to us here belong to the two large classes, Insecta and Arachnida. The class Insecta contains four important orders, Diptera (*flies*), Siphonaptera (*fleas*), Mallophaga (*biting lice*) and Siphunculata (*sucking lice*). The class Arachnida contains the order, Acarina, in which *ticks and mites* are classified. For information on biological characters and classification, reference should be made to texts on entomology.

Many **arthropod bites or stings** go unreported and are of minimal consequence. The type and number of arthropods inflicting the bite or sting and the individual host response determine the severity of the injury. In general, most arthropod bites initially appear as circular, erythematous lesions, 0.5–2.0 cm in diameter. Lesions may progress to focal areas of necrosis with ulceration, alopecia and crust formation. Histologically, the area of necrosis and inflammation may have a triangular outline with one point of the triangle in the deep dermis or panniculus. In early lesions, the inflammation is perivascular to diffuse and includes variable numbers of eosinophils, neutrophils, lymphocytes, and macrophages. Edema and hemorrhage may be present. As the lesion ages, the area may become nodular to form "*arthropod-bite granuloma*" comprised of macrophages, lymphocytes, mast cells, eosinophils and plasma cells. Lymphoid follicles may form. More specific details concerning injury inflicted by various arthropods, if known, are discussed in the following sections.

Bibliography

Bowman DD. Arthropods. In: Georgi's Parasitology for Veterinarians. 7th ed. Philadelphia, PA: WB Saunders, 1999:1–78.

Gross TL, Ihrke PJ. Nodular and diffuse diseases of the dermis with prominent eosinophils or plasma cells. In: Gross TL, et al., eds. Veterinary Dermatopathology. A Macroscopic and Microscopic Evaluation of Canine and Feline Skin Disease. St. Louis, MO: Mosby Year Book, 1992:207–210.

Steen CJ, et al. Arthropods in dermatology. J Am Acad Dermatol 2004;50:819–842.

Wall R, Shearer D. Veterinary Entomology. Arthropod Ectoparasites of Veterinary Importance. London: Chapman and Hall, 1997.

Flies

Flies belong to the insect order, Diptera. Different species have various degrees of adaptation to a parasitic existence. Adult flies feed on blood, sweat, tears, saliva, feces, urine, and other body secretions. Non-biting, nuisance flies accomplish this by feeding only at the body surface on wounds or natural body orifices, whereas biting flies puncture the skin to feed. *Musca* are facultative feeders. Some, such as the Simuliidae and parasitic species of Culicidae and Ceratopogonidae, are obligate bloodsuckers, although usually only the females draw blood. At the other end of the spectrum are the Oestridae, whose larvae are obligate parasites, and some members of the Hippoboscidae that are obligate parasites in the adult stage.

Because of the variety of parasitic modes, it is not possible to generalize on the effects of flies on domestic animals nor, with the exception of a few obligate parasites, is it possible to be specific because there is little information available on primary pathogenicity. Flies adversely affect domestic animals by *causing annoyance*, by *direct toxicity* that may be fatal following massive insect attack, by *indirect toxicity* due to the deposition of larva into damaged skin (myiasis), by *local irritant effects* causing dermatitis that may predispose to secondary bacterial infection or to myiasis, by *injection of antigens* that induce hypersensitivity reactions, by *blood-feeding activities* that cause anemia, and by the biological or mechanical *transmission of other pathogens*. It has been estimated that tabanid flies could transmit 35 pathogens including *Equine infectious anemia virus* and trypanosomes. *Musca* spp. have been implicated in the mechanical transmission of anthrax, mastitis, and conjunctivitis in animals. *Stomoxys calcitrans*, the stable fly, is thought to be the primary transmitter of habronemiasis in horses.

Animal annoyance, so-called "*fly-worry*," is an important source of economic loss to the cattle, sheep and, to a lesser extent, swine industries. Fly worry refers to the behavioral disturbances in animals brought about by the attempted feeding of flies. Biting flies inflict pain whereas non-biting flies cause annoyance by clustering around the eyes and nostrils where they feed on lacrimal or nasal secretions (*Musca autumnalis* and *Hydrotaea irritans*) or by other means such as simulating the sound of a bumble bee (*Hypoderma* spp.). Fly-worry occasionally induces such apprehension that the animals run aimlessly ("*gadding*"), and severe injury or death may result from misadventure. Deaths are usually sporadic but high levels of mortality have been reported. Of much greater economic importance is the *loss of production* associated with fly worry. When the insects are numerous, they cause very considerable annoyance to livestock, interfere with feeding and resting and cause reduced milk production and reduced weight gain. Fly worry has been attributed to biting flies such as the horn fly (*Haematobia (Lyperosia) irritans*), the stable fly (*Stomoxys calcitrans*), and horse flies (several genera in the family Tabanidae), and to non-biting species such as house flies (*Musca* spp.), *Hypoderma* spp. and the sheep-head fly (*Hydrotaea irritans*). *Culicoides* spp. biting midges can cause pruritus and restlessness in horses. Horses that develop a hypersensitivity response to *Culicoides* spp. insect bites may suffer weight loss as a result of severe pruritus and irritation (see Immune-mediated dermatoses).

Mortality may arise from direct toxic effect as well as from misadventure. Death may be the result of urticarial swelling of the head and neck or of shock. Many flies are attracted to exhaled carbon dioxide and can occasionally cause *death by suffocation* of cattle, horses, or other animals when large numbers of flies are inhaled. Mosquitoes, especially aggressive species such as *Aedes vigilex*, may cause significant mortality amongst piglets and puppies. The Simuliidae (black flies or buffalo gnats) are responsible for massive animal mortalities, particularly in temperate latitudes and river valleys following extensive flooding when the insect population expands. They feed on cattle, horses, sheep, goats, poultry, wild mammals and birds. *Simuliid flies exert systemic effects through inoculation of a heat-stable toxin*, which causes increased vascular permeability and abnormalities in cardiorespiratory function, which may cause death.

The hematophagous flies seldom cause serious loss of blood, however anemia may result from heavy infestations by *Haematobia irritans*, mosquitoes, the sheep ked *Melophagus ovinus* and *Stomoxys calcitrans*, which may ingest as much as 16 mg blood per feeding.

In dogs, stable flies (*Stomoxys calcitrans*) typically attack the face and tips or folded edges of the pinnae producing erythematous to hemorrhagic dermatitis with variable pruritus. *Simuliidae* spp. can also feed on small animals. Lesions are most often found on the head, ears, legs, or hairless areas of the abdomen and appear as papules, ulcers, or circumscribed areas of necrosis. Occasionally annular macular lesions with a central puncture surrounded by an edematous zone with a peripheral erythematous rim may be evident.

Local irritant effect results from *injection of salivary fluids into the host*. Very little is known of the nature of the cutaneous lesions produced in animals by these insects. The character and severity of the local lesions vary. Pruritus is often intense, resulting in secondary traumatic lesions. The primary lesions are usually erythematous papules or wheals often surrounding a central bleeding point (mosquitoes) or small puncture wounds (biting flies). The wheals are usually transient but may persist for several weeks. The puncture wounds often develop an exudative crust. Some flies (Simuliidae) feed by lacerating the skin until a pool of blood forms on the surface from which they feed. Histologically, there may be intraepithelial eosinophilic spongiform pustules or focal areas of epidermal necrosis indicating the penetration point. The dermal reaction is superficial perivascular in pattern and contains predominantly eosinophils, lymphocytes and plasma cells. Occasionally there is acute necrosis of the surface of the papules, including both dermis and epidermis.

The injected salivary substances are irritant and many are allergenic, and hypersensitivity reactions probably contribute to the severity of the local lesions caused by a variety of biting flies. Hypersensitivity reactions to *S. calcitrans* are recognized in cattle; affected animals develop coalescing blisters on the forelimbs. An important allergic dermatitis of horses is caused by hypersensitivity to *Culicoides* spp.

Rather more important than the bloodsucking or biting flies are those species whose larvae are highly destructive facultative or obligate parasites. Infestations with such larvae cause *myiasis*, which is discussed below.

Bibliography

Foil L, Foil C. Dipteran parasites of horses. Eq Pract 1988;10:21–38.

Foil LD, et al. The role of horn fly feeding and the management of seasonal equine ventral midline dermatitis. Eq Pract 1990;12:6–14.

Scott DW, et al. Diptera (flies). In: Scott DW, et al., ed. Muller and Kirk's Small Animal Dermatology. 5th ed. Philadelphia, PA: WB Saunders, 1995:457–459.

Yeruham I, et al. Skin lesions in dogs, horses and calves caused by the stable fly *Stomoxys calcitrans* (L.) (Diptera: Muscidae). Rev Elev Med Vet Pays Trop 1995;48:347–349.

Myiasis

Myiasis is the infestation of the tissue of living animals with the larvae of dipterous flies. The larvae are referred to as *maggots* or *grubs* and may be facultative or obligate parasites. The important families are Cuterebridae, Sarcophagidae (*Wohlfahrtia* spp.), Gasterophilidae (stomach bots of horses), Oestridae (nasal bots, warbles), and Calliphoridae (blowflies). Only those flies whose larvae cause cutaneous or subcutaneous lesions are discussed here. Nasal and stomach bots are described elsewhere. Agents of facultative myiasis affecting the skin live in decaying organic matter, and the females oviposit in wounded, infected, or heavily soiled skin of warm-blooded vertebrate hosts. The larvae feed on host tissues and eventually drop to the

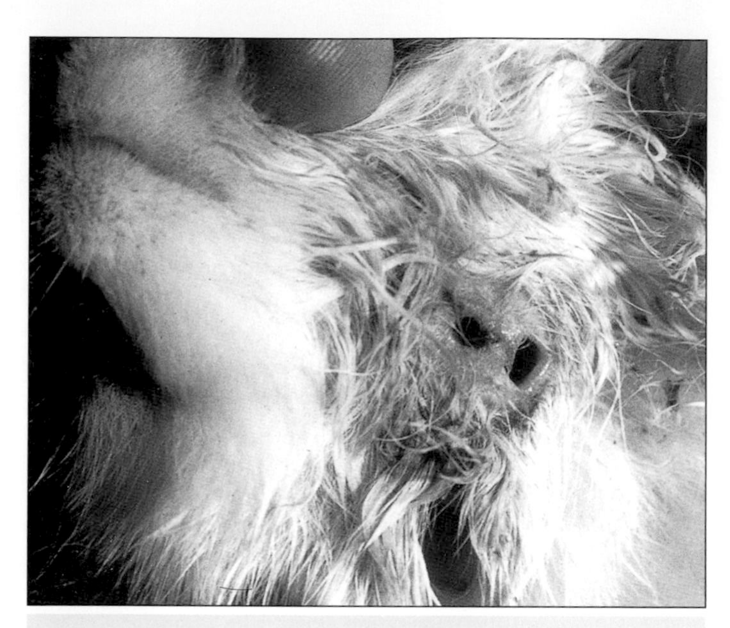

Figure 5.104 ***Cuterebra* infestation** with draining lesions in a cat.

ground to pupate. *Cochliomyia hominovorax,* the screwworm fly, produces larvae that are obligatory parasites and are discussed separately.

Cuterebra

The larvae of ***Cuterebra*** spp. (Diptera; Family: Oestridae; sub-family: Cuterebrinae) are obligate parasites of rodents and rabbits but occasionally aberrant infestations occur in cats and rarely in dogs, pigs, and humans. Larvae attach to the host's fur and either enter via ingestion through grooming, direct skin penetration or through natural orifices to migrate to the subcutaneous tissues to produce an initially firm, then fluctuant, cyst-like subcutaneous abscess in which the larvae mature. The larvae breathe through a fistulous pore in the skin through which they are visible, and feed off tissue debris. Wounds heal slowly after larvae are removed or released and secondary bacterial infection may occur. The majority of infections occur in late summer or fall. *In cats, the larvae have a predilection for the neck area* (Fig. 5.104), often over the submandibular salivary gland, but swellings also occur in the scrotal region. Larvae may locate in aberrant locations such as the pharynx, nasal cavity, eye, and brain.

In South and Central America, ***Dermatobia hominis*** (Diptera; Oestridae; sub-family: Cuterebrinae) affects cattle, sheep, goats, pigs and people and, rarely dogs and cats. It is also known as the *human bot fly*. The adult fly captures another carrier insect to which it attaches its eggs. The eggs hatch when the carrier insect visits a host. The larvae then attach to the host and penetrate the skin to form local cutaneous nodules that can be pruritic. The mature larvae exit the nodule through holes that leave the host susceptible to fly strike. A case report of an infected dog from the Netherlands described lesions as painful, erythematous, exudative nodules with a central pore.

Wohlfahrtia

Wohlfahrtia magnifica (Diptera; Superfamily: Oestoidea; Family: Sarcophagidae) is an *obligate larval parasite of warm-blooded vertebrates* in the Mediterranean basin, eastern and central Europe and Asia minor. The female fly deposits larvae on the host near body orifices or in wounds. Larvae mature and drop to the ground to pupate in 5–7 days. *W. magnifica* causes myiasis in sheep, camels, poultry and to a lesser extent in cattle, horses, pigs, and dogs. Fecal soiling in sheep is a predisposing condition. *W. vigil* is a parasite of mink, foxes, rabbits, and occasionally dogs and cats in North America. The larvae can penetrate the tender skin of young animals, hence the young are most often affected. *W. nubia* is a secondary facultative invader of wounds in camels in North Africa and the Middle East.

Bibliography

Farkas R, Kepes G. Traumatic myiasis of horses caused by *Wohlfahrtia magnifica*. Acta Vet Hung 2001;49:311–318.

Glass EN, et al. Clinical and clinicopathologic features in 11 cats with *Cuterebra* larvae myiasis of the central nervous system. J Vet Intern Med 1998;12:365–368.

Rodriguez JM, Perez M. Cutaneous myiasis in three obese cats. Vet Q 1996;18:102–103.

Roosje PJ, et al. A case of a *Dermatobia hominis* infection in a dog in the Netherlands. Vet Dermatol 1992;3:183–185.

Williams KJ, et al. Cerebrospinal cuterebriasis in cats and its association with feline ischemic encephalopathy. Vet Pathol 1998;35:330–343.

Warbles

Warbles caused by ***Hypoderma bovis*** and ***Hypoderma lineatum*** (Diptera; Family: Oestridae; sub-family: Hypodermatinae) *occur chiefly in cattle*, although the parasite is not host specific; horses, sheep and humans are affected occasionally. *H. bovis, H. lineatum*, and *H. sinense* are present in Europe and Asia. Intensive eradication programs have eliminated *Hypoderma* spp. from the UK and Ireland and have greatly reduced their populations in much of the USA and Canada. *Przhevalskiana silensus* affects sheep and goats in Asia and Eastern Europe. *H. diana* is an important parasite of deer and possibly sheep in the Palaearctic. *H. tarandi* parasitizes reindeer in northern Eurasia and North America. There are no warble flies in Australia.

Warble flies are also known as heel flies because the eggs are deposited predominantly on the hair of the legs. Larvae emerge 4–6 days later and burrow directly into the skin or into hair follicles causing minimal irritation. Larvae migrate along fascial planes leaving tracks of green gelatinous material known as "butcher's jelly." The first instar larvae of *H. bovis* overwinter in the epidural fat, whereas those of *H. lineatum* develop in the esophageal submucosa. In the esophageal lesions, collagen bundles around the first instar larvae of *H. lineatum* appear fragmented, as if undergoing enzymatic digestion. A collagenase has been isolated from *H. lineatum*. In the epidural lesions of *H. bovis*, it is the fat tissue that appears necrotic. In the spring, the larvae migrate dorsally to the subcutaneous tissue of the back to form subcutaneous nodules ~3 cm diameter with a central pore for respiration. The lesions, which are known as "warbles," last for 4–6 weeks, during which the larvae undergo 2 molts. The mature third-instar larvae emerge from the breathing hole and pupate in the soil. In horses, the lesions occur in the saddle region and are often "blind" in that the larvae do not complete their development. Fatalities resulting from aberrant migration into the central nervous system are reported in horses.

Histologically, the cellular reaction is predominantly eosinophilic and lymphocytic. It is the eosinophilic infiltrate that gives "butcher's jelly" its green coloration. However, the most intense inflammatory reactions occur at sites of previous migration rather than around the viable larvae, suggesting that in naive hosts the parasites depress any effective host responses. Proteinases with the capacity to cleave the third component of bovine complement have been isolated from the first instar larvae of *H. lineatum*. Such enzymes could well ablate the host's inflammatory responses. The actual "warble" is lined by a wall of granulation tissue that matures to form a connective tissue capsule in which lie islands of eosinophils. The cystic cavity between the cuticle of the parasite and the granulation tissue fills with fibrin and a few inflammatory cells, chiefly eosinophils. Cuticle sloughed during ecdysis, or remnants of dead larva, incite a marked foreign body giant cell reaction. Once the larvae emerge, the cavity is repaired by fibrosis, but small foreign body granulomas may persist for months.

Warbles are economically important. The buzzing of the adult *H. bovis* (*H. lineatum* is silent) disturbs cattle causing considerable loss in milk and meat production. Larval tracks in the tissues decrease carcass value and the larval-induced holes markedly depreciate the value of the hide. Larval rupture, either accidental or deliberate, may induce a fatal anaphylactic reaction. This may result from systemic effects of the warble toxin, from type I hypersensitivity reactions, or a combination of both.

Bibliography

Baron RW. Cleavage of purified bovine complement component C_3 in larval *Hypoderma lineatum* (Diptera: Oestridae) hypodermins. J Med Entomol 1990;27:899–904.

Faliero SM, et al. Goat warble fly infestation by *Przhevalskiana silenus* (Diptera: Oestridae): immuno-epidemiologic survey in the Basilicata region (southern Italy). Parassitologia 2001;43:131–134.

Guo RM, Fu GZ. Report on the infestation of *Hypoderma lineatum* infestation in sheep. Chin J Vet Med 1986;12:16–17.

Hadlow WJ, et al. Intracranial myiasis by *Hypoderma bovis* (Linnaeus) in a horse. Cornell Vet 1977;67:272–281.

Otranto D, et al. A third species of *Hypoderma* (Diptera: Oestridae) affecting cattle and yaks in China: molecular and morphological evidence. J Parasitol 2004;90:958–965.

Panciera RJ, et al. Eosinophilic mediastinitis, myositis, pleuritis, and pneumonia of cattle associated with migration of first-instar larvae of *Hypoderma lineatum*. J Vet Diagn Invest 1993;5:226–231.

Calliphorine myiasis

This occurs in all animal species but is *most common in sheep*, particularly in Australia where it is of major economic importance. The flies involved are members of the subfamily Calliphoridae (**blowflies**). Important blowfly genera are *Lucilia, Calliphora, Protophormia, Phormia* and *Chrysomia*. The larvae (*maggots*) adopt a *facultative parasitic mode*, which is an adaptation of their beneficial and important role in the breakdown of carrion. Adult flies lay eggs on moist, warm skin of weakened or debilitated animals, in wounds or areas of heavy soiling with feces, urine or other body fluids. Hence, any species of animal can be susceptible.

Moisture, whether provided by rain, dew, urine, sweat or inflammatory exudate, predisposes to bacterial proliferation. These bacteria are often of fecal or urinary origin. The odor induced by the bacterial proliferation and resultant inflammatory exudate attracts the primary flies, which deposit batches of 50–200 ova. The larvae of primary flies emerge within 12–24 hours and grow rapidly, feeding on inflammatory exudates. *The primary larvae secrete proteolytic enzymes*, including collagenases, which liquefy the host tissues and provide predigested nutrients. The *cutaneous necrosis* that results attracts the secondary flies to oviposit. The resulting larvae *tunnel into the adjacent viable tissue* and markedly expand the lesion. The putrefactive odor attracts more flies, and the process is further exacerbated. The lesions of fly strike are often extensive and *leave large areas of undermined skin with punched-out holes*. The subcutaneous tissues may become cavitated. Muscle may be destroyed and body cavities invaded. Lesions may result in death from *shock, debilitation, toxemia or bacterial septicemia*.

The species of fly involved in fly strike differs with geographic location: *Lucilia cuprina* is the most important primary fly in Australia, *Phormia regina* in USA and Canada, and *Lucilia sericata* in Great Britain. Several different species of flies are involved in the development of the lesion of cutaneous myiasis. Primary flies, such as *L. cuprina*, are capable of initiating a strike on living sheep. Secondary flies, such as *Chrysomia rufifaces*, are not able to initiate a strike, but greatly exacerbate the lesions initiated by the primary fly. They may also displace the maggots developing from the eggs laid by the primary fly. Tertiary flies, such as the housefly *Musca domestica*, attack at a later stage and do not contribute significantly to the skin damage.

The development of fly strike in sheep depends upon abundance of primary flies, susceptible sheep, and moisture. The prevalence of the disease tends to follow the rise and fall in the population of primary flies, which in turn depends upon the climatic zone. In general, the flies require warm and moist but not hot conditions. Thus there is usually a double wave of primary flies, peaking in the spring and autumn. Certain breeds of sheep, in particular the fine-wooled Merino, have an inherent predisposition to attract fly strike. The character of the fleece and conformational features, such as skin wrinkling, allow retention of moisture or predispose to fecal or urinary soiling which are all initiating factors in fly strike. *Pseudomonas aeruginosa* (of "fleece rot") proliferation in soiled wool of sheep is of major importance. *Dermatophilus congolensis* may be involved occasionally.

In sheep, the lesions are most common in the perineum ("*breech strike*"), particularly in sheep with a narrow conformation and/or marked skin wrinkling which favor urine or fecal soiling. Lesions may affect the preputial orifice ("*pizzle strike*") particularly in animals with narrow urethral orifices, which predispose to urine soiling. Rams with deep head folds may develop "*poll strike*," possibly predisposed to by fight wounds. "*Wound strike*" occasionally follows castration or tail docking and "*body strike*" follows prolonged wetting, which in turn predisposes to "fleece rot" or dermatophilosis.

The initial *gross lesion* is a patch of dark-brown, moist wool, which has a foul smell. The wool is often very hot as a result of putrefaction and inflammation caused by the larvae. As the process advances, the maggots burrow under the skin causing irregular ulcers with scalloped edges. The lesions are irritating and pruritic. Occasionally the maggots migrate deeper into the muscle.

The economic losses of fly strike in sheep result from death, disfigurement, and depreciation of the fleece and costs associated with prevention and treatment.

Bibliography

Colditz IG, et al. Production of antibodies to recombinant antigens from *Lucilia cuprina* following cutaneous immunisation of sheep. Vet Parasitol 2002;104:345–350.

Hall MJ. Traumatic myiasis of sheep in Europe: a review. Parasitologia 1997;39:409–413.

Hendrix CM. Facultative myiasis in dogs and cats. Compend Contin Educ Pract Vet 1991;13:86–93.

Tellam RL, Bowles VM. Control of blowfly strike in sheep: current strategies and future prospects. Int J Parasitol 1997;27:261–273.

Watts JE, et al. The significance of certain skin characters of sheep in resistance and susceptibility to fleece-rot and body strike. Aust Vet J 1980;56:57–63.

Screwworm myiasis

Members of the Calliphoridae also cause myiasis; however, they differ from the blowflies in that *screwworm fly larvae are obligate parasites, invading edges of fresh, uncontaminated wounds on live animals*. The American species of screwworm flies are ***Cochliomyia hominivorax*** and ***Cochliomyia macellaria*** (the secondary screwworm fly), which is usually a carrion breeder but can act as a secondary invader of fly strikes. The African and Asian screwworm fly is *Chrysomyia bezziana*. The disease occurs in Africa, Asia, Central and South America and Mexico but has been virtually eradicated from the USA and Mexico, following a program in which release of massive numbers of irradiated male flies rendered the annual breeding a sterile one. An outbreak of screwworm in Libya in 1988, seen as a major threat to the livestock of southern Europe and Africa, was dealt with in a similar fashion. International air travel proffers a source of spread to susceptible countries.

Screwworm myiasis affects all domestic animals and humans and is an important cause of mortality in wildlife. The flies oviposit in cutaneous wounds, such as those caused by castration, dehorning, branding or accidental injuries. The navel of neonatal calves, the perineum of recently calved cows and tick bites are also favorable sites for oviposition. The larvae feed in groups, to penetrate and liquefy fresh, live host tissue with the aid of proteolytic enzymes. Blood-stained fluid, often containing incompletely digested shreds of tissue, oozes from the wound, which contains clusters of voraciously feeding larvae. A distinctive and particularly evil odor emanates from the lesion. The lesions are extremely painful and may expand rapidly, leading to death in untreated animals. Screwworm infestation is a reportable condition in many countries.

Bibliography

Hendrix CM. Facultative myiasis in dogs and cats. Compend Contin Educ Pract Vet 1991;13:86–93.

Litjens P, et al. Characterization of the screwworm flies *Cochliomyia hominivorax* and *Cochliomyia macellaria* by PCR-RFLP of mitochondrial DNA. Med Vet Entomol 2001;15:183–188.

Rajapaksa N, Spradbery JP. Occurrence of the Old World screw-worm fly *Chrysomyia bezziana* on livestock vessels and commercial aircraft. Aust Vet J 1989;66:21–23.

Wyss JH. Screwworm eradication in the Americas. Ann N Y Acad Sci 2000;916:186–193.

Sheep ked infestation

Melophagus ovinus (Diptera: Hippoboscidae) *is a wingless fly that causes a chronic, pruritic dermatitis of sheep*. Goats are also affected. Of worldwide distribution, the disease's chief economic importance is the associated *loss of wool production*.

Melophagus ovinus is an obligate ectoparasite. The eggs develop into larvae within the female until they are ready to pupate. After parturition, the female attaches its larva to wool fibers with the aid of a sticky substance. The immotile larva transforms into a chestnut-brown pupa ~3–4 mm long. The pupal stage lasts 3–5 weeks and the adult keds live 4–5 months. They prefer the sides of the neck and body and are difficult to detect in fully-fleeced animals. The adults feed actively on blood. While anemia may develop in severe ked infestations, the more significant lesions are the result of the *severe pruritus*, which causes the sheep to rub and bite, and thus damage the fleece. The adult fly's excreta stains the wool, further reducing its value. Wool loss and vertical ridging of the skin leads to a condition referred to as "cockle." The irritation induced by the bites also affects weight gain. The US sheep industry has estimated losses attributed to sheep keds to be about $40 million per year.

Histologic lesions reported are superficial and deep perivascular dermatitis with eosinophils and lymphocytes predominating. Fibrinoid necrosis of small arterioles is also described.

Bibliography

Arundel JH, Sutherland AK. Animal Health in Australia. Volume 10. Ectoparasitic Diseases of Sheep, Cattle, Goats and Horses. Australian Government Publishing Service, 1988:69–72.

Mehlhorn H, et al. *In vivo* and *in vitro* effects of imidacloprid on sheep keds (*Melophagus ovinus*): a light and electron microscopic study. Parasitol Res 2001;87:331–336.

Nelson WA, Bainborough AR. Development in sheep of resistance to the ked *Melophagus ovinus* (L.). III. Histopathology of sheep skin as a clue to the nature of resistance. Exp Parasitol 1963;13:118–127.

Hornfly dermatitis

While mainly an obligate parasite of cattle, the **horn fly (*Haematobia irritans*)** is one cause of *seasonal ventral midline dermatitis in the horse*. In **cattle**, the flies feed in groups primarily on the back, withers, and head. They leave the animal only briefly to mate and lay eggs. Horn flies require fresh bovine feces to lay eggs. Large numbers of horn flies in cattle can result in significant loss of blood, wounds that attract other flies, and in loss of production. *H. irritans* is also thought to transmit the skin parasitic nematode of cattle, *Stephanofilaria stilesi*.

In **horses**, horn flies, cluster on the ventral abdomen (and occasionally on the neck or periocular region), producing bites marked by tiny drops of dried blood. A few days later pruritic, scaling, alopecic patches develop. These become lichenified and heal with either leukoderma or melanosis. The lesions are often single, usually well-circumscribed and occur near the umbilicus. Histologically, lesions are perivascular and eosinophilic, typical of many insect bite-induced dermatopathies. If ulcerated, lesions predispose to infection by *Habronema* spp. nematodes. Lesions of *Culicoides* hypersensitivity (see Immune-mediated dermatoses) and onchocerciasis may also occur on the ventrum, but these are diffuse, often extending from the axillae to the groin. Both *Culicoides* hypersensitivity and onchocerciasis are sporadic diseases whereas up to 80% of horses in a group may be affected with horn-fly bite dermatitis.

Bibliography

Barros AT. Dynamics of *Haematobia irritans irritans* (Diptera: Muscidae) infestation on Nelore cattle in the Pantanal, Brazil. Mem Inst Oswaldo Cruz 2001;96:445–450.

Perris EE. Parasitic dermatoses that cause pruritus in horses. Vet Clin N Am: Eq Pract 1995;11:14–15.

Mosquito-bite dermatitis

Mosquito bites in animals are common and the bite itself is of little consequence most of the time. Mosquitoes serve as *vectors* for a number of important diseases, including malaria in humans, canine and feline heartworm disease, equine viral encephalitis and equine infectious anemia, and rabbit myxomatosis. In **cats**, mosquito bites can induce a severe papular, crusting dermatitis characterized by dense eosinophilic infiltrates. Experimental studies in cats utilizing intradermal skin tests and Prausnitz–Kustner tests indicate that these lesions develop only in cats hypersensitive to mosquito bite antigens and are initiated by a type I hypersensitivity reaction. The disease is seasonal and often pruritic. Clinically, cats initially develop wheals progressing to erythematous papules and plaques that eventuate into crusted, ulcerated and sometimes hypopigmented lesions (Fig. 5.105). Sparsely haired regions of the body are most often affected such as the bridge of the nose, the pinnae, and footpad margins. The pinnae may develop symmetrical lesions of miliary dermatitis. The severity of lesions varies by individual, leading to scar formation in the more severe cases.

Histologic lesions include intraepidermal eosinophilic microabscessation and perivascular to diffuse interstitial infiltrates of eosinophils, mast cells, macrophages and lymphocytes. The epidermis is often spongiotic and acanthotic. Eosinophilic granulomas around focal areas of collagen degeneration, and perifollicular to intrafollicular eosinophilic infiltrates with furunculosis, may be present. Cats may have regional lymphadenopathy and peripheral eosinophilia. *Clinical differential diagnoses* include lesions of the eosinophilic granuloma complex, other cutaneous hypersensitivities such as atopy or food allergy, actinic dermatitis or squamous cell carcinoma, and pemphigus foliaceus. *Histologic differentials* include *Felid herpesvirus-1*-associated dermatitis, other cutaneous hypersensitivities mentioned above, and feline eosinophilic granulomas. Eosinophilic folliculitis and furunculosis are not usually seen in feline eosinophilic granulomas and are less prominent in food allergy than in mosquito bite hypersensitivity. Ballooning degeneration, viral inclusions, and marked necrosis are usually present in herpesvirus-induced lesions. Careful evaluation of histologic lesions and circumstantial evidence are essential keys to the diagnosis.

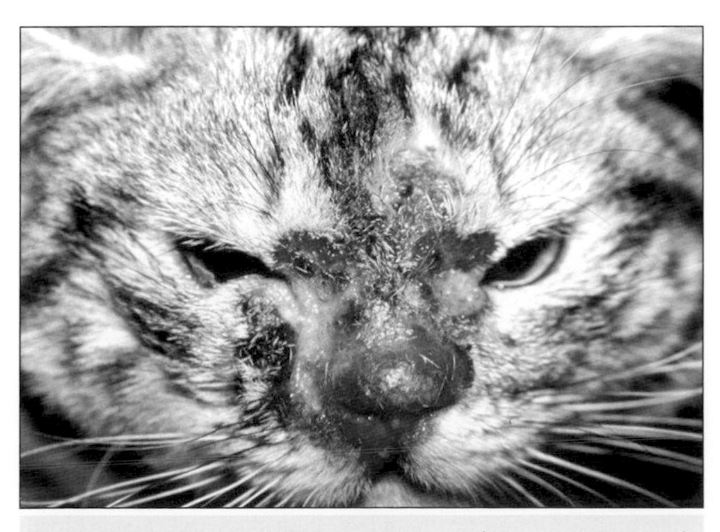

Figure 5.105 Mosquito-bite dermatitis in a cat. (Courtesy of B Dunstan.)

Bibliography

Nagata M, Ishida T. Cutaneous reactivity to mosquito bites and its antigens in cats. Vet Dermatol 1997;8:19–26.

Power HT, Ihrke PJ. Selected feline eosinophilic skin diseases Vet Clin N Am: Small Anim Pract 1995;25:838–840.

Lice

Lice are host specific, obligate parasites of the class Insecta. Two orders of lice are recognized. The Mallophaga are *biting lice,* which have mouth parts specially adapted for chewing the epithelial scales, feathers, and sebaceous secretions of birds and mammals. The Anoplura have piercing mouth parts and are the *blood-sucking lice* of mammals. Lice cannot live away from their hosts for more than a few days. Consequently, spread of infestation occurs mainly by direct contact among hosts. Pigs and humans are parasitized only by sucking lice, birds and cats are parasitized only by biting lice, and both types parasitize other domestic animals. Because various species of lice have adapted to different microenvironments within the host pelage, it is possible for an animal to carry several species at once.

Infestation with lice is called **pediculosis**. It tends to be a seasonal problem, being worse in winter. The signs associated with pediculosis are extremely variable. In most instances, lice do not pose a significant threat to the host. *Heavy infestations signal an underlying contributing condition such as poor sanitation, overcrowding, ill thrift, or poor nutrition.* Low infestations may be unaccompanied by clinical signs in carrier animals. *Most lesions result from skin irritation and resultant pruritus.* They include alopecia, papules, crusts, and damage to wool or hide caused by rubbing or biting. *Sucking lice may induce anemia,* which is occasionally fatal in heavily infested animals. Weight loss and decreased milk production are associated with the constant irritation seen in some lice infestations.

Lice are almost always host specific, but *Heterodoxus longitarsus*, normally parasitic on kangaroos, has become an important ectoparasite of Australian dogs. *Phthirus pubis*, the human crab louse, has been reported to infest dogs living with infested humans. Because of host specificity, it is advantageous to consider pediculosis of the different hosts in turn.

Louse infestation occurs in **cattle** more often than in other domestic species. *Haematopinus eurysternus*, the short-nosed louse; *H. quadripertusus*, the tail-switch louse; *H. tuberculatis*, the buffalo louse; *Linognathus vituli*, the long-nosed louse; and *Solenoptes capillatus* are sucking lice of cattle. *Damalinia bovis* is the one biting species. The various species have preferred habitats. *Damalinia bovis* tend to cluster about the poll, forehead, neck, back, and rump; *Linognathus* and *Solenoptes* prefer the head, neck, and dewlap. There may be antagonism between the species; in dual infestation with *D. bovis* and *L. vituli*, the former tends to occupy the dorsal half and the latter the ventral areas. Some lice are widely distributed, others tend to cluster in groups. Infestations are quite common, particularly in colder weather or seasons, but, unless heavy, are not particularly deleterious. Poorly fed, overcrowded, and unthrifty animals are more susceptible to heavy infestations. Conversely, heavy infestations may indicate underlying disease as debilitated or ill animals cease normal grooming activities. Lesions reflect pruritus. Heavy periorbital infestation of heifers by *Haematopinus quadripertusus* has caused keratoconjunctivitis and periorbital papillomatosis. Bovine pediculosis usually has little deleterious effect on weight gain and other production parameters. Economic consequences are due to deterioration of hide quality, damage to fences, and costs of treatment. The exception is *Hematopinus eurysternus* infestation, which may cause anemia and death in some uniquely susceptible cattle. *H. eurysternus* feed most often around the poll, neck, brisket, and tail but may become generalized.

The species of sucking lice affecting **sheep** include *Linognathus ovillus* (the face or blue louse), *L. africanus* (also called the blue louse) and *L. pedalis* (the foot louse). *L. ovillus* is not very pathogenic. *L. pedalis* characteristically infests the hairy skin on the legs. Infestations are frequently light and may be confined to one limb, as the lice form localized clusters. Rarely, heavy infestations spread to adjacent scrotal or abdominal skin, causing irritation and dermatitis secondary to self-trauma. While goat and sheep lice are considered host specific, there are reports of naturally occurring transmission of the goat louse *Damalinia caprae* to sheep and experimental transmission of *D. ovis* to goats.

Damalinia ovis, a biting louse, is a common and serious ectoparasite in sheep. Populations of *D. ovis*, on an individual or in a flock, can build up very quickly. The numbers of lice fluctuate with the season, increasing usually in late winter and early summer. The population declines in the summer probably because the lice, which are sensitive to heat and low humidity, cannot survive in the body fleece where temperatures at the tip of the staple may reach 48°C. There are also unexplained individual differences amongst sheep in their susceptibility but, in general, unthrifty sheep carry the heaviest infestation. The size of louse populations may be in part regulated by the sheep's immune response. The lice feed on loose skin scales and sebaceous secretion and there is a correlation between the degree of scurf and the size of the louse population. The highest concentration of lice occurs along the dorsal midline, chiefly over the withers, but the parasites range over the entire body. Eggs are attached to the wool fibers close to the body surface. The infestation has serious consequences because of the *marked pruritus* it induces. The cause of the pruritus is unknown but is thought to be more than simple mechanical irritation. Affected sheep rub, scratch and bite at the skin resulting in severe damage to the fleece. Focal crusting may be associated with some louse infestations. Economic loss is due to reduced fleece quality, cost of prevention, and mortality from secondary myiasis. There is, however, no evidence to support the claim that sheep louse infestation leads to unthriftiness.

In **goats**, the sucking louse, *Linognathus stenopsis*, is more pathogenic than the biting lice, *Damalinia caprae*, *D. limbata* and *Holokartikos crassipes*. The haircoat of Angora goats may be seriously damaged by the irritation induced by pediculosis.

Two species of lice occur on **horses**, namely *Haematopinus asini*, a sucking louse, and *Damalinia equi*, a biting louse. The populations of lice fluctuate considerably, being highest when the hair is long as in winter or in debilitated animals which have not shed their hair. In warm weather, the populations decline but some lice persist in the long hair of the mane and tail. Both species of louse induce skin irritation. The lesions of pediculosis, rough coat, variable alopecia and self-excoriation, result from the animal rubbing or biting at the irritated areas.

One species, *Haematopinus suis*, a sucking louse is parasitic on **pigs**. Preferential sites include the ears and skin folds of the neck, axillae and inguinal areas. Infestations are often severe but, with the exception of nursing piglets, anemia is not severe. In white-skinned animals, numerous small puncta may be seen, especially in scalded carcasses. Constant irritation from lice also interferes with growth rate and efficiency of food conversion. The lice are vectors for *Swinepox virus*, *African swine fever virus*, and *Eperythrozoon suis*.

Linognathus setosus is a sucking louse and *Trichodectes canis* and *Heterodoxus spiniger* are biting lice of **dogs**. *Trichodectes canis* may serve as an intermediate host for the tapeworm, *Dipylidium caninum*. Pediculosis is a rare disease in pet dogs. Breeds with moderately long, fine hair may provide a more favorable environment for lice, and the disease is more prevalent in the cooler winter months. The biting lice cause pruritus, which may be associated with mild to moderately severe dermatitis with papules and crusts or with patchy alopecia. Infestation in the absence of pruritus may be an incidental finding.

Only one species, the biting louse, *Felicola subrostratus*, occurs on **cats**. Infestation may be an incidental finding or it may be associated with mild pruritus in the absence of lesions. Occasionally there is generalized scaling (seborrhea sicca) or multifocal or generalized papular, crusting dermatitis.

Bibliography

James PJ. Do sheep regulate the size of their mallophagan louse populations? Int J Parasitol 1999;29:869–875.

Sinclair AN, et al. Feeding of the chewing louse *Damalinia ovis* (Schrank) (Phthiraptera: Trichodectidae) on sheep. Vet Parasitol 1989;30:233–251.

Yeruham I, et al. Keratoconjunctivitis and periorbital papillomatosis associated with heavy periorbital infestation by the tail louse *Haematopinus quadripertusus* in heifers. J Vet Med B Infect Dis Vet Public Health 2001;48:133–136.

Fleas

Fleas are ubiquitous and obligate parasites. They are intermittent parasites and their survival depends upon temporary episodes of feeding and a habitat where the host is periodically available. Fleas primarily parasitize hosts that return on a regular basis to a nest, burrow, bedding, or lair. Hence, animals such as ungulates rarely have fleas and carnivores, rabbits, rodents, and bats often do. Most fleas can parasitize a range of hosts. An exception to this general rule, is the more recent finding that cat fleas spend more of their lifetime on the cat than fleas infesting other species. Fleas are chiefly a problem in cats, dogs, pigs, and humans. Flea bites damage the host from the irritation, pruritus, blood loss, and possible transmission of infectious agents. *Ctenocephalides felis*, the cat flea, *Ctenocephalides canis*, the dog flea, and *Pulex irritans*, the human flea, are vectors for the dog tapeworm, *Dipylidium caninum*. Fleas are also vectors of tularemia, bubonic plague, and rabbit myxomatosis. Flea saliva is injected into the host as the flea feeds leading to hypersensitivity reactions in some animals.

Fleas are the most common ectoparasites of **cats** and **dogs**. The most important species are *Ctenocephalides felis*, the cat flea, and *Ctenocephalides canis*, the dog flea. However, infestations also occur with *Pulex irritans* (human flea), *Leptopsylla segnis* (rat flea), *Echidnophaga gallinacea* (chicken stick-tight flea), *Spilopsyllus cuniculi* (European rabbit flea), and *Ceratophyllus* spp. (bird and hedgehog fleas). *C. felis* is the most common flea found on both dogs and cats in North America and northern Europe.

The clinical manifestations of flea infestation are highly variable. Some animals, despite heavy infestations, remain asymptomatic carriers. Some animals may develop **flea bite dermatitis**, which is a reaction to the many irritant substances in the flea's saliva, but the vast majority of animals that develop lesions do so because of hypersensitivity reactions to allergenic components of the flea saliva. **Flea allergy dermatitis** is an extremely common and very important disease of the dog and cat; it is discussed in detail under Immune-mediated dermatoses. Finally the blood-sucking activities of fleas may induce blood-loss, iron deficiency anemia in heavily infested animals, particularly in kittens, puppies or debilitated adults.

Lesions affecting the pinna of cats may be caused by *Spilopsyllus cuniculi*, the flea of rabbits and hares. Typically, hunting cats acquire the infestation from their prey. Macroscopic lesions are crusted, alopecic patches on both aspects of the pinna. Histologically, eosinophils are prominent in the dermal inflammatory cell infiltrate.

The two fleas most commonly associated with **swine** are the human flea (*P. irritans*) and the chicken stick-tight flea (*E. gallinacea*). Infestation with *C. felis* and *C. canis* have also been reported. In Africa, *Tunga penetrans*, the chigoe flea, has been associated with swine infestations although it is chiefly a human parasite. The female flea burrows into the skin causing ulcerative lesions. The skin around the coronary band, on the scrotum and snout are favored sites. Infestations of the teat canal have been associated with agalactia in sows. Fleas may act as vectors for *Swinepox virus*. Heavy infestations with *Ctenocephalides* spp. in Africa lead to anemia, reduced weight gain and even death in **sheep** and **goats**, particularly in the young. Fleas may also trigger allergic dermatitis in sheep. *C. felis* has been rarely reported in **cattle**. Heavy infestation with C. *felis* was reported to cause mortality in calves, lambs and kids in Israel. Rarely, **horses** may become infested with *Echidnophaga gallinacea* or *Tunga penetrans*. Papules, crusts, pruritus, and alopecia may develop.

Bibliography

Fagbemi BO. Effect of *Ctenocephalides felis strongylus* infestation on the performance of West African dwarf sheep and goats. Vet Q 1982;4:92–95.

Logas DB. The cat, the flea, and pesticides. Vet Clinics N Am 1995;25:801–811.

Studdert VP, Arundel JH. Dermatitis of the pinnae of cats in Australia associated with the European rabbit flea (*Spilopsyllus cuniculi*). Vet Rec 1988;123:624–625.

Visser M, et al. Species of flea (siphonaptera) infesting pets and hedgehogs in Germany. J Vet Med B Infect Dis Vet Public Health 2001;48:197–202.

Yeruham L, et al. Mortality in calves, lambs and kids caused by severe infestation with the cat flea *Ctenocephalides felis* (Bouché, 1835) in Israel. Vet Parasitol 1989;30:351–356.

Yeruham I, et al. Seasonal allergic dermatitis in sheep associated with *Ctenocephalides* and *Culicoides* bites. Vet Dermatol 2004;15:377–380.

Mites

Sarcoptic mange

Sarcoptes scabiei (Acarina: Sarcoptidae) is responsible for scabies in man and sarcoptic mange in domestic animals worldwide. Scabies has also been reported to cause severe disease in a number of wildlife species. *It is a common ectoparasite in swine*. The disease occurs in *cattle* and goats but is not as important as psoroptic mange. The disease is rare in horses and sheep. Ovine sarcoptic mange has not been reported in North America. Sarcoptic mange is *common in the dog* and may be underdiagnosed. It occurs rarely in the cat. So-called feline scabies is caused by *Notoedres*. The economic importance of sarcoptic mange in food-producing animals is due to depressed growth rate and decreased rates of food conversion. Production studies in experimentally infected pigs and sheep demonstrating the effect of therapy, support the contention that *the disease is of economic significance*. Sarcoptic mange is a notifiable disease in many countries.

Through host-adaptation, *S. scabiei* has become divided into morphologically indistinguishable varieties, which rarely cross infect. Each variety is named for its host; thus *S. scabiei* var *equi* is usually confined to the horse but may live temporarily on cattle or humans. People are quite readily parasitized by most of the animal-adapted varieties. However, in most cross-infestations, the parasites remain on the skin surface and do not complete their life cycle.

In the normal host, the parasite completes it life cycle in tunnels burrowed into and under the stratum corneum. After mating in a "molting pocket" close to the surface, the female burrows through the stratum corneum to feed on cells of the stratum granulosum and stratum spinosum. Cutting mouthparts and tarsal claws on the legs of the mite achieve the excavation. In swine, this phase of infestation takes ~3 weeks. Epidermal cell damage induces proliferative changes in the surrounding keratinocytes so that the surface openings of the tunnels become sealed with thick parakeratotic scale-crust. In swine this process takes a further 3–4 weeks. After 7 weeks of infestation, the crust falls off and the mites vacate the tunnels. Approximately 40–50 ova are laid in the burrows at a rate of 1–3 per day. They develop through the larval and nymphal stages in the same tunnel or in new ones, to reach maturity in 10–15 days depending on the host species. In general, both parasites and ova have poor viability in the external environment, however, low temperature and high humidity may allow some mites and nymphs to persist in the environment up to 21 days. The disease, which is *highly contagious*, is transmitted largely by direct contact, but may occur following indirect contact with contaminated objects such as bedding.

The *pathogenesis* of lesions in *S. scabiei* infestation is due to *direct damage* inflicted by the parasite mechanically, by the *irritant effects* of its secretions and excreta, and by an *allergic reaction* developed against components of the mite or one or more of the extracellular products of the parasite. Evidence for an allergic pathogenesis in animals comes chiefly from experimental infestations of swine. Initial lesions in pigs are due to parasite invasion and are localized and non-pruritic. After 7–11 weeks, there is generalized urticarial eruption associated with extreme pruritus. This eruption coincides with the development of immediate and delayed hypersensitivity reactions and peripheral eosinophilia. The delayed hypersensitivity response is dependent on antigen dose, whereas the immediate hypersensitivity response is independent of the degree of antigen exposure. Lesions regress between 12–18 weeks after the initial infestation.

The variability of the clinical manifestations of sarcoptic mange probably reflects individual variations in the duration and intensity of the hypersensitivity reaction and in the related capacity of the host to limit parasitic multiplication. Asymptomatic carriers exist. Most *S. scabiei*-related diseases are caused chiefly by the allergic reaction, and the lesions are the result of self-trauma induced by severe pruritus. However, animals with a weak hypersensitivity reaction may exhibit severe crusting dermatitis characterized by the presence of large numbers of mites. This type of disease is typically seen in poorly nourished animals or animals debilitated by coexisting disease. An

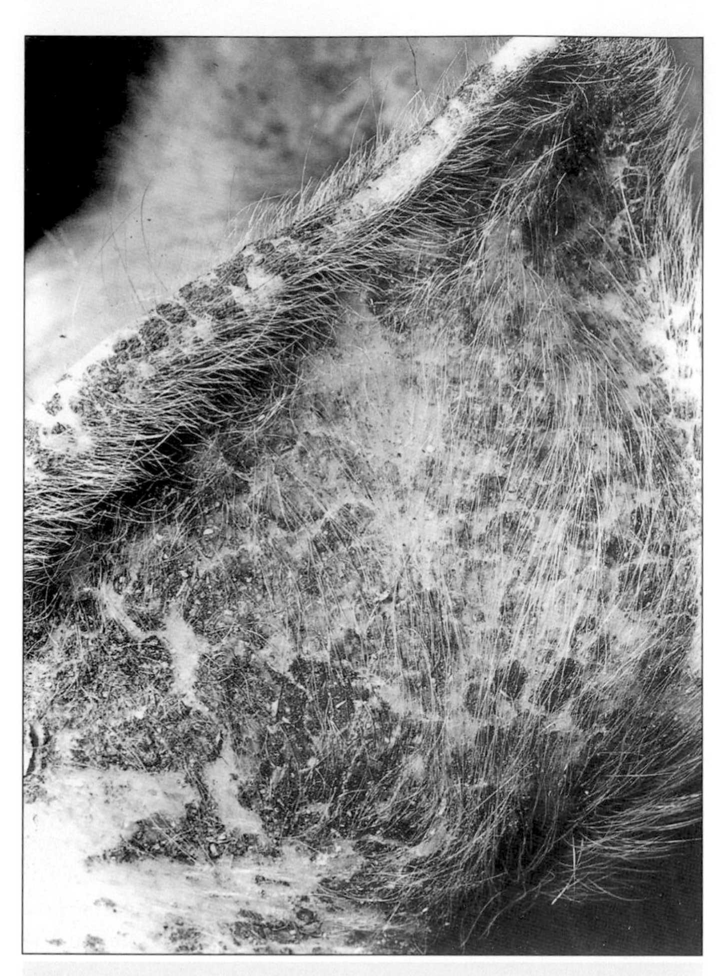

Figure 5.106 Sarcoptic mange in a pig.

example is the chronic form of scabies in dogs associated with long-term corticosteroid therapy. This has been referred to as *Norwegian-type scabies*, following the human nomenclature for severe scabies in immunosuppressed people. Diminished levels of hypersensitivity are correlated also with the development of chronic infestations in swine, known as *hyperkeratotic mange*. This manifestation of mange is sporadic and chiefly affects breeding adults.

The primary parasite-related lesions of sarcoptic mange are erythematous macules or papules, which develop a local scale-crust in reaction to the burrowing mites. The thickness of the overlying scale-crust is proportional to the number of tunnels beneath. In poorly nourished or immunosuppressed animals, which develop massive mite infestations, the lesions are characterized by alopecia, marked lichenification, accumulation of thick gray scale-crust and fissuring. Excoriations, hemorrhagic crusts and patchy alopecia follow the early lesions of erythematous papules. Chronic hypersensitivity lesions include marked alopecia, scaling and lichenification.

The distribution of the lesions is characteristic in the various species. In **pigs**, the mites have a predilection for the *inner surface of the pinna* where they cause primary lesions (Fig. 5.106). The papular lesions associated with the allergic reactions are located chiefly on the rump, flank and abdomen, and the secondary changes due to chronic self trauma follow a similar pattern. In the chronic hyperkeratotic form of the disease, heavily crusted lesions develop over the whole body but are most severe on the head, neck, and legs. In **dogs**, the preferred sites are the lateral elbows, hocks, ventral thorax, and lateral margin of the pinna. There may be an associated peripheral lymphadenopathy. The lesions may become generalized in untreated dogs or dogs inappropriately treated with corticosteroids. In **cattle**, the lesions chiefly affect the neck, head and sacral areas but may become generalized. The disease in **goats** also has a predilection for the head but may involve the whole body. In **sheep**, only the haired areas develop lesions, particularly the lips, nostrils, external surface of the pinna and occasionally the legs. Generalized lesions occur in the more hairy desert sheep of the Sudan. Lesions in the **horse** begin on the head and neck and may extend to involve most of the body, but seldom the legs or mane.

Histologically the lesions vary with the balance between allergic reaction and parasitic infestation and chronicity. *Definitive diagnosis requires demonstration of the parasite.* Rarely, sections of mites or ova may be present within the epidermis or surface crusts. Lesions consist of a mild to severely acanthotic epidermis with variable orthokeratosis to patchy parakeratosis. In fully developed lesions, there is marked spongiosis, mixed leukocytic exocytosis, serocellular crusts, and possibly intraepidermal eosinophilic pustules. Vasodilation, endothelial swelling, and edema may also be present. Immunosuppressed animals with large numbers of adult mites in epidermal burrows often have a markedly parakeratotic stratum corneum. Dermal lesions consist of a mild-to-moderate superficial to mid-level perivascular infiltrate with a variable ratio of lymphohistiocytic cells and eosinophils. The chronic allergic lesions reflect continued trauma with dermal fibrosis, epidermal hyperplasia with prominent rete ridge formation, hyperpigmentation and a predominantly mononuclear cell perivascular infiltrate.

Diagnosis of the typical allergic form of the disease depends chiefly on the clinical signs of extreme pruritus and the nature and distribution of the cutaneous lesions. Mites are characteristically difficult to demonstrate, either in skin scrapings or in microscopic section. Approximately two-thirds of affected dogs fail to yield parasites even when multiple scrapings are performed. Mites are more commonly recovered from puppies than adult dogs. *The microscopic lesions are not diagnostic, being indistinguishable from other allergic dermatoses.* The most useful diagnostic procedure is response to appropriate therapy. In the chronic form of sarcoptic mange associated with poorly developed hypersensitivity reactions, mites are plentiful in scrapings and in tissue section. *Clinical differential diagnoses* include other causes of pruritic dermatitis such as atopy, contact, food, or flea-bite hypersensitivity, infestation by other parasites, *Malassezia* dermatitis, or superficial pyoderma.

Bibliography

Arlian LG. Biology, host relations, and epidemiology of *Sarcoptes scabiei*. Annu Rev Entomol 1989;34:139–161.

Davis DP, Moon RD. Dynamics of swine mange: A critical review of the literature. J Med Entomol 1990;27:727–737.

Elbers AR, et al. Production performance and pruritic behaviour of pigs naturally infected by *Sarcoptes scabiei var. suis* in a contact transmission experiment. Vet Q 2000;22:145–149.

Fthenakis GC, et al. Effects of sarcoptic mange on the reproductive performance of ewes and transmission of *Sarcoptes scabiei* to newborn lambs. Vet Parasitol 2001;95:63–71.

Hollanders W, Vercruysse J. Sarcoptic mite hypersensitivity: A cause of dermatitis in fattening pigs at slaughter. Vet Rec 1990;126:308–310.

Jackson PGG, et al. Sarcoptic mange in goats. Vet Rec 1983;112:330.

Kershaw A. *Sarcoptes scabiei* infestation in a cat. Vet Rec 1989;124:537–538.
Little SE, et al. Responses of red foxes to first and second infection with *Sarcoptes scabiei*. J Wildl Dis 1998;34:600–611.
Martineau G, et al. Pathophysiology of sarcoptic mange in swine – Part I and II. Compend Contin Educ Pract Vet 1987;9:F51–F57, F93–F97.
Morris DO, Dunstan RW. A histomorphological study of sarcoptic acariasis in the dog: 19 cases. J Am Anim Hosp Assoc 1996;32:119–124.
Morsy GH, et al. Scanning electron microscopy of sarcoptic mange lesions in swine. Vet Parasitol 1989;31:281–288.
Scott DW, et al., eds. Parasitic skin diseases. In: Small Animal Dermatology. 5th ed. Philadelphia, PA: WB Saunders, 1995:434–443.

Notoedric mange

Notoedres cati (Acarina: Sarcoptidae) is the cause of *feline scabies* and is also a parasite of the rabbit, and occasionally foxes, dogs, and humans. *The disease in cats is uncommon to rare,* although there are some endemic areas of higher prevalence. The mite has a life cycle similar to that of *S. scabiei*. The infestation is *highly contagious*, with transmission chiefly by direct contact. The major clinical sign is *pruritus*. The lesions in cats commence on the head and ears, particularly on the margin of the pinna but may extend to the neck, paw or become generalized. Lesions include partial alopecia, thickening and wrinkling of the skin and, in chronic cases, the formation of tightly adherent yellow-gray crusts (Fig. 5.107A). There may be accompanying regional lymphadenopathy. Lesions in dogs are indistinguishable from sarcoptic mange. Histologically, the lesion is a hyperplastic, eosinophil-rich, superficial perivascular dermatitis with focal parakeratosis. *The diagnosis is based on history, clinical signs and demonstration of typical mites in section* (Fig. 5.107B) *or skin scrapings*. Mites are readily found in skin scrapings and histologic sections from cats.

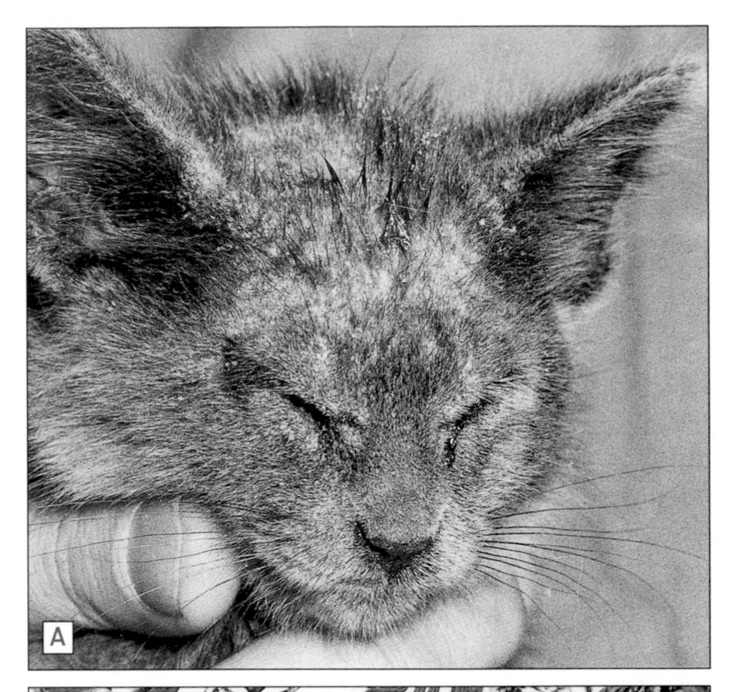

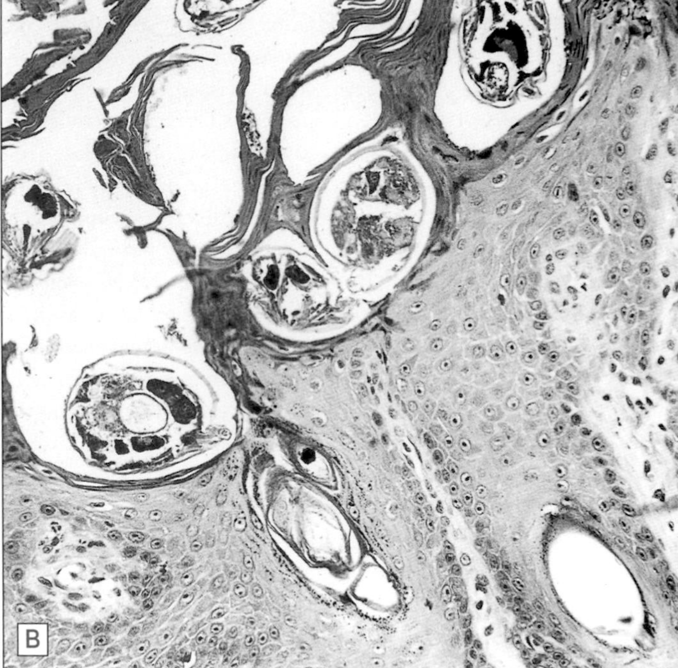

Figure 5.107 Notoedric mange in a cat. **A.** Gross photo **B.** Mites embedded in the surface keratin of the hyperplastic epidermis.

Bibliography

Scott DW, et al., eds. Parasitic skin diseases. In: Small Animal Dermatology. 5th ed. Philadelphia, PA: WB Saunders, 1995:434–443.

Psoroptic mange

The psoroptic mites (Acarina: Psoroptidae) infest *sheep, cattle, horses, rabbits, and goats* as well as other nondomestic species. Human beings are not susceptible. There are actually fewer species of ***Psoroptes* mites** than originally thought, as mites from one host can often infect another host, and morphologic distinctions overlap. Based on critical literature review and molecular genetic analyses, the *Psoroptes* mites are conspecific, and, by rule of priority, belong to the one genus *P. equi* (Hering, 1838). Traditionally, *Psoroptes ovis* infests sheep, cattle and horses; *P. natalensis* infects cattle in South Africa, South America, and Europe; and *P. cuniculi* affects the ears of several species including rabbit, horse, donkey, goat and sheep.

Psoroptic mange is a serious disease in cattle and sheep and is a reportable disease in several countries. Bovine psoroptic mange showed a recrudescence in North America during the 1970s and early 1980s but has been brought under control by the effective use of ivermectin. Ovine psoroptic mange has been eradicated from many countries including Australia and New Zealand. The *economic importance* in sheep and cattle results from a marked decrease in weight gain, reduced milk production, reduced fleece weight and quality, occasional mortality and costs related to prevention and eradication campaigns.

Psoroptic mites do not burrow into the outer epidermis, as do the sarcoptic mites, but instead complete their life cycle on the skin surface. Lipids from the stratum corneum provide a major source of nutrients in the early stages of infestation, probably supplemented by serous and hemorrhagic inflammatory exudates in the later stages.

Psoroptic mange is characterized by *intensely pruritic dermatitis*. The pathogenicity of the mite has been attributed to its local irritant effect on the epidermis, but this does not readily explain the marked loss of condition induced by *Psoroptes* infestation in some species, particularly cattle. The detrimental systemic effects may derive directly or indirectly from a *chronic hypersensitivity reaction* rather than from local dermatitis. The histologic lesions, in which the predominant inflammatory cells in the superficial dermis are eosinophils, mast cells, and lymphocytes, are consistent with an *allergic pathogenesis*. Constant pruritus resulting from allergy markedly reduces feed intake, and secondary bacterial infection or myiasis may further contribute to loss of condition. There is little evidence to support the hypothesis that the mites inoculate a toxic compound along with their saliva.

Histologically, the lesions are similar in all species. The pattern of inflammation is superficial perivascular dermatitis with predominantly spongiotic, exudative or hyperplastic reactions depending on chronicity. The eosinophil is the most numerous of the infiltrating leukocytes, followed by lymphocytes, other mononuclear cells and mast cells. Dermal edema is usually marked. Mites are present both on top of and under the surface scale-crust. Sebaceous gland hyperplasia has been described in lesions in sheep and cattle.

Psoroptic mange in **sheep**, also known as "*sheep scab*," may occur as a latent infection in which mites persist in the ears, infraorbital fossae, inguinal and perineal folds and at the base of the horns. In rams, mites may be found on the scrotum or prepuce in small, dry lesions. Latency occurs in the summer months when the fleece microclimate is less favorable to parasite proliferation. In autumn and winter or with debilitation of the host, the parasitic population explodes and lesions are induced. The withers and sides are particularly affected. The initial lesions are papules ~0.5 cm in diameter covered with a yellow serous crust, which may mat the fleece. The individual lesions expand at the periphery and may coalesce to become diffuse over most of the body surface. The main damage to the fleece is caused by self-trauma induced by the severe pruritus. Affected sheep scratch, kick, rub and tear out the fleece with their teeth.

In **cattle**, psoroptic mange is sometimes referred to as "*cattle scabies*." Lesions also diminish in the summer months as a result of decreasing mite populations, attributable to increased self-grooming. Previous exposure to mites, while not conferring solid resistance to reinfection, also limits the mite population, chiefly by reducing the rate of oviposition in the females. Lesions in reinfested cattle, while occurring earlier, progress more slowly, reflecting the decreased mite population. Lesions in naturally affected cattle usually commence about the poll, withers or at the base of the tail (Fig. 5.108) and chiefly result from persistent licking, rubbing and scratching induced by pruritus. Infested areas are fairly well defined as areas of alopecia. Alopecic areas become lichenified and covered by dry gray crusts and scales. Severely affected calves may develop mild anemia, lymphopenia and marked neutropenia.

In **goats**, *P. cuniculi* is known as the *"ear canker" mite* because of its predilection for the external auditory meatus. Mite infestation induces head shaking and occasionally crusted lesions on the inner surface, and alopecia on the outer surface of the pinna. In debilitated or stressed animals, thick brown-yellow, dry scale-crust accumulates on the inner aspect of the pinna and, rarely, spreads to involve the poll, body and the legs. Concurrent *Mycoplasma* and *P. cuniculi* infections have been described in the ears of goats; however, *Mycoplasma* may be cultured from the ears of clinically normal animals, placing some doubt on the significance of the finding.

In **horses**, *P. cuniculi* is found quite frequently in the ear. Infestations have been associated with "head shakers" in the United Kingdom and Australia, but are often subclinical. *Psoroptes ovis* infestations are rare; lesions are crusted papules with alopecia and the preferred sites are at the base of the mane, forelock and tail.

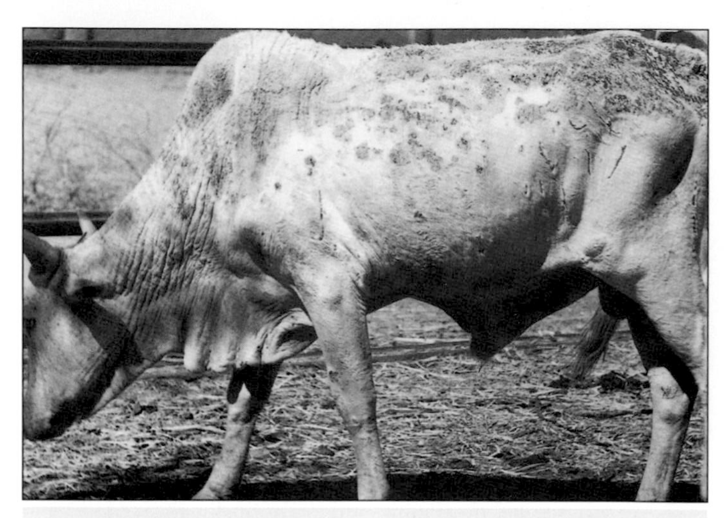

Figure 5.108 Psoroptic mange in a cow. (Courtesy of FI Awad.)

Bibliography

Abu-Samra MT, et al. Five cases of psoroptic mange in the domestic donkey (*Equus asinus asinus*) and treatment with ivermectin. Eq Vet J 1987;19:143–144.

Cook RW. Ear mites (*Raillieta manfredi* and *Psoroptes cuniculi*) in goats in New South Wales. Aust Vet J 1981;57:72–75.

Corke MJ, Broom DM. The behaviour of sheep with sheep scab, *Psoroptes ovis* infestation. Vet Parasitol 1999;83:291–300.

Fourie LJ, et al. The growth of sheep scab lesions in relation to sheep breed and time of the year. Exp Appl Acarol 2002;27:277–281.

Losson B, et al. Haematological and immunological response of unrestrained cattle to *Psoroptes ovis*, the sheep scab mite. Res Vet Sci 1988;44:197–201.

Perris EE., Parasitic dermatoses that cause pruritus in horses. Vet Clin North Am: Eq Pract 1995;11:11–28.

Ramey RR, et al. Phylogeny and host specificity of psoroptic mange mites (Acarina: Psoroptidae) as indicated by ITS sequence data. J Med Entomol 2000;37:791–796.

Sinclair AN, Filan SJ. Lipid ingestion from sheep epidermis by *Psoroptes ovis* (Acari: Psoroptidae). Vet Parasitol 1989;31:149–164.

Stromberg PC, Guillot FS. Pathogenesis of psoroptic scabies in Hereford heifer calves. Am J Vet Res 1989;50:594–601.

Wilson GI, et al. Infectivity of scabies mites, *Psoroptes ovis* (Acarina: Psoroptidae), to sheep in naturally contaminated enclosures. Res Vet Sci 1977;22:292–297.

Zahler M, et al. Species of the genus *Psoroptes* (Acari: Psoroptidae): a taxonomic consideration. Exp Appl Acarol 2000;24:213–225.

Chorioptic mange

Chorioptic mange, caused by ***Chorioptes bovis*** *(Acarina: Psoroptidae), affects horses, cattle, sheep, and goats. Not host specific, C. bovis is an obligate parasite that lives on the surface of the skin.* The mite populations tend to fluctuate considerably as a result of host and environmental factors. Inapparent infections allow persistence in the population. Clinically affected animals are pruritic and have papular, crusted, scaly, alopecic and/or lichenified lesions depending upon the duration of the disease and the degree of self-trauma inflicted.

The disease in **cattle** predominantly affects *housed dairy cows* and is most prevalent in winter. Subclinical infections are probably quite common. The major clinical sign is *pruritus*, but this is not as severe as in sarcoptic or psoroptic mange. Chorioptic mange is, in general, a less serious condition than psoroptic mange in cattle, although a syndrome of highly irritant coronitis was associated with falling milk production. The typical distribution of lesions is perineum, tail, scrotum, udder, and caudal areas of thigh, hindlimbs and rump. Lesions are predominantly alopecia, erythema, lichenification, and wrinkling of the skin.

The disease in **horses** is uncommon. As indicated by the colloquial name "leg mange," lesions occur preferentially on the lower limb around the fetlock but may extend proximally to the thigh and ventral abdomen. Draft horses, with thick-feathered fetlocks are affected more often. The lesions are most severe in winter, as in cattle.

In **goats**, lesions originally were described as commencing on the neck and spreading to the back, base of tail, and lateral body. Another pattern, in which lesions affect the coronet, pasterns, and lower limbs, appears to be more typical. The face, udder, and scrotum also may be affected.

In **sheep**, *C. bovis* mites prefer the distal extremities, particularly the pastern and interdigital skin of the hind limbs. The scrotum may be affected and the resultant scrotal dermatitis may lead to temporary infertility. Chorioptic mange has been eradicated from the sheep population in the United States. It is a reportable disease in some countries.

Bibliography

Cremers HJ. The incidence of *Chorioptes bovis* (Acarina: Psoroptidae) on the feet of horses, sheep, and goats in the Netherlands. Vet Q 1985;7:283–289.

Heath ACG. The scrotal mange mite, *Chorioptes bovis* (Hering 1845) on sheep: seasonality, pathogenicity and intraflock transfer. N Z Vet J 1978;26:299–300, 309–310.

Sargison ND, et al. Chorioptic mange in British Suffolk rams. Vet Rec 2000;147:135–136.

Otodectic mange

Otodectes cynotis (Acarina: Psoroptidae) is an obligate parasite of the external skin surface of *dogs and cats*. While the mite may be found at several body sites, its preferred habitat is the *external ear canal*. The major lesion is thus *otitis externa* (see Vol. 1, Eye and ear). Focal, erythematous, alopecic, or excoriated lesions occur occasionally on the face, feet, neck, or tailhead. Self-trauma and head shaking can lead to aural hematomas. The mites are contagious, particularly in young animals and can live off the host for extended periods of time. *Diagnosis is by direct visualization*; however, mites may be difficult to demonstrate in some cases.

Cheyletiellosis

Members of the genus ***Cheyletiella*** (Acarina: Cheyletidae) affect *dogs, cats, rabbits, wild animal species, and, incidentally, humans*. There are three species involved: *C. parasitivorax* is chiefly a parasite of rabbits although formerly considered as a canine pathogen; C. *yasguri* is the major canine cheyletiellid; and, the species most commonly associated with feline infestation is *C. blakei*. Host specificity is weak and cross infestations are not uncommon. The mites are obligate parasites, completing their life cycle on the skin surface in ~35 days. The infestation is transmitted by direct contact, frequently from a carrier female to her litter. The mites originally were thought to survive for only 1–2 days away from the host, but more recent observations suggest longer survival may permit indirect transmission.

The pathogenicity of cheyletiellid infestation is controversial. The presence of the mite on naive hosts usually, but not always, induces hyperkeratosis, which may or may not be associated with pruritus. Adults, possibly because of acquired immunity, usually have asymptomatic infestations.

The gross lesions in both the dog and cat reflect the mite's *predilection for the dorsal midline*. Lesions often commence over the caudal back and progress cranially but may become generalized. The typical lesion is a moderate to marked exfoliation of small, dry, white scales (seborrhea sicca). The mites crawl in "pseudotunnels" in the loose keratin debris and their movement has produced the colloquial name "*walking dandruff*" for cheyletiellosis. Cats may develop, in addition, focal, multifocal or generalized erythematous papules or crusted lesions. Occasionally animals show pruritus in the absence of scaling. *Diagnosis depends upon demonstration of the mites* via skin scraping, acetate tape, vacuum cleaning, or brush techniques. Biopsy, which shows a spongiotic hyperplastic superficial perivascular dermatitis with variable numbers of eosinophils, is nondiagnostic since mites are usually not demonstrable. *Clinical differentials* should include other pruritic dermatoses and idiopathic or primary seborrhea. Humans in contact with affected animals often develop a pruritic maculopapular rash on the arms and trunk. As the mites do not complete their life cycle on human skin, these lesions regress once the animal is treated.

Bibliography

Paradis M, et al. Efficacy of ivermectin against *Cheyletiella blakei* infection in cats. J Am Anim Hosp 1990;26:125–128.

Saevik BK, et al. *Cheyletiella* infestation in the dog: observations on diagnostic methods and clinical signs. J Small Anim Pract 2004;45:495–500.

Sotiraki ST. Factors affecting the frequency of ear canal and face infestation by *Otodectes cynotis* in the cat. Vet Parasitol 2001;96:309–315.

Wagner R, Stallmeister N. *Cheyletiella* dermatitis in humans, dogs and cats. Br J Dermatol 2000;143:1110–1112.

Psorergatic mange

Psorergates ovis (Acarina: Cheyletidae) is a parasite of the integument of *sheep*. The disease occurs in Australia, New Zealand, South Africa, and South America. It is thought to have been eradicated from the USA and has not been reported in Europe. The mite, which is much smaller than sarcoptid mites, is an *obligate parasite and goes through its life cycle on the skin surface in the loose keratin debris*. The mite does not penetrate deeper than the stratum corneum. Infestations occur predominantly *on the dorsum*. Seasonal influences greatly affect mite populations, with lowest numbers occurring in the summer and highest in the spring.

Mite infestations induce *pruritus*; the pathogenesis of which is not known, although hypersensitivity reactions have been postulated. Lesions result from the sheep biting and pulling at the fleece. Fleece damage is more severe in the fine-wooled Merino than in the coarse-wooled breeds. The lesions occur on the flanks, thighs and lateral body wall, and comprise bleached, twisted tufts which give the fleece a ragged, tasselled appearance.

A mite named *P. bos* has been isolated from nonpruritic, scaling and alopecic lesions in cattle in the USA, Canada, Australia, New Zealand, and South America.

Bibliography

Johnson PW. The effect of host nutrition on itch mite, *Psorergates ovis*, populations and fleece derangement in sheep. Med Vet Entomol 1996;10:121–128.

Oberem PT, Malan FS. A new cause of cattle mange in South Africa: *Psorergates bos* Johnston. J S Afr Vet Assoc 1984;55:121–122.

Sinclair A. The epidermal location and possible feeding site of *Psorergates ovis*, the sheep itch mite. Aust Vet J 1990;67:59–62.

Demodectic mange

Demodex mites *(Acarina: Demodicidae) are normal inhabitants of the hair follicles and sebaceous glands in most species of domestic animals and in humans*. The cat also hosts a species of *Demodex*, *Demodex felis*, that lives in the superficial stratum corneum rather than in the follicles. The mites found in the different hosts are regarded as separate species, although they are similar morphologically. The mites are generally named for the host species, as in *D. canis* of dogs and *D. bovis* of cattle. *D. phylloides* of swine, *D. ghanensis* of cattle, *D. caballi* of horses and *D. aries* of sheep are exceptions in the nomenclature. A short form of Demodex species mite is also reported in dogs. It has been considered unusual for an animal to host more than one species of *Demodex*, but synhospitality may in fact be the rule rather than the exception.

Demodex spp. are *obligate parasites*, completing their life cycle in the hair follicle or its adnexae. They are rapidly killed by desiccation on the surface of the skin, but mites move from follicle to follicle and it is probably at this time that transmission to another host takes place. Transmission usually occurs by direct contact from the dam to her offspring during nursing in the neonatal period.

Demodex mites are part of the normal fauna of the skin in most, if not all, mammalian species. This implies that small numbers of mites exist in harmony with the host, and it is only when the equilibrium between the host and parasite is altered in favor of the mite that excessive proliferation occurs and lesions of demodectic mange are produced. The most severe expression of demodectic mange is seen in the dog as *generalized dermatitis* (Fig. 5.109A), which is, on occasion, fatal. Multiple lesions occur commonly in cattle, less commonly in pigs and goats, but with no systemic consequences. The demodectic mites of sheep rarely assume pathogenicity.

Demodicosis is one of the most common skin disorders of **dogs** *in North America*. In active infections, mites are first observed on skin scraping from the muzzles or feet of newly infected animals. Lesions may remain localized and self-limiting or become generalized. Generalized demodicosis is more prevalent in particular breeds of purebred dogs and often affects successive litters of certain clinically normal bitches or sires. *It has been postulated that puppies genetically predisposed to develop demodectic mange have a form of cell-mediated immune dysfunction that alters the body's recognition and reaction to the mites allowing massive proliferation of the mite population*. Immunophenotypic and histopathologic studies in the dog indicate active lesions of demodicosis produce *mural lymphocytic folliculitis with infiltration of the follicular wall by primarily CD3+ and CD8+ T lymphocytes*. The mural folliculitis is often associated with apoptosis or degeneration of keratinocytes and perifollicular pigmentary incontinence consistent with a lichenoid tissue reaction similar to epidermal lesions of lupus erythematosus or graft vs. host disease. Current research suggests lymphocyte-mediated follicular wall injury may be directed against keratinocytes expressing either altered self-antigens or *Demodex* antigens. It is not known whether or not the presence of cytotoxic T lymphocytes indicates an appropriate host reaction to eliminate the parasite or if it represents an inappropriate and self-damaging host response. *The disease itself, in its complicated form, appears to induce a secondary immunodeficiency state*, especially in the presence of *S. intermedius*. Dogs with chronic generalized pustular demodicosis show reduced cell-mediated immune responsiveness as measured by depressed lymphocyte blastogenesis reactivity. Evidence of humoral immunosuppressive factors also exists in dogs with generalized demodicosis. It is not yet clear whether this change is attributable to the secondary bacterial infection or to the mite infestation itself. A dog exhibiting generalized demodicosis at the time of rabies vaccination later developed rabies after exposure to a rabid skunk. This dog also failed to receive the recommended rabies vaccine booster but nevertheless suggests the dog may not have been able to mount an appropriate immune response to the vaccine.

Demodicosis in the dog has two forms, *squamous or pustular* and may be *localized or generalized*. Erythema, alopecia, scaling, and comedones characterize the squamous form. *Pustular demodicosis* occurs when secondary bacterial infection ensues and furunculosis and cellulitis develop. Papules, pustules, draining tracts, and edema may be evident. Perifollicular hypermelanosis manifest as pinpoint hyperpigmentation is suggestive of demodicosis.

Localized demodicosis (limited to one body region) occurs in young dogs 3–10 months of age and is usually self-limiting. These dogs do not have depressed cell-mediated immune responsiveness and can respond to intradermal challenge with a crude *Demodex* antigen. The lesions are single or multiple, well-circumscribed, erythematous, scaly, and alopecic patches usually affecting the head around the lips, eyes, ear canals, or on the extremities. Approximately 10% of cases of localized juvenile demodicosis progress to the generalized form of the disease.

The *generalized form* may be of juvenile onset (dogs 3–18 months of age) or adult onset (dogs >12–18 months of age). *Juvenile-onset generalized demodicosis* is familial in many breeds. *Adult-onset generalized demodicosis* has no breed predispositions. Adult-onset, severe demodicosis has been reported to occur concurrently with hyperadrenocorticism, corticosteroid administration, hypothyroidism, and chemotherapy and other serious internal or infectious diseases. It is not known if these conditions predispose the dog to generalized demodicosis or if the affected dogs were initially already immunologically predisposed to develop demodicosis. The lesions of generalized demodicosis may be particularly severe on the face, forelimbs and feet. In some dogs, lesions may be confined to the feet (Fig. 5.109B). Lesions include patchy to diffuse alopecia, erythema, scaling and crusting, with or without lesions of secondary bacterial pyoderma. Peripheral lymphadenopathy occurs in ~50% of affected dogs. Often the dogs with generalized pustular demodicosis are depressed, febrile and debilitated, and may die.

Histologically, demodicosis has a variable appearance depending on the stage of the disease and presence of secondary bacterial infection. Early, uncomplicated lesions are characterized by a predominantly *lymphocytic mural interface folliculitis*. Lymphocytic infiltration of the isthmus and infundibulum accompanied by various degrees of vacuolar degeneration and apoptosis of keratinocytes of the outer root sheath, follicular melanosis or pigment clumping in the outer root sheath, and perifollicular pigmentary incontinence are present.

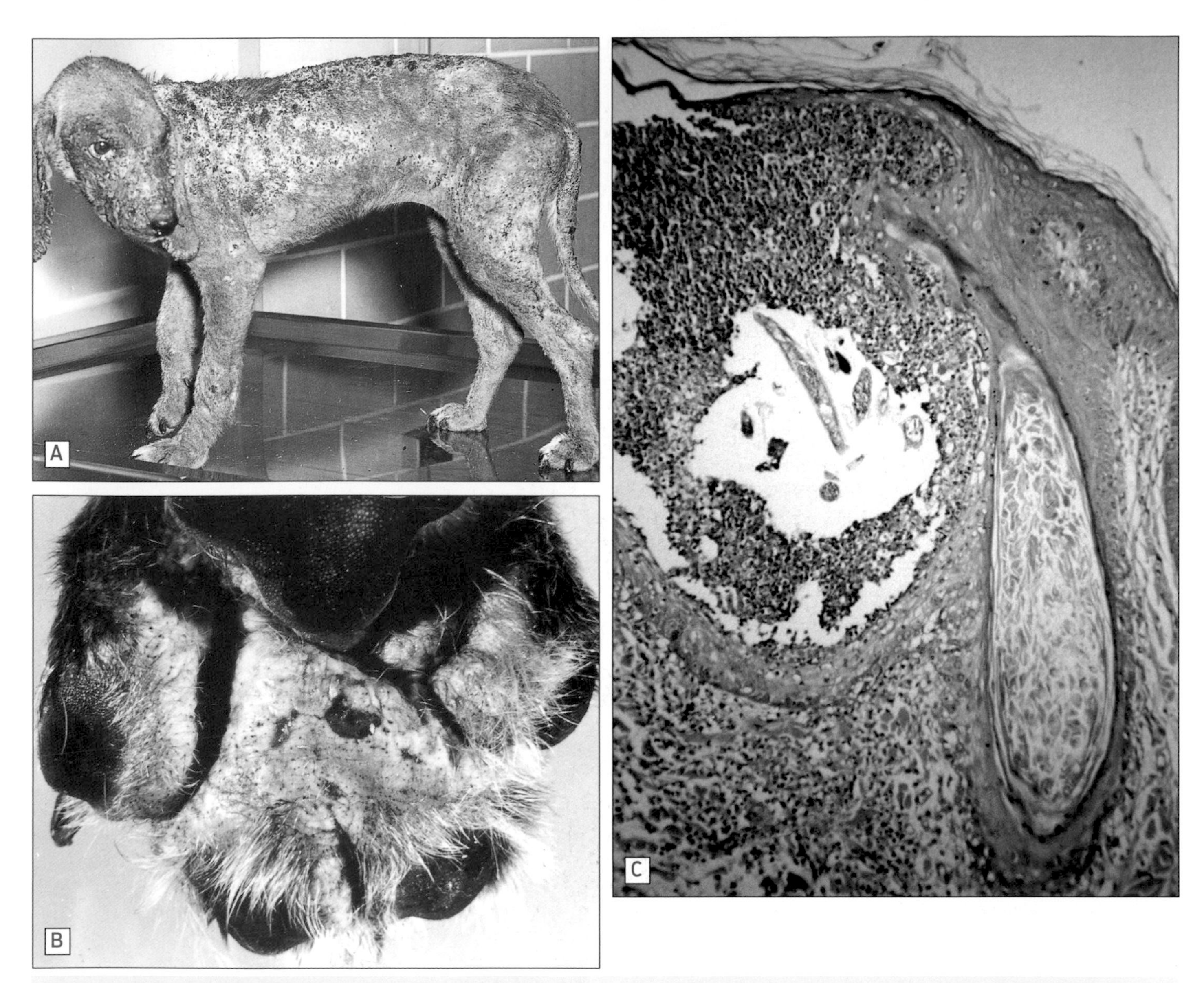

Figure 5.109 Demodicosis in a dog. **A.** Generalized demodectic mange. **B. Pododermatitis** in demodicosis. **C.** Folliculitis and **furunculosis** releasing *Demodex* mites into the dermis.

Immunophenotyping has identified infiltrating lymphocytes as CD8+ cytotoxic T cells, while the perifollicular infiltrates was found to be comprised of approximately equal numbers of CD4+ and CD8+ lymphocytes. The external root sheath may be hyperplastic. *Perifolliculitis* is also a consistent feature with infiltrates of plasma cells, macrophages, and lymphocytes in periadnexal regions. Mast cells and eosinophils may be present in smaller numbers. Marked follicular hyperkeratosis is associated with variable numbers of mites in the upper third of the follicle. Mural folliculitis is also consistently present at later stages and in cases with secondary bacterial infection but may not be the predominant pattern. In some cases, follicles may contain numerous mites but have no evidence of folliculitis of any type. This is especially true in cats. *Suppurative folliculitis and furunculosis* may be present depending on the presence and extent of secondary bacterial infection and the generation of deep pyoderma. Typically, large numbers of mites occupy the hair follicles at all levels and also occlude the opening of the sebaceous gland into the pilar canal. Marked follicular hyperkeratosis and build up of mite products causes follicular plugging. Bacterial proliferation within the plugged follicle often induces neutrophilic folliculitis. The combined effects of *follicular keratosis*, mite proliferation and folliculitis lead to *follicular rupture* and release of mites, bacteria, keratin, sebum, and other irritant products into the dermis (Fig. 5.109C). The bacteria, chiefly *Staphylococcus* spp., induce neutrophilic dermatitis often with abscessation. The keratin and other irritant substances stimulate a granulomatous reaction, chiefly of epithelioid macrophages, but a few multinucleated giant cells may be present. This *pyogranulomatous furunculosis* of demodectic mange differs from most other types of furunculosis in that eosinophils are rare or absent in the reaction. Epidermal lesions include hyperplasia, orthokeratotic and parakeratotic hyperkeratosis and variable spongiosis, neutrophilic exocytosis, ulceration and inflammatory crusting. Longer-standing lesions consist of perifollicular mid-to-deep dermal or occasionally subcuticular granulomas sometimes containing remnants of mites. Chronic lesions also have marked dermal fibrosis, often with obliteration of adnexa. Mites or fragments of mites are found in the subcapsular zone of regional lymph nodes associated with a local granulomatous inflammatory response. These do not indicate active invasion but rather passive transport to the node, via lymphatic channels.

Demodectic mange in **cattle** occurs worldwide. Three species are responsible: *D. bovis, D. ghanensis,* and *D. tauri*. Economic significance lies largely in the damage that mite infestation produces in hides. In some parts of Africa and Madagascar, demodectic mange in cattle may become generalized and fatal, this outcome contributed to by other debilitating conditions such as malnutrition, tick-worry and tropical heat.

Typical gross lesions are *multiple cutaneous papules or nodules*, usually between 2–4 mm diameter and occasionally reaching 1 cm or more. Nodules vary in number from a few to several hundred (Fig. 5.110A, B). The nodules are visible in smooth-coated cattle, often indicated by overlying tufts of erect hairs. In rough-coated cattle such as Herefords, detection usually requires palpation. The preferred sites are the shoulders, neck, dewlap, and muzzle but, in heavy infestations, nodules may be present over most of the body. The content of the nodules is thick, waxy or caseous material, sometimes stained with blood. The contents may liquefy and discharge to the surface forming a thick crust, or rupture of the nodule into the dermis may generate an abscess or a granulomatous reaction.

Histologically, the nodules are follicular cysts lined by a flattened squamous epithelium and filled with keratin squames and large numbers of demodicid mites. Adult parasites occur occasionally in sebaceous glands and rarely in apocrine sweat glands. A mild mononuclear cell infiltrate may occur around the epithelial lining. Rupture of a follicular cyst induces a marked nodular granulomatous reaction in which degenerating and occasionally mineralized segments of parasites and keratin debris are surrounded by epithelioid macrophages, multinucleated giant cells, lymphocytes, plasma cells and eosinophils.

The lesions in **goats**, caused by *D. caprae,* are similar to those described for cattle in both distribution and morphology. Some affected goats are mildly depressed, inappetent and have decreased milk production. Generally, the chief economic significance of caprine demodicosis lies in damage to the hides.

Demodectic mange is rare in **sheep**. *D. ovis* infestation is probably not uncommon in the medium to coarse-wooled sheep, affecting the Meibomian glands of the eyelid and the sebaceous glands of the primary follicles on the body, particularly the neck, flank and shoulders. *D. aries* infests the large sebaceous glands of the vulva, prepuce and nostrils. Grossly, lesions may be papular, nodular and rarely pustular. *D. ovis* infestation has been associated with matted fleece ("stringy wool"). Histologically, the mites are present in sebaceous glands or the pilar canal, occasionally inciting folliculitis or furunculosis.

While *Demodex* spp. are found commonly in the eyelid glands of the **horse**, demodectic mange is a very rare disease. *D. caballi* parasitizes the pilosebaceous units of the eyelids and muzzle, while *D. equi* infestation occurs over the body. Lesions associated with the latter occur on the head, neck and shoulder but may become generalized. They include papules, nodules and occasionally pustules. A patchy to diffuse alopecia with marked scaling occurs in the "squamous" form of the disease.

Demodex phylloides of **pigs** is not uncommon but is relatively unimportant in comparison to sarcoptic mange. The mites reside in the pilosebaceous units on the eyelids and snout with no clinical

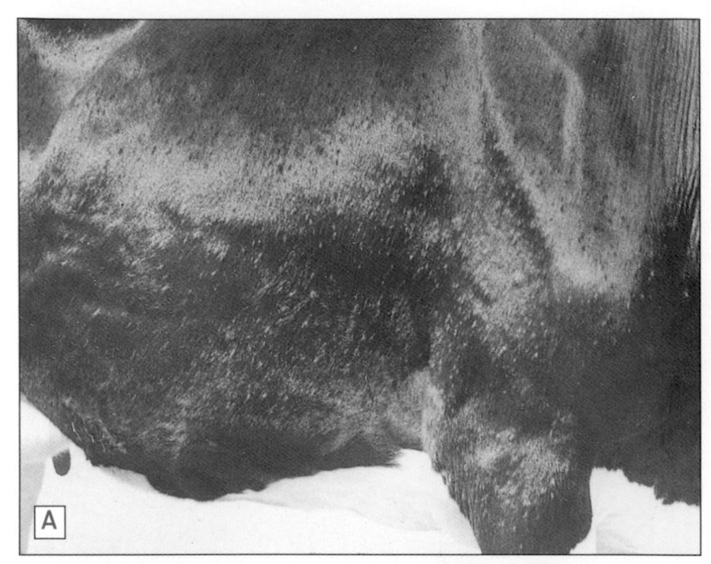

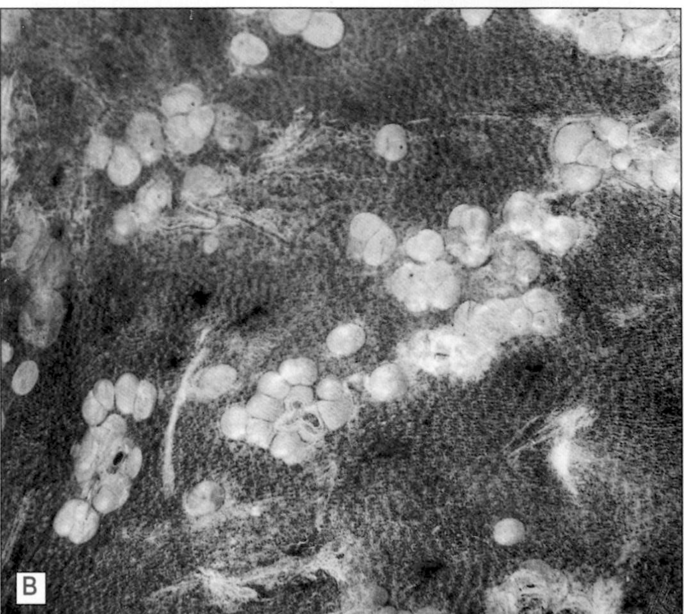

Figure 5.110 Demodectic mange in a cow. **A.** Multiple cutaneous nodules. **B.** *Demodex bovis* nodules beneath the hide.

effect. The principal economic loss results from extensive trimming of affected carcasses. The lesions typically involve the ventral abdomen, ventral neck, eyelids, and snout. They commence as small red macules, developing into cutaneous nodules covered by surface scale. Incision of the nodules releases thick white caseous debris that is full of mites. The histologic lesions are as described in cattle.

Cats may develop demodectic mange. Two species of *Demodex* mites have been associated with feline demodicosis. One is *D. cati* that resides in the hair follicles and sebaceous glands; the other, *D. gatoi*, is found on the skin surface in pits in the stratum corneum. *D. gatoi* is shorter and broader than *D. cati*. Unlike dogs, there is no age or clear breed predisposition.

Demodex gatoi is associated with alopecia, scaling, hyperpigmentation, erythema, and excoriations due to pruritus and excessive grooming. Lesions are most often on the head, neck, groin, and extremities. Ceruminous otitis may be present. Clinical reports suggest this species of mite may be transmitted horizontally between cats. *Differentials* include atopy, food allergy, flea-bite hypersensitivity, dermatophytosis, feline psychogenic alopecia, or other ectoparasitism.

Demodex cati infestation results in single or multiple areas of alopecia, erythema and scaling that resemble the localized form of canine demodicosis. Lesions have a predilection for the chin, eyelid, head, and neck. Generalized lesions may occur in association with systemic disease, such as feline leukemia virus or feline immunodeficiency virus infection, hyperadrenocorticism, or diabetes mellitus, which presumably suppress normal cell-mediated immune responses. *D. cati* infestation of lesions of multicentric squamous cell carcinoma in situ (Bowen's disease) suggest that a localized alteration in the cutaneous immune response may allow mite proliferation. The lesions of *D. cati* are multifocal to generalized areas of alopecia and erythema, with variable degrees of scaling, and papules and crusts. Secondary pyoderma is not a common accompaniment. A third syndrome, otitis externa, has also been associated with *D. cati* infestation.

Histologic lesions tend to be limited to follicular and surface hyperkeratosis, sometimes with follicular atrophy. Inflammatory cell infiltration is minimal in *D. cati* lesions. Some eosinophil, mast cell and neutrophil infiltrates have been described in infestations with *D. gatoi,* but the reaction was never severe and concurrent allergic disease could not be ruled out.

Bibliography

Barriga OO, et al. Evidence of immunosuppression by *Demodex canis*. Vet Immunol Immunopathol 1992;32:37–46.

Briggs DJ, et al. Rabies in a vaccinated canine exhibiting generalized demodicosis. J Vet Diagn Invest 1993;5:248–249.

Bukva V. *Demodex tauri* sp. n. (Acari: Demodicidae), a new parasite of cattle. Folia Parasitol (Praha) 1986;33:363–369.

Bukva V. Three species of the hair follicle mites (Acari: Demodicidae) parasitizing the sheep, *Ovis aries* L. Folia Parasitol (Praha) 1990;37:81–91.

Burrows AK. Generalised demodicosis in the dog: the unresponsive or recurrent case. Aust Vet J 2000;78:244–246.

Caswell JL, et al. A prospective study of the immunophenotype and temporal changes in the histologic lesions of canine demodicosis. Vet Pathol 1997;34:279–287.

Chesney CJ. Short form of *Demodex* species mite in the dog: occurrence and measurements. J Small Anim Pract 1999;40:58–61.

Day MJ. An immunohistochemical study of the lesions of demodicosis in the dog. J Comp Pathol 1997;116:203–216.

Desch CE. *Demodex aries* sp. nov., a sebaceous gland inhabitant of the sheep, *Ovis aries*, and a redescription of *Demodex ovis* Hirst, 1919. NZ J Zool 1986;13:367–375.

Desch CE Jr, Nutting WB. Redescription of *Demodex caballi* (=*D. folliculorum var. equi* Railliet, 1895) from the horse, *Equus caballus*. Acarologia 1979;20:235–240.

Desch CE, Stewart TB. *Demodex gatoi*: new species of hair follicle mite (Acari: Demodecidae) from the domestic cat (Carnivora: Felidae). J Med Entomol 1999;36:167.

Dorny P, et al. Survey on the importance of mange in the aetiology of skin lesions in goats in Peninsular Malaysia. Trop Anim Health Prod 1994;26:81–86.

Foley RH. Feline demodicosis. Compend Cont Ed: Small Anim 1995;17:481–486.

Guague're E, et al. *Demodex cati* infection in association with feline cutaneous squamous cell carcinoma in situ: a report of five cases. Vet Dermatol 1999;10:61–67.

Harland EC, et al. Demodectic mange of swine. J Am Vet Med Assoc 1971;159:1752.

Hillier A, Desch CE. Large-bodied *Demodex* mite infestation in 4 dogs. J Am Vet Med Assoc 2002;220:623–627.

Lemarie' SL, et al. A retrospective study of juvenile- and adult-onset generalized demodicosis in dogs (1986–91). Vet Dermatol 1996;7:3–10.

Matthes HF. Investigations of pathogenesis of cattle demodicosis: sites of predilection, habitat and dynamics of demodectic nodules. Vet Parasitol 1994;53:283–291.

Morris DO. Contagious demodicosis in three cats residing in a common household. J Am Anim Hosp Assoc 1996;32:350–352.

Rapp J, Koch F. Demodicosis in the pig. Vet Med Rev 1979;1:67–69.

Saridomichelakis M, et al. Adult-onset demodicosis in two dogs due to *Demodex canis* and a short-tailed demodectic mite. J Small Anim Pract 1999;40:529–532.

Williams JF, Williams CF. Demodicosis in dairy goats. J Am Vet Med Assoc 1982;180:168–169.

Trombiculiasis

The nymphs and adults of the trombiculid mites are free-living or parasitize plants or other arthropods; the larvae are parasitic and are known as "harvest mites," "chiggers," or "red bugs." The parasitic larvae are six-legged and resemble minute red or yellow spiders just visible to the naked eye. The mites attach themselves to the skin and make a channel into the epidermis, called a *stylostome*, through which salivary enzymes are injected and digested tissue fluids are withdrawn. The mites engorge to twice their original size over a period of 3–5 days, after which they drop off and complete their life cycle in the soil. *Intensely pruritic dermatitis* develops at the sites of attachment, probably as a result of an allergic reaction to the salivary secretions delivered through the stylostome; the allergic reaction caused by larval trombiculid mites is known as *trombidiosis*.

Wild vertebrates are the usual hosts for the trombiculid mite larvae, but food-producing domestic animals, pets and people may be accidentally infested. The disease tends to have a seasonal incidence, occurring in the *late summer and autumn* when climatic conditions favor an expansion of the mite population. Factors such as soil-type also influence the prevalence of trombiculiasis in different geographical regions. Animals exposed to fields and woodlands are more often infested.

Trombicula autumnalis, the European harvest mite, attacks most domestic species. *T. sarcina*, an Australian species known as the leg-itch mite, is an important parasite of sheep although its principal host is the gray kangaroo. *T. alfreddugesi* (North American chigger), and *T. splendens* are some of the species implicated in trombiculiasis in cats, dogs and horses. *Straelensia cynotis* normally reside on foxes, but can infest dogs.

Lesions tend to occur in areas close to ground contact in animals exposed to wild or semi-wild areas. Lesions are extremely pruritic. In **sheep**, the larvae attach preferentially on the skin of the caudal pastern. The interdigital web is the predilection site in the **dog**. In a massive infestation reported in two dogs, temporary hindlimb paresis developed. The mite in **horses** is known as the "heel-bug" because of its tendency to parasitize the feathered area of the pastern. Lesions may also occur along the mane and at the tail-head. Face, particularly lip, involvement is not infrequent. The lesions are intensely pruritic. In **cats**, lesions affect the paws, head and ears, but an atypical generalized form of the disease may occur in association with *W. americana* infestation.

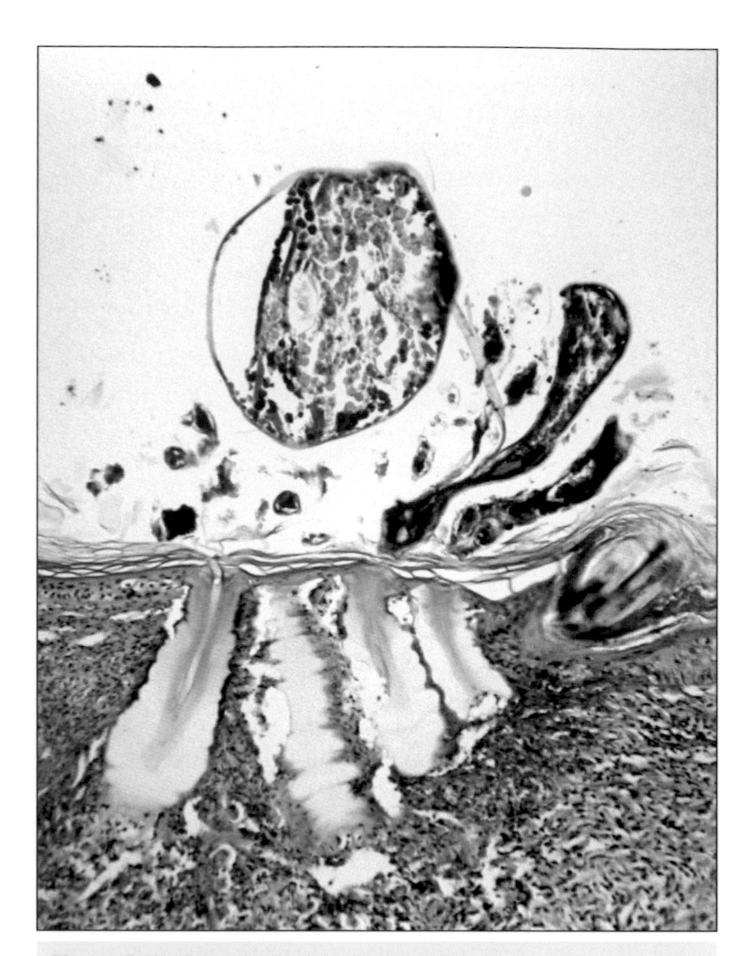

Figure 5.111 Trombiculiasis in a black bear. Section of skin showing mites within the surface keratin and multiple stylostomes oriented vertical to the skin's surface and extending into the dermis.

The gross lesions in all species are small, erythematous papules on which are clustered tiny (0.2–0.4 mm) bright red, orange or yellow mites. The mites leave a small, shallow ulceration that oozes a serous discharge and becomes crusted. Pruritus induces marked self-trauma, which may incite secondary bacterial infection. Histologically, *the mite is present in tunnels within the stratum spinosum or in the stratum corneum*. The presence of the mites induces both hyperplastic and degenerative changes in the epidermis. The stylostome appears as a pale staining, hyalinized tube with undulating margins oriented vertical to the skin's surface and extending into the dermis (Fig. 5.111). A large zone of necrotic cellular debris usually surrounds the stylostome. The surrounding dermis has a superficial perivascular infiltrate, with eosinophils and mast cells predominating.

Bibliography

Flemming EJ, Chastain CB. Miliary dermatitis associated with *Eutrombicula* infestation in a cat. J Am Vet Med Assoc 1991;27:529–531.

Goff ML, McKown RD. The genus *Hexidionis* (Acari:Trombiculidae) with the description of a new species from Texas. J Med Entomol 1997;34:438–440.

Le Net JL, et al. Straelensiosis in dogs: a newly described nodular dermatitis induced by *Straelensia cynotis*. Vet Rec 2002;150:205–209.

Little SE, et al. Trombidiosis-induced dermatitis in white-tailed deer (*Odocoileus virginianus*). Vet Pathol 1997;34:350–352.

Mair TS. Headshaking associated with *Trombicula autumnalis* larval infestation in two horses. Eq Vet J 1994;26:244–245.

Prosl H, et al. *Neotrombicula autumnalis* (harvest mite) in veterinary medicine. Nervous symptoms in dogs following massive infestation. Tierarztliche Praxis 1985;13:57–64.

Spalding MG, et al. Dermatitis in young Florida sandhill cranes (*Grus canadensis pratensis*) due to infestation the chigger, *Blankaartia sinnamaryi*. J Parasitol 1997;83:768–771.

White B. Early *Trombicula autumnalis* infection. Vet Rec 2001;148:188.

Other mite-induced dermatoses

The **cat fur mite**, *Lynxacarus radovsky*, infests cats in the USA, Australia, Fiji, South America, and the Caribbean. The mite attaches to the hair shafts rather than to the skin surface. Predilection sites include the tail tip, tail head, and perineum. The mite infestation mimics seborrhea sicca, giving the coat a characteristic "salt and pepper" appearance. The infestation is not usually associated with lesions, although crusted, exudative and pruritic lesions and alopecia have been described.

The **straw-itch mite** (*Pyemotes tritici*) is normally found in straw or grain where it parasitizes the larvae of soft-bodied grain insects. The parasite may occasionally infest humans and other mammals causing pruritic dermatitis. Mildly pruritic lesions may develop in horses fed infested hay. Multiple papules and wheals may occur on the neck, withers and thorax. *Acarus (Tyroglyphus) farinae* and *A. (Tyroglyphus) longior* may cause a pruritic, exudative, crusting and alopecic dermatosis in horses exposed to contaminated grain or hay.

Cats and dogs may be infested on rare occasions with the **poultry mite**, *Dermanyssus gallinae*. The infestation resembles that of cheyletiellosis but pruritic eruptions have been described.

Sheep may, on rare occasions, become infested with the **stored product mite**, *Sancassania berlesei*. These mites cannot infest dry skin; infestations are secondary to other conditions such as myiasis.

Bibliography

Arundel JH, Sutherland AK. Animal Health in Australia. Vol 10. Ectoparasitic Diseases of Sheep, Cattle, Goats and Horses. Australian Government Publishing Service, 1988.

Barton NJ, et al. Infestation of sheep with the stored product mite *Sancassania berlesei* (Acaridae). Aust Vet J 1988;65:140–143.

Craig TM, et al. *Lynxacarus radovskyi* infection in a cat. J Amer Vet Med Assoc 1993;202:613–614.

Foley RH. Parasitic mites of dogs and cats. Compend Contin Educ Pract Vet 1991;13:783–798.

Kunkle GA, Greiner EC. Dermatitis in horses and man caused by the straw itch mite. J Am Vet Med Assoc 1982;181:467–469.

Norvall J, McPherson EA. Dermatitis in the horse caused by *Acarus farinae*. Vet Rec 1983;112:385–386.

Ticks

Ticks belong to the class Arachnida, sub-class Acari. They are divided into two families, the Argasidae and the Ixodidae. *The*

Argasidae are the so-called soft ticks, lacking the scutum that characterizes the Ixodidae. Included in this group is *Argas persicus*, a complex of tick species that are important parasites of birds. *Otobius megnini*, known as the "spinose ear-tick," is parasitic to all domestic animals causing severe parasitic otitis externa and predisposing to bacterial infection or myiasis. Most of the pathogenic species of tick are found in the Ixodidae.

Ticks are most important as vectors for a large number of serious viral, bacterial and protozoal diseases of domestic animals. Babesiosis, Rocky Mountain spotted fever, Lyme borreliosis, heartwater disease, Q fever, louping ill, and anaplasmosis are a few examples of tick-transmitted diseases. Ticks also are small, attach firmly to their hosts, utilize multiple hosts, live for prolonged periods of time, and can often survive without feeding for long periods of time. These factors make ticks important in the possible transport and transmission of diseases from one host to another and between countries or continents. Importation of animals harboring ticks can pose a threat to animals in areas free of certain diseases. Ticks also harm their hosts more directly by causing *local injury* at the site of attachment. If infestation is heavy, fatalities may result. The local injury may predispose to myiasis and secondary bacterial infection, particularly to staphylococcal cutaneous abscesses or septicemia. Heavy infestations are also capable of causing *anemia* as a result of the bloodsucking activities of the ticks, but the Ixodidae, which engorge only once at each instar, are much less important in this respect than are the argasid ticks, which as adults engorge repeatedly. Tick bites may also induce hypersensitivity reactions. Several species of ixodid ticks have neurotoxins in salivary secretions that can cause *paralysis* of the host. These species include *Ixodes rubicundus* and *Rhipicephalus evertsi* of South Africa, *I. holocyclus* of Australia, *Dermacentor andersoni* in western North America, and *D. variabilis* in eastern North America.

The *local reaction to ticks is variable*, depending on properties of the tick, for example its ability to secrete prostaglandins, and on host factors such as the level of tick resistance. Primary tick bite lesions are papules and wheals, which proceed to focal areas of necrosis with crusts, erosions and ulcers and lead to focal alopecia. In contrast, tick-sensitized hosts produce extremely erythematous reactions. Histologically, the primary lesions are less severe and develop more slowly than those of sensitized animals. For example, in experimental *Ixodes holocyclus* infestations of cattle, the inflammatory cell reaction to the tick mouthparts embedded deeply into the dermis is not marked, even at 40 hr post-attachment. The lesions are restricted to the immediate feeding site and are predominantly neutrophilic. By contrast, previously sensitized cattle show epidermal spongiosis and vesiculation at some distance from the actual point of penetration as early as 1 hour post-attachment. By 12 hours, intraepidermal vesicles, bullae and microabscesses containing basophils with eosinophils and neutrophils are prominent. Basophils, many degranulated, are numerous in the edematous dermis from 1 hour post-attachment, reflecting the important role cutaneous basophil hypersensitivity plays in tick immunity. Severe hypersensitivity reactions to *Boophilus microplus* have been described in horses in Australia. Within 30 min of reinfestation, sensitized horses develop intensely pruritic papules and wheals, chiefly on the lower legs and muzzle. As tick bite lesions progress, they are often typified by the "arthropod-bite granuloma" described earlier in this section.

Tick infestation in lambs leading to secondary staphylococcal septicemia can result in high mortality.

Bibliography

Allen JR, et al. Histology of bovine skin reactions to *Ixodes holocyclus* Neumann. Can J Comp Med 1977;41:26–35.

Atwell RB, et al. Prospective survey of tick paralysis in dogs. Aust Vet J 2001;79:412–418.

Brown SJ. Highlights of contemporary research on host immune responses to ticks. Vet Parasitol 1988;28:321–334.

Burridge MJ. Ticks (Acari: Ixodidae) spread by the international trade in reptiles and their potential roles in dissemination of diseases. Bull Entomol Res 2001;91:3–23.

Falcone FH, et al. Do basophils play a role in immunity against parasites? Trends Parasitol 2001;17:126–129.

Madigan JE, et al. Muscle spasms associated with ear tick (*Otobius megnini*) infestations in five horses. J Am Vet Med Assoc 1995;207:74–76.

McLaren DJ, et al. Cutaneous basophil associated resistance to ectoparasites (ticks). Electron microscopy of *Rhipicephalus appendiculatus* larval feeding sites in actively sensitized guinea pigs and recipients of immune serum. J Pathol 1983;139:291–308.

Schleger AV, et al. *Boophilus microplus*: Cellular responses to larval attachment and their relationship to host resistance. Aust J Biol Sci 1976;29:499–512.

Shaw SE, et al. Tick-borne infectious diseases of dogs. Trends Parasitol 2001;17:74–80.

HELMINTH DISEASES OF SKIN

The skin is the natural portal of entry of a number of metazoan parasites that have their final habitat in the gastrointestinal tract or elsewhere. As a rule, those infective larvae that can invade percutaneously are not host specific, thus infection of aberrant hosts occurs. Such parasites are quite varied in their nature and include infective larvae of trematodes such as *Schistosoma*, and of the nematodes of various genera including *Strongyloides, Gnathostoma, Ancylostoma, Bunostomum, Uncinaria*, and others. Infective larvae of the filariids such as *Dirofilaria* and *Setaria* are deposited in the skin by the biting insects that are their vectors. The first percutaneous invasion of one of these parasites in its natural hosts takes place very quickly (for example, the larvae of *Strongyloides* and *Bunostomum* reach the dermis in 15 min) and provokes little reaction. Repeated invasions in a natural host or single invasion in an unnatural host are met with some resistance that is manifested as acute dermatitis limited to the invaded area. The cutaneous lesions are, except under experimental circumstances, seldom observed in animals. It is on the glabrous nonpigmented skin of people that they are easily observed and well recognized as the so-called "creeping eruption." There the larvae produce acutely inflamed, serpiginous, vesicular to papular tracts that may advance several centimeters a day. Usually, aberrant larvae die in the skin, but some enter the vessels and become lodged in the lungs or other tissues. Nematode larvae most often incriminated are *Ancylostoma braziliense* and *A. caninum*, the canine hookworm larvae. *Uncinaria stenocephala, Bunostomum phlebotomum, Gnathostoma spinigerum, Dirofilaria* sp., *Strongyloides procyonis,* and *Strongyloides westeri* are nematode parasites of other domestic and wild animals that have also been reported to cause cutaneous larval migration in humans.

Hookworm dermatitis occurs in dogs kept on grass or dirt and subjected to poor sanitation. Lesions consist of pruritic red papules on parts of the body exposed to the ground. The footpads and interdigital regions of the feet may be erythematous, edematous and painful. Claw deformities may occur. Histologically, hyperplastic spongiotic perivascular dermatitis with eosinophils and neutrophils is present. Larval tracts may be present in the epidermis or dermis lined by degenerating leukocytes. Inflammation is thought to be due to hypersensitivity reaction to migrating larvae.

The cutaneous lesions produced by the blood flukes and those nematodes that pass through the skin on the way to the gut are discussed elsewhere with the mature parasites (Vol. 2, Alimentary system). To be discussed in more detail here are those helminthic infestations that remain more or less localized to the dermis. The dermatitis produced by the larvae of *Elaeophora* is discussed in Vol. 3, Cardiovascular system.

Cutaneous habronemiasis

The aberrant deposition of the larvae of the spirurid nematodes *Habronema majus* (*microstoma*), *H. muscae* and *H. megastoma* by transmitting flies at cutaneous or mucocutaneous sites causes this *common disease of* **horses**. The adult worms normally develop in the stomach of horses following the ingestion of infective larva (see Vol. 2, Alimentary system). The cutaneous disease occurs sporadically in horse populations in temperate or tropical climates during the summer when the transmitting flies, *Musca* spp. and *Stomoxys calcitrans*, are active. Horses with a hypersensitivity response to the larvae are affected and the condition is recurrent each summer, hence the term, "*summer sores*." Lesions are consistently pruritic.

The location of the lesions is in the moist exposed areas of the body that attract flies. The most common sites are the *medial canthus of the eye* (Fig. 5.112A), *the glans penis and prepuce, and any cutaneous wound*. Since lacerations are more common on the distal extremities, these too are predilection sites for habronemiasis. Fly bites alone are sufficient to initiate an infestation. Ulcerative diseases initiated by other causes can be complicated by habronemiasis.

The gross lesions are rapidly progressive and proliferative in nature, comprising *ulcerated, tumorous masses of red-brown granulation tissue*. The surface is friable and hemorrhages readily. Lesions may be single or multiple and range in size from 5–15 cm in diameter and from 0.5–1.5 cm in depth. They are often irregular in shape in the early stages but become circular as they enlarge. On cut section, multiple small (1–5 mm) yellow-white, caseous, and occasionally gritty foci are scattered through the granulation tissue. These are often confused with the "kunkers" of pythiosis, but lack the characteristic branching pattern of the true kunker. In the deeper parts of the lesion, the more mature connective tissue has a dense, white appearance. The lesions on the conjunctiva and eyelids do not usually exceed 2 cm. Commencing with a serous conjunctivitis, small ulcerated, proliferative nodular lesions develop on the mucous membrane of the third eyelid and at the medial canthus. Lacrimal duct involvement characteristically produces a lesion 2–3 cm below the medial canthus. The entire conjunctiva may be affected resulting in profuse lacrimation, photophobia, chemosis, and inflammation of the eyelid. On cut section, *the nodular lesions of brown-red granulation tissue contain the typical caseous or mineralized foci*. Involvement of the penis and prepuce may cause prolapse of the urethral process and dysuria. On rare occasions, *Habronema* granulomas are found in the lung.

Histologically, multiple aggregates of degenerate eosinophils are scattered randomly throughout a collagenous connective tissue stroma of variable maturity. Epithelioid macrophages, multinucleated giant cells and degenerating eosinophils often surround longitudinal or cross-sections of degenerating larvae, which may be mineralized (Fig. 5.112B). However, *larvae may be rare or absent in many caseous foci*. The fibrous connective tissue is heavily and diffusely infiltrated with eosinophils and with fewer numbers of mast cells, lymphocytes and plasma cells. The surface of the lesion is usually covered with fibrinonecrotic exudate overlying highly vascular granulation tissue infiltrated with neutrophils.

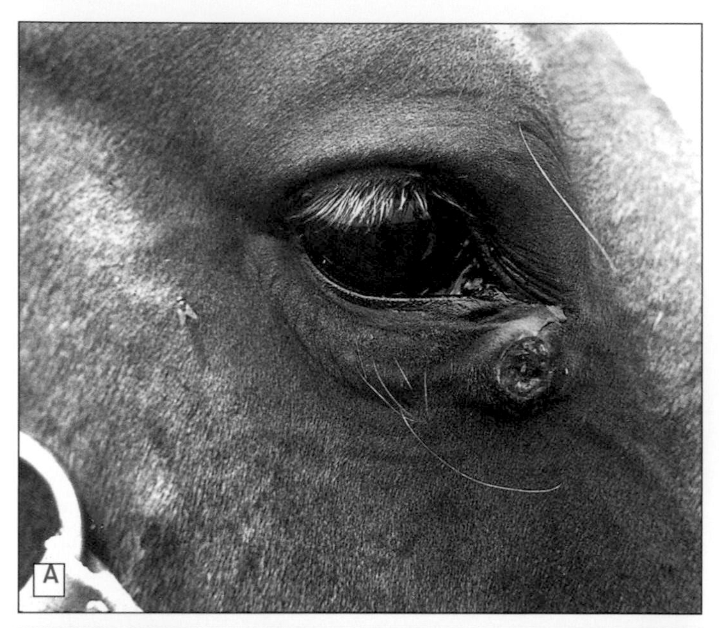

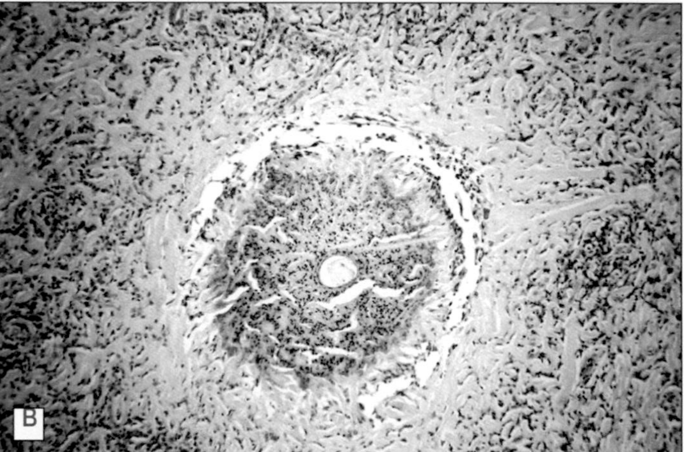

Figure 5.112 Cutaneous habronemiasis in a horse. **A.** Ulcerated nodule below medial canthus. **B.** Clusters of degranulating eosinophils surround a cross section of a *Habronema* sp. larva.

Since the gross lesions of cutaneous habronemiasis may resemble those of exuberant granulation tissue, botryomycosis, pythiosis, equine sarcoid and squamous cell carcinoma, the diagnosis requires biopsy and histologic evaluation. Squamous cell carcinoma and equine sarcoid are readily distinguished histologically. Exuberant granulation tissue lacks the caseous foci of degenerating eosinophils and larvae. Special stains will reveal the causative agents in botryomycosis (see Bacterial diseases of skin) and pythiosis (see Fungal diseases of skin). Nodular collagenolytic granuloma (nodular necrobiosis) presents a different clinical appearance but may be confused histologically with habronemiasis (see Miscellaneous skin conditions). Habronemiasis may complicate a pre-existing lesion; secondary *Habronema* infestations occur with pythiosis, *Corynebacterium pseudotuberculosis* infection and in skin tumors, particularly squamous cell carcinoma of the penis.

Cutaneous habronemiasis has been reported in a **dog**. Lesions developed on the face but, unlike the equine disease, were not characterized by rapid proliferation of granulation tissue. The dog was housed under unsanitary conditions in the company of several heavily parasitized ponies.

Bibliography

Hendrix CM, et al. Cutaneous larva migrans and enteric hookworm infections. J Am Vet Med Assoc 1996;209:1763–1767.

Mathison PT. Eosinophilic nodular dermatoses. Vet Clin N Am Eq Pract 1995;11:83–85.

Pusterla N, et al. Cutaneous and ocular habronemiasis in horses: 63 cases (1988–2002). J Am Vet Med Assoc 2003;222:978–982.

Sanderson TP, Niyo Y. Cutaneous habronemiasis in a dog. Vet Pathol 1990;27:208–209.

Scott DW, et al., eds. Muller and Kirk's Small Animal Dermatology. 5th ed. Philadelphia, PA: WB Saunders, 1995:393–394.

Stephanofilariasis

Members of the genus ***Stephanofilaria*** (Spirurida: Setariidae) are parasites of **cattle**. All stephanofilarid parasites cause similar cutaneous lesions, but the species are geographically separated and the lesions occur on different parts of the host's body. *Stephanofilaria stilesi* occurs in North America, affecting the abdominal skin near the midline; in Australian cattle, initial lesions develop at the medial canthus of the eye; *S. dedoesi* in Indonesia causes dermatitis, known locally as "cascado," on the sides of the neck, dewlap, withers and around the eyes; *S. assamensis* causes "hump-sore" of Zebu cattle in India and the Soviet Union; S. *kaeli* causes dermatitis of the legs of cattle from the Malay Peninsula; *S. dinniki* affects the shoulder of black rhinoceros; *S. boomkeri* causes severe dermatitis in pigs in Zaire; *S. zaheeri* causes dermatitis of the ears of buffalo, and *S. okinawaensis* causes lesions on the teats and muzzle of cattle in Japan. *Stephanofilaria kaeli, S. assamensis,* and *S. dedoesi* cause crusting dermatitis in **goats.**

Flies transmit stephanofilariasis. The hornfly, *Haematobia irritans*, is the vector of *S. stilesi* and the buffalo fly, *Haematobia irritans exigua*, is the major vector for stephanofilariasis in Australia. *Musca conducens* transmits *S. assamensis* and *S. kaeli*. The flies ingest microfilariae when feeding on cutaneous lesions. After a period of development in the fly, the infective larva is deposited on the skin by the biting species of fly or onto cutaneous wounds in the case of the nonbiting vectors such as *M. conducens*. The adults of *S. stilesi* live in cystic diverticula off the base of the hair follicles. The parasites are very small, with males reaching 3 mm and females 8 mm in length.

The *initial macroscopic lesions* in *S. stilesi* infections are circular patches 1 cm or less in diameter in the skin of the ventral midline, in which the hairs are moist and erect and the underlying epidermis is spotted with small hemorrhages and droplets of serum. These initial foci enlarge and coalesce, sometimes to produce a lesion 25 cm or more in diameter. As the foci enlarge, new spots of hemorrhage and exudation develop at the periphery while, in the central areas, the hair is shed and the exudate builds up into scabs or rough dry crusts through which the few remaining hairs penetrate (Fig. 5.113). The lesions are mildly pruritic and rubbing may aggravate them. In the healing stage, the affected areas remain as alopecic, lichenified plaques (Fig. 5.114).

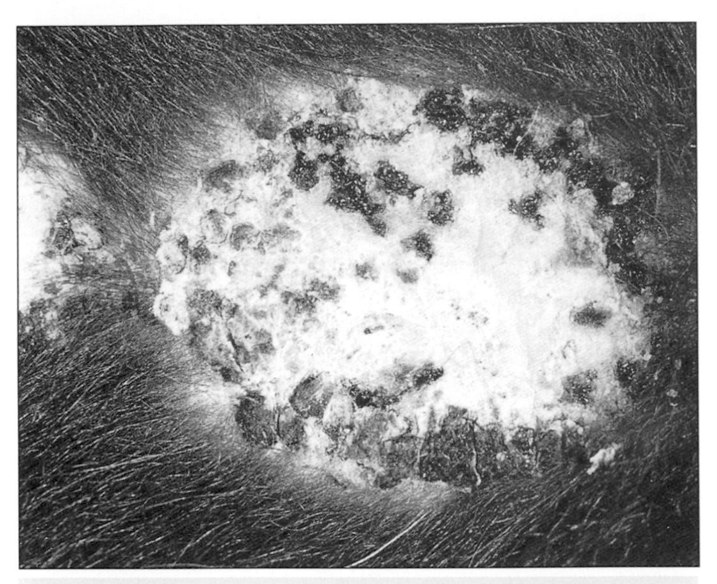

Figure 5.113 Early lesion on the ventral midline in **stephanofilariasis** in a cow.

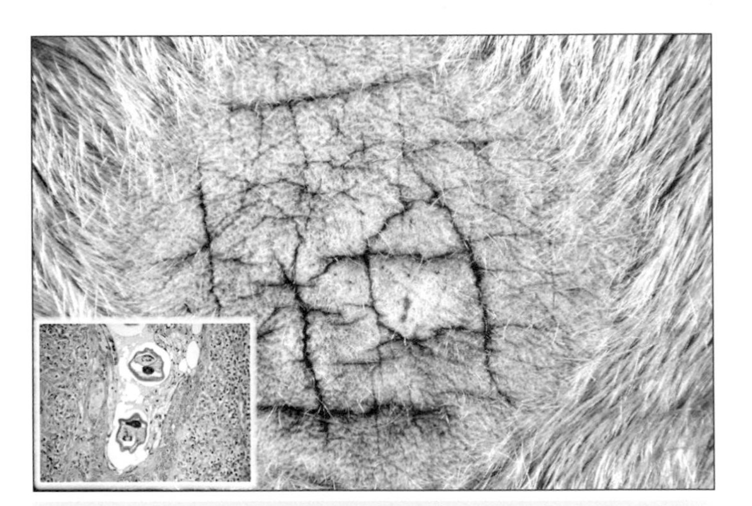

Figure 5.114 Chronic lesion of lichenified, alopecic plaque in **stephanofilariasis**. Nematode within a hair follicle (inset).

Histologically, sections of adult parasites may be seen in the cystic diverticula from hair follicles or lying free in the adjacent dermis. They may be identified as *Stephanofilaria* spp. with some confidence if microfilariae are seen in the uteri of females since this parasite is viviparous; if ova rather than larvae are found, it is more likely for the parasite to be of the genus Rhabditis. Microfilariae occur free in the dermis or in dermal lymphatics, enclosed within their own vitelline membranes (*S. stilesi*), or may be found free or unhatched in surface exudate (*S. kaeli*). There is little dermal reaction to the microfilariae or to the adults enclosed in cystic hair follicles, but the presence of adults in the dermis stimulates a mononuclear inflammatory reaction. There is accompanying superficial and deep perivascular dermatitis characterized by accumulations of eosinophils and mononuclear cells, chiefly lymphocytes. The epidermis is hyperplastic, spongiotic and often covered by orthokeratotic and parakeratotic hyperkeratosis and inflammatory crust. Spongiform microabscesses containing eosinophils and mononuclear cells are also described; such lesions are more typically associated with the bites of arthropod ectoparasites. It is difficult to assess the relative contributions made to the lesion by the stephanofilarial parasite and by the bites of the fly that acts as the vector.

Diagnosis is usually made on the basis of the typical gross lesions, by histologic examination of biopsy specimens or by demonstration of microfilariae by deep scrapings.

Bibliography

Agrawal MC, Shah HL. Stephanofilarial dermatitis in India. Vet Res Commun 1984;8:93–102.

Bain O, et al. *Stephanofilaria boomkeri* n. sp., as a cause of severe skin disease in pigs in Zaire. Parasite 1996;3:377–381.

Dies KH, Pritchard J. Bovine stephanofilarial dermatitis in Alberta. Can Vet J 1985;26:361–362.

Johnson SJ. Stephanofilariasis – a review. Helminthol Abst 1987;56:287–289.

Johnson SJ, Toleman MA. Prevalence of stephanofilariasis in young *Bos indicus* cattle in northern Australia. Vet Parasitol 1988;29:333–339.

Onchocerciasis

Onchocerca spp. are filarial nematodes (Spirurida: Onchocercidae) which affect cattle, horses, sheep, goats and man. *The adult worms reside in various connective tissue locations*, chiefly ligaments, tendons and subcutaneous nodules, but also perimysial sheaths, cartilage and the aorta. The microfilariae migrate to the dermis where they lie free in tissue spaces or lymphatics. In man, blindness caused by migration of microfilariae into the chambers of the eye has been a serious health concern in Africa and Central America. Microfilariae in the dermis of any host are aspirated by the intermediate hosts, which are insects of the families Simuliidae (black flies, buffalo gnats) and Ceratopogonidae (biting midges). The prevalence of infection is very high in cattle and horses, ranging up to 100% in some studies.

Onchocerca cervicalis occurs worldwide and is the major species affecting the horse in North America; adults reside in the ligamentum nuchae and range from 27–75 mm in length. *Onchocerca reticulata* occurs in horses in Europe and Asia; adults live in the flexor tendons and suspensory ligaments, particularly of the forelimbs. *Onchocerca cervicalis* and *O. reticulata* are primarily transmitted by *Culicoides* sp.

Onchocerca gutturosa more commonly affects cattle but also is recovered from horses. *Onchocerca gibsoni* infects cattle in Australia, Asia, and Africa; *O. ochengi* infests cattle in Africa. *Onchocerca armillata* occurs in cattle, sheep, and goats in Africa and Asia; the adults live in the aorta.

Most animals show no reaction to the presence of living microfilariae in the dermis. The reason for the lack of host reaction to the living microfilariae is unknown. Dead microfilariae are, however, highly phlogistic and an intense inflammatory reaction may occur after treatment with microfilaricides in some animals. *Onchocerca* microfilariae cause cutaneous lesions in some horses; in cattle, the adults cause the cutaneous lesions.

In dogs, onchocerciasis has been reported involving the palpebral conjunctiva, third eyelid, sclera, cornea, and retrobulbar space. Dogs were presented for evaluation of periocular or ocular masses. Degenerating or mineralized adult *Onchocerca* spp. parasites were found in the center of pyogranulomas comprising the masses.

Equine cutaneous onchocerciasis

The pathogenicity of *Onchocerca cervicalis* and *O. reticulata* microfilariae, originally questioned because the parasites could be readily demonstrated in the skin of clinically normal horses, became accepted when it was shown that ivermectin treatment induces rapid and concurrent disappearance of cutaneous lesions and microfilariae. The prevalence of adult parasites in horses has not diminished despite the widespread use of avermectins. It has been postulated that individual hypersensitivity to microfilarial antigens is the reason for the sporadic occurrence of equine skin lesions.

Areas affected are the face, neck, medial aspects of the forelimbs, ventral thorax, and abdomen. Lesions on the face may be diffuse, periorbital or central. *The central lesions, which often involve the facial markings, are very characteristic of onchocerciasis.* The lesions on the neck are focal and tend to occur at the base of the mane. Lesions on the ventral thorax and abdomen are often diffuse, in comparison with the localized lesions of horn fly-induced ventral midline dermatitis. The ventral lesions are indistinguishable grossly from those of *Culicoides* hypersensitivity, but onchocerciasis does not cause lesions at the base of the tail. It is likely that onchocerciasis and *Culicoides* hypersensitivity can exist simultaneously.

Cutaneous lesions include partial or complete alopecia, scaling, crusting, and leukoderma. Secondary excoriations or ulcerative dermatitis are induced by self-trauma in pruritic animals. Ocular lesions are discussed in Vol. 1, Eye and ear. The microscopic lesions associated with microfilarial infection vary from none to superficial and deep perivascular lymphocytic and eosinophilic dermatitis. Microfilariae may be present in large numbers or may be very sparse. They are best recovered from unfixed biopsies that are minced and incubated in saline at 37°C. *Differential diagnoses* include other fly-bite-associated dermatitides, staphylococcal folliculitis, occult sarcoid, and infestation with lice, mites, or ticks. Lesion distribution should be helpful.

Viable adult parasites in the nuchal ligament are not associated with significant lesions; in older horses, there is an increased frequency of caseated, mineralized and granulomatous lesions, associated with death of the parasite. *Onchocerca gutturosa* is also found in the nuchal ligament of horses in Australia. Histologic examination revealed that this parasite does not penetrate the elastic tissue of the ligament and the inflammatory reaction is localized around the worm. Mineralization is the fate of degenerate *Onchocerca gutturosa* worms, in contrast to caseation with *O. cervicalis*.

Bovine cutaneous onchocerciasis

Cattle can be infected by three species of *Onchocerca*. Cattle infested with *O. gibsoni* develop multiple subcutaneous papules and nodules of ~2 cm diameter, although lesions up to 9 cm are recorded. Lesions may be hard or soft depending on the degree of mineralization and fibrosis or the degree of caseation and suppuration. Lesions predominantly affect the brisket but also the stifle and hip. Histologic assessment of *O. gibsoni* nodules revealed dead worms and associated degenerative changes such as mineralization in ~30% of nodules. Eosinophilic infiltration was more marked around viable worms, with eosinophils apparently adherent to the cuticle. In *O. gutturosa* infections, the worm is found in the nuchal ligament and connective tissue around tendons and ligaments of the shoulder, hip, and stifle. It does not form nodules and is thus easily overlooked. In *O. ochengi* infections, scrotum, udder, flanks, lateral thorax, and head are affected.

Bibliography

Abraham D, et al. Immunity to *Onchocerca* spp. in animal hosts. Trends Parasitol 2002;18:164–171.

Achukwi MD, et al. *Onchocerca ochengi* transmission dynamics and the correlation of *O. ochengi* microfilaria density in cattle with the transmission potential. Vet Res 2000;31:611–621.

Collobert C, et al. Prevalence of *Onchocerca* species and *Thelazia lacrimalis* in horses examined post mortem in Normandy. Vet Rec 1995;136:463–465.

Eberhard ML, et al. Ocular *Onchocerca* infections in two dogs in western United States. Vet Parasitol 2000;90:333–338.

Ferenc SA, et al. *Onchocerca gutturosa* and *Onchocerca lienalis* in cattle: Effect of age, sex, and origin on prevalence of onchocerciasis in subtropical and temperate regions of Florida and Georgia. Am J Vet Res 1986;47:2266–2268.

Foil L, Foil C. Parasitic skin diseases. Vet Clin N Am Eq Pract 1986;2:403–437.

Folkard SG, et al. Eosinophils are the major effector cells of immunity to microfilariae in a mouse model of onchocerciasis. Parasitol 1996;112 (pt 3):323–329.

Lyons ET, et al. Prevalence of selected species of internal parasites in equids at necropsy in central Kentucky (1995–1999). Vet Parasitol 2000;92:51–62.

Mtei BJ, Sanga HJ. Aortic onchocercosis and elaeophorosis in traditional TSZ-cattle in Tabora (Tanzania): prevalence and pathology. Vet Parasitol 1990; 36:165–170.

Ottley ML, et al. Equine onchocerciasis in Queensland and the Northern Territory of Australia. Aust Vet J 1983;60:200–203.

Slocombe JOD. Pathogenesis of helminths in equines. Vet Parasitol 1985;18:139–153.

Szell Z, et al. Ocular onchocercosis in dogs: aberrant infection in an accidental host or lupi onchocercosis? Vet Parasitol 2001;101:115–125.

Wahl G, et al. Bovine onchocercosis in north Cameroon. Vet Parasitol 1994; 52:297–311.

Wildenburg G, et al. Distribution of mast cells and their correlation with inflammatory cells around *Onchocerca gutturosa*, *O. tarsicola*, *O. ochengi*, and *O. flexuosa*. Parasitol Res 1997;83:109–120.

Pinworms

Oxyuris equi infection of the equine large intestine can be associated with *pruritic dermatitis of the perineal region* leading to self-induced excoriations and alopecia of the tail known as "*rat tail*." The adult parasite crawls out of the anus to deposit eggs on the hair and skin using a gelatinous material that can induce pruritus. *Diagnosis* is made by using the tape method in the perianal region for identification of characteristic operculated eggs.

Bibliography

Perris E. Parasitic dermatoses that cause pruritus in horses. Vet Clin N Am Eq Pract 1995;11:27.

Parafilariasis

Parafilaria multipapillosa occurs in horses in Eastern Europe. *Parafilaria bovicola* is endemic in cattle in Africa, India, and parts of Europe. *Parafilaria bassoni* has been reported in African buffalo and springbok in Namibia. The parasites are thin, thread-like worms, 2–7 cm long. The adults inhabit subcutaneous and intermuscular connective tissues producing nodules 1–2 cm in diameter. In the spring and summer, the nodules rapidly enlarge, burst open, hemorrhage, and heal. This coincides with the migration of the fully gravid female into the more superficial dermis to oviposit and to release the infective microfilariae. The vectors, flies such as *Haematobia atripalpis* in Russia and *Musca* spp., are infected when they feed from these bleeding points, known as "blood nodules." Secondary subcutaneous abscesses may occur.

Bibliography

Chambers PG. Prevalence of *Parafilaria* lesions in slaughter cattle in Zimbabwe. Vet Rec 1991;129:431–432.

Chirico J. Prehibernating *Musca autumnalis* (Diptera: Muscidae) – an overwintering host for parasitic nematodes. Vet Parasitol 1994;52:279–284.

Gibbons LM, et al. Redescription of *Parafilaria bovicola* Tubangui, 1934 (Nematoda: Filarioidea) from Swedish cattle. Acta Vet Scand 2000;41:85–91.

Keet DF, et al. Parafilariosis in African buffaloes (*Syncerus caffer*). Onderstepoort J Vet Res 1997;64:217–225.

Kretzmann PM, et al. Manifestations of bovine parafilariasis. J S Afr Vet Assoc 1984;55:127–129.

Pelodera dermatitis

Some of the biological characteristics of the Rhabditidae have been discussed with the principal parasitic genus, *Strongyloides*, in Vol. 2, Alimentary system. Here it is necessary only to describe the cutaneous lesions produced occasionally by the small free-living worms of this family. Those worms that are found in the lesions are usually classified as ***Pelodera (Rhabditis) strongyloides***.

Pelodera dermatitis occurs most commonly in dogs, occasionally in cattle and rarely in horses and sheep. The condition has been reported in humans. The development of dermatitis to a clinical degree probably requires exposure to many larvae. These worms live as saprophytes in warm moist soil that is rich in organic matter, and significant infections probably require that the host's skin should be continually moist and filthy. The lesions develop on contact areas, particularly at the margins of areas caked with dirt. Affected **dogs** often have a history of being bedded on straw. Acute dermatitis develops, commonly with neutrophilic folliculitis and is due to the combined stimuli of the parasites, bacterial folliculitis, and of the scratching, rubbing, and licking prompted by severe pruritus, probably induced by an allergic reaction to the parasite. The gross lesions include erythema, papules, excoriations, scaling, exudation and crusting with partial to complete alopecia. Pustules may occur, particularly in dogs. Histologically, the worms are in the lumina of the hair follicles or in the dermis, surrounded by an intense eosinophilic inflammatory reaction (Fig. 5.115). *Differential diagnoses* based on gross lesions in dogs include hookworm dermatitis, dirofilarial dermatitis, dermatophytosis, demodicosis, bacterial folliculitis, scabies, strongyloidiasis and contact dermatitis. Definitive diagnosis is based upon environmental history and deep skin scrapings or biopsy. *Pelodera* dermatitis in **sheep** may result in complete loss of wool, hyperkeratosis and lichenification in affected areas.

Bibliography

Horton ML. Rhabditic dermatitis in dogs. Mod Vet Pract 1980;61:158–159.

Ramos JJ, et al. *Pelodera* dermatitis in sheep. Vet Rec 1996;138:474–475.

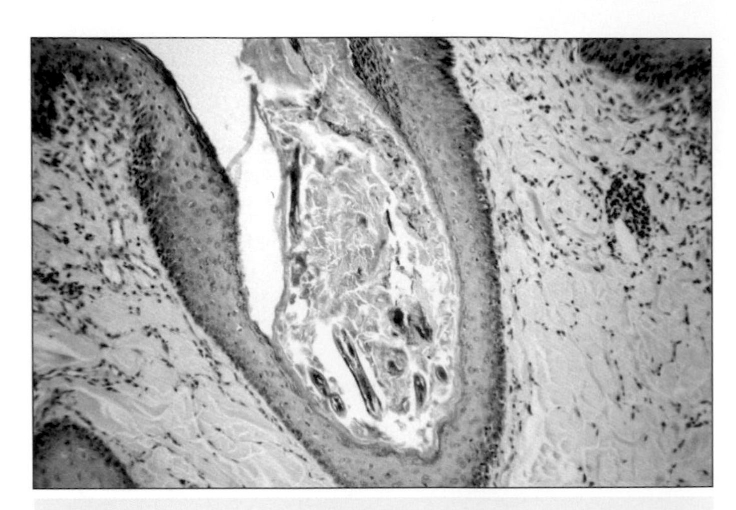

Figure 5.115 ***Pelodera (Rhabditis) strongyloides*** **folliculitis** in a dog. Adult rhabditiform parasites within distended hair follicle.

Rashmir-Raven AM, et al. Papillomatous pastern dermatitis with spirochetes and *Pelodera strongyloides* in a Tennessee Walking Horse. J Vet Diagn Invest 2000;12:287–291.

Miscellaneous helminths

Dracunculus medinensis (Spirurida: Dracunculidae) is the "guinea worm" of humans in Asia and Africa. It has been introduced into America, the West Indies, and Fiji. The parasite has been reported in *dogs, cats, horses, and cattle* as well as other species in endemic areas. *Dracunculus insignis* is the species of the nematode that occurs in dogs and wild carnivores in North America. Infection is particularly prevalent in raccoons and mink that appear to be the natural definitive species. The intermediate host is a crustacean copepod but frogs may act as paratenic hosts. Ingesting the intermediate host, infected frogs, or water containing infected copepods infects the final host. The larvae are released during digestion and proceed to migrate through the body. The adult worms mature in the connective tissue of the host in approximately 1 year. The parasite occurs typically in the subcutaneous tissues of the limbs. The mature female may measure up to 70 cm in length, resulting in the formation of a 2–4 cm nodule. The gravid female produces an intraepidermal bulla with her anterior end by means of toxin secretion. Rupture of the bulla forms a shallow ulcer from which a milky exudate drains. When these lesions contact water, the worm is stimulated to release very large numbers of larvae that are ingested by copepods in the water. Fine needle aspiration of the cutaneous nodules reveals rhabditiform *Dracunculus* larvae, approximately 500 μm long and covered by a striated cuticle. The adults lie in a pseudocyst lined by fibrous connective tissue and infiltrated with eosinophils, lymphocytes and multinucleated giant cells. Ulcerated lesions are seen as draining fistulae that may be painful or pruritic. *Differentials* include foreign body, neoplasia, infected wound, or cutaneous dirofilariasis. The parasite can be identified by morphologic features.

Dirofilaria immitis microfilariae can occasionally lead to cutaneous lesions in dogs harboring the adult parasite. A series of five cases document a scabies-like, papular to nodular, variably ulcerated, pruritic dermatitis of the skin of the head, trunk, and extremities in dogs infected with *D. immitis*. Histologic examination of affected skin revealed angiocentric and pyogranulomatous dermatitis with intralesional microfilariae. A type II hypersensitivity response was proposed as a pathogenic mechanism based on positive immunoreaction of microfilariae with anti-IgG serum. Lesions resolved with antiparasitic treatment. Ectopic adult *D. immitis* have been recovered from cutaneous abscesses and interdigital cysts in parasitized dogs. In addition, a generalized cutaneous syndrome characterized by a pruritic papular and crusting dermatitis without intralesional microfilariae has been apparently associated with infection with *D. immitis* and was thought to be a manifestation of an unusual hypersensitivity reaction. Parasites are not present in the cutaneous tissues. Lesions also resolved with antiparasitic treatment. *Dirofilaria repens* occurs in the subcutaneous connective tissues of dogs in Mediterranean countries and tropical parts of the Orient. The intermediate hosts are probably mosquitoes. The microfilariae occur in dermal lymphatics. This parasite is not known to be pathogenic. *Dipetalonema reconditum* occurs in the subcutis of dogs and coyotes. Its only significance is in the differential diagnosis of *D. immitis* infections by identification of microfilariae in peripheral blood.

Dermatitis associated with nematode microfilariae of **undetermined species** has been associated with a pruritic, papular, or plaque-like dermatitis of the head and limbs in dogs determined by multiple assays to be free of adult *Dirofilaria immitis* and *Dipetalonema reconditum*. Lesions were single to multiple, erythematous, alopecic, ulcerated, and crusted. Histologic changes included ulceration and perivascular, periglandular, or interstitial mixed inflammatory cell infiltrates with variable eosinophils and plasma cells. Microfilariae were free within the dermis or subcutis and within microgranulomas. No microfilariae were present within vessels. One adult nematode was also present in the cutaneous tissues and was determined to be *Acanthocheilonema* sp.

Incidental subcutaneous parasitism by the free-living form of the helminth, ***Gordius robustus*** has been reported in the cat. The cat developed a 1–2 cm firm subcutaneous nodule on the back. Histologically, the nodule consisted of an adult nematomorph surrounded by granulation tissue and pyogranulomatous to eosinophilic to lymphoplasmacytic infiltrates. *G. robustus* has a free-living adult form as well as a parasitic larval form that resides in the body cavity of freshwater or terrestrial insects. *Differentials* include many causes of solitary cutaneous nodules. Definitive diagnosis is dependent upon recognizing morphologic features of the parasite.

Suifilaria suis occurs in pigs in South Africa. The worms are 2–4 cm long and live in the subcutaneous and intermuscular connective tissues, sometimes producing small white nodules. The female is oviparous and the eggs are released to the surface via small vesicular eruptions in the epidermis. The remainder of the life cycle is unknown.

Parelaphostrongylus tenuis, a common parasite of white-tailed deer, is an occasional cause of neurological disease in goats. Some affected goats also develop an unusual dermatitis, often restricted to one side of the body. Lesions are vertically oriented, alopecic, ulcerated, crusted or scarred, linear tracks on the shoulder, thorax or flanks. The lesions have been explained tentatively on the basis of ganglioneuritis leading to irritation of dermatomes. Histologically, the lesion is a fibrosing dermatitis with focal areas of basal keratinocyte hydropic degeneration.

Bibliography

Beyer TA, et al. Massive *Dracunculus insignis* infection in a dog. J Am Vet Med Assoc 1999;214:366–368.

Coles LD, et al. Adult *Dirofilaria immitis* in hind leg abscesses of a dog. J Am Anim Hosp Assoc 1988;24:363–365.

Cornegliani L, et al. Two cases of cutaneous nodular dirofilariasis in the cat. J Small Anim Pract 2003;44:316–318.

Elkins AD, Berkenblit M. Interdigital cyst in the dog caused by an adult *Dirofilaria immitis*. J Am Anim Hosp Assoc 1990;26:71–72.

Hargis AM, et al. Dermatitis associated with microfilariae (Filarioidea) in 10 dogs. Vet Dermatol 1999;10:95–107.

Moisan PG. Incidental subcutaneous gordiid parasitism in a cat. J Vet Diag Invest 1996;8:270–272.

Seavers A. Cutaneous syndrome possibly caused by heartworm infestation in a dog. Aust Vet J 1997;76:18–20.

MISCELLANEOUS SKIN CONDITIONS

Canine juvenile cellulitis

Canine juvenile cellulitis (juvenile sterile granulomatous dermatitis, puppy strangles, juvenile pyoderma) is an idiopathic disease typically affecting puppies less than 4 months of age. The condition can affect one or more puppies from a litter of any breed but golden and yellow Labrador Retrievers, Dachshunds, Lhasa Apsos, and Gordon Setters are most often reported. A condition clinically and histopathologically identical to juvenile cellulitis has also been reported in adult dogs. Immunologic, infectious, traumatic, parasitic and environmental conditions have all been proposed as possible etiologies. The fact that the lesions are sterile when cultured, nontransmissible, and respond to corticosteroids better than antibiotics alone eliminates infectious agents as probable causes. Special stains and electron microscopy have also failed to identify intralesional infectious agents. Immune system tests have not revealed abnormalities in affected animals. Depressed in vitro lymphocyte blastogenesis responses have been reported but likely represent the result not the cause of the disease.

Cutaneous lesions comprise papules, pustules, crusts, alopecia, and very marked edema (Fig. 5.116). Skin of the muzzle, face, ears, and occasionally the feet, abdomen, vulva, prepuce, and anus are affected. Otitis externa is common. Lymphadenopathy of the mandibular nodes is common and may precede the onset of the skin lesions. Lymphadenitis may also occur in nodes distant to the skin lesions and may occur in the absence of skin lesions. The cutaneous lesions are bilaterally symmetric, painful but not pruritic. Anorexia, fever, malaise and arthritis affecting multiple joints are not uncommon. *Histologically, the lesions are pyogranulomatous nodular to diffuse dermatitis with furunculosis and pyogranulomatous lymphadenitis.* Inflammation often extends into the panniculus. The differential diagnoses include severe bacterial dermatitis, demodicosis, and adverse drug reactions or other cause of angioedema. The condition resolves with proper treatment in 1.5–6 weeks and rarely recurs.

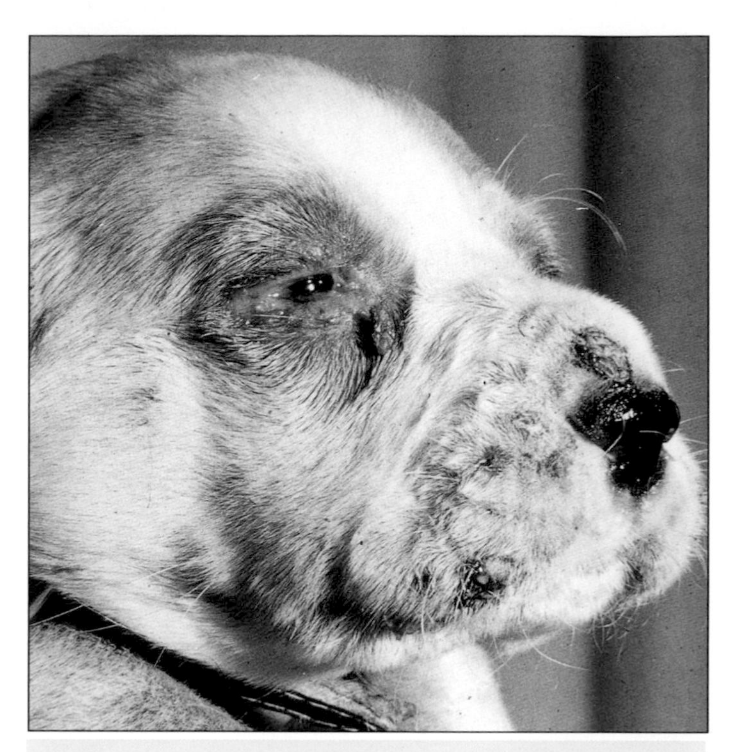

Figure 5.116 Marked soft tissue swelling in **juvenile cellulitis** in a puppy.

Bibliography

Neuber AE, et al. Dermatitis and lymphadenitis resembling juvenile cellulitis in a four-year-old dog. J Small Anim Pract 2004;45:254–258.

Reimann KA, et al. Clinicopathologic characterization of canine juvenile cellulitis. Vet Pathol 1989;26:499–504.

White SD, et al. Juvenile cellulitis in dogs: 15 cases (1979–1988). J Am Vet Med Assoc 1989;195:1609–1611.

Cutaneous paraneoplastic syndromes

Cutaneous paraneoplastic syndromes are dermatoses associated with internal neoplasms. The neoplasms may be malignant or benign but are most often malignant. In keeping with the definition of a paraneoplastic syndrome, *these conditions cannot be directly attributed to the anatomic location of the neoplasm.* The skin or mucosal lesions may precede, concur with, or follow the diagnosis of the underlying neoplasm. Removal or elimination of the tumor should alleviate the cutaneous lesions, while relapse of the dermatosis signals recurrence of the underlying neoplasm. The majority of cutaneous paraneoplastic syndromes in animals do not have a defined pathogenesis and often have only been reported a limited number of times. These syndromes are better documented in humans, but the increased recognition and clinical significance in domestic animals warrants mention in this chapter. The well-recognized cutaneous lesions seen with functional pituitary, adrenal or testicular tumors are discussed elsewhere (see Endocrine diseases of skin). Cutaneous lesions associated with the cryoglobulinemia associated with multiple myelomas have been discussed elsewhere (see Other immune-mediated dermatoses).

A unique dermatosis reported in aged cats is characterized by symmetrical ventrally distributed alopecia affecting the trunk and limbs (Fig. 5.117A) has been reported to be associated with a concurrent **pancreatic carcinoma** or **bile duct carcinoma**. The alopecia is due to *marked follicular atrophy* (Fig. 5.117B). Adnexal structures are also markedly atrophic. The epidermis lacks a stratum

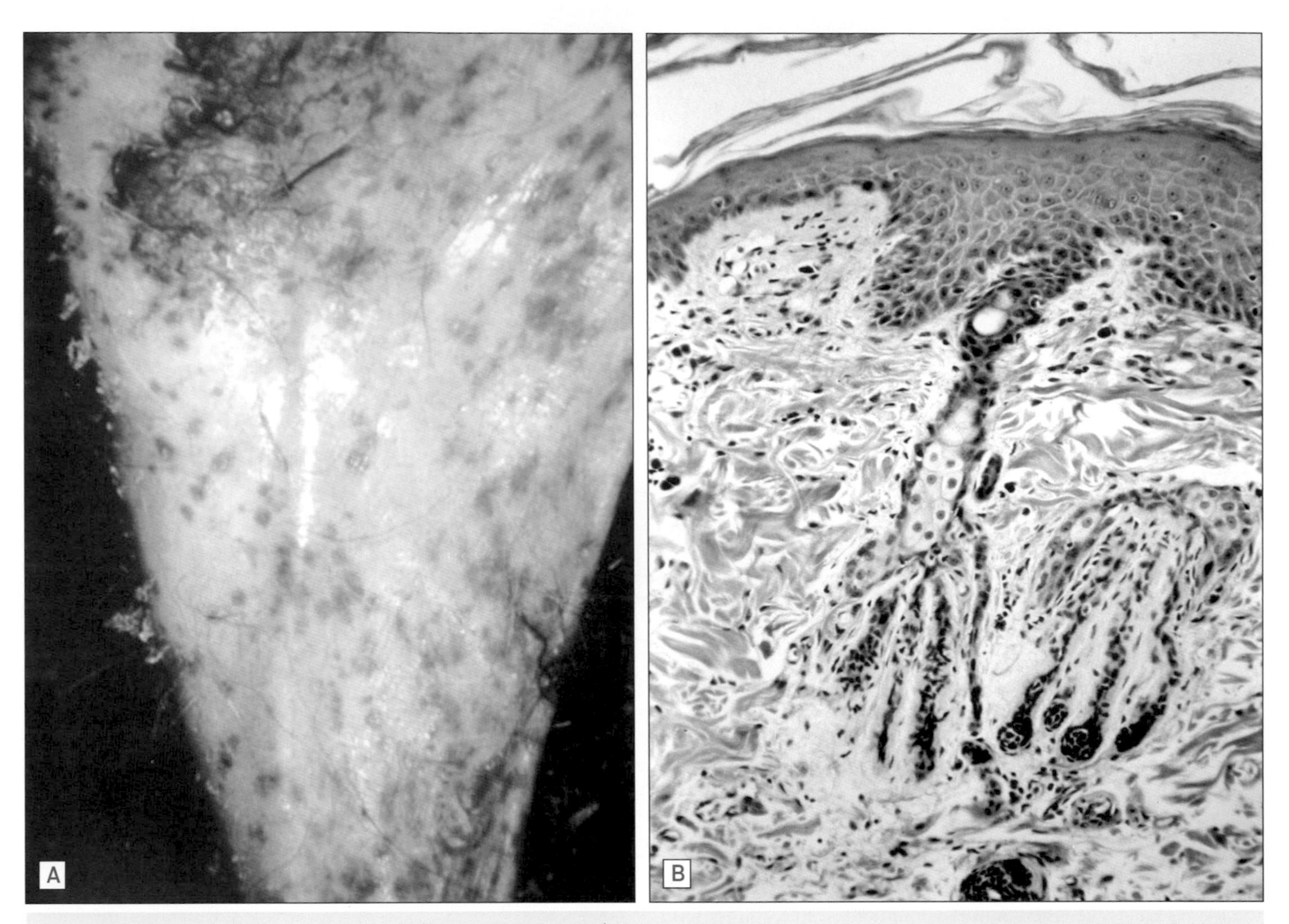

Figure 5.117 Feline paraneoplastic alopecia. (Courtesy of B Dunstan.) **A.** Glistening appearance of the skin on the medial aspect of the limb. **B.** Marked follicular atrophy.

corneum, giving the regions of affected skin the characteristic "glistening" or moist appearance. The lack of the stratum corneum may be due to licking by the cat. Inflammation is not a feature unless complicated by secondary infection. Footpads may be softened and hyperkeratotic. The pancreatic carcinoma is usually in an advanced stage, often with hepatic metastasis at the time of diagnosis and the prognosis is grave. The condition must be differentiated from hyperadrenocorticism and feline psychogenic alopecia.

Thymoma and concurrent **exfoliative dermatitis** has been reported in cats. Cats are usually aged and have signs such as dyspnea and coughing referable to an intrathoracic mass. Cutaneous lesions may be well developed prior to onset of respiratory signs. The cutaneous lesions consist of generalized, dry exfoliative dermatitis with multifocal ulceration, easily epilated hairs and variable pruritus. Histologically, marked orthokeratotic hyperkeratosis with patchy parakeratosis is usually present. The epidermis is hyperplastic with multifocal spongiosis and exocytosis of lymphocytes and variable neutrophils into the surface and follicular epithelium. The dermal component has been reported as either a perivascular mixed infiltrate or a lichenoid, lymphocytic dermatitis with hydropic changes in the basal epidermis and outer follicular root sheath. Epidermal and follicular keratinocyte apoptosis with lymphocytic satellitosis may be present. Some cases have been reported to also have a overgrowth of *Malassezia pachydermatis* and bacteria. It has been speculated that the presence of a thymoma initiates abnormal immunological responses responsible for the dermatitis, which at times can resemble erythema multiforme or graft vs. host dermatitis histologically.

Superficial necrolytic dermatitis (hepatocutaneous syndrome) has been reported in dogs and occasionally the cat. The condition is sometimes associated with **endocrine tumors of the pancreas** (see Nutritional diseases of skin).

Multiple **nodular dermatofibromas** of the distal limbs have been reported in middle-aged German Shepherd Dogs and occasionally other breeds (Golden Retriever, Boxer, Belgian Shepherd, mixed breed) in association with **renal cysts**, **renal cystadenocarcinomas** and/or **uterine leiomyomas** in the bitch. Both kidneys are often affected. The cutaneous lesions range from 2 mm to several centimeters and are comprised of mature, sparsely cellular bundles of collagen within the subcutis or occasionally the dermis (Fig. 5.118A, B). Animals may be presented for examination of the cutaneous lesions prior to signs referable to the internal neoplasms. Death occurs most often due to complications of the renal lesions. Nodular dermatofibrosis is suspected to be inherited in an autosomal dominant manner in German Shepherd Dogs.

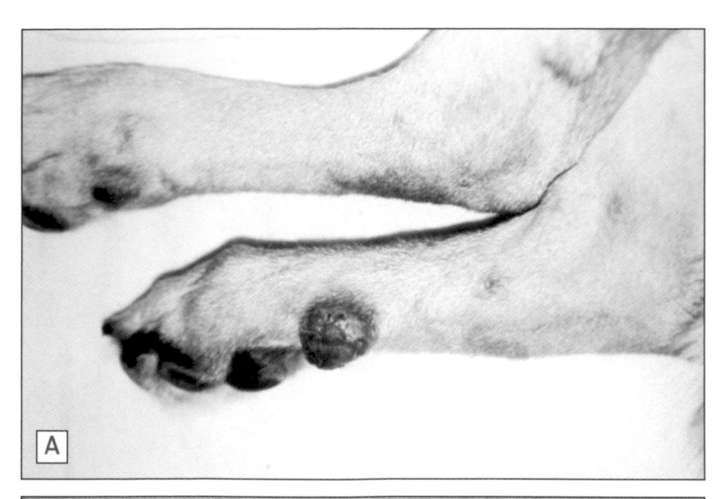

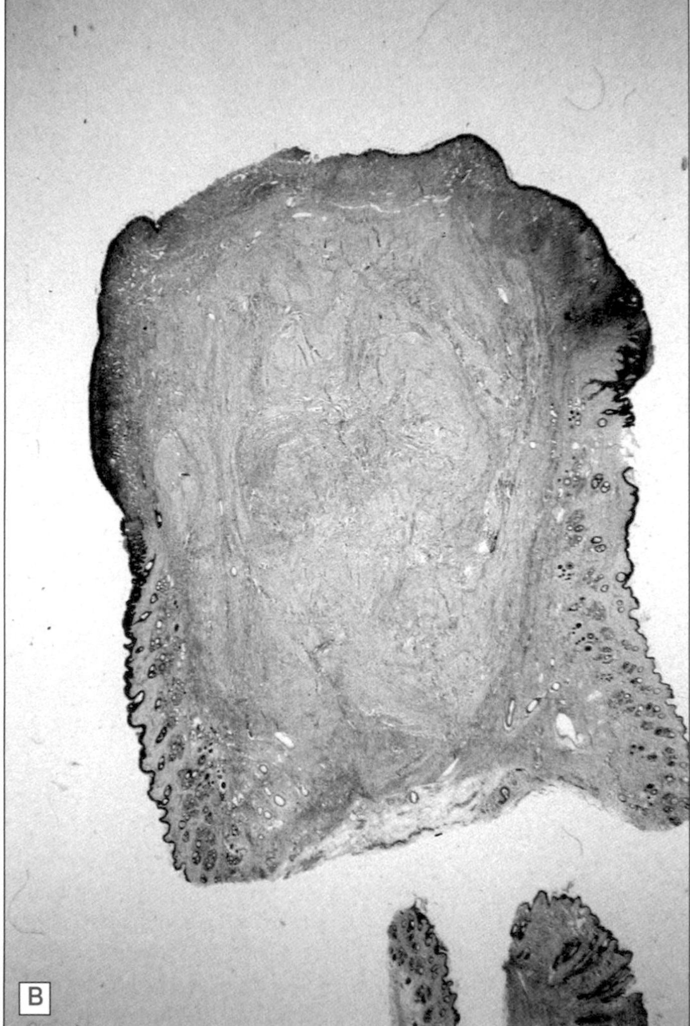

Figure 5.118 Dermatofibrosis in a German Shepherd Dog. (Courtesy of University of Florida Clinical Dermatology Service.) **A.** Protruding fibrous nodule on the distal limb. **B.** Nodule from (**A**) comprises sparsely cellular bundles of mature collagen.

Severe **generalized pruritus** without primary gross or histologic cutaneous lesions or other identifiable cause for pruritus has been reported in the dog and horse in association with underlying **malignant lymphoma**. Self-trauma can lead to extensive excoriations and secondary infection. This condition is also reported in humans with lymphoma and a variety of other internal malignancies. The mechanism of the development of pruritus is not understood but is speculated to be related to tumor-induced release of chemical mediators. Pruritus can only be relieved by successful treatment of the malignancy.

Paroxysmal **cutaneous flushing** of extensive areas of the skin without pruritus has been reported in a German Shepherd Dog with an intrathoracic mast cell tumor and pulmonary adenocarcinoma. Functional pheochromocytomas upon rare occasion can lead to cutaneous flushing in the dog. Flushing is due to vasodilation and is usually caused by vasoactive mediators.

Occasionally, vesicular, pustular or bullous dermatoses virtually identical to idiopathic autoimmune skin diseases may be associated with an underlying malignancy. The tumor is suspected to trigger the production of autoantibodies. These types of paraneoplastic dermatoses must be differentiated from true autoimmune skin diseases as the prognosis may vary. Differentiation is based on ruling out the presence of an underlying neoplasm and resolution of the skin lesions with tumor removal. A **subepidermal bullous stomatitis** microscopically identical to bullous pemphigoid has been reported in a horse in association with a hemangiosarcoma. Immunoprecipitation studies indicated the horse had antibodies to desmoplakin I and II, the bullous pemphigoid 230 antigen, and a 190 kDa antigen. This immunoprecipitation profile was consistent with that reported for **paraneoplastic pemphigus** as reported in humans and the dog. Paraneoplastic pemphigus is a form of pemphigus that is sometimes associated with an underlying malignancy and has been previously discussed (see Immune-mediated dermatoses).

Bibliography

Anderson RK, Carpenter JL. Severe pruritus associated with lymphoma in a dog. J Am Vet Med Assoc 1995;207:455–456.

Anhalt GJ, et al. An autoimmune mucocutaneous disease associated with neoplasia. New Engl J Med 1990;323:1729–1735.

Brooks DG, et al. Pancreatic paraneoplastic alopecia in three cats. J Am Anim Hosp Assoc 1994;30:557–563.

Castellano MC, et al. Generalized nodular dermatofibrosis and cystic renal disease in five German Shepherd dogs. Canine Pract 2000;25:18–21.

Day MJ. Review of thymic pathology in 30 cats and 36 dogs. J Small Anim Pract 1997;38:393–403.

Finley MR, et al. Paraneoplastic pruritus and alopecia in a horse with diffuse lymphoma. J Am Vet Med Assoc 1998;213:102–104.

Forster-van Hufte MA, et al. Resolution of exfoliative dermatitis and *Malassezia pachydermatis* overgrowth in a cat after surgical thymoma resection. J Small Anim Pract 1997;38:451–454.

Godfrey DR. A case of feline paraneoplastic alopecia with secondary *Malassezia*-associated dermatitis. J Small Anim Pract 1998;39:394–396.

Lemmens P, et al. Paraneoplastic pemphigus in a dog. Vet Dermatol 1998; 9:127–134.

Miller WH. Cutaneous flushing associated with intrathoracic neoplasia in the dog. J Am Anim Hosp Assoc 1992;28:217–219.

Pascal-Tenoria A, et al. Paraneoplastic alopecia associated with internal malignancies in the cat. Vet Dermatol 1997;7:221–226.

Scott DW, et al. Exfoliative dermatitis in association with thymoma in three cats. Feline Pract 1995;23:8–13.

Turek MM. Cutaneous paraneoplastic syndromes in dogs and cats: a review of the literature. Vet Dermatol 2003;14:279–296.

White SD, et al. Nodular dermatofibrosis and cystic renal disease in three mixed-breed dogs and a boxer dog. Vet Dermatol 1998;9:119–126.
Williams AA, et al. Paraneoplastic bullous stomatitis in a horse. J Am Vet Med Assoc 1995;207:331–334.

Eosinophilic and collagenolytic dermatitides

The presence of eosinophils in inflammation is usually considered to be an indication of a hypersensitivity reaction or parasitic infestation, however eosinophils can be seen in many diseases and complete understanding of the role of this leukocyte remains to be elucidated. Eosinophils produce lipid mediators that contribute to an acute allergic response, and also TGF-β that is associated with chronic inflammation and fibrosis. Eosinophil cytoplasmic granules contain four cationic proteins that are essential in host defense against parasites, however in the process of this defense the contents of the granules also cause severe tissue damage and contribute to the collagen degeneration and collagenolysis which are so common in many eosinophilic dermatitides. Eosinophilic inflammation in the horse and cat is a common tissue reaction and it seems that the chemotactic stimuli that attract neutrophils in most species attract both eosinophils and neutrophils in these two species.

Feline eosinophilic dermatoses

Cats have several distinct eosinophilic dermatitides, some of which have been previously collected under the term **eosinophilic granuloma complex**. These conditions include *feline eosinophilic granuloma, eosinophilic plaque, and indolent ulcer*. The collective term has been useful as a grouping since these conditions respond to similar treatments. Histologically these three conditions are distinct, although occasionally the features overlap. In addition, allergic dermatitis in cats, such as hypersensitivity to ectoparasites, atopy, and food allergic dermatitis, can demonstrate overlapping features, especially with eosinophilic plaque and occasionally with feline eosinophilic granuloma. Indeed eosinophilic plaque has been established as a hypersensitivity, and although not as yet fully characterized, eosinophilic granuloma and indolent ulcer may well eventually be shown to have an allergic basis. Cats with eosinophilic granuloma can also have eosinophilic plaque or indolent ulcer.

Feline eosinophilic plaque *is a common condition in cats and is a hypersensitivity reaction to food, fleas, or may be associated with atopy*. The condition can occur alone or together with miliary dermatitis, and in some cases the two conditions can form a continuum. It occurs most commonly in the inguinal, axillary, perineal or lateral thigh areas, although it can occur anywhere. *Lesions are pruritic, and affected cats lick them constantly*, resulting in raised, red, ulcerated plaques and patches that can develop peracutely. *Histologically the lesions are characterized by epidermal acanthosis and spongiosis with exocytosis of eosinophils* (Fig. 5.119A, B). In some cases there is epidermal and follicular epithelial mucinosis characterized by pale basophilic or gray mucin between keratinocytes. Inflammation in the dermis is diffuse or perivascular, markedly eosinophilic, and may extend into the subcutis. Mast cells, lymphocytes, and macrophages are present in smaller numbers.

Feline eosinophilic granuloma (feline collagenolytic granuloma, linear granuloma) is a common condition in cats. It can occur at any age, however is *more common in young cats*. Spontaneous regression can occur. An underlying hypersensitivity has been suggested as the cause however the condition may also occur in cats with no other evidence of allergic disease. A genetic predisposition has been documented in some cases. The lesions can be nodular or linear, and occur on the skin, footpads, mucocutaneous junctions, and in the oral cavity. Linear lesions are more common on the caudal or medial thigh and nodular lesions are more common on the lips, chin, oral cavity and face. The lesions are raised, pink and frequently alopecic. Histologically the lesions are characterized by *diffuse dermal inflammation composed primarily of eosinophils*, with fewer mast cells, macrophages, and occasional lymphocytes. *Within the inflammation are large irregular foci of collagen fibers and degranulated an degenerating eosinophils (flame figures)* (Fig. 5.120). These foci may be surrounded by macrophages and multinucleated giant cells. The epidermis may be acanthotic or ulcerated.

Indolent ulcer (rodent ulcer) is a common and clinically distinct condition in cats. The cause of these lesions is unknown. In

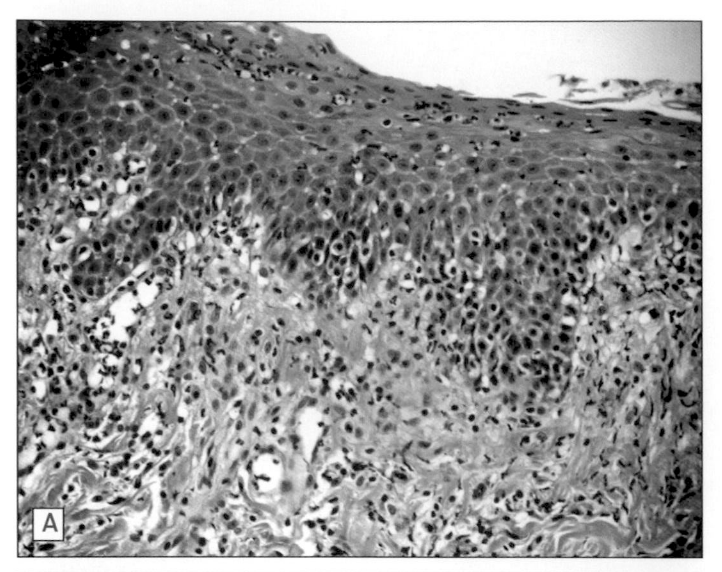

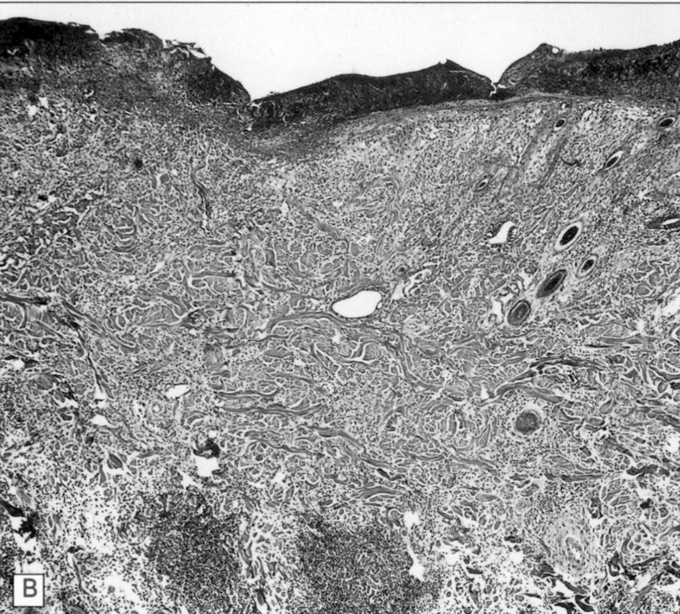

Figure 5.119 Feline eosinophilic plaque. A. Hyperplastic, spongiotic epidermis. **B.** Dermal infiltrate of eosinophils and mast cells.

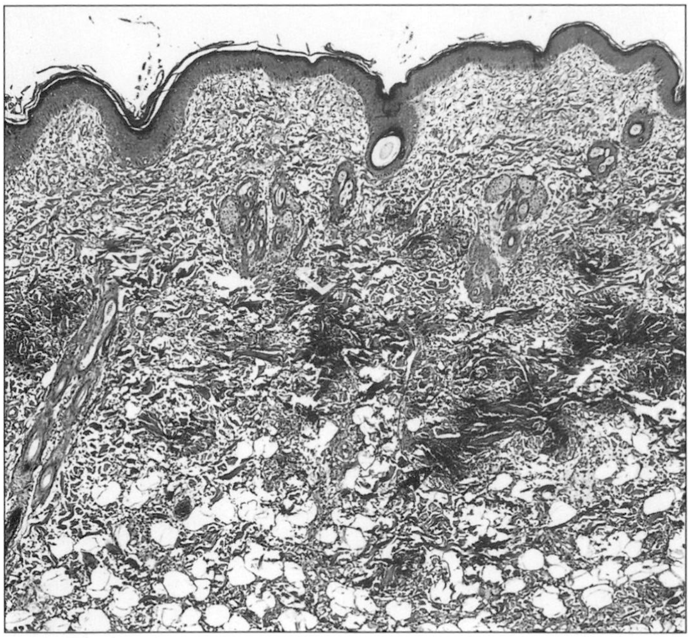

Figure 5.120 Eosinophilic granuloma in a cat. The dermis contains multiple foci of collagen fibers (arrow) surrounded by degranulated and degenerating eosinophils and mononuclear leukocytes (flame figures).

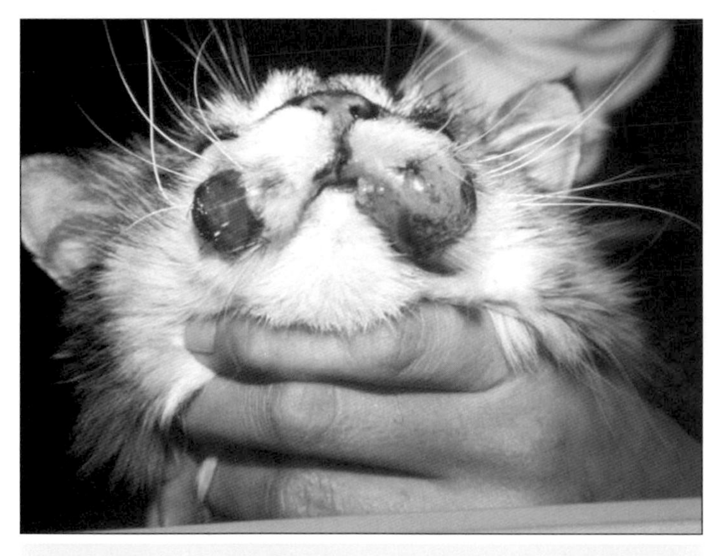

Figure 5.121 Feline indolent ulcer. Ulcerated lesions on the upper lips. (Courtesy of B Dunstan.)

some cats they are reported to be a manifestation of allergic disease, although in other cases an allergic etiology cannot be found. Affected cats can have concurrent eosinophilic granuloma or eosinophilic plaque, increasing the index of suspicion of an allergic etiology. *Clinically the condition is characterized by an ulcerated lesion on the upper lip adjacent to the philtrum that can be unilateral or bilateral* (Fig. 5.121). The ulcers are not pruritic or painful. Histologically the acute lesions are characterized by diffuse infiltrates of eosinophils with neutrophils, mast cells, and macrophages, however the lesions are more often biopsied in the chronic phase when the inflammation is composed almost entirely of lymphocytes, plasma cells, macrophages and neutrophils, together with fibrosis. The numbers of neutrophils vary according to the degree of ulceration.

Bibliography

Bardagi M, et al. Ultrastructural study of cutaneous lesions in feline eosinophilic granuloma complex. Vet Dermatol 2003;14:297–303.

Gross TL, Ihrke PJ. Nodular and diffuse diseases of the dermis with prominent eosinophils or plasma cells. In: Gross TL, et al., eds. Veterinary Dermatopathology. St. Louis, MO: Mosby Year Book, 1992:213–218.

Power HT, Ihrke PJ. Selected feline eosinophilic skin diseases. Vet Clin North Am: Small Anim Pract 1995;25:833–850.

Scott DW, et al. In: Muller and Kirk's Small Animal Dermatology. 6th ed. Philadelphia, PA: WB Saunders, 2001:1148–1153.

Yager JA, Wilcock BP. Color Atlas and Text of Surgical Pathology of the Dog and Cat: Dermatopathology and Skin Tumors. London: Wolfe M, 1994:146–149.

Canine eosinophilic granuloma

This is a *rare condition in dogs* that histologically has many similarities to feline eosinophilic granuloma. Any breed and age can be affected, however the condition appears to be more common in Siberian Huskies, in dogs under 3 years of age, and males. There may be a genetic basis for the disease in Siberian Huskies and Cavalier King Charles Spaniels. The etiology is unknown although a hypersensitivity has been proposed, due to the fact that the lesions are corticosteroid-responsive, the eosinophilic nature of the lesions, and that there is occasionally circulating eosinophilia. *The lesions can be nodules or plaques, and occur most commonly in the mouth and on the tongue*. Cutaneous lesions can be multiple and there is one report of a single lesion occurring in the external ear canal. *Histologically the lesions are composed of diffuse dermal eosinophilic inflammation within which are foci of degranulating eosinophils and degenerating collagen sometimes surrounded by epithelioid macrophages*. The overlying epithelium or epidermis may be acanthotic or ulcerated.

Bibliography

Bredal WP, et al. Oral eosinophilic granuloma in three Cavalier King Charles spaniels. J Small Anim Pract 1996;37:499–504.

Potter KA, et al. Oral eosinophilic granuloma of Siberian huskies. J Am Anim Hosp Assoc 1980;16:595–600.

Poulet FM, et al. Focal proliferative eosinophilic dermatitis of the external ear canal in four dogs. Vet Pathol 1991;28:171–173.

Equine eosinophilic nodular diseases

Eosinophilic inflammation is a common reaction pattern in the horse, and cutaneous nodules, either single or multiple, are common skin lesions in the horse. Nodular conditions of unknown etiology and pathogenesis include collagenolytic granuloma (nodular necrobiosis), axillary nodular necrosis, and unilateral papular dermatosis. Other eosinophilic nodular conditions with known etiologies, such as cutaneous habronemiasis, can look histologically similar (see Helminth diseases of skin). Cutaneous mast cell tumors in the horse can also be seen clinically as cutaneous nodular lesions, and, as histologically they may contain significant numbers of eosinophils and areas of necrosis, care should be taken to differentiate this tumor from an inflammatory eosinophilic lesion.

Collagenolytic granuloma (nodular necrobiosis, equine eosinophilic granuloma) is the *most common* of the equine cutaneous eosinophilic nodular diseases. The etiology is unknown. Hypersensitivity, especially to insect bites, has been suggested,

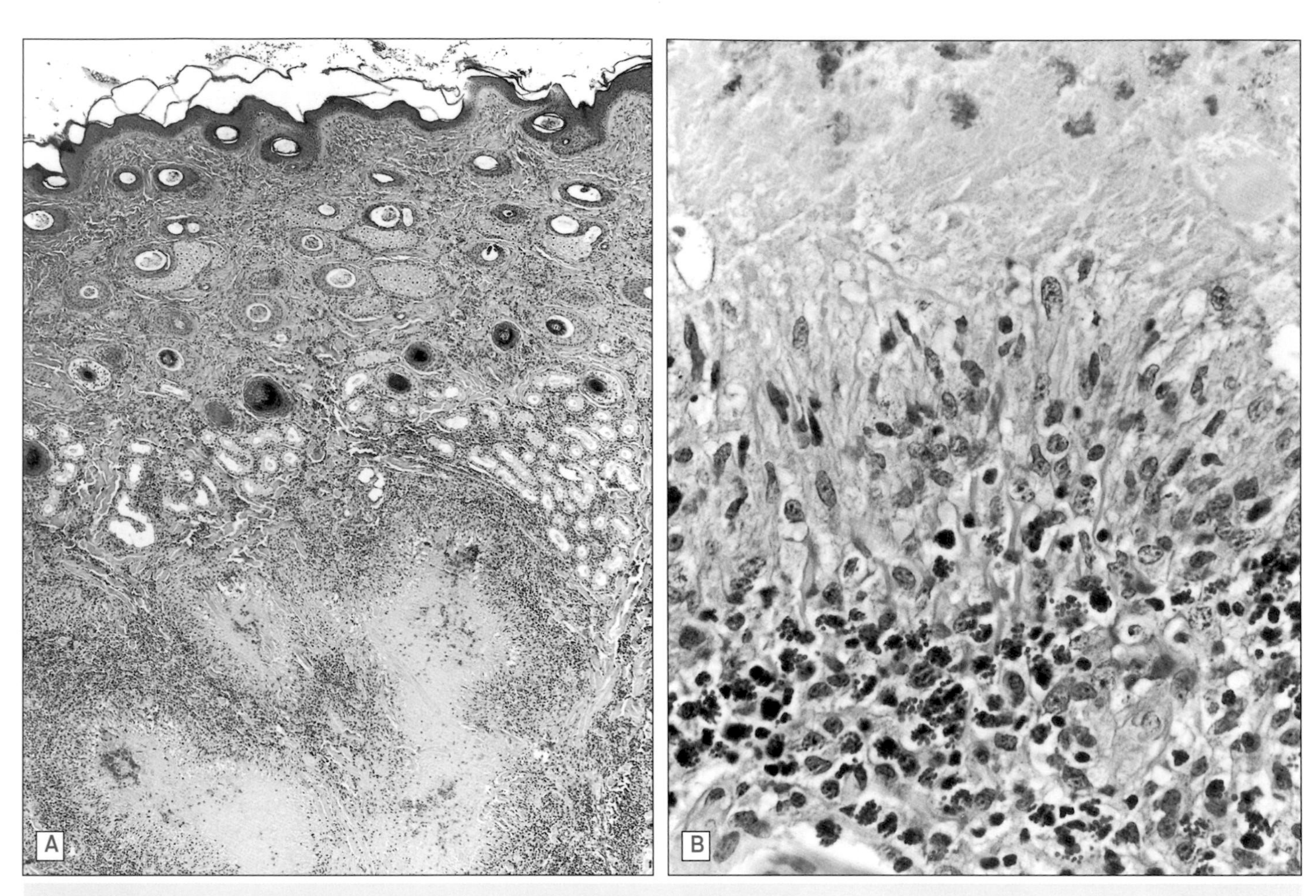

Figure 5.122 Equine nodular collagenolytic granuloma. A. Foci of collagen degeneration deep in the dermis. **B.** Degenerating collagen and degranulating eosinophils are surrounded by epithelioid macrophages and additional eosinophils.

however this has not been fully established. The lesions occur as single or multiple firm nodules measuring 0.5–5 cm in diameter, most commonly on the withers and back but can occur anywhere on the body, and can be generalized. *Histologically the dermal lesions are characterized by foci of dermal collagen degeneration that are surrounded by granulomatous inflammation, sometimes forming a palisading granuloma, and inflammation that is markedly eosinophilic* (Fig. 5.122A, B). Eosinophilic granulomas have also been reported associated with the silicone coating on needles at injection sites, however these lesions are clinically distinct as they tend to be linear, and can usually be documented to be at an injection site.

Axillary nodular necrosis is considerably less common than collagenolytic granuloma. The cutaneous and subcutaneous nodules are 1–5 cm in diameter and can be single or multiple. They are usually unilateral and occur on the trunk behind the axilla, which explains the colloquial term "girth galls." Trauma from tack can explain the ulceration of nodules but is not considered to the cause, which is currently unknown. *Histologically the lesions are characterized by foci of coagulative necrosis that may contain eosinophils, surrounded by eosinophilic and granulomatous inflammation.* Eosinophilic vasculitis can sometimes be found. The collagen degeneration that is a feature of collagenolytic granuloma is not usually a feature of axillary nodular necrosis.

Unilateral papular dermatosis is an uncommon condition in horses seen primarily in the United States, and is more common in spring and summer. It has been seen in many breeds although Quarter Horses appear to be over-represented. *Clinically the lesions are multiple cutaneous nodules and papules, measuring 2–10 mm, which occur in a unilateral distribution, usually on the trunk.* The etiology is unknown, however the seasonality of the lesions together with the eosinophilic nature of the histologic findings *suggests ectoparasite hypersensitivity*. It has further been suggested that the unilateral distribution may indicate direct contact hypersensitivity to an ectoparasite. *The histologic lesions are characterized by small foci of eosinophilic coagulative necrosis that are often folliculocentric, surrounded by eosinophilic dermal inflammation.* Histologic differentiation of this condition from the two preceding nodular diseases in horses, especially in the absence of folliculocentricity, can be problematic without a clinical description of the lesions.

Bibliography

Mathison PT. Eosinophilic nodular dermatoses. Vet Clin North Am: Equine Pract 1995;11:75–89.

Rothwell TL, Birch CB. Unilateral papular dermatitis in a horse. Aust Vet J 1991;68:122–123.

Slovis NM, et al. Injection site eosinophilic granulomas and collagenolysis in 3 horses. J Vet Intern Med 1999;13:606–612.

von Tscharner C, et al. Stannard's illustrated equine dermatology notes. Nodular diseases. Vet Dermatol 2000;11:179–186.

Multisystemic, eosinophilic, epitheliotropic disease in the horse

This rare disease typically occurs in young horses and is characterized by eosinophilic infiltration of many organs, with intestine and skin being most commonly affected. The cause of multisystemic, eosinophilic, epitheliotropic disease is unknown. Proposed etiologies have included viral, bacterial, and toxic mechanisms, however none of these has been confirmed. Recurrent episodes of type I hypersensitivity due to dietary, inhaled or parasitic antigens has been suggested in several reports. There is one report of this condition occurring concurrently with intestinal lymphosarcoma, and several other unpublished cases that appear identical to the case described; the authors suggest that the clonal proliferation of T lymphocytes triggers proliferation of eosinophils by secretion of cytokines such as IL-5. This mechanism has also been proposed in humans who have concurrent abnormal T-lymphocyte proliferations and hypereosinophilic syndrome. Affected horses are presented clinically with weight loss, pitting edema, and often with exudative, exfoliative dermatitis that usually originates at the coronary bands or head and becomes generalized. Eosinophilia is generally absent. Histologically the condition is characterized by *eosinophilic and lymphoplasmacytic infiltration of multiple organs, sometimes with eosinophilic granuloma formation.* Organs most commonly affected include pancreas, gastrointestinal tract, salivary glands, and skin. In the skin the inflammation may be perivascular and interstitial, with epidermal acanthosis and hyperkeratosis, and sometimes with spongiosis and eosinophilic exocytosis into eosinophilic subcorneal pustules.

Bibliography

Hillyer MH, Mair TS. Multisystemic eosinophilic epitheliotropic disease in a horse: attempted treatment with hydroxyurea and dexamethasone. Vet Rec 1992;130:392–395.

La Perle KMD, et al. Multisystemic, eosinophilic, epitheliotropic disease with intestinal lymphosarcoma in a horse. Vet Pathol 1998;35:144–146.

Schumacher J, et al. Chronic idiopathic inflammatory bowel diseases of the horse. J Vet Intern Med 2000;14:258–265.

Sterile eosinophilic folliculitis and furunculosis (eosinophilic furunculosis of the face)

This is an uncommon condition in **dogs** characterized by the sudden onset of painful folliculocentric nodules and papules with erosion or ulceration. The etiology of this condition has not been fully characterized, but *a hypersensitivity reaction to arthropod bites is strongly suspected.* The condition is most common in young, large breed dogs, and lesions are primarily seen on the dorsal muzzle, around the eyes, ears, and less commonly in the axillae, inguinal areas, and ventrum. Histologic lesions are characterized by predominantly folliculocentric eosinophilic inflammation. Eosinophilic luminal inflammation can lead to furunculosis, with free hair shafts surrounded by eosinophils and degranulating eosinophils. The dermal inflammation may be accompanied by edema and mucin deposition, and occasionally dermal collagen necrosis is present.

In **cats**, sterile eosinophilic folliculitis and furunculosis may be seen as a bystander lesion in any allergic dermatitis, however is more commonly seen in mosquito-bite hypersensitivity and feline herpesvirus dermatitis, both of which are most commonly located on the face and head. In **horses**, sterile eosinophilic folliculitis and furunculosis can be seen in any of the eosinophilic nodular conditions or hypersensitivities. However, other than unilateral papular dermatosis, the follicles are affected secondarily and the lesions are not folliculocentric. Sterile eosinophilic folliculitis has been reported in **cattle** and is characterized by multiple crusting or alopecic lesions primarily on the head, neck, and trunk.

Bibliography

Gross TL, Ihrke PJ. Feline mosquito-bite hypersensitivity. In: Gross TL, et al., eds. Veterinary Dermatopathology. St. Louis, MO: Mosby Year Book, 1992:210–212.

Guaguere E, et al. Eosinophilic furunculosis. A study of 12 dogs. Prat Med Chirurg Anim Cie 1996;31:413–419.

Hargis AM, et al. Ulcerative facial and nasal dermatitis and stomatitis in cats associated with feline herpesvirus 1. Vet Dermatol 1999;10:267–274.

Scott DW, et al. Sterile eosinophilic folliculitis in cattle. Agri-Pract 1986;7:8–14.

Scott DW, et al. Sterile eosinophilic folliculitis in the cat: an unusual manifestation of feline allergic skin disease? Comp Anim Pract 1989;19:6–11.

Eosinophilic dermatitis with edema

This is a rare condition in dogs. The cause is unknown, although hypersensitivity to drugs, arthropods, or diet is suspected. *It is characterized by erythematous macules and plaques primarily involving the ventral abdomen and ears*, and has been compared to Wells' syndrome (eosinophilic cellulitis) in humans. The histologic lesions are marked perivascular to diffuse eosinophilic dermatitis with edema, and occasional foci of collagen degeneration.

Bibliography

Holm KS, et al. Eosinophilic dermatitis with edema in nine dogs, compared with eosinophilic cellulitis in humans. J Am Vet Med Assoc 1999;215:649–653.

Feline relapsing polychondritis

Feline relapsing polychondritis is a rare condition in the cat characterized by bilateral dorsal or medial curling of the pinnae. The pinnae are discolored purple and markedly edematous. Histologically, lymphoplasmacytic infiltrates surround areas of necrosis of the auricular cartilage. The condition was named after a similar human condition thought to be an immune-mediated attack directed against type II collagen and known to affect other cartilaginous sites such as the nose, trachea, and cardiac valves. The pathogenesis in cats is not defined and despite the name, the condition in cats is not known to be recurrent. Too few cases have been studied to accurately document the clinical course or define association with other diseases.

Bibliography

Gerber B, et al. Feline relapsing polychondritis: two cases and a review of the literature. J Feline Med Surg 2002;4:189–194.

Rest JR. Floppy pinnae in Siamese cats. Vet Rec 1998;143:568.

Follicular lipidosis

Regional alopecia of areas of mahogany-colored points of the hair of the feet and face of young Rottweilers has been reported. Histologically, the lesions are characterized by vacuolation and nuclear pyknosis of the hair matrix cells of primary anagen hair follicles. Matrix cells of the bulb are most severely affected while cells of the internal and external root sheath are affected to a lesser degree. The vacuoles are clear or contain fine granular or clumped melanin. Hair shafts also contain occasional vacuoles and have irregular, thickened, or frayed cuticles. Ultrastructural examination and oil-red-O staining of additional sections confirm the vacuoles to be lipid. *This condition may represent yet another type of color-associated follicular dysplasia.* Too few cases have been recognized to clearly predict the clinical course of the alopecia, or to identify associated abnormalities or the mode of inheritance, if any. The cause has not been determined.

Bibliography

Gross TL, et al. Follicular lipidosis in three Rottweilers. Vet Dermatol 2001;8: 33–40.

Follicular mucinosis (alopecia mucinosa)

Follicular mucinosis is characterized by collections of mucin in the outer root sheath of the follicular epithelium and of sebaceous glands. Intraepithelial cysts filled with mucin may form. Grossly, the lesions consist of patchy alopecia and scaling. A disease resembling follicular mucinosis in humans has been described in the **cat** and **dog**. The condition described in 2 cats chiefly affected the head, neck, and shoulders. Histologically, there was mucinous degeneration of the outer root sheath of the follicular infundibulum. Both cats developed epitheliotropic lymphoma within several months of the initial biopsy. Follicular mucinosis has been reported in a 10-year-old male Labrador Retriever. The skin of the head, limbs, and some areas of the trunk were affected. In addition to the histologic lesions described above, there was a perivascular and perifollicular lymphocytic to plasmacytic infiltrate. The epidermis was mildly acanthotic with compact orthokeratosis and multifocal spongiosis with lymphocytic exocytosis. The basal cell layer demonstrated hydropic degeneration, mild apoptosis and prominent pigmentary incontinence. No follow-up information was available. In humans, follicular mucinosis can resolve spontaneously or become a chronic relapsing condition. Some cases are thought to progress to epitheliotropic lymphoma, but this is controversial. It should be noted that epidermal and epithelial mucinosis can be seen in various allergic dermatitides of the cat.

Bibliography

Bell A, Oliver F. Alopecia mucinosa (follicular mucinosis) in a dog. Vet Dermatol 1995;6:221–226.

Mehregan DA, et al. Follicular mucinosis: histopathologic review of 33 cases. Mayo Clin 1991;66:387–390.

Scott DW. Feline dermatology 1983–1985: "The secret sits". J Am Anim Hosp Assoc 1987;23:255–274.

Laminitis

The hoof wall is a complex structure composed of an epidermis and dermis that attaches to the underlying distal phalanx. The distal phalanx is held in place by interdigitation of the epidermal lamina of the inner hoof wall and the dermal lamina of the corium that is attached to the third phalanx. When these laminae fail, the forces of body weight, motion, and tendons lead to sinking and rotation of P3, shearing of vessels that supply these tissues, and damage to the corium of the sole and coronet. *The separation of the distal phalanx (coffin bone, P3) from the inner hoof wall is responsible for the severe clinical signs in laminitis*, rather than a primary inflammatory process. Laminitis occurs in all hoofed species, but particularly affects horses and cattle. *Laminitis is one of the most devastating of equine diseases, often leading to chronic debilitation or euthanasia.*

Precipitating events include trauma and generalized metabolic disturbances. In the horse, laminitis is sporadic, although fat, underexercised ponies are especially predisposed. Colic, sepsis, toxemia, episodes of diarrhea or shock, excessive water (after exercise), or lush pasture intake, carbohydrate overload, drug therapy, and intense training with repeated foot trauma ("road founder") have all been implicated as precipitating events in the horse. Black walnut (*Juglans nigra*) heartwood shavings toxicity causes natural disease in the horse.

Laminitis occurs sporadically in *dairy cows, heifers, fattening cattle, and young bulls*. In cattle, carbohydrate overload is also an important predisposing cause of laminitis. Others include metritis, mastitis, and ketosis. A heritable form has been reported in Jersey cattle in South Africa, the USA, and the UK. *Laminitis, not related to traumatic and metabolic episodes, occurs in all species but is important only in ungulates.* Erysipelas in lambs, the various causative types of footrot in pigs, sheep, and cattle, and bluetongue in sheep are examples of diseases in which degenerative and inflammatory changes occur in the laminae of the hoof.

The *pathogenesis* of metabolic laminitis remains incompletely understood although progress has been made. Past studies suggested that a *primary ischemic event* precipitated laminitis. Recent studies using an equine model of carbohydrate overload-induced laminitis indicate that degeneration of primary epidermal laminae and the basement membrane are responsible for the architectural changes in the hoof wall and the onset of clinical signs. Vascular events leading to ischemia also play an important role in laminitis but are now thought to occur as a consequence of the initial laminar degenerative changes. Events triggering the degeneration are still not completely defined, however bacterial-derived soluble factors generated in the equine large intestine have been shown in vitro to activate laminar enzymes capable of lysing components of the epidermal laminae. Two of these enzymes, metalloproteinase-2 (MMP-2) and metalloproteinase-9 (MMP-9) are present in normal laminar tissues and levels are increased in laminar tissues affected by laminitis. MMP-2, MMP-9, and inhibitors of MMP enzymes are thought to work in concert to regulate epidermal cell-to-cell detachment/attachment and cell-to-basement-membrane attachment during regular growth and maintenance of the laminar tissues. Cultured human keratinocytes increase production of MMP enzymes under the influence of TNF, IL-1 and TFG-1. Factors leading to increased production of MMP-2 and MMP-9 in the epidermal laminae during laminitis are not yet known.

The earliest changes evident in the laminar tissue anatomy during acute laminitis are elongation and disorganization of basal and parabasal keratinocytes and attenuation of the tips of the secondary epidermal laminae. The basement membrane of the secondary laminae detaches first in the region of parabasal cell attachment and subsequently in the region of the basal cells leaving aggregates of degenerating basement membrane components within the connective tissue space between the laminae. *Loss of the basement membrane leads to separation of the dermal and epidermal laminae of the hoof wall and is key in loss of structural integrity of the P3/hoof wall attachment.* Collapse of secondary laminae leads to loss of capillaries normally present within the connective tissue between the epidermal laminae. The loss of capillaries leads to increased resistance to blood flow, arteriovenous shunting, and eventual ischemic damage. This early stage is characterized clinically by a bounding digital pulse. Current research suggests that the progression of laminitis in the very early stages prior to degeneration of the epidermal laminae and basement membrane may possibly be slowed or halted by attempts to produce vasoconstriction in the foot (ice-packing). This slowing of circulation would theoretically decrease the delivery of cytokines or other factors responsible for induction of MMP activity.

Acute laminitis is seen as sudden lameness and severe pain affecting most commonly the forefeet but may affect all feet, or just the hind feet. An increase in the hoof wall temperature and a bounding digital pulse indicate marked vascular engorgement in the hoof tissues. In horses, pain is often severe enough to provoke systemic disturbances. A section through an acutely affected hoof reveals little gross alteration beyond congestion of the laminar dermis and occasionally hemorrhage. There is no hoof deformity, although the skin above the coronary band may be swollen. Horses with diffuse swelling and depression along the coronary band are often found to have acute separation and displacement of P3 and are referred to as "sinkers," a manifestation of acute laminitis. Microscopic changes are as described above. In addition, the dermis may be congested, edematous, and have mild hemorrhage and mild infiltrates of mononuclear cells. In time, coagulative necrosis of the secondary laminae may be evident.

Chronic laminitis is defined clinically as the phase commencing after several days of lameness or when *rotation of the third phalanx is first radiographically evident.* The rotation has been attributed to loss of the interlocking force normally supplied by the epidermal laminae. In chronic cases, the ventral deviation is caused also by irregular hyperplasia of epidermal laminae placing a wedge of epidermis between the phalanx and the immovable hoof wall. The weight of the animal, the leverage forces placed on the toe and the pulling forces of the deep digital flexor tendon contribute mechanically to the rotation. *In severely affected animals, the third phalanx may penetrate the sole,* which becomes convex. A mid-sagittal section through the hoof wall at this point will show obvious separation of P3 from the dorsal hoof wall, sinking and various degrees of rotation of P3. The corium at the coronary band and sole may be edematous or hemorrhagic. In long-standing cases, the space between the dorsal hoof wall and P3 is filled with firm white tissue (proliferative epidermis). The toe usually turns up and the cranial aspect of the hoof becomes concave and wrinkled by encircling horizontal ridges.

The chief microscopic lesion in chronic equine laminitis is marked irregular hyperplasia of the epidermal laminae. The regenerating secondary laminae may not regain their orderly arrangement and instead form irregular and anastomosing epidermal cords. The epidermal laminae, both primary and secondary, become markedly hyperkeratotic. The reason for the hyperkeratosis is not known. Both physical and physiologic influences on keratogenesis are likely altered in chronic laminitis. Similar epidermal lesions occur in chronic bovine laminitis, although parakeratotic hyperkeratosis develops in addition to the orthokeratotic hyperkeratosis. Alterations in the dermal vasculature are most prominent in cattle. Moderate-to-marked arteriolosclerosis and arteriosclerosis occur in chronic bovine laminitis, especially in the solar dermis. Other changes in laminitis in cattle include chronic dermal granulation tissue, organized and recanalized vascular thrombi, perineural fibrosis and perivascular accumulations of macrophages, often containing hemosiderin.

Bibliography

Bailey SR, et al. Current research and theories on the pathogenesis of acute laminitis in the horse. Vet J 2004;167:129–142.
Budras KD, et al. Light and electron microscopy of keratinization on the laminar epidermis of the equine hoof with reference to laminitis. Amer J Vet Res 1989;50:50–60.
Cripps PJ, Eustace RA. Factors involved in the prognosis of equine laminitis in the UK. Equine Vet J 1999;31:433–442.
Galey FD, et al. Black walnut (*Juglans nigra*) toxicosis: A model for equine laminitis. J Comp Pathol 1991;104:313–326.
Hood DM. The pathophysiology of developmental and acute laminitis. Vet Clin North Am Eq Pract 1999;15:321–343.
Johnson PJ, et al. Glucocorticoids and laminitis in the horse. Vet Clin North Am Equine Pract 2002;18:219–236.
Mungall BA, et al. *In vitro* evidence for a bacterial pathogenesis of equine laminitis. Vet Microbiol 2001;79:209–223.
Pollitt CC. Basement membrane pathology: a feature of acute equine laminitis. Equine Vet J 1996;28:38–46.
Pollitt CC. Equine laminitis: A revised pathophysiology. Proc Am Assoc Eq Pract 1999;45:188–192.
Sloet van Oldruitenborgh-Oosterbaan MM. Laminitis in the horse: A review. Vet Quart 1999;21:121–127.

Localized scleroderma

Localized scleroderma (morphea) is a rare disease of dogs and cats. *Asymptomatic, well-demarcated, sclerotic plaques that are alopecic, smooth and shiny characterize the condition.* Lesions tend to be linear and occur on the trunk, limbs, and head. Diffuse fibrosing dermatitis is seen histologically. Dense collagen bundles replace the entire dermis and subcutis. Pilosebaceous units are essentially absent. A mild superficial and deep perivascular accumulation of lymphohistiocytic cells is present. The pathogenesis is not defined. Affected animals are otherwise healthy and lesions have been reported to regress spontaneously in some cases.

Bibliography

Bensignor E, et al. Morphea-like lesion in a cat. J Small Anim Pract 1998;39:538–540.
Scott DW. Localized scleroderma (morphea) in two dogs. J Am Anim Hosp Assoc 1986;22:207–211.

Porcine juvenile pustular psoriasiform dermatitis

This disease of weanling pigs was originally named **pityriasis rosea**. Because the clinical signs and gross lesions bear little relationship to those of the human disease for which it was originally named, the new designation, porcine juvenile pustular psoriasiform dermatitis, has been suggested. *The disease is of no significance, except esthetic. The cause is not known.* A hereditary predisposition has been suggested but not proven, particularly in Landrace pigs. Lesions develop most often in weaned pigs 3–14 weeks of age. Entire litters or just a few piglets may be affected.

The disease begins with nonpruritic, small scaly, erythematous papules on the skin of the abdomen and inner thighs. The papules expand centrifugally to produce at first scaly plaques and later, when the central areas return to normal, ring-shaped, erythematous lesions (Fig. 5.123). As the rings expand, they coalesce to produce mosaic patterns and may extend to the sides and perineum. *The clinical differential diagnoses include swinepox, dermatosis vegetans, and ringworm.* The acute histologic lesion is superficial and deep perivascular dermatitis with eosinophils, neutrophils and mononuclear cells. Spongiosis and leukocytic exocytosis lead to the formation of spongiform pustules, and there is superficial dermal mucinous degeneration. Superficial epidermal necrosis may extend into the ostia of the hair follicles. As the lesions heal, marked psoriasiform hyperplasia and parakeratotic scale-crusts are predominant. The condition spontaneously resolves within about 4 wk.

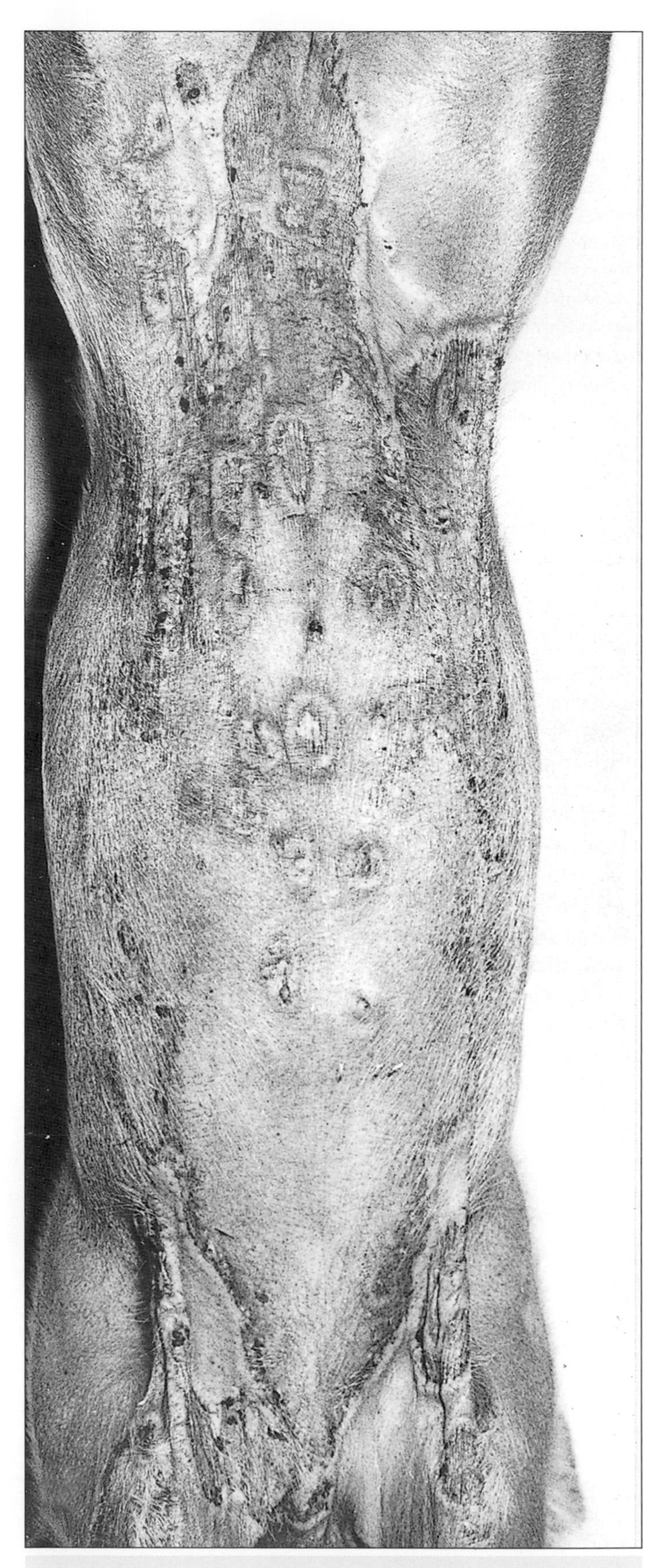

Figure 5.123 Porcine juvenile pustular dermatitis. Circular, ring, and coalescing lesions of the ventral abdomen and proximal limbs. (Courtesy of JA Flatla.)

Bibliography

Dunstan RW, Rosser EJ. Does a condition like human pityriasis rosea occur in pigs? Am J Dermatopathol 1986;8:86–89.

Kimura T, Doi K. Clinical and histopathological findings in pustular psoriaform dermatitis (pityriasis rosea) in pigs. J Vet Med Sci 2004;66:1147–1150.

Straw BE, et al., eds. Skin. In: Diseases of Swine. 8th ed. Ames, IA: Iowa State University Press, 1999:955.

Spiculosis

Spiculosis is a dysplastic and dyskeratotic condition of the hair follicle that results in 1–2 mm diameter and 0.5–2.0 cm long brittle spicules (hair shafts) protruding from hair follicles. The condition has been reported in humans and Kerry Blue Terriers. Clinically, the condition is characterized by coarse, brittle, and long hair shafts and pruritus, scaling, and alopecia of the skin of various areas of the body. Histologically, hair follicles have enlarged hair bulbs that may have two dermal papilla. Enlargement of the hair bulb is due to collections of heavily pigmented matrix cells that keratinize prematurely to form hyperpigmented keratinized amorphous masses or columns of unpigmented keratin in place of normal hairs.

Bibliography

McKeever PJ, et al. Spiculosis. J Am Anim Hosp Assoc 1992;28:257–261.

Sterile granulomas and pyogranulomas

Sterile granulomatous or pyogranulomatous dermatoses have been reported in dogs, cats, and less commonly in horses. Absence of microbial agents and foreign material and good response to glucocorticoid therapy has suggested an *immune-mediated pathogenesis*.

Sterile pyogranuloma syndrome

The sterile granuloma/pyogranuloma syndrome (idiopathic periadnexal multinodular granulomatous dermatitis) occurs in **dogs** of all ages and sexes but Collies, Boxers, Great Danes, Weimaraners, English Bulldogs, Doberman Pinschers, Dachshunds, and Golden Retrievers appear to be predisposed. The condition is clinically and, in many respects, histologically very similar to cutaneous reactive histiocytosis as described in dogs (see Histiocytic proliferative disorders). Future studies may indicate that these two entities are a single disorder. Most dogs have multiple asymptomatic haired to partially alopecic papules, nodules or plaques on the face and/or feet. Pedal lesions are frequently secondarily infected, ulcerative and fistulous. The pinnae, periocular region, trunk and abdomen may also be affected and lymphadenopathy may be present. Dogs are not systemically ill and the condition may spontaneously resolve or wax and wane. Histologic findings include *large perifollicular granulomas or pyogranulomas* that are elongated and vertically oriented that track hair follicles but do not invade them. Older lesions may become diffuse; obliterating adnexal structures and extending extend into the subcutis. Histiocytes, lymphocytes and neutrophils predominate, with occasional plasma cells or multinucleated giant cells.

Sterile granulomatous or pyogranulomatous dermatitis has also been reported in **cats**. Older male cats had multiple, pruritic, erythematous-to-violaceous papules, nodules and plaques, especially on the head and pinnae. Histologically these lesions were characterized by perifollicular pyogranulomatous dermatitis. Middle-aged female cats had pruritic, bilaterally symmetric, erythematous-to-purpuric plaques in the temporal regions. Histologically these lesions were characterized by nodular-to-diffuse granulomatous inflammation wherein multinucleated histiocytic giant cells, unexplained purpura and erythrophagocytosis, and a superficial dermal Grenz zone were prominent features.

The histologic differential diagnoses includes inflammation due to the presence of infectious agents or foreign material, sarcoidosis, sebaceous adenitis, and cutaneous reactive histiocytosis. Negative special stains for bacterial and fungal organisms, negative cultures, lack of polarization of foreign material on microscopic examination and failure to respond to antibiotics are supportive. Sebaceous glands are clearly the target of inflammation in sebaceous adenitis leading to somewhat regular and mid-dermal perifollicular location of inflammatory nodules. Lesions of cutaneous histiocytosis may be difficult to distinguish and both conditions may have a waxing and waning course. Distinct, organized granulomas are typically not present in cutaneous reactive histiocytosis whereas they may be present in sterile nodular pyogranuloma syndrome. Histiocytes are often larger, possibly atypical and may have numerous mitotic figures in cutaneous reactive histiocytosis.

"Sarcoidal" granulomatous disease

Sarcoidosis in humans is a systemic granulomatous disease of undetermined etiology. The granulomas are characteristic, being composed predominantly of epithelioid macrophages with few lymphocytes ("naked" granulomas).

A sterile "sarcoidal" granulomatous dermatitis has been described in **dogs** and **horses**. Dogs develop multiple erythematous papules, nodules and plaques that were neither pruritic nor painful. The lesions most commonly affected the neck and trunk. Nodular-to-diffuse sarcoidal granulomatous inflammation was present histologically.

Equine generalized granulomatous disease is characterized by exfoliative dermatitis, wasting, and sarcoidal granulomatous inflammation in multiple organ systems and is discussed in more detail in Vetch toxicosis and vetch-like diseases.

Bibliography

Carpenter JL, et al. Idiopathic periadnexal multinodular granulomatous dermatitis in twenty-two dogs. Vet Pathol 1987;24:5–10.

Scott DW, et al. Idiopathic sterile granulomatous and pyogranulomatous dermatitis in cats. Vet Dermatol 1991;1:129–137.

Scott DW, Noxon JO. Sterile sarcoidal granulomatous skin disease in three dogs. Canine Pract 1990;15:11–18.

Torres SMF. Sterile nodular dermatitis in dogs. Vet Clin North Am 1999;29:1311–1323.

Yager JA, Wilcock BP. Nodular and /or diffuse dermatitis. In: Color Atlas and Text of Surgical Pathology of the Dog and Cat. Spain: Mosby-Year Book, 1994: 141–143.

Sterile nodular panniculitis

Panniculitis refers to inflammation of the subcutaneous adipose tissue. Panniculitis has many causes, most of which have been discussed in previous sections (bacteria, fungi, immune-mediated disease, trauma, injection of irritant substances, foreign bodies, nutritional disorders, adverse reactions to vaccines or other injections, pancreatic disease). *The syndrome of sterile nodular panniculitis currently is considered to be idiopathic and the diagnosis is largely based on elimination of known causes of panniculitis, particularly panniculitis due to infectious agents.* It is likely that future studies will provide insight into the pathogenesis of lesion formation and define specific diseases now grouped within this syndrome.

In sterile nodular panniculitis, adipose tissue is the primary target of inflammation. Excisional biopsy is necessary to establish the diagnosis as the lesions are often confined to the subcutis and deep dermis. It is a rare condition affecting **dogs, cats**, and **horses**. There is no age or breed predisposition in cats or horses but, in dogs, affected animals are usually young (<1 yr) and Dachshunds and Poodles are over-represented.

The gross lesions are subcutaneous nodules that may become cystic, ulcerate or develop fistulous tracts. The exudate may be oily, serosanguineous, or hemorrhagic. Lesions are often multiple, 0.5 to several centimeters in diameter and may be grouped or distributed widely (Fig. 5.124). There is a tendency for the canine lesions to affect the trunk. Lesions in the horse are most often found on the neck, thorax, abdomen, and proximal limbs and may elicit pain upon palpation. *The microscopic lesion is lobular panniculitis that varies from necrotizing, to pyogranulomatous or granulomatous, to fibrotic, depending on the stage of the lesion.* Lipid released from damaged

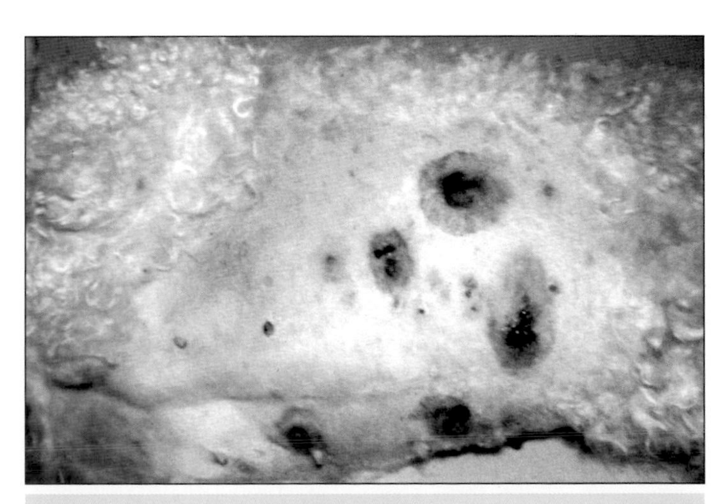

Figure 5.124 Sterile nodular panniculitis. Note multiple draining lesions on the trunk.

lipocytes hydrolyzes to glycerol and fatty acids. Fatty acids incite further inflammation that perpetuates the lesions. Affected animals with single lesions may be asymptomatic while animals with multiple lesions often have pyrexia, lethargy, and anorexia. A normochromic, normocytic nonregenerative anemia is seen in chronically affected animals with multiple extensive lesions. *Sterile panniculitis is indistinguishable histologically from the panniculitides of infectious cause.* The lesions fail to respond to antibiotics but resolve with corticosteroid therapy, sometime leaving residual scars. Some cases spontaneously regress. The condition can be recurrent.

Necrotizing panniculitis

Panniculitis secondary to pancreatitis and pancreatic neoplasia is well-recognized in humans. *Necrotizing cutaneous lesions are rare complications of pancreatic disease in the dog.* Cases have been reported in a dog with pancreatic carcinoma and one with pancreatic nodular hyperplasia. The pathogenesis likely pertains to the release of pancreatic lipases.

The lesions are multifocal, erythematous, nonpruritic cutaneous nodules, which may ulcerate centrally and discharge seropurulent exudate. Histologically, the lesion is necrotizing panniculitis in which mineralization of the lipocytes is a predominant feature. The initial inflammatory reaction is neutrophilic but may become granulomatous with time.

Bibliography

Bassage LH, et al. Sterile nodular panniculitis associated with lameness in a horse. J Am Vet Med Assoc 1996;209:1242–1244.

Dagleish MP, et al. Serum alpha-1-proteinase inhibitor concentration in 2 Quarter Horse foals with idiopathic pyogranulomatous panniculitis. Equine Vet J 2000;32:449–452.

German AJ, et al. Sterile nodular panniculitis and pansteatitis in three weimaraners. J Small Anim Pract 2003;44:449–455.

Hughes D, et al. Serum alpha1-antitrypsin concentration in dogs with panniculitis. J Am Vet Med Assoc 1996;209:1582–1584.

Mason KV. Disseminated necrotizing panniculitis associated with pancreatic carcinoma in a dog. Proc Amer Acad Vet Derm 1989:61.

Menzies-Gow NJ, et al. Chronic nodular panniculitis in a three-year-old mare. Vet Rec 2002;151:416–419.

Rothstein E, et al. Sterile pyogranuloma syndrome. J Am Anim Hosp Assoc 1997;33:540–543.

Torres SMF. Sterile nodular dermatitis in dogs. Vet Clin 1999;29:1311–1323.

Symmetrical lupoid onychodystrophy

Symmetrical lupoid onychodystrophy (SLO) is a degenerative disease of the nailbed in **dogs**. A wide variety of breeds and both male and females are affected. Dogs between 1–8 years are more commonly affected. German Shepherd Dogs, Rottweilers, Miniature Schnauzers, Golden and Labrador Retrievers, Boxers, and Greyhounds may be predisposed. The condition is characterized initially by brown discoloration of the proximal nailbed followed by separation and sloughing of one or more of the claws of multiple feet in otherwise healthy dogs. The condition is painful and often leads to lameness. Amputation of the third phalanx of affected digits to include nailbed epithelium is often needed to establish the diagnosis. Histologic lesions are most pronounced on the dorsal aspect of the claw. *The most common changes are a lichenoid interface dermatitis with lymphocytic exocytosis and spongiosis and multifocal hydropic degeneration of the basal epidermis.* Pigmentary incontinence may be severe and there may be dermal hemorrhage or fibrosis and mucinosis of the deep dermis. Direct immunofluorescence for deposits of immunoglobulin have not revealed specific labeling. Nails regrow but are misshapen, dry, soft or brittle and discolored. Secondary bacterial infection may occur. *The pathogenesis of SLO is not known* and, in fact, the possibility that SLO is not a specific disease entity but merely an inflammatory reaction typical for the nailbed has not been ruled out. Amputation of the third phalanx and histopathological evaluation of this tissue is a relatively new procedure. *The clinical differential diagnoses includes pemphigus, lupus erythematosus, vasculitis, keratinization disorders, and bacterial or fungal infection.*

Bibliography

Ovrebo Bohnhorst J, et al. Antinuclear antibodies (ANA) in Gordon setters with symmetrical lupoid onychodystrophy and black hair follicular dysplasia. Acta Vet Scand 2001;42:323–329.

Scott DW, et al. Symmetrical lupoid onychodystrophy in dogs: A retrospective analysis of 18 cases (1989–1993). J Am Anim Hosp Assoc 1995;31:194–201.

NEOPLASTIC AND REACTIVE DISEASES OF THE SKIN AND MAMMARY GLANDS

Epithelial tumors of the skin

Epithelial tumors of the skin are classified according to the predominant pattern of differentiation and the biological behavior. Recent refinements of the classification of a number of these tumors according to the World Health Organization International Histological Classification of Tumors of Domestic Animals have led to changes in nomenclature. These changes may not be widely accepted, as justification for reclassification based on prognosis or response to therapy has not been forthcoming. The decision to classify a given tumor as one or another of the epidermal or adnexal tumors is often quite arbitrary. A neoplasm of the multipotential germinal cells of the epidermis may differentiate into a number of types of epithelial cells characteristic of mature cells of the various components of the epidermis or adnexa. Sometimes the differentiation results in a distinctive group of tumor cells, making precise identification unequivocal. At other times, the tumor cells may differentiate toward several skin structures forming squamous cells, sebaceous cells or components of the hair follicle. The tumor can then be named according to the most aggressive or dominant cell type within the tumor. Other than squamous cell carcinomas, the majority of tumors derived from the epidermis or adnexa exhibit benign behavior.

Tumors of the epidermis include squamous papilloma, squamous cell carcinoma, and basal cell tumors. *Adnexal tumors of follicular origin* include infundibular keratinizing acanthoma (intracutaneous cornifying epithelioma, keratoacanthoma), tricholemmoma, trichoblastoma, trichoepithelioma, and pilomatricoma. *Adnexal tumors arising from glandular structures* include sebaceous gland tumors, apocrine gland tumors, and eccrine gland tumors. Also included in this section are varieties of tumor-like or keratin-filled cystic lesions that can be confused with true neoplasms. Mention will be made also of tumors that metastasize to the skin.

Cysts, hamartomas, and tumor-like lesions

Cysts

Infundibular cysts (epidermoid cyst, epidermal cyst, epidermal inclusion cyst) are seen as single or multiple, smooth, most often unilocular, spherical dermal nodules seldom larger than 1 cm in diameter. *Each nodule consists of an orderly wall of stratified squamous epithelium identical to epidermis, with gradual keratinization at its luminal surface* (Fig. 5.125A, B). *The cyst lumen is filled with concentric laminations of keratin.* There is usually neither mineralization nor inflammation within the cyst. The basal layer of the cyst wall abuts dermal collagen in a smooth line analogous to the normal dermal–epidermal junction. In longstanding lesions, the epithelial wall may become very thin, and *rupture may release entrapped keratin to stimulate pyogranulomatous dermal inflammation*. Infundibular cysts may arise from dilatation of the infundibulum of occluded hair follicles, and indeed occasionally one can detect superficial dermal scarring that may support this hypothesis. As well, such cysts may contain fragments of mature hair shafts. Other cysts arise from traumatic, developmental or surgical implantation of epidermal fragments into dermis or subcutis. Penetrating grass seeds cause implantation of epidermal fragments in **sheep**. Occasionally, an epidermal inclusion cyst (*subungual epidermal inclusion cyst*) can be found within the bone of the third phalanx of the **dog**. One report in the dog documents multiple squamous cell carcinomas arising from multiple infundibular cysts in a dog. In the **horse**, epidermal inclusion cysts are most commonly reported to occur in the nasal diverticulum (*atheromas*) or at the base of the ear (*dentigerous cysts*).

Isthmus cyst is a cyst lined by a keratinizing epithelium that lacks a granular layer. The inner layers of the epidermis lining the cyst have large amounts of pale eosinophilic cytoplasm and inconspicuous intercellular bridges.

Panfollicular cyst (trichoepitheliomatous cyst, hybrid cyst) is lined by stratified squamous epithelium that includes areas resembling both the infundibular cyst and isthmus cyst. In addition, areas of squamous epithelium comprised of primitive basal cells with abrupt keratinization to shadow cells may be present.

Dilated pore of Winer is a flask-shaped epidermal cyst on the head or neck of middle-aged or old cats and rarely, dogs. It is connected to the skin surface by a pore. It differs from the infundibular cyst in that the stratified keratinizing epithelium of the cyst wall near its base is hyperplastic with very regular rete ridges in parallel columns. For practical purposes, *it is yet another variant of epidermal/follicular cyst.*

Keratoma (horn cyst, horn tumor, keratin cyst) is a keratin-filled cyst arising from the coronary band. They are seen in cloven-hoofed animals and have been most often reported in the **horse**. The cysts are 1–5 cm in diameter and grow distally, between the third phalanx and the hoof wall. Keratomas are painful, causing lameness and bulging of the affected area of the hoof wall. *Histologically, the cyst is lined by squamous epithelium of the primary epidermal lamellae and filled with laminated keratin that in some cases may mineralize.* Trauma to the hoof wall and infection have been suggested, though not proven, causes of keratomas.

Dermoid cysts (dermoid sinus) are congenital lesions found in young animals along the dorsal midline. They arise by developmental failure of epidermal closure along embryonic fissures that

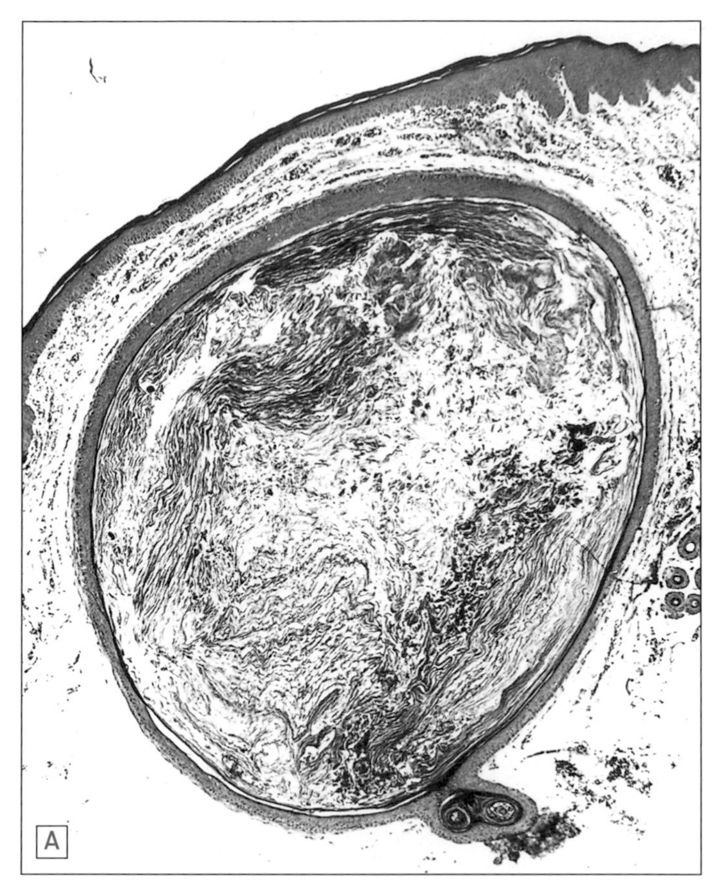

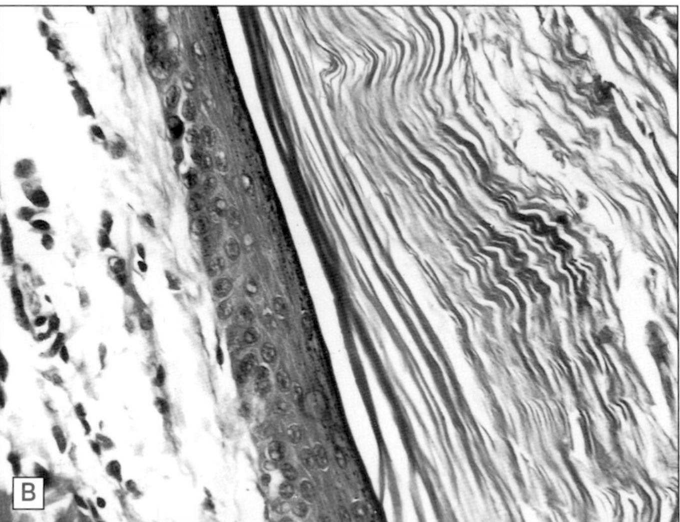

Figure 5.125 Infundibular cyst. A. Cyst filled with laminated keratin. **B.** Simple wall formed by an epidermis with gradual keratinization.

maroons an island of multipotential ectoderm within the subcutis. Some dermoid cysts may extend deep into the tissue and be connected to the dura mater of the spinal cord. Some, such as those occurring in Rhodesian Ridgeback **dogs**, actually retain a sinus pore to the skin surface (see Congenital and hereditary diseases of skin). Dermoid cysts are common in some families of Boxer dogs and affected animals have multiple cysts along the midline of the skin over the forehead. In the **horse**, dermoid cysts occur most often on the midline between the withers and the rump. Dermoid cysts contain keratin and hair fragments and sometimes sebaceous secretions. The dermis abutting the cyst wall has numerous hair follicles, sebaceous glands and occasionally, apocrine glands. Specimens with only hair follicle differentiation may be confused with unilocular trichoepitheliomas, but the dermoid cyst has gradual keratinization rather than abrupt trichilemmal keratinization.

Apocrine cysts may be single or multiple and are filled with clear secretions and lined by a single layer of apocrine cells. The lining may form intraluminal papillary projections. In some animals, particularly dogs, apocrine cysts can be multiple and numerous. The observation of very orderly proliferation, especially if in multiple sites, should lead to a diagnosis of hyperplasia. This condition is referred to as *apocrine gland cystomatosis* (cystic hyperplasia of apocrine glands) and currently is of undetermined etiology. It is most common in middle aged to older male dogs. Expression of epidermal growth factor was detected in the epithelial cyst lining in one case of apocrine gland cystomatosis in an Old English Sheepdog.

Hamartomas

Hamartomas are *disorganized and excessive amounts, or enlarged components, of mature tissue elements indigenous to the site in which they arise.* Most hamartomas are congenital. Hamartomas grow independent of the growth of the animal and hence may enlarge later in life and become a problem. **Epidermal hamartomas** (pigmented epidermal nevus) grossly appear as focal hyperkeratotic and hyperpigmented plaques. Histologically, there is epidermal papillary hyperplasia and hyperpigmentation of the lower epidermis. The stratum granulosa has enlarged keratohyaline granules. In the dog, an association with papilloma virus infection has been documented in some cases. **Follicular hamartomas** have been reported in the dog and consist of collections of very large primary hair follicles and associated glands surrounded by variable amounts of collagen. The hair follicles extend into the subcutis. Clinically, the lesions may be focal or form rugose, disfiguring nodular to plaque-like lesions with large protruding hairs. **Fibroadnexal hamartomas** (adnexal nevus, focal adnexal dysplasia, folliculosebaceous hamartoma) consist of aggregates of markedly distorted and variably inflamed folliculosebaceous units surrounded by dense collagen and lacking a connection to the skin surface. Some pathologists believe this type of lesion is a result of trauma and is not a true hamartoma.

Tumor-like lesions

Idiopathic squamous papillomas *(warts) are 1–5 mm papillary masses comprised of hyperplastic stratified squamous epithelium supported by dermal projections.* The maturation of the epidermis is orderly and does not show viral-induced cytopathic effects as seen in viral papillomas. These lesions are most often seen on the eyelids, face, conjunctiva, or footpads of older dogs and occasionally cats.

Cutaneous horns *are exophytic cylindrical formations of compact keratin* a few millimeters in diameter and 1–2 cm in length formed by an underlying markedly hyperplastic epithelium. Orthokeratotic hyperkeratosis predominates. Cutaneous horns may arise from squamous papillomas, infundibular keratinizing acanthomas, or dilated pores of Winer. Cutaneous horns of the footpad of cats have been associated with feline leukemia virus infection. One report in a cat cites a concurrent cutaneous horn and multiple squamous cell carcinoma in situ.

Warty dyskeratoma is an endophytic growth comprised of a markedly hyperplastic epidermis demonstrating extensive dyskeratosis and suprabasilar acantholysis.

Xanthomas (*xanthogranulomas*) are single to multiple nodular lesions occurring most often in the cat and occasionally in the dog. Clinically, the lesions are *asymptomatic yellow to white nodules, plaques or dermal papules.* In cats, xanthogranulomas are most often found on the face, legs, trunk, or footpads while in the dog the lesions appear on the face, ears, and ventrum. Histologically, the xanthogranulomas are dermal to subcutaneous collections of large foamy macrophages and multinucleated giant cells interspersed among deposits of cholesterol and triglycerides that appear as arrays of clear lenticular clefts and lakes of extracellular pale staining material. Disorders of metabolism such as hyperlipidemia, diabetes mellitus, or high cholesterol diets lead to the formation of xanthogranulomas in most cases, while other cases, particularly solitary xanthomas, are idiopathic. *The histologic differential diagnosis includes granulomatous inflammation associated with infectious agents, such as feline leprosy.* The presence of cholesterol clefts and free lipid and lack of detection of infectious agents should lead to the diagnosis of xanthogranuloma.

Bibliography

Fadok VA. Overview of equine papular and nodular dermatoses. Vet Clin N Amer 1995;11:69–70.

Goldschmidt MH, et al. Histological classification of epithelial and melanocytic tumors of the skin of domestic animals. Washington DC: Armed Forces Institute of Pathology, 1998.

Goldschmidt MH, Shofer FS. Skin Tumors of the Dog and Cat. Oxford, England: Pergamon Press, 1992.

Gross TL, et al. Veterinary Dermatopathology: A Macroscopic and Microscopic Evaluation of Canine and Feline Skin Disease. St. Louis, MO: Mosby-Year Book, 1992.

Hamir AN, et al. Equine keratoma. J Vet Diagn Invest 1992;4:99–100.

Scott DW, et al., eds. Muller and Kirk's Small Animal Dermatology. 6th ed. Philadelphia, PA: WB Saunders, 2001.

Scott DW, Teixeira EAC. Multiple squamous cell carcinomas arising from multiple cutaneous follicular cysts in a dog. Vet Dermatol 1995;6:27–31.

Vilafranca M, et al. Generalized apocrine gland cystomatosis in an Old English sheepdog. Vet Dermatol 1994;3:83–87.

Tumors of the epidermis

Papilloma and fibropapilloma

Cutaneous papillomas are benign proliferative epithelial neoplasms that have a complex etiology and pathogenesis. The differences in site preference, clinical course and histology of such lesions have been made more understandable by the discovery that *most papillomas are caused by infection with a host- and often site-specific papillomavirus* of the family Papovaviridae.

Not all papillomas are caused by or contain viruses. The nonviral lesion is considered to be an idiopathic squamous papilloma and is described in tumor-like lesions. Papillomaviruses are associated with skin papillomas in all domestic and many nondomestic species. Immunocompromised animals have increased susceptibility to papillomavirus infection. Cattle, horses and dogs are most frequently affected. In each species, there are several viruses distinguishable by gene sequencing, and in most instances each identified virus type has a preferred site for replication and, except for bovine papillomaviruses, seems highly species-specific. *In general, papillomaviruses induce two types of cutaneous lesions – squamous papilloma and fibropapilloma* – but lesions of intermediate type are common. While some of the variation in anatomic localization or histologic pattern appears to result from management practices and routes of inoculation, the different viral strains themselves seem to have site preferences and typically induce one or the other histologic reaction (papilloma or fibropapilloma).

Advances in immunohistochemical localization of the viral antigens or detection via gene probes has greatly increased the sensitivity of viral detection, permitting retrospective studies on fixed tissues for the presence of the viral genome. Viral papillomas may regress due to cell-mediated immune attack, may persist, or may progress to squamous cell carcinomas. While some viral and host factors are known to influence the behavior of viral-induced papillomas and fibropapillomas, many other factors are not yet defined.

The typical papilloma is a 1–2 cm wart-like, filiform, exophytic, and hyperkeratotic mass composed of hyperplastic epidermis supported by thin, inconspicuous dermal stalks with dilated capillaries. Lesions can be anatomically extensive and multiple (Fig. 5.126A). The stratum corneum exhibits variable degrees of ortho- to parakeratotic hyperkeratosis. Most of the hyperplasia is due to marked expansion of stratum spinosum cells, which have pale basophilic cytoplasm (Fig. 5.126B). Cells of the spinous and/or granular layer have ballooning degeneration of their cytoplasm and eccentric pyknotic nuclei (*koilocytes*). Degenerating keratinocytes may have condensed *eosinophilic cytoplasmic inclusions that represent aggregates of keratin*, a result of the viral cytopathic effect. These inclusions should not be confused with the cytoplasmic inclusions associated with poxvirus infections. The stratum granulosum has large, irregularly shaped eosinophilic keratohyalin granules. Cells of the stratum spinosum and granulosum may have vesicular nuclei with intranuclear pale basophilic viral inclusions that contain virus particles visible with electron microscopy and viral antigen detectable by immunohistochemistry, but these may not be numerous. A variant of the typical squamous papilloma is the **inverted papilloma** that shares the same morphological features, as the typical squamous papilloma except the lesion is endophytic, residing in an invagination of the epidermis. Inverted papillomas have been described as arising in the nailbed of dogs as well as on the skin.

Fibropapillomas *appear as nodules or plaques covered by a variably hyperplastic and hyperkeratotic epidermis.* Classic examples of fibropapillomas are the *equine sarcoid* and *feline fibropapilloma* (see Spindle cell tumors). Microscopic lesions typical of fibropapillomas include the features of acanthosis, hyperkeratosis and downgrowth of rete ridges, but the dermal proliferation predominates. The proliferating cell is a large, plump fibroblast. The cells are arranged in haphazard whorls and fascicles rather than in perpendicular sheets as in granulation tissue. In some the epidermal proliferation is minimal and is seen only as slight acanthosis and accentuation of rete pegs, while in others the hyperplasia resembles full-fledged papillomas.

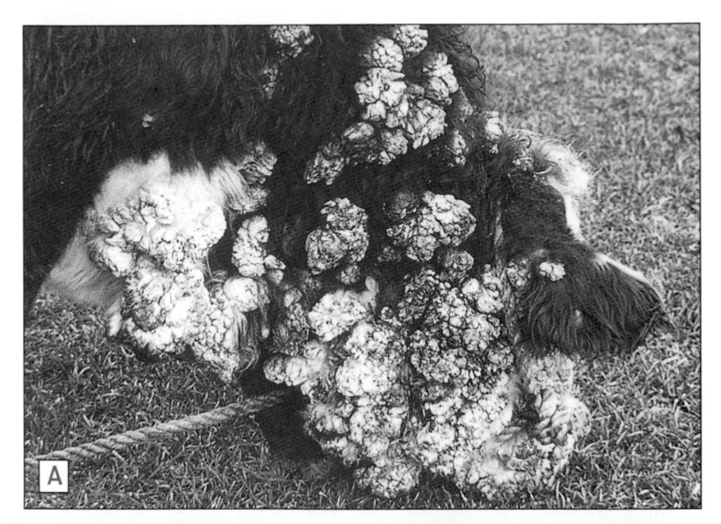

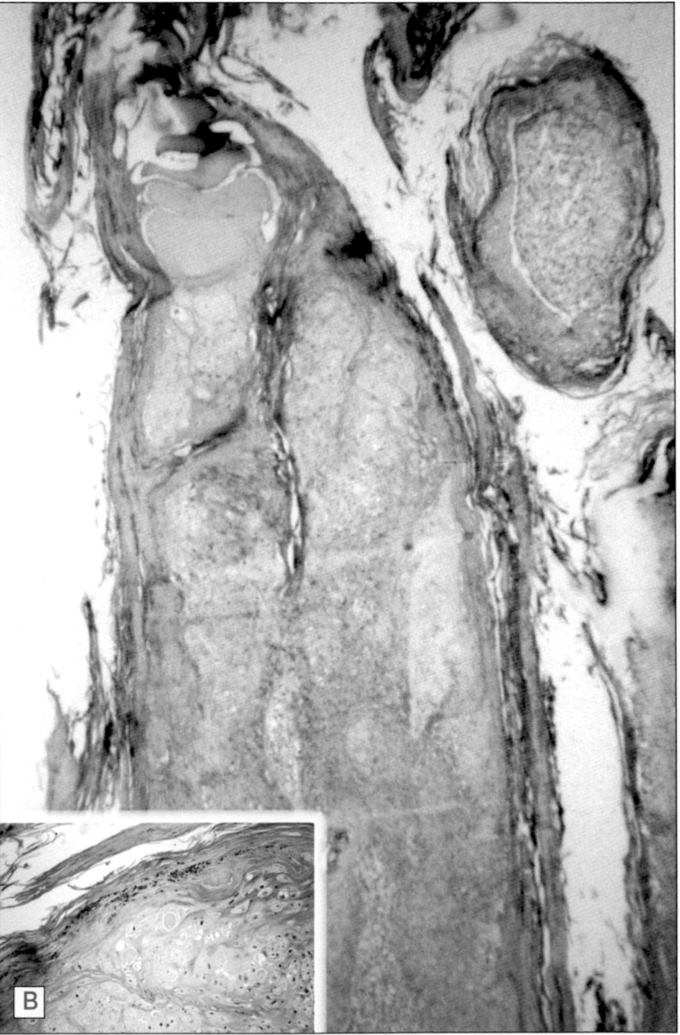

Figure 5.126 A. Multiple **papillomas (warts)** in a steer. **B. Papilloma** in a puppy. Marked hyperplasia is due to marked expansion of stratum spinosum cells. Cells of the spinous and/or granular layer have ballooning degeneration of their cytoplasm (see inset).

Cattle

Six different papillomaviruses occur in cattle. Three (*Bovine papillomavirus* (BPV) types 1, 2, and 5) cause cutaneous fibropapillomas, whereas the other three (BPV-3, -4, -6) cause papillomas of skin (BPV-3, -6) or alimentary tract (BPV-4). For both lesion types, affected cattle are less than 2 years of age and have single or multiple lesions that usually spontaneously regress within a year of appearance. Bovine papillomatosis may be a herd problem in that the virus is easily transmitted by animal-to-animal contact and by fomites. *BPV-1, -2, and -5 cause "teat frond" warts, common cutaneous warts, and "rice grain" fibropapillomas.* These three conditions are characterized by a fibrous core with an overlying variably hyperplastic stratified squamous epithelial lining and occur most often on the udder, teats, head, neck, shoulders and to a lesser extent on the omasum, vagina, vulva, penis, and anus. Lesions may be small nodules or large cauliflower-like lesions subject to trauma and possibly fly strike. Teat papillomas that appear during lactation and regress during the nonlactating period are not uncommon. Interdigital papillomas can lead to lameness. *BPV-3, -4, and -6 cause lesions that are grossly flattened and sessile.* Histologically there is epithelial hyperplasia but not fibroblast proliferation. These lesions tend to be more persistent. In some parts of Scotland and England, BPV-4 causes lesions in the alimentary tract and urinary bladder that may progress to squamous papillomas. Ingested bracken fern (*Pteridium aquilinum*) acts as a co-carcinogen in the progression from benign papilloma of the bladder mucosa to an invasive squamous cell carcinoma. Infection with papillomavirus and repeated exposure to strong sunlight appears to accelerate the development of squamous carcinomas arising in the sclera and lid margins of cattle, particularly those with poorly pigmented periocular skin such as Simmental and Hereford cattle. Papilloma viral infection is therefore one of the contributing factors in the development of the condition known as *cancer-eye*. BPV-1 and BPV-2 have a broader host range and tissue tropism than other papillomaviruses in that they are responsible for both bovine cutaneous fibropapillomas and equine sarcoids.

Horses

Horses develop *typical viral squamous papillomas*. They occur as single or multiple masses in young horses and usually regress within a year (Fig. 5.127). *Muzzle* is the most prevalent site, but tumors may occur anywhere including genital mucous membranes. They are histologically identical to squamous papillomas in calves. Two different viral genome sequences have been described in horses. Unlike the bovine viral strains, however, *the equine virus appears to be species specific. Congenital papillomas* have been reported in foals, and may be hamartomatous rather than viral induced.

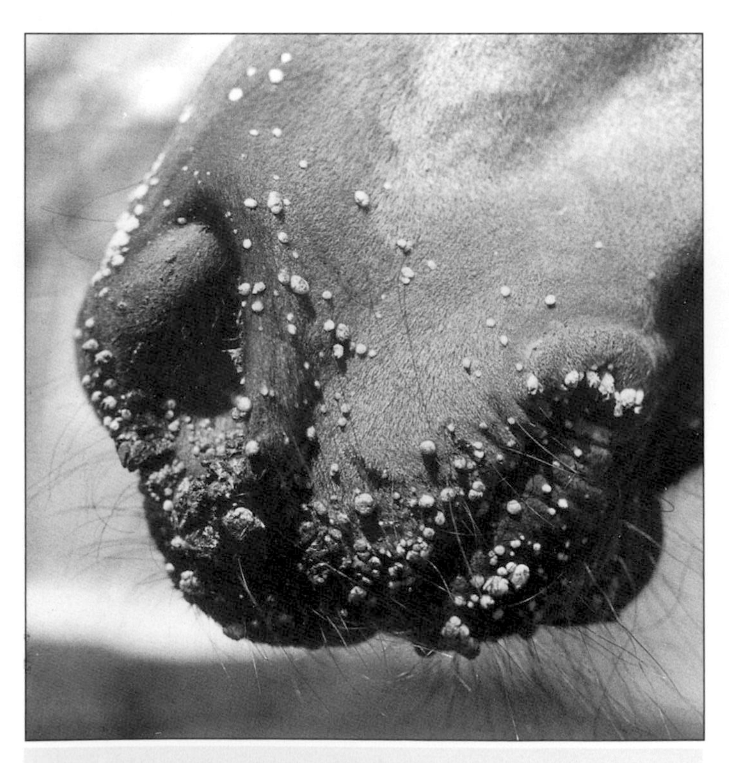

Figure 5.127 Multiple viral papillomas on an equine muzzle.

The most important papillomavirus-induced lesion in the horse is the *sarcoid,* known to be caused by BPV-1 and BPV-2. The lesions are primarily fibroblastic (see Spindle cell tumors) and have not been shown to be transmissible by direct contact.

Sheep and goats

Ovine papillomavirus 1 causes *fibropapillomas* in sheep. There is one report of multiple cutaneous papillomas in a sheep in England in which papilloma-like virus was observed and subsequently transmitted to other sheep. Multiple cutaneous papillomas have been described in goats but circumstantial evidence points towards an actinic rather than viral cause. No virus has been demonstrated by immunofluorescence, electron microscopy or in situ hybridization.

Dogs

Papillomaviruses in dogs cause papillomas of the oral, ocular and genital mucous membranes and of haired skin. Studies indicate that more than one papillomavirus infects the dog and that each virus is responsible for papillomas at a specific body site. *Canine oral papillomavirus* (COPV) has been cloned and characterized and is known to be responsible for canine oral papillomatosis, a contagious and self-limiting condition of young dogs. Occasionally, young dogs with this condition will also develop papillomas on the esophagus, conjunctiva or cornea. Idiopathic sporadic and solitary papillomas can occur on the haired skin of dogs of any age. Eyelid papillomas may appear as part of juvenile papillomatosis or as solitary lesions in older dogs. A report documenting COPV as the cause of multiple papillomas of the haired skin and oral cavity of a dog with corticosteroid-induced immunosuppression suggests that the tissue tropism of the various papillomaviruses is influenced by the immune system. Generalized cutaneous papillomatosis has also been reported in a dog with chemotherapy-induced immunosuppression. A novel papillomavirus was also documented as the cause of multiple foci of endophytic epidermal hyperplasia in a dog on long-term corticosteroid therapy. The lesions resolved with cessation of corticosteroid therapy. Only the oral papillomatosis has been well studied. *The typical transient squamous papillomas contain virus-like basophilic intranuclear inclusions* that are typical of papillomavirus with electron microscopy and immunohistochemistry. The virus is similar to *Bovine papillomavirus 1*. Evidence of viral pathogenesis for the other papilloma-like lesions is not as strong. Some solitary cutaneous papillomas and venereal papillomas contain papillomaviral genome, but the relationship of the viral genetic material to lesion development or to the virus of oral papillomatosis are unknown. Oral or ocular papillomas in young dogs have been reported to progress to squamous cell carcinoma in situ or to invasive squamous cell carcinomas upon rare occasion. A variant of the typical papilloma, the **inverted papilloma** has been reported in the dog. The tumors were single-to-multiple and grossly resembled intracutaneous cornifying epitheliomas (keratoacanthomas). They were keratin-filled cyst-like structures lined by stratified squamous epithelium. The epithelium, however, had intraluminal papillary projections and typical keratinocyte viral cytopathic effects, intranuclear inclusions, and papillomavirus virions present ultrastructurally. Molecular studies suggested the virus was different from COPV.

Cats

Feline fibropapillomas with features virtually identical to the equine sarcoid have been described and found to be associated with papillomavirus DNA via PCR. The implicated virus is most similar to *Bovine papillomavirus* (see Spindle cell tumors). Papillomavirus antigens have also been detected in a large number of cases of multicentric squamous cell carcinoma in situ in cats and in non-neoplastic, proliferative lesions of the epidermis and outer root sheath of hair follicles in immunosuppressed cats. One cat with the non-neoplastic proliferative lesions was infected with FIV and the others were Persians with coat color characteristics suggestive of Chediak–Higashi syndrome. Progression to overt neoplasia and malignancy of these lesions has not been established. At least eight feline papillomaviruses infect the oral cavity and skin of domestic and wild felids.

Rabbits

Domestic **rabbits** develop oral papillomatosis due to infection with *Rabbit oral papillomavirus*. Papillomas, which are multiple and found most often under the tongue, are grossly and histologically typical of viral-induced squamous papillomas.

Bibliography

Anderson DE, Badzioch M. Association between solar radiation and ocular squamous cell carcinoma in cattle. Am J Vet Res 1991;52:784–788.

Campbell KL, et al. Cutaneous inverted papillomas in dogs. Vet Pathol 1988;25:67–71.

Desrochers A, et al. Congenital cutaneous papillomatosis in a one-year-old Holstein. Can Vet J 1994;35:646–647.

Ghim S, et al. Spontaneously regressing oral papillomas induce systemic antibodies that neutralize canine oral papillomavirus. Exp Mol Pathol 2000;68:147–151.

LeClerc SM, et al. Papillomavirus infection in association with feline cutaneous squamous cell carcinoma in situ. Proc Am Assoc Vet Derm/Am Coll Vet Derm 1997;13:125–126.

Le Net JL, et al. Multiple pigmented cutaneous papules associated with a novel canine papillomavirus in an immunosuppressed dog. Vet Pathol 1997;34:8–14.

Lucroy MD, et al. Cutaneous papillomatosis in a dog with malignant lymphoma following long-term chemotherapy. J Vet Diagn Invest 1998;10:369–371.

Murphy FA, et al., eds. Papovaviridae. In: Veterinary Virology. 3rd ed. San Diego, CA: Academic Press, 1999:335–342.

Nicholls PK, et al. Regression of canine oral papillomas is associated with infiltration of CD4+ and CD8+ lymphocytes. Virology 2001;283:31–39.

Nicholls PK, Stanley MA. The immunology of animal papillomaviruses. Vet Immunol Immunopathol 2000;73:101–127.

Rutten VP, et al. Search for bovine papilloma virus DNA in bovine ocular squamous cell carcinomas (BOSCC) and BOSCC-derived cell lines. Am J Vet Res 1992;53:1477–1481.

Schulman FY, et al. Feline cutaneous fibropapillomas: clinicopathologic findings and association with papillomavirus infection. Vet Pathol 2001;38:291–296.

Shimada A, et al. Cutaneous papillomatosis associated with papillomavirus infection in a dog. J Comp Pathol 1993;108:103–107.

Sundberg JP, et al. Involvement of canine oral papillomavirus in generalized oral and cutaneous verrucosis in a Chinese Shar pei dog. Vet Pathol 1994;31:183–187.

Sundberg JP, et al. Feline papillomas and papillomaviruses. Vet Pathol 2000; 37:1–10.

Vanselow BA, Spradbrow PB. Papillomaviruses, papillomas and squamous cell carcinomas in sheep. Vet Rec 1982;110:561–562.

White KS, et al. Equine congenital papilloma: pathological findings and results of papillomavirus immunohistochemistry in five cases. Vet Dermatol 2004; 15:240–244.

Squamous cell carcinoma

Squamous cell carcinoma *is a relatively common, locally invasive and occasionally metastatic neoplasm of most domestic species*. The behavior of squamous cell carcinoma of the skin is usually that of locally destructive spread. Its metastatic potential is low, with certain qualifications depending on location. Those initiated by sunlight are slow to metastasize, then usually only to local lymph nodes. In contrast, those originating on the canine digit may be more prone to metastasize, but even these are cured by amputation in virtually all but the most neglected cases.

Sunlight is probably the most important carcinogenic stimulus for these tumors and accounts for the preference of squamous cell carcinoma for the eyelid and conjunctiva of cattle and horses, the ear pinna of cats and sheep, and the vulva of cattle, goats, and recently sheared sheep (Fig. 5.128A, B). Chronic exposure to sunlight has also been proven to cause squamous cell carcinoma of the relatively hairless, poorly pigmented abdominal and juxtanasal skin of dogs (see Actinic diseases of skin). The progression from solar keratosis to carcinoma occurs over several years and in many instances never attains the full status of carcinoma. The action of sunlight may be related to overexpression of p53 protein as a result of UV-induced mutations of the *p53* tumor suppressor gene.

In addition to sunlight, *carcinogens* contained in tobacco, coal tar and soot, arsenic, and smegma have been shown experimentally or by epidemiologic inference to cause squamous cell carcinoma of skin and other tissues. *Genetic factors and papillomaviruses* also influence the occurrence of squamous cell carcinomas. The influence of *epidermal injury* per se in the initiation of cancer is still unsettled, but there is support for this theory in the greater risk of squamous carcinoma at sites of ear notching, branding, burns, and chronic inflammation. Squamous cell carcinomas of the nasal planum arising in chronic cutaneous lesions of discoid lupus erythematosus have been reported in dogs.

Squamous cell carcinomas are usually firm, white, poorly demarcated dermal masses that are ulcerated and streaked with red. In some locations (eye, penis) they are raised and papillary even though the surface is ulcerated. Chronic inflammation accompanies many of these tumors, particularly those of the ear pinna and nail bed. In these instances, the reddening, crusting and ulceration of the inflammatory lesion may hide the tumor. Microscopic examination of such lesions is often dominated by hyperkeratosis, parakeratosis, ulceration, acanthosis and superficial dermal scarring, with only a few foci of unequivocal neoplasia in which atypical squamous cells have invaded across the basal lamina of the hyperplastic rete pegs. The precancerous plaque and papilloma lesions of ocular squamous cell carcinoma are described under Ocular neoplasia (Vol. 1, Eye and ear).

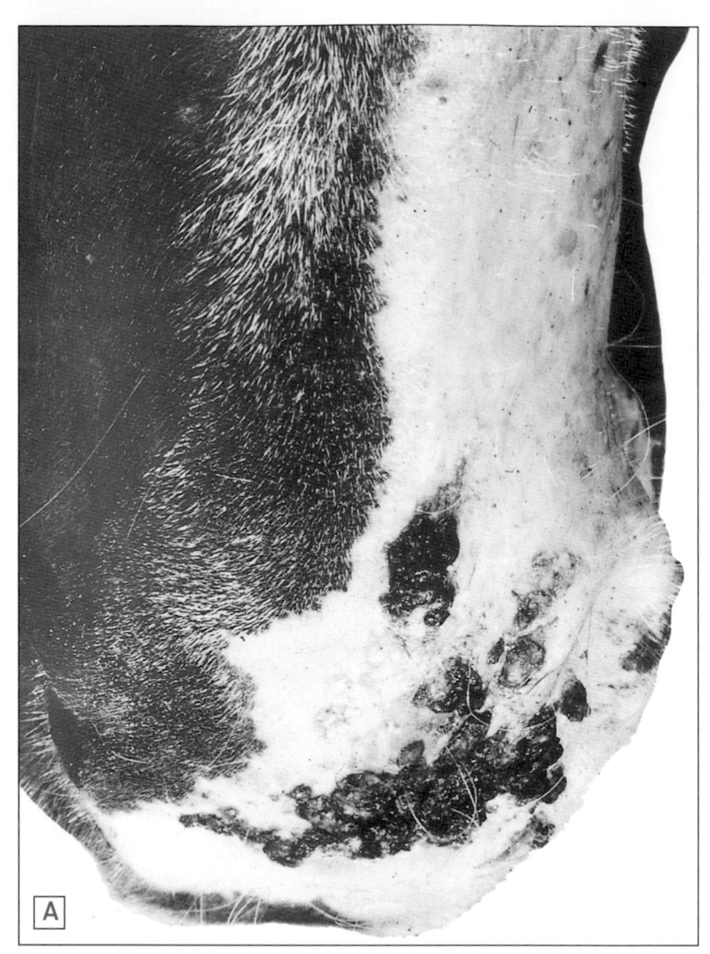

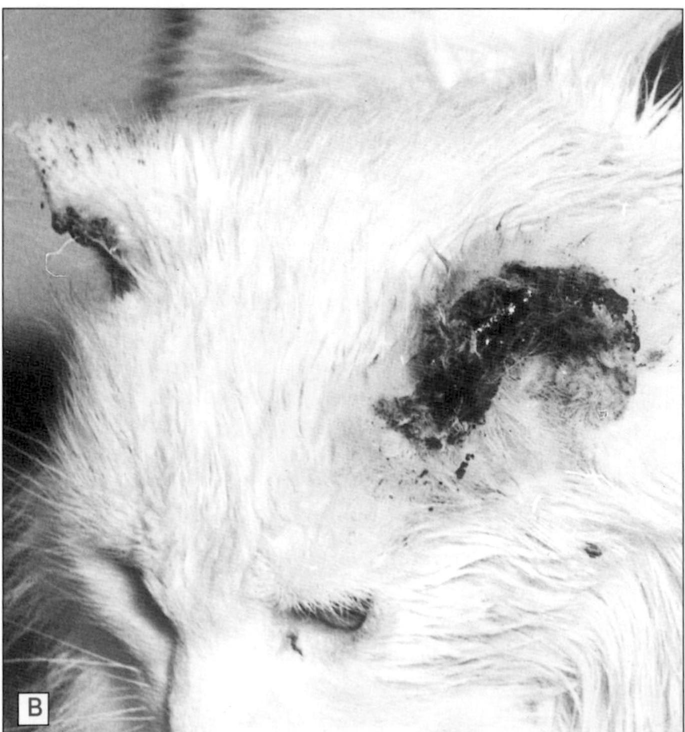

Figure 5.128 Squamous cell carcinoma. A. Involving the unpigmented skin of a horse's nose. **B.** Involving the unpigmented skin of a cat's ears.

Squamous cell carcinomas are recognized microscopically by identifying malignant epithelial cells demonstrating various degrees of differentiation towards keratinocytes. **Squamous cell carcinoma in situ** refers to a malignant tumor of cells with squamous differentiation that is *confined by the basement membrane.* These tumors are often seen in association with ultraviolet light exposure and are interpreted by some pathologists as marked dysplasia (solar keratosis, actinic keratosis), a precancerous stage in the process of malignant transformation of cells. In **invasive squamous cell carcinomas**, *tumor cells breach the basement membrane* to form trabeculae, nests and cords within the dermis that are usually contiguous with the epidermis in at least one area. The tumor cells most resemble those of normal stratum spinosum but have vesicular nuclei with one or multiple very prominent nucleoli. Cytoplasm is usually abundant and eosinophilic. Keratinization within such cords or islands results in laminated keratin "pearls" surrounded by tumor cells. With increasing anaplasia, tumors exhibit wide variation in nuclear size, decreasing cytoplasmic mass, increased basophilia, and disappearance of intercellular bridges. Keratinization may be limited to only individual tumor cells and mononuclear or even multinucleated giant tumor cells may be present. In the typical squamous cell carcinoma, the tumor cells spread through the dermis as slender anastomosing cords, with some cells falling off the cords to remain as apparently isolated islands in the dermal stroma. Tumor cell invasion is usually associated with marked desmoplasia. Mitotic figures are usually numerous and are in proportion to the degree of anaplasia. Some tumors, especially those of actinic origin with a long precancerous phase, are accompanied by abundant mononuclear leukocytic inflammation. Others, such as those of the digit, are both inflamed and very scirrhous. In such tumors, the neoplastic cells may be obscured by inflammatory cell influx, difficult to distinguish from the reactive fibroblasts, or largely destroyed by the ulceration of the inflamed mass.

Acantholytic squamous cell carcinomas are histologic variants demonstrating marked dyscohesion and degeneration of neoplastic keratinocytes resulting in pseudocyst formation within the tumor. This type of tumor must be carefully distinguished from an adenocarcinoma by identifying tumor cell keratinization. **Spindle cell squamous cell carcinomas**, in which the neoplastic epithelium is distinguishable from the desmoplastic stroma only by immunohistochemistry, have been reported. **Basosquamous carcinomas** are low-grade malignant tumors comprised primarily of dermal lobules of basaloid cells with centralized foci of atypical abruptly keratinized cells. The basaloid population may have foci of dyskeratosis or melanization. Tumor lobules may or may not be connected with the epidermis.

Subungual squamous cell carcinomas in **dogs** may be multiple and are seen most often in black dogs, particularly, Labrador Retrievers and Standard Poodles. **Carcinoma of the horn of cattle** is almost exclusive to castrated male adult cattle in India and neighboring countries. The tumor gradually infiltrates and destroys the horn core and may invade adjacent sinuses and cranial bone. The histology is of well-differentiated squamous cell carcinoma but neither the site of origin nor the reason for its peculiar site and sex preference is understood. Theories about chronic trauma to the huge horns are not now in vogue.

Multicentric squamous cell carcinoma in situ (Bowen-like disease) is a type of squamous cell carcinoma confined by the basement membrane. These lesions may progress to invasive squamous cell carcinomas. This tumor is not associated with exposure to ultraviolet light but instead has been associated with papillomavirus infection. The condition has been described in middle-aged to older mixed-breed **cats**. One case reports an association with a cutaneous horn in a cat with no evidence of a viral infection. Tumors appear as 0.5–5 cm in diameter, single to multiple irregular, slightly elevated plaque or papillary lesions of haired pigmented skin. Microscopically, sharply demarcated areas of the epidermis and follicular outer root sheath are irregularly thickened and disorganized by neoplastic keratinocytes. The basal and spinous layers are most affected. Mitotic activity is present in all layers of the epidermis and keratin pearl formation may be present. Tumor cells often have large hyperchromatic nuclei and may have vacuolated cytoplasm, cytoplasmic pallor, or occasionally are multinucleated. The tumors are often pigmented and may have papillomatous epidermal projections with marked hyperkeratosis.

Bibliography

Baer KE, Helton K. Multicentric squamous cell carcinoma in situ resembling Bowen's disease in cats. Vet Pathol 1993;30:535–543.

Goldschmidt MH, et al. Histological classification of epithelial and melanocytic tumors of the skin of domestic animals. Washington DC: Armed Forces Institute of Pathology, 1998.

Lascelles BD, et al. Squamous cell carcinoma of the nasal planum in 17 dogs. Vet Rec 2000;147:473–476.

LeClerc SM, et al. Papillomavirus infection in association with feline cutaneous squamous cell carcinoma in situ. Proc Am Assoc Vet Derm/Am Coll Vet Derm 1997;13:125–126.

Mozos E, et al. Ovine cutaneous squamous cell carcinoma: immunohistochemical expression of CD3, CD4, CD8 and MHC class II antigens in the associated inflammatory infiltrate. Vet Immunol Immunopathol 1998;61:221–228.

Murakami Y, et al. Immunohistochemical analysis of cyclin A, cyclin D1 and P53 in mammary tumors, squamous cell carcinomas and basal cell tumors of dogs and cats. J Vet Med Sci 2000;62:743–750.

Nikula KJ, et al. Ultraviolet radiation, solar dermatosis, and cutaneous neoplasia in beagle dogs. Radiat Res 1992;129:11–18.

O'Brien MG, et al. Treatment by digital amputation of subungual squamous cell carcinoma in dogs: 21 cases (1987–1988). J Am Vet Med Assoc 1992;201:759–761.

Rees CA, Goldschmidt MH. Cutaneous horn and squamous cell carcinoma in situ (Bowen's disease) in a cat. J Am Anim Hosp Assoc 1998;34:485–486.

Sironi G, et al. p53 protein expression in conjunctival squamous cell carcinomas of domestic animals. Vet Ophthalmol 1999;2:227–231.

Basal cell tumor

Basal cell tumors are *common in dogs and cats but are rare in other domestic species. They are the most common skin tumor of cats.* Current classification schemes limit the category of basal cell tumors to tumors *comprised only of proliferations of undifferentiated basaloid cells.* Those that exhibit differentiation towards basal cell-derived structures such as sebaceous glands, hair follicles or even keratinized epidermis are given a wide variety of names depending on the predominant direction of such differentiation. This new reclassification of cutaneous tumors has now placed some of the tumors that used to be considered basal cell tumors in the category of trichoblastomas (see Tumors with adnexal differentiation). Human basal cell tumors most frequently occur in lightly pigmented skin exposed to sunlight, the latter known to favor the development of the tumor. No such predilection is proven for dogs and cats.

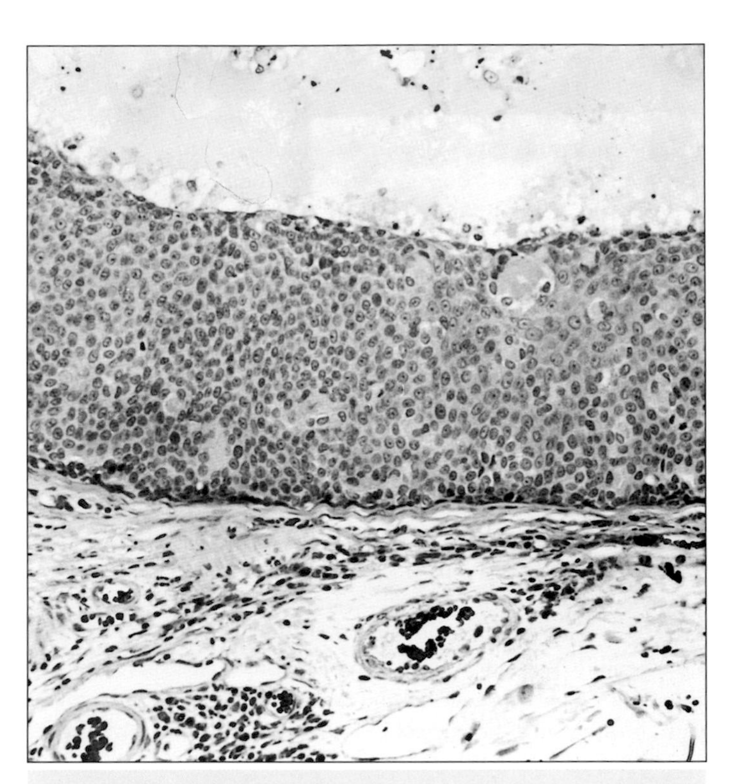

Figure 5.129 Cystic basal cell tumor.

Histologically, basal cell tumors are composed of cords or nests of cells resembling those of normal stratum germinativum. Each has an oval, deeply basophilic nucleus, a single nucleolus, and scant, eosinophilic cytoplasm with indistinct cell boundaries. In contrast to normal stratum germinativum, there are no intercellular bridges. The cells extend into the dermis as islands, or grow expansively as solid sheets, multiple small cysts lined by basal cells, or less frequently as a single large cyst (Fig. 5.129). The latter form is most common in the cat. Several layers of undifferentiated basal cells with no inner limiting membrane and no adnexal or squamous differentiation form each cyst. The cysts are usually filled with eosinophilic debris, and most probably form by central necrosis of an initially solid mass of basal cells. The islands of tumor cells may or may not connect with the overlying epidermis. Mitotic figures and nuclear pleomorphism are variable. Benign tumors have no stromal invasion or associated desmoplasia. Tumor cells may contain melanin, and melanophages may be present in the intervening stroma.

Basal cell carcinomas have two subtypes. **Infiltrative basal cell carcinomas** are comprised of cords of primitive basaloid cells that penetrate the surrounding dermis and possibly subcutis. Mitotic figures may be numerous. The tumor is usually associated with desmoplasia. **Clear cell basal carcinomas** are more rare and consist of large, polygonal cells with clear or finely granular cytoplasm. Nuclei lack pleomorphism and mitoses may be variable.

Tumors with adnexal differentiation

Tumors arising from hair follicles

Hair follicle (pilar) neoplasms are common in dogs but apparently are very rare in other domestic species. Their classification is rather complex; however, the majority of tumors arising in animals share a benign biological behavior. Exceptions exist as described below.

Intracutaneous cornifying epithelioma (*infundibular keratinizing acanthoma*) is a benign cystic tumor of the skin of dogs. Common sites are the dorsum of the neck and back. Usually there is only a single tumor, but in Norwegian Elkhounds, a breed predisposed to these tumors, they may be multiple or occur in succession. Tumors of this description arising in the subungual region are called **keratoacanthomas**.

The gross lesion is a slightly raised firm 1–3 cm nodule that may have a central craterous pore representing the follicular isthmus or infundibulum from which keratin can be expressed. *The histologic lesion is a simple or multiloculated cavity filled with keratin and lined by squamous epithelium with large, pale eosinophilic squamous cells multifocally containing keratohyaline granules.* The periphery of the cyst wall consists of basal cells (Fig. 5.130A, B). The basal cells have gradual and complete maturation to stratum corneum, but may become somewhat disoriented and form keratin pearls within the cyst wall as well as shedding keratin into the lumen. The basilar layer is orderly, and while it may show blunt cord-like expansion into surrounding compressed dermis and anastomosing cords of epithelial cells forming small horn cysts in the wall of the central cyst, there is no breach of the basement membrane by tumor cells. Focal rupture is common, inciting a granulomatous or pyogranulomatous reaction in surrounding dermis.

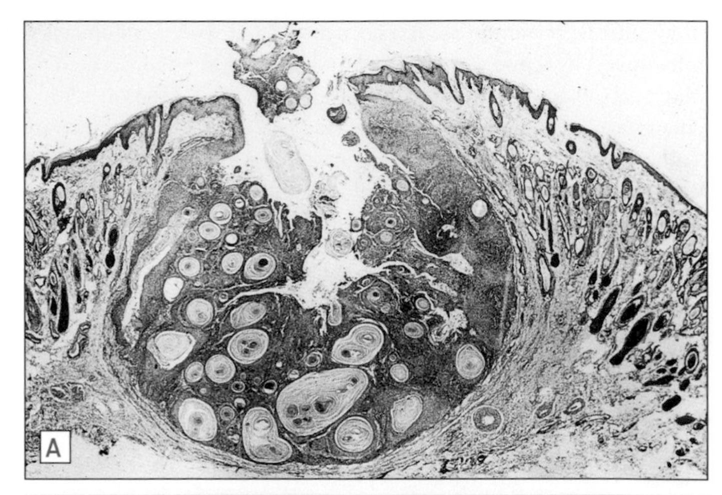

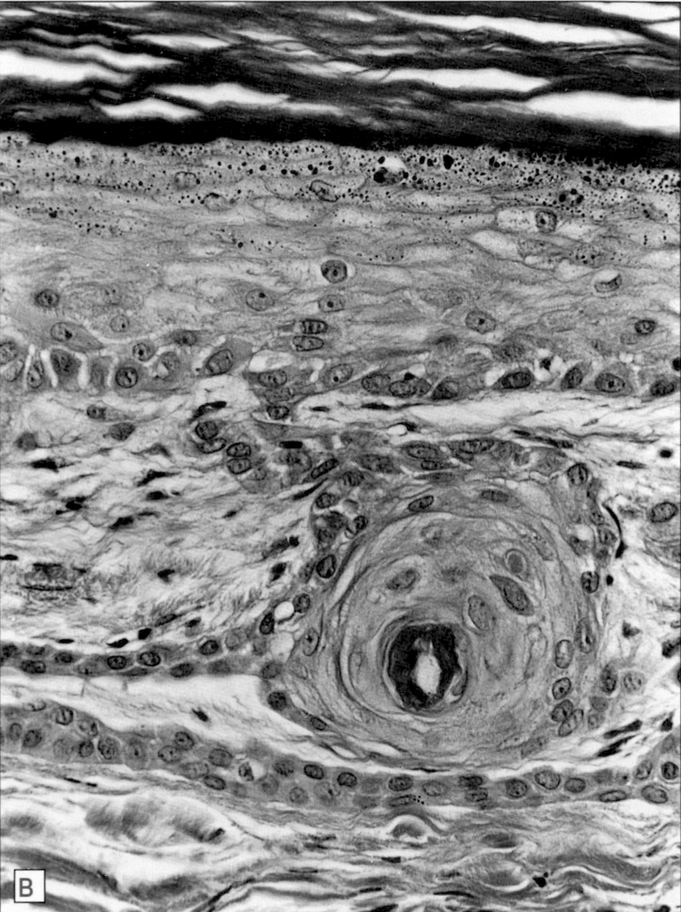

Figure 5.130 Intracutaneous cornifying epithelioma. **A.** With pore opening to the surface of the skin. **B.** Detail of wall showing gradual keratinization and keratin pearl formation.

Trichoepithelioma is *a tumor of primitive hair germ that exhibits rudimentary differentiation towards all three segments of the follicle: the infundibulum, isthmus, and the inferior segment.* Trichoepitheliomas are single or multiple skin tumors occurring anywhere on the body with a slight preference for the back. The typical macroscopic appearance is of a very firm, white, multilobulated and encapsulated tumor that may infrequently be mineralized. Histologically, the usual pattern consists of multiple islands of basal cells with differentiation into the external or internal sheath surrounded by a thickened basement membrane; the center of each island undergoes abrupt keratinization without interposition of a granular layer (Fig. 5.131A, B). Occasional tumor cells containing trichohyaline granules and foci of matrical keratinization are present.

The outer layer of basal cells may abut the fibrous stroma or send out basal cell ribbons into a mucinous stroma. Some trichoepitheliomas have several large primary cystic areas surrounded by many smaller cysts. Rupture of some of the keratinaceous cysts stimulates pyogranulomatous inflammation within the stroma and even within the cyst, sometimes accompanied by mineralization and foreign-body giant cells. Mineralization and inflammation are more typical of the closely related pilomatricoma. **Malignant trichoepitheliomas** have the additional features of mitotic activity, cystic degeneration and necrosis, and invasion of subcutis sometimes accompanied by desmoplasia. Lymphatic invasion is considered an essential finding to confirm malignancy by some pathologists. Regional and pulmonary metastasis is possible. *Trichoepitheliomas are distinguished from all other epidermal or appendage tumors by the abrupt (matrical) keratinization and the follicle-like basal cell nests that surround it.* Other tumors or cysts simulating trichoepithelioma lack one or both of these features.

Tricholemmoma (also trichilemmoma) is a rare, *benign and nonrecurring,* pilar tumor of dogs in which tumor cells differentiate into cells characteristic of either the inferior segment of the hair follicle (**inferior tricholemmoma**), external root sheath, or the isthmic (**isthmic tricholemmoma**) section of the external root sheath. In *inferior tricholemmomas*, tumor cells form nests separated by a fine collagenous stroma. The tumor cells have abundant eosinophilic cytoplasm that is pale (clear cells) peripherally and more intensely eosinophilic toward the center of the nests (Fig. 5.132). Pallor of the outermost layer of cells is due to marked cytoplasmic glycogen storage, seen in histologic section as cytoplasmic clearing. These are thought to represent differentiation toward

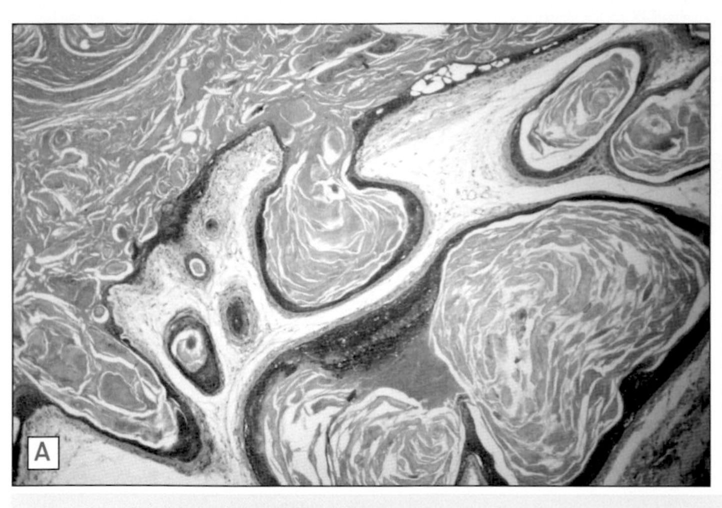
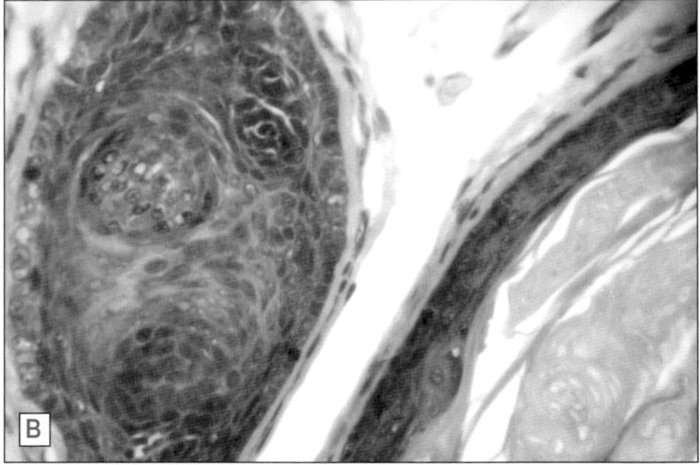

Figure 5.131 Trichoepithelioma. **A.** Note multiple keratin-filled cysts. **B.** Note rudimentary hair follicle formation.

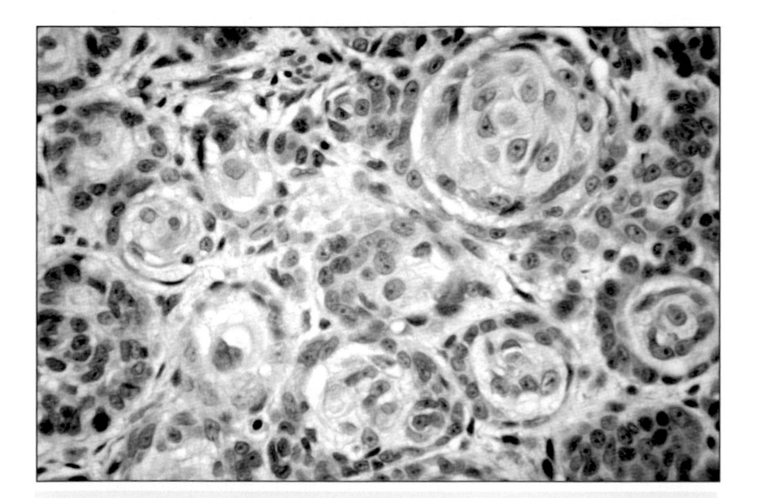

Figure 5.132 Tricholemmoma. Tumor cells have abundant eosinophilic cytoplasm that is pale (clear cells) peripherally and more intensely eosinophilic toward the center of the nests.

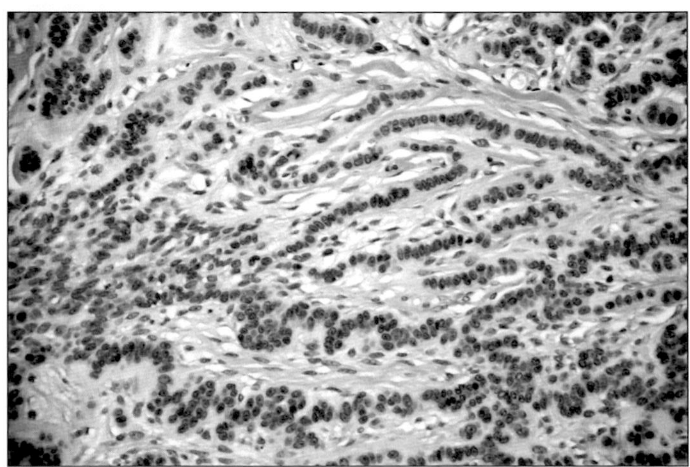

Figure 5.133 Trichoblastoma. Long ribbons of pale epithelial cells extend into the dermis.

outer root-sheath cells. Each tumor follicle is surrounded by a thick, homogeneous basal lamina resembling the vitreous sheath of the normal follicle. The epithelial cells in the *isthmic tricholemmoma* are arranged as islands and radiating cords that may intersect or be associated with the epidermis. The tumor cells show central trichilemmal keratinization.

Trichoblastoma is *a benign tumor derived from the primitive hair germ of embryonic follicular development*. There are ribbon, trabecular, granular, and spindle cell trichoblastomas. In dogs, these tumors were formerly classified as basal cell tumors.

- The **ribbon trichoblastoma** is a dermal to subcutaneous tumor formed by long, narrow, branching cords of pale eosinophilic epithelial cells (Fig. 5.133) that may join or radiate from a large central aggregate (medusoid pattern). A mucinous stroma is frequently associated with the medusoid pattern. Cell borders are indistinct. Nuclei of tumors arranged in cords often palisade perpendicular to the long axis of the cord. Mitotic figures may be numerous. Abundant collagen that may appear hyalinized accompanies the tumor cells.
- **Trabecular trichoblastomas** occur in the dermis and consist of multiple lobules of pale eosinophilic epithelial cells with scant poorly demarcated cytoplasm and euchromatic nuclei. The cells at the periphery of the lobules palisade while centrally located cells have more abundant cytoplasm.
- **Granular trichoblastoma** tumor cells have large numbers of intracytoplasmic eosinophilic granules and eccentrically placed nuclei.
- **Spindle cell trichoblastomas** are most often seen in cats and consist of trabeculae and lobules of elongated, streaming, basaloid epithelial cells within a fibrous stroma. Tumor cells have scant cytoplasm, oval nuclei with inconspicuous nucleoli, and rare mitoses. Melanin may be present in the tumor cells and accompanying melanophages.

Pilomatricoma (*pilomatrixoma, epithelioma of Malherbe, necrotizing and calcifying epithelioma*), macroscopically resembles trichoepithelioma (Fig. 5.134A) but is often more heavily mineralized and consists of fewer, larger cysts than does trichoepithelioma. Pilomatricomas are believed to be derived from primitive hair

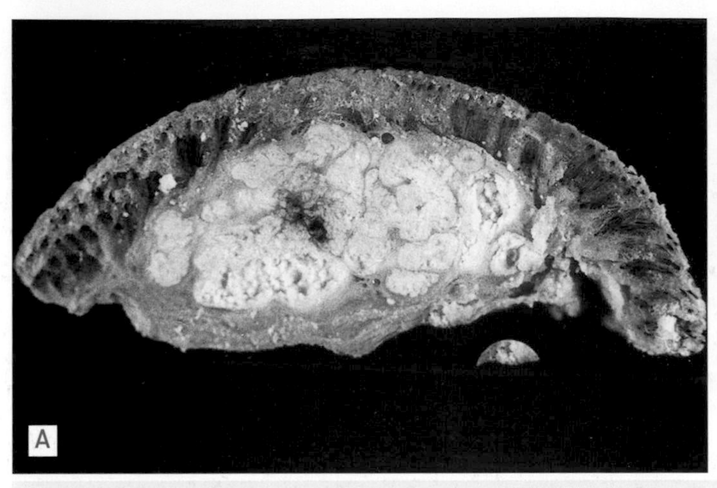

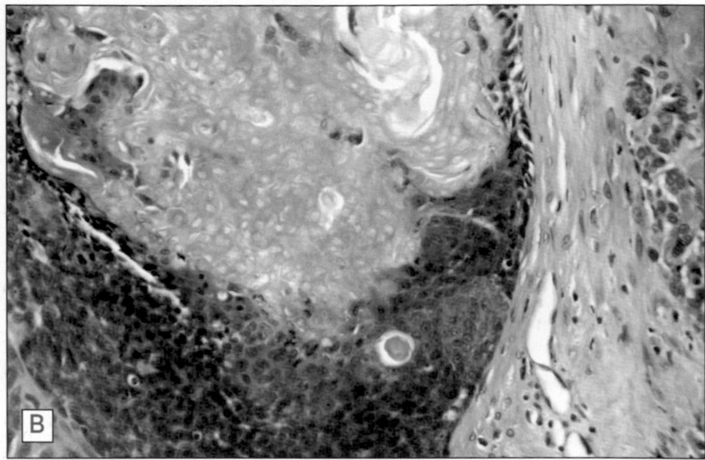

Figure 5.134 Pilomatricoma in a dog. **A.** Multilobulated, mineralized, and well-demarcated keratinizing dermal tumor. **B.** Multiple lobules of basal cells with abrupt keratinization. Note shadow cells in the center of the lobules.

matrix and thus show incomplete differentiation towards hair cortex. *The typical microscopic morphology is of one or more large, thick-walled cysts partially filled with so-called shadow or ghost cells* (Fig. 5.134B) *typical of matrical differentiation.* These cells are flattened eosinophilic epithelial cells with a central empty halo in place of the lysed nucleus. The cyst wall is composed of multiple layers of basal cells, showing a sudden zonal degeneration to form the central laminations of shadow cells. Mitoses may be present. Mineralization of shadow cells is very common, and cyst rupture results in the pyogranulomatous inflammation that is very typical of these tumors. Foci of necrosis within the tumor are frequently seen, and mineralization or even ossification within the stroma occurs occasionally.

Pilomatricomas are almost always single and benign. They occur most often on the back, neck and tail. One report indicates that Miniature Poodles and Kerry Blue Terriers develop these tumors more frequently than other breeds. The very few reports of behaviorally malignant tumors describe tumors with greater mitotic activity and nuclear pleomorphism; however, some of these tumors were not readily distinguished at initial presentation from benign tumors and the diagnosis of malignancy was made in retrospect after documented metastasis. Metastases to the regional lymph nodes, lung and bone have been documented.

Tumors arising from sebaceous or modified sebaceous glands

Sebaceous glands give rise to *sebaceous gland hyperplasia, sebaceous adenoma, sebaceous epithelioma, and sebaceous carcinoma.* **Modified sebaceous glands** include the Meibomian glands of the eyelid, which give rise to *Meibomian gland adenomas, epitheliomas, and carcinomas* that are histologically identical to the corresponding sebaceous gland lesion and will not be described separately. The **hepatoid (perianal) glands** are also modified sebaceous glands that give rise to hepatoid gland adenomas, epitheliomas, and carcinomas. *Epitheliomas are considered to be lesions intermediate between an adenoma and carcinoma.*

Sebaceous gland hyperplasia is seen as single or multiple, raised, multilobulated masses within the superficial dermis below focally hyperplastic, hyperkeratotic epidermis. Many are ulcerated by continued tumor growth or by trauma. Most are less than 1 cm in diameter and are most frequently submitted with clinical diagnoses of "multiple papillomas." Histologically, each tumor consists of rather symmetrical hyperplasia of a single sebaceous gland clustered about a keratinized sebaceous duct. In some specimens, more than one gland is involved. The sebaceous cells (sebocytes) are fully mature and the peripheral rim of basal (reserve) cell population is inconspicuous. Surrounding dermis and adnexa are compressed. The hyperplasia is multiple in about 40% of affected dogs.

Sebaceous adenoma is *comprised primarily of mature sebaceous cells, but differs from hyperplasia in that there are more basal (reserve) cells than in hyperplasia, and the lobular proliferation is greater, less symmetrical, and not necessarily related to a single sebaceous duct.* The lesion compresses adjacent structures. Melanin within tumor cells, and stromal melanocytes and melanophages may be present and cause the tumor to be grossly pigmented. **Sebaceous ductal adenomas** are similar tumors but are comprised primarily of large numbers of haphazardly arranged ducts with intervening clusters of sebocytes and reserve cells.

Sebaceous epithelioma *is a term used by some to refer to sebaceous gland tumors of low-grade malignancy.* These tumors have mostly basaloid reserve cells with numerous mitoses and only scattered single or small clusters of well-differentiated sebocytes. Horn cysts suggesting ductal differentiation may be present (Fig. 5.135). Melanocytes and melanophages may be present within the intervening stroma and the basaloid cells may contain melanin also.

Sebaceous carcinomas are occasionally encountered in dogs and rarely in cats. *Sebaceous carcinomas are locally infiltrative, solitary, poorly circumscribed tumors made up of pleomorphic cells that show some evidence of sebaceous differentiation.* The sebaceous carcinoma lacks complete or orderly sebaceous cell maturation, and distinct reserve cell populations are not present. Lobule formation is often present but is not prominent. Mitotic figures, anisocytosis, anisokaryosis and hyperchromasia are present as the cytologic counterparts of malignancy. The prognosis following wide surgical excision seems to be good, although no large series has been published. Differentiation from liposarcomas and balloon cell melanomas may be difficult.

Perianal gland adenomas (*hepatoid gland tumor, circumanal gland tumor*) are common in intact, aged male dogs. They occur occasionally in females and rarely in castrated males. They have not

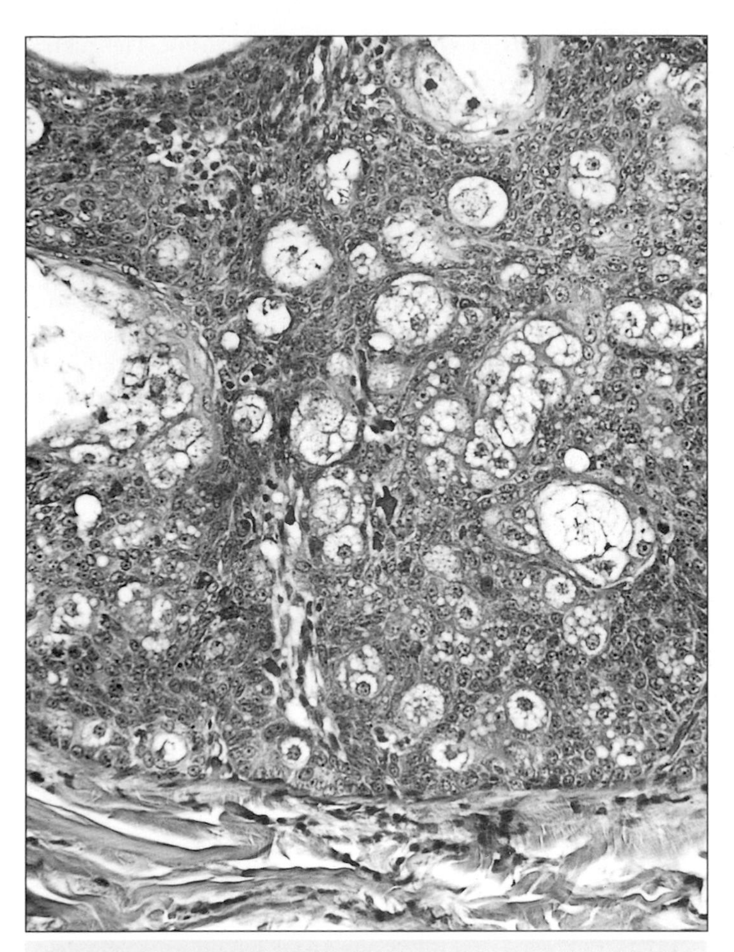

Figure 5.135 Sebaceous epithelioma in a dog.

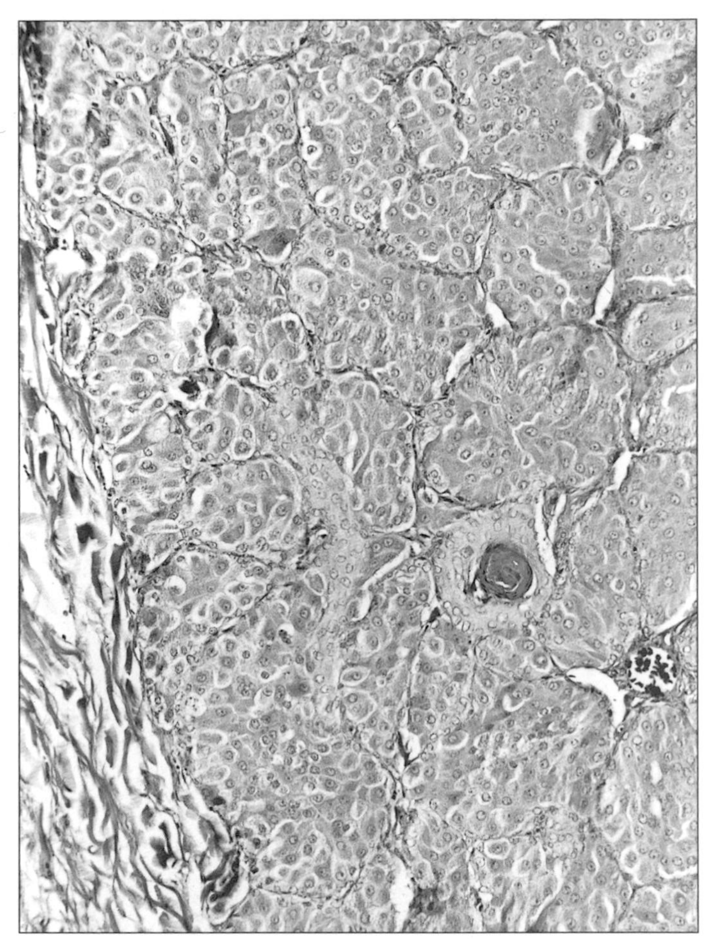

Figure 5.136 Perianal gland adenoma. Lobular arrangement of hepatoid cells and foci of squamous metaplasia.

been reported in other domestic species. *Most perianal gland tumors are called adenomas, even though the lobular development is so uniform that the tumor is more likely to be hormone-dependent hyperplasia.* The strong predilection for intact male dogs and the regression of about 95% of these tumors following castration also points to hyperplasia rather than true neoplasia. Nonetheless, "perianal adenoma" seems firmly entrenched and the difference in terminology is of no practical importance. The tumor growths most commonly occur in the perianal area, but about 10% occur in sites of ectopic perianal gland tissue such as tail, flank, back, prepuce and even chin. Of these, the ventral skin of the tail is the most frequent location.

The *gross appearance* of perianal gland adenomas is of one or more raised rubbery masses that may grow to 10 cm or more in diameter. Ulceration and secondary infection are common, and can serve to confuse the diagnosis. The typical tumor consists of multiple tan lobules separated by a delicate but definite collagenous stroma. *The histologic lesion is similar to normal perianal gland.* Well-differentiated tumors consist of islands, cords, and lobules of polygonal cells with abundant, finely vacuolated eosinophilic cytoplasm and a central, small, round, vesicular nucleus. The cells resemble hepatocytes and these tumors are sometimes called "hepatoid gland" tumors (Fig. 5.136). At the periphery of each lobule is a rim of basal reserve cells, and in some tumors these cells may predominate over the fully differentiated hepatoid cells. Mitotic activity of reserve cell, necrosis, hemorrhage, secondary inflammation, squamous metaplasia and squamous pearl formation (ductal differentiation) are common and are no cause for concern. Some cells may resemble sebocytes. Aggregates of tumor cells are separated by a fine fibrovascular stroma and tumors are often encapsulated. *Local excision and castration is curative and prevents the development of new perianal gland tumors.*

Perianal gland epitheliomas are tumors of low-grade malignancy comprised of mostly reserve cells. Mitotic activity is increased in comparison to the adenomas but nuclear atypia is not present.

Perianal gland carcinomas account for no more than 5% of all perianal tumors if rigorous diagnostic criteria are used. They are relatively more common in castrated males and in females. They exhibit the usual features of malignancy: variation in nuclear and cytoplasmic mass, poor cytoplasmic differentiation, frequent mitotic figures, and lack of organized lobule formation. Local tissue invasion should be evident. Lymphatic invasion must be diagnosed with caution since compression of reserve cells by lobular expansion may simulate a tumor embolus surrounded by lymphatic endothelium. Direct extension into the pelvic canal or metastasis to regional lymph nodes occurs as a late event in chronically neglected tumors. Castration has no demonstrated effect on tumor behavior.

Tumors arising from apocrine and modified apocrine glands

Tumors of the *apocrine (paratrichial) sweat glands* are the least frequent of the adnexal skin tumors in dogs. They are relatively more common

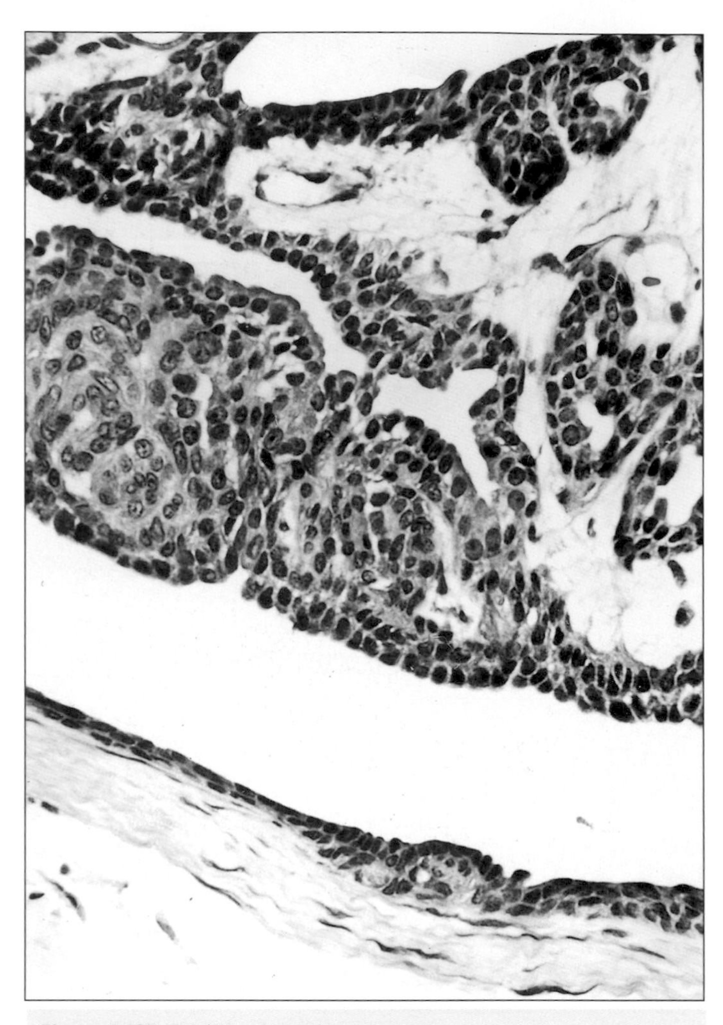

Figure 5.137 Papillary apocrine adenoma.

in cats. There is a single report of a mixed sweat gland tumor in a bull. Tumors of the eccrine sweat glands are rare but histologically distinctive tumors occurring in the footpads.

Apocrine gland adenomas include *cystic and papillary types*, the latter merely a variant of the former. The cystic lesion consists of one or more cavities lined by well-differentiated cuboidal-to-columnar epithelium with eosinophilic cytoplasm and basally located nuclei, often with the apical secretory blebs typical of normal apocrine glands. Many tumors have at least some tubules lined by an orderly bi-layer of cuboidal epithelium, perhaps an effort by the tumor cells to recreate the structure of the duct of the normal gland (Fig. 5.137). Proliferation of epithelium may result in intraluminal papillary growths supported by a delicate fibrous stroma. The proliferation may fill the cyst lumen, or lumens may contain eosinophilic secretions.

Apocrine gland carcinomas include *solid, cystic or tubular types*, the latter clearly predominating. The cystic tumors have intraluminal papillary growths. Apocrine carcinomas are locally aggressive growths, spreading through the dermis, subcutis and muscle from the primary focus. Invasive tumor cells are often accompanied by desmoplasia. Lymphatic invasion and regional lymph node and pulmonary metastasis are common. The histology of carcinomas differs from their benign counterparts primarily in the criteria of loss of polarity and local stromal invasion, as mitotic figures and nuclear and cellular pleomorphism may be variable. The tubular carcinomas have focal cystic or solid areas and are typically very scirrhous. Identification is based upon tubules retaining differentiation to resemble sweat glands, particularly the presence of secretory blebs at the luminal surface. The sweat gland carcinoma is the only primary tubular adenocarcinoma of skin.

Complex and mixed apocrine gland tumors are rare. The proliferation involves both epithelial cells and the periglandular myoepithelial sheath, and may be analogous to the mixed mammary tumor of dogs. Mucinous, chondroid and osseous metaplasia within the tumor stroma is allegedly of myoepithelial origin. The malignant version of this tumor varies from the benign tumor in that the glandular epithelial component demonstrates features of anaplasia and stromal invasion. On rare occasions, both glandular and myoepithelial components demonstrate features of malignancy and the tumor is referred to as an **apocrine gland carcinosarcoma** or **mixed malignant apocrine gland tumor**.

Benign and malignant tumors with differentiation towards apocrine ducts may occur. **Apocrine ductal adenomas** and **ductal carcinomas** are characterized by multilobular and sometimes cystic dermal-to-subcutaneous masses formed by a double layer of basophilic epithelial cells with scant, clear cytoplasm. Cells adjacent to the basement membrane zone may be fusiform. Squamous differentiation may be present. Malignant tumors have nuclear and cellular pleomorphism and stromal invasion. Lymphatic invasion and metastasis are not common.

Ceruminous glands *can give rise to adenomas, complex and mixed adenomas and the malignant versions of these tumors*. Morphologic features are very similar to those described for the apocrine gland counterpart with the additional distinguishing feature of *brown luminal secretions* on H&E-stained sections. In addition, foci of tumor cells may be found within the overlying epithelium and secondary inflammation is more common.

Carcinoma of the apocrine glands of the anal sac is an uncommon but very malignant tumor of *old female dogs*. Males are rarely affected. The tumor histologically varies from solid, rosette, to tubular types. The solid form consists of sheets of relatively monomorphic polygonal cells with scant eosinophilic cytoplasm and round-to-oval hyperchromatic nuclei. In the rosette form, tumor cells with peripheral nuclei are arranged radially, sometimes surrounding small amounts of eosinophilic secretory material. The tubular arrangement has larger cells with abundant eosinophilic cytoplasm and hyperchromatic nuclei. Tubules are filled with eosinophilic secretions. These tumors are invasive, induce a desmoplastic response, and almost invariably spread to regional lymph nodes and then various viscera. Over half have already metastasized prior to diagnosis. Tumor growth is often directed inward through the pelvic canal so that a grossly visible perianal mass is seen in only about 50% of cases. The unusual feature of the tumor is its ability regularly to *induce hypercalcemia in affected dogs* (see Vol. 3, Endocrine glands).

Tumors of **atrichial (eccrine) glands** are rare but do occur as *adenomas or scirrhous tubular carcinomas* within the loose connective tissue of the pad of dogs and cats. Tumor cells have very pale eosinophilic cytoplasm and basally located nuclei. **Eccrine gland carcinomas** are morphologically similar to apocrine gland carcinomas. Differentiation is dependent upon knowing the site of origin.

Bibliography

Abramo F, et al. Survey of canine and feline follicular tumours and tumour-like lesions in central Italy. J Small Anim Pract 1999;40:479–481.

Goldschmidt MH, et al. Histological classification of epithelial and melanocytic tumors of the skin of domestic animals. Washington DC: Armed Forces Institute of Pathology, 1998.

Goldschmidt MH, Shofer FS. Skin Tumors of the Dog and Cat. Oxford, England: Pergamon Press, 1992.

Marino DJ, et al. Evaluation of dogs with digit masses: 117 cases (1981–1991). J Am Vet Med Assoc 1995;207:726–728.

Scott DW, Anderson WI. Canine hair follicle neoplasms: a retrospective analysis of 80 cases (1986–1987). Vet Dermatol 1991;2:143–150.

Melanocytic tumors

Tumors derived from melanocytes or melanoblasts are of *neuroectodermal origin*. They have been reported in most species of domestic animals and many wildlife species, although they are most common in dogs, horses, and some breeds of swine. There are some species differences in melanocytic tumors. In **dogs**, *melanomas in the oral cavity and non-haired skin of the lip are almost invariably malignant.* Those of the nailbeds also are frequently malignant, whereas cutaneous tumors are more commonly benign. In **horses**, melanomas occasionally occur as congenital tumors, however they are most common in *older gray horses with a site predilection for the perineum, genital area, and distal limbs* (Fig. 5.138). The behavior of melanomas in horses is difficult to predict based on histologic features. They can be clinically malignant and aggressive from the outset, or they may demonstrate slow growth for years with a sudden onset of malignant behavior, or growth can be slow for many years without evidence of metastasis. In some breeds of **swine**, such as Sinclair miniature swine and Hormel crosses (MeLiM), melanomas can occur as *congenital tumors*, and these breeds have been extensively used in biomedical research. Melanomas are uncommon in **cats** and are often *amelanotic*. Melanomas in **cattle** may occur as a congenital lesion, or they may occur at any age. Most are benign in cattle, although occasional tumors are malignant. Melanocytic tumors are uncommon in **goats** and **sheep** and are generally pigmented.

The *histologic diagnosis* of melanocytic tumors is complicated by the fact that they can display various degrees of pigmentation, from heavily pigmented to amelanotic. In addition, neoplastic melanocytes can be pleomorphic, and melanocytic tumors can display a variety of cell shapes, including *spindle cell, balloon cell (clear cell), epithelioid cell, and signet-ring cell*, thus making them difficult to distinguish from poorly differentiated sarcomas and carcinomas. *Junctional activity can be helpful in identification* (Fig. 5.139), as the only other tumors to display this activity are epitheliotropic lymphoma, and rarely, cutaneous histiocytomas. The advances in development of immunohistochemical detection of melanocytic markers has aided greatly in diagnosis of these tumors, particularly in the diagnosis of amelanotic melanomas. While antibodies against vimentin, S-100, and neuron-specific enolase are sensitive for tumors of melanocytic origin, they are not specific for these tumors and react with many other tumors. Currently *Melan A is the most specific immunohistochemical marker for melanomas*, albeit not 100% sensitive, and has been shown to be useful in many species, including the dog, cat, and horse.

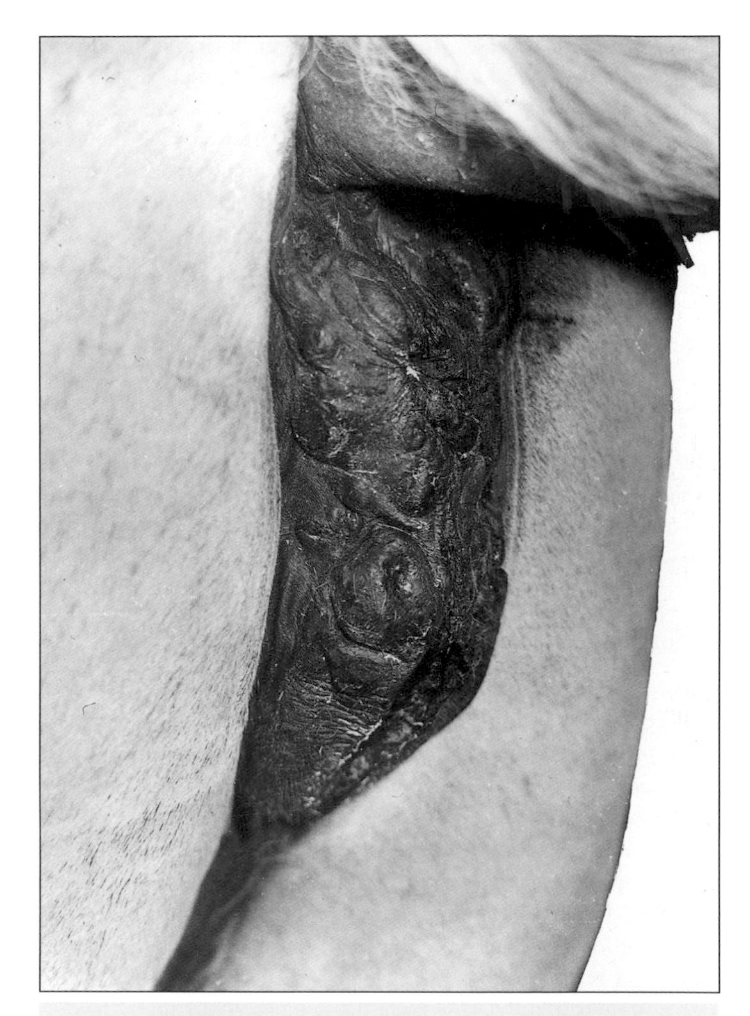

Figure 5.138 Melanoma of the perineum in a gray mare.

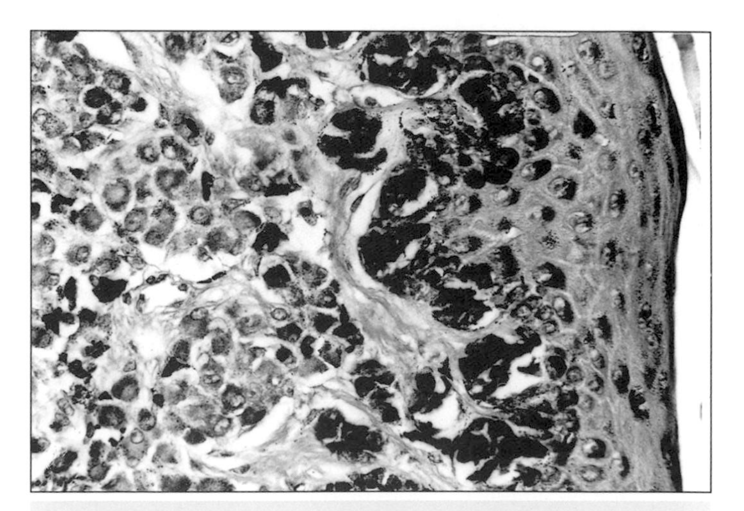

Figure 5.139 Benign melanoma demonstrating junctional activity.

Various studies on canine melanomas have attempted to establish criteria on which to base the prediction of biologic behavior of melanomas. These studies suggest *that the most significant factor predicting the clinical behavior of a melanocytic tumor in the dog is mitotic index* (total number of mitotic figures in ten randomly selected high-power (×40) fields). In one study, a mitotic index of three or greater, notwithstanding the cytologic features, was regarded as indication of malignancy, whereas in another study mitotic activity together with atypical cytologic features was regarded as predictive of clinical behavior. Several proliferation markers have been examined as an aid in predicting survival. It is reported that Ki67, but not PCNA, is a useful prognostic factor in melanomas of dogs and cats, however Ki67 is not useful in predicting clinical behavior in equine melanomas. The degree of pigmentation and cell type are reported not to be associated with prognosis.

Benign melanocytic tumors

Lentigo (lentigo simplex)

A lentigo is a proliferation of melanocytes that is usually confined to the epidermis, resulting clinically in a pigmented circumscribed macule. This lesion is considered to be a hyperplastic melanocytic lesion rather than neoplastic (see Disorders of pigmentation).

Melanocytoma (benign melanoma, melanocytic nevus)

Cutaneous melanocytomas are usually solitary, black, brown, or gray cutaneous nodules. Histologically, melanocytomas can be *junctional* (confined to the epidermis and dermoepidermal junction), *compound* (involving both epidermis and dermis), or *dermal*. Of these, the most common in domestic animals are compound and dermal melanocytomas. They are moderately circumscribed but not encapsulated and may be composed of any melanocytic cell type, i.e., spindle, epithelioid, balloon cell (clear cell), or signet ring. Most commonly they are composed of spindle cells, epithelioid cells, or a mixture of these cell types. The epithelioid cells often occur in nests in the dermis or in the epidermis and along the dermoepidermal junction, or in follicular epithelium. The spindle cell component may form whorls and fingerprint patterns in the dermis. The degree of pigmentation can vary, with the epithelioid cells commonly being darkly pigmented, and the spindle cells lightly pigmented or amelanotic. Mitotic figures are rare, and in the dog a mitotic index of less than three is reported to predict benign behavior.

Balloon-cell melanocytoma is a well-recognized variant in which the circumscribed dermal mass is composed of large epithelioid to polygonal cells with plentiful pale amphophilic to eosinophilic cytoplasm that has a faintly granular appearance. Fine melanin granules can sometimes be detected in low numbers of tumor cells. The nuclei are small, hyperchromatic, and uniform.

Melanocytoma-acanthoma

This tumor is composed of both melanocytic and epithelial cells. It is well described in humans but is rare in domestic animals and has been reported only in dogs. The tumors are seen as solitary pigmented nodules, generally 1 cm or less in diameter. Histologically, the tumor is a *combination of a junctional melanocytoma together with a benign epithelial tumor.* The epithelial population forms a mass in the dermis composed of cords and nests with occasional small cystic structures containing keratin. Melanocytic cells form nests in the epidermis and sometimes in the cords of epithelial cells within the dermal mass; melanocytic spindle cells can form whorls and bundles between the epithelial cords and nests.

Malignant melanoma (melanosarcoma)

Malignant melanomas are generally tumors of older animals, however they have been reported in juvenile animals of many species. Criteria for malignancy and prognosis are described in the introduction to this section; *in the dog, a mitotic index of 3 or greater appears to be the most accurate predictor of a poor prognosis.* In addition, several studies have indicated that *the degree of pigmentation and the histologic pattern are not correlated with prognosis.* Malignant melanomas can be composed of a variety of cell morphologies including spindle cells, epithelioid cells, a mixture of spindle cells and epithelioid cells, signet-ring cells, or balloon cells (clear cells). In addition, the cells can be heavily pigmented or amelanotic and form bundles, sheets, nests, and whorled patterns. Focal areas of chondroid or osseous metaplasia within the tumor may be seen on rare occasion. The most common types of malignant melanoma are composed of epithelioid cells, a mixture of epithelioid and spindle cells, or spindle cells alone, forming an unencapsulated mass in the dermis or subcutis. Various degrees of junctional activity may be present in the epithelioid cell form and in the mixed epithelioid-spindle cell form. The epithelioid cells tend to form clusters and nests, and the spindle cells tend to form sheets, bundles, or whorls. The neoplastic cells have variable nuclear pleomorphism, usually single prominent basophilic nucleoli, three or more mitotic figures per ten high-power (×400) fields, and mitotic atypia (Fig. 5.140A). Cytoplasm is generally moderate to abundant, and the degree of pigmentation is highly variable, from darkly pigmented to amelanotic. An infrequent form of spindle cell melanoma, composed entirely of amelanotic spindle cells, can be impossible to distinguish from fibrosarcoma or neurofibrosarcoma without the aid of immunohistochemistry. While the epithelioid and spindle cell forms of melanoma are usually pigmented to some degree, the uncommon balloon cell form and signet-ring cell form are usually unpigmented or poorly pigmented.

Balloon cell melanosarcomas (Fig. 5.140B) are dermal masses that are sometimes multilobulated, and exhibit no junctional activity. The cells are large, with large vesicular nuclei, prominent nucleoli, a relatively low mitotic index, and plentiful clear cytoplasm without visible melanin. Rare cells may have fine pale cytoplasmic dust-like granules. Occasional multinucleated cells can be present.

Signet-ring melanosarcomas (Fig. 5.140C) are composed of round to polygonal cells, that have eccentric nuclei compressed by abundant faintly eosinophilic or amphophilic cytoplasm that is not visibly pigmented. Occasional cells have fine pale brown granules. Nucleoli are prominent. Occasional multinucleated cells can be present.

Bibliography

Aronsohn MG, Carpenter JL. Distal extremity melanocytic nevi and malignant melanomas in dogs. J Am Anim Hosp Assoc 1990;26:605–612.

Bolon B, et al. Characteristics of canine melanomas and comparison of histology and DNA ploidy to their biologic behavior. Vet Pathol 1990;27:96–102.

Chenier S, Dore M. Oral malignant melanoma with osteoid formation in a dog. Vet Pathol 1999;36:74–76.

Espinosa de Los Monteros A, et al. Immunohistopathologic characterization of a dermal melanocytoma-acanthoma in a German Shepherd dog. Vet Pathol 2000;37:268–271.

Fleury C, et al. The study of cutaneous melanomas in Camargue-type gray-skinned horses (1): Clinical-pathological characterization. Pigment Cell Res 2000;13:39–46.

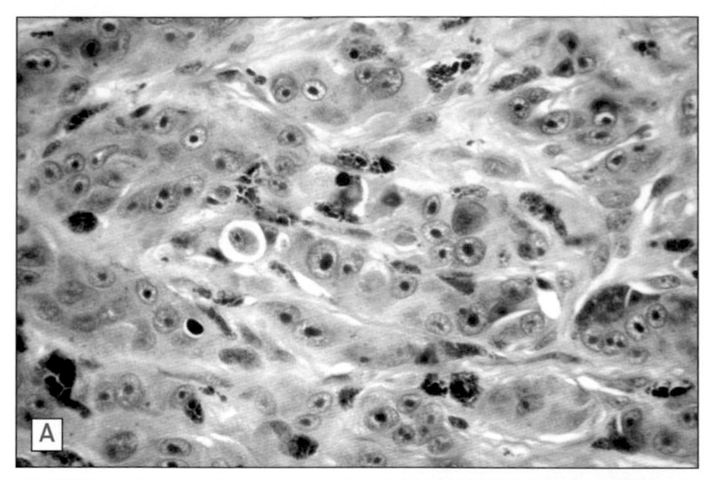

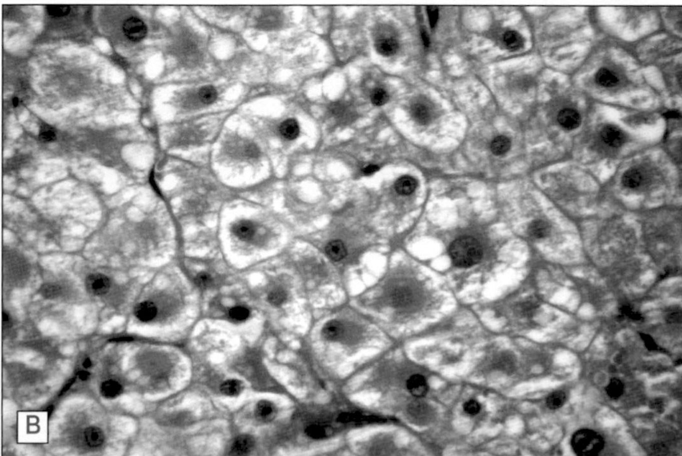

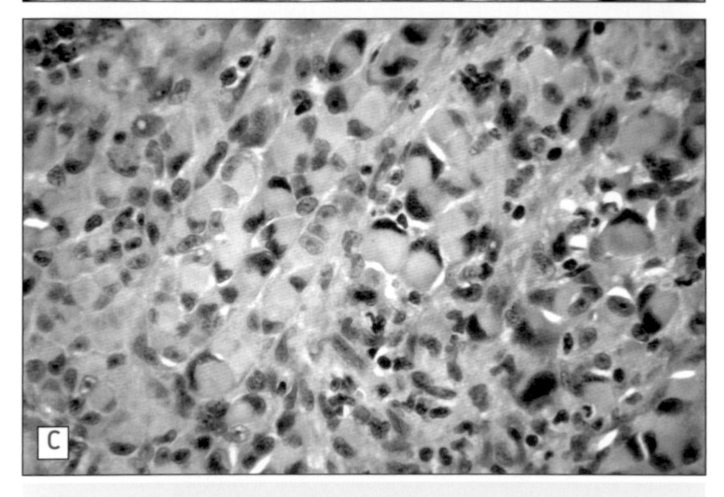

Figure 5.140 Malignant melanoma (melanosarcoma). **A.** Note large prominent nuclei and cellular atypia. **B.** Balloon cell type. **C.** Signet-ring cell type.

Hook RR, et al. Sinclair swine melanoma. Am J Pathol 1982;108:130–133.

Horak V, et al. Hereditary melanoblastoma in miniature pigs and its successful therapy by devitalization technique. Cell Mol Biol 1999;45:1119–1129.

Miller MA, et al. Cutaneous melanocytomas in 10 young cattle. Vet Pathol 1995;32:479–484.

Miller WH, et al. Feline cutaneous melanocytic neoplasms: a retrospective analysis of 43 cases (1979–1991). Vet Dermatol 1993;4:19–26.

Patnaik AK, Mooney S. Feline melanoma: a comparative study of ocular, oral, and dermal neoplasms. Vet Pathol 1988;25:105–112.

Ramos-Vara JA, et al. Retrospective study of 338 canine oral melanomas with clinical, histologic, and immunohistochemical review of 129 cases. Vet Pathol 2000;37:597–608.

Roels S, et al. PCNA and Ki67 proliferation markers as criteria for prediction of clinical behaviour of melanocytic tumours in cats and dogs. J Comp Pathol 1999;121:13–24.

Roels S, et al. Proliferation, DNA ploidy, p53 overexpression and nuclear DNA fragmentation in six equine melanocytic tumours. J Vet Med 2000;47:439–448.

Smith SH, et al. A comparative review of melanocytic neoplasms. Vet Pathol 2002;39:651–678.

Valentine BA. Equine melanocytic tumors: a retrospective study of 53 horses (1988 to 1991). J Vet Intern Med 1995;9:291–297.

van der Linde-Sipman JS, et al. Cutaneous malignant melanomas in 57 cats: identification of (amelanotic) signet-ring and balloon cell types and verification of their origin by immunohistochemistry, electron microscopy, and in situ hybridisation. Vet Pathol 1997;34:31–38.

Walder EJ, Gross TL. Melanocytic tumors. In: Gross TL, et al., eds. Veterinary Dermatopathology. St. Louis, MO: Mosby Year Book, 1992.

Yeruham I, et al. Congenital skin neoplasia in cattle. Vet Dermatol 1999;10:149–156.

Spindle cell tumors

Tumors arising from spindle-shaped cells of the skin are common in dogs and cats, sporadic in horses, and uncommon to rare in other domestic species. *Classification of these tumors may be difficult and the nomenclature is inconsistent and controversial.* The tumors are classified according to the mature tissue they resemble but histologic differences are frequently subtle and morphologic appearance may not be specific enough to reflect histogenesis, particularly for malignant spindle cell tumors. Consequently, *accurate diagnosis by morphologic features alone may not be possible for many tumors.* An immunohistochemical study of canine cutaneous fibrosarcoma, hemangiopericytoma, and schwannoma found poor correlation between morphologic diagnosis and tumor cell differentiation. Although electron microscopy and immunohistochemistry may be helpful in determining the line of differentiation exhibited by tumor cells, some tumors defy identification because of conflicting results owing to loss or alteration in antigens normally present or acquisition of novel antigens. Classification of neoplasms is considered important because of the expectation that it will provide a prediction of the biologic behavior of the tumor. Exact identification of spindle cell sarcomas of the skin may not be essential, however, because *most soft tissue spindle cell tumors exhibit similar behavior and prognosis. They are typically locally invasive, recur frequently after surgical excision, but metastasize infrequently.* The *mitotic index* is more important than the tumor type in predicting the biologic behavior of most soft tissue sarcomas in dogs. Although soft tissue sarcomas may appear well-circumscribed or even encapsulated, *finger-like microextensions of tumor commonly infiltrate into the surrounding tissue to give rise to satellite lesions not visible grossly.* The apparent tumor circumscription commonly results in incomplete excision, leaving microscopic foci of tumor tissue that result in recurrence. Wide surgical excision may be curative, however. Because determination of adequacy of excision is prognostic, *surgical margins should be marked.*

Benign spindle cell tumors

Skin tags (*fibrovascular papilloma, acrochordon, skin polyp*) are benign, fibrovascular lesions of middle-aged and older dogs that may be a *proliferative response to trauma or inflammation rather than actual neoplasms.* They are solitary or multiple soft, polypoid or filiform hairless masses up to 1 cm in diameter and 2–3 cm long that occur most commonly on the *trunk, sternum, and bony prominences* of the limbs. Microscopically, skin tags are composed of mature collagenous tissue that is more highly vascular than normal dermis and covered by an irregularly hyperplastic, hyperkeratotic and hyperpigmented epidermis. Adnexal structures are absent and mononuclear inflammatory cells may be present in low numbers. Ulceration and neutrophilic inflammation are common sequelae to trauma.

Collagen nevi *are focal nodular accumulations of excessive dermal collagen that are relatively common in middle-aged and older dogs.* They are typically solitary, alopecic, firm, dome-shaped nodules up to 1 cm in diameter. Microscopically, they are composed of haphazardly arranged bundles of collagen and low numbers of mature fibroblasts that entrap adnexal structures and result in their distortion or atrophy. Collagen nevi are usually located in the dermis but large masses may extend into the subcutis. The primary differential is fibroma, which tends to be larger and located deeper in the dermis, displaces and compresses adjacent structures, and is more cellular than a collagen nevus. Some veterinary pathologists believe that collagen nevi are actually fibromas of low cellularity. A syndrome called **nodular dermatofibrosis**, characterized by *multiple cutaneous collagenous nodules*, has been reported as *a marker of renal epithelial neoplasia in German Shepherd Dogs.* The condition is thought to be inherited in an autosomal dominant manner. Affected dogs are adults and most have bilateral renal cystadenocarcinomas. Nodules may number in the hundreds and are located anywhere on the body. Individual cases in several other breeds have also been reported. Histologically the lesions are similar to collagen nevi and are differentiated primarily on the basis of the large number of lesions present and the breed affected.

Fibromas *are uncommon benign tumors of fibroblasts and collagen that occur in adult and aged animals of all species.* Fibromas are usually solitary, soft-to-firm, well-circumscribed, round, dome-shaped or pedunculated masses that vary from 1 to 50 cm in diameter. They are usually alopecic and may be hyperpigmented. Large tumors may be ulcerated secondary to trauma. Microscopically, fibromas are well-circumscribed, nonencapsulated dermal or subcutaneous nodules composed of fibroblasts and abundant collagen. The fibroblasts have uniform, oval-to-elongate bland nuclei that may be slightly larger than fibroblasts in the normal dermis and have fine chromatin, inconspicuous nucleoli, and rare mitotic figures. The cytoplasm merges imperceptibly with collagen that is arranged in whorls and interwoven bundles that are thicker and more dense than those in the normal dermis. Adnexal structures are usually displaced and compressed peripherally. Some tumors contain substantial amounts of *mucinous or myxomatous matrix material in addition to the collagen*, in which case the term **fibromyxoma** may be used. In contrast to collagen nevi, fibromas are typically larger, more highly cellular, and displace rather than incorporate adnexal structures.

Myxomas (myxofibromas) are *rare cutaneous neoplasms arising from fibroblasts or multipotential mesenchymal cells and containing abundant glycosaminoglycan stroma.* They usually occur in adult or aged animals as solitary, infiltrative soft masses that are poorly circumscribed and may extend along fascial planes. The tissue is pale and exudes a clear viscous fluid on cut surface. A report of a myxoma developing at the site of a subcutaneously implanted pacemaker in a dog raised the question of whether the implant may have induced the tumor. Microscopically, myxomas are nonencapsulated dermal or subcutaneous masses composed of small stellate to spindle cells randomly distributed within abundant basophilic mucinous stroma with scant, fine collagen fibers. Cellularity is typically low and the cells have small hyperchromatic nuclei and rare mitotic figures. *Recurrence is common because of the infiltrative growth pattern.* Myxomas are difficult to differentiate from myxosarcomas because both are poorly circumscribed, locally infiltrative, and have low mitotic activity. However, nuclear and cellular pleomorphism is more apparent and atypical mitotic figures may be seen in myxosarcomas.

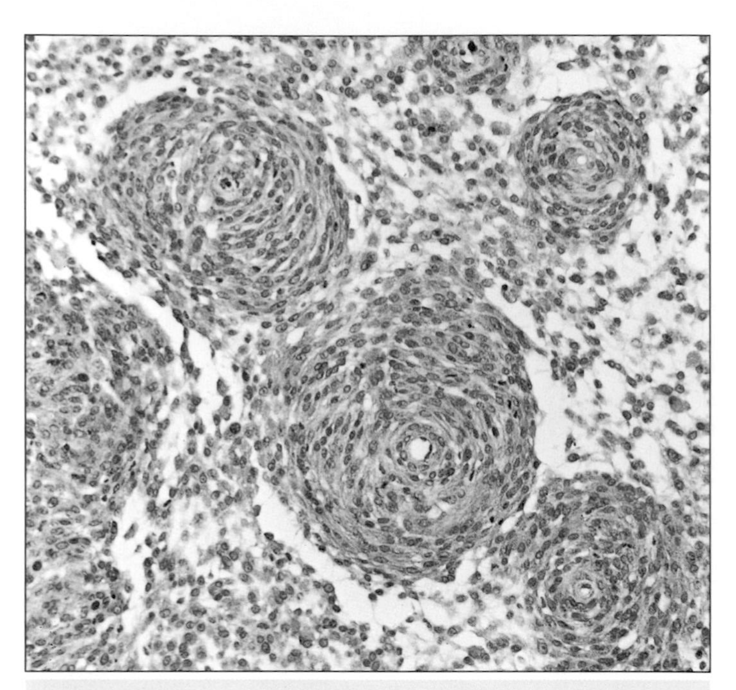

Figure 5.141 Hemangiopericytoma from a dog. Concentric whorls of plump spindle cells around capillary lumina.

Locally infiltrative or malignant spindle cell tumors

Hemangiopericytomas *are relatively common, histologically distinctive, spindle cell tumors of dogs.* Occasional tumors with similar microscopic features are seen in horses and cats. Some ultrastructural and immunohistochemical findings have supported a pericyte origin for this tumor in dogs but *histogenesis is still uncertain.* They usually occur on the *limbs of older dogs* of either sex and any breed but are most common in large breed (>30 kg) dogs. They are usually solitary, slow growing multinodular masses that appear grossly well circumscribed and measure up to 25 cm in diameter. The tissue is usually pale and the consistency varies from soft to very firm. The tumors *frequently recur following excision* owing to the difficulty in identifying tumor margins and inability to perform wide surgical excision because of anatomic constraints. *Metastasis is uncommon*, however.

Hemangiopericytomas are usually located in the dermis and subcutis and are primarily composed of uniform plump spindle cells with oval nuclei, fine chromatin, and small central nucleoli. The characteristic microscopic feature of hemangiopericytoma is *plump spindle cells arranged in concentric layers to form whorls, sometimes with small vessels within the centers* (Fig. 5.141). Sheets and interlacing bundles of similar spindle cells, occasional polygonal cells and multinucleated cells, and variable amounts of collagen also comprise most tumors. Densely cellular areas alternate with loose, myxomatous-appearing areas. Aggregates of lymphocytes may be scattered within some tumors and are usually most prominent along the periphery. At the margins of the tumor, *finger-like microextensions* of tumor cells commonly infiltrate along fascial planes and are the reason many tumors are incompletely excised despite the clinical impression that they are well circumscribed. The mitotic index is usually low but it may not be a reliable prognostic indicator of metastasis. Recurrent tumors may exhibit more prominent pleomorphism and a higher mitotic index. *Tumor cells typically express vimentin intermediate filament and are also frequently positive for actin but are negative for desmin.* A small number of tumors has been positive for S-100 protein, suggesting that some tumors diagnosed as hemangiopericytoma by morphologic features may actually be of neural origin.

Cutaneous tumors of neural origin are uncommon in domestic animals but are likely under-diagnosed because of their histologic similarity to other more common tumors of the skin. They can be composed of one or more elements of a nerve, i.e., axon, Schwann cell, and perineurial fibroblast. Consequently, these tumors are histologically heterogeneous and the histogenesis is frequently uncertain, resulting in varied and confusing classification and terminology in the literature. They have been called neurofibromas/neurofibrosarcomas, neurilemmomas, neurinomas, and schwannomas/malignant schwannomas. The name **peripheral nerve sheath tumor** is a broad term proposed to include all tumors arising from peripheral nerves; however, since most tumors are composed of Schwann cells, the term **schwannoma** is appropriate for the majority of the tumors. Both benign and malignant forms occur; however, tumors that appear histologically benign commonly recur. Schwannomas are common in **cattle** but occur primarily in the heart and rarely involve the skin. A condition termed **neurofibromatosis** has been observed in cattle of all ages and may occur congenitally. It is characterized by multiple neural tumors that usually involve deep nerves and viscera but sometimes also the skin.

Cutaneous peripheral nerve sheath tumors are usually solitary, well-circumscribed, slow growing, soft to firm nodules in middle-aged to aged animals. In cats, the head and distal limbs may be involved most frequently. Schwannomas are usually subcutaneous in dogs; in cats they may be confined to the dermis. Microscopically, *schwannomas are most commonly composed of small spindle cells characterized by oval, spindle-shaped, or wavy nuclei, fine chromatin, small inconspicuous nucleoli, and pale indistinct cytoplasm. The spindle cells form whorls, interlacing fascicles, and palisades reminiscent of nerve* (Fig. 5.142). A delicate collagenous stroma is moderately abundant and a mucinous matrix may be prominent in some tumors. Delicate finger-like projections of tumor cells commonly extend into adjacent tissues and between fascial planes, accounting for frequent recurrences. Cellularity is increased, cellular pleomorphism is more prominent, and there is a decreased tendency to form whorls and palisades in malignant tumors. Mitotic figures are uncommon in benign tumors but may be moderately numerous in malignant peripheral nerve sheath tumors. Histologically and behaviorally, peripheral nerve sheath tumors may be difficult to differentiate from fibromas, well differentiated fibrosarcomas, and hemangiopericytomas. However, *neural tumors express S-100 protein, myelin basic protein, neuron-specific enolase, and glial fibrillary acidic protein, whereas the other more common cutaneous tumors do not.* Immunohistochemical staining of **granular cell tumors** (granular cell myoblastomas) has demonstrated S-100 protein, myelin basic protein, and neuron-specific enolase within tumor cells, suggesting that they also represent a form of peripheral nerve sheath tumor.

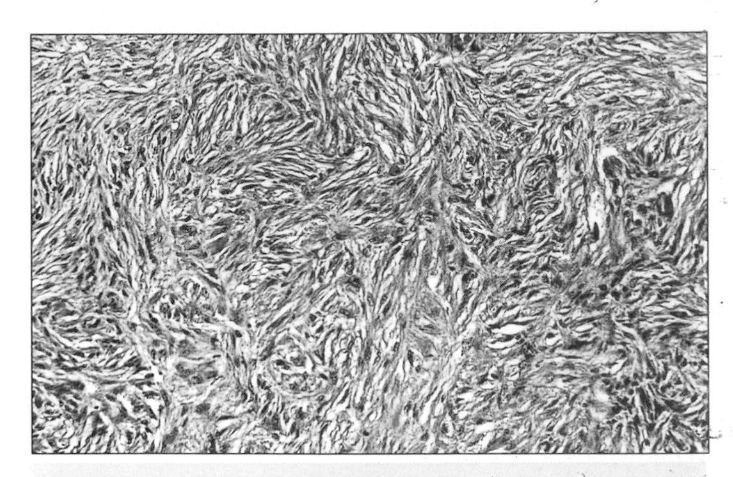

Figure 5.142 Peripheral nerve sheath tumor.

Traumatic neuroma (*tail dock neuroma, amputation neuroma*) is considered an exuberant but non-neoplastic proliferation of the proximal nerve stump occurring in response to injury or surgery. In veterinary medicine, this lesion is rare and occurs most frequently as a result of tail docking in **dogs**. The tumors develop in young dogs, usually within 1 year after caudectomy. They are typically painful, self-traumatized, alopecic, hyperpigmented, lichenified lesions adherent to the underlying deep tissues at the tip of the tail. Microscopically, traumatic neuromas are well-circumscribed nodules composed of *haphazardly arranged myelinated nerve bundles of varying size randomly distributed within a relatively abundant connective tissue stroma.*

Sarcoids *are locally aggressive, non-metastatic fibroblastic skin tumors of horses, mules, and donkeys.* They are the *most common skin tumor of horses*, accounting for up to 30% of tumors, and occur in any breed, sex, or age. However, there appears to be a higher incidence in Quarter Horses, Arabians, and Appaloosas and a lower incidence in Standardbreds. Young adult horses 3–6 yr of age are most commonly affected. A combination of factors appears to be involved in development of the tumors, including *exposure to a viral agent, cutaneous trauma, and a genetic predilection.* Viral etiology has been deduced based on reports of epizootics of cases, transmission studies, detection of virus particles in cultured tumor cells, and demonstration of DNA sequences very similar or identical to that of *Bovine papillomavirus-1* or *-2* genome in tumor cells but not in normal tissues, granulation tissue, or other tumors of horses and donkeys. Sarcoids frequently develop in areas subjected to trauma or at sites of wounds 6 to 8 months after wound healing. A genetically determined predisposition is suggested since an association between susceptibility to sarcoid and certain major histocompatibility complex (MHC) alleles has been found.

Sarcoids develop anywhere but are most common on the *head, legs, and ventral trunk.* They may be single or multiple. The tumors are classified according to their gross appearance as verrucous, fibroblastic, mixed, or occult. The *verrucous type* is a small wart-like growth, usually measuring less than 6 cm in diameter, with a dry, rough surface and variable alopecia. The *fibroblastic type* of sarcoid is more

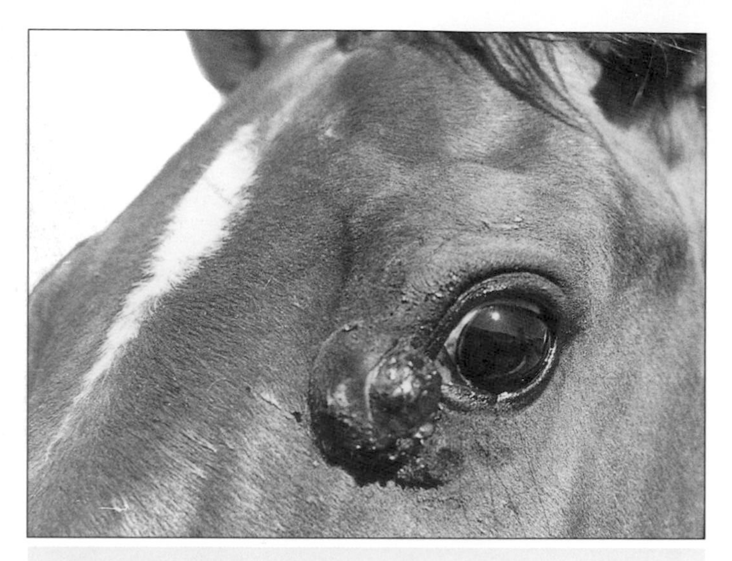

Figure 5.143 Sarcoid from a horse.

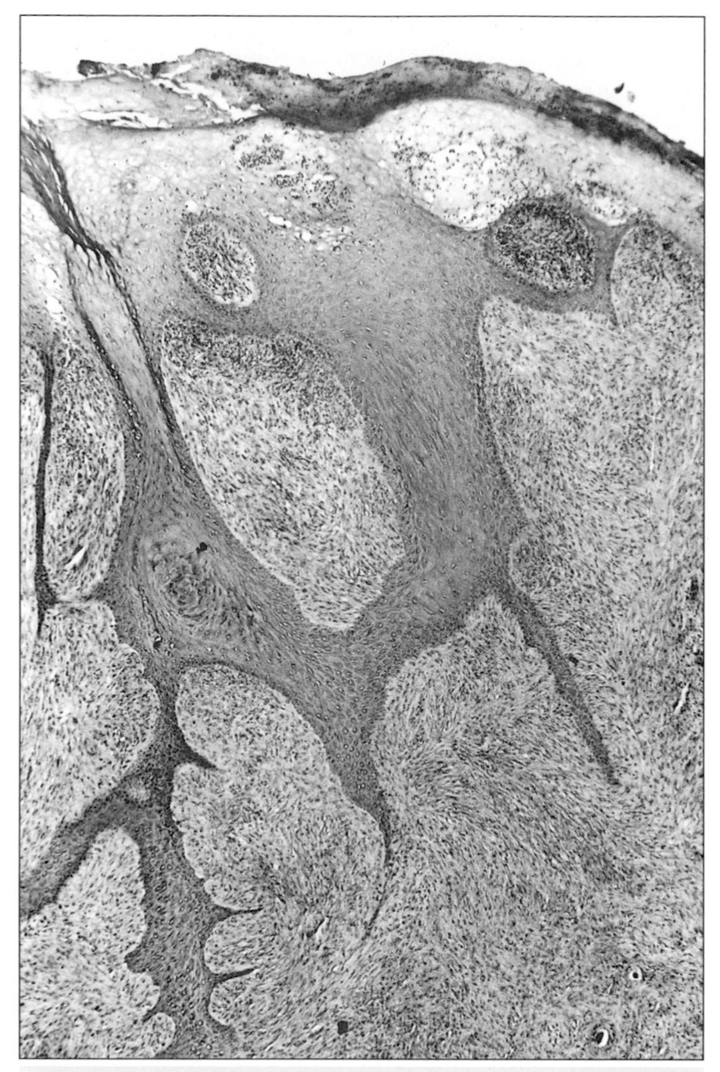

Figure 5.144 Sarcoid from a horse. Note epithelial proliferation and associated dermal fibroblastic proliferation.

variable in appearance and may range from a well-circumscribed firm nodule with intact surface to large masses, greater than 25 cm in diameter, with an ulcerated surface prone to hemorrhage and resembling exuberant granulation tissue. The *mixed type* is a transitional form in which a verrucous sarcoid becomes a fibroblastic type as a result of trauma or biopsy. The *occult form* consists of a slow-growing, slightly thickened area of skin with slight surface roughening and alopecia that remains static for long periods. *Spontaneous remission* may occur after several years in up to 30% of cases. The tumors are characterized by a high rate of recurrence, up to 50%, following surgical excision.

Grossly, sarcoids may resemble many inflammatory and neoplastic diseases including bacterial and fungal granulomas, exuberant granulation tissue, habronemiasis, papilloma, squamous cell carcinoma, fibroma, and other less frequent mesenchymal tumors (Fig. 5.143). Consequently, *histopathology is necessary for definitive diagnosis of a sarcoid.* Wide surgical excision is preferable to a biopsy because the lesions are frequently associated with ulceration, inflammation, and granulation tissue proliferation and the diagnosis may be missed in a small biopsy. Additionally, the trauma associated with obtaining a biopsy of a sarcoid may dramatically stimulate the growth rate and aggressiveness of the tumor. Sarcoids are typically *biphasic tumors composed of both epidermal and dermal components.* The epidermal component may be minimal or absent in some tumors, however. When the epidermis is intact, hyperkeratosis, parakeratosis, and acanthosis with thin rete pegs extending deep into the dermis are common features (Fig. 5.144). The dermal component consists of fibroblasts and collagen in various proportions. The fibroblasts have plump nuclei and nucleoli may be prominent. The mitotic index is usually low. *Fibroblasts at the dermal-epidermal junction are frequently oriented perpendicular to the basement membrane in a "picket fence" pattern, which is a distinctive histologic feature seen in most sarcoids.* The cells are arranged in whorls, interlacing bundles, or haphazard arrays of variable density. Tumor margins are typically indistinct and adequacy of excision is frequently difficult to determine. When the tumor is ulcerated, it may not be possible to differentiate a sarcoid from granulation tissue, fibroma, well-differentiated fibrosarcoma, and peripheral nerve sheath tumor. Immunohistochemical staining for S-100 protein may be useful in confirming a peripheral nerve sheath tumor. Additional biopsies to include intact epidermis may be required to make a diagnosis.

A tumor with histologic features similar to equine sarcoid has been described in cats and termed **feline fibropapilloma**. The cats are frequently young, 5 years or less, and have one or several tumors that may be ulcerated. The tumors have been reported in various sites, including the lip, nose, digits, pinna, tail, and gingiva. Recurrence was common but metastasis has not been documented. As in equine sarcoids, papillomavirus DNA has been identified in some of the feline tumors by polymerase chain reaction testing. The nucleotide sequence was similar to a bovine papillomavirus and many of the affected cats had known exposure to cattle.

Fibrosarcomas are malignant tumors of fibroblasts that show no other evidence of cell differentiation. They commonly recur and may metastasize. *Fibrosarcomas are undoubtedly over-diagnosed*, as virtually any anaplastic highly cellular spindle cell sarcoma containing collagen is diagnosed as a fibrosarcoma when more specific histogenesis is not apparent. However, as *immunohistochemistry* has become a routine technique in most diagnostic laboratories, fibrosarcoma can be separated from other spindle cell tumors such as peripheral nerve sheath tumor, leiomyosarcoma, rhabdomyosarcoma, amelanotic malignant melanoma, spindle cell carcinoma, and others.

Fibrosarcomas are common in dogs and cats and uncommon in other domestic species. In **dogs**, they usually occur in older animals and are most common on the trunk and limbs. They usually arise in the subcutis and are poorly circumscribed masses of variable size that may be soft to firm in consistency. Large tumors are often ulcerated and alopecic. Most canine fibrosarcomas are low-grade malignancies that commonly recur locally and metastasize infrequently. Similarities have been noted between canine fibrosarcomas from presumed injection sites and feline post-vaccinal fibrosarcomas, suggesting that post-injection sarcomas may also occur in dogs.

Fibrosarcoma is the most common malignant mesenchymal tumor of **cats**, and three forms of fibrosarcoma have been recognized – virus-induced, solitary in older cats, and post-vaccinal.

Virus-induced fibrosarcoma is rare. *Feline sarcoma virus* (FeSV) is the cause of multicentric fibrosarcoma in cats usually less than 5 years of age. FeSV is a replication-defective retrovirus that requires *Feline leukemia virus* (FeLV) as a helper virus. The genetic recombination of the two viruses produces an acutely transforming virus that induces multiple simultaneous rapidly growing fibrosarcomas after a short incubation period. FeSV-induced fibrosarcomas are typically locally invasive and metastasize to lung and other sites.

Solitary fibrosarcomas in older cats are much more common that virus-induced multicentric tumors. These may arise in the dermis or subcutis. Subcutaneous tumors are usually on the trunk and limbs; dermal tumors primarily involve the digits and pinnae. The clinical appearance and behavior of this type of fibrosarcoma are similar to those in dogs.

Epidemiologic evidence supports a relationship between vaccine administration in cats and the development of *post-vaccinal fibrosarcomas* and, to a lesser extent, other sarcomas in the injection sites. The interval between vaccination and tumor development is 3 months to 3.5 years. The mechanism of tumor development is unknown but persistent injection-site induced inflammation leading to deranged fibrous connective tissue repair response and eventual neoplastic transformation in genetically predisposed cats has been postulated. Alterations in oncogene and growth factor expression may be involved in the pathogenesis. Post-vaccinal fibrosarcomas typically develop in the subcutis of the dorsal cervical and interscapular area, dorsal and lateral thorax, flank, and musculature of the thigh, locations that are all *common vaccination sites*. These tumors arise in cats that are younger (median age, 8 years) than those with fibrosarcomas at nonvaccination sites (median age, 10.5 years) and are larger than nonvaccination site fibrosarcomas. The masses frequently have cystic centers, firm attachments to dorsal spinous processes or other deep structures, and ill-defined margins. *They are biologically aggressive and commonly recur multiple times within a period of weeks to months when removed.* The metastatic rate is not well characterized, but was found to be as high as 24% in one study. The lungs and regional lymph nodes are the most common sites of metastasis. Wide surgical excision prolongs the interval to recurrence but often fails to remove the tumor completely. Radiation therapy and chemotherapy are under evaluation as adjunctive treatment to prevent local recurrence and systemic spread, respectively.

Microscopically, *fibrosarcomas consist of interlacing and intersecting bundles of immature fibroblastic cells.* The tumors show a great deal of variation with respect to cellular pleomorphism and density, mitotic activity, and amount and maturity of collagen. Multinucleated giant cells are seen in many fibrosarcomas but are not numerous. The tumors are dermal, subcutaneous, or both. They are usually nonencapsulated, and local invasion is evident as finger-like projections of tumor cells extending along fascial planes and into surrounding tissues. These microscopic extensions of the tumor account for the difficulty in excising the tumor completely and resultant recurrences. Although collagen is the primary stromal element, mucin may also be produced in small amounts. Immunohistochemical staining is *positive for vimentin* only. *Retrospective studies have found only the mitotic index* (total number of mitotic figures in ten high-power (×400) fields) *to be significant in predicting tumor behavior.* In dogs, a mitotic index less than 9 was associated with greater survival than a mitotic index of 9 or greater. Likewise, cats with solitary fibrosarcomas with a mitotic index of 5 or less had significantly greater survival time than cats with tumors with mitotic index of 6 or greater. Poorly differentiated fibrosarcomas may be difficult to differentiate from a number of other mesenchymal and nonmesenchymal tumors including malignant schwannoma, malignant fibrous histiocytoma, leiomyosarcoma, and spindle cell forms of amelanotic melanoma and squamous cell carcinoma. In such cases, immunohistochemical staining is necessary to exclude other tumors by showing lack of immunoreactivity to antigens typical of other cell types. In small biopsies with a limited amount of tissue to evaluate, it may be difficult to differentiate fibrosarcoma from reactive granulation tissue.

Post-vaccinal fibrosarcomas are typically subcutaneous and have large cavitated centers as a result of extensive necrosis. An inflammatory reaction, consisting of lymphocytes and macrophages that sometimes contain gray-brown or blue globular material typical of a vaccine reaction, is commonly present at the periphery of the tumor. Mitotic activity and cellular pleomorphism tend to be high; however, histologic grade does not appear to be associated with outcome. Tumor cells of vaccination-site fibrosarcomas have been reported to be consistently strongly immunoreactive for platelet-derived growth factor and its receptor, epidermal growth factor and its receptor, and transforming growth factor-β, while nonvaccine-associated fibrosarcomas are negative or only slightly positive.

Malignant fibrous histiocytoma *(giant cell tumor of soft parts, extraskeletal giant cell tumor) is an uncommon tumor of controversial histogenesis.* It was originally believed to be derived from malignant cells of monocyte-macrophage origin capable of acting as "facultative" fibroblasts. Ultrastructural and immunohistochemical findings, however, indicate that malignant fibrous histiocytoma may not be a distinct entity but rather a *collection of anaplastic mesenchymal and nonmesenchymal tumors.* Nevertheless, the diagnosis of malignant fibrous histiocytoma is made for those neoplasms characterized histologically by the *combination of fibroblast-like spindle cells, vacuolated histiocyte-like cells, and variable numbers of pleomorphic multinucleated giant cells along with a collagenous stroma.* The tumor is uncommon to rare in dogs and cats and has been reported in horses and an adult cow. Most cases occur in older animals. They occur on the *legs and shoulders* most commonly. The tumor is usually solitary, firm, and poorly circumscribed and the skin surface may be ulcerated. *The tumors typically have a moderate rate of growth, exhibit locally invasive growth, and recur commonly after surgical excision.* The potential for metastasis is disputed but has been found to be low in most reports. Microscopically, the giant cell type of malignant fibrous histiocytoma is most common and is composed of fibroblastic-like spindle cells arranged in a storiform (or cartwheel) pattern or in interwoven bundles with variable amounts of collagen resembling a fibrosarcoma. Polygonal cells that resemble histiocytes are distributed throughout the tumor or form focal aggregates. Multinucleated giant cells with 30 or more nuclei and abundant eosinophilic cytoplasm usually form aggregates rather than being diffusely distributed throughout the tumor. The giant cells resemble osteoclasts but are not associated with any osteoid production. Mitotic activity is variable but usually moderate to high and atypical mitotic figures are common. There is no immunohistochemical profile unique to malignant fibrous histiocytoma and, in fact, immunohistochemical staining may result in classification of tumors diagnosed as malignant fibrous histiocytoma by light microscopy as various other malignant tumors.

Other mesenchymal tumors

Tumors arising from subcutaneous lipocytes occur in all species. **Lipomas** are most common in dogs and may be multiple. In all species, they usually occur in adult and aged animals and are most commonly located on the trunk and proximal limbs. *Lipomas are masses of well-differentiated lipocytes indistinguishable from normal fat* except for a compressed boundary of delicate stroma that normally serves to delineate the margin between tumor and adjacent normal adipose tissue. Some lipomas contain cartilage, bone, collagen, or blood vessels. In addition, some mesenchymal tumours contain roughly equal proportions of adipose tissue mixed with other mesenchymal components. These form distinctive variants such as *angiolipomas*, *fibrolipomas* and *leiomyolipomas*. Occasionally hemangiosarcomas and mast cell tumours may be found arising within lipomatous masses, suggesting that lipomas may sometimes provide a local environment suitable for the emergence of these more sinister neoplasms. Necrosis, hemorrhage, fibrosis, and mild macrophage inflammation may occur as a result of trauma to lipomas.

Infiltrative lipomas are uncommon tumors of dogs. *They are usually large, poorly delineated, deep subcutaneous masses composed of well differentiated lipocytes that infiltrate subcutaneous muscle and fascia.* They may cause pain or interfere with limb function and may invade through the body wall.

Liposarcomas are malignant tumors of lipocytes and are uncommon in all species. Liposarcomas in cats have been associated with retrovirus infection and with vaccination sites; a liposarcoma in a dog was associated with a glass foreign body. *Liposarcomas may recur but rarely metastasize. They are usually well-circumscribed, nonencapsulated, highly cellular masses of round to polyhedral cells primarily and fewer stellate, spindle, and multinucleated cells.* Lipocyte origin is recognized by the presence of *cytoplasmic vacuolation* that may be numerous fine vacuoles or a single large clear vacuole that displaces the nucleus peripherally. Mitotic figures are generally infrequent. *Myxoid liposarcomas* have prominent mucinous ground substance. Liposarcomas may be difficult to differentiate from anaplastic sebaceous carcinomas and balloon cell or clear cell melanomas. The tumor cells of liposarcoma are usually arranged in solid sheets of vacuolated cells while in sebaceous carcinoma the cells tend to be subdivided into nests and lobules. The presence of rare cells with cytoplasmic dusting of very fine brown granules can differentiate melanoma from the other two tumors; however, immunohistochemical staining for cytokeratin, vimentin, and a melanocytic marker (such as Melan A) may be needed to differentiate the tumors.

Tumors originating from muscle are rare in the skin of animals. Smooth muscle tumors, **leiomyomas** and **leiomyosarcomas**, can arise from arrector pili muscles (*piloleiomyomas*), cutaneous blood vessels (*angioleiomyomas*), and specialized muscles of genital skin. These tumors are usually solitary, firm, and well-circumscribed in animals. In humans, piloleiomyomas are commonly multiple; and multiple piloleiomyomas have been reported in an old cat. Microscopically, leiomyomas are small, well-circumscribed dermal masses adjacent to and surrounding hair follicles. They are composed of uniform long spindle cells in whorling and interlacing bundles. The cells have bland elongate nuclei with blunt ends ("cigar-shaped") and moderately abundant pale eosinophilic cytoplasm. Mitotic figures are rare. Leiomyosarcomas exhibit nuclear pleomorphism and low to moderate mitotic activity. Angioleiomyomas consist of interlacing bundles of smooth muscle cells between numerous vascular channels. Smooth muscle tumors may be confused with fibromas, fibrosarcomas, or malignant schwannomas. In such cases, *immunohistochemical staining for actin and desmin can confirm muscle origin.*

Cutaneous tumors of skeletal muscle, **rhabdomyomas** and **rhabdomyosarcomas**, are extremely rare. Rhabdomyomas of the ear pinna have been reported in four white-eared cats. The tumors were thinly haired, red-purple, nonulcerated discoid nodules 1–2 cm in diameter on the convex surface of the pinna. Histologically, they were well-circumscribed masses composed of whorls and bundles of long spindle cells with cross-striations evident in a few tumor cells. Mitotic figures were rare. Surgical excision was curative.

Bibliography

Bostock DE, Dye MT. Prognosis after surgical excision of canine fibrous connective tissue sarcomas. Vet Pathol 1980;17:581–588.

Carr EA, et al. Bovine papillomavirus DNA in neoplastic and nonneoplastic tissues obtained from horses with and without sarcoids in the western United States. Am J Vet Res 2001;62:741–745.

Chambers G, et al. Association of bovine papillomavirus with the equine sarcoid. J Gen Virol 2003;84(Pt 5):1055–1062.

Esplin DG, et al. Metastasizing liposarcoma associated with a vaccination site in a cat. Fel Pract 1996;24:20–23.

Finnie JW, et al. Multiple piloleiomyomas in a cat. J Comp Pathol 1995;113:201–204.

Hendrick MJ. Feline vaccine-associated sarcomas. Cancer Invest 1999;17:273–277.

Jones BR, et al. Nerve sheath tumours in the dog and cat. N Zealand Vet J 1995;43:190–196.

Kim DY, et al. Malignant peripheral nerve sheath tumor with divergent mesenchymal differentiations in a dog. J Vet Diagn Invest 2003;15:174–178.

Kuntz CA, et al. Prognostic factors for surgical treatment of soft-tissue sarcomas in dogs: 75 cases (1986–1996). J Am Vet Med Assoc 1997;211:1147–1151.

Kuwamura M, et al. Canine peripheral nerve sheath tumor with eosinophilic cytoplasmic globules. Vet Pathol 1998;35:223–226.

Martens A, et al. Polymerase chain reaction analysis of the surgical margins of equine sarcoids for bovine papilloma virus DNA. Vet Surg 2001;30:460–467.

McCarthy PE, et al. Liposarcoma associated with a glass foreign body in a dog. J Am Vet Med Assoc 1996;209:612–614.

Miller MA, et al. Cutaneous neoplasia in 340 cats. Vet Pathol 1991;28:389–395.

Nasir L, Reid SWJ. Bovine papillomaviral gene expression in equine sarcoid tumours. Virus Res 1999;61:171–175.

Pace LW, et al. Immunohistochemical staining of feline malignant fibrous histiocytomas. Vet Pathol 1994;31:168–172.

Pérez J, et al. Immunohistochemical characterization of hemangiopericytomas and other spindle cell tumors in the dog. Vet Pathol 1996;33:391–397.
Roth L. Rhabdomyoma of the ear pinna in four cats. J Comp Pathol 1990;103:237–240.
Rowland PH, et al. Myxoma at the site of a subcutaneous pacemaker in a dog. J Am Anim Hosp Assoc 1991;27:649–651.
Sartin EA, et al. Invasive malignant fibrous histiocytoma in a cow. J Am Vet Med Assoc 1996;208:1709–1710.
Schulman FY, et al. Feline cutaneous fibropapillomas: Clinicopathologic findings and association with papillomavirus infection. Vet Pathol 2001;38:291–296.
Vascellari M, et al. Fibrosarcomas at presumed sites of injection in dogs: characteristics and comparison with non-vaccination site fibrosarcomas and feline post-vaccinal fibrosarcomas. J Vet Med A Physiol Pathol Clin Med 2003;50:286–291.
Waters CB, et al. Giant cell variant of malignant fibrous histiocytoma in dogs: 10 cases (1986–1993). J Am Vet Med Assoc 1994;205:1420–1424.
Williamson MM, Middleton DJ. Cutaneous soft tissue tumours in dogs: classification, differentiation, and histogenesis. Vet Dermatol 1998;9:43–48.

Vascular tumors

Cutaneous vasoformative tumors are common in dogs, occasional in cats and horses, and uncommon in other species. The majority are benign in dogs and horses whereas malignant tumors are more common in cats. Vascular tumors may be associated with thrombocytopenia, disseminated intravascular coagulation, and other hemostatic abnormalities.

Hemangioma *is a benign neoplasm of blood vessel endothelium that can originate in the dermis or subcutis.* The tumor is usually a solitary, well-circumscribed, fluctuant to firm, blue to red-black, slow-growing mass. Cutaneous hemangioma in **dogs** usually occurs in older animals (mean, 9–10 years) without apparent sex predilection. The tumor can occur anywhere but lightly pigmented, sparsely haired ventral abdominal and inguinal skin may be predisposed. Chronic solar damage has been suggested as a cause of dermal hemangiomas in this location and they may be multiple. Surgical excision is curative.

Benign cutaneous vascular lesions in **horses** frequently occur in animals less than 1 year of age and some are congenital, raising the question of whether the lesions are true neoplasms or vascular malformations (hamartoma or nevus). The confusion in categorizing these vascular lesions in young horses has resulted in *inconsistent nomenclature* and they have been referred to as **lobular capillary hemangioma** and **vascular nevus** in the literature. The lesions are most commonly located on the limbs and present as a cauliflower or nodular mass or diffuse skin thickening which may become alopecic and ulcerated. The lesions may recur following excision. In some instances they are too extensive to be excised, necessitating euthanasia of the affected animal. Cutaneous hemangiomas usually occur in adult and aged **cattle**; congenital hemangiomas have been reported also and these are frequently multiple.

Microscopically, hemangiomas consist of nonencapsulated dermal or subcutaneous masses composed of blood-filled channels lined by a single layer of flattened, mature endothelium (Fig. 5.145). Mitotic figures are rare. Subcutaneous tumors are usually well-circumscribed, while those in the dermis may not be as well defined and may incorporate adnexal structures within the mass. The tumors are classified as *capillary* or *cavernous* depending on the size of the vascular spaces. The cavernous type is more common in dogs. The vascular channels are usually separated by collagenous septa that contain variable numbers of mast cells, lymphoid cells, and hemosiderin-laden macrophages. Occasional vascular channels contain fibrin thrombi. *Solar-induced dermal hemangiomas* of glabrous skin are located in the superficial dermis and may be associated with solar elastosis. A variant of hemangioma, called **angiokeratoma**, is a raised superficial dermal hemangioma with prominent, irregular hyperplasia of the epidermis which extends down to separate and partially surround the vascular channels. The *lobular capillary hemangioma/vascular nevus of young horses* consists of multiple discrete dermal lobules of closely packed, haphazardly arranged vascular structures of small caliber. The vessels are lined by endothelial cells with plump oval nuclei and low mitotic activity. **Cutaneous angiomatosis** is a multinodular hemangioma with intervening inflamed connective tissue stroma that extends above the skin surface and bleeds spontaneously. It occurs in cattle and horses most commonly and also in cats and goats. This lesion has been compared to the human "pyogenic granuloma."

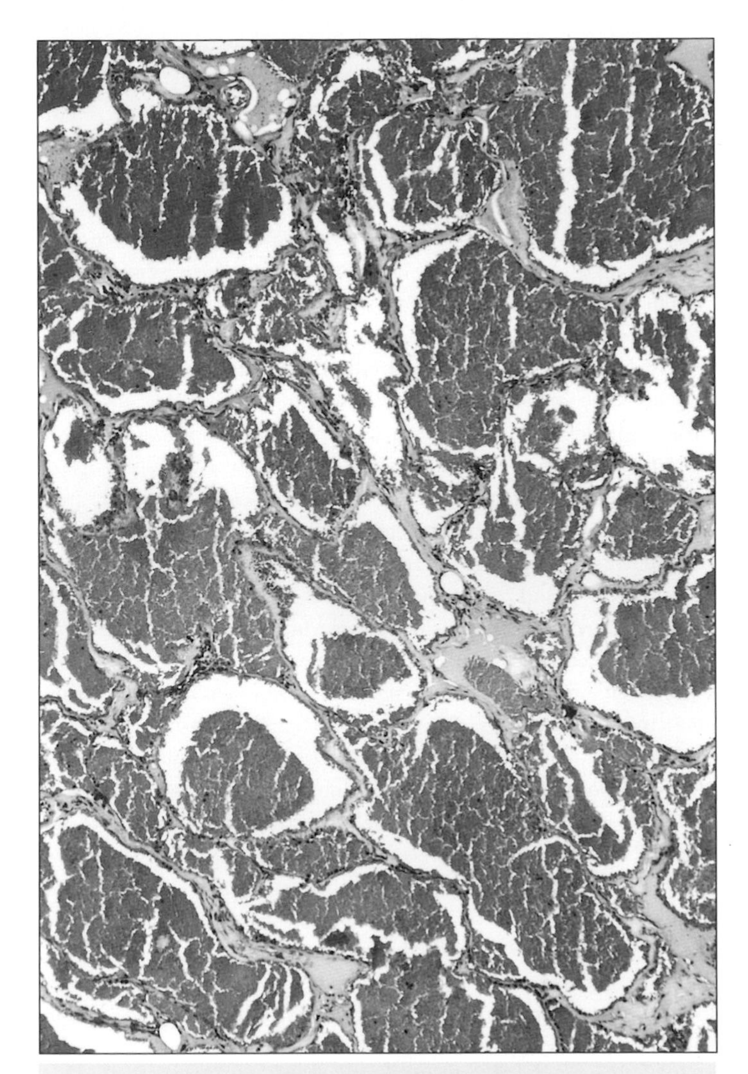

Figure 5.145 Cutaneous hemangioma from a dog.

Hemangiosarcoma, the malignant form of a tumor of blood vessel endothelium, can occur in the skin as a primary site or as a result of metastatic disease from a primary visceral tumor. These tumors usually occur in adult and aged animals. In one study of cutaneous vascular tumors of cats, hemangiosarcomas occurred most frequently in white-haired sites and most commonly involved the pinnae and head. Cutaneous hemangiosarcoma commonly recurs following excision and has the potential for widespread local invasion and metastasis; but in general it appears to be less aggressive, has a longer clinical course, and prolonged survival when compared to visceral hemangiosarcomas. In contrast to the subcutaneous form, dermal hemangiosarcoma may be cured by wide surgical excision alone.

The degree of differentiation is extremely variable, ranging from well-differentiated tumors with well-defined vascular channels to poorly differentiated tumors with minimal lumen formation. *Usually hemangiosarcomas consist of plump pleomorphic endothelial cells arranged in single or multiple layers along trabeculae of collagen or preexisting dermal collagen fibers to form a poorly circumscribed meshwork of blood-filled spaces.* Collagenous trabeculae lined by endothelial cells commonly protrude blindly into the vascular spaces. Mitotic activity may be high. Frequently, portions or entire tumors are composed entirely of sheets or intersecting and anastomosing bundles of pleomorphic spindle cells and they may be indistinguishable from fibrosarcoma or other poorly differentiated spindle cell sarcomas. The presence of slit-like spaces containing erythrocytes between tumor cells may be the only clue to the diagnosis. Immunohistochemical staining may be required to identify the cells in anaplastic tumors. Endothelial cells express vimentin, factor VIII-related antigen (von Willebrand factor), and CD31 (platelet-endothelial cell adhesion molecule/PECAM). However, *immunostaining must be interpreted with knowledge of limitations of the procedure*; in poorly differentiated tumors, very anaplastic cells may not express typical antigens and immature reactive stromal endothelial cells may be mistaken for tumor cells.

Tumors arising from endothelium of lymphatic vessels are rare in domestic animals. Both the benign, **lymphangioma**, and malignant, **lymphangiosarcoma**, forms occur in young animals and it has been suggested that they represent lymphatic malformations resulting from a failure of connection between lymph vessels and the venous system rather than being true neoplasms. *The skin and subcutis appear to be the most common site of tumors of lymphatic endothelium and the caudal ventral abdomen and inguinal areas appear to be predisposed.* They typically present as poorly defined fluctuant or edematous masses that are present for many months and drain clear serous to milky fluid. Rarely they occur as multiple clear turgid vesicles or bullae. It may be difficult to distinguish between lymphangioma and lymphangiosarcoma histologically as the histologic appearance may not correlate well with the biologic behavior of the tumor. Tumors that appear histologically benign commonly recur and may be locally invasive. Lymphangiosarcomas commonly invade local tissues extensively and metastasize to distant sites. They are poorly defined and difficult to remove completely, resulting in poor wound healing and recurrence. In contrast to tumors of vascular endothelium, *lymphangiomas/lymphangiosarcomas are composed of spaces largely devoid of material.* They may contain only small amounts of proteinaceous fluid and low numbers of erythrocytes and/or lymphoid cells. The connective tissue stroma separating the vascular spaces is loose or edematous and may contain aggregates of lymphoid cells. These tumors have been reported to be immunoreactive for factor VIII-related antigen (von Willebrand factor); CD31 reactivity is variable. Ulceration, hemorrhage, granulation tissue proliferation, and inflammation are frequently present because of the chronic clinical course and may result in misdiagnosis when a small biopsy is taken. It may not be possible to differentiate a poorly differentiated lymphangiosarcoma from hemangiosarcoma. Further complicating diagnosis is a condition called **lymphangiomatosis**, which is considered a developmental disorder composed of bland dilated lymph channels involving skin, soft tissue, bone, and parenchymal organs.

Bibliography

Belanger MC, et al. Invasive multiple lymphangiomas in a young dog. J Am Anim Hosp Assoc 1999;35:507–509.

Berry WL, et al. Lymphangiomatosis of the pelvic limb in a Maltese dog. J Small Anim Pract 1996;37:340–343.

Diessler ME, et al. Cutaneous lymphangiosarcoma in a young dog: clinical, anatomopathological and lectinhistochemical description. J Vet Med A Physiol Pathol Clin Med 2003;50:452–456.

Ferrer L, et al. Immunohistochemical detection of CD31 antigen in normal and neoplastic canine endothelial cells. J Comp Pathol 1995;112:319–326.

Hargis AM, et al. A retrospective clinicopathologic study of 212 dogs with cutaneous hemangiomas and hemangiosarcomas. Vet Pathol 1992;29:316–328.

Hinrichs U, et al. Lymphangiosarcomas in cats: a retrospective study of 12 cases. Vet Pathol 1999;36:164–167.

Johnson GC, et al. Histologic and immunohistochemical characterization of hemangiomas in the skin of seven young horses. Vet Pathol 1996;33:142–149.

Miller MA, et al. Cutaneous vascular neoplasia in 15 cats: clinical, morphologic, and immunohistochemical studies. Vet Pathol 1992;29:329–336.

Ward H, et al. Cutaneous hemangiosarcoma in 25 dogs: A retrospective study. J Vet Intern Med 1994;8:345–348.

Histiocytic proliferative disorders

Proliferations of histiocytic cells in the dog comprise a complex and incompletely understood category of disease. Fortunately, advancement in the characterization of the canine histiocytic proliferative disorders in terms of morphologic characteristics, clinical behavior, and phenotype has led to enhanced diagnostic and prognostic capabilities. The cause and pathogenesis of these conditions remain largely undetermined. Currently, histiocytic proliferative disorders in the dog comprise the entities of **cutaneous histiocytoma, cutaneous histiocytosis, localized histiocytic sarcoma**, and **disseminated histiocytic sarcoma** (formerly known as malignant histiocytosis). These conditions have only been well characterized in the dog.

Histiocytes arise from a CD34+ precursor cell found in the bone marrow and differentiate into cells of the mononuclear-phagocyte system or the dendritic cell system. Dendritic cells and macrophages have overlapping functions in that both can function as antigen-presenting cells and can act as effector cells. *Macrophages* are primarily effector cells and act as elements of the innate immune system, whereas *dendritic cells* function primarily in antigen presentation and hence provide a strong influence on the adaptive immune system. The morphological features of neoplastic or abnormally reactive histiocytes are similar and can mimic tumor cells of different histogenic origin or be confused with granulomatous inflammation. Differentiation often requires immunophenotyping and sometimes ultrastructural characterization.

Canine cutaneous histiocytoma

Canine cutaneous histiocytomas (CCH) (Langerhans cell histiocytosis) are tumors arising from proliferations of the intra-epidermal dendritic cell, the Langerhans cell. Langerhans cells acquire and process foreign cutaneous antigens, migrate to regional lymph nodes and present the antigen to T cells. Immunophenotypic markers of Langerhans cells and therefore cells comprising CCH include MHC I and II, CD1a, CD1c, CD11a, CD11b, CD11c, CD18, CD44, CD45, CD45R, CD49d, ICAM-1, and E-cadherin. Expression of the above markers may vary with the state of activation of the tumor cells and clinical stage of the tumor. CCH should also express vimentin. Lysozyme is a useful but not a reliable marker for these tumors. Histiocytoma cells are negative for Thy-1 and CD4. Unfortunately, at the time of writing, the majority of the above markers are not commercially available and/or require the use of cryopreserved tissues. Establishing the diagnosis may rely on attempting to rule out other round cell neoplasms for which commercially available antibodies for formalin-fixed specimens are available.

Canine cutaneous histiocytomas are most often solitary, benign tumors but can be multiple and on very rare occasion have been noted to lead to regional and distant metastasis. Greater than 70% of CCH occur in *dogs <4 years of age* and are most often found on the *head (pinna), or limbs* but can occur anywhere on the body. There is no sex predilection. Grossly, the tumors are raised, red, frequently ulcerated, 0.5–4 cm nodules that grow rapidly. The tumors are well demarcated but unencapsulated and located primarily in the dermis with the base of the tumor smaller in configuration than the more superficial aspect ("top heavy"). Microscopically, *tumor cells form diffuse sheets that displace adnexal structures and dermal collagen, and extend from the dermoepidermal junction into the subcutis.* Epidermotropism may be evident in some CCH. A clear zone usually surrounds intra-epidermal tumor cells. Care must be taken to differentiate the lesion from an epidermotropic lymphoma. The epidermis is often attenuated or ulcerated and associated edema may lead to *vertical rowing of tumor cells* near the surface. Ulceration is associated with infiltrates of neutrophils. The intact epidermis may be hyperplastic. Individual tumor cells are round to oval with moderate to abundant eosinophilic, slightly foamy cytoplasm. Cell borders are fairly distinct in areas of low density but obscure when cells are arranged in diffuse sheets. Nuclei are centrally located, oval, to indented and vesicular with most often a single nucleolus that may be inconspicuous. *Mitotic figures are variable but most often numerous* with up to 10–15/hpf. The base of the tumor may have infiltrates of CD8+ cytotoxic T lymphocytes, a sign of *host-mediated spontaneous tumor regression.* Infiltrates of lymphocytes may also be found in perivascular or periadnexal regions. In older lesions, the lymphocytic infiltrates may be more extensive than the remaining tumor cell infiltrates, leading to a misinterpretation of primary inflammatory process. *Tumor cell apoptosis and zones of necrosis are common findings,* particularly in regressing lesions but are not present in all CCH. As the function of Langerhans cells is to capture antigen and migrate to regional lymph nodes, regional lymph nodes may be enlarged but are not painful and should regress to normal size after tumor removal. Histologic changes in regional lymph nodes have not been well documented but in rare cases have been shown to be due to infiltrates of Langerhans cells.

The histologic appearance of tumors in dogs with *multiple cutaneous histiocytomas* is the same as described above, however spontaneous regression may be delayed and secondary bacterial infection may be a complication. Shar-Peis, Shar-Pei crosses and the English Cocker Spaniel are reported to have a higher incidence of multiple cutaneous histiocytomas. At least one author has proposed the term; "*progressive Langerhans cell histiocytosis*" for cases characterized by multiple, treatment-refractory canine cutaneous histiocytomas shown to be of Langerhans cell origin.

The overwhelming majority of CCH are benign and cured by surgical excision or by the spontaneous regression that usually occurs within a few weeks. Immunosuppressive drugs are contraindicated as this may delay natural regression of the lesions. Morphological features that suggest possible malignant behavior of a CCH include aggregates of tumor cells that are primarily in the deep dermis and subcutis, lack of lymphocytic infiltration, presence of plasma cells, and plugging of lymphatic vessels by tumor cells. The histologic differential diagnosis includes inflammatory lesions and other round cell neoplasms such as lymphomas, plasma cell tumors, and mast cell tumors. The deep dermal lymphocytic infiltrates, presence of typical histiocytes in the superficial regions, high mitotic index, infrequent presence of eosinophils, signalment and anatomical location are useful features in confirming the diagnosis of a histiocytoma. Immunophenotyping may be needed in some cases to distinguish CCH from other round cell tumors such as cutaneous lymphoma, particularly if epidermotropism is present.

Cutaneous reactive histiocytosis and systemic reactive histiocytosis

Cutaneous reactive histiocytosis (CRH) is *a reactive disorder targeting the skin that is characterized by single to multiple, non-painful plaques or nodules comprised of proliferations of histiocytes accompanied by lymphocytes and neutrophils.* **Systemic reactive histiocytosis** (SRH) is *the term used to designate a similar condition that affects not only the skin, but also lymph nodes and other body organs.* Cutaneous reactive histiocytosis does not necessarily lead to systemic reactive histiocytosis and not all cases of systemic histiocytosis have cutaneous lesions. The histiocytic cells in CRH and SRH are immunophenotypically CD1+, CD11b+, CD11c+, MHCII+, CD4+, and CD90+ (Thy-1+), ICAM-1+ activated dendritic cells. The lymphocytes are CD3+, CD8+, TCRαβ+ T lymphocytes, and the neutrophils label for CD11b+. Cultures and special stains fail to reveal causative agents and the condition responds favorably, at least for a time, with immunomodulatory therapy, hence it is thought to be the result of immune dysregulation.

Gross lesions of CRH are restricted to the skin and subcutis, may be alopecic or haired, and are most often on the *head, neck, perineum, scrotum, and extremities* (Fig. 5.146). The condition occurs in dogs 2–11 years of age with no sex or breed predilection. Systemic histiocytosis can have similar cutaneous lesions in addition to infiltrates of other tissues and organs such as the nasal cavity, sclera, retrobulbar tissues, lung, spleen, liver, lymph nodes, and bone marrow. Systemic reactive histiocytosis can occur in any breed, but Bernese Mountain Dogs, Rottweilers, Golden and Labrador Retrievers are predisposed. The age range for SRH is 1–9 years.

Histologically, cutaneous lesions are *"bottom heavy" multinodular infiltrates of large round-to-oval, rather bland histiocytes* mixed with

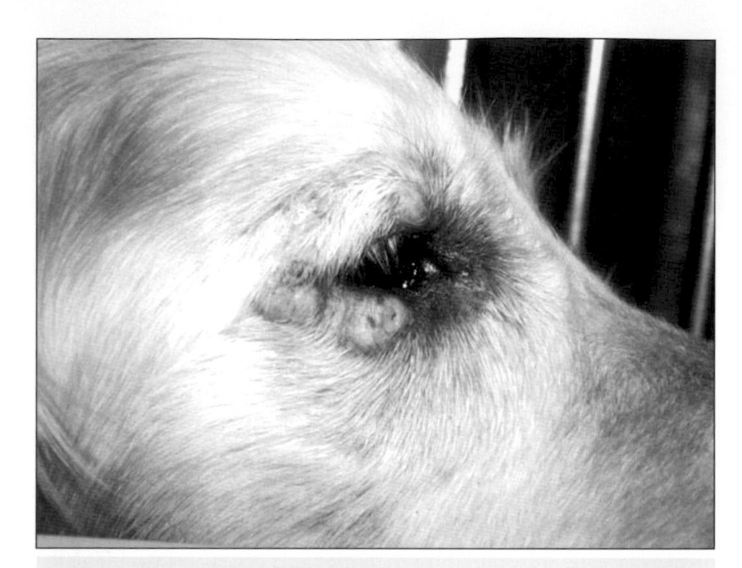

Figure 5.146 Cutaneous histiocytosis from a dog.

lymphocytes and neutrophils in the deep dermis and subcutis. In some cases, the histiocytes may be vacuolated, giving the infiltrate a lipomatous appearance. Lymphocytes may comprise 50% of the infiltrate. Eosinophils and rare plasma cells may occasionally be present. Vessels are often surrounded and invaded by the infiltrate leading to thrombosis and tissue necrosis. Older lesions extend into the more superficial dermis and may have a periadnexal distribution. Epitheliotropism is not a feature. Infiltrates of other tissues and organs in SRH are morphologically similar to the cutaneous infiltrates.

The *histologic differential diagnoses* include a response to infectious agents, other causes of periadnexal granulomas such as idiopathic sterile pyogranulomas, drug reactions, cutaneous histiocytoma, and lymphomatoid granulomatosis.

The prognosis for CRH and SRH is guarded. Lesions may wax and wane and the minority of cases of CRH may spontaneously regress. Many times, the lesions are slowly progressive and require long term management with immunosuppressive therapy and often lead to death, particularly if there is systemic involvement.

Localized histiocytic sarcoma

Localized histiocytic sarcomas are rapidly growing malignant neoplasms occurring most often in the skin, subcutis, and associated soft tissues of the extremities. The tumors are often found in periarticular regions and invade the joint capsule, tendons and muscles of the region. Other reported sites for LHS include the spleen, brain, liver, gastric wall, and tongue. LHS are most often reported in Bernese Mountain Dogs, Golden, Labrador, and Flat-coated Retrievers, and Rottweilers, but can occur in any breed. There is no sex predilection and reported age range is 2–11 years.

Immunophenotypically, the histiocytic cells comprising these lesions are variable but most consistent with a *dendritic cell origin or occasionally a macrophage origin (hemophagocytic histiocytic splenic sarcoma)*. Splenic histiocytic sarcomas are comprised of cells phenotypically characteristic of interdigitating dendritic cells of the white pulp (CD1+, CD11c+, MHCII+) while histiocytic sarcomas arising in periarticular regions have phenotypic evidence of interstitial dendritic cell origin.

Grossly, the tumors are comprised of white, multinodular tissue that invades and destroys surrounding tissues. Metastasis to regional lymph nodes has been reported. Splenic histiocytic sarcomas metastasize to the liver. Histologically, histiocytic sarcomas consist of a mixture of pleomorphic, anaplastic, plump, round histiocytic cells and pleomorphic spindle-shaped cells. Tumor cells have abundant eosinophilic cytoplasm and large oval-to-indented or twisted vesicular nuclei. Multinucleated giant cells are common. Neutrophils and CD8+ lymphocytes may be present as well. Mitotic activity is high and phagocytosis may be evident. Immunophenotyping reveals positive labeling for CD1, CD11c, MHCII, ICAM-1, variable reactivity to CD90 (Thy-1) and negative reactivity for CD4. Histologic differential diagnoses include a wide variety of other sarcomas. Definitive diagnosis often requires immunohistochemistry. The prognosis is guarded but best when early, wide resection is performed (amputation) and the regional lymph nodes are determined to be uninvolved.

Disseminated histiocytic sarcoma

Disseminated histiocytic sarcoma is the term now used to refer to the previously described condition of malignant histiocytosis. Disseminated histiocytic sarcoma is a term used to reflect the multicentric form of histiocytic sarcoma described above. Histologically and immunophenotypically, the lesions are identical. It is unclear whether the disseminated histiocytic sarcoma represents metastasis of a primary lesion or multicentric malignant transformation of histiocytes. The condition was originally described in Bernese Mountain Dogs but has since been documented in Golden and Labrador Retrievers and Rottweilers. It is likely that cases in other breeds will be reported as well. The condition has been reported in the spleen, lung, liver, lymph nodes, bone marrow, central nervous system, kidneys, skeletal muscle, stomach, vertebral bodies, and adrenal glands. Cutaneous involvement is rare. The age at presentation ranges from 3–11 years and there is no sex predilection. The prognosis is extremely poor and the condition is rapidly progressive and there no known successful therapy.

Histiocytic diseases in cats

Histiocytic diseases in cats are inadequately characterized at this time to provide details regarding morphologic features, immunophenotyping, and clinical behavior. To date, a small number of cases of epitheliotropic cutaneous histiocytic proliferative conditions identified as Langerhans cell histiocytosis, histiocytic sarcomas, and an angiocentric pleocellular dendritic antigen presenting cell proliferative disorder have been documented. Further studies are needed before conclusions regarding histiocytic proliferative disorders in cats can be drawn.

Bibliography

Affolter VK, Moore PF. Localized and disseminated histiocytic sarcoma of dendritic cell origin in dogs. Vet Pathol 2002;39:74–83.

Baines SJ, et al. Maturation states of dendritic cells in canine cutaneous histiocytoma. Vet Dermatol 2000;11(Suppl 1):9–10.

Day MJ, et al. Multiple cutaneous histiocytomas in a cat. Vet Dermatol 2000;11:305–310.

Goldschmidt MH, Shofer FS. Skin tumors of the dog and cat. Oxford: Pergamon Press, 1992:222–230.
Kerlin RL, Hendrick MJ. Malignant fibrous histiocytoma and malignant histiocytosis in the dog-convergent or divergent phenotypic differentiation? Vet Pathol 1996;33:713–716.
Moore PF. Canine histiocytic diseases: Proliferation of dendritic cells is key. Proc Am Coll Vet Pathol 2000:180–185.
Moore PF, et al. Canine cutaneous histiocytoma is an epidermotropic Langerhans cell histiocytosis that expresses CD1 and specific beta 2 integrin molecules. Am J Pathol 1996;148:1699–1708.
Nagata M, et al. Progressive Langerhans' cell histiocytosis in a puppy. Vet Dermatol 2000;11:241–246.
Spangler WL, Kass PH. Pathologic and prognostic characteristics of splenomegaly in dogs due to fibrohistiocytic nodules: 98 cases. Vet Pathol 1998;35:488–498.
Spangler WL, Kass PH. Splenic myeloid metaplasia, histiocytosis, and hypersplenism in the dog (65 cases). Vet Pathol 1999;36:583–593.

Mast cell tumors

Single or multiple nodular dermal proliferations of mast cells occur in all domestic species but are *most common in dogs* (Fig. 5.147A). When the mast cells are present in large numbers and as an essentially pure population, a diagnosis of mast cell tumor (*mastocytoma*) is usually made. Some, more cautiously, consider such growths as *cutaneous mastocytosis* until invasive growth or morphologic evidence of anaplasia confirms their neoplastic nature. As heavy accumulations of mast cells may occur in a variety of parasitic, mycotic, allergic and idiopathic inflammatory syndromes, such caution is warranted; however, sheets of mast cells are not present in these other conditions. Multiple spontaneously regressing mast cell tumors have been reported in young dogs, cats, pigs, calves, foals, and humans suggesting the underlying process may have been mast cell hyperplasia rather than a true neoplasm. Diffuse dermal and subcutaneous infiltrates of well-differentiated mast cells occurring over large areas of the body have been reported in cats, dogs and a foal. The condition has been compared to *urticaria pigmentosa* described in humans.

The histologic lesion is seldom a diagnostic challenge except in the very poorly differentiated tumors. *The mast cells form diffuse loose sheets or densely packed cords of round cells with a central round nucleus, abundant granular basophilic cytoplasm, and distinct cell membrane* (Fig. 5.147B). Scattered diffusely among the tumor cells are mature eosinophils. Even solid tumors tend to have some areas composed of cords of tumor cells alternating with collagen bundles, particularly at the infiltrative border of the tumor. They are never encapsulated or even well demarcated except at their superficial edge. A Grenz zone typically separates them from an intact epidermis. Ulceration in large or traumatized tumors may bring the skin surface in contact with the tumor. Eosinophils are few to numerous. Edema may be very severe, giving the tumor an appearance that macroscopically and microscopically resembles acute inflammation. Foci of tumor necrosis, eosinophilic or mononuclear leukocytic vasculitis, vascular necrosis, mineralization, mucinous extracellular matrix, collagen degeneration or tumor cells with giant or multiple nuclei are all occasionally encountered. Degenerating collagen may incite granulomatous inflammation.

In **dogs**, *mast cell tumors account for 15–20% of skin tumors and are the most frequent malignant or potentially malignant tumor of the skin.* The mean age of affected dogs is ~9 years with a range of 3 weeks

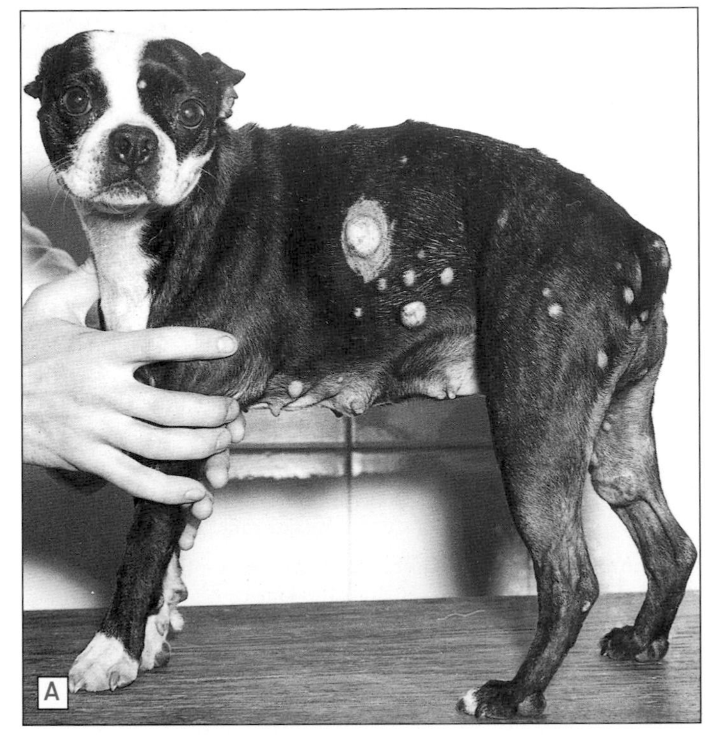

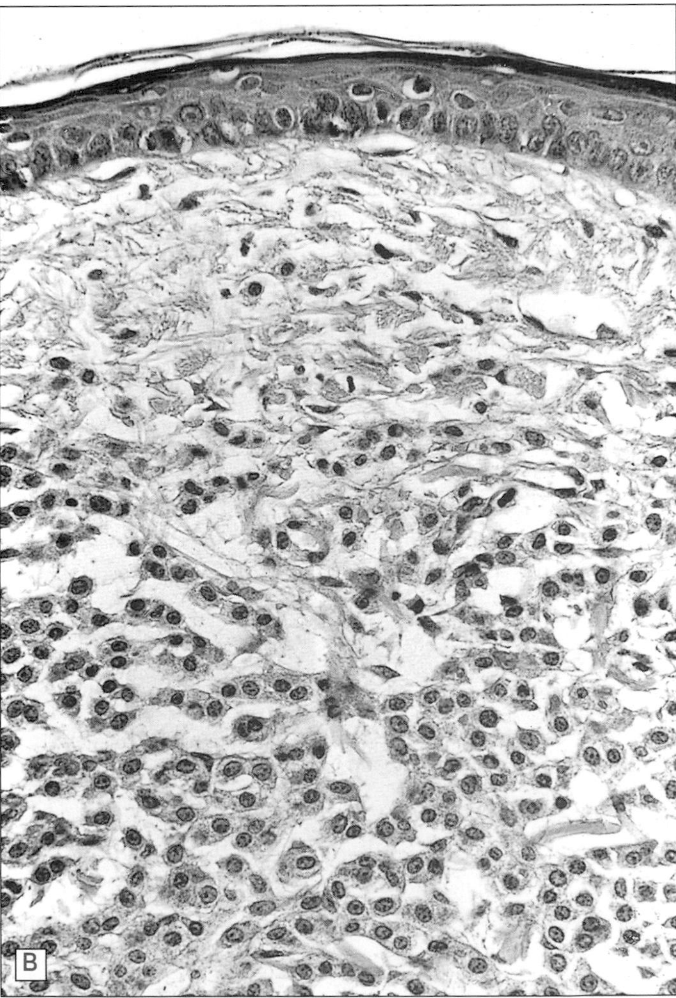

Figure 5.147 Cutaneous mast cell tumors. A. Multiple tumors in a Boston Terrier. **B.** Well-differentiated cutaneous mast cell tumor from a dog. Short cords of uniform round cells with sparing of the superficial dermis.

to 19 years. Boxers, Terriers, Boston Terriers, Labrador Retrievers, Beagles, and Schnauzers are reportedly predisposed. Shar-Peis are also predisposed and in this breed, mast cell tumors often occur at an earlier age than in other breeds. Site predilections vary with the breed. Studies investigating mast cell tumors in the dog have attempted to correlate clinical outcome with histologic grade, breed, tumor location, growth rate, clinical stage, argyrophilic nucleolar organizer region (AgNOR) counts, DNA ploidy, *p53* tumor suppressor gene product alterations, and proliferating cell nuclear antigen reactivity. Analysis of matrix metalloproteinases and expression of stem cell factor receptor and their correlation with histologic grade has also been investigated. Alterations in stem cell factor receptor expression are postulated to contribute to the proliferation of mast cells. To date, the most reliable criterion upon which to base a prognosis remains the histologic grade, however, establishing the histologic grade is subjective and less useful in tumors determined to be of intermediate differentiation. All mast cell tumors in the dog maintain a degree of unpredictability and should be regarded as potentially malignant.

There are currently two accepted grading systems for canine mast cell tumors, *the Patnaik system* (most commonly used) and *the Bostock system*. Well-differentiated tumors are considered Patnaik grade 1, while well-differentiated tumors in the Bostock system are considered grade 3. To avoid confusion, it is best to designate mast cell tumors as *well-differentiated, intermediate, or poorly differentiated.* Well-differentiated tumors carry an approximate metastatic potential of 10% while poorly differentiated mast cell tumors have a 55–96% rate of possible metastasis. Mast cell tumors metastasize first to regional lymph nodes and then most often to the liver and spleen. Mast cells may be detected in the peripheral blood and bone marrow in cases of widespread dissemination. Some mast cells may be present in the blood, bone marrow, and peripheral lymph nodes in the absence of disseminated disease, in normal animals and in animals with other diseases and these findings must be interpreted with caution.

- The **well-differentiated mast cell tumor** consists of round cells with a central small nucleus with a single inconspicuous nucleolus, and abundant, well-granulated cytoplasm. Cytoplasmic borders are distinct. There is very little cellular variation and mitotic figures are almost never seen. Tumor cells are arranged in rows or nests separated by collagen bundles. The tumor is confined to the dermis. Tumors of this type account for ~50% of the mast cell tumors of dogs and their behavior is usually benign. Excision is usually curative, with over 90% of affected dogs surviving >4 years.
- **Mast cell tumors of intermediate grade** are comprised of closely packed cells with distinct cytoplasmic boundaries, an increased nuclear-to-cytoplasmic ratio and fewer granules than a well-differentiated tumor. Giant, binucleate or occasional spindle-shaped cells may be present. Mitotic figures may be present in small numbers. The tumor cells are arranged in rows or nests separated by a collagenous stroma that may be thick or hyalinized with areas of edema and necrosis. The tumor may infiltrate the lower dermis and subcutis. The 3.5 year survival rate is ~55%.
- The cells of **undifferentiated (anaplastic) mast cell tumors** exhibit poor cytoplasmic granulation, large nucleus in relationship to cytoplasmic volume, irregular nuclear shape, moderate variation in nuclear size, several nucleoli and occasional binucleate, multinucleated or giant cell. Mitotic figures may be numerous. The cytoplasmic granulation may be inapparent or visible only as fine cytoplasmic dusting, and may require staining with Giemsa or toluidine blue to demonstrate the metachromatic granules. Tumor cells infiltrate the subcutis and deeper tissues. About 20% of the canine tumors fall into this prognostic category. Dogs with poorly differentiated tumors have a 3.5 year survival rate of approximately 15%.

The *macroscopic appearance* of canine mast cell tumors varies widely with their stage of progression and degree of histologic differentiation. Well-differentiated tumors most often appear as a rubbery, nodular nonencapsulated variably alopecic dermal mass 1–4 cm in diameter that clinically resembles a lipoma. Poorly differentiated tumors tend to achieve a large size more quickly, are less circumscribed and often associated with inflammation and edema of the surrounding dermis and possible satellite lesions. Tumors of intermediate grade have a gross appearance that varies between those described above.

Other clinical signs may occasionally result from the release of histamine or other vasoactive products from the mast cells. *Gastroduodenal ulceration* is relatively frequent in dogs with disseminated disease, occurring in 35–83% of cases. Histamine release stimulates the specific H2 gastric parietal cell receptors, resulting in increased acid secretion and perhaps local mucosal ischemia. Ulceration follows and may lead to fatal exsanguination. *Hypotensive shock* from massive synchronous degranulation, as may occur with cryosurgery, is a rarely reported complication.

Mast cell tumors in **cats** exist as *primary cutaneous mast cell tumors* and as *visceral mastocytosis*. They are separate diseases. Mast cell tumors are the second most common cutaneous neoplasm in the cat and account for 20% of skin tumors of cats in the USA. The metastatic potential of feline cutaneous mast cell tumors is very low (~5%) and those destined for behavioral malignancy are easily detected by anisocytosis, hyperchromasia and mitotic activity. Apparent recurrence at the surgical site or elsewhere in the skin is seen in 25–50% of the cases, but most of these probably represent multicentric origin. Cats with multiple mast cells tumors are often FIV positive. There is *no widely accepted grading system* for feline mast cell tumors.

Mast cell tumors in cats appear as one or several firm, raised pink, alopecic papules varying in size from millimeters to several centimeters. Less commonly, the tumor appears as a poorly defined area of swelling due to an infiltrative rather than nodular lesion. The head and neck are preferred sites. Histologically the cells are usually extraordinarily uniform, polygonal to round, and grow in a diffuse sheet interrupted only by small clusters of lymphocytes and rare eosinophils. The cytoplasm is clear, eosinophilic or only faintly basophilic. Obvious granularity is infrequent. The nucleus is round, central and relatively hyperchromatic in comparison to that of canine mast cells. Even with metachromatic stains such as Giemsa or toluidine blue, cytoplasmic granules may stain poorly, yet ultrastructurally they are abundant. Occasionally, binucleate, multinucleated or cells with giant nuclei measuring up to 25 μm may be seen. Eosinophils are seen in only a small number of feline mast cell tumors. The tumor is not encapsulated and is most often confined to the dermis. Collagen degeneration and stromal proliferation are rare. Much less frequent is a *second histologic type* seen most often in young cats as multiple, simultaneous or sequential, tumors located at the junction of the dermis and subcutis. Siamese cats are predisposed. The tumor mast cells resemble histiocytes and the lesion may be mistaken for granulomatous inflammation. Toluidine blue or Giemsa staining may be equivocal. The cells are confirmed as mast cells on electron microscopic examination. Eosinophils, lymphoid aggregates, well-circumscribed growth habit and benign behavior are similar to the more usual mast cell tumor of cats described above.

Mast cell tumors in **horses** have been cautiously termed *cutaneous mastocytosis*, but the growths are comparable to the cutaneous tumors of other species. They most commonly present as solitary nodules on the head, trunk, neck, and limbs. The tumors may be hyperpigmented, alopecic or ulcerated. Collagen degeneration, large aggregates of eosinophils, necrosis, and focal mineralization are more prominent. While in some respects resembling such lesions as cutaneous onchocerciasis, habronemiasis or collagenolytic granulomas, none of these three is characterized by sheets of mast cells. Multiple congenital mast cell tumors that spontaneously regress have been reported. There are no reports of metastasis of mast cell tumors in the horse.

Mast cell tumors in **ferrets** resemble the well-differentiated feline mast cell tumor grossly, histologically and in terms of biological behavior.

In **pigs**, mast cell nodules have been described as tumors and as multifocal inflammatory aggregates, perhaps in response to *Eperythrozoon*. Their morphology resembles that of well-differentiated feline tumors. In the pigs with multiple skin lesions, visceral aggregates were also found.

In **cattle**, scant data suggest the cutaneous tumors are usually multiple and are associated with visceral mast cell aggregates, although purely cutaneous tumors have been reported. Congenital cutaneous mast cell tumors consisting of well-circumscribed 1–7 cm nodules randomly distributed all over the body have also been reported. Histologically, the tumors had features of well-differentiated mast cell tumors. There are more reports of cutaneous metastases of multicentric visceral tumors than there are of primary skin disease. Cattle of any age, including calves, may be affected.

Bibliography

Ayl RD, et al. Correlation of DNA ploidy to tumor histologic grade, clinical variables, and survival in dogs with mast cell tumors. Vet Pathol 1992;29:386–390.

Bundza A, Dukes TW. Cutaneous and systemic porcine mastocytosis. Vet Pathol 1982;19:453–455.

Ginn PE, et al. Immunohistochemical detection of p53 tumor-suppressor protein is a poor indicator of prognosis for canine cutaneous mast cell tumors. Vet Pathol 2000;37:33–39.

Goldschmidt MH, Shofer FS. Mast cell tumors. In: Goldschmidt MH, ed. Skin Tumors of the Dog and Cat. New York: Pergamon Press, 1992:231–251.

Hendrick MJ, et al. Histological classification of mesenchymal tumors of skin and soft tissues of domestic animals. Armed Forces Institute of Pathology 1998;2:28–29.

Hill JE, et al. Prevalence and location of mast cell tumors in slaughter cattle. Vet Pathol 1991;28:449–450.

Jaffe MH, et al. Immunohistochemical and clinical evaluation of p53 in canine mast cell tumors. Vet Pathol 2000;37:40–46.

Jeromin AM, et al. Urticaria pigmentosa-like disease in the dog. J Amer Anim Hosp Assoc 1993;29:508–513.

Leibman NF, et al. Identification of matrix metalloproteinases in canine cutaneous mast cell tumors. J Vet Intern Med 2000;14:583–586.

Lopez A. Cutaneous mucinosis and mastocytosis in a Shar-pei. Can Vet J 1999;40:881–883.

Mathison PT. Eosinophilic nodular dermatoses. Vet Clin N Amer 1995;11:86–88.

McManus PM. Frequency and severity of mastocytemia in dogs with and without mast cell tumors: 120 cases (1995–1997). J Am Vet Med Assoc 1999;215:355–357.

Molander-McCrary H, et al. Cutaneous mast cell tumors in cats: 32 cases (1991–1994). J Am Anim Hosp Assoc 1998;34:281–284.

Patnaik AK, et al. Canine cutaneous mast cell tumor: morphologic grading and survival time in 83 dogs. Vet Pathol 1984;21:469–474.

Reguera MJ, et al. Canine mast cell tumors express stem cell factor receptor. Am J Dermatopathol 2000;22:49–54.

Shaw DP, et al. Multicentric mast cell tumor in a cow. Vet Pathol 1991;28:450–452.

Simoes PC, Shoning P. Canine mast cell tumors: a comparison of staining techniques. J Vet Diag Invest 1994;6:458–465.

Simoes JPC, et al. Prognosis of canine mast cell tumors: a comparison of three methods. Vet Pathol 1994;31:637–647.

Vail DM. Mast cell tumors. In: Withrow SJ, MacEwen EG, eds. Small Animal Clinical Oncology. 2nd ed. Philadelphia, PA: WB Saunders, 1996:192–210.

Vitale CB, et al. Feline urticaria pigmentosa in three related Sphinx cats. Vet Dermatol 1996;7:227–233.

Whitler WA, et al. Equine mast cell tumor. Eq Pract 1994;16:16–21.

Wilcock BP, et al. The morphology and behavior of feline cutaneous mastocytomas. Vet Pathol 1986;23:320–324.

Yeruham I, et al. Congenital skin neoplasia in cattle. Vet Dermatol 1999;10:149–156.

Cutaneous lymphoma

Lymphomas in the skin can be a primary cutaneous neoplasm or can be part of a multicentric lymphocytic neoplasm. Cutaneous lymphomas have been reported in most domestic animals and in many wildlife species, however the tumor has been most closely studied in the dog, cat, horse, and in cattle. The body of information about cutaneous lymphomas in veterinary dermatopathology has expanded rapidly in recent years, and is still a subject under close study. The development of *monoclonal antibodies directed against lymphocyte antigens* has greatly enhanced immunophenotypic analysis of tissue sections and needle aspirate preparations of these tumors. There are currently several antibodies that are routinely used in formalin-fixed tissue to characterize cutaneous lymphomas. As in humans, *T lymphocytes* in many domestic species consistently express the cell surface antigen CD3, and *B lymphocytes* can be identified in fixed tissues in many species by expression of CD79a. Many other monoclonal antibodies have been developed to identify lymphocyte subsets and others to identify lymphocyte antigens in fresh-frozen tissue. A description of these is beyond the scope of this chapter and the reader is referred to more detailed information on this topic in the bibliography. Classification schemes to predict behaviour of cutaneous lymphomas have been controversial. Several classification schemes devised for human lymphomas have been used, however they were based on lymphomas in lymph nodes. These schemes have included Rappaport, Lukes-Collins, Kiel, National Cancer Institute working formulation; and more recently, the Revised European-American Classification of Lymphoid Neoplasms (REAL). Since primary cutaneous lymphomas differ histologically and immunophenotypically from primary nodal lymphomas and often carry a better prognosis, *classification of primary cutaneous lymphomas using lymph node schemes has been difficult and unsatisfactory*. A new classification scheme devised for primary cutaneous human lymphomas has been

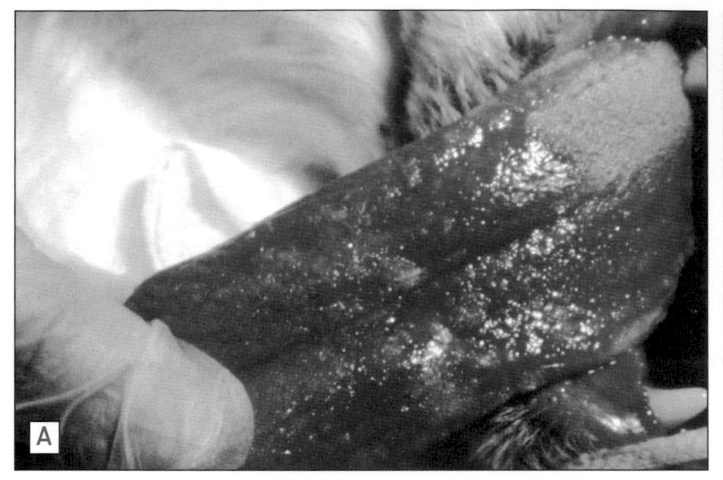

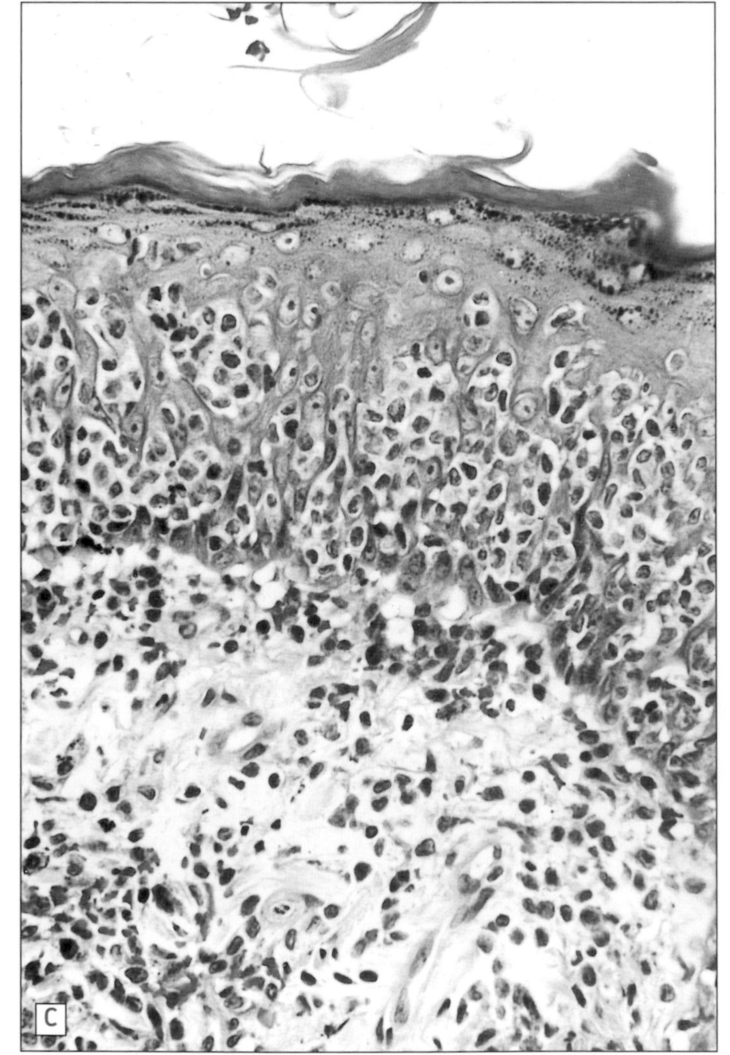

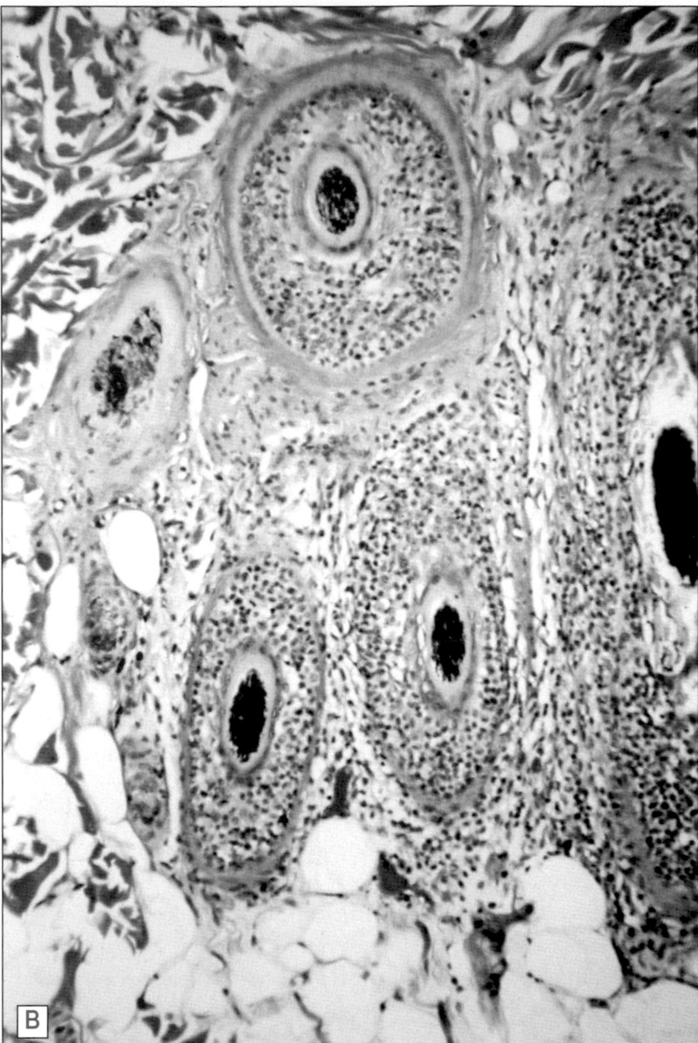

Figure 5.148 Mycosis fungoides in a dog. **A.** Ulceration of the tongue. (Courtesy of B Dunstan.) **B.** Marked follicular infiltration. (Courtesy of B Dunstan.) **C.** Diffuse infiltration of the epidermis by neoplastic lymphocytes.

proposed by the European Organization for Research and Treatment of Cancer (EORTC). It is based on a combination of clinical, histologic, immunophenotypic, and genetic criteria. The EORTC and REAL schemes use similar terminology, and these two systems may allow for recognition and comparison of similar tumors in cutaneous and non-cutaneous sites. Currently there have been no studies using the EORTC system on primary cutaneous lymphomas in domestic animals.

Cutaneous lymphomas in domestic animals are usually divided into two groups; *epitheliotropic cutaneous lymphomas*, in which the neoplastic lymphocytes invade the epidermis and/or adnexal epithelium, and *nonepitheliotropic lymphomas* that involve the dermis and subcutis. With the increasing use of immunohistochemical characterization of cutaneous lymphomas in domestic animals, division into *T-cell cutaneous lymphomas* (which would include mycosis fungoides, Pagetoid reticulosis, and angiocentric lymphomas/lymphomatoid granulomatosis), and *B-cell lymphomas*, will become more useful.

Epitheliotropic cutaneous lymphoma in domestic animals is represented primarily by **mycosis fungoides**. Mycosis fungoides has been reported in the *dog, cat, horse, rabbit, and cattle*. Mycosis fungoides is a disease of *older animals* and frequently there is a history of chronic erythematous, exfoliative dermatitis or multiple plaques and nodules. Lesions can be anywhere, however mucocutaneous junctions of the mouth, nose, eyes, anus, vulva, or the gingiva and palate are often involved (Fig. 5.148A). Histologically the neoplastic lymphoid infiltrate involves epidermis but can also involve the epithelium of adnexal structures (Fig. 5.148B). The lymphoid infiltrate in the epithelium can be diffuse (Fig. 5.148C), scattered, or form aggregates ("*Pautrier's microabscesses*") (see Fig. 5.10). Dermal involvement varies from a mixed perivascular cellular component that contains low numbers of neoplastic lymphocytes to a more fulminating diffuse monomorphic neoplastic infiltrate. Epidermotropic cutaneous lymphomas frequently ulcerate and verification of the epitheliotropic nature of the neoplasm can be difficult, however, a neoplastic lymphocytic component that abuts the ulcerated epidermis suggests epidermotropism. The neoplastic lymphocytes can vary from a small cell type, with a low mitotic index, hyperchromatic nucleus and scant cytoplasm, to a large cell type with moderate mitotic index together with moderate amounts of pale basophilic to clear cytoplasm. Although less well characterized than the human form of mycosis fungoides, epitheliotropic lymphomas in domestic animals also express T-cell surface antigens such as CD3. However, in contrast to human epitheliotropic lymphomas, which are reported to express CD4 in approximately 90% of cases, 80% of epitheliotropic lymphomas in domestic animals express CD8. Mycosis fungoides with a leukemic blood component (**Sezary syndrome**) has been reported in the dog, cat, horse, and cow. **Pagetoid reticulosis (Woringer–Kolopp disease)** is a localized solitary plaque form of epidermotropic lymphoma that is well recognized in humans and has been reported rarely in the dog. In this form, the neoplastic lymphocytes are confined primarily to the epidermis and the dermal component is a mixture of mature lymphocytes and macrophages.

Angiocentric lymphoma (lymphomatoid granulomatosis) in the skin is usually a cutaneous manifestation of pulmonary lymphoma, however, it is thought to occur rarely as a primary cutaneous disease. Although well described in humans, this form of lymphoma has been reported infrequently in domestic animals. It is characterized by *angiocentric, angioinvasive, and angiodestructive neoplastic lymphocytes in the dermis and subcutis, resulting in intramural and extravascular neoplastic infiltrates*, in contrast to the luminal accumulations of lymphocytes in malignant angioendotheliomatosis. The neoplastic cells are medium- to large-sized lymphoid cells that can have a histiocytic appearance, with a cleaved or reniform nucleus. Inflammatory cells such as eosinophils, plasma cells, and small lymphocytes may accompany the neoplastic cells. In the small number of cases reported, the neoplastic lymphocytes have been identified as T lymphocytes by immunophenotyping. Clinically the presentation is one of multiple alopecic and frequently ulcerated dermal or subcutaneous nodules. The angiodestructive nature of the neoplasm can result in multifocal necrotic or infarctive lesions.

Nonepitheliotropic cutaneous lymphomas appear to be less common than epitheliotropic lymphomas in most domestic animal species. Clinically the animals have multiple dermal and subcutaneous nodules that infrequently ulcerate. Histologically the neoplastic cells form *"bottom-heavy" nodules in the dermis and subcutis*, often with a Grenz zone. The neoplastic cells may be large cells with a histiocytic appearance, and immunophenotyping is often necessary to distinguish them from the histiocytic proliferative diseases. The neoplastic cells can efface adnexal structures, but invasion into the epidermis or adnexal epithelium is very unusual.

Nonepitheliotropic lymphomas that have been studied are usually of B-lymphocyte origin, with the exception of the angiocentric lymphomas discussed previously. An interesting form of nonepitheliotropic lymphoma is the **T-cell-rich B-cell lymphoma,** which is well recognized in humans and has now been reported in the *cat, pig, dog, and horse*. In the horse, it appears to be the most common form of cutaneous lymphoma. In this form, the nodular masses are composed of neoplastic large B lymphocytes accompanied by a background population of smaller reactive T lymphocytes that usually comprise the majority of the cell population. The large neoplastic B cells exhibit cellular atypia, with large vesicular nuclei and numerous mitotic figures that are often atypical. Since the neoplastic population is often the minority population, mitotic index should be evaluated carefully taking into account the fact that the majority population is non neoplastic small T lymphocytes with normal morphology and low mitotic index. These tumors also usually contain variable numbers of macrophages, epithelioid macrophages, and occasionally multinucleated giant cells. The mixed nature of the population can lead to this tumor being mistaken for inflammation, or a neoplasm of T lymphocytes. T-cell-rich B-cell lymphomas in the horse appear to be histologically the same as the neoplasm referred to in the older literature as *equine cutaneous histiolymphocytic lymphosarcoma*.

Intravascular lymphoma (malignant angioendotheliomatosis, intravascular lymphomatosis, angiotropic large-cell lymphoma) is *characterized by intravascular neoplastic lymphocytes in the vessels of the skin and other organs in the absence of a primary mass or circulating neoplastic cells*. This condition is rare in humans and was originally thought to be a proliferation of endothelial cells, which lead to the original name of malignant angioendotheliomatosis. At present it has been reported rarely in the dog and cat. Clinically the skin lesions appear as plaques and nodules, and histologically vessels in the dermis and subcutis are partially or completely filled with *large atypical lymphoid cells*. In humans, the intravascular neoplastic cells are of B-lymphocyte origin, however in dogs the majority of cases so far have been of T-lymphocyte origin.

Cutaneous pseudolymphomas *are benign reactive proliferations of lymphocytes that mimic cutaneous lymphomas histologically and sometimes clinically*. These proliferations are poorly characterized in the veterinary literature, but are well recognized in humans as forming both a band-like infiltrate in the superficial dermis (*T-cell pattern*) and nodular to diffuse infiltrates in the dermis and subcutis (*B-cell pattern*). Pseudolymphomas in humans can be due to many antigenic stimuli, such as drug eruptions, arthropod or tick-bite reactions, and contact dermatitis. *Differentiation between benign inflammatory lesions and early cutaneous lymphoma can be extremely difficult.* Although immunophenotyping can distinguish between T-cell and B-cell lymphomas, methods to distinguish between inflammatory and malignant lymphocyte proliferations are unreliable at present.

Bibliography

Caniatti M, et al. Canine lymphoma: immunocytochemical analysis of fine-needle aspiration biopsy. Vet Pathol 1996;33:204–212.

Harris NL, et al. A revised European-American classification of lymphoid neoplasms: A proposal from the International Lymphoma Study Group. Blood 1994;84:1361–1392.

Kelley LC, Mahaffey EA. Equine malignant lymphomas: morphologic and immunohistochemical classification. Vet Pathol 1998;35:241–252.

Kiupel M, et al. Prognostic factors for treated canine malignant lymphomas. Vet Pathol 1999;36:292–300.

Latimer KS, Rakich PM. Sezary syndrome in a dog. Comp Haematol International 1996;6:115–119.

Moore PF, et al. Canine cutaneous lymphoma (mycosis fungoides) is a proliferative disorder of CD8+ T-cells. Am J Pathol 1994;144:421–429.

Moore PF, Olivry T. Cutaneous lymphomas in companion animals. Clin Dermatol 1994;12:499–505.

Murphy KM, Olivry T. Comparison of T-lymphocyte proliferation in canine epitheliotropic lymphosarcoma and benign lymphocytic dermatoses. Vet Dermatol 2000;11:99–105.

Non-Hodgkin's lymphoma pathologic classification project: National Cancer Institute sponsored study of classifications of non-Hodgkin's lymphomas. Cancer 1982;49:2112–2135.

Peleteiro MC, et al. Two cases of cutaneous T cell lymphoma in Friesian cows in the Azores. Vet Dermatol 2000;11:299–304.

Ploysangam T, et al. Cutaneous pseudolymphomas. J Am Acad Dermatol 1998;38:877–895.

Potter K, Anez D. Mycosis fungoides in a horse. J Am Vet Med Assoc 1998;212:550–552.

Schick RO, et al. Cutaneous lymphosarcoma and leukaemia in a cat. J Am Vet Med Assoc 1993;203:1155–1158.

Smith KC, et al. Canine lymphomatoid granulomatosis: an immunophenotypic analysis of three cases. J Comp Pathol 1996;115:129–138.

Steele KE, et al. T-cell rich B-cell lymphoma in a cat. Vet Pathol 1997;34:47–49.

Tanimoto T, Ohtsuki Y. T-cell-rich B-cell lymphoma in a pig. Vet Pathol 1998;35:147–149.

Vangessel YA, et al. Cutaneous presentation of canine intravascular lymphoma (malignant angioendotheliomatosis). Vet Dermatol 2000;11:291–297.

White SD, et al. Lymphoma with cutaneous involvement in three domestic rabbits (*Oryctolagus cuniculus*). Vet Dermatol 2000;11:61–67.

Willemze R, et al. EORTC classification for primary cutaneous lymphomas: A proposal from the cutaneous lymphoma study group of the European Organization for Research and Treatment of Cancer. Blood 1997;90:354–371.

Cutaneous plasmacytoma

Cutaneous plasmacytomas are common in dogs and rare in cats. Most cases are benign however malignant cutaneous plasmacytomas demonstrating local invasion and tissue destruction do occur. It has not been described in other species. It occurs most often in *middle-aged or old dogs* with a marked predilection for *feet, ear canal, and mouth.* The typical tumor is a small spherical mass grossly similar to benign cutaneous histiocytoma, but its histology is distinctive. *Sheets of pleomorphic round cells are divided into solid lobules by a fine fibrous stroma.* The cells often have marked variation in nuclear size and degree of basophilia, with binucleation or multinucleation and numerous mitotic figures. *At least some of the cells retain a perinuclear halo (suggesting a Golgi zone), "clockface" nucleus, and basophilic cytoplasm considered typical of plasma cells.* Russell bodies are sometimes seen even in very atypical cells, and the cytoplasm of most cells is pyroninophilic. Cells recognizable as plasma cells are most easily found near the periphery (Fig. 5.149). A Grenz zone is usually present and there is no epithelial invasion. Electron microscopy or immunohistochemistry for canine immunoglobulin confirms the diagnosis but seldom are these tests necessary. Occasionally a particularly anaplastic example must be distinguished from amelanotic epithelioid melanoma or lymphoma. The distinction is critical, since even bizarre plasmacytomas are cured by excision. Extracellular amyloid (AL) is found in a small percentage (perhaps up to 10% of plasmacytomas). They bear no apparent relationship to multiple myeloma. Multiple tumors, rarely > 2–3, have been reported, as has a very low prevalence (~5%) of local recurrence.

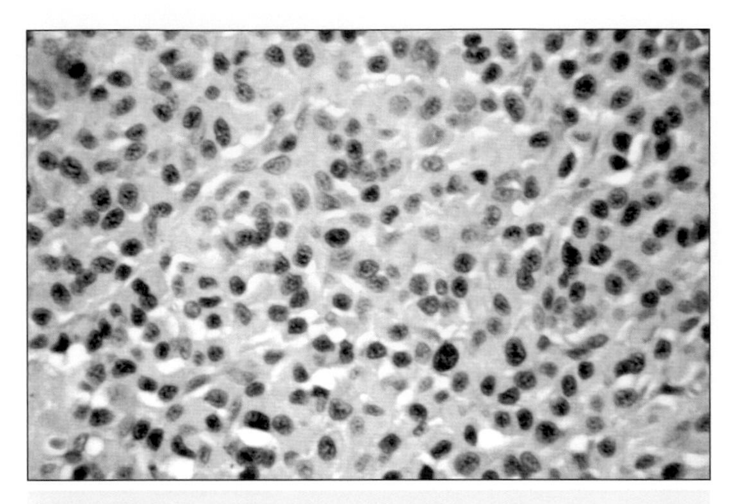

Figure 5.149 Cutaneous plasmacytoma from a dog.

Bibliography

Cangul IT, et al. Clinico-pathological aspects of canine cutaneous and mucocutaneous plasmacytomas. J Vet Med A Physiol Pathol Clin Med 2002;49:307–312.

Clark GN, et al. Extramedullary plasmacytomas in dogs: Results of surgical excision in 131 cases. J Am Anim Hosp Assoc 1992;28:106–111.

Platz SJ, et al. Prognostic value of histopathological grading in canine extramedullary plasmacytomas. Vet Pathol 1999;36:23–27.

Rakich PM, et al. Mucocutaneous plasmacytomas in dogs: 75 cases (1980–1987). J Am Vet Med Assoc 1989;194:803–810.

Merkel cell tumor

Merkel cell tumors have rarely been reported in the **dog**. Clinically, the tumors appear as nodular lesions that may resemble a histiocytoma. Too few cases have been reported to establish age, site or sex predilections. Microscopically, the tumors are comprised of *dermal infiltrates of round cells arranged as solid nests or clusters separated by collagenous stroma.* Individual tumor cells are reported to have indistinct margins and moderate amounts of pale cytoplasm. The nuclei are oval or spherical with dispersed chromatin. The nucleolus is not conspicuous. A small number of mitotic figures may be present. *Differential diagnoses* include cutaneous plasmacytoma and basal cell epithelioma. Definitive diagnosis requires ultrastructural examination or immunohistochemistry. Merkel cell tumors label for cytokeratin and chromogranin A and do not label for immunoglobulins.

Electron microscopic evaluation demonstrates *electron dense-core granules typical of neuroendocrine cells*. Merkel cell tumors in the dog are most often benign with only one report documenting metastasis. A malignant neuroendocrine carcinoma of the skin (Merkel cell tumor) has been reported in a Maine coon **cat**.

Bibliography

Konno A, et al. Immunohistochemical diagnosis of a Merkel cell tumor in a dog. Vet Pathol 1998;35:538–540.

Patnaik AK, et al. Clinicopathologic and electron microscopic study of cutaneous neuroendocrine (Merkel cell) carcinoma in a cat with comparisons to human and canine tumors. Vet Pathol 2001;38:553–556.

Tumors of the mammary gland

Mammary masses are *very common in dogs and to a lesser extent cats*, but are rare in other domestic species. In the dog, mammary tumors vary greatly in their morphologic appearance and biological behaviour. The high prevalence of canine mammary tumors, the need to identify dogs that would benefit from aggressive therapy, and the potential usefulness as an animal model has led to many investigations into the factors governing mammary tumor development and behavior in the dog. These studies have attempted to correlate histologic features and clinical outcome with characteristics such as hormone receptor expression, oncogene and tumor suppressor gene alterations, intratumoral vessel density, argyrophilic nucleolar organizer counts, tumor cell kinetics and intermediate filament expression. Results of these studies have added to the current state of knowledge regarding mammary gland tumors in the dog but have not completely defined parameters upon which to base a prognosis. **Invasion** *by the tumor into surrounding tissue is considered one of the most important predictors of behavioral malignancy*. In dogs, 80% of animals with invasive tumors will have a survival time of <2 years. Metastases to lung and lymph nodes are frequently found at necropsy. Conversely, 80% of dogs with non-invasive tumors – regardless of any other histologic features – will be alive at 2 years post-diagnosis. *The presence of tumor emboli in lymphatics or veins is absolute evidence for local invasion and metastatic potential*. In its absence, care must be taken to ensure that the invasion is really into surrounding normal tissue and not just into the abundant stroma accompanying the tumor itself.

Classification schemes for mammary tumors may be based on histogenesis of the neoplastic cells, morphologic appearance, or prognostic factors. *No scheme is completely satisfactory, and correlation of histopathological diagnosis and clinical outcome vary*. The scheme utilized in this text follows that outlined by the current World Health Organization International Histological Classification of Tumors of Domestic Animals, and considers both morphologic features and known indicators of prognosis for the dog. One exception to the WHO classification scheme that is included here is the findings of a recent study documenting the morphologic features and biological behavior of all mammary neoplasms occurring during the lifespans of 1343 Beagles. This study found a specific tumor type, the **ductular carcinoma** (arising from interlobular or intralobular ductules) had a higher fatality rate than other types of adenocarcinomas arising in the mammary gland. The ductular carcinoma is not a specific morphological subtype currently recognized by the WHO classification scheme but it will be included in this discussion as *it carries a poorer prognosis that other types of mammary gland adenocarcinomas*. The Beagle study also found that there was no difference in the frequency of metastasis between simple and complex carcinomas or between these tumors and adenocarcinomas in mixed tumors. They also reported that carcinosarcomas metastasized more frequently than adenocarcinomas in mixed tumors.

In **cats**, *mammary tumors are 85–90% behaviorally malignant* and are classified as subtypes of carcinomas based on morphologic features alone. Hyperplastic and dysplastic lesions of the mammary gland will also be considered here.

Mammary hyperplasia and dysplasia

Mammary ductal hyperplasia occurs frequently in bitches and occasionally in queens. Single or multiple extralobular ducts are distended with proteinaceous fluid and some cellular debris. Their leakage may induce sterile granulomatous inflammation rich in ceroid-laden macrophages. Histologically, the lesion consists of *patchy intraductal hyperplasia of epithelial cells*. Papillary proliferations of epithelium may fill the duct lumens. Proliferative cells are small, uniform and associated with an orderly myoepithelial layer. They may spontaneously regress, and ovariectomy reliably causes their regression, whereas progestogen administration induces their development. It is not known whether they predispose to, or even progress to neoplasia although neoplastic transformation would seem likely.

Mammary lobular hyperplasia *consists of patchy hyperplasia of secretory acini indistinguishable from the normal lactating gland*. Proliferation involves intralobular ductular epithelium, myoepithelium, and fibrous tissue in varying proportions. The lobular architecture of the gland is maintained. It occurs in intact, nonpregnant and non-lactating bitches, and occasionally in queens. Serial sectioning of the mammary glands reveals numerous small (1–4 mm diameter) hyperplastic foci in 50% of clinically normal bitches even at 3 years of age. They are most numerous in the caudal two glands, paralleling the greater prevalence of neoplasia in these glands. Circumstantial evidence supports the view that such lesions should be considered *preneoplastic changes*. Indeed, many hyperplastic lobules contain dysplastic foci with some degree of epithelial disorganization and hyperchromasia, blurring the distinction between hyperplasia, dysplasia and in situ neoplasia.

Mammary fibroepithelial hyperplasia *(fibroadenomatous change) occurs in young cycling, or pregnant cats*. It also can be induced in old unspayed females and males by treatment with *megestrol acetate*. Progesterone receptors are present in high concentrations. The condition appears most often 1–2 weeks post-estrus, usually affects one or more glands, and may regress spontaneously or require ovariectomy. Grossly, the mammary tissue is markedly swollen and erythematous. Necrosis and ulceration may be present. Edema may involve the rear limbs. Histologically there is *branching and proliferation of mammary ducts lined by simple columnar epithelium, surrounded by massive and concentric proliferation of edematous stroma compatible with myoepithelium* (Fig. 5.150). The prominence of the stroma is in sharp contrast to mammary neoplasia in cats, which almost always is solid or alveolar carcinoma with little stroma.

Mammary neoplasia in dogs and cats

Mammary tumors have been reported to comprise 50% of all neoplasms in the **bitch**. They occur most often in bitches 10–11 years old and are

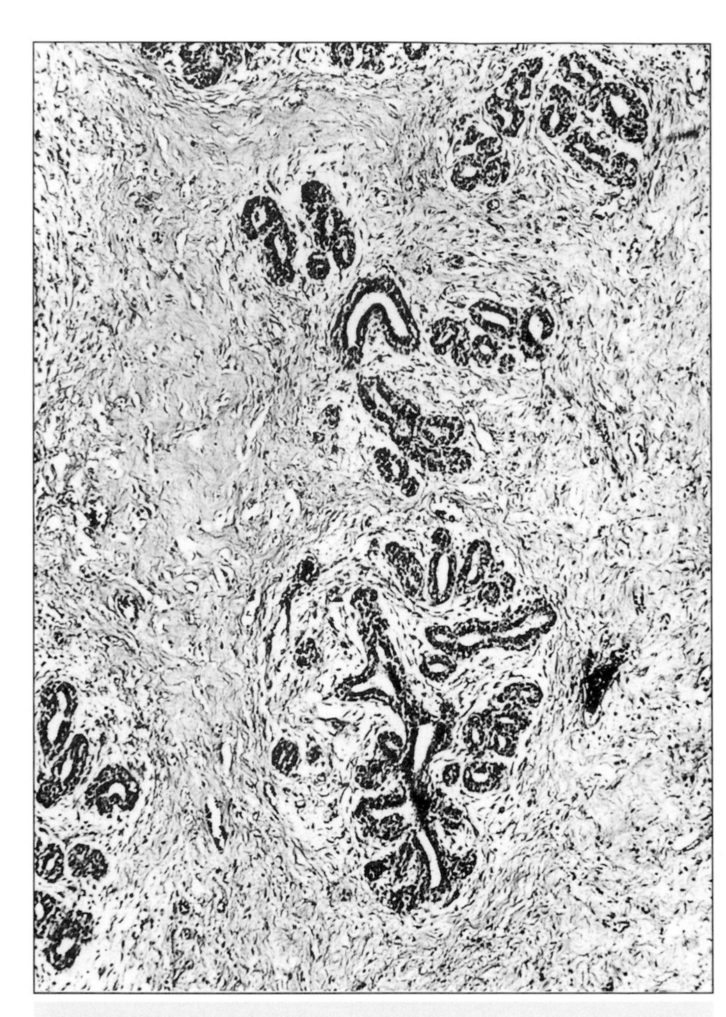

Figure 5.150 Fibroepithelial hyperplasia in the mammary gland of a cat.

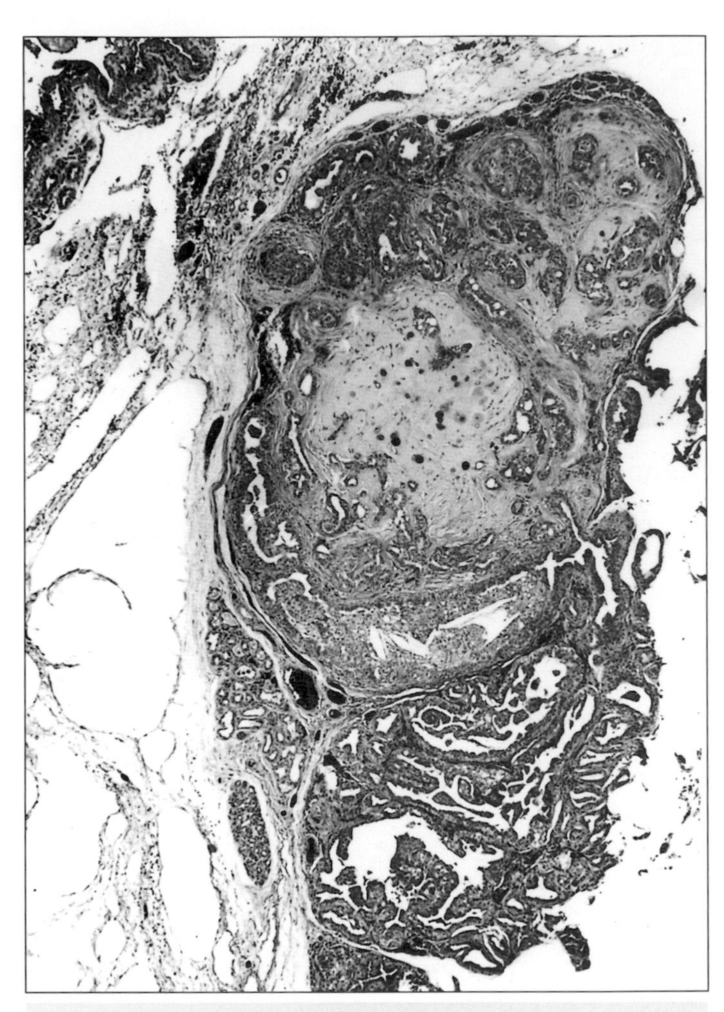

Figure 5.151 Benign mixed mammary tumor with typical mixture of tubular, papillary, and cartilaginous elements.

very rare in dogs less than 5 years of age. Dogs have five pairs of glands and 70% of all tumors develop in glands 4 and 5. Tumors can involve the lobular tissue or the nipple. Mammary tumors in the dog are hormonally dependent. Ovariohysterectomy at or prior to first estrus dramatically decreases the risk of development of mammary tumors. Between 41–53% of mammary tumors in the dog are considered malignant. *Metastasis occurs via hematogenous or lymphatic routes to seed the lung and regional nodes, respectively*. Carcinomas that metastasize to the inguinal lymph nodes may spread to the internal iliac nodes and lead to colonic compression. Many tumors with histologic criteria of malignancy such as cellular atypia or invasion, do not exhibit malignant biological behavior. In addition, the morphologic appearance of the tumor can vary significantly within the section and the lack of consensus regarding criteria for the diagnosis of malignancy leads to a variation in interpretation of lesions.

Benign tumors of the canine mammary gland include simple adenomas, complex adenomas, basaloid adenomas, fibroadenomas, and benign mixed tumors. The *malignant tumors* include ductular carcinoma, carcinoma in situ, complex carcinoma, simple carcinoma, spindle cell carcinoma, squamous cell carcinoma, mucinous carcinoma, lipid-rich carcinoma, and a variety of sarcomas.

- **Simple adenomas** are comprised of either well-differentiated luminal epithelium arranged as simple acini with or without secretions, or as solid nodules of spindle cells (**myoepithelioma**).
- Tumor comprised of both myoepithelium and secretory epithelium that are encapsulated and demonstrate no cellular atypia are classified as **complex adenomas**.
- **Basaloid adenomas** are comprised of solid lobules of monomorphic basaloid epithelium that palisade against a basement membrane. Central cells may show squamous or secretory epithelial differentiation.
- **Fibroadenomas** are tumors comprised of luminal epithelium and possible myoepithelium mixed with stromal elements. The stroma may be sparsely cellular or highly cellular.
- **Benign mixed tumors** are comprised of well-differentiated luminal and/or myoepithelial cells accompanied by a mesenchymal population that has produced cartilage, bone, or fat in combination with a fibrous component (Fig. 5.151).

Carcinomas occurring in the mammary glands of dogs will be discussed in order of increasing malignancy.

- **Carcinomas in situ** (noninfiltrating carcinoma) consist of cerebriform or solid clusters of neoplastic epithelium confined by the basement membrane of a duct, lobule, or cyst. The tumor may be necrotic in the center. These lesions are often multicentric.
- **Complex carcinomas** are comprised of both luminal epithelium and myoepithelium. Complex carcinomas demonstrate

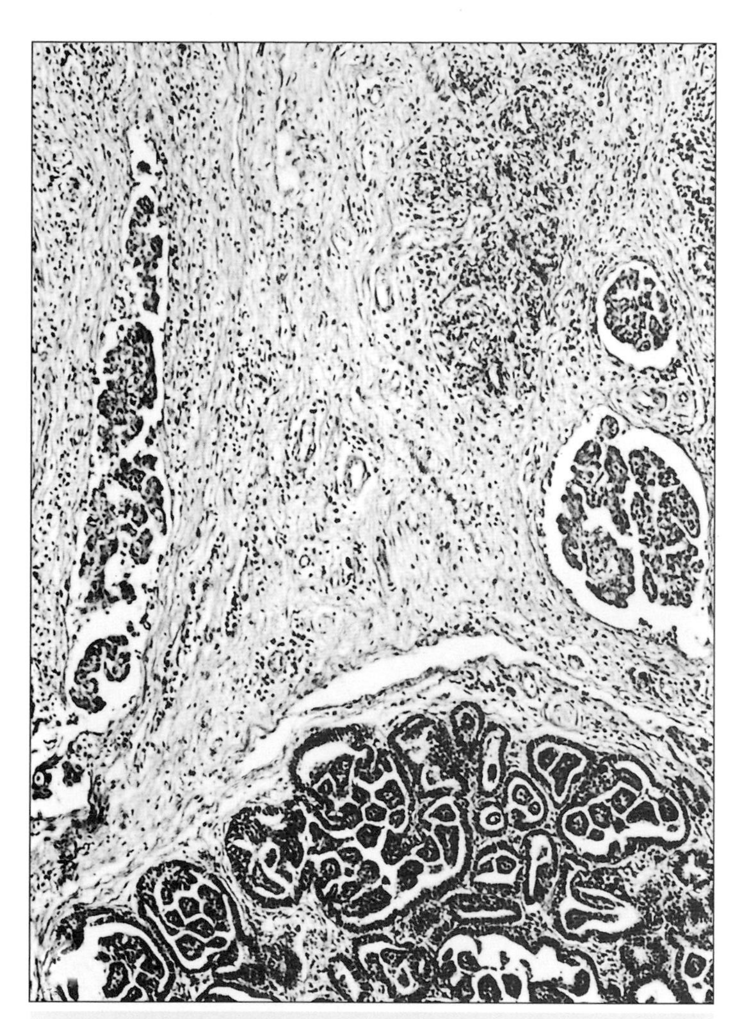

Figure 5.152 Mammary gland papillary adenocarcinoma with lymphatic invasion from a bitch.

infiltrative growth, lack of encapsulation, high cellularity, necrosis and numerous mitotic figures. Squamous metaplasia is frequently present. Lymphatic invasion is present in about 10% of the tumors.

- **Simple carcinomas** are comprised of luminal epithelium **or** myoepithelium. They may have a tubulopapillary or solid arrangement (Fig. 5.152). If the tumor cells are highly pleomorphic and defy histologic recognition as luminal or myoepithelium, the tumors are classified as **anaplastic carcinomas**. Anaplastic carcinomas may be positive for vimentin and cytokeratin with immunohistochemistry. Simple carcinomas are highly invasive and frequently metastasize.
- **Spindle cell carcinomas** are rare malignant tumors comprised of spindle cells arranged as solid or tubular patterns, and are thought to arise from myoepithelium as the cells label for vimentin and cytokeratin.
- **Ductular carcinomas** are comprised of branching duct-like structures filled with solid sheets, papillary projections or cystic aggregates of neoplastic epithelium. They may be simple or complex.
- **Squamous cell carcinomas** arising in the mammary gland are usually highly invasive and frequently invade lymphatics. The periphery of the tumor has predominantly basal cells with cellular atypia. Care must be taken to distinguish these tumors from cutaneous squamous cell carcinomas as the former are more aggressive.
- **Mucinous carcinomas** are of the simple or complex type and produce large amounts of mucin.
- **Lipid-rich carcinomas** are comprised of highly vacuolated epithelial cells that are positive for neutral lipids.

Primary mammary sarcomas *are infrequent in dogs and very rare in cats*. They presumably arise from the fibrous stroma of the gland or of the adjacent subcutaneous tissue. Histologic changes that suggest malignancy are occasionally seen in the myoepithelial stroma, or in the metaplastic bone or cartilage of mixed mammary tumors (so-called malignant mixed tumors). If such tumors metastasize, it is usually the epithelial component that spreads. **Osteosarcomas, chondrosarcomas, liposarcomas, fibrosarcomas,** and **carcinosarcomas** (malignant luminal or myoepithelial cells admixed with malignant stromal cells) have all been reported to arise in the mammary gland.

Mammary tumors in the **cat** represent the third most commonly reported tumor in the cat. Tumors develop most often in intact female cats with a mean age of 10–12 years. Tumors occasionally develop in spayed females or male cats. Spaying decreases the incidence of tumors but does not have the dramatic protective effect as seen in dogs. *At least 85–90% of the tumors are malignant* (Fig. 5.153A, B) *and metastasis to regional lymph nodes, lungs, pleura, liver, adrenal glands, and kidneys is common*. Tumors are firm, nodular and may be ulcerated. Any gland may be affected and tumors are usually multiple. Differences in biological behavior based on histologic subtype of mammary gland carcinomas in the cat have not been shown. **Carcinoma in situ, tubulopapillary carcinoma, solid carcinoma, squamous cell carcinoma, mucinous carcinoma,** and **carcinosarcomas** have all been reported in the cat. These tumors are morphologically similar to the same tumor described in the dog. In addition, a subtype referred to as a **cribriform carcinoma** comprised of malignant epithelial cells arranged in a solid pattern with many small apertures is common in the cat.

Mammary tumors in other species

In **mares**, the few reported tumors have been *scirrhous solid carcinomas* that have been extremely invasive locally, and all have had widespread metastasis.

In **cows**, the literature is old and of variable quality in that many diagnoses had no histologic confirmation. Most descriptions are of fibropapilloma-like growths in the teat canal or large ducts, but everything from fibroma, squamous cell carcinoma, osteoma to fibrosarcoma has been diagnosed. Many of the polypoid teat or cisternal growths were probably hyperplastic inflammatory polyps. **Goats** and water buffalo are cited in review articles as having a very low prevalence of mammary neoplasia.

Bibliography

Ahern TE, et al. Expression of the oncogene c-erbB-2 in canine mammary cancers and tumor-derived cell lines. Am J Vet Res 1996;57:693–696.

Benjamin SA, et al. Classification and behavior of canine mammary epithelial neoplasms based on life-span observations in beagles. Vet Pathol 1999;36:423–436.

Center SA. Lactation and spontaneous remission of feline mammary hyperplasia following pregnancy. J Am Anim Hosp Assoc 1985;21:56–58.

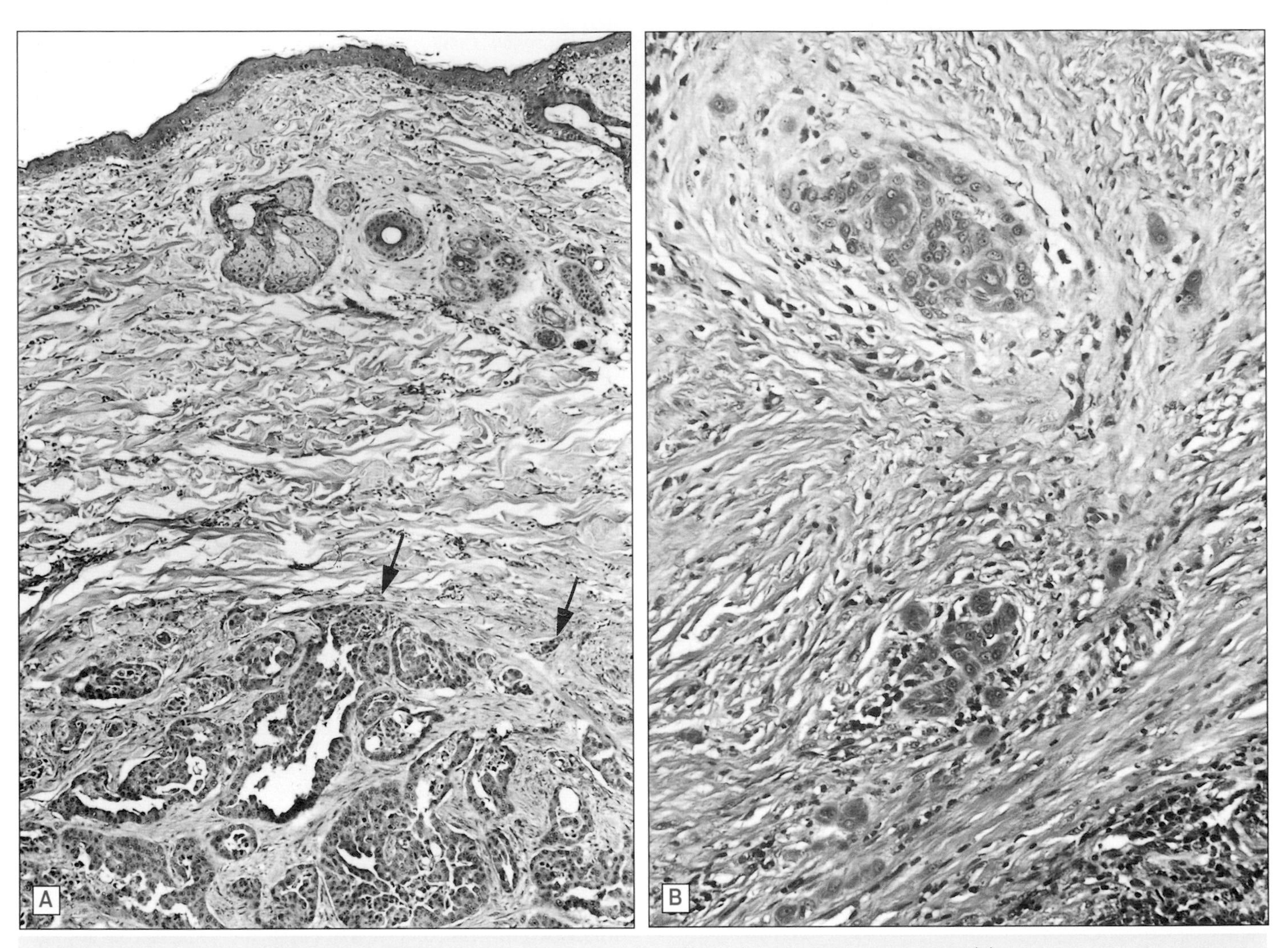

Figure 5.153 Mammary gland carcinoma from a cat. **A.** Note stromal invasion (arrows). **B.** Higher magnification of (**A**) showing poorly cohesive islands of malignant epithelial cells invading the dermis.

Destexhe E, et al. Comparison of argyrophilic nucleolar organizer regions by counting and image analysis in canine mammary tumors. Am J Vet Res 1995;56:185–187.

Donnay I, et al. Comparison of estrogen and progesterone receptor expression in normal and tumor mammary tissues from dogs. Am J Vet Res 1995;56:1188–1194.

Foreman JH. Pleural effusion secondary to thoracic metastatic mammary adenocarcinoma in a mare. J Am Vet Med Assoc 1990;197:1193–1195.

Griffey SM, et al. Computer-assisted image analysis of intratumoral vessel density in mammary tumors from dogs. Am J Vet Res 1998;10:1238–1242.

Hahn KA, et al. Canine malignant mammary neoplasia: biological behavior, diagnosis, and treatment alternatives. J Am Anim Hosp Assoc 1992;28:253–256.

Hayden DW, et al. Feline mammary hypertrophy/fibroadenoma complex: clinical and hormonal aspects. Am J Vet Res 1981;42:1699–1703.

Hellmen E, Lindgren A. The expression of intermediate filaments in canine mammary glands and their tumors. Vet Pathol 1989;26:420–428.

Ivanyi D, et al. Cytokeratins as markers of initial stages of squamous metaplasia in feline mammary carcinomas. Am J Vet Res 1993;54:1095–1102.

MacEwen EG, Withrow SJ. Tumors of the mammary gland. In: Withrow SJ, MacEwen EG, eds. Small Animal Clinical Oncology. 2nd ed. Philadelphia, PA: WB Saunders, 1996:356–372.

Misdorp W, et al. Histological classification of mammary tumors of the dog and cat. Armed Forces Institute of Pathology 1999;7:9–27.

Moulton JE. Tumors of the mammary gland. In: Moulton JE, ed. Tumors of Domestic Animals. 3rd ed. Berkeley, CA: University of California Press, 1990.

Muto T, et al. P53 gene mutations occurring in spontaneous benign and malignant mammary tumors of the dog. Vet Pathol 2000;37:248–253.

Nieto A, et al. Immunohistologic detection of estrogen receptor alpha in canine mammary tumors: clinical and pathologic associations and prognostic significance. Vet Pathol 2000;37:239–247.

Povey RC, Osborne AD. Mammary gland neoplasia in the cow. A review of the literature and report of a fibrosarcoma. Pathol Vet 1969;6:502–512.

Restucci B, et al. Evaluation of angiogenesis in canine mammary tumors by quantitative platelet endothelial cell adhesion molecule immunohistochemistry. Vet Pathol 2000;37:297–301.

Tumors metastatic to the skin

A variety of tumors can metastasize to the skin, but *the process is uncommon*. The usual routes of lymphatic, hematogenous, or implantation from a surgical procedure apply. A thorough search for a primary tumor, knowledge of prior history of a tumor, and an awareness of a few unique tumor patterns of metastasis are necessary to help establish the condition as a metastatic process.

Pulmonary carcinomas in the **cat** have a propensity to metastasize to the digits, often prior to onset of clinical signs referable to the primary tumor. Clinically, the lesions are suggestive of paronychia. Histologically, nests, solid sheets and glandular structures formed by malignant epithelial cells are found in the dermis and subcutis. Bony lysis of the third phalanx may be evident radiographically and histologically. Tumor cells have abundant eosinophilic cytoplasm, basally oriented nuclei and, frequently, apical cilia. Squamous differentiation is also common. Desmoplasia is usually present.

Visceral **hemangiosarcomas** may metastasize to the subcutis in the dog. Subcutaneous hemangiosarcomas, particularly if multiple, should prompt the clinician to search for a primary visceral tumor. Metastatic tumors may be fairly well-differentiated or anaplastic.

Mammary gland carcinomas in the dog may metastasize to the dermis of the inner thigh. Spread of tumor cells occurs via direct invasion of dermal lymphatics or from retrograde metastasis of tumor cells from the external inguinal lymph node. Mammary gland carcinomas in the cat may also metastasize to the ventral abdominal tissues using similar pathways. Primary apocrine gland carcinoma of the skin may be difficult to distinguish.

Abdominal surgeries to remove **transitional cell, colonic** or **prostatic carcinomas** have the potential for implantation of tumor cells in the skin at the surgical site. Tumor cells may also reach the skin via retrograde lymphatic metastasis.

Index

Entries in **boldface** represent major discussions, those followed by 'f' and 't' refer to figures and tables, respectively. The volume number of the entry is indicated in *italics* at the beginning of the page number.

A

B

C

D

E

F

G

H

I

J

K

L

M

O

P

Q

R

S

T

U

V

W